CONTENTS

Seventh Edition

UNDERSTANDING
PATHOPHYSIOLOGY

Sue E. Huether, MS, PhD
Professor Emerita
College of Nursing
University of Utah
Salt Lake City, Utah

Kathryn L. McCance, MS, PhD
Professor Emerita
College of Nursing
University of Utah
Salt Lake City, Utah

SECTION EDITOR

Valentina L. Brashers, MD, FACP, FNAP
Professor Emerita
University of Virginia
Charlottesville, Virginia

ELSEVIER

Elsevier
3251 Riverport Lane
St. Louis, Missouri 63043

Notices

Knowledge and best practice in this field are constantly changing. As new research and experience broaden our understanding, changes in research methods, professional practices, or medical treatment may become necessary.

Practitioners and researchers must always rely on their own experience and knowledge in evaluating and using any information, methods, compounds, or experiments described herein. In using such information or methods they should be mindful of their own safety and the safety of others, including parties for whom they have a professional responsibility.

With respect to any drug or pharmaceutical products identified, readers are advised to check the most current information provided (i) on procedures featured or (ii) by the manufacturer of each product to be administered, to verify the recommended dose or formula, the method and duration of administration, and contraindications. It is the responsibility of practitioners, relying on their own experience and knowledge of their patients, to make diagnoses, to determine dosages and the best treatment for each individual patient, and to take all appropriate safety precautions.

To the fullest extent of the law, neither the Publisher nor the authors, contributors, or editors assume any liability for any injury and/or damage to persons or property as a matter of products liability, negligence or otherwise, or from any use or operation of any methods, products, instructions, or ideas contained in the material herein.

International Standard Book Number 978-0-323-63908-8

Director, Traditional Nursing Program: Tamara Myers
Senior Content Development Manager: Luke Held
Senior Content Development Specialist: Jennifer Wade
Publishing Services Manager: Julie Eddy
Senior Project Manager: Richard Barber
Designer: Maggie Reid

Printed in Canada

Last digit is the print number: 9 8 7 6 5 4 3 2 1

Working together
to grow libraries in
developing countries

www.elsevier.com • www.bookaid.org

CONTRIBUTORS

Barbara J. Boss, RN, PhD, CFNP, CANP
Professor of Nursing Retired
University of Mississippi
Jackson, Mississippi

Valentina L. Brashers MD, FACP, FNAP
Professor Emerita
University of Virginia
Charlottesville, Virginia

Lois E. Brenneman MSN, FNP
Adjunct Faculty
Fairleigh Dickinson University
Florham Park, New Jersey

Russell J. Butterfield, MD, PhD
Assistant Professor
Neurology and Pediatrics
University of Utah
Salt Lake City, Utah

**Sara J. Fidanza, MS, RN, CNS-BC,
CPNP-PC, DHI**
Digestive Health Institute Advanced Practice
    Nurse
Children's Hospital Colorado
Aurora, Colorado

Diane P. Genereux, PhD
Research Scientist
Vertebrate Genome Biology
Broad Institute of MIT and Harvard
Cambridge, Massachusetts

Sue E. Huether MS, PhD
Professor Emerita
Nursing
University of Utah
Salt Lake City, Utah

Lynn B. Jorde, PhD
Mark and Kathie Miller Presidential
    Professor and Chair
Department of Human Genetics
University of Utah School of Medicine
Salt Lake City, Utah

Lauri A. Linder, PhD, APRN, CPON
Assistant Professor
College of Nursing
University of Utah
Salt Lake City, Utah
Clinical Nurse Specialist
Cancer Transplant Center
Primary Children's Hospital
Salt Lake City, Utah

Kathryn L. McCance MS, PhD
Professor Emerita
Nursing
University of Utah
Salt Lake City, Utah

Sue Ann McCann, MSN, RN
Programmatic Nurse Specialist
Nursing
University of Pittsburgh Medical Center
Pittsburgh, Pennsylvania
Clinical Research Coordinator
Dermatology
University of Pittsburgh Medical Center
Pittsburgh, Pennsylvania

Noreen Heer Nicol, PhD, RN, FNP, NEA-BC
Associate Professor
College of Nursing
University of Colorado
Denver, Colorado

Jennifer Peterson, PhD, RN, CCNS
Sue and Bill Gross School of Nursing
University of California, Irvine
Irvine, California

Nancy Pike, PhD, CPNP-PC/AC, FAAN
Associate Professor
UCLA School of Nursing
Los Angeles, California
Pediatric Nurse Practitioner
Cardiothoracic Surgery
Children's Hospital Los Angeles
Los Angeles, California

Geri C. Reeves, PhD, APRN, FNP-BC
Assistant Professor
School of Nursing
Vanderbilt University
Nashville, Tennessee

Patricia Ring, RN, MSN, PNP, BC
Retired
Renal/Voiding Improvement Program
Children's Hospital Wisconsin
Milwaukee, Wisconsin

George W. Rodway, PhD, APRN
Associate Clinical Professor
UC Davis School of Nursing
Sacramento, California

Neal S. Rote, PhD
Academic Vice-Chair and Director of
    Research
Department of Obstetrics and Gynecology
University Hospitals Case Medical Center
Case Western Reserve University School of
    Medicine
Cleveland, Ohio

**Sharon Sables-Baus, PhD, RN, MPA,
PCNS-BC, CPPS, FAAN**
Associate Professor
University of Colorado College of Nursing
    and
School of Medicine, Department Pediatrics
Denver, Colorado

Benjamin A. Smallheer, PhD
Assistant Professor
School of Nursing
Duke University, Durham
North Carolina
Acute Care Nurse Practitioner
Critical Care Medicine
Duke Raleigh Hospital
Raleigh, North Carolina

Lorey K. Takahashi, PhD
Professor of Psychology
Department of Psychology
University of Hawaii at Manoa
Honolulu, Hawaii

Karen Turner, BS
Freelance Editor
Editorial
TurnKey Content
Melbourne, Florida

REVIEWERS

Jennifer B. Drexler, MSN, RN, CCRN
Clinician Faculty Educator
College of Nursing
University of New Mexico College of Nursing
Albuquerque, New Mexico

Linda Phillips, FNP-C
Clinical Associate Professor
Herzing University
Brookfield, Wisconsin

Shawn Theobald, EdD(c), MS(N), MBA, RN
Assistant Professor
College of Health Sciences - Nursing
University of Arkansas – Fort Smith
Fort Smith, Arkansas

Linda Turchin, MSN, CNE
Associate Professor of Nursing
Fairmont State University
Fairmont, West Virginia

The updates for the seventh edition of *Understanding Pathophysiology*, include a simplification of the content to make it less complex and easier for student comprehension. The primary focus of the text is the pathophysiology associated with the most common diseases. Some of the molecular and cellular content has been rewritten into more general explanations of disease processes. The text has also been written to assist students with the translation of the concepts and processes of pathophysiology into clinical practice and to promote lifelong learning. For preparatory knowledge, students need to have a good understanding of human organ system anatomy and physiology. Because of the rapidly evolving discovery of disease mechanisms and treatment at the molecular and cellular level, students also need to have a working understanding of cell structure and function. We continue to include discussions of the following interconnected topics to highlight their importance for clinical practice:

- Pathophysiologic alterations of organ and cell function related to mechanisms of disease
- A life-span approach that includes special sections on aging and separate chapters on children
- Epidemiology and incidence rates showing regional and worldwide differences that reflect the importance of environmental and lifestyle factors on disease initiation and progression
- Sex differences that affect epidemiology and pathophysiology
- Clinical manifestations, summaries of treatment, and health promotion/risk reduction strategies

ORGANIZATION AND CONTENT FOR THE SEVENTH EDITION

The book is organized into two parts: Part One, Basic Concepts of Pathophysiology, and Part Two, Body Systems and Diseases. All content has been updated and includes the most common content related to mechanisms of disease.

Part One: Basic Concepts of Pathophysiology

Part One introduces basic principles and processes that are important for a contemporary understanding of the pathophysiology of common diseases. The concepts include descriptions of cell structure, cellular transport and communication; forms of cell injury; genes and genetic disease; epigenetics; fluid and electrolytes and acid and base balance; immunity, inflammation and wound healing; mechanisms of infection; stress, coping, and illness; tumor biology and cancer epidemiology. We separated the content on infection into a new chapter, Chapter 9.

Part Two: Body Systems and Diseases

Part Two presents the pathophysiology of the most common alterations according to body system. To promote readability and comprehension, we have used a logical sequence and uniform approach in presenting the content of the units and chapters. Each unit focuses on a specific organ system and contains chapters related to anatomy and physiology, the pathophysiology of the most common diseases, and common alterations in children. The anatomy and physiology content is presented as a review to enhance the learner's understanding of the structural and functional changes inherent in pathophysiology. A brief summary of normal aging effects is included at the end of these review chapters. The general organization of each disease/disorder discussion includes an introductory paragraph on relevant risk factors and epidemiology, a significant focus on pathophysiology and clinical manifestations, and

then a brief review of evaluation and treatment. A new chapter was added with content related to obesity, starvation, and anorexia of aging, Chapter 21.

FEATURES TO PROMOTE LEARNING

A number of features are incorporated into this text that guide and support learning and understanding, including:

- *Chapter Outlines* including page numbers for easy reference
- *Quick Check* questions strategically placed throughout each chapter to help readers confirm their understanding of the material; answers are included on the textbook's Evolve website
- *Risk Factors* boxes for selected diseases
- *Did You Know* boxes
- End-of-chapter *Summary Reviews* that condense the major concepts of each chapter into an easy-to-review list format; printable versions of these are available on the textbook's Evolve website
- *Key Terms* set in blue boldface in text and listed, with page numbers, at the end of each chapter
- Special boxes for *Aging* and *Pediatrics* content that highlight discussions of life-span alterations

ART PROGRAM

All of the figures and photographs have been carefully reviewed, revised, or updated. This edition features approximately 100 new or heavily revised illustrations and photographs with a total of approximately 1000 images. The figures and algorithms are designed to help students visually understand sometimes difficult and complex material. High-quality photographs show actual pathologic features of disease. Micrographs show normal and abnormal cellular structure. The combination of illustrations, algorithms, photographs, and use of color for tables and boxes allows a more complete understanding of essential information.

TEACHING/LEARNING PACKAGE

For Students

The free electronic **Student Resources** on Evolve include review questions and answers, numerous animations, answers to the Quick Check questions in the book, chapter summary reviews, and bonus case studies with questions and answers. These electronic resources enhance learning options for students. Go to http://evolve.elsevier.com/Huether.

The newly rewritten **Study Guide** includes many different question types, aiming to help the broad spectrum of student learners. Question types include the following:
Choose the Correct Words
Complete These Sentences
Categorize These Clinical Examples
Explain the Pictures
Teach These People about Pathophysiology
Plus many more…

Answers are found in the back of the **Study Guide** for easy reference for students.

For Instructors

The electronic **Instructor Resources** on Evolve are available free to instructors with qualified adoptions of the textbook and include the following: TEACH Lesson Plans with case studies to assist with clinical application; a Test Bank of more than 1200 items; PowerPoint Presentations for each chapter, with integrated images, audience response questions, and case studies; and an Image Collection of approximately 1000 key figures from the text. All of these teaching resources are also available to instructors on the book's Evolve site. Plus the *Evolve Learning System* provides a comprehensive suite of course communication and organization tools that allow you to upload your class calendar and syllabus, post scores and announcements, and more. Go to http://evolve.elsevier.com/Huether.

The most exciting part of the learning support package is **Pathophysiology Online**, a complete set of online modules that provide thoroughly developed lessons on the most important and difficult topics in pathophysiology supplemented with illustrations, animations, interactive activities, interactive algorithms, self-assessment reviews, and exams. Instructors can use it to enhance traditional classroom lecture courses or for distance and online-only courses. Students can use it as a self-guided study tool.

ACKNOWLEDGMENTS

This book would not be possible without the knowledge and collaboration of our contributing authors, both those who have worked with us through previous editions and the new members of our team. Their reviews and synthesis of the evidence and clear concise presentation of information is a strength of the text. We thank them.

The reviewers for this edition provided excellent recommendations for focus of content and revisions. We appreciate their insightful work.

Tina Brashers, MD, is our section editor and a contributing author. Tina is a distinguished teacher and has received numerous awards for her teaching and work with nursing and medical students and faculty. She is nationally known for her leadership and development in promoting and teaching interprofessional collaboration and is the founder of the Center for Academic Strategic Partnerships for Interprofessional Research and Education (ASPIRE) at the University of Virginia. Tina brings innovation and clarity to the subject of pathophysiology. Her contributions to the online course continue to be intensive and creative, and a significant learning enhancement for students. Thank you, Tina, for the outstanding quality of your work.

Karen Turner joined our team with a new role for this edition. She assisted with the editing of several chapters, managed the revision of artwork, and organized the flow of content for the Summary Reviews. She is an experienced and dedicated editor and made significant contributions to this edition. Thank you, Karen.

Kellie White was our Executive Content Strategist for the first year of the revision until she was promoted to another position. We appreciate her helpful leadership and guidance not only for this edition but, for the past years that she has worked with us. Thank you, Kellie. Jennifer Wade was our Content Development Specialist. Jennifer kept us on track and managed the multiple tasks of acquiring images and getting the manuscript ready for copy editing and page proofs. Thank you, Jennifer.

We are particularly grateful to Cassie Carey who jumped into the copy edit process and kept us going when Beth Welch, our long time copy editor, had to take medical leave. We appreciate the work you both contributed to this edition.

The internal layout, selection of colors, and design of the cover were done by our Designer, Maggie Reid. Great work, Maggie! Thanks to the team from Graphic World, who created many new images and managed the cleanup and scanning of artwork obtained from many resources.

Rich Barber was our Senior Project Manager and brought us into the home stretch and took us through copy edit to final page proofs. Thank you, Rich.

Tamara Meyers, Director of Traditional Nursing Programs, provided the oversight for the entire 7th edition revision. We are thankful for her exceptional leadership, coordination and problem solving in bringing this project to completion.

We thank the Department of Dermatology at the University of Utah School of Medicine, which provided numerous photos of skin lesions. Thank you to our many colleagues and friends at the University of Utah College of Nursing and Health Sciences Center for their suggestions and content critiques.

We extend gratitude to those who contributed to the book supplements. Linda Felver has created an all new inventive and resourceful Study Guide. Thank you, Linda, for your very astute edits. A special thanks to Amber Ballard and Karen Turner for their thorough approach in preparing the materials for the Evolve website. Tina Brashers, Amber Ballard, and Linda Turchin also updated the interactive online lessons and activities for *Pathophysiology Online*.

Sincerely and with great affection we thank our families, especially Mae and John. Always supportive, you make the work possible!

Sue E. Huether
Kathryn L. McCance

We dedicate this book to Sue Anne Meeks, who has been our manuscript manager since the first edition of *Understanding Pathophysiology* and for all of the editions of our more extensive book, *Pathophysiology: The Biologic Basis of Disease in Adults and Children*. The behind-the-scene processes for the development and revision of a major textbook is extensive and requires coordination, attention to detail, organizational skills, good communication, and lots of laughter. Sue is prodigious; she has been a tireless, dedicated, and exceptionally fun person. She is now ready for retirement. We will forever be grateful for her colossal work. We could not have done it without her at our side for the past 30 years. We wish her continuing joy and happiness as she begins her next life adventure.

INTRODUCTION TO PATHOPHYSIOLOGY

The word root *"patho"* is derived from the Greek word *pathos,* which means suffering. The Greek word root *"logos"* means discourse or, more simply, system of formal study, and *"physio"* refers to functions of an organism. Altogether, pathophysiology is the study of the underlying changes in body physiology (molecular, cellular, and organ systems) that result from disease or injury. Important, however, is the inextricable component of suffering and the psychological, spiritual, social, cultural, and economic implications of disease.

The science of pathophysiology seeks to provide an understanding of the mechanisms of disease and to explain how and why alterations in body structure and function lead to the signs and symptoms of disease. Understanding pathophysiology guides healthcare professionals in the planning, selection, and evaluation of therapies and treatments.

Knowledge of human anatomy and physiology and the interrelationship among the various cells and organ systems of the body is an essential foundation for the study of pathophysiology. Review of this subject matter enhances comprehension of pathophysiologic events and processes. Understanding pathophysiology also entails the utilization of principles, concepts, and basic knowledge from other fields of study including pathology, genetics, epigenetics, immunology, and epidemiology. A number of terms are used to focus the discussion of pathophysiology; they may be used interchangeably at times, but that does not necessarily indicate that they have the same meaning. Those terms are reviewed here for the purpose of clarification.

Pathology is the investigation of structural alterations in cells, tissues, and organs, which can help identify the cause of a particular disease. Pathology differs from **pathogenesis**, which is the pattern of tissue changes associated with the *development* of disease. **Etiology** refers to the study of the *cause* of disease. Diseases may be caused by infection, heredity, gene–environment interactions, alterations in immunity, malignancy, malnutrition, degeneration, or trauma. Diseases that have no identifiable cause are termed **idiopathic**. Diseases that occur as a result of medical treatment are termed **iatrogenic** (for example, some antibiotics can injure the kidney and cause renal failure). Diseases that are acquired as a consequence of being in a hospital environment are called **nosocomial**. An infection that develops as a result of a person's immune system being depressed after receiving cancer treatment during a hospital stay would be defined as a nosocomial infection.

Diagnosis is the naming or identification of a disease. A diagnosis is made from an evaluation of the evidence accumulated from the presenting signs and symptoms, health and medical history, physical examination, laboratory tests, and imaging. A **prognosis** is the expected outcome of a disease. **Acute disease** is the sudden appearance of signs and symptoms that last only a short time. **Chronic disease** develops more slowly and the signs and symptoms last for a long time, perhaps for a lifetime. Chronic diseases may have a pattern of remission and exacerbation. **Remissions** are periods when symptoms disappear or diminish significantly. **Exacerbations** are periods when the symptoms become worse or more severe. A **complication** is the onset of a disease in a person who is already coping with another existing disease (for example, a person who has undergone surgery to remove a diseased appendix may develop the complication of a wound infection or pneumonia). **Sequelae** are unwanted outcomes of having a disease or are the result of trauma, such as paralysis resulting from a stroke or severe scarring resulting from a burn.

Clinical manifestations are the signs and symptoms or *evidence* of disease. **Signs** are objective alterations that can be observed or measured by another person, measures of bodily functions such as pulse rate, blood pressure, body temperature, or white blood cell count. Some signs are **local**, such as redness or swelling, and other signs are **systemic**, such as fever. **Symptoms** are subjective experiences reported by the person with disease, such as pain, nausea, or shortness of breath; and they vary from person to person. The **prodromal period** of a disease is the time during which a person experiences vague symptoms such as fatigue or loss of appetite before the onset of specific signs and symptoms. The term **insidious symptoms** describes vague or nonspecific feelings and an awareness that there is a change within the body. Some diseases have a **latent period**, a time during which no symptoms are readily apparent in the affected person, but the disease is nevertheless present in the body; an example is the incubation phase of an infection or the early growth phase of a tumor. A **syndrome** is a group of symptoms that occur together and may be caused by several interrelated problems or a specific disease; severe acute respiratory syndrome (SARS), for example, presents with a set of symptoms that include headache, fever, body aches, an overall feeling of discomfort, and sometimes dry cough and difficulty breathing. A **disorder** is an abnormality of function; this term also can refer to an illness or a particular problem such as a bleeding disorder.

Epidemiology is the study of tracking patterns or disease occurrence and transmission among populations and by geographic areas. **Incidence** of a disease is the number of new cases occurring in a specific time period. **Prevalence** of a disease is the number of existing cases within a population during a specific time period.

Risk factors, also known as **predisposing factors**, increase the probability that disease will occur, but these factors are not the *cause* of disease. Risk factors include heredity, age, gender, race, environment, and lifestyle. A **precipitating factor** is a condition or event that *does* cause a pathologic event or disorder. For example, asthma is precipitated by exposure to an allergen, or angina (pain) is precipitated by exertion.

Pathophysiology is an exciting field of study that is ever-changing as new discoveries are made. Understanding pathophysiology empowers healthcare professionals with the knowledge of how and why disease develops and informs their decision making to ensure optimal healthcare outcomes. Embedded in the study of pathophysiology is understanding that suffering is a personal, individual experience and a major component of disease.

CONTENTS

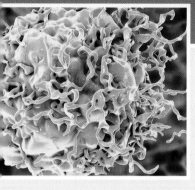

Cellular Biology

Kathryn L. McCance

EVOLVE WEBSITE

http://evolve.elsevier.com/Huether/
Student Review Questions
Audio Key Points

Case Studies
Animations
Quick Check Answers

CHAPTER OUTLINE

All body functions depend on the integrity of cells. Therefore an understanding of cellular biology is increasingly necessary to comprehend disease processes. An overwhelming amount of information reveals how cells behave as a multicellular "social" organism. At the heart of it all is cellular communication (cellular "crosstalk")—how messages originate and are transmitted, received, interpreted, and used by the cell. Streamlined conversation between, among, and within cells maintains cellular function and specialization. Cells must demonstrate a "chemical fondness" for other cells to maintain the integrity of the entire organism. When they no longer tolerate this fondness, the conversation breaks down, and cells either adapt (sometimes altering function) or become vulnerable to isolation, injury, or disease.

PROKARYOTES AND EUKARYOTES

Living cells generally are divided into eukaryotes and prokaryotes. The cells of higher animals and plants are eukaryotes, as are the single-celled organisms, fungi, protozoa, and most algae. Prokaryotes include cyanobacteria (blue-green algae), bacteria, and rickettsiae. Prokaryotes traditionally were studied as core subjects of molecular biology. Today emphasis is on the eukaryotic cell; much of its structure and function have no counterpart in bacterial cells.

Eukaryotes (*eu* = good; *karyon* = nucleus; also spelled "eucaryotes") are larger and have more extensive intracellular anatomy and organization than prokaryotes. Eukaryotic cells have a characteristic set of membrane-bound intracellular compartments, called *organelles,* that includes a well-defined nucleus. The prokaryotes contain no organelles, and their nuclear material is not encased by a nuclear membrane. Prokaryotic cells are characterized by lack of a distinct nucleus.

Besides having structural differences, prokaryotic and eukaryotic cells differ in chemical composition and biochemical activity. The *nuclei* of prokaryotic cells carry genetic information in a single circular chromosome, and they lack a class of proteins called *histones,* which in eukaryotic cells bind with deoxyribonucleic acid (DNA) and are involved in the supercoiling of DNA. Eukaryotic cells have several or many chromosomes. Protein production, or synthesis, in the two classes of cells also differs because of major structural differences in ribonucleic acid (RNA)–protein complexes. Other distinctions include differences in mechanisms of transport across the outer cellular membrane and in enzyme content.

CELLULAR FUNCTIONS

Cells become specialized through the process of differentiation, or maturation, so that some cells eventually perform one kind of function and other cells perform other functions. Cells with a highly developed function, such as movement, often lack some other property, such as hormone production, which is more highly developed in other cells.

The eight chief cellular functions are as follows:

1. *Movement.* Muscle cells can generate forces that produce motion. Muscles that are attached to bones produce limb movements, whereas those muscles that enclose hollow tubes or cavities move or empty contents when they contract (e.g., the colon).
2. *Conductivity.* Conduction as a response to a stimulus is manifested by a wave of excitation, an electrical potential that passes along the surface of the cell to reach its other parts. Conductivity is the chief function of nerve cells.
3. *Metabolic absorption.* All cells can take in and use nutrients and other substances from their surroundings.
4. *Secretion.* Certain cells, such as mucous gland cells, can synthesize new substances from substances they absorb and then secrete the new substances to serve, as needed, elsewhere.
5. *Excretion.* All cells can rid themselves of waste products resulting from the metabolic breakdown of nutrients. Membrane-bound sacs (lysosomes) within cells contain enzymes that break down, or digest, large molecules, turning them into waste products that are released from the cell.
6. *Respiration.* Cells absorb oxygen, which is used to transform nutrients into energy in the form of adenosine triphosphate (ATP). Cellular respiration, or oxidation, occurs in organelles called *mitochondria.*
7. *Reproduction.* Tissue growth occurs as cells enlarge and reproduce themselves. Even without growth, tissue maintenance requires that new cells be produced to replace cells that are lost normally through cellular death. Not all cells are capable of continuous division. (see Chapter 4).
8. *Communication.* Communication is vital for cells to survive as a society of cells. Appropriate communication allows the maintenance of a dynamic steady state.

STRUCTURE AND FUNCTION OF CELLULAR COMPONENTS

Fig. 1.1, *A,* shows a "typical" eukaryotic cell, which consists of three components: an outer membrane called the **plasma membrane**, or **plasmalemma**; a fluid "filling" called **cytoplasm** (see Fig. 1.1, *B*); and

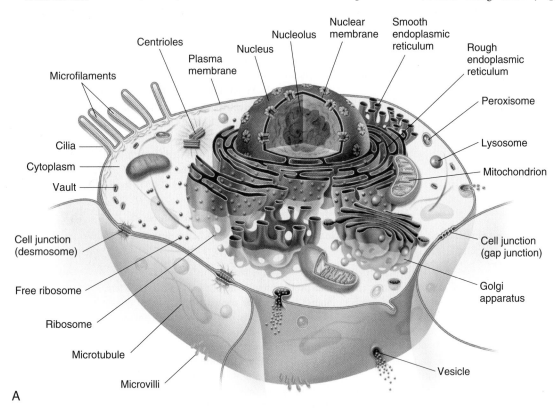

A

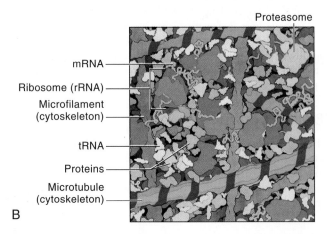

B

FIGURE 1.1 Typical Components of a Eukaryotic Cell and Structure of the Cytoplasm. A, Artist's interpretation of cell structure. Note the many mitochondria known as the "power plants" of the cell. Note, too, the innumerable dots bordering the endoplasmic reticulum. These are ribosomes, the cell's "protein factories." **B,** Color-enhanced electron micrograph of a cell showing the cell is crowded. (*B,* from Patton KT, Thibodeau GA: *Anatomy & physiology,* ed 8, St Louis, 2013, Mosby.)

the "organs" of the cell—the membrane-bound intracellular organelles, among them the nucleus.

Nucleus

The nucleus, which is surrounded by the cytoplasm and generally is located in the center of the cell, is the largest membrane-bound organelle. Two pliable membranes compose the nuclear envelope (Fig. 1.2, A). The nuclear envelope is pockmarked with pits, called nuclear pores, which allow chemical messages to exit and enter the nucleus (see Fig. 1.2, B). The outer membrane is continuous with membranes of the endoplasmic reticulum (see Fig. 1.1). The nucleus contains the nucleolus (a small dense structure composed largely of RNA), most of the cellular DNA, and the DNA-binding proteins (i.e., the histones) that regulate its activity. The DNA "chain" in eukaryotic cells is so long that it is easily broken. Therefore the histones that bind to DNA cause DNA to fold into chromosomes (see Fig. 1.2, C), which decreases the risk of breakage and is essential for cell division in eukaryotes.

The primary functions of the nucleus are cell division and control of genetic information. Other functions include the replication and repair of DNA and the transcription of the information stored in DNA.

Genetic information is transcribed into RNA, which can be processed into messenger, transport, and ribosomal RNAs and introduced into the cytoplasm, where it directs cellular activities. Most of the processing of RNA occurs in the nucleolus. (The roles of DNA and RNA in protein synthesis are discussed in Chapter 2.)

Cytoplasmic Organelles

Cytoplasm is an aqueous solution (cytosol) that fills the cytoplasmic matrix—the space between the nuclear envelope and the plasma membrane. The cytosol represents about half the volume of a eukaryotic cell. It contains thousands of enzymes involved in intermediate metabolism and is *crowded* with ribosomes making proteins (see Fig. 1.1, B). Newly synthesized proteins remain in the cytosol if they lack a signal for transport to a cell organelle.[1] The organelles suspended in the cytoplasm are enclosed in biologic membranes, so they can simultaneously carry out functions requiring different biochemical environments. Many of these functions are directed by coded messages carried from the nucleus by RNA. The functions include synthesis of proteins and hormones and their transport out of the cell, isolation and elimination of waste products from the cell, performance of metabolic processes,

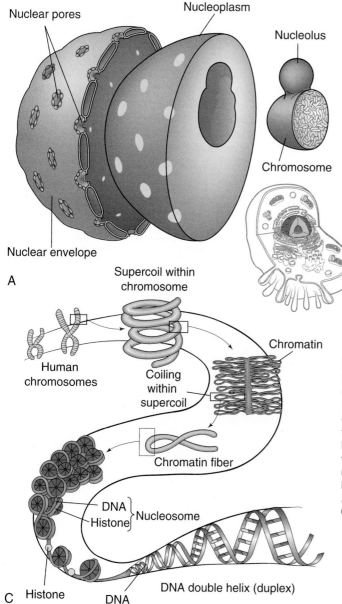

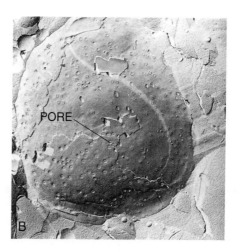

FIGURE 1.2 The Nucleus. The nucleus is composed of a double membrane, called a nuclear envelope, which encloses the fluid-filled interior, called *nucleoplasm*. The chromosomes are suspended in the nucleoplasm (illustrated here much larger than actual size to show the tightly packed deoxyribonucleic acid [DNA] strands). Swelling at one or more points of the chromosome, shown in **A**, occurs at a nucleolus where genes are being copied into ribonucleic acid (RNA). The nuclear envelope is studded with pores. **B**, The pores are visible as dimples in this freeze-etch of a nuclear envelope. **C**, Histone-folding DNA in chromosomes. (**A, C**, from McCance KL, Huether S: *Pathophysiology: the biologic basis for disease in adults and children*, St. Louis, 2019, Elsevier. **B**, from Raven PH, Johnson GB: *Biology*, St Louis, 1992, Mosby.)

breakdown and disposal of cellular debris and foreign proteins (antigens), and maintenance of cellular structure and motility. The cytosol is a storage unit for fat, carbohydrates, and secretory vesicles. Table 1.1 lists the principal cytoplasmic organelles.

✔ QUICK CHECK 1.1

1. Why is the process of differentiation essential to specialization? Give an example.
2. Describe at least two cellular functions.

Plasma Membranes

Every cell is contained within a membrane with gates, channels, and pumps. Membranes surround the cell or enclose an intracellular organelle and are exceedingly important to normal physiologic function because they control the composition of the space, or compartment, they enclose. Membranes can allow or exclude various molecules, and because of selective transport systems, they can move molecules in or out of the space (Fig. 1.3). By controlling the movement of substances from one compartment to another, membranes exert a powerful influence on metabolic pathways. Directional transport is facilitated by polarized domains, distinct apical and basolateral domains. Cell polarity, the direction of cellular transport, maintains normal cell and tissue structure for numerous functions (e.g., movement of nutrients in and out of the cell) and becomes altered with diseases (Fig. 1.4). The plasma membrane also has an important role in cell-to-cell recognition. Other functions of the plasma membrane include cellular mobility and the maintenance of cellular shape (Table 1.2).

Membrane Composition

The basic structure of cell membranes is the lipid bilayer, composed of two apposing leaflets and proteins that span the bilayer or interact with the lipids on either side of the two leaflets (Fig. 1.5). Lipid research is growing and principles of membrane organization are being overhauled. In short, the main constituents of cell membranes are lipids and proteins. Historically, the plasma membrane was described as a fluid lipid bilayer (fluid mosaic model) composed of a *uniform* lipid distribution with inserted moving proteins. Although the notion is controversial, it now appears that the lipid bilayer is a much more complex structure where lipids and proteins are not uniformly distributed but may separate into discrete units called *microdomains*, differing in their protein and lipid compositions. Different membranes have varying percentages of lipids and proteins. Intracellular membranes may have a higher percentage of proteins than do plasma membranes, presumably because most enzymatic activity occurs within organelles. The membrane organization is achieved through noncovalent bonds that allow different physical states called phases (solid gel, fluid liquid–crystalline, and liquid ordered). These phases can change under physiologic factors, such as temperature and pressure fluctuations. Carbohydrates are mainly associated with plasma membranes, in which they are chemically combined with lipids, forming glycolipids, and with proteins, forming glycoproteins (see Fig. 1.5).

The outer surface of the plasma membrane in many types of cells, especially endothelial cells and adipocytes, is not smooth but dimpled with flask-shaped invaginations known as *caveolae* ("tiny caves"). Caveolae are thought to serve as a storage site for many receptors, provide a route for transport into the cell and may act as the initiator for relaying signals from several extracellular chemical messengers into the cell's interior.

Lipids. Each lipid molecule is said to be polar, or amphipathic, which means that one part is hydrophobic (uncharged, or "water hating") and another part is hydrophilic (charged, or "water loving") (see Fig. 1.5, *B*). The membrane spontaneously organizes itself into two layers because of these two incompatible solubilities. The hydrophobic region (hydrophobic tail) of each lipid molecule is protected from water, whereas the hydrophilic region (hydrophilic head) is immersed in it. The bilayer

---

TABLE 1.1 Principal Cytoplasmic Organelles

Organelle	Characteristics and Description
Ribosomes	Ribonucleic acid (RNA)–protein complexes (nucleoproteins) synthesized in nucleolus and secreted into cytoplasm. Provide sites for cellular protein synthesis.
Endoplasmic reticulum	Network of tubular channels (cisternae) that extend throughout outer nuclear membrane. Specializes in synthesis, folding, and transport of protein and lipid components of most organelles. A new role is sensing cellular stress.

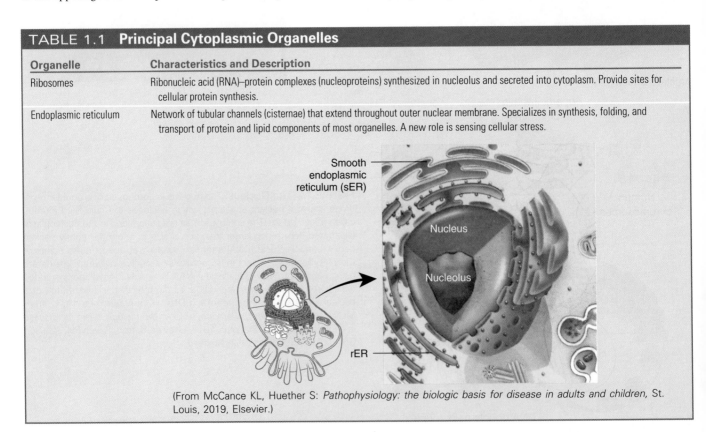

Smooth endoplasmic reticulum (sER)

Nucleus

Nucleolus

rER

(From McCance KL, Huether S: *Pathophysiology: the biologic basis for disease in adults and children*, St. Louis, 2019, Elsevier.)

TABLE 1.1   Principal Cytoplasmic Organelles—cont'd

Organelle	Characteristics and Description
Golgi complex	Network of smooth membranes and vesicles located near nucleus. Responsible for processing and packaging proteins onto secretory vesicles that break away from the complex and migrate to various intracellular and extracellular destinations, including plasma membrane. Best-known vesicles are those that have coats largely made of the protein *clathrin*. Proteins in the complex bind to the cytoskeleton, generating tension that helps organelle function and keep its stretched shape intact. The complex is a refining plant and directs traffic. 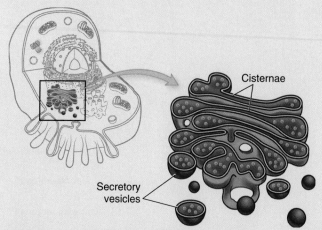 (From McCance KL, Huether S: *Pathophysiology: the biologic basis for disease in adults and children*, St. Louis, 2019, Elsevier.)
Lysosomes	Sac-like structures that contain enzymes for digesting most cellular substances to their basic form, such as amino acids, fatty acids, and carbohydrates (sugars). Cellular injury leads to release of lysosomal enzymes that cause cellular self-destruction. A new function of lysosomes is signaling hubs of a sophisticated network for cellular adaptation. 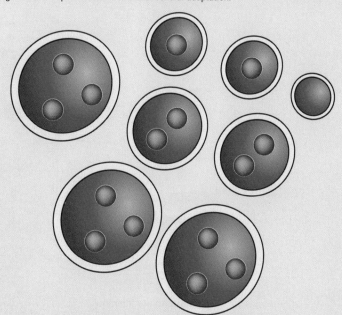 (From McCance KL, Huether S: *Pathophysiology: the biologic basis for disease in adults and children*, St. Louis, 2019, Elsevier.)
Peroxisomes	Similar to lysosomes in appearance but contain several oxidative enzymes (e.g., catalase, urate oxidase) that produce hydrogen peroxide; reactions detoxify various wastes (see Fig. 1.1, *A*).

Continued

TABLE 1.1   Principal Cytoplasmic Organelles—cont'd

Organelle	Characteristics and Description
Mitochondria	Contain metabolic machinery needed for cellular energy metabolism. Enzymes of respiratory chain (electron-transport chain), found in inner membrane of mitochondria, generate most of cell's adenosine triphosphate (ATP) (oxidative phosphorylation). Have a role in osmotic regulation, pH control, calcium homeostasis, and cell signaling.

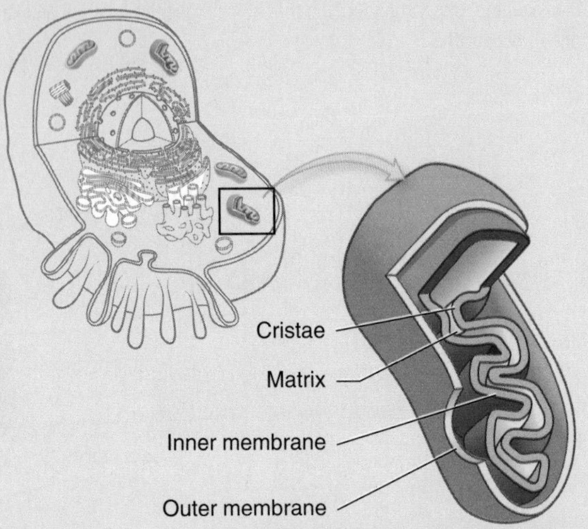

Cristae

Matrix

Inner membrane

Outer membrane

(From McCance KL, Huether S: *Pathophysiology: the biologic basis for disease in adults and children*, St. Louis, 2019, Elsevier.)

| Cytoskeleton | "Bone and muscle" of cell. Composed of a network of protein filaments, including microtubules and actin filaments (microfilaments); forms cell extensions (microvilli, cilia, flagella). Intermediate filaments bridge the cytoplasm from one cell junction to another strengthening and supporting the sheet of epithelium. |

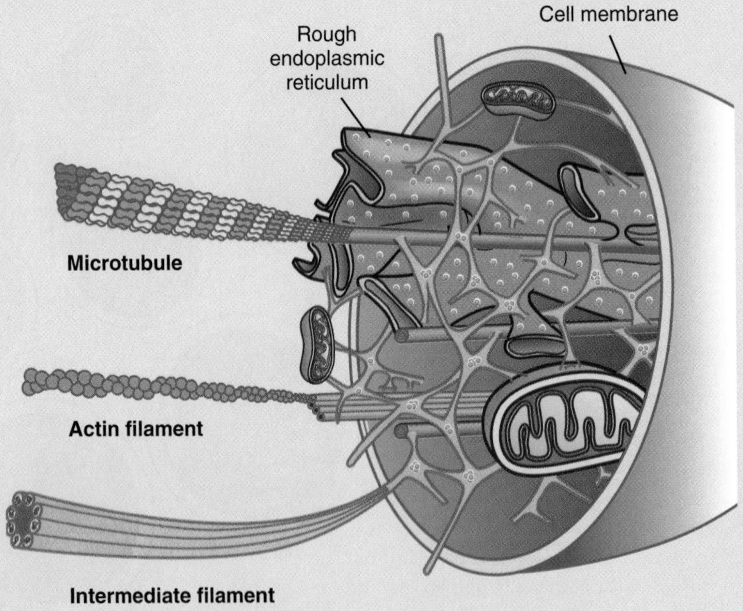

Cell membrane

Rough endoplasmic reticulum

Microtubule

Actin filament

Intermediate filament

(From McCance KL, Huether S: *Pathophysiology: the biologic basis for disease in adults and children*, St. Louis, 2019, Elsevier.)

serves as a barrier to the diffusion of water and hydrophilic substances, while allowing lipid-soluble molecules, such as oxygen (O_2) and carbon dioxide (CO_2), to diffuse through the membrane readily.

A major component of the plasma membrane is a bilayer of lipid molecules—glycerophospholipids, sphingolipids, and sterols (e.g., cholesterol). The most abundant lipids are phospholipids. Phospholipids

have a phosphate-containing hydrophilic head connected to a hydrophobic tail. Phospholipids and glycolipids form self-sealing lipid bilayers. Lipids along with protein assemblies act as "molecular glue" for the structural integrity of the membrane. Investigators are studying the concept of *lipid rafts*, which may be structurally and functionally distinct regions of the plasma membrane.

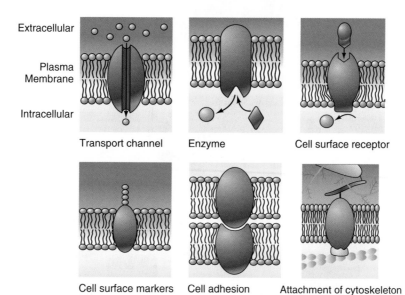

Extracellular

Plasma Membrane

Intracellular

Transport channel   Enzyme   Cell surface receptor

Cell surface markers   Cell adhesion   Attachment of cytoskeleton

FIGURE 1.3 Functions of Plasma Membrane Proteins. The plasma membrane proteins illustrated here show a variety of functions performed by the different types of plasma membranes. (From Raven PH, Johnson GB: *Understanding biology*, ed 3, Dubuque, IA, 1995, Brown.)

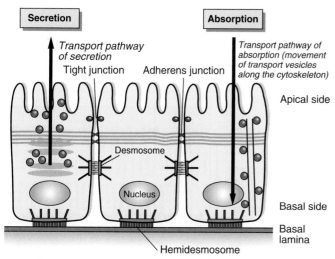

Secretion   Absorption

Transport pathway of secretion
Tight junction   Adherens junction
Transport pathway of absorption (movement of transport vesicles along the cytoskeleton)
Apical side

Desmosome

Nucleus

Basal side

Basal lamina

Hemidesmosome

FIGURE 1.4 Cell Polarity of Epithelial Cells. Schematic of cell polarity (cell direction) of epithelial cells. Shown are the directions of the basal side and the apical side. Organelles and cytoskeleton are also arranged directionally to enable, for example, intestinal cell secretion and absorption. (Adapted from *Life science web textbook,* The University of Tokyo.)

Proteins. Proteins perform most of the plasma membrane's tasks. A **protein** is made from a chain of amino acids, known as **polypeptides**. There are 20 types of amino acids in proteins and each type of protein has a unique sequence of amino acids. After translation (the synthesis of protein from RNA, see Chapter 2) of a protein, **posttranslational modifications (PTMs)** are the methods used to diversify the limited numbers of proteins generated. These modifications alter the activity and functions of proteins and have become very important in understanding diseases. Researchers have known for decades that pathogens interfere with the host's PTMs. New approaches are being used to understand changes in proteins—a field called **proteomics** is the study of the **proteome**, or entire set of proteins expressed by a genome from synthesis, translocation, and modification (e.g., folding), and the analysis of the roles of proteomes in a staggering number of diseases.

TABLE 1.2	Plasma Membrane Functions
Cellular Mechanism	**Membrane Functions**
Structure	Usually thicker than membranes of intracellular organelles
	Containment of cellular organelles
	Maintenance of relationship with cytoskeleton, endoplasmic reticulum, and other organelles
	Maintenance of fluid and electrolyte balance (ion channels)
	Outer surfaces of plasma membranes in many cells are not smooth but are dimpled with cave-like indentations called *caveolae;* they are also studded with cilia or even smaller cylindrical projections called *microvilli;* both are capable of movement
Protection	Barrier to toxic molecules and macromolecules (proteins, nucleic acids, polysaccharides)
	Barrier to foreign organisms and cells
Activation of cell	Hormones (regulation of cellular activity)
	Mitogens (cellular division; see Chapter 2)
	Antigens (antibody synthesis; see Chapter 7)
	Growth factors (proliferation and differentiation; see Chapter 11)
Storage	Storage site for many receptors
	Transport (e.g., sodium [Na$^+$] pump)
	Diffusion and exchange diffusion
	Endocytosis (pinocytosis, phagocytosis)
	Exocytosis (secretion)
	Active transport
Cell-to-cell interaction	Communication, anchors (integrins), and attachment at junctional complexes
	Symbiotic nutritive relationships
	Release of enzymes and antibodies to extracellular environment
	Relationships with extracellular matrix

Modified from King DW, Fenoglio CM, Lefkowitch JH: *General pathology: principles and dynamics,* Philadelphia, 1983, Lea & Febiger.

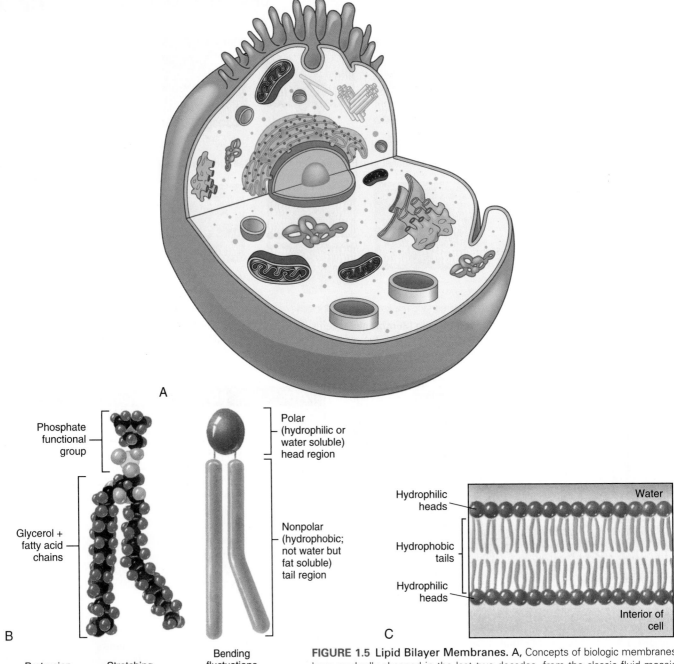

A

Phosphate functional group

Polar (hydrophilic or water soluble) head region

Glycerol + fatty acid chains

Nonpolar (hydrophobic; not water but fat soluble) tail region

B

Hydrophilic heads

Water

Hydrophobic tails

Hydrophilic heads

Interior of cell

C

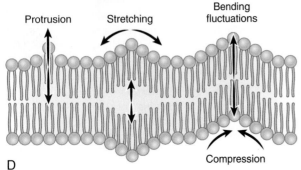

Protrusion

Stretching

Bending fluctuations

Compression

D

FIGURE 1.5 Lipid Bilayer Membranes. A, Concepts of biologic membranes have markedly changed in the last two decades, from the classic fluid mosaic model to the current model that lipids and proteins are not evenly distributed but can isolate into microdomains, differing in their protein and lipid composition. Important for pathophysiology is the proposal that protein–lipid interactions can be critical for correct insertion, folding, and orientation of membrane proteins. For example, diseases related to lipids that interfere with protein folding are becoming more prevalent. **B,** Each phospholipid molecule consists of a phosphate functional group and two fatty acid chains attached to a glycerol molecule. **C,** The fatty acid chains and glycerol form nonpolar, hydrophobic "tails," and the phosphate functional group forms the polar, hydrophilic "head" of the phospholipid molecule. When placed in water, the hydrophobic tails of the molecule face inward, away from the water, and the hydrophilic head faces outward, toward the water. **D,** The cell membrane is not static but is always moving. Observed for the first time from measurements taken at the National Institute of Standards and Technology (NIST) and France's Institute Laue-Langevin (ILL). (A & D, adapted from Bagatolli LA et al: An outlook on organization of lipids in membranes: searching for a realistic connection with the organization of biological membranes, *Prog Lipid Res* 49[4]:378–389, 2010; Contreras FX et al: Specificity of intramembrane protein-lipid interactions, *Cold Spring Harb Perspect Biol* 3[6]:pii a004705, 2011; Cooper GM: *The cell—a molecular approach,* ed 2, Sunderland, MA, 2000, Sinauer Associates; Defamie N, Mesnil M: *Biochim Biophys Acta* 1818(8):1866–1869, 2012; Woodka AC et al: *Phys Rev Lett* 9(5):058102, 2012. B & C, from Raven PH, Johnson GB: *Understanding biology,* ed 3, Dubuque, IA, 1995, Brown.)

Membrane proteins associate with the lipid bilayer in different ways (Fig. 1.6), including:

1. Transmembrane proteins that extend across the bilayer and exposed to an aqueous environment on both sides of the membrane (see Fig. 1.6, *A*)
2. Proteins located almost entirely in the cytosol and associated with the cytosolic half of the lipid bilayer by an α helix exposed on the surface of the protein (see Fig. 1.6, *B*)
3. Proteins that exist outside the bilayer, on one side or the other, and attached to the membrane by one or more covalently attached lipid groups (see Fig. 1.6, *C*)
4. Proteins bound indirectly to one or the other bilayer membrane face and held in place by their interactions with other proteins (see Fig. 1.6, *D*).[1].

Proteins directly attached to the membrane bilayer can be removed by dissolving the bilayer with detergents called integral membrane proteins. The remaining proteins that can be removed by gentler procedures that interfere with protein–protein interactions but do not dissolve the bilayer are known as peripheral membrane proteins.

Proteins exist in densely folded molecular configurations rather than straight chains; thus most hydrophilic units are at the surface of the molecule, and most hydrophobic units are inside. Membrane proteins, like other proteins, are synthesized by the ribosome and translocate, called *trafficking*, to different membrane locations of a cell. Trafficking puts unique demands on membrane proteins for folding, translocation, and stability. Therefore much research is now being done to understand misfolded proteins (e.g., as a cause of disease; Box 1.1).

Although membrane structure is determined by the lipid bilayer, membrane functions are determined largely by proteins. Proteins act as:

1. Recognition and binding units (receptors) for substances moving into and out of the cell
2. Pores or transport channels for various electrically charged particles, called ions or *electrolytes*, and specific carriers for amino acids and monosaccharides
3. Specific enzymes that drive active pumps to promote concentration of certain ions, particularly potassium (K^+), within the cell while keeping concentrations of other ions (e.g., sodium [Na^+]), less than concentrations found in the extracellular environment;
4. Cell surface markers, such as glycoproteins (proteins attached to carbohydrates), which identify a cell to its neighbor
5. Cell adhesion molecules (CAMs), or proteins that allow cells to hook together and form attachments of the cytoskeleton for maintaining cellular shape
6. Catalysts of chemical reactions (e.g., conversion of lactose to glucose (see Fig. 1.3).

Membrane proteins are key components of energy transduction, converting chemical energy into electrical energy, or electrical energy into either mechanical energy or synthesis of ATP. Investigators are studying ATP enzymes and the changes in shape of biologic membranes, particularly mitochondrial membranes, and their relationship to aging and disease.

In animal cells, the plasma membrane is stabilized by a meshwork of proteins attached to the underside of the membrane called the cell cortex. Human red blood cells have a cell cortex that maintains their flattened biconcave shape.[1]

Protein regulation in a cell: proteostasis. The cellular protein pool is in constant change or flux. Proteostasis is a state of cell balance of the processes of protein synthesis, folding, and dehydration. It is vital to health. This adaptable system depends on how quickly proteins are made, how long they survive, or when they are broken down. The proteostasis network comprises ribosomes (makers); chaperones (helpers); and two protein breakdown systems or proteolytic systems—lysosomes and the ubiquitin–proteasome system (UPS). These systems regulate protein homeostasis under a large variety of conditions, including variations in nutrient supply, the existence of oxidative stress or cellular differentiation, changes in temperature, and the presence of heavy metal ions and other sources of stress. Malfunction or failure of the proteostasis network is associated with human (Fig. 1.7).

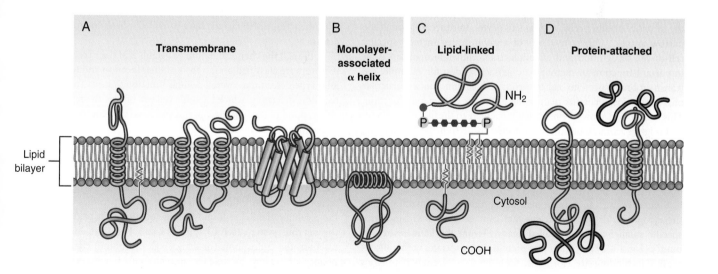

FIGURE 1.6 Proteins Attach to the Plasma Membrane in Different Ways. **A,** Transmembrane proteins extend through the membrane as a single α helix, as multiple α helices, or as a rolled-up barrel-like sheet called a β barrel. **B,** Some membrane proteins are anchored to the cytosolic side of the lipid bilayer by an amphipathic α helix. **C,** Some proteins are linked on either side of the membrane by a covalently attached lipid molecule. **D,** Proteins are attached by weak noncovalent interactions with other membrane proteins. (**D,** adapted from Alberts B et al: *Essential cell biology,* ed 4, New York, 2014, Garland.)

BOX 1.1   Endoplasmic Reticulum, Protein Folding, and Endoplasmic Reticulum Stress

Protein folding in the endoplasmic reticulum (ER) is critical for humans. As the biologic workhorses, proteins perform vital functions in every cell. To do these tasks, proteins must fold into complex three-dimensional structures (see figure). Most secreted proteins *fold* and are modified in an error-free manner, but ER or cell stress, mutations, or random (stochastic) errors during protein synthesis can decrease the folding amount or the rate of folding. Pathophysiologic processes, such as viral infections, environmental toxins, and mutant protein expression, can perturb the sensitive ER environment. Natural processes also can perturb the environment, such as the large protein-synthesizing load placed on the ER. These perturbations cause the accumulation of immature and abnormal proteins in cells, leading to **ER stress**. Fortunately, the ER is loaded with protective ways to help folding, for example, protein so-called *chaperones* that facilitate folding and prevent the formation of off-pathway types. Because specialized cells produce large amounts of secreted proteins, the movement or flux through the ER is tremendous. Therefore misfolded proteins not repaired in the ER are observed in some diseases and can initiate apoptosis, or cell death. It has recently been shown that the ER mediates intracellular signaling pathways in response to the accumulation of unfolded or misfolded proteins; collectively, the adaptive pathways are known as the **unfolded-protein response (UPR)**. Investigators are studying UPR-associated inflammation and how the UPR is coupled to inflammation in health and disease. Specific diseases include Alzheimer disease, Parkinson disease, prion disease, amyotrophic lateral sclerosis, diabetes mellitus, and sepsis. Additionally being studied is ER stress and how it may accelerate age-related dysfunction. Overall, ER is a major organelle for protein quality control.

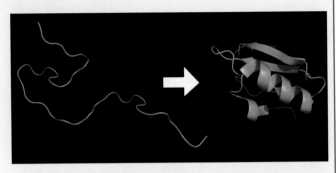

Protein Folding. Each protein exists as an unfolded polypeptide *(left)* or random coil after the process of translation from a sequence of messenger ribonucleic acid (mRNA) to a linear string of amino acids. From amino acids interacting with each other they produce a three-dimensional structure called the folded protein *(right)* that is its native state.

Data from Alberts B et al: *Molecular biology of the cell,* ed 6, New York, 2015; Brodsky J, Skach WR: *Curr Opin Cell Biol* 23:464–475, 2011; Jäger R et al: *Biol Cell* 104(5):259–270, 2012; Khan MM, Yang VVL, Wang P: *Shock* 44(4):294–304, 2015; Shah SZ et al: *J Mol Neurosci* 57(4):529–537, 2015.

Carbohydrates. The short chains of sugars or carbohydrates *(oligosaccharides)* contained within the plasma membrane are mostly bound to membrane proteins (glycoproteins) and lipids (glycolipids). Long polysaccharide chains attached to membrane proteins are called *proteoglycans*. All of the carbohydrate on the glycoproteins, proteoglycans, and glycolipids is located on the outside of the plasma membrane and the carbohydrate coating is called the glycocalyx. The glycocalyx helps protect the cell from mechanical damage.[1] Additionally, the layer of carbohydrate gives the cell a slimy surface that assists the mobility of other cells, such as leukocytes, to squeeze through the narrow spaces.[1] Other functions of carbohydrates include specific cell-to-cell recognition and adhesion. Intercellular recognition is an important function of membrane oligosaccharides; for example, the transmembrane proteins called *lectins*, which bind to a particular oligosaccharide, recognize neutrophils at the site of bacterial infection. This recognition allows the neutrophil to adhere to the blood vessel wall and migrate from blood into the infected tissue to help eliminate the invading bacteria.[1]

Cellular Receptors

Cellular receptors are protein molecules on the plasma membrane, in the cytoplasm, or in the nucleus that can recognize and bind with specific smaller molecules called ligands (from the Latin *ligare,* "to bind") (Fig. 1.8). The region of a protein that associates with a ligand is called its binding site. Hormones, for example, are ligands. Numerous receptors are found in most cells, and ligand binding to receptors activates or inhibits the receptor's associated signaling or biochemical pathway (see the Cellular Communication and Signal Transduction section). Recognition and binding depend on the chemical configuration of the receptor and its smaller ligand, which must fit together somewhat like the pieces of a jigsaw puzzle (see Chapter 19). Binding selectively to a protein receptor with high affinity to a ligand depends on formation of weak, noncovalent interactions—hydrogen bonds, electrostatic attractions, and van der Waals attractions—and favorable hydrophobic forces.[1]

Plasma membrane receptors protrude from or are exposed at the external surface of the membrane and are important for cellular uptake of ligands (see Fig. 1.8). The ligands that bind with membrane receptors include hormones, neurotransmitters, antigens, complement components, lipoproteins, infectious agents, drugs, and metabolites. Many new discoveries concerning the specific interactions of cellular receptors with their respective ligands have provided a basis for understanding disease.

Although the chemical nature of ligands and their receptors differs, receptors are classified on the basis of their location and function. Cellular type determines overall cellular function, but plasma membrane receptors determine which ligands a cell will bind with and how the cell will respond to the binding. Specific processes also control intracellular mechanisms.

Receptors for different drugs are found on the plasma membrane, in the cytoplasm, and in the nucleus. Membrane receptors have been found for certain anesthetics, opiates, endorphins, enkephalins, antibiotics, cancer chemotherapeutic agents, digitalis, and other drugs. Membrane receptors for endorphins, which are opiate-like peptides isolated from the pituitary gland, are found in large quantities in pain pathways of the nervous system (see Chapters 14 and 15). With binding to the receptor, the endorphins (or drugs, e.g., morphine) change the cell's permeability to ions, increase the concentration of molecules that regulate intracellular protein synthesis, and initiate molecular events that modulate pain perception.

Receptors for infectious microorganisms, or antigen receptors, bind bacteria, viruses, and parasites to the cell membrane. Antigen receptors on white blood cells (lymphocytes, monocytes, macrophages, granulocytes) recognize and bind with antigenic microorganisms and activate the immune and inflammatory responses (see Chapter 6).

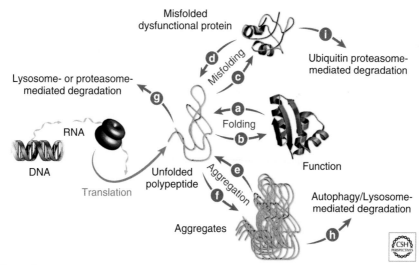

FIGURE 1.7 Protein Homeostasis System and Outcomes. A main role of the protein homeostasis network *(proteostasis)* is to minimize protein misfolding and protein aggregation. The network includes ribosome-mediated protein synthesis, chaperone (folding helpers in the ER) and enzyme mediated folding, breakdown systems of lysosome and proteasome-mediated protein degradation, and vesicular trafficking. The network integrates biologic pathways that balance folding, trafficking, and protein degradation depicted by arrows *a, b, c, d, e, f, g, h,* and *i. ER,* Endoplasmic reticulum. (Adapted from Lindquist SL, Kelly JW: *Cold Spring Harb Perspect Biol* 3[12]:pii: a004507, 2011.)

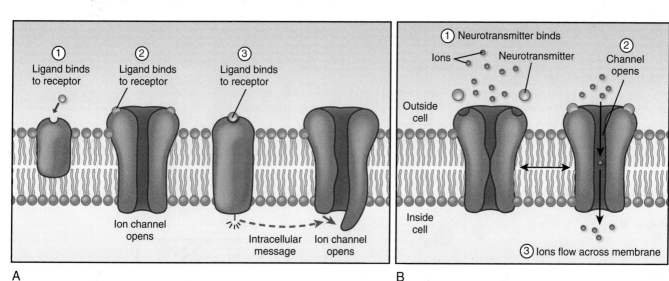

A   B

FIGURE 1.8 Cellular Receptors. A, 1. Plasma membrane receptor for a ligand (here, a hormone molecule) on the surface of an integral protein. A neurotransmitter can exert its effect on a postsynaptic cell by means of two fundamentally different types of receptor proteins. **2.** Channel-linked receptors. **3.** Non–channel-linked receptors. Channel-linked receptors are also known as *ligand-gated channels.* **B,** Example of ligand-gated ion channels. The channel structure is changed when, for example, a neurotransmitter binds and ions can now enter.

CELL-TO-CELL ADHESIONS

Cells are small and squishy, *not* like bricks. They are enclosed only by a flimsy membrane, yet the cell depends on the integrity of this membrane for its survival. How can cells be connected strongly, with their membranes intact, to form a muscle that can lift this textbook? Plasma membranes not only serve as the outer boundaries of all cells but also allow groups of cells to be held together robustly, in **cell-to-cell adhesions,** to form tissues and organs (Box 1.2). Once arranged, cells are linked by three different means: (1) cell adhesion molecules in the cell's plasma membrane, (2) the extracellular matrix (ECM), and (3) specialized cell junctions.

BOX 1.2   Cell Adhesion Molecules

Cell adhesion molecules (CAMs) are cell surface proteins that bind the cell to an adjacent cell and to components of the extracellular matrix (ECM). CAMs include four protein families: (1) the integrins, (2) the cadherins, (3) the selectins, and (4) the **immunoglobulin superfamily CAMs** (IgSF CAMs). **Integrins** are receptors within the ECM and regulate cell-ECM interactions with collagen. **Cadherins** are calcium (Ca^{++})–dependent glycoproteins throughout tissue, for example, epithelial (E-cadherin). **Selectins** are proteins that bind some carbohydrates, for example, mucins. The IgSF CAMs bind integrins and other IgSF CAMs.

Extracellular Matrix and Basement Membrane

Cells can be united by attachment to one another or through the ECM (including the basement membrane), which the cells secrete around themselves. The extracellular matrix (ECM) is an intricate meshwork of fibrous proteins embedded in a watery, gel-like substance composed of complex carbohydrates (Fig. 1.9). The basement membrane (BM) (also known as basal lamina) is a specialized type of ECM. This sheet of matrix is very thin, tough, and flexible; lies beneath epithelial cells; occurs between two cell sheets (kidney glomerulus); and surrounds individual muscle cells, fat cells, and Schwann cells (which wrap around peripheral nerve cell axons) (Fig. 1.10). The ECM is similar to glue; however it provides a pathway for diffusion of nutrients, wastes, and other water-soluble substances between the blood and tissue cells. Interwoven within the matrix are three groups of large molecules or macromolecules: (1) fibrous structural proteins, including collagen and elastin; (2) adhesive glycoproteins, such as fibronectin; and (3) proteoglycans and hyaluronic acid.

1. Collagen forms cable-like fibers or sheets that provide tensile strength or resistance to longitudinal stress. Collagen breakdown, such as occurs in osteoarthritis, destroys the fibrils that give cartilage its tensile strength.
2. Elastin is a rubber-like protein fiber most abundant in tissues that must be capable of stretching and recoiling, such as found in the lungs.
3. Fibronectin, a large glycoprotein, promotes cell adhesion and cell anchorage. Reduced amounts have been found in certain types of cancerous cells; this allows cancer cells to travel, or metastasize, to other parts of the body. All of these macromolecules occur in intercellular junctions and cell surfaces and may assemble into two different components: interstitial matrix and BM (see Fig. 1.9).

The ECM is secreted by fibroblasts ("fiber formers") (Fig. 1.11), local cells that are present in the matrix. The matrix and the cells within it are known collectively as *connective tissue* because they interconnect cells to form tissues and organs. Human connective tissues are enormously varied. They can be hard and dense, for example, bone; flexible, for example, tendons or the dermis of the skin; resilient and shock absorbing, for example, cartilage; or soft and transparent, similar to the jelly-like substance that fills the eye. In all these examples, the majority of the tissue is composed of ECM, and the cells that produce the matrix are scattered within it like raisins in a pudding (see Fig. 1.11).

The matrix is not just passive scaffolding for cellular attachment but also helps regulate the function of the cells with which it interacts. The matrix helps regulate important functions, such as cell growth and differentiation.

Specialized Cell Junctions

Cells in direct physical contact with neighboring cells are often interconnected at specialized plasma membrane regions called cell junctions. Cell junctions are classified by their function:

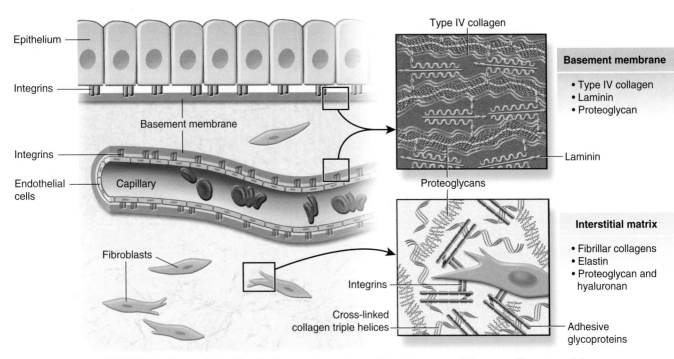

FIGURE 1.9 Extracellular Matrix. Tissues are not just cells but also extracellular space. The extracellular space is an intricate network of macromolecules called the *extracellular matrix (ECM).* The macromolecules that constitute the ECM are secreted locally (by mostly fibroblasts) and assembled into a meshwork in close association with the surface of the cell that produced them. Two main classes of macromolecules include proteoglycans, which are bound to polysaccharide chains called *glycosaminoglycans;* and fibrous proteins (e.g., collagen, elastin, fibronectin, and laminin), which have structural and adhesive properties. Together the proteoglycan molecules form a gel-like ground substance in which the fibrous proteins are embedded. The gel permits rapid diffusion of nutrients, metabolites, and hormones between blood and the tissue cells. Matrix proteins modulate cell–matrix interactions, including normal tissue remodeling (which can become abnormal, for example, with chronic inflammation). Disruptions of this balance result in serious diseases such as arthritis, tumor growth, and other pathologic conditions. (Adapted from Kumar V et al: *Robbins and Cotran pathologic basis of disease,* ed 9, Philadelphia, 2015, Saunders.)

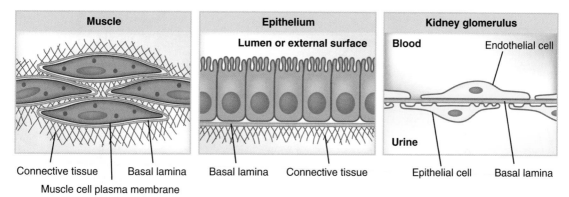

FIGURE 1.10 Three Ways Basement Membranes (Basal Laminae) Are Organized. Basal laminae (yellow) surround certain cells like skeletal cells, underlie epithelia, and occur between two cell sheets (kidney glomerulus). (Adapted from Alberts B et al: *Essential cell biology*, ed 4, New York, 2014, Garland.)

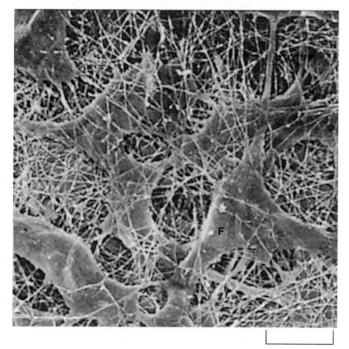

0.1 μm

FIGURE 1.11 Fibroblasts in Connective Tissue. This micrograph shows tissue from the cornea of a rat. The extracellular matrix surrounds the fibroblasts *(F)*. (From Nishida T et al: The extracellular matrix of animal connective tissues, *Invest Ophthalmol Vis Sci* 29:1887–1880, 1998.)

1. To hold cells together and form a tight seal (tight junctions)
2. To provide strong mechanical attachments (adherens junctions, desmosomes, hemidesmosomes)
3. To provide a special type of chemical communication (e.g., inorganic ions and small water-soluble molecules to move from the cytosol of one cell to the cytosol of another cell), such as those causing an electrical wave (gap junctions)
4. To maintain apico-basal polarity of individual epithelial cells (tight junctions) (Fig. 1.12)

In summary, cell junctions make the epithelium leak-proof and mediate mechanical attachment of one cell to another, allow communicating tunnels and maintaining cell polarity.

Cell junctions can be classified as symmetric and asymmetric. Symmetric junctions include tight junctions (zonula occludens), the belt desmosome (zonula adherens), desmosomes (macula adherens),

and gap junctions (also called *intercellular channel* or *communicating junctions*). An asymmetric junction is the hemidesmosome (see Fig. 1.12, *A*). Together they form the junctional complex. Desmosomes unite cells either by forming continuous bands or belts of epithelial sheets or by developing button-like points of contact. Desmosomes also act as a system of braces to maintain structural stability. Tight junctions are barriers to diffusion, prevent the movement of substances through transport proteins in the plasma membrane, and prevent the leakage of small molecules between the plasma membranes of adjacent cells. Gap junctions are clusters of communicating tunnels or connexons that allow small ions and molecules to pass directly from the inside of one cell to the inside of another. Connexons are hemichannels that extend outward from each of the adjacent plasma membranes (see Fig. 1.12, *C*).

Multiple factors regulate gap junction intercellular communication, including voltage across the junction, intracellular pH, intracellular calcium (Ca^{++}) concentration, and protein phosphorylation.

The junctional complex is a highly permeable part of the plasma membrane where permeability is controlled by a process called gating. Increased levels of cytoplasmic calcium cause decreased permeability at the junctional complex. Gating enables uninjured cells to protect themselves from injured neighbors. Calcium is released from injured cells.

CELLULAR COMMUNICATION AND SIGNAL TRANSDUCTION

Cells need to communicate with each other to maintain a stable internal environment, or homeostasis; to regulate their growth and division; to oversee their development and organization into tissues; and to coordinate their functions. Cells communicate by using hundreds of kinds of signal molecules, for example, insulin-like growth factor 1. Cells communicate in three main ways:

1. They display plasma membrane–bound signaling molecules (receptors) that affect the cell itself and other cells in direct physical contact (Fig. 1.13, *A*).
2. They affect receptor proteins *inside* the target cell and the signal molecule has to enter the cell to bind to them (see Fig. 1.13, *B*).
3. They form protein channels (gap junctions) that directly coordinate the activities of adjacent cells (see Fig. 1.13, *C*). Alterations in cellular communication affect disease onset and progression. In fact, if a cell cannot perform gap junctional intercellular communication, normal growth control and cell differentiation is compromised, thereby favoring cancerous tumor development (see Chapter 11).

Secreted chemical signals involve communication locally and at a distance. Primary modes of intercellular signaling are contact-dependent, paracrine,

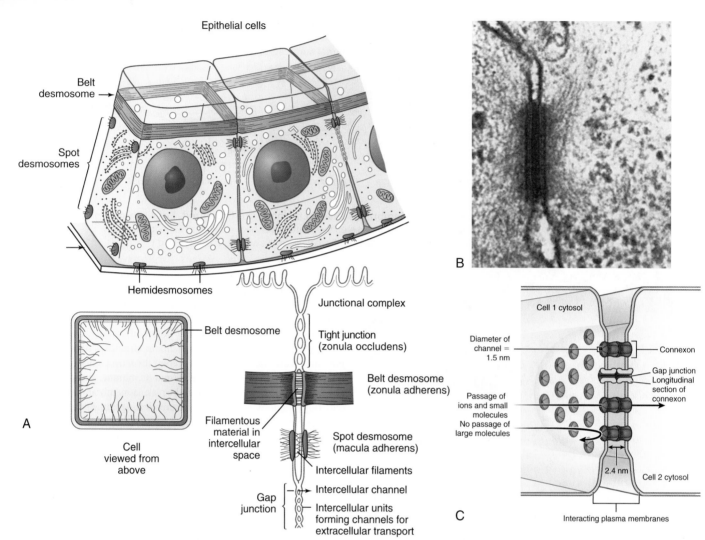

FIGURE 1.12 Junctional Complex. A, Schematic drawing of a belt desmosome between epithelial cells. This junction, also called *zonula adherens*, encircles each interacting cell. The spot desmosomes and hemidesmosomes, like the belt desmosomes, are adhering junctions. The tight junction is an impermeable junction that holds cells together but seals them in such a way that molecules cannot leak between them. The gap junction, as a communicating junction, mediates the passage of small molecules from one interacting cell to the other. **B,** Electron micrograph of desmosomes. **C,** Connexons. The connexin gap junction proteins have four transmembrane domains and they play a vital role in maintaining cell and tissue function and homeostasis. Cells connected by gap junctions are considered ionically (electrically) and metabolically coupled. Gap junctions coordinate the activities of adjacent cells; for example, they are important for synchronizing contractions of heart muscle cells through ionic coupling and for permitting action potentials to spread rapidly from cell to cell in neural tissues. The reason gap junctions occur in tissues that are not electrically active is unknown. Although most gap junctions are associated with junctional complexes, they sometimes exist as independent structures. (**A and B,** from Raven PH, Johnson GB: *Biology,* St Louis, 1992, Mosby; **C** adapted from Gartner LP, Hiatt JL: *Color textbook of histology,* ed 3, St Louis, 2006, Saunders Elsevier; Sherwood L: *Learning,* ed 8, Belmont, California, 2013, Brooks/Cole CENGAGE.)

hormonal, neurohormonal, and neurotransmitter. Autocrine stimulation occurs when the secreting cell targets itself (Fig. 1.14).

Contact-dependent signaling requires cells to be in close membrane-to-membrane contact. In **paracrine signaling**, cells secrete local chemical mediators that are quickly taken up, destroyed, or immobilized. Paracrine signaling usually involves different cell types; however cells also can produce signals to which they alone respond, and this is called **autocrine signaling** (see Fig. 1.14). For example, cancer cells use this form of signaling to stimulate their survival and proliferation. The mediators act only on nearby cells. **Hormonal signaling** involves specialized endocrine cells that secrete chemicals called *hormones;* hormones are released by one set of cells and travel through the bloodstream to produce a response in other sets of cells (see Chapter 19). In **neurohormonal signaling** hormones are released into blood by neurosecretory neurons. Like endocrine cells, neurosecretory neurons release blood-borne chemical messengers, whereas ordinary neurons secrete short-range neurotransmitters into a small discrete space (i.e., synapse). Neurons communicate directly with the cells they innervate by releasing chemicals or **neurotransmitters** at specialized junctions called **chemical synapses;** the neurotransmitter diffuses across the synaptic cleft and acts on the postsynaptic target cell (see Fig. 1.14). Many of these same signaling molecules are receptors used in hormonal, neurohormonal, and paracrine

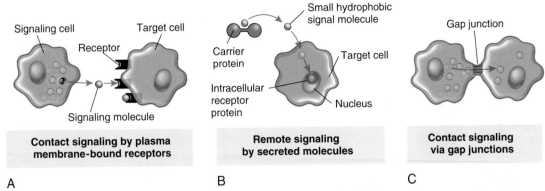

A

B

C

FIGURE 1.13 Cellular Communication. Three primary ways (A–C) cells communicate with one another. (B, adapted from Alberts B et al: *Molecular biology of the cell,* ed 5, New York, 2008, Garland.)

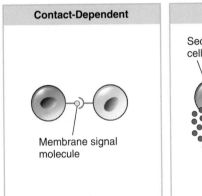

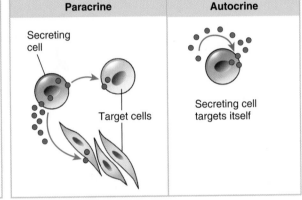

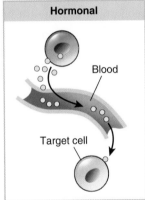

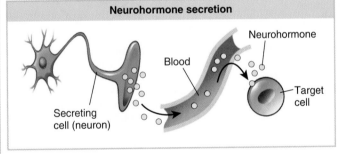

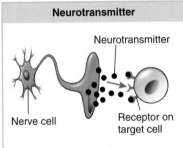

FIGURE 1.14 Primary Modes of Chemical Signaling. Five forms of signaling mediated by secreted molecules. Hormones, paracrines, neurotransmitters, and neurohormones are all intercellular messengers that accomplish communication between cells. Autocrines bind to receptors on the same cell. Not all neurotransmitters act in the strictly synaptic mode shown; some act in a contact-dependent mode as local chemical mediators that influence multiple target cells in the area.

signaling. Important differences lie in the speed and selectivity with which the signals are delivered to their targets.[1]

Plasma membrane receptors belong to one of three classes that are defined by the signaling (transduction) mechanism used. Table 1.3 summarizes these classes of receptors. Cells respond to external stimuli by activating a variety of **signal transduction pathways**, which are communication pathways, or signaling cascades (Fig. 1.15). Signals are passed between cells when a particular type of molecule is produced by one cell—the **signaling cell**—and received by another—the **target cell**—by means of a **receptor protein** that recognizes and responds specifically to the signal molecule (see Fig. 1.15, A and B). In turn, the

signaling molecules activate a pathway of intracellular protein kinases that results in various responses, such as growing and reproducing, dying, surviving, or differentiating (see Fig. 1.15). If deprived of appropriate signals, most cells undergo a form of cell suicide known as *programmed cell death*, or *apoptosis* (see Chapter 4).

Binding of the extracellular signaling messenger (i.e., ligand), or **first messenger**, to the membrane receptors causes (1) opening or closing of specific channels in the membrane to regulate the movement of ions into or out of the cell; and (2) transfer of the signal to an intracellular messenger or **second messenger**, which triggers a cascade of biochemical events within the cell (Fig. 1.16).

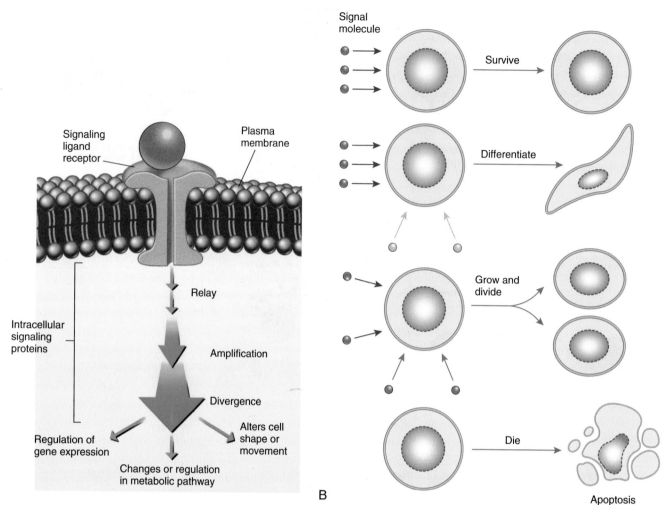

FIGURE 1.15 Schematic of a Signal Transduction Pathway. Like a telephone receiver that converts an electrical signal into a sound signal, a cell converts an extracellular signal. **A,** An extracellular signal molecule (ligand) binds to a receptor protein located on the plasma membrane, where it is transduced into an intracellular signal. This process initiates a signaling cascade that relays the signal into the cell interior, amplifying and distributing it during transit. Amplification is often achieved by stimulating enzymes. Steps in the cascade can be modulated by other events in the cell. **B,** Different cell behaviors rely on multiple extracellular signals.

TABLE 1.3	Classes of Plasma Membrane Receptors
Type of Receptor	**Description**
Channel linked	Also called *ligand-gated channels;* involve rapid synaptic signaling between electrically excitable cells. Channels open and close briefly in response to neurotransmitters, changing ion permeability of plasma membrane of postsynaptic cell.
Catalytic	Once activated by ligands, function directly as enzymes. Composed of transmembrane proteins that function intracellularly as tyrosine-specific protein kinases.
G-protein linked	Indirectly activate or inactivate plasma membrane enzyme or ion channel; interaction mediated by guanosine triphosphate (GTP)–binding regulatory protein (G protein). When activated, a chain of reactions occurs that alters concentration of intracellular messengers, such as cyclic adenosine monophosphate (cAMP) and calcium, or signaling molecules. Behaviors of other target proteins are also altered. May also interact with inositol phospholipids, which are significant in cell signaling, and molecules involved in the inositol–phospholipid transduction pathway. A G-protein–linked receptor activates the enzyme phosphoinositide-specific phospholipase, which, in turn, generates two intracellular messengers: (1) inositol triphosphate (IP$_3$) releases calcium (Ca^{++}), and (2) diacylglycerol remains in the plasma membrane and activates protein kinase C. Protein kinase C further activates various cell proteins. Several different plasma membrane receptors are known to use the inositol–phospholipid transduction pathway.

Data from Alberts B et al: *Molecular biology of the cell,* ed 5, New York, 2008, Garland.

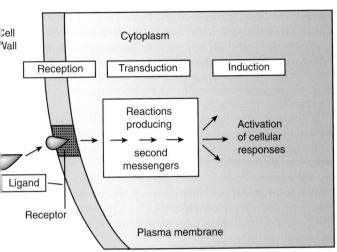

FIGURE 1.16 First and Second Messengers. The first messenger or ligand attaches to the membrane receptor relaying the message across the membrane and intracellular messengers or second messengers trigger the cascade of intracellular events. The two major second-messenger pathways are cyclic adenosine monophosphate (cAMP) and calcium (Ca++). A large number of human disorders involve problematic signaling.

CELLULAR METABOLISM

All of the chemical tasks of maintaining essential cellular functions are referred to as cellular metabolism. The energy-using process of metabolism is called anabolism (*ana* = upward), and the energy-releasing process is known as catabolism (*kata* = downward). Metabolism provides the cell with the energy it needs to produce cellular structures.

Dietary proteins, fats, and starches (i.e., carbohydrates) are hydrolyzed in the intestinal tract into amino acids, fatty acids, and glucose, respectively. These constituents are then absorbed, circulated, and incorporated into the cell, where they may be used for various vital cellular processes, including the production of ATP. The process by which ATP is produced is one example of a series of reactions called a metabolic pathway. A metabolic pathway involves several steps whose end products are not always detectable. A key feature of cellular metabolism is the directing of biochemical reactions by protein catalysts or enzymes. Each enzyme has a high affinity for a substrate, a specific substance converted to a product of the reaction.

Role of Adenosine Triphosphate

What is best known about ATP is its role as a universal "fuel" *inside* living cells. This fuel or energy drives biologic reactions necessary for cells to function. For a cell to function, it must be able to extract and use the chemical energy in organic molecules. When 1 mole (mol) of glucose metabolically breaks down in the presence of oxygen into CO_2 and water, 686 kilocalories (kcal) of chemical energy are released. The chemical energy lost by one molecule is transferred to the chemical structure of another molecule by an energy-carrying or energy-transferring molecule, such as ATP. The energy stored in ATP can be used in various energy-requiring reactions and in the process is generally converted to adenosine diphosphate (ADP) and inorganic phosphate (Pi). The energy available as a result of this reaction is about 7 kcal/mol of ATP. The cell uses ATP for muscle contraction and active transport of molecules across cellular membranes. ATP not only stores energy but also *transfers* it from one molecule to another. Energy stored by carbohydrate, lipid, and protein is catabolized and transferred to ATP.

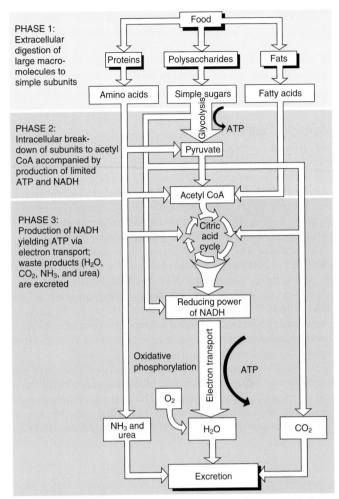

FIGURE 1.17 Three Phases of Catabolism, Which Lead From Food to Waste Products. These reactions produce adenosine triphosphate (ATP), which is used to power other processes in the cell.

Emerging understandings are the role of ATP *outside* cells—as a messenger. In animal studies, using the newly developed ATP probe, ATP has been measured in pericellular spaces. New research is clarifying the role of ATP as an extracellular messenger and its role in many physiologic processes, including inflammation.[2,3]

Food and Production of Cellular Energy

Catabolism of the proteins, lipids, and polysaccharides found in food can be divided into the following three phases (Fig. 1.17):

Phase 1: Digestion. Large molecules are broken down into smaller subunits: proteins into amino acids, polysaccharides into simple sugars (i.e., monosaccharides), and fats into fatty acids and glycerol. These processes occur outside the cell and are activated by secreted enzymes.

Phase 2: Glycolysis and oxidation. The most important part of phase 2 is glycolysis, the splitting of glucose. Glycolysis produces two molecules of ATP per glucose molecule through oxidation, or the removal and transfer of a pair of electrons. The total process is called *oxidative cellular metabolism* and involves 10 biochemical reactions (see Fig. 1.17).

Phase 3: Citric acid cycle (Krebs cycle, tricarboxylic acid cycle). Most of the ATP is generated during this final phase, which begins with the citric acid cycle and ends with oxidative phosphorylation. About two-thirds of the total oxidation of carbon compounds in most cells is accomplished during this phase. The major end products are CO_2 and two dinucleotides—reduced nicotinamide adenine dinucleotide (NADH) and the reduced form of flavin adenine dinucleotide ($FADH_2$)—both of which transfer their electrons into the electron-transport chain.

Oxidative Phosphorylation

Oxidative phosphorylation occurs in the mitochondria and is the mechanism by which the energy produced from carbohydrates, fats, and proteins is transferred to ATP. During the breakdown (catabolism) of foods, many reactions involve the removal of electrons from various intermediates. These reactions generally require a coenzyme (a nonprotein carrier molecule), such as nicotinamide adenine dinucleotide (NAD), to transfer the electrons and thus are called transfer reactions.

Molecules of NAD and flavin adenine dinucleotide (FAD) transfer electrons they have gained from the oxidation of substrates to molecular O_2. The electrons from reduced NAD and FAD, NADH and $FADH_2$, respectively, are transferred to the electron-transport chain on the inner surfaces of the mitochondria with the release of hydrogen ions. Some carrier molecules are brightly colored, iron-containing proteins known as cytochromes, which accept a pair of electrons. These electrons eventually combine with molecular oxygen.

If oxygen is not available to the electron-transport chain, ATP will not be formed by the mitochondria. Instead, an anaerobic (without oxygen) metabolic pathway synthesizes ATP. This process, called substrate phosphorylation or anaerobic glycolysis, is linked to the breakdown (glycolysis) of carbohydrate (Fig. 1.18). Because glycolysis occurs in the cytoplasm of the cell, it provides energy for cells that lack mitochondria. The reactions in anaerobic glycolysis involve the conversion of glucose to pyruvic acid (pyruvate) with the simultaneous production of ATP. With the glycolysis of one molecule of glucose, two ATP molecules and two molecules of pyruvate are liberated. If oxygen is present, the two molecules of pyruvate move into the mitochondria, where they enter the citric acid cycle (Fig. 1.19).

If oxygen is absent, pyruvate is converted to lactic acid, which is released into the extracellular fluid (ECF). The conversion of pyruvic acid to lactic acid is reversible; therefore once oxygen is restored, lactic acid is quickly converted back to either pyruvic acid or glucose. The anaerobic generation of ATP from glucose through glycolysis is not as efficient as the aerobic generation process. Adding an oxygen-requiring stage to the catabolic process (phase 3; see Fig. 1.18) provides cells with a much more powerful method for extracting energy from food molecules.

MEMBRANE TRANSPORT: CELLULAR INTAKE AND OUTPUT

Cell survival and growth depend on the constant exchange of molecules with their environment. Cells continually import nutrients, fluids, and chemical messengers from the extracellular environment and expel metabolites, or the products of metabolism, and end products of lysosomal digestion. Cells also must regulate ions in their cytosol and organelles. Simple diffusion across the lipid bilayer of the plasma membrane occurs for such important molecules as O_2 and CO_2. However the majority of molecular transfer depends on specialized membrane transport proteins that span the lipid bilayer and provide private conduits for select molecules.[1] Membrane transport proteins occur in many forms

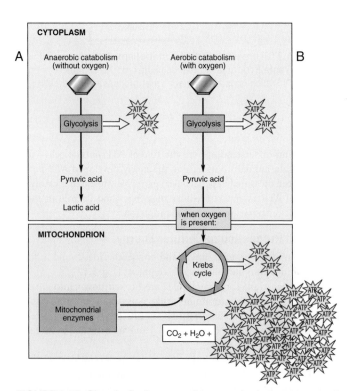

FIGURE 1.18 Glycolysis. Sugars are important for fuel or energy and they are oxidized in small steps to carbon dioxide (CO_2) and water. Glycolysis is the process for oxidizing sugars or glucose. Breakdown of glucose. **A,** Anaerobic catabolism, to lactic acid and little ATP. **B,** Aerobic catabolism, to carbon dioxide, water, and lots of ATP. (From Herlihy B: *The human body in health and illness*, ed 5, St Louis, 2015, Saunders.)

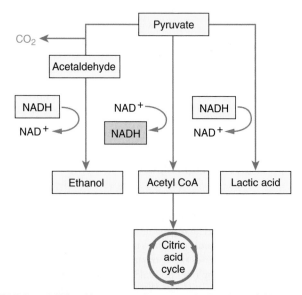

FIGURE 1.19 What Happens to Pyruvate, the Product of Glycolysis? In the presence of oxygen, pyruvate is oxidized to acetyl coenzyme A *(Acetyl CoA)* and enters the citric acid cycle. In the absence of oxygen, pyruvate instead is reduced, accepting the electrons extracted during glycolysis and carried by reduced nicotinamide adenine dinucleotide *(NADH).* When pyruvate is reduced directly, as it is in muscles, the product is lactic acid. When carbon dioxide (CO_2) is first removed from pyruvate and the remainder is reduced, as it is in yeasts, the resulting product is ethanol.

and are present in all cell membranes.[1] Transport by membrane transport proteins is sometimes called mediated transport. Most of these transport proteins allow selective passage (e.g., Na^+ but not K^+, or K^+ but not Na^+). Each type of cell membrane has its own transport proteins that determine which solute can pass into and out of the cell or organelle.[1] The two main classes of membrane transport proteins are *transporters* and *channels*. These transport proteins differ in the type of solute—small particles of dissolved substances—they transport. A transporter is specific, allowing only those ions that fit the unique binding sites on the protein (Fig. 1.20, *A*). A transporter undergoes conformational changes to enable membrane transport. A channel, when open, forms a pore across the lipid bilayer that allows ions and selective polar organic molecules to diffuse across the membrane (see Fig. 1.20, *B*). Transport by a channel depends on the size and electrical charge of the molecule. Some channels are controlled by a gate mechanism that determines which solute can move into it. Ion channels are responsible for the electrical excitability of nerve and muscle cells and play a critical role in the membrane potential.

The mechanisms of membrane transport depend on the characteristics of the substance to be transported. In passive transport, water and small, electrically uncharged molecules move easily through pores in the plasma membrane's lipid bilayer (see Fig. 1.20). This process occurs naturally through any semipermeable barrier. Molecules will easily flow "downhill" from a region of high concentration to a region of low concentration; this movement is called *passive* because it does not require expenditure of energy or a driving force. It is driven by osmosis, hydrostatic pressure, and diffusion, all of which depend on the laws of physics and do not require life.

Other molecules are too large to pass through pores or are ligands bound to receptors on the cell's plasma membrane. Some of these molecules are moved into and out of the cell by active transport, which requires life, biologic activity, and the cell's expenditure of metabolic energy (Fig. 1.21). Unlike passive transport, active transport occurs across only living membranes that have to drive the flow "uphill" by coupling it to an energy source). Movement of a solute against its concentration gradient occurs by special types of transporters called *pumps* (see Fig. 1.21). These transporter pumps must harness an energy source to power the transport process. Energy can come from ATP hydrolysis, a transmembrane ion gradient, or sunlight (see Fig. 1.21). The best-known energy source is the Na^+-K^+–dependent adenosine

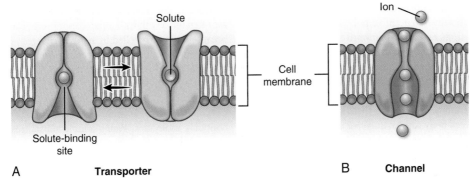

A   **Transporter**   B   **Channel**

FIGURE 1.20 Inorganic Ions and Small, Polar Organic Molecules Can Cross a Cell Membrane Through Either a Transporter or a Channel. (Adapted from Alberts B et al: *Essential cell biology*, ed 4, New York, 2014, Garland.)

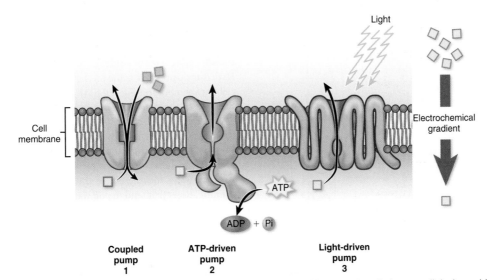

Coupled pump 1   ATP-driven pump 2   Light-driven pump 3

FIGURE 1.21 Pumps Carry Out Active Transport in Three Ways. 1. *Coupled pumps* link the uphill transport of one solute to the downhill transport of another solute. **2.** *ATP-driven pumps* drive uphill transport from hydrolysis of ATP. **3.** *Light-driven pumps* are mostly found in bacteria and use energy from sunlight to drive uphill transport. (Adapted from Alberts B et al: *Essential cell biology*, ed 4, New York, 2014, Garland.)

triphosphatase (ATPase) pump (see Fig. 1.26 later in the chapter). It continuously regulates the cell's volume by controlling leaks through pores or protein channels and maintaining the ionic concentration gradients needed for cellular excitation and membrane conductivity (see the Active Transport of Na^+ and K^+ section). The maintenance of intracellular K^+ concentrations is required also for enzyme activity, including enzymes involved in protein synthesis. Large molecules (macromolecules), along with fluids, are transported by endocytosis (taking in) and exocytosis (expelling) (see the Transport by Vesicle Formation section). Receptor-macromolecule complexes enter the cell by means of receptor-mediated endocytosis.

Mediated transport systems can move solute molecules singly or two at a time. Two molecules can be moved simultaneously in one direction (a process called symport; e.g., sodium–glucose in the digestive tract) or in opposite directions (called antiport; e.g., the sodium–potassium pump in all cells), or a single molecule can be moved in one direction (called uniport; e.g., glucose) (Fig. 1.22).

Electrolytes as Solutes

Body fluids are composed of electrolytes, which are electrically charged and dissociate into constituent ions when placed in solution, and nonelectrolytes, such as glucose, urea, and creatinine, which do not dissociate. Electrolytes account for approximately 95% of the solute molecules in body water. Electrolytes exhibit polarity by orienting themselves toward the positive or negative pole. Ions with a positive charge are known as cations and migrate toward the negative pole, or cathode, if an electrical current is passed through the electrolyte solution. Anions carry a negative charge and migrate toward the positive pole, or anode, in the presence of electrical current. Anions and cations are located in both the intracellular fluid (ICF) and the ECF compartments, although their concentration depends on their location. (Fluid and electrolyte balance between body compartments is discussed in Chapter 5.) For example, Na^+ is the predominant extracellular cation, and K^+ is the principal intracellular cation. The difference in ICF and ECF concentrations of these ions is important to the transmission of electrical impulses across the plasma membranes of nerve and muscle cells.

Electrolytes are measured in milliequivalents per liter (mEq/L) or milligrams per deciliter (mg/dL). The term *milliequivalent* indicates the chemical-combining activity of an ion, which depends on the electrical charge, or valence, of its ions. In abbreviations, valence is indicated by the number of plus or minus signs. One milliequivalent of any cation can combine chemically with 1 mEq of any anion: one monovalent anion will combine with one monovalent cation. Divalent ions combine more strongly than monovalent ions. To maintain electrochemical balance, one divalent ion will combine with two monovalent ions (e.g., $Ca^{++} + 2Cl^-$ {ReversReact} Calcium dichloride [$CaCl_2$]).

Passive Transport: Diffusion, Filtration, and Osmosis

Diffusion. Diffusion is the movement of a solute molecule from an area of greater solute concentration to an area of lesser solute concentration. This difference in concentration is known as a concentration gradient. Although particles in a solution move randomly in any direction, if the concentration of particles in one part of the solution is greater than that in another part, the particles distribute themselves evenly throughout the solution. According to the same principle, if the concentration of particles is greater on one side of a *permeable membrane* than on the other side, the particles diffuse spontaneously from the area of greater concentration to the area of lesser concentration until equilibrium is reached. The higher the concentration on one side, the greater is the diffusion rate.

The diffusion rate is influenced by differences of electrical potential across the membrane (see the Movement of Electrical Impulses: Membrane Potentials section). Because the pores in the lipid bilayer are often lined with Ca^{++}, other cations (e.g., Na^+ and K^+) diffuse slowly because they are repelled by positive charges in the pores.

The rate of diffusion of a substance depends also on its size (diffusion coefficient) and its lipid solubility (Fig. 1.23). Usually, the smaller the molecule and the more soluble it is in oil, the more hydrophobic or nonpolar it is and the more rapidly it will diffuse across the bilayer. O_2, CO_2, and steroid hormones (e.g., androgens and estrogens) are all nonpolar molecules. Water-soluble substances, such as glucose and inorganic ions, diffuse very slowly, whereas uncharged lipophilic ("lipid-loving") molecules, such as fatty acids and steroids, diffuse rapidly. Ions and other polar molecules generally diffuse across cellular membranes more slowly compared with lipid-soluble substances.

Water readily diffuses through biologic membranes because water molecules are small and uncharged. The dipolar structure of water allows it to rapidly cross the regions of the bilayer containing the lipid head groups. The lipid head groups constitute the two outer regions of the lipid bilayer.

Filtration: hydrostatic pressure. Filtration is the movement of water and solutes through a membrane because of a greater pushing pressure (force) on one side of the membrane than on the other side. Hydrostatic pressure is the mechanical force of water pushing against cellular membranes (Fig. 1.24, *A*). In the vascular system, hydrostatic pressure is the *blood pressure* generated in vessels when the heart contracts. Blood reaching the capillary bed has a hydrostatic pressure of 25 to 30 millimeters of mercury (mm Hg), which is sufficient force to push water across the thin capillary membranes into the interstitial space. Hydrostatic pressure is partially balanced by osmotic pressure, whereby water moving *out* of the capillaries is partially balanced by osmotic forces that tend to *pull* water *into* the capillaries (see Fig. 1.24, *B*). Water that is not osmotically attracted back into the capillaries moves into the lymph system (see the discussion of Starling forces in Chapter 5).

Osmosis. Osmosis is the movement of water "down" a concentration gradient—that is, across a semipermeable membrane from a region of higher water concentration to one of lower concentration. For osmosis to occur, (1) the membrane must be more permeable to water than to solutes, and (2) the concentration of solutes on one side of the membrane must be greater than that on the other side so that water moves more

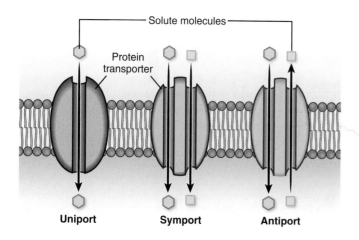

FIGURE 1.22 Mediated Transport. Illustration shows simultaneous movement of a single solute molecule in one direction *(Uniport)*, of two different solute molecules in one direction *(Symport)*, and of two different solute molecules in opposite directions *(Antiport)*.

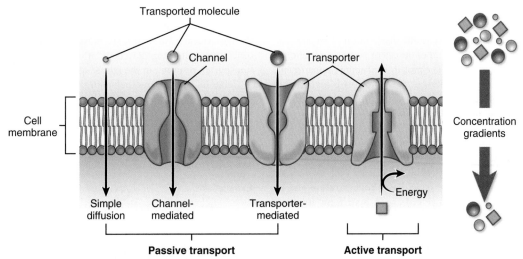

FIGURE 1.23 Passive Diffusion of Solute Molecules Across the Plasma Membrane. Oxygen, nitrogen, water, urea, glycerol, and carbon dioxide can diffuse readily down the concentration gradient. Macromolecules are too large to diffuse through pores in the plasma membrane. Ions may be repelled if the pores contain substances with identical charges. If the pores are lined with cations, for example, other cations will have difficulty diffusing because the positive charges will repel one another. Diffusion can still occur, but it occurs more slowly.

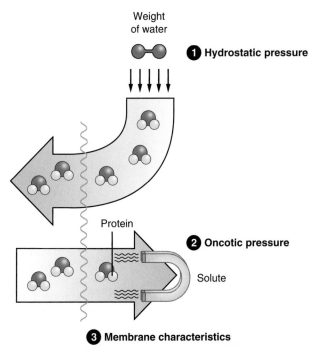

FIGURE 1.24 Hydrostatic Pressure and Oncotic Pressure in Plasma. 1. Hydrostatic pressure in plasma. **2.** Oncotic pressure exerted by proteins in the plasma usually tends to *pull* water into the circulatory system. **3.** Individuals with low protein levels (e.g., starvation) are unable to maintain a normal oncotic pressure; therefore water is not reabsorbed into the circulation and, instead, causes body edema.

easily. Osmosis is directly related to both hydrostatic pressure and solute concentration but *not* to particle size or weight. For example, particles of the plasma protein albumin are small but are more concentrated in body fluids compared with the larger and heavier particles of globulin. Therefore albumin exerts a greater osmotic force compared with globulin.

Osmolality controls the distribution and movement of water between body compartments. The terms *osmolality* and *osmolarity* often are used interchangeably in reference to osmotic activity, but they define different measurements. Osmolality measures the number of milliosmoles per kilogram (mOsm/kg) of water, or the concentration of molecules per *weight* of water. Osmolarity measures the number of milliosmoles per liter of solution, or the concentration of molecules per *volume* of solution.

In solutions that contain only dissociable substances, such as Na and chloride (Cl⁻), the difference between the two measurements is negligible. When considering all the different solutes in plasma (e.g., proteins, glucose, lipids), however, the difference between osmolality and osmolarity becomes more significant. Less of plasma's weight is water, and the overall concentration of particles is therefore greater. The osmolality will be greater than the osmolarity because of the smaller proportion of water. Osmolality is thus preferred in human clinical assessment.

The normal osmolality of body fluids ranges from 280 to 294 mOsm/kg. The osmolalities of ICF and ECF tend to equalize, providing a measure of body fluid concentration and thus the body's hydration status. Hydration is affected also by hydrostatic pressure because the movement of water by osmosis can be opposed by an equal amount of hydrostatic pressure. The amount of hydrostatic pressure required to oppose the osmotic movement of water is called the osmotic pressure of the solution. Factors that determine osmotic pressure are the type and thickness of the plasma membrane, the size of the molecules, the concentration of molecules or the concentration gradient, and the solubility of molecules within the membrane.

Effective osmolality is sustained osmotic activity and depends on the concentration of solutes remaining on one side of a permeable membrane. If the solutes penetrate the membrane and equilibrate with the solution on the other side of the membrane, the osmotic effect will be diminished or lost.

Plasma proteins influence osmolality because they have a negative charge (see Fig. 1.24, *B*). The principle involved is known as *Gibbs-Donnan equilibrium*; it occurs when the fluid in one compartment contains small, diffusible ions, such as Na⁺ and Cl⁻, together with large, nondiffusible, charged particles, such as plasma proteins. Because the body tends to maintain an electrical equilibrium, the nondiffusible protein molecules cause asymmetry in the distribution of small ions. Anions such as Cl⁻ are thus driven out of the cell or plasma, and cations, such as Na⁺, are attracted to the cell. The protein-containing compartment maintains a state of electroneutrality, but the osmolality is higher. The overall osmotic effect of colloids, such as plasma proteins, is called the **oncotic pressure**, or **colloid osmotic pressure**.

Tonicity describes the effective osmolality of a solution. (The terms *osmolality* and *tonicity* may be used interchangeably.) Solutions have relative degrees of tonicity. An isotonic solution (or isosmotic solution) has the same osmolality or concentration of particles (285 mOsm) as ICF or ECF. A hypotonic solution has a lower concentration and is thus more dilute than body fluids (Fig. 1.25). A hypertonic solution has a concentration of more than 285 to 294 mOsm/kg. The concept of tonicity is important when correcting water and solute imbalances by administering different types of replacement solutions (see Fig. 1.25 and Chapter 5).

✔**QUICK CHECK 1.2**
1. What does glycolysis produce?
2. Define membrane transport proteins.
3. What are the differences between passive and active transport?
4. Why do water and small, electrically charged molecules move easily through pores in the plasma membrane?

Active Transport of Na⁺ and K⁺

The active transport system for Na⁺ and K⁺ is found in virtually all mammalian cells. The Na⁺-K⁺–antiport system (i.e., Na⁺ moving out of the cell and K⁺ moving into the cell) uses the direct energy of ATP to transport these cations. The transporter protein is ATPase, which requires Na⁺, K⁺, and magnesium (Mg⁺⁺) ions. The concentration of ATPase in plasma membranes is directly related to Na⁺-K⁺–transport activity. Approximately 60% to 70% of the ATP synthesized by cells, especially muscle and nerve cells, is used to maintain the Na⁺-K⁺–transport system. Excitable tissues have a high concentration of Na⁺-K⁺ ATPase, as do other tissues that transport significant amounts of Na⁺. For every ATP molecule hydrolyzed, three molecules of Na⁺ are transported out of the cell, whereas only two molecules of K⁺ move into the cell. The process leads to an electrical potential and is called *electrogenic,* with the inside of the cell more negative than the outside. Although the exact

mechanism for this transport is uncertain, it is possible that ATPase induces the transporter protein to undergo several conformational changes, causing Na⁺ and K⁺ to move short distances (Fig. 1.26). The conformational change lowers the affinity for Na⁺ and K⁺ to the ATPase transporter, resulting in the release of the cations after transport.

Table 1.4 summarizes the major mechanisms of transport through pores and protein transporters in the plasma membranes. Many disease states are caused or manifested by loss of these membrane transport systems.

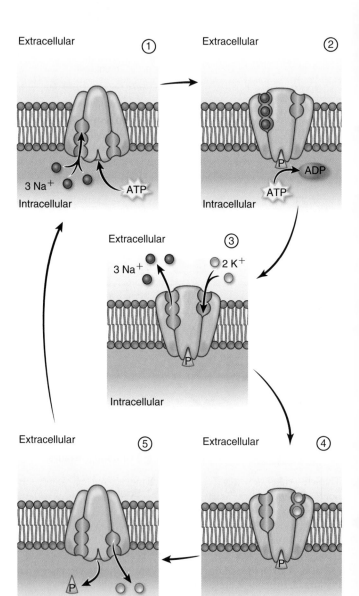

FIGURE 1.26 Active Transport and the Sodium–Potassium (Na⁺–K⁺) Pump. 1. Three sodium (Na⁺) ions bind to Na-binding sites on the carrier's inner face. **2.** At the same time, an energy-containing adenosine triphosphate *(ATP)* molecule produced by the cell's mitochondria binds to the carrier. Adenosine triphosphate (ATP) dissociates, transferring its stored energy to the carrier, and changes shape. **3 and 4.** The ATP releases the three Na⁺ ions to the outside of the cell, and attracts two potassium *(K⁺)* ions to its potassium-binding sites. **5.** The carrier then returns to its original shape, releasing the two K⁺ ions and the remnant of the ATP molecule to the inside of the cell. The carrier is now ready for another pumping cycle.

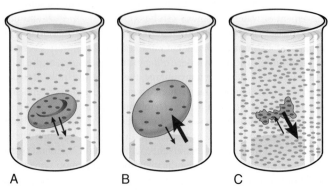

FIGURE 1.25 Tonicity. Tonicity is important, especially for red blood cell function. **A,** Isotonic solution. **B,** Hypotonic solution. **C,** Hypertonic solution. (From Waugh A, Grant A: *Ross and Wilson anatomy and physiology in health and illness,* ed 12, London, 2012, Churchill Livingstone.)

TABLE 1.4   Major Transport Systems in Mammalian Cells

Substance Transported	Mechanism of Transport*	Tissues
Carbohydrates		
Glucose	Passive: protein channel Active: symport with Na^+	Most tissues
Fructose	Active: symport with Na^+ Passive	Small intestines and renal tubular cells Intestines and liver
Amino Acids		
Amino acid specific transporters	Coupled channels	Intestines, kidney, and liver
All amino acids except proline	Active: symport with Na^+	Liver
Specific amino acids	Active: group translocation Passive	Small intestine
Other Organic Molecules		
Cholic acid, deoxycholic acid, and taurocholic acid	Active: symport with Na^+	Intestines
Organic anions (e.g., malate, α-ketoglutarate, glutamate)	Antiport with counter-organic anion	Mitochondria of liver cells
ATP-ADP	Antiport transport of nucleotides; can be active	Mitochondria of liver cells
Inorganic Ions		
Na^+	Passive	Distal renal tubular cells
Na^+/H^+	Active antiport, proton pump	Proximal renal tubular cells and small intestines
Na^+/K^+	Active: ATP driven, protein channel	Plasma membrane of most cells
Ca^{++}	Active: ATP driven, antiport with Na^+	All cells, antiporter in red cells
H^+/K^+	Active	Parietal cells of gastric cells secreting H^+
Cl^-/HCO_3 (perhaps other anions)	Mediated: antiport (anion transporter–band 3 protein)	Erythrocytes and many other cells
Water	Osmosis passive	All tissues

*NOTE: The known transport systems are listed here; others have been proposed. Most transport systems have been studied in only a few tissues and their sites of activity may be more limited than indicated.

ADP, Adenosine diphosphate; *ATP*, adenosine triphosphate; *Ca⁺⁺*, calcium; *Cl⁻/HCO₃*, chloride/bicarbonate; *H⁺*, hydrogen; *K⁺*, potassium; *Na⁺*, sodium.

Data from Alberts B et al: *Molecular biology of the cell*, ed 4, New York, 2001, Wiley; Alberts B et al: *Essential cell biology*, ed 4, New York, 2014, Garland; Devlin TM, editor: *Textbook of biochemistry: with clinical correlations*, ed 3, New York, 1992, Wiley; Raven PH, Johnson GB: *Understanding biology*, ed 3, Dubuque, IA, 1995, Brown.

Transport by Vesicle Formation

Endocytosis and Exocytosis

The active transport mechanisms by which the cells move large proteins, polynucleotides, or polysaccharides (macromolecules) across the plasma membrane are very different from those that mediate small solute and ion transport. Transport of macromolecules involves the sequential formation and fusion of membrane-bound vesicles.

In endocytosis, a section of the plasma membrane enfolds substances from outside the cell, invaginates (folds inward), and separates from the plasma membrane, forming a vesicle that moves into the cell (Fig. 1.27, A). Two types of endocytosis are designated based on the size of the vesicle formed. Pinocytosis (cell drinking) involves the ingestion of fluids, bits of the plasma membrane, and solute molecules through formation of small vesicles; and phagocytosis (cell eating) involves the ingestion of large particles, such as bacteria, through formation of large vesicles (vacuoles).

Because most cells continually ingest fluid and solutes by pinocytosis, the terms *pinocytosis* and *endocytosis* often are used interchangeably. In pinocytosis, the vesicle containing fluids, solutes, or both fuses with a lysosome, and lysosomal enzymes digest the vesicle's contents for use by the cell. Vesicles that bud from membranes have a particular protein coat on their cytosolic surface and are called coated vesicles. The best studied are those that have an outer coat of bristle-like structures—the protein clathrin. Pinocytosis occurs mainly by the clathrin-coated pits and vesicles (Fig. 1.28). After the coated pits pinch off from the plasma membrane, they quickly shed their coats and fuse with an endosome. An endosome is a vesicle pinched off from the plasma membrane from which its contents can be recycled to the plasma membrane or sent to lysosomes for digestion. In phagocytosis, the large molecular substances are engulfed by the plasma membrane and enter the cell so that they can be isolated and destroyed by lysosomal enzymes (see Chapter 6). Substances that are not degraded by lysosomes are isolated in residual bodies and released by exocytosis. Both pinocytosis and phagocytosis require metabolic energy and often involve binding of the substance with plasma membrane receptors before membrane invagination and fusion with lysosomes in the cell. New data are revealing that endocytosis has an even larger and more important role than previously known (Box 1.3). Exosomes are small membrane vesicles of endocytic origin containing protein, lipid, and RNA species in a single unit. Exosomes are secreted by many cell types and confer messages between cells as mediators of cell-to-cell communication. Researchers are revealing this communication through exosomes, including those released from cancer cells, taken up by neighboring cells, and capable of inducing pathways involved in cancer initiation and progression (Fig. 1.29).[4]

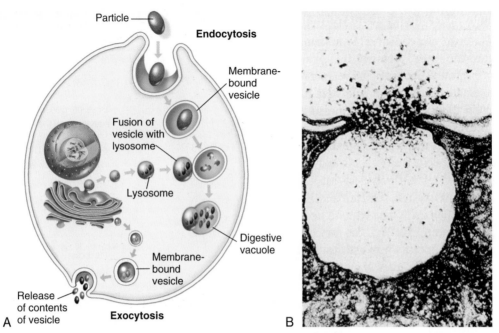

FIGURE 1.27 Endocytosis and Exocytosis. A, Endocytosis and fusion with lysosome and exocytosis. **B,** Electron micrograph of exocytosis. (**B,** from Raven PH, Johnson GB: *Biology,* ed 5, New York, 1999, McGraw-Hill.)

FIGURE 1.28 Ligand Internalization by Means of Receptor-Mediated Endocytosis. A, The ligand attaches to its surface receptor (through the bristle coat or clathrin coat **(1)** and receptor-mediated endocytosis), invagination **(2)** and coated pit **(3)**, and enters the cell. The ingested material fuses **(4)** with an endosome and lysosomes **(6)** and is processed by hydrolytic lysosomal enzymes **(7)**. Processed molecules can then be transferred to other cellular components **(8 and 9)**. **B,** Electron micrograph of a coated pit showing different sizes of filaments of the cytoskeleton (×82,000). (**B,** from Erlandsen SL, Magney JE: *Color atlas of histology,* St Louis, 1992, Mosby.)

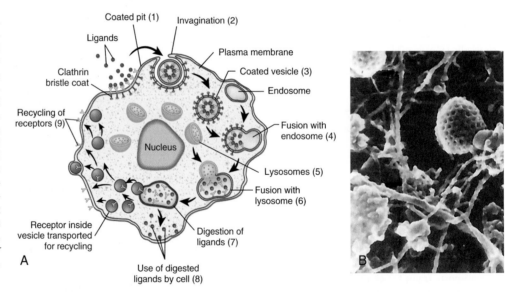

In eukaryotic cells, secretion of macromolecules almost always occurs by exocytosis (see Fig. 1.27). Exocytosis has two main functions: (1) replacement of portions of the plasma membrane that have been removed by endocytosis and (2) release of molecules synthesized by the cells into the ECM.

Receptor-Mediated Endocytosis

The internalization process, called receptor-mediated endocytosis (ligand internalization), is rapid and enables the cell to ingest large amounts of receptor-macromolecule complexes in clathrin-coated vesicles without ingesting large volumes of extracellular fluid (see Fig. 1.28). The cellular uptake of cholesterol, for example, depends on receptor-mediated endocytosis. Additionally, many essential metabolites (e.g.,

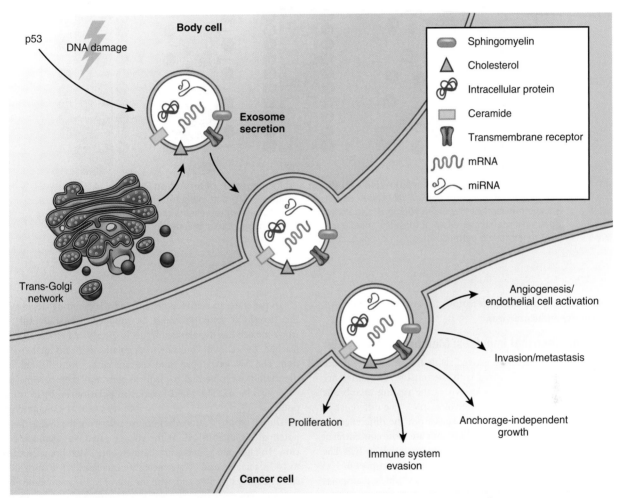

FIGURE 1.29 Exosomes and Cell Signaling: Cancer. From a model of cancer cell signaling, exosomes are secreted with characteristic protein and ribonucleic acid (RNA) components. Exosomes are released from cancer cells and taken up by neighboring cells and are capable of inducing pathways in cancer initiation and progression. A growing interest in defining the clinical relevance of exosomes in cancers is based partially on their ability to alter tumor microenvironment by regulating immunity, angiogenesis, and metastasis. (From Henderson M, Azorsa D: The genomic and proteomic content of cancer cell-derived exosomes, *Front Oncol* 2:38, 2012.)

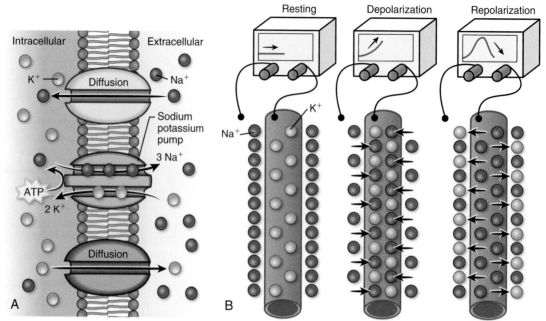

FIGURE 1.30 Sodium–Potassium (Na⁺–K⁺) Pump and Propagation of an Action Potential. **A,** Concentration difference of sodium *(Na⁺)* and potassium *(K⁺)* intracellularly and extracellularly. The direction of active transport by the Na⁺–K⁺ pump is also shown. **B,** The left diagram represents the polarized state of a neuronal membrane when at rest. The middle and right diagrams represent changes in sodium and potassium membrane permeabilities with depolarization and repolarization.

vitamin B_{12} and iron) depend on receptor-mediated endocytosis and, unfortunately, the influenza virus.

Movement of Electrical Impulses: Membrane Potentials

All body cells are electrically polarized, with the inside of the cell more negatively charged compared with the outside. The difference in electrical charge, or voltage, is known as the **resting membrane potential** and is about −70 to −85 millivolts (mV). The difference in voltage across the plasma membrane results from the differences in ionic composition of ICF and ECF. Sodium ions are more concentrated in ECF, and potassium ions are in greater concentration in ICF. The concentration difference is maintained by the active transport of Na^+ and K^+ (the sodium–potassium [Na^+-K^+] pump), which transports Na^+ outward and K^+ inward (Fig. 1.30). Because the resting plasma membrane is more permeable to K^+ than to Na^+, K^+ diffuses easily from ICF to ECF. Because both Na^+ and K^+ are cations, the net result is an excess of anions inside the cell, resulting in the resting membrane potential.

Nerve and muscle cells are excitable and can change their resting membrane potential in response to electrochemical stimuli. Changes in resting membrane potential convey messages from cell to cell. When a nerve or muscle cell receives a stimulus that exceeds the membrane threshold value, a rapid change occurs in the resting membrane potential, known as the **action potential**. The action potential carries signals along the nerve or muscle cell and conveys information from one cell to another in a domino-like fashion. Nerve impulses are described in Chapter 14. When a resting cell is stimulated through voltage-regulated channels, the cell membranes become more permeable to Na^+, so a net movement of Na^+ into the cell occurs and the membrane potential decreases, or moves forward, from a negative value (in mV) to zero. This decrease is known as **depolarization**. The depolarized cell is more positively charged, and its polarity is neutralized.

To generate an action potential and the resulting depolarization, the **threshold potential** must be reached. Generally this occurs when the cell has depolarized by 15 to 20 mV. When the threshold is reached, the cell will continue to depolarize with no further stimulation. The Na^+ gates open, and sodium rushes into the cell, causing the membrane potential to drop to zero and then become positive (depolarization). The rapid reversal in polarity results in the action potential.

During **repolarization**, the negative polarity of the resting membrane potential is reestablished. As the voltage-gated Na^+ channels begin to close, voltage-gated potassium channels open. Membrane permeability to Na^+ decreases and K^+ permeability increases, so K^+ ions leave the cell. The Na^+ gates close and, with the loss of K^+ the membrane potential, becomes more negative. The Na^+-K^+ pump then returns the membrane to the resting potential by pumping K^+ back into the cell and Na^+ out of the cell.

During most of the action potential, the plasma membrane cannot respond to an additional stimulus. This time is known as the **absolute refractory period** and is related to changes in permeability to Na^+. During the latter phase of the action potential, when permeability to K^+ increases, a stronger-than-normal stimulus can evoke an action potential; this time is known as the **relative refractory period**.

When the membrane potential is more negative than normal, the cell is in a **hyperpolarized state** (less excitable: decreased K^+ levels within the cell). A stronger-than-normal stimulus is then required to reach the threshold potential and generate an action potential. When the membrane potential is more positive than normal, the cell is in a **hypopolarized state** (more excitable than normal: increased K^+ levels within the cell) and a weaker-than-normal stimulus is required to reach the threshold potential. Changes in the intracellular and extracellular concentrations of ions or a change in membrane permeability can cause these alterations in membrane excitability.

CELLULAR REPRODUCTION: THE CELL CYCLE

Humans must make millions of cells every second to just survive.[5] In most tissues, new cells are created as fast as old cells die. Continuity of life depends on constant rounds of cell growth and division; the cycle of repeated rounds of duplication and division is called the cell cycle. Reproduction of gametes (sperm and egg cells) occurs through a process called *meiosis*, which is described in Chapter 2. The reproduction, or

division, of other body cells (somatic cells) involves two sequential phases—mitosis, or nuclear division, and cytokinesis, or cytoplasmic division. Before a cell can divide, however, it must double its mass and duplicate all its contents. Most of the work preparing for division occurs during the growth phase, called interphase. The cell cycle drives the alternation between mitosis and interphase in all tissues with cellular turnover (Fig. 1.31).

The four designated phases of the cell cycle (Fig. 1.32) are (1) the G₁ phase (G = gap), which is the period between the M phase and the start of DNA synthesis; (2) the S phase (S = synthesis), in which DNA is synthesized in the cell nucleus; (3) the G₂ phase, in which RNA and protein synthesis occurs, the period between the completion of DNA synthesis and the next phase (M); and (4) the M phase (M = mitosis), which includes both nuclear and cytoplasmic division.

Phases of Mitosis and Cytokinesis

Interphase (the G₁, S, and G₂ phases) is the longest phase of the cell cycle. During interphase, the chromatin consists of very long, slender rods jumbled together in the nucleus. Late in interphase, strands of

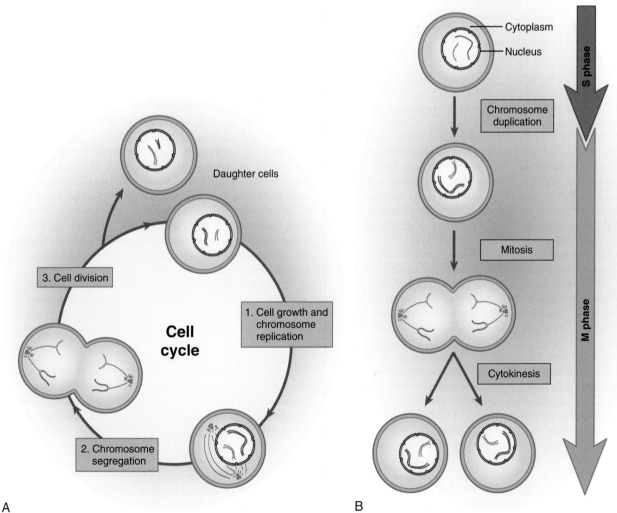

A

B

FIGURE 1.31 The Cell Cycle. A, Simplified figure of schematic cell with one green chromosome and one yellow chromosome to show how two genetically identical daughter cells are produced in each cycle. **B,** Cell cycle events: mitosis and cytokinesis. (Adapted from Alberts B et al: *Molecular biology of the cell*, ed 6, New York, 2015, Garland Science.)

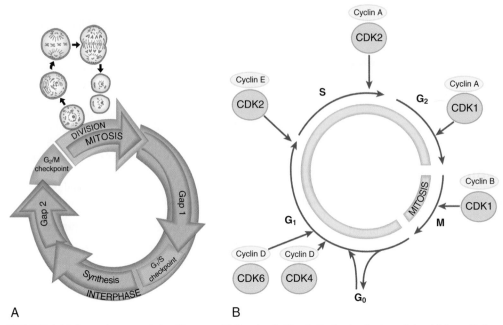

FIGURE 1.32 Interphase and the Phases of Mitosis. A, The G_1/S checkpoint is to "check" for cell size, nutrients, growth factors, and deoxyribonucleic acid (DNA) damage. See text for resting phases. The G_2/M checkpoint checks for cell size and DNA replication. **B,** The orderly progression through the phases of the cell cycle is regulated by *cyclins* (so called because levels rise and fall) and *cyclin-dependent protein kinases* (CDKs) and their inhibitors. When cyclins are complexed with CDKs, cell cycle events are triggered.

chromatin (the substance that gives the nucleus its granular appearance) begin to coil, causing shortening and thickening.

The M phase of the cell cycle, mitosis and cytokinesis, begins with prophase, the first appearance of chromosomes. As the phase proceeds, each chromosome is seen as identical halves called chromatids, which lie together and are attached by a spindle site called a centromere. (The two chromatids of each chromosome, which are genetically identical, are sometimes called *sister chromatids.*) The nuclear membrane, which surrounds the nucleus, disappears. Spindle fibers are microtubules formed in the cytoplasm. They radiate from two centrioles located at opposite poles of the cell and pull the chromosomes to opposite sides of the cell, beginning the metaphase. Next, the centromeres become aligned in the middle of the spindle, which is called the equatorial plate (or metaphase plate) of the cell. In this stage, chromosomes are easiest to observe microscopically because they are highly condensed and arranged in a relatively organized fashion.

The anaphase begins when the centromeres split and the sister chromatids are pulled apart. The spindle fibers shorten, causing the sister chromatids to be pulled, centromere first, toward opposite sides of the cell. With sister chromatid separation, each is considered to be a chromosome. Thus the cell has 92 chromosomes during this stage. By the end of the anaphase, there are 46 chromosomes lying at each side of the cell. Barring mitotic errors, each of the two groups of 46 chromosomes is identical to the original 46 chromosomes present at the start of the cell cycle.

During the telophase, the final stage, a new nuclear membrane is formed around each group of 46 chromosomes, the spindle fibers disappear, and the chromosomes begin to uncoil. Cytokinesis causes the cytoplasm to divide into almost equal parts during this phase. At the end of the telophase, two identical diploid cells, called daughter cells, have been formed from the original cell.

Control of Cell Division and Cell Growth: Mitogens, Growth Factors, and Survival Factors

Organ size and body size are determined by three main processes: (1) cell growth, (2) cell division, and (3) cell survival.[5] These processes are tightly regulated by intracellular programs and extracellular signal molecules, usually soluble proteins, proteins bound to cells, or molecules of the ECM. The molecules comprise three main classes: (1) mitogens, (2) growth factors, and (3) survival factors. A mitogen is a chemical agent that induces or stimulates mitosis (cell division). Mitogens act as an extracellular signal and they usually come from another neighboring cell. Mitogens can stimulate cell growth, differentiation, migration, and survival.[5]

Growth factors (also called *cytokines*) stimulate an increase in cell mass or cell growth by fostering the synthesis of proteins and other macromolecules and inhibiting their breakdown (Table 1.5), including examples of mitogens and growth factors. Survival factors promote cell survival by inhibiting programmed cell death, or *apoptosis* (see Chapter 4).

DNA Damage Response: Blocks Cell Division

The DNA damage response occurs when DNA is damaged with recruitment of protein kinases to the site of damage and signaling that promotes a stop to the progression of the cell cycle, called cell cycle arrest (Fig. 1.33).

TISSUES

Cells of common structure and function are organized into tissues, of which there are four primary types: *muscle, neural, epithelial,* and *connective.* Epithelial, connective, and muscle tissues are summarized in Tables 1.6, 1.7, and 1.8, respectively. Different types of neurons have special characteristics that depend on their distribution and function within the nervous system (see Chapter 14). Different types of tissues

TABLE 1.5   Examples of Mitogens and Growth Factors and Their Actions

Growth Factor	Physiologic Actions
Platelet-derived growth factor (PDGF)	Stimulates proliferation of connective tissue cells and neuroglial cells
Epidermal growth factor (EGF)	Stimulates proliferation of epidermal cells and other cell types
Insulin-like growth factor 1 (IGF-1)	Collaborates with PDGF and EGF; stimulates proliferation of fat cells and connective tissue cells
Insulin-like growth factor 2 (IGF-2)	Collaborates with PDGF and EGF; stimulates proliferation of fat cells and connective tissue cells
Transforming growth factor-beta (TGF-β)	Stimulates or inhibits response of most cells to other growth factors; regulates differentiation of some cell types (e.g., cartilage)
Fibroblast growth factor (FGF)	Stimulates proliferation of fibroblasts, endothelial cells, myoblasts, and other cell types
Interleukin-2 (IL-2)	Stimulates proliferation of T lymphocytes
Nerve growth factor (NGF)	Promotes axon growth and survival of sympathetic and some sensory and CNS neurons
Hematopoietic cell growth factors (IL-3, GM-CSF, M-CSF, G-CSF, erythropoietin)	Promotes growth of white and red blood cells

CNS, Central nervous system; *CSF,* colony-stimulating factor; *G,* granulocyte; *GM,* granulocyte-macrophage; *M,* macrophage.

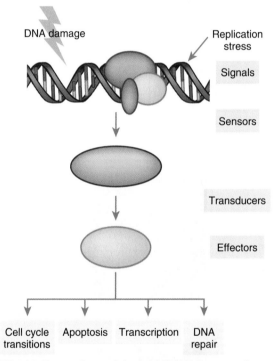

FIGURE 1.33 Deoxyribonucleic Acid (DNA) Damage Response. Several injurious agents can damage DNA. These include exogenous agents such as ultraviolet light; ionizing radiation; chemicals; and endogenous agents; oxidative damage; and replicative stress. Protein kinases are activated and serve as sensors and transducers causing many effector responses. The cell cycle arrest prevents entry into mitosis and several cell fates occur including DNA repair and apoptosis or cell death.

compose organs. Finally, organs are integrated to perform complex functions as tracts or systems.

All cells are in contact with a network of extracellular macromolecules known as the ECM (see the Extracellular Matrix and Basement Membrane section). This matrix not only holds cells and tissues together but also provides an organized latticework within which cells can migrate and interact with one another.

Tissue Formation and Differentiation

To form tissues, cells must exhibit intercellular recognition and communication, adhesion, and memory. Specialized cells sense their environment through signals, such as growth factors, from other cells. This type of communication ensures that new cells are produced only when and where they are required. Different cell types have different adhesion molecules in their plasma membranes, sticking selectively to other cells of the same type. They can also adhere to the ECM components. Because cells are tiny and squishy and enclosed by a flimsy membrane, it is remarkable that they form a strong human being. Strength can occur because of the ECM and the strength of the cytoskeleton with cell-to-cell adhesions to neighboring cells. Cells have memory because of specialized patterns of gene expression evoked by signals that acted during embryonic development. Memory allows cells to autonomously preserve their distinctive character and pass it on to their progeny.[1]

Fully specialized, or **terminally differentiated,** cells that are lost are regenerated from proliferating *precursor cells.* These precursor cells have been derived from a smaller number of stem cells.[1] **Stem cells** are cells with the potential to develop into many different cell types during early development and growth. In many tissues, stem cells serve as an internal repair and maintenance system, dividing indefinitely. These cells can maintain themselves over very long periods, an ability that is referred to as **self-renewal,** and can generate all the differentiated cell types of the tissue or **multipotency.** This stem cell–driven tissue renewal is very evident in the epithelial lining of the intestine, stomach, blood cells, and skin, which is continuously exposed to environmental factors. When a stem cell divides, each daughter cell has a choice: It can remain as a stem cell, or it can follow a pathway that results in terminal differentiation (Fig. 1.34).

QUICK CHECK 1.4
1. What is the cell cycle?
2. Describe the DNA damage response
3. Discuss the five types of intracellular communication.
4. Why is the ECM important for tissue cells?

Text continued on p. 36

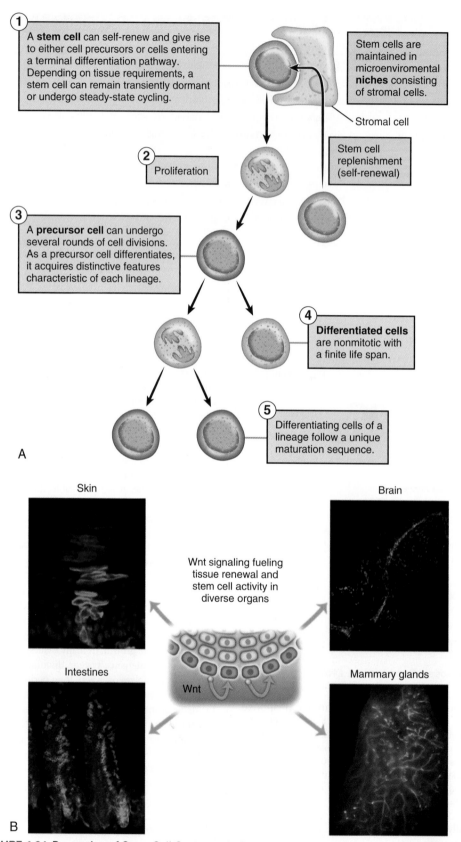

① A **stem cell** can self-renew and give rise to either cell precursors or cells entering a terminal differentiation pathway. Depending on tissue requirements, a stem cell can remain transiently dormant or undergo steady-state cycling.

Stem cells are maintained in microenviromental **niches** consisting of stromal cells.

Stromal cell

② Proliferation

Stem cell replenishment (self-renewal)

③ A **precursor cell** can undergo several rounds of cell divisions. As a precursor cell differentiates, it acquires distinctive features characteristic of each lineage.

④ **Differentiated cells** are nonmitotic with a finite life span.

⑤ Differentiating cells of a lineage follow a unique maturation sequence.

A

Skin

Brain

Wnt signaling fueling tissue renewal and stem cell activity in diverse organs

Intestines

Mammary glands

Wnt

B

FIGURE 1.34 Properties of Stem Cell Systems. A, Stem cells have three characteristics: *self-renewal, proliferation,* and *differentiation* into mature cells. Stem cells are housed in *niches* consisting of *stromal cells* that provide factors for their maintenance. Stem cells of the embryo can give rise to cell precursors that generate all the tissues of the body. This property defines stem cells as *multipotent.* Stem cells are difficult to identify anatomically. Their identification is based on specific *cell surface markers* (cell surface antigens recognized by specific monoclonal antibodies) and on the lineage they generate following *transplantation.* **B,** Wnt signaling fuels tissue renewal. (**A,** from Kierszenbaum A: *Histology and cell biology: an introduction to pathology,* ed 3, St Louis, 2012, Elsevier. **B,** from Clevers H, et al: *Science* 346(6205):1248012, 2014.)

TABLE 1.6 Characteristics of Epithelial Tissues

Simple Squamous Epithelium

Structure

Single layer of cells

Location and Function

Lining of blood vessels leads to diffusion and filtration

Lining of pulmonary alveoli (air sacs) leads to separation of blood from fluids in tissues

Bowman's capsule (kidney), where it filters substances from blood, forming urine

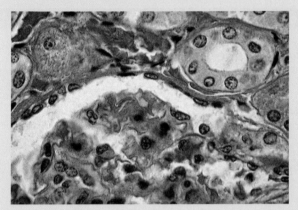

Simple Squamous Epithelial Cell. Photomicrograph of simple squamous epithelial cell in parietal wall of Bowman's capsule in kidney. (From Erlandsen SL, Magney JE: *Color atlas of histology,* St Louis, 1992, Mosby.)

Stratified Squamous Epithelium

Structure

Two or more layers, depending on location, with cells closest to basement membrane tending to be cuboidal

Location and Function

Epidermis of skin and linings of mouth, pharynx, esophagus, and anus provide protection and secretion

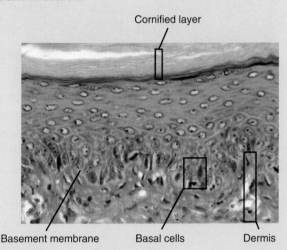

Cornified layer

Basement membrane   Basal cells   Dermis

Cornified Stratified Squamous Epithelium. Diagram of stratified squamous epithelium of skin. (Copyright Ed Reschke. Used with permission.)

Transitional Epithelium

Structure

Vary in shape from cuboidal to squamous depending on whether basal cells of bladder are columnar or are composed of many layers; when bladder is full and stretched, the cells flatten and stretch like squamous cells

Location and Function

Linings of urinary bladder and other hollow structures stretch, allowing expansion of the hollow organs

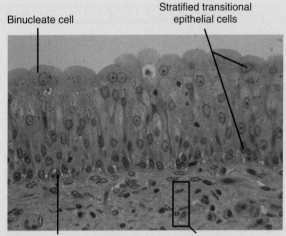

Binucleate cell

Stratified transitional epithelial cells

Basement membrane   Connective tissue

Stratified Squamous Transitional Epithelium. Photomicrograph of stratified squamous transitional epithelium of urinary bladder. (Copyright Ed Reschke. Used with permission.)

Simple Cuboidal Epithelium

Structure

Simple cuboidal cells; rarely stratified (layered)

Location and Function

Glands (e.g., thyroid, sweat, salivary) and parts of the kidney tubules and outer covering of ovary secrete fluids

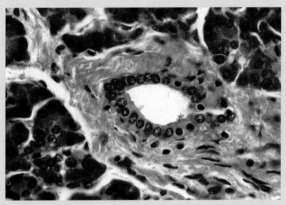

Simple Cuboidal Epithelium. Photomicrograph of simple cuboidal epithelium of pancreatic duct. (From Erlandsen SL, Magney JE: *Color atlas of histology,* St Louis, 1992, Mosby.)

Continued

TABLE 1.6   Characteristics of Epithelial Tissues—cont'd

Simple Columnar Epithelium

Structure

Large amounts of cytoplasm and cellular organelles

Location and Function

Ducts of many glands and lining of digestive tract allow secretion and absorption from stomach to anus

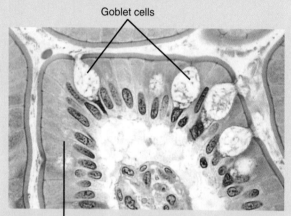

Goblet cells

Columnar epithelial cell

Simple Columnar Epithelium. Photomicrograph of simple columnar epithelium. (Copyright Ed Reschke. Used with permission.)

Ciliated Simple Columnar Epithelium

Structure

Same as simple columnar epithelium but ciliated

Location and Function

Linings of bronchi of lungs, nasal cavity, and oviducts allow secretion, absorption, and propulsion of fluids and particles

Stratified Columnar Epithelium

Structure

Small and rounded basement membrane (columnar cells do not touch basement membrane)

Location and Function

Linings of epiglottis, part of pharynx, anus, and male urethra provide protection

Pseudostratified Ciliated Columnar Epithelium

Structure

All cells in contact with basement membrane

Nuclei found at different levels within cell, giving stratified appearance

Free surface often ciliated

Location and Function

Linings of large ducts of some glands (parotid, salivary), male urethra, respiratory passages, and eustachian tubes of ears transport substances

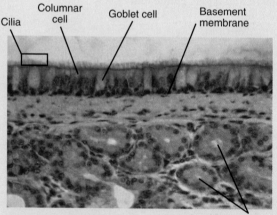

Cilia   Columnar cell   Goblet cell   Basement membrane

Mucous glands

Pseudostratified Ciliated Columnar Epithelium. Photomicrograph of pseudostratified ciliated columnar epithelium of trachea. (Copyright Robert L. Calentine. Used with permission.)

TABLE 1.7   Connective Tissues

Loose or Areolar Tissue

Structure

Unorganized; spaces between fibers

Most fibers collagenous, some elastic and reticular

Includes many types of cells (fibroblasts and macrophages most common) and large amount of intercellular fluid

Location and Function

Attaches skin to underlying tissue; holds organs in place by filling spaces between them; supports blood vessels

Intercellular fluid transports nutrients and waste productsFluid accumulation causes swelling (edema)

Bundle of collagenous fibers

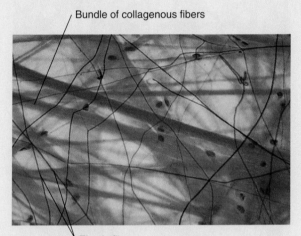

Elastic fibers

Loose Areolar Connective Tissue. (Copyright Ed Reschke. Used with permission.)

Dense Irregular Tissue

Structure

Dense, compact, and areolar tissue, with fewer cells and greater number of closely woven collagenous fibers than in loose tissue

Location and Function

Dermis layer of skin; acts as protective barrier

Fibroblast   Collagenous fibers

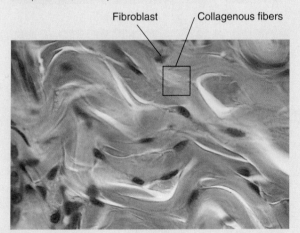

Dense, Irregular Connective Tissue. (Copyright Ed Reschke. Used with permission.)

Dense, Regular (White Fibrous) Tissue

Structure

Collagenous fibers and some elastic fibers, tightly packed into parallel bundles, with only fibroblast cells

Location and Function

Forms strong tendons of muscle, ligaments of joints, some fibrous membranes, and fascia that surrounds organs and muscles

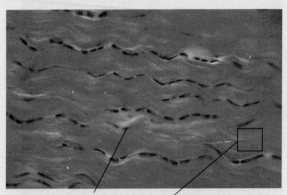

Fibroblast   Collagenous fibers

Dense, Regular (White Fibrous) Connective Tissue. (Copyright Phototake. Used with permission.)

Elastic Tissue

Structure

Elastic fibers, some collagenous fibers, fibroblasts

Location and Function

Lends strength and elasticity to walls of arteries, trachea, vocal cords, and other structures

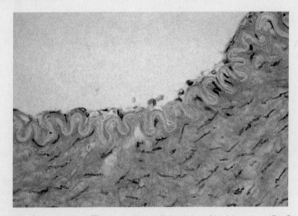

Elastic Connective Tissue. (From Erlandsen SL, Magney JE: *Color atlas of histology*, St Louis, 1992, Mosby.)

Continued

TABLE 1.7   Connective Tissues—cont'd

Adipose Tissue

Structure

Fat cells dispersed in loose tissues; each cell containing a large droplet of fat flattens nucleus and forces cytoplasm into a ring around cell's periphery

Location and Function

Stores fat, which provides padding and protection

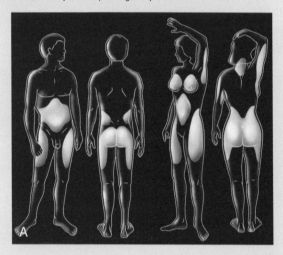

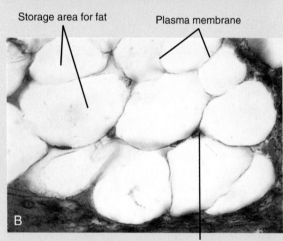

Adipose Tissue. **A,** Fat storage areas—distribution of fat in male and female bodies. **B,** Photomicrograph of adipose tissue. (**A** from Thibodeau GA, Patton KT: *Anatomy & physiology,* ed 6, St Louis, 2007, Mosby; **B** copyright Ed Reschke. Used with permission.)

Cartilage (Hyaline, Elastic, Fibrous)

Structure

Collagenous fibers embedded in a firm matrix (chondrin); no blood supply

Location and Function

Gives form, support, and flexibility to joints, trachea, nose, ear, vertebral disks, embryonic skeleton, and many internal structures

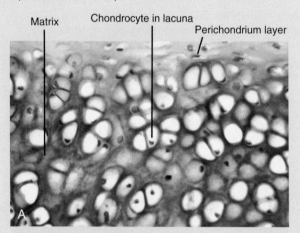

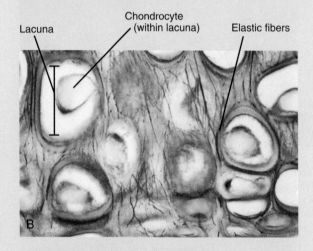

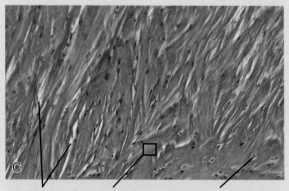

Cartilage. **A,** Hyaline cartilage. **B,** Elastic cartilage. **C,** Fibrous cartilage. (**A and C,** copyright Robert L. Calentine. **B,** copyright Ed Reshke. Used with permission.)

TABLE 1.7   Connective Tissues—cont'd

Bone
Structure
Rigid connective tissue consisting of cells, fibers, ground substances, and minerals

Location and Function
Lends skeleton rigidity and strength

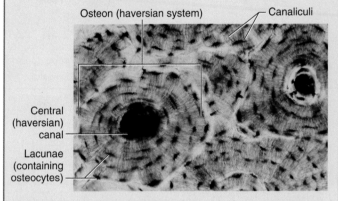

Bone. (From Patton KT, Thibodeau GA: *Anatomy & physiology*, ed 10, St. Louis, 2019, Elsevier.)

Special Connective Tissues
Plasma
Structure
Fluid

Location and Function
Serves as matrix for blood cells

Macrophages in Tissue, Reticuloendothelial, or Macrophage System
Structure
Scattered macrophages (phagocytes) called *Kupffer cells* (in liver), alveolar macrophages (in lungs), microglia (in central nervous system)

Location and Function
Facilitate inflammatory response and carry out phagocytosis in loose connective, lymphatic, digestive, medullary (bone marrow), splenic, adrenal, and pituitary tissues

TABLE 1.8   Muscle Tissues

Skeletal (Striated) Muscle
Structure Characteristics of Cells
Long, cylindrical cells that extend throughout length of muscles

Striated myofibrils (proteins)

Many nuclei on periphery

Location and Function
Attached to bones directly or by tendons and provide voluntary movement of skeleton and maintenance of posture

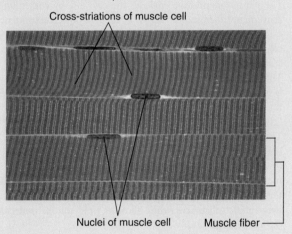

Skeletal (Striated) Muscle. (From Thibodeau GA, Patton KT: *Anatomy & physiology*, ed 6, St Louis, 2007, Mosby.)

Cardiac Muscle
Structure Characteristics of Cells
Branching networks throughout muscle tissue

Striated myofibrils

Location and Function
Cells attached end-to-end at intercalated disks with tissue forming walls of heart (myocardium) to provide involuntary pumping action of heart

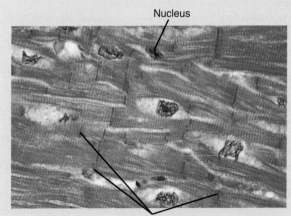

Cardiac Muscle. (Copyright Ed Reschke. Used with permission.)

Continued

TABLE 1.8   Muscle Tissues—cont'd

Smooth (Visceral) Muscle
Structure Characteristics of Cells
Long spindles that taper to a point

Absence of striated myofibrils

Location and Function
Walls of hollow internal structures, such as digestive tract and blood vessels (viscera), provide voluntary and involuntary contractions that move substances through hollow structures

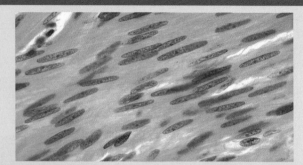

Smooth (Visceral) Muscle. (From Young B, Woodford P: *Wheater's functional histology*, ed 6, Philadelphia, 2014, Churchill Livingstone.)

SUMMARY REVIEW

Prokaryotes and Eukaryotes

1. Eukaryotes are the cells of higher animals and plants, fungi, protozoa, and most algae. These cells are larger and have membrane bound intracellular compartments (organelles) and a well-defined nucleus. Genetic information is contained in several or many chromosomes.
2. Prokaryotes include blue-green algae, bacteria, and rickettsiae. They contain no organelles and their nucleus is not well defined. Genetic information is contained in a single circular chromosome.

Cellular Functions

1. Cells become specialized through the process of differentiation, or maturation, so that they perform one kind of function.
2. The eight specialized cellular functions are movement, conductivity, metabolic absorption, secretion, excretion, respiration, reproduction, and communication.

Structure and Function of Cellular Components

1. The eukaryotic cell consists of three general components: the plasma membrane, the cytoplasm, and the intracellular organelles.
2. The nucleus is the largest membrane-bound organelle and is found usually in the cell's center. The chief functions of the nucleus are cell division and control of genetic information.
3. Cytoplasm, or the cytoplasmic matrix, is an aqueous solution (cytosol) that fills the space between the nucleus and the plasma membrane. It represents about half of the volume of the cell.
4. The organelles are suspended in the cytoplasm and are enclosed in biologic membranes.
5. Ribosomes are RNA-protein complexes that provide sites for cellular protein synthesis.
6. The endoplasmic reticulum is a network of tubular channels (cisternae) that extend throughout the outer nuclear membrane. It specializes in the synthesis, folding, and transport of protein and lipid components of most of the organelles, as well as in sensing cellular stress.
7. The Golgi complex is a network of smooth membranes and vesicles located near the nucleus. The Golgi complex is responsible for processing and packaging proteins into secretory vesicles that break away from the Golgi complex and migrate to a variety of intracellular and extracellular destinations, including the plasma membrane.
8. Lysosomes are saclike structures that contain digestive enzymes. These enzymes are responsible for digesting most cellular substances to their basic form, such as amino acids, fatty acids, and carbohydrates (sugars). Cellular injury leads to a release of the lysosomal enzymes, causing cellular self-digestion. They also serve as signaling hubs in a network for cellular adaptation.
9. Peroxisomes appear similar to lysosomes but contain several enzymes that either produce or use hydrogen peroxide and their reactions detoxify waste products.
10. Mitochondria contain the metabolic machinery necessary for cellular energy metabolism. The enzymes of the respiratory chain (electron-transport chain), found in the inner membrane of the mitochondria, generate most of the cell's ATP.
11. The cytoskeleton is the "bone and muscle" of the cell. The internal skeleton is composed of a network of protein filaments, including microtubules and actin filaments (microfilaments). They also form cell extensions (microvilli, cilia, flagella).
12. The plasma membrane encloses the cell and, by controlling the movement of substances across it, exerts a powerful influence on metabolic pathways. Other important functions include cell-to-cell recognition, cellular mobility, and maintenance of cellular shape.
13. The basic structure of plasma membrane is the lipid bilayer, which is studded with various proteins. Carbohydrates contained within the plasma membrane are generally bound to membrane proteins (glycoproteins) and lipids (glycolipids).
14. The lipid bilayer determines the structure of the membrane. Each lipid molecule is polar, or amphipathic: the head is hydrophilic ("water loving") and the tail is hydrophobic ("water hating"). The membrane is organized in two layers, with the tails inward and the heads outward. This provides a barrier to the diffusion of hydrophilic substances, while allowing lipid-soluble molecules to diffuse through readily.
15. Membrane proteins can extend across the bilayer, be in the bilayer but primarily on one side or the other, or can exist outside of the bilayer. Membrane proteins, like other proteins, are synthesized by the ribosome and then translocate, called trafficking, to different locations in the cell. Trafficking places unique demands on membrane proteins for folding, translocation, and stability. Misfolded proteins are emerging as an important cause of disease.

16. Proteins determine the functions of the membrane. Proteins perform most of the plasma membrane's tasks. Proteins act as recognition and binding units for substances moving in and out of the cell, pores and transport channels, enzymes that drive pumps or maintain ion concentrations, cell surface markers, cell adhesion molecules, and catalysts of chemical reactions. Proteins form cellular receptors that recognize and bind with smaller molecules called ligands.

17. Proteostasis is the state of cell balance of the processes of protein synthesis, folding, and dehydration (protein homeostasis). The proteostasis network is composed of ribosomes (makers), chaperones (helpers), and protein breakdown or proteolytic systems. Malfunction of these systems is associated with disease.

18. The carbohydrates on the outside of the plasma membrane form a coating (glycocalyx) that protects the cell from mechanical damage and creates a slimy surface that assists in mobility. Carbohydrates also function in cell-cell recognition and adhesion.

Cell-to-Cell Adhesions

1. Cell-to-cell adhesions are formed on plasma membranes, thereby allowing the formation of tissues and organs. Cells are held together by three different means: (1) the extracellular membrane, (2) cell adhesion molecules in the cell's plasma membrane, and (3) specialized cell junctions.

2. The extracellular matrix (ECM) is secreted by cells and is a meshwork of fibrous proteins in a gel-like substance. It provides a pathway for diffusion of nutrients, wastes, and other water-soluble substances. The ECM includes three groups of macromolecules: (1) fibrous structural proteins (collagen and elastin), (2) adhesive glycoproteins, and (3) proteoglycans and hyaluronic acid. The matrix helps regulate cell growth, movement, and differentiation.

3. Basement membrane is a specialized type of ECM that is very thin, tough, and flexible. It lies under the epithelium of many organs and is also called the basal lamina.

4. Cell junctions are the contacts between neighboring cells. They can hold cells together with a tight seal, provide strong mechanical attachments, provide a chemical communication, and maintain polarity of cells. Cell junctions can be classified as symmetric and asymmetric. Symmetric junctions include tight junctions, the belt desmosome, desmosomes, and gap junctions. An asymmetric junction is the hemidesmosome.

Cellular Communication and Signal Transduction

1. Cells communicate in three main ways: (1) they form protein channels (gap junctions); (2) they display receptors that affect intracellular processes or other cells in direct physical contact; and (3) they use receptor proteins inside the target cell.

2. Primary modes of intercellular signaling include contact-dependent, paracrine, hormonal, neurohormonal, and neurotransmitter.

3. Signal transduction involves signals or instructions from extracellular chemical messengers that are conveyed to the cell's interior for execution. If deprived of appropriate signals, cells undergo a form of cell suicide known as programmed cell death or apoptosis.

4. Binding of the extracellular signaling messenger (first messenger) to the membrane receptors causes 1) the opening or closing of channels that regulate ion movement and 2) the transfer of the signal to an intracellular messenger (second messenger) that triggers a cascade of events in the cell.

Cellular Metabolism

1. The chemical tasks of maintaining essential cellular functions are referred to as cellular metabolism. Anabolism is the energy-using process of metabolism, whereas catabolism is the energy-releasing process.

2. Adenosine triphosphate (ATP) functions as an energy-transferring molecule. It is fuel for cell survival. Energy is stored by molecules of carbohydrate, lipid, and protein, which, when catabolized, transfers energy to ATP. The phases of catabolism are digestion, glycolysis and oxidation, and the citric acid cycle.

3. Oxidative phosphorylation occurs in the mitochondria and is the mechanism by which the energy produced from carbohydrates, fats, and proteins is transferred to ATP.

Membrane Transport: Cellular Intake and Output

1. Cell survival and growth depends on the constant exchange of molecules with their environment. The majority of molecular transfer depends on specialized membrane transport proteins. The two main classes of membrane transport proteins are transporters and channels.

2. Passive transport does not require the expenditure of energy; rather, it is driven by physical effects. Passive transport mechanisms include diffusion, filtration, and osmosis. Water and small, electrically uncharged molecules move through pores in the plasma membrane's lipid bilayer via passive transport.

3. Diffusion is the passive movement of a solute from an area of greater solute concentration to an area of lesser solute concentration, a difference known as the concentration gradient.

4. Filtration is the movement of water and solutes through a membrane because of a greater pushing pressure on one side. Hydrostatic pressure is the force of water pushing against a cellular membrane.

5. Osmosis is the movement of water across a semipermeable membrane from a region of lower solute concentration to a region of higher solute concentration. The amount of hydrostatic pressure required to oppose the osmotic movement of water is called the osmotic pressure of solution. The overall osmotic effect of colloids, such as plasma proteins, is called the oncotic pressure or colloid osmotic pressure.

6. Active transport requires expenditure of metabolic energy by the cell by means of ATP. Larger molecules and molecular complexes are moved into the cell by active transport.

7. The active transport of Na^+ and K^+ is found in virtually all cells. Around 60-70% of ATP synthesized by cells is used to maintain the transport of Na^+ and K^+.

8. The largest molecules (macromolecules) and fluids are transported by membrane-bound vesicles through the processes of endocytosis (ingestion) and exocytosis (expulsion).

9. Endocytosis, or vesicle formation, is when the substance to be transported is engulfed by a segment of the plasma membrane, forming a vesicle that moves into the cell. Pinocytosis is a type of endocytosis in which fluids and solute molecules are ingested through formation of small vesicles. Phagocytosis is a type of endocytosis in which large particles, such as bacteria, are ingested through formation of large vesicles, called vacuoles.

10. In receptor-mediated endocytosis, the plasma membrane receptors are clustered, along with bristlelike structures, in specialized areas called coated pits. Endocytosis occurs when the coated pits invaginate, internalizing ligand-receptor complexes in coated vesicles.

11. Inside the cell, lysosomal enzymes process and digest material ingested by endocytosis.

12. In exocytosis, a membrane bound vesicle carries macromolecules to the outer cell membrane. It has two main functions: it releases molecules synthesized by the cells into the extracellular matrix and replaces portions of the plasma membrane that have been removed by endocytosis.

13. Two types of solutes exist in body fluids: electrolytes and nonelectrolytes. Electrolytes are electrically charged and dissociate into constituent ions when placed in solution. Nonelectrolytes do not dissociate when placed in solution.

14. All body cells are electrically polarized, with the inside of the cell more negatively charged than the outside. The difference in voltage across the plasma membrane is the resting membrane potential.

15. When an excitable (nerve or muscle) cell receives an electrochemical stimulus, cations enter the cell and cause a rapid change in the resting membrane potential known as the action potential. The action potential "moves" along the cell's plasma membrane and is transmitted to an adjacent cell. This is how electrochemical signals convey information from cell to cell.

Cellular Reproduction: The Cell Cycle

1. Cellular reproduction in body tissues involves mitosis (nuclear division) and cytokinesis (cytoplasmic division).

2. Only mature cells are capable of division. Maturation occurs during a stage of cellular life called interphase (growth phase).

3. The cell cycle is the reproductive process that begins after interphase in all tissues with cellular turnover. There are four phases of the cell cycle: (1) the G_1 phase (G = gap), the period between the M phase and the start of DNA synthesis; (2) the S phase (S = synthesis), during which DNA synthesis takes place in the cell nucleus; (3) the G_2 phase, the period between the completion of DNA synthesis and the next phase in which RNA and protein synthesis occurs; and (4) the M phase (M = mitosis), which involves both nuclear and cytoplasmic division.

4. The M phase (mitosis) involves four stages: prophase, metaphase, anaphase, and telophase.

5. Cellular division and growth are regulated by intracellular programs and several extracellular signal molecules. Mitogens induces or simulates mitosis. Growth factors stimulate an increase in cell mass or cell growth. Survival factors inhibit the programmed cell death called apoptosis.

Tissues

1. Cells of one or more types are organized into tissues, and different types of tissues compose organs. Organs are organized to function as tracts or systems.

2. Three key factors that maintain the cellular organization of tissues are (1) recognition and cell communication, (2) selective cell-to-cell adhesion, and (3) memory.

3. Fully specialized or terminally differentiated cells that are lost are generated from proliferating precursor cells and they, in turn, have been derived from a smaller number of stem cells. Stem cells are cells with the potential to develop into many different cell types during early development and growth. In many tissues, stem cells serve as an internal repair and maintenance system dividing indefinitely. These cells can maintain themselves over very long periods of time, called self-renewal, and can generate all the differentiated cell types of the tissue or multipotency.

4. The four basic types of tissues are epithelial, muscle, nerve, and connective tissues.

5. Neural tissue is composed of highly specialized cells called neurons that receive and transmit electrical impulses rapidly across junctions called synapses.

6. Epithelial tissue covers most internal and external surfaces of the body. The functions of epithelial tissue include protection, absorption, secretion, and excretion.

7. Connective tissue binds various tissues and organs together, supporting them in their locations and serving as storage sites for excess nutrients.

8. Muscle tissue is composed of long, thin, highly contractile cells or fibers. Muscle tissue that is attached to bones enables voluntary movement. Muscle tissue in internal organs enables involuntary movement, such as the heartbeat.

KEY TERMS

Absolute refractory period, 26
Action potential, 26
Active transport, 19
Amphipathic, 4
Anabolism, 17
Anaphase, 28
Anion, 20
Antiport, 20
Autocrine signaling, 14
Basal lamina, 12
Basement membrane (BM), 12
Binding site, 10
Cadherin, 11
Catabolism, 17
Cation, 20
Cell adhesion molecule (CAM), 9
Cell cortex, 9
Cell cycle, 27
Cell cycle arrest, 28
Cell junction, 12
Cell polarity, 4
Cell-to-cell adhesion, 11
Cellular metabolism, 17

Cellular receptor, 10
Centromere, 28
Channel, 19
Chemical synapse, 14
Chromatid, 28
Chromatin, 28
Citric acid cycle (Krebs cycle, tricarboxylic acid cycle), 17
Clathrin, 23
Coated vesicle, 23
Collagen, 12
Concentration gradient, 20
Connexons, 13
Contact-dependent signaling, 14
Cytokinesis, 27
Cytoplasm, 2
Cytoplasmic matrix, 3
Cytochrome, 18
Cytosol, 3
Daughter cell, 28
Depolarization, 26
Desmosome, 13
Differentiation, 1
Diffusion, 20

Digestion, 17
DNA damage response, 28
Effective osmolality, 21
Elastin, 12
Electrolyte, 20
Electron-transport chain, 18
Endocytosis, 23
Endosome, 23
Equatorial plate (metaphase plate), 28
ER stress, 10
Eukaryote, 1
Exocytosis, 24
Exosome, 23
Extracellular matrix (ECM), 12
Fibroblast, 12
Fibronectin, 12
Filtration, 20
First messenger, 15
G_1 phase, 27
G_2 phase, 27
Gap junction, 13
Gating, 13
Glycocalyx, 10

Glycolipid, 4
Glycolysis, 17
Glycoprotein, 4, 9
Growth factor, 28
Homeostasis, 13
Hormonal signaling, 14
Hydrostatic pressure, 20
Hyperpolarized state, 26
Hypopolarized state, 26
Immunoglobulin superfamily (CAM), 11
Integral membrane protein, 9
Integrin, 11
Interphase, 27
Ion, 9, 20
Junctional complex, 13
Ligand, 10
Lipid bilayer, 4
M phase, 27
Macromolecule, 12
Mediated transport, 19
Membrane transport protein, 18
Metabolic pathway, 17

REFERENCES

1. Alberts B, et al: *Essential cell biology*, ed 4, New York, 2014, Garland.
2. Ramdani G, Langsley G: ATP, an extracellular signaling molecule in red blood cells: a messenger for malaria?, *Biomed J* 37(5):284-292, 2014.
3. Dou L, et al: Extracellular ATP signaling and clinical relevance, *Clin Immunol* 188:67-73, 2018.
4. Soung YH, et al: Exosomes in cancer diagnostics, *Cancers (Basel)* 9(1):2017.
5. Alberts B, et al: *Molecular biology of the cell*, ed 6, New York, 2015, Garland Science.

2

Genes and Genetic Diseases

Lynn B. Jorde

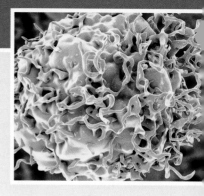

EVOLVE WEBSITE

CHAPTER OUTLINE

Genetics is the study of biologic inheritance. An understanding of genetics is essential to study human, animal, plant, or microbial life. In the nineteenth century, microscopic studies of cells led scientists to suspect the nucleus of the cell contained the important mechanisms of inheritance. Scientists found chromatin, the substance giving the nucleus a granular appearance, is observable in nondividing cells. Just before the cell divides, the chromatin condenses to form discrete, dark-staining organelles, which are called chromosomes. (Cell division is discussed in Chapter 1.) With the rediscovery of Mendel's important breeding experiments at the turn of the twentieth century, it soon became apparent the chromosomes contained genes, the basic units of inheritance (Fig. 2.1).

The primary constituent of chromatin is deoxyribonucleic acid (DNA). Genes are composed of sequences of DNA. By serving as the blueprints of proteins in the body, genes ultimately influence all aspects of body structure and function. Humans have approximately 20,000 protein-coding genes and at least an additional 9000 to 10,000 genes that encode various types of ribonucleic acid (RNA; see below) that are not translated into proteins. An error in one of these genes often leads to a recognizable genetic disease.

To date, more than 20,000 genetic traits and diseases have been identified and cataloged. As infectious diseases continue to be more effectively controlled, the proportion of beds in pediatric hospitals occupied by children with genetic diseases has risen. In addition to genetic diseases in children, many common diseases primarily affecting adults, such as hypertension, coronary heart disease, diabetes, and cancer, are now known to have important genetic components.

Great progress is being made in the diagnosis of genetic diseases and in the understanding of genetic mechanisms underlying them.

With the huge strides being made in molecular genetics, "gene therapy"—the utilization of normal genes to correct genetic disease—has begun.

DNA, RNA, AND PROTEINS: HEREDITY AT THE MOLECULAR LEVEL

Definitions

Composition and Structure of DNA

Genes are composed of DNA, which has three basic components: the five-carbon monosaccharide deoxyribose; a phosphate molecule; and four types of nitrogenous bases. Two of the bases, cytosine and thymine, are single carbon-nitrogen rings called pyrimidines. The other two bases, adenine and guanine, are double carbon-nitrogen rings called purines. The four bases are commonly represented by their first letters: A (adenine), C (cytosine), T (thymine), and G (guanine).

Watson and Crick demonstrated how these molecules are physically assembled as DNA, proposing the double-helix model, in which DNA appears like a twisted ladder with chemical bonds as its rungs (Fig. 2.2). The two sides of the ladder consist of deoxyribose and phosphate molecules, united by strong phosphodiester bonds. Projecting from each side of the ladder, at regular intervals, are the nitrogenous bases. The base projecting from one side is bound to the base projecting from the other by a weak hydrogen bond. Therefore the nitrogenous bases form the rungs of the ladder; adenine pairs with thymine, and guanine pairs with cytosine. Each DNA subunit—consisting of one deoxyribose molecule, one phosphate group, and one base—is called a nucleotide.

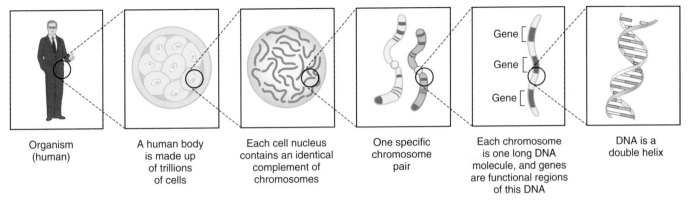

FIGURE 2.1 Successive Enlargements From a Human to the Genetic Material.

DNA as the Genetic Code

DNA directs the synthesis of all the body's proteins. Proteins are composed of one or more polypeptides (intermediate protein compounds), which in turn consist of sequences of amino acids. The body contains 20 different types of amino acids; they are specified by the four nitrogenous bases. To specify (code for) 20 different amino acids with only four bases, different combinations of bases, occurring in groups of three (triplets), are used. These triplets of bases are known as codons. Each codon specifies a single amino acid in a corresponding protein. Because there are 64 ($4 \times 4 \times 4$) possible codons but only 20 amino acids, there are many cases in which several codons correspond to the same amino acid.

The genetic code is universal: *all* living organisms use precisely the same DNA codes to specify proteins except for mitochondria, the cytoplasmic organelles in which cellular respiration takes place (see Chapter 1)—they have their own extranuclear DNA. Several codons of mitochondrial DNA encode different amino acids, compared with the same nuclear DNA codons.

Replication of DNA

DNA replication consists of breaking the weak hydrogen bonds between the bases, leaving a single strand with each base unpaired (Fig. 2.3). The consistent pairing of adenine with thymine and of guanine with cytosine, known as complementary base pairing, is the key to accurate replication. The unpaired base attracts a free nucleotide only if the nucleotide has the proper complementary base. When replication is complete, a new double-stranded molecule identical to the original is formed. The single strand is said to be a template, or molecule on which a complementary molecule is built, and is the basis for synthesizing the new double strand.

Several different proteins are involved in DNA replication. The most important of these proteins is an enzyme known as DNA polymerase. This enzyme travels along the single DNA strand, adding the correct nucleotides to the free end of the new strand and checking to ensure that its base is actually complementary to the template base. This mechanism of DNA proofreading substantially enhances the accuracy of DNA replication.

Mutation

A mutation is any alteration of genetic material. One type of mutation is the base pair substitution, in which one base pair replaces another. This replacement *can* result in a change in the amino acid sequence. However, because of the redundancy of the genetic code, many of these mutations do not change the amino acid sequence and thus have no consequence. Such mutations are called silent mutations. Base pair substitutions altering amino acids consist of two basic types: missense mutations, which produce a change (i.e., the "sense") in a single amino acid; and nonsense mutations, which produce one of the three stop codons (UAA, UAG, or UGA) in the messenger RNA (mRNA) (Fig. 2.4). Missense mutations (see Fig. 2.4, *A*) produce a single amino acid change, whereas nonsense mutations (see Fig. 2.4, *B*) produce a premature stop codon in the mRNA. Stop codons terminate translation of the polypeptide.

The frameshift mutation involves the insertion or deletion of one or more base pairs of the DNA molecule. As Fig. 2.5 shows, these mutations change the entire "reading frame" of the DNA sequence because the deletion or insertion is not a multiple of three base pairs (the number of base pairs in a codon). Frameshift mutations can thus greatly alter the amino acid sequence. (*In-frame* insertions or deletions, in which a multiple of three bases is inserted or lost, tend to have less severe disease consequences than do frameshift mutations.)

Agents known as mutagens increase the frequency of mutations. Examples include radiation and chemicals, such as nitrogen mustard, vinyl chloride, alkylating agents, formaldehyde, and sodium nitrite.

Mutations are rare events. The rate of spontaneous mutations (those occurring in the absence of exposure to known mutagens) in humans is about 10^{-4} to 10^{-7} per gene per generation. This rate varies from one gene to another. Some DNA sequences have particularly high mutation rates and are known as mutational hot spots.

From Genes to Proteins

DNA is formed and replicated in the cell nucleus, but protein synthesis takes place in the cytoplasm. The DNA code is transported from nucleus to cytoplasm, and subsequent protein is formed through two basic processes: transcription and translation. These processes are mediated by ribonucleic acid (RNA), which is chemically similar to DNA except the sugar molecule is ribose rather than deoxyribose, and uracil rather than thymine is one of the four bases. The other bases of RNA, as in DNA, are adenine, cytosine, and guanine. Uracil is structurally similar to thymine, so it also can pair with adenine. DNA usually occurs as a double strand, whereas RNA usually occurs as a single strand.

Transcription

In transcription, RNA is synthesized from a DNA template, forming messenger RNA (mRNA). RNA polymerase binds to a promoter site, a sequence of DNA that specifies the beginning of a gene. RNA polymerase then separates a portion of the DNA, exposing unattached DNA bases. One DNA strand then provides the template for the sequence of mRNA nucleotides.

The sequence of bases in the mRNA is thus complementary to the template strand, and except for the presence of uracil instead of thymine, the mRNA sequence is identical to that of the other DNA strand.

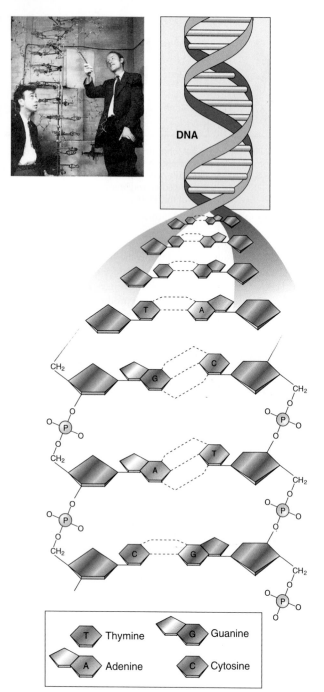

DNA

CH₂

CH₂

CH₂

FIGURE 2.2 Watson-Crick Model of the Deoxyribonucleic Acid (DNA) Molecule. The DNA structure illustrated here is based on that published by James Watson *(photograph, left)* and Francis Crick *(photograph, right)* in 1953. Note that each side of the DNA molecule consists of alternating sugar and phosphate groups. Each sugar group is bonded to the opposing sugar group by a pair of nitrogenous bases (adenine–thymine or cytosine–guanine). The sequence of these pairs constitutes a genetic code that determines the structure and function of a cell. (Illustration from Herlihy B: *The human body in health and illness,* ed 5, St Louis, 2015, Saunders.)

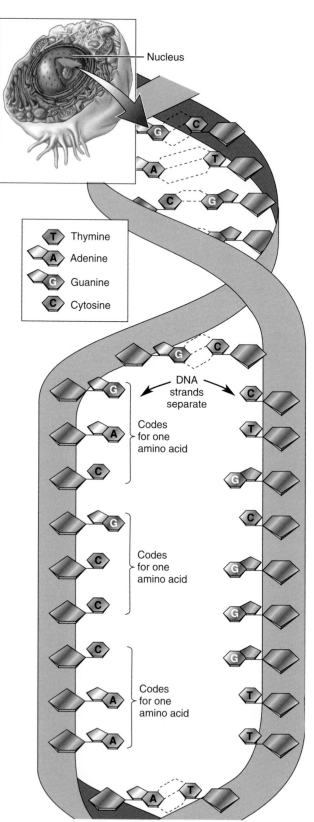

FIGURE 2.3 Replication of Deoxyribonucleic Acid (DNA). The two chains of the double helix separate and each chain serves as the template for a new complementary chain. (From Herlihy B: *The human body in health and illness,* ed 5, St Louis, 2015, Saunders.)

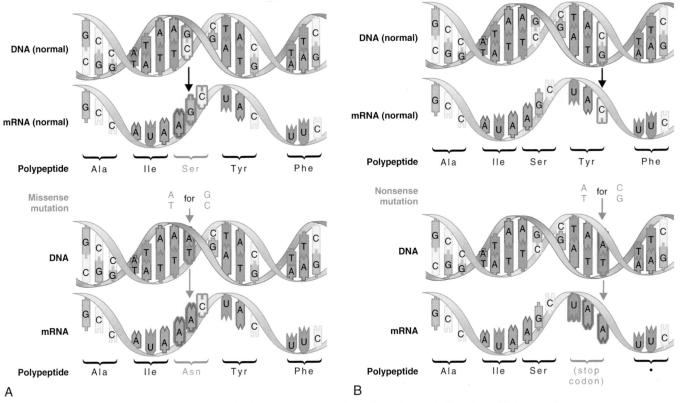

FIGURE 2.4 Base Pair Substitution. Missense mutations (**A**) produce a single amino acid change, whereas nonsense mutations (**B**) produce a stop codon in the messenger ribonucleic acid (mRNA). Stop codons terminate translation of the polypeptide. (From Jorde L et al: *Medical genetics,* ed 4, St Louis, 2010, Mosby.)

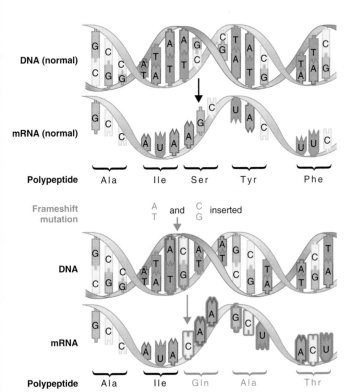

FIGURE 2.5 Frameshift Mutations. Frameshift mutations result from the addition or deletion of a number of bases that is not a multiple of 3. This mutation alters all of the codons downstream from the site of insertion or deletion. (From Jorde L et al: *Medical genetics,* ed 4, St Louis, 2010, Mosby.)

Transcription continues until a **termination sequence**, codons that act as signals for the termination of protein synthesis, is reached. Then the RNA polymerase detaches from the DNA, and the transcribed mRNA is freed to move out of the nucleus and into the cytoplasm (Figs. 2.6 and 2.7).

Gene Splicing

When the mRNA is first transcribed from the DNA template, it reflects exactly the base sequence of the DNA. In eukaryotes, many RNA sequences are removed by nuclear enzymes, and the remaining sequences are spliced together to form the functional mRNA that migrates to the cytoplasm. The excised sequences are called **introns** (intervening sequences), and the sequences that are left to code for proteins are called **exons**.

Translation

In **translation**, RNA directs the synthesis of a polypeptide (see Fig. 2.7), interacting with **transfer RNA (tRNA)**, a cloverleaf-shaped strand of about 80 nucleotides. The tRNA molecule has a site where an amino acid attaches. The three-nucleotide sequence at the opposite side of the cloverleaf is called the **anticodon**. It undergoes complementary base pairing with an appropriate codon in the mRNA, which specifies the sequence of amino acids through tRNA.

The site of actual protein synthesis is in the **ribosome**, which consists of approximately equal parts of protein and **ribosomal RNA (rRNA)**. During translation, the ribosome first binds to an initiation site on the mRNA sequence and then binds to its surface, so that base pairing can occur between tRNA and mRNA. The ribosome then moves along the mRNA sequence, processing each codon and translating an amino acid by way of the interaction of mRNA and tRNA.

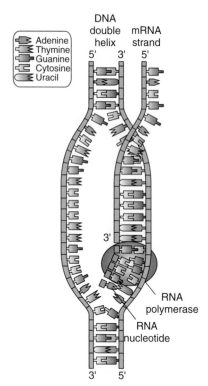

FIGURE 2.6 General Scheme of Ribonucleic Acid (RNA) Transcription. In transcription of messenger RNA (mRNA), a deoxyribonucleic acid (DNA) molecule "unzips" in the region of the gene to be transcribed. RNA nucleotides already present in the nucleus temporarily attach themselves to exposed DNA bases along one strand of the unzipped DNA molecule according to the principle of complementary pairing. As the RNA nucleotides attach to the exposed DNA, they bind to each other and form a chainlike RNA strand called a messenger RNA (mRNA) molecule. Note that the new mRNA strand is an exact copy of the base sequence on the opposite side of the DNA molecule. As in all metabolic processes, the formation of mRNA is controlled by an enzyme—in this case, the enzyme is called RNA polymerase. (From Ignatavicius DD, Workman LD: *Medical-surgical nursing,* ed 6, St Louis, 2010, Saunders.)

The ribosome provides an enzyme that catalyzes the formation of covalent peptide bonds between the adjacent amino acids, resulting in a growing polypeptide. When the ribosome arrives at a termination signal on the mRNA sequence, translation and polypeptide formation cease; the mRNA, ribosome, and polypeptide separate from one another; and the polypeptide is released into the cytoplasm to perform its required function.

CHROMOSOMES

Human cells can be categorized into **gametes** (sperm and egg cells) and **somatic cells**, which include all cells other than gametes. Each somatic cell nucleus has 46 chromosomes in 23 pairs (Fig. 2.8). These are **diploid cells**, and the individual's father and mother each donate one chromosome per pair. New somatic cells are formed through **mitosis** and **cytokinesis**. Gametes are **haploid cells**: They have only 1 member of each chromosome pair, for a total of 23 chromosomes. Haploid cells are formed from diploid cells by **meiosis** (Fig. 2.9).

In 22 of the 23 chromosome pairs, the two members of each pair are virtually identical in microscopic appearance: thus they are **homologous** (Fig. 2.10, *B*). These 22 chromosome pairs are homologous in both males and females and are termed **autosomes**. The remaining pair

of chromosomes, the sex chromosomes, consists of two homologous X chromosomes in females and a nonhomologous pair, X and Y, in males.

Fig. 2.10, *A,* illustrates a **metaphase spread**, which is a photograph of the chromosomes as they appear in the nucleus of a somatic cell during metaphase. (Chromosomes are easiest to visualize during this stage of mitosis.) In Fig. 2.10, *A,* the chromosomes are arranged according to size, with the homologous chromosomes paired. The 22 autosomes are numbered according to length, with chromosome 1 being the longest and chromosome 22 the shortest. A **karyotype**, or **karyogram**, is an ordered display of chromosomes. Some natural variation in relative chromosome length can be expected from person to person, so it is not always possible to distinguish each chromosome by its length. Therefore the position of the centromere (region of DNA responsible for movement of the replicated chromosomes into the two daughter cells during mitosis and meiosis) also is used to classify chromosomes (see Fig. 2.10, *B,* and Fig. 2.11).

The chromosomes in Fig. 2.10 were stained with Giemsa stain, resulting in distinctive **chromosome bands**. These form various patterns in the different chromosomes so that each chromosome can be distinguished easily. Using banding techniques, researchers can number chromosomes and study individual variations. Missing or duplicated portions of chromosomes, which often result in serious diseases, also are readily identified. More recently, techniques have been devised permitting each chromosome to be visualized with a different color.

Chromosome Aberrations and Associated Diseases

Chromosome abnormalities are the leading known cause of intellectual disability and miscarriage. Estimates indicate that a major chromosome aberration occurs in at least 1 in 12 conceptions. Most of these fetuses do not survive to term; about 50% of all recovered first-trimester spontaneous abortuses have major chromosome aberrations.[1] The number of live births affected by these abnormalities is, however, significant; approximately 1 in 150 has a major diagnosable chromosome abnormality.[1]

Polyploidy

Cells with a multiple of the normal number of chromosomes are **euploid cells** (Greek *eu* = good or true). Because normal gametes are haploid and most normal somatic cells are diploid, they are both euploid forms. When a euploid cell has more than the diploid number of chromosomes, it is said to be a **polyploid cell**. Several types of body tissues, including some liver, bronchial, and epithelial tissues, are normally polyploid. A zygote that has three copies of each chromosome, rather than the usual two, has a form of polyploidy called **triploidy**. Nearly all triploid fetuses are spontaneously aborted or stillborn. The prevalence of triploidy among live births is approximately 1 in 10,000. **Tetraploidy**, a condition in which euploid cells have 92 chromosomes, has been found primarily in early abortuses, although occasionally affected infants have been born alive. Like triploid infants, however, they do not survive. Triploidy and tetraploidy are relatively common conditions, accounting for approximately 10% of all known miscarriages.[2]

Aneuploidy

A cell that does not contain a multiple of 23 chromosomes is an **aneuploid cell**. A cell containing three copies of one chromosome is said to be trisomic (a condition termed **trisomy**) and is aneuploid. Monosomy, the presence of only one copy of a given chromosome in a diploid cell, is the other common form of aneuploidy. Among the autosomes, monosomy of any chromosome is lethal, but newborns with trisomy of chromosomes 13, 18, 21, or X can survive. This difference illustrates an important principle: *In general, loss of chromosome material*

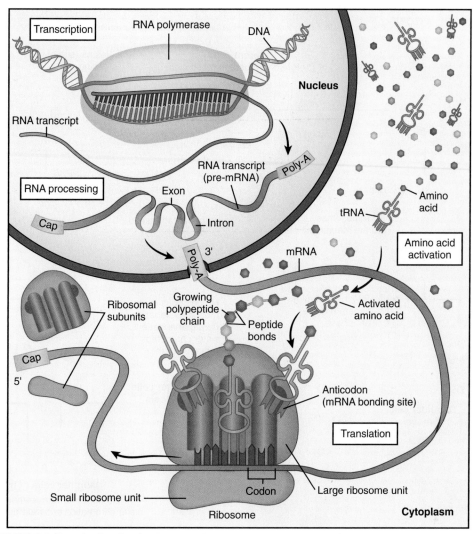

FIGURE 2.7 Protein Synthesis. The site of transcription is the nucleus and the site of translation is the cytoplasm. See the text for details.

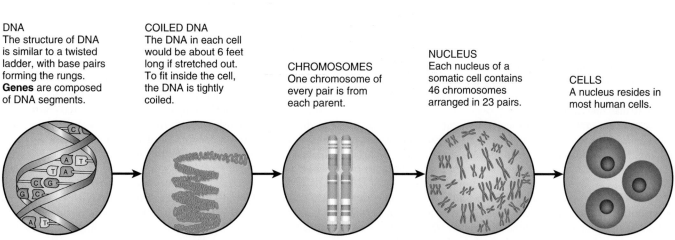

DNA
The structure of DNA is similar to a twisted ladder, with base pairs forming the rungs. **Genes** are composed of DNA segments.

COILED DNA
The DNA in each cell would be about 6 feet long if stretched out. To fit inside the cell, the DNA is tightly coiled.

CHROMOSOMES
One chromosome of every pair is from each parent.

NUCLEUS
Each nucleus of a somatic cell contains 46 chromosomes arranged in 23 pairs.

CELLS
A nucleus resides in most human cells.

FIGURE 2.8 From Molecular Parts to the Whole Somatic Cell.

has more serious consequences than duplication of chromosome material.

Aneuploidy of the sex chromosomes is less serious than that of the autosomes. Very little genetic material—only about 40 genes—is located on the Y chromosome. For the X chromosome, inactivation of extra chromosomes (see the X-linked Inheritance section) largely diminishes their effect. A zygote bearing *no* X chromosome, however, will not survive.

Aneuploidy is usually the result of **nondisjunction**, an error in which homologous chromosomes or sister chromatids fail to separate normally

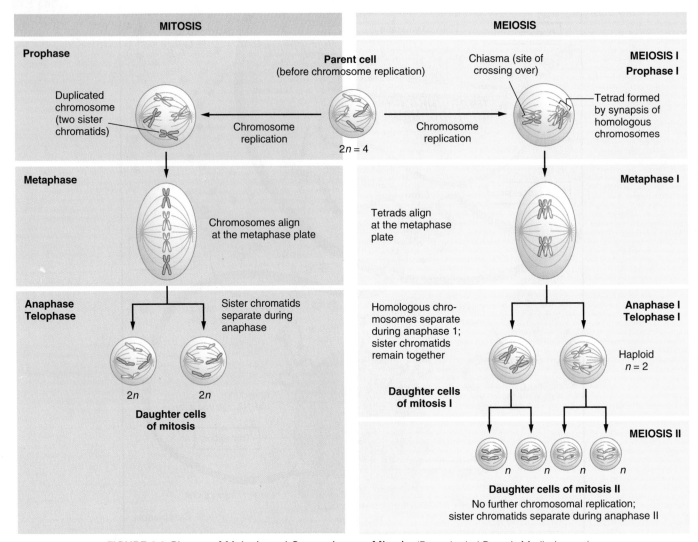

FIGURE 2.9 Phases of Meiosis and Comparison to Mitosis. (From Jorde LB et al: *Medical genetics,* ed 5, St Louis, 2016, Elsevier.)

during meiosis or mitosis (Fig. 2.12). Nondisjunction produces some gametes that have two copies of a given chromosome and others that have no copies of the chromosome. When such gametes unite with normal haploid gametes, the resulting zygote is monosomic or trisomic for that chromosome. Occasionally, a cell can be monosomic or trisomic for more than one chromosome.

Autosomal aneuploidy. Trisomy can occur for any chromosome, but fetuses with other trisomies of chromosomes (other than 13, 18, 21, or X) do not survive to term. Trisomy 16, for example, is the most common trisomy among abortuses, but it is not seen in live births.

Partial trisomy, in which only an extra portion of a chromosome is present in each cell, can occur also. The consequences of partial trisomies are not as severe as those of complete trisomies. Trisomies may occur in only some cells of the body. Individuals thus affected are said to be chromosomal mosaics, meaning that the body has two or more different cell lines, each of which has a different karyotype. Mosaics are often formed by early mitotic nondisjunction occurring in one embryonic cell but not in others.

The best-known example of aneuploidy in an autosome is trisomy of chromosome 21, which causes Down syndrome (named after J. Langdon Down, who first described the syndrome in 1866).

Down syndrome is seen in approximately 1 in 800 to 1 in 1000 live births; its principal features are shown and outlined in Fig. 2.13 and Table 2.1.

The risk of having a child with Down syndrome increases greatly with maternal age. As Fig. 2.14 demonstrates, women younger than 30 years of age have a risk ranging from about 1 in 1000 births to 1 in 2000 births. The risk begins to rise substantially after age 35 years, and reaches 3% to 5% for women older than 45 years of age. This dramatic increase in risk is caused by the age of maternal egg cells, which are held in an arrested state of prophase I from the time they are formed in the female embryo until they are shed in ovulation. Thus an egg cell formed by a 45-year-old woman is itself 45 years old. This long suspended state causes defects to accumulate in the cellular proteins responsible for meiosis, leading to nondisjunction. The risk of Down syndrome, as well as other trisomies, does not increase with paternal age.

Sex chromosome aneuploidy. The incidence of sex chromosome aneuploidies is fairly high. Among live births, about 1 in 500 males and 1 in 900 females have a form of sex chromosome aneuploidy. Because these conditions are generally less severe than autosomal aneuploidies, all forms except complete absence of any X chromosome material allow at least some individuals to survive.

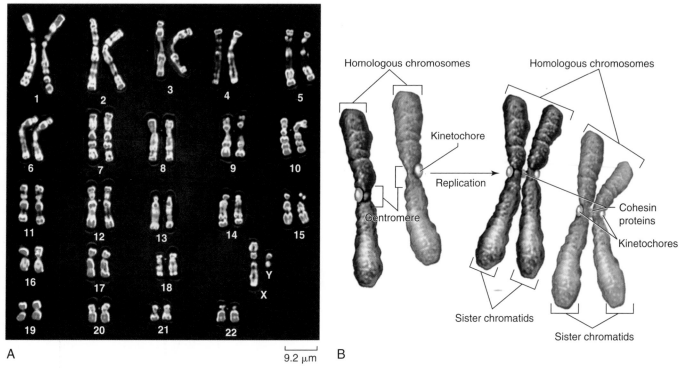

FIGURE 2.10 Karyogram of Chromosomes. A, Human karyogram. **B,** Homologous chromosomes and sister chromatids. (From Raven PH et al: *Biology,* ed 8, New York, 2008, McGraw-Hill.)

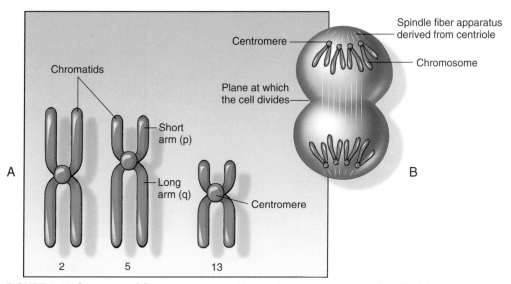

FIGURE 2.11 Structure of Chromosomes. A, Human chromosomes 2, 5, and 13. Each is replicated and consists of two chromatids. Chromosome 2 is a metacentric chromosome because the centromere is close to the middle; chromosome 5 is submetacentric because the centromere is set off from the middle; chromosome 13 is acrocentric because the centromere is at or very near the end. **B,** During mitosis, the centromere divides and the chromosomes move to opposite poles of the cell. At the time of centromere division, the chromatids are designated as chromosomes.

One of the most common sex chromosome aneuploidies, affecting about 1 in 1000 newborn females, is trisomy X. Instead of two X chromosomes, these females have three X chromosomes in each cell. Most of these females have no overt physical abnormalities, although sterility, menstrual irregularity, or intellectual disability is sometimes seen. Some females have four X chromosomes, and they are more often intellectually disabled. Those with five or more X chromosomes generally have more severe intellectual disability and various physical defects.

A condition that leads to somewhat more serious problems is the presence of a single X chromosome and no homologous X or Y chromosome, so that the individual has a total of 45 chromosomes. The karyotype is usually designated 45,X, and it causes a set of symptoms known as Turner syndrome (Fig. 2.15; see Table 2.1). Individuals with at least two X chromosomes and one Y chromosome in each cell (47,XXY karyotype) have a disorder known as Klinefelter syndrome (Fig. 2.16; see Table 2.1).

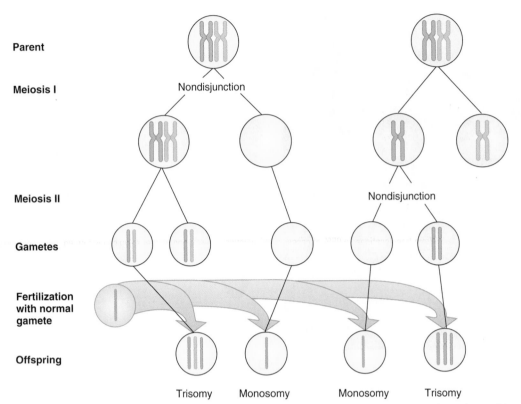

FIGURE 2.12 Nondisjunction. Nondisjunction causes aneuploidy when chromosomes or sister chromatids fail to divide properly. (From Jorde LB et al: *Medical genetics*, ed 5, St Louis, 2016, Elsevier.)

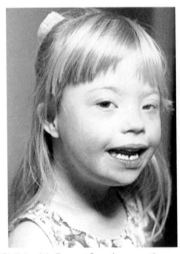

FIGURE 2.13 Child with Down Syndrome. (Courtesy Drs. A. Olney and M. MacDonald, University of Nebraska Medical Center, Omaha, Neb.)

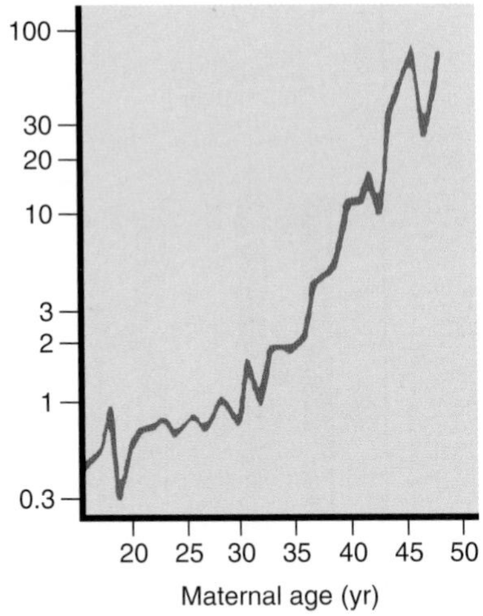

FIGURE 2.14 Down Syndrome Increases With Maternal Age. Rate is per 1000 live births related to maternal age.

Abnormalities of Chromosome Structure

In addition to the loss or gain of whole chromosomes, parts of chromosomes can be lost or duplicated as gametes are formed, and the arrangement of genes on chromosomes can be altered. Unlike aneuploidy and polyploidy, these changes sometimes have no serious consequences for an individual's health. Some of them can even remain entirely unnoticed, especially when very small pieces of chromosomes are involved. Nevertheless, abnormalities of chromosome structure can also produce serious disease in individuals or their offspring.

During meiosis and mitosis, chromosomes usually maintain their structural integrity, but chromosome breakage occasionally occurs.

Mechanisms exist to "heal" these breaks and usually repair them perfectly with no damage to the daughter cell. However, some breaks remain or heal in a way that alters the chromosome's structure. The risk of chromosome breakage increases with exposure to harmful agents called clastogens (e.g., ionizing radiation, viral infections, or some types of chemicals).

Deletions. Broken chromosomes and lost DNA cause deletions (Fig. 2.17). Usually, a gamete with a deletion unites with a normal gamete to form a zygote. The zygote thus has one chromosome with the normal complement of genes and one with some missing genes. Because many genes can be lost in a deletion, serious consequences result, even though one normal chromosome is present. The most often

TABLE 2.1 Characteristics of Various Chromosome Disorders

Disease/Disorder	Features
Down Syndrome *Trisomy of Chromosome 21*	
Intelligence quotient (IQ)	Usually ranges from 20 to 70 (intellectual disability)
Male/female findings	Virtually all males are sterile; some females can reproduce
Face	Distinctive: low nasal bridge, epicanthal folds, protruding tongue, low-set ears
Musculoskeletal system	Poor muscle tone (hypotonia), short stature
Systemic disorders	Congenital heart disease (one-third to half of cases), reduced ability to fight respiratory tract infections, increased susceptibility to leukemia—overall reduced survival rate; by age 40 years usually develop symptoms similar to those of Alzheimer disease
Mortality	About 75% of fetuses with Down syndrome abort spontaneously or are stillborn; 20% of infants die before age 10 years; those who live beyond 10 years have life expectancy of about 60 years
Causative factors	97% caused by nondisjunction during formation of one of parent's gametes or during early embryonic development; 3% result from translocations; in 95% of cases, nondisjunction occurs when mother's egg cell is formed; remainder involve paternal nondisjunction; 1% are mosaics—these have a large number of normal cells, and effects of trisomic cells are attenuated and symptoms are generally less severe
Turner Syndrome *(45,X) Monosomy of X Chromosome*	
IQ	Not considered to be intellectually disabled, although some impairment of spatial and mathematical reasoning ability is found
Male/female findings	Found only in females
Musculoskeletal system	Short stature common, characteristic webbing of neck, widely spaced nipples, reduced carrying angle at elbow
Systemic disorders	Coarctation (narrowing) of aorta, edema of feet in newborns, usually sterile and have gonadal streaks rather than ovaries; streaks are sometimes susceptible to cancer
Mortality	About 15%-20% of spontaneous abortions with chromosome abnormalities have this karyotype, most common single-chromosome aberration; highly lethal during gestation, only about 0.5% of these conceptions survive to term
Causative factors	75% inherit X chromosome from mother, thus caused by meiotic error in father; frequency low compared with other sex chromosome aneuploidies (1 : 5000 newborn females); 50% have simple monosomy of X chromosome; remainder have more complex abnormalities; combinations of 45, X cells with XX or XY cells common
Klinefelter Syndrome *(47,XXY) XXY Condition*	
IQ	Moderate degree of mental impairment may be present
Male/female findings	Have a male appearance but usually sterile; 50% develop female-like breasts (gynecomastia); occurs in 1 : 1000 male births
Face	Voice somewhat high pitched
Systemic disorders	Sparse body hair, sterile, small testicles
Causative factors	50% of cases the result of nondisjunction of X chromosomes in mother, frequency rises with increasing maternal age; also involves XXY and XXXY karyotypes with degree of physical and mental impairment increasing with each added X chromosome; mosaicism fairly common with most prevalent combination of XXY and XY cells

cited example of a disease caused by a chromosomal deletion is the cri du chat syndrome. The term literally means "cry of the cat" and describes the characteristic cry of the affected child. Other symptoms include low birth weight, severe intellectual disability, microcephaly (smaller than normal head size), and heart defects. The disease is caused by a deletion of part of the short arm of chromosome 5.

Duplications. A deficiency of genetic material is more harmful than an excess, so duplications usually have less serious consequences than deletions. For example, a deletion of a region of chromosome 5 causes cri du chat syndrome, but a duplication of the same region causes intellectual disability, but less serious physical defects.

Inversions. An inversion occurs when two breaks take place on a chromosome, followed by the reinsertion of the missing fragment at its original site but in inverted order. Therefore a chromosome symbolized as ABCDEFG might become ABEDCFG after an inversion.

Unlike deletions and duplications, no loss or gain of genetic material occurs, so inversions are "balanced" alterations of chromosome structure,

and they often have no apparent physical effect. Some genes are influenced by neighboring genes, however, and this position effect, a change in a gene's expression caused by its position, sometimes results in physical defects in these persons. Inversions can cause serious problems in the offspring of individuals carrying the inversion because the inversion can lead to duplications and deletions in the chromosomes transmitted to the offspring.

Translocations. The interchange of genetic material between nonhomologous chromosomes is called translocation. A reciprocal translocation occurs when breaks take place in two different chromosomes and the material is exchanged (Fig. 2.18, *A*). As with inversions, the carrier of a reciprocal translocation is usually normal, but his or her offspring can have duplications and deletions.

A second and clinically more important type of translocation is Robertsonian translocation. In this disorder, the long arms of two nonhomologous chromosomes fuse at the centromere, forming a single chromosome. Robertsonian translocations are confined to chromosomes

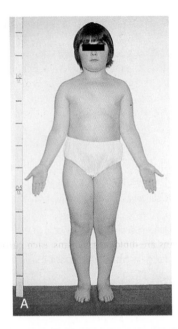

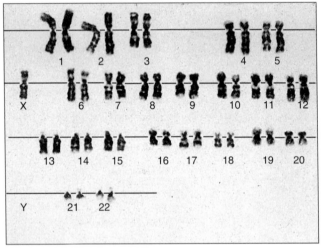

B

FIGURE 2.15 Turner Syndrome. A, A sex chromosome is missing, and the person's chromosomes are 45,X. Characteristic signs are short stature, female genitalia, webbed neck, shield-like chest with underdeveloped breasts and widely spaced nipples, and imperfectly developed ovaries. **B,** As this karyotype shows, Turner syndrome results from monosomy of sex chromosomes (genotype XO). (From Patton KT, Thibodeau GA: *Anatomy & physiology,* ed 8, St Louis, 2013, Mosby. Courtesy Nancy S. Wexler, PhD, Columbia University.)

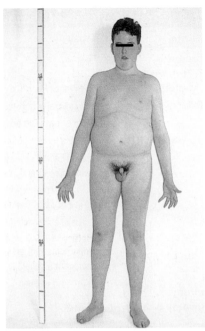

FIGURE 2.16 Klinefelter Syndrome. This young man exhibits many characteristics of Klinefelter syndrome: small testes, some development of the breasts, sparse body hair, and long limbs. This syndrome results from the presence of two or more X chromosomes with one Y chromosome (genotypes XXY or XXXY, for example). (From Patton KT, Thibodeau GA: *Anatomy & physiology,* ed 9, St Louis, 2016, Mosby. Courtesy Nancy S. Wexler, PhD, Columbia University.)

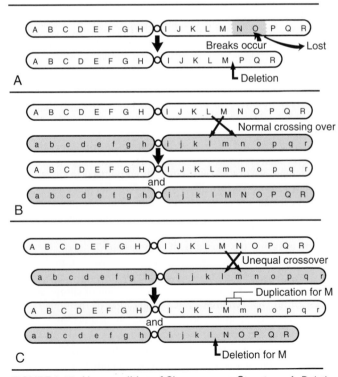

FIGURE 2.17 Abnormalities of Chromosome Structure. A, Deletion occurs when a chromosome segment is lost. **B,** Normal crossing over. **C,** The generation of duplication and deletion through unequal crossover.

13, 14, 15, 21, and 22 because the short arms of these chromosomes are very small and contain no essential genetic material. The short arms are usually lost during subsequent cell divisions. Because the carriers of Robertsonian translocations lose no important genetic material, they are unaffected, although they have only 45 chromosomes in each cell. Their offspring, however, may have serious monosomies or trisomies. For example, a common Robertsonian translocation involves the fusion of the long arms of chromosomes 21 and 14. An offspring who inherits a gamete carrying the fused chromosome can receive an extra copy of the long arm of chromosome 21 and develop Down syndrome. Robertsonian translocations are responsible for approximately 3% to 5% of Down syndrome cases. Parents who carry a Robertsonian translocation

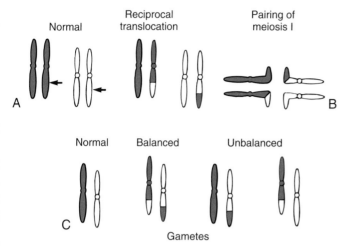

FIGURE 2.18 Normal and Abnormal Chromosome Translocation. **A,** Normal chromosomes and reciprocal translocation. **B,** Pairing at meiosis. **C,** Consequences of translocation in gametes; unbalanced gametes result in zygotes that are partially trisomic and partially monosomic and consequently develop abnormally.

involving chromosome 21 have an increased risk for producing multiple offspring with Down syndrome.

Fragile sites. A number of areas on chromosomes develop distinctive breaks and gaps (observable microscopically) when the cells are cultured. Most of these fragile sites do not appear to be related to disease. However, one fragile site, located on the long arm of the X chromosome, is associated with *fragile X syndrome.* The most important feature of this syndrome is intellectual disability. With a relatively high population prevalence (affecting approximately 1 in 4000 males and 1 in 8000 females), fragile X syndrome is the second most common genetic cause of intellectual disability (after Down syndrome).

In fragile X syndrome, females who inherit the mutation do not necessarily express the disease condition, but they can pass it on to descendants who do express it. Ordinarily, a male who inherits a disease gene on the X chromosome expresses the condition because he has only one X chromosome. An uncommon feature of this disease is that about one-third of carrier females are affected, although less severely than males. Unaffected transmitting males have been shown to have more than about 50 repeated DNA sequences near the beginning of the fragile X gene. These trinucleotide sequences, which consist of CGG sequences duplicated many times, cause fragile X syndrome when the number of copies exceeds 200.[3] The number of these repeats can increase from generation to generation. More than 20 other genetic diseases, including Huntington disease and myotonic dystrophy, also are caused by this mechanism.[4]

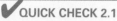**QUICK CHECK 2.1**
1. What is the major composition of DNA?
2. Define the terms *mutation, autosomes,* and *sex chromosomes.*
3. What is the significance of mRNA?
4. What is the significance of chromosomal translocation?

ELEMENTS OF FORMAL GENETICS

The mechanisms by which an individual's set of paired chromosomes produces traits are the principles of genetic inheritance. Mendel's work with garden peas first defined these principles. Later geneticists have

refined Mendel's work to explain patterns of inheritance for traits and diseases that appear in families.

Analysis of traits that occur with defined, predictable patterns has helped geneticists assemble the pieces of the human gene map. Current research focuses on determining the RNA or protein products of each gene and understanding the way they contribute to disease. Eventually, diseases and defects caused by single genes can be traced and therapies to prevent and treat such diseases can be developed.

Traits caused by single genes are called mendelian traits (after Gregor Mendel). Each gene occupies a position along a chromosome, known as a locus. The genes at a particular locus can have different forms (i.e., they can be composed of different nucleotide sequences) called alleles. A locus that has two or more alleles that each occur with an appreciable frequency in a population is said to be polymorphic (or to have a polymorphism).

Because humans are diploid organisms, each chromosome is represented twice, with one member of the chromosome pair contributed by the father and one by the mother. At a given locus, an individual has one allele whose origin is paternal and one whose origin is maternal. When the two alleles are identical, the individual is homozygous at that locus. When the alleles are not identical, the individual is heterozygous at that locus.

Phenotype and Genotype

The composition of genes at a given locus is known as the genotype. The outward appearance of an individual, which is the result of both genotype and environment, is the phenotype. For example, an infant who is born with an inability to metabolize the amino acid phenylalanine has the single-gene disorder known as phenylketonuria (PKU) and thus has the PKU genotype. If the condition is left untreated, abnormal metabolites of phenylalanine will begin to accumulate in the infant's brain and irreversible intellectual disability will occur. Intellectual disability is thus one aspect of the PKU phenotype. By imposing dietary restrictions to exclude food that contains phenylalanine, however, intellectual disability can be prevented. Foods high in phenylalanine include proteins found in milk, dairy products, meat, fish, chicken, eggs, beans, and nuts. Although the child still has the PKU genotype, a modification of the environment (in this case, the child's diet) produces an outwardly normal phenotype.

Dominance and Recessiveness

In many loci, the effects of one allele mask those of another when the two are found together in a heterozygote. The allele whose effects are observable is said to be dominant. The allele whose effects are hidden is said to be recessive (from the Latin root for "hiding"). Traditionally, for loci having two alleles, the dominant allele is denoted by an uppercase letter and the recessive allele is denoted by a lowercase letter. When one allele is dominant over another, the heterozygote genotype *Aa* has the same phenotype as the dominant homozygote *AA*. For the recessive allele to be expressed, it must exist in the homozygote form, *aa.*

A carrier is an individual who has a disease gene but is phenotypically normal. Many genes for a recessive disease occur in heterozygotes, who carry one copy of the gene but do not express the disease. When recessive genes are lethal in the homozygous state, they are eliminated from the population when they occur in homozygotes. By "hiding" in carriers, however, recessive genes for diseases are passed on to the next generation.

TRANSMISSION OF GENETIC DISEASES

The pattern in which a genetic disease is inherited through generations is termed the mode of inheritance. Knowing the mode of inheritance can reveal much about the disease-causing gene itself, and members of families with the disease can be given reliable genetic counseling.

The known single-gene diseases can be classified into four major modes of inheritance: autosomal dominant, autosomal recessive, X-linked dominant, and X-linked recessive. The first two types involve genes known to occur on the 22 pairs of autosomes. The last two types occur on the X chromosome; very few disease-causing genes occur on the Y chromosome.

The pedigree chart summarizes family relationships and shows which members of a family are affected by a genetic disease (Fig. 2.19). Generally the pedigree begins with one individual in the family, the proband. This individual is usually the first person in the family diagnosed or seen in a clinic.

Autosomal Dominant Inheritance
Characteristics of Pedigrees
Diseases caused by autosomal dominant genes are rare, with the most common occurring in fewer than 1 in 500 individuals. Therefore it is uncommon for two individuals who are both affected by the same autosomal dominant disease to produce offspring together. Fig. 2.20, *A,* illustrates this unusual pattern. Affected offspring are usually produced by the union of a normal parent with an affected heterozygous parent. The Punnett square in Fig. 2.20, *B,* illustrates this mating. The affected parent can pass either a disease-causing allele or a normal allele to the next generation. On average, half the children will be heterozygous and will express the disease, and half will be normal.

The pedigree in Fig. 2.21 shows the transmission of an autosomal dominant allele. Several important characteristics of this pedigree support the conclusion that the trait is caused by an autosomal dominant gene:

1. The two sexes exhibit the trait in approximately equal proportions; males and females are equally likely to transmit the trait to their offspring.
2. No generations are skipped. If an individual has the trait, one parent must also have it. If neither parent has the trait, none of the children will have it (with the exception of new mutations, as discussed later).
3. Affected heterozygous individuals transmit the trait to approximately half their children, and because gamete transmission is subject to chance fluctuations, all or none of the children of an affected parent may have the trait. When large numbers of matings of this type are studied, however, the proportion of affected children closely approaches one-half.

Recurrence Risks
Parents at risk for producing children with a genetic disease nearly always ask the question, "What is the *chance* that our child will have this disease?" The probability that an individual will develop a genetic disease is termed the recurrence risk. When one parent is affected by an autosomal dominant disease (and is a heterozygote) and the other is unaffected, the recurrence risk for each child is one-half.

An important principle is that each birth is an independent event, much like a coin toss. Thus even though parents may have already had a child with the disease, their recurrence risk remains one-half. Even if they have produced several children, all affected (or all unaffected) by the disease, the law of independence dictates that the probability their next child will have the disease is still one-half. Parents' misunderstanding of this principle is a common problem encountered in genetic counseling.

If a child is born with an autosomal dominant disease and there is no history of the disease in the family, the child is probably the product of a new mutation. The gene transmitted by one of the parents has thus undergone a mutation from a normal allele to a disease-causing allele. The alleles at this locus in most of the parent's other germ cells

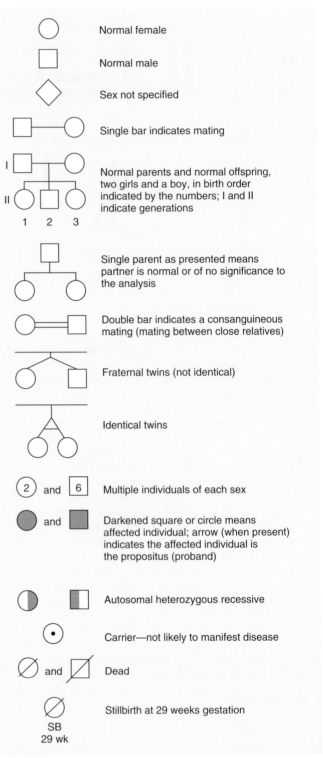

FIGURE 2.19 Symbols Commonly Used in Pedigrees. (From Jorde LB et al: *Medical genetics,* ed 5, St Louis, 2016, Elsevier.)

are still normal. In this situation, the recurrence risk for the parent's subsequent offspring is not greater than that of the general population. The offspring of the affected child, however, will have a recurrence risk of one-half (probability of 0.5). Because these diseases often reduce the potential for reproduction, many autosomal dominant diseases result from new mutations.

A

		Affected parent: D	Affected parent: d
Affected parent	D	DD Homozygous affected (usually rare)	Dd Heterozygous affected
	d	Dd Heterozygous affected	dd Homozygous normal

B

		Normal parent: d	Normal parent: d
Affected parent	D	Dd Heterozygous affected	Dd Heterozygous affected
	d	dd Homozygous normal	dd Homozygous normal

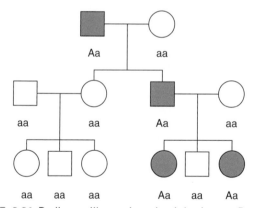

FIGURE 2.20 Punnett Square and Autosomal Dominant Traits. **A,** Punnett square for the mating of two individuals with an autosomal dominant gene. Here both parents are affected by the trait. **B,** Punnett square for the mating of a normal individual with a carrier for an autosomal dominant gene.

FIGURE 2.21 Pedigree Illustrating the Inheritance Pattern of Postaxial Polydactyly, an Autosomal Dominant Disorder. Affected individuals are represented by shading. (From Jorde LB et al: *Medical genetics,* ed 5, St Louis, 2016, Elsevier.)

Delayed Age of Onset

One of the best-known autosomal dominant diseases is Huntington disease, a neurologic disorder whose main features are progressive dementia and increasingly uncontrollable limb movements (chorea; discussed further in Chapter 16). A key feature of this disease is its **delayed age of onset**: Symptoms usually are not seen until 40 years of age or later. Thus those who develop the disease often have borne children before they become aware that they have the disease-causing mutation. If the disease was present at birth, nearly all affected persons would die before reaching the reproductive age, and the occurrence of the disease-causing allele in the population would be much lower. An individual whose parent has the disease has a 50% chance of developing it during middle age. He or she is thus confronted with a torturous question: Should I have children, knowing that there is a 50:50 chance that I may have this disease-causing gene and will pass it to half my children? A DNA test can now be used to determine whether an individual has inherited the trinucleotide repeat mutation that causes Huntington disease.

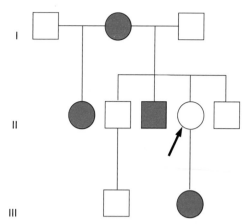

FIGURE 2.22 Pedigree for Retinoblastoma Showing Incomplete Penetrance. Female with marked arrow in line II must be heterozygous, but she does not express the trait.

Penetrance and Expressivity

The **penetrance** of a trait is the percentage of individuals with a specific genotype who also exhibit the expected phenotype. Incomplete penetrance means individuals who have the disease-causing genotype may not exhibit the disease phenotype at all, even though the genotype and the associated disease may be transmitted to the next generation. A pedigree illustrating the transmission of an autosomal dominant mutation with incomplete penetrance is provided in Fig. 2.22. Retinoblastoma, the most common malignant eye tumor affecting children, typically exhibits incomplete penetrance. About 10% of the individuals who are **obligate carriers** of the disease-causing mutation (i.e., those who have an affected parent and affected children and therefore must themselves carry the mutation) do not have the disease. The penetrance of the disease-causing genotype is then said to be 90%.

The gene responsible for retinoblastoma is a **tumor-suppressor gene**: The normal function of its protein product is to regulate the cell cycle so cells do not divide uncontrollably. When the protein is altered because of a genetic mutation, its tumor-suppressing capacity is lost and a tumor can form[5] (see Chapters 11 and 18).

Expressivity is the extent of variation in phenotype associated with a particular genotype. If the expressivity of a disease is variable, penetrance may be complete but the severity of the disease can vary greatly. A good example of variable expressivity in an autosomal dominant disease is neurofibromatosis type 1, or von Recklinghausen disease. As in retinoblastoma, the mutations that cause neurofibromatosis type 1 occur in a tumor-suppressor gene.[6] The expression of this disease varies from a few harmless café-au-lait (light brown) spots on the skin to numerous neurofibromas, scoliosis, seizures, gliomas, neuromas, malignant peripheral nerve sheath tumors, hypertension, and learning disorders (Fig. 2.23).

Several factors cause variable expressivity. Genes at other loci sometimes modify the expression of a disease-causing gene. Environmental (i.e., nongenetic) factors also can influence expression of a disease-causing gene. Finally, different mutations at a locus can cause variation in severity. For example, a mutation that alters only one amino acid of the factor VIII gene usually produces a mild form of hemophilia

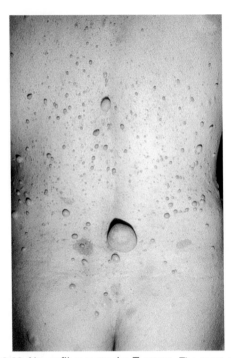

FIGURE 2.23 Neurofibromatosis: Tumors. The most common is sessile or pedunculated. Early tumors are soft, dome-shaped papules or nodules that have a distinctive violaceous hue. Most are benign. (From Habif et al: *Skin disease: diagnosis and treatment,* ed 2, St Louis, 2005, Mosby.)

A, whereas a "stop" codon (premature termination of translation) usually produces a more severe form of this blood coagulation disorder.

Epigenetics and Genomic Imprinting

Although this chapter focuses on DNA sequence variation and its consequence for disease, there is increasing evidence that the same DNA sequence can produce dramatically different phenotypes because of chemical modifications altering the *expression* of genes (these modifications are collectively termed epigenetic; see Chapter 3). An important example of such a modification is DNA methylation, the attachment of a methyl group to a cytosine base followed by a guanine base in the DNA sequence (Fig. 2.24). These sequences, which are common near many genes, are termed CpG islands. When the CpG islands located near a gene become heavily methylated, the gene is less likely to be transcribed into mRNA. In other words, the gene becomes transcriptionally inactive. One study showed that identical (monozygotic) twins accumulate different methylation patterns in the DNA sequences of their somatic cells as they age, causing increasing numbers of phenotypic differences. Intriguingly twins with more differences in their lifestyles (e.g., smoking versus nonsmoking) accumulated larger numbers of differences in their methylation patterns. The twins, despite having identical DNA sequences, become more and more different as a result of epigenetic changes, which, in turn, affect the expression of genes (see Fig. 3.5).

Epigenetic alteration of gene activity can have important disease consequences. For example, a major cause of one form of inherited colon cancer (termed *hereditary nonpolyposis colorectal cancer [HNPCC]*) is the methylation of a gene whose protein product repairs damaged DNA. When this gene becomes inactive, damaged DNA accumulates, eventually resulting in colon tumors. Epigenetic changes are also discussed in Chapters 3, 11, and 12.

Approximately 100 human genes are thought to be methylated differently, depending on which parent transmits the gene. This epigenetic modification, characterized by methylation and other changes, is termed genomic imprinting. For each of these genes, one of the parents *imprints* the gene (inactivates it) when it is transmitted to the offspring. An example is the insulin-like growth factor 2 gene *(IGF2)* on chromosome 11, which is transmitted by both parents, but the copy inherited from the mother is normally methylated and inactivated (imprinted). Thus only one copy of *IGF2* is active in normal individuals. However the maternal imprint is occasionally lost, resulting in two active copies of *IGF2*. This causes excess fetal growth and contributes to a condition known as *Beckwith-Weidemann syndrome* (see Chapter 3).

A second example of genomic imprinting is a deletion of part of the long arm of chromosome 15 (15q11–q13), which, when inherited from the father, causes the offspring to manifest a disease known as *Prader-Willi syndrome* (short stature, obesity, hypogonadism). When the same deletion is inherited from the mother, the offspring develop *Angelman syndrome* (intellectual disability, seizures, ataxic gait). The two different phenotypes reflect the fact that different genes are normally active in the maternally and paternally transmitted copies of this region of chromosome 15.

Autosomal Recessive Inheritance
Characteristics of Pedigrees

Like autosomal dominant diseases, diseases caused by autosomal recessive genes are rare in populations, although there can be numerous carriers. Cystic fibrosis, the most common lethal recessive disease in white children, occurs in about 1 in 2500 births. Approximately 1 in 25 whites carries a copy of a mutation that causes cystic fibrosis (see Chapter 30). Carriers are phenotypically unaffected. Some autosomal recessive diseases are characterized by delayed age of onset, incomplete penetrance, and variable expressivity.

Fig. 2.25 shows a pedigree for cystic fibrosis. The gene responsible for cystic fibrosis encodes a chloride ion channel in some epithelial cells. Defective transport of chloride ions leads to a salt imbalance, which results in secretions of abnormally thick, dehydrated mucus. Some digestive organs, particularly the pancreas, become obstructed, causing malnutrition, and the lungs become clogged with mucus, making them highly susceptible to bacterial infections. Death from lung disease or heart failure occurs before age 40 years in about half the individuals with cystic fibrosis.

The important criteria for discerning autosomal recessive inheritance include the following:
1. Males and females are affected in equal proportions.
2. Consanguinity (marriage between related individuals) is sometimes present, especially in cases of rare recessive diseases.
3. The disease may be seen in siblings of affected individuals but usually not in their parents.
4. On average, one-fourth of the offspring of carrier parents will be affected.

Recurrence Risks

In most cases of recessive disease, both of the parents of affected individuals are heterozygous carriers. On average, one-fourth of their offspring will be normal homozygotes, half will be phenotypically normal carrier heterozygotes, and one-fourth will be homozygotes with the disease (Fig. 2.26). Thus the recurrence risk for the offspring of carrier parents is 25%. However, in any given family, there are chance fluctuations.

If two parents have a recessive disease, they each must be homozygous for the disease. Therefore all their children also must be affected. This distinguishes recessive from dominant inheritance because two parents both affected by a dominant gene are nearly always both heterozygotes, and thus one-fourth of their children will be unaffected.

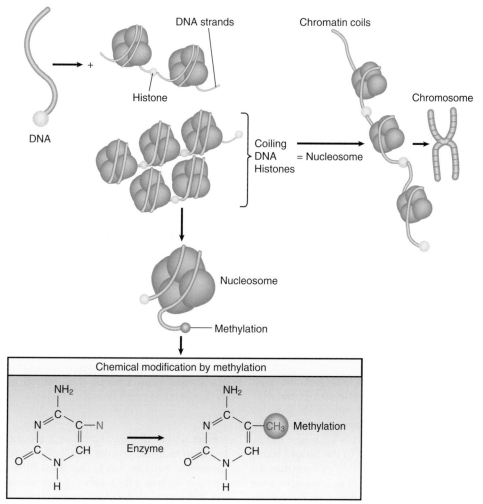

FIGURE 2.24 Epigenetic Modifications. Because deoxyribonucleic acid (DNA) is a long molecule, it needs packaging to fit in the tiny nucleus. Packaging involves *coiling* of the DNA in a "left-handed" spiral around spools, made of four pairs of proteins individually known as *histones* and collectively termed the *histone octamer*. The entire spool is called a nucleosome (also see Fig. 1.2). Nucleosomes are organized into chromatin, the repeating building blocks of a chromosome. Histone modifications are correlated with methylation, are reversible, and occur at multiple sites. Methylation occurs at the 5 position of cytosine and provides a "footprint" or signature as a unique epigenetic alteration *(red)*. When genes are expressed, chromatin is open or active; however, when chromatin is condensed because of methylation and histone modification, genes are inactivated.

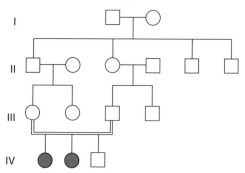

FIGURE 2.25 Pedigree for Cystic Fibrosis. Cystic fibrosis is an autosomal recessive disorder. The double bar denotes a consanguineous mating. Because cystic fibrosis is relatively common in European populations, most cases do not involve consanguinity.

	D	d
D	DD Homozygous normal	Dd Heterozygous carrier
d	Dd Heterozygous carrier	dd Homozygous affected

FIGURE 2.26 Punnett Square for the Mating of Heterozygous Carriers Typical of Most Cases of Recessive Disease.

Because carrier parents usually are unaware that they both carry the same recessive allele, they often produce an affected child before becoming aware of their condition. Carrier detection tests can identify heterozygotes by analyzing the DNA sequence to reveal a mutation. Some recessive diseases for which carrier detection tests are routinely used include PKU, sickle cell disease, cystic fibrosis, Tay-Sachs disease, hemochromatosis, and galactosemia.

Consanguinity

Consanguinity and inbreeding are related concepts. Consanguinity refers to the mating of two related individuals, and the offspring of such matings are said to be *inbred*. Consanguinity is sometimes an important characteristic of pedigrees for recessive diseases because relatives share a certain proportion of genes received from a common ancestor. The proportion of shared genes depends on the closeness of their biologic relationship. Consanguineous matings produce a significant increase in recessive disorders and are seen most often in pedigrees for rare recessive disorders.

X-Linked Inheritance

Some genetic conditions are caused by mutations in genes located on the sex chromosomes, and this mode of inheritance is termed sex linked. Only a few diseases are known to be inherited as X-linked dominant or Y chromosome traits, so only the more common X-linked recessive diseases are discussed here.

Because females receive two X chromosomes, one from the father and one from the mother, they can be homozygous for a disease allele at a given locus, homozygous for the normal allele at the locus, or heterozygous. Males, having only one X chromosome, are hemizygous for genes on this chromosome. If a male inherits a recessive disease gene on the X chromosome, he will be affected by the disease because the Y chromosome does not carry a normal allele to counteract the effects of the disease gene. Because a single copy of an X-linked recessive gene will cause disease in a male, whereas two copies are required for disease expression in females, more males are affected by X-linked recessive diseases than are females.

X Inactivation

In the late 1950s, Mary Lyon proposed that one X chromosome in the somatic cells of females is permanently inactivated, a process termed X inactivation.[7] This proposal, the Lyon hypothesis, explains why most gene products coded by the X chromosome are present in equal amounts in males and females, even though males have only one X chromosome and females have two X chromosomes. This phenomenon is called dosage compensation. The inactivated X chromosomes are observable in many interphase cells as highly condensed intranuclear chromatin bodies, termed Barr bodies (after Barr and Bertram, who discovered them in the late 1940s). Normal females have one Barr body in each somatic cell, whereas normal males have no Barr bodies.

X inactivation occurs very early in embryonic development—approximately 7 to 14 days after fertilization. In each somatic cell, one of the two X chromosomes is inactivated. In some cells, the inactivated X chromosome is the one contributed by the father; in other cells, it is the one contributed by the mother. Once the X chromosome has been inactivated in a cell, all the descendants of that cell have the same chromosome inactivated (Fig. 2.27). Thus inactivation is said to be random but *fixed*.

Some individuals do not have the normal number of X chromosomes in their somatic cells. For example, males with Klinefelter syndrome typically have two X chromosomes and one Y chromosome. These males do have one Barr body in each cell. Females whose cell nuclei have three X chromosomes have two Barr bodies in each cell, and

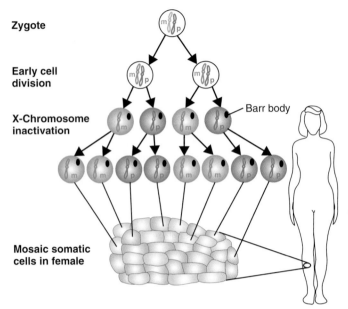

FIGURE 2.27 The X Inactivation Process. The maternal *(m)* and paternal *(p)* X chromosomes are both active in the zygote and in early embryonic cells. X inactivation then takes place, resulting in cells having either an active paternal X or an active maternal X. Females are thus X chromosome mosaics, as shown in the tissue sample at the bottom of the page. (From Jorde LB et al: *Medical genetics*, ed 5, St Louis, 2016, Elsevier.)

females whose cell nuclei have four X chromosomes have three Barr bodies in each cell. Females with Turner syndrome have only one X chromosome and no Barr bodies. Thus the number of Barr bodies is always one less than the number of X chromosomes in the cell. All but one X chromosome are always inactivated.

Persons with abnormal numbers of X chromosomes, such as those with Turner syndrome or Klinefelter syndrome, are not physically normal. This situation presents a puzzle because they presumably have only one active X chromosome, the same as individuals with normal numbers of chromosomes. This is probably because the distal tips of the short and long arms of the X chromosome, as well as several other regions on the chromosome arm, are not inactivated. Thus X inactivation is also known to be *incomplete*.

The inactivated X chromosome DNA is heavily methylated. Inactive X chromosomes can be at least partially reactivated in vitro by administering 5-azacytidine, a demethylating agent.

Sex Determination

The process of sexual differentiation, in which the embryonic gonads become either testes or ovaries, begins during the sixth week of gestation. A key principle of mammalian sex determination is that one copy of the Y chromosome is sufficient to initiate the process of gonadal differentiation that produces a male fetus. The number of X chromosomes does not alter this process. For example, an individual with two X chromosomes and one Y chromosome in each cell is still phenotypically a male. Thus the Y chromosome contains a gene that begins the process of male gonadal development.

This gene, termed *SRY* (for "sex-determining region on the Y"), has been located on the short arm of the Y chromosome.[8] The *SRY* gene lies just outside the pseudoautosomal region (Fig. 2.28), which pairs with the distal tip of the short arm of the X chromosome during meiosis and exchanges genetic material with it (crossover), just as autosomes do. The DNA sequences of these regions on the X and Y chromosomes

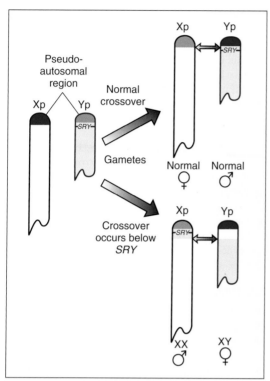

FIGURE 2.28 Distal Short Arms of the X and Y Chromosomes Exchange Material During Meiosis in the Male. The region of the Y chromosome in which this crossover occurs is called the *pseudoautosomal region*. The *SRY* gene, which triggers the process leading to male gonadal differentiation, is located just outside the pseudoautosomal region. Occasionally, the crossover occurs on the centromeric side of the *SRY* gene, causing it to lie on an X chromosome instead of a Y chromosome. An offspring receiving this X chromosome will be an XX male, and an offspring receiving the Y chromosome will be an XY female.

are highly similar. The rest of the X and Y chromosomes, however, do not exchange material and are not similar in DNA sequence.

Other genes that contribute to male differentiation are located on other chromosomes. Thus *SRY* triggers the action of genes on other chromosomes. This concept is supported by the fact that the *SRY* protein product is similar to other proteins known to regulate gene expression.

Occasionally, the crossover between X and Y occurs closer to the centromere than it should, placing the *SRY* gene on the X chromosome after crossover. This variation can result in offspring with an apparently normal XX karyotype but a male phenotype. Such XX males are seen in about 1 in 20,000 live births and resemble males with Klinefelter syndrome. Conversely, it is possible to inherit a Y chromosome that has lost the *SRY* gene (the result of either a crossover error or a deletion of the gene). This situation produces an XY female. Such females have gonadal streaks rather than ovaries and have poorly developed secondary sex characteristics.

✔ **QUICK CHECK 2.2**
1. Why is the influence of environment significant to phenotype?
2. Discuss the differences between a dominant allele and a recessive allele.
3. Why are the concepts of variable expressivity, incomplete penetrance, and delayed age of onset so important in relation to genetic diseases?
4. What is the recurrence risk for autosomal dominant inheritance and recessive inheritance?

Characteristics of Pedigrees

X-linked pedigrees show distinctive modes of inheritance. The most striking characteristic is that females seldom are affected. To express an X-linked recessive trait fully, a female must be homozygous: either both her parents are affected, or her father is affected and her mother is a carrier. Such matings are rare.

The following are important principles of X-linked recessive inheritance:
1. The trait is seen much more often in males than in females.
2. Because a father can give a son only a Y chromosome, the trait is never transmitted from father to son.
3. The gene can be transmitted through a series of carrier females, causing the appearance of one or more "skipped generations."
4. The gene is passed from an affected father to all his daughters, who, as phenotypically normal carriers, transmit it to approximately half their sons, who are affected.

A relatively common X-linked recessive disorder is Duchenne muscular dystrophy (DMD), which affects approximately 1 in 3500 males. As its name suggests, this disorder is characterized by progressive muscle degeneration. Affected individuals usually are unable to walk by age 10 or 12 years. The disease affects the heart and respiratory muscles, and death caused by respiratory or cardiac failure usually occurs before age 20 years. Identification of the disease-causing gene (on the short arm of the X chromosome) has greatly increased our understanding of the disorder.[9] The *DMD* gene is the largest gene ever found in humans, spanning more than 2 million DNA bases. It encodes a previously undiscovered muscle protein, termed **dystrophin**. Extensive study of dystrophin indicates that it plays an essential role in maintaining the structural integrity of muscle cells: it may also help regulate the activity of membrane proteins. When dystrophin is absent, as in DMD, the cell cannot survive, and muscle deterioration ensues. Most cases of DMD are caused by frameshift deletions of portions of the *DMD* gene and thus involve alterations of the amino acids encoded by the DNA following the deletion.

Recurrence Risks

The most common mating type involving X-linked recessive genes is the combination of a carrier female and a normal male (Fig. 2.29, *A*). On average, the carrier mother will transmit the disease-causing allele to half her sons (who are affected) and half her daughters (who are carriers).

The other common mating type is an affected father and a normal mother (see Fig. 2.29, *B*). In this situation, all the sons will be normal because the father can transmit only his Y chromosome to them. Because all the daughters must receive the father's X chromosome, they will all be heterozygous carriers. Because the sons *must* receive the Y chromosome and the daughters *must* receive the X chromosome with the disease gene, these are precise outcomes and not probabilities. None of the children will be affected.

The final mating pattern, less common than the other two, involves an affected father and a carrier mother (see Fig. 2.29, *C*). With this pattern, on average, half the daughters will be heterozygous carriers, and half will be homozygous for the disease allele and thus affected. Half the sons will be normal, and half will be affected. Some X-linked recessive diseases, such as DMD, are fatal or incapacitating before the affected individual reaches reproductive age, and therefore affected fathers are rare.

Sex-Limited and Sex-Influenced Traits

A **sex-limited trait** can occur in only one sex, often because of anatomic differences. Inherited uterine and testicular defects are two obvious examples. A **sex-influenced trait** occurs much more often in one sex than in the other. For example, male-pattern baldness occurs in both males and females but is much more common in males. Autosomal dominant breast cancer, which is much more commonly expressed in females than in males, is another example of a sex-influenced trait.

LINKAGE ANALYSIS AND GENE MAPPING

Locating genes on specific regions of chromosomes has been one of the most important goals of human genetics. The location and identification of a gene can tell much about the function of the gene, the interaction of the gene with other genes, and the likelihood that certain individuals will develop a genetic disease.

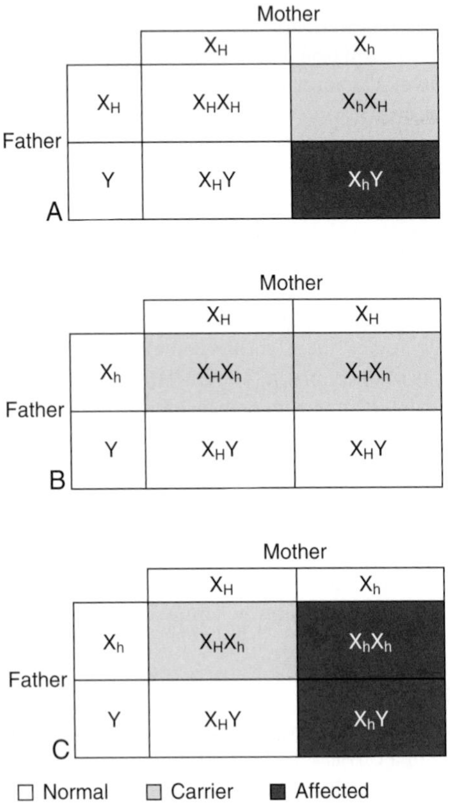

☐ Normal   ☐ Carrier   ■ Affected

FIGURE 2.29 Punnett Square and X-Linked Recessive Traits. A, Punnett square for the mating of a normal male (X_HY) and a female carrier of an X-linked recessive gene (X_HX_h). **B,** Punnett square for the mating of a normal female (X_HX_H) with a male affected by an X-linked recessive disease (X_hY). **C,** Punnett square for the mating of a female who carries an X-linked recessive gene (X_HX_h) with a male who is affected with the disease caused by the gene (X_hY).

Classic Pedigree Analysis

During the first meiotic stage, the arms of homologous chromosome pairs intertwine and sometimes exchange portions of their DNA (Fig. 2.30) in a process known as **crossover**. During crossover, new combinations of alleles can be formed. For example, two loci on a chromosome have alleles A and a and alleles B and b. Alleles A and B are located together on one member of a chromosome pair, and alleles a and b are located on the other member. The genotype of this individual is denoted as $AB/a0b$.

As Fig. 2.30, A, shows, the allele pairs would be transmitted together when no crossover occurs. However, when crossover occurs (see Fig. 2.30, B), all four possible pairs of alleles can be transmitted to the offspring. The process of forming such new arrangements of alleles is called **recombination**. Loci that are located very close to one another are unlikely to experience recombination and are said to demonstrate **linkage**. The frequency of recombination can be assessed in families and is used to determine the relative positions of loci on chromosomes (the gene map, discussed below).

Complete Human Gene Map: Prospects and Benefits

The major goals of the Human Genome Project were to find the locations of all human genes (the "gene map") and to determine the entire human DNA sequence. These goals have now been accomplished, and the genes responsible for approximately 5000 mendelian conditions have been identified[1,10] (Fig. 2.31). This has greatly increased our understanding of the mechanisms that underlie many diseases, such as retinoblastoma, cystic fibrosis, neurofibromatosis, and Huntington disease. The project also has led to more accurate diagnosis of these conditions and, in some cases, more effective treatment.[11]

DNA sequencing has become much less expensive and more efficient in recent years. Consequently hundreds of thousands of individuals have now been sequenced, leading, in some cases, to the identification of disease-causing genes[10] (see *Did You Know?* Gene Therapy).

DID YOU KNOW?

Gene Therapy

Thousands of subjects are currently enrolled in gene therapy clinical trials, and several gene therapy treatments have been approved by the U.S. Food and Drug Administration (FDA). Most trials and treatments involve the genetic alteration of cells to combat various types of cancer. Others involve the treatment of inherited diseases, such as β-thalassemia, hemophilia B, severe combined immunodeficiency, and retinitis pigmentosa.

Data from: Dunbar CE et al: *Science* 359(6372), 2018.

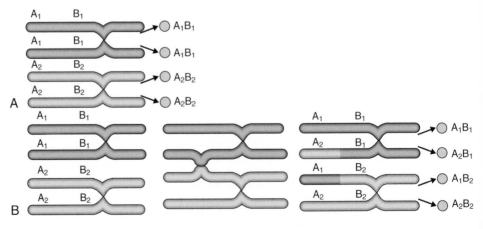

FIGURE 2.30 Genetic Results of Crossover. A, No crossing over. **B,** Crossing over with recombination.

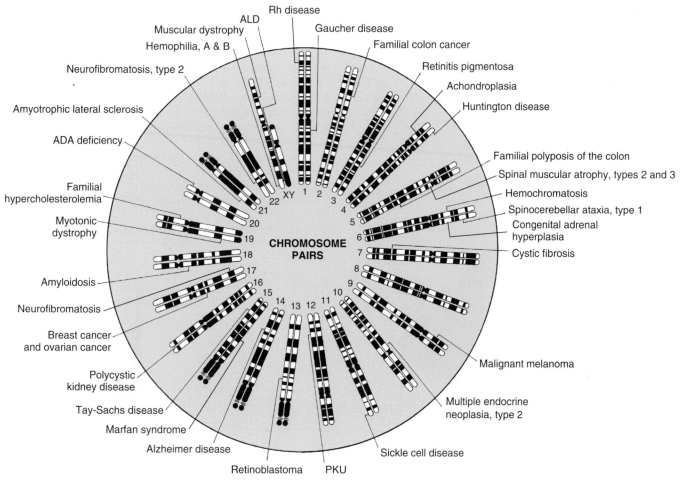

FIGURE 2.31 Example of Diseases: A Gene Map. *ADA,* Adenosine deaminase; *ALD,* adrenoleukodystrophy; *PKU,* phenylketonuria.

MULTIFACTORIAL INHERITANCE

Not all traits are produced by single genes; some traits result from several genes acting together. These are called **polygenic traits**. When environmental factors influence the expression of the trait (as is usually the case), the term **multifactorial inheritance** is used. Many multifactorial and polygenic traits tend to follow a normal distribution in populations (the familiar bell-shaped curve). Fig. 2.32 shows how three loci acting together can cause grain color in wheat to vary in a gradual way from white to red, exemplifying multifactorial inheritance. If both alleles at each of the three loci are white alleles, the color is pure white. If most alleles are white but a few are red, the color is somewhat darker; if all are red, the color is dark red.

Other examples of multifactorial traits include height and intelligent quotient (IQ). Although both height and IQ are determined, in part, by genes, they are also influenced by environment. For example, the average height of many human populations has increased by 5 to 10 cm in the past 100 years because of improvements in nutrition and health care. Also, IQ scores can be improved by exposing individuals (especially children) to enriched learning environments. Thus both genes and environment contribute to variation in these traits.

A number of diseases do not follow the bell-shaped distribution. Instead they appear to be either present in or absent from an individual. Yet they do not follow the patterns expected of single-gene diseases. Many of these are probably polygenic or multifactorial, but a certain **threshold of liability** must be crossed before the disease is expressed.

Below the threshold the individual appears normal; above it, the individual is affected by the disease (Fig. 2.33).

A good example of such a threshold trait is pyloric stenosis, a disorder characterized by a narrowing or obstruction of the pylorus, the area between the stomach and small intestine. Chronic vomiting, constipation, weight loss, and electrolyte imbalance can result from the condition, but it is easily corrected with surgery. The prevalence of pyloric stenosis is about 3 in 1000 live births in whites. This disorder is much more common in males than in females, affecting 1 in 200 males and 1 in 1000 females. The apparent reason for this difference is the threshold of liability is much lower in males than females, as shown in Fig. 2.33. Thus fewer defective alleles are required to generate the disorder in males. This situation also means the offspring of affected females are more likely to have pyloric stenosis because affected females necessarily carry more disease-causing alleles compared with most affected males.

A number of other common diseases are thought to correspond to a threshold model. They include cleft lip and cleft palate, neural tube defects (anencephaly, spina bifida), clubfoot (talipes), and some forms of congenital heart disease.

Although recurrence risks can be given with confidence for single-gene diseases (e.g., 50% for autosomal dominant diseases, 25% for autosomal recessive diseases), it is considerably more difficult to do so for multifactorial diseases. The number of genes contributing to the disease is not known, the precise allelic constitution of the biologic parents is not known, and the extent of environmental effects can vary from one population to another. For most multifactorial diseases, **empirical risks** (i.e., those based on direct observation) have been derived. To determine empirical risks, a large sample of biologic families in which one child has developed the disease is examined. The siblings of each child are then surveyed to calculate the percentage who also develop the disease.

Another difficulty is distinguishing polygenic or multifactorial diseases from single-gene diseases having incomplete penetrance or variable expressivity. Large data sets and good epidemiologic data often are

necessary to make the distinction. Box 2.1 lists the criteria commonly used to define multifactorial diseases.

The genetics of common disorders, such as hypertension, heart disease, and diabetes, is complex and often confusing. Nevertheless, the public health impact of these diseases, together with the evidence for hereditary factors in their etiology, demands that genetic studies be pursued. Thousands of genes contributing to susceptibility for these diseases have been discovered, and the next decade will undoubtedly witness substantial advancements in our understanding of these disorders.

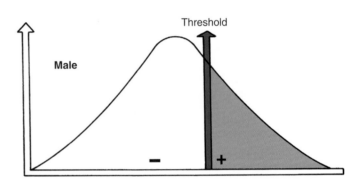

FIGURE 2.32 Multifactorial Inheritance. Analysis of mode of inheritance for grain color in wheat. The trait is controlled by three independently assorted gene loci.

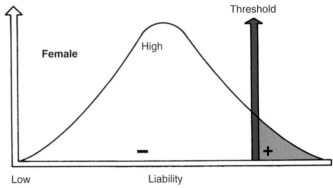

FIGURE 2.33 Threshold of Liability for Pyloric Stenosis in Males and Females.

BOX 2.1   Criteria Used to Define Multifactorial Diseases

1. The recurrence risk becomes higher if more than one family member is affected. For example, the recurrence risk for neural tube defects in a family increases to 10% if two siblings have been born with the disease. By contrast, the recurrence risk for single-gene diseases remains the same regardless of the number of siblings affected.
2. If the expression of the disease is more severe, the recurrence risk is higher. This is consistent with the liability model; a more severe expression indicates that the individual is at the extreme end of the liability distribution. Relatives of the affected individual are thus at a higher risk for inheriting disease genes. Cleft lip or cleft palate is a condition in which this has been shown to be true.
3. Relatives of probands of the less commonly affected are more likely to develop the disease. As with pyloric stenosis, this occurs because an affected individual

of the less susceptible sex is usually at a more extreme position on the liability distribution.
4. Generally, if the population frequency of the disease is f, the risk for offspring and siblings of probands is approximately $\sqrt{f}$. This does not usually hold true for single-gene traits.
5. The recurrence risk for the disease decreases rapidly in more remotely related relatives. Although the recurrence risk for single-gene diseases decreases by 50% with each degree of relationship (e.g., an autosomal dominant disease has a 50% recurrence risk for siblings, 25% for uncle–nephew relationship, 12.5% for first cousins), the risk for multifactorial inheritance decreases much more quickly.

SUMMARY REVIEW

DNA, RNA, and Proteins: Heredity at the Molecular Level

1. Genes, the basic units of inheritance, are composed of sequences of deoxyribonucleic acid (DNA) and are located on chromosomes.
2. Each subunit of DNA, called a nucleotide, is composed of one deoxyribose, a phosphate molecule, and one of four types of nitrogenous bases. The physical structure of DNA is a double helix. The two strands connect by the nitrogenous bases, with thymine bonding to adenine, and guanine bonding to cytosine.
3. The four DNA bases code for amino acids, which in turn make up proteins. The amino acids are specified by triplet sets of nitrogenous bases in specific orders, called codons. Several codons correspond to the same amino acid in many cases.
4. DNA replication is based on complementary base pairing, in which a single strand of DNA serves as the template for attracting complementary bases that form a new strand of DNA.
5. DNA polymerase is the primary enzyme involved in replication. It adds bases to the new DNA strand and performs "proofreading" functions.
6. A mutation is an alteration of genetic material (e.g., base pair substitution, frameshift mutation). Substances that cause mutations are called mutagens.
7. Mutations are rare events, and the rate of mutations varies from gene to gene. Mutational hot spots are DNA sequences with particularly high mutation rates.
8. Transcription and translation, the two basic processes in which proteins are specified by DNA, both involve ribonucleic acid (RNA). RNA is chemically similar to DNA, but it is single stranded, has a ribose sugar molecule, and has uracil rather than thymine as one of its four nitrogenous bases (uracil pairs with the base adenine).
9. Transcription is the process by which a DNA template synthesizes a RNA, thus forming messenger RNA (mRNA).
10. Much of the RNA sequence is spliced from the mRNA before the mRNA leaves the nucleus. The excised sequences are called introns, and those that remain to code for proteins are called exons.
11. Translation is the process by which RNA directs the synthesis of polypeptides. This process takes place in the ribosomes, which consist of proteins and ribosomal RNA (rRNA).
12. During translation, mRNA interacts with transfer RNA (tRNA), a molecule that has an attachment site for a specific amino acid and an anticodon, a region that matches up with a 3-base codon on the mRNA. The ribosome moves along the mRNA, matching different tRNAs to codons on the mRNA, and forming a growing chain of amino acids called a polypetide.

Chromosomes

1. Human cells consist of diploid somatic cells (body cells with 23 pairs of chromosomes, 46 total) and haploid gametes (sperm and egg cells with 23 total chromosomes).
2. Humans have 23 pairs of chromosomes. Twenty-two of these pairs are autosomes, ones that appear virtually identical (homologous) between males and females). The remaining pair consists of the sex chromosomes. Females have two homologous X chromosomes as their sex chromosomes; males have an X and a Y chromosome.
3. A karyogram is an ordered display of chromosomes arranged according to length and the location of the centromere. The karyogram is the visual representation of the individual's chromosome karyotype.
4. Various types of stains can be used to make chromosome bands more visible. Chromosome bands can be used to identify chromosomes and identify variations.

5. About 1 in 150 live births has a major diagnosable chromosome abnormality. Chromosome abnormalities are the leading known cause of intellectual disability and miscarriage.
6. Euploid cells are ones with the normal number of chromosomes. Polyploidy is a condition in which a cell has some multiple of the normal number of chromosomes. Humans have been observed to have triploidy (three copies of each chromosome) and tetraploidy (four copies of each chromosome); both conditions are lethal.
7. Aneuploidy is when a cell does not have a multiple of 23 chromosomes: there is an extra or missing single chromosome. Trisomy is a type of aneuploidy in which one chromosome is present in three copies. A partial trisomy is one in which only part of a chromosome is present in three copies. Monosomy is a type of aneuploidy in which one chromosome is present in only one copy.
8. In general, monosomies cause more severe physical defects than do trisomies, illustrating the principle that the loss of chromosome material has more severe consequences than the duplication of chromosome material.
9. Down syndrome, a trisomy of chromosome 21, is the best-known disease caused by a chromosome aberration. It affects 1 in 800 to 1 in 1000 live births.
10. Most aneuploidies of the sex chromosomes have less severe consequences than those of the other chromosomes.
11. The most commonly observed sex chromosome aneuploidies are the 47,XXX karyotype, 45,X karyotype (Turner syndrome), 47,XXY karyotype (Klinefelter syndrome), and 47,XYY karyotype.
12. Abnormalities of chromosome structure include deletions, duplications, inversions, and translocations.

Elements of Formal Genetics

1. Mendelian traits are caused by single genes, each of which occupies a position, or locus, on a chromosome.
2. Alleles are different forms of genes located at the same locus on a chromosome.
3. At any given locus in a somatic cell, an individual has two genes, one from each parent. An individual may be homozygous (alleles are identical) or heterozygous (alleles are different) for a locus.
4. An individual's genotype is his or her genetic makeup, and the phenotype reflects the interaction of genotype and environment.
5. In a heterozygote, a dominant gene's effects mask those of a recessive gene. The recessive gene is expressed only when it is present in two copies.

Transmission of Genetic Diseases

1. Genetic diseases caused by single genes usually follow autosomal dominant, autosomal recessive, X-linked dominant, or X-linked recessive modes of inheritance. Pedigree charts are important tools in the analysis of modes of inheritance.
2. Autosomal dominant inheritance affects males and females are equally likely and the two sexes are equally likely to transmit to their offspring. Skipped generations are not seen in classic autosomal dominant pedigrees. Affected heterozygous individuals transmit the trait to approximately half their children.
3. Recurrence risks specify the probability that future offspring will inherit a genetic disease. For single-gene diseases, recurrence risks remain the same for each offspring, regardless of the number of affected or unaffected offspring.
4. Many genetic diseases have a delayed age of onset: symptoms are not seen until some time after birth.

5. The penetrance of a trait is the percentage of individuals with a specific genotype who also exhibit the expected phenotype. A gene that is not always expressed phenotypically is said to have incomplete penetrance.
6. Expressivity is the extent of variation in phenotype associated with a particular genotype. If the expressivity of a disease is variable, penetrance may be complete but the severity of the disease can vary greatly.
7. Epigenetics involves changes, such as the methylation of DNA bases, that do not alter the DNA sequence but can alter the expression of genes.
8. Genomic imprinting, which is associated with methylation, results in differing expression of a disease gene, depending on which parent transmitted the gene.
9. Autosomal recessive inheritance affect males are females in equal proportions. Consanguinity (mating of related individuals) is sometimes present in families with autosomal recessive diseases, and it becomes more prevalent with rarer recessive diseases. The disease may be seen in siblings but not their parents. The recurrence risk for autosomal recessive diseases is 25%.
10. Most commonly, biologic parents of children with autosomal recessive diseases are both heterozygous carriers of the disease gene.
11. Carrier detection tests for autosomal recessive diseases are routinely available.
12. In each normal female somatic cell, one of the two X chromosomes is inactivated early in embryonic development. X inactivation is random, fixed, and incomplete (i.e., only part of the chromosome is actually inactivated) and involves methylation.
13. Gender is determined embryonically by the presence of the *SRY* gene on the Y chromosome. Embryos that have a Y chromosome (and thus the *SRY* gene) become males, whereas those lacking the Y chromosome become females. When the Y chromosome lacks the *SRY* gene, an XY female can be produced. Similarly, an X chromosome that contains the *SRY* gene can produce an XX male.
14. Sex linked inheritance is caused by mutations in genes on sex chromosomes. X-linked genes are those that are located on the X chromosome. Nearly all known X-linked diseases are caused by X-linked recessive genes.
15. Males are hemizygous for genes on the X chromosome. If a male inherits a recessive disease gene on the X chromosome, he will be affected by the disease because the Y chromosome does not carry a normal allele to counteract the effects.
16. X-linked recessive inheritance produces traits more often in males than in females because males need only one copy of the gene to express the disease. Because a father can give a son only a Y chromosome, biologic fathers cannot pass X-linked genes to their sons. Skipped generations often are seen in X-linked recessive disease pedigrees because the gene can be transmitted through carrier females. The gene is passed from an affected father to his daughters, who transmit to approximately half of their sons.
17. Recurrence risks for X-linked recessive diseases depend on the carrier and affected status of the mother and father.
18. A sex-limited trait is one that occurs only in one sex (gender). A sex-influenced trait is one that occurs more often in one sex than in the other.

Linkage Analysis and Gene Mapping
1. During meiosis I, crossover occurs and can cause recombinations of alleles located on the same chromosome. Loci that are located very close to one another are unlikely to experience recombination and are said to demonstrate linkage.
2. The major goals of the Human Genome Project were to find the locations of all human genes (the "gene map") and to determine the entire human DNA sequence. These goals have now been accomplished and the genes responsible for approximately 5000 mendelian conditions have been identified.

Multifactorial Inheritance
1. Traits that result from the combined effects of several loci are polygenic. When environmental factors also influence the trait, it is multifactorial.
2. Many multifactorial traits have a threshold of liability. Once the threshold of liability has been crossed, the disease may be expressed.
3. Recurrence risks are difficult to determine for multifactorial inheritance. Empirical risks, which are based on direct observation of large numbers of families, are used to estimate recurrence risks.

KEY TERMS

Adenine, 40
Allele, 51
Amino acid, 41
Aneuploid cell, 44
Anticodon, 43
Autosome, 44
Barr body, 56
Base pair substitution, 41
Carrier, 51
Carrier detection test, 56
Chromosomal mosaic, 46
Chromosome, 40
Chromosome band, 44
Chromosome breakage, 48
Clastogen, 48
Codon, 41
Complementary base pairing, 41
Consanguinity, 56
CpG islands, 54
Cri du chat syndrome, 49

Crossover, 58
Cytokinesis, 44
Cytosine, 40
Delayed age of onset, 53
Deletion, 48
Deoxyribonucleic acid (DNA), 40
Diploid cell, 44
DNA methylation, 54
DNA polymerase, 41
Dominant, 51
Dosage compensation, 56
Double-helix model, 40
Down syndrome, 46
Duplication, 49
Dystrophin, 57
Empirical risk, 59
Epigenetic, 54
Exon, 43

Expressivity, 53
Fragile site, 51
Frameshift mutation, 41
Gamete, 44
Gene, 40
Genetics, 40
Genomic imprinting, 54
Genotype, 51
Guanine, 40
Haploid cell, 44
Hemizygous, 56
Heterozygote, 51
Heterozygous, 51
Homologous, 44
Homozygote, 51
Homozygous, 51
Inbreeding, 56
Intron, 43
Inversion, 49
Karyotype (karyogram), 44

Klinefelter syndrome, 47
Linkage, 58
Locus, 51
Meiosis, 44
Messenger RNA (mRNA), 41
Metaphase spread, 44
Methylation, 54
Missense, 41
Mitosis, 44
Mode of inheritance, 51
Multifactorial inheritance, 59
Mutagen, 41
Mutation, 41
Mutational hot spot, 41
Nondisjunction, 45
Nonsense, 41
Nucleotide, 40
Obligate carrier, 53
Partial trisomy, 46
Pedigree, 52

REFERENCES

1. Jorde LB, et al: *Medical genetics*, ed 5, St Louis, 2016, Elsevier.
2. Gardner RJM, Amor DJ: *Gardner and Sutherland's chromosome abnormalities and genetic counseling*, ed 5, Oxford, 2018, Oxford University Press.
3. Mila M, et al: Fragile X syndrome: an overview and update of the FMR1 gene, *Clin Genet* 93(2):197-205, 2017.
4. Hannan AJ: Tandem repeats mediating genetic plasticity in health and disease, *Nat Rev Genet* 19(5):286-298, 2018.
5. Rahman N: Realizing the promise of cancer predisposition genes, *Nature* 505(7483):302-308, 2014.
6. Kresak JL, Walsh M: Neurofibromatosis: a review of NF1, NF2, and schwannomatosis, *J Pediatr Genet* 5(2):98-104, 2016.
7. Lee JT, Bartolomei MS: X-inactivation, imprinting, and long noncoding RNAs in health and disease, *Cell* 152(6):1308-1323, 2013.
8. Larney C, et al: Switching on sex: transcriptional regulation of the testis-determining gene *Sry*, *Development* 141(11):2195-2205, 2014.
9. Flanigan KM: The muscular dystrophies, *Semin Neurol* 32(3):255-263, 2012.
10. Boycott KM, et al: International cooperation to enable the diagnosis of all rare genetic diseases, *Am J Hum Genet* 100(5):695-705, 2017.
11. Rehm HL: Evolving health care through personal genomics, *Nat Rev Genet* 18(4):259-267, 2017.

3

Epigenetics and Disease

Diane P. Genereux

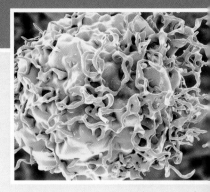

EVOLVE WEBSITE

CHAPTER OUTLINE

Human beings exhibit great diversity in physical and behavioral features. Much of this diversity is because of genetic variation. Epigenetic ("upon genetic") information is another contributor. This information, which is encoded by chemical modifications to DNA and associated histone proteins, helps determine which of an individual's genes are active in which cells. Epigenetic information is critical for normal human development. Abnormal changes in epigenetic information can occur spontaneously or through environmental exposures. Some of these changes lead to disease.

EPIGENETIC MECHANISMS

DNA Methylation

DNA methylation (Fig. 3.1) occurs when a methyl group (CH_3) is attached to a cytosine. Methylation within a gene generally renders it inactive. Methylation usually occurs only at cytosines that are followed by a guanine base known as a CpG dinucleotide, and the fraction of CpG dinucleotides that are methylated is variable across the genome. In human embryonic stem cells, methylation also can occur at cytosines outside of the CpG context (see Fig. 2.24).

DNA methylation plays a prominent role in human development and disease. For example, in each cell of a normal human female, one of the two X chromosomes is silenced by dense methylation and associated molecular marks, whereas the other X chromosome is transcriptionally active and largely devoid of methylation (see Chapter 2). During early embryonic development, one of the two X chromosomes in each cell is inactivated. Random inactivation of the X chromosome inherited from the mother or the father occurs independently in each cell of the embryo, and the methylation state is inherited by all subsequent copies. If a woman's two X chromosomes carry different alleles at a given locus, random X inactivation can lead to cells with different traits. Striking examples include the patchy coloration of calico cats and *anhidrotic ectodermal dysplasia*, a condition characterized by patchy presence and absence of sweat glands in the skin of human females. Abnormal changes to DNA methylation are involved in several human cancers, including cancers of the breast and ovary (Box 3.1).

Histone Modifications

Histone modifications (see Fig. 3.1) are chemical changes to the histone proteins around which DNA is coiled. The coiling, or extreme compaction of DNA, enables it to fit into the nucleus of a cell. Histone modifications can up-regulate or down-regulate nearby gene expression by increasing or decreasing the tightness of the interaction between DNA and histones. The material made of DNA in association with histones is called *chromatin.*

Histone modifications of a given region of DNA can undergo dramatic changes during cellular differentiation and organismal development. Certain modifications characterize specific cell types. Accrual of specific sets of histone modifications enable diverse types of differentiated cells to differentiate from a founder stem cell. Mutations that impair histone modification have been implicated in congenital

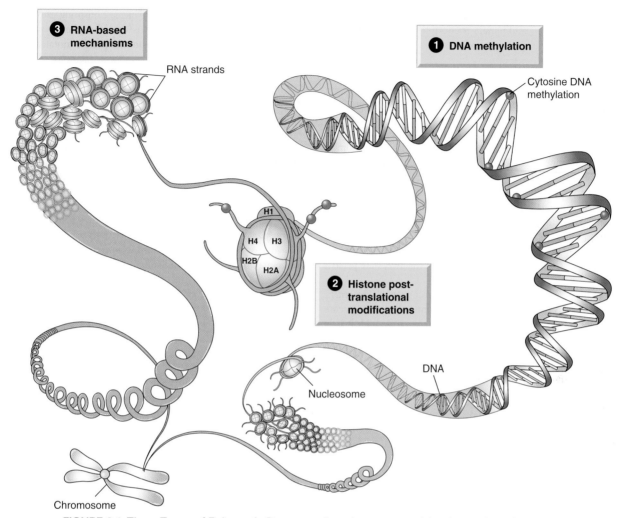

FIGURE 3.1 Three Types of Epigenetic Processes. Investigators are studying three epigenetic mechanisms: **(1)** DNA methylation. **(2)** Histone modifications. **(3)** RNA based-mechanisms. See text for discussion.

BOX 3.1   Cancer of Ovary and Breast Can Arise Through Epigenetic Silencing of Tumor-Suppressor Gene *BRCA1*.

Inherited mutations in the coding region of the *BRCA1* and *BRCA2* genes are known to increase risk of breast, ovarian, and prostate cancer. Such mutations, however, cannot explain all cases of breast cancer. Many families have a high incidence of breast cancer but no known pathogenic variants in the coding regions of the *BRCA1* gene. Researchers sought to identify epimutations (errors in epigenetic gene repression) that could potentially account for breast cancer in these families.

Evans et al. used bisulfite sequencing to examine the promoter region of the *BRAC1* or *BRCA2* genes in 49 women who had breast or ovarian cancer but did not have mutations in the coding regions of either gene. Abnormal, dense DNA methylation in the *BRCA1* promoter was found in two of these women. Both women also had a single mutation in the promoter of the gene. Examination of DNA from other women in the families of these women revealed that the point mutation was strongly associated with DNA methylation and transcriptional silencing of the *BRCA1* gene.

In conclusion, point mutations in the promoter region of the *BRCA1* gene can increase the probability of dense methylation. This dense methylation can lead to gene inactivation, indicating that epigenetic mechanisms driven by noncoding mutations can lead to breast cancer through loss of *BRCA1* function.

Data from Evans GR et al: Inherited BRCA1 epimutation as a novel cause of breast and ovarian cancer. Available at: https://doi.org/10.1101/246934, 2018; Garett D et al: A dominantly inherited 5′ UTR variant causing methylation-associated silencing of BRCA1 as a cause of breast and ovarian cancer, *Am J Human Genet* 103:213-220, 2018.

---

heart disease, thus highlighting histone modification states as critical for normal development.

In contrast to the vast majority of other cell types, including oocytes, sperm cells do not have histones. Instead, they have closely related proteins called **protamines**. DNA coils on the right side or more "rightly" around protamines, making sperm-cell nuclei smaller, and facilitate sperm movement.

EPIGENETICS AND HUMAN DEVELOPMENT

Each of the cells in the early embryo has the potential to give rise to a somatic cell of any type. These **embryonic stem cells** are therefore said to be *totipotent* ("possessing all powers"). Epigenetic modifications that arise during development ensure that specific genes are expressed only in the cells and tissue types in which their gene products normally function. Only a small percentage of genes, termed **housekeeping genes**, escape *epigenetic silencing* and remain transcriptionally active in all or nearly all cells.

EPIGENETICS IN GENOMIC IMPRINTING

For every gene not encoded on a sex chromosome, a child inherits two copies: one from the mother and one from the father. For a large subset of these, expression is **biallelic**, meaning that both copies contribute to phenotype. For a few genes, expression is stochastically (randomly) **monoallelic**, meaning that the maternal copy is randomly chosen for inactivation in some somatic cells and the paternal copy is randomly chosen for inactivation in other somatic cells. As discussed earlier, the process whereby monoallelic expression is established is much like that of random inactivation of the X chromosomes. For a third and smaller subset of autosomes (about 1%), either the maternal copy or the paternal copy is **imprinted**, meaning that either the sperm or the egg carries an inactive copy (see Chapter 2). This *imprinted,* or inactive, state persists in all of the somatic cells of the individual.

Many of the genes subject to imprinting regulate growth. The *genetic conflict hypothesis* is useful to explain the imprinting pattern. Because a mother makes a large physiologic investment in each child, it is in her evolutionary best interest to limit the flow of energetic resources to any given child, thus preserving her ability to have subsequent children. Contrarily, it is in the best biologic interests of the father for his child to extract maximal resources from the mother. In general, imprinting of maternally inherited genes tends to reduce offspring size; imprinting of paternally inherited genes tends to increase offspring size. One hallmark of imprinting-associated disease is that the phenotype of affected individuals is critically dependent on whether the mutation is inherited from the mother or from the father. Some examples are included in the following syndromes.

Prader-Willi and Angelman Syndromes

When a deletion of about 4 million base (Mb) pairs of the long arm of chromosome 15 is inherited from the father, a child manifests **Prader-Willi syndrome**. The characteristics of this syndrome include short stature, hypotonia, small hands and feet, obesity, mild to moderate intellectual disability, and hypogonadism (Fig. 3.2, *A*). The same 4-Mb deletion, when inherited from the mother, causes **Angelman syndrome**, which is characterized by severe intellectual disability, seizures, and an ataxic gait (see Fig. 3.2, *B*). These diseases are each observed in about 1 of every 15,000 live births; chromosome deletions are responsible for about 70% of cases of both diseases. The deletions that cause Prader-Willi and Angelman syndromes are indistinguishable at the DNA sequence level.

The 4-Mb deletion (the *critical region*) contains several genes that are normally transcribed only on the copy of chromosome 15 that is inherited from the father. These genes are transcriptionally inactive (imprinted) on the copy of chromosome 15 inherited from the mother. Similarly, other genes in the critical region are transcriptionally active only on the chromosome copy inherited from the mother and are inactive on the chromosome inherited from the father. Thus several genes in this region are normally active on only one chromosome copy (Fig. 3.3). If the single active copy of one of these genes is lost because

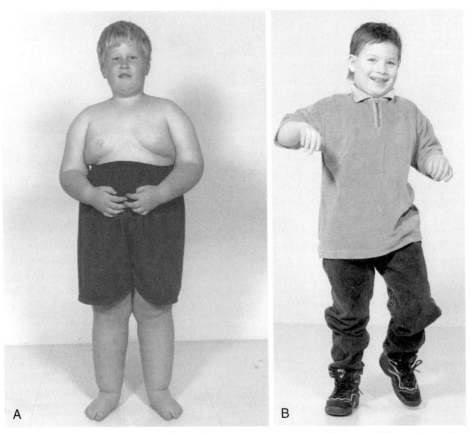

FIGURE 3.2 Prader-Willi and Angelman Syndromes. A, A child with Prader-Willi syndrome (truncal obesity, small hands and feet, inverted V-shaped upper lip). **B,** A child with Angelman syndrome (characteristic posture, ataxic gait, bouts of uncontrolled laughter). (From Jorde LB, Carey JC, Bamshad MJ: *Medical genetics,* ed 4, Philadelphia, 2010, Mosby.)

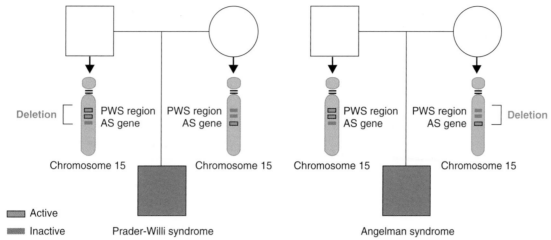

Active

Inactive   Prader-Willi syndrome   Angelman syndrome

FIGURE 3.3 Prader-Willi Syndrome Pedigrees. These pedigrees illustrate the inheritance patterns of Prader-Willi syndrome, which can be caused by a 4-million base pairs (Mb) deletion of chromosome 15q when inherited from the father. In contrast, Angelman syndrome can be caused by the same deletion but only when it is inherited from the mother. The reason for this difference is that different genes in this region are normally imprinted (inactivated) in the copies of 15q transmitted by the mother and the father. (From Jorde LB, Carey JC, Bamshad MJ: *Medical genetics*, ed 4, Philadelphia, 2010, Mosby.)

of a chromosome deletion, then no gene product is produced, resulting in disease.

Beckwith-Wiedemann Syndrome

Another well-known example of imprinting is Beckwith-Wiedemann syndrome, an overgrowth condition accompanied by an increased predisposition to cancer. **Beckwith-Wiedemann syndrome** is usually identifiable at birth by the large size for gestational age, neonatal hypoglycemia, large tongue, creases on the earlobe, and birth defects of the intestines. Children with Beckwith-Wiedemann syndrome have an increased risk of developing Wilms tumor or hepatoblastoma. Both these tumors can be treated effectively if they are detected early; thus screening at regular intervals is an important part of management. Some children with Beckwith-Wiedemann syndrome also develop asymmetric overgrowth of a limb or one side of the face or trunk (hemihyperplasia).

As in Angelman syndrome, in some individuals, Beckwith-Wiedemann syndrome (about 20%–30%) is caused by the inheritance of two copies of a chromosome from the father and no copy of the chromosome from the mother (*uniparental disomy*, in this case affecting chromosome 11). Several genes on the short arm of chromosome 11 are imprinted on either the paternally or the maternally transmitted chromosome. These genes are found in two separate, differentially methylated regions (DMRs). In DMR1, the gene that encodes insulin-like growth factor 2 (*IGF2*) is inactive on the maternally transmitted chromosome but active on the paternally transmitted chromosome. Thus a normal individual has only one active copy of *IGF2*. When two copies of the paternal chromosome are inherited (i.e., paternal uniparental disomy) or there is loss of imprinting on the maternal copy of *IGF2*, an active *IGF2* gene is present in double dose. These changes produce increased levels of IGF2 during fetal development, contributing to the overgrowth features of Beckwith-Wiedemann syndrome. Note that in contrast to Prader-Willi and Angelman syndromes, which are produced by a missing gene product, Beckwith-Wiedemann syndrome is caused, in part, by overexpression of a gene product.

Russell-Silver Syndrome

Characteristics of **Russell-Silver syndrome** include growth retardation, proportionate short stature, leg length discrepancy, and a small, triangular face. About one-third of Russell-Silver syndrome cases are caused by imprinting abnormalities of chromosome 11p15.5 that lead to down-regulation of *IGF2* and therefore diminished growth. Another 10% of cases are caused by maternal uniparental disomy. Thus whereas up-regulation, or extra copies, of active *IGF2* causes overgrowth in Beckwith-Wiedemann syndrome, down-regulation of *IGF2* causes the diminished growth seen in Russell-Silver syndrome.

> ### ✓ QUICK CHECK 3.1
> 1. Define epigenetics.
> 2. What are the two types of epigenetic mechanisms?
> 3. What is meant by the genetic conflict hypothesis?
> 4. Compare and contrast the molecular and phenotypic features of Prader-Willi and Angelman syndromes.

ENVIRONMENTAL IMPACTS ON EPIGENETIC INFORMATION

Imprinted genes are not the only loci for which epigenetic modifications persist over time. Conditions encountered in utero, during childhood, and even during adolescence or later can have long-term impacts on epigenetic states, sometimes with impacts that can be transmitted across generations. A few such examples are listed below.

Epigenetics and Nutrition

During the winter of 1943, millions of people in the Netherlands suffered starvation conditions as a result of a Nazi blockade that interfered with the shipping of food. This era is now called "The Dutch Hunger Winter." Researchers found individuals who were in utero during the Dutch Hunger Winter were more likely to suffer from obesity and diabetes as adults compared with those who had not experienced nutritional deprivation during gestation. More recent work has identified similar consequences in mice exposed to famine conditions in utero.

The specific molecular mechanisms that may mediate these apparent relationships between nutritional deprivation and disease are largely

BOX 3.2   Epigenetics Could Explain Correlation Between Birth Month and Body Mass Index (BMI).

It has long been observed that people conceived during cold times of the year tend to have lower body mass index (BMI) compared with people conceived during warmer times of the year. Sun et al. exposed male and female mice to cold temperatures before mating, then assessed the body mass and gene expression in their offspring.

Their findings confirmed data from human populations. Offspring of male mice exposed to cold before mating tend to have larger amounts of brown adipose, a tissue with very high metabolic rate, as well as a lower overall probability of diet-induced obesity. Exposing female mice to cold before mating had no impact on brown adipose or obesity risk in their offspring. Exploration

of DNA methylation in the sperm of cold-exposed male mice revealed methylation in the promoters of several genes involved in the production of brown adipose tissue.

In conclusion, the sperm of male mice exposed to cold have reduced methylation in several genes relevant to the development of brown adipose tissue by a yet unknown mechanism. The offspring of these cold-exposed males have higher expression of these genes, resulting in higher amounts of brown adipose tissue, higher metabolic rate, and lowering risk of diet-induced obesity. Future work could focus on potential applications of cold exposure in the treatment or prevention of obesity.

Data from Sun W et al: Cold-induced epigenetic programming of the sperm enhances brown adipose tissue activity in offspring, *Nat Med* 24(9):1372-1383, 2018.

unknown. From some animal models, it seems that the *IGF2* gene is a possible target of epigenetic modifications. Exposure in utero and through lactation to some chemicals also seems to lead to epigenetic modifications similar to those that arise through nutritional deprivation in early life. Effects on offspring epigenetics also can arise through parental exposure to chemicals, including bisphenol A (a constituent of plastics sometimes used in food preparation and storage), and cold temperatures (Box 3.2).

Epigenetics and Maternal Care

It is increasingly clear that parenting style can affect epigenetic states and that this information can be transmitted from one generation to the next. Mice and other rodents can exhibit two alternative styles of nursing behavior: (1) frequent arched-back nursing with a high level of licking and grooming behavior or (2) infrequent arched-back nursing with reduced licking and grooming behavior. Offspring of rodent mothers that engage in frequent arched-backed nursing have significantly lower methylation levels and higher transcription activity of a glucocorticoid receptor–encoding locus. Because the glucocorticoid receptor is involved in a pathway that intensifies fearfulness and response to stress, these findings suggest that alteration to methylation states could help explain how stress early in life can impact behavior in adulthood. These findings also highlight the concept that epigenetic processes can help store information about the environment with lasting consequences.

Epigenetics and Ethanol Exposure in Utero

The impact of ethanol exposure in utero on skeletal and neural development was first reported in 1973 and led to broad awareness of fetal alcohol syndrome. Recently population-based and molecular-level studies began to clarify the epigenetic signals that mediate these impacts. Culturing neural stem cells in the presence of ethanol leads to dense methylation and inactivation of loci typically active in neurons. One possible explanation is that maternal ethanol exposure alters fetal expression of the DNA methyltransferases (DNMTs).

Epigenetics and Genetic Abnormalities

In some diseases, both genetic and epigenetic factors contribute to abnormal phenotypes. For example, a range of abnormal phenotypes can arise in individuals with mutations at the fragile X locus *FMR1* (Fig. 3.4, *A*). Some of these phenotypes arise in individuals for whom epigenetic changes are coincident with genetic changes. The promoter of the *FMR1* genes contains a series of cytosine–guanine (CGG) dinucleotide repeats. Normal individuals have ≈35 CGG repeats. Females with >35 repeats are at risk for fragile X–associated primary ovarian insufficiency, which can lead to early menopause. Males with moderate

expansions are at risk of fragile X tremor ataxia syndrome (FXTAS), which is characterized by a late-onset intention tremor. Both conditions seem to arise through accumulation of excess *FMR1* messenger RNAs (mRNAs) in cellular nuclei. Individuals with 200 repeats increase the risks of dense methylation of the region and fragile X syndrome. These risks are characterized by reduced intelligence quotient (IQ) and various behavioral abnormalities. Although excessive CGG repeats in the *FMR1* promoters increase the probability of fragile X syndrome, the presence of an atypically large number of repeats does not, itself, lead to the syndrome. For example, fragile X syndrome also can be present in a male with excessive repeats but absent in brothers who also inherited the full mutation allele. How can this be? Methylation-based silencing at *FMR1* is stochastic, meaning that a large number of CGG repeats increases the probability of silencing but does not guarantee it. It remains to be seen whether dietary or environmental factors shape the probability of fragile syndrome in individuals who inherit the full-length allele.

In another genetic-epigenetic disease, fascioscapulohumeral muscular dystrophy (FSHMD) (see Fig. 3.4, *B*), the disease phenotype arises through a genetic deletion, not expansion, in the *DUX4* gene. This eventually leads to loss of methylation in a region that is densely methylated in normal individuals (see Fig. 3.4, *A*). Symptoms include adverse impacts on skeletal musculature. Although life span is not typically decreased, wheelchair use eventually becomes necessary for some individuals. Together, fragile X syndrome and FSHMD highlight that both abnormal gain and abnormal loss of epigenetic modifications can result in disease.

Twin Studies Provide Insights on Epigenetic Modification

Identical (monozygotic) twins, whose DNA sequences are essentially the same, offer a unique opportunity to isolate and examine the impacts of epigenetic modifications. As twins age, they accrue substantial genetic differences in their somatic cells. Twins—especially those with significant lifestyle differences, such as smoking versus nonsmoking—tend to accumulate differences in their methylation patterns. These results suggest that changes in epigenetic patterns may be an important part of the aging process (Fig. 3.5).

Molecular Approaches to Understand Epigenetic Disease

Epigenetic information is not encoded by DNA sequences but instead by chemical modifications. As a result, conventional genome sequencing approaches are not sufficient to screen epigenetic states and to identify differences between normal individuals and those with disease. To collect information on DNA methylation states of individual nucleotides, DNA

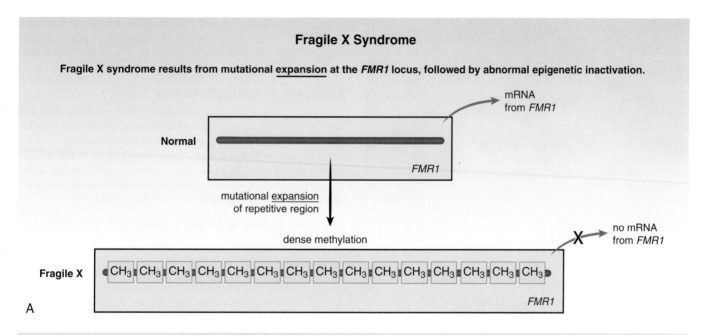

Fragile X Syndrome

Fragile X syndrome results from mutational <u>expansion</u> at the *FMR1* locus, followed by abnormal epigenetic inactivation.

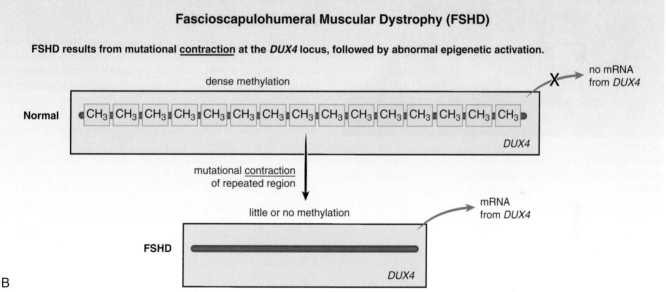

Fascioscapulohumeral Muscular Dystrophy (FSHD)

FSHD results from mutational <u>contraction</u> at the *DUX4* locus, followed by abnormal epigenetic activation.

FIGURE 3.4 Comparing the Molecular Mechanisms of Fragile X and Facioscapulohumeral Muscular Dystrophy (FSHD). **A,** *FMR1* in normal, expanded permutation, and full-mutation states. **B,** *DUX4* in normal and contracted states.

is typically subjected to bisulfite conversion before sequencing. Bisulfite treatment deaminates unmethylated, but not methylated, cytosines to uracil. Because uracil complements adenine, not guanine, methylated and unmethylated cytosines can be distinguished in resulting sequence data as long as the genetic sequence is known. Histone modification states can be assayed through the use of antibodies specific for histones with various modifications.

> ✔ **QUICK CHECK 3.2**
> 1. Evaluate the statement: "Epigenetic information is highly dynamic in early development."
> 2. How does the epigenetic regulation of imprinted genes compare with that of the rest of the genome?
> 3. Compare and contrast the molecular mechanisms leading to FX syndrome and to FSHMD.

EPIGENETICS AND CANCER

DNA Methylation and Cancer

Some of the most extensive evidence for the role of epigenetic modification in human disease comes from studying cancer (Fig. 3.6). Tumor cells often exhibit two abnormalities of DNA: (1) methylation hypomethylation in the promoters genes that promote cell division and cancer, leading to their silencing; and (2) hypermethylation in the promoter regions of the tumor-suppressor genes that work to keep cell division in check. For example, hypermethylation of the promoter region of the *RB1* gene is often seen in retinoblastoma; hypermethylation of the *BRCA1* gene is seen in some cases of inherited breast cancer (see Box 3.1 for data on epigenetics and breast cancer, and Chapter 35)

Colon cancer cells often have the hypermethylation in the promoter region of the *MLH1* gene that encodes a protein that repairs DNA

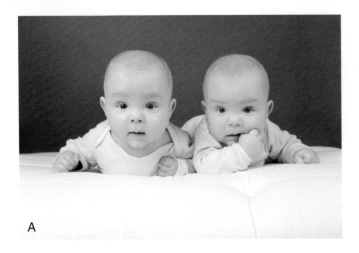

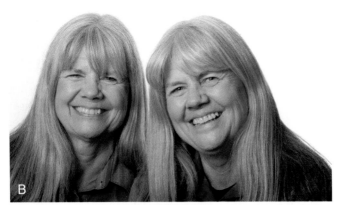

FIGURE 3.5 Twins and Aging. A, Twins as babies look very much alike but, **B,** as adults, have slight differences in appearance, possibly because of epigenetics. (**A,** vgm/Shutterstock. **B,** Stacey Bates/Shutterstock.)

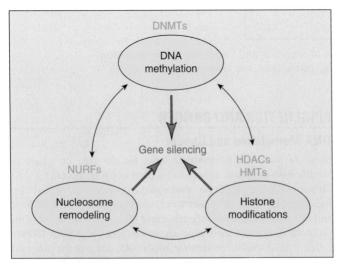

FIGURE 3.6 Global Changes in Three Processes Relevant to Cancer. Three processes—DNA cytosine methylation, histone modification, and nucleosomal remodeling—are intimately linked. Alterations in these processes result in permanent silencing of cancer-relevant genes. (From Jones PA, Baylin SB: The epigenomics of cancer, *Cell* 128(4):683-692, 2007.)

damage. When *MLH1* becomes inactive, DNA damage accumulates, giving rise to colon tumors.[1,2] Abnormal methylation of tumor-suppressor genes also is common in Barrett esophagus, a condition in which the lining of the esophagus is replaced by abnormal cells.

Epigenetic Screening for Cancer

The finding that epigenetic alterations are common in tumors raises the possibility that epigenetic screening approaches could be useful for detecting cancer. For example, in some cases, epigenetic screening could be done by using bodily fluids (e.g., urine or sputum), eliminating the need for the more invasive, costly, and risky strategies currently in place. Other epigenetics-based screening approaches have shown promise for detection of cancers of the bladder, lung, and prostate.

Emerging Strategies for the Treatment of Epigenetic Disease

Epigenetic modifications are potentially reversible: DNA can be demethylated, and histones can be modified to change the transcriptional state of nearby DNA. This raises the prospect of treating epigenetic disease with pharmaceutical agents that directly reverse the changes associated with disease. In recent years, such interventions have shown considerable promise for the treatment of disease.

DNA Demethylating Agents

5-Azacytidine (Fig. 3.7) has been used as a therapeutic drug in the treatment of leukemia and myelodysplastic syndrome. The cytosine analogue 5-azacytidine is incorporated into DNA opposite its complementary nucleotide, guanine. 5-Azacytidine differs from cytosine because it has nitrogen, instead of carbon, in the fifth position of its cytidine ring. As result, the DNMTs cannot add methyl groups to 5-azacytidine, and DNAs that contain 5-azacytidine decline in their methylation density

Cytosine → DNMT1+S-Adenosylmethionine → **5-Methylcytosine**

A

5-Azacytosine → DNMT1+S-Adenosylmethionine → **5-Azacytosine**

B

FIGURE 3.7 5-Azacytosine as Demethylating Agent. A, Unmethylated cytosines in DNA are typically subject to the addition of methyl groups by DNA methyltransferase 1 (DNMT1), a DNA methyltransferase, using methyl groups supplied by the methyl donor S-adenosylmethionine. **B,** In 5-azacytosine, the 5′ carbon of cytosine is replaced with a nitrogen. This chemical difference is sufficient both to block the addition of a methyl group and to confer irreversible binding to DNMT1. Incorporation of 5-azacytosine into DNA is therefore sufficient to drive passive loss of methylation from replicating DNA and thus to reactivate hypermethylated loci. 5-Azacytosine, bound to a sugar, can be integrated into DNA, and has been administered with some success in treating epigenetic diseases that arise through hypermethylation of individual loci.

over successive rounds of DNA replication. Administration of 5-azacytidine is associated with various side effects, including digestive disturbance, but it has shown promise in the treatment of diseases, including pancreatic cancer and myelodysplastic syndromes.

Histone Deacetylase Inhibitors

The activity of the histone deacetylases (HDACs) increases chromatin compaction, decreasing transcriptional activity (see Fig. 3.7). In many cases, excessive activity of HDACs results in transcriptional inactivation of tumor-suppressor genes, leading ultimately to the development of tumors. Treatment with HDAC inhibitors, either alone or in combination with other drugs, has shown promise in the treatment of cancers of the breast and prostate but only very limited success in the treatment of pancreatic cancer.

> ✓ QUICK CHECK 3.3
> 1. Assess the statement that cancer is, in many cases, an epigenetic disease.
> 2. Describe a potential strategy for the treatment of epigenetic disease.

FUTURE DIRECTIONS

Emerging experimental data are clarifying the role of epigenetics in determining cell fates and disease phenotypes. The well-documented involvement of epigenetic abnormalities in carcinogenesis and the mounting evidence for these epigenetic changes in other common diseases (discussed in other chapters) will likely elucidate possibilities for reversing the epigenetic abnormalities and possibly preventing their establishment in utero.

SUMMARY REVIEW

Epigenetic Mechanisms

1. Epigenetic ("upon genetic") information is encoded by chemical modifications to DNA and associated histone proteins. It helps determine which of an individual's genes are active in which cells.
2. DNA methylation, which results from attachment of a methyl group to a cytosine, generally renders a gene inactive. One of the two X chromosomes in a female is silenced by methylation. Abnormal changes to DNA methylation are involved in several human cancers.
3. Histone modifications are chemical changes to the histone protein around which DNA is coiled for extreme compaction. This alters gene expression by increasing or decreasing the tightness of the interaction between DNA and histones.

Epigenetics and Human Development

1. Embryonic stem cells have the potential to give rise to any type of somatic cell.
2. Epigenetic modifications that arise during early development ensure that specific genes are expressed only in the cells and tissue types in which their gene products normally function.
3. Housekeeping genes escape epigenetic silencing and remain active.

Epigenetics in Genomic Imprinting

1. In biallelic expression, both inherited copies of a gene contribute to phenotype. In monoallelic expression, one copy of a gene (from either the mother or father) is randomly inactivated in some somatic cells.
2. For some human genes, one copy of an inherited chromosome is transcriptionally inactive: either the sperm or the egg carries the inactive copy. This process of gene silencing, in which genes are silenced depending on which parent transmits them, is known as imprinting; the transcriptionally silenced genes are said to be "imprinted." The imprinted state persists in all somatic cells of the individual.
3. Many genes subject to imprinting regulate growth. Generally, imprinting of maternally inherited genes tends to reduce offspring size; imprinting of paternally inherited genes tends to increase offspring size.
4. The phenotype of individuals affected by imprinting is critically dependent on whether the mutation is inherited from the mother or from the father. When the deletion of about 4 million base pairs (Mb) of the long arm of chromosome 15 is inherited from the father, the child manifests Prader-Willi syndrome. The same

4 Mb deletion, when inherited from the mother, causes Angelman syndrome.
5. Beckwith-Wiedemann syndrome is an overgrowth condition caused by imprinting that is accompanied by an increased predisposition to cancer.
6. Up-regulation, or extra copies, of active *IGF2* causes overgrowth in Beckwith-Wiedemann syndrome. Down-regulation of *IGF2* causes the diminished growth seen in Russell-Silver syndrome.

Environmental Impacts on Epigenetic Information

1. Events encountered in utero, in childhood, and in adolescence can result in specific epigenetic changes that yield a wide range of phenotypic abnormalities, and can be transmitted across generations.
2. Widespread nutritional deprivation (such as during times of war) has been shown to increase obesity and diabetes in the next generation due to epigenetic changes to individuals who were *in utero* during the deprivation.
3. Fetal alcohol syndrome, which results from ethanol exposure *in utero*, may be mediated by the repressive impact of ethanol on the DNA methyltransferases.
4. Both abnormal gain of methylation, as in the case of fragile X syndrome, and abnormal loss of methylation, as in the case of FSHMD, can produce disease phenotypes. Both phenotypes arise through epigenetic abnormalities that occur secondary to a genetic mutation.
5. Identical twins have DNA sequences that are essentially the same. As twins age, they accrue substantial genetic in their somatic cells, especially when they have significantly different lifestyles (e.g., smoking versus nonsmoking).
6. Epigenetic information is encoded by chemical modifications, not DNA sequences, so conventional genome sequencing approaches cannot screen for epigenetic states.

Epigenetics and Cancer

1. The best evidence for epigenetic effects on disease risk comes from studies of human cancer.
2. Methylation densities change as tumors progress. These changes can increase the activity of oncogenes and decrease the activity of tumor-suppressor genes, causing tumors to progress to malignancy.
3. Epigenetics-based screening approaches have shown promise for the detection of some cancers.
4. Epigenetic modifications can be reversed through pharmaceutical intervention. For example, 5-azacytidine, a demethylating agent, has been used as a therapeutic drug in the treatment of leukemia and

myelodysplastic syndrome. Histone deacetylase inhibitors have shown promise in treating cancers of the breast and prostate.

Future Directions

1. Emerging experimental data are clarifying the roles of epigenetic states in determining cell fates and disease phenotypes.

2. The well-documented involvement of epigenetic abnormalities in cancer and the mounting evidence for these epigenetic changes in other common diseases will likely elucidate new therapies with the possibilities of reversing the epigenetic abnormalities.

KEY TERMS

5-Azacytidine, 70
Angelman syndrome, 66
Beckwith-Wiedemann syndrome, 67
Biallelic, 66
CpG dinucleotide, 64

DNA methylation, 64
Embryonic stem cell, 65
Epigenetic, 64
Fascioscapulohumeral muscular dystrophy (FSHMD), 68
Fragile X, 68

Histone modification, 64
Housekeeping genes, 66
Imprinted, 66
Monoallelic, 66
Prader-Willi syndrome, 66

Protamine, 65
Russell-Silver syndrome, 67

REFERENCES

1. Lynch HT, de la Chapelle A: Hereditary colorectal cancer, *N Engl J Med* 348:919-932, 2003.
2. Pino MS, Chung DC: Microsatellite instability in the management of colorectal cancer, *Expert Rev Gastroenterol Hepatol* 5(3):385-399, 2011.

ADDITIONAL READINGS

Feinberg AP: The key role of epigenetics in human disease prevention and mitigation, *N Engl J Med* 378(14):1323-1334, 2018.
Sillanpää E, et al: Leisure-time physical activity and DNA methylation age—twin study, *Clin Epigenetics* 11(1):12, 2019.
Wang J, et al: DNA methylation patterns of adult survivors of adolescent/young adult Hodgkin lymphoma compared to their unaffected monozygotic twin, *Leuk Lymphoma* 22:1-9, 2019.
Wang Y, et al: Epigenetic influences on aging: a longitudinal genome-wide methylation study in old Swedish twins, *Epigenetics* 13(9):975-987, 2018.
Webster AP, et al: Increased DNA methylation variability in rheumatoid arthritis-discordant monozygotic twins, *Genome Med* 10(1):64, 2018.

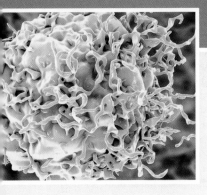

4

Altered Cellular and Tissue Biology

Kathryn L. McCance, Lois E. Brenneman

EVOLVE WEBSITE

http://evolve.elsevier.com/Huether/
Student Review Questions
Audio Key Points

Case Studies
Animations
Quick Check Answers

CHAPTER OUTLINE

The majority of diseases are caused by multiple factors acting together (*multifactorial*) or a single factor interacting with a genetically susceptible person. Injury to cells or their surrounding environment, the *extracellular matrix (ECM)*, leads to tissue and organ damage. Although the normal cell is characterized by a narrow range of structural and functional constraints, cells can *adapt* to increased demands and stress so as to maintain a steady state, called *homeostasis*. Adaptation is a reversible response involving structural or functional modifications to accommodate both physiologic (normal) demands and pathologic (adverse) conditions. For example, the uterus adapts to pregnancy—a normal physiologic state—by enlarging. Pregnancy triggers an increase in the size and number of cells to accommodate a growing fetus. Adaptation to a pathologic condition occurs with high blood pressure or hypertension. Myocardial cells become enlarged, resulting in a larger, thicker left ventricle to accommodate the increased workload of the heart. Cellular adaptations to pathologic conditions are usually only temporarily successful. Severe or long-term stressors commonly overwhelm the adaptive processes, resulting in cellular injury or death. Common sources of cell stress include structural damage, neoplasia, fluid/solute accumulations, genetic

influences, and aging. Altered cellular and tissue biology can result from adaptation.

Cellular injury can result from any factor that disrupts cellular structures or deprives the cell of oxygen and essential nutrients. Resultant injury may be *sublethal* (reversible) or *lethal* (irreversible). Common sources of cell injury are classified broadly as ischemic–hypoxic (lack of sufficient oxygen), ischemia–reperfusion, free radical, immunologic, infectious, intentional or unintentional, and inflammatory. Clinical manifestations and alteration to normal physiology will vary with the type of injury. Stress from metabolic derangements is linked to intracellular excessive *accumulations* of carbohydrate, protein, and lipids. Cell death can result in calcium accumulation within surrounding tissue, a condition referred to as *pathologic calcification*. The two main types of cell death are *necrosis* and *apoptosis*. A third process, *autophagy*, occurs during times of cellular stress and is typically triggered by deficiency of nutrients or growth factors. The various forms of cell death are discussed in greater detail later in this chapter.

Cellular aging causes structural and functional changes that may result in decreased capacity to recover from injury and, ultimately, cell death. The exact mechanisms governing cellular aging is unclear; distinguishing pathologic changes from age-associated physiologic changes can be challenging. Aging clearly results in alterations to cellular structure and function, yet *senescence* (growing old) is both inevitable and normal.

CELLULAR ADAPTATION

Cells adapt to their environment to avoid injury. An adapted cell is neither normal nor injured; its status falls somewhere between these two states. Adaptations are reversible changes affecting the size, number, phenotype, metabolic activity, or function of cells.[1] Adaptive responses have limits; additional stress can compromise essential cell functions leading to cell injury or death. Cell adaptation may be the central component in many disease states. In the early stages of successful adaptation, cells may have enhanced function making it difficult to distinguish a pathologic response from vigorous adaptation. Over time, the adaptive response may fail and pathology will ensue. The most significant adaptive changes in cells include the following:

- Atrophy—decrease in cell size
- Hypertrophy—increase in cell size
- Hyperplasia—increase in cell number
- Metaplasia—reversible replacement of one mature cell type by another, less mature cell type or a change in cell phenotype
- Dysplasia—or deranged cellular growth, is not considered a true cellular adaptation but rather atypical hyperplasia
These changes are shown in Fig. 4.1.

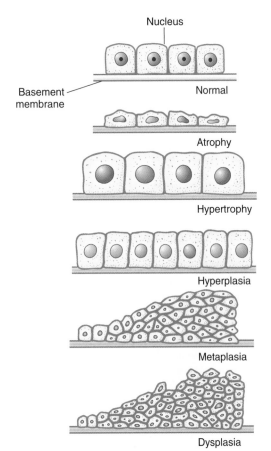

FIGURE 4.1 Adaptive and Dysplastic Alterations in Simple Cuboidal Epithelial Cells.

Atrophy

Atrophy refers to decrease in cell size. If atrophy affects a sufficient number of cells, the affected organ shrinks in size and is said to be atrophic. Atrophy can affect any organ, but it occurs most commonly in skeletal muscle, heart muscle, secondary sex organs, and the brain. Atrophy is classified as either *physiologic* or *pathologic,* depending on the underlying cause. Identical changes to cellular structure will occur regardless of whether atrophy results from normal or pathologic conditions. Physiologic atrophy occurs with early development, such as the thymus gland during early childhood; the atrophy is a normal event. Age-related atrophic changes to the gonads occur secondary to decreases in hormonal stimulation. The ovaries atrophy in postmenopausal women secondary to a lack of estrogenic stimulation. Aging results in atrophic changes to brain cells.

Pathologic atrophy occurs in organs as a result of decreases in workload, pressure, use, blood supply, nutrition, hormonal stimulation, or neural stimulation (Fig. 4.2). Pathologic atrophy to muscle will occur when a limb is placed in a cast. This form of atrophy, known as disuse atrophy, also occurs with prolonged bed rest or other immobilization.

Atrophic muscle cells contain less endoplasmic reticulum (ER), fewer mitochondria, and fewer myofilaments (the contractile components of the muscle fiber) compared with normal cells. Muscle atrophy, caused by decreased neural stimulation, results in reduced oxygen consumption and decreased amino acid uptake. The mechanisms of atrophy for such changes include a decrease in protein synthesis, an increase in protein degradation, or both. The degradation of proteins occurs mainly by the ubiquitin–proteosome pathway (see Chapter 1). Current research emphasis is related to misfolded proteins, abnormalities in protein degradation, and a host of diseases, especially neurodegenerative diseases.

Atrophy, secondary to chronic malnutrition, is associated with a process called *autophagy* ("self-eating"), where self-destructive autophagic vacuoles are created within the cell. These membrane-bound vesicles contain cellular debris and hydrolytic enzymes that degrade substances into simple units of fat, carbohydrate, or protein. Isolation of these enzymes within autophagic vacuoles prevents uncontrolled cell destruction in neighboring cells and tissue. Some substances contained within autophagic vacuole may resist destruction, persisting as membrane-bound

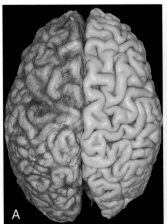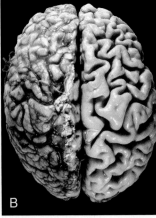

FIGURE 4.2 Atrophy. A, Normal brain of a young adult. B, Atrophy of the brain in an 82-year-old male with atherosclerotic cerebrovascular disease, resulting in reduced blood supply. Note that loss of brain substance narrows the gyri and widens the sulci. The meninges have been stripped from the right half of each specimen to reveal the surface of the brain. (From Kumar V et al, editors: *Robbins and Cotran pathologic basis of disease,* ed 9, Philadelphia, 2015, Elsevier.)

residual bodies within tissues. **Lipofuscin** refers to yellow-brown pigmented granules; lipid-containing residue that persists after lysosomal destruction. These granules tend to accumulate in liver, myocardial, renal, retinal, adrenal, and neural tissues as individuals age. When they accumulate in the skin, they are the basis of the so-called age spots appearing in older individuals.

Hypertrophy

Hypertrophy is a compensatory increase in the *size* of cells, occurring in response to mechanical load or stress, and results in increased size of the affected organ. Common triggers include repetitive stretching, chronic pressure, and volume overload (Fig. 4.3). The cells of the heart and kidneys are particularly prone to enlargement. Hypertrophy, as an adaptive response, occurs in the striated muscle cells of both the heart and skeletal muscles. It presents clinically as muscle enlargement. In the case of cardiac muscle hypertrophy, typically left ventricular hypertrophy (LVH), an increased synthesis of cardiac muscle proteins follows, allowing muscle fibers to do more work. Hypertrophy may be *physiologic* or *pathologic*. **Physiologic hypertrophy** results from increased demand, stimulation by hormones, and growth factors. An example of physiologic hypertrophy is enlargement secondary to aerobic exercise or a "runner's heart." In this case, no pathology is present and normal structure and function is preserved. **Pathologic hypertrophy** results from chronic hemodynamic overload, such as from hypertension or heart valve dysfunction. When LVH occurs secondary to hypertension, it represents *pathologic hypertrophy*. The initial adaptation, in the form of cardiac enlargement with dilated ventricles, is short lived. Prolonged cardiac hypertrophy progresses to contractile dysfunction and, finally, heart failure. In contrast to physiologic hypertrophy, where the myocardial matrix is preserved, pathologic hypertrophy is associated with increased interstitial fibrosis, cell death, and abnormal cardiac function (see Fig. 4.3). After a unilateral nephrectomy (removal of one kidney), compensatory hypertrophy occurs in the remaining kidney, which preserves renal structure and function.

Hyperplasia

Hyperplasia is an increase in the *number* of cells, resulting from an increased rate of cellular division. As a response to injury, hyperplasia occurs when the damage is severe or prolonged or when it results in cell death. Hyperplasia requires that cells undergo mitosis, a process wherein a single cell divides into two identical cells. The main mechanism

for hyperplasia is the production of growth factors, which stimulate the remaining cells after injury or cell loss to synthesize new cell components and, ultimately, to divide. Another mechanism is increased output of new cells from tissue stem cells. For example, if liver cells are injured, new cells can regenerate from intrahepatic stem cells.[2] Mature cells have differing capacity for hyperplastic (mitotic) growth. Although hyperplasia and hypertrophy have distinct processes, they can occur together within the same tissue.

Two types of physiologic (normal) hyperplasia occur: *compensatory hyperplasia* and *hormonal hyperplasia*. **Compensatory hyperplasia** is an adaptive mechanism that enables organs to regenerate. Removal of part of the liver leads to rapid hyperplasia of the remaining hepatocytes (liver cells). Even with removal of 70% of liver mass, regeneration is complete in about 2 weeks. Significant compensatory hyperplasia readily occurs in epidermal and intestinal epithelia, hepatocytes, bone marrow cells, and fibroblasts. Loss of cells within an organ triggers deoxyribonucleic acid (DNA) synthesis, mitotic division, and hyperplasia. To a lesser extent, hyperplasia occurs in bone, cartilage, and smooth muscle cells. A **callus**, or thickening of the skin, is an example of compensatory hyperplasia. It occurs in response to injury from a mechanical stimulus. Another example is the response to wound healing secondary to the inflammation process.

Hormonal hyperplasia occurs in organs that respond to endocrine hormonal stimulation. For example, during the follicular phase of the menstrual cycle, estrogen secretion by the ovary results in hyperplasia and endometrial proliferation. Hormonal secretion from a variety of endocrine organs maintains normal structure and function of target organs. (Hormone function is discussed further in Chapters 19, 20, 34, and 35.)

Pathologic hormonal hyperplasia is the abnormal proliferation of normal cells, usually in response to excessive hormonal stimulation or to the action of growth factors on target cells (Fig. 4.4). A common example is pathologic hyperplasia of the uterine endometrium (lining of the uterus) that occurs from an imbalance between estrogen and progesterone levels (see Chapter 35). The resulting endometrial hyperplasia commonly presents as erratic or excessive uterine bleeding, known as *dysfunctional uterine bleeding*. Left unchecked, the regular growth-inhibiting control mechanisms can fail over time, producing malignant transformation or endometrial cancer. Benign prostatic hyperplasia (BPH) is another example of pathologic hyperplasia. The incidence of BPH increases with age, secondary to age-related hormonal imbalances

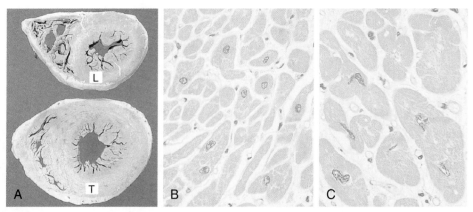

FIGURE 4.3 Hypertrophy of Cardiac Muscle in Response to Valve Disease. A, Transverse slices of a normal heart and a heart with hypertrophy of the left ventricle (*L,* normal thickness of left ventricular wall; *T,* thickened wall from heart in which severe narrowing of aortic valve caused resistance to systolic ventricular emptying). **B,** Histology of cardiac muscle from the normal heart. **C,** Histology of cardiac muscle from a hypertrophied heart. (From Stevens A, Lowe J: *Pathology: illustrated review in color,* ed 2, Edinburgh, 2000, Mosby.)

that result in epithelial and stromal proliferation or impaired apoptosis. Similarly, thyroid enlargement, including thyroid goiters, can result from excessive levels of pituitary thyroid-stimulating hormone (TSH). In the absence of malignant transformation, when the predisposing factors are corrected, pathologic hyperplasia will typically regress.

Dysplasia: Not a True Adaptive Change

Dysplasia refers to abnormal changes in the size, shape, and organization of mature cells (Fig. 4.5). Dysplasia is not considered a true adaptive process but is related to hyperplasia and is often referred to as atypical hyperplasia. Although dysplastic tissue appears disorderly, the term *dysplasia* does not refer to cancer. Dysplastic changes are common in the epithelial tissue of the uterine cervix, the endometrium, and the gastrointestinal and respiratory tract mucosa. Dysplasias that do not involve the entire thickness of epithelium may be completely reversible.[2] When dysplastic changes penetrate the basement membrane, it is considered an invasive neoplasm. Dysplasia is described as "low grade" or "high grade," depending on the degree of variation from normal. If the triggering stimulus is removed—for example, certain hormonal stimuli—dysplastic transformation may be reversible. (Dysplasia is discussed further in Chapter 11.)

Metaplasia

Metaplasia is the *reversible* replacement of one mature cell type (epithelial or mesenchymal) by another cell type, frequently one less differentiated. It is found in association with tissue damage, repair, and regeneration.[2] It is thought to develop as an adaptive response wherein the new cell type may be better suited to withstand an adverse environment. Usually, however, the change is not beneficial. For example, in the long-term cigarette smoker, the chronic irritation from smoke causes the normal ciliated columnar epithelial cells of the trachea and bronchi to become replaced by stratified squamous epithelial cells (Fig. 4.6). The newly

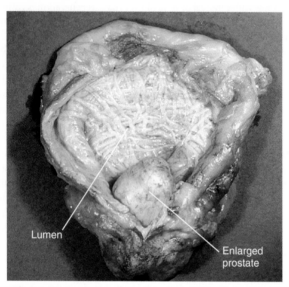

FIGURE 4.4 Hyperplasia of the Prostate With Secondary Thickening of the Obstructed Urinary Bladder (Bladder Cross-Section). The enlarged prostate is seen protruding into the lumen of the bladder, which appears trabeculated. These "trabeculae" result from hypertrophy and hyperplasia of smooth muscle cells that occur in response to increased intravesical pressure caused by urinary obstruction. (From Damjanov I: *Pathology for the health professions,* ed 4, St Louis, 2012, Saunders.)

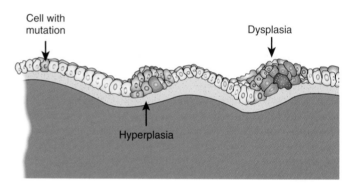

FIGURE 4.5 Dysplasia. Abnormal changes in the size, shape, and organization of cells. Dysplasia is related to hyperplasia and called atypical hyperplasia. (Adapted from Biology of Cancer modules, Boston University, School of Public Health. Available at sphweb.bumc.bu.edu.)

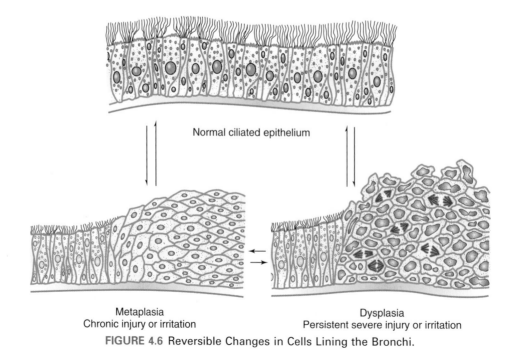

FIGURE 4.6 Reversible Changes in Cells Lining the Bronchi.

formed squamous epithelial cells do not secrete mucus or have cilia, causing a loss of a critical protective mechanism.

Metaplasia results from a reprogramming of *stem cells* present in most epithelia or of undifferentiated mesenchymal (tissue from embryonic mesoderm) cells present in connective tissue.[2] These precursor cells mature along a different pathway with metaplastic change. Differentiation of stem cells from a particular cell lineage responds to signals generated by growth factors, cytokines, and ECM components in the cell's environment.

CELLULAR INJURY

Injury to cells and to the ECM leads to injury of tissues and organs and ultimately determines the structural patterns of disease. Cellular injury occurs when the cell is unable to maintain homeostasis (a normal or adaptive steady state). The injury may be reversible injury (the cell can recover) or irreversible injury (cellular death). Loss of function is the result of cell and ECM injury and cell death. Cellular injury may occur secondary to a variety of factors: chemical agents, lack of sufficient oxygen (hypoxia), free radicals, infectious agents, physical and mechanical factors, immunologic reactions, genetic factors, and nutritional imbalances. Types of injuries and their responses are summarized in Table 4.1 and Fig. 4.7.

The extent of cellular injury is a function of cell type, level of differentiation, and adaptive mechanisms of the cell. Also important is the nature, severity, and duration of the injury. Fully differentiated, mature cells are more susceptible to injury than are cell precursors. Two individuals exposed to an identical stimulus may incur varying degrees of cellular injury. Individual differences, including genetics, nutritional status, and immunologic competency, can profoundly influence the extent of cell injury. The precise "point of no return" with respect to cell death remains unclear. Once changes to the nucleus have occurred or cell membranes are disrupted, or both, irreversible injury and cell death are inevitable.

General Mechanisms of Cell Injury

Regardless of the cause of injury, a host of biochemical events result in cell injury and death. Such events include adenosine triphosphate (ATP) depletion, damage from oxygen-derived free radicals, and alterations in calcium level. Injury to cell components includes membrane damage, protein folding defects, mitochondrial compromise, and DNA damage (Table 4.2). The most common forms of cell injury include (1) ischemic and hypoxic injury, (2) ischemia–reperfusion injury, (3) oxidative stress or accumulation of oxygen-derived free radicals-induced injury, and (4) chemical injury.

Ischemic and Hypoxic Injury

Hypoxia, or the lack of sufficient oxygen within cells, is the single most common cause of cellular injury (Fig. 4.8). Hypoxia can result from a number of circumstances, such as reduced oxygen content in the ambient air, loss of hemoglobin, decreased red blood cell (RBC) production, respiratory and cardiovascular diseases, and poisoning of the cellular oxidative enzymes (cytochromes). The most common cause of hypoxia is ischemia or a reduced supply of blood and therefore oxygen. Hypoxia negatively impacts normal physiologic processes: differentiation, angiogenesis, proliferation, erythropoiesis, and overall cell viability. Mitochondria are the primary consumers of oxygen. Hypoxia triggers the mitochondrial complex to produce *reactive oxygen species* (ROS). From a physiologic perspective, ROS can be both beneficial and harmful, for example, by promoting *oxidative stress,* which can damage cells (oxidative stress is discussed in the next section). The relationship between hypoxia and inflammation has been linked to inflammatory bowel disease, certain cancers, and infection (Fig. 4.9). Ongoing research seeks to clarify how tumors adapt to low oxygen levels, including

TABLE 4.1 Types of Progressive Cell Injury and Responses

Type	Responses
Adaptation	Atrophy, hypertrophy, hyperplasia, metaplasia
Active cell injury	Immediate response of "entire" cell
Reversible	Loss of ATP, cellular swelling, detachment of ribosomes, autophagy of lysosomes
Irreversible	"Point of no return" structurally when severe vacuolization of mitochondria occurs and Ca^{++} moves into cell
Necrosis	Common type of cell death with severe cell swelling and breakdown of organelles
Apoptosis, or programmed cell death	Cellular self-destruction for elimination of unwanted cell populations
Autophagy	Eating of self, cytoplasmic vesicles engulf cytoplasm and organelles, recycling factory
Chronic cell injury (subcellular alterations)	Persistent stimuli response may involve only specific organelles or cytoskeleton (e.g., phagocytosis of bacteria)
Accumulations or infiltrations	Water, pigments, lipids, glycogen, proteins
Pathologic calcification	Dystrophic and metastatic calcification

ATP, Adenosine triphosphate; *Ca++,* calcium.

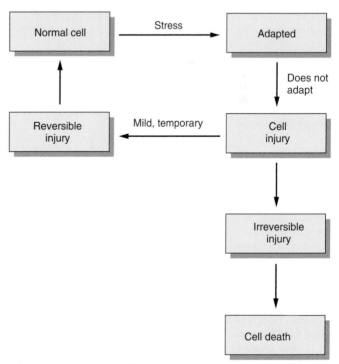

FIGURE 4.7 Stages of Cellular Adaptation, Injury, and Death. The normal cell responds to physiologic and pathologic stresses by adapting (atrophy, hypertrophy, hyperplasia, metaplasia). Cell injury occurs if the adaptive responses are exceeded or compromised by injurious agents, stress, and mutations. The injury is reversible if it is mild or transient, but if the stimulus persists, the cell suffers irreversible injury and eventually death.

TABLE 4.2 Common Themes in Cell Injury and Cell Death

Theme	Comments
ATP depletion	Loss of mitochondrial ATP and decreased ATP synthesis; results include cellular swelling, decreased protein synthesis, decreased membrane transport, and lipogenesis, all changes that contribute to loss of integrity of plasma membrane
Reactive oxygen species ($\uparrow$ROS)	Lack of oxygen is key in progression of cell injury in ischemia (reduced blood supply); activated oxygen species (ROS, O_2^-, H_2O_2, OH^-) cause destruction of cell membranes and cell structure
Ca^{++} entry	Normally intracellular cytosolic calcium concentrations are very low; ischemia and certain chemicals cause an increase in cytosolic Ca^{++} concentrations; sustained levels of Ca^{++} continue to increase with damage to plasma membrane; Ca^{++} causes intracellular damage by activating a number of enzymes
Mitochondrial damage	Can be damaged by increases in cytosolic Ca^{++}, ROS; two outcomes of mitochondrial damage are loss of membrane potential, which causes depletion of ATP and eventual death or necrosis of cell, and activation of another type of cell death (apoptosis) (see p. 102)
Membrane damage	Early loss of selective membrane permeability found in all forms of cell injury, lysosomal membrane damage with release of enzymes causing cellular digestion
Protein misfolding, DNA damage	Proteins may misfold, triggering *unfolded protein response* that activates corrective responses; if overwhelmed, response activates cell suicide program or apoptosis; DNA damage (genotoxic stress) also can activate apoptosis (see p. 102)

ATP, Adenosine triphosphate; *Ca^{++}*, calcium; *DNA*, deoxyribonucleic acid; *H$_2$O$_2$*, hydrogen peroxide; *O$_2^-$*, superoxide radical; *OH$^-$*, hydroxyl radical; *ROS*, reactive oxygen species.

angiogenesis, increasing glucose consumption, and promoting the metabolic state of glycolysis.

Arteriosclerosis (narrowing of blood vessels) and thrombus (blood clots within vessels) can result in localized tissue ischemia. Progressive hypoxia, caused by gradual arterial narrowing, is better tolerated than the acute anoxia (total lack of oxygen) caused by an acute obstruction, or a thrombus. An acute obstruction in a coronary artery can result in a rapidly evolving *myocardial infarction* ("heart attack") if the blood supply is not restored. Irreversible myocardial cell death, with loss of heart function, will follow. Gradual onset of ischemia, however, usually results in myocardial adaptation. Myocardial infarction and stroke are frequent causes of mortality in the United States. These events typically result from ischemia.

Cellular responses to hypoxic injury occur rapidly. Within 1 minute after the blood supply to the myocardium is interrupted, the heart becomes pale and dysfunctional and unable to contract normally. Within 3 to 5 minutes, mitochondrial compromise occurs, resulting in insufficient ATP production. At this point, the compromised portion of the myocardium ceases to contract. The abrupt lack of contraction is caused by a rapid decrease in mitochondrial phosphorylation, which results in insufficient ATP production. Lack of ATP leads to an increase in

anaerobic metabolism, which generates ATP from glycogen when there is insufficient oxygen. When glycogen stores are depleted, even anaerobic metabolism ceases.

Ischemia-induced reduction in ATP levels causes a failure of the plasma membrane's sodium–potassium (Na^+-K^+) pump and sodium–calcium (Na^+-Ca^{++}) exchange mechanisms. Sodium and calcium influx into and accumulate in the cell. Potassium (K^+) diffuses out of the cell. Without the pump mechanism, sodium and water can freely enter the cell resulting in cellular swelling and dilation of the ER. With dilation, ribosomes detach from the rough ER, reducing protein synthesis. If hypoxia persists, the entire cell becomes markedly swollen. These disruptions are reversible if oxygen (O_2) is restored. If oxygen is not restored, vacuolation (formation of vacuoles) occurs within the cytoplasm (see Manifestations of Cellular Injury section). The damaged outer membrane causes lysosomes to swell; marked swelling occurs to the mitochondria. With continued hypoxia, cell death rapidly follows as calcium accumulates within the cell, essential metabolic processes cease, and cell membranes become dysfunctional (see Figs. 4.8, *C*, and, late in the chapter, Fig. 4.21). Influx of calcium into the cell activates enzymes that trigger apoptosis (see Figs. 4.23 and 4.28 later in the chapter). Restoration of blood flow and oxygen can actually result in additional injury known as *ischemia–reperfusion injury*.

Ischemia–Reperfusion Injury

Restoration of blood flow and oxygen to ischemic tissues can increase recovery of cells reversibly injured, but paradoxically result in additional injury known as ischemia–reperfusion injury (reperfusion [reoxygenation] injury) and cause cell death (Fig. 4.10). Reperfusion is a serious complication and an important mechanism of injury in instances of tissue transplantation and other ischemic syndromes (e.g., hepatic, intestinal, renal). Several mechanisms are proposed for reperfusion injury, including the following:

- *Oxidative stress:* Reoxygenation induces *oxidative stress* by generating highly ROS and nitrogen species. Reactive oxygen intermediates include hydroxyl radical (OH^-), superoxide radical (O_2^-), and hydrogen peroxide (H_2O_2). Nitrogen-based free radicals present mostly in the form of nitric oxide (NO) and are generated by endothelial cells, macrophages, neurons, and other cells. The radicals further damage the already compromised membrane and facilitate calcium overload within the mitochondria. Additionally, reperfusion injury promotes proinflammatory neutrophil adhesion to the endothelium where they release toxic oxidants and harmful proteases. Antioxidant agents, such as vitamin C and vitamin E, reverse neutrophil adhesion. They also reverse neutrophil-mediated reperfusion injury in cardiac muscle.[3,4]
- *Increased intracellular calcium concentration*: Intracellular and mitochondrial calcium accumulate within the cell during acute ischemia. Reperfusion results in even more calcium influx because of damaged cell membranes and ROS-mediated injury to the sarcoplasmic reticulum. The increased calcium enhances mitochondrial permeability; damaged mitochondria have decreased or ceased production of ATP.
- *Inflammation*: Ischemic injury promotes inflammation. Dead cells stimulate immune cells to release cytokine-mediated danger signals, thus initiating an inflammatory response.
- *Complement activation*: Complement activation may exacerbate damage which has occurred secondary to reperfusion injury.[2]

✓ **QUICK CHECK 4.1**

1. When does a cell become irreversibly injured?
2. Discuss the pathogenesis of hypoxic injury?
3. What are the mechanisms of ischemia–reperfusion injury?

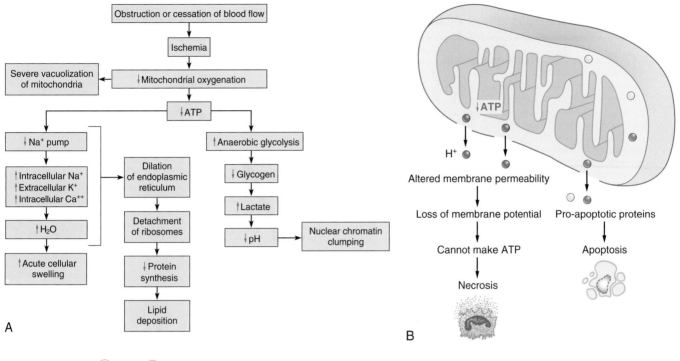

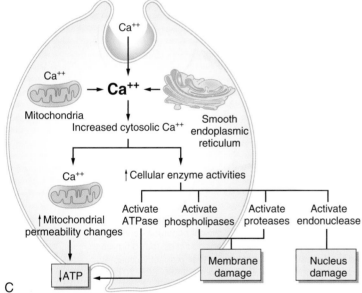

FIGURE 4.8 Hypoxic Injury Induced by Ischemia. A, Consequences of decreased oxygen delivery or ischemia with decreased adenosine triphosphate (ATP). The structural and physiologic changes are reversible if oxygen is delivered quickly. Significant decreases in ATP result in cell death, mostly by necrosis. **B,** Mitochondrial damage can result in changes in membrane permeability, loss of membrane potential, and decrease in ATP concentration. Between the outer and inner membranes of the mitochondria are proteins that can activate the cell's suicide pathways, called *apoptosis*. **C,** Calcium ions are critical mediators of cell injury. Calcium ions (Ca++) are usually maintained at low concentrations in the cell's cytoplasm; thus ischemia and certain toxins can initially cause an increase in the release of Ca++ from intracellular stores and later an increased movement (influx) across the plasma membrane. (Adapted from Kumar V et al, editors: *Pathology*, St Louis, 2014, Elsevier.)

Free Radicals and Reactive Oxygen Species— Oxidative Stress

Free radicals are an important mechanism of cellular injury, especially injury caused by ROS. This form of injury is called oxidative stress. Reactive oxygen species (ROS) are reactive molecules from molecular oxygen formed as a natural oxidant species in cells during mitochondrial respiration and energy generation. Oxidative stress is caused by an increase in different reactive species, depletion of antioxidant defense, or both. Oxidative stress results in detrimental oxidation of different molecules, including proteins, lipids, nucleic acids, and others. Oxidative stress can activate several intracellular signaling pathways because ROS can regulate enzymes and transcription factors. This process is an important mechanism of cell damage in many conditions.

A free radical is an electrically uncharged atom, or group of atoms, which has an unpaired electron. Having one unpaired electron makes the molecule unstable; the molecule becomes stabilized either by donating or by accepting an electron from another molecule. The free radical has the potential to form a damaging chemical bond with proteins, lipids, and carbohydrates found within the cell membrane. Free radicals are highly reactive. They have low chemical specificity—that is, they can react with most molecules in their proximity. Reactions involving free radicals are difficult to control, and they initiate chain reactions. Free radicals are generated in a variety of conditions, including chemical and radiation injury, ischemia–reperfusion injury, cellular aging, and microbial destruction by phagocytes.

Free radicals are generated within cells by a number of mechanisms. These mechanisms are as follows:

1. *Reduction–oxidative reactions* (redox reactions): An oxidative-reduction reaction is a type of biochemical reaction involving the transfer of elections between two species (molecule, atom, or ion).

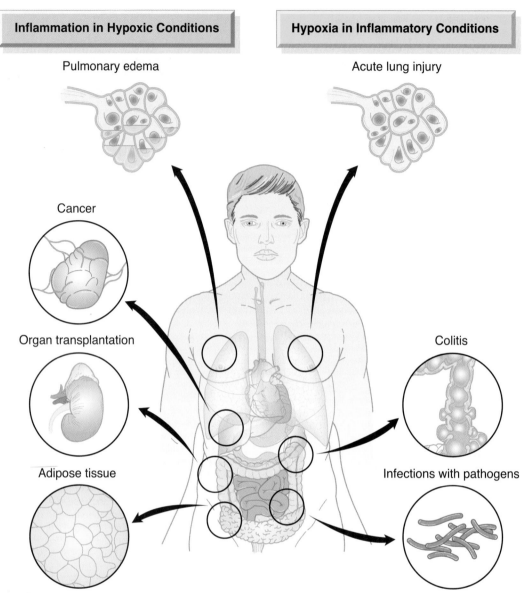

Inflammation in Hypoxic Conditions

Hypoxia in Inflammatory Conditions

Pulmonary edema

Acute lung injury

Cancer

Organ transplantation

Adipose tissue

Colitis

Infections with pathogens

FIGURE 4.9 Hypoxia and Inflammation. Shown is a simplified drawing of clinical conditions character-ized by tissue hypoxia that causes inflammatory changes *(left)* and inflammatory diseases that ultimately lead to hypoxia *(right)*. These diseases and conditions are discussed in more detail in their respective chapters. (Adapted from Eltzschig HK, Carmeliet P: Hypoxia and inflammation, *N Engl J Med* 364:656–665, 2011.)

A species may either gain or lose an electron. All biologic membranes contain redox systems, which serve to support cellular activity.

2. *Absorption of extreme energy sources* (ultraviolet light, radiation) produces free radicals.

3. *Enzymatic metabolism of exogenous chemicals or drugs:* Many exogenous (outside the body) substances within the environment readily generate free radicals. As an example, CCL_3, a byproduct of carbon tetrachloride [CCl_4]), forms free radicals known to damage the liver, predisposing this organ to cancer. Accordingly, CCL_4 is classified by the International Agency for Research on Cancer (IARC; Group 2B) as a possible carcinogenic and by the Environmental Protection Agency (EPA) as a probable human car-cinogen. Many reported cases of CCL_4 toxicity are associated with drinking alcohol.

4. *Transition metals* (iron and copper) donate or accept free electrons during intracellular reactions, generating free radicals in the process.

As an example, the Fenton reaction, involving iron and H_2O_2, produces the potentially damaging hydroxyl radical and higher oxidation states of the iron. It has been implicated in iron accumulation disease.

5. *NO,* a colorless gas, acts as an intermediate in reactions involving endothelial cells, neurons, macrophages, and other cell types. NO can act as a free radical and convert to highly reactive compounds, including peroxynitrite anion ($ONOO^-$), nitrogen dioxide (NO_2), and nitrate (NO_3). Table 4.3 describes the most significant free radicals. Free radicals also cause several damaging effects, such as the following:

1. Lipid peroxidation—the destruction of polyunsaturated lipids, which leads to membrane damage and increased permeability. This same process causes fats to become rancid.

2. Protein alteration—a process whereby polypeptide chains become fragmented leading to protein loss, protein misfolding, and alters protein–protein interaction.

3. DNA damage—results in mutations (Fig. 4.11; also see Chapter 2).

4. Mitochondrial effects—mitochondria are organelles that generate ATP. They can become damaged by ROS compromising available energy for the cell. Increases in intracellular calcium also damage mitochondria (see Fig. 4.8). Box 4.1 summarizes the major types of mitochondrial damage. Cell damage from ROS can extend to neighboring cells.

The toxicity of certain drugs and chemicals can be attributed to free radicals. The drug/chemical may be converted to a free radical or it may generate oxygen-derived metabolites. Free radicals have been either directly or indirectly linked with a growing number of diseases and disorders (Box 4.2). The body has various mechanisms to eliminate

TABLE 4.3	Biologically Relevant Free Radicals
Reactive oxygen species (ROS) Superoxide radical $O_2^{\cdot-}$ $O_2 \xrightarrow{Oxidase} O_2^{\cdot-}$	Generated either (1) directly during autoxidation in mitochondria or (2) enzymatically by enzymes in cytoplasm, such as xanthine oxidase or cytochrome p450; once produced, it can be inactivated spontaneously or more rapidly by enzyme superoxide dismutase (SOD): $O_2^{\cdot-} + O_2^{\cdot-} + -H_2^{\cdot} \xrightarrow{SOD} H_2O_2 + O_2$
Hydrogen peroxide (H_2O_2) $O_2^{\cdot-} + O_2^{\cdot-} + -H \xrightarrow{SOD} H_2O_2 + O_2$ Or Oxidases present in peroxisomes O_2 peroxisome $O_2^{\cdot-} \xrightarrow{SOD} H_2O_2$	Generated by SOD or directly by oxidases in intracellular peroxisomes (NOTE: SOD is considered an antioxidant because it converts superoxide to H_2O_2); catalase (another antioxidant) can then decompose H_2O_2 to $O_2 + H_2O$.)
Hydroxyl radicals (OH^-) $H_2O \rightarrow H \cdot + OH \cdot$ Or $Fe^{++} + H_2O_2 \rightarrow Fe^{++} + OH \cdot + OH^-$ Or $H_2O_2 + O_2^{\cdot-} \rightarrow OH \cdot + OH^- + O_2$	Generated by hydrolysis of water caused by ionizing radiation or by interaction with metals—especially iron (Fe) and copper (Cu); iron is important in toxic oxygen injury because it is required for maximal oxidative cell damage
Nitric oxide (NO) $NO \cdot + O_2^{\cdot-} \rightarrow ONOO^- + H^+$	NO by itself is an important mediator that can act as a free radical; it can be converted to another radical—peroxynitrite anion ($ONOO^-$), as well as nitrogen dioxide ($NO_2^{\cdot}$) and carbonate radical ($CO_3^{\cdot-}$)

Data from Cotran RS et al: *Robbins pathologic basis of disease,* ed 6, Philadelphia, 1999, Saunders.

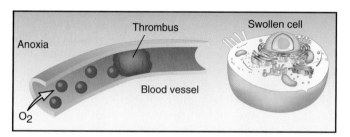
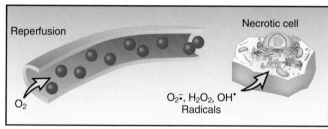

FIGURE 4.10 Reperfusion Injury. Without oxygen, or in anoxia, the cells display hypoxic injury and become swollen. With reoxygenation, risk of reperfusion injury increases because of the formation of reactive oxygen radicals that can cause cell necrosis. (Redrawn from Damjanov I: *Pathology for the health professions,* ed 3, St Louis, 2006, Saunders.)

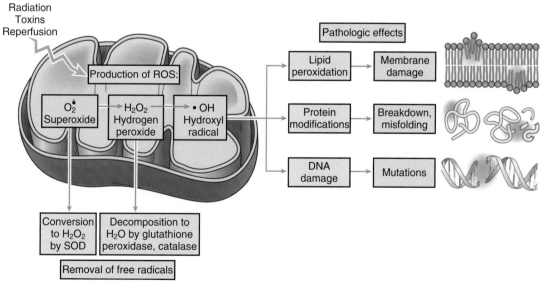

FIGURE 4.11 The Role of Reactive Oxygen Species (ROS) in Cell Injury. The production of ROS can be initiated by many cell stressors, such as radiation, toxins, and reperfusion of oxygen. Free radicals are removed by normal decay and enzymatic systems. ROS accumulates in cells because of insufficient removal or excess production leading to cell injury, including lipid peroxidation, protein modifications, and DNA damage or mutations. (Adapted from Kumar V et al, editors: *Robbins and Cotran pathologic basis of disease,* ed 9, Philadelphia, 2015, Elsevier.)

BOX 4.1   Three Major Types and Consequences of Mitochondrial Damage

1. Damage to the mitochondria results in the formation of the *mitochondrial permeability transition pore,* a high-conductance channel or pore. The opening of this channel results in the loss of mitochondrial membrane potential, causing failure of oxidative phosphorylation, depletion of adenosine triphosphate (ATP), and damage to **mitochondrial DNA (mtDNA)**, leading to necrosis of the cell.
2. Altered oxidative phosphorylation leads to the formation of reactive oxygen species (ROS) that can damage cellular components.
3. Because mitochondria store several proteins between their membranes, increased permeability of the outer membrane may result in leakage of proapoptotic proteins and cause cell death by apoptosis.

Data from Kumar V et al, editors: *Robbins and Cotran pathologic basis of disease,* ed 9, Philadelphia, 2015, Elsevier.

BOX 4.2   Diseases and Disorders Linked to Oxygen-Derived Free Radicals

Deterioration noted in aging
  Atherosclerosis
  Ischemic brain injury
  Alzheimer disease
Neurotoxins
Cancer
Cardiac myopathy
Chronic granulomatous disease
Diabetes mellitus
Eye disorders
  Macular degeneration
  Cataracts
Inflammatory disorders
Iron overload

Lung disorders
  Asbestosis
  Oxygen toxicity
  Emphysema
Nutritional deficiencies
Radiation injury
Reperfusion injury
Rheumatoid arthritis
Skin disorders
Toxic states
  Xenobiotics (tetrachloride [CCl₄],
    paraquat, cigarette smoke, etc.)
  Metal irons (nickel [Ni], copper
    [Cu], iron [Fe], etc.)

TABLE 4.4   Methods Contributing to Inactivation or Termination of Free Radicals

Method	Process
Antioxidants	Endogenous or exogenous; either blocks synthesis or inactivates (e.g., scavenges) free radicals; includes vitamin E, vitamin C, cysteine, glutathione, albumin, ceruloplasmin, transferrin, γ-lipoacid, others
Enzymes	Superoxide dismutase,* which converts superoxide to hydrogen peroxide (H_2O_2); catalase* (in peroxisomes) decomposes H_2O_2; glutathione peroxidase* decomposes hydroxyl radical (OH^-) and H_2O_2

*These enzymes are important in modulating the cellular destructive effects of free radicals; also released in inflammation.

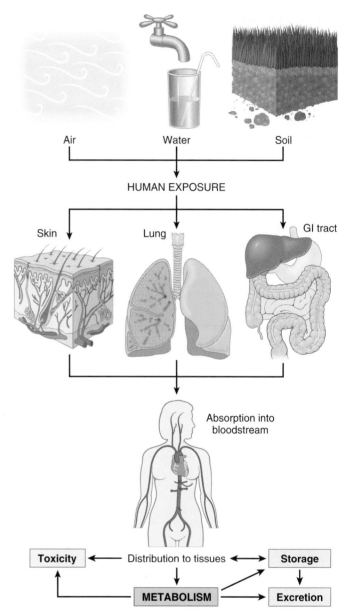

FIGURE 4.12 Human Exposure to Pollutants. Pollutants contained in air, water, and soil are absorbed through the lungs, gastrointestinal tract, and skin. In the body, the pollutants may act at the site of absorption but are generally transported through the bloodstream to various organs where they can be stored or metabolized. Metabolism of xenobiotics may result in the formation of water-soluble compounds that are excreted, or a toxic metabolite may be created by activation of the agent. (From Kumar V et al, editors: *Robbins and Cotran pathologic basis of disease,* ed 9, Philadelphia, 2015, Elsevier).

free radicals. As an example, the oxygen free radical *superoxide* may spontaneously decay into oxygen and hydrogen peroxide. Table 4.4 summarizes other methods that contribute to inactivation or termination of free radicals.

Chemical or Toxic Injury

Humans are exposed to thousands of chemicals that have insufficient toxicologic data.[5] Time, cost, and an interest in reducing animal testing dictate the need to develop new methods for toxicity testing. In an effort to meet public health concerns, many agencies have partnered to investigate how chemicals interact with biologic systems. Investigators are aided by advances in molecular and systems biology, computational toxicology, and bioinformatics. Mechanisms of cell stress from chemical agents include oxidative stress, ER stress, heat shock response, DNA damage response, mental stress, inflammation, and osmotic stress (sudden change in solute concentration). Chemicals are being classified under these types of cell stress mechanisms.

Xenobiotics (from Greek *xenos,* "foreign"; *bios,* "life") are compounds and chemicals that have toxic, mutagenic, or carcinogenic properties (Fig. 4.12). Some of these chemicals are found in the human diet, for example, the fungal mycotoxin, aflatoxin B₁. Many xenobiotics are hepatotoxic (toxic to the liver). The liver is the initial site of contact for many ingested compounds—xenobiotics, drugs, and alcohol—predisposing this organ to chemically induced injury. Once absorbed by the gastrointestinal (GI) tract, the liver is the initial site of contact. This dynamic is called *first-pass effect.* A frequent cause for withdrawing medications from the market is hepatotoxicity. Herbal products are less subject to regulation by the U.S. Food and Drug Administration (FDA). The compounds chaparral and ma huang, marketed as herbal medicines, are potent hepatotoxins.[6] Many chemical compounds used in household cleaning, insect control, outdoor maintenance, or chemical manufacturing are potential carcinogens. Many such agents are absorbed in the body through the skin or by inhalation; ubiquitous in the environment, some agents have been linked with liver and other organ damage. The extent of chemically induced liver injury varies from minor liver injury to acute liver failure, cirrhosis, and liver cancer.[7]

Hepatic detoxification occurs through enzyme-mediated biotransformation and antioxidant systems. Biotransformation is a process whereby enzymatic reactions convert one chemical into a less toxic or nontoxic compound. The liver has the highest supply of biotransformation enzymes of all organs and plays a key role in protecting the host from chemical toxicity (Fig. 4.13). Fig. 4.14 provides a summary of chemically induced liver injury.

Antioxidants are molecules that inhibit the oxidation of other molecules, thereby preventing the formation of free radicals. Antioxidants often terminate a chain reaction, which would otherwise result in free radical formation. *Endogenous antioxidants* are antioxidants produced by the body. The five most powerful endogenous antioxidants are *superoxide dismutase (SOD), alpha lipoic acid (ALA), catalase, coenzyme Q 10 (CoQ10),* and *glutathione peroxidase (GPX).* Exogenous antioxidants are antioxidants that originate from outside the body, typically from dietary sources, such as vitamin C. Foods rich in antioxidants are appropriately encouraged as part of a healthy diet.

Chemical Agents Including Drugs

Numerous chemical agents cause cellular injury. Minute amounts of some, such as arsenic and cyanide, can rapidly destroy cells and cause death of the individual. Chronic exposure to air pollutants, insecticides, and herbicides can cause cell injury (see Fig. 4.12). Carbon tetrachloride, alcohol, and social drugs can significantly alter cellular function and injure cellular structures. Over-the-counter (OTC) and prescribed drugs are an important cause of cellular injury. The abuse and addiction to opioids, such as heroin, morphine, and fentanyl, and other prescription pain relievers are a serious global problem that affects all societies. Millions of people abuse opioids worldwide. The issue has become a public health crisis. In the United States, drug overdoses have dramatically increased over the last two decades, with deaths more than tripling between 1999 and 2016; and approximately 72,000 deaths in 2017.[8] The leading cause of poisoning in children is medications, including inappropriate administration of OTC preparations containing acetaminophen (paracetamol). Acetaminophen is one of the most common causes of poisonings worldwide when used as an analgesic. The liver is the most common site for chemically induced injury. Common drugs of abuse are listed in Table 4.5 and social or street drugs in Table 4.6.

Common Environmental Toxins

Air pollution. The world's largest single environmental health risk is air pollution.[9] According to the *State of Global Air 2018,* which provides evidence as part of the Global Burden of Disease (GBD) project,[10] seven billion people, or more than 95% of the world's population, live in areas of unhealthy air. Air pollution is the leading environmental cause of death worldwide.[10] Air pollution from both indoor and outdoor exposure contributed to 6.1 million premature deaths from stroke, heart attack, lung cancer, and chronic lung disease.[10] For the first time, worldwide estimates of exposure to and health effects of indoor pollution or burning solid fuel in homes resulted in a total of 2.5 billion people, or one in three global persons, exposed to household pollution from the use of solid fuels (e.g., coal, charcoal, wood, dung, or other biomass) for heating and

TABLE 4.5 Common Drugs of Abuse

Class	Molecular Target	Example
Opioid narcotics	Mu (μ) opioid receptor (agonist)	Heroin, hydromorphone (Dilaudid) Oxycodone (Percodan, Percocet, OxyContin) Fentanyl Methadone (Dolophine) Meperidine (Demerol)
Sedative-hypnotics	GABA$_A$ receptor (agonist)	Barbiturates Ethanol Methaqualone (Quaalude) Glutethimide (Doriden) Ethchlorvynol (Placidyl)
Psychomotor stimulants	Dopamine transporter (antagonist) Serotonin receptors (toxicity)	Cocaine Amphetamines 3,4-Methylenedioxymethamphetamine (MDMA, ecstasy)
Phencyclidine-like drugs	NMDA glutamate receptor channel (antagonist)	Phencyclidine (PCP, angel dust) Ketamine
Cannabinoids	CB₁ cannabinoid receptors (agonist)	Marijuana Hashish
Hallucinogens	Serotonin 5-HT₂ receptors (agonist)	Lysergic acid diethylamide (LSD) Mescaline Psilocybin

CB₁, Cannabinoid receptor type 1; *GABA,* γ-aminobutyric acid; *5-HT₂,* 5-hydroxytryptamine; *NMDA,* N-methyl-ᴅ-aspartate.
From Kumar V et al: Cellular responses to stress and toxic insults: adaptation, injury, and death. In Kumar V et al, editors: *Robbins and Cotran pathologic basis of disease,* ed 9, St Louis, 2014, Saunders; Hyman SE: A 28-year-old man addicted to cocaine. *JAMA* 286:2586, 2001.

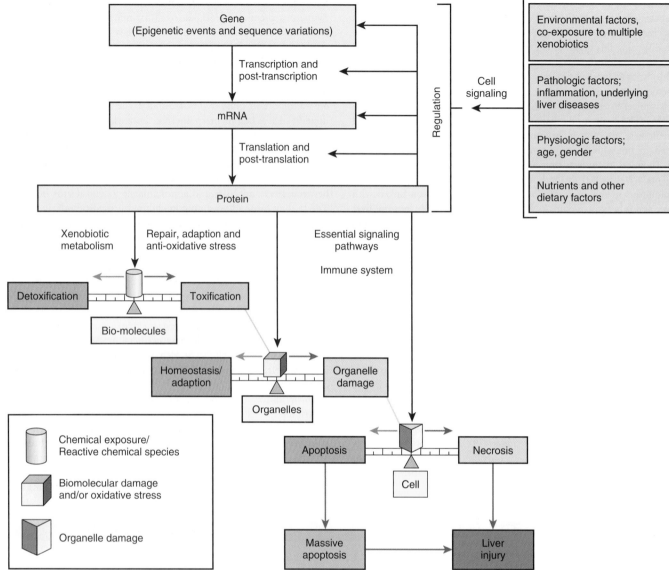

FIGURE 4.13 Chemical Liver Injury. Liver injury is a result of genetic, environmental, biologic, and dietary factors. Certain chemicals can form toxic or chemically reactive metabolites. The risk of liver injury also can increase with increasing doses of a toxicant. Xenobiotic enzyme induction can lead to altered metabolism of chemicals, and drugs can either inhibit or induce drug-metabolizing enzymes. These changes can lead to greater toxicity. The dose at the site of action is controlled by phase I to III xenobiotic metabolites and metabolizing enzymes are encoded by numerous different genes. Therefore the metabolism and toxicity outcomes can vary greatly among individuals. Additionally all aspects of xenobiotic metabolism are regulated by certain transcription factors (cellular mediators of gene regulation). Overall the extent of cell damage depends on the balance between reactive chemical species and protective responses aimed at decreasing oxidative stress, repairing macromolecular damage, or preserving cell health by inducing apoptosis or cell death. Significant clinical outcomes of chemical-induced liver injury occur with necrosis and the immune response. Covalent binding of reactive metabolites to cellular proteins can produce new antigens (haptens) that initiate autoantibody production and cytotoxic T-cell responses. Necrosis, a form of cell death (see the Cellular Death section), can result from extensive damage to the plasma membrane with altered ion transport, changes of membrane potential, cell swelling, and eventual dissolution. Altogether the pathogenesis of chemically induced liver injury is determined by genetics, environmental factors, and other underlying pathologic conditions. Green arrows are pathways leading to cell recovery; red arrows indicate pathways to cell damage or death; black arrows are pathways leading to chemically induced liver injury. (Adapted from Gu X, Manautou JE: Molecular mechanisms underlying chemical liver injury, *Exp Rev Mol Med* 14:e4, 2013.)

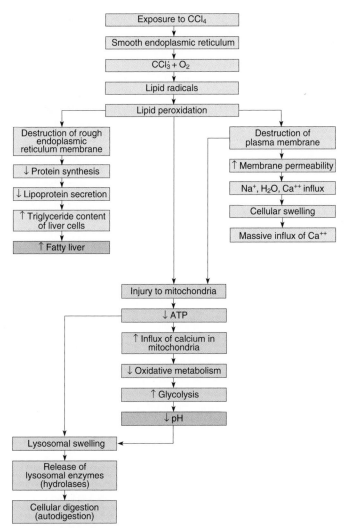

FIGURE 4.14 Chemical Injury of Liver Cells Induced by Carbon Tetrachloride (CCl₄) Poisoning. Light blue boxes are mechanisms unique to chemical injury, purple boxes involve hypoxic injury, and green boxes are clinical manifestations.

cooking. These people live mostly in low- and middle-income countries and together with outdoor pollution face a double health burden[10] Fig. 4.15. Over half of the total global attributable deaths were found to be from China and India together.[10] India is now similar to China for the highest air pollution health burdens worldwide with both countries having 1.1 million deaths from outdoor air pollution.[10]

Ambient particulate matter is particulate matter less than or equal to 2.5 micrometers in aerodynamic matter, or $PM_{2.5}$ Fig. 4.16. Ambient particulate matter is ranked as the sixth highest risk factor for early death. Another component of outdoor air pollution is **ozone**, a special form of oxygen in a deep layer in the stratosphere, whose levels are increasing around the world and contributes to 234,000 deaths from chronic lung disease.[10]

Heavy Metals as Environmental Pollutants

The most common heavy metals associated with harmful effects in humans include lead, mercury, arsenic, and cadmium. Damage from metals includes involvement of DNA repair mechanisms, tumor suppressor functions, and interference with signal transduction pathways.

Lead. **Lead (Pb)** is a heavy toxic metal present in paint of older homes, the environment, and the workplace. The organ systems most

affected by lead include the nervous, hematopoietic (organs and tissues that produce blood cells), reproductive, GI, cardiovascular, musculoskeletal systems and the kidneys. Exposure occurs through inhalation, ingestion, and, less frequently, skin contact. Lead induces cellular damage by increasing oxidative stress.[11] The key underlying effects of lead exposure in humans is disruption of cellular ion status, and disruption of protein function from displacement of metal enzyme cofactors. Lead inhibits several enzymes involved in hemoglobin synthesis and causes a microcytic, hypochromic anemia. Renal lesions can cause tubular dysfunction resulting in glycosuria (glucose in the urine), aminoaciduria (amino acids in the urine), and hyperphosphaturia (excess phosphate in urine). GI symptoms are less severe and include nausea, loss of appetite, weight loss, and abdominal cramping. Low lead levels can increase the levels of other metals and also may be a risk factor for hypertension.[12]

Lead may be found in hazardous concentrations in food, water, and air, and is one of the most common sources of overexposures injuries found in industry. Older buildings, where lead-based paint is peeling from the walls, is a particular hazard to children (see *Did You Know? CDC Update: Primary Prevention of Lead Exposures for Children*). Lead-based paint has a sweet taste and toddlers are prone to find paint chips on the floor and put them into their mouths.

The neurologic effect of lead in exposed children is the driving force for reducing lead levels in the environment. Children are more susceptible than adults to the effects of lead for several reasons:

1. Children have increased hand-to-mouth behavior and thus are prone to putting objects found in their environment into their mouths.
2. The blood–brain barrier in children is immature during fetal development, contributing to greater accumulation in the developing brain.
3. Infant absorption of lead is greater than that in adults. In adults, the body burden of lead is found in bone. In children, growth results in a rapid turnover in skeletal bone causing a continuous leaching of lead into blood.[13,14] In cases of compromised nutrition, where dietary intake of iron and calcium is insufficient, children are more likely to have elevated blood lead levels.[13]

Elevated blood lead levels in children are linked to cognitive deficits and behavioral changes, including antisocial behavior, acting out in school, and attention deficits.[13] These deficits can persist even after the individuals are no longer exposed to lead within their environment. Lead interferes with the normal remodeling of cartilage and bone in children (remodeling increases lead reintroduction). Radiologic studies often reveal *lead lines* in children. Lead accumulates in gums, causing hyperpigmentation. Particularly worrisome is lead exposure during pregnancy because the developing fetal nervous system is especially vulnerable to lead toxicity. Lead exposure in utero can result in significant cognitive impairment and subsequent learning disabilities. Main methods of treatment are removal of the source of exposure and for those with high blood lead levels, chelation therapy. Additional treatment may include correcting deficiencies for iron, calcium, and zinc; irrigating the bowel; removing strategic bullets or shrapnel; and medications for seizures.

Cadmium and arsenic. See Table 4.7 for a summary of the toxic effects of cadmium and arsenic.

Mercury. Mercury (quicksilver) is a neurotoxic elemental metal liquid at room temperature and widely present in the environment. Mercury is a global threat to human and environmental health. It can be released into the air, water, and soil through industrial processes, including mining, metal and cement production, fuel extraction, and combustions of fossil fuels. Sources of exposure include natural geologic sources, vehicle emissions, consumer products, industrial waste, and landfills and disposal sites. Mercury also is found in dental amalgam; some vaccine preservatives; food products (e.g., rice); and terrestrial

TABLE 4.6   Social or Street Drugs and Their Effects

Type of Drug	Description and Effects
Marijuana (pot)	*Active substance:* Δ9-Tetrahydrocannabinol (THC), found in resin of *Cannabis sativa* plant. With smoking (e.g., "joints"), about 5%–10% is absorbed through lungs; with heavy use, the following adverse effects have been reported: alterations of sensory perception; impairment of cognitive and psychomotor judgments (e.g., inability to judge time, speed, distance); increases in heart rate and blood pressure; increases susceptibility to laryngitis, pharyngitis, bronchitis; causes cough and hoarseness; may contribute to lung cancer (dosages levels not determined); contains large number of carcinogens; data from animal studies only indicate reproductive changes include reduced fertility, decreased sperm motility, and decreased levels of circulatory testosterone; fetal abnormalities include low birth weight; increased frequency of infectious illness is thought to be result of depressed cell-mediated and humoral immunity; beneficial effects include decreased nausea secondary to cancer chemotherapy and decreased pain in certain chronic conditions.
Methamphetamine ("meth")	An amine derivation of amphetamine ($C_{10}H_{15}N$) used as crystalline hydrochloride CNS stimulant; in large doses causes irritability, aggressive (violent) behavior, anxiety, excitement, auditory hallucinations, and paranoia (delusions and psychosis); mood changes are common and abuser can swiftly change from being friendly to being hostile; paranoiac swings can result in suspiciousness, hyperactive behavior, and dramatic mood swings. Appeals to abusers because body's metabolism is increased and produces euphoria, alertness, and perception of increased energy Stages: *Low intensity:* User is not psychologically addicted and uses methamphetamine by swallowing or snorting. *Binge and high intensity:* User has psychological addiction and smokes or injects to achieve a faster, stronger high. *Tweaking:* Most dangerous stage; user is continually under the influence, not sleeping for 3–15 days, extremely irritated, and paranoid.
Cocaine and crack	Extracted from leaves of cocoa plant and sold as a water-soluble powder (cocaine hydrochloride) liberally diluted with talcum powder or other white powders; extraction of pure alkaloid from cocaine hydrochloride is "free-base" called *crack* because it "cracks" when heated. Crack is more potent than cocaine; cocaine is widely used as an anesthetic, usually in procedures involving oral cavity; it is a potent CNS stimulant, blocking reuptake of neurotransmitters norepinephrine, dopamine, and serotonin; also increases synthesis of norepinephrine and dopamine; dopamine induces sense of euphoria, and norepinephrine causes adrenergic potentiation, including hypertension, tachycardia, and vasoconstriction; cocaine can therefore cause severe coronary artery narrowing and ischemia; reason cocaine increases thrombus formation is unclear; other cardiovascular effects include dysrhythmias, sudden death, dilated cardiomyopathy, rupture of descending aorta (i.e., secondary to hypertension); effects on fetus include premature labor, retarded fetal development, stillbirth, hyperirritability.
Heroin	Opiate closely related to morphine, methadone, and codeine Highly addictive, and withdrawal causes intense fear ("I'll die without it"); sold "cut" with similar-looking white powder; dissolved in water it is often highly contaminated; feeling of tranquility and sedation lasts only a few hours and thus encourages repeated intravenous or subcutaneous injections; acts on the receptors enkephalins, endorphins, and dynorphins, which are widely distributed throughout body with high affinity to CNS; effects can include infectious complications, especially *Staphylococcus aureus* infections, granulomas of lung, septic embolism, and pulmonary edema—in addition, viral infections from casual exchange of needles and HIV; sudden death is related to overdosing secondary to respiratory depression, decreased cardiac output, and severe pulmonary edema.
Fentanyl	Synthetic opioid analgesic similar to morphine but is 50-100 times more potent. The synthetic opioid fentanyl and its analogs have risen across the United States in a variety of forms. Currently, it is documented in connection with a growing number of overdoses and overdose deaths.

CNS, Central nervous system; *HIV,* human immunodeficiency virus.
Data from Kumar V, Abbas A, Aster J: *Robbins and Cotran pathologic basis of disease,* ed 9, Philadelphia, 2015, Saunders; Nahas G et al: Review of marihuana and medicine, *N Engl J Med* 343(7):514, 2000.

and marine animals, some of which are consumed by humans. The previously common practice of allowing school children to handle mercury in chemistry classes is no longer permitted. Similarly, the once ubiquitous mercury-filled household thermometer is being phased out of production. There is debate among experts as to exactly how much direct mercury ingestion from the food supply or environmental vapor inhalation results in health hazards to humans or animals. There is little debate, however, concerning the hazards of mercury exposure during pregnancy. Mercury negatively impacts fetal brain development, so pregnant women are well advised to avoid dietary sources of mercury. Climate change and thawing of enormous areas of frozen lands may release long-stored mercury into lakes, rivers, and oceans.[15]

Ethanol. Alcohol (ethanol) is the primary choice of mood-altering drugs available in the United States. It is estimated there are more than 10 million chronic alcoholics in the United States. Alcohol contributes to more than 100,000 deaths annually, with 50% of these deaths resulting from drunk driving accidents, alcohol-related homicides, and suicides.[2] A blood concentration of 80 mg/dL is the legal definition for driving while intoxicated in the United States. The amount of alcohol intake required to achieve this blood level will vary, depending on age, sex, percent body fat, metabolic rate, and genetically controlled factors influencing alcohol metabolism.

A large intake of alcohol has implications for nutritional status. Major nutritional deficiencies associated with alcohol abuse include those of magnesium, vitamin B_6, thiamine, folic acid, and phosphorus. Folic acid deficiency, in particular, is problematic in persons consuming large quantities of alcohol. Ethanol alters folic acid (folate) homeostasis by decreasing intestinal absorption of folate, increasing liver retention of folate, and increasing the loss of folate through urinary and fecal excretion. Folic acid deficiency becomes especially serious when alcohol is consumed during pregnancy and may contribute to *fetal alcohol*

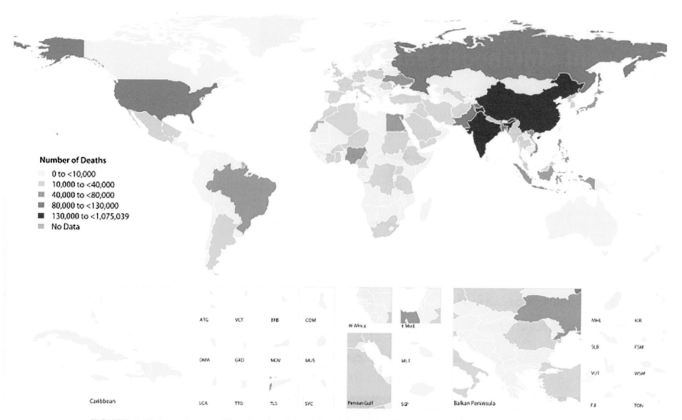

FIGURE 4.15 Numbers of Deaths Attributable to Ambient PM$_{2.5}$. (From GDB 2016 Risk Factors Collaborators: Global, regional, and national comparative risk assessment of 84 behavioural, environmental and occupational, and metabolic risks or clusters of risks, 1990–2016: a systematic analysis for the Global Burden of Disease Study 2016, *Lancet* 390(10100):1345–1422, 2017. Available at: https://www.ncbi.nlm.nih.gov/pubmed/28919119.

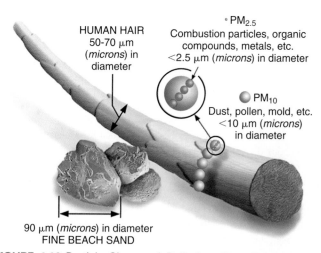

FIGURE 4.16 Particle Sizes and Pollution. (From Environmental Protection Agency: *Particulate matter updated March 18, 2013*, Washington, DC, 2013, Author.)

syndrome. Thiamine deficiencies result in major neurologic sequela, common in persons with alcohol abuse.

Most of the alcohol ingested is metabolized to *acetaldehyde* in the liver. Acetaldehyde is a highly toxic substance and known carcinogen, with particular implications for head and neck cancer. It is responsible for both the acute effects of alcohol ingestion and for numerous disease processes associated with chronic alcohol consumption.

The major effects of acute alcoholism involve the central nervous system (CNS). After alcohol is ingested, it is absorbed, unaltered, from the stomach and small intestine. Fatty foods and milk slow absorption. After absorption, alcohol is distributed to all body tissues and fluids in direct proportion to blood concentration levels. Individuals differ widely in their capability to metabolize alcohol. Genetic differences in the hepatic metabolism of alcohol are related to levels of hepatic aldehyde dehydrogenases. There is considerable variability in alcohol tolerance among different ethnic groups. Persons with chronic alcoholism tend to develop an increased tolerance because of the enhanced production of metabolic enzymes.

Numerous studies have validated the so-called *J-curve* or *U-shaped* inverse association between alcohol and overall or cardiovascular mortality, including myocardial infarction and ischemic stroke. Both irregular and chronic heavy drinking has a detrimental impact on most cardiovascular diseases. Among light to moderate drinkers, in the absence of binge drinking, mortality rates tend to be lower than in nondrinkers;

Prevent Childhood Lead Poisoning

Exposure to lead can seriously harm a child's health.

Damage to the brain and nervous system

Slowed growth and development

Learning and behavior problems

Hearing and speech problems

This can cause:

- **Lower IQ**

- **Decreased ability to pay attention**

- **Underperformance at school**

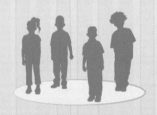

Lead can be found throughout a child's environment.

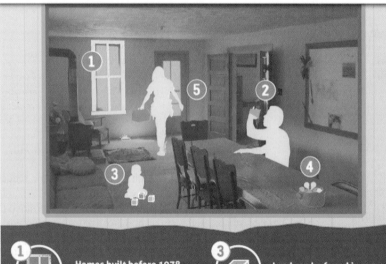

 1 Homes built before 1978 (when lead-based paints were banned) probably contain lead-based paint.

When the paint peels and cracks, it makes lead dust. Children can be poisoned when they swallow or breathe in lead dust.

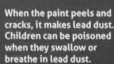 **2** Certain water pipes may contain lead.

 3 Lead can be found in some products such as toys and toy jewelry.

 4 Lead is sometimes in candies imported from other countries or traditional home remedies.

 5 Certain jobs and hobbies involve working with lead-based products, like stain glass work, and may cause parents to bring lead into the home.

In 2012, the Centers for Disease Control and Prevention (CDC) updated recommendations on children's blood lead levels. The shift is to focus on primary prevention of lead exposure to reduce or eliminate dangerous and toxic sources in children's environments. At least 4 million households have children living in houses where they are being exposed to high levels of lead. Experts now use a reference level of 5 micrograms per deciliter (mcg/dL) to identify children with blood lead levels that are much higher than most children's levels. (This new level is based on the US population of children ages 1 to 5 years who are in the highest percentile [2.5% of children] when tested for lead.) The CDC will update the reference value every 4 years using the most recent National Health and Nutrition Examination Survey (NHANES) based on the 97.5th percentile of blood lead distribution in children.

The recommendation for when medical treatment is advised for children with high blood lead levels has not changed. Chelation therapy is recommended in a child with blood lead test result showing ≥ 45 mcg/dL.

Data from Centers for Disease Control and Prevention (CDC): *Lead,* Atlanta, GA, 2017, Centers for Disease Control and Prevention, U.S. Department of Health and Human Services, updated February 9, 2017; Centers for Disease Control and Prevention (CDC): *Lead: what do parent's need to know to protect their children?* Atlanta, GA, Author, updated March 15, 2016.

TABLE 4.7   Summary of Toxic Effects of Cadmium and Arsenic

Metals	Key Concepts
Arsenic	Arsenic salts were the poison of choice during the Renaissance in Italy.
	Deliberate poisoning by arsenic is rare today; however, its exposure is an important health concern in many areas worldwide.
	Arsenic is found naturally in soils and water and used in products (wood preservers, herbicides, agricultural products).
	It can be released from mines and smelting industries and may be present in some Chinese and Indian herbal medicines.
	Inorganic arsenic may be present in ground water with large concentrations found in Bangladesh, Chile, and China.
	Most toxic forms are the trivalent compounds arsenic trioxide, sodium arsenite, and arsenic trichloride.
	Arsenic trioxide is used as a therapy for acute promyelocytic leukemia; ingestion of large quantities of arsenic causes acute gastrointestinal, cardiovascular, and CNS toxicities that often are fatal.
	These effects are partially attributed to replacement of phosphates in ATP and interference of mitochondrial oxidative phosphorylation and the function of some proteins.
	Chronic exposure causes skin lesions (hyperpigmentation, hyperkeratosis) and the development of cancers (lung, bladder, skin).
	The mechanism for arsenic carcinogenesis has not been fully defined.
	Arsenic present in drinking water has been correlated with nonmalignant respiratory disease.
Cadmium	Compared with the other metals discussed, cadmium poisoning is a more modern problem.
	Pollution in the environment and occupationally is from mining, electroplating, and production of nickel-cadmium batteries, which are often disposed of in household waste.
	Food is an important source of cadmium because cadmium can contaminate soil and plants directly or from fertilizers and irrigation water.
	The most probable mechanism of toxicity is the generation of ROS.
	The main toxic effects of excess cadmium is obstructive lung disease and renal tubular damage.
	It also can cause skeletal abnormalities associated with calcium loss.
	In Japan, cadmium-containing water used to irrigate rice fields caused a disease in postmenopausal women known as "Itai-Itai" (ouch-ouch), a combination of osteoporosis and osteomalacia associated with renal disease.
	Cadmium is associated with higher risk of lung cancer in populations living near zinc smelters.

ATP, adenosine triphosphate; *CNS,* central nervous system; *ROS,* reactive oxygen species.
Data from Kumar V, Abbas A, Aster J, editors: *Robbins & Cotran pathologic basis of disease,* ed 9, Philadelphia, 2015, Saunders.

mortality rates are higher among heavy drinkers. These findings, however, may be confounded by medical care and social relationships. Experts hold that further research is indicated. They also recommend that people who do not consume alcohol should not be encouraged to start drinking for purposes of health maintenance.

The proposed mechanisms for observed cardiovascular benefit includes one or more of the following effects: increased levels of high-density lipoprotein–cholesterol (HDL-C), decrease in levels of low-density lipoprotein (LDL), prevention of clot formation, reduction in platelet aggregation, decrease in blood pressure, increase in coronary vessel vasodilation, increase in coronary blood flow, decrease in coronary inflammation, decrease in atherosclerosis, limited ischemia–reperfusion injury, and decreased diabetic vessel pathology. The American Heart Association recommends no more than two drinks per day for men and no more than one drink per day for women. One drink is defined as 12 oz beer, 4 oz of wine, 1.5 oz of 80-proof spirits, or 1 oz of 100-proof spirits. Consuming alcohol in greater than recommended amounts is associated with numerous health hazards, including increased risk for alcoholism, high blood pressure, obesity, stroke, breast cancer, suicide, and accidents.

Acute alcohol intoxication (drunkenness) primarily affects the CNS, causing dose-related CNS depression. Alcohol consumption induces varying levels of sedation, drowsiness, loss of motor coordination, delirium, altered behavior, and loss of consciousness. Toxic blood levels (300–400 mg/dL) result in a lethal coma or respiratory arrest caused by medullary center depression. Additionally, acute alcoholism may induce reversible hepatic and gastric changes.[1].

Binge drinking, defined as four standard alcoholic drinks on one occasion for women and five drinks for men, has significant health hazards. Chronic drinking and binge drinking cause alcoholic liver disease (ALD) with the spectrum ranging from *hepatic steatosis* (fatty change) and *steatohepatitis* (fatty and inflammatory changes) to cirrhosis of the liver. These alterations can lead to hepatocellular carcinoma. Alcohol can induce damage to mitochondrial DNA, lipid accumulation, and oxidative stress. Additionally, there is evidence that alcohol drinking in adolescents, especially binge drinking, can result in neurocognitive changes affecting both gray and white brain matter and may result in risk-taking behaviors.

Chronic alcoholism causes structural alterations in practically all organs and tissues in the body. The most significant changes, however, occur in the liver. Alcohol is the leading cause of liver-related morbidity and mortality.[16] Hepatic changes, initiated by acetaldehyde, are far reaching and include inflammation, fat deposition, and liver enlargement. On the cellular level, changes include protein transport malfunctions, increased intracellular water, decreased mitochondrial fatty acid oxidation, excessive membrane rigidity, and liver cell necrosis. Chronic, excessive alcohol consumption typically results in cirrhosis of the liver and the associated portal hypertension (Fig. 4.17). Other disorders associated with chronic alcoholism include alcoholic cardiomyopathy; increased risk of hypertension, gastritis, and pancreatitis; regressive changes in skeletal muscle; and an increased risk for oral, liver, esophageal and breast cancer. Ethanol is implicated in the onset of a variety of immune defects, including cytokine production, inflammation, increased susceptibility to infection, and enhanced progression of human immunodeficiency disease.[17]

Alcohol ingestion during pregnancy is associated with *cognitive deficiencies* and *neurobehavioral disorders,* including fetal alcohol syndrome (FAS). Fetal alcohol spectrum disorders (FASDs) are a range of health effects or disorders of prenatal alcohol exposure with FAS at the more severe end of the spectrum. FAS syndrome is characterized by growth retardation, facial anomalies, cognitive impairment, and ocular malformations (Fig. 4.18). Research suggests that alcohol-induced

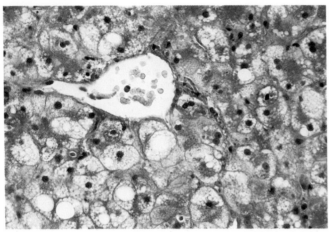

FIGURE 4.17 Alcoholic Hepatitis. Chicken-wire fibrosis extending between hepatocytes (Mallory trichrome stain). (From Damjanov I, Linder J, editors: *Anderson's pathology*, ed 10, St Louis, 1996, Mosby.)

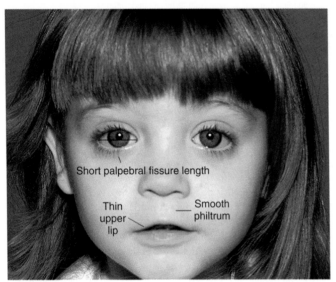

Short palpebral fissure length

Thin upper lip

Smooth philtrum

FIGURE 4.18 Diagnostic Facial Features of Fetal Alcohol Syndrome (FAS). Three diagnostic facial features of FAS: (1) short palpebral fissure lengths, (2) smooth philtrum, and (3) thin upper lip. (© 2017 Susan Astley, PhD, University of Washington.)

epigenetic alterations may be carried through the male germline for multiple generations.[18] Alcohol readily crosses the placenta, reaching the fetus in 1 to 2 hours, and produces fetal blood levels that are equivalent to maternal alcohol levels.[19] Amniotic fluid acts as a reservoir for alcohol, prolonging fetal exposure.[19] Overall, maternal ingestion of alcohol can be catastrophic for the developing fetus.

✔ QUICK CHECK 4.2

1. Why are children more susceptible to the toxic effects of lead exposure?
2. Discuss the nutritional implications of chronic alcoholism.
3. Discuss the mechanisms of cell injury related to chronic alcoholism.
4. What are the sources of mercury exposure?
5. Why has air pollution become a leading cause of morbidity and mortality?

Social or Street Drugs

The social or recreational use of psychoactive and narcotic drugs is a major problem in many parts of the world. Popular drugs are methamphetamine ("meth"); marijuana; cocaine, heroin; and, increasingly, fentanyl. Many of these drugs have a high risk for addiction and dependence, and some can cause respiratory distress and death. Opiates both prescription and illicit are the main causes of drug overdose deaths.[20] Opiates were involved in 42,249 deaths in 2016; opiate overdose deaths were five times higher in 2016 than in 1999[20] (see Table 4.6 for a summary of the effects of these drugs).

Unintentional and Intentional Injuries

Unintentional and intentional injuries are an important health problem in the United States. In 2016, there were 231,991 injury deaths, an injury death rate of 71.8 per 100,000.[21] The number of deaths because of poisoning was 68,995, at a rate of 21.4 deaths per 100,000. Motor vehicle accident–related deaths accounted for 38,804, with a rate of 12 deaths per 100,000. Deaths caused by all firearms were 38,658, with a rate of 12 deaths per 100,000. From data reported in 2016, drug poisoning deaths occurred at a rate of 19.7 per 100,000.[21] Rates of drug overdose deaths continues to increase. The 10 drugs most frequently involved in overdose deaths included the following opioids: heroin, oxycodone, methadone, morphine, hydrocodone, and fentanyl; the following benzodiazephines: alprazolam and diazepam; and the following stimulants: cocaine and methamphetamine. The rate of drug overdose deaths involving fentanyl more than doubled in a single year (from 2013 to 2014).[22] Increases in drug overdose deaths are seen for both males and females and the largest percentage increase is for adults aged 55 to 64. Rates had a fivefold increase in this age group. Overall, 70,237 drug overdose deaths occurred in the United States in 2017. The opioid epidemic continues to worsen because of the continuing increase in deaths from synthetic opioids.[23] Death rates because of falls increased 30%.[24] Each year 3 million older people are treated in emergency departments for fall injuries. More than 95% of hip fractures are caused by falls and falls are the leading cause of traumatic brain injuries (TBI). Sexual violence affects millions of people each year in the United States. Specifically, 1 in 3 women and 1 in 4 men experience sexual violence.[25] Sports- and recreation-related injury account for an estimated 3.2 million visits to emergency rooms each year for children 5 to 14 years. Injuries from organized and unorganized sports account for 775,000 emergency room visits annually for this same age group. Sports-related injuries are the leading cause of emergency room visits in 12- to 17-year-olds.[26] Death from all injury is significantly more common among men than among women. Significant racial differences are noted in mortality rates, with mortality rate of whites at 64.85 per 100,000, that of blacks at 56.20 per 100,000, and that of other racial groups at a combined rate of 28.96 per 100,000. There also is a bimodal age distribution for injury-related deaths, with peaks in the young adult and elderly age groups.

Unintentional injury is the leading cause of death among those between ages 1 and 34 years; intentional injury (suicide, homicide) ranks between the second and fourth leading causes of death in these age groups. A 1999 report published by the Institute of Medicine (IOM) indicated that 44,000 to 98,000 unnecessary deaths per year occurred in hospitals alone as a result of errors made by health care professionals. Death and injury from medical care itself is a very important issue and a main concern is the lack of a comprehensive, nationwide system for estimating premature deaths and unintentional injury associated with preventable harm to people.[27] Subsequent data to the IOM report suggest that the magnitude of the problem may have been underestimated and that hospital-acquired infections alone explained more than 90,000 deaths per year.[28] In 2013, a review of studies estimated that the true number of premature deaths associated with preventable harm to individuals was far higher than the IOM report with an estimate of more than 400,000 per year.[29] From the Agency for Health Care Research and Quality (AHRQ) on hospital-acquired conditions approximately 75,000 preventable hospital deaths occurred in 2013.[27] Getting close to the real number is absolutely necessary to assist educators, clinicians, administrators, and boards of trustees to guarantee a culture of safety for individuals. The more common terms used to describe and classify unintentional and intentional injuries and brief descriptions of important features of these injuries are presented in Table 4.8.

Asphyxiation

Asphyxial injuries are caused by the failure of cells to receive or use oxygen. Deprivation of oxygen may be partial (*hypoxia*) or total (*anoxia*). Asphyxiation can be grouped into four general categories: *suffocation, strangulation, chemical asphyxiants,* and *drowning.*

Suffocation. Suffocation, or the process of dying as a result of lack of oxygen, can result from either a *lack of oxygen in the environment* or from a *blockage of the respiratory airways* (see Choking Asphyxiation section below). Persons can become entrapped in an enclosed space that is lacking in adequate oxygen. This scenario would occur if a child becomes trapped in an abandoned refrigerator or if a toddler's head becomes entangled in a plastic bag. Both scenarios have been linked to fatalities. Suffocation also can occur when another gas displaces oxygen in the environment. Methane, the largest component of sewer gas, has caused fatal asphyxiation when it has displaced atmospheric oxygen. Children have died from methane asphyxiation shortly after falling into a pit containing sewage; rescue workers have a very narrow time frame in which to save the child. Volcanos have been known to belch carbon dioxide (CO_2) gas in amounts sufficient to displace the normal oxygen level in the atmosphere for several miles, resulting in widespread death of humans and animals within the area. Normal ambient oxygen level in the atmosphere is 21%. A reduction to a level of 16% poses immediate danger. If the level drops below 5%, death can ensue within minutes.

TABLE 4.8 Unintentional and Intentional Injuries

Type of Injury	Description
BLUNT-FORCE INJURIES 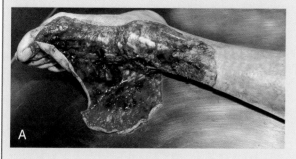 A	Mechanical injury to body resulting in tearing, shearing, or crushing; most common type of injury seen in healthcare settings; caused by blows or impacts; motor vehicle accidents and falls most common cause (see Photo A) *Contusion (bruise):* Bleeding into skin or underlying tissues; initial color will be red-purple, then blue-black, then yellow-brown or green (see Fig. 4.22); duration of bruise depends on extent, location, and degree of vascularization; bruising of soft tissue may be confined to deeper structures; *hematoma* is collection of blood in soft tissue; *subdural hematoma* is blood between inner surface of dura mater and surface of brain; can result from blows, falls, or sudden acceleration/deceleration of head as occurs in *shaken baby syndrome; epidural hematoma* is collection of blood between inner surface of skull and dura; is most often associated with a skull fracture *Laceration:* Tear or rip resulting when tensile strength of skin or tissue is exceeded; is ragged and irregular with abraded edges; an extreme example is *avulsion,* where a wide area of tissue is pulled away; lacerations of internal organs are common in blunt-force injuries; lacerations of liver, spleen, kidneys, and bowel occur from blows to abdomen; thoracic aorta may be lacerated in sudden deceleration accidents; severe blows or impacts to chest may rupture heart with lacerations of atria or ventricles *Fracture:* Blunt-force blows or impacts can cause bone to break or shatter (see Chapter 40)
SHARP-FORCE INJURIES 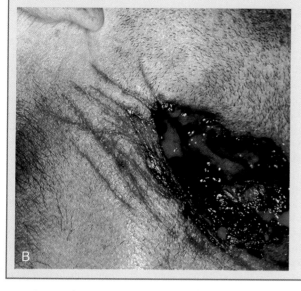 B	Cutting and piercing injuries accounted for 2734 deaths in 2007; men have a higher rate (1.37/100,000) compared with women (0.44/100,000); differences by race are as follows: whites 0.71/100,000; blacks 2.12/100,000; and other groups 0.80/100,000 *Incised wound:* A wound that is *longer* than it is *deep;* wound can be straight or jagged with sharp, distinct edges without abrasion; usually produces significant external bleeding with little internal hemorrhage; these wounds are noted in sharp-force injury suicides; in addition to a deep, lethal cut, there will be superficial incisions in same area called *hesitation marks* (see Photo B) *Stab wound:* A penetrating sharp-force injury that is *deeper* than it is *long;* if a sharp instrument is used, depths of wound are clean and distinct but can be abraded if object is inserted deeply and wider portion (e.g., hilt of a knife) impacts skin; depending on size and location of wound, external bleeding may be surprisingly small; after an initial spurt of blood, even if a major vessel or heart is struck, wound may be almost completely closed by tissue pressure, thus allowing only a trickle of visible blood despite copious internal bleeding *Puncture wound:* Instruments or objects with sharp points but without sharp edges produce puncture wounds; classic example is wound of foot after stepping on a nail; wounds are prone to infection, have abrasion of edges, and can be very deep *Chopping wound:* Heavy, edged instruments (axes, hatchets, propeller blades) produce wounds with a combination of sharp- and blunt-force characteristics

Continued

TABLE 4.8   Unintentional and Intentional Injuries—cont'd

Type of Injury	Description
GUNSHOT WOUNDS 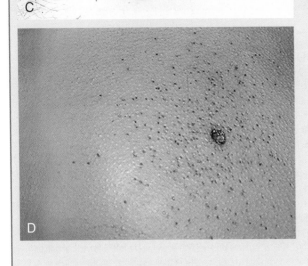	Accounted for > 33,636 deaths in the United States in 2015; men more likely to die compared with women (18.16 vs. 2.73/100,000); black men ages 15 to 24 years have greatest death rate (86.95/100,000); gunshot wounds are either penetrating (bullet remains in body) or perforating (bullet exits body); bullet also can fragment; most important factors or appearances are whether it is an entrance or exit wound and range of fire *Entrance wound:* All wounds share some common features; overall appearance is most affected by range of fire *Contact range entrance wound:* Distinctive type of wound when gun is held so muzzle rests on or presses into skin surface; there is searing of edges of wound from flame and soot or smoke on edges of wound in addition to hole; hard contact wounds of head cause severe tearing and disruption of tissue (because of thin layer of skin and muscle overlying bone); wound is gaping and jagged, known as *blow back;* can produce a patterned abrasion that mirrors weapon used (see Photo C) *Intermediate (distance) range entrance wound:* Surrounded by gunpowder tattooing or stippling; *tattooing* results from fragments of burning or unburned pieces of gunpowder exiting barrel and forcefully striking skin; *stippling* results when gunpowder abrades but does not penetrate skin (see Photo D) *Indeterminate range entrance wound:* Occurs when flame, soot, or gunpowder does not reach skin surface but bullet does; *indeterminate* is used rather than *distant* because appearance may be same regardless of distance; for example, if an individual is shot at close range through multiple layers of clothing the wound may look the same as if the shooting occurred at a distance *Exit wound:* Has the same appearance regardless of range of fire; most important factors are speed of projectile and degree of deformation; size cannot be used to determine whether hole is an exit or entrance wound; usually has clean edges that can often be reapproximated to cover defect; skin is one of toughest structures for a bullet to penetrate; thus it is not uncommon for a bullet to pass entirely through body but stopped just beneath skin on "exit" side *Wounding potential of bullets:* Most damage done by a bullet is a result of amount of energy transferred to tissue impacted; speed of bullet has much greater effect than increased size; some bullets are designed to expand or fragment when striking an object, for example, *hollow-point* ammunition; lethality of a wound depends on what structures are damaged; wounds of brain may not be lethal; however, they are usually immediately incapacitating and lead to significant long-term disability; a person with a "lethal" injury (wound of heart or aorta) also may not be immediately incapacitated

History and forensic examination are important in diagnosing suspected asphyxiation, because even autopsy may not demonstrate specific physical findings in such cases.

Choking asphyxiation occurs when there is an obstruction of the pulmonary airways. An object may become lodged in a large airway, directly obstructing breathing. Injury or disease also may result from soft tissue swelling surrounding the airway, leading to a partial or complete obstruction and subsequent asphyxiation. Treatment requires locating and removing the obstructing object immediately or, in the case of airway swelling, reversing the swelling before asphyxiation occurs. *Compressional asphyxiation* occurs when mechanical compression of the chest or abdomen prevents normal respiratory movements. Usual signs and symptoms include florid facial congestion and *petechiae* (pinpoint hemorrhages) of the eyes and face. An individual entrapped beneath a heavy object, which impairs chest expansion, may become asphyxiated.

Strangulation. Strangulation is caused by compression of the blood vessels and air passages resulting from external pressure on the neck. The compression causes hypoxia from impaired blood flow to the brain. The amount of force needed to compress the jugular veins (2 kg) or carotid arteries (5 kg) is significantly less than the force required to crush the trachea (15 kg). Injury or death, which occurs secondary to strangulation results from the impaired cerebral blood flow, not from lack of airflow. With a complete blockage of the carotid arteries, unconsciousness will typically occur within 10 to 15 seconds.

Hanging strangulation occurs when a noose or similar object is placed around the neck after which the support under the victim's feet is suddenly removed so that the body falls freely. Death or severe injury results as the noose tightens, cutting off air flow through the trachea. Hanging strangulation is usually an intentional event, such as suicide, homicide, or a judicial hanging. However it can also be accidental. This form of strangulation typically produces severe soft tissue injury and cervical spinal trauma. The body does not need to be completely suspended for death to occur. Hanging may cause petechiae in the eyes or face; however this finding is uncommon. More typically, an inverted V–shaped ligature mark about the neck is seen at autopsy.

Ligature strangulation does not require suspension. Instead some form of cord encircles and tightens about the neck. This event may be intentional, as in the case of homicide with use of a garrote from behind the victim. It also may be accidental, as when a child becomes accidentally entangled in cords of window blinds. Autopsy will reveal a horizontal mark about the neck, without an inverted V pattern. Petechiae are more common in this scenario because intermittent opening and closure of the blood vessels may occur as a result of the victim's struggle. Internal injuries of the neck are rare.

Manual strangulation occurs when an assailant's hands compress the neck of the victim to the point where death by asphyxiation occurs. There is evidence of variable amounts of external trauma to the neck. Contusions and abrasions are either caused directly by the assailant or by the victim clawing at their own neck in an attempt to remove the assailant's hands. Internal damage can be quite severe; bruising of deep structures, including fractures of the hyoid bone, the tracheal cartilage, and the cricoid cartilages, are seen. Petechiae are common.

Chemical asphyxiants. A number of substances can act as **chemical asphyxiants.** They either prevent the delivery of oxygen to the tissues or block oxygen utilization. Carbon monoxide is the most common chemical asphyxiant. **Carbon monoxide (CO)** is an odorless, colorless, nonirritating, and undetectable gas; it is often mixed with a visible or odorous compound. CO is produced by incomplete combustion of fuels, such as gasoline. CO produces hypoxic injury, specifically, oxygen deprivation. As a systemic asphyxiant, CO causes death by inducing CNS depression. Normally, oxygen molecules are carried to tissues bound to the hemoglobin in RBCs. Because the affinity of CO for hemoglobin is 300 times greater than that of oxygen, CO quickly binds with hemoglobin, preventing oxygen molecules from binding to hemoglobin, and they are thus transported to tissues. Minute amounts of CO can produce a significant percentage of *carboxyhemoglobin* (carbon monoxide bound with hemoglobin). With increasing levels of carboxyhemoglobin, hypoxia occurs insidiously, evoking widespread ischemic changes in the CNS. Individuals are often unaware of exposure. Death may occur in an individual who believes he is simply feeling sleepy, thus no evasive action is taken. The use of CO monitors in homes is therefore strongly recommended. Diagnosis can be made from the measurement of carboxyhemoglobin levels in blood. Victims of CO poisoning may have a cherry red coloration to the skin and mucous membranes.

Symptoms related to CO poisoning include headache, giddiness, tinnitus (ringing in the ears), chest pain, confusion, nausea, weakness, and vomiting. CO is an environmental air pollutant found in combustion fumes produced by cars and trucks, small gasoline engines, stoves, gas ranges, gas refrigerators, heating systems, lanterns, burning charcoal or wood, and cigarette smoke. Chronic exposure can occur in people working in confined spaces, such as underground garages and tunnels. Fumes can accumulate in enclosed or semi-enclosed spaces. Individuals most susceptible to CO poisoning are fetuses, infants, and people with chronic heart disease, respiratory problems, and anemia.

Cyanide is an extremely toxic salt. Cyanide acts as an asphyxiant by combining with the ferric (iron) ion in hemoglobin, facilitating its transport to tissues. When present in tissues, cyanide inhibits the formation of cytochrome oxidase by interrupting the electron transport chain within the mitochondria. As a result, the mitochondria can no longer aerobically generate ATP, and oxygen can no longer bind to the final molecule in the electron transport chain. The host dies from oxygen deprivation, even though abundant oxygen may be present. As with CO poisoning, victims of cyanide poisoning may have a cherry red coloration to the skin and mucus membranes. With the presence of cyanide, an odor of bitter almonds may be detected; however the ability to smell cyanide is a genetic trait that is present in only 20% to 40% of the general population.

Hydrogen sulfide, one of several sewer gases, is a chemical asphyxiant and neurotoxin; it interferes with the body's ability to carry oxygen. It has a characteristic "rotten egg" odor that is detectable even at very low levels. Victims of hydrogen sulfide poisoning may have brown-tinged blood, in addition to the nonspecific signs of asphyxiation. **Methane,** another sewer gas, is nontoxic but readily causes asphyxiation by displacing oxygen. Because of the presence of asphyxiant gases, caution is indicated when working in areas containing septic tanks, cesspools, and manure pits. Numerous fatalities have occurred in persons working in these environments.

Drowning. **Drowning** is death from inhalation of and suffocation by a liquid, usually water. The CDC has reported that between 2005 and 2014, an average of 3536 fatal, unintentional drownings occurred annually. The major mechanism of injury is hypoxemia (low blood oxygen levels). Contrary to previous prevailing views, there is no evidence that drowning deaths result from fluid and electrolyte disturbances or from blood hemolysis. In freshwater drownings, large amounts of water can pass through the alveolar–capillary interface. Even in this setting, there is no evidence that an increase in blood volume results in either hemolysis or electrolyte derangements. With drowning, airway obstruction is the more important consideration because in as many as 15% of drownings, little or no water enters the lungs. Vagal-mediated laryngospasms may close off the airway producing a phenomenon known as **dry-lung drowning.**

Regardless of the mechanism, cerebral hypoxia leads to unconsciousness in a matter of minutes. Whether this status progresses to death depends on a number of factors, including the age and the health of the individual. One of the most important determinants is water temperature. Irreversible injury develops much more rapidly in warm water than in cold water. Survival after up to 1 hour has been reported in children who were submerged in very cold water. Complete submersion is not enough to cause drowning. An incapacitated or helpless individual (e.g., persons with epilepsy or alcoholism, infants) may drown in water that is only a few inches deep.

No specific or diagnostic findings *prove* that a person, recovered from the water, is actually a drowning victim. In cases where water has entered the lung, there may be large amounts of foam exiting the nose and mouth. This same phenomenon, however, could occur with other causes of death, including drug overdoses. A body recovered from water could have been that of a victim of some other type of fatal injury. Drowning may represent an effort to obscure the actual cause of death. When treating a living victim recovered from water, it is essential to keep an index of suspicion for any underlying condition that may have predisposed the person to become incapacitated, causing him or her to fall into the water.

✔ **QUICK CHECK 4.3**
1. Give examples of intentional and unintentional asphyxia cases in the United States.
2. What are common chemical asphyxiants, and why are they lethal?
3. How does CO cause death?
4. What is the major mechanism of injury with drowning?

Infectious Injury

The pathogenicity (virulence) of microorganisms lies in their ability to survive and proliferate within the host. The disease-producing potential of a microorganism is a function of its ability to (1) invade and destroy cells, (2) produce toxins, and (3) produce damaging hypersensitivity reactions. (Chapter 8 contains a description of infection and infectious microorganisms.)

Immunologic and Inflammatory Injury

Cellular membranes are injured as a result of direct contact with immune or inflammatory-mediated responses, such as phagocytes (lymphocytes and monocytes) and biochemical substances generated during an inflammatory response. Potentially injurious biochemical agents include histamine, antibodies, lymphokines, complement system products, and proteases (see Chapter 6). A variety of mechanisms for potential cellular injury exist. The complement system is responsible for several membrane alterations associated with immunologic injury. Membrane alterations can facilitate a rapid leakage of potassium out of the cell, along with an influx of water. Antibodies can bind and occupying receptor molecules located on the plasma membrane, interfering with its function. Antibodies also can block or destroy cellular junctions, obstructing intercellular communication. Other mechanisms include genetic and epigenetic factors, nutritional imbalances, and physical agents. These are summarized in Table 4.9.

MANIFESTATIONS OF CELLULAR INJURY

Cellular Manifestations: Accumulations

Metabolic disturbances can result from cell injury, particularly where there is excessive intracellular accumulation of biochemical substances. Cellular accumulations, also known as infiltrations, can occur with both sustained cell injury and with normal but inefficient cell function. Two categories of substances can produce infiltrations:

1. *Normal cellular substances*—excess water, proteins, lipids, and carbohydrates
2. *Abnormal substances*—including *endogenous* substances (products of abnormal metabolism and synthesis) and *exogenous* substances (infectious agents or minerals)

Products can accumulate transiently or permanently, and can be toxic or harmless. Infiltrations may occur in the cytoplasm, typically within the lysosomes, and they also can occur in the nucleus. Most accumulations

TABLE 4.9	**Mechanisms of Cellular Injury**	
Mechanism	**Characteristics**	**Examples**
Genetic factors	Alter cell's nucleus and plasma membrane's structure, shape, receptors, or transport mechanisms	Sickle cell anemia, Huntington disease, muscular dystrophy, abetalipoproteinemia, familial hypercholesterolemia
Epigenetic factors	Induction of mitotically heritable alterations in gene expression without changing DNA	Gene silencing in cancer
Nutritional imbalances	Pathophysiologic cellular effects develop when nutrients are not consumed in diet and transported to body's cells *or* when excessive amounts of nutrients are consumed and transported	Protein deficiency, protein-calorie malnutrition, glucose deficiency, lipid deficiency (hypolipidemia), hyperlipidemia (increased lipoproteins in blood causing deposits of fat in heart, liver, and muscle), vitamin deficiencies
Physical Agents		
Temperature extremes	*Hypothermic injury* results from chilling or freezing of cells, creating high intracellular sodium concentrations; abrupt drops in temperature lead to vasoconstriction and increased viscosity of blood, causing ischemic injury, infarction, and necrosis; reactive oxygen species (ROS) are important in this process	Frostbite
	Hyperthermic injury is caused by excessive heat and varies in severity according to nature, intensity, and extent of heat	Burns, burn blisters, heat cramps usually from vigorous exercise with water and salt loss; heat exhaustion with salt and water loss causes heme contraction; heat stroke is life-threatening with a clinical rectal temperature of 106° F
	Tissue injury caused by compressive waves of air or fluid impinging on body, followed by sudden wave of decreased pressure; changes may collapse thorax, rupture internal solid organs, and cause widespread hemorrhage: carbon dioxide and nitrogen that are normally dissolved in blood precipitate from solution and form small bubbles (gas emboli), causing hypoxic injury and pain	Blast injury (air or immersion), decompression sickness (caisson disease or "the bends"); recently reported in a few individuals with subdural hematomas after riding high-speed roller coasters
Ionizing radiation	Refers to any form of radiation that can remove orbital electrons from atoms; source is usually environment and medical use; damage is to DNA molecule, causing chromosomal aberrations, chromosomal instability, and damage to membranes and enzymes; also induces growth factors and extracellular matrix remodeling; uncertainty exists regarding effects of low levels of radiation	X-rays, γ-rays, and α- and β-particles cause skin redness, skin damage, chromosomal damage, cancer
Illumination	Fluorescent lighting and halogen lamps create harmful oxidative stresses; ultraviolet light has been linked to skin cancer	Eyestrain, obscured vision, cataracts, headaches, melanoma
Mechanical stresses	Injury is caused by physical impact or irritation; they may be overt or cumulative	Faulty occupational biomechanics, leading to overexertion disorders
Noise	Can be caused by acute loud noise or cumulative effects of various intensities, frequencies, and duration of noise; considered a public health threat	Hearing impairment or loss; tinnitus, temporary threshold shift (TTS), or loss can occur as a complication of critical illness, from mechanical trauma, ototoxic medications, infections, vascular disorders, and noise

result from four types of mechanisms, all of which are abnormal (Fig. 4.19). The four mechanisms are:

1. Insufficient removal of the normal substance because of altered configuration or transport. Example: *steatosis*, fatty changes in the liver.
2. Accumulation of abnormal substance because of defects in protein folding, transport, or abnormal degradation. Such occurrences are usually secondary to gene mutation.
3. Inadequate metabolism of an endogenous (physiologic) substance, usually because of a lack of a lysosomal enzyme. Example: *storage diseases.*
4. Harmful exogenous materials. Example: heavy metals and mineral dust inhalation and ingestion or the presence of pathogenic microorganisms.

In all storage diseases, the cells attempt to digest, or catabolize, the "stored" substances resulting in excessive amounts of metabolites accumulating within the cells. These metabolites are expelled into the ECM where they are attacked by phagocytic cells, usually macrophages (see Chapter 6). Some of these scavenger cells circulate throughout the body; others remain fixed in tissues, particularly in liver or spleen tissue. Affected tissues swell resulting in organ enlargement as increasing numbers of phagocytes migrate to tissues. Hepatomegaly or splenomegaly occurs in many storage diseases.

Water

Cellular swelling is the most common degenerative change; it results from a shift of extracellular water into the cells. In hypoxic injury, the movement of fluid and ions into the cell is associated with acute metabolic failure and the loss of ATP production. The energy-dependent sodium pump, which transports sodium ions out of the cell, requires ATP. Adenosine triphosphatase (ATPase) is the active transport enzyme; it is reduced with hypoxia. Inadequate levels of ATP and ATPase permit sodium to accumulate within the cell while potassium diffuses outward. Increased intracellular sodium concentration raises osmotic pressure, drawing yet more water into the cell. The cisternae of the ER become distended and are predisposed to rupture. Once ruptured, the cisternae reunite, forming large vacuoles that isolate water, a process called *vacu-olation*. Progressive vacuolation results in cytoplasmic swelling, termed oncosis (*hydropic degeneration*) or vacuolar degeneration (Fig. 4.20). Where cellular swelling affects the majority of cells within an organ, the affected organ becomes expanded; the weight of the organ increases and it takes on a pale appearance.

Cellular swelling is reversible or sublethal. It is an early manifestation of almost all types of cellular injury, including injuries that are severe or lethal. Cellular swelling is associated with high fever, hypokalemia (decreased blood potassium), and certain infections.

Lipids and Carbohydrates

Certain metabolic disorders result in an abnormal intracellular accumulation of carbohydrates and lipids. These substances may accumulate throughout the body, but they are found primarily in the spleen, liver, and CNS. Accumulations within CNS cells are associated with neurologic deficits and severe intellectual impairment. Lipids accumulate in Tay-Sachs disease, Niemann-Pick disease, and Gaucher disease. When carbohydrates accumulate, mucopolysaccharide diseases (mucopolysaccharidoses) result. Mucopolysaccharidoses are progressive disorders, typically affecting multiple organs and, particularly, the liver, spleen, heart, and blood vessels. Mucopolysaccharides accumulate at a variety of sites throughout the body: reticuloendothelial cells, endothelial cells, intimal smooth muscle cells, and fibroblasts. Carbohydrate accumulations are associated with cataracts (corneal clouding), joint stiffness,

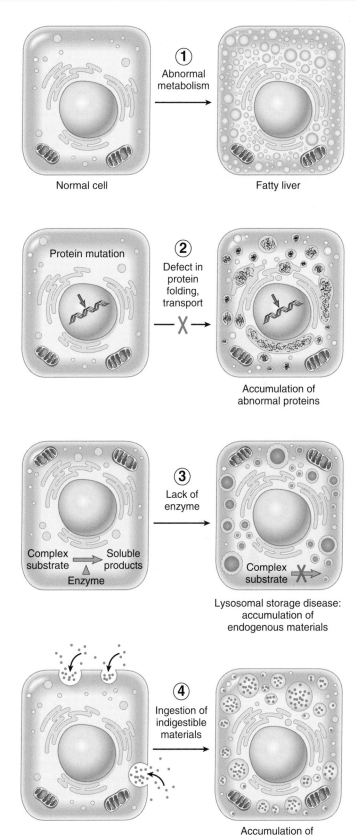

FIGURE 4.19 Mechanisms of Intracellular Accumulations. (From Kumar V et al, editors: *Robbins and Cotran pathologic basis of disease,* ed 9, Philadelphia, 2015, Elsevier.)

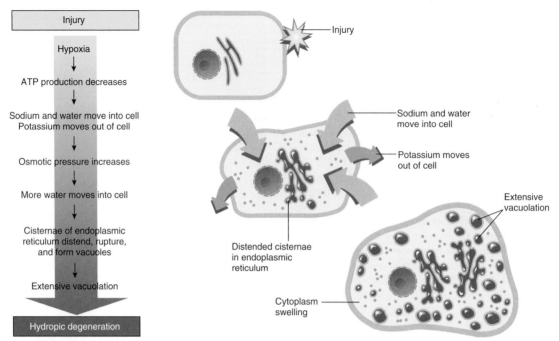

FIGURE 4.20 The Process of Oncosis (Formerly Referred to as "Hydropic Degeneration"). *ATP,* Adenosine triphosphate.

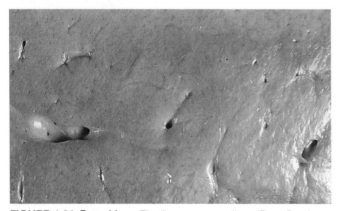

FIGURE 4.21 Fatty Liver. The liver appears yellow. (From Damjanov I, Linder J: *Pathology: a color atlas,* St Louis, 2000, Mosby.)

intellectual deficits, and the characteristic eye changes seen in Graves disease (hyperthyroidism).

The most common site of intracellular lipid accumulation is the liver where **steatosis** or fatty changes of the liver occur (Fig. 4.21). Other sites include heart, muscle, and kidney cells. Lipid accumulation in the liver results in deficits to hepatic functioning. As lipids accumulate in the cells, increased vacuolation pushes the nucleus and other organelles aside. The outward appearance of the liver becomes yellow and greasy. In developed countries, the most common cause of fatty changes to the liver is alcohol abuse. Other causes include diabetes mellitus, protein malnutrition, toxins, anoxia, and obesity. Mechanisms for lipid accumulation in the liver include the following:

1. Increased movement of free fatty acids into the liver (for example, starvation increases triglyceride metabolism in adipose tissue and fatty acids are released and enter liver cells)
2. Failure to convert fatty acids to phospholipids results in (preferential) conversion into triglycerides
3. Increased synthesis of triglycerides from fatty acids
4. Decreased synthesis of apoproteins (lipid-acceptor proteins)
5. Failure of lipids to bind with apoproteins to form lipoproteins
6. Failure of mechanisms that transport lipoproteins out of the cell
7. Direct damage to the ER by free radicals released by alcohol's toxic effects

Many pathologic states show accumulation of cholesterol and cholesterol esters. Atherosclerosis is characterized by plaques containing lipids, cholesterol, calcium, macrophages, and other substances. The coronary and carotid arteries are particularly prone to plaques. Their presence in these vessels can result in myocardial infarction and stroke. Cholesterol-rich deposits in the gallbladder commonly lead to obstruction from cholelithiasis (gall stones). Niemann-Pick disease is characterized by lipid accumulation in the spleen, liver, lungs, bone marrow, and brain, secondary to a genetic lack of sphingomyelinase, an enzyme that affects cholesterol transport.

Glycogen

Glycogen is the storage form of glucose, with 90% found in the liver. Glycogen serves as a readily available source of energy needed for normal cell function. Intracellular accumulations of glycogen are seen in a large group of genetic disorders called *glycogen storage diseases.* Accumulations also are noted disorders affecting glucose and glycogen metabolism. Glycogen storage diseases have profound detrimental effects on growth and development, and they negatively impact a variety of organ and body system functions. As with water and lipid accumulation, glycogen accumulation results in excessive vacuolation in the cytoplasm. Excess glycogen accumulation is evident in 80% of persons with diabetes. The high levels of blood glucose and excess glycogen cause a multiplicity of problems in the individual with diabetes (see Chapter 20).

Proteins

Proteins provide cellular structure and account for most of the cell's dry weight. Proteins are synthesized on ribosomes from the essential amino acids. Intracellular accumulation of excess protein damages cells in two ways. First, protein metabolism results in the release of lysosomal enzymes, which can damage cellular organelles. Second, excessive amounts of protein in the cytoplasm crowd cell organelles, disrupting their function and intracellular communication.

Protein excess accumulates primarily in two locations: in the epithelial cells of the renal convoluted tubules and in the antibody-producing B lymphocytes. A variety of renal disorders result in excessive excretion of protein molecules into urine (proteinuria). Normally, protein is conserved with little or no protein escaping into urine. Proteinuria suggests cellular injury or altered cellular function, or both. As a function of the immune response, protein complexes are elaborated as B lymphocytes (plasma cells) synthesize antibodies. Excess protein aggregates, called *Russell bodies,* have been identified in multiple myeloma, which is a cancer of the plasma cells.

A number of disease states result from mutations, which impair protein folding; partially folded intermediates accumulate within the cell. Emphysema, without a history of smoking, can result from α_1-antitrypsin deficiency, a genetic mutation that impairs protein folding. Cell injury also is associated with the accumulation of cytoskeleton proteins. The *neurofibrillary tangle* found in the brain in Alzheimer disease contains these types of proteins.

Pigments

Pigment accumulations may be normal or abnormal, endogenous (produced within the body), or exogenous (produced outside the body). Endogenous pigments, derived from amino acids (tyrosine, tryptophan), include melanin and blood proteins (porphyrins, hemoglobin, and hemosiderin). Lipofuscin, a lipid-rich pigment, known as the "aging pigment," imparts a yellow-brown color to cells, which are undergoing slow, regressive, or atrophic changes. The most common exogenous pigment is carbon black (coal dust), a pervasive air pollutant in urban areas. Inhaled carbon black interacts with lung macrophages. Lymphatics transport it to regional pulmonary lymph nodes where it accumulates. This accumulation blackens lung tissues and pulmonary nodes causing a variety of respiratory disorders. Other exogenous pigments include mineral dusts: silica, iron particles, lead, silver salts, and dyes used for tattoos.

Melanin

Melanin is a brown-black pigment derived from the amino acid *tyrosine.* Melanin is synthesized by epidermal cells called *melanocytes* and is stored in membrane-bound cytoplasmic vesicles, called *melanosomes.* It accumulates in epithelial cells (keratinocytes) of the skin and retina, where it serves to protect the tissue from the harmful effects of prolonged exposure to sunlight. Melanin is essential in the prevention of skin cancer. Persons with absent or low levels of melanin (lighter-skinned persons) are more susceptible to skin cancer (see Chapters 12 and 43). Particularly hazardous are episodes of sunburn during the early years of life because these events increase the life-long risk for developing skin cancer. Ultraviolet radiation from nonnatural sources (tanning salon lamps) also is associated with an increased risk for skin cancer. Individuals who have more darkly pigmented skin because of the presence of higher levels of melanin are proportionately less susceptible to skin cancers.

Ultraviolet light, from sunlight and other sources, stimulates the synthesis of melanin. Melanin absorbs ultraviolet rays during subsequent exposures. Melanin also may serve to trap harmful free radicals, derived by the action of ultraviolet light on skin. Melanin accounts for the brown to black coloration seen in *pigmented nevi,* benign skin moles. Melanin also is found in cancerous skin lesions, particularly *malignant melanoma,* a highly aggressive and lethal form of skin cancer. It is characterized by irregular black skin lesions, which rapidly metastasize to other organs.

Albinism is a congenital inherited disorder characterized by the complete or partial absence of melanin. These individuals are extremely predisposed to developing skin cancer because they experience sunburn upon even minimal exposure to sunlight. In humans, the disorder is inherited as either an autosomal recessive or a sex-linked recessive genetic disorder, depending on the type of albinism involved. The mechanism for albinism is a defect in tyrosinase, a copper-containing enzyme, which catalyzes the production of melanin from the amino acid tyrosine.

Hemoproteins

Hemoproteins are essential endogenous pigments. They include hemoglobin and oxidative enzymes, the cytochromes. Numerous disorders result from abnormalities involving these pigments, particularly, iron uptake, metabolism, excretion, and storage (see Chapter 22). Excessive intracellular iron storage results from accumulations of hemoprotein, originating when this substance is transferred from the bloodstream into cells. Iron enters blood from three primary sources: (1) tissue stores, (2) the intestinal mucosa, and (3) macrophages. Macrophages remove and destroy dead or defective RBCs. The amount of iron in blood plasma also depends on the metabolism of the major iron-transport protein, *transferrin.*

Iron is stored in tissue cells in two forms: ferritin, the major vehicle for iron storage and, with greater levels of iron present, as hemosiderin, an intracellular, yellow-brown pigment. Excess accumulation of hemosiderin usually occurs in the mononuclear phagocyte systems (MPSs) and, to a lesser extent, in the liver, kidneys, lungs, spleen, lymph nodes, and bone marrow. Iron overload, also known as hemochromatosis, refers to an accumulation of iron within the body and results from a variety of mechanisms (see Chapter 23).

In contrast to hemochromatosis, a chronic and systemic disorder, hemosiderosis is a transient, localized deposition of iron. It usually does not result in tissue damage. Transient hemosiderin accumulation within tissues can be seen in bruising where ruptured blood vessels result in RBCs exiting the circulatory system. The RBCs diffuse into tissues surrounding the site of injury. A local hemorrhage (bruise) forms after a contusion. The skin surrounding the site of impact injury first appears red or dark blue, or both, or, in lay terminology, "black and blue" as blood accumulates under the skin. Depending on the nature of the trauma, the color change can be quite profound (deep, blackish blue) and extend over a large area. Over the course of a few days to several weeks, the blue coloration is gradually replaced by characteristic color changes—green, yellow, and brown-pigmentation to the skin. The colors reflect the sequential degradation of hemoglobin (red–blue) to biliverdin (green) to bilirubin (yellow) and, finally, to hemosiderin (golden brown) (Fig. 4.22). Eventually the abnormal pigmentation resolves, and the normal skin color returns.

Bilirubin is a normal, yellow-to-green pigment of bile derived from the porphyrin structure of hemoglobin. Excess bilirubin within cells and tissues causes jaundice (icterus), a yellowing of the skin and sclera of eye. Jaundice occurs when the bilirubin level exceeds 1.5 to 2 mg/dL of plasma, compared with the normal values of 0.4 to 1 mg/dL. Hyperbilirubinemia develops because of one of several mechanisms: (1) destruction of RBCs causing *hemolytic jaundice;* (2) diseases affecting the metabolism and excretion of bilirubin in the liver; and (3) diseases causing obstruction of the common bile duct, such as gallstones or pancreatic tumors. Various drugs can cause the obstruction of normal bile flow through the liver, increasing blood levels of bilirubin.

Calcium

Calcium salts accumulate in both injured and dead tissues (Fig. 4.23), a process that results in *cellular calcification.* An important mechanism for cellular calcification is the influx of extracellular calcium of the mitochondria. Another mechanism involves the excretion of acid leading to the production of hydroxyl ions. These hydroxyl irons precipitate calcium hydroxide ($Ca[OH]_2$) and hydroxyapatite ($Ca_3[PO_4]_2)_3•Ca(OH)_2$) into a mixed salt. Injury occurs when clustered calcium salts harden, interfering with normal structure and function of the cell. This process is often identified in the pulmonary alveoli, gastric epithelium, and renal tubules.

Dystrophic calcification refers to calcification occurring in dying or necrotic tissues. This form of calcification is commonly noted in chronic pulmonary tuberculosis. Other sites affected include lymph nodes, advanced atherosclerotic cardiovascular plaques, and injured heart valves (Fig. 4.24). Calcification impedes the smooth opening or closing of heart valves and presents clinically as a heart murmur (see Chapter 26). Dystrophic calcification is frequently found in the center of tumors. Over time, necrosis and subsequent calcification occurs in the inner regions of growing tumors as they are progressively deprived of oxygen. Calcium salts appear as gritty, clumped granules that can become stone-like. Psammoma bodies (named for the Greek word denoting "sand") are laminated, calcified structures, which resemble grains of sand. They are concentric and commonly found within tumors; however the exact mechanism responsible for their formation remains unclear.

Metastatic calcification consists of mineral deposits that occur in undamaged, normal tissues secondary to hypercalcemia (excess calcium in the blood). Frequent causes of hypercalcemia include hyperparathyroidism, toxic levels of vitamin D, hyperthyroidism, Addison disease (adrenocortical insufficiency), and excess calcium supplementation. Hypercalcemia can develop secondary to the increased bone demineralization, resulting from bone tumors, leukemia, and disseminated cancers. It also may occur in advanced renal failure with phosphate retention.

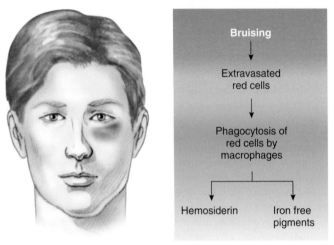

FIGURE 4.22 Hemosiderin Accumulation Is Noted as the Color Changes in a "Black Eye."

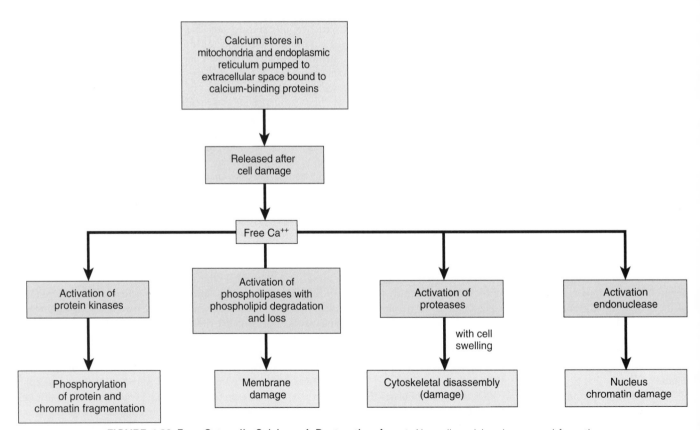

FIGURE 4.23 Free Cytosolic Calcium: A Destructive Agent. Normally, calcium is removed from the cytosol by adenosine triphosphate (ATP)–dependent calcium pumps. In normal cells, calcium is bound to buffering proteins, such as calbindin or parvalbumin, and is contained in the endoplasmic reticulum and the mitochondria. If there is abnormal permeability of calcium ion channels, direct damage to membranes, or depletion of ATP (i.e., hypoxic injury), calcium increases in the cytosol. If the free calcium cannot be buffered or pumped out of cells, uncontrolled enzyme activation takes place, causing further damage. Uncontrolled entry of calcium into the cytosol is an important final common pathway in many causes of cell death.

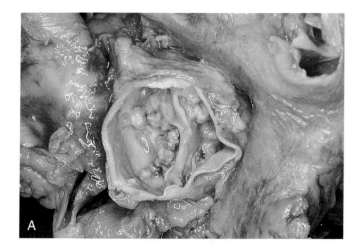

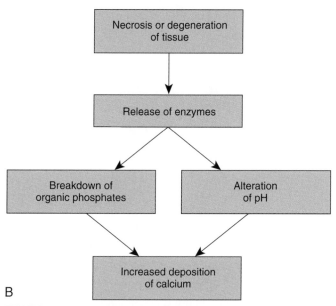

B

FIGURE 4.24 Aortic Valve Calcification. A, This calcified aortic valve is an example of dystrophic calcification. **B,** This algorithm shows the dystrophic mechanism of calcification. (**A,** from Damjanov I: *Pathology for the health professions,* ed 4, St Louis, 2012, Saunders.)

TABLE 4.10 Systemic Manifestations of Cellular Injury

Manifestation	Cause
Fever	Release of endogenous pyrogens (interleukin-1, tumor necrosis factor-α, prostaglandins) from bacteria or macrophages; acute inflammatory response
Increased heart rate	Increase in oxidative metabolic processes resulting from fever
Increase in leukocytes (leukocytosis)	Increase in total number of white blood cells because of infection; normal is 5000–9000/mm³ (increase is directly related to severity of infection)
Pain	Various mechanisms, such as release of bradykinins, obstruction, pressure
Presence of cellular enzymes	Release of enzymes from cells of tissue* in extracellular fluid
Lactate dehydrogenase (LDH) (LDH isoenzymes)	Release from red blood cells, liver, kidney, skeletal muscle
Creatine kinase (CK) (CK isoenzymes)	Release from skeletal muscle, brain, heart
Aspartate aminotransferase (AST/ serum glutamic-oxaloacetic transaminase [SGOT])	Release from heart, liver, skeletal muscle, kidney, pancreas
Alanine aminotransferase (ALT/ serum glutamic pyruvic transaminase [SGPT])	Release from liver, kidney, heart
Alkaline phosphatase (ALP)	Release from liver, bone
Amylase	Release from pancreas
Aldolase	Release from skeletal muscle, heart

*The rapidity of enzyme transfer is a function of the weight of the enzyme and the concentration gradient across the cellular membrane. The specific metabolic and excretory rates of the enzymes determine how long levels of enzymes remain elevated.

As phosphate levels increase, the activity of the parathyroid gland increases resulting in higher levels of circulating calcium.

Urate

In humans, uric acid (**urate**) is the major end product of purine catabolism. Humans lack the enzyme urate oxidase present in most other mammals. This enzyme is needed to convert uric acid to allantoin. Because urate crystals are not degraded by lysosomal enzymes, they persist in dead cells. Normally, serum urate concentration is stable measuring approximately 5 mg/dL in postpubertal males and 4.1 mg/dL in postpubertal females. With elevated serum urate levels, sodium urate crystals accumulate in tissues, leading to a group of painful disorders collectively called **gout**. These disorders include acute arthritis, chronic gouty arthritis, tophi (firm, nodular, subcutaneous deposits of urate crystals surrounded by fibrosis), and nephritis (inflammation of the nephron). In all of these disorders, cell injury and inflammation are characteristic findings (see Chapter 41).

Systemic Manifestations of Cellular Injury

Dead and injured cells initiate local inflammation and, with more severe injury, cause systemic inflammation. Inflammation promotes systemic manifestations of cellular injury, including fatigue, malaise, altered appetite, and fever. Fever may occur because of endogenous pyrogens (fever-inducing substances) released during the inflammatory response. Table 4.10 summarizes the most significant systemic manifestations of cellular injury.

CELLULAR DEATH

With sufficient structural or physiologic damage, cell injury becomes irreversible and cells die. Historically, cell death has been attributed to either necrosis or apoptosis (Fig. 4.25 and Table 4.11). Necrosis is a form of cell destruction characterized by rapid loss of plasma membrane structure, swelling of organelles, mitochondrial dysfunction, and the lack of typical features of apoptosis.[30] Apoptosis is known as a regulated

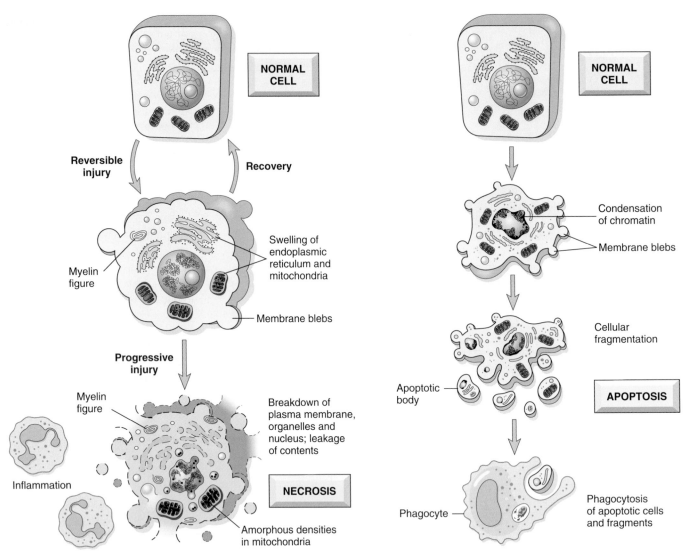

FIGURE 4.25 Schematic Illustration of the Morphologic Changes in Cell Injury Culminating in Necrosis or Apoptosis. Myelin figures come from degenerating cellular membranes and are noted within the cytoplasm or extracellularly. (From Kumar V et al, editors: *Robbins and Cotran pathologic basis of disease,* ed 9, Philadelphia, 2015, Elsevier.)

or programmed cell process discussed below. Until recently, necrosis was considered passive or accidental, occurring after severe and sudden injury. It is now understood that necrosis can be driven by *regulated* or *programmed* molecular pathways. Hence the new term is programmed necrosis, or necroptosis.

Necrosis

Cellular death leads to necrosis, the dissolution of cellular components. Necrosis is the sum of cellular changes occurring after local cell death. It is characterized by autolysis or *autodigestion,* a process of cellular self-digestion (see Fig. 4.25). Cellular death is initiated long before any necrotic changes can be detected by light microscopy.[31] Dense clumping of nuclear material and the progressive disruption of plasma and organelle membranes portend irreversible injury, and necrosis follows. As membrane integrity is lost, necrotic cell contents leak into the surrounding intracellular spaces, where they trigger an inflammatory response within the tissue. In the later stages of necrosis, when most organelles are disrupted, karyolysis (enzymatic hydrolysis of nuclear chromatin) is well underway. In some cells, pyknosis, a process where the nucleus shrinks into a small, dense mass of genetic material, occurs. Eventually,

lysosomal enzymes break up the pyknotic nucleus. Karyorrhexis is fragmentation of the nucleus into small particles or "nuclear dust."

Different types of necrosis tend to occur in different organs or tissues, sometimes indicating the mechanism or cause of cellular injury. The four major forms of necrosis are *coagulative, liquefactive, caseous,* and *fatty* (Fig. 4.26). Another form, *gangrenous necrosis,* is not a distinctive type of cell death but, instead, refers to large areas of tissue death. These forms of necrosis occur mostly in the kidneys, heart, and adrenal glands. Necrosis commonly results from hypoxia secondary to severe ischemia or chemical injury. Necrosis also is particularly common after the ingestion of mercuric chloride.

Coagulative necrosis occurs as a result of protein denaturation, where albumin is transformed from a gelatinous, transparent state into a firm, opaque substance (see Fig. 4.26, *A*). The area of coagulative necrosis is called an infarct.

Liquefactive necrosis commonly results from ischemic injury to neurons and glial cells in the brain (see Fig. 4.26, *B*). Dead brain tissue is readily subjected to liquefactive necrosis because brain cells are rich in digestive hydrolytic enzymes and lipids. Additionally the brain contains little connective tissue. Cells are digested by their own hydrolases as

TABLE 4.11 Features of Necrosis and Apoptosis

Feature	Necrosis	Apoptosis
Cell size	Enlarged (swelling)	Reduced (shrinkage)
Nucleus	Pyknosis → karyorrhexis → karyolysis	Fragmentation into nucleosome-size fragments
Plasma membrane	Disrupted	Intact; altered structure, especially orientation of lipids
Cellular contents	Enzymatic digestion; may leak out of cell	Intact; may be released in apoptotic bodies
Adjacent inflammation	Frequent	No
Physiologic or pathologic role	Invariably pathologic (culmination of irreversible cell injury)	Often physiologic, means of eliminating unwanted cells; may be pathologic after some forms of cell injury, especially deoxyribonucleic acid (DNA) damage

From Kumar V et al: Cellular responses to stress and toxic insults: adaptation, injury, and death. In Kumar V et al, editors: *Robbins and Cotran pathologic basis of disease,* ed 9, Philadelphia, 2015, Elsevier.

the tissue becomes soft and liquefied. In response, cysts form segregating this material from healthy tissue. Liquefactive necrosis is often triggered by bacterial infection, especially staphylococci, streptococci, and *Escherichia coli.*

Caseous necrosis commonly results from pulmonary tuberculosis or infection caused by *Mycobacterium tuberculosis* (see Fig. 4.26, *C*). It combines elements of both coagulative and liquefactive necrosis. Dead cells disintegrate, but the debris is not completely hydrolyzed. Instead a granulomatous inflammatory response ensues. Soft and granular tissues form the end-product, resembling clumped cheese. An inflammatory wall encloses the areas of caseous necrosis forming the characteristic *granulomas* of pulmonary tuberculosis (see Chapter 29).

Fatty necrosis is cellular dissolution caused by lipases, potent enzymes found in the breast and abdominal structures, especially within the pancreas (see Fig. 4.26, *D*). Lipases break down triglycerides, releasing free fatty acids. The fatty acids combine with calcium, magnesium, and sodium ions creating soaps, a process known as *saponification.* The necrotic tissue formed appears opaque and chalky white.

Gangrenous necrosis refers to tissue death but does not denote a specific pattern of cell death. It results from severe hypoxic injury, commonly secondary to the blockage of major arterial vessels supplying a region of the body. Gangrenous necrosis is particularly common with severely compromised circulation of the lower leg, either from acute or chronic disorders. With hypoxia, bacterial invasion, which enters a wound, can readily result in gangrenous necrosis. *Dry gangrene* typically results from coagulative necrosis. The skin becomes very dry and shriveled, and skin coloration in such cases is brown or black. *Wet gangrene,* the

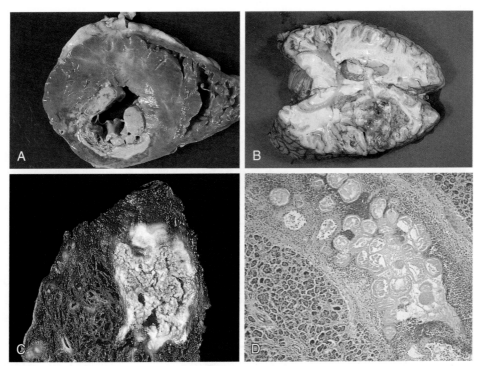

FIGURE 4.26 Types of Necrosis. A, Coagulative necrosis of myocardium of posterior wall of left ventricle of heart. A large anemic *(white)* infarct is readily apparent; note also the necrosis of papillary muscle. **B,** Liquefactive necrosis of the brain. The area of infarction is softened as a result of liquefactive necrosis. **C,** Caseous necrosis. Tuberculosis of the lung, with a large area of caseous necrosis containing yellow-white and cheesy debris. **D,** Fat necrosis of pancreas. Interlobular adipocytes are necrotic; these are surrounded by acute inflammatory cells. **(A and D,** from Damjanov I, Linder J, editors: *Anderson's pathology,* ed 10, St Louis, 1996, Mosby. **B,** from Damjanov I: *Pathology for the health professions,* ed 5, St Louis, 2016, Saunders. **C,** from Kumar V et al, editors: *Robbins and Cotran pathologic basis of disease,* ed 9, Philadelphia, 2015, Elsevier.)

more lethal form, develops secondary to necrotizing bacterial infections, particularly infection with gram-positive cocci, gram-negative rods, or anaerobic microorganisms, especially *Clostridium* spp. These microorganisms invade the site, causing a liquefactive necrosis. Wet gangrene causes the affected tissues to become cold, swollen, and black, and a foul odor is present. Wet gangrene also can affect internal organs, usually secondary to hypoxia. The presentation is similar regardless of the site involved. Wet gangrene is an aggressive disorder, which spreads rapidly to surrounding tissue. Left untreated, it rapidly can progress to death.

Gas gangrene refers to a type of wet gangrene caused by tissue infection with *Clostridium* spp., most commonly *Clostridium perfringens*. These microorganisms are widely present in soil and proliferate under conditions of low oxygen tension. Deep puncture wounds from soil-contaminated objects are common sources of infection. Once established at the site of infection, the microorganisms produce hydrolytic enzymes and toxins, which destroy tissue and cause bubbles of gas to form in the affected region. The infection progresses rapidly, spreading to adjacent tissue. Untreated, death typically occurs within 12 hours secondary to overwhelming sepsis, shock, and renal shutdown

Apoptosis

Apoptosis ("dropping off") is a distinct type of cell death that differs from necrosis in several ways (see Fig. 4.25 and Table 4.11). Apoptosis is an active process of cellular self-destruction, resulting in *programmed cell death*. It has been implicated in both normal and pathologic tissue changes. Cells die as a part of a normal physiologic process. Were it otherwise, endless cell proliferation would result in large and unwieldy

anatomy. In the average adult, 10 billion new cells may be created every day, and the same number of cells are destroyed daily. Death by apoptosis also causes loss of cells in many pathologic states, including the following:

- *Severe cell injury:* When cell injury exceeds the capacity for repair mechanisms, cell signaling triggers apoptosis.
- *Accumulation of misfolded proteins:* This condition results from either genetic mutations or free radicals. Excessive accumulation of misfolded proteins in the ER leads to a condition known as endoplasmic reticulum stress (ER stress) (see Chapter 1). ER stress culminates in cell death secondary to apoptosis. This mechanism has been linked to several degenerative diseases of the CNS and other organs (Fig. 4.27).
- *Infections (particularly viral infections):* Apoptosis may be the result of the host's immune response to the presence of a virus infecting the cell. Cytotoxic T lymphocytes respond to viral infections by inducing apoptosis, thus eliminating infectious cells. This process, however, can result in tissue damage. The same mechanism can result in cell death in tumor-related disease and organ transplant rejection.
- *Obstruction in tissue ducts:* Obstruction of blood flow to an organ results in pathologic atrophy, a process commonly noted in the pancreas, kidney, or parotid gland.

Excessive or insufficient apoptosis is known as *dysregulated apoptosis*. A low rate of apoptosis can encourage survival of abnormal cells, particularly mutated cells, which predispose the individual to developing cancer. Similarly, defective apoptosis may fail to eliminate lymphocytes implicated in attacking host tissue (self-antigens), thus leading to autoimmune disorders. Excessive apoptosis occurs in several neurodegenerative diseases

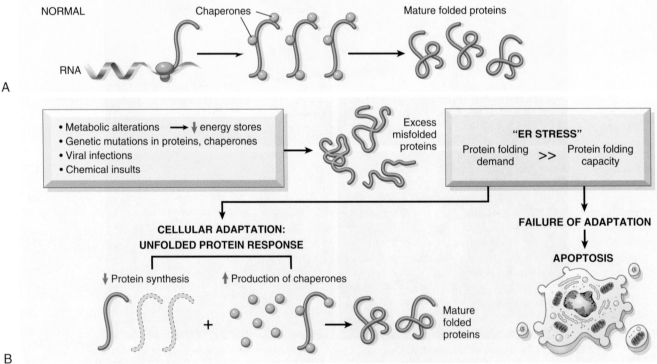

FIGURE 4.27 The Unfolded Protein Response, Endoplasmic Stress, and Apoptosis. **A,** In normal or healthy cells the newly made proteins are folded with help from chaperones and then incorporated into the cell or secreted. **B,** Various stressors can cause endoplasmic reticulum (ER) stress whereby the cell is challenged to cope with the increased load of misfolded proteins. The accumulation of the protein load initiates the *unfolded protein response* in the ER; if restoration of the protein fails, the cell dies by apoptosis. An example of a disease caused by misfolding of proteins is Alzheimer disease. (From Kumar V et al, editors: *Robbins and Cotran pathologic basis of disease,* ed 9, Philadelphia, 2015, Elsevier.)

MITOCHONDRIAL (INTRINSIC) PATHWAY   DEATH RECEPTOR (EXTRINSIC) PATHWAY

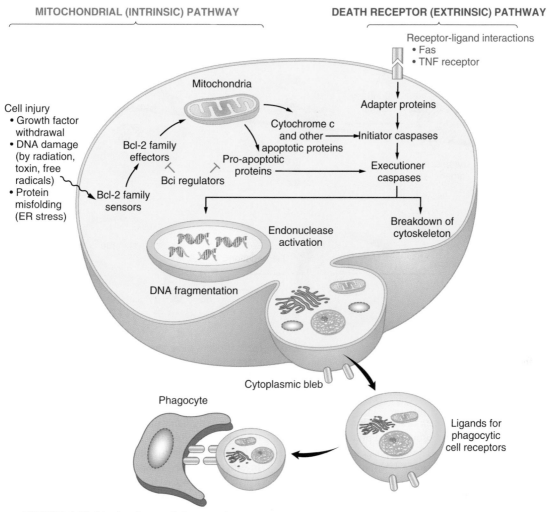

FIGURE 4.28 Mechanisms of Apoptosis. The two pathways of apoptosis differ in their induction and regulation, and both culminate in the activation of "executioner" caspases. The induction of apoptosis by the mitochondrial pathway involves the Bcl-2 family, which causes leakage of mitochondrial proteins. The regulators of the death receptor pathway involve the proteases, called *caspases.* (Adapted from Kumar V et al, editors: *Robbins and Cotran pathologic basis of disease,* ed 9, Philadelphia, 2015, Elsevier.)

and with ischemic injury, such as with myocardial infarction and stroke, and in the context of virus-infected cells.

Initiation of apoptosis requires tightly regulated cell signaling. Key components involve proteases, enzymes that divide other proteins. Caspases are a family of aspartic acid–specific enzymes that trigger proteolytic activity in response to signals, which induce apoptosis. Specifically, activated caspases cleave other proteins within the system, initiating a series of sequential reactions known as the "suicide" cascade. The cascade results in a rapid and contained cell death. Caspase activation triggers two different but convergent pathways: the *mitochondrial (intrinsic) pathway* and the *death receptor (extrinsic) pathway* (Fig. 4.28). Cells undergoing apoptosis release chemical factors, which recruit phagocytes. The phagocytes quickly engulf cellular remnants, reducing their potential to induce damaging inflammation. Cell death secondary to necrosis is less contained because injured cells swell and burst spilling their contents into the extracellular spaces, triggering an inflammatory response.

Autophagy

The Greek term autophagy means "eating of self." Autophagy is a "recycling factory" as well as a survival mechanism. It is a self-destructive

---

BOX 4.3 The Major Forms of Autophagy

Macroautophagy, the most common term to refer to autophagy, involves the sequestration and transportation of parts (cargo) of the cytosol in an autophagic vacuole (autophagosome).

Microautophagy is the inward invagination of the lysosomal membrane for cargo delivery.

Chaperone-mediated autophagy is the chaperone-dependent proteins that direct cargo across the lysosomal membrane.

---

process that delivers cytoplasmic contents to the lysosome for degradation. Box 4.3 includes terminology used to describe autophagy.

When cells are starved or nutrient deprived, autophagy initiates a "cannibalization response," which digests the cell and recycles the contents. Autophagy can maintain cellular metabolism under conditions of starvation. Under conditions of stress, autophagy removes damaged organelles, thus enhancing the likelihood of survival. Autophagy also has been implicated in cancer, heart disease, neurodegeneration diseases, inflammation, and infection.[32] Although somewhat controversial, the process is thought to begin with a cup-shaped, curved membrane known

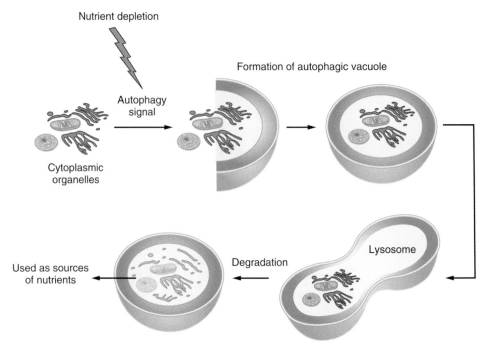

FIGURE 4.29 Autophagy. Cellular stresses, such as nutrient deprivation, activate autophagy genes that create vacuoles in which cellular organelles are sequestered and then degraded following fusion of the vesicles with lysosomes. The digested materials are recycled to provide nutrients for the cell. (Adapted from Mexcelom Bioscience Collometer.)

as a *phagophore* (Fig. 4.29). This membrane expands and engulfs intracellular contents—organelles, ribosomes, and proteins—forming a double membrane *autophagosome*. The autophagosome fuses with the lysosome, forming an *autophagolysosome*. Lysosomal acid proteases then degrade the autophagosome into amino acids and other elemental substances. These end-products are transported out of the cytoplasm, where they are subsequently utilized for the synthesis of macromolecules or for fueling metabolism.

Autophagy holds promise for formulating new therapeutic strategies in treating disease. Evidence also suggests that autophagy may be the last immune defense against infectious microorganisms that have invaded the intracellular environment.[33] The "garbage collecting" and recycling functions, characterizing autophagy, becomes less efficient and less discriminating in aging individuals. Consequently harmful agents accumulate and cause increasing cell damage as people age. Failure to clear protein products in neurons of the CNS has been linked with dementia. Similarly failure to clear mitochondria, which generates ROS, can lead to nuclear DNA mutations and cancer. These processes may even partially define normal aging. Enhancing autophagy may serve to decrease the incidence of cancer and prevent the development of particular degenerative diseases.

✔ **QUICK CHECK 4.4**

1. Why is an increase in the concentration of intracellular calcium injurious?
2. Compare and contrast necrosis and apoptosis.
3. Why is apoptosis significant?
4. Autophagy may become less efficient with aging. Why is this harmful?

AGING AND ALTERED CELLULAR AND TISSUE BIOLOGY

Aging is defined as a normal physiologic process, which is universal and inevitable. **Life span** is the period from birth to death and its study offers

insight into the aging process. Aging is associated with a gradual loss of homeostatic mechanisms. It is a complex process involving a multiplicity of factors; however the underlying cause of aging is not entirely clear. Investigators have focused on genetic, inflammatory, oxidative, and metabolic parameters of aging. Active investigation includes the study of genetic signatures in humans with exceptional longevity. Current research is focused on epigenetic mechanisms that modulate gene expression and the role of intrauterine environment. Lifelong patterns of health, the effects of personality, behavioral patterns, and social support also are thought to be relevant. Investigators have studied the influence of biochemical factors believed to impact aging, particularly the role of insulin and insulin-like growth factor 1 (IGF-1) signaling on senescence; mitochondrial dysfunction; and an inflammatory microenvironment leading to chronic disease, frailty, and decreased lifespan. Coagulation is part of the inflammatory response and may be responsible for thickening (hypercoagulable) blood with aging leading to arterial and venous clot formation in the elderly. The microbiota plays a role in the induction of the immune system, adaptive immunity declines with age, and innate immunity may result in mild hyperactivity.[34]

Senescence is a process leading to permanent proliferative arrest of cells in response to various stressors. Senescent cells accumulate with time and contribute to tissue dysfunction. A recent study in immune factors in identical twins found increasing differences between identical twins, suggesting the influence of nonheritable factors or environmental factors.[35] Diet is believed to play a major role on both the development and the prevention of age-related diseases. A major research challenge has been to separate the causes of cell and tissue aging from the changes that characterize it. Understanding the physiology of aging supports public health efforts to promote healthy aging and delay the progression to vulnerability and frailty.

Traditionally aging has not been considered a disease; rather it has been regarded as a normal process. Disease has been defined as deviation from the normal state secondary to injury or abnormal function. Conceptually this distinction has been clear; however issues

TABLE 4.12 Aging: Degenerative Extracellular Changes, Cellular Changes, and Tissue and Systemic Aging

Degenerative extracellular changes	Binding of collagen; increase in free radicals; alterations of tendons, ligaments, bones and joints; development of peripheral vascular disease, particularly, arteriosclerosis Extracellular matrix with increased cross-linking, decreased synthesis, and increased degradation of collagen Oxidative stress damages cellular function Development of cardiovascular diseases with endothelial cell shifts to proinflammatory, proproliferative, and procoagulative state
Cellular aging	Atrophy, decreased function, loss of cells possibly by apoptosis Compensatory mechanisms of hypertrophy and hyperplasia can lead to metaplasia, dysplasia, and neoplasia deoxyribonucleic acid (DNA), ribonucleic acid (RNA), and cellular proteins and membranes susceptible to injuries Lack of DNA repair leads to increase in mutations Increased production of reactive oxygen species (ROS) Cumulative damage to mitochondrial DNA (mtDNA) Progression of common diseases (diabetes, cancer, heart failure
Tissue and Systemic Aging	Progressive stiffness or rigidity affects many systems (arterial, pulmonary, musculoskeletal) Peripheral resistance to blood flow Thymus atrophy occurs at puberty causing a decreased response to T-dependent antigens (foreign proteins), increased formation of autoantibodies and immune complexes decreasing effectiveness of immune function later in life Reproductive system loss of ova and spermatogenesis decreased in men Responsiveness to hormones decreases in the breast and endometrium Stomach decreases in the rate of emptying and secretion of hormones and hydrochloric acid Muscular atrophy decreases motor tone and contractility Sarcopenia or loss of muscle mass and strength Decrease in height Reduction in circumference of the neck, thighs, and arms; widening of the pelvis; lengthening of the nose and ears Increase in body weight in middle age followed by a decrease in stature, weight, fat-free mass, and body mass As the amount of fat increases, the percentage of total body water decreases. Increased body fat distribution (abdominal) is associated with non-insulin-dependent diabetes and heart disease. Total body potassium concentration decreases

BOX 4.4 Life Expectancy Differences Across the United States

- Improved public health strategies and health advances in the United States between the years 1900 and 2000 added about 30 years to life expectancy
- The increase in life expectancy, however, does not apply to all Americans.
- Women outnumber men in each successive age group from 65 years and older.
- The historic advances in life expectancy resulted in a larger older adult population and, for some, problems of disability, disease, and socioeconomic hardship.
- Although U.S. spending on health care far exceeds that of other countries, rates of life expectancy and key measures of health lag behind those of other high-income countries.
- The National Center for Health Statistics has reported that Americans, on average, have a life expectancy of 78.8 years, a decline from 78.9 in 2014.

- The decline in life expectancy is attributed to rising fatalities from heart disease and stroke; diabetes; drug overdoses; accidents, including unintentional injuries; and other conditions.
- Chronic health problems associated with modifiable risk factors, such as smoking, poor nutrition, overweight, and lack of physical activity, represent 6 of the 10 costliest in terms of health care burden.
- The preventable conditions lead to injuries and diseases and cause soaring medical and labor costs that burden U.S. employers and bankrupt families.
- All of these conditions are highly amenable to population-based preventive strategies.
- The current generation of children and young adults in the United States could become the first generation to have shorter life spans, multiple medical conditions, and fewer years of healthy life.

involving cellular injury or damage challenge traditional views. Life span can be altered in animals. But extending life span is not equivalent to delaying aging.[36] For example, death can be prevented through treatment of an acute infection, but the *rate* of aging continues. What is critical is extending a person's *health span*, which results in an increase in life span and a decrease in time spent in a frail state.[37] The passage of time cannot be stopped (*chronologic aging*), but it may be possible to delay the decline in health, or *biologic aging*. Table 4.12 presents degenerative changes, cellular changes, and tissue and systemic aging.

Studies have suggested the possibility of altering the "aging clock" by changing the cell's differentiation program. Causes of aging may be largely epigenetic or influences on gene expression.

Normal Life Span and Life Expectancy

The maximal life span of humans is 80 to 100 years, and it does not vary significantly among populations. Life expectancy is the *average* number of years of life remaining at a given age (Box 4.4).

Frailty

Frailty, a common clinical syndrome in older adults, is characterized by overall weakness, decreased stamina, and functional decline. The individual is susceptible to falls, disability, disease, and death. This presentation is often described as frailty syndrome. Criteria indicating compromised functioning include low grip strength, slowed walking speed, low physical activity, and unintentional weight loss.[38] The

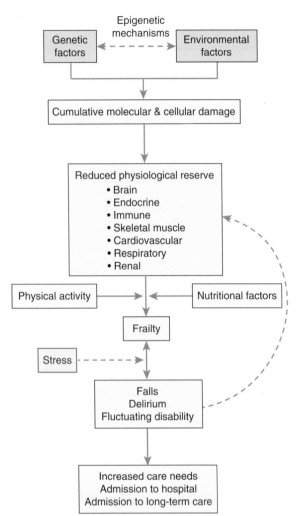

FIGURE 4.30 Frailty. Frailty is a disorder of multiple interrelated physiologic systems. A gradual decline progresses with aging, but in frailty this decline becomes accelerated. Homeostatic mechanisms begin to fail, and vulnerability becomes disproportionate to changes in health status after a relatively minor stressor event. (From Clegg A et al: Frailty in elderly people, *Lancet* 381[9868]:752–762, 2013.)

pathophysiology of frailty includes several interrelated physiologic systems (Fig. 4.30). It is complex, with multiple aging mechanisms influenced by genetic factors, epigenetic factors, or both, as well as environmental factors. Frailty also can involve such alterations as osteopenia, cognitive impairment, and anemia. Differences between men and women in presentation include the following: (1) Higher baseline levels of muscle mass in men may be protective against frailty; (2) testosterone and growth hormone can provide advantages to men in muscle mass maintenance; (3) cortisol is more dysregulated, especially in older women; (4) alterations in immune function and immune responsiveness to sex steroids make men more susceptible to sepsis and infection and make women more susceptible to chronic inflammatory conditions and loss of muscle mass; and (5) lower levels of activity and caloric intake may increase the risk of frailty in women. Sarcopenia and cachexia are common sequelae of aging and also occur secondary to many chronic illnesses.

SOMATIC DEATH

Somatic death is systemic death of the entire body. Unlike the changes that follow cellular death, **postmortem change** is diffuse and does not involve an inflammatory response. Within minutes after death, postmortem changes appear, and it becomes readily evident that death has occurred. The most immediate manifestations are the complete cessation of respiration and circulation, followed rapidly by a host of other changes. The surface of the skin becomes pale and yellowish, marking the first stage after death known as **pallor mortis**. In instances of death secondary to carbon monoxide poisoning, drowning, or chloroform poisoning, this phenomenon may not be apparent; instead, a lifelike coloration of the cheeks and lips may persist even after death has occurred.[39]

The second stage after death, **algor mortis**, is defined as a decrease in body temperature after death. Body temperature falls gradually, immediately after death, then decreases more rapidly (approximately 1.0° F–1.5° F/hr) until body temperature equals environmental temperature.[40] In cases of death caused by certain infective diseases, body temperature may transiently rise for a short time.

The third stage after death, **rigor mortis**, is characterized by stiffening of muscles. Within 6 hours after death, acidic compounds accumulate within the muscles secondary to degradation of carbohydrates and the depletion of ATP. With lack of ATP, the detachment of myosin from actin (contractile proteins) fails, resulting in muscle rigidity. The smaller muscles are usually affected first, particularly the muscles of the jaws. Many factors affect the onset of rigor mortis, which begins 0 to 8 hours after death and peaks at approximately 8 to 12 hours from onset. The body remains stiff for another 12 to 24 hours, after which the rigor begins to dissipate with muscle flexibility returning after 24 to 36 hours.

Livor mortis is the fourth stage after death. Gravity causes blood to settle in dependent (anatomically low areas) tissues, resulting in a prominent blue-purple discoloration of the skin over these regions. During this stage, blood pressure within the retinal vessels decreases, causing muscle tension to decrease and the pupils to dilate. The face, nose, and chin become sharp or peaked-looking as blood and fluids drain from these areas.[39] The process begins immediately after death but is not readily apparent to the human eye until 2 hours after death. It reaches a maximum peak 8 to 12 hours after death. Incisions made during this time frame usually will not cause bleeding. The skin loses elasticity and transparency. Appreciation of the changes that occur during this stage is very useful to forensic pathologists because it enables them to determine the approximate time of death and whether the body has been moved or repositioned.

Putrefaction is the fifth stage after death when tissues and organs of the body lose cohesiveness as they break down into gaseous and liquid matter. This process is largely driven by the action of bacteria present both within the body and in the external environment. Visible signs of putrefaction are generally obvious about 24 to 48 hours after death. The rate at which putrefactive changes occur varies, depending on the environmental temperature surrounding the body. Changes will occur more rapidly in warm environments (e.g., hot summer days or nights). Putrefaction occurs most rapidly in ambient air. The rate is sequentially slower in water and earth. The first sign is usually a greenish discoloration of the skin, particularly over the abdomen. Discoloration is thought to occur because of the diffusion of hemolyzed blood into tissues and the production of denatured hemoglobin derivatives. Slippage or loosening of the skin from underlying tissues occurs during this phase. Black discoloration to the tissues follow, and gases with characteristic noxious odors are released. As the process progresses, gas builds within body structures resulting in swelling or bloating. Gas buildup will eventually lead to bursting of organs and body cavity openings. Liquefactive changes occur as internal organs begin to liquefy.

Decomposition is the sixth stage after death. It occurs when the organic matter of the body is broken down into elemental matter and recycled into the earth's biosphere. The body's own enzymes and chemicals drive this process. Putrification may be ongoing simultaneously.

Skeletonization, the seventh and final stage after death, occurs when the various tissues of the body have degraded and decayed to the point of exposing the skeleton. When all of the organic matter of the body is gone, the process is complete, and only disarticulated bones will remain. Depending on the environment surrounding the skeleton, bones can persist for periods lasting from several years to relatively indefinitely. Under rare circumstances, an eighth stage, **fossilization**, may occur. At this stage, the bones are infiltrated and replaced with inorganic mineral deposits. If this process transpires, the fossilized bones will have the permanence of rocks, thus accounting for many museum specimens. Fossilization is uncommon and only occurs under select and relatively unusual environmental conditions.

> **✔ QUICK CHECK 4.5**
> 1. Aging is a complex process. Discuss the many mechanisms of aging.
> 2. What are the body composition changes that occur with aging?
> 3. Define frailty and possible endocrine–immune system involvement.

SUMMARY REVIEW

Cellular Adaptation

1. Cellular adaptation is a reversible event involving a structural or functional response to both physiologic (normal) conditions and to pathologic (adverse) conditions. Cells adapt to meet physiologic demands and stress in an effort to maintain a steady state called homeostasis.
2. The most significant *adaptive* changes include atrophy, hypertrophy, hyperplasia, metaplasia, and dysplasia.
3. Atrophy is a decrease in cellular size caused by aging, disuse, or insufficient blood supply. Insufficient hormonal or neural stimulation also can cause atrophy. Endoplasmic reticulum, mitochondria, and microfilaments decrease with atrophy. Mechanisms predisposing the cell to atrophy include decreased protein synthesis or increased protein catabolism, or both.
4. Hypertrophy is an increase in the size of cells in response to mechanical stimuli (e.g., stretching, pressure, or volume overload) and results in increased size of the affected organ. Hypertrophy can be either physiologic or pathologic, depending on the circumstances.
5. Hyperplasia is an increase in the number of cells caused by an increased rate of mitosis (cell division). Hyperplasia can be physiologic (compensatory and hormonal) or pathologic hormonal.
6. Metaplasia is the reversible replacement of one mature cell type with another less mature cell type. It is found in association with tissue damage, repair, and regeneration.
7. Dysplasia, or atypical hyperplasia, is an abnormal change in the size, shape, and organization of mature tissue cells. It is considered an atypical rather than a true adaptation response.

Cellular Injury

1. Injury to cells and to the extracellular matrix leads to tissue and organ injury. This injury affects the structural patterns of disease. Cellular injury occurs when the cell fails to maintain homeostasis (normal or adaptive steady state) secondary to insult or stress. Injured cells may recover (reversible injury) or die (irreversible injury).
2. Biochemical events result in characterize cell injury and death, including: (1) ATP depletion, resulting in mitochondrial damage; (2) accumulation of oxygen and radical oxygen species (ROS) which cause membrane damage;(3) increased intracellular calcium concentration and the loss of calcium steady state; (4) mitochondrial damage causing loss of membrane potential and activation of cell death; (5) membrane damage; and (6) protein folding defects.
3. The most common forms of cell injury include ischemic and hypoxic injury, ischemia-reperfusion injury, oxidative stress or accumulation of oxygen-derived free radical-induced injury, and chemical injury.
4. Hypoxia is the lack of sufficient oxygen in cells and is the most common cause of cellular injury. The most common cause of hypoxia is ischemia, or a reduced supply of blood.
5. Restoration of oxygen in ischemic states can result in additional injury, called reperfusion injury. The mechanisms for such injury include oxidative stress, increased intracellular calcium concentration, inflammation, and complement activation.
6. Free radicals have an unpaired electron making the molecule unstable. Seeking stability, they may form chemical bonds with proteins, lipids, and carbohydrates located within membranes and nucleic acids (DNA), causing injury. The damaging effects of free radicals is termed oxidative stress. Mechanisms include (1) peroxidation of lipids, (2) alteration of ion pumps and transport mechanisms, (3) fragmentation of DNA, and (4) damage to mitochondria, releasing calcium into the cytosol.
7. Humans are exposed to thousands of chemicals for which there is inadequate toxicologic data. Potential mechanisms for injury include oxidative stress, heat shock proteins, DNA damage, hypoxia, ER stress, mental stress, inflammation, and osmotic stress.
8. The world's largest single environmental health risk is air pollution. Millions of deaths and diseases occur because of indoor and outdoor air pollution.
9. The most common heavy metals associated with cell injury include lead, mercury, arsenic, and cadmium. Damage from metals affects DNA repair mechanisms, tumor suppressor functions, and signal transduction pathways.
10. Alcohol contributes to cell injury by altering nutritional status, causing the metabolism of acetaldehyde (toxic and known carcinogen), and effecting the liver, CNS, and other body tissues. Chronic alcoholism and binge drinking have significant health hazards including alcoholic liver disease, cirrhosis, and hepatocellular carcinoma.
11. Fetal alcohol spectrum disorders are a range of health effects or disorders of prenatal alcohol exposure. Maternal ingestion of alcohol can be catastrophic for the developing fetus.
12. The use of psychoactive and narcotic drugs is a major problem in many parts of the world. Both prescription and illicit opiates are the main causes of drug overdose deaths.
13. Unintentional and intentional injuries are a major health problem in the United States. Death as a result of these injuries is more common for men than women and there are differences among ethnic/racial groups.
14. Injuries by blunt force are the result of the application of mechanical energy to the body, resulting in tearing, shearing, or crushing of tissues. These include contusions (bruises), lacerations (tears or rips in the skin), and fractures of bone. The most common causes of blunt-force injuries include motor vehicle accidents and falls.
15. Injuries by sharp force are the result of cutting or piercing. Examples of this include incised, stab, puncture, and chopping wounds.
16. Gunshot wounds may be either penetrating (bullet is retained in the body) or perforating (bullet exits the body). The most important factors determining the appearance of a gunshot injury are whether

it is an entrance or an exit wound and the range at which the bullet was fired.

17. Asphyxial injuries are caused by mechanisms that prevent oxygen from entering the body and reaching the cells. These injuries can be grouped into four general categories: suffocation, strangulation, chemical asphyxiation, and drowning.

18. Activation of inflammation and immunity that follows cell injury or infection produces powerful biochemical reactions and proteins capable of damaging normal cells.

19. Genetic disorders result in cellular injury by altering the nucleus and the plasma membrane (structure, shape, receptors, or transport mechanisms).

20. Deprivation and excessive consumption of essential nutrients (proteins, carbohydrates, lipids, vitamins) can result in cellular injury by altering cellular structure and function.

21. Environmental factors can result in cellular injury. Common triggers include temperature extremes, changes in atmospheric pressure, ionizing radiation, illumination, mechanical stresses, and excessive noise.

Manifestations of Cellular Injury

1. Metabolic derangements can trigger cellular injury, especially cellular accumulations. Intracellular accumulation of substances is called infiltration. Infiltrations include (1) excess accumulation of normal cellular substances (water, proteins, lipids, and carbohydrate excesses), and (2) concentration or accumulation of abnormal substances which can be either endogenous (produced within the body, such as from abnormal metabolism) or exogenous (derived from outside the body, like a virus).

2. Most accumulations occur secondary to one of four mechanisms: (1) a normal substances that is insufficiently removed due to altered transport; (2) an abnormal substance, often secondary to a gene mutation, accumulates; (3) an endogenous substance that is inadequately catabolized; and (4) an inhaled or ingested harmful exogenous substance accumulates or is produced secondary to an infection.

3. Protein accumulations injure cells by "crowding" the organelles and producing potentially harmful metabolites. Metabolites are released into the cytoplasm or expelled in the extracellular matrix. They may be abnormal substances or normal metabolites produced in excessive amounts.

4. Oncosis is a type of cell death that occurs secondary to cellular swelling with water. It is seen in many types of cellular injury and occurs as a result of a failure of the transport mechanisms to regulate water flow into and out of the cell.

5. Certain metabolic disorders result in abnormal intracellular accumulations of carbohydrates and lipids, primarily in the spleen, liver, and CNS.

6. Glycogen (the storage form of glucose) is an important source of energy in normal cell function, but intracellular accumulations of it can have detrimental effects on growth and development.

7. Protein accumulations primarily occur in epithelial cells of renal convoluted tubules and in the antibody B-lymphocytes.

8. Pigment accumulations can be endogenous (e.g., melanin and blood proteins) or exogenous (e.g., coal dust and other mineral dusts).

9. Dystrophic calcification is the accumulation of calcium salts in injured or dead cells, and is a sign of pathologic change. Metastatic calcification occurs in uninjured cells secondary to hypercalcemia.

10. Gout, a very common and painful disorder, results from disturbances in urate metabolism. It occurs secondary to hyperuricemia where sodium urate crystals are deposited into tissues.

11. Systemic manifestations of cellular injury initiate inflammation with associated manifestations, including fever, leukocytosis, increased heart rate, pain, and serum elevations of plasma enzymes.

12. Inflammation promotes systemic manifestations of cellular injury, including fever, fatigue, malaise, pain, altered appetite, increased heart rate, increased number of leukocytes, or the presence of cellular enzymes.

Cellular Death

1. Historically, cell death has been classified as either necrosis or apoptosis. Necrosis is characterized by a rapid loss of the plasma membrane structure, organelle swelling, mitochondrial dysfunction, and the lack of any hallmark features of apoptosis. Apoptosis is known as regulated or programmed cell death and is characterized by the "dropping off" of cellular fragments, called apoptotic bodies.

2. It is now understood that under certain conditions, necrosis is regulated or programmed, hence, the new term programmed necrosis or necroptosis.

3. There are four major types of necrosis: coagulative, liquefactive, caseous, and fatty. Different types of necrosis occur in different tissues and under differing disease circumstances.

4. Gangrenous necrosis, or gangrene, is not a type of cell death but rather refers to large areas of tissue death. It is tissue necrosis caused by hypoxia and subsequent infection with anaerobic bacteria.

5. Structural signs which indicate irreversible injury with subsequent progression to necrosis are (1) dense clumping and disruption of nuclear genetic material and (2) disruption of plasma and organelle membranes.

6. Apoptosis is a distinct type of selective cellular self-destruction that occurs in both normal and pathologic tissue changes. Death by apoptosis results in the loss of cells and occurs in many pathologic states: (1) severe cell injury, (2) accumulation of misfolded proteins, (3) infections, and (4) obstruction in tissue ducts.

7. Excessive or insufficient apoptosis is known as dysregulated apoptosis.

8. Autophagy, defined as the "eating of self," is a self-destructive process. It serves as a survival mechanisms and has been compared to a "recycling factory." When cells are starved or nutrient deprived, autophagy initiates cannibalization to recycle digested contents. Autophagy can maintain cellular metabolism under conditions of starvation and can remove damaged organelles under stress conditions. Autophagy declines and becomes less efficient as cells age, a dynamic, which contributes to the aging process.

Aging and Altered Cellular and Tissue Biology

1. It is difficult to distinguish physiologic (normal) from pathologic (abnormal) changes associated with aging. Investigators are focused on genetic, inflammatory, oxidation, and metabolic origins of aging.

2. Important factors in aging include increased damage to cells, reduced capacity for mitosis, reduced ability to repair DNA damage, and defective nitrogen balance.

3. Frailty is a common clinical syndrome in older adults characterized by overall weakness, decreased stamina, and functional decline. This leaves the individual vulnerable to falls, functional decline, disability, disease, and, eventually, death. Sarcopenia and cachexia are common sequela of aging.

Somatic Death

1. Somatic death is death of the entire organism. Postmortem changes are diffuse, predictable, and do not involve an inflammatory response.

2. Manifestations of somatic death are progressive, occurring in a sequenced manner. Death typically begins with the cessation of respiration and circulation and characteristic dilation of the pupils and culminates with the skeletonization of the body. The seven stages of death are (1) pallor mortis, (2) algor mortis, (3) rigor mortis, (4) livor mortis, (5) putrefaction, (6) decomposition, and (7) skeletonization.

3. Depending on the environment surrounding the bones, a rare eighth stage, fossilization, may occur.

KEY TERMS

Adaptation, 73
Aging, 104
Albinism, 97
Algor mortis, 106
Ambient particulate matter, 85
Anoxia, 78
Antioxidant, 83
Apoptosis, 102
Asphyxial injury, 91
Atrophy, 74, 74
Autolysis, 100
Autophagic vacuole, 74
Autophagy, 103
Bilirubin, 97
Binge drinking, 89
Biotransformation, 83
Callus, 75
Carbon monoxide (CO), 93
Caseous necrosis, 101
Caspase, 103
Cellular accumulation (infiltration), 94
Cellular swelling, 95
Chemical asphyxiant, 93
Choking asphyxiation, 92
Coagulative necrosis, 100
Compensatory hyperplasia, 75
Cyanide, 93
Cytochrome, 97
DNA damage, 80
Decomposition, 106

Disuse atrophy, 74
Drowning, 93
Dry-lung drowning, 93
Dysplasia (atypical hyperplasia), 74, 76
Dystrophic calcification, 98
Endoplasmic reticulum stress (ER stress), 102
Ethanol, 86
Fatty necrosis, 101
Ferritin, 97
Fetal alcohol spectrum disorder (FASD), 89
Fetal alcohol syndrome (FAS), 89
Fossilization, 107
Frailty, 105
Frailty syndrome, 105
Free radical, 79
Gangrenous necrosis, 101
Gas gangrene, 102
Gout, 99
Hanging strangulation, 92
Hemochromatosis, 97
Hemoprotein, 97
Hemosiderin, 97
Hemosiderosis, 97
Hormonal hyperplasia, 75
Hydrogen sulfide, 93
Hyperplasia, 74, 75
Hypertrophy, 74, 75

Hypoxia, 77
Infarct, 100
Irreversible injury, 77
Ischemia, 77
Ischemia-reperfusion injury (reperfusion [reoxygenation] injury), 78
Karyolysis, 100
Karyorrhexis, 100
Lead (Pb), 85
Life expectancy, 105
Life span, 104
Ligature strangulation, 92
Lipid peroxidation, 80
Lipofuscin, 75
Liquefactive necrosis, 100
Livor mortis, 106
Manual strangulation, 93
Maximal life span, 105
Melanin, 97
Mesenchymal (tissue from embryonic mesoderm) cell, 77
Metaplasia, 74, 76
Metastatic calcification, 98
Mercury (quicksilver), 85
Methane, 93
mitochondrial DNA (mtDNA), 82
Mitochondrial effect, 81
Necrosis, 100

Oncosis (vacuolar degeneration), 95
Oxidative stress, 79
Ozone, 85
Pallor mortis, 106
Pathologic atrophy, 74
Pathologic hormonal hyperplasia, 75
Pathologic hypertrophy, 75
Physiologic atrophy, 74
Physiologic hypertrophy, 75
Postmortem change, 106
Programmed necrosis (necroptosis), 100
Protein alteration, 80
Psammoma body, 98
Putrefaction, 106
Pyknosis, 100
Reactive oxygen species (ROS), 79
Reversible injury, 77
Rigor mortis, 106
Senescence, 104
Skeletonization, 107
Somatic death, 106
Strangulation, 92
Steatosis, 96
Suffocation, 91
Urate, 99
Vacuolation, 78
Xenobiotic, 82

REFERENCES

1. Kumar V, et al, editors: *Pathology*, St Louis, 2014, Elsevier.
2. Kumar V, Abbas A, Fausto N, editors: *Robbins & Cotran pathologic basis of disease*, ed 9, Philadelphia, 2015, Saunders.
3. Wang ZJ, et al: The effect of intravenous vitamin C infusion on periprocedural myocardial injury for patients undergoing elective percutaneous coronary intervention, *Can J Cardiol* 30(1):96-101, 2014.
4. Rodrigo R, et al: The effectiveness of antioxidant vitamins C and E in reducing myocardial infarct size in patients subjected to percutaneous coronary angioplasty (PREVEC Trial): study protocol for a pilot randomized double-blind controlled trial, *Trials* 15:192, 2014.
5. Tice RR, et al: Improving the human hazard characterization of chemicals: a TOX21 update, *Environ Health Perspect* 121:756-765, 2013.
6. Seeff LB: Herbal hepatotoxicity, *Clin Liver Dis* 11:577-596, 2007.
7. Carithers RL, Jr, McClain CJ: Alcoholic liver disease. In Sleisenger MH, et al, editors: *Sleisenger and Fordtran's gastrointestinal and liver disease:*

pathophysiology, diagnosis, management, ed 9, Philadelphia, 2010, Saunders/Elsevier, pp 1383-1400.
8. Centers for Disease Control and Prevention (CDC): *Confronting opioids*, Atlanta GA, 2018, National Center for Injury Prevention and Control, Division of Unintentional Injury Prevention, Centers for Disease Control and Prevention. Available at: https://www.cdc.gov/drugoverdose/data/statedeaths.html. (Accessed 29 September 2018).
9. World Health Organization (WHO): *Air pollution*, Geneva, 2016, Author. Available at: http://www.who.int/topics/air_pollution/en/. (Accessed September 3, 2016).
10. GDB 2016 Risk Factors Collaborators: Global, regional, and national comparative risk assessment of 84 behavioural, environmental and occupational, and metabolic risks or clusters of risks, 1990–2016: a systematic analysis for the Global Burden of Disease Study 2016, *Lancet* 390(10100):1345-1422, 2017. Available at: https://www.ncbi.nlm.nih.gov/pubmed/28919119.
11. Jomova K, Valko M: Advances in metal-induced oxidative stress and human disease, *Toxicology* 283:65-87, 2011.

12. Abadin H, et al: *Toxicological profile for lead*, Atlanta, GA, 2007, Agency for Toxic Substances and Disease Registry (US).
13. Neal AP, Guilarte TR: Mechanisms of lead and manganese neurotoxicity, *Toxicol Res* 2:99-114, 2013.
14. Centers for Disease Control and Prevention (CDC): *Blood lead levels in children aged 1-5 years—United States, 1999-2010*, Atlanta, GA, 2013, Author.
15. United Nations Environmental Programme (UNEP): *Global mercury assessment 2013: sources, emissions, releases and environmental transport*, Geneva, Switzerland, 2013, UNEP Chemicals Branch.
16. Nassir F, Ibdah JA: Role of mitochondria in alcoholic liver disease, *World J Gastroenterol* 20(9):2136-2142, 2014.
17. Curtis BJ, et al: Epigenetic targets for reversing immune defects caused by alcohol exposure, *Alcohol Res* 35(1):97-113, 2013.
18. Govorko D, et al: Male germline transmits fetal alcohol adverse effect on hypothalamic proopiomelanocortin gene across generations, *Biol Psychiatry* 72:378-388, 2012.
19. Burd L, et al: Prenatal alcohol exposure, blood alcohol concentrations and alcohol elimination

rates for the mother, fetus and newborn, *J Perinatol* 32(9):652-659, 2012.

20. Centers for Disease Control and Prevention (CDC): *Drug overdose death data*, Atlanta GA, 2017, Centers for Disease Control and Prevention, National Center for Injury Prevention and Control, Division of Unintentional Injury Prevention, U.S. Department of Health & Human Services. Available at: https://www.cdc.gov/drugoverdose/data/statedeaths.html. (Accessed 8 March 2018).

21. Centers for Disease Control and Prevention (CDC): CDC 24/7: saving lives, protecting people. In *All injuries. Health, United States*, 2013.

22. Warner M, et al: Drugs most frequently involved in drug overdose deaths: United States, 2010-2014, *Natl Vital Stat Rep* 65(10):2016.

23. Centers for Disease Control and Prevention (CDC): *Drug overdose deaths*, Atlanta, GA, 2018, Centers for Disease Control and Prevention, National Center for Injury Prevention and Control, U.S. Department of Health & Human Services.

24. Centers for Disease Control and Prevention (CDC): *Important facts about falls*, Atlanta, GA, 2017, National Center for Injury Prevention and Control, U.S. Department of Health & Human Services.

25. Centers for Disease Control and Prevention (CDC): *Preventing sexual violence*, Atlanta, GA, 2019, Centers for Disease Control and Prevention, National Center for Injury Prevention and Control, U.S. Department of Health & Human Services.

26. Centers for Disease Control and Prevention (CDC): *Sports and recreation-related injuries*, Atlanta, GA, 2017, Centers for Disease Control and Prevention, National Center for Injury Prevention and Control, U.S. Department of Health & Human Services.

27. Abbasi J: Headline-grabbing study brings attention back to medical error, *J Am Med Assoc* 316(7):698-700, 2016.

28. Leape LL, Berwick DM: Five years after to err is human: what have we learned?, *J Am Med Assoc* 293(19):2384-2390, 2005.

29. James JT: A new, evidence-based estimate of patient harms associated with hospital care, *J Patient Saf* 9(3):122-128, 2013.

30. Hitomi J, et al: Identification of a molecular signaling network that regulates a cellular necrotic cell death pathway by a genome wide siRNA screen, *Cell* 135(7):1311-1323, 2008.

31. Moquin D, Chan F: The molecular regulation of programmed necrotic cell injury, *Trends Biochem Sci* 35(8):434-441, 2010.

32. Ge L, et al: The protein-vesicle network of autophagy, *Curr Opin Cell Biol* 29:18-24, 2014.

33. Levine B, et al: Autophagy in immunity and inflammation, *Nature* 469:323-335, 2011.

34. Belkaid Y, Hand TW: Role of the microbiota in immunity and inflammation, *Cell* 157(1):121-141, 2014.

35. Brodin P, et al: Variation in the human immune system is largely driven by non-heritable influences, *Cell* 160(1-2):37-47, 2015.

36. Rando TA, Chang HY: Aging rejuvenation, and epigenetic reprogramming: resetting the aging clock, *Cell* 148:46-57, 2012.

37. Bansal A, et al: Uncoupling lifespan and healthspan in Caenorhabditis elegans longevity mutants, *Proc Natl Acad Sci USA* 112(3):E277-E286, 2015.

38. Walston JD: Frailty. Preface, *Clin Geriatr Med* 27(1):xi, 2011.

39. Shennan T: *Postmortems and morbid anatomy*, ed 3, Baltimore, 1935, William Wood.

40. Riley MW: Foreword: the gender paradox. In Ory MG, Warner HR, editors: *Gender, health, and longevity: multidisciplinary perspectives*, New York, 1990, Springer.

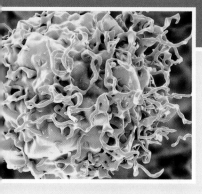

5

Fluids and Electrolytes, Acids and Bases

Lois E. Brenneman, Sue E. Huether

EVOLVE WEBSITE

http://evolve.elsevier.com/Huether/
Student Review Questions
Audio Key Points

Case Studies
Animations
Quick Check Answers

CHAPTER OUTLINE

The cells of the body live in a fluid environment where electrolyte and acid–base concentrations are maintained within a narrow range. Changes in electrolyte concentration affect the electrical activity of nerve and muscle cells, resulting in fluid shifts from one compartment to another. Alterations in acid–base balance disrupt cell functions. Fluid fluctuations also affect blood volume. Disturbances in these functions are common and can be life-threatening. Understanding how alterations occur and how the body compensates for the disturbance is key to understanding many pathophysiologic conditions.

DISTRIBUTION OF BODY FLUIDS AND ELECTROLYTES

The sum of all fluids within body compartments constitutes the total body water (TBW)—about 60% of body weight in adults (Table 5.1). The volume of TBW is usually expressed as a percentage of body weight in kilograms. One liter of water weighs 2.2 lb (1 kg). The remainder of the body weight is composed of fat and fat-free solids, particularly bone. The total volume of body water for a person weighing 154 lb (70 kg) is about 42 liters.

Body fluids are distributed among functional compartments, sometimes called *spaces*, and provide a transport medium for cellular and tissue function. Intracellular fluid (ICF) is all the fluid within cells and comprises about two-thirds of TBW. The distribution of intracellular water in females is less due to larger amounts of subcutaneous tissue and smaller muscle mass. Extracellular fluid (ECF) is all the fluid outside the cells and comprises about one-third of TBW. ECF includes the interstitial fluid, the intravascular fluid, and the various transcellular fluids (Table 5.2). The interstitial fluid is the fluid found in the spaces between cells but not within the blood vessels. The intravascular fluid is the fluid found within blood vessels; it is more commonly known as the blood plasma. The transcellular fluids, the smallest component of extracellular fluids, are the fluids contained within epithelial-lined cavities of the body. Examples of transcellular fluid include synovial fluid, cerebral spinal fluid, gastrointestinal fluids, pleural fluids, pericardial fluids, peritoneal fluids, and urine. *Sweat* is yet another component of the extracellular fluid. Derived directly from the interstitial fluid, sweat is released through pores onto the skin in varying amounts as a function of physiologic and environmental conditions. Sweating and lung ventilation are two major sources of insensible fluid loss. Insensible losses must be replaced regularly, usually by drinking fluids, to maintain fluid balance.

Electrolytes and other solutes are distributed throughout the intracellular and extracellular fluids (Table 5.3). Note that the extracellular fluid contains a large amount of *sodium* and *chloride* and smaller amounts of *potassium*. Intracellular fluid contains larger amounts of potassium with smaller amounts of sodium and chloride. An active energy-requiring physiologic pump maintains these differences in the electrolyte concentration. The concentrations of *phosphates* and *magnesium* are greater in the intracellular fluid; the concentration of *calcium* is greater in the extracellular fluid. These differences in electrolyte concentration are important in maintaining several physiologic functions: *electroneutrality* between the extracellular and intracellular compartments, the

TABLE 5.1 Total Body Water as a Percentage of Body Weight

Body Build	Adult Male	Adult Female	Child (1–10 yr)	Infant (1 mo–1 yr)	Newborn (Up to 1 mo)
Normal	60	50	65	70	70–80
Lean	70	60	50–60	80	
Obese	50	42	50	60	

TABLE 5.2 Distribution of Body Water (70-kg Adult)

Fluid Compartment	% of Body Weight	Volume (L)
Intracellular fluid (ICF)	40 (males)	28
	30 (females)	21
Extracellular fluid (ECF)	20 male and female	14
Interstitial	15	11
Intravascular	5	3
Total body water (TBW)	60 (males)	42
	50 (females)	35

TABLE 5.3 Representative Distribution of Electrolytes in Body Compartments*

Electrolytes	ECF (mEq/L)	ICF (mEq/L)
Cations		
Sodium	142	12
Potassium	4.2	150
Calcium	5	0
Magnesium	2	24
TOTAL	*153.2*	*186*
Anions		
Bicarbonate	24	12
Chloride	103	4
Phosphate	2	100
Proteins	16	65
Other anions	8	6
TOTAL	*153*	*187*

*Values may vary slightly among different laboratories.
ECF, Extracellular fluid; *ICF,* intracellular fluid.

TABLE 5.4 Normal Water Gains and Losses (70-kg Adult)

	Daily Intake (mL)		Daily Output (mL)
Drinking	1400–1800	Urine	1400–1800
Water in food	700–1000	Stool	100
Water of oxidation	300–400	Skin	300–500
		Lungs	600–800
TOTAL	2400–3200	**TOTAL**	2400–3200

and ingesting foods and from secondary to oxidative metabolism are the primary sources of body water. Most water is lost through renal excretion; relatively smaller amounts are lost through stool and through insensible loss from perspiration and ventilation (Table 5.4).

Water Movement Between Plasma and Interstitial Fluid

The distribution of water and the movement of nutrients and waste products between the capillary and interstitial spaces occur as a result of changes in hydrostatic pressure and osmotic/oncotic pressure. Hydrostatic pressure pushes water out of the capillaries; osmotic/oncotic pressure pulls water into the capillaries (see Fig. 1.24). Water, sodium, and glucose readily move across the capillary membrane. Under normal conditions, proteins (particularly albumin) do not cross the capillary membrane. They maintain physiologic osmolality by generating oncotic pressure within the plasma.

Filtration refers to fluid movement out of the capillary and into the interstitial space. *Reabsorption* refers to fluid movement into the capillary from the interstitial space. As plasma flows from the arterial to the venous end of the capillary, four forces determine whether the net effect is filtration or reabsorption. These forces, acting in concert, are described as **net filtration** or **Starling forces**:

1. **Capillary hydrostatic pressure (blood pressure)** facilitates the movement of water from the capillary into the interstitial space.
2. **Capillary (plasma) oncotic pressure** osmotically attracts water from the interstitial space into the capillary.
3. **Interstitial hydrostatic pressure** facilitates the inward movement of water from the interstitial space into the capillary.
4. **Interstitial oncotic pressure** osmotically attracts water from the capillary into the interstitial space.

The forces controlling the movement of fluid across the capillary wall are summarized by these equations:

$$Net\ filtration = (Forces\ favoring\ filtration)\ - (Forces\ opposing\ filtration)$$

$$Forces\ favoring\ filtration = Capillary\ hydrostatic\ pressure\ and\ interstitial\ oncotic\ pressure$$

$$Forces\ opposing\ filtration = Capillary\ oncotic\ pressure\ and\ interstitial\ hydrostatic\ pressure$$

At the *arterial end* of the capillary, hydrostatic pressure exceeds capillary oncotic pressure; thus fluid moves into the interstitial space (filtration). At the *venous end* of the capillary, oncotic pressure within the capillary exceeds capillary hydrostatic pressure; thus fluids move into the capillary to enter into the circulation (reabsorption). Interstitial hydrostatic pressure promotes the movement of approximately 10% of the interstitial fluid, along with small amounts of protein, into the lymphatics. Once the fluid enters the lymphatic system, it travels through

transmission of electrical impulses, and the movement of water among body compartments (see Chapter 1).

Although the amount of fluid within the various compartments is relatively constant, solutes and water are exchanged between compartments to maintain their unique compositions. The percentage of TBW varies with the amount of body fat and age. Fat is *hydrophobic* (water repelling), and very little water is contained in adipose (fat) cells. Individuals with more body fat have proportionately less TBW and tend to be more susceptible to dehydration.

The distribution and the amount of TBW change with age (see the *Pediatric Considerations* and *Geriatric Considerations* boxes). Although daily fluid intake may fluctuate widely, the body regulates water volume within a relatively narrow range. Water obtained from drinking fluids

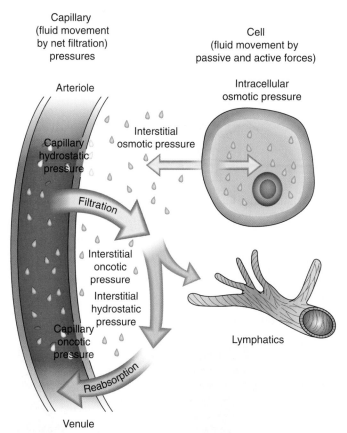

Capillary
(fluid movement
by net filtration)
pressures

Cell
(fluid movement by
passive and active forces)

Arteriole

Intracellular
osmotic pressure

Interstitial
osmotic pressure

Capillary
hydrostatic
pressure

Filtration

Interstitial
oncotic
pressure

Interstitial
hydrostatic
pressure

Capillary
oncotic
pressure

Lymphatics

Reabsorption

Venule

FIGURE 5.1 Net Filtration—Fluid Movement Between Plasma and Interstitial Space. The movement of fluid between the vascular, interstitial spaces and the lymphatics is the result of net filtration of fluid across the semipermeable capillary membrane. Capillary hydrostatic pressure is the primary force for fluid movement out of the arteriolar end of the capillary and into the interstitial space. At the venous end, capillary oncotic pressure (from plasma proteins) attracts water back into the vascular space. Interstitial hydrostatic pressure promotes the movement of fluid and proteins into the lymphatics. Osmotic pressure accounts for the movement of fluid between the interstitial space and the intracellular space. Normally intracellular and extracellular fluid osmotic pressures are equal (280 to 294 mOsm), and water is equally distributed between the interstitial and intracellular compartments.

progressively larger lymphatic vessels until it enters the systemic circulation. These two systems, the lymphatic and circulatory systems, connect at a location near the left internal jugular vein where the lymphatic thoracic duct joins the left subclavian vein. Because albumin does not normally cross the capillary membrane, interstitial oncotic pressure normally is minimal. Fig. 5.1 illustrates net filtration.

Water Movement Between ICF and ECF

Water moves between ICF and ECF compartments primarily as a function of osmotic forces (see Chapter 1). Water moves freely by diffusion through the lipid bilayer cell membrane and through aquaporins, a class of water channel proteins that are permeable to water.[1] Sodium is responsible for the osmotic balance of the ECF, and potassium maintains the ICF osmotic balance. The osmotic force of ICF proteins and other nondiffusible substances is balanced by the active transport of ions out of the cell. Water crosses cell membranes freely, thus the osmolality of TBW normally is at equilibrium. Under normal conditions, the ICF is not subject to rapid changes in osmolality; however, when the ECF osmolality changes, water moves from one

compartment to another until osmotic equilibrium is reestablished (see Fig. 5.8).

ALTERATIONS IN WATER MOVEMENT

Edema

Edema is the excessive accumulation of fluid within the interstitial spaces. It results from a shift of fluid from the capillaries (intravascular fluid) or lymphatic vessels into the tissues (Fig. 5.2). Physiologic conditions that promote fluid flow into the tissues include (1) increased capillary hydrostatic pressure, (2) decreased plasma oncotic pressure, (3) increased capillary membrane permeability, and (4) lymphatic channel obstruction.

PATHOPHYSIOLOGY *Capillary hydrostatic pressure* increases as a direct result of either venous obstruction or salt and water retention. *Venous obstruction* results in an increased hydrostatic pressure behind the obstruction, pushing fluid from the capillaries into the interstitial spaces. Common causes of venous obstruction include thrombophlebitis (inflammation of veins), hepatic obstruction, tight clothing around the extremities, and prolonged standing. Similarly, *excessive salt and water retention* results in edema secondary to plasma volume overload. The overload produces an increased capillary hydrostatic pressure. Common predisposing causes include congestive heart failure, renal failure, and cirrhosis of the liver.

Decreased plasma oncotic pressure occurs when production of plasma proteins, especially albumin, is lost or diminished. Plasma albumin functions to attract and hold water within blood vessels. Decreased albumin—commonly seen in liver disease or protein malnutrition—results in a decrease of plasma oncotic pressure. Fluid remains in the interstitial spaces instead of filtering into the systemic circulation through the capillaries. As fluid accumulates within the tissues, edema worsens. Common causes of plasma protein loss include glomerular diseases of the kidney, serous drainage from open wounds, hemorrhage, burns, and cirrhosis of the liver.

Increased capillary membrane permeability, resulting in edema, occurs with inflammation and immune responses. The increased vessel permeability permits proteins to escape from within blood vessels (the vascular space) into the interstitial space, producing edema. This edema results from decreased capillary oncotic pressure and interstitial fluid protein accumulation. Common triggers include trauma, especially burns or crushing injuries; neoplastic disease; and allergic reactions. Inflammation invariably results in some measure of increased vascular permeability with edema at the site of the injury. The extent of the edema typically is a function of the amount of tissue damage. Allergic reactions can produce profound edema, including life-threatening laryngeal edema (closed-off airway), depending on the extent of vascular permeability.

Lymphatic channel obstruction, causing edema, occurs when lymphatic channels are blocked.[2] The lymphatic system normally absorbs interstitial fluid, along with small amounts of protein. These substances travel through a *one-way system* of progressively larger lymphatic vessels until they are returned to the systemic circulation. When lymphatic channels are blocked or surgically removed, proteins and fluid accumulate within the interstitial space, causing lymphedema. Lymphedema of the arm or, less commonly, the leg can occur after surgical removal of axillary or femoral lymph nodes, a procedure commonly performed during resection (cutting out) of malignant tumors (Fig. 5.3). Other causes of lymphedema include radiation therapy, obstruction from malignant tumors, and infection.

CLINICAL MANIFESTATIONS Edema can be can be identified by pressing on tissues overlying bony prominences. An indentation or pit left in

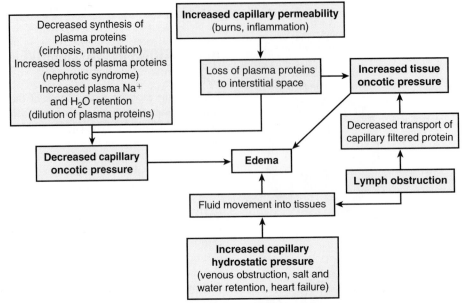

FIGURE 5.2 Mechanisms of Edema Formation.

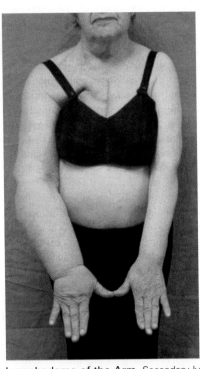

FIGURE 5.3 **Lymphedema of the Arm.** Secondary lymphedema of the upper extremity in an 82-year-old female with right upper extremity lymphedema 2 years after mastectomy, radiation therapy, and lymphadenectomy for breast cancer. (From Slavin SA, Schook CC, Greene AK: Lymphedema management. In Davis MP et al, editors: *Supportive oncology,* Philadelphia, 2011, Elsevier/Saunders, pp 211-210. Available at www.sciencedirect.com: http://dx.doi.org/10.1016/B978-1-4377-1015-1.00021-7.)

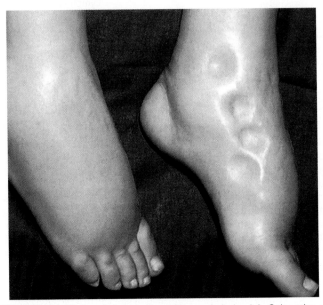

FIGURE 5.4 **Pitting Edema.** (From Bloom A, Ireland J: *Color atlas of diabetes,* ed 2, St Louis, 1992, Mosby.)

the skin indicates the presence of edema, hence the term *pitting edema* (Fig. 5.4). Edema may be localized or generalized. *Localized edema* usually is limited to a single body region, often at the site where trauma has occurred, as might be seen with a sprained ankle. Localized edema also may occur within an organ of the body. Common examples include cerebral, pulmonary, and laryngeal edema. Fluid accumulation within a body cavity or space is referred to as an *effusion.* Examples include a

pleural effusion (fluid accumulation in the pleural space) and a *pericardial effusion* (fluid accumulation within the membrane surrounding the heart). Localized edema can be life-threatening when vital organs are involved (e.g., the brain, lung, or larynx). *Generalized edema* is characterized by a more uniform distribution of fluid within the interstitial spaces throughout the body. *Anasarca* refers to a severe generalized edema. *Dependent edema* occurs when fluid accumulates in gravity-dependent areas of the body and may be a precursor to more generalized edema. Dependent edema appears in the feet and legs when standing and in the sacral area and buttocks when supine.

Edema is associated with weight gain, swelling and puffiness, tight-fitting clothes or shoes, and limited movement of affected joints. It usually presents along with symptoms associated with the underlying pathologic condition. Fluid accumulations increase the distance required for nutrients and waste products to travel between capillaries and tissues. Blood flow may be impaired. Accordingly, wounds heal more slowly, and the risk of infection or decubiti (pressure sores) increase. The region where edematous fluid accumulates is referred to as a *third space (interstitial space);* the term *third spacing* sometimes is used to refer to the process of edema formation. Fluid trapped in such spaces is unavailable for metabolic processes or perfusion. Common third space sites include interstitial regions, pleural membranes (pleural effusion), and the space between the heart the pericardial membrane (pericardial effusion). Although the person with generalized edema appears swollen because of excess fluid, dehydration can develop as a result of the fluid sequestering. When severe edema is treated with *diuretics* (a drug or drug class that promotes kidney excretion of sodium and water), it is not uncommon for an individual to appear *cachectic* (severe loss of weight and muscle mass) after the excess fluid has been eliminated. With severe burns, large amounts of vascular fluid are lost into the interstitial spaces and shock often occurs secondary to the resulting reduced blood volume (see Chapter 26).

Clinically, lymphedema presents differently from edema secondary to fluid accumulation from the capillaries. With edema from capillary sources, the edematous tissue is easily compressed (i.e., pitting edema). By contrast, lymphedema is firm and noncompressible. In severe cases, lymphedema can be profound and causes gross enlargement and distortion of the body parts affected.

EVALUATION AND TREATMENT Medical treatment for edema varies, depending on the underlying conditions that cause fluid retention. Edema may be treated symptomatically, commonly with diuretics, until the underlying disorder has been corrected. In addition to diuretics, symptomatic treatment includes elevating edematous limbs, applying compression stockings, avoiding prolonged standing, and restricting salt intake. Administration of intravenous (IV) albumin may be required in severe cases.

✔ **QUICK CHECK 5.1**
1. How does an increase in capillary hydrostatic pressure cause edema?
2. How does a decrease in capillary oncotic pressure cause edema?
3. What are possible consequences of edema? How is edema treated?

SODIUM, CHLORIDE, AND WATER BALANCE

The combined influences of the renal and endocrine systems have a central role in maintaining sodium and water balance. Because water follows the osmotic gradients established by changes in salt concentration, the sodium concentration and water balance are integrally related. The sodium concentration is regulated by the renal effects of *aldosterone* (see Fig. 31.9). Water balance is regulated primarily by **antidiuretic hormone (ADH)**, also known as *vasopressin*, and is discussed in the Water Balance section.

Sodium (Na^+) accounts for 90% of the ECF cations (positively charged ions) (see Table 5.3). Sodium in concert with chloride and bicarbonate, the two major anions (negatively charged ions), acts to regulate water balance by contributing to extracellular osmotic forces. Sodium has an important role in several other physiologic functions, including nerve impulse conduction (see Fig. 1.31), regulation of the acid–base balance, cellular biochemistry, and the transport of substances across the cellular membrane.

The serum sodium concentration normally is maintained within a narrow range (135 to 145 mEq/L) by renal tubular reabsorption within the kidney in response to neural and hormonal influences. Hormonal regulation of sodium (and potassium) balance is mediated by **aldosterone**, a mineralocorticoid synthesized and secreted from the adrenal cortex. Aldosterone is a component of the **renin-angiotensin-aldosterone**

system (see Chapters 19 and 31). Aldosterone secretion is influenced by a number of factors, including circulating blood volume, blood pressure, and plasma concentrations of sodium and potassium. When the circulating blood volume or blood pressure is reduced, **renin**, an enzyme secreted by the juxtaglomerular cells of the kidney, is released. Renin also is released when sodium levels are depressed or potassium levels are increased. Once released, renin stimulates the formation of **angiotensin I**, an inactive polypeptide, from *angiotensinogen*, a substance secreted by the liver. *Angiotensin-converting enzyme (ACE)*, found primarily in pulmonary vessels and to a lesser extent in endothelial and renal epithelial cells, converts angiotensin I to **angiotensin II**, a potent vasoconstrictor. Vasoconstriction elevates blood pressure and restores renal perfusion. Restoring renal perfusion inhibits further release of renin. Angiotensin II also stimulates both the secretion of aldosterone from the adrenal cortex and antidiuretic hormone from the posterior pituitary. Aldosterone promotes sodium and water reabsorption, in addition to the excretion of potassium within the renal tubules. The net effect is to increase blood volume (Fig. 5.5; also see Fig. 31.9).

Drugs used for the treatment of hypertension include angiotensin-converting enzyme (ACE) inhibitors and angiotensin receptor blockers, which are well-tolerated. Both of these classes of drugs inhibit the renin-angiotensin-aldosterone system and lower blood pressure. Direct renin inhibitors are a third class of antihypertensive drugs. They are used less commonly because of their less favorable safety profile.

Natriuretic peptides are hormones primarily produced by the myocardium. Atrial natriuretic hormone (ANH) is produced by the atria. B-type natriuretic peptide (BNP) is produced by the ventricles. Urodilatin (an ANP analogue) is synthesized within the kidney. Natriuretic peptides are released when the transmural atrial pressure increases (increased volume), which commonly occurs with congestive heart failure or when the mean arterial pressure increases (Fig. 5.6). Measurement of BNP is used as a means to assist with the initial diagnosis and management of people with congestive heart failure.[3] These hormones are natural antagonists to the renin-angiotensin-aldosterone system. Natriuretic peptides cause vasodilation and increase sodium and water excretion, decreasing blood pressure. Natriuretic peptides sometimes are called a "third factor" in sodium regulation. An increased glomerular filtration rate is considered to be the first factor, and aldosterone is considered to be the second factor.

Chloride (Cl^-) is the major anion in the ECF and provides electroneutrality, particularly in relation to sodium. Chloride transport generally is passive and follows the active transport of sodium. Increases or decreases in chloride concentration are proportional to changes in sodium concentration. Chloride concentration tends to vary inversely with changes in the concentration of bicarbonate (HCO_3^-), the other major anion.

Water balance is regulated by the secretion of ADH, also known as **vasopressin**. ADH is produced in the posterior pituitary and secreted when plasma osmolality increases or circulating blood volume decreases, causing a drop in blood pressure (Fig. 5.7). Increased Plasma osmolality occurs when there is a decrease in water or an excess concentration of sodium in relation to total body water. The increased osmolality stimulates hypothalamic **osmoreceptors**, resulting in thirst. Thirst, in turn, stimulates the individual to consume liquids, thus increasing total body water. In addition to stimulating thirst, the osmoreceptors signal the posterior pituitary gland to release ADH, a hormone that increases water reabsorption from the renal distal tubules and collecting ducts into the plasma (see Chapter 31). The net effect of both increased water intake and increased renal reabsorption of water is to decrease plasma osmolality, returning it to a normal status. Urine concentration increases as less water is excreted into the urine.

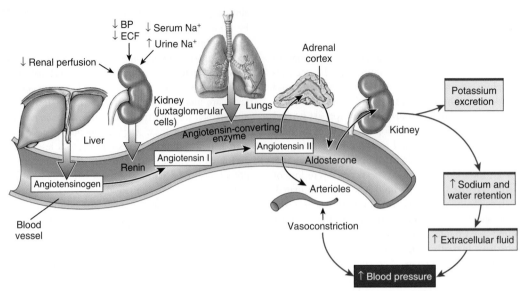

FIGURE 5.5 **The Renin-Angiotensin-Aldosterone System.** *BP,* blood pressure; *ECF,* extracellular fluid; *Na+,* sodium ion. (Modified from Herlihy B, Maebius N: *The human body in health and disease,* ed 4, Philadelphia, 2011, Saunders. Borrowed from Lewis SL et al: *Medical-surgical nursing: assessment and management of clinical problems,* ed 9, St Louis, 2014, Mosby.)

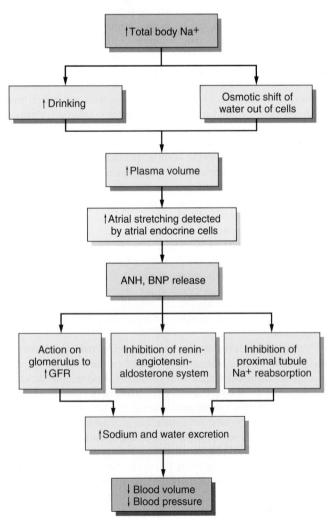

FIGURE 5.6 **The Natriuretic Peptide System.** *ANH,* Atrial natriuretic hormone; *BNP,* brain natriuretic peptide; *GFR,* glomerular filtration rate; *Na+,* sodium ion.

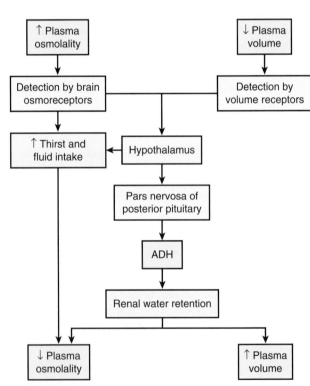

FIGURE 5.7 **The Antidiuretic Hormone (ADH) System.**

With dehydration (fluid loss) secondary to vomiting, diarrhea, or excessive sweating, a decrease in systemic blood volume and blood pressure often follows. **Volume-sensitive receptors** and **baroreceptors,** both of which are nerve endings sensitive to changes in blood volume and pressure, also stimulate thirst and the release of pituitary ADH, which prompts fluid consumption. The volume receptors are located in the right and left atria and in the thoracic vessels; baroreceptors are found in the aorta, pulmonary arteries, and carotid sinus. Additionally, ADH secretion is increased when atrial pressure drops. Such pressure drops occur with a decrease in blood volume (see Fig. 31.9).

ADH-mediated reabsorption of water follows, restoring normal status for plasma volume and blood pressure (see Fig. 5.7).

✔ QUICK CHECK 5.2

1. What forces promote net filtration?
2. How do hormones regulate salt and water balance?
3. Where are volume and baroreceptors located and how do they function?

ALTERATIONS IN SODIUM, CHLORIDE, AND WATER BALANCE

Alterations in sodium and water balance are closely related. Sodium imbalances occur with gains or losses of body water. Water imbalances develop with gains or losses of salt. These alterations can be classified as changes in *tonicity* (i.e., the change in the concentration of solutes in relation to the amount of water present). Normal plasma osmolality is 280 milliosmoles [mOsm]/kg. Solutions are classified as isotonic, hypertonic, or hypotonic as a function of the solute concentration compared with that of normal body cells (Table 5.5 and Fig. 5.8; also see Fig. 1.25. *Isotonic solutions* have solute concentrations that are equal to that of normal cells; *hypertonic* or *hypotonic* solutions have more or less solute concentration, respectively. Changes in tonicity (solute concentration) affect the volume of water within the intracellular and

TABLE 5.5	**Water and Solute Imbalances**
Tonicity	**Mechanism**
Isotonic (isoosmolar) imbalance Serum osmolality = 280–294 mOsm/kg	Gain or loss of ECF resulting in concentration equivalent to 0.9% sodium chloride solution (normal saline); no shrinking or swelling of cells
Hypertonic (hyperosmolar) imbalance Serum osmolality >294 mOsm/kg	Imbalances that result in ECF concentration >0.9% salt solution (i.e., water loss or solute gain); cells shrink in hypertonic fluid
Hypotonic (hypoosmolar) imbalance Serum osmolality <280 mOsm/kg	Imbalance that results in ECF <0.9% salt solution (i.e., water gain or solute loss); cells swell in hypotonic fluid
Formula for calculating serum osmolarity	$(2 \times [Na] + [Glu])/18 + BUN/2.8$

BUN, Blood serum urea nitrogen level (mg/dl); *ECF*, extracellular fluid; *[Glu]*, serum glucose concentration (mg/dl); *[Na]*, serum sodium concentration (mEq/dL).

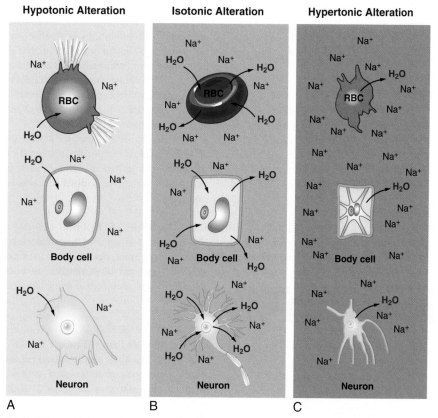

Hypotonic Alteration   **Isotonic Alteration**   **Hypertonic Alteration**

A   B   C

FIGURE 5.8 Effects of Alterations in Extracellular Sodium Concentration in RBC, Body Cell, and Neuron. A, Hypotonic alteration: Decrease in ECF sodium (Na⁺) concentration (hyponatremia) results in ICF osmotic attraction of water with swelling and potential bursting of cells. **B,** Isotonic alteration: Normal concentration of sodium in the ECF and no change in shifts of fluid into or out of cells. **C,** Hypertonic alteration: Increase in ECF sodium concentration (hypernatremia) results in osmotic attraction of water out of cells with cell shrinkage. *ECF,* Extracellular fluid; *H₂O,* water; *ICF,* intracellular fluid; *Na⁺,* sodium ion; *RBC,* red blood cell.

extracellular compartments, resulting in *isovolemia*, *hypervolemia*, or *hypovolemia*—that is, normal volume, excess volume, or less than normal volume in the blood, respectively.

Isotonic Fluid Alterations

Isotonic fluid alterations are the most common and occur when TBW changes are accompanied by proportional changes in the concentrations of electrolytes (see Fig. 5.8). Isotonic fluid loss causes hypovolemia. Causes include hemorrhage, severe wound drainage, excessive diaphoresis (sweating), and inadequate fluid intake. Clinically the person has a loss of extracellular fluid volume with weight loss, dry skin and mucous membranes, decreased urine output, and symptoms of hypovolemia. Indicators of hypovolemia include a rapid heart rate, flattened neck veins, and normal or decreased blood pressure. In severe states, hypovolemic shock can occur (see Chapter 26). Treatment includes fluid replacement with isotonic solutions, given either intravenously or orally. IV replacements include 0.9% normal saline solution (NS solution), 5% dextrose in normal saline solution (D5NS solution) or Ringer's lactate (RL) solution. A variety of sports oral replacement beverages and pediatric oral replacement solutions are available, without a prescription, for oral fluid replacement with isotonic solutions.

Isotonic fluid excess causes hypervolemia. Common causes include excessive administration of IV fluids, hypersecretion of aldosterone, or the effects of drugs such as cortisone (which causes renal reabsorption of sodium and water). As plasma volume expands, hypervolemia with weight gain develops. The diluting effect of excess plasma volume leads to a decreased hematocrit and decreased plasma protein concentration. The neck veins may distend, and the blood pressure increases. Increased capillary hydrostatic pressure leads to edema formation. Pulmonary edema and heart failure frequently develop. These presentations may be acute or chronic, depending on the underlying pathophysiology causing the fluid overload. Diuretics are commonly used for treatment.

Hypertonic Fluid Alterations

Hypertonic fluid alterations develop when the osmolality of the ECF is elevated above normal (>294 mOsm). The most common causes are hypernatremia (increased concentration of ECF sodium) or a deficit of ECF water, or both. In either case, the ECF hypertonicity attracts water from the intracellular space, causing ICF dehydration (see Fig. 5.8). Dehydration refers to water deficit.[4] The symptoms are summarized in Box 5.1.

Hypernatremia

PATHOPHYSIOLOGY   Hypernatremia occurs when serum sodium levels exceed 145 mEq/L. Increased levels of serum sodium cause hypertonicity.[5] Water is redistributed osmotically to the hypertonic extracellular space, causing intracellular dehydration. Hypernatremia can be isovolemic, hypovolemic, or hypervolemic, depending on the accompanying ECF water volume.

Isovolemic (euvolemic) hypernatremia is the most common presentation. It occurs when a deficit of free water is accompanied by normal or near-normal body sodium concentration. The most common causes include inadequate water intake, excessive sweating (sweat is hypotonic), fever, vomiting, diarrhea, burns, or respiratory tract infections. Both fever and respiratory infections result in an increased ventilatory rate with enhanced water loss from rapid breathing. A less common cause of isovolemic hypernatremia is diabetes insipidus, which results from a central lack of ADH (e.g., it is not released from the posterior pituitary), or nephrogenic diabetes insipidus (an inadequate renal response to ADH). Infants with severe diarrhea are vulnerable and at increased risk because they cannot communicate thirst. Insufficient water intake occurs particularly in individuals who are comatose, confused, or immobilized and in those who are receiving gastric feedings.

Hypovolemic hypernatremia occurs when a loss of sodium is accompanied by a relatively greater loss of body water. Common causes include use of loop diuretics (diuretics that inhibit sodium and chloride reabsorption in the kidney loop of Henle) or renal failure in which the kidneys fail to concentrate urine and excrete a large volume of urine. Osmotic diuresis from diabetes-induced hyperglycemia or the use of mannitol (an osmotic diuretic) also can result in hypovolemic hypernatremia.

Hypervolemic hypernatremia is rare. It occurs when an increase in total body water is accompanied by a greater increase in total body sodium level, resulting in hypervolemia. One cause is infusion of hypertonic saline solutions in an effort to replace sodium in cases of salt depletion. The salt depletion might occur with renal impairment, heart failure, or gastrointestinal losses. Other causes include oversecretion of adrenocorticotropic hormone (ACTH) or aldosterone, as might occur with Cushing syndrome or adrenal hyperplasia. High amounts of dietary sodium rarely cause hypernatremia in a healthy individual because the sodium is eliminated by the kidneys.

Because chloride follows sodium, hyperchloremia, defined as an elevation of serum chloride concentration greater than 105 mEq/L, often accompanies hypernatremia.[6] Plasma bicarbonate deficits, as would occur with metabolic acidosis (discussed later in this chapter), also occur.

CLINICAL MANIFESTATIONS   Central nervous system signs are the most serious signs of hypernatremia and are related to alterations in membrane potentials and shrinking of brain cells (sodium cannot cross brain capillaries because of their tight endothelial junctions). Clinical manifestations of hypernatremia are summarized in Table 5.6.

EVALUATION AND TREATMENT   With hypernatremia, serum sodium levels are greater than 145 mEq/L and urine specific gravity is greater than 1.030. The history and physical examination provide information about underlying disorders and events. Treatment for isovolemic hyponatremia is to give oral water, IV dextrose 5% in water, or 0.45% normal saline. Treatment for hypovolemic hypernatremia is to give oral fluids or isotonic salt-free IV fluid (5% dextrose in water) until the serum sodium level returns to normal. Fluid replacement must be given slowly to prevent cerebral edema. Treatment for hypervolemic hypernatremia is to administer loop diuretics. Serum sodium levels must be monitored throughout treatment. The underlying clinical condition also must be addressed.

BOX 5.1   Signs and Symptoms of Dehydration

Increased serum sodium concentration (hypernatremia due to water loss)	Elevated temperature
Thirst	Soft eyeballs
Headache	Sunken fontanels in infants
Weight loss	Prolonged capillary refill time
Oliguria and concentrated urine	Tachycardia
Hard stools	Weak pulses
Decreased skin turgor	Low blood pressure
Dry mucous membranes	Postural hypotension
Decreased sweating and tears	Hypovolemic shock
	Confusion
	Coma

TABLE 5.6 Signs and Symptoms of Sodium Imbalance

Isovolemic Hypernatremia	Isovolemic Hyponatremia
Thirst; tongue and mucosa are dry and sticky	Anorexia, nausea, cramps
Weakness, lethargy, agitation	Fatigue, lethargy, muscle weakness
Edema	Headache, confusion, seizures
Elevated blood pressure	Decreased blood pressure
Hypervolemic Hypernatremia	**Hypervolemic Hyponatremia**
Thirst	Nausea and vomiting
Weight gain	Diarrhea
Increased blood pressure	Abdominal cramping
Peripheral edema	Weight gain
Pulmonary edema	Increased blood pressure
Restlessness	Headache
Agitation	Apathy
Muscle twitching	Confusion
Seizures	Muscle twitching
Coma	Seizures
	Coma
Hypovolemic Hypernatremia	**Hypovolemic Hyponatremia**
Thirst	Dry mucous membranes
Dry, sticky mucous membranes	Postural hypotension
Postural hypotension	Tachycardia, thread pulse
Weakness	Irritability, apprehension
Lethargy	Confusion
	Dizziness
	Tremors
	Seizures
	Coma

Hypotonic Fluid Alterations

Hypotonic fluid imbalances occur when the osmolality of the ECF is less than 280 mOsm (see Fig. 5.8). The most common causes are sodium deficit or water excess. Either problem leads to *intracellular overhydration* (cellular edema) and cellular swelling. When there is a sodium deficit, the osmotic pressure of the ECF decreases; water moves into the cell, where the higher osmotic pressure pulls it in. As water leaves the ECF, plasma volume decreases, resulting in symptoms of hypovolemia. Excess water results in increases in both the ICF and ECF fluid volume, causing symptoms of hypervolemia and water intoxication; cerebral and pulmonary edema can occur in such scenarios.

Hyponatremia

PATHOPHYSIOLOGY Hyponatremia develops when the serum sodium concentration falls below 135 mEq/L. Hyponatremia results from a loss of sodium, inadequate intake of sodium, or sodium dilution secondary to excess water. Sodium depletion usually causes a decrease in osmolality with an associated movement of water into cells. Cell membrane rupture may then occur.

Isovolemic hyponatremia occurs when there is loss of sodium without a significant loss of water (pure sodium deficit). Causes include water retention secondary to the *syndrome of inappropriate antidiuretic*

hormone (SIADH) (see Chapter 20), hypothyroidism, pneumonia, and glucocorticoid deficiency. Inadequate intake of dietary sodium is rare but possible in individuals on low-sodium diets, particularly when diuretics also are used.

Hypervolemic hyponatremia occurs when the total body sodium level increases. The increased sodium leads to an increase in total body water and the dilution of sodium in the extracellular space. Causes include congestive heart failure, cirrhosis of the liver, and nephrotic syndrome. Edema typically is present in these cases.

Hypovolemic hyponatremia occurs with a loss of total body water and a greater loss of body sodium. The extracellular volume is decreased. Causes include prolonged vomiting, severe diarrhea, inadequate secretion of aldosterone (adrenal insufficiency), and renal losses from diuretics.

Dilutional hyponatremia (water intoxication) occurs with an oral intake of a large amount of free water or with inappropriate IV administration of 5% dextrose in water (D5W) to replace fluid loss. The net effect in either case is to dilute sodium. The glucose from the D5W is metabolized to carbon dioxide and water, resulting in a dilutional effect. Excessive sweating stimulates thirst. If large amounts of free water are consumed orally, sodium dilution can occur. This scenario can occur with endurance sports in which the athlete consumes large amounts of water instead of sports drinks containing electrolytes. Individuals with psychogenic disorders have developed water intoxication from compulsive water drinking. Other causes can include tap water enemas, near-drowning in fresh water, and the use of selective serotonin reuptake inhibitors (SSRIs). When the body is functioning normally, producing an excess of TBW is almost impossible because water balance is regulated by the kidneys.

Hypochloremia, a serum chloride level of less than 97 mEq/L, usually occurs secondary to hyponatremia or an elevated bicarbonate concentration. This scenario might occur with metabolic alkalosis (discussed later in this chapter). Sodium deficits related to restricted intake, use of diuretics, vomiting, or nasogastric suction is accompanied by a chloride deficiency. Cystic fibrosis may present with hypochloremia (see Chapter 30). Treatment is aimed at addressing the underlying cause.

CLINICAL MANIFESTATIONS Serum sodium concentration is less than 135 mEq/L, and with severe sodium deficits, the concentration is less than 120 mEq/L. Sodium depletion usually causes a decreased serum osmolality. The high concentration of intracellular solutes, compared to the low concentration of extracellular solutes (hyponatremia), causes an osmotic shift of water into the cells, and cell swelling occurs. A decrease in the sodium concentration changes the cell's ability to depolarize and repolarize normally, altering the action potential in neurons and muscle (see Chapter 1). Clinical manifestations are related to impaired nerve conduction and neurologic changes (see Table 5.6). The most life-threatening consequence is cerebral edema and increased intracranial pressure. Hyponatremia is a major cause of morbidity and mortality among individuals hospitalized in intensive care units and in the elderly.

Hyponatremia among the elderly is the most common of the electrolyte disorders, and the prevalence is highest among elderly hospitalized individuals. Isovolemic hyponatremia, resulting from SIADH, is thought to be the most common cause. Predisposing factors include central nervous system injury, pulmonary disease, malignancies, nausea, pain, and changes related to aging. Other contributing factors include use of thiazide diuretics, use of proton pump inhibitors, dehydration secondary to an age-related decrease in thirst, and diminished urine concentrating ability. Common consequences of hyponatremia include cognitive deficits, gait disturbances, falls with fractures, the need for long-term care, and death. Assessing for risk factors and implementing preventive strategies are particularly important for the elderly; early intervention is the key to preventing the serious consequences of hyponatremia.

EVALUATION AND TREATMENT   Treatment includes identifying and correcting the underlying etiology of the hyponatremia. Small amounts of IV hypertonic sodium chloride (3% sodium chloride) can be given when neurologic manifestations are severe; however, it must be administered slowly to avoid osmotic demyelination syndrome in the brain. This occurs when the serum sodium concentration is 120 mEq/L or less and sodium is replaced too fast. Brain cells shrink, and the myelin sheath is destroyed, particularly in the pons. Symptoms include tremor and ataxia (loss of control of body movements). Water restriction is required in most cases of dilutional hyponatremia. ADH receptor antagonists (vaptans) are a class of drugs used for the treatment of hypervolemic and euvolemic hyponatremia.[7] The serum sodium concentration must be closely monitored throughout treatment.

✔ **QUICK CHECK 5.3**
1. What are the causes of isotonic fluid imbalance?
2. What are some causes of hypernatremia?
3. What is the most severe complication of hyponatremia? Who is most at risk?

ALTERATIONS IN POTASSIUM AND OTHER ELECTROLYTES

Potassium

Potassium (K^+) is the major intracellular electrolyte. It is essential for normal cellular functions. The total body potassium content is about 4000 mEq, with 98% located in the cells. The ICF concentration of potassium is 150 to 160 mEq/L; the ECF potassium concentration is 3.5 to 5.0 mEq/L. This concentration gradient is maintained by an *active transport system,* the sodium-potassium adenosinetriphosphatase pump (Na^+-K^+ ATPase pump) (see Fig. 1.26. As with all active transport pumps, the system requires energy derived from adenosine triphosphate (ATP).

As the predominant ICF ion, potassium exerts a major influence on the regulation of ICF osmolality and fluid balance. Potassium also influences the intracellular electrical status in relation to hydrogen (H^+) and sodium. Potassium maintains the resting membrane potential, as reflected in the conduction of nerve impulses (see Fig. 1.30). Other physiologic functions of potassium include facilitating glycogen and glucose deposition in liver and skeletal muscle cells, maintaining normal cardiac rhythm, and having a role in the contraction of both skeletal and smooth muscle (see *Did You Know? Potassium Intake: Hypertension and Stroke*).

- Dietary potassium moves rapidly into the cells after ingestion; however, the distribution of potassium between the intracellular and extracellular fluids is influenced by several factors. Insulin, aldosterone, epinephrine, and alkalosis all facilitate the shift of potassium into cells. Insulin deficiency, aldosterone deficiency, acidosis, cell lysis, and strenuous exercise promote a shift of potassium out of cells. Glucagon blocks entry of potassium into cells; glucocorticoids promote potassium excretion. Potassium also moves out of cells, along with water, with an increased ECF osmolarity.

Although potassium is found in most body fluids, the kidney is the most significant regulator of potassium balance. Potassium is freely filtered by the renal glomerulus; 90% is reabsorbed by the proximal tubule and loop of Henle. In the distal tubules, *principal cells* secrete

---

DID YOU KNOW?
Potassium Intake: Hypertension and Stroke

An adequate dietary intake of potassium (3500 mg per day) is associated with a lower risk of hypertension and stroke. The American diet often exceeds recommendations for sodium intake but is deficient in potassium intake. The risk for hypertension, cardiovascular disease, and mortality increases with a high plasma ratio of sodium to potassium concentration. Potassium attenuates the effects of high dietary salt, and blood pressure decreases, as does the risk for stroke and cardiovascular disease. The exact mechanism of this dynamic is unclear. Likely mechanisms include renal management of sodium, endothelial cell functioning, decreased vascular resistance, and reduced oxidative stress. Lower mortality rates were demonstrated for all women with a higher potassium intake. In the absence of compromised renal function, increased dietary potassium is recommended for most individuals.

Data from Hunt BD, Cappuccio FP: *Stroke* 45(5):1519-1522, 2014; Seth A et al: *Stroke* 45(10):2874-2880, 2014; Vinceti M et al: *J Am Heart Assoc* 5(10), 2016.

---

potassium and *intercalated cells* reabsorb potassium. The net effect of secretion and reabsorption determines the amount of potassium excreted from the body. Evidence suggests that the gut also may sense the amount of K^+ ingested and stimulate renal K^+ excretion, independent of aldosterone.[8]

The potassium concentration in the distal tubular cells is determined primarily by the plasma concentration of potassium in the *peritubular capillaries.* When the plasma potassium concentration increases secondary to increased dietary intake, potassium is secreted into the urine by the distal tubules. Potassium also is secreted into the urine when potassium shifts from the ICF to the ECF. Decreased levels of plasma potassium result in decreased distal tubular secretion, although approximately 5 to 15 mEq per day will continue to be lost. Changes in the rate of filtrate (urine) flow through the distal tubule also influence the concentration gradient for potassium secretion. When the urine flow rate is high (e.g., with diuretic use), the potassium concentration in the distal tubular urine is lower; potassium subsequently is secreted into the urine.

Changes in pH (hydrogen ion concentration) also affect the potassium balance. During acute acidosis, hydrogen ions accumulate in the ICF. To maintain ionic balance, potassium shifts out of the cell and into the ECF. This shift occurs, in part, because of a decrease in the sodium–potassium ATPase pump activity. Decreased ICF potassium results in decreased potassium secretion by the distal tubular cells, increasing the potential for hyperkalemia. In acute alkalosis, hydrogen ions within the ICF decrease, resulting in a shift of potassium into the cell. Additionally, potassium secretion increases within the distal tubular cells, increasing the potential for hypokalemia.

In addition to conserving sodium, *aldosterone* regulates the potassium concentration. An elevated plasma potassium concentration causes the release of renin by the renal juxtaglomerular cells. Aldosterone is secreted through the renin-angiotensin-aldosterone system; it stimulates the secretion of potassium into the urine by the distal renal tubules. Aldosterone also increases the secretion of potassium from sweat glands.

Insulin, which is released after eating, drives potassium into liver and muscle cells by stimulating the sodium–potassium ATPase pump. Clinically insulin is used to treat hyperkalemia. In cases of hyperglycemia, dangerously low levels of plasma potassium can result when insulin is administered to treat elevated glucose levels. Particularly in emergency settings, it is crucial to check potassium levels before administering insulin to treat elevated glucose levels. The potassium status is a key factor in any diabetic treatment regimen involving the administration of insulin.

Potassium adaptation refers to the ability of the body to adapt to increased levels of potassium intake over time. A sudden increase in potassium may be fatal. If the potassium intake is increased slowly, renal excretion increases, maintaining the potassium balance.

Hypokalemia

PATHOPHYSIOLOGY Potassium deficiency, or hypokalemia, develops when the serum potassium concentration falls to less than 3.5 mEq/L. Because cellular and total body stores of potassium are difficult to measure, changes in the potassium balance are reflected—although not always accurately—by the plasma concentration. Generally a decreased serum potassium level indicates loss of total body potassium. When potassium is lost from the ECF, the concentration gradient favors the movement of potassium from within the cell into the ECF. The ICF/ECF concentration ratio is maintained, but the total body potassium has been decreased. Factors contributing to the development of hypokalemia include a reduced intake of potassium, an increased movement of potassium into the cells, and increased losses of potassium. A dietary deficiency of potassium is more common in elderly individuals because of both a low protein intake and an inadequate consumption of fruits and vegetables. Hypokalemia also is prevalent in individuals with alcoholism or anorexia nervosa. A reduced potassium intake generally becomes problematic when accompanied by other causes of potassium depletion.[9]

ECF hypokalemia can develop during the treatment of individuals with diabetic ketoacidosis (DKA). In acidosis potassium moves from the ICF to the ECF in exchange for hydrogen ion in order to maintain the plasma acid-base balance. The individual may present with normokalemia or hyperkalemia despite potassium continuing to be excreted by the kidney. Insulin promotes the cellular uptake of potassium, and insulin administration may cause an ECF potassium deficit and hypokalemia. Accordingly, in the treatment of DKA, it is important to monitor serum potassium levels.

Potassium loss from total body stores can also be caused by gastrointestinal and renal disorders. Diarrhea, intestinal drainage tubes, fistulae, and laxative abuse all can result in hypokalemia. Normally only 5 to 10 mEq of potassium and 100 to 150 ml of water are excreted in the stool daily. With diarrhea, fluid and electrolyte losses can be voluminous; several liters of fluid and 100 to 200 mEq of potassium may be lost daily. Vomiting or continuous nasogastric suctioning often is associated with potassium depletion. The loss occurs, in part, because of potassium lost from the gastric fluid. However, the loss principally is caused by renal compensation for volume depletion and metabolic alkalosis, which occurs secondary to losses of sodium, chloride, and hydrogen ions. The loss of fluid and sodium stimulates the secretion of aldosterone which in turn results in renal excretion of potassium.

Renal potassium loss occurs with increased secretion of potassium at the distal tubule. Predisposing factors include the use of potassium-wasting diuretics, excessive aldosterone secretion, an increased distal tubular flow rate, and a low plasma magnesium concentration. Alkalosis results in increased renal potassium excretion. Many diuretics inhibit the reabsorption of sodium chloride, resulting in increased urine production. With enhanced fluid excretion, the increased flow through the distal tubule also promotes potassium excretion. If sodium loss is severe, the compensating aldosterone secretion may further deplete potassium stores. Primary hyperaldosteronism, typically from an adrenal adenoma (tumor), results in potassium wasting. Many renal diseases impair the kidney's ability to conserve sodium. The

decreased sodium reabsorption produces a diuretic effect. As a result, the increased flow through the distal tubule promotes the secretion of potassium. Magnesium deficits increase renal potassium secretion, promoting hypokalemia. Certain antibiotics (carbenicillin disodium and amphotericin B) are associated with hypokalemia by increasing the rate of potassium excretion. Rare hereditary defects in renal potassium transport (Bartter and Gitelman syndromes) also can result in hypokalemia.

CLINICAL MANIFESTATIONS Mild losses of potassium usually are asymptomatic. Severe potassium loss results in neuromuscular and cardiac disorders. Neuromuscular excitability decreases, causing skeletal muscle weakness, smooth muscle atony, cardiac dysrhythmias, glucose intolerance, and impaired urinary concentrating ability.

Symptoms occur in proportion to the rate of potassium depletion. The body can accommodate slow losses of potassium. Decreases in the ECF potassium concentration may facilitate a shift in potassium away from the intracellular space and into the ICF. This dynamic promotes the return of the potassium concentration gradient toward a more normal status, reducing neuromuscular symptoms. With acute and severe potassium loss, the changes in neuromuscular excitability are more profound. Skeletal muscle weakness initially occurs in the larger muscles of the legs and arms and ultimately affects the diaphragm, compromising ventilation. With severe losses, paralysis and respiratory arrest may occur. Loss of smooth muscle tone may result in a variety of gastrointestinal manifestations, such as constipation, intestinal distention, anorexia, nausea, vomiting, and paralytic ileus (paralysis of the intestinal muscles).

The cardiac effects of hypokalemia are related to changes in membrane excitability. As the ECF potassium concentration decreases, the resting membrane potential becomes more negative (i.e., *hyperpolarized*). A hyperpolarized membrane requires a greater stimulus to trigger an action potential. Potassium also contributes to the repolarization phase of the action potential; hypokalemia delays ventricular repolarization. Consequently, hypokalemia may result in various dysrhythmias, including sinus bradycardia, atrioventricular block, and paroxysmal atrial tachycardia. The characteristic changes in the electrocardiogram (ECG) reflect *delayed repolarization*. For instance, the amplitude of the T wave decreases, the amplitude of the U wave increases, and the ST segment is depressed (Fig. 5.9). In severe states of hypokalemia, P waves peak, the QT interval is prolonged, and T-wave inversions may be seen. Hypokalemia enhances the therapeutic effect of digitalis and increases the risk of digitalis toxicity.

A wide range of metabolic dysfunctions may result from potassium deficiency (Table 5.7). Carbohydrate metabolism is affected. Hypokalemia depresses insulin secretion and alters hepatic and skeletal muscle glycogen synthesis. Renal function is impaired, resulting in a decreased ability to concentrate urine. Polyuria (increased urine output) and polydipsia (increased thirst) result from a decreased responsiveness to ADH. Long-term potassium deficits (i.e., lasting longer than 1 month) may damage renal tissue, and interstitial fibrosis and tubular atrophy can result.

EVALUATION AND TREATMENT Hypokalemia can result from disorders associated with potassium loss or from shifts of extracellular potassium into the intracellular space. Treatment involves replacing lost potassium to restore normal levels and correcting the associated acid–base imbalances. Once these have been corrected, further potassium loss should be prevented by correcting the underlying mechanism. In particular, individuals should be encouraged to eat potassium-rich foods. With normal renal function, the maximal rate of oral replacement is 40 to 80 mEq/day. A maximal safe rate of IV replacement is 20 mEq/hr.

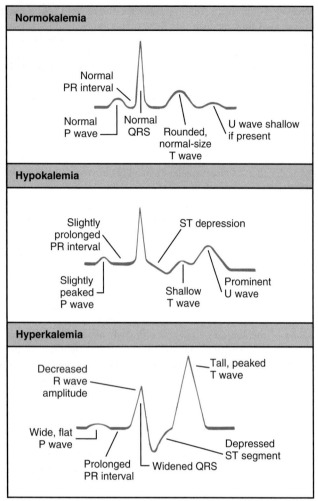

FIGURE 5.9 Electrocardiogram Changes With Potassium Imbalance.

TABLE 5.7 Clinical Manifestations of Potassium Level Alterations

Organ System	Hypokalemia	Hyperkalemia
Cardiovascular	Dysrhythmias Electrocardiograph (ECG) changes (flattened T waves, U waves, ST depression, peaked P wave, prolonged QT interval) Cardiac arrest Weak, irregular pulse rate Postural hypotension	Dysrhythmias ECG changes (peaked T waves, prolonged PR interval, absent P wave with widened QRS complex) Bradycardia Heart block Cardiac arrest
Nervous	Lethargy Fatigue Confusion Paresthesias	Anxiety Tingling Numbness
Gastrointestinal	Nausea and vomiting Decreased motility Distention Decreased bowel sounds Ileus	Nausea and vomiting Diarrhea Colicky pain
Kidney	Water loss Thirst Inability to concentrate urine Increased tubular production of ammonia and ammonium Kidney damage	Oliguria Kidney damage
Skeletal and smooth muscle	Weakness Flaccid paralysis Respiratory arrest Constipation Bladder dysfunction	Early: hyperactive muscles Late: weakness and flaccid paralysis

Potassium is irritating to blood vessels and can result in considerable pain for the individual. Accordingly, IV infusions containing potassium should not exceed 40 mEq/L. Replacement therapy requires close monitoring of the plasma potassium concentration.

Hyperkalemia

PATHOPHYSIOLOGY   Hyperkalemia is defined as an ECF potassium concentration greater than 5.5 mEq/L. Increases in the total body potassium level are relatively rare, largely because of efficient renal excretion. Acute increases in the serum potassium level are handled quickly through increased cellular uptake and renal excretion of potassium excesses.

Hyperkalemia may be caused by an increased intake, a shift of potassium from cells to the ECF, decreased renal excretion, or drugs that decrease renal potassium excretion. Such drugs include ACE inhibitors, angiotensin receptor blockers, and aldosterone antagonists. With normal renal function, gradual increases in potassium, including long-term persistent increases, usually are well tolerated; renal excretion can compensate. Short-term potassium loading, however, can exceed renal excretion rates. Dietary excesses of potassium are uncommon, but accidental ingestion of potassium salt substitutes can cause toxicity. Administration of stored whole blood and IV boluses of potassium

penicillin G or potassium replacement solutions also can precipitate hyperkalemia, particularly in the setting of impaired renal function. With cell trauma or changes to cell membrane permeability, potassium moves from the ICF to the ECF. Similar changes occur with acidosis, insulin deficiency, or cell hypoxia. Burns, massive crushing injuries, and extensive surgeries can cause the release of potassium to the ECF secondary to cell trauma. With intact renal function, this excess ECF potassium is excreted.

With acidosis, ECF hydrogen ions shift into cells in exchange for ICF potassium and sodium. As a result, hyperkalemia and acidosis often occur simultaneously. Insulin also facilitates the movement of potassium into the cell. Accordingly, insulin deficit often is accompanied by hyperkalemia. Diabetic ketoacidosis commonly presents with hyperkalemia, and potassium is lost through the urine secondary to an osmotic diuresis. Hypoxia can lead to hyperkalemia by inhibiting the active transport mechanisms within the cell membrane; potassium escapes into the ECF. Hyperkalemia may result secondary to digitalis toxicity. High levels of digitalis also inhibit the Na^+-K^+ ATPase transport pump, allowing potassium to remain outside the cell.

Compromised renal function, particularly decreased renal excretion of potassium, is commonly associated with hyperkalemia. Oliguria (urine output of 30 ml/hr or less) secondary to renal failure typically presents with elevations of the serum potassium level. The severity of the hyperkalemia is a function of the amount of potassium intake, the degree of acidosis, and the rate of renal cell damage. Decreased secretion of aldosterone can result in decreased renal potassium excretion. Addison disease, characterized by adrenal cortical insufficiency, often presents with hyperkalemia secondary to decreased aldosterone secretion.

CLINICAL MANIFESTATIONS Symptoms vary with the severity of the hyperkalemia. With a mild presentation, increased neuromuscular irritability may manifest as restlessness, intestinal cramping, and diarrhea. Severe hyperkalemia decreases the resting membrane potential from −90 to −70 millivolts, resulting in muscle weakness, loss of muscle tone, and paralysis. With mild hyperkalemia, repolarization is more rapid. This is reflected in characteristic ECG changes, such as narrow, taller T waves and a shortened QT interval. Severe hyperkalemia causes delayed cardiac conduction, preventing repolarization of heart muscle. Inactivated sodium channels result in a decrease in conduction velocity. Severe hyperkalemia depresses the ST segment, prolongs the PR interval, and widens the QRS complex related to the associated decreased conduction velocity (see Fig. 5.9). Bradydysrhythmias and delayed conduction are common in hyperkalemia; severe hyperkalemia can cause ventricular fibrillation or cardiac arrest.

Changes in the ratio of intracellular to extracellular potassium concentration contribute to the clinical presentation of hyperkalemia (see Table 5.7). The neuromuscular changes seen with hyperkalemia are related both to the increased rate of repolarization and to the effects of acidosis and calcium balance. Prolonged increases in the ECF potassium concentration result in a movement of potassium into the cell, which maintains the normal ICF to ECF potassium ratio. Acute elevations of the extracellular potassium concentration produce neuromuscular irritability because the normal ratio is disrupted. Calcium, another cation, also affects the threshold potential; an increased extracellular calcium concentration can override the neuromuscular effects of hyperkalemia (see Chapter 1).

EVALUATION AND TREATMENT Hyperkalemia is a common finding in many clinical settings (e.g., renal disease, massive trauma, insulin deficiency, Addison disease, use of potassium salt substitutes, and metabolic acidosis). How rapidly symptoms evolve often is a function of the underlying cause.

Management of hyperkalemia includes both treating the underlying cause and reversing the excessive potassium concentration. When serum potassium levels are dangerously high, calcium gluconate can decrease the negativity of the threshold potential. This action restores normal neuromuscular irritability and stabilizes the resting cardiac membrane potential. Administration of glucose, an *insulin secretagogue* (a substance that causes another substance to be secreted), facilitates the movement of potassium into the cells. For the diabetic individual, presenting with ketoacidosis and hyperkalemia (this occurs more commonly when there is diminished renal function), treatment with fluids and insulin facilitates the movement of potassium back into the cell. In this case potassium levels should be monitored to assess for the development of hypokalemia. Sodium bicarbonate corrects metabolic acidosis and lowers the serum potassium concentration. Oral or rectal administration of potassium-binding agents (i.e., drugs that exchange sodium for potassium or calcium in the intestine) can be effective. Dialysis may be needed to remove excess potassium in cases of renal failure.

QUICK CHECK 5.4
1. What is the role of potassium in the body? What metabolic dysfunctions occur in potassium deficiency? What occurs in potassium excess?
2. Explain how a person can have normal total body potassium levels but still exhibit hypokalemia.
3. What is the most prominent ECG change associated with hyperkalemia? What are the changes with hypokalemia?

Other Electrolytes—Calcium, Phosphate, and Magnesium

The specific dynamics governing the balance for other major electrolytes—calcium (Ca^{++}), phosphate (PO_4^{3+}), and magnesium (Mg^{++})—are summarized in Table 5.8. Parathyroid hormone, vitamin D, and calcitonin also are important for the regulation of these minerals[10] (see Chapter 19).

ACID–BASE BALANCE

The acid–base balance must be regulated within a narrow range for normal physiologic functioning. Slight changes in amounts of hydrogen and changes in pH can significantly alter biologic processes in cells and tissues. Hydrogen ions are required to maintain membrane integrity and metabolic enzyme reactions. Many alterations to normal physiology disturb the acid–base balance, producing complications that are arguably more harmful than the disease process itself.[11]

Hydrogen Ion and pH

The concentration of hydrogen ions in body fluids is very small—approximately 0.0000001 mg/L. This number is expressed as the negative logarithm 10^{-7} mg/L and is indicated on the pH scale as pH 7.0, a neutral status. Values less than 7.0 are more acid. Values more than 7.0 are more alkaline. Accordingly, the pH number indicates the acidity or alkalinity of a solution. The pH scale is logarithmic, not linear, meaning the difference between numbers on the scale is not constant. Each number on the scale is 10 times more acid or more alkaline than the preceding number. Accordingly, a pH of 5 is 10 times more acid than a pH of 6; a pH of 4 is 10 times more acid than a pH of 5 and 100 times more acid than a pH of 6. As the pH changes by one unit from a pH 7 to a pH 6, the H^+ increases tenfold, making the solution much more acid than a neutral solution with a pH of 7.0. Solutions with an excess of hydrogen ions are acidic in nature; solutions with an excess of hydroxide ions (OH^-) are basic, or alkaline, in nature. In biologic fluids, a pH of 7.40 is defined as neutral. Accordingly, a pH less than 7.40 is defined as acidic, and a pH greater than 7.40 is defined as alkaline, or basic (Table 5.9).

Body acids form as the end products of protein, carbohydrate, and fat metabolism; these acids can release hydrogen ion. Acids must be balanced by base substances within the body to maintain a normal pH. A base is a substance that accepts hydrogen ions; an acid is a substance that donates hydrogen ions. The two must be in balance to maintain a physiologic neutral status (pH 7.40). Body acids exist in two forms: **volatile acids** (substances that can be eliminated as carbon dioxide [CO_2] gas) and **nonvolatile acids** (substances that can be eliminated only by the kidney). The sole volatile acid formed in the body is carbonic acid (H_2CO_3), a *weak acid*, which means that it does not easily release its hydrogen ion. In the presence of the enzyme carbonic anhydrase, it readily dissociates into CO_2 and water (H_2O). The carbon dioxide is eliminated by pulmonary ventilation. The rest of the body acids are nonvolatile acids, such as lactic acid, phosphoric acid, sulfuric acid,

TABLE 5.8 Alterations in Calcium, Phosphate, and Magnesium

Parameter	Calcium	Phosphate	Magnesium
Normal values	Serum: 8.8–10.5 mg/dL (total), 4.5–5.6 mg/dL (ionized); 99% in bone as hydroxyapatite; remainder in plasma and body cells with 50% bound to plasma proteins; 40% free or ionized; ionized form most important physiologically	Serum: 2.5–5.0 mg/dL, but may be as high as 6.0–7.0 mg/dL in infants and young children; mainly in bone with some in ICF and ECF; exists as phospholipids, phosphate esters, and inorganic phosphate (ionized form)	Serum: 1.8–3.0 mEq/L; 40%–60% stored in bone, 33% bound to plasma proteins; primary intracellular divalent cation
Function	Needed for fundamental metabolic processes; major cation for structure of bone and teeth; enzymatic cofactor for blood clotting; required for hormone secretion and function of cell receptors; directly related to plasma membrane stability and permeability, transmission of nerve impulses, and contraction of muscles; parathyroid hormone, vitamin D_3, and calcitonin act together to control calcium absorption and excretion (see Chapter 19)	Intracellular and extracellular anion buffer in regulation of acid–base balance; provides energy for muscle contraction (as ATP); parathyroid hormone, vitamin D_3, and calcitonin act together to control phosphate absorption and excretion (see Chapter 19)	Cofactor in intracellular enzymatic reactions and causes neuromuscular excitability; often interacts with calcium and potassium in reactions at cellular level and has important role in smooth muscle contraction and relaxation; magnesium is absorbed in the intestine and eliminated by the kidney
Excess	Hypercalcemia (serum concentrations >10–12 mg/dL)	Hyperphosphatemia (serum concentrations >4.7 mg/dL)	Hypermagnesemia (serum concentrations >3.0 mEq/L)
Causes	Hyperparathyroidism; bone metastases with calcium resorption from breast, prostate, renal, and cervical cancer; sarcoidosis; excess vitamin D; many tumors that produce PTH	Acute or chronic renal failure with significant loss of glomerular filtration; treatment of metastatic tumors with chemotherapy that releases large amounts of phosphate into serum; long-term use of laxatives or enemas containing phosphates; hypoparathyroidism	Usually renal insufficiency or failure; also excessive intake of magnesium-containing antacids, adrenal insufficiency
Effects	Many nonspecific; fatigue, weakness, lethargy, anorexia, nausea, constipation; impaired renal function, kidney stones; dysrhythmias, bradycardia, cardiac arrest; bone pain, osteoporosis	Symptoms primarily related to low serum calcium levels (caused by high phosphate levels) similar to results of hypocalcemia; when prolonged, calcification of soft tissues in lungs, kidneys, joints	Skeletal smooth muscle contraction; excess nerve function; loss of deep tendon reflexes; nausea and vomiting; muscle weakness; hypotension; bradycardia; respiratory distress
Deficit	Hypocalcemia (serum calcium concentration <8.5 mg/dL)	Hypophosphatemia (serum phosphate concentration <2.0 mg/dL)	Hypomagnesemia (serum magnesium concentration <1.5 mEq/L)
Causes	Related to inadequate intestinal absorption, deposition of ionized calcium into bone or soft tissue, blood administration, or decreases in PTH and vitamin D; nutritional deficiencies occur with inadequate sources of dairy products or green leafy vegetables	Most commonly by intestinal malabsorption related to vitamin D deficiency, use of magnesium- and aluminum-containing antacids, long-term alcohol abuse, and malabsorption syndromes; respiratory alkalosis; increased renal excretion of phosphate associated with hyperparathyroidism	Malnutrition, malabsorption syndromes, alcoholism, urinary losses (renal tubular dysfunction, loop diuretics)
Effects	Increased neuromuscular excitability; tingling, muscle spasm (particularly in hands, feet, and facial muscles), intestinal cramping, hyperactive bowel sounds; severe cases show convulsions and tetany; prolonged QT interval, cardiac arrest	Conditions related to reduced capacity for oxygen transport by red blood cells and disturbed energy metabolism; leukocyte and platelet dysfunction; deranged nerve and muscle function; in severe cases, irritability, confusion, numbness, coma, convulsions; possibly respiratory failure (because of muscle weakness), cardiomyopathies, bone resorption (leading to rickets or osteomalacia)	Behavioral changes, irritability, increased reflexes, muscle cramps, ataxia, nystagmus, tetany, convulsions, tachycardia, hypotension

ATP, Adenosine triphosphate; *ECF*, extracellular fluid; *ICF*, intracellular fluid; *PTH*, parathyroid hormone.

acetoacetic acid, and beta-hydroxybutyric acid. Many nonvolatile acids are *strong acids;* they readily release their hydrogen ions. Nonvolatile acids are secreted into the urine by the renal tubules in amounts of approximately 60 to 100 mEq of hydrogen per day, or about 1 mEq per kilogram of body weight.

Mechanisms to Maintain Normal pH

The body has three mechanisms, or lines of defense, to maintain the acid–base balance: (1) physiologic (chemical) buffer systems (bicarbonate, phosphate, hemoglobin, and protein), the first line of defense; (2) respiratory acid–base control, the second line of defense; and (3) renal acid–base control, the third line of defense. The physiologic buffers are primarily intracellular and function instantaneously to correct alterations in the acid–base balance. The lungs and the kidneys work in concert to maintain a normal pH, as is discussed below. The lungs respond relatively quickly (within seconds to minutes), but the kidneys require more time (hours to days) to bring the system into balance. Although the lungs respond more quickly, mechanisms involving the kidney are more long term in restoring the acid–base balance.

Buffer Systems

Buffer systems resist changes in pH and maintain pH within the normal range. Physiologic processes generate H^+ (acid) or OH^- (base) ions. Unchecked these ions would alter the pH of the body. Buffer systems are located in both the ECF and the ICF compartments and function at different rates (Table 5.10). The most important are the *plasma buffer systems*, which have two components: carbonic acid–bicarbonate and the protein hemoglobin (Fig. 5.10). The important intracellular buffers are phosphate and protein. Ammonia and phosphate can attach hydrogen ions and are important renal buffers.

Carbonic Acid-Bicarbonate Buffering

As mentioned previously, cellular respiration results in the production of CO_2, which combines with water to form carbonic acid (H_2CO_3).

H_2CO_3 dissociates, forming one hydrogen (H^+) ion and one bicarbonate ion (HCO_3^-) in the blood. The bicarbonate ion is a base component of the buffer system, and the hydrogen ion is the acid component. These reactions are readily reversible, depending on whether an acid or a base environment exists. The reactions can move in one or the other direction to maintain a neutral pH. Accordingly, these reactions can correct for imbalances in pH by releasing hydrogen ions or absorbing hydrogen ions as the need arises. If excess H^+ ions are present, the buffer absorbs these ions. If excess bicarbonate ions are present, the buffer releases H^+ ions. The relationship between bicarbonate (HCO_3^-) and carbonic acid (H_2CO_3) usually is expressed as a ratio. Under normal conditions, the bicarbonate level is about 24 mEq/L and the carbonic acid level is about 1.2 mEq/L when the arterial CO_2 (Pa_{CO_2}) is 40 mm Hg. Therefore the ratio of bicarbonate to carbonic acid is 20:1 (24/1.2). This ratio maintains a normal pH of 7.40 (Fig. 5.11).

Both the lungs and the kidneys augment the action of the bicarbonate–carbonic acid buffer system. The lungs eliminate CO_2 and can increase the amount of CO_2 eliminated by increasing the rate and depth of ventilation. Although the lungs do not respond as rapidly as the physiologic buffering system, they have twice the ability to correct for pH imbalances compared to all the chemical buffering systems combined. Similarly, the kidneys augment the carbonic acid–bicarbonate buffer system by reabsorbing or regenerating bicarbonate in the renal tubules or excreting hydrogen into the urine. The renal response takes considerably longer than does the respiratory response. However, the kidneys ability to regulate and maintain a normal pH is necessary because the kidneys are the only organs that can excrete fixed acids.

Protein Buffering

In a manner similar to the bicarbonate–carbonic acid buffer system, *proteins* also function as buffers. All proteins can attach or release a hydrogen ion. Most proteins are inside cells; hence protein-based buffering is primarily an intracellular buffer system. Hemoglobin (Hb) is an excellent protein buffer in the blood. As the pH increases, hemoglobin loses hydrogen ions, and the reverse happens when the pH decreases. Hemoglobin also affects the pH through a different mechanism when it binds carbon dioxide to form carbaminohemoglobin ($HHbCO_2$). The bound CO_2 is transported to the lungs, where it is released from the body through ventilation. This dynamic is important because CO_2 is a *potential acid*. Unbound CO_2 can dissociate in water to form H_2CO_3, a weak acid. Carbonic acid releases hydrogen ion, lowering the pH. By binding carbon dioxide, the hemoglobin is preventing CO_2 from dissociating into carbonic acid; it thereby prevents the release of excess

TABLE 5.9 pH of Body Fluids

Body Fluid	pH	Factors Affecting pH
Gastric juices	1.0–3.0	Hydrochloric acid production
Urine	5.0–6.0	H^+ ion excretion from waste products
Arterial blood	7.35–7.45	pH is slightly higher because there is less carbonic acid (H_2CO_3)
Venous blood	7.37	pH is slightly lower because there is more carbonic acid
Cerebrospinal fluid	7.32	Decreased bicarbonate and higher carbon dioxide content decrease pH
Pancreatic fluid	7.8–8.0	Contains bicarbonate produced by exocrine cells
Bile	7.0–8.0	Contains bicarbonate
Small intestine fluid	6.5–7.5	Contains alkaline fluid from pancreas, liver, and gallbladder

TABLE 5.10 Buffer Systems

Buffer Pairs	Buffer System	Chemical Reaction	Rate
HCO_3^-/H_2CO_3	Bicarbonate	$H^+ + HCO_3^- \rightleftharpoons H_2CO_3 \rightleftharpoons H_2O + CO_2$	Instantaneously
Hb^-/HHb	Hemoglobin	$HHb \rightleftharpoons H^+ + Hb^-$	Instantaneously
$HPO_4^-/H_2PO_4^-$	Phosphate	$H_2PO_4^- + H^+ + HPO_4^-$	Instantaneously
Pr^-/HPr	Plasma proteins	$HPr \rightleftharpoons H^+ + Pr^-$	Instantaneously

Organs	Physiologic Mechanism	Rate
Lung ventilation	Regulates retention or elimination of CO_2 and therefore H_2CO_3 concentration	Minutes to hours
Ionic shifts	Exchange of intracellular potassium and sodium for hydrogen	2–4 hours
Kidney tubules	Bicarbonate reabsorption and regeneration; ammonium formation, phosphate buffering to eliminate hydrogen	Hours to days
Bone	Exchanges of calcium and phosphate and release of carbonate	Hours to days

CO_2, Carbon dioxide; *Hb*, hemoglobin; HCO_3^-, bicarbonate; H_2CO_3, carbonic acid; *HHb*, hydrogenated hemoglobin; HPO_4^-, dibasic phosphate; $H_2PO_4^-$, monobasic phosphate; *HPr*, hydrogenated protein; Pr^+, protein.

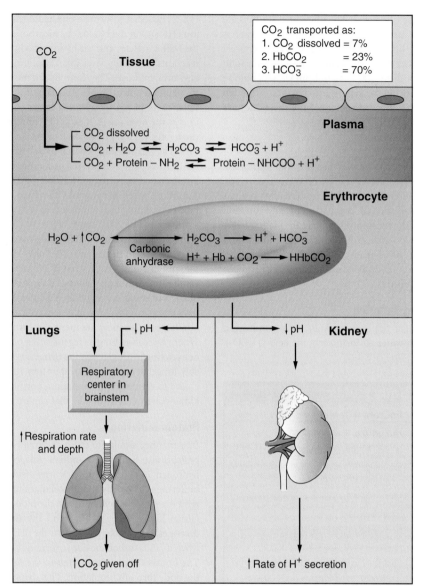

FIGURE 5.10 Integration of pH Control Mechanisms (Example for Acidosis). CO_2 is produced in tissue cells and diffuses to plasma, where it is transported as dissolved CO_2; or it combines with water to form carbonic acid (H_2CO_3); or it combines with protein from which hydrogen has been released. Most of the CO_2 diffuses into the red blood cells and combines with water to form H_2CO_3. The H_2CO_3 dissociates to form hydrogen ion (H^+) and bicarbonate (HCO_3^-). Hydrogen combines with hemoglobin that has released its oxygen to form HHb, which buffers the hydrogen and makes venous blood slightly more acidic than arterial blood. The increase in H^+ coupled with elevated CO_- levels results in $HHbCO_3$ and an increase in the ventilatory rate and secretion of H^+ by the kidneys.

H^+ ions into the environment. The pH control mechanism is illustrated in Fig. 5.10.

Renal Buffering

The kidneys have a major role in maintaining the acid–base balance. The bicarbonate–carbonic acid buffer system is functional within the kidney. Two additional buffer systems are active in the renal tubules, the *phosphate buffer* and the *ammonia buffer*. Once H^+ has reacted with all available HCO_3^-, any additional H^+ ions react with either the phosphate or the ammonia buffer systems. The *phosphate buffer* functions both in the renal tubules and in the intracellular fluid. The two components of this system, monobasic phosphate ($H_2PO_4^-$) and dibasic phosphate ($HPO_4^=$), usually function in association with sodium to form a sodium

salt. As with any buffer, these components bind or release H^+ to maintain physiologic neutrality (pH 7.40). The *ammonia buffer* functions within the renal tubules. The components for this system are ammonia (NH_3) and ammonium (NH_4^+). These components reversibly bind or release hydrogen ion to maintain a neutral pH.

Although various physiologic buffers can compensate for excess acids and bases on a moment-to-moment basis, the kidneys have a far more potent effect in maintaining a neutral pH. They actually can rid the body of excess acids by excreting hydrogen ions into the urine. Monobasic phosphate ($H_2PO_4^-$) and ammonium (NH_4^+) are secreted into the urine as they have attached hydrogen ions. Renal tubules also can reabsorb bicarbonate into the plasma using a mechanism that involves the bicarbonate-carbonic acid buffer. Carbonic anhydrase, an

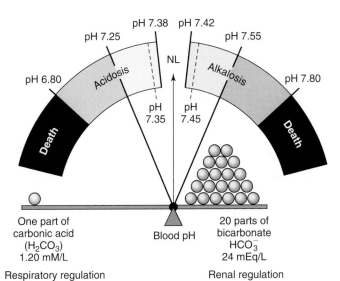

FIGURE 5.11 Ratio of Carbonic Acid and Bicarbonate Concentration in Maintaining pH Within Normal Limits An increase in H_2CO_3 or a decrease in HCO_3^- concentration causes acidosis. A decrease in H_2CO_3 or increase in HCO_3^- concentration causes alkalosis. H_2CO_3, Carbonic acid; HCO_3^-, bicarbonate. (From Monahan FD: *Medical-surgical nursing: health and illness perspectives*, ed 8, St Louis, 2007, Mosby.)

enzyme, catalyzes the reaction of carbon dioxide (CO_2) and water (H_2O) to form carbonic acid (H_2CO_3). The hydrogen in the carbonic acid is secreted from the tubular cell and buffered in the tubular lumen by dibasic phosphate ($HPO_4^=$) or ammonia (NH_3), or both, leaving a bicarbonate ion. The remaining bicarbonate ion is reabsorbed from the tubule, adding a new bicarbonate ion to the plasma when it is needed to maintain a neutral pH (Fig. 5.12).

Acid–Base Imbalances

Pathophysiologic changes in the concentration of hydrogen ion in the blood lead to acid–base imbalances.[12,13] **Acidemia** refers to arterial blood with a pH less than 7.40. A systemic increase in the hydrogen ion concentration or a loss of base is termed **acidosis**. **Alkalemia** refers to arterial blood with a pH greater than 7.40. A systemic decrease in the hydrogen ion concentration or an excess of base is termed **alkalosis**. These changes may be caused by either *respiratory* or *metabolic* processes. If the altered pH occurs secondary to biochemical processes within the body, it is said to be *metabolic*. If the alteration in pH is secondary to an issue with breathing, it is said to be *respiratory*. In clinical settings, the terms *acidosis* and *alkalosis* is usually are accompanied by the source of the problem (i.e., whether the derangement is caused by metabolic or respiratory factors). Accordingly, four clinical alterations in the acid–base status can be seen: *respiratory acidosis, metabolic acidosis, respiratory alkalosis,* and *metabolic alkalosis*. Arterial blood gases are measured to determine which of the four alterations is present. This measurement typically includes four parameters: the blood pH, Pa_{O_2} (oxygen), Pa_{CO_2} (carbon dioxide), and HCO_3^- (bicarbonate). The Pa_{O_2} provides information about the person's oxygenation status, but it does not provide information about the acid–base status. The blood pH, Pa_{CO_2}, and bicarbonate level, when evaluated together, provide information about whether an individual is experiencing acidosis or alkalosis and whether the cause is respiratory or metabolic. Fig. 5.13 summarizes the relationships among pH, Pa_{CO_2}, and bicarbonate during different acid–base alterations. Fig. 5.11 summarizes the relationship among pH, the partial pressure of carbon dioxide (respiratory regulation), and the concentration of bicarbonate (renal regulation) during alkalosis and

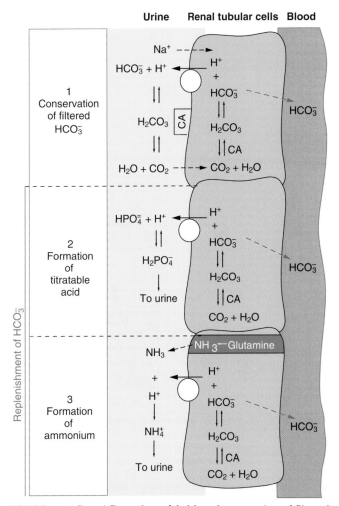

FIGURE 5.12 Renal Excretion of Acid. **1, Conservation of filtered bicarbonate.** Filtered bicarbonate combines with secreted hydrogen ion in the presence of carbon anhydrase *(CA)* to form carbonic acid (H_2CO_3), which then dissociates to water (H_2O) and carbon dioxide (CO_2); both diffuse into the epithelial cell. The CO_2 and H_3O combine to form H_2CO_3 in the presence of CA, and the resulting bicarbonate ion (HCO_3^-) is reabsorbed into the capillary. **2, Formation of titratable acid.** Hydrogen ion is secreted and combines with dibasic phosphate ($HPO_4^=$) to form monobasic phosphate ($H_2PO_4^-$). The secreted hydrogen ion is formed from the dissociation of H_2CO_3, and the remaining HCO_3^- is reabsorbed into the capillary. **3, Formation of ammonium.** Ammonia (NH_3) is produced from glutamine in the epithelial cell and diffuses to the tubular lumen, where it combines with H^+ to form ammonium ion (NH_4^+). Once NH_4^+ has been formed, it cannot return to the epithelial cell (diffusional trapping), and the bicarbonate remaining in the epithelial cell is reabsorbed into the capillary. **NOTE:** The white circles with the arrows on top represent a renal tubular cell active transport pump.

acidosis. An individual can experience both metabolic and respiratory disorders at the same time. In such cases the person may have a mixed acid–base alteration.

Renal and respiratory adjustments in response to primary changes in the pH are known as **compensation**. The respiratory system compensates for changes in the pH by altering the rate and depth of ventilation to increase or decrease the concentration of retained carbon dioxide. Carbon dioxide is referred to as a *potential acid* because it is readily converted to carbonic acid. Breathing more shallowly retains CO_2; breathing more rapidly and deeply blows off CO_2. In this manner, the lungs compensate for excess acidity or alkalinity of the blood. The

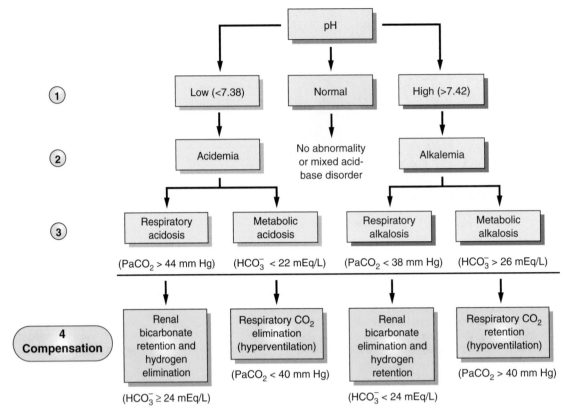

FIGURE 5.13 Primary and Compensatory Acid–Base Changes. A systematic approach can be used to interpret the cause of an acid–base imbalance. **1,** Is the pH low or high? **2,** If the pH is low (acidemia), is the cause respiratory (high $PaCO_2$) or metabolic (low HCO_3^-)? **3,** If the pH is high (alkalemia), is the cause respiratory (low $PaCO_2$) or metabolic (high HCO_3^-)? **4,** Is there compensation for the primary acid–base disorder? *(a)* HCO_3^- will be ≥24 mEq/L if there is renal compensation for a primary respiratory acidosis; *(b)* $PaCO_2$ will be <40 mm Hg if there is respiratory compensation of a primary metabolic acidosis; *(c)* HCO_3^- will be <24 mEq/L if there is renal compensation for primary respiratory alkalosis; *(d)* $PaCO_2$ will be >40 mm Hg if there is respiratory compensation for primary metabolic alkalosis. **NOTE**: Examine the pH first to determine whether acidemia or alkalemia is present. Then examine the changes in HCO_3^- and $PaCO_2$. **1,** HCO_3^- will be elevated with primary metabolic alkalosis or renal compensation for primary respiratory acidosis. **2,** HCO_3^- will be decreased with primary metabolic acidosis or renal compensation for primary respiratory alkalosis. **3,** $PaCO_2$ will be elevated with primary respiratory acidosis or respiratory compensation for primary metabolic alkalosis. **4,** $PaCO_2$ will be decreased with primary respiratory alkalosis or respiratory compensation for metabolic acidosis. *H_2CO_3*, Carbonic acid; *HCO_3^-*, bicarbonate; *$PaCO_2$*, arterial partial pressure of carbon dioxide.

$Paco_2$ and bicarbonate levels provide information on the source of the altered pH and also indicate whether any compensation is ongoing. A low blood pH signals acidosis. If the $Paco_2$ is high, the source of the problem is respiratory (i.e., retained CO_2). Such a scenario might occur with an opioid overdose, in which respirations are depressed and CO_2 is retained. This individual is described as having a primary *respiratory acidosis*. If the pH is low and the $Paco_2$ is normal or low, the acidosis is not caused by respiratory factors. Instead, it is caused by metabolic processes within the body. In this case, the individual is described as having a primary *metabolic acidosis*. An example of a primary metabolic acidosis is an individual experiencing DKA from a lack of insulin secretion or administration. The diabetic individual, lacking insulin, cannot metabolize glucose. The body metabolizes fat stores, and as a result, acid byproducts are released into the blood, causing *metabolic acidosis*.

In cases of primary *respiratory acidosis*, the kidneys attempt to compensate for abnormal pH levels by resorbing bicarbonate ions into the plasma and excreting H^+ ions into the urine, as described previously. This dynamic is referred to as *renal compensation*. Similarly, with a primary *metabolic acidosis*, the lungs attempt to compensate by breathing deeply and rapidly (Kussmaul respirations) in an attempt to rid the body of CO_2, a potential acid. This dynamic is referred to as *respiratory compensation*. In cases of metabolic acid–base imbalance, respiratory compensation occurs rapidly, within minutes of an abnormal pH. Renal compensation occurs more slowly; however, the kidneys have a far greater capacity to restore the normal pH. Renal compensation typically requires hours to days to correct for an abnormal pH. As the kidneys compensate, the values for bicarbonate and $Paco_2$ vary from their normal 20 : 1 ratio. Similar dynamics occur with primary respiratory alkalosis and metabolic alkalosis. The kidneys attempt to compensate for a primary respiratory alkalosis by decreasing the rate of H^+ ions excreted into the urine and reducing the resorption of bicarbonate ions into the plasma. The lungs attempt to compensate for a primary metabolic alkalosis by retaining CO_2 with slower and shallower ventilation. The measured values (laboratory values) of pH, $Paco_2$, and HCO_3^- can identify three parameters:

- the nature of the alteration in pH: acidosis (pH <7.40) or alkalosis (pH >7.40);
- the source of the abnormality—respiratory or metabolic; or
- whether any compensation has developed.

With respect to compensation, the pH abnormality may be compensated, partially compensated, or uncompensated. As an example, an individual with *respiratory acidosis* (pH <7.40) has an elevated Pa_{CO_2} level. The kidneys attempt to compensate for the acidosis by retaining bicarbonate ions (HCO_3^-); therefore the *plasma bicarbonate* level will be elevated. If the pH is normal and the bicarbonate level is elevated, the respiratory acidosis is described as *compensated respiratory acidosis.* If the pH is near normal and the bicarbonate level is elevated, the respiratory acidosis is described as *partially compensated respiratory acidosis.* If the pH is low and the bicarbonate level is normal, the respiratory acidosis is described as *uncompensated respiratory acidosis* because the kidneys have not had sufficient time to compensate for the problem. In all three cases, the Pa_{CO_2} level will be elevated because the source of the acidosis is respiratory. Correction occurs when the values for both components of the buffer pair (bicarbonate and Pa_{CO_2} [carbonic acid]) return to normal levels.

Metabolic Acidosis

In metabolic acidosis, the concentrations of nonvolatile (noncarbonic) acids increase. Less commonly, this condition can result if bicarbonate either is lost from extracellular fluid or cannot be regenerated by the kidney (Table 5.11). This scenario can occur quickly, as in lactic acidosis secondary to poor perfusion or hypoxemia. It also can occur slowly, over an extended time, as in renal failure, diabetic ketoacidosis, or starvation (anion gap acidosis).[14] The buffering systems normally compensate for excess acid and maintain the arterial pH within the normal range. When acidosis is severe, buffers become depleted and cannot compensate; the ratio of the concentrations of bicarbonate to carbonic acid decreases to less than 20:1 (see Fig. 5.11). An increase in the plasma concentration of chloride, out of proportion to sodium, causes hyperchloremic acidosis (non–anion gap acidosis). The specific type of acidosis can be determined by examining the serum anion gap (see Table 5.11). This evaluation helps guide treatment.

TABLE 5.11 **Causes of Metabolic Acidosis**	
Increased Non–Carbonic Acids (Elevated Anion Gap*)	**Bicarbonate Loss or Hyperchloremic Acidosis (Normal Anion Gap)**
Increased H⁺ load	Diarrhea
Ketoacidosis (e.g., diabetes mellitus, starvation)	Ureterosigmoidoscopy (chloride absorbed in excess of sodium in small intestine)
Lactic acidosis (e.g., shock, hypoxemia)	Early renal failure (loss of bicarbonate)
Ingestion (e.g., ammonium chloride, ethylene glycol, methanol, salicylates, paraldehyde)	Proximal renal tubular acidosis (loss of more renal sodium in relation to chloride)
Decreased renal H⁺ excretion	
Advanced renal failure	
Distal renal tubular acidosis	

*Anion gap refers to anions not usually measured in laboratory reports (e.g., sulfate, phosphate, and lactate). The anions usually measured are chloride (Cl^-) and bicarbonate (HCO_3^-). When the sum of the concentrations of measured anions (e.g., chloride and bicarbonate) is subtracted from the sum of the concentrations of measured cations (e.g., sodium and potassium), there is a "gap" of approximately 10 to 12 mEq/L; this is the normal anion gap. An elevated anion gap provides clues to the cause of the acidosis (i.e., to the addition of endogenously or exogenously generated acids). In a normal anion gap acidosis, chloride is retained to replace lost bicarbonate.

Metabolic acidosis is manifested by changes in the function of the neurologic, respiratory, gastrointestinal, and cardiovascular systems. Early symptoms include headache and lethargy, which progress to confusion and coma in severe acidosis. The respiratory system's efforts to compensate for the increase in metabolic acids result in what are termed *Kussmaul respirations,* a form of hyperventilation in which ventilations are deep and rapid. This represents the body's attempt to increase the pH by expelling carbon dioxide (respiratory compensation), which in turn decreases the carbonic acid concentration. Other symptoms include anorexia, nausea, vomiting, diarrhea, and abdominal discomfort. Death can result in the most severe and prolonged cases, preceded by dysrhythmias and hypotension. Treatment varies, depending on the underlying condition.

Metabolic Alkalosis

When excessive loss of metabolic acids occurs, the bicarbonate concentration increases, causing metabolic alkalosis (see Fig. 5.13). When acid loss is caused by vomiting, renal compensation is not very effective because loss of chloride (an anion) in hydrochloric acid (HCl) stimulates renal retention of bicarbonate (an anion). The result is known as hypochloremic metabolic alkalosis. Hyperaldosteronism also can lead to alkalosis as a result of sodium bicarbonate retention and loss of hydrogen and potassium. Diuretics may produce a mild alkalosis because they promote greater excretion of sodium, potassium, and chloride than of bicarbonate.

Common signs and symptoms of metabolic alkalosis are weakness, muscle cramps, hyperactive reflexes, tetany, confusion, convulsions, and atrial tachycardia. Respirations may be shallow, with slow ventilation, as the lungs attempt to compensate by increasing carbon dioxide retention. Manifestations vary with the cause and severity of the alkalosis. Symptoms of hyperactive reflexes and tetany occur because alkalosis increases the binding of Ca^{++} to plasma proteins, thus decreasing the ionized calcium concentration. The decreased ionized calcium concentration causes hyperpolarization of excitable cells, initiating an action potential more easily and resulting in muscle contraction. This is known as *low calcium tetany.*

Treatment is related to the underlying cause. Hypochloremic alkalosis or contraction alkalosis with volume depletion requires a sodium chloride solution; chloride must be replaced before bicarbonate can be excreted by the kidney.

Respiratory Acidosis

Respiratory acidosis occurs with alveolar hypoventilation, resulting in hypercapnia (an excess of carbon dioxide in the blood). The arterial carbon dioxide pressure (Pa_{CO_2}) is greater than 45 mm Hg and the pH is less than 7.35 (see Fig. 5.13). Decreased alveolar ventilation, in relation to the metabolic production of carbon dioxide, produces an increased concentration of carbonic acid, which results in respiratory acidosis. Respiratory acidosis can be acute or chronic. Common causes include depression of the respiratory center (e.g., from drugs or head injury), paralysis of the respiratory muscles, disorders of the chest wall (e.g., kyphoscoliosis or broken ribs), and disorders of the lung parenchyma (e.g., pneumonia, pulmonary edema, emphysema, asthma, bronchitis). Intracellular buffers, particularly hemoglobin and phosphates, provide compensation for acute respiratory acidosis. Renal compensation for chronic respiratory acidosis occurs within 3 to 4 days with increased retention of bicarbonate.

Clinical presentations may include headache, blurred vision, breathlessness, restlessness, and apprehension, followed by lethargy, disorientation, muscle twitching, tremors, convulsions, and coma. The respiratory rate initially is rapid, then gradually becomes depressed as the respiratory center adapts to increasing levels of carbon dioxide.

The skin may be warm and flushed from vasodilation secondary to an elevated carbon dioxide concentration. Treatment involves restoring adequate alveolar ventilation to remove the excess CO_2 ($\downarrow H_2CO_3$).

Respiratory Alkalosis

Respiratory alkalosis follows alveolar hyperventilation (deep, rapid respirations). Hypocapnia (decreased plasma carbon dioxide) decreases the carbonic acid concentration. Laboratory analysis reveals a Pa_{CO_2} less than 35 mm Hg and an elevated pH (see Fig. 5.13). Respiratory alkalosis can be acute or chronic. Hyperventilation can result from a variety of causes, including hypoxemia (pulmonary disease, congestive heart failure, or high altitudes), hypermetabolic states (fever, anemia, thyrotoxicosis), early salicylate intoxication, hysteria, cirrhosis, and gram-negative sepsis. Improper settings on mechanical ventilators result in iatrogenic (treatment-related) respiratory alkalosis. Secondary alkalosis may result from hyperventilation triggered by metabolic acidosis (a mixed acid–base disorder). In acute respiratory alkalosis, the intracellular buffer hemoglobin releases hydrogen. Renal compensation occurs with chronic respiratory alkalosis and is characterized by decreased hydrogen excretion and decreased bicarbonate reabsorption.

Respiratory alkalosis stimulates the central and peripheral nervous systems, resulting in dizziness, confusion, tingling of the extremities (paresthesias), convulsions, and coma. Cerebral vasoconstriction reduces the cerebral blood flow. As with metabolic acidosis, symptoms of hypocalcemia are common, including carpopedal spasm (spasm of muscles in the fingers and toes) and tetany (see Table 5.8). Treatment is aimed at correcting the underlying disturbance, particularly in reversing hypoxemia.

> ### ✔ QUICK CHECK 5.5
> 1. What is the difference between compensation and correction of acid–base disturbances?
> 2. What two chemicals are altered in metabolic acid–base disturbances?
> 3. How do alterations in the carbon dioxide concentration influence acid–base status?

PEDIATRIC CONSIDERATIONS

Distribution of Body Fluids

Newborn Infants
At birth, total body water (TBW) represents 75% to 80% of body weight. This decreases to approximately 67% during the first year of life. Physiologic loss of body water, amounting to 5% of body weight, occurs as the infant adjusts to a new environment. Infants are particularly susceptible to significant changes in TBW because of their high metabolic rate and greater body surface area compared to adults. Consequently, infants have greater fluid intake and output in relation to their body size. Dehydration poses a significant risk because the infant's renal mechanisms for fluid and electrolyte conservation may not be sufficiently mature to compensate for abnormal losses through vomiting or diarrhea. Symptoms of dehydration include increased thirst, decreased urine output, decreased body weight, decreased skin elasticity, sunken fontanels, absent tears, dry mucous membranes, increased heart rate, constipation, and irritability.

Children and Adolescents
TBW slowly decreases to 60% to 65% of body weight. At adolescence, the percentage of TBW approaches adult levels and sex differences appear. Males have a greater percentage of body water because of their increased muscle mass. Females have less body water secondary to the influence of estrogen, which results in a higher percentage of body fat.

GERIATRIC CONSIDERATIONS

Distribution of Body Fluids

The further decline in the percentage of TBW in the elderly occurs as a result of a decrease in both free fat and muscle mass. Additionally, older adults have a reduced ability to regulate sodium and water balance. The kidneys are less efficient at producing either a concentrated or a diluted urine, and sodium conservation responses are sluggish. Thirst perception may be impaired, and loss of cognitive function can influence fluid intake. Healthy older adults can adequately maintain their hydration status. When disease is present, a decrease in TBW, dehydration, and hypernatremia can become life-threatening.

▮ SUMMARY REVIEW

Distribution of Body Fluids

1. The sum of all fluids is the total body water (TBW). Body fluids are distributed among functional compartments. They are classified as intracellular fluid (ICF), or within cells, and extracellular fluid (ECF), or outside of cells. ECF includes interstitial, intravascular, and transcellular fluids.
2. TBW varies with age and the amount of body fat. At birth, TBW is 75%–80% of body weight. Through childhood and adolescence, TBW decreases to 60%–65%. Males have a greater percentage because of increased muscle mass. Females have a lesser percentage due to the effects of estrogen, resulting in a higher percentage of body fat.
3. TBW continues to decline in elderly people due to decreases in free fat and muscle mass, less efficient kidney function, and impairments in thirst perception.

4. Water moves between the plasma and interstitial fluid by osmosis (pulling of water) and hydrostatic pressure (pushing of water), which occur across the capillary membrane.
5. Movement across the capillary wall is called net filtration and is described according to Starling law (the balance between hydrostatic and osmotic forces).
6. Water moves between the ICF and ECF compartments principally with osmotic forces.

Alterations in Water Movement

1. Edema is a problem of fluid distribution that results in accumulation of fluid within the interstitial spaces.
2. The pathophysiologic process that leads to edema is related to an increase in forces favoring fluid filtration from the capillaries or from lymphatic channels into the tissues.

3. Physiologic conditions that promote edema include: (1) increased capillary hydrostatic pressure, (2) decreased plasma oncotic pressure, (3) increased capillary membrane permeability, and (4) lymphatic channel obstruction.

4. Edema may be localized or generalized. It is usually is associated with weight gain, swelling and puffiness, tighter-fitting clothes and shoes, and limited movement of the affected area.

Sodium, Chloride, and Water Balance

1. There is an integral relationship between the balance of sodium and water levels; chloride levels are generally proportional to changes in sodium levels. Sodium balance is regulated by aldosterone, a hormone which increases reabsorption of sodium from the renal filtrate into the blood, at the distal tubule of the kidney.

2. Renin and angiotensin are enzymes that promote secretion of aldosterone and thus regulate sodium and water balance.

3. Natriuretic peptides are hormones involved in decreasing tubular reabsorption and promoting urinary excretion of sodium.

4. Water balance is regulated by the sensation of thirst and by antidiuretic hormone (ADH), which is secreted in response to an increase in plasma osmolality or a decrease in circulating blood volume.

Alterations in Sodium, Water, and Chloride Balance

1. Alterations in sodium and water balance may be classified as isotonic, hypertonic, or hypotonic.

2. Isotonic alterations occur when changes in TBW are accompanied by proportional changes in electrolytes. Isotonic fluid loss—hemorrhage, severe wound drainage, excessive sweating, and inadequate fluid intake—causes hypovolemia. Isotonic fluid excess—excessive administration of intravenous fluids, hypersecretion of aldosterone, or the effects of drugs such as cortisone—causes hypervolemia.

3. Hypertonic alterations develop when the osmolality (the concentration of the solution) of the ECF is elevated above normal, usually because of an increased concentration of ECF sodium (hypernatremia) or a deficit of ECF water.

4. Hypernatremia (serum sodium greater than 145 mEq/L) may be caused by an acute increase in sodium level or a loss of water. Hypernatremia can be isovolemic, hypovolemic, or hypervolemic, depending on accompanying changes in the level of body water. Hypernatremia, with marked water deficit, is manifested by hypovolemia and dehydration. Hyperchloremia (serum chloride greater than 105 mEq/L) is caused by an excess of sodium or a deficit of bicarbonate. This often accompanies hypernatremia because chloride follows sodium.

5. Hypotonic alterations occur when the osmolality of the ECF is less than normal. Hyponatremia is a result of hypotonic alterations.

6. Hyponatremia (serum sodium of less than 135 mEq/L) usually causes movement of water into cells. Hyponatremia may be caused by sodium loss, inadequate sodium intake, or dilution of the body's sodium level with excess water. Hyponatremia can be isovolemic, hypervolemic or hypovolemic, or dilutional depending on accompanying changes in the amount of body water.

7. Hypochloremia (serum chloride less than 97 mEq/L) is usually the result of hyponatremia or elevated bicarbonate concentrations.

Alterations in Potassium and Other Electrolytes

1. Potassium is the predominant ICF ion; it regulates ICF osmolality and maintains the resting membrane potential. Potassium is required for deposition of glycogen and glucose in liver and skeletal muscle cells, maintenance of normal cardiac rhythm, and contraction of muscles.

2. Potassium balance is regulated by the kidney, by aldosterone and insulin secretion, and by changes in pH.

3. Potassium adaptation allows the body to slowly accommodate increased levels of potassium intake.

4. Hypokalemia (serum potassium less than 3.5 mEq/L) indicates loss of total body potassium. Hypokalemia may result from reduced potassium intake, a shift of potassium into cells, and increased losses of potassium. ECF hypokalemia can develop without losses of total body potassium; plasma potassium levels may be normal or elevated when total body potassium is depleted.

5. Hyperkalemia (serum potassium greater than 5.5 mEq/L) may be caused by increased potassium intake, a shift of potassium from the ICF to the ECF, decreased renal excretion, or drugs that decrease renal potassium excretion.

6. Calcium, phosphate, and magnesium concentrations are rigidly controlled by parathyroid hormone (PTH), vitamin D, and calcitonin.

7. Calcium is an ion necessary for bone and teeth formation, blood coagulation, hormone secretion and cell receptor function, and membrane stability.

8. Hypercalcemia (serum calcium greater than 10–12 mg/dl) can be caused by hyperparathyroidism, bone metastases, sarcoidosis, and excess vitamin D. Hypocalcemia (serum calcium less than 8.5 mg/dl) is related to inadequate intestinal absorption, deposition of calcium into bone or soft tissue, blood administration, or decreased PTH and vitamin D levels.

9. Phosphate acts as a buffer in acid–base regulation and provides energy for muscle contraction.

10. Hyperphosphatemia (serum phosphate greater than 4.7 mg/dl) develops with acute or chronic renal failure when there is significant loss of glomerular filtration. Hypophosphatemia (serum phosphate less than 2.0 mg/dl) is usually caused by intestinal malabsorption and increased renal excretion of phosphate.

11. Magnesium functions in enzymatic reactions and often interacts with calcium at the cellular level.

12. Hypermagnesemia (serum magnesium greater than 3.0 mEq/L) is usually caused by renal failure. Hypomagnesemia (serum magnesium less than 1.5 mEq/L) may be caused by malnutrition, malabsorption syndromes, and alcoholism.

Acid–Base Balance

1. Acid–base balance must be regulated within a narrow range for normal physiologic functioning. This balance maintains membrane integrity and the speed of enzymatic reactions. Many alterations to physiology disturb acid–base balances, producing complications that are often more harmful than the disease process itself.

2. Hydrogen ion concentration $[H^+]$, is expressed as pH, which represents the negative logarithm (i.e., 10^{-7}) of hydrogen ions in solution (i.e., 0.0000001 mg/L).

3. Different body fluids have different pH values. In biologic fluids, values less than 7.40 are more acidic and values greater than 7.40 are more basic.

4. The renal and respiratory systems, together with the body's buffer systems, are the principal regulators of acid–base balance.

5. Buffers are substances that can absorb excessive acid or base ions without a significant change in pH, thus maintaining pH within a normal range.

6. Buffers exist as acid–base pairs. The principal plasma buffers are carbonic acid-bicarbonate and the protein hemoglobin. The important intracellular buffers are phosphate and protein.

7. The lungs and kidneys act to compensate for primary changes in pH by increasing or decreasing ventilation and by producing more acidic or more alkaline urine.

8. Acid–base imbalances are caused by changes in the concentration of hydrogen ion in the blood. An increase in hydrogen ions causes acidosis; a decrease causes alkalosis. These changes may be either respiratory or metabolic processes.

9. An abnormal increase or decrease in bicarbonate concentration causes metabolic alkalosis or metabolic acidosis. Changes in the rate of alveolar ventilation and the associated removal of carbon dioxide result in respiratory acidosis or respiratory alkalosis.

10. Metabolic acidosis is caused by an increase in the levels of non–carbonic acids or by the loss of bicarbonate from the extracellular fluid.

11. Metabolic alkalosis occurs with an increase in bicarbonate concentration or from a loss of metabolic acids, such as through vomiting.

12. Respiratory acidosis occurs with decreased alveolar ventilation resulting in hypercapnia (increased carbon dioxide concentration) and increased carbonic acid concentration.

13. Respiratory alkalosis occurs with alveolar hyperventilation resulting in hypocapnia (low carbon dioxide levels) from excessive elimination of carbon dioxide or from decreases in carbonic acid concentration.

14. Renal and respiratory adjustments, in response to primary changes in pH, are known as compensation. Correction occurs when the values for both components of the buffer pair return to normal as the primary disorder is treated or resolves.

KEY TERMS

Acidemia, 127
Acidosis, 127
Aldosterone, 115
Alkalemia, 127
Alkalosis, 127
Angiotensin I, 115
Angiotensin II, 115
Anion gap, 129
Antidiuretic hormone (ADH), 115
Aquaporin, 113
Baroreceptor, 116
Blood plasma, 111
Buffer system, 125
Capillary hydrostatic pressure (blood pressure), 112
Capillary (plasma) oncotic pressure, 112
Chloride (Cl⁻), 115
Compensation, 127
Correction, 129
Dehydration, 118

Dilutional hyponatremia (water intoxication), 119
Edema, 113
Extracellular fluid (ECF), 111
Hypercalcemia, 124 in Table 5.8
Hypercapnia, 129
Hyperchloremia, 118
Hyperkalemia, 122
Hypermagnesemia, 124 in Table 5.8
Hypernatremia, 118
Hyperphosphatemia, 124 in Table 5.8
Hypertonic fluid alteration, 118
Hypervolemic hypernatremia, 118
Hypervolemic hyponatremia, 119
Hypocalcemia, 124
Hypocapnia, 130
Hypochloremia, 119
Hypochloremic metabolic alkalosis, 129

Hypokalemia, 121
Hypomagnesemia, 124
Hyponatremia, 119
Hypophophatemis, 124
Hypotonic fluid imbalance, 119
Hypovolemic hypernatremia, 118
Hypovolemic hyponatremia, 119
Interstitial fluid, 111
Interstitial hydrostatic pressure, 112
Interstitial oncotic pressure, 112
Intracellular fluid (ICF), 111
Intravascular fluid, 111
Isotonic fluid alteration, 000
Isotonic fluid excess, 118
Isotonic fluid loss, 118
Isovolemic (euvolemic) hypernatremia, 118
Isovolemic (euvolemic) hyponatremia, 119
Metabolic acidosis, 129
Metabolic alkalosis, 129

Natriuretic peptide, 115
Net filtration, 112
Nonvolatile acids, 123
Osmoreceptor, 115
Potassium (K⁺), 120
Potassium adaptation, 121
Renin, 115
Renin-angiotensin-aldosterone system, 115
Respiratory acidosis, 129
Respiratory alkalosis, 130
Sodium (Na⁺), 115
Starling force, 112
Total body water (TBW), 111
Transcellular fluid, 111
Vasopressin, 115
Volatile acids, 123
Volume-sensitive receptor, 116
Water balance, 115

REFERENCES

1. Li C, Wang W: Molecular biology of aquaporins, *Adv Exp Med Biol* 969:1-34, 2017.
2. Grada AA, Phillips TJ: Lymphedema: pathophysiology and clinical manifestations, *J Am Acad Dermatol* 77(6):1009-1020, 2017.
3. Abuzaanona A, Lanfear D: Pharmacogenomics of the natriuretic peptide system in heart failure, *Curr Heart Fail Rep* 14(6):536-542, 2017.
4. Armstrong LE, et al: Diagnosing dehydration? Blend evidence with clinical observations, *Curr Opin Clin Nutr Metab Care* 19(6):434-438, 2016.
5. Braun MM, Barstow CH, Pyzocha NJ: Diagnosis and management of sodium disorders: hyponatremia and hypernatremia, *Am Fam Physician* 91(5):299-307, 2015.
6. Nagami GT: Hyperchloremia—why and how, *Nefrologia* 36(4):347-353, 2016.
7. Gankam Kengne KF: Physiopathology, clinical diagnosis, and treatment of hyponatremia, *Acta Clin Belg* 71(6):359-372, 2016.
8. McDonough AA, Youn JH: Potassium homeostasis: the knowns, the unknowns, and the health benefits, *Physiology (Bethesda)* 32(2):100-111, 2017.
9. Elliott TL: Electrolytes: potassium disorders, *FP Essent* 459:21-28, 2017.
10. Allgrove J: Physiology of calcium, phosphate, magnesium and vitamin D, *Endocr Dev* 28:7-32, 2015.
11. Hamm LL, Nakhoul N, Hering-Smith KS: Acid-base homeostasis, *Clin J Am Soc Nephrol* 10(12):2232-2242, 2015.
12. Berend K, de Vries AP, Gans RO: Physiological approach to assessment of acid-base disturbances, *N Engl J Med* 371(15):1434-1445, 2014. Erratum in: *N Engl J Med* 371(20):1948.
13. Seifter JL, Chang HY: Disorders of acid-base balance: new perspectives, *Kidney Dis (Basel)* 2(4):170-186, 2017.
14. Sharma S, Aggarwal S: Hyperchloremic acidosis, *StatPearls [Internet]*. Treasure Island, FL, 2018, StatPearls Publishing. Available from: http://www.ncbi.nlm.nih.gov/books/NBK482340/.

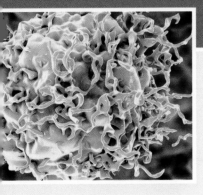

6

Innate Immunity: Inflammation and Wound Healing

Valentina L. Brashers, Lois E. Brenneman

EVOLVE WEBSITE

http://evolve.elsevier.com/Huether/
Student Review Questions
Audio Key Points

Case Studies
Animations
Quick Check Answers

CHAPTER OUTLINE

The human body is continually exposed to a large variety of conditions that result in damage, such as sunlight, pollutants, agents that can cause physical trauma, and infectious agents (viruses, bacteria, fungi, and parasites). Damage can also come from within, such as with cancers. The damage may be at the level of a single cell, which can be easily repaired, or may be at the level of multiple cells, tissues, or organs, which can result in disease and death. In response, the human body has developed a highly sophisticated system of interactive immune defense mechanisms. *Innate immunity* refers to defense mechanisms that are present at birth and provide the initial response to invasion and injury. *Adaptive (or acquired) immunity* refers to immunity that develops over the lifetime of the individual and provides long-term protection against specific invaders.

HUMAN DEFENSE MECHANISMS

The human body has several ways to protect itself from injury and infection. Innate immunity includes natural barriers and inflammation. Innate barriers form the first line of defense at the body's surfaces. They serve to prevent damage by the environment and thwart infection by pathogenic microorganisms. If the surface barriers are breached, the second line of defense, the inflammatory response, is activated to protect the body from further injury, fight infection, and promote healing. The third line of defense, adaptive immunity (also known as *acquired* or *specific immunity*), is induced through a slower and more specific process and targets particular invaders and diseased tissues for the purpose of eradicating them. Adaptive immunity also involves "memory,"

which results in a more rapid response during future exposure to the same invader. Comparisons among defense mechanisms are described in Table 6.1. The information presented in this chapter introduces the components and processes of innate immunity and sets the stage for Chapter 7, which presents an overview of adaptive immunity; Chapter 8, which discusses alterations in immunity; and Chapter 9, which reviews infection. Innate immunity in the newborn and changes associated with aging are reviewed in the Pediatric Considerations and Geriatric Considerations boxes at the end of the chapter.

INNATE IMMUNITY

First Line of Defense: Physical and Biochemical Barriers and the Human Microbiome

Innate barriers form the first line of defense at the body's surfaces. These barriers can be physical, mechanical, and biochemical. Surface barriers also may house a group of beneficial microorganisms known as the "normal microbiome" that can protect us from pathogenic microorganisms.

Physical Barriers

The physical barriers offer considerable protection from tissue damage and infection. These barriers comprise tightly associated epithelial cells of the skin and of the linings of the gastrointestinal, genitourinary, and respiratory tracts (Fig. 6.1). When pathogens attempt to penetrate such barriers, they may be removed by mechanical means. Such

TABLE 6.1   **Overview of Human Defenses**

| Characteristics | INNATE IMMUNITY | | Adaptive Immunity |
	Barriers	Inflammatory Response	
Level of defense	First line of defense against infection and tissue injury	Second line of defense; occurs as response to tissue injury or infection (inflammatory response)	Third line of defense; initiated when innate immune system signals cells of adaptive immunity
Timing of defense	Constant	Immediate response	Delay between first exposure to antigen and maximal response; immediate against secondary exposure to same antigen
Specificity	Broadly specific	Broadly specific	Response is very specific toward target
Cells	Epithelial cells	Mast cells, granulocytes (neutrophils, eosinophils, basophils), monocytes/macrophages, natural killer (NK) cells, platelets, endothelial cells	T lymphocytes, B lymphocytes, macrophages, dendritic cells
Memory	No memory involved	No memory involved	Specific immunologic memory by T and B lymphocytes
Active molecules	Defensins, collectins, lactoferrin, bacterial toxins	Activation of complement, clotting factors, kinins, cytokines	Antibodies, complement, cytokines
Protection	Protection includes anatomic barriers (i.e., skin and mucous membranes), cells and secretory molecules (e.g., lysozymes, low pH of stomach and urine), and ciliary activity	Protection includes vascular responses, cellular components (e.g., mast cells, neutrophils, macrophages), secretory molecules or cytokines, and activation of plasma protein systems	Protection includes activated T and B lymphocytes, cytokines, and antibodies

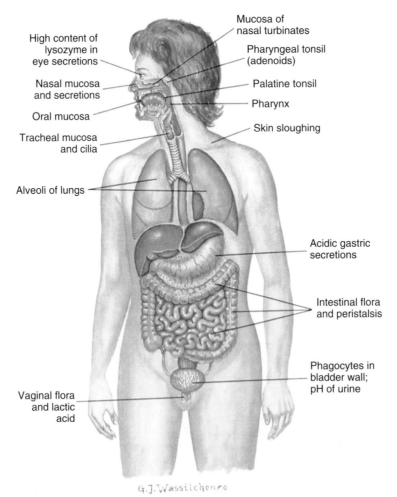

G.J.Wassilchenro

FIGURE 6.1 Protection at Body Surfaces. (From Grimes DE: *Infectious diseases,* St. Louis, 1991, Mosby.)

microorganisms may be sloughed off with dead skin cells (which can then be replaced). Epithelial cells of the upper respiratory tract can trap microorganisms through the production of mucus and remove them through the action of hair-like cilia which move the mucus upward where it is expelled through coughing or sneezing. Invading microorganisms can be removed from the gastrointestinal (GI) tract through vomiting or defecation and from the urinary tract through urination. Other protective mechanisms of innate barriers include the relatively low temperature present on the skin and the low pH found in the stomach, both of which inhibit the growth of pathogenic microorganisms.

Cell-Derived Chemicals

Several cells participate in innate immune defenses.[1] Epithelial cells secrete an array of substances that protect against infection, including mucus, perspiration, saliva, tears, and earwax. These substances trap potential invaders and contain substances that are lethal to microorganisms. Perspiration, tears, and saliva contain the enzyme lysozyme which attacks the cell walls of gram-positive bacteria. Sebaceous glands in the skin secrete fatty acids and lactic acid, substances which kill bacteria and fungi. These secretions also create an acidic environment on the skin surface (pH 3 to pH 5) which is inhospitable to most bacteria. Epithelial cell secretions contain antimicrobial peptides, substances that kill or inhibit the growth of disease-causing bacteria, fungi, and viruses. Defensins are antimicrobial peptides produced by neutrophils and epithelial cells that defend against bacterial infection by disrupting bacterial membranes. Collectins are soluble glycoproteins that facilitate the ability of macrophages to recognize and kill pathogenic microorganisms and can activate the lectin pathway of the complement system (see the Plasma Protein Systems and Inflammation section). They are produced by various organs, including the lung (i.e., surfactant is a type of collectin).

The Normal Microbiome

The body's surfaces are colonized with an array of microorganisms, called the normal microbiome (previously referred to as normal flora).[2] Body surfaces that have their own types of microbiome include the skin; mucous membranes of the eye, nose, and mouth; upper and lower GI tracts; upper respiratory tract; urethra; and vagina. These surfaces are colonized by a combination of bacteria and fungi unique to the anatomic location and the particular individual. The microorganisms in the microbiome do not normally cause disease. Their relationship with the human body may be *commensal* (benefitting the microorganism without affecting the body), or it may be *mutualistic* (benefitting both the microorganism and the body). The normal microbiome benefits the human body in a number of ways, and the human body provides an ideal environment for the microbiome to grow. For example, the human colon and lower gut are relatively sterile at birth, but colonization with bacteria begins quickly and progressively increases during the first year of life. During this time frame, the diversity and concentration of microorganisms increase forming the normal microbiome of the gut. The normal microbiome:

1. Produces enzymes which facilitate digestion of fatty acids and large polysaccharides
2. Synthesizes essential metabolites (e.g., vitamins K and B)
3. Releases antibacterial substances that are toxic to pathogenic microorganisms (e.g., ammonia, phenols, and indoles)
4. Competes with pathogens for nutrients and blocks attachment of the pathogens to the epithelium, an obligatory first step in the infectious process
5. Fosters adaptive immunity by inducing the growth of gut-associated lymphoid tissue, an important site in the development of both local and adaptive immunity

6. Contributes to bidirectional communication between the brain and the GI tract (brain–gut axis) which has implications for cognitive function, behavior, pain modulation, stress responses, and disease

Prolonged treatment with broad-spectrum antibiotics can alter the normal microbiome, decreasing its protective activity, and leads to an overgrowth of pathogenic microorganisms. In the intestine, for example, overgrowth of the yeast *Candida albicans* or the bacterium *Clostridioides difficile* (the cause of pseudomembranous colitis) may occur with antibiotic use.

The physical integrity of the skin and mucosal epithelium act in concert with other protective mechanisms to shield the microbiome from immune and inflammatory responses. Some members of the normal bacterial microbiome are opportunistic pathogens—that is, they are harmless under normal conditions but can cause disease in immunocompromised individuals who lack the usual defense mechanisms. For example, *Pseudomonas aeruginosa* is a member of the normal microbiome of the skin, where it produces a toxin that protects the skin from infections caused by pathologic bacteria. With severe burns, where the integrity of the skin is compromised, *Pseudomonas* may enter the bloodstream and cause life-threatening systemic infections.

✔ QUICK CHECK 6.1

1. How do physical and mechanical barriers contribute to defense mechanisms?
2. What are antimicrobial peptides?
3. What is the microbiome? What is its role in defense?
4. What are opportunistic microorganisms?

Second Line of Defense: Inflammation

Inflammation is a protective response that supports recovery from injury and disease. Fig. 6.2 summarizes the process. When cellular or tissue damage occurs, inflammatory mediators are released, causing a number of changes in the microcirculation. The ultimate result of these changes is the migration of leukocytes, plasma proteins, and other biochemical mediators from the circulation into the nearby damaged tissue, where they can work together to destroy invaders, limit tissue injury, and promote healing. Uncontrolled or chronic inflammation plays a role in virtually all diseases, including heart and lung disease, cancer, neurodegenerative disorders, and rheumatologic disease.

Inflammation is a dynamic process programmed to respond to cellular or tissue damage irrespective of the location or condition of the tissue. There is a *rapid* initiation of an interactive system of humoral (soluble in the blood) and cellular responses. Inflammation functions to destroy pathogens, trigger the adaptive immune response, limit the extent of tissue damage, and initiate the healing process.

The inflammatory response is characterized by the following:

1. The process occurs in vascularized tissues (i.e., tissues with a blood supply).
2. Activation is rapid (within seconds) after damage occurs.
3. The response includes both *cellular and chemical components*.
4. The response is *nonspecific*—that is, it takes place in approximately the same way regardless of the type of injury (stimulus) and whether or not the same stimulus has occurred in the past.

Vascular Response

Inflammation is activated by virtually any injury to vascularized tissues. Triggers include infection and tissue damage (e.g., ischemia, trauma, physical or chemical injury, foreign bodies, and immune reactions). The classic or cardinal signs of acute inflammation were

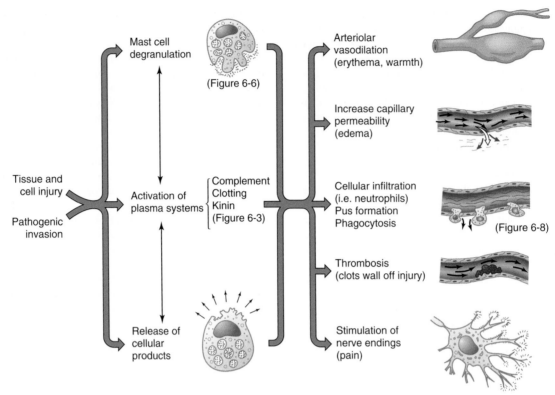

FIGURE 6.2 Acute Inflammatory Response. Inflammation is usually initiated by cellular injury and may be complicated by infection. The inflammatory response involves mast cell degranulation, the activation of three plasma protein systems, and the activation of macrophages that release numerous cytokines. These systems are interdependent so that induction of one (e.g., mast cell degranulation) can result in the induction of the other two. The result is the development of the characteristic microscopic and clinical hallmarks of inflammation. The figure numbers refer to additional figures in which more detailed information may be found on that portion of the response.

described in the first century by a Roman named Celsus. They include the following:

1. **Rubor** (redness, erythema)
2. **Calor** (heat)
3. **Tumor** (swelling)
4. **Dolor** (pain)
5. **Functio laesa (loss of function)**

All of these signs occur because of microscopic inflammatory changes that happen within seconds of the injury in the microcirculation (arterioles, capillaries, and venules) surrounding the site of an injury. They include the following processes:

1. **Hemostasis (coagulation):** Injury to blood vessels initiates the clotting cascade and activates platelets. Clotting slows blood flow, walls off injury, and provides a meshwork for healing.
2. **Vasodilation:** Increased diameter of blood vessels that increases the volume of blood delivered to the injured site and slows the velocity of blood flow, and this allows more time for the movement of fluids, chemicals, and cells into surrounding tissues, resulting in erythema (redness) and warmth in the area of injury.
3. **Increased vascular permeability:** Blood vessels become porous, secondary to contraction of endothelial cells, thus enlarging the spaces between these cells. This results in exudation (the leaking of fluid from vessels) and edema (tissue swelling from fluid leakage) of the area surrounding the injury.
4. **White blood cell adhesion:** White blood cells (WBCs) adhere to the inner walls of vessels, where they migrate through the enlarged spaces between endothelial cells and into the surrounding tissue. Accordingly,

there is an influx of **phagocytes** (neutrophils and macrophages) to the injured tissue, where they target foreign microorganisms.

These vascular changes deliver leukocytes (particularly neutrophils), plasma proteins, and other biochemical mediators to the site of injury. Chemical mediators activate pain fibers, producing the characteristic pain associated with injury. The tissue injury, pain, and swelling contribute to loss of function. Lymphatic vessels, which drain the extravascular fluid to lymph nodes, may become secondarily inflamed. The resulting **lymphangitis** (inflammation of lymph vessels) or **lymphadenitis** (inflammation of nodes) can present as enlarged and painful lymph nodes. For example, in an individual with a sore throat, the infected and inflamed pharynx can result in enlarged and painful lymph nodes, which are readily palpable in the neck region.

Inflammation, although producing pain and functional limitations in the individual so affected, also results in numerous physiologic benefits. Protective functions of inflammation include the following:

1. *Prevention of infection and further damage caused by invading microorganisms:* Inflammatory exudates dilute the toxins produced by both bacteria and dying cells. The activation of plasma protein systems (e.g., complement and clotting systems) serves to contain and destroy invading microorganisms. The influx of phagocytes (neutrophils and macrophages) removes toxic cellular debris and pathogenic microorganisms, preventing them from further harming the body.
2. *Limitation of the scope of the inflammatory process:* The influx of plasma protein systems (e.g., clotting system, plasma enzymes, and

specific blood or tissue cells) prevents the inflammatory response from spreading to areas of healthy tissue.

3. *Preparation of injury for healing and repair:* This involves removal of bacterial microorganisms, dead cells, and other physiologic debris through the epithelial channels and the lymphatic vessels that drain the region.

4. *Facilitation of the development of adaptive immunity:* As fluid and cellular debris drain through the lymphatic vessels and nodes, microbial antigens encounter macrophages and lymphocytes concentrated in these nodes. Adaptive immunity is initiated and helps fight off invaders and protect the body from future exposures to particular pathogens (see Chapter 7).

✔ **QUICK CHECK 6.2**
1. Why are innate immunity and inflammation described as "nonspecific"?
2. What are the five classic symptoms of acute inflammation?
3. Describe the basic steps in acute inflammation.
4. What are the benefits of inflammation?

Plasma Protein Systems and Inflammation

Three key plasma protein systems are essential to an effective inflammatory response, the complement system, the clotting system, and the kinin system (Fig. 6.3). Although each system has a unique role in inflammation, all these systems have many similarities as well. Each system consists of multiple proteins and enzymes usually present in blood as inactive forms. The proteins are activated early in inflammation by enzymes, which circulate as proenzymes until some form of tissue damage triggers the system initiating the sequence. Activation of the first components results in sequential activation of other components of the system, leading to a protective biologic function. This sequential activation is referred to as a *cascade,* hence the common terminology that references the complement cascade, the clotting cascade, or the kinin cascade.

Complement system. The complement system intensifies or complements the capacity of antibodies and phagocytes to clear pathogens and damaged cells and activate inflammation. The complement system consists of a large number of proteins (sometimes called *complement factors*), which, together, constitute about 10% of the total circulating serum protein. Factors activated during the complement cascade are among the body's most potent defenses, particularly in the context of bacterial infection. Activation of the complement system produces several substances that can destroy pathogens directly or can eradicate pathogens through enhancing the activity of other components of the immune response.[3] The activation of C3 and C5, two important components of the complement cascade, results in three potent molecules critical to the immune response:

1. C3b—along with antibodies, serves as opsonins which coat the surface of bacteria increasing their susceptibility to phagocytosis by inflammatory cells (i.e., phagocytes [neutrophils and macrophages]).

2. C5a—functions as a chemotactic factor by diffusing from a site of inflammation and, like a magnet, attracting leukocytes to that site.

3. C3a and C5a—sometimes called anaphylatoxins, induce rapid degranulation of mast cells to release histamine, a substance which induces vasodilation and increased capillary permeability.

Another important component of the complement system is the membrane attack complex (MAC), composed of elements C6 through C9. The MAC leads to bacterial destruction and tissue injury by creating pores in the outer membranes of cells or bacteria. These pores facilitate the infusion of water into the cells culminating in cellular death.

Three major pathways or cascades control the activation of complement (see Fig. 6.3, *A*): the classical pathway, the alternative pathway, and the lectin pathway. The classical pathway is activated by antibodies, which are components of the adaptive immune system. Antibodies bind to their targets, antigens, which are typically proteins or carbohydrates produced by infectious microorganisms. Such antibodies activate the first complement component, C1, which, in turn, leads to the sequential activation of other components of the complement cascade, specifically, C3 and C5, triggering inflammation.

The alternative pathway is activated directly by substances found on the surface of infectious microorganisms. These substances would include lipopolysaccharides (endotoxins) found on bacterial membranes and carbohydrates (zymosan) found on yeast cell walls. This pathway uses unique proteins (factor B, factor D, and properdin) to form a complex that sequentially activates the complement proteins C3 and C5. At this point, the process converges with the classical pathway. The alternative pathway provides a mechanism whereby the complement system can be activated in the absence of antibodies.

The lectin pathway, like the alternative pathway, is independent of antibodies and is activated by several plasma proteins, particularly mannose-binding lectin (MBL). MBL binds to bacterial polysaccharides that contain the carbohydrate mannose and activates the complement cascade. Infectious agents that do not activate the alternative pathway may still be susceptible to the complement system through the lectin pathway.

In summary, the complement pathway or cascade is a sequential series of cellular events that serve as defense mechanisms for the body. It can be activated by at least three different pathways, resulting in one or more of four protective functions: *opsonization* (C3b), *anaphylatoxic activity* from mast cell degranulation (C3a, C5a), *leukocyte chemotaxis* (C5a), and *cell lysis* (C5b–C9; membrane attack complex).

Clotting. The clotting system (also known as the coagulation system) is a group of plasma proteins, which, when activated sequentially, form a blood clot (see Fig. 6.3, *B*). The clotting system can be activated by a variety of substances, such as collagen, enzymes, and bacterial toxins, released during tissue injury or infection. A blood clot is a meshwork of fibrin strands and platelets, the primary cellular initiator of clotting. Clots serve to plug damaged vessels and stop bleeding (hemostasis), trap microorganisms, prevent their spread to adjacent tissues, and provide a framework for future repair and healing.

When the wall of a blood vessel is injured, two converging pathways lead to clot formation (see Fig. 6.3, *B*):

1. The tissue factor (extrinsic) pathway is activated by tissue factor (TF), also called tissue thromboplastin, a substance released by damaged endothelial cells of the blood vessels. It reacts with activated factor VII (VIIa).

2. The contact activation (intrinsic) pathway is activated when vessel wall damage causes negatively charged subendothelial substances to come into contact with Hageman factor (factor XII) found in plasma.

Both pathways converge at factor X, forming a common pathway leading to activation of fibrin. Fibrin, in turn, comes together to form a fibrin clot. Activation of the clotting system produces protein fragments known as fibrinopeptides (FPs), which attract neutrophils (chemotaxis) and increase vascular permeability. Additional details concerning the clotting system are discussed in Chapter 22.

Kinin system. The third plasma protein system, the kinin system (see Fig. 6.3, *C*), interacts closely with the clotting system. Both the clotting and kinin systems can be initiated through activation of Hageman factor (factor XII), which, in turn, results in the formation of factor XIIa, also known as *prekallikrein activator.* Factor XIIa activates *prekallikrein,* the first component of the kinin system. The next product in

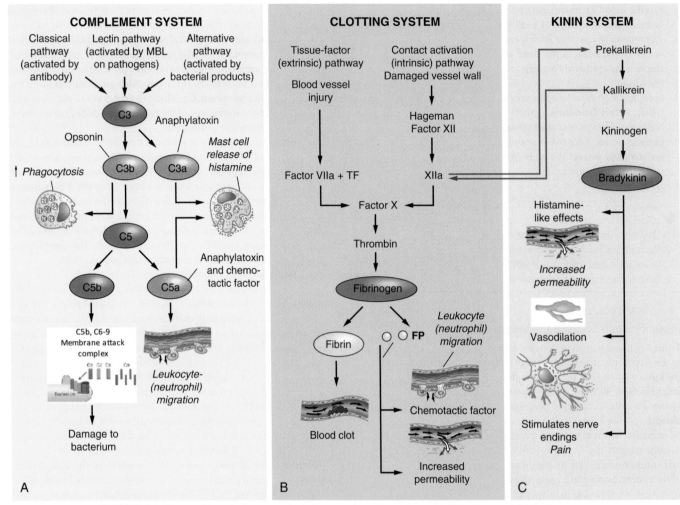

FIGURE 6.3 Plasma Protein Systems in Inflammation: Complement, Clotting, and Kinin Systems.
Each plasma protein system consists of a family of proteins that are activated in sequence to create potent
biologic effects. **A,** The complement system can be activated by three mechanisms, each of which results
in proteolytic activation of C3. The fragments of C3 activation, C3a and C3b, are major components of inflammation. C3a is a potent anaphylatoxin, which induces degranulation of mast cells. C3b can bind to the surface
or cells, such as bacteria, and either serve as an opsonin for phagocytosis or proteolytically activate the next
component of the complement cascade, C5. The smaller fragment of C5 activation is C5a, a powerful anaphylatoxin, and is also chemotactic for neutrophils, attracting them to the site of inflammation. The larger
fragment, C5b, activates the components of the membrane attack complex (C5b–C9), which damage the
bacterial membrane and kill the bacteria. **B,** The clotting system can be activated by the tissue factor (extrinsic)
pathway and the contact activation (intrinsic) pathway. All routes of clotting initiation lead to activation of
factor X and thrombin. Thrombin is an enzyme that activates fibrinogen to form fibrin and small FPs. Fibrin
comes together to form a clot, and the FPs are highly active as chemotactic factors and cause increased
vascular permeability. **C,** Factor XIIa produced by the clotting system can also be activated by kallikrein of
the kinin system *(red arrow)*. Prekallikrein is enzymatically converted to kininogen, which activates bradykinin.
Bradykinin functions similar to histamine and increases vascular permeability. Bradykinin can also stimulate
nerve endings to cause pain. *FP,* Fibrinopeptide; *MBL,* mannose binding lectin; *TF,* tissue factor.

the cascade is *kallikrein,* followed by *kininogen,* a precursor molecule,
and then bradykinin, the final product of the kinin system. **Bradykinin**
causes dilation of blood vessels. Bradykinin also acts in concert with
prostaglandins to induce pain, trigger smooth muscle cell contraction
(i.e., bronchoconstriction), and increase vascular permeability.

Control and interaction of plasma protein systems. The three
plasma protein systems are highly interactive. The activation of one
system results in the production of a large number of biologically
active substances that activate other systems. Tight regulation of these
processes is essential for two reasons. First the inflammatory process

is critical for an individual's survival; therefore efficient activation
must occur regardless of the cause of tissue injury. The interaction among the three systems means that the entire inflammatory
response may be activated regardless of which system initially triggers
the sequence. Second the biochemical mediators released during the
inflammatory response are potent and potentially harmful to the
individual. Their actions must be controlled and confined to injured or
infected tissues.

Multiple mechanisms are available to regulate the plasma protein
systems, activating or inactivating the reactions to maintain balance,

and contain the inflammatory response. Plasma entering the tissues during inflammation contains enzymes that destroy the mediators of inflammation and downregulate the inflammatory response. These enzymes include protease inhibitors (e.g., C1-inhibitor), which inhibit activation of the complement system; carboxypeptidase, which inactivates the toxic activities of C3a and C5a; kininase, which degrades kinins; and histaminase, which degrades histamine and kallikrein. The formation of clots activates a fibrinolytic system. This system serves to limit the size of the clot and degrade the clot after bleeding has ceased. In this system thrombin activates plasminogen, forming the enzyme plasmin, which degrades the fibrin polymers in clots.

Defects in these mechanisms can be genetic or acquired. For example, a genetic defect in the protease C1 inhibitor (C1-inh) results in hereditary angioedema, a self-limiting edema of cutaneous and mucosal layers. Acquired defects in plasminogen activation, which is seen in severe infection, can result in widespread clotting.

✔ QUICK CHECK 6.3
1. What are the three most important products of the complement system?
2. How is the clotting cascade activated? How is it related to the plasma kinin cascade?
3. Why is the control of the plasma protein systems of inflammation essential?

Cellular Components of Inflammation

Cells of both the innate and the adaptive immune systems respond to molecules produced at a site of cellular damage and are recruited to that site to help with the protective response. These molecules originate from destroyed or damaged cells, microorganisms, activation of the plasma protein systems, or secretions by other cells of the innate or adaptive immune systems. Each cell has a set of cell surface receptors that specifically bind these molecules, resulting in intracellular signaling pathways and activation of the cell itself. Most of these inflammatory cells and protein systems, along with the substances they produce, act at the site of tissue injury to confine the extent of damage, kill microorganisms, remove the cellular debris, and activate healing (tissue regeneration or repair).

Many different types of cells and cellular components are involved in the inflammatory process, including mast cells, endothelial cells, platelets, phagocytes (neutrophils and macrophages), and lymphocytes. Inflammatory cells and cellular mediators are critical components of an effective innate immune response

Vascular Tissues and Cells

Inflammation is a process occurring in vascular tissue, where numerous protective cells reside, both in blood and within the tissues surrounding blood vessels (Fig. 6.4). Blood vessels are lined with endothelial cells, which actively maintain blood flow. During inflammation, the vascular

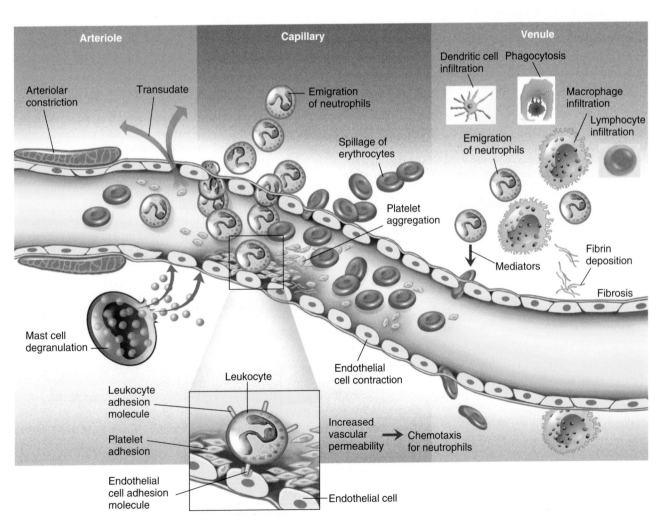

FIGURE 6.4 Cellular Components and Sequences of Events in the Acute Inflammatory Response.

endothelium becomes a principal coordinator of blood clotting and facilitates the passage of cells and fluid into the surrounding tissue. The tissues surrounding the vessels contain mast cells, the most important mediators of inflammation. Also present are macrophages and dendritic cells (a type of macrophage), which connect the innate and adaptive immune responses.

Blood cells are divided into erythrocytes (red blood cells [RBCs]), platelets, and leukocytes (WBCs). Erythrocytes, which carry oxygen to tissues and platelets, are small cell fragments involved in blood clotting. Leukocytes are subdivided into granulocytes (containing many enzyme-filled cytoplasmic granules), monocytes, and lymphocytes. Granulocytes are the most common leukocytes and are classified by the type of stains needed to visualize enzyme-containing granules in their cytoplasm (basophils, eosinophils, and neutrophils). Monocytes are precursors of macrophages that are found in the tissue. Various forms of lymphocytes participate in the innate immune response (e.g., natural killer [NK] cells) and the adaptive immune response (B and T cells).

Cells of both the innate and the adaptive immune systems respond to molecules (chemotaxins) produced at sites of cellular injury, where they mediate both the innate and the adaptive immune responses. Triggers include dead or damaged cells, infectious microorganisms, plasma protein system mediators, or secretions from cells involved in the immune response. Each cell has a set of cell surface receptors that specifically bind these molecules. Binding results in *cellular activation* through intracellular signaling pathways. Activation may result in the cell gaining a function critical to the inflammatory response and releasing additional cellular mediators to support the response.

Cellular Receptors

Cells involved in initiating the innate immune response have evolved a set of receptors referred to as *pattern recognition receptors (PRRs)* (Table 6.2). PRRs are generally expressed on cells in tissues near the body's surfaces (skin, respiratory tract, GI tract, genitourinary tract), where they monitor the environment for products of cellular damage and infectious microorganisms. PRRs recognize two types of molecular patterns:

1. Pathogen-associated molecular patterns (PAMPs), which are molecules expressed by infectious agents found either on their surface or released as soluble molecules
2. Damage-associated molecular patterns (DAMPs), which are products of cellular damage

Accordingly cells of the innate immune system can respond to both sterile tissue damage (DAMPs) and septic tissue damage (PAMPs and DAMPs). It is estimated that at least 100 different PRRs are found on innate immune cells, rendering them capable of recognizing more than 1000 different molecules.

An important group of PRRs are toll-like receptors (TLRs), which recognize a large variety of PAMPs located on the cell wall or surface of microorganisms (e.g., bacterial lipopolysaccharide, peptidoglycans, lipoproteins, yeast zymosan, flagellin, bacterial or viral nucleic acid, and viral coat proteins). TLRs are expressed on the surface of many cells that have direct and early contact with potential pathogens. Such cells include mucosal epithelial cells, mast cells, neutrophils, macrophages, dendritic cells, and lymphocytes. Activation of TLRs leads to the release of numerous *inflammatory cytokines,* such as tumor necrosis factor (TNF) and interleukin-6 (IL-6), which have a key role in the destruction of many pathogenic microorganisms.

C-type lectin receptors (CLRs) are a group of PRRs that bind to both PAMPs and DAMPs. There are many types of CLRs, such as macrophage mannose, Dectin 1 and 2, and mannose-binding lectin receptors. They are particularly important in recognizing fungal antigens and subsequent activation of innate immune cells.

Nucleotide-binding-like receptors (NLRs) and nucleotide oligo-merization domain–like (NOD-like) receptors are cytoplasmic (intracellular) receptors in lymphocytes, macrophages, and dendritic cells. At least 22 NLRs have been identified in humans. They recognize PAMPs and DAMPs and initiate the production of proinflammatory mediators. NOD-like receptors help control the inflammatory response.

Complement receptors are found on many cells involved in the immune response, as well as on some epithelial cells. These receptors recognize several fragments produced through activation of the complement system, particularly C3a, C5a, and C3b. This results in chemotaxis and activation of innate immune cells.

Scavenger receptors are membrane receptors primarily expressed on macrophages, where they facilitate recognition and phagocytosis of bacterial pathogens, damaged cells, and soluble lipoproteins, such as high-density lipoprotein (HDL), low-density lipoprotein (LDL), and oxidized LDL. Ten classes of receptors have been identified, including receptors that function to remove senescent erythrocytes and cells undergoing apoptosis (normal cell death).

Cellular Mediators and Products

To elicit an effective inflammatory or adaptive immune response, intercellular communication and cooperation are necessary. Cytokines constitute a large family of small soluble *intercellular-signaling molecules.* They are secreted by a variety of cells and bind to specific cell membrane receptors, where they regulate innate or adaptive immunity (Fig. 6.5). Cytokines may be either *proinflammatory* or *antiinflammatory,* depending

TABLE 6.2 **Pattern Recognition Receptors (PRRs)**			
Receptors	**Number of Receptors**	**What They Recognize**	**Where They Are Found**
Toll-like receptors (TLRs)	10	PAMPs such as microbial surface structures and nucleic acids	Outer membrane of phagocytic cells with early contact with infectious microorganisms especially macrophages and dendritic cells
C-type lectin receptors (CLRs)	Multiple	PAMPS (especially fungi) and DAMPs	Outer membrane of phagocytic cells
NOD-like receptors and NLR receptors	~22	PAMPs and DAMPs	Cytoplasm of innate immune cells
Complement receptors	Multiple	C3a, C3b, C5a	Outer membrane of innate immune cells, platelets, epithelial cells, vascular smooth muscle
Scavenger receptors	~8	Cell membrane phospholipid phosphatidylserine (PS)	Outer membrane of macrophages

DAMP, Damage-associated molecular patterns; *NOD,* nucleotide oligomerization domain-like receptors; *NRL,* nucleotide-binding-like receptors; *PAMP,* pathogen-associated molecular patterns.

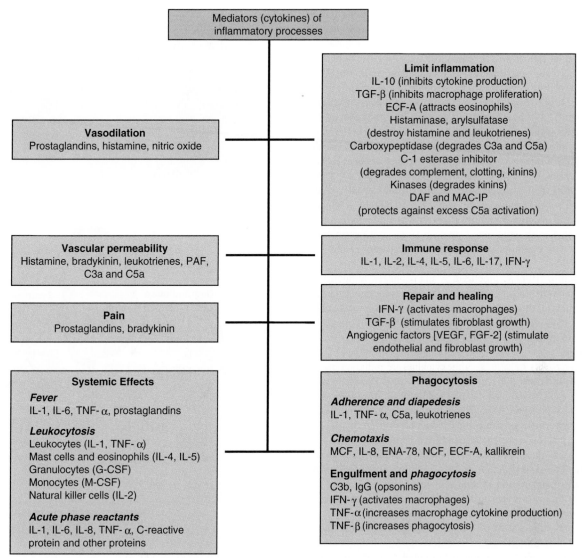

FIGURE 6.5 Principal Mediators of Inflammatory Processes. *C3b,* Large fragment produced from complement component C3; *C3a,* small fragment produced from complement component C3; *C5a,* small fragment produced from complement component C5; *DAF,* (complement) decay accelerating factor; *ECF-A,* eosinophil chemotactic factor of anaphylaxis; *FGF,* fibroblast growth factor; *IFN,* interferon; *IgG,* immunoglobulin G (predominant class of antibody in the blood); *IL,* interleukin; *MAC-IP,* membrane attack complex-inhibitory protein; *MCF,* monocyte chemotactic factor; *NCF,* neutrophil chemotactic factor; *PAF,* platelet-activating factor; *TGF,* T-cell growth factor; *TNF,* tumor necrosis factor; *VEGF,* vascular endothelial growth factor.

on whether they tend to induce or inhibit the inflammatory response. These molecules usually diffuse over short distances; however, some have systemic effects, such as fever induced by particular cytokines known as *endogenous pyrogens.*

A large number of cytokines have been described and classified into several families based on structural differences. Cytokines are small signaling proteins secreted by a variety of cell types. The terms lymphokines and monokines refer to cytokines secreted from lymphocytes or monocytes, respectively. Chemokines are members of a special family of cytokines that are chemotactic (i.e., they attract leukocytes to the sites of inflammation). Chemokines also are synthesized by many cell types, including macrophages, fibroblasts, and endothelial cells. To date, more than 50 different human chemokines have been described.

Interleukins (ILs) are produced predominantly by macrophages and lymphocytes in response to stimulation of PRRs or by other cytokines

and serve to alter the behavior of cells. More than 30 interleukins have been identified. Their effects include the following:

1. Regulation of cell adhesion molecules (CAMs), proteins that facilitate cells to bind with other cells or with the extracellular matrix
2. Attraction of leukocytes to a site of inflammation (chemotaxis)
3. Induction, proliferation, and maturation of leukocytes in bone marrow
4. General enhancement or suppression of inflammation and the adaptive immune response

Proinflammatory cytokines. There are many proinflammatory cytokines, of which TNF-α is one of the most important. It interacts closely with two major proinflammatory interleukins, that is, IL-1 and IL-6.

Tumor necrosis factor-alpha (TNF-α) is primarily secreted by activated macrophages but is also released by mast cells, neutrophils, and lymphocytes. When PRRs on the surface of macrophages bind to PAMPs or DAMPs, an intracellular protein complex, called *nuclear factor-kappa B (NF-κB)*, is activated, which induces a multitude of proinflammatory effects, such as chemotaxis and adherence of neutrophils, phagocytosis, and inflammatory and adaptive immune cell proliferation. TNF-α plays a role in the response to virtually any injury or infection. It also contributes to the damaging effects of chronic inflammation. TNF-α has systemic effects, including the induction of fever, increased liver synthesis of inflammation-related serum proteins (acute phase proteins), muscle wasting (cachexia), and intravascular thrombosis. These effects can be deleterious in cases of severe or chronic infection and cancer.

Interleukin-1 (IL-1) is produced mainly by macrophages and activates monocytes, other macrophages, and lymphocytes, thereby enhancing both innate and adaptive immunity. It also acts as a growth factor for many cells. IL-1 is an endogenous pyrogen (fever-causing cytokine) which reacts with receptors on cells of the hypothalamus resulting in fever.

Interleukin-6 (IL-6) is produced by macrophages, lymphocytes, fibroblasts, and other cells. IL-6 directly induces hepatocytes in the liver to produce many of the proteins needed for inflammation (acute phase proteins). IL-6 also stimulates growth and differentiation of blood cells in the bone marrow and the growth of fibroblasts required for wound healing.

Antiinflammatory cytokines. Some cytokines are antiinflammatory and diminish and control the inflammatory response. Two of the most important are IL-10 and TNF-β. **Interleukin-10 (IL-10)** is primarily produced by lymphocytes. It suppresses the activation and proliferation of other lymphocytes and limits the production of proinflammatory cytokines by macrophages. The result is a downregulation of both the inflammatory and the adaptive immune responses. **Transforming growth factor-beta (TGF-β)** is produced by many cells in response to inflammation. Its primary role in immunity is to suppress the activity of lymphocytes and downregulate the production of proinflammatory cytokines by macrophages.

Interferons. **Interferons (IFNs)** are members of a unique family of cytokines that protect against viral infections and modulate the immune response. They are considered essential components of both innate and adaptive immunity. Type I interferons (primarily IFN-α, IFN-β) are produced and released by virally infected cells. These IFNs do not kill viruses; rather they induce antiviral proteins and protection in neighboring healthy cells. Type II interferon (IFN-γ) is produced primarily by lymphocytes. It activates macrophages and increases their capacity to detect and process invaders and abnormal cells so that they can be removed by the adaptive immune system.

Immunoreactive Cells

Mast cells. **Mast cells** are significant and potent activators of the inflammatory response. They have abundant granules containing biochemical mediators, which are released in instances of tissue injury (Fig. 6.6). They also can be activated by components of the complement cascade and by immunoglobulin E (IgE) antibodies produced in allergies. Located in connective tissue and close to vessels, they can be found near the body's surfaces (skin, GI, and respiratory tract linings). A variety of stimuli associated with tissue injury can induce inflammation by triggering the release of potent soluble substances from mast cells. These substances are released in two ways:

1. *Degranulation*—release of the contents of mast cell granules
2. *Synthesis*—the new production and release of mediators in response to a stimulus

Degranulation. Mast cells release biochemical mediators from their granules into the surrounding tissues within seconds of a stimulus,

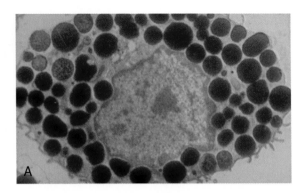

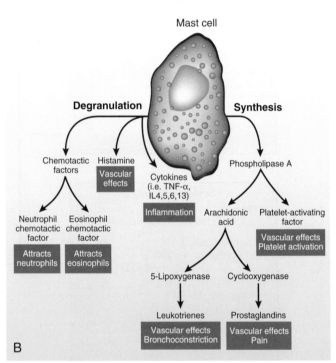

FIGURE 6.6 Mast Cell and Mast Cell Degranulation and Synthesis of Biologic Mediators During Inflammation. A, Colorized photomicrograph of mast cell; dense red granules contain biologically active substances. Among these are histamine, which is a major initiator of vascular changes, and a variety of chemotactic factors. **B,** Mast cell degranulation *(left)* and synthesis *(right)*. Histamine and other biologically active substances are released immediately after stimulation of mast cells. (A, from Roitt IM et al: *Immunology,* ed 3, St Louis, 1993, Mosby.)

resulting in tissue injury. Substances within the granules include histamine, chemotactic factors, and cytokines. Their effects occur immediately. **Histamine** is a small-molecular-weight molecule with potent effects on many other cells, particularly those that control the circulation. Histamine binds to *histamine receptors* (H1 and H2) on the target cell surface (Fig. 6.7). The binding of histamine to the *H1 receptor* is proinflammatory. Histamine and serotonin (not found in mast cells but released from platelets) are called *vasoactive amines.* These molecules cause a rapid, temporary constriction of smooth muscle, along with dilation of the postcapillary venules. The net result of these two effects is increased blood flow within the microcirculation. Histamine also causes increased vascular permeability, secondary to the retraction of endothelial cells lining the capillaries, and increased leukocyte adherence to the endothelial walls. **Antihistamines** are drugs that block the binding of histamine to its receptors, resulting in decreased vascular effects. The

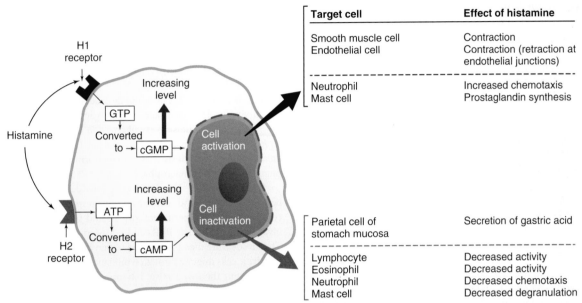

FIGURE 6.7 Effects of Histamine Through H1 and H2 Receptors. The effects depend on (1) the density and affinity of H1 or H2 receptors on the target cell and (2) the identity of the target cell. *ATP,* Adenosine triphosphate; *cAMP,* cyclic adenosine monophosphate; *cGMP,* cyclic guanosine monophosphate; *GTP,* guanosine triphosphate.

H1 receptor also is present on smooth muscle cells, especially smooth muscle within the bronchi. H1 stimulation results in bronchial smooth muscle contraction and bronchoconstriction often seen in asthma.

In contrast, binding to the *H2 receptor* is generally antiinflammatory because it results in the suppression of leukocyte function. Both H1 and H2 receptors are distributed among many cells and are often present on the same immune cells where they may act in an antagonistic fashion. For example, stimulation of H1 receptors on neutrophils results in an augmentation of neutrophil chemotaxis, whereas stimulation of the H2 receptor results in its inhibition. The role of histamine receptors and hypersensitivity is discussed in Chapter 8. The H2 receptor also is abundant on parietal cells of the stomach mucosa, where stimulation induces the secretion of gastric acid as part of the normal physiology of the stomach. **H2 blockers** are an important group of medications that reduce gastric acidity in individuals prone to peptic ulcers or gastroesophageal reflux disorder (GERD), or both.

Mast cell granules also contain chemotactic factors. **Chemotaxis** is directional movement of cells along a chemical gradient formed by a chemotactic factor. Two important factors are **neutrophil chemotactic factor (NCF)** and **eosinophil chemotactic factor of anaphylaxis (ECF-A)**. Neutrophils are the predominant cell which destroys bacteria in the early stages of inflammation. Eosinophils help regulate the inflammatory response. Both cells are discussed in more detail later in this chapter.

Synthesis of mediators. Activated mast cells initiate synthesis of other mediators of inflammation. These mediators include leukotrienes, prostaglandins, and platelet-activating factor.

1. **Leukotrienes (slow-reacting substances of anaphylaxis [SRS-A])** are lipids that induce smooth muscle contraction (especially bronchoconstriction) and increased vascular permeability. Leukotrienes appear to be important in the later stages of the inflammatory response because they stimulate slower and more prolonged inflammatory responses than does the rapid-acting histamine.
2. **Prostaglandins** cause increased vascular permeability, neutrophil chemotaxis, and pain. Pain results from direct effects on nerves. They are long-chain, unsaturated fatty acids produced by the action of

cyclooxygenase (COX). COX exists in two different forms: COX-1, which activates platelets and protects the stomach lining, and COX-2, which is associated with inflammation. Particular drugs can have inhibitory effects on one or both COX entities. The inhibition of COX-1 is associated with a number of undesirable side effects. Among the most serious of such side effect involves the GI system, where the use of these agents can result in GI bleeding and ulcers. Aspirin and other nonsteroidal antiinflammatory drugs (NSAIDs) inhibit both COX-1 and COX-2. Their use to suppress inflammation is associated with GI tract bleeding. **Selective COX-2 inhibitors** are available and may offer an improved GI effect profile. However, all COX inhibitors have been associated with an increased risk for cardiovascular disease because of their effects on blood vessels and clotting.

3. **Platelet-activating factor (PAF)** molecules can be produced by neutrophils, monocytes, endothelial cells, mast cells, and platelets. The biologic activity of PAF is similar to that of leukotrienes. It causes endothelial cell retraction, which results in increased vascular permeability, leukocyte adhesion to endothelial cells, and platelet activation and can activate mast cells.

Endothelial cells. The lining of blood vessels consists of a layer of **endothelial cells**. Endothelial cells regulate circulation through the microvessels and control the movement of water and solutes between blood and tissues. They maintain normal blood flow by preventing spontaneous activation of platelets and other members of the clotting system when no tissue injury has occurred. Endothelial cells play a key role in inflammation. Damage to the endothelial cell lining of the vessel exposes the *subendothelial connective tissue matrix,* which is prothrombogenic. Platelet activation and formation of clots are initiated through the contact activation (intrinsic) pathway. During episodes of tissue injury, endothelial cells promote the recruitment and invasion of leukocytes. During inflammation, proinflammatory mediators, such as histamine and bradykinin, stimulate endothelial cell contraction and increases capillary permeability and the efflux of plasma and nutrients into the injured tissue. Endothelial cells also promote angiogenesis and facilitate wound healing.

Platelets. Platelets are anucleated (containing no nucleus), cytoplasmic fragments formed from megakaryocytes. They circulate in the bloodstream until activated by a vascular injury. Platelets may be activated through a variety of byproducts of tissue destruction and inflammation, including collagen, thrombin, and PAF. In addition to interacting with components of the coagulation cascade to stop bleeding, platelets degranulate and release biochemical mediators, such as serotonin, which has vascular effects similar to those of histamine to accelerate inflammation. They also synthesize thromboxane A_2 (TXA_2), a potent vasoconstrictor and inducer of platelet aggregation. Finally, platelets can recognize and kill pathogens and release growth factors and proangiogenic factors that promote wound healing.[4] Platelet function is described in further detail in Chapter 22.

Neutrophils. The neutrophil, or polymorphonuclear neutrophil (PMN), is a granulocyte named for its characteristic staining pattern as well as its multilobed nucleus. Neutrophils are the predominant phagocytes in early inflammation, arriving at the inflammatory site within 6 to 12 hours after the initial injury.[5] Several inflammatory mediators (bacterial proteins, complement fragments, and other chemotactic factors) specifically attract and activate circulating neutrophils. The primary role of the neutrophil is to phagocytize pathogenic microbes and remove cellular debris and dead cells from lesions. The neutrophil is a mature cell incapable of division and is sensitive to the acidic environment found at inflammatory sites. Accordingly, it is short lived and rapidly becomes a component of the purulent exudate (pus) removed from the body through the epithelium or drained from the infected site through the lymphatic system. They are present in sterile lesions, which drain "sterile pus," as well as in septic (nonsterile) lesions found in bacterial infections.

Eosinophils. Another type of granulocyte is the eosinophil. Although eosinophils are only mildly phagocytic, they serve as the body's primary defense against *parasites* and regulate *vascular mediators* released from mast cells. Lysosomal granules within the eosinophil contain enzymes that degrade vasoactive substances from mast cells, thus limiting and controlling the vascular effects of inflammation. Eosinophils also are important components of allergic conditions and can contribute to tissue damage; these effects are discussed in Chapter 8.

Basophils. The basophil is the least prevalent granulocyte in the blood. It is similar to mast cells with respect to the contents of its granules. Basophilic granules also contain heparin, a naturally occurring anticoagulation product. Basophils release histamine which, as discussed previously, has potent vasoactive properties. Basophils are an important source of cytokines involved in the adaptive immune response, particularly responses associated with allergies and asthma.

Monocytes and macrophages. Monocytes are the largest of the white blood cells (14–20 μm in diameter). As with other blood cell types, they are produced in bone marrow and enter into the circulation. Monocytes migrate to the site of inflammation where they transform into macrophages. Monocytes also are the precursors of specific *tissue macrophages,* including Kupffer cells (liver), alveolar macrophages (lungs), and microglia (brain). Tissue macrophages are important initial mediators of the inflammatory response.

Monocyte-derived macrophages from the circulation begin appearing at the inflammatory site as soon as 24 hours after the initial neutrophil infiltration but do not arrive in large numbers until 3 to 7 days later. They are attracted by chemotactic factors released by the neutrophils that are already present at the site. Macrophage activation results in two subpopulations, M1 and M2 macrophages, each with specialized functions. *M1 macrophages* have greater bactericidal activity, whereas *M2 macrophages* are primarily involved in tissue healing and repair. Macrophages can survive and divide in the acidic environment of the inflammatory site and so are capable of conducting prolonged phagocytosis of microorganisms and damaged cells. They play an essential role in removing debris and promoting the formation of new blood vessels (angiogenesis) and secretion of growth factors that prepare the tissue for healing.[6] Macrophages are important for the resolution of inflammation.

Several bacteria are resistant to destruction by granulocytes and also can survive inside macrophages. Microorganisms, such as *Mycobacterium tuberculosis* (tuberculosis), *Mycobacterium leprae* (leprosy), *Salmonella typhi* (typhoid fever), *Brucella abortus* (brucellosis), and *Listeria monocytogenes* (listeriosis), can remain dormant or multiply inside the phagolysosomes of macrophages.

Dendritic cells. Dendritic cells provide one of the major links between the innate and adaptive immune responses. They are phagocytic cells located in the peripheral organs and skin, where they recognize invaders through their PRRs and release proinflammatory mediators. The invaders are then internalized within the cell through phagocytosis. Dendritic cells migrate through lymphatic vessels to lymph nodes, where they present the invaders to T lymphocytes resulting in an adaptive immune response.

Lymphocytes and natural killer cells. Lymphocytes, a type of WBC, activate macrophages and initiate specific, protective immune responses against pathogens and cancer. B lymphocytes produce antibodies, and T lymphocytes regulate other immune cells and kill viruses and cancer cells (see Chapter 7). Natural killer (NK) cells, a type of lymphocyte, eliminate virally infected and cancerous cells. NK cells have inhibitory and activating receptors that allow differentiation between infected or tumor cells and normal cells. If the NK cell binds to a target cell through activating receptors, it produces several cytokines and toxic molecules, which, in turn, kill the target cell.

Phagocytosis

Phagocytosis is the ingestion of microbes, foreign particles, or cell fragments[7] (Fig. 6.8). The two most important phagocytes for phagocytizing pathogens or damaged cells are neutrophils and macrophages. Neutrophils circulate in the blood in large numbers and are attracted to the area of injury by chemotactic factors, such as mast cell cytokines, chemokines, and complement. Activated neutrophils and endothelial cells express *adhesion molecules,* which increase the "stickiness" of the cells, causing these neutrophils to more readily adhere to the endothelial cell wall of the capillaries and venules. This process of increased adhesion is called margination, or pavementing. Neutrophil-endothelial interactions lead to diapedesis, the emigration of the cells through the interendothelial junctions.

Once the phagocytic cell enters the inflammatory site inside the tissue, phagocytosis of the invader or damaged cells begins.[8] Phagocytosis, at the inflammatory site, involves four steps:

1. Recognition and adherence of the phagocyte to its target through PRRs and opsonization
2. Engulfment (ingestion or endocytosis) and formation of phagosomes
3. Fusion of the phagosome with lysosomal granules within the phagocyte
4. Destruction of the target

Throughout the process, the digestive enzymes are isolated within membrane-bound vesicles. This isolation protects the phagocyte from harm secondary to the phagocyte's own enzymes.

Opsonization greatly enhances adherence of the phagocyte to the target microorganism or cell. Opsonins that coat the target bacteria or cell act as a "glue" tightening the affinity between the phagocyte and the target making phagocytosis more effective. The most efficient opsonins are C3b of the complement system and antibodies produced during the adaptive immune response.

A. **Tissue**

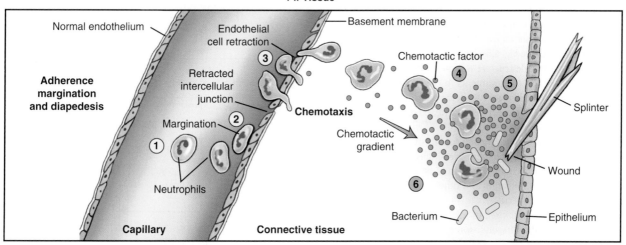

B. **Phagocytosis**

C. **Example of phagocytosis**

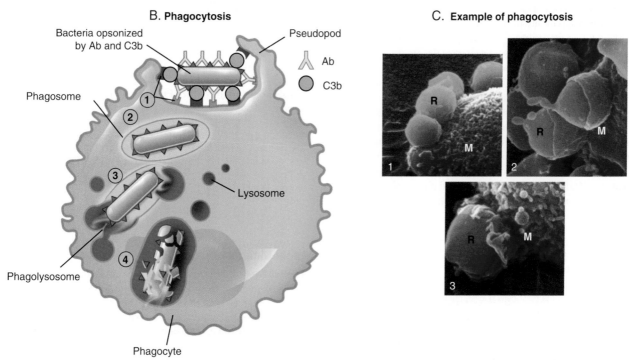

FIGURE 6.8 Process of Phagocytosis. The process that results in phagocytosis is characterized by three interrelated steps: adherence and diapedesis, tissue invasion by chemotaxis, and phagocytosis. **A,** Tissue damage. *Adherence, margination, diapedesis, and chemotaxis.* The primary phagocyte in the blood is the neutrophil, which usually moves freely within the vessel (1). At sites of inflammation, the neutrophil progressively develops increased adherence to the endothelium, leading to accumulation along the vessel wall (margination or pavementing) (2). At sites of endothelial cell retraction the neutrophil exits the blood by means of diapedesis (3). *Chemotaxis.* In the tissues, the neutrophil detects chemotactic factor gradients through surface receptors (4) and migrates toward higher concentrations of the factors (5). The high concentration of chemotactic factors at the site of inflammation immobilizes the neutrophil (6). **B,** Phagocytosis. Opsonized microorganisms are recognized and bind to the surface of a phagocyte through specific receptors (1). The microorganism is engulfed (ingested) into a phagocytic vacuole, or phagosome (2). Lysosomes fuse with the phagosome, resulting in the formation of a phagolysosome (3). During this process, the microorganism is exposed to products of the lysosomes, including a variety of enzymes and products of the hexose-monophosphate shunt (e.g., H_2O_2, O_2^-). The microorganism is killed and digested (4). **C,** Phagocytosis of a red blood cell. The scanning electron micrographs show the progressive steps in phagocytosis. (1) Red blood cells (R) attach to the surface of a macrophage (M). (2) Part of the macrophage membrane starts to enclose the red cell. (3) The red blood cells are almost totally engulfed by the macrophage. (Modified from King DW et al: *General pathology: principles and dynamics,* Philadelphia, 1983, Lea & Febiger.) *Ab,* Antibody; *C3b,* complement component C3b.

Engulfment (**endocytosis**) is a process whereby the microorganism is drawn into the interior of a phagocytic cell. Engulfment is carried out by small pseudopods that extend from the plasma membrane of the phagocyte to surround the target, forming an intracellular **phagocytic vacuole**, or **phagosome** (see Fig. 6.8). Upon formation of a phagosome, the lysosomes (containing destructive enzymes) converge, fuse with the phagosome, and discharge their contents to create a **phagolysosome**. Destruction of the target takes place within the phagolysosome. Destruction is accomplished by both oxygen-dependent and oxygen-independent mechanisms.

Oxygen-dependent killing mechanisms result from the production of toxic oxygen species (e.g., hydrogen peroxide, singlet oxygen, or hydroxyl radicals). Phagocytosis is accompanied by a burst of oxygen uptake by the phagocyte. Chemical mediators and other reactive oxygen species are highly damaging to bacteria.

Oxygen-independent mechanisms of microbial killing include (1) the acidic pH (3.5–4.0) of the phagolysosome, (2) cationic proteins that bind to and damage target cell membranes, (3) enzymatic attack of the microorganism's cell wall by lysozyme and other enzymes, and (4) inhibition of bacterial growth by lactoferrin binding of iron (iron is essential for bacterial growth).

Dying phagocytes can cause tissue damage at the site of inflammation. When a phagocyte dies at an inflammatory site, it frequently lyses (breaks open), releasing its enzymatic contents into the tissue. These enzymes can cause inflammation-associated tissue destruction. The destructive effects of enzymes released by dying phagocytes are minimized by natural inhibitors found in blood. Examples of such inhibitors would include **catalase**, which breaks down hydrogen peroxide, and **alpha1-antitrypsin** (α1-antitrypsin), a protease inhibitor produced by the liver. An inherited deficiency of α_1-antitrypsin, a disease known as **alpha1 antitrypsin deficiency**, results in a loss of lung elasticity and pulmonary emphysema secondary to chronic pulmonary inflammation, even in nonsmokers

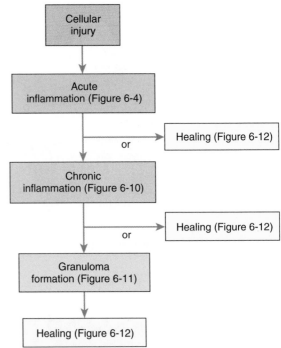

FIGURE 6.9 Inflammatory Phases and Healing. Cellular injury leads to acute inflammation and may result in resolution and healing of the injured site or may progress into chronic inflammation. Chronic inflammation in turn may result in healing or progress to development of a granuloma. The final step of the inflammatory process is usually healing and reconstruction of the damaged tissue. (The figure numbers refer to those in which more detailed information on that portion of the process may be found.)

✔ **QUICK CHECK 6.4**
1. What are PRRs?
2. What are cytokines? How do cytokines promote inflammation?
3. What products do the mast cells release during inflammation, and what are their effects?
4. What phagocytic cell types are involved in the acute inflammatory response? What is the role of each?
5. What is the function of opsonins?
6. What are the four steps in the process of phagocytosis?

ACUTE AND CHRONIC INFLAMMATION

Injury causes inflammation. Inflammation can be divided into two phases: acute inflammation and chronic inflammation (Fig. 6.9). The acute inflammatory response is self-limiting; it continues only until the threat to the body is eliminated. The process usually takes 8 to 10 days from onset of injury to healing. If the acute inflammatory response proves inadequate, a chronic inflammation may develop and persist for weeks or months. If healing has not been initiated, inflammation may progress to a *granulomatous* response. This process isolates the cause of tissue damage so that it no longer poses a threat to the body. The characteristics of the acute (early) inflammatory response differ from those of a chronic (later) response. Each phase involves different biochemical mediators and cells, all of which function in a coordinated manner. Depending on the successful containment of tissue damage and infection, both the acute and chronic phases lead to healing.[1]

Local Manifestations of Acute Inflammation

The cells and plasma protein systems involved in the inflammatory response interact to produce the characteristic changes of inflammation, whether local or systemic. They also determine the duration of inflammation, either acute or chronic. The characteristic signs of **acute inflammation** result from cellular and vascular changes and include *swelling, pain, heat, redness,* and, in some injuries, *loss of function.*

Inflammatory **exudates** result from increased vascular permeability and the leakage of fluid into tissues. Exudates vary in composition, depending on the stage of inflammation, and, to a lesser extent, the triggering event. In early or mild inflammation, the exudate may be a **serous exudate** (watery) with very few plasma proteins or leukocytes (e.g., fluid in a blister). In more severe or advanced inflammation, the exudate may be a **fibrinous exudate** (thick and clotted) (e.g., the fluid exudates in the lungs of an individual with pneumonia). A **purulent exudate (pus)** is the accumulation of a large number of leukocytes, as occurs in persistent bacterial infections. A purulent exudate is characteristic of walled-off lesions, known as **cysts** or **abscesses**. When bleeding occurs, the exudate is filled with erythrocytes and is described as a **hemorrhagic exudate**.

Systemic Manifestations of Acute Inflammation

Three primary systemic changes are associated with an acute inflammatory response: fever, leukocytosis (a transient increase in the levels of circulating leukocytes), and increased levels of circulating plasma proteins.

Fever

Fever is partially induced by specific cytokines (e.g., TNF-α and IL-1) released from neutrophils and macrophages. These cytokines are known as endogenous pyrogens to differentiate them from pathogen-produced exogenous pyrogens. Pyrogens act directly on the hypothalamus, the portion of the brain which controls the body's thermostat. A fever can be beneficial, as many microorganisms are sensitive to small increases in body temperature. For example, the microorganisms causing syphilis or gonococcal urethritis are highly sensitive to small increases in body temperature. However, fever may have harmful side effects when it enhances the body's susceptibility to the endotoxins associated with gram-negative bacterial infections when bacteria die or are destroyed.

Leukocytosis

Leukocytosis is an increase in the number of circulating white blood cells beyond the upper limit of normal (11,000/mL³ in adults). During many infections, the leukocytosis may be accompanied by a *left shift*, a term that denotes an increase in the ratio of immature to mature neutrophils. The term dates back to the 1920s and may have its origin in early cell counting devises or from left to right cell counting on printed reports. Inflammation stimulates the proliferation and release of granulocyte and monocyte precursors in bone marrow. The cells migrate into the systemic circulation resulting in both an increase in the total number of circulating leukocytes and an increased ratio of immature to mature cell forms. In particular, increased numbers of immature neutrophil forms, band cells, metamyelocytes, and (rarely) myelocytes are released from the marrow into blood causing an abnormal complete blood count (CBC), a common laboratory analysis of blood cells. The differential count is a measure of the ratio or proportion of each of the various blood cell types circulating in the blood. An increase in the total number of white blood cells in combination with an abnormal differential count (i.e., the "shift to the left") is a clue that there may be an ongoing infection.

Plasma Protein Synthesis

The synthesis of many plasma proteins, typically produced by the liver, is increased during inflammation. These proteins, which can be either proinflammatory or antiinflammatory in nature, are referred to as acute-phase reactants (proteins). Acute-phase reactants reach maximal circulating levels within 10 to 40 hours after the onset of inflammation.

Laboratory tests that measure levels of acute-phase reactants are available. For example, an increase in blood levels of acute-phase reactants, primarily fibrinogen, is associated with an increased adhesiveness of erythrocytes. Erythrocytes adhere to one another under these circumstances, forming large clumps that are buoyant and slow to settle to the bottom of a test tube of blood. This results in an increased value for the laboratory test referred to as erythrocyte sedimentation rate (ESR) or, as it is more commonly known, the "sed rate." Although this increased ESR is a nonspecific reaction, persons found to have an elevated ESR will likely have an inflammatory process going on somewhere within the body. Another common laboratory measure of inflammation is the cross-reactive protein (CRP, produced by the liver), a laboratory measurement which also is increased during an inflammatory response. CRP is used to look for subclinical inflammation in individuals at risk for heart disease and to estimate the severity of infectious and autoimmune diseases.

Chronic Inflammation

In its simplest terms, the difference between acute and chronic inflammation is duration. Chronic inflammation lasts 2 weeks or longer, regardless of cause, and is sometimes preceded by an unsuccessful acute inflammatory response (Fig. 6.10). For example, if bacterial contamination or foreign objects (dirt, wood splinter, silica, glass, etc.) persist in a wound, an acute response may be prolonged beyond 2 weeks. Pus formation, suppuration (purulent discharge), and incomplete wound healing may characterize this type of chronic inflammation.

Chronic inflammation also can occur as a distinct process without a previous episode of acute inflammation. Virtually all chronic diseases are characterized by a component of chronic inflammation. Although the cause of the persistent inflammatory response is often unknown, some common conditions associated with chronic inflammation include cardiac and neurologic disorders, malignancy, autoimmune disorders (see Chapter 8), and chronic infection (see Chapter 9). Some microorganisms are resistant to killing by the acute inflammatory response or may produce toxins which damage tissue and cause persistent inflammation, even after the original microorganism is killed.

Chronic inflammation is characterized by a dense infiltration of lymphocytes and macrophages. If macrophages are unable to protect the body from tissue damage, the body attempts to wall off and isolate the infected area forming a granuloma (Fig. 6.11). Infections caused by certain bacteria (tuberculosis, listeriosis, brucellosis), fungi (histoplasmosis, coccidioidomycosis), and parasites (leishmaniasis, schistosomiasis, toxoplasmosis) commonly result in granuloma formation. Retained foreign objects also commonly result in granulomas. Finally, many autoimmune conditions also are associated with granulomatous tissue changes. Granuloma formation is mediated by TNF-α and other proinflammatory cytokines. Macrophages are called to the area of persistent inflammation, where some differentiate into large epithelioid cells, which specialize in taking up debris and other small particles. Other macrophages fuse into multinucleated giant cells, which are active phagocytes, which can engulf particles larger than those that can be engulfed by a single macrophage. These two types of specialized cells form the center of the granuloma and are surrounded by lymphocytes. The granuloma itself is often encapsulated by fibrous deposits of collagen. It may become cartilaginous or even calcified by deposits of calcium carbonate and calcium phosphate.

The classic granuloma associated with tuberculosis is characterized by a wall of lymphocytes and epithelioid cells surrounding the mycobacteria. Death of cells within the granuloma results in the release of acids and enzymatic lysosomal contents from dead phagocytes forming a cheese-like proteinaceous center which consists of decaying tissue (caseous necrosis). In this inhospitable environment, the cellular debris is broken down into its basic constituents, forming a clear fluid within the granuloma (liquefaction necrosis). Eventually, this fluid diffuses out leaving a hollow, thick-walled structure that has replaced normal tissue resulting in the reduced lung function seen with tuberculosis infections.

> ✔ **QUICK CHECK 6.5**
> 1. Describe how acute inflammation differs from chronic inflammation. What characteristics do they share?
> 2. List the types of exudate produced in inflammation.
> 3. Describe a granuloma including how a granuloma forms.

WOUND HEALING

The conclusion of inflammation is healing and repair.[9] The most favorable outcome is a return to normal structure and function. If the damage is minor, with no complications, complete healing and restoration of function may occur. Some destroyed tissues are capable of regeneration, a process where damaged tissue is replaced with healthy tissue of the original type. Regeneration occurs within the epithelia of the skin and

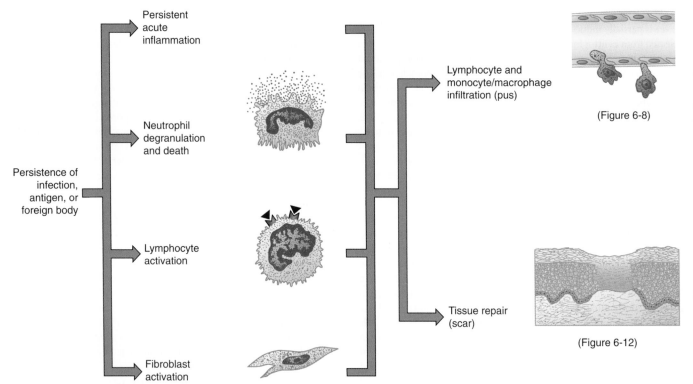

FIGURE 6.10 **The Chronic Inflammatory Response.** Inflammation usually becomes chronic because of the persistence of an infection, an antigen, or a foreign body in the wound. Chronic inflammation is characterized by the persistence of many of the processes of acute inflammation. In addition, large amounts of neutrophil degranulation and death, the activation of lymphocytes, and the concurrent activation of fibroblasts result in the release of mediators that induce the infiltration of more lymphocytes and monocytes/macrophages and the beginning of wound healing and tissue repair. (For more detailed information on each portion of the response, see the figures referenced in this illustration.)

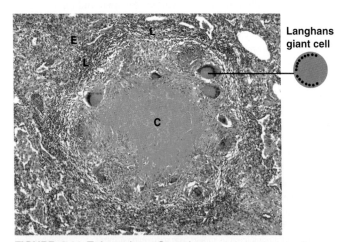

FIGURE 6.11 **Tuberculous Granuloma.** A central area of amorphous caseous necrosis *(C)* is surrounded by a zone of lymphocytes *(L)* and enlarged epithelioid macrophage cells *(E)*. Activated macrophages frequently fuse to form multinucleated cells (Langerhans giant cells). In tuberculoid granulomas the nuclei of the giant cells move to the cellular margins in a horseshoe-like formation. (From Kumar V, Abbas AK, Aster JC: *Robbins basic pathology*, ed 9, Philadelphia, 2013, Saunders.)

intestines as well as in some organs, notably the liver. This restoration is called **resolution** (or *maturation*), and the process may take up to 2 years.

Resolution does not always follow inflammation and may not be possible when extensive damage has occurred, at sites where the original tissue is not capable of regeneration, in areas where an infection has resulted in abscess or granuloma formation, or in cases where fibrin persists in the lesion. Where resolution is not possible, tissue repair occurs. **Repair** refers to the replacement of destroyed tissue with scar tissue. **Scar tissue** is composed primarily of collagen, a substance which fills in the lesion, restoring tissue integrity and strength. Collagen, however, cannot carry out the physiologic functions of the tissue it has replaced. Scar tissue then results in a loss of function.

A clean incision, such as a paper cut or a sutured surgical wound, heals primarily through the process of **primary intention**. Because this type of wound has minimal tissue loss and close apposition of the wound edges, healing can occur quickly. (Fig. 6.12).

Other wounds do not heal as readily. Healing of an open wound, such as a severe burn, requires a great deal of tissue replacement. In these cases, healing occurs through **secondary intention** (see Fig. 6.12). Healing by either primary or secondary intention may occur at different rates for different types of tissue injury.

Epidermal wounds that heal by secondary intention and unsutured internal lesions are not completely restored by healing. At best, repaired tissue regains 80% of its original tensile strength. Only epithelial, hepatic (liver), and bone marrow cells are capable of complete mitotic regeneration of the normal tissue, a process known as *compensatory hyperplasia*.

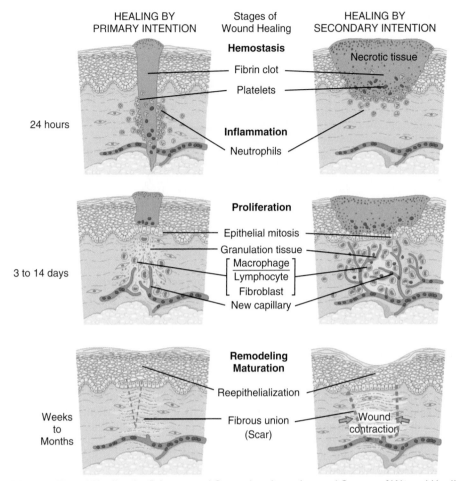

FIGURE 6.12 Wound Healing by Primary and Secondary Intention and Stages of Wound Healing. Phases of wound healing (coagulation, inflammation, proliferation/tissue formation, remodeling, and maturation) and steps in wound healing by primary intention *(left)* and secondary intention *(right)*. Note the large amounts of granulation tissue and wound contraction in healing by secondary intention. (From Roberts JR, Custalow CB: *Roberts and Hedges' clinical procedures in emergency medicine,* ed 6, Philadelphia, 2013, Saunders.)

In fibrous connective tissue, such as joints and ligaments, normal healing results in replacement of the original tissue with new tissue which does not exactly replicate the structure or function of the original. Some tissues heal without replacement of any functional cells. For example, damage resulting from myocardial infarction heals with fibrous scar tissue rather than with cardiac muscle. Accordingly, cardiac function is not restored completely and the individual surviving the infarction will have varying amounts of impaired cardiac function depending on the size of the scar.

Wound healing occurs in four overlapping phases or stages: (1) *hemostasis (coagulation),* (2) *inflammation,* (3) *proliferation with new tissue formation,* and, (4) *remodeling and maturation* (Fig. 6.13).

Phase I: Hemostasis (Coagulation)

Tissue injury damages capillaries and blood vessels and causes bleeding into the wound. Damage to blood vessels causes immediate vasoconstriction followed by vasodilation and initiates the coagulation cascade and activation of platelets. The fibrin mesh of the blood clot acts as a scaffold for cells that participate in healing. Platelets contribute to clot formation. As the platelets degranulate, they release factors which cause increased capillary permeability and promote growth factors which initiate proliferation in undamaged cells. In addition to activation of clotting there is activation of complement and kinins.

Phase II: Inflammation

The **inflammatory phase** begins within minutes.[10] As has been described in detail previously, macrophages and mast cells release numerous vasoactive cytokines that increase blood flow to the wound and bring needed cells and proteins to the area of injury. Neutrophils infiltrate the area of injury and initiate the process of clearing the wound of debris and bacteria. Lymphocytes initiate an immune response.

Phase III: Proliferation and New Tissue Formation

The proliferative phase begins 3 to 4 days after the injury and continues for as long as 2 weeks. The wound is sealed and the fibrin clot is replaced by normal tissue or scar tissue during this phase. The **proliferative phase** is characterized by an invasion of macrophage cells. Macrophages are essential to the later stages of wound healing, serving several functions essential to the healing process.[11] They clear debris, release growth factors, recruit fibroblasts, and promote collagen synthesis and **angiogenesis** (the formation of a new blood vessels). The cleanup of the lesion, which also involves dissolution of fibrin clots (or scabs), is called débridement. After débridement, the remaining debris is drained away by blood and lymphatic vessels and the vascular dilation and permeability associated with early inflammation are reversed, thus preparing the lesion for either regeneration or repair.

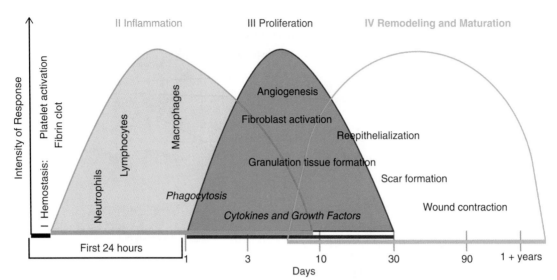

FIGURE 6.13 Phases of Wound Healing and Time Course.

As wound healing progresses, **granulation tissue** grows into the wound from surrounding healthy connective tissue. It consists of invasive cells, new lymphatic vessels, and new capillaries, all derived from the analogous structures found in the surrounding healthy tissue. These components lend a red and granular appearance to the newly formed granulation tissue. Capillary buds sprout from vascular endothelial cells around the wound and extend into the débrided areas. Loops form when the young capillaries join (anastomose). The loops are more fragile and permeable than mature vessels, resulting in leakage of erythrocytes and neutrophils. The erythrocytes are phagocytosed by macrophages, and the neutrophils assist in further débridement of the inflammatory lesion. Many of the new capillaries differentiate into larger vessels as repair continues, promoting influx of nutrients and removal of metabolic wastes. New lymphatic vessels also grow into the granulation tissue by a similar process.

During this process, the healing wound must be protected. **Epithelialization** is the process by which epithelial cells grow into the wound from surrounding healthy tissue. Epithelial cells migrate under the clot or scab using matrix metalloproteinases to unravel the collagen. The migrating epithelial cells connect with similar cells from all sides of the wound and seal it. The epithelial cells remain active, undergoing differentiation to give rise to the various epidermal layers. Epithelialization of a skin wound can be hastened if the wound is kept moist, preventing the fibrin clot from becoming a scab.

Fibroblasts are important cells during healing because they secrete collagen and other connective tissue proteins. Fibroblasts deposit connective tissue proteins in débrided areas, about 6 days after they have entered a lesion. **Collagen** is the most abundant protein in the body. It contains high concentrations of the amino acids glycine, proline, and lysine, many of which are enzymatically modified during the healing process. Additionally, wound healing requires iron, ascorbic acid (vitamin C), and molecular oxygen (O_2). The absence of any of these components results in impaired wound healing. As healing progresses, collagen molecules form collagen fibrils which further modify to form collagen fibers. The complete process takes several months.

In granulation tissue, some fibroblasts transition into **myofibroblasts,** specialized cells responsible for wound contraction. Myofibroblasts have features of both smooth muscle cells and fibroblasts. **Wound**

contraction occurs as extensions from the plasma membrane of myofibroblasts establish connections between neighboring cells. They anchor themselves to the wound bed then contract their fibers so as to exert tension on the neighboring cells. Wound contraction is necessary for closure of all wounds, especially those that heal by secondary intention. Contraction is noticeable 6 to 12 days after injury.

Phase IV: Remodeling and Maturation

Tissue remodeling and **maturation** is a process that begins several weeks after injury and is normally completed within 2 years. Tissue regeneration and wound contraction continue in this phase, a phase for recovering normal tissue structure. During this phase, there is a continuation of cellular differentiation, scar formation, and scar remodeling. The fibroblast is the major cell involved in tissue remodeling, where it functions to deposit collagen into an organized matrix. For wounds that heal by scarring, scar tissue is remodeled and capillaries disappear, resulting in an avascular scar. Within 2 to 3 weeks after maturation has begun, the scar tissue has gained about two-thirds of its eventual maximal strength.

Dysfunctional Wound Healing

Dysfunctional wound healing and impaired epithelialization may occur during any phase of the healing process. The cause of dysfunctional wound healing includes ischemia; excessive bleeding; excessive fibrin deposition; a predisposing disorder, such as diabetes mellitus; obesity; wound infection; inadequate nutrition; use of certain drugs; and tobacco smoking.

Ischemic (oxygen-deprived) *tissue* is susceptible to cellular death and infection, which prolongs inflammation and delays healing. Ischemia reduces energy production and impairs collagen synthesis as well as the tensile strength of regenerating connective tissue.

Excessive bleeding delays healing. Large clots increase the amount of space that granulation tissue must fill. Clots also serve as mechanical barriers to oxygen diffusion. Accumulated blood is an excellent growth medium for bacteria. Bacteria predispose the wound to infection and prolong inflammation through increased exudation and pus formation.

Under normal conditions, vessels dilate, delivering inflammatory cells, nutrients, and oxygen to the site of injury. Decreased blood volume, associated with bleeding, inhibits inflammation secondary to vessel constriction.

Excessive fibrin deposition is detrimental to healing. Fibrin released in response to injury must eventually be reabsorbed to prevent the formation of **fibrous adhesions**. Adhesions that form in the pleural, pericardial, or abdominal cavities can bind together forming fibrous bands. Such bands distort, impinge on, or strangulate the affected organs. An adhesion, so formed, may bind an organ to an adjacent organ resulting in both pain and/or impaired organ function (Fig. 6.14).

Obesity delays wound healing through impairing leukocyte function, which, in turn, predisposes the wound to infection, decreased growth factor production, and increases in proinflammatory cytokines. Additionally, there is a dysregulation of collagen synthesis and a decrease in angiogenesis.

Persons with *diabetes* are at risk for prolonged wound healing and wound infection if they have persistent hyperglycemia. Wounds in an individual with diabetes tend to be ischemic because of the prevalence of small-vessel diseases and impaired blood flow. The hyperglycemia increases the level of glycosylated hemoglobin, a form of hemoglobin with an increased affinity for oxygen. The tightly bound oxygen, characteristic of glycosylated hemoglobin, is not as readily released into the tissues. The hyperglycemia of diabetes also suppresses macrophage function, further predisposing the tissue to wound infection. Additionally, leukocytes require glucose to produce adenosine 5′-triphosphate (5′-adenosine triphosphate [ATP]), an energy source needed for physiologic functioning. The insulin resistance of persons with diabetes results in deficient glucose within the leukocytes, limiting their function and impairing their role in wound healing.

Wound infection is caused by the infiltration of pathogens into the injured or compromised tissues. Such pathogens damage cells, stimulate the continued release of inflammatory mediators, consume nutrients, and delay wound healing.

Optimal *nutrition* is important during all phases of healing because of the increased metabolic needs of the affected tissues. The hyperglycemia of diabetes impairs wound healing through the mechanisms noted above. Hypoproteinemia impairs fibroblast proliferation and collagen synthesis. Prolonged lack of vitamins A and C, which are cofactors required for collagen synthesis, results in poorly formed connective tissue and significantly impaired healing. Other cofactors for collagen synthesis include iron, zinc, manganese, and copper. Accordingly, malnutrition results in an increased risk for wound infection, delayed healing, and reduced wound tensile strength.

Medications associated with delayed or dysfunctional wound healing include antineoplastic (anticancer) agents, NSAIDs, and steroids. Antineoplastic agents slow cell division and inhibit angiogenesis. NSAIDs suppress acute inflammation and inhibit prostaglandin production, resulting in delayed wound healing, especially healing involving bone tissue. NSAIDs also have been associated with excessive scarring. Steroids disrupt wound healing by preventing macrophages from migrating to the site of injury and through inhibiting the release of both collagenase and plasminogen activator. Steroids also inhibit fibroblast migration into the wound during the proliferative phase, thus delaying epithelialization.

Toxic agents in *tobacco smoke* (carbon monoxide and hydrogen cyanide) delay wound healing. Nicotine is a potent vasoconstrictor that compromises wound healing by predisposing the tissue to ischemia and infection.

Dysfunctional collagen synthesis may involve excessive production of collagen, leading to a hypertrophic scar or keloid. A **hypertrophic scar** is

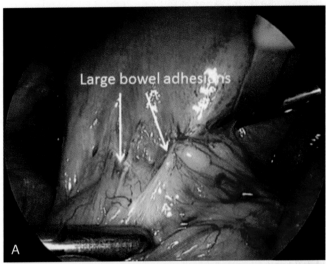

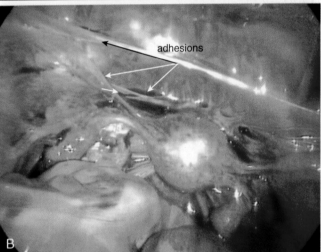

FIGURE 6.14 Fibrous Adhesions. Large bowel adhesion (**A**). Uterine adhesion (**B**) and adhesions that extend from the liver to the inner lining (peritoneum) of the abdominal wall. (**A,** from *International Journal of Surgery Case Reports* Volume 16, 2015, Pages 146–149. https://doi.org/10.1016/j.ijscr.2015.09.039; **B,** from *Nursing for Women's Health* Volume 16, Supplement 1, February–March 2012, Pages S3-S11. https://doi.org/10.1111/j.1751-486X.2012.01707.x).

raised but remains within the original boundaries of the wound. It tends to regress over time (Fig. 6.15, *A*). A **keloid** is a raised scar that extends beyond the original boundaries of the wound, invading surrounding tissue. It is likely to recur after surgical removal (see Fig. 6.15, *B*). A familial tendency to keloid formation has been observed, with a greater incidence in persons with darker skin pigmentation, especially African Americans.

Wound Disruption

A potential complication of wounds that are closed with sutures is **dehiscence**, a scenario where the wound pulls apart at the suture line. Dehiscence generally occurs 5 to 12 days after suturing, at a time when collagen synthesis is at its peak. Approximately half of dehiscence occurrences are associated with wound infection. Other instances result from suture rupture caused by excessive strain. Adipose tissue

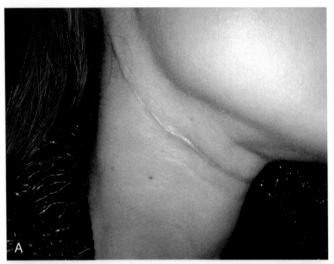

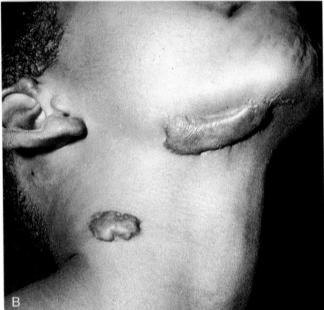

FIGURE 6.15 Hypertrophic Scar and Keloid Scar Formation. Hypertrophic scar (**A**) and keloid scar (**B**) caused by excessive synthesis of collagen at suture sites. (**A**, from Flint PW et al: *Cummings otolaryngology: head & neck surgery*, ed 6, Philadelphia, 2015, Mosby; **B**, from Damjanov I, Linder J: *Anderson's pathology*, ed 10, St Louis, 1996, Mosby.)

is difficult to suture, increasing the risk of dehiscence in individuals who are obese. Wound dehiscence is usually heralded by an increased serous drainage from the wound; there often is a perception by the individual that "something gave way." Prompt surgical attention is required.

Contracture

Wound contraction, necessary for healing, may become excessive where it results in an anatomic deformity or contracture of scar tissue. Burns of the skin are especially prone to contracture, particularly at joints with a resultant loss of joint function. Internal contractures include duodenal strictures, caused by dysfunctional healing of a peptic ulcer; esophageal strictures, caused by chemical burns, such as lye ingestion; or abdominal adhesions, caused by surgery, infection, or radiation. Contracture may occur in cirrhosis of the liver, where constricted vascular flow contributes to the development of portal hypertension and esophageal varices. Proper positioning, range-of-motion exercises, compression, and surgery are among the strategies used to prevent or treat skin contractures. Internal contractures, such as fibrous adhesions between loops of bowel, cause pain or result in a loss of function and are released with surgery.

✔ **QUICK CHECK 6.6**
1. How does regeneration of tissue differ from repair of tissue?
2. What does "healing by primary intention" mean?
3. What is the role of fibroblasts in wound healing?
4. Describe various ways wound healing may be dysfunctional.

PEDIATRIC CONSIDERATIONS

Age-Related Factors Affecting Innate Immunity in the Newborn Child

Newborn innate immune function is limited.
- Newborn physiologic immunity is acquired from the mother through the placenta and breast milk.
- Newborns have transiently depressed inflammatory responses with limited production of inflammatory cytokines.
- Neutrophils in the newborn are incapable of chemotaxis. They lack fluidity in the plasma membrane.
- Complement levels in the newborn are diminished, especially components of the alternative pathways (factor B). This status is particularly common in premature newborns.
- Monocyte/macrophage numbers are normal in the newborn, but chemotaxis of monocytes is delayed.

- Newborns are predisposed to infections associated with chemotactic defects, especially cutaneous abscesses caused by staphylococci or cutaneous candidiasis.
- Newborns have compromised oxidative and bactericidal responses in cases of in utero infection or respiratory insufficiency.
- Newborns are predisposed to develop severe overwhelming sepsis and meningitis when infected by bacteria against which there are no circulating maternal antibodies.
- The establishment of the gut microbiome is facilitated by breast milk.
- Newborns delivered via cesarean section have reduced gut microbial diversity.

Data from Collins A, Weitkamp JH, Wynn JL: Why are preterm newborns at increased risk of infection? *Arch Dis Child Fetal Neonatal Ed* 103(4):F391-F394, 2018; Kumar SK, Bhat BV: Distinct mechanisms of the newborn innate immunity, *Immunol Lett* 173:42-54, 2016.

GERIATRIC CONSIDERATIONS

Age-Related Factors Affecting Innate Immunity in the Elderly

- The elderly have normal numbers of cells associated with innate immunity, but there may be diminished cellular function to include decreased phagocytic activity, decreased antibody production, and altered cytokine synthesis.
- The elderly are at increased risk for chronic inflammation, possibly secondary to increased production of proinflammatory mediators.
- The elderly are at increased risk for decreased phagocytic function, infection, and impaired wound healing. Predisposing causes include chronic illness, such as diabetes mellitus, peripheral vascular disease, or cardiovascular disease.
- The elderly have increased use of medications known to impair healing, notably nonsteroidal antiinflammatory drugs (NSAIDs) and steroid use.

- The elderly have decreased subcutaneous fat which diminishes layers of protection against injury.
- The elderly have atrophied epidermis, including the underlying capillaries, and this results in decreased perfusion and an increased risk of hypoxia in wound beds.
- The normal aging process of the immune system diminishes the effectiveness of vaccines. For this reason, the flu vaccine for the elderly is given in a higher dose.

Data from: Fuentes E et al: Immune system dysfunction in the elderly, *An Acad Bras Cienc* 89(1):285-299, 2017.

SUMMARY REVIEW

Human Defense Mechanisms

1. Innate defenses are the first line of defense, are present at birth, and include the surface barriers skin and mucous membranes.
2. Inflammation is the second line of defense and is activated with injury or infectious disease.
3. Adaptive (acquired) immunity is the third line of defense, is specific to particular antigens, and has memory.

Innate Immunity

1. Neonates often have transiently depressed inflammatory function, particularly neutrophil chemotaxis and alternative complement pathway activity.
2. Elderly persons are at risk for impaired wound healing, usually because of chronic illnesses.
3. There are three layers of human defense: physiologic barriers, the inflammatory response, and adaptive (acquired) immunity.
4. Physical barriers are the first lines of defense functioning to prevent damage to the individual and thwart the entrance of pathogens. These barriers include the skin and mucous membranes.
5. Antibacterial peptides are found in mucous secretions, perspiration, saliva, tears, and other secretions. They provide a biochemical barrier against pathogenic microorganisms.
6. The skin, mucous membranes, and the lining of the gastrointestinal (GI) tract are colonized by commensal or mutualistic microorganisms. These microorganisms provide protection by releasing biochemical compounds which facilitate immune responses and prevent colonization by pathogens. Within the gut, they also facilitate digestion in the GI tract.
7. The second line of defense is the *inflammatory response*, a rapid and nonspecific protective response to cellular injury resulting from any cause. It can occur only in vascularized tissues.
8. The macroscopic hallmarks of inflammation are redness, swelling, heat, pain, and loss of function for the inflamed tissues.
9. The microscopic hallmarks of inflammation are vasodilation, increased capillary permeability, and an accumulation of fluid and cells at the inflammatory site.
10. Inflammation is mediated by three key plasma protein systems: the complement system, the clotting system, and the kinin system. The components of all three systems are a series of inactive proteins which are activated sequentially in the presence of tissue injury.
11. The complement system can be activated by antigen–antibody reactions (through the classical pathway) or by other products,

especially bacterial polysaccharides (through the lectin pathway or the alternative pathway). The lectin and alternative pathways do not require antibody activation to recruit phagocytes, activate mast cells, and destroy pathogens.
12. The most biologically potent products of the complement system are C3b (opsonin), C3a (anaphylatoxin), and C5a (anaphylatoxin, chemotactic factor).
13. The clotting system stops bleeding, localizes microorganisms, and provides a meshwork for repair and healing.
14. Bradykinin is the most important product of the kinin system and causes vascular permeability, smooth muscle contraction, and pain.
15. Control of inflammation regulates inflammatory cells and enzymes and localizes the inflammatory response to the area of injury or infection.
16. Carboxypeptidase, histaminase, kinase, and C1 inhibitor are inactivating enzymes. The fibrinolytic system and plasmin facilitate clot degradation after bleeding is stopped.
17. Many different types of cells are involved in the inflammatory process, including mast cells, endothelial cells, platelets, phagocytes (neutrophils, eosinophils, monocytes and macrophages, dendritic cells), lymphocytes, and natural killer (NK) cells,.
18. Most cells express plasma membrane pattern recognition receptors (PRRs) which recognize molecules produced by infectious microorganisms. These molecules include pathogen-associated molecular patterns (PAMPs) and damage-associated molecular patterns (DAMPs). Toll-like receptors (TLRs) are transmembrane receptors and nucleotide-binding-like receptors (NLR-like), and nucleotide oligomerization domain-like (NOD-like) receptors are cytoplasmic receptors. They are expressed by many inflammatory cells and recognize both PAMPs and DAMPs. Upon recognition, they promote the release of cytokines and inflammatory mediators, which, in turn, eliminate damaged cells and protect against invasion by microbes.
19. The cells of the innate immune system secrete many biochemical mediators (cytokines), which are responsible for activating other cells and regulating the inflammatory response. These cytokines include chemokines, interleukins, interferons, and other molecules.
20. Chemokines induce chemotaxis (attraction) of leukocytes, fibroblasts, and other cells to promote phagocytosis and wound healing.
21. Interleukins are produced primarily by lymphocytes and macrophages. They either promote or inhibit inflammation by activating the growth and differentiation of leukocytes especially lymphocytes.

22. The most important proinflammatory interleukins are interleukin-1 (IL-1), interleukin-6 (IL-6), and tumor necrosis factor-alpha (TNF-α). IL-6 and IL-10 downregulate the inflammatory response.

23. Interferons are produced by cells that are infected by viruses. Once released from infected cells, interferons can stimulate neighboring healthy cells to produce substances that prevent viral infection.

24. The most important activator of the inflammatory response is the mast cell, located in connective tissue near capillaries. Mast cells initiate inflammation by releasing biochemical mediators (histamine and chemotactic factors) from cytoplasmic granules. They also synthesize other mediators (prostaglandins, leukotrienes, and platelet-activating factor [PAF]) in response to stimuli. Basophils, found in blood, function in a manner that is similar to mast cells.

25. Histamine is the major vasoactive amine released from mast cells. It increases vascular permeability through dilation of capillaries and retraction of endothelial cells lining the capillaries.

26. The endothelial cells lining the circulatory system (vascular endothelium) regulate circulating components of the inflammatory system, maintaining normal blood flow. They function in this capacity by preventing spontaneous activation of platelets and other elements of the clotting system.

27. During inflammation, the endothelium expresses receptors that stimulate leukocytes to exit the vessel. The endothelium also retracts to allow fluid to pass into the tissues.

28. Platelets interact with the coagulation cascade to stop bleeding. They release mediators which facilitate and control inflammation.

29. The polymorphonuclear neutrophil (PMN), the predominant phagocytic cell in the early inflammation, exits the circulation, through retracted endothelial junctions, by diapedesis. On exiting, it moves to the inflammatory site by chemotaxis.

30. Eosinophils release products that control the inflammatory response, and they are the principal cells that destroy parasitic organisms.

31. The macrophage, the predominant cell in the late inflammatory response, is highly phagocytic. Additionally, it is responsive to cytokines, which promote wound healing.

32. Dendritic cells function as messengers between the innate and acquired (adaptive) immune systems. They process antigens at the site of inflammation and transport the antigen to lymph nodes and spleen, where they present these antigens to the resident T cells. The result of this process is the formation of antibodies.

33. Phagocytosis is a multistep cellular process, which usually results in the destruction of pathogens and foreign debris. The steps include recognition and attachment, engulfment, formation of a phagosome, formation of a phagolysosome, and eventual destruction of the pathogen or foreign debris. Phagocytic cells engulf microorganisms, enclosing them within phagocytic vacuoles (phagolysosomes). The vacuoles contain toxins (especially metabolites of oxygen) and/or enzymes that kill and digest the microorganisms.

34. Opsonins are molecules which enhance phagocytosis by coating the antigen. This activity results in a stronger attraction between the microorganism and the phagocyte ("marking" the organism). It also enhances the affinity with which the phagocyte binds to the microorganism. Examples include antibodies and the complement component C3b.

Acute and Chronic Inflammation

1. *Acute inflammation* is self-limiting and usually resolves within 8 to 10 days.

2. *Local* manifestations of inflammation include the classic signs of redness, heat, swelling, pain, and loss of function. They are the result of vascular changes associated with the inflammatory process, including vasodilation and increased capillary permeability.

3. The principal *systemic effects* of inflammation are fever, leukocytosis (increased levels of circulating leukocytes), and an increase in plasma proteins, primarily the acute-phase reactants, IL-1, and IL-6.

4. *Chronic inflammation* can be a continuation of acute inflammation that lasts 2 weeks or longer, or it can occur as a distinct process without significant preceding acute inflammation.

5. Chronic inflammation is characterized by a dense infiltration of lymphocytes and macrophages. *Granuloma* formation is a process wherein the body walls off and isolates infectious microorganisms. It serves to protect the body from further tissue damage.

Wound Healing

1. *Resolution* (regeneration) is the return of tissue to nearly normal structure and function. *Repair* is healing by scar tissue formation.

2. Resolution occurs when little tissue has been lost or where the injured tissue is capable of regeneration. This type of healing is called *healing by primary intention.*

3. Tissues that have sustained extensive damage or tissue types that are incapable of regeneration heal by repair, a process which results in the formation of a scar. This process is called *healing by secondary intention.*

4. Resolution and repair occur in two separate phases. The *reconstructive phase* occurs when the wound begins to heal. The *maturation phase* occurs when the healed wound is remodeled. Cellular activity decreases and the blood vessels regress.

5. Dysfunctional wound healing can be secondary to ischemia, excessive bleeding, excessive fibrin deposition, predisposing disorders (e.g., diabetes mellitus), wound infection, inadequate nutrients, use of NSAIDs and steroids, or altered collagen synthesis.

6. *Dehiscence* is a disruption where the wound pulls apart at the suture line.

7. A *contracture* is a structural deformity caused by the excessive shortening of collagen in scar tissue.

▌ KEY TERMS

REFERENCES

1. Sugimoto MA, et al: Resolution of inflammation: what controls its onset?, *Front Immunol* 7:160, 2016.
2. Lloyd-Price J, Abu-Ali G, Huttenhower C: The healthy human microbiome, *Genome Med* 8(1):51, 2016.
3. Lubbers R, et al: Production of complement components by cells of the immune system, *Clin Exp Immunol* 88(2):183-194, 2017.
4. Kim SJ, Davis RP, Jenne CN: Platelets as modulators of inflammation, *Semin Thromb Hemost* 44(2):91-101, 2018.
5. Teng TS, et al: Neutrophils and immunity: from bactericidal action to being conquered, *J Immunol Res* 2017:2017. 9671604.
6. Krzyszczyk P, et al: The role of macrophages in acute and chronic wound healing and interventions to promote pro-wound healing phenotypes, *Front Physiol* 9:419, 2018.
7. Rosales C, Uribe-Querol E: Phagocytosis: a fundamental process in immunity, *Biomed Res Int* 2017:2017. 9042851.
8. Kaufmann SHE, Dorhoi A: Molecular determinants in phagocyte-bacteria interactions, *Immunity* 44(3):476-491, 2016.
9. Sorg H, et al: Skin wound healing: an update on the current knowledge and concepts, *Eur Surg Res* 58(1-2):81-94, 2017.
10. Landén NX, Li D, Ståhle M: Transition from inflammation to proliferation: a critical step during wound healing, *Cell Mol Life Sci* 73(20):3861-3885, 2016.
11. Kotwal GJ, Chien S: Macrophage differentiation in normal and accelerated wound healing, *Results Probl Cell Differ* 62:353-364, 2017.

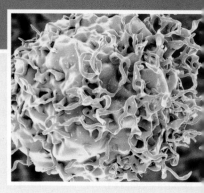

7

Adaptive Immunity

Valentina L. Brashers, Kathryn L. McCance

EVOLVE WEBSITE

CHAPTER OUTLINE

The third line of defense in the human body is adaptive (acquired) immunity, often called the immune response or immunity. Adaptive immunity consists of lymphocytes (Fig. 7.1) and serum proteins called *antibodies*. Once external barriers have been compromised and inflammation (innate immunity; see Chapter 6) has been activated, the adaptive immune response is mobilized. Inflammation is the "first responder" that contains the initial injury and slows the spread of infection, whereas adaptive immunity *slowly* augments the initial defenses against infection and promotes processes against reinfection.

OVERVIEW OF ADAPTIVE IMMUNITY

Inflammation and adaptive immunity differ in several key ways. First the components of innate immunity and inflammation are activated immediately after tissue damage. Adaptive immunity is *inducible;* the effectors of the immune response, lymphocytes and antibodies, do not preexist in large numbers but are produced in response to infection or other abnormal molecules. Thus adaptive immunity develops more slowly than inflammation.

Second the inflammatory response is similar regardless of differences in the cause of tissue damage or whether the inflammatory site is sterile or contaminated with infectious microorganisms. The adaptive immune response is exquisitely *specific.* For example, the lymphocytes and antibodies induced in response to infection are extremely specific to the infecting microbe.

Third the residual mediators of inflammation must be removed quickly to limit damage to surrounding healthy tissue and allow healing.

The effectors of the adaptive immune response are *long-lived* and systemic, providing long-term protection against specific invaders.

Finally, the inflammatory responses to both recurrent tissue damage and infection are identical. The adaptive immune response has *memory.* For example, if reinfected with the same microbe, protective lymphocytes and antibody are produced immediately, thus providing permanent long-term protection against infection.

Despite the differences, the innate and adaptive immune systems are highly interactive and complementary. Many components of innate resistance are necessary for the development of the adaptive immune response. Conversely products of the adaptive immune response activate components of innate resistance. Thus both systems are essential for complete protection against infectious disease.

The mechanisms underlying the adaptive immune response will be discussed in this chapter. As with Chapter 6, a complete description of all the important components and processes of an effective immune response would require far more space than available. Therefore this chapter will focus on the basic concepts and the most important, or well-studied, mediators of the adaptive immune response.

The adaptive immune response has its own vocabulary (Fig. 7.2). Antigens are the molecular targets of antibodies and lymphocytes. Antigens are generally small molecules (usually within proteins, carbohydrates, or lipids) found on the surface of microbes, infected cells, or abnormal tissues, although this definition is expanded with immunologic diseases in Chapter 8. In the fetus, well before exposure to any foreign antigens, lymphocytes have undergone extensive differentiation. Some lymphoid stem cells enter the thymus and differentiate into T

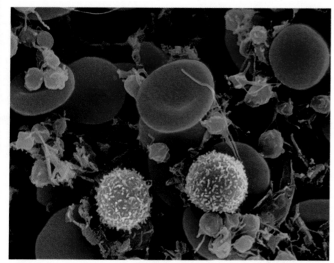

FIGURE 7.1 **Lymphocytes.** A scanning electron micrograph showing lymphocytes (yellow, like cotton candy), red blood cells, and platelets. (Copyright Dennis Kunkel Microscopy, Inc.)

lymphocytes (T cells, *T* refers to thymus derived), whereas others enter specific regions of the bone marrow and differentiate into **B lymphocytes** (**B cells**, B refers to bone marrow derived). Each type of cell develops cell surface proteins that identify them as T or B cells. Both B and T cells also develop cell surface antigen receptors. The receptors are remarkable because an individual lymphocyte is programmed to recognize only one specific antigen. It is estimated that before birth each individual has produced a population of B and T lymphocytes capable of recognizing at least 10^8 different antigens. This process is called generation of **clonal diversity** and refers to the process by which the extensive diversity of antigen receptors on B and T cells is established (see Fig. 7.2).

B and T lymphocytes leaving the primary lymphoid organs (bone marrow and thymus) are **immunocompetent** (able to respond to antigens) but have not been exposed to antigen and thus are **naïve**. These cells enter the blood and lymphatic vessels and migrate to the **secondary lymphoid organs** (e.g., lymph nodes, spleen) of the systemic immune system (Fig. 7.3). Some take up residence in B cell and T cell rich areas of those organs, and others reenter the circulation. Approximately 60% to 70% of circulating lymphocytes are immunocompetent T cells, and 10% to 20% are immunocompetent B cells.

A second process, *clonal selection,* is initiated when exposure to an antigen occurs. This process requires the cooperation among a variety of cells in the secondary lymphoid organs. Antigen needs to be *processed* by phagocytic cells which then express the processed antigen on their surfaces and *present* the antigen to lymphocytes. Thus begins a symphony of cellular interactions, referred to as **clonal selection**, involving:

- Several subsets of B and T cells
- Intercellular adhesion through specific antigen receptors and intercellular adhesion molecules
- Production and response to multiple cytokines
- Activation and regulation of the immune response by helping the clonal selection process (T-helper cells [Th cells])
- Differentiation of immunocompetent B and T cells into highly specialized effector cells (B cells developing into **plasma cells** that become factories for the production of antibody and T cells developing into **T-cytotoxic (Tc) cells** that can identify and kill a target cell.)
- Suppression of inappropriate immune responses (**T-regulatory cells** [**Treg cells**]);
- Differentiation of T and B cells into very long-lived **memory cells** that exist for decades or, in some cases, for the life of the individual

- Activation of memory cells if a second exposure occurs with the same antigen

Antibodies circulate in the blood and defend against extracellular antigens, such as microbes and microbial toxins. This is referred to as *humoral immune response,* or **humoral immunity**. Effector T cells are found in the blood and tissues and defend against intracellular pathogens (e.g., viruses) and abnormal cells, such as cancer cells. This is referred to as *cellular immune response,* or **cellular immunity** (also *cell-mediated immunity*).

The preceding overview describes what is termed **active immunity** (**active acquired immunity**), which develops in response to antigen. In certain clinical situations, preformed antibody or lymphocytes may be administered to an individual, termed **passive immunity** (**passive acquired immunity**). Examples include individuals exposed to an infectious agent without having a preexisting vaccine-induced immunity (e.g., hepatitis A virus or rabies virus) (Table 7.1). Passive immunization with specific T cells has been used to treat several forms of cancer. Active acquired immunity is long lived, whereas passive immunity is only temporary because the donor's antibodies or T cells are eventually destroyed.

ANTIGENS AND IMMUNOGENS

The terms *antigen* and *immunogen* are commonly used as synonyms. More specifically, the term **antigen** describes a molecule that can *bind with* antibodies or antigen receptors on B and T cells. A molecule that binds to receptors and will *induce* an immune response is an **immunogen**. Thus all immunogens are antigens but not all antigens are immunogens. Despite these specific definitions, the term *antigen* is used most often to describe molecules that are foreign to the host and cause an immune response. Common antigens include infectious agents, allergens, chemical agents (including some medications), and abnormal molecules on the surface of cells (cancers and infected cells). The ability of an antigen to induce an immune response is frequently related to the size of the antigen. In general, large molecules (those > 10,000 daltons), such as proteins and polysaccharides, are the most immunogenic antigens. Many low-molecular-weight molecules can function as **haptens**; they are too small to induce an immune response by themselves but become immunogenic after combining with larger molecules that function as carriers for the hapten. For example, poison ivy contains an oily sap called *urushiol* (molecular weight approximately 1500 daltons), that is an antigen, which, upon contact with the skin, is chemically altered, binds to large proteins in the skin, and becomes immunogenic, resulting in a T-cell response and onset of a classic poison ivy rash. Similar conditions will be discussed in Chapter 8.

> 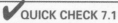 **QUICK CHECK 7.1**
> 1. Distinguish between innate immunity and acquired immunity.
> 2. Distinguish between humoral immunity and cell-mediated immunity.
> 3. Define clonal selection.
> 4. What is antigen?

IMMUNE RESPONSE: COLLABORATION OF B CELLS AND T CELLS

Generation of Clonal Diversity

The immune response occurs in two phases: generation of clonal diversity and clonal selection (Table 7.2; and see Fig. 7.2). **Clonal diversity** is the production of a large population of B cells and T cells before birth and throughout life that have the capacity to recognize almost any foreign antigen found in the environment. This process mostly occurs

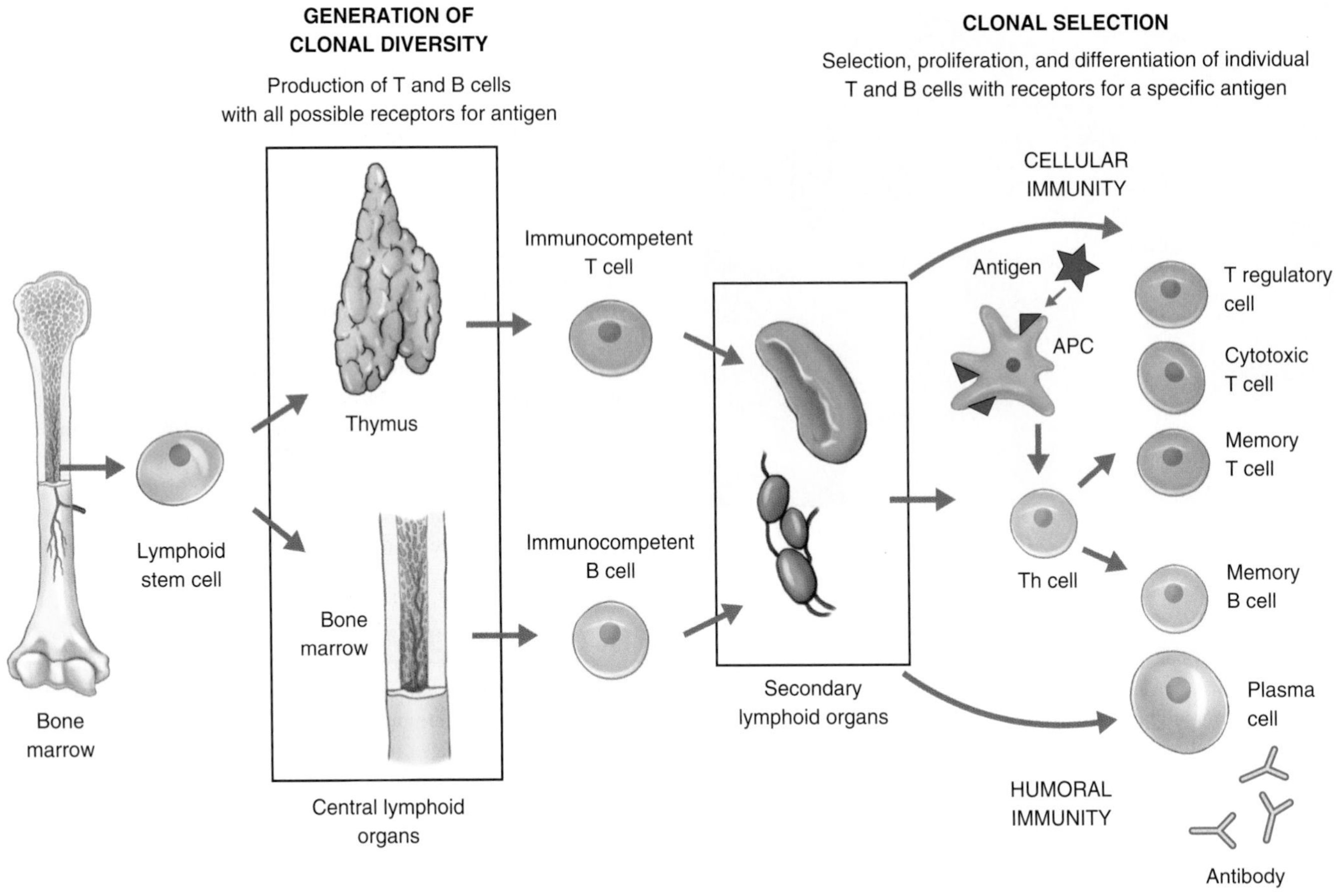

GENERATION OF
CLONAL DIVERSITY

Production of T and B cells
with all possible receptors for antigen

FIGURE 7.2 Overview of the Immune Response. The immune response can be separated into two phases: the *generation of clonal diversity* and *clonal selection*. During the generation of clonal diversity, lymphoid stem cells from the bone marrow migrate to the central lymphoid organs (the thymus or regions of bone marrow), where they undergo a series of cellular division and differentiation stages resulting in either immunocompetent T cells from the thymus or immunocompetent B cells from the bone marrow. These cells are still naïve in that they have never encountered a foreign antigen. The immunocompetent cells enter the circulation and migrate to the secondary lymphoid organs (e.g., spleen and lymph nodes), where they establish residence in B and T cell–rich areas. The clonal selection phase is initiated by exposure to foreign antigen. The antigen is usually processed by antigen-presenting cells (APCs) for presentation to T-helper cells (Th cells). The intercellular cooperation among APCs, Th cells, and immunocompetent T and B cells results in a second stage of cellular proliferation and differentiation. Because antigen has "selected" those T and B cells with compatible antigen receptors, only a small population of T and B cells undergo this process at one time. The result is an active cellular immunity or humoral immunity, or both. Cellular immunity is mediated by a population of *effector* T cells that can kill targets (T-cytotoxic cells) or regulate the immune response (T-regulatory [Treg] cells), as well as a population of memory cells (T-memory cells) that can respond more quickly to a second challenge with the same antigen. Humoral immunity is mediated by a population of soluble proteins (antibodies) produced by plasma cells and by a population of memory B cells that can produce more antibody rapidly to a second challenge with the same antigen.

in specialized lymphoid organs (the **primary [central] lymphoid organs**): **bone marrow** for B cells and the **thymus** for T cells. The result is the differentiation of **lymphoid stem cells** into B and T lymphocytes with the ability to react against almost any antigen that will be encountered throughout life. It is estimated that B and T cells can collectively recognize more than 10^8 different antigenic determinants. Lymphocytes are released from these organs into the circulation as immunocompetent cells that have the capacity to react with antigens and migrate to the circulation and other (secondary) lymphoid organs in the body.

Development of B Lymphocytes

Lymphocyte stem cells destined to become B cells circulate through the specialized regions of bone marrow, where they are exposed to

hormones and cytokines that induce proliferation and differentiation into B cells (see Fig. 7.2). As the stem cell begins to mature, it progressively develops a variety of necessary surface markers important for the further differentiation and proliferation of the B cell. The next stage in development is formation of the B-cell receptor (BCR).

The **B-cell receptor (BCR)** is a complex of antibody bound to the cell surface and other molecules involved in intracellular signaling (Fig. 7.4). Its role is to recognize an antigen and communicate that information to the cell's nucleus. The BCRs in immunocompetent cells are membrane-associated immunoglobulin M (mIgM) with or without IgD (mIgD) antibodies that have identical specificities for antigen.

The enormous repertoire of BCR specificities is made possible by rearrangement of existing deoxyribonucleic acid (DNA) during B-cell

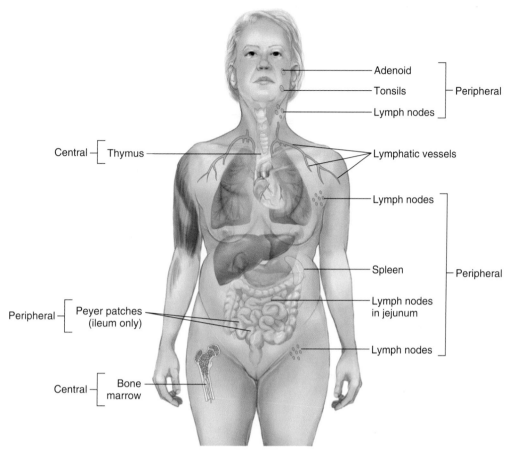

FIGURE 7.3 Lymphoid Tissues: Sites of B-Cell and T-Cell Differentiation. Immature lymphocytes migrate through central (primary) lymphoid tissues: the bone marrow (central lymphoid tissue for B lymphocytes) and the thymus (central lymphoid tissue for T lymphocytes). Mature lymphocytes later reside in the T and B lymphocyte–rich areas of the peripheral (secondary) lymphoid tissues.

TABLE 7.1	**Clinical Use of Antigen or Antibody**			
Use of Antigen or Antibody				
Antigen Source	**Protection: Combat Active Disease**	**Protection: Vaccination**	**Diagnosis**	**Therapy**
Infectious agents	Neutralize or destroy pathogenic microorganisms (e.g., antibody response against viral infections)	Induce safe and protective immune response (e.g., recommended childhood vaccines)	Measure circulating antigen from infectious agent or antibody (e.g., diagnosis of hepatitis B infection)	Passive treatment with antibody to treat or prevent infection (e.g., administration of antibody against hepatitis A)
Cancers	Prevent tumor growth or spread (e.g., immune surveillance to prevent early cancers)	Prevent cancer growth or spread (e.g., vaccination with cancer antigens)	Measure circulating antigen (e.g., circulating PSA for diagnosis of prostate cancer)	Immunotherapy (e.g., treatment of cancer with antibodies against cancer antigens)
Environmental substances	Prevent entrance into body (e.g., secretory IgA limits systemic exposure to potential allergens)	No clear example	Measure circulating antigen or antibody (e.g., diagnosis of allergy by measuring circulating IgE)	Immunotherapy (e.g., administration of antigen for desensitization of individuals with severe allergies)
Self-antigens	Immune system tolerance to self-antigens, which may be altered by an infectious agent leading to autoimmune disease (see Chapter 8)	Some cases of vaccination alter tolerance to self-antigens, leading to autoimmune disease	Measure circulating antibody against self-antigen for diagnosis of autoimmune disease (see Chapter 8)	No clear example

IgA, Immunoglobulin A; *IgE,* Immunoglobulin E; *PSA,* Prostate-specific antigen.

TABLE 7.2   Generation of Clonal Diversity Versus Clonal Selection

	Generation of Clonal Diversity	Clonal Selection
Purpose?	To produce large numbers of T and B lymphocytes with maximum diversity of antigen receptors	Select, expand, and differentiate clones of T and B cells against specific antigen
When does it occur?	Primarily in fetus	Primarily after birth and throughout life
Where does it occur?	Central lymphoid organs: thymus for T cells, bone marrow for B cells	Peripheral lymphoid organs, including lymph nodes, spleen, and other lymphoid tissues
Is foreign antigen involved?	No	Yes, antigen determines which clones of cells will be selected
What hormones or cytokines are involved?	Thymic hormones, IL-7, others	Many cytokines produced by Th cells and APCs
Final product?	Immunocompetent T and B cells that can react with antigen but have not seen antigen, and migrate to secondary lymphoid organs	Plasma cells that produce antibody, effector T cells that help (Th cells), kill targets (Tc cells), or regulate immune responses (Treg cells); memory B and T cells

APCs, Antigen-presenting cells; *IL,* interleukin; *Tc,* T-cytotoxic cells; *Th,* T-helper cells; *Treg cells,* T-regulatory cells.

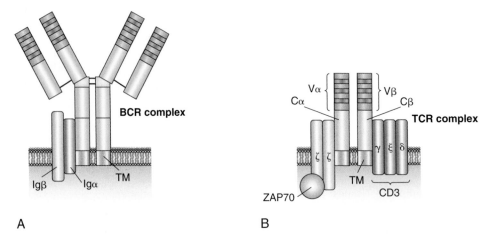

FIGURE 7.4 B-cell Antigen Receptor and T-cell Antigen Receptor. **A,** The antigen receptor on the surface of B cells (B-cell receptor [BCR] complex) is a monomeric (single) antibody with a structure similar to that of circulating antibody, with an additional transmembrane region *(TM)* that anchors the molecule to the cell surface. The active BCR complex contains molecules *(Igα* and *Igβ)* that are responsible for intracellular signaling after the receptor has bound antigen. **B,** The T-cell receptor *(TCR)* consists of an α- and a β-chain joined by a disulfide bond. Each chain consists of a constant region *(Cα* and *Cβ)* and a variable region *(Vα* and *Vβ).* Each variable region contains CDRs and FRs in a structure similar to that of antibody. The active TCR is associated with several molecules that are responsible for intracellular signaling after antigen binding. These include the CD3, which is a complex of γ (gamma), ε (epsilon); and δ (delta) subunits and a complex of two ζ (zeta) molecules. The ζ molecules are attached to a cytoplasmic protein kinase *(ZAP70)* that is critical to intracellular signaling.

development in the primary lymphoid organs, a process known as **somatic recombination.** Multiple loci in the DNA that encode for BCRs are recombined to generate receptors that collectively can recognize and bind to any possible antigen. A single lymphocyte will synthesize antibodies that can recognize the identical antigen as the BCR on that cell. (Antibody synthesis is discussed in the Humoral Immunity (Antibodies) section.)

Somatic rearrangement will frequently result in a BCR that recognizes the individual's own antigens, which may result in an inadvertent attack on "self" antigens expressed on various tissues causing autoimmune disease or hypersensitivities. Many of these "autoreactive" B cells are eliminated in bone marrow, where they undergo apoptosis. It is estimated that > 90% of developing B cells are eliminated in this way. This process is referred to as **clonal deletion** or **central tolerance,** so that the remaining pool of immunocompetent B cells target foreign antigens and are "tolerant" to *self-antigens.* **Peripheral**

tolerance occurs in the tissues and is discussed in the T-Regulatory Lymphocytes section.

B-cell differentiation also is characterized by the development of a variety of important surface molecules that are markers for B cells. These include CD21 (a complement receptor) and CD40 (adhesion molecule required for later interactions with T cells). The designation "CD" refers to **cluster of differentiation,** specific cell surface proteins that are assigned a unique number (e.g. CD21 and CD40).

Development of T Lymphocytes

The process of T-cell proliferation and differentiation is similar to that for B cells (see Fig. 7.2). The primary lymphoid organ for T-cell development is the thymus. Lymphoid stem cells journey through the thymus, where, under influence of thymic hormones and the cytokine IL-7, they are driven to undergo cell division and gain receptors (**T-cell receptors [TCRs]**) against the diversity of antigens the individual will encounter throughout life. They exit the thymus through the blood vessels and lymphatics as mature (immunocompetent) T cells with antigen-specific receptors on the cell surface and establish residence in secondary lymphoid organs.

The most common TCR consists of two protein chains, α- and β-chains, each of which has a variable region and a constant region and a complex of signaling molecules called CD3 (see Fig. 7.4). As with BCR generation, each T cell expresses only one type of TCR and the diversity of TCRs generated through somatic recombination collectively can recognize and bind to any possible antigen.

Differentiation of T cells in the thymus also results in expression of other important surface molecules. Initially proteins called CD4 and CD8 are concurrently expressed on the developing cells. As the cells mature, they retain either the CD4 molecule or the CD8 molecule, but not both. Those that retain the CD4 molecule develop into Th cells, whereas those that retain the CD8 molecule become T-cytotoxic (Tc) cells. Approximately 60% of immunocompetent T cells in the circulation express CD4, and 40% express CD8.

Central tolerance also occurs in the thymus where > 95% of developing T cells are clonally deleted because they are potentially autoreactive.

> ✔ QUICK CHECK 7.2
> 1. How is clonal diversity generated?
> 2. Describe the importance of BCRs and TCRs.
> 3. How is central tolerance achieved, and why is it important?

Clonal Selection

Antigens initiate the second phase of the immune response, clonal selection. Clonal selection is the processing of antigen for a specific immune response. This process involves a complex interaction among cells in the secondary lymphoid organs (see Fig. 7.2). Clonal selection usually begins at birth and continues throughout the life of an individual as new antigens are experienced. It can begin as early as week 8 of gestation in humans if foreign antigens are encountered in utero. Most of these in utero antigens are related to fetal infection during the last third period of gestation.

To initiate an effective immune response, most antigens must be processed because they cannot react directly with most cells of the immune system and they must be shown or presented to the immune cells in a specific manner. This is the job of antigen-processing (antigen-presenting) cells (APCs) (usually dendritic cells, macrophages, and B cells), generally referred to as APCs. The interaction among APCs, subpopulations of T cells that facilitate immune responses (T-helper cells [Th cells]), and immunocompetent B or T cells results in differentiation of B cells into active antibody-producing cells (plasma cells) and T cells into T-cytotoxic (Tc) effector cells. Both lines also develop into memory cells that respond even faster when that antigen enters the body again. Thus activation of the immune system produces a long-lasting protection against specific antigens (see Fig. 7.2). Defects in any aspect of cellular collaboration will lead to defects in cell-mediated immunity, humoral immunity, or both and, depending on the particular defect (see Chapter 8).

Antigen Processing and Presentation

Antigens that enter the body and circulate in blood and lymph undergo phagocytosis and destruction by APCs. These are referred to as exogenous antigens. Other antigens, called endogenous antigens, are intracellular antigens that have been generated when the cell has become abnormal because of injury, infection by a microorganism (e.g., viruses), or mutation of its DNA like occurs in cancer. Both exogenous and endogenous antigens undergo processing and presentation.

Processing results in the presentation of antigens on the surface of APCs and abnormal cells by molecules of the major histocompatibility complex (MHC). MHC molecules in humans also are called human leukocyte antigens (HLAs) when they are identified for organ transplantation (discussed in more detail in Chapter 8). Major histocompatibility complex (MHC) molecules are glycoproteins found on the surface of all human cells except red blood cells. They are divided into two general classes, class I and class II, based on their molecular structure, distribution among cell populations, and function in antigen presentation. MHC class I molecules are found on all nucleated cells and are composed of a large alpha (α) chain along with a smaller chain called β2-microglobulin. MHC class II molecules are found only on APCs and are composed of α- and β-chains that differ from the ones used for MHC class I. The α- and β-chains of the MHC molecules are encoded from different genetic loci located as a large complex of genes on human chromosome 6 (Fig. 7.5). MHC genes are highly polymorphic; therefore no two individuals, except identical twins, will have a complete set of identical MHC molecules.

MHC class I molecules present endogenous (intracellular) antigens, which are primarily recognized by Tc cells. Because MHC class I molecules are expressed on all cells, except red blood cells, any change in that cell that renders it abnormal (as occurs with viral infection or malignancy) may result in foreign antigens being presented by MHC class I molecules. MHC class II molecules present exogenous antigens (Fig. 7.6) and are found only on cells that have APC function, including macrophages, dendritic cells, and B lymphocytes. Antigens presented by MHC class II molecules are preferentially recognized by Th cells. Thus antigen presentation to Tc cells is MHC class I restricted and presentation to Th cells is MHC class II restricted. Because APCs have both MHC I and MCH II molecules, they can present both endogenous and exogenous antigens that can then be recognized by Tc and Th cells, respectively.

In summary, the term antigen processing and antigen presentation refers to the process by which large exogenous and endogenous antigens are cut up by enzymes into small antigenic fragments and then presented to Tc cells (MCH class I) or Th cells (MCH class II). Lipid antigens are frequently presented by a molecule unrelated to the MHC, known as CD1, and are not discussed here.

Cellular Interactions in the Immune Response

The second step in clonal selection is a finally tuned set of intercellular collaborations that result in the production of effector cells (plasma cells, Th cells, Tc cells) and memory cells. Each collaboration requires three complementary intracellular signaling events: antigen-specific recognition through the TCR or BCR complex, activation of intercellular communication, and the response to specific groups of cytokines. Without each signaling event, a protective immune response will not be produced.

T-helper lymphocytes. To induce an optimal cellular or humoral immune response, APCs must present antigens to Th cells. The APC presents antigen held by the variable regions (α1 and β1) of the α- and β-chains of MHC class II molecules. Activation of the Th cell then requires six steps:

1. The presented antigen is recognized and bound by the TCR on a Th cell (see Fig. 7.4).
2. Intercellular antigen binding is strengthened by the binding of the CD4 on the Th cell with the β2 region of the MHC class II molecule.
3. The cytoplasmic portions of CD3 and CD4 interact to activate intracellular signaling pathways.
4. Intercellular communication through adhesion molecules and co-stimulatory signals further activates the Th cell; the most critical being the B7 protein on the APC and CD28 on the Th cell.

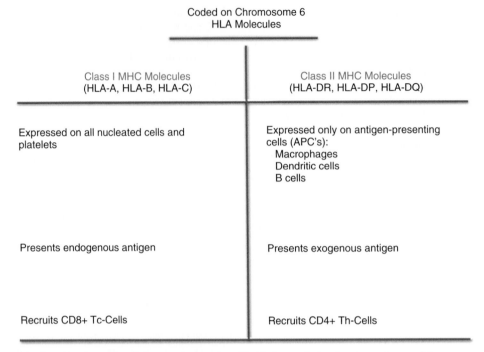

Coded on Chromosome 6
HLA Molecules

Class I MHC Molecules (HLA-A, HLA-B, HLA-C)	Class II MHC Molecules (HLA-DR, HLA-DP, HLA-DQ)
Expressed on all nucleated cells and platelets	Expressed only on antigen-presenting cells (APC's): Macrophages Dendritic cells B cells
Presents endogenous antigen	Presents exogenous antigen
Recruits CD8+ Tc-Cells	Recruits CD4+ Th-Cells

T cells recognize antigenic fragments complexed to HLA-encoded molecules as "non-self."

FIGURE 7.5 Antigen-Presenting Molecules. *HLA-A, HLA-B, HLS-C, isotypes of class I MCH molecules; HLA-DR, HLA-DP, HLA-DQ, isotypes of class II MCH molecules.*

5. Interleukin-1 (IL-1) is secreted by the APC and provides an additional signal through the IL-1 receptor on the Th cell (Fig. 7.7).
6. IL-2 is secreted by the Th cell and acts in an autocrine (self-stimulating) fashion to induce further maturation and proliferation of the Th cell. Without IL-2 production, the Th cell cannot efficiently mature into a functional helper cell.

Depending on the predominant cytokines in the immediate environment, activated Th cells undergo differentiation into one of several subsets: Th1, Th2, Th17, or Treg cells. These subsets have different functions: **Th1 cells** preferentially provide help in developing Tc cells (cell-mediated immunity); **Th2 cells** provide more help for developing B cells (humoral immunity); **Th17 cells** are lymphokine-secreting cells that activate macrophages; and **Treg cells** limit the immune response (discussed later in this chapter). The Th subsets differ considerably in the spectrum of cytokines they produce. Additionally, Th1 and Th2 cells may suppress each other so that the immune response may favor either antibody formation, with suppression of a cell-mediated response, or the opposite. For example, antigens derived from viral pathogens and those derived from cancer cells seem to induce a greater number of Th1 cells relative to Th2 cells, whereas antigens derived from multicellular parasites and allergens may result in production of more Th2 cells. Many antigens (e.g., tetanus vaccine), however, will produce excellent humoral and cell-mediated responses simultaneously. Th cells are necessary for development of most humoral and cellular immune responses; therefore the virus that causes acquired immunodeficiency syndrome (AIDS) results in life-threatening infections because it specifically infects and destroys Th cells (see Chapter 8).

Superantigens. Some viruses and bacteria can manipulate the normal interaction between APCs and Th cells to the detriment of the individual and the benefit of the microbe. The normal antigen-specific recognition between Th cells and APCs results in activation of relatively few cells—only those cells with specific TCRs against that antigen. In contrast, a group of microbial molecules called superantigens (SAGs) bind to the TCR and MHC II molecules outside of their normal

antigen-specific binding sites (Fig. 7.8). SAGs can therefore activate a large population of Th cells, regardless of antigen specificity, and induce excessive production of cytokines, including IL-2, interferon-gamma (IFN-γ), and tumor necrosis factor-alpha (TNF-α). The overproduction of inflammatory cytokines results in symptoms of a systemic inflammatory reaction, including fever, low blood pressure, and, potentially, fatal shock. Some examples of SAGs are the bacterial toxins produced by *Staphylococcus aureus* and *Streptococcus pyogenes* (SAGs that cause toxic shock syndrome and food poisoning).[1]

T-cytotoxic lymphocytes. The differentiation of immunocompetent T cells into effector Tc cells requires similar intercellular communications as described for Th cells. The Tc cell TCR recognizes antigen presented by MHC class I molecules on the surface of the APC and on virus-infected or cancerous cells (Fig. 7.9). The Tc cell CD8 binds to the MHC class I molecule and, as with Th cell differentiation, the proximity of the CD3 and CD8 cytoplasmic portions activates intercellular signaling pathways. Cytokine signals, especially IL-2, are produced by Th1 cells and activate cytokine receptors on the Tc cells.

B-cell clonal selection. Additional cellular interactions are required to produce an effective antibody response. The immunocompetent B cell is also an APC and expresses surface mIgM and mIgD BCRs (Fig. 7.10). Unlike the TCR, which can only *see* processed and presented antigens, the BCR can react with soluble antigens that have not been processed. B cells also express surface CD21, which is a receptor for opsonins produced by complement activation. Antigen binding through the BCR and CD21 activates the B cell, resulting in internalization, processing, and presentation of antigen fragments. Although B cells have MHC class I molecules on their surface, they preferentially present processed antigen on their MHC class II molecules and therefore activate Th cells. Intercellular communication between the B cell and the Th cell induces Th2 cell differentiation and the secretion of cytokines (particularly IL-4) that initiate B-cell proliferation and maturation into plasma cells. **Plasma cells** are activated B cells that produce antibodies that are capable of detecting the identical antigen as the BCR.

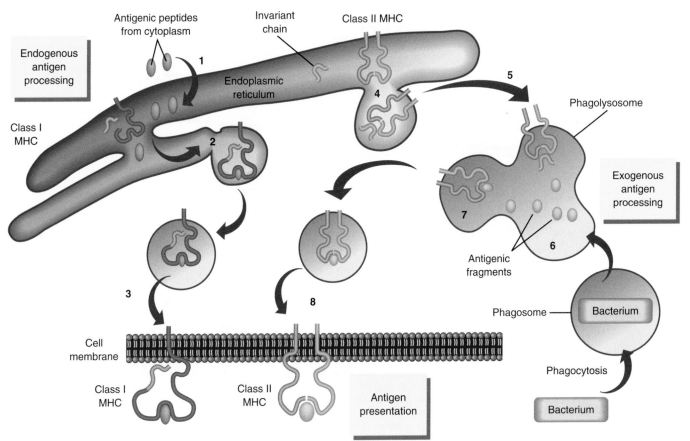

FIGURE 7.6 Antigen Processing and Presentation. Antigen processing and presentation are required for initiation of most immune responses. Foreign antigen may be either endogenous (cytoplasmic protein) or exogenous (e.g., bacterium). Endogenous antigenic peptides are transported into the endoplasmic reticulum (ER) (1), where the major histocompatibility complex (MHC) molecules are being assembled. In the ER, antigenic peptides bind to the α-chains of the MHC class I molecule (2), and the complex is transported to the cell surface (3). The α- and β-chains of the MHC class II molecules are also being assembled in the ER (4), but the antigen-binding site is blocked by a small molecule (invariant chain) to prevent interactions with endogenous antigenic peptides. The MHC class II–invariant chain complex is transported to phagolysosomes (5), where exogenous antigenic fragments have been produced as a result of phagocytosis (6). In the phagolysosomes, the invariant chain is digested and replaced by exogenous antigenic peptides (7), after which the MHC class II–antigen complex is inserted into the cell membrane (8).

Although most antigens require B cells to interact with Th cells, a few antigens can bypass the need for cellular interactions and can directly stimulate B-cell maturation and proliferation. These are called *T-cell–independent antigens* (Fig. 7.11). They are mostly bacterial products that are large and are capable of cross-linking several BCRs. T cell–independent antigens usually induce plasma cells to secrete only IgM.

Memory cells. During the clonal selection process, both B cells and T cells differentiate and proliferate into an extremely large population of long-lived memory cells. Memory cells remain inactive until subsequent exposure to the same antigen. Upon reexposure, these memory cells do not require much further differentiation and will therefore rapidly become new plasma cells or effector T cells without the cellular interactions described previously.

HUMORAL IMMUNITY (ANTIBODIES)

The terms **antibody** and **immunoglobulin (Ig)** are frequently used interchangeably. However, the term *antibody* is used more frequently in health care settings. When a B cell matures in response to antigen exposure, it becomes a plasma cell capable of producing antibodies.

Classes of Antibodies

There are five classes of antibodies (IgG, IgA, IgM, IgE, and IgD) which are characterized by differences in structure and function (Fig. 7.12). Both IgG and IgA have subclasses (Table 7.3).

IgG is the most abundant class of antibody, constituting 80% to 85% of the antibodies in the blood and accounting for most of the protective activity against infections. During pregnancy maternal IgG is transported across the placenta and protects the newborn child during the first 6 months of life.

IgM is the largest antibody and usually exists as a pentamer (a molecule consisting of five identical smaller molecules) that is stabilized by a J chain. It is the first antibody produced during the initial, or primary, response to antigens. IgM is usually synthesized early in neonatal life but may be increased as a response to infection in utero.

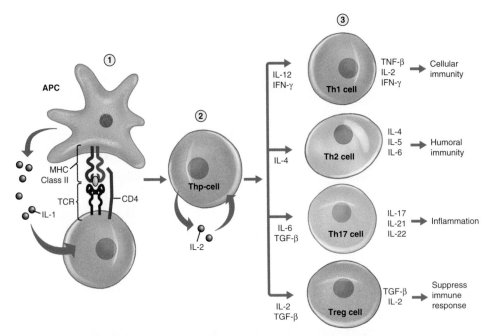

FIGURE 7.7 Development of T-Cell Subsets. The most important step in clonal selection is the production of populations of T-helper (Th) cells (Th1, Th2, and Th17) and T-regulatory (Treg) cells that are necessary for the development of cellular and humoral immune responses. In this model, antigen-presenting cells (APCs) (1) (probably multiple populations) may influence whether a precursor Th cell (Thp cell) (2) will differentiate into a Th1, Th2, Th17, or Treg cell (3). Differentiation of the Thp cell is initiated by three signaling events. The antigen signal is produced by the interaction of the T-cell receptor (TCR) and CD4 with antigen presented by major histocompatibility complex (MHC) class II molecules. A set of costimulatory signals is produced from interactions between adhesion molecules (not shown). A third signal is produced by the interactions of cytokines (particularly interleukin-1 [IL-1]) with appropriate cytokine receptors (IL-1R) on the Thp cell. The Thp cell up-regulates IL-2 production and expression of the IL-2 receptor (IL-2R), which acts in an autocrine fashion to accelerate Th cell differentiation and proliferation. Commitment to a particular phenotype results from the relative concentrations of other cytokines. IL-12 and interferon-gamma (IFN-γ) produced by some populations of APCs favor differentiation into the Th1 cell phenotype; IL-4, which is produced by a variety of cells, favors differentiation into the Th2 cell phenotype; IL-6 and transforming growth factor-beta (TGF-β) (T-cell growth factor) facilitate differentiation into Th17 cells; IL-2 and TGF-β induce differentiation into Treg cells. The Th1 cell is characterized by the production of cytokines that assist in the differentiation of T-cytotoxic (Tc) cells, leading to cellular immunity, whereas the Th2 cell produces cytokines that favor B-cell differentiation and humoral immunity. Th1 and Th2 cells affect each other through the production of inhibitory cytokines: IFN-γ will inhibit development of Th2 cells, and IL-4 will inhibit the development of Th1 cells. Th17 cells produce cytokines that affect phagocytes and increase inflammation. Treg cells produce immunosuppressive cytokines that prevent the immune response from being excessive.

TABLE 7.3 Properties of Antibodies

Class	Subclass	Adult Serum Levels (mg/dL)	Present in Secretions	Complement Activation	Opsonin	Agglutinin	Mast Cell Activation	Placental Transfer
IgG	IgG1	800–900	+	++	++	+	−	+++
	IgG2	280–300	+	+	−	+	−	+
	IgG3	90–100	+	+++	++	+	−	+++
	IgG4	50	−	−	−	+	+	++
IgM		120–150	+	++++	−	++++	−	−
IgA	IgA1	280–300	+	−	−	+	−	−
	IgA2	50	+	−	−	+	−	−
	sIgA	5	++++	−	−	+	−	−
IgD		3	−	−	−	−	−	−
IgE		0.03	+	−	−	−	+++	−

sIgA, Secretory immunoglobulin A; − indicates lack of activity; + to ++++ indicate relative activity or concentration.

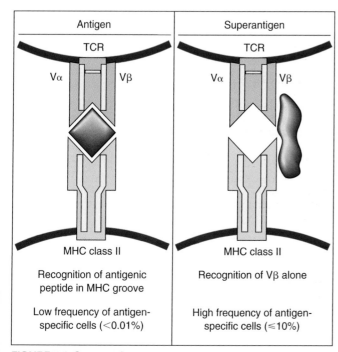

FIGURE 7.8 **Superantigens.** The T-cell receptor (TCR) and major histocompatibility complex (MHC) class II molecule are normally held together by processed antigen. Superantigens, such as some bacterial exotoxins, bind directly to the variable region of the TCR β-chain and the MHC class II molecule. Each superantigen activates sets of Vβ chains independently of the antigen specificity of the TCR.

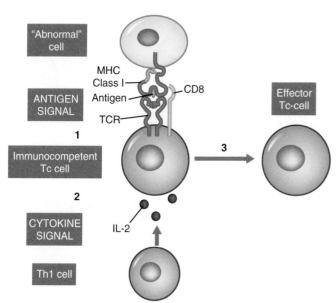

FIGURE 7.9 **T-Cytotoxic (Tc)-Cell Clonal Selection.** The immunocompetent Tc cell can react with antigen but cannot yet kill target cells. During clonal selection, this cell reacts with antigen presented by major histocompatibility complex (MHC) class I molecules on the surface of a virally infected or cancerous *abnormal* cell. (1) The antigen–MHC class I complex is recognized simultaneously by the T-cell receptor (TCR), which binds to antigen, and CD8, which binds to the MHC class I molecule. (2) A separate signal is provided by cytokines, particularly IL-2 from T-helper 1 (Th1) cells. (3) In response to these signals, the Tc cell develops into an effector Tc cell with the ability to kill abnormal cells.

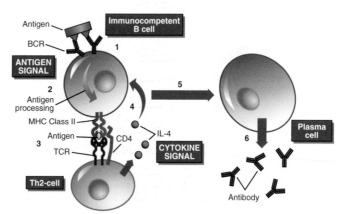

FIGURE 7.10 **B-Cell Clonal Selection.** Immunocompetent B cells undergo proliferation and differentiation into antibody-secreting plasma cells. Multiple signals are necessary (1). The B cell itself can directly bind soluble antigen through the B-cell receptor (BCR) and act as an antigen-processing cell. Antigen is internalized, processed (2), and presented (3) to the TCR on a T-helper 2 (Th2) cell by major histocompatibility complex (MHC) class II molecules (4). A cytokine signal is provided by the Th2 cell cytokines (e.g., interleukin-4 [IL-4]) that react with the B cell (5). The B cell differentiates into plasma cells that secrete antibody specific to the antigen (6).

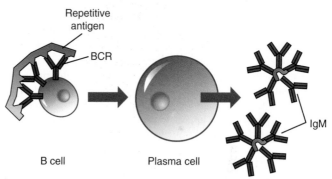

FIGURE 7.11 **Activation of a B Cell by a T Cell–Independent Antigen.** Molecules containing repeating identical antigenic determinants may interact simultaneously with several receptors on the surface of the B cell and induce the proliferation and production of immunoglobulins. Because T-helper 2 (Th2) cells do not participate, class switch does not occur and the resultant antibody response is immunoglobulin M (IgM).

IgA is found in blood and in bodily secretions as secretory IgA (subclass IgA2). **Secretory IgA** is a *dimer* consisting of two IgA2 molecules held together through a J chain and secretory piece. The secretory piece is attached to dimeric IgA during transportation through mucosal epithelial cells to protect against degradation by enzymes also found in secretions.

IgD functions as a part of the BCR antigen receptor on the surface of early B cells.

IgE is normally at low concentrations in the circulation. It has very specialized functions as a mediator of many common allergic responses (see Chapter 8) and as a defense against parasitic infections.

A major component of B-cell maturation is **class switch**, the process that results in the change in antibody production from one class to another (e.g., IgM to IgG). Antibody diversification is essential for the immune system to produce protective humoral responses. Before exposure to antigens and Th2 cells, the B cell produces IgM and IgD, which are used as cell membrane receptors. During the clonal selection process, a B cell proliferates and develops into antibody-secreting

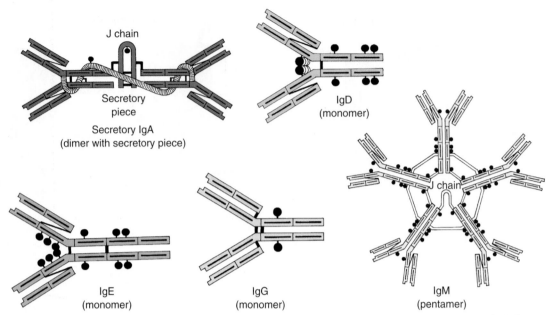

FIGURE 7.12 Structures of Different Immunoglobulins. Secretory immunoglobulin A (IgA), IgD, IgE, IgG, and IgM. The black circles attached to each molecule represent carbohydrate residues.

plasma cells, and each B cell has the option of becoming a secretor of IgM or changing the class of antibody to a secreted form of IgG, IgA, or IgE. The antigenic specificity of the antibody remains unchanged. Thus during clonal selection, a B cell may produce a population of plasma cells that are capable of producing many different classes of antibodies against the same antigen. The type of antibody produced is under the control of Th cytokines. For instance, the Th2 cytokines IL-4 and IL-13 appear to preferentially stimulate switch to IgE secretion.

Molecular Structure

There are three parts to an antibody molecule (Fig. 7.13). Two identical fragments have the ability to bind antigen and are termed **antigen-binding fragments (Fab)**. The third fragment is termed the **crystalline fragment (Fc)**. The Fab portions contain the recognition sites (receptors) for antigens and confer the molecule's specificity toward a particular antigen. The Fc portion is responsible for most of the biologic functions of antibodies.

An antibody molecule consists of four polypeptide chains: two identical light (L) chains and two identical heavy (H) chains. The light and heavy chains are held together by noncovalent bonds and covalent disulfide linkages. The class of antibody is determined by the different amino acid sequences in the heavy chains that make up the Fc portion of the antibody. The Fab portion of the antibody is sometimes called the **variable region** or **complementary determining region (CDR)**. Its specificity for a particular antigen corresponds to the BCR on the B cell that produced the antibody (see Fig. 7.13).

Antigen–Antibody Binding

Because antigens are relatively small, a large molecule (e.g., protein, polysaccharide, nucleic acid) usually contains multiple and diverse antigens. The precise area of the antigen that is recognized by a particular antibody is called its **antigenic determinant, or epitope**. The matching Fab portion on the antibody is sometimes referred to as the **antigen-binding site, or paratope**. The antigen fits into the antigen-binding site of the antibody with the specificity of a key into a lock and is held there by noncovalent chemical interactions.

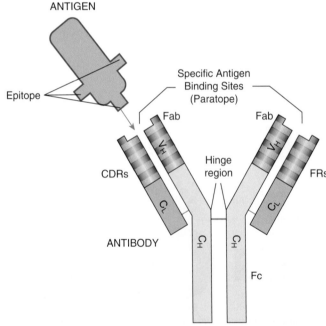

FIGURE 7.13 Antigen–Antibody Binding. C_H, Constant region heavy chain; V_L, Variable region light chain; V_H, Variable region heavy chain; C_L, Constant region light chain; Fab, Fragment antigen binding; Fc, Crystalline fragment; CDRs, Complementary determining regions; FRs, Framework regions. Red lines are disulfide linkages.

Function of Antibodies

The chief function of antibodies is to protect against infection. The mechanism can be either *direct*—through the action of antibody alone or *indirect*—requiring activation of other components of the innate immune response (Fig. 7.14). Directly, antibodies can affect infectious agents or their toxic products by **neutralization** (inactivating or blocking the binding of antigens to receptors). For instance, the influenza virus must attach to specific receptors on respiratory tract epithelial cells,

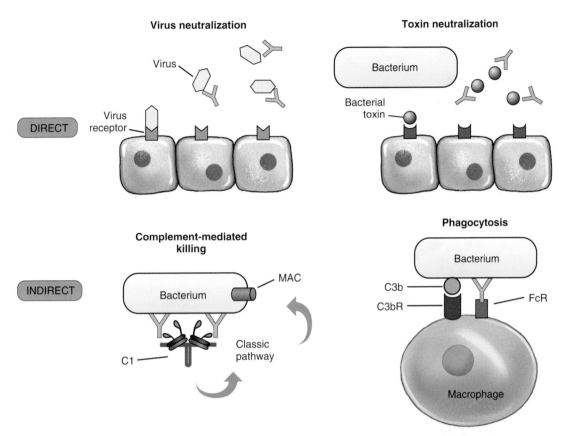

FIGURE 7.14 Direct and Indirect Functions of Antibody. Protective activities of antibodies can be direct (through the action of antibody alone) or indirect (requiring activation of other components of the innate immune response, usually through the Fc region). *Direct* means include neutralization of viruses or bacterial toxins before they bind to receptors on the surface of the host's cells. *Indirect* means include activation of the classical complement pathway through C1, resulting in formation of the membrane attack complex (MAC), or increased phagocytosis of bacteria opsonized with antibody and complement components bound to appropriate surface receptors (FcR and C3bR).

and *Neisseria gonorrhoeae* (causes gonorrhea) must attach to specific sites on urogenital epithelial cells. Antibodies may protect the host by covering sites on the microorganism that are needed for attachment, thereby preventing infection. Many viral infections can be prevented by vaccination with inactivated or attenuated (weakened) viruses designed to induce neutralizing antibody production. Antibodies also can protect against infection through **agglutination** (clumping insoluble particles that are in suspension) or **precipitation** (making a soluble antigen into an insoluble precipitate).

Some bacteria secrete toxins that harm individuals. For instance, bacterial toxins cause the symptoms of tetanus or diphtheria. Most toxins are proteins that bind to surface molecules on cells and damage those cells. Protective antibodies produced against the toxin, known as **antitoxins**, can bind to the toxins, prevent their interaction with host cells, and neutralize their biologic effects (see Chapter 8).

Indirectly, through the Fc portion, antibodies activate components of innate immunity, including complement and phagocytes (Fig. 7.15). Through the classical pathway, complement component C1 will be activated by binding simultaneously to the Fc regions of two adjacent antibodies bound to a microbe, resulting in activation of the entire cascade. Phagocytic cells express receptors that bind the Fc portion of antibody; thus antibody is an **opsonin** that facilitates phagocytosis of bacteria. IgM is the best complement-activating antibody, and IgG is the best opsonin. Some antibodies are more protective than others. It is now a common procedure to clone the "best" antibodies

(monoclonal antibodies) for use in diagnostic tests and for therapy (Box 7.1).

Immunoglobulin E

IgE is a special class of antibody that protects the individual from infection by large parasitic worms (helminths). However, when IgE is produced against relatively innocuous environmental antigens, it is also the primary cause of common allergies (e.g., hay fever, dust allergies, bee stings). The role of IgE in allergies is discussed in Chapter 8.

Large multicellular parasites usually invade mucosal tissues. IgG, IgM, and IgA bind to the surface of parasites, activate complement, generate chemotactic factors for neutrophils and macrophages, and serve as opsonins for those phagocytic cells. This response, however, does not greatly damage parasites. The only inflammatory cell that can adequately damage a parasite is the eosinophil because of the special contents of its granules. These contents include major basic protein, eosinophil cationic protein, eosinophil peroxidase, and eosinophil neurotoxin, each of which can damage infectious worms. IgE is designed to specifically initiate an inflammatory reaction that preferentially attracts eosinophils to the site of parasitic infection; thus elevated levels of IgE are commonly found in parasitic infection.

Mast cells in the tissues have Fc receptors that bind IgE to the mast cell surface. Soluble antigen molecules from the parasite bind to multiple IgE antibodies and initiate a cascade of effects that can ultimately kill the parasite. The steps of the cascade are presented in Fig. 7.15.

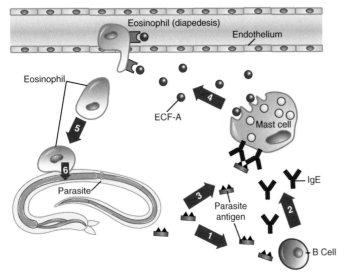

FIGURE 7.15 Immunoglobulin E (IgE) Function. (1) Soluble antigens from a parasitic infection cause production of IgE antibody by B cells. **(2)** Secreted IgE binds to IgE-specific receptors on the mast cell. **(3)** Additional soluble parasite antigen cross-links the IgE on the mast cell surface, **(4)** leading to mast cell degranulation and release of many proinflammatory products, including eosinophil chemotactic factor of anaphylaxis (ECF-A). **(5)** ECF-A attracts eosinophils from the circulation. **(6)** The eosinophil attaches to the surface of the parasite and releases potent lysosomal enzymes that damage microorganisms.

BOX 7.1   Monoclonal Antibodies

Most humoral immune responses are polyclonal—that is, a mixture of antibodies produced from multiple B lymphocytes. Most antigenic molecules have multiple antigenic determinants, each of which induces a different group of antibodies. Thus a polyclonal response is a mixture of antibody classes, specificities, and function, some of which are more protective than others.

Monoclonal antibody is produced in the laboratory from one B cell that has been cloned; thus the entire antibody is of the same class, specificity, and function. The advantages of monoclonal antibodies are that (1) a single antibody of known antigenic specificity is generated rather than a mixture of different antibodies; (2) monoclonal antibodies have a single, constant binding affinity; (3) monoclonal antibodies can be diluted to a constant titer (concentration in fluid) because the actual antibody concentration is known; and (4) the antibody can be easily purified. Thus a highly concentrated antibody with optimal function has been used to develop extremely specific and sensitive laboratory tests (e.g., home and laboratory pregnancy tests) and therapies, such as infections and cancer. In fact, monoclonal antibodies have become important immunotherapies for some cancers that are resistant to standard chemotherapy treatments.

Secretory Immune System

Immunocompetent lymphocytes migrate among secondary lymphoid organs and tissue as part of the systemic immune system. Another, partially independent, immune system protects the external surfaces of the body through lacrimal and salivary glands and a network of lymphoid tissues residing in the breasts, bronchi, intestines, and genitourinary tract. This system is called the secretory (mucosal) immune system (Fig. 7.16). Plasma cells in those sites secrete antibodies in bodily secretions, such as tears, sweat, saliva, mucus, and breast milk, to prevent pathogenic microorganism from infecting the body's surfaces and possibly penetrating to cause systemic disease.

IgA is the dominant secretory immunoglobulin, although IgM and IgG also are present in secretions. The primary role of IgA is to prevent the attachment and invasion of pathogens through mucosal membranes, such as those of the gastrointestinal, pulmonary, and genitourinary tracts. Dimeric IgA antibodies are produced by plasma cells of the mucosa. Mucosal epithelium expresses a cell surface antibody receptor that binds and internalizes IgA. The IgA, along with the epithelial receptor (secretory piece), is secreted as secretory IgA (sIgA).

The lymphoid tissues of the secretory immune system are connected; thus many foreign antigens in a mother's gastrointestinal tract (e.g., polio virus) induce secretion of specific antibodies into breast milk. Colostral antibodies (i.e., those found in the colostrum of breast milk) may protect the nursing newborn against infectious disease agents that enter through the gastrointestinal tract. Although colostral antibodies provide the newborn with passive immunity against gastrointestinal infections, they do not provide systemic immunity because transport across the newborn's gut into the bloodstream is discontinued after the first 24 hours of life. Maternal antibodies that pass across the placenta into the fetus before birth provide passive systemic immunity.

Primary and Secondary Immune Responses

The immune response to antigen has classically been divided into two phases—primary and secondary responses. Although these two phases occur in cellular immune responses, this process is most easily demonstrated by measuring concentrations of circulating antibodies over time (Fig. 7.17). After a single initial exposure to most antigens, there is a latent period, or lag phase, during which clonal selection occurs. After approximately 5 to 7 days, IgM antibody is detected in the circulation. This is the primary immune response, characterized typically by initial production of IgM followed by production of IgG against the same antigen. The quantity of IgG may be about equal to or less than the amount of IgM. The amount of antibody in a serum sample is frequently referred to as the titer; a higher titer indicates more antibodies. If no further exposure to the antigen occurs, the circulating antibody is catabolized (broken down) and titers fall. The individual's immune system, however, has been primed.

A second challenge by the same antigen results in the secondary immune response, which is characterized by the more rapid production of a larger amount of antibody compared with the primary response. The rapidity of the secondary immune response is the result of memory cells that require less further differentiation. IgM may be transiently produced in the secondary response, but IgG production is increased considerably making it the predominant antibody class. Natural infection (e.g., rubella) may result in measurable levels of protective IgG for the life of the individual. Some vaccines (e.g., polio) also may produce extremely long-lived protection, although most vaccines require boosters at specified intervals.

✔ **QUICK CHECK 7.4**
1. What are the major classes of antibodies?
2. What are the major functions of antibodies?
3. What is the difference between the secretory and systemic immune systems?
4. What is meant by the terms primary and secondary immune response?

CELL-MEDIATED IMMUNITY

The function of effector T cells is complex and utilizes the principles of intercellular recognition necessary for clonal selection.

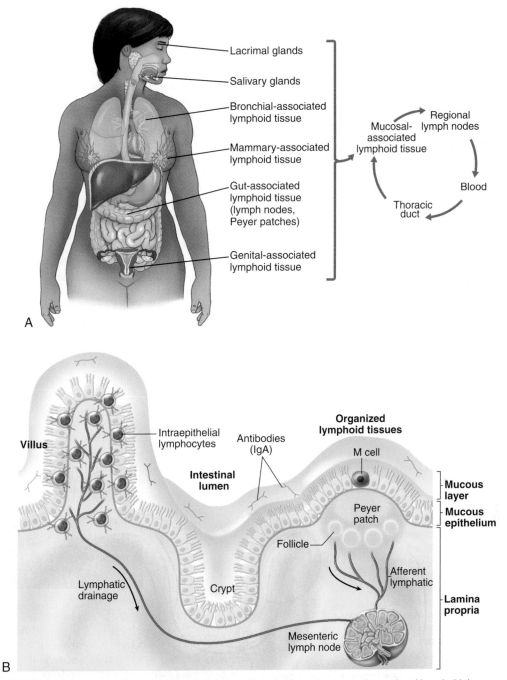

FIGURE 7.16 Secretory Immune System. A, Lymphocytes from the mucosal-associated lymphoid tissues (MALTs) circulate throughout the body in a pattern separate from other lymphocytes. For example, lympho-cytes from the gut-associated lymphoid tissue circulate through the regional lymph nodes, the thoracic duct, and the blood and return to other MALTs rather than to lymphoid tissue of the systemic immune system. **B,** Lymphoid tissue associated with mucous membranes is referred to as MALT.

T-Lymphocyte Function

The clonal selection process produces several subsets of effector T cells. Th cells and T memory cells have already been discussed. Other effector T cells include Tc cells that attack and destroy cells expressing antigens from intracellular (endogenous) origins, Treg cells that limit (suppress) the immune response, and T lymphokine–producing cells that secrete cytokines that activate other cells.

T-Cytotoxic Lymphocytes

Tc cells are responsible for the cell-mediated destruction of abnormal cells, such as tumor cells or cells infected with viruses. Similar to intercellular recognition during the clonal selection process, the Tc cell must directly adhere to the target cell through antigen presented by MHC class I molecules and CD8 (Fig. 7.18). Because of the broad cellular distribution of MHC class I molecules, Tc cells can recognize

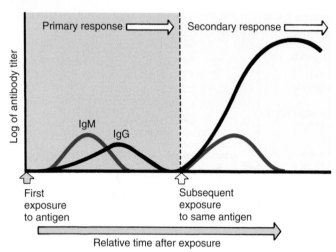

FIGURE 7.17 Primary and Secondary Immune Responses. The initial administration of antigen induces a primary response during which IgM is initially produced, followed by Immunoglobulin G (IgG). Another administration of the antigen induces the secondary response in which IgM is transiently produced and larger amounts of IgG are produced over a longer period.

antigens on the surface of almost any type of cell that has become abnormal. Attachment to a target cell activates multiple killing mechanisms through which the Tc cell induces the target cell to undergo apoptosis.

Various other cells kill targets in a fashion similar to Tc lymphocytes. Prominent among these cells are natural killer cells. **Natural killer (NK) cells** are a special group of lymphoid cells that are important components of both innate and adaptive immunity. They are similar to T cells but lack antigen-specific receptors. Instead, they express a variety of cell surface activation receptors (similar to pattern recognition receptors; see Chapter 6), which identify protein changes on the surface of cells infected with viruses or that have become cancerous. After attachment, the NK cell kills its target in a manner similar to that of Tc cells. Unlike Tc cells, NK cells lack CD8, and binding to MHC class I molecules results in inactivation of the NK cell. Thus if MHC class I antigen presentation has occurred, Tc cells provide the target cell killing. But in some instances, a virus-infected or cancerous cell will "protect" itself from Tc cells by downregulating MHC class I molecule expression. In these instances, the lack of MHC class I inhibition allows NK cells to become activated and kill the target cell.

NK cells, as well as some macrophages, also can specifically target abnormal cells through use of antibodies. NK cells express Fc receptors for IgG. If antigens on the infected or cancerous cell bind IgG, the NK cell can attach through Fc receptors and activate its normal killing mechanisms. This is referred to as **antibody-dependent cellular cytotoxicity (ADCC).**

FIGURE 7.18 Cellular Killing Mechanisms. Several cells have the capacity to kill abnormal (e.g., virally infected, cancerous) target cells. **(1)** T-cytotoxic (Tc) cells recognize endogenous antigen presented by major histocompatibility complex (MHC) class I molecules. The Tc cell mobilizes multiple killing mechanisms that induce apoptosis of the target cell. **(2)** Natural killer (NK) cells identify and kill target cells through receptors that recognize abnormal surface changes. NK cells specifically kill targets that do not express surface MHC class I molecules. **(3)** Several cells, including macrophages and NK cells, can kill by antibody-dependent cellular cytotoxicity (ADCC). IgG antibodies bind to foreign antigen on the target cell, and cells involved in ADCC bind IgG through Fc receptors (FcRs) and initiate killing. The insert is a scanning electron microscopic view of Tc cells *(L)* attacking a much larger tumor cell *(Tu).* (Insert from Abbas A, Lichtman A: *Cellular and molecular immunology*, ed 5, Philadelphia, 2003, Saunders.)

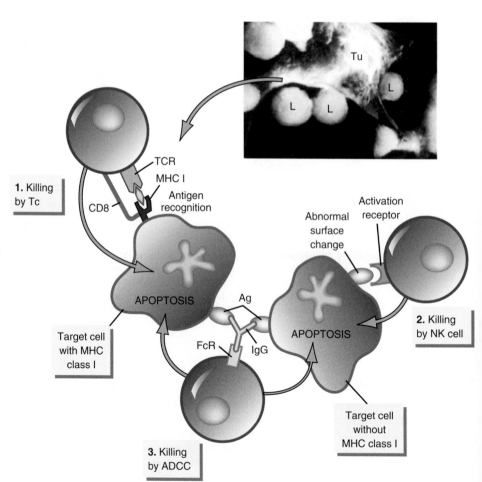

Lymphokine-Secreting T Cells

Two subsets of Th cells amplify inflammation. Th1 cells, in addition to assisting Tc-cell clonal selection, secrete cytokines that activate M1 macrophages to increase phagocytic and microbial killing functions (described in Chapter 6). The most important Th1 cytokine for macrophage activation is interferon-γ (IFN-γ). Th2 cells, in addition to assisting B-cell clonal selection, secrete cytokines (e.g., IL-4, IL-13) that activate M2 macrophages for healing and repair of damaged tissue (described in Chapter 6). Th17 cells secrete a set of cytokines (e.g., IL-17, IL-22, chemokines) that recruit phagocytic cells to a site of inflammation. Th17-cell cytokines also activate epithelial cells, to produce antimicrobial proteins in defense against certain bacterial and fungal pathogens.

T-Regulatory Lymphocytes

T-regulatory (Treg) cells are a diverse group of T cells that control the immune response, usually suppressing the response and maintaining tolerance against self-antigens. Many Treg cells develop in the thymus and suppress the maturation of autoreactive T cells. Other Treg cells are derived from Th cells in response to excessive inflammation and autoimmunity. This process occurs in the secondary lymphoid organs and is known as peripheral tolerance. Treg cells produce very high levels of immunosuppressive cytokines TGF-β and IL-10, which decrease Th1 and Th2 activity by suppressing antigen recognition and Th-cell proliferation.

✔ QUICK CHECK 7.5

1. What are the functions of T cytotoxic cells?
2. How do NK cell differ from T cytotoxic cells?
3. What is the role of Treg cells?

Age-related mechanisms of self-defense in the newborn and in the elderly are summarized in the *Pediatric Considerations* and *Geriatric Considerations* boxes.

PEDIATRIC CONSIDERATIONS

Age-Related Factors Affecting Mechanisms of Self-Defense in the Newborn Child

Normal human newborns are immunologically immature with deficient antibody production, phagocytic activity, and complement activity, especially components of alternative pathways (e.g., factor B).

The newborn cannot produce all classes of antibody; IgM is produced by the newborn (develops in the last trimester) to in utero infections (e.g., cytomegalovirus, rubella virus, and *Toxoplasma gondii*); only limited amounts of IgA are produced in the newborn; IgG production begins after birth and rises steadily throughout the first year of life.

Maternal antibodies provide protection within the newborn's circulation (see figure below).

Deficits in specific maternal transplacental antibody may lead to a tendency to develop severe, overwhelming sepsis and meningitis in the newborn.

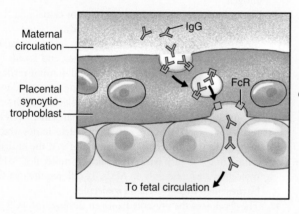

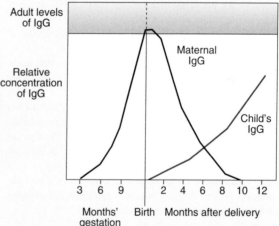

Antibody Levels in Umbilical Cord Blood and in Neonatal Circulation. Early in gestation, maternal IgG begins active transport across the placenta and enters the fetal circulation. At birth, the fetal circulation may contain nearly adult levels of IgG, which is almost exclusively from the maternal source. The fetal immune system has the capacity to produce IgM and small amounts of IgA before birth *(not shown)*. After delivery, maternal IgG is rapidly destroyed and neonatal IgG production increases.

GERIATRIC CONSIDERATIONS

Age-Related Factors Affecting Mechanisms of Self-Defense in the Elderly

Immune function decreases with age; diminished T-cell function and reduced antibody responses to antigenic challenge occur with age.

The thymus reaches maximum size at sexual maturity and then undergoes involution until it is a vestigial remnant by middle age; by age 45 to 50 years, the thymus is only 15% of its maximum size.

With age there is a decrease in thymic hormone production and the organ's ability to mediate T-cell differentiation.

SUMMARY REVIEW

Overview of Adaptive Immunity

1. Adaptive immunity is a state of protection, primarily against infectious agents, that differs from inflammation by being slower to develop, being more specific, and having memory that makes it much longer lived.

2. The adaptive immune response is most often initiated by cells of the innate system. These cells process and present portions of invading pathogens (i.e., antigens) to lymphocytes in peripheral lymphoid tissue.

3. The adaptive immune response is mediated by two different types of lymphocytes—B lymphocytes and T lymphocytes. Each has distinct functions. B cells are responsible for humoral immunity that is mediated by circulating antibodies, whereas T cells are responsible for cell-mediated immunity, in which they kill targets directly or stimulate the activity of other leukocytes.

4. Adaptive immunity can be either active or passive depending on whether immune response components originated in the host or came from a donor.

5. B and T lymphocytes leaving the primary lymphoid organs are immunocompetent but have not been exposed to antigen, thus are naïve.

6. Clonal selection is initiated when exposure to an antigen occurs.

Antigens and Immunogens

1. Antigens are molecules that bind and react with components of the immune response, such as antibodies and receptors on B and T cells. Most antigens can induce an immune response, and these antigens are called *immunogens*.

2. All immunogens are antigens, but not all antigens are immunogens.

3. Some pathogens are successful because they mimic "self" antigens but avoid inducing an immune response.

4. Common antigens include infectious agents, allergens, chemical agents, and abnormal molecules on the surface of cells.

5. Large molecules, such as proteins, polysaccharides, and nucleic acids, are most immunogenic. Thus molecular size is an important factor for antigen immunogenicity.

6. Haptens are antigens too small to be immunogens by themselves but become immunogenic after combining with larger molecules.

7. The antigenic determinant, or epitope, is the precise chemical structure with which an antibody or B-cell/T-cell receptor (BCR/TCR) reacts.

8. Self-antigens are antigens on an individual's own cells. The individual's immune system does not normally recognize self-antigens as immunogenic, a condition known as *tolerance*.

Immune Response: Collaboration of B Cells and T Cells

1. The generation of clonal diversity results in production of B and T lymphocytes with receptors against millions of antigens that possibly will be encountered in an individual's lifetime occurs in the fetus in the primary lymphoid organs: the thymus for T cells and portions of bone marrow for B cells..

2. The generation of clonal diversity is the differentiation of lymphoid stem cells into B and T lymphocytes. Lymphoid stem cells interact with stromal cells through a variety of adhesion factors. As the stem cell matures it develops a variety of surface markers or receptors, one of the earliest is interleukin-7 (IL-7) receptor. IL-7, produced by stromal cells is critical for driving differentiation and proliferation of the B cell.

3. The next stage in development is formation of the BCR. The role of the BCR is to recognize antigen and communicate that information to the cell's nucleus.

4. The enormous repertoire of BCR specificities is made possible by rearrangement of existing deoxyribonucleic acid (DNA) during B-cell development in the primary lymphoid organs, a process called *somatic recombination*.

5. Somatic rearrangement of the antibody variable regions will frequently result in a BCR that recognizes the individual's own antigens, which may result in attack on "self" antigens expressed on various tissue and organs. Many of these "autoreactive" B cells are eliminated in the bone marrow. Most of the developing B cells undergo apoptosis. This entire process is referred to as clonal deletion or central tolerance.

6. The process of T-cell proliferation and differentiation is similar to that for B cells. The primary lymphoid organ for T-cell development is the thymus. Lymphoid stem cells travel through the thymus, where thymic hormones and the cytokine IL-7 promote lymphoid stem cell division and the production of receptors. They exit the thymus as mature immunocompetent T cells with antigen-specific receptors on the cell surface.

7. TCR proceeds in a manner similar to BCR. Initially proteins called *CD4* and *CD8* are expressed on the developing cells. As the cell matures they retain either the CD4 molecule or the CD8 molecule but not both. Eventually CD4 cells develop into T-helper cells (Th cells) and CD 8 cells become T-cytotoxic cells (Tc cells). Other mature T cells include T-regulatory cells (Treg cells) and memory cells.

8. The generation of clonal diversity concludes when immunocompetent T and B cells migrate from the primary lymphoid organs into the circulation and secondary lymphoid organs to await antigen.

9. The induction of an immune response, or clonal selection, begins when antigen enters the individual's body.

10. Most antigens must first interact with antigen-presenting cells (APCs) (e.g., dendritic cells, macrophages, and B cells).

11. To induce an optimal cellular or humoral immune response, APCs must present antigens to Th cells. Antigen is processed in the APCs and presented on the cell surface by molecules of the major histocompatibility complex (MHC). The particular MHC molecule (class I or class II) that presents antigen determines which cell will respond to that antigen. Th cells require that the antigen be presented in a complex with MHC class II molecules. MHC class II molecules are found only on APCs. Tc cells require that the antigen be presented by MHC class I molecules.

12. The T cell sees the presented antigen through the TCR and accessory molecules: CD4 or CD8. CD4 is found on Th cells and reacts specifically with MHC class II. CD8 is found on Tc cells and reacts specifically with MHC class I.

13. Th cells consist of Th1 cells, which help Tc cells respond to antigen; Th2 cells, which help B cells develop into plasma cells; and Th17 cells, which help activate macrophages.

14. Tc cells bind to and kill cellular targets, such as cells infected with viruses or cancer cells.

15. The natural killer (NK) cell has some characteristics of the Tc cells and is important for killing target cells in which viral infection or malignancy has resulted in the loss of cellular MHC molecules.

Humoral Immunity (Antibodies)

1. The humoral immune response consists of molecules (antibodies) produced by B cells. B cells are lymphocytes.

2. Antibodies are plasma glycoproteins that can be classified by chemical structure and biologic activity as immunoglobulin G (IgG), IgM, IgA, IgE, or IgD.

3. A typical antibody molecule is constructed of two identical heavy chains and two identical light chains (either κ or λ) and has two Fab portions that bind antigen and an Fc portion that interacts with complement or receptors on cells.
4. The protective effects of antibodies may be *direct* through the action of antibody alone or *indirect* requiring activation of other components of the innate immune response.
5. IgE is a special class of antibody produced against environmental antigens that are the primary cause of common allergies. It also protects the individual from infection by large parasitic worms (helminths).
6. The secretory immune system protects the external surfaces of the body through secretion of antibodies in bodily secretions, such as tears, sweat, saliva, mucus, and breast milk. IgA is the dominant secretory immunoglobulin.

Cell-Mediated Immunity
1. Other effector T cells include Tc cells that attack and destroy cells expressing antigens from intracellular origins, Treg cells that suppress the immune response, and T lymphokine–producing cells that secrete cytokines that activate other cells.
2. Tc cells are responsible for cell-mediated destruction of abnormal cells, such as tumor cells or cells infected with viruses.
3. Attachment to a target cell activates multiple killing mechanisms through which the Tc cell induces the target cell to undergo apoptosis.
4. Two subsets of Th cells amplify inflammation. Th1 cells, in addition to assisting Tc-cell clonal selection, secrete cytokines that activate M1 macrophages to increase phagocytic and microbial killing functions. Th2 cells, in addition to assisting B-cell clonal selection, secrete cytokines that activate M2 macrophages for healing and repair of damaged tissue.

5. Th17 cells secrete a set of cytokines that recruit phagocytic cells to a site of inflammation. Th17-cell cytokines also activate epithelial cells to produce antimicrobial proteins in defense against certain bacterial and fungal pathogens.
6. Treg cells are a diverse group of T cells that control the immune response, usually suppressing the response and maintaining tolerance against self-antigens. Treg cells produce very high levels of immunosuppressive cytokines, which decrease Th1 and Th2 activity by suppressing antigen recognition and Th-cell proliferation.

Pediatric Considerations: Age-Related Factors Affecting Mechanisms of Self-Defense in the Newborn Child
1. Neonates often have transiently depressed inflammatory function, particularly neutrophil chemotaxis and alternative complement pathway activity.
2. The T cell–independent immune response is adequate in the fetus and neonate, but the T cell–dependent immune response develops slowly during the first 6 months of life.
3. Maternal IgG antibodies are transported across the placenta into the fetal blood and protect the neonate for the first 6 months, after which they are replaced by the child's own antibodies.

Geriatric Considerations: Age-Related Factors Affecting Mechanisms of Self-Defense in the Elderly
1. Elderly persons are at risk for impaired wound healing, usually because of chronic illnesses.
2. T-cell function and antibody production are somewhat deficient in elderly persons. Elderly individuals also tend to have increased levels of circulating autoantibodies (antibodies against self-antigens).

KEY TERMS

REFERENCES
1. Ramachandran G: Gram-positive and gram-negative bacterial toxins in sepsis, *Virulence* 5(1):213-218, 2014.

8

Alterations in Immunity

Valentina L. Brashers, Sue E. Huether

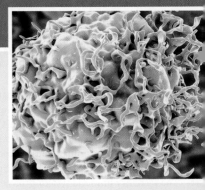

EVOLVE WEBSITE

CHAPTER OUTLINE

The defensive system protecting the body from infection or foreign antigens is a fine-tuned network, but it is not perfect. Immunity is the protective responses to antigens expressed by disease causing agents. Inappropriate responses or hypersensitivity reactions may be (1) exaggerated against noninfectious environmental substances (allergy); (2) misdirected against the body's own cells (autoimmunity); (3) directed against beneficial foreign issues, such as transfusions or transplants (alloimmunity); or (4) insufficient to protect the host against pathogens and abnormal or foreign cells (immune deficiency). Several of these inappropriate responses can be serious or life-threatening. This chapter will describe the mechanisms of hypersensitivity reactions with examples of allergy, autoimmunity, and alloimmunity. This will be followed by a summary of immune deficiency diseases and acquired immune deficiency syndrome (AIDS) caused by human immunodeficiency virus (HIV).

HYPERSENSITIVITY REACTIONS

A hypersensitivity reaction is an altered immunologic response to an antigen that results in disease or damage to the individual. Hypersensitivity reactions can be classified in two ways: by the immunologic mechanism that causes disease (types I, II, II, and IV), and by the source of the antigen that the immune system is attacking (allergy, autoimmunity, and alloimmunity (also termed *isoimmunity*). The mechanism that initiates the onset of hypersensitivity reactions is not completely understood. It is generally accepted that genetic, infectious, and environmental agents are contributing factors.

    Hypersensitivity reactions can be characterized by the particular immune mechanism that results in the disease (Table 8.1). These mechanisms are apparent in most hypersensitivity reactions and have been divided into four distinct types: *type I* (IgE-mediated reactions), *type II* (tissue-specific reactions), *type III* (immune complex–mediated reactions), and *type IV* (cell-mediated reactions). This classification is an artificial one, and a particular disease is seldom associated with only a single mechanism. The four mechanisms are interrelated, and in most hypersensitivity reactions, several mechanisms can be functioning simultaneously or sequentially.

IMMUNOLOGIC MECHANISMS OF HYPERSENSITIVITY REACTIONS

As with all immune responses, hypersensitivity reactions require *sensitization* against a particular antigen that results in a primary immune response. This occurs when the immune system first encounters an antigen and forms antigen-specific memory B cells and T cells (immunologic memory). Disease symptoms appear after secondary exposure to the offending antigen when memory cells are rapidly activated against the same antigen (see Chapter 7). Hypersensitivity reactions are immediate or delayed, depending on the time required to elicit clinical symptoms after *reexposure* to the antigen. Reactions that occur within minutes to a few hours after exposure to antigen are termed **immediate hypersensitivity reactions**. **Delayed hypersensitivity reactions** may take several hours to appear and are at maximal severity days after reexposure to the antigen. Generally, immediate reactions are caused by antibody, whereas delayed reactions are caused by cells (e.g., T cells, natural killer [NK] cells, macrophages).

    The most rapid and severe immediate hypersensitivity reaction is **anaphylaxis**. Anaphylaxis occurs within minutes of reexposure to the antigen and can be either systemic (generalized) or cutaneous (localized). Symptoms of systemic anaphylaxis include pruritus, erythema, vomiting, abdominal cramps, diarrhea, and breathing difficulties, and the most severe reactions may include contraction of bronchial smooth muscle, edema of the throat, and decreased blood pressure that can lead to shock and death. Examples of systemic anaphylaxis are allergic reactions

TABLE 8.1 Immunologic Mechanisms of Hypersensitivity Reactions

Type	Name	Rate of Development	Class of Antibody Involved	Principal Effector Cells Involved	Participation of Complement	Examples of Disorders
I	Immunoglobulin E (IgE)–mediated reaction	Immediate	IgE	Mast cells	No	Seasonal allergic rhinitis Asthma
II	Tissue-specific reaction	Immediate	IgG IgM	NK cells, macrophages, neutrophils	Frequently	Autoimmune thrombocytopenic purpura, Graves disease, autoimmune hemolytic anemia
III	Immune complex–mediated reaction	Immediate	IgG IgM	Neutrophils	Yes	Systemic lupus erythematosus
IV	Cell-mediated reaction	Delayed	None	Lymphocytes Macrophages	No	Contact sensitivity to poison ivy, metals (jewelry), and latex

to bee stings, peanuts, shellfish, or eggs. Cutaneous anaphylaxis results in local symptoms related to inflammation, such as pain, swelling, and redness, which occur at the site of exposure to an antigen (e.g., a painful local reaction to an injected vaccine or drug).

Mechanisms of Hypersensitivity Reactions

Type I: IgE-Mediated Hypersensitivity Reactions

Type I hypersensitivity reactions are mediated by antigen-specific immunoglobulin E (IgE) and the products of tissue mast cells (Fig. 8.1). Most common allergic reactions are type I reactions against environmental antigens. Because of this strong association, many health care professionals use the term *allergy* to indicate only IgE-mediated reactions. However, IgE can contribute to some autoimmune and alloimmune diseases.

Mechanisms of type I, IgE-mediated hypersensitivity reactions. IgE has a relatively short life span in blood because it rapidly binds to Fc receptors (antibody receptors) on mast cells. The Fc receptors on mast cells specifically bind IgE that has not previously interacted with antigen. After a large amount of IgE has bound to the mast cells, an individual is considered *sensitized*. When there is a secondary or reexposure of a sensitized individual to the allergen, the IgE antibodies signal the mast cells to release mediators.

Histamine is the most potent preformed mediator of IgE-mediated hypersensitivity. Histamine acts immediately (within 15-30 minutes) and affects several key target cells. The tissues most commonly affected by type I responses contain large numbers of mast cells and are sensitive to the effects of histamine released from them. These tissues are found in the gastrointestinal tract, the skin, and the respiratory tract (Fig. 8.2 and Table 8.2). Acting through histamine 1 (H1) receptors, histamine contracts bronchial smooth muscles (bronchial constriction), increases vascular permeability (edema), and causes vasodilation (increased blood flow) (see Chapter 6 and Fig. 6.7). The interaction of histamine with H2 receptors results in increased gastric acid secretion.

Mast cells also synthesize secondary mediators, such as leukotrienes, prostaglandins, and platelet activating factor, which act more slowly (within hours) and have effects similar to that of histamine. These newly formed mediators also attract other immune cells (e.g., eosinophils, neutrophils, basophils, monocytes) and activate kinins and complement. These mediators are responsible for a late phase reaction that sets in 2 to 24 hours later even without additional exposure to antigen and may last for several days.

Gastrointestinal allergy is caused by allergens that enter through the mouth—usually foods or medicines—and results in increased fluid secretion and increased peristalsis. Symptoms include vomiting, diarrhea, or abdominal pain. Foods most often implicated in gastrointestinal allergies are milk, chocolate, citrus fruits, eggs, wheat, nuts, peanut butter, and fish (see *Did You Know? Peanut Allergy in Children*). The most common food allergy in adults is a reaction to shellfish, which may initiate an anaphylactic response and death. When food is the source of an allergen, the active immunogen may be an unidentifiable product of how the food is processed during manufacture or broken down by digestive enzymes. Sometimes the allergen is a drug, an additive, or a preservative in the food. For example, cows treated for mastitis with penicillin yield milk containing trace amounts of this antibiotic. Thus hypersensitivity apparently caused by milk proteins may, instead, be the result of an allergy to penicillin.

DID YOU KNOW?

Peanut Allergy in Children

Peanut allergy affects as many as 2% of children in the United States and is the leading cause of death related to food-induced anaphylaxis. For many years, parents were advised to avoid exposing infants to peanuts in an effort to reduce the likelihood of sensitization to peanut allergens. However, peanuts are contained in many processed foods and often contaminate food processing machines used to make other food products, so it is difficult for an individual to avoid accidental exposure. A study published in 2015 found that exposure to peanut butter in the first year of life creates tolerance to peanut allergens, resulting in a 70% reduction in the risk for later peanut allergy. Later studies demonstrated that mothers who consumed peanuts while breast feeding and then introduced peanuts into their infant's diets during the first year of life further reduced the risk of future allergy. It is postulated that peanut antigens are delivered to the infant along with maternal immunoglobulins and immune cells, cytokines, and microbiota, which prime the infant immune system to develop tolerance. Guidelines published in 2017 recommend that infants 4 to 6 months of age should be given age-appropriate peanut-containing foods (along with other solid foods). In high-risk children (history of severe eczema or egg allergy) peanuts should be administered only after testing for peanut-specific IgE levels or performing skin-prick tests with peanut allergen. If strong sensitivity to peanuts is found on these tests, peanut exposure should occur under supervision of a specialist.

Data from Bunyavanich S et al: *J Allergy Clin Immunol* 134:753–755, 2014; Du Toit G et al: *N Engl J Med* 372:803–813, 2015; Du Toit G et al: *N Engl J Med* 374:1435–1443, 2016; Togias A et al: *Ann Allergy Asthma Immunol* 118:166–173, 2017.

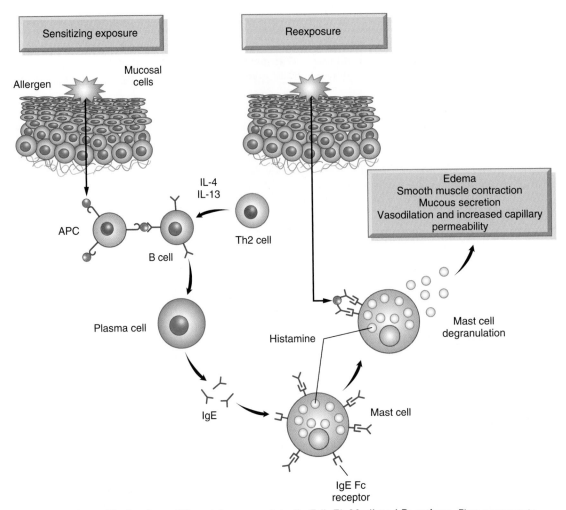

FIGURE 8.1 Mechanism of Type I, Immunoglobulin E (IgE)–Mediated Reactions. First exposure to an allergen leads to antigen processing and presentation of antigen by an antigen-presenting cell (APC) to B lymphocytes, which is under the direction of T-helper 2 (Th2) cells. Th2 cells produce specific cytokines (e.g., interleukin 4 [IL-4], IL-13, and others) that favor maturation of the B lymphocytes into plasma cells that secrete IgE. The IgE is adsorbed to the surface of the mast cell by binding with IgE-specific Fc receptors. When an adequate amount of IgE is bound, the mast cell is sensitized. During a reexposure, the allergen cross-links the surface-bound IgE and causes degranulation of the mast cell. Contents of the mast cell granules, primarily histamine, induce local edema, smooth muscle contraction, mucous secretion, and other characteristics of an acute inflammatory reaction. (See Chapter 6 for more details on the role of mast cells in inflammation.)

Urticaria, or **hives,** is a dermal (skin) manifestation of allergic reactions (see Fig. 8.2). The underlying mechanism is the localized release of histamine and increased vascular permeability, resulting in limited areas of edema. Urticaria is characterized by white fluid-filled blisters (wheals) surrounded by areas of redness (flares). This **wheal and flare reaction** is usually accompanied by pruritus. Not all urticarial symptoms are caused by immunologic reactions. Some, termed *nonimmunologic urticaria,* result from exposure to cold temperatures, emotional stress, medications, systemic diseases, or malignancies (e.g., lymphomas).

Effects of allergens on the mucosa of the eyes, nose, and respiratory tract include conjunctivitis (inflammation of the membranes lining the eyelids) (see Fig. 8.2), rhinitis (inflammation of the mucous membranes of the nose), and asthma (constriction of the bronchi). Symptoms are caused by vasodilation, hypersecretion of mucus, edema, and swelling of the respiratory mucosa. Because the mucous membranes lining the respiratory tract are continuous, they are all adversely affected. The degree to which each is affected determines the symptoms of the disease.

One of the most common type I reactions is asthma. It is presented in detail in Chapters 29 and 30. The central problem in allergic diseases

of the lung is obstruction of the large and small airways (bronchi) of the lower respiratory tract by bronchospasm (constriction of smooth muscle in airway walls), edema, and thick secretions. This leads to ventilatory insufficiency, wheezing, and difficult or labored breathing.

Certain individuals are genetically predisposed to develop allergies and are described as being **atopic.** In families in which one parent has an allergy, allergies develop in about 40% of the offspring. If both parents have allergies, the incidence may be as high as 80%. Atopic individuals tend to produce higher quantities of IgE and have more Fc receptors for IgE on their mast cells. The airways and the skin of atopic individuals have increased responsiveness to a wide variety of both specific and nonspecific stimuli.

Evaluation and treatment of IgE hypersensitivity. Allergic reactions can be life-threatening; therefore it is essential that individuals with severe allergies be informed of the specific allergen against which they are sensitized and instructed to avoid contact with that material. Several tests are available to evaluate individuals with allergies. These include food challenges, skin tests with allergens, and laboratory tests for total IgE and allergen-specific IgE. Treatment can include the use

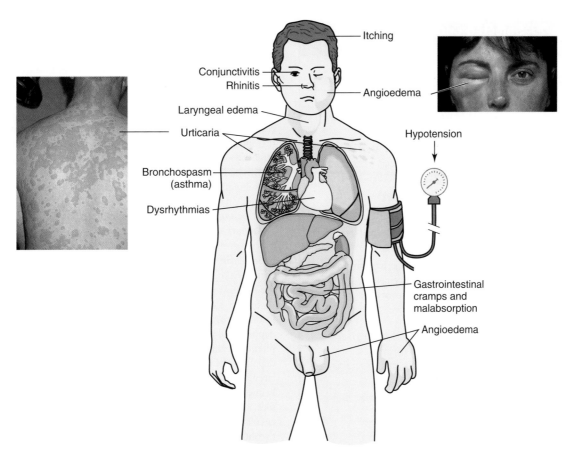

FIGURE 8.2 Type I Hypersensitivity Reactions. Manifestations of allergic reactions as a result of type I hypersensitivity include pruritus, angioedema (swelling caused by exudation), edema of the larynx, urticaria (hives), bronchospasm (constriction of airways in the lungs), hypotension (low blood pressure), and dysrhythmias (irregular heartbeat) because of anaphylactic shock, and gastrointestinal cramping caused by inflammation of the gastrointestinal mucosa. Photographic inserts show a diffuse allergy-like eye and skin reaction on an individual. The skin lesions have raised edges and develop within minutes or hours, with resolution occurring after about 12 hours. (Inserts from Male D et al: *Immunology*, ed 8, St Louis, 2013, Mosby.)

of antihistamines or other drugs that block the action of synthesized mediators involved in the type I reaction (e.g., corticosteroids, leukotriene receptor inhibitor, platelet activating receptor inhibitor).

Type II: Tissue-Specific Hypersensitivity Reactions

Type II hypersensitivities are generally immune reactions against a specific cell or tissue. Cells express a variety of antigens on their surfaces, some of which are called tissue-specific antigens because they are expressed on the plasma membranes of only certain cells. Platelets, for example, have groups of antigens that are found on no other cells of the body. The symptoms of many type II diseases are determined by which tissue or organ expresses the particular antigen. Environmental antigens (e.g., drugs or their metabolites) may bind to the plasma membranes of specific cells (especially erythrocytes and platelets) and function as targets of type II reactions. The five general mechanisms by which type II hypersensitivity reactions can affect cells are shown in Fig. 8.3. Each mechanism begins with antibody binding to tissue-specific antigens or antigens present on particular tissues.

Mechanisms of type II, tissue-specific reactions. The cell may be destroyed by antibody and complement (see Fig. 8.3, *A*). Antibodies (IgM or IgG) react with an antigen on the surface of the cell, causing activation of the complement cascade through the classical pathway (see Fig. 6.3). Formation of the membrane attack complex (C5-9)

damages the membrane and may result in lysis of the cell. For example, erythrocytes are destroyed by complement-mediated lysis in individuals with autoimmune hemolytic anemia (see Chapters 23 and 24) or as a result of an alloimmune reaction to mismatched transfused blood cells (see the section on Alloimmunity).

Antibody may cause cell destruction through phagocytosis by macrophages (see Fig. 8.3, *B*). Antibodies may additionally activate complement, resulting in the deposition of C3b on the cell surface. Receptors on the macrophage recognize and bind these opsonins (antibody and C3b) and increase phagocytosis of the target cell. For example, antibodies against platelet-specific antigens or against red blood cell antigens of the Rh system cause their removal by phagocytosis in the spleen.

Toxic products produced by neutrophils may cause tissue damage (see Fig. 8.3, *C*). Soluble antigens, such as medications, molecules released from infectious agents, or molecules released from an individual's own cells, may enter the circulation. In some instances, the antigens are deposited on the surface of tissues, where they are bound by antibodies. These antibodies may activate complement, resulting in the release of C3a and C5a, which are chemotactic for neutrophils, and the deposition of complement component C3b. Neutrophils are attracted, bind to the tissues through receptors for the Fc portion of antibody (Fc receptor) or for C3b, and release their granules onto the healthy tissue. The components of neutrophil granules, as well as the toxic oxygen products produced by these cells, will damage the tissue contributing

TABLE 8.2   Selected Causes of Clinical Allergic Reactions

Typical Allergen	Mechanism of Hypersensitivity	Clinical Manifestation
Ingestants		
Foods	Type I	Gastrointestinal allergy, anaphylaxis
Drugs	Types I, II, III	Urticaria, anaphylaxis, immediate drug reaction, hemolytic anemia, serum sickness
Inhalants		
Pollens, dust, molds	Type I	Allergic rhinitis, bronchial asthma
Fungi	Types I, III, IV	Allergic bronchopulmonary aspergillosis, extrinsic allergic alveolitis
Injectants		
Drugs	Types I, II, III	Immediate drug reaction, anaphylaxis hemolytic anemia, serum sickness
Bee venom	Type I	Anaphylaxis
Vaccines	Type III	Localized Arthus reaction
Serum	Types I, III	Anaphylaxis, serum sickness
Contactants		
Poison ivy, metals	Type IV	Contact dermatitis
Latex	Type I, IV	Contact dermatitis, anaphylaxis

Modified from Bellanti JA: *Immunology III*, Philadelphia, 1985, Saunders.

to complication such as acute respiratory distress syndrome, sepsis, and multiple organ failure.

Antibody-dependent cell-mediated cytotoxicity (ADCC) involves NK cells (see Fig. 8.3, *D*) or phagocytes. Antibodies on the target cell are recognized by Fc receptors on NK cells, macrophages or neutrophils, which release toxic substances that destroy the target cell. Examples include acute transplant rejection and immune reactions against neoplasms.

The last mechanism does not destroy the target cell but rather *causes the cell to malfunction* (see Fig. 8.3, *E*). The antibodies are directed against specific cell surface receptors. They change the function of the receptor by blocking, appropriately stimulating, or destroying the receptor. For example, in the hyperthyroidism (excessive thyroid activity) of Graves disease, autoantibodies bind to and activate receptors for thyroid-stimulating hormone (TSH) (a pituitary hormone that controls the production of the hormone thyroxine [T_4] by the thyroid). In this way, the antibody stimulates the thyroid cells to abnormally produce thyroxine (see Chapter 20).

Type III: Immune Complex–Mediated Hypersensitivity Reactions

Most type III hypersensitivity disease reactions are caused by antigen–antibody (immune) complexes that are formed in the circulation and are deposited in vessel walls or other tissues (Fig. 8.4).

The primary difference between type II and type III mechanisms is that in type II hypersensitivity, antibody binds to antigen on the cell surface, whereas in type III, antibody binds to soluble antigen that was released into blood or body fluids. The immune complex is then deposited in the tissues. Type III reactions are not organ specific and most commonly result in a vasculitis in the skin, kidney, or lungs. The harmful effects of immune complex deposition are caused by complement activation and by neutrophils attempting to phagocytose the immune complexes. During the attempted phagocytosis, large quantities of lysosomal enzymes are released into the inflammatory site instead of into phagolysosomes. The attraction of neutrophils and the subsequent release of lysosomal enzymes cause most of the resulting tissue damage.

Mechanisms of type III, immune-mediated hypersensitivity reactions

Immune complex disease. Two prototypic models of type III hypersensitivity help explain the variety of diseases in this category. Serum sickness is a model of systemic type III hypersensitivities, and the Arthus reaction is a model of localized or cutaneous reactions.

Serum sickness–type reactions are caused by the formation of immune complexes in the blood and their subsequent generalized deposition in target tissues. A form of serum sickness is Raynaud phenomenon, a condition caused by the temperature-dependent deposition of immune complexes in the capillary beds of the peripheral circulation. Certain immune complexes precipitate at temperatures below normal body temperature, particularly in the tips of the fingers, toes, and nose, and are called cryoglobulins. The precipitates block the circulation and cause localized pallor and numbness, followed by cyanosis (a bluish tinge resulting from oxygen deprivation) and eventually gangrene if the circulation is not restored.

Arthus reaction is vasculitis caused by repeated local exposure to an antigen that reacts with preformed antibody and forms immune complexes in the walls of the local blood vessels. Symptoms of Arthus reaction begin within 1 hour of exposure and peak 6 to 12 hours later. The lesions are characterized by a typical inflammatory reaction, with increased vascular permeability, an accumulation of neutrophils, edema, hemorrhage, clotting, and tissue damage. For example, gluten-sensitive enteropathy (celiac disease), follows ingestion of antigen, usually gluten from wheat products (see Chapter 39). Allergic alveolitis (farmer lung disease, pigeon breeder disease) is Arthus-like acute hemorrhagic inflammation of the air sacs (alveoli) of the lungs, resulting from inhalation of fungal antigens, usually particles from moldy hay or pigeon feces (see Chapter 29).

Type IV: Cell-Mediated Hypersensitivity Reactions

Types I, II, and III hypersensitivity reactions are mediated by antibodies, whereas type IV hypersensitivity reactions are mediated by T lymphocytes and do not involve antibodies (Fig. 8.5). Type IV mechanisms occur through either cytotoxic T lymphocytes (Tc cells) or T-helper cells (Th cells) producing Th1 and Th17 cytokines (see Chapter 7). Tc cells attack and destroy cellular targets directly. Th1 and Th17 cytokines recruit and activate phagocytic cells, especially macrophages. Destruction of the tissue is usually caused by direct killing by Tc cells or the release of soluble factors, such as lysosomal enzymes and toxic reactive oxygen species from activated macrophages. The response is delayed, occurring 24 to 72 hours after antigen reexposure, compared with an immediate type I reaction, which occurs within minutes. The response is delayed because of the time it takes for sensitized T cells to travel to the site of antigen reexposure and the time needed to produce cytokines that activate other cells including macrophages.

Mechanisms of type IV cell-mediated hypersensitivity reactions. Clinical examples of type IV hypersensitivity reactions include

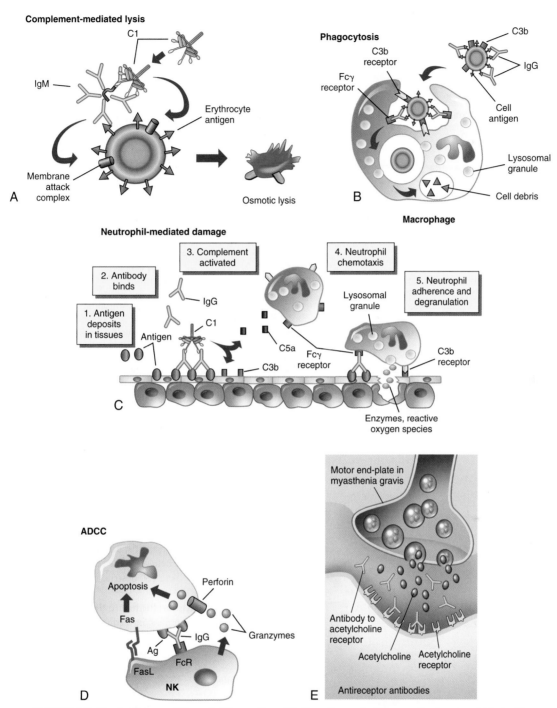

FIGURE 8.3 Mechanisms of Type II, Tissue-Specific Reactions. Antigens on the target cell bind with antibody and are destroyed or prevented from functioning by one of the following mechanisms: **A,** Complement-mediated lysis (an erythrocyte target is illustrated here). **B,** Clearance (phagocytosis) by macrophages in the tissue. **C,** Neutrophil-mediated immune destruction. **D,** Antibody-dependent cell-mediated cytotoxicity (ADCC) (apoptosis of target cells is induced by natural killer [NK] cells by two mechanisms: by the release of granzymes and perforin, which is a molecule that creates pores in the plasma membrane, and enzymes [granzymes] that enter the target through the perforin pores; and by the interactions of Fas ligand [FasL; a molecule similar to tumor necrosis factor-alpha (TNF-α)] on the surface of NK cells with Fas [the receptor for FasL] on the surface of target cells). **E,** Or modulation or blocking of the normal function of receptors by antireceptor antibody. This example of mechanism **(E)** depicts myasthenia gravis in which acetylcholine receptor antibodies block acetylcholine from attaching to its receptors on the motor end plates of skeletal muscle, thereby impairing neuromuscular transmission and causing muscle weakness. *C1,* Complement component C1; *C3b,* complement fragment produced from C3, which acts as an opsonin; *C5a,* complement fragment produced from C5, which acts as a chemotactic factor for neutrophils; *Fcγ receptor,* cellular receptor for the Fc portion of IgG; *FcR,* Fc receptor.

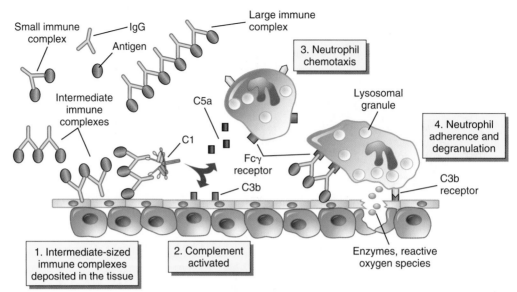

FIGURE 8.4 Mechanism of Type III, Immune Complex–Mediated Reactions. Immune complexes form in the blood from circulating antigen and antibody. Both small and large immune complexes are removed successfully from the circulation and do not cause tissue damage. Intermediate-sized complexes are deposited in certain target tissues in which the circulation is slow or filtration of blood occurs. The complexes activate the complement cascade through C1 and generate fragments, including C5a and C3b. C5a is chemotactic for neutrophils, which migrate into the inflamed area and attach to the IgG and C3b in the immune complexes. The neutrophils attempt unsuccessfully to phagocytose the tissue and in the process release a variety of degradative enzymes that destroy the healthy tissues. Fcγ receptor is the cellular receptor for the Fc portion of immunoglobulin G (IgG).

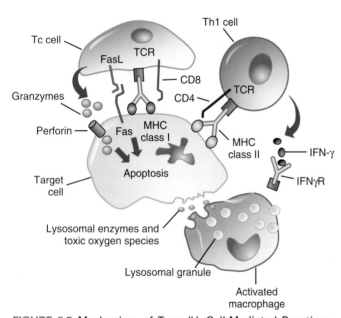

FIGURE 8.5 Mechanism of Type IV, Cell-Mediated Reactions. Antigens from target cells stimulate T cells to differentiate into T-cytotoxic cells *(Tc cells)*, which have direct cytotoxic activity, and T-helper cells *(Th1 cells)* involved in delayed hypersensitivity. The Th1 cells produce lymphokines (especially interferon-γ [*IFN-γ*]) that activate the macrophage through specific receptors (e.g., IFN-γ receptor [*IFNγR*]). The macrophages can attach to targets and release enzymes and reactive oxygen species that are responsible for most of the tissue destruction.

graft rejection, reaction on the skin test for tuberculosis, and allergic reactions resulting from skin contact with some substances, such as poison ivy and metals. A type IV component also may be present in many autoimmune diseases. For example, T cells against type II collagen (a protein present in joint tissues) contribute to the destruction of joints in rheumatoid arthritis, and T cells against an antigen on the surface of pancreatic beta cells (the cell that normally produces insulin) are responsible for beta-cell destruction in insulin-dependent (type 1) diabetes mellitus.

In 1891, Ehrlich was the first to thoroughly describe type IV hypersensitivity reaction in the skin, leading to the development of a diagnostic skin test for tuberculosis. The reaction follows an intradermal injection of tuberculin antigen into an individual who has latent or active tuberculosis and is therefore sensitized (has developed adaptive immune cells against tuberculosis antigen). This test is called a delayed hypersensitivity skin test because of its slow onset—24 to 72 hours to reach maximal intensity. The reaction site is infiltrated with T lymphocytes and macrophages, resulting in a clear hard center (induration) and a reddish surrounding area (erythema). The reaction is referred to as a positive skin test result for tuberculosis infection.

Allergic type IV reactions are elicited by some environmental antigens that are haptens and become immunogenic after binding to larger (carrier) proteins in the individual (see Chapter 7). In allergic contact dermatitis, the carrier protein is in the skin. The best-known example is the reaction to poison ivy (Fig. 8.6). The antigen is a plant catechol, urushiol, which reacts with normal skin proteins and evokes a cell-mediated immune response. Skin reactions to industrial chemicals, cosmetics, detergents, clothing, food, metals, and topical medicines (such as penicillin) are elicited by the same mechanism. Contact dermatitis consists of lesions only at the site of contact with the allergen, as in metal allergy to jewelry.

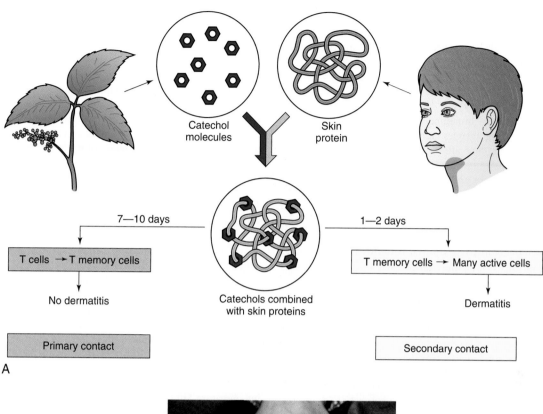

Catechol molecules

Skin protein

7—10 days

1—2 days

| T cells → T memory cells |

| T memory cells → Many active cells |

No dermatitis

Catechols combined with skin proteins

Dermatitis

Primary contact

Secondary contact

A

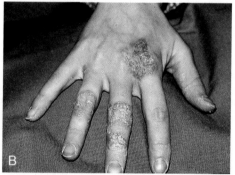

B

FIGURE 8.6 Development of Allergic Contact Dermatitis. A, The development of type IV hypersensitivity to poison ivy. The first (primary) contact with allergen sensitizes (produces reactive T cells) the individual but does not produce a rash (dermatitis). Secondary contact activates a type IV cell-mediated reaction that causes dermatitis. **B,** Contact dermatitis caused by a delayed hypersensitivity reaction leading to vesicles and scaling at the sites of contact. (From Damjanov I, Linder J: *Anderson's pathology*, ed 10, St Louis, 1996, Mosby.)

Developments of allergic contact dermatitis

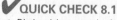

> **QUICK CHECK 8.1**
> 1. Distinguish among the four types of hypersensitivity mechanisms.
> 2. What is the mechanism of anaphylaxis?
> 3. What are some clinical examples of type IV hypersensitivity?

Allergy

Allergy (atopy) refers to hypersensitivity to environmental antigens. These can include medicines, natural products (e.g., pollens, bee stings), infectious agents, and any other antigen that is not naturally found in the individual. Allergies are the most common hypersensitivity reactions. The majority of allergies are type I reactions that lead to annoying symptoms, including rhinitis, sneezing, and other relatively mild reactions. In some individuals, however, these reactions can be excessive and life-threatening (anaphylaxis). Antigens that cause allergic responses are called allergens. It is not known why some antigens are allergens and others are not. Typical allergens include pollens (e.g., ragweed), molds and fungi (e.g., *Penicillium chrysogenum*), foods (e.g., milk, eggs, fish), animals (e.g., cat dander, dog dander), cigarette smoke, and components of house dust (e.g., fecal pellets of house mites).

Allergic Disease: Bee Sting Allergy

Bee venoms contain a mixture of enzymes and other proteins that may serve as allergens and cause a type I hypersensitivity reaction. About 1% of children may have an anaphylactic reaction to bee venom. Within minutes, they may develop excessive swelling (edema) at the bee sting site, followed by generalized hives, pruritus, and swelling in areas distal from the sting (e.g., eyes, lips), and other systemic symptoms, including flushing, sweating, dizziness, and headache. The most severe symptoms may include gastrointestinal (e.g., stomach cramps, vomiting), respiratory (e.g., tightness in the throat, wheezing, difficulty breathing), and vascular (e.g., low blood pressure, shock) reactions. Severe respiratory tract and vascular reactions may lead to death.

For an individual with known bee sting hypersensitivity, lifestyle changes include avoidance of stinging or biting insects. If a child has experienced a previous anaphylactic reaction, the chance of having another is about 60%. The primary life-threatening symptoms result from contraction of respiratory tract smooth muscle as a result of the effects of mast cell–derived histamine and leukotrienes. Thus most individuals with bee sting allergies carry self-injectable epinephrine (EpiPen), which reverses these effects causing bronchodilation. The administration of antihistamines has little effect because histamine has already bound H1 receptors and initiated severe bronchial smooth muscle contraction.

Clinical desensitization to allergens can be achieved in some individuals. Minute quantities of the allergen are injected in increasing doses over a prolonged period. The procedure may reduce the severity of the allergic reaction in the treated individual. However, this form of therapy may trigger systemic anaphylaxis, which can be severe and life-threatening. This approach works best for routine respiratory tract allergens and biting insect allergies. Food allergies have been very difficult to suppress, but some promising trials are underway to evaluate desensitization by oral or sublingual administration of increasing amounts of allergen.

Autoimmunity

Autoimmunity is a disturbance in the immunologic tolerance of *self-antigens*. The immune system normally does not strongly recognize the individual's own antigens. Healthy individuals of all ages may produce low quantities of antibodies against their own antigens *(autoantibodies)* without developing overt autoimmune disease. Therefore the presence of low quantities of autoantibodies does not necessarily indicate a disease state. Autoimmune diseases occur when the immune system reacts against self-antigens to such a degree that autoantibodies or autoreactive T cells damage the individual's tissues. Many clinical disorders are associated with autoimmunity and are collectively referred to as autoimmune diseases. Table 8.3 presents a review of autoimmune diseases.

Examples of Autoimmune Diseases

Autoimmune diseases originate from an initiating event in a genetic predisposed individual. Most often, the initiating event is unrecognized but is hypothesized to be an environmental factor or some change in neurologic, endocrine, and/or immune status. Although most autoimmune diseases appear as isolated events without a positive family history, susceptibility for developing such diseases appears to be linked to a combination of multiple genes. Some autoimmune diseases can be familial and attributed to the presence of a very small number of susceptibility genes; affected family members may not all develop the same disease but have different disorders characterized by a variety of hypersensitivity reactions. Autoimmune diseases are more common among women.

Breakdown of Tolerance

An individual is usually tolerant to his or her own antigens. Tolerance is a state of immunologic control so that the individual does not make a detrimental immune response against his or her own cells and tissues. Autoimmune disease results from a breakdown of this tolerance.

The initiating event that breaks tolerance is unclear for most autoimmune diseases. Potential infectious initiators of autoimmune disease are implicated for many autoimmune disorders, including type 1 diabetes, multiple sclerosis, and rheumatoid arthritis. One example of documented infection-related autoimmunity is acute rheumatic fever. In a small number of individuals with group A streptococcal sore throat, the M proteins in the bacterial capsule mimic *(antigenic mimicry)* normal heart antigens and induce antibodies that also react with proteins in the heart valve, causing inflammation and damaging the valve. The joints (migratory polyarthritis), skin (erythema and nodules), and nervous system (chorea) also can be affected. Thus acute rheumatic fever is a type II autoimmune hypersensitivity. Additionally, some streptococcal skin or throat infections release bacterial antigens into the blood that form circulating immune complexes. The complexes may deposit in the kidneys and initiate an immune complex–mediated glomerulonephritis (inflammation of the kidney). Thus streptococcal antigens (an environmental antigen) may also cause a type III allergic hypersensitivity (poststreptococcal glomerulonephritis) (see Chapter 33).

Autoimmune Disease: Systemic Lupus Erythematosus

Systemic lupus erythematosus (SLE) is the most common, complex, and serious of the autoimmune disorders. SLE is characterized by the production of a large variety of antibodies (autoantibodies) against self-antigens, including nucleic acids, erythrocytes, coagulation proteins, phospholipids, lymphocytes, platelets, and many other self-components. The most characteristic autoantibodies are against nucleic acids (e.g., single-stranded deoxyribonucleic acid [ssDNA], double-stranded DNA [dsDNS]), histones, ribonucleoproteins, and other nuclear materials. The blood normally contains many of these products of cellular turnover and breakdown so that autoantibodies react with the circulating antigen and form circulating immune complexes. The deposition of circulating DNA/anti-DNA complexes in the kidneys can cause severe kidney inflammation. Similar reactions can occur in other systems, such as the brain, heart, spleen, lung, gastrointestinal tract, peritoneum, and skin. Thus some of the symptoms of SLE result from a type III hypersensitivity reaction. Other symptoms are related to type II hypersensitivity reactions and include destruction of red blood cells (anemia), lymphocytes (lymphopenia), and platelets (thrombocytopenia).

SLE, like most autoimmune diseases, occurs more often in women (approximately a 9:1 predominance of females), especially in the 20- to 40-year-old age group. Blacks are affected more often compared with whites (about an eightfold increased risk). A genetic predisposition for the disease has been implicated on the basis of increased incidence in twins and the existence of autoimmune disease in the families of individuals with SLE.

As with many autoimmune diseases, clinical manifestations of SLE may wax and wane; the individual may go through periods of remission and be relatively disease free until the onset of a *flare* (exacerbated disease activity). Symptoms include arthralgias or arthritis (90% of individuals), vasculitis, and rash (70%–80% of individuals) (see the section Discoid Lupus Erythematosus in Chapter 43), renal disease (40%–50% of individuals), hematologic abnormalities (50% of individuals, with anemia being the most common complication), and cardiovascular diseases (30%–50% of individuals). Because the signs and symptoms affect almost every body system and tend to vacillate, SLE can be difficult to diagnose. This has led to the development of a list of common clinical findings, such as rash, photosensitivity, arthritis, serositis, renal dysfunction, neurologic disorders, and hematologic manifestations, which, when they occur together, are highly suggestive of SLE. The presence of antinuclear antibodies further supports the diagnosis.

Laboratory diagnosis is usually based on a positive antinuclear antibody (ANA) screening test; about 98% of individuals with SLE are positive, but a substantial number of false-positive results occur in healthy individuals and those with other diseases. Because SLE is a progressive and slowly developing disease, some laboratory tests, including the ANA test, may yield positive results years before the onset of clinical symptoms. Detection of ANAs is usually followed by one or more specific

TABLE 8.3 Examples of Autoimmune Diseases

System Disease	Organ or Tissue	Probable Self-Antigen
Endocrine System		
Hyperthyroidism (Graves disease)	Thyroid gland	Receptors for thyroid-stimulating hormone
Hashimoto hypothyroidism	Thyroid gland	Thyroid cell surface antigens, thyroglobulin
Insulin-dependent diabetes	Pancreas	Islet cells, insulin, insulin receptors on pancreatic cells
Addison disease	Adrenal gland	Surface antigens on steroid-producing cells; microsomal antigens
Male infertility	Testis	Surface antigens on spermatozoa
Skin		
Pemphigus vulgaris	Skin	Intercellular substances in stratified squamous epithelium
Bullous pemphigoid	Skin	Basement membrane
Vitiligo	Skin	Surface antigens on melanocytes (melanin-producing cells)
Neuromuscular Tissue		
Multiple sclerosis	Neural tissue	Surface antigens of nerve cells
Myasthenia gravis	Neuromuscular junction	Acetylcholine receptors; striations of skeletal and cardiac muscle
Rheumatic heart disease	Heart	Cardiac tissue antigens that cross-react with group A streptococcal antigen
Cardiomyopathy	Heart	Cardiac muscle
Gastrointestinal System		
Ulcerative colitis	Colon	Mucosal cells
Pernicious anemia	Stomach	Surface antigens of parietal cells; intrinsic factor
Primary biliary cirrhosis	Liver	Cells of bile duct
Chronic active hepatitis	Liver	Surface antigens of hepatocytes, nuclei, microsomes, smooth muscle
Eye		
Sjögren syndrome	Lacrimal gland	Antigens of lacrimal gland, salivary gland, thyroid, and nuclei of cells
Connective Tissue		
Ankylosing spondylitis	Joints	Sacroiliac and spinal apophyseal joint
Rheumatoid arthritis	Joints	Collagen, immunoglobulin G (IgG)
Systemic lupus erythematosus	Multiple sites	Numerous antigens in nuclei, organelles, and extracellular matrix
Renal System		
Immune complex glomerulonephritis	Kidney	Numerous immune complexes deposited in glomerular vessels
Goodpasture syndrome	Kidney	Glomerular basement membrane
Hematologic System		
Idiopathic neutropenia	Neutrophil	Surface antigens on polymorphonuclear neutrophils
Idiopathic lymphopenia	Lymphocytes	Surface antigens on lymphocytes
Autoimmune hemolytic anemia	Erythrocytes	Surface antigens on erythrocytes
Autoimmune thrombocytopenic purpura	Platelets	Surface antigens on platelets
Respiratory System		
Goodpasture syndrome	Lung	Septal membrane of alveolus

tests (e.g., antibodies against Smith antigen [Sm], and dsDNA). Further diagnostic testing may be indicated for specific clinical findings, such as renal or joint disorders.

There is no cure for SLE or most other autoimmune diseases. Fatalities resulting from SLE are usually related to infection, organ failure, or cardiovascular disease. The goals of treatment are to control symptoms and prevent further damage by suppressing the autoimmune response. Nonsteroidal antiinflammatory drugs (NSAIDs), such as aspirin, ibuprofen, or naproxen, reduce inflammation and relieve pain. Corticosteroids are often prescribed for more serious active disease. Immunosuppressive drugs (e.g., methotrexate, azathioprine, or mycophenolate mofetil) are used to treat severe symptoms involving internal organs and new drugs are under investigation. Antimalarial medications (e.g., hydroxychloroquine) are preferred treatments for individuals with stable disease. Ultraviolet light may initiate flares and protection from sun exposure is helpful. Prolonged use of certain drugs can cause transient SLE-like symptoms, and the medication history is important for differential diagnosis.[1]

Alloimmunity

Alloimmunity (isoimmunity) occurs when the immune system of one individual produces an immunologic reaction against tissues of another individual. Alloimmunity can be observed during immunologic reactions against blood transfusions, transplanted tissue, or the fetus during pregnancy. Alloantigens (isoantigens) are nonself antigens from members of the same species. Two types of alloantigen are blood group antigens and histocompatibility antigens (e.g., human leucocyte antigen [HLA]).

Genetic diversity is observed among self-antigens so that two individuals have different antigens on their tissues and therefore make an immune response against each other's tissues. Some self-antigens, such as the ABO blood group, have limited diversity with very few different antigens being expressed in the population, whereas others, such as the HLA system, have tremendous diversity.

Alloimmune Disease: Transfusion Reactions

Red blood cells (erythrocytes) express several important surface antigens, which are known collectively as the blood group antigens and can be targets of alloimmune reactions. More than 80 different red blood cell antigens are grouped into several dozen blood group systems. The most important of these, because they provoke the strongest humoral alloimmune response, are the ABO and Rh systems.

The ABO blood group consists of two major carbohydrate antigens, labeled A and B (Fig. 8.7), that are expressed on virtually all cells. These are codominant so that both A and B can be simultaneously expressed, resulting in an individual having any one of four different blood types. The erythrocytes of blood type A express the type A carbohydrate antigen, those with blood type B express the B antigen, those with blood type AB express both A and B antigens on the same cell, and those of blood type O express neither the A nor the B antigen. A person with type A blood also has circulating antibodies to the B carbohydrate antigen. If

this person receives blood from a type AB or B individual, a severe transfusion reaction occurs, and the transfused erythrocytes are destroyed by agglutination or complement-mediated lysis. Similarly, a type B individual (whose blood contains anti-A antibodies) cannot receive blood from a type A or AB donor. Type O individuals, who have neither antigen but have both anti-A and anti-B antibodies, cannot accept blood from any of the other three types. These naturally occurring antibodies, called isohemagglutinins, are IgM antibodies developed early in life because of the presence of similar antigens expressed on naturally occurring bacteria in the intestinal tract.

ABO blood types. Harmful transfusion reactions can be prevented by complete and careful ABO matching between donor and recipient. Because individuals with type O blood lack both types of antigens, they are considered universal donors—that is, anyone can accept their red blood cells. Similarly, type AB individuals are considered universal recipients because they lack both anti-A and anti-B antibodies and can be transfused with any ABO blood type.

The Rh blood group is a group of antigens also expressed on red blood cells. This is the most diverse group of red blood cell antigens, consisting of at least 45 separate antigens, although only one is considered of major importance: the D antigen. Individuals who express the D antigen on their red blood cells are Rh positive, whereas individuals who do not express the D antigen are Rh negative. About 85% of North Americans are Rh positive. Rh-negative individuals can make an IgG antibody to the D antigen (anti-D) if exposed to Rh-positive erythrocytes.

A disease called *hemolytic disease of the newborn* was most commonly caused by IgG anti-D alloantibody produced by Rh-negative mothers against erythrocytes of their Rh-positive fetuses (see Chapter 24). The

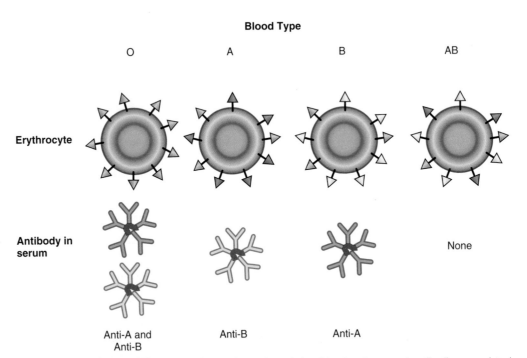

FIGURE 8.7 ABO Blood Types. This figure shows the relationship of antigens and antibodies associated with the ABO blood groups. The surfaces of erythrocytes of individuals with blood group O have a core carbohydrate that is present on cells of all ABO blood groups (H antigen). The sera of blood group O individuals contain IgM antibodies against both A and B carbohydrates. In individuals of the blood group A, some of the H antigens have been modified into A antigens. The sera of these individuals have IgM antibodies against the B antigen. In individuals with blood group B, some of the H antigens have been modified into B antigens. These individuals have IgM antibodies against the A antigen in their sera. In individuals of the blood group AB, some of the H antigens have been modified into both the A and B antigens. These individuals do not have antibody to either A or B antigens.

mother's antibody crossed the placenta and destroyed the red blood cells of the fetus. The occurrence of this particular form of the disease has decreased dramatically because of the use of prophylactic anti-D immunoglobulin (i.e., RhoGAM). Administration of anti-D antibody within a few days of exposure to RhD-positive erythrocytes prevents sensitization against the D antigen. Because hemolytic disease of the newborn related to the D antigen has been controlled, alloantibodies against the other Rh antigens have become more important. In general, these alloantibodies are associated with a less severe hemolytic disease.

Alloimmune Disease: Transplant Rejection

Molecules of the major histocompatibility complex (MHC) were discussed in Chapter 7 as antigen-presenting molecules (see Fig. 7.5). MHC molecules are also a major target of transplant rejection. As a result of studies on transplantation, the human MHC molecules are also referred to as human leukocyte antigens (HLAs). The different MHC genetic loci are identified as class I: HLA-A, HLA-B, and HLA-C, and class 2: HLA-DR, HLA-DQ, and HLA-DP (Fig. 8.8). The class I (HLA-A, -B, and -C) and class II MHC loci (HLA-DR, -DQ, and -DP) are the most genetically diverse (polymorphic) of any human genetic loci. Additional genes encoding complement components (e.g., C4, factor B) are also contained in the MHC region and are referred to as *class III loci*. Within the human population, the number of possible different alleles (i.e., forms of the gene) expressed by each locus is astounding. For example, > 300 different HLA-A molecules are expressed in the population.

Human leukocyte antigens (HLAs). Clearly, not every allele is expressed in the same individual. Humans have two copies of each MHC locus (one inherited from each parent) that are codominant so that molecules encoded by each parent's genes are expressed on the surface of every cell, except erythrocytes (Fig. 8.9). The tremendous number of possible alleles that can be expressed throughout the population makes it highly unlikely that any two unrelated individuals will have the same MHC antigens.

Inheritance of HLA. The diversity of MHC molecules becomes clinically relevant during organ transplantation. The recipient of a transplant can mount an immune response against the foreign HLA antigens on the donor tissue, resulting in rejection. To minimize the chance of tissue rejection, the donor and recipient are often tissue-typed beforehand to identify differences in HLA antigens. It is highly unlikely that a perfect match can be found between someone who needs a transplant and a potential donor from the general population, but the more similar the two individuals are in their HLA tissue type, the more

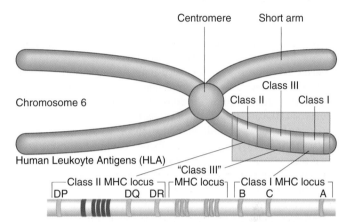

FIGURE 8.8 Human Leukocyte Antigens (HLAs). The major histocompatibility complex *(MHC)* is located on the short arm of chromosome 6 and contains genes (genetic loci) that code for class I antigens (found mostly on nucleated cells), class II antigens (found mostly on dendritic cells, macrophages and B lymphocytes), and class III proteins (i.e., complement proteins and cytokines). (From Peakman M, Vergani D: *Basic and clinical immunology,* ed 2, London, 2009, Churchill Livingstone; and Abbas AK, Lichtman AH, Pillai S: *Basic Immunology,* ed 4, St Louis, 2014, Elsevier.)

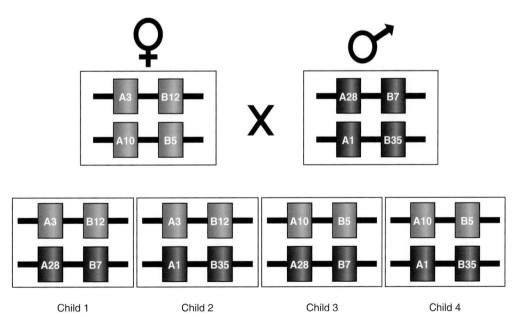

FIGURE 8.9 Inheritance of Human Leukocyte Antigen (HLA). HLA alleles are inherited in a codominant fashion; both maternal and paternal antigens are expressed. Specific HLA alleles are commonly given numbers to indicate different antigens. In this example, the mother has linked genes for HLA-A3 and HLA-B12 on one chromosome 6 and genes for HLA-A10 and HLA-B5 on the second chromosome 6. The father has HLA-A28 and HLA-B7 on one chromosome and HLA-A1 and HLA-B35 on the second chromosome. The children from this pairing may have one of four possible combinations of maternal and paternal HLA.

likely it is that transplantation will be successful. The chance of finding a match among siblings is much higher (25%) than the general population and, clearly, the most successful transplants would be between identical twins because they are identical genetically.

Transplant rejection may be classified as hyperacute, acute, or chronic, depending on the amount of time that elapses between transplantation and rejection. Hyperacute rejection is immediate and rare. Hyperacute rejection occurs because of the presence of preexisting antibodies (type II reaction) to HLA antigens on the vascular endothelial cells in the grafted tissue. These preexisting antigens are usually found in individuals who have received multiple blood transfusions or previous transplants. When the circulation is reestablished to the grafted area, the graft may immediately turn white (the so-called *white graft*) instead of a normal pink color. Hyperacute rejection can be avoided by testing the recipient for preexisting antibodies prior to transplantation.

Acute rejection is a cell-mediated immune response that occurs within days to months after transplantation. This type of rejection occurs when the recipient develops an immune response against unmatched HLA antigens after transplantation. A biopsy of the rejected organ usually shows an infiltration of lymphocytes and macrophages characteristic of a type IV reaction, although antibodies to the graft vasculature also occur. Acute rejection is treated with a combination of corticosteroids and antirejection drugs which block adaptive immune function.

Chronic rejection may occur after a period of months or years of normal function. It is characterized by slow, progressive organ failure. Chronic rejection usually results from chronic inflammation and a weak cell-mediated (type IV) reaction against minor histocompatibility antigens on the grafted tissue. It occurs most often in recipients who were poorly matched to their donor, have comorbidities (e.g., diabetes, hypertension), who received a graft that was damaged during the transplantation procedure, or who have required treatment for multiple acute rejection episodes. Once chronic rejection is well established, there are few effective treatments, and it may be necessary to replace the graft with a new transplanted organ.

> ✔ **QUICK CHECK 8.2**
> 1. Why do certain drugs become immunogenic to the host?
> 2. Why is an individual with type O blood considered a universal blood donor?
> 3. Why is SLE considered an autoimmune disease?
> 4. Define the different types of graft rejection.

DEFICIENCIES IN IMMUNITY

Immune deficiency is the failure of the immune or inflammatory response to function normally, resulting in increased susceptibility to infections. Primary (congenital) immune deficiency is caused by a genetic defect, whereas secondary (acquired) immune deficiency is caused by another condition, such as cancer, infection, or normal physiologic changes, such as aging. Acquired forms of immune deficiency are far more common than the congenital forms.

Initial Clinical Presentation

The clinical hallmark of immune deficiency is a tendency to develop unusual or recurrent, severe infections. The most severe primary immune deficiencies develop in young children 2 years of age and younger. Potential immune deficiencies should be considered if the individual has experienced severe, documented bouts of pneumonia, otitis media, sinusitis (sinus infection), bronchitis, septicemia (blood infection), or meningitis or infections with rare opportunistic microorganisms (e.g.,

Pneumocystis jiroveci). Infections are generally recurrent, and multiple simultaneous infections are common. Invasive fungal infections are rare in healthy individuals and strongly indicate a defective immune system. Children frequently present with failure to thrive because of chronic diarrhea and other chronic symptoms. A familial history of immune deficiency may be found in some types of primary deficiency.

Routine care of individuals with immune deficiencies must be tempered with the knowledge that the immune system may be totally ineffective. Prolonged antibiotic use is commonly ineffective by oral or injected routes and may necessitate intravenous administration. It is unsafe to administer many conventional immunizing agents to many of these individuals because of the risk of causing an uncontrolled infection. Infection is a particular problem when attenuated vaccines that contain live but weakened microorganisms are used (e.g., live polio vaccine; vaccines against measles, mumps, and rubella).

The type of recurrent infections may indicate the type of immune defect. Deficiencies in T-cell immune responses are associated with recurrent infections caused by certain viruses (e.g., varicella herpes, cytomegalovirus), fungi, and yeasts (e.g., *Candida*, *Histoplasma*), or atypical microorganisms (e.g., *P. jiroveci*). B-cell deficiencies and phagocyte deficiencies, however, are suggested if the individual has documented, recurrent infections with microorganisms that require opsonization (e.g., encapsulated bacteria, such as *Pneumococcus*) or those with viruses against which humoral immunity is normally effective (e.g., rubella virus). Some complement deficiencies resemble defects in antibody or phagocyte function, but others are associated with disseminated infections with bacteria of the genus *Neisseria* (*Neisseria meningitides* and *Neisseria gonorrhoeae*).

Primary (Congenital) Immune Deficiencies

Most primary immune deficiencies are the result of *single gene defects*. Generally the mutations are sporadic and not inherited: a family history exists in only about 25% of individuals. The sporadic mutations occur before birth, but the onset of symptoms may be early or later, depending on the particular syndrome. In some instances, symptoms of immune deficiency appear within the first 2 years of life. Other immune deficiencies are progressive, with the onset of symptoms appearing in the second or third decade of life.

Individually, primary immune deficiencies are rare. The prevalence of primary immune deficiency diseases was approximately 30 to 50 new cases per year in the United States from 2001 to 2007.[2] However, 354 inborn errors of immunity were identified as of February 2017.[3] Together, primary immune deficiencies are more common than cystic fibrosis, hemophilia, childhood leukemia, or many other well-known diseases. Many are subtle with minor deficiencies, but several result from major defects and lead to recurrent life-threatening infections. Sex distribution is about even, although some specific diseases have a male or female predominance. The three most commonly diagnosed deficiencies are common variable immune deficiency (34% of individuals with primary immune deficiencies), selective IgA deficiency (24%), and IgG subclass deficiency (17%).

Primary immune deficiencies have recently been reclassified into nine groups, based on the principal component of the immune or inflammatory systems that is defective.[3] Of these nine groups, the most common disorders are included within combined immunodeficiencies (affecting both cellular and humoral immunity), with or without associated or syndromic features. They are predominantly antibody deficiencies, defects in phagocyte number or function, defects in innate immunity, and complement defects. To provide a better understanding of the diversity and severity of primary immune deficiencies, a few select examples will be discussed.

Combined Deficiencies

Combined deficiencies include the most life-threatening disorders and result from defects that directly affect the development of both T and B lymphocytes. However, the severity depends on the degree to which B and T cells are affected. The most severe disorders are called severe combined immunodeficiencies (SCIDs). Most individuals with SCIDs have few detectable lymphocytes in the circulation and secondary lymphoid organs (spleen, lymph nodes). The thymus usually is underdeveloped because of the absence of T cells. Immunoglobulin levels, especially IgM and IgA, are absent or greatly reduced. Several forms of SCID are caused by autosomal recessive enzymatic defects that result in the accumulation of toxic metabolites, and rapidly dividing cells, such as lymphocytes, are especially sensitive. For instance, deficiency of adenosine deaminase (ADA deficiency) results in the accumulation of toxic purines. X-linked SCID results from a common defect in most of the important interleukin (IL) receptors needed for lymphocyte maturation (e.g., IL-2, IL-4, IL-7, and others).

Even if nearly adequate numbers of B and T cells are produced, their cooperation may be defective. Bare lymphocyte syndrome is the immune deficiency characterized by the inability of lymphocytes and macrophages to produce MHC class I or class II molecules. Without MHC molecules, antigen presentation and intercellular cooperation cannot occur effectively. Children with this deficiency develop serious, life-threatening infections and usually die before age 5 years.

Some combined immune deficiencies are associated with other features. Wiskott-Aldrich syndrome (WAS), an X-linked recessive disorder, is a condition in which IgM antibody production is greatly depressed. Antibody responses against antigens that primarily elicit an IgM response, such as polysaccharide antigens from bacterial cell walls (e.g., *P. aeruginosa*, *S. pneumoniae*, *Haemophilus influenzae*, and other microorganisms with polysaccharide outer capsules), are deficient. WAS results from a mutation of the *WAS* gene that also affects the actin cytoskeleton, which is important for platelet function. Thus WAS is a combined immune deficiency with an associated major defect in platelet function. Clinical manifestations include bleeding secondary to thrombocytopenia (low platelet counts), eczema, and recurrent infections (e.g., otitis media, pneumonia, herpes simplex, cytomegalovirus).

DiGeorge syndrome (22q11.2 deletion syndrome) is a combined immunodeficiency with syndromic features. It is caused by the lack or partial lack of the thymus, resulting in greatly decreased T-cell numbers and function. Defective development of the third and fourth pharyngeal pouches during embryonic development results in thymic defects and the absence of the parathyroid gland (causing inability to regulate calcium concentration). Low blood calcium levels cause the development of tetany or involuntary rigid muscular contraction. DiGeorge syndrome is frequently associated with abnormal development of facial features that are controlled by the same embryonic pouches; these include low-set ears, fish-shaped mouth, and other altered features (Fig. 8.10). There are numerous other combined immune deficiencies, including defects in CD3 resulting in the loss of T-cell receptor intracellular signaling, defective somatic gene rearrangement of variable region genes or constant region genes, IL-2 receptor defects, and defects in DNA repair.

Predominantly Antibody Deficiencies

Predominantly antibody deficiencies result from defects in B-cell maturation or function and are the most common of immune deficiencies. T-cell immune responses are not affected in pure B-lymphocyte deficiencies. The results are lower levels of circulating immunoglobulins (hypogammaglobulinemia) or occasionally totally or nearly absent immunoglobulins (agammaglobulinemia).

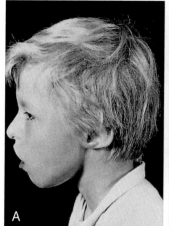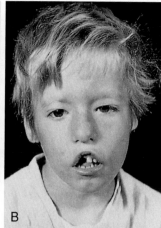

FIGURE 8.10 Facial Anomalies Associated With DiGeorge Syndrome. Note the wide-set eyes (**B**), low-set ears (**A and B**), shortened structure of the upper lip (**B**), and underdeveloped chin (**A and B**). (From Male D et al: *Immunology*, ed 8, Philadelphia, 2013, Mosby.)

Some defects may involve a particular class of antibody, such as selective IgA deficiency, in which only IgA is suppressed. This occurs in 1 in 700 to 1 in 400 individuals and may result from failure to class-switch to IgA and mature into IgA-producing plasma cells. Many individuals are asymptomatic, although others have a history of recurring sinus, pulmonary, and gastrointestinal infections. Individuals with IgA deficiency often have chronic intestinal candidiasis (infection with *C. albicans*). Complications of IgA deficiency include severe allergic disease and autoimmune diseases. Secretory IgA normally may prevent the uptake of allergens from the environment; therefore IgA deficiency may lead to a more intense challenge to the immune system by environmental antigens.

Bruton agammaglobulinemia (X-linked agammaglobulinemia) is caused by blocked development of mature B cells in bone marrow. There are few or no circulating B cells, although T-cell number and function are normal, resulting in repeated bacterial infections, such as otitis media, streptococcal sore throat, and conjunctivitis, as well as more serious conditions, such as septicemia.

Other predominantly antibody deficiencies include severe reduction in particular classes or subclasses of antibody; defects in B-cell surface receptors, such as CD21 and CD40; and defects in class-switch, which may result in hyper-IgM syndrome.

Phagocyte Defects

Phagocyte defects range from inadequate numbers of phagocytes (e.g., severe congenital neutropenia) to defects in phagocyte function that can result in recurrent infections with the same group of microorganisms (encapsulated bacteria). Chronic granulomatous disease (CGD) is a severe defect in the myeloperoxidase–hydrogen peroxide system—a major means of bacterial destruction using the enzyme myeloperoxidase, halides (e.g., chloride ion), and hydrogen peroxide (H_2O_2). Deficient production of hydrogen peroxide and other oxygen products needed for phagocytic killing results in recurrent severe pneumonias; tumor-like granulomata in the lungs, skin, and bones; and other infections with some opportunistic microorganisms, such as *Staphylococcus aureus*, *Serratia marcescens*, and *Aspergillus* species. Other phagocytic deficiencies include defects in various leukocyte adhesion molecules, defects in the phagocytosis process or bacterial killing, and defects in cytokine receptors.

Defects in Innate Immunity

Some immune deficiencies are characterized by a defect in the capacity to produce an immune response against a particular antigen. In chronic mucocutaneous candidiasis, interaction between the Th17 lymphocytes and macrophages is ineffective related to a specific infectious agent, *C. albicans*. Thus the macrophage cannot be activated, and these individuals usually have mild to extremely severe recurrent *Candida* infections involving the mucous membranes and skin. Other defects in innate immunity include defects in Toll-like receptors and NK cells. Other primary defects in innate immunity result in susceptibility to infections with mycobacteria, salmonella, and viruses (Epstein Barr, Herpes, influenza viruses).

Complement Deficiencies

Many complement deficiencies have been described. C3 deficiency is the most severe defect because of its central role in the complement cascade. Loss of C3b and C3a production and the inability to activate C5 result in recurrent life-threatening infections with encapsulated bacteria (e.g., *Haemophilus influenzae* and *Streptococcus pneumoniae*) at an early age. Deficiencies of any of the terminal components of the complement cascade (C5, C6, C7, C8, or C9 deficiencies) are associated with increased infections with only one group of bacteria—those of the genus *Neisseria* (*Neisseria meningitides* or *N. gonorrhoeae*). *Neisseria* species usually cause localized infections (meningitis or gonorrhea), but terminal pathway defects result in an 8000-fold increased risk for systemic infections with atypical strains of these microorganisms.

Mannose-binding lectin (MBL) deficiency is the primary defect of the lectin pathway of complement activation. This defect, as well as defects in the alternative pathway, results in increased risk of infection with microorganisms that have polysaccharide capsules rich in mannose, particularly the yeast *Saccharomyces cerevisiae* and encapsulated bacteria, such as *N. meningitidis* and *S. pneumoniae*. Other complement deficiencies include defects in the components C1, C4, C2, C5, C1 inhibitor, factor B, factor D, properdin, complement control factors, MASP, or complement receptors.

Evaluation and Care of Those With Primary Immune Deficiency

A review of clinical characteristics can help select the appropriate tests. A basic screening test is a complete blood count (CBC) with a differential. The CBC provides information on the numbers of red blood cells, white blood cells, and platelets, and the differential indicates the quantities of lymphocytes, granulocytes, and monocytes in blood. Quantitative determination of immunoglobulins (IgG, IgM, IgA) is a screening test for antibody production, and an assay for total complement (total hemolytic complement, CH_{50}) is useful if a complement defect is suspected.

Replacement Therapies for Primary Immune Deficiencies

Many primary immune deficiencies can be successfully treated by replacing the missing component of the immune system. Individuals with B-cell deficiencies that cause hypogammaglobulinemia or agammaglobulinemia are usually treated by administration of intravenous immunoglobulin (IVIG), antibody-rich fractions prepared from plasma pooled from large numbers of donors. Administration of IVIG replaces the individual's antibodies temporarily; these antibodies have a half-life of 3 to 4 weeks. Thus individuals must be treated repeatedly to maintain a protective level of antibodies in blood. Gene therapy would provide long-term replacement of specific immune factors. Trials have verified immune reconstitution in individuals with ADA deficiency, X-linked SCID, CGD, and WAS and progress is promising for this form of treatment.[4]

Defects in lymphoid cell development in the primary lymphoid organs (e.g., SCID, WAS) can sometimes be treated by replacement of stem cells through transplantation of bone marrow, umbilical cord cells, or other cell populations that are rich in stem cells. Thymic defects (e.g., DiGeorge syndrome, chronic mucocutaneous candidiasis) may be treated with transplantation of fetal thymus tissue or thymic epithelial cells (the cells that produce thymic hormones). However, in most cases, improvement is only temporary.

Enzymatic defects that cause SCID (e.g., adenosine deaminase deficiency) have been treated successfully with transfusions of glycerol frozen-packed erythrocytes. The donor erythrocytes contain the needed enzyme and can, at least temporarily, provide sufficient enzyme for normal lymphocyte function.

Bone marrow transplants containing hematopoietic stem cells are routinely used to treat SCID. However, individuals with SCID are at risk for graft-versus-host disease (GVHD). This occurs if T cells in a transplanted graft (e.g., transfused blood, bone marrow transplants) are mature and therefore capable of cell-mediated immunity against the recipient's HLA. The primary targets for GVHD are the skin (e.g., rash, loss or increase of pigment, thickening of skin), liver (e.g., damage to bile duct, hepatomegaly), mouth (e.g., dry mouth, ulcers, infections), eyes (e.g., burning, irritation, dryness), and gastrointestinal tract (e.g., severe diarrhea) and the disease may lead to death from infections. The risk of GVHD can be diminished by removing mature T cells from tissue used to treat individuals with immune deficiencies. Mesenchymal stem cells (MSCs) are present in all adult tissues and may be useful in treating GVHD. MSCs have potent immunosuppressive properties. Several clinical trials have demonstrated complete suppression of GVHD in a large number of recipients of MSCs.[5]

Secondary (Acquired) Immune Deficiencies

Secondary, or acquired, immune deficiencies are far more common than primary deficiencies. These deficiencies are complications of other physiologic or pathophysiologic conditions. Some conditions that are known to be associated with acquired deficiencies are summarized in Box 8.1.

Some Conditions Known to Be Associated With Secondary (Acquired) Immune Deficiencies

Although secondary deficiencies are common, many are not clinically relevant. In many cases, the degree of the immune deficiency is relatively minor and without any apparent increased susceptibility to infection. Alternatively, the immune system may be substantially suppressed, but only for a short duration, thus minimizing the incidence of clinically relevant infections. Some secondary immune deficiencies (e.g., malignancy, immunosuppressive treatments, AIDS), however, can be severe and may result in recurrent life-threatening infections.

Malignancies. Virtually all malignancies are complicated by immunosuppression, either through the effect of the disease itself on the body's defense mechanisms or as the result of treatment. Cancer cells are capable of protecting themselves by directly suppressing T lymphocytes. T lymphocytes seek to destroy cancer cells through a variety of inhibitory signals and secreted immunosuppressive chemicals (see Chapter 11). Virtually all late-stage malignancies result in generalized deficiency of the immune response and greatly increased susceptibility to developing life-threatening infections. Mechanisms include replacement of bone marrow by cancer cells, decreased NK and T lymphocyte function, and the release of soluble immunosuppressive chemicals. In fact, many people with malignancies die as a result of infections rather than of the direct effects of the tumor. Some malignancies (e.g., lymphomas, leukemias, plasmacytomas) present with an early and specific immune depression through a direct effect on B cells.

BOX 8.1 Some Conditions Known to Be Associated With Acquired Immunodeficiencies

Normal Physiologic Conditions
Pregnancy
Infancy
Aging

Psychologic Stress
Emotional trauma
Eating disorders

Dietary Insufficiencies
Malnutrition caused by insufficient intake of large categories of nutrients, such as protein or calories
Insufficient intake of specific nutrients, such as vitamins, iron, or zinc

Infections
Congenital infections, such as rubella, cytomegalovirus, hepatitis B
Acquired infections, such as acquired immunodeficiency syndrome (AIDS)

Malignancies
Malignancies of lymphoid tissues, such as Hodgkin disease, acute or chronic leukemia, or myeloma
Malignancies of nonlymphoid tissues, such as sarcomas and carcinomas

Physical Trauma
Burns

Medical Treatments
Stress caused by surgery
Anesthesia
Immunosuppressive treatment with corticosteroids or antilymphocyte antibodies
Splenectomy
Cancer treatment with cytotoxic drugs or ionizing radiation

Other Diseases or Genetic Syndromes
Diabetes
Alcoholic cirrhosis
Sickle cell disease
Systemic lupus erythematosus (SLE)
Chromosome abnormalities, such as trisomy 21

Immunosuppressive treatments. The list of medications that affect the immune response is ever increasing and includes anesthetics, analgesics, antithyroid medications, anticonvulsants, antihistamines, antimicrobial agents, antilymphocyte antibodies, and tranquilizers. The most profound immunosuppressive treatments are those that are intentionally used to suppress the immune system to manage immune-mediated disease, to treat malignancy, or to prevent rejection of transplanted tissues.

Corticosteroids are intentionally used to control hypersensitivity diseases (especially autoimmune disease) or to prevent rejection of transplants. They predominantly inhibit T cell function, prevent lymphocyte proliferation, inhibit production of critical cytokines, and suppress monocyte/macrophage functions but do not affect neutrophils. Because of their nonspecific activity, however, immune responses against infectious agents also can be suppressed, increasing an individual's susceptibility to infection.

Many drugs and other treatments that are used to treat cancer (e.g., chemotherapeutic agents, irradiation) are not specific for cancer cells but are designed to attack cells at susceptible stages in their cell cycles or to attack rapidly proliferating cells, including the cells of the immune system as well as malignant cells. Depending on the dose of chemotherapy and/or irradiation administered, the entire immune system may be depleted.

Antirejection drugs are used to prevent immune-mediated rejection of transplanted tissue. Although more targeted treatments are becoming available, most antirejection regimens still cause generalized immune suppression and increase the likelihood of infection and even cancer. A careful therapeutic balance must be maintained between protecting the graft and preventing these complications.

Acquired immunodeficiency syndrome. AIDS is secondary immune deficiency that develops in response to viral infection. **Human immunodeficiency virus (HIV)** infects and destroys the CD4-positive (CD4+) Th cells, which are necessary for the development of both B cells (humoral immunity) and cytotoxic T cells (cellular immunity). There are two types of HIV: HIV-1 (the most common [95% of HIV infections]) and HIV-2 (less common and less infectious). The discussion in this section

is related to HIV-1 and will be referred to as "HIV." HIV suppresses the immune response against itself and secondarily creates a generalized immune deficiency by suppressing the development of immune responses against other pathogens and opportunistic microorganisms. **Acquired immunodeficiency syndrome (AIDS)** is the most advanced stage of HIV infection.

Despite major efforts by health care agencies around the world, the number of cases and deaths from HIV infection and AIDS (HIV/AIDS) remains a major health concern. In 2017, 36.9 million people were living with HIV/AIDS, including 1.8 million children. Approximately 70% of these people live in Sub-Saharan Africa in middle and low income countries. An estimated 1.8 million people became infected worldwide in 2016. About 75% of people with HIV know their status. By the end of 2017, 21.7 million people in the world were accessing antiretroviral therapy.[6] With the advent of effective therapy to stabilize progression of the disease in the mid-1990s, HIV infection has become a chronic disease in the United States, with fewer deaths. An estimated 1.1 million people in the United States were reported to be living with HIV at the end of 2015.[7]

HIV infection is a bloodborne infection, with typical routes of transmission: blood or blood products, intravenous drug abuse, sexual activity, and maternal–child transmission before or during birth. Although the disease first gained attention in the United States related to sexual transmission between males, the most common route worldwide and in the United States is through heterosexual activity. Worldwide, women constitute more than half of those living with HIV/AIDS. Hundreds of thousands of cases of HIV/AIDS have been reported in children who contracted the virus from their mothers across the placenta, through contact with infected blood during delivery, or through the milk during breastfeeding.

Pathogenesis of AIDS. HIV is a member of a family of viruses called *retroviruses*, which carry genetic information in the form of two identical copies of single-stranded ribonucleic acid RNA rather than DNA. RNA—along with the viral enzymes reverse transcriptase, integrase, and protease—is packaged within the viral particle inside a capsid. The capsid is encased in an envelope which displays glycoprotein 120 (gp120) on its surface connected to a transmembrane glycoprotein 41 (gp41) (Fig. 8.11).

HIV-1 structure. The first step in the life cycle of HIV is attachment to the target cell (Fig. 8.12). After transmission from one person to another, the virus attaches to dendritic cells, which then carry the virus into the lymph nodes, where it can infect its primary target cell, the Th lymphocyte. For both dendritic cells and Th cells, the process of viral attachment begins with the binding of gp120 to CD4 molecules

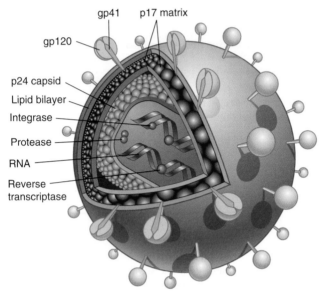

gp41   p17 matrix
gp120
p24 capsid
Lipid bilayer
Integrase
Protease
RNA
Reverse transcriptase

FIGURE 8.11 Human Immunodeficiency Virus-1 (HIV-1) Structure. The HIV-1 virion consists of a core of two identical strands of viral ribonucleic acid (RNA) molecules of viral enzymes (reverse transcriptase [RT], protease [PR], integrase [IN]) enveloped in a core capsid structure consisting primarily of the structural viral protein p24. The capsid is further encased in a matrix consisting primarily of viral protein p17. The outer surface is an envelope consisting of the plasma membrane of the cell from which the virus budded (lipid bilayer) and two viral glycoproteins: a transmembrane glycoprotein, gp41, and a noncovalently attached surface glycoprotein, gp120 (site of viral attachment). (Modified from Kumar V et al, editors: *Robbins and Cotran pathologic basis of disease,* ed 9, Philadelphia, 2015, Saunders.)

present on the surface of these cells. Further viral attachment requires binding to chemokine coreceptors. The coreceptor is CCR5 on macrophages and dendritic cells. On T-helper cells, the coreceptor is CCR4. Fusion of the virus to the cellular membrane requires that the gp120/CD4 molecule complex undergoes conformational changes that allow the transmembrane gp41 to fuse with the target cell. At this point, the viral envelope and the cellular membrane are fully fused and the viral capsid is released into the target cell cytoplasm. A group of antiretroviral medications are used to block these steps in viral attachment and fusion (see Fig. 8.12).Once the virus has been released into the target cell cytoplasm, the viral enzyme HIV reverse transcriptase converts RNA into dsDNA. Using a second viral enzyme, HIV integrase, the new DNA is inserted into the infected cell's genetic material. If the cell is activated, transcription and translation of the viral information are initiated, resulting in the production of a long strand of viral components which is then processed by the viral enzyme HIV protease. Assembly of the virion core follows. Antiretroviral medications have been developed that prevent the action of all three HIV enzymes (see Fig. 8.12).

The final step in the HIV lifecycle is the formation and release of new virions. As the virus buds, it takes some of the host cell membrane with it, making the virus less vulnerable to adaptive immune attack. New viruses infect mature Th cells in the circulation, as well as bone marrow precursor cells and lymphoid cells in the gastrointestinal tract. T cytotoxic cells target these infected cells leading to a gradual loss of Th cells over time. When Th cells are lost, they can no longer be replaced by healthy Th cells from bone marrow and the thymus. The result is immunosuppression. If an infected Th cell is relatively dormant (e.g., memory cells), then few new viruses are made and the cell survives the HIV infection. In these cells, the viral genetic material remains in the cell's chromosomes for the life of the individual, and new viruses will be made when that Th cell is activated at a later time.

Clinical manifestations of AIDS. The clinical manifestations of HIV infection and AIDS are primarily the result of depletion of Th cells, and this has a profound effect on the immune system, causing a severely diminished response to a wide array of infectious pathogens and cancers (Box 8.2). At the time of diagnosis, the individual may present with one of several different conditions: serologically negative (no detectable antibody), serologically positive (positive for antibody against HIV proteins) but asymptomatic, early stages of HIV disease, or AIDS (Fig. 8.13).

BOX 8.2   **AIDS-Defining Opportunistic Infections and Neoplasms Found in Individuals With HIV Infection**

Infections
Protozoal and Helminthic Infections
Cryptosporidiosis or isosporiasis (enteritis)
Pneumocystosis (pneumonia or disseminated infection)
Toxoplasmosis (pneumonia or CNS infection)

Fungal Infections
Candidiasis (esophageal, tracheal, or pulmonary)
Coccidioidomycosis (disseminated)
Cryptococcosis (CNS infection)
Histoplasmosis (disseminated)

Bacterial Infections
Mycobacteriosis ("atypical," e.g., *Mycobacterium avium-intracellulare,* disseminated or extrapulmonary

M. tuberculosis, disseminated or extrapulmonary)
Nocardiosis (pneumonia, meningitis, disseminated)
Salmonella infections (septicemia, recurrent)

Viral Infections
Cytomegalovirus (pulmonary, intestinal, retinitis, or CNS)
Herpes simplex virus (localized or disseminated)
Progressive multifocal leukoencephalopathy
Varicella-zoster virus (localized or disseminated)

Neoplasms
Invasive cancer of the uterine cervix
Kaposi sarcoma
Non-Hodgkin lymphomas (Burkitt, immunoblastic)
Primary lymphoma of brain

AIDS, Acquired immunodeficiency syndrome; *CNS,* Central nervous system; *HIV,* human immunodeficiency virus.
From Kumar V et al: *Robbins and Cotran pathologic basis of disease,* ed 9, Philadelphia, 2015, Saunders.

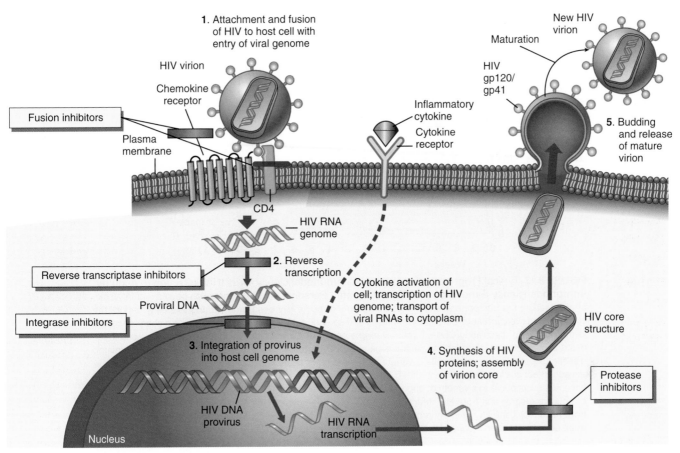

FIGURE 8.12 **Human Immunodeficiency Virus-1 (HIV-1) Life Cycle and Sites of Drug Intervention.** The HIV virion consists of a core of two identical strands of viral ribonucleic acid (RNA) enveloped in a protein structure with viral glycoproteins gp41 and gp120 on its surface (envelope). (1) HIV infection begins when a virion attaches to CD4 and chemokine co-receptors (e.g., CCR5) on dendritic and T-helper cells. (2) Conformational changes in the gp120/CD4 complex allow for fusion of the virus to the cell membrane and entry into a cell. (3) Reverse transcription (a deoxyribonucleic acid [DNA] copy of the viral RNA). (4) Integration into the nucleus. (5) Synthesis of HIV proteins (protease) and viral assembly. (6) Budding and release from the cell. The HIV life cycle is susceptible to blockage at several sites (see the text for further information), including attachment and fusion inhibitors, reverse transcriptase inhibitors, integrase inhibitors, and protease inhibitors. (Modified from Kumar V et al, editors: *Robbins and Cotran pathologic basis of disease,* ed 9, Philadelphia, 2015, Saunders.)

Current CDC recommendations for screening of HIV infection in all health care settings should be performed routinely for all persons 13 to 64 years of age after the individual is notified orally or in writing that testing will be performed unless the individual declines (known as *opt-out screening*). Screening also is recommended for men who have sex with men (MSM), pregnant women, and those with other sexually transmitted diseases (STDs) or tuberculosis (TB).[8]

HIV is diagnosed by the measurement of both HIV antibodies and HIV p24 antigen in blood. If positive, these tests are confirmed by HIV DNA (nucleic acid tests [NATs]). The amount of virus in the blood (viral load) and the Th cell count are used to determine what is called the "set point," which describes the severity of infection and the level of risk for rapid progression to AIDS.

Those with the early stages of HIV disease (early-stage disease) usually initially present with relatively mild and nonspecific symptoms resembling influenza, such as headaches, fever, or fatigue. These symptoms disappear after 1 to 6 weeks, and although the infection appears to be in clinical latency, it is actively proliferating in lymph nodes.

As the disease progresses, more serious symptoms and signs appear. The diagnosis of AIDS is made when the HIV infection becomes associated with various clinical conditions (Fig. 8.14; also see Box 8.2). These conditions include atypical or opportunistic infections and cancers, as well as indications of debilitating chronic disease (e.g., wasting syndrome, recurrent fevers). Most commonly, new cases of AIDS are diagnosed initially by decreased CD4+ T cell numbers. A diagnosis of AIDS can be made if the CD4+ T cell numbers decrease to < 200/mm³. Without treatment, the average time from infection to development of AIDS is just over 10 years.

Treatment and prevention of AIDS. HIV/AIDS treatment guidelines are published by the National Institutes of Health (NIH) and are revised frequently as new antiretroviral medications are approved.[9] Approved AIDS medications are classified by mechanism of action: **chemokine receptor inhibitors** (CCR5 antagonist prevents viral attachment), **HIV fusion inhibitors** (prevent CD4-gp 120 conformational changes during binding), **reverse transcriptase inhibitors** (nucleoside and nonnucleoside inhibitors of reverse transcriptase), **HIV integrase inhibitors** (inhibitors of viral integration into host genome), and **HIV protease inhibitors** (inhibitors of the proteases HIV uses for assembly of new virus) (see Fig. 8.12). The current regimen for the

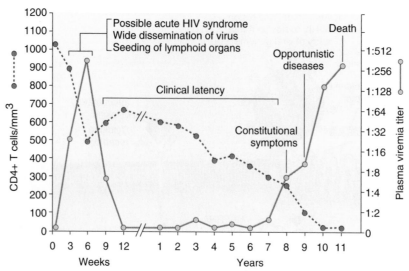

FIGURE 8.13 Typical Progression From Human Immunodeficiency Virus (HIV) Infection to Acquired Immunodeficiency Syndrome (AIDS) in Untreated Persons. Clinical progression begins within weeks after infection; the person may experience symptoms of acute HIV syndrome. During this early period, the virus progressively infects T cells and other cells and spreads to the lymphoid organs, with a sharp decrease in the number of circulating CD4+ T cells. During a period of clinical latency, the virus replicates and T-cell destruction continues, although the person is generally asymptomatic. The individual may develop HIV-related disease (constitutional symptoms)—a variety of symptoms of acute viral infection that do not involve opportunistic infections or malignancies. When the number of CD4+ cells is critically suppressed, the individual becomes susceptible to a variety of opportunistic infections and cancers with a diagnosis of AIDS. The length of time for progression from HIV infection to AIDS may vary considerably from person to person. (Redrawn from Fauci AS, Lane HC: Human immunodeficiency virus disease: AIDS and related conditions. In Fauci AS et al, editors: *Harrison's principles of internal medicine*, ed 14, New York, 1997, McGraw-Hill; Saunders.)

treatment of HIV infection is a combination of drugs, termed antiretroviral therapy (ART). ART protocols require a combination of synergist drugs from different classes, and specific regimens (e.g., timing of drug administration, doses, drug combinations) are adapted on the basis of the age of the individual, secondary clinical symptoms (renal or hepatic insufficiency), CD4+ T-cell levels, viral load, specific coinfections, preexisting cardiac risk factors, past history of treatment failure, suspected drug resistance, and other parameters. The clinical benefits of ART are profound. Death resulting from AIDS-related diseases has been reduced significantly since the introduction of ART. However, resistant variants to these drugs are increasing and may be found even in individuals

when they are first diagnosed with HIV infection. The U.S. Food and Drug Administration (FDA) recently approved the first humanized monoclonal antibody for the treatment of multidrug-resistant HIV-1/ AIDS (see *Did You Know?* Iblaizumab-Uiyk and Multidrug-Resistant Human Immunodeficiency Virus-1). Drug therapy for AIDS is not curative because HIV incorporates into the genetic material of the host, particularly CD4+ T memory cells, and may never be removed by antimicrobial therapy. Therefore drug administration to control the virus may have to continue for the lifetime of the individual. Additionally HIV may persist in organs where the antiviral drugs are not as effective, such as the central nervous system (CNS).

DID YOU KNOW?

Iblaizumab-Uiyk and Multidrug-Resistant Human Immunodeficiency Virus-1

The U.S. Food and Drug Administration (FDA) has recently approved ibalizumab-uiyk (Trogarzo) in combination with other antiretrovirals for treatment of multidrug-resistant human immunodeficiency virus (HIV). Ibalizumab is a drug that blocks HIV-1 entry into CD4+ T cells while preserving normal immunologic function. It is the first CD4-directed postattachment HIV-1 inhibitor and the first humanized monoclonal antibody for the treatment of HIV infection and acquired immunodeficiency syndrome (HIV/AIDS). It has a unique specificity for domain 2 of CD4 and leads to conformational changes of the CD4 T cell receptor–glycoprotein 120 (gp120) complex and prevents HIV fusion and entry. Thus this antibody potently blocks HIV-1 infection by inhibiting a critical step required for viral entry, but

without interfering with major histocompatibility complex class II (MHC II)–mediated T-helper cell activation. In clinical trials, for individuals with *drug-resistant HIV-1*, ibalizumab has demonstrated anti–HIV-1 activity without causing immunosuppression. A potential life-threatening side effect is immune reconstitution inflammatory syndrome (IRIS). IRIS can occur when the immune system is recovering after treatment for HIV, and there is an overwhelming inflammatory response. For example, pulmonary IRIS is associated with opportunistic infections, such as *Mycobacterium tuberculosis* and *Pneumocystis jiroveci* infections, with high morbidity and mortality.

Data from: Food and Drug Administration (FDA): *FDA approves new HIV treatment for patients who have limited treatment options.* March 6, 2018. Available at: https://www.fda.gov/NewsEvents/Newsroom/PressAnnouncements/ucm599657.htm; Gopal R, Rapaka RR, Kolls JK: Immune reconstitution inflammatory syndrome associated with pulmonary pathogens, *Eur Respir Rev* 26(143):160042, 2017; Kaplon H, Reichert JM: Antibodies to watch in 2018, *MAbs* 10(2):183-203, 2018; Markham A. Ibalizumab: first global approval, *Drugs* 78(7):781–785, 2018.

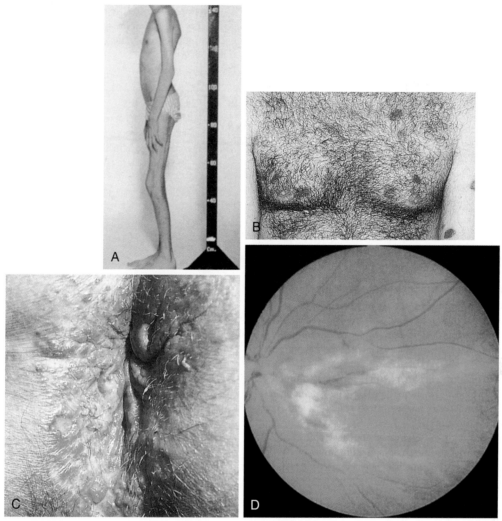

FIGURE 8.14 Clinical Symptoms of Acquired Immunodeficiency Syndrome (AIDS). A, Severe weight loss and anorexia. B, Kaposi sarcoma lesions. C, Perianal lesions of herpes simplex infection. D, Deterioration of vision from cytomegalovirus retinitis leading to areas of infection, which can lead to blindness. (A and D, from Taylor PK: *Diagnostic picture tests in sexually transmitted diseases,* London, 1995, Mosby; B and C, from Morse SA et al, editors: *Atlas of sexually transmitted diseases and AIDS,* ed 4, London, 2011, Saunders.)

The chronic nature of HIV/AIDS resulting from successful ART has led to additional concerns. Long-term toxicity of ART drugs has resulted in increased risk for cardiovascular disease, metabolic disorders, and organ failure. Some individuals receiving treatment fail to fully reconstitute their immune system or develop chronic immune activation characterized by activation of monocytes and T cells, production of proinflammatory cytokines, and depletion of Th17 cells and CD4+ T-cells.[10] Chronic immune activation tends to exacerbate clinical disease in adults and neonates.

Pediatric AIDS and central nervous system involvement. HIV can be transmitted from mother to child during pregnancy, at the time of delivery, or through breastfeeding, although the risk of mother-to-child transmission has dropped precipitously since the introduction of ART in pregnant women. The clinical diagnosis of HIV infection in young children born to HIV-infected mothers is very often a difficult task because the presence of maternal antibodies may result in a misleading false-positive result on tests for antibodies against HIV for as long as 18 months after birth. Testing for antibody against HIV

can be performed recurrently from birth until 18 months; if the test results become negative and remain so after 12 months, the child can be considered uninfected.

The protocol for diagnosis of HIV infection in infants and children younger than 18 months of age has been published by the Panel on Antiretroviral Therapy and Medical Management of Children Living with HIV.[11] HIV infection in babies is generally more aggressive than in adults; on average, an untreated child will die by his or her second birthday. Neurologic involvement occurs more commonly in children than in adults and results from CNS involvement, rather than from the effects on peripheral portions of the CNS. HIV encephalopathy occurs with varying degrees of severity and is a clinical component in the diagnosis of AIDS in children. Most newborns with HIV infection appear normal but may progressively develop signs of CNS involvement. These usually appear as failure to attain, or loss of, developmental milestones or loss of intellectual ability, verified by standard developmental scale or neuropsychological tests; acquired symmetric motor deficits, seen in children older than 1 month of age;

impaired brain growth or acquired microcephaly, demonstrated by head circumference measurements; or brain atrophy, demonstrated by serial imaging and required in children younger than 2 years of age.

It may be difficult to completely differentiate the effect of HIV infection on the CNS from other risk factors, including prenatal drug exposure, prematurity, chronic illness, and chaotic social conditions. The pathogenesis of HIV encephalopathy in children is poorly understood, but the presence of inflammatory mediators may be a contributing factor.

Because HIV infection in infants progresses very rapidly, treatment must begin at the diagnosis of infection. In older children, the criteria for treatment are similar to those used in adults. A growing number of investigational protocols are available for treatment of children with HIV infection. In general, treatment is focused on the preservation and maintenance of the immune system, aggressive response to opportunistic infections, support and relief of symptomatic occurrences, and administration of ART.

✔ QUICK CHECK 8.3

1. Why is the development of recurrent or unusual infections the clinical hallmark of immunodeficiency?
2. Compare and contrast the most common infections in individuals with defects in cell-mediated immune response and those with defects in humoral immune response.
3. How does HIV cause immune suppression?

SUMMARY REVIEW

Hypersensitivity: Allergy, Autoimmunity, and Alloimmunity

1. Hypersensitivity is an immune response misdirected against the host's own tissues (autoimmunity) or directed against beneficial foreign tissues, such as transfusions or transplants (alloimmunity); or it can be exaggerated responses against environmental antigens (allergy).
2. Mechanisms of hypersensitivity are classified as type I (immunoglobulin E [IgE]–mediated) reactions, type II (tissue-specific) reactions, type III (immune complex–mediated) reactions, and type IV (cell-mediated) reactions.
3. Hypersensitivity reactions can be immediate (developing within seconds or hours) or delayed (developing within hours or days).
4. Anaphylaxis, the most rapid immediate hypersensitivity reaction, is an explosive reaction that occurs within minutes of reexposure to the antigen and can lead to shock.
5. Type I (IgE-mediated) reactions occur after antigen reacts with IgE on mast cells, leading to mast cell degranulation and the release of histamine and other inflammatory substances.
6. Type II (tissue-specific) reactions are caused by four possible mechanisms: complement-mediated lysis, opsonization and phagocytosis, antibody-dependent cell-mediated cytotoxicity, and modulation of cellular function.
7. Type III (immune complex–mediated) reactions are caused by the formation of immune complexes that are deposited in target tissues, where they activate the complement cascade, generating chemotactic fragments that attract neutrophils into the inflammatory site.
8. Immune complex disease can be a systemic reaction, such as serum sickness (e.g., Raynaud phenomenon), or localized, such as the Arthus reaction.
9. Type IV (cell-mediated) reactions are caused by specifically sensitized T cells, which either kill target cells directly or release lymphokines that activate other cells, such as macrophages.
10. Allergens are antigens that cause allergic responses, usually a type I hypersensitivity response.
11. Autoimmune disease is loss of tolerance to self-antigens. There can be a genetic predisposition, and the diseases can be a type II or type III hypersensitivity reaction.
12. Alloimmunity is the immune system's reaction against antigens on the tissues of other members of the same species.
13. Alloimmune disorders include transient neonatal disease, in which the maternal immune system becomes sensitized against antigens expressed by the fetus; and transplant rejection and transfusion reactions, in which the immune system of the recipient of an organ transplant or blood transfusion reacts against foreign antigens on the donor's cells.

Deficiencies in Immunity

1. Immunodeficiency is the failure of mechanisms of self-defense to function in their normal capacity.
2. Immunodeficiencies are either primary or secondary. Congenital immunodeficiencies are caused by genetic defects that disrupt lymphocyte development, whereas acquired immunodeficiencies are secondary to disease or other physiologic alterations.
3. The clinical hallmark of immunodeficiency is a propensity to unusual or recurrent severe infections. The type of infection usually reflects the immune system defect.
4. The most common infections in individuals with defects of cell-mediated immune response are fungal and viral, whereas infections in individuals with defects of the humoral immune response or complement function are primarily bacterial.
5. Severe combined immunodeficiency (SCID) is a total lack of T-cell function and a severe (either partial or total) lack of B-cell function.
6. Wiskott-Aldrich syndrome (WAS) is caused by decreased production of IgM antibody.
7. DiGeorge syndrome is characterized by complete or partial lack of the thymus (resulting in depressed T-cell immunity), frequently associated with diminished or absent parathyroid gland activity (resulting in hypocalcemia) and cardiac anomalies.
8. Antibody deficiencies result from defects in B-cell maturation or function and range from a complete lack of the human bursal equivalent, the lymphoid organs required for B-cell maturation (as in Bruton agammaglobulinemia), to deficiencies in a single class of immunoglobulins (e.g., selective IgA deficiency).
9. Phagocyte defects include inadequate numbers or alteration in function, such as inadequate adhesion to bacteria or ineffective killing.
10. Complement and mannose-binding lectin deficiencies also are rare causes of increased risk for infection.
11. Primary immunodeficiency syndromes are usually treated with replacement therapy. Deficient antibody production is treated by replacement of missing immunoglobulins with commercial gamma-globulin preparations. Lymphocyte deficiencies are treated by the replacement of host lymphocytes with transplants of bone marrow, fetal liver, or fetal thymus from a donor. There are ongoing trials for gene therapy.

12. Acquired immunodeficiencies are caused by superimposed conditions, such as malnutrition, malignancy, medical therapies, physical or psychologic trauma, or infections.
13. Malignancy is associated with both local and generalized immune suppression that can result in life-threatening infections.
14. Treatments for hypersensitivity disorders, malignancy, and transplant rejection cause profound immune suppression and the

benefits of these treatments must be carefully balanced with the risks.
15. Acquired immunodeficiency syndrome (AIDS) is acquired dysfunction of the immune system caused by a retrovirus (HIV) that infects and destroys CD4+ lymphocytes (T-helper cells).

KEY TERMS

ABO blood group, 184
Acquired immunodeficiency syndrome (AIDS), 189
Acute rejection, 186
Adenosine deaminase (ADA deficiency), 187
Agammaglobulinemia, 187
Allergen, 181
Allergy (atopy), 181
Alloantigen, 184
Alloimmunity (isoimmunity), 183
Anaphylaxis, 174
Antiretroviral therapy, (ART), 192
Arthus reaction, 178
Atopic, 176
Autoimmune disease, 182, 182
Autoimmunity, 182
Bare lymphocyte syndrome, 187
Blood group antigen, 184
Bruton agammaglobulinemia, 187
C3 deficiency, 188
Chemokine receptor inhibitor, 191

Chronic granulomatous disease (CGD), 187
Chronic mucocutaneous candidiasis, 188
Chronic rejection, 186
Combined deficiency, 187
Complement deficiency, 188
Contact dermatitis, 180
Cryoglobulin, 178
Delayed hypersensitivity reaction, 174
Delayed hypersensitivity skin test, 180
Desensitization, 182
DiGeorge syndrome, 187
Erythema, 180
Graft-versus-host disease (GVHD), 188
HIV fusion inhibitor, 191
HIV integrase, 190
HIV integrase inhibitor, 191
HIV protease, 190
HIV protease inhibitor, 191
HIV reverse transcriptase, 190
Human immunodeficiency virus (HIV), 189

Human leukocyte antigen (HLA), 185
Hyperacute rejection, 186
Hypogammaglobulinemia, 187
Immediate hypersensitivity reaction, 174
Immune deficiency, 186
Induration, 180
Isohemagglutinin, 184
Major histocompatibility complex (MHC), 185
Mannose-binding lectin (MBL) deficiency, 188
Mesenchymal stem cell (MSC), 188
Phagocyte defect, 187
Predominantly antibody deficiency, 187
Primary (congenital) immune deficiency, 186
Raynaud phenomenon, 178
Reverse transcriptase inhibitor, 191
Rh blood group, 184
Secondary (acquired) immune deficiency, 186

Selective IgA deficiency, 187
Serum sickness, 178
Severe combined immunodeficiency (SCID), 187
Severe congenital neutropenia, 187
Systemic lupus erythematosus (SLE), 182
Tissue-specific antigen, 177
Tolerance, 182
Type I hypersensitivity, 175
Type II hypersensitivity, 177
Type III hypersensitivity, 178
Type IV hypersensitivity, 178
Universal donor, 184
Universal recipient, 184
Urticaria (hives), 176
Wheal and flare reaction, 176
Wiskott-Aldrich syndrome (WAS), 187
X-linked SCID, 187

REFERENCES

1. Thong B, Olsen NJ: Systemic lupus erythematosus diagnosis and management, *Rheumatology (Oxford)* 56(suppl_1):i3-i13, 2017.
2. Kobrynski L, Powell RW, Bowen S: Prevalence and morbidity of primary immunodeficiency diseases, United States 2001-2007, *J Clin Immunol* 34(8):954-961, 2014.
3. Picard C, et al: International Union of Immunological Societies: 2017 Primary Immunodeficiency Diseases Committee report on inborn errors of immunity, *J Clin Immunol* 38(1):96-128, 2018.
4. Kuo CY, Kohn DB: Gene therapy for the treatment of primary immune deficiencies, *Curr Allergy Asthma Rep* 16(5):39, 2016.

5. Dunavin N, et al: Mesenchymal stromal cells: what is the mechanism in acute graft-versus-host disease, *Biomedicines* 5(3):E39, 2017.
6. World Health Organization: HIV/AIDS, Data and statistics. Accessed 27 June 2019. Available at https://www.who.int/hiv/data/en/.
7. Centers for Disease Control and Prevention (CDC): HIV/AIDS, basic statistics. Last updated March 13, 2019. Available at: https://www.cdc.gov/hiv/basics/statistics.html.2017a.
8. Centers for Disease Control and Prevention (CDC): HIV testing guidelines. Page last reviewed March 16, 2018. Available at: https://www.cdc.gov/hiv/guidelines/testing.html.
9. National Institutes of Health: NIH guidelines for antiretroviral agents in adults and adolescents. Last updated October 15, 2018. Available at: https://

aidsinfo.nih.gov/contentfiles/lvguidelines/AA_Recommendations.pdf.
10. Paiardini M, Müller-Trutwin M: HIV-associated chronic immune activation, *Immunol Rev* 254(1):78-101, 2013.
11. U.S. Department of Health and Human Services (DHHS): AIDSinfo: guidelines for the use of antiretroviral agents in pediatric HIV infection: diagnosis of HIV infection in infants and children, U.S. Department of Health and Human Services, Last updated December 14, 2018. Available at: https://aidsinfo.nih.gov/guidelines/html/2/pediatric-arv/55/diagnosis-of-hiv-infection-in-infants-and-children.

9

Infection

Valentina L. Brashers, Sue E. Huether

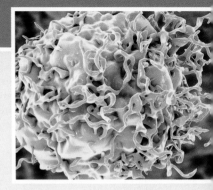

EVOLVE WEBSITE

http://evolve.elsevier.com/Huether/
Student Review Questions
Audio Key Points

Case Studies
Animations
Quick Check Answers

Modern health care has shown great progress in preventing and treating infectious diseases. However, infectious disease continues to be a threat to human health because of the emergence of previously unknown infections, the reemergence and spread of old infections that were thought to be under control, and the development of infectious agents that are resistant to multiple antibiotics. Endemic diseases, such as chronic hepatitis, human immunodeficiency virus (HIV) infection, other sexually transmitted infections, and foodborne infections, remain major challenges in the United States. Most deaths related to infections occur in individuals whose immune systems are compromised (young children, the elderly, and those with chronic disease).

MICROORGANISMS AND HUMANS: A DYNAMIC RELATIONSHIP

For many microorganisms, the human body is a hospitable site in which to grow and flourish because of sufficient nutrients and appropriate conditions of temperature and moisture. Only a small number of microorganisms are capable of causing disease. The relationship between humans and microorganisms is summarized in Box 9.1. The symbiotic microorganisms make up the normal human microbiome—the resident microorganisms found in different parts of the body, including the skin, mouth, gastrointestinal tract, respiratory tract, and genital tract. For instance, the normal bacterial microbiome of the human gut is provided with nutrients from ingested food and produces enzymes that facilitate the digestion and use of many of the more complex molecules found in the human diet. It also produces antibacterial factors that prevent colonization by pathogenic microorganisms and produces usable metabolites (e.g., vitamins K and B).

The symbiotic relationship between the body and the human microbiome is maintained by physical barriers (e.g., skin and lining of

respiratory, intestinal and genital tracts) and the complex interaction of the microbiome and inflammatory and immune systems. Microorganisms that may cause infection if the protective barriers are breached or defensive systems are weakened are referred to as *opportunistic microorganisms*. For example, alterations in the microbiome by antibiotics may allow local overgrowth of opportunistic microorganisms that can cause disease (e.g., *Clostridium difficile, Candida albicans*). Individuals with immune deficiencies also become easily infected with opportunistic microorganisms. The concepts and processes of infection are presented in this chapter. Specific infections are presented in Part Two of the book with the organ system chapters (i.e., infections that occur in the cardiovascular, pulmonary, genitourinary tract, gastrointestinal tract, and skin).

The Process of Infection

Infectious diseases are caused by pathogenic microorganisms. Classes of pathogenic microorganisms and their characteristics are summarized in Table 9.1. The process of infection includes encounter and transmission, colonization, invasion, dissemination, and cellular or tissue damage by the pathogenic microorganisms. There are several different ways that an individual can encounter or come in contact with microorganisms. *Endogenous microorganisms* are already present in the body and part of the normal microbiome. *Exogenous microorganisms* are transmitted from an external source (e.g., contaminated water, food, or from another human, animals or insects).

Transmission of microorganisms can occur in several different ways: *Direct transmission or contact:* Vertical transmission from mother to child across the placenta (e.g., *Listeria monocytogenes*, cytomegalovirus [CMV]), during delivery from the birth canal (e.g., group B *Streptococcus, Escherichia coli, Chlamydia trachomatis*), or from breast milk (e.g., *Staphylococcus aureus*); horizontal transmission from one person to another through exposure to blood and body fluids (e.g., HIV, *Neisseria gonorrhoeae*); or zoonotic infections directly transmitted from animals (e.g., giardiasis, toxoplasmosis).

Indirect transmission: Occurs from contact with infected materials, such as towels, toys, bandages and contact lenses (e.g., cellulitis, conjunctivitis); inhalation or droplet infection (e.g., common cold, pneumonia); ingestion of contaminated food or water (e.g., gastroenteritis, cholera); or inoculation (e.g., malaria, tetanus).

Colonization is the ability of a pathogenic microorganism to survive and multiply on or within the human environment. They must be able to compete with the symbiotic microorganisms and resist local defenses. Table 9.2 summarizes mechanisms used by pathogens to resist immune defenses. The multiple layers of defense against pathogens are described in Chapters 6 and 7. The estimated minimum number of microorganisms needed to cause infection (minimum infective dose) varies greatly with the particular pathogen: *Vibrio cholerae* (103-108 microorganisms), norovirus and rotavirus (10-100), *Giardia lamblia* parasitic diarrhea (10), and *Mycobacterium tuberculosis* (<10). *Adherence* helps protect the microorganism from removal by mechanical,

BOX 9.1 Relationships Between Humans and Microorganisms

Symbiosis: Benefits only the human; no harm to the microorganism
Mutualism: Benefits the human and the microorganism
Commensalism: Benefits only the microorganism; no harm to the human
Pathogenicity: Benefits the microorganism; harms the human
Opportunism: A situation in which benign microorganisms become pathogenic because of decreased human host resistance or translocation to other body sites.

TABLE 9.1 Classes of Microorganisms Infectious to Humans

Class	Size	Site of Reproduction	Example
Virus	20-300 nm	Intracellular	Human immunodeficiency virus, hepatitis A and B, chicken pox, measles
Bacteria	0.8-15 mcg	Skin	Staphylococcal wound infection
		Mucous membranes	Cholera
		Extracellular	Streptococcal pneumonia *Mycoplasma* pneumonia
		Intracellular	Tuberculosis, chlamydiasis
Fungi	2-200 mcg	Skin	Tinea pedis (athlete's foot)
		Mucous membranes	Candidiasis (e.g., thrush)
		Extracellular	Sporotrichosis
		Intracellular	Histoplasmosis
Protozoa	1-50 mm	Mucosal	Giardiasis
		Extracellular	African trypanosomiasis (sleeping sickness)
Helminths	3 mm to 10 m	Intracellular	Trichinosis
		Extracellular	Filariasis

TABLE 9.2 Examples of Mechanisms Used by Pathogens to Resist the Immune System

Mechanisms	Effect on Immunity	Example of Specific Microorganisms
Destroy or Block Component of Immune System		
Produce toxins	Kills phagocyte or interferes with chemotaxis. Prevents phagocytosis by inhibiting fusion between phagosome and lysosomal granules	*Staphylococcus* *Streptococcus* *Mycobacterium tuberculosis*
Produce antioxidants (e.g., catalase, superoxide dismutase) Produce protease to digest immunoglobulin A (IgA)	Prevents killing by oxygen-dependent mechanisms Promotes bacterial attachment	*Mycobacterium* sp. *Salmonella typhi* *Neisseria gonorrhoeae* (urinary tract infection), *Haemophilus influenzae*, and *Streptococcus pneumoniae* (pneumonia)
Produce surface molecules that mimic Fc receptors and bind antibody	Prevents activation of complement system Prevents antibody functioning as opsonin	*Staphylococcus* Herpes simplex virus
Mimic Self-Antigens		
Produce surface antigens (e.g., M protein, red blood cell antigens) that are similar to self-antigens	Pathogen resembles individual's own tissue; in some individuals, antibodies can be formed against self-antigen, leading to hypersensitivity disease (e.g., antibody to M protein also reacts with cardiac tissue, causing rheumatic heart disease; antibody to red blood cell antigens can cause anemia)	Group A *Streptococcus* (M protein) *Mycoplasma pneumoniae* (red cell antigens)
Change Antigenic Profile		
Undergo mutation of antigens or activate genes that change surface molecules	Immune response delayed because of failure to recognize new antigen	Influenza virus Human immunodeficiency virus (HIV) Some parasites

nonspecific forces, such as coughing of respiratory mucus. Adherence occurs between receptors on the microorganism and on the surface of cells, the specificity of which results in localization of an infectious agent to particular sites, such as the confinement of common cold viruses to the respiratory tract.

One of the ways microorganism overcome defenses is by the formation of biofilms. Biofilms consist of mixed species of microorganisms, including bacteria and fungi, immersed in a highly organized extracellular matrix produced by the microorganisms. Microorganisms in biofilms become tolerant and resistant to antibiotics and immune responses, making them difficult to treat. Biofilms form on implanted medical devises (e.g., catheters, pacemakers, implanted heart valves, prosthetic joints, dentures) and are associated with chronic infections (e.g., persistent nasopharyngeal colonization with staphylococci; otitis media; diabetes-associated foot ulcers; infected burns; or pneumonia associated with cystic fibrosis).

Invasion or penetration is the ability of pathogens to cross surface barriers including the skin and mucous membranes. This requires penetration (e.g., mosquito bite) or a break in the integrity of the barrier (e.g., trauma). Normal protective barriers are described in Chapter 6. Dissemination or spread of infection can occur by direct extension through surrounding tissue or through the blood or lymphatic vessels. Tissue damage or cellular alterations can occur directly by the production of toxins or indirectly as a result of an immune response with inflammation, swelling, scarring, or necrosis. Table 9.3 contains examples of mechanisms used by pathogens to cause tissue damage.

Several factors also influence the capacity of a microorganism to cause infection. These factors include:

Communicability: The ability to spread from one individual to others and cause disease (measles and pertussis spread very easily; HIV is of lower communicability)

Immunogenicity: The ability to induce an immune response

Infectivity: The ability to invade and multiply in the host

Mechanism of action: How the microorganism damages tissue

Pathogenicity: The ability to produce disease—success depends on communicability, infectivity, extent of tissue damage, and virulence

Portal of entry: The route by which a microorganism infects the host (e.g., direct contact, inhalation, ingestion, or bites of an animal or insect)

Toxigenicity: The ability to produce soluble toxins or endotoxins, factors that greatly influence the degree of virulence

Virulence: The capacity to cause severe disease, for example, measles virus is of low virulence; rabies virus is highly virulent

Infectious diseases also are classified by their prevalence and spread within the community:

Endemic: Diseases with relatively high but constant rates of infection in a particular population

Epidemic: The number of new infections in a particular population greatly exceeds the number usually observed

Pandemic: An epidemic that spreads over a large area, such as a continent or worldwide

Stages of Infection

The clinical process of infection occurs in the following four distinct stages:

Incubation period: The period from initial exposure to the infectious agent and the onset of the first symptoms; during this time, the microorganisms have entered the individual, undergone initial colonization, and begun multiplying but are at insufficient numbers to cause symptoms; this period may last from several hours to years.

TABLE 9.3   Examples of Mechanisms Used by Pathogens to Cause Tissue Damage

Pathogens That Directly Cause Tissue Damage	
Produce Exotoxin	
Streptococcus pyogenes	Tonsillitis, scarlet fever
Staphylococcus aureus	Boils, toxic shock syndrome, food poisoning
Corynebacterium diphtheria	Diphtheria
Clostridium tetani	Tetanus
Vibrio cholerae	Cholera
Produce Endotoxin	
Escherichia coli	Gram-negative sepsis
Haemophilus influenzae	Meningitis, pneumonia
Salmonella typhi	Typhoid
Shigella	Bacillary dysentery
Pseudomonas aeruginosa	Wound infection
Yersinia pestis	Plague
Cause Direct Damage With Invasion	
Variola	Smallpox
Varicella-zoster	Chickenpox, shingles
Hepatitis B virus	Hepatitis
Poliovirus	Poliomyelitis
Measles virus	Measles, subacute sclerosing panencephalitis
Influenza virus	Influenza
Herpes simplex virus	Cold sores
Pathogens That Indirectly Cause Tissue Damage	
Produce Immune Complexes	
Hepatitis B virus	Kidney disease
Streptococcus pyogenes	Glomerulonephritis
Treponema pallidum	Kidney damage in secondary syphilis
Most acute infections	Transient renal deposits
Cause Cell-Mediated Immunity	
Mycobacterium tuberculosis	Tuberculosis
Mycobacterium leprae	Tuberculoid leprosy
Lymphocytic choriomeningitis virus	Aseptic meningitis
Borrelia burgdorferi	Lyme arthritis
Herpes simplex virus	Herpes stromal keratitis

Data modified from Janeway CA et al: *Immunobiology: the system in health and disease*, ed 5, New York, 2001, Garland.

Prodromal stage: The occurrence of initial symptoms, which are often very mild and include a feeling of discomfort and tiredness; pathogens continue to multiply during this stage.

Invasion or acute illness period: The pathogen is multiplying rapidly, invading farther and affecting the tissues at the site of initial colonization as well as other areas; the immune and inflammatory responses have been triggered; symptoms may be specifically related to the pathogen or to the inflammatory response

Convalescence: In most instances, the individual's immune and inflammatory systems successfully remove the infectious agent and symptoms decline; alternatively, the disease may be fatal or enter a latency phase with resolution of symptoms until pathogen reactivation at a later time.

Infectious disease can be contagious during all stages of infection.

> ✔ **QUICK CHECK 9.1**
> 1. What are the steps involved in the process of infection?
> 2. List four mechanisms that a pathogens can use to cause tissue damage.
> 3. What are the four stages of infection?

INFECTIOUS DISEASE

Bacterial Infection

Bacteria are prokaryocytes (lack a discrete nucleus), are relatively small, and are a common cause of disease (see Fig. 9.1, *A*). They can be aerobic or anaerobic and motile or immotile. Spherical bacteria are called *cocci*, rod-like forms are called *bacilli*, and spiral forms are termed *spirochetes*. Gram staining differentiates the microorganisms as gram-positive or gram-negative bacteria (see Fig. 9.1, *B* and *C*). Gram-positive bacteria have teichoic acid and peptidoglycan in their outer membranes

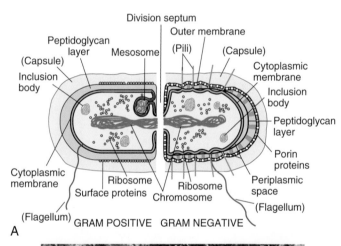

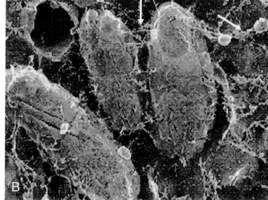

FIGURE 9.1 General Structure of Bacteria. A, The structure of the bacterial cell wall determines its staining characteristics with Gram staining. A gram-positive bacterium has a thick layer of peptidoglycan *(left)*. A gram-negative bacterium has a thick peptidoglycan layer and an outer membrane *(right)*. **B,** Scanning electron micrograph of *Escherichia coli* (*orange*) showing pili (arrows) attached to bladder epithelium (*blue*). (**A,** from Murray PR et al: *Medical microbiology,* ed 7, Philadelphia, 2013, Saunders; **B,** modified from Wein A et al: *Campbell-Walsh urology,* ed 9, Philadelphia, 2007, Saunders.)

causing them to appear dark purple on Gram stain. Gram-negative bacteria have a lipopolysaccharide (LPS) in the outer membrane causing them to appear light pink on Gram staining. LPS also is known as *endotoxin*.

Bacteria can survive in an extracellular or intracellular environment.[1] Extracellular bacteria use virulence mechanisms to proliferate in the body fluids of the extracellular environment. The presence of extracellular bacterial antigens induces the formation of humoral antibodies. Intracellular bacteria can enter and survive in cells (including immune, epithelial, and endothelial cells), where they evade humoral antibodies and can only be eliminated by a cellular immune response. Intracellular microbes can persist for long periods (e.g., *C. trachomatis, M. tuberculosis,* and *Mycobacterium leprae*) and cause disease by disrupting cellular structure and function. Virulence factors that help bacteria cause infection include:

Pili (fimbria): Hair-like projections that express adhesion molecules to attach to cells and invade tissue

Flagella: A rotary structure that provides motility and expresses adhesion molecules

Capsules: An outer covering of the cell wall that prevents phagocytosis and resists host immunity

Enzymes: Proteins that promote tissue invasion (e.g., proteases and lipases)

Toxins: Poisonous substances that cause injury, such as exotoxins (direct injury), endotoxins (indirect injury)

Microorganisms also can compete for iron and nutrients to support their metabolism and growth. Examples of human diseases caused by specific bacteria are listed in Table 9.4. The general structure of bacteria is reviewed in Fig. 9.1.

Many bacteria use toxins as virulence factors, including exotoxins and endotoxins (Table 9.5). Exotoxins are secreted molecules, mostly protein enzymes. They directly injure cells by damaging cell membranes or by entering cells and changing their function. Exotoxins are immunogenic eliciting production of antibodies known as antitoxins (important for vaccine development) (see the section Vaccines and Protection Against Infection). The most poisonous exotoxin yet discovered is botulinum neurotoxin produced by *Clostridium botulinum,* which causes paralysis and respiratory compromise. Different strains of *S. aureus* are capable of producing a wide array of exotoxins (see Did You Know? *Staphylococcus aureus* Infections). Some damage the cell membrane and others cause blood clots (coagulase); break down clots (staphylokinase); cause separation of the epidermis, resulting in scalded skin syndrome (exfoliative toxins); secrete enzymes, which degrade lipids on the skin surface and facilitate abscess formation (lipases); produce enterotoxins, which cause food poisoning; or produce superantigens (a type of exotoxin), which stimulate a profound immune response (discussed in Chapter 7). Endotoxins cause a profound immune and inflammatory response.

Gram-negative microbes produce endotoxin (lipopolysaccharide [LPS]), a structural portion of the cell wall that is released during growth, lysis, or destruction of the bacteria or during treatment with antibiotics. Bacteria that produce endotoxins are called *pyrogenic bacteria* because they activate the inflammatory process and produce fever (see Chapter 15). Antibiotics cannot prevent the toxic effects of endotoxins.

Bacteremia occurs when bacteria are present in the blood. Sepsis, or septicemia, occurs when bacteria are growing in the blood and release large amounts of toxins causing clinical symptoms and signs. Released endotoxin from gram-negative bacteria and exotoxins from gram-positive bacteria induces the overproduction of proinflammatory cytokines, particularly tumor necrosis factor-alpha (TNF-α), interleukin-1 (IL-1), interleukin-6 (IL-6), and reactive oxygen species

TABLE 9.4   Examples of Common Bacterial Infections

Microorganism	Gram Stain	Respiratory Pathway	Intracellular or Extracellular
Respiratory Tract Infections			
Upper Respiratory Tract Infections			
Corynebacterium diphtheriae (diphtheria)	Gram +	Facultative anaerobic	Extracellular
Haemophilus influenzae	Gram −	Facultative anaerobic	Extracellular
Streptococcus pyogenes (group A)	Gram +	Facultative anaerobic	Extracellular
Otitis Media			
Haemophilus influenzae	Gram −	Facultative anaerobic	Extracellular
Streptococcus pneumoniae	Gram +	Facultative anaerobic	Extracellular
Lower Respiratory Tract Infections			
Bacillus anthracis (pulmonary anthrax)	Gram +	Facultative anaerobic	Extracellular
Bordetella pertussis (whooping cough)	Gram −	Aerobic	Extracellular
Chlamydia pneumonia	Not stainable	Aerobic	Obligate intracellular
Escherichia coli	Gram −	Facultative anaerobic	Extracellular
Haemophilus influenzae	Gram −	Facultative anaerobic	Extracellular
Legionella pneumophila	Gram −	Aerobic	Facultative intracellular
Mycobacterium tuberculosis	Gram + (weakly)	Aerobic	Extracellular
Mycoplasma pneumoniae	Not stainable	Aerobic	Extracellular
Neisseria meningitidis (develops into meningitis)	Gram −	Aerobic	Extracellular
Pseudomonas aeruginosa	Gram −	Aerobic	Extracellular
Streptococcus agalactiae (group B; develops to meningitis)	Gram +	Facultative anaerobic	Extracellular
Streptococcus pneumoniae	Gram +	Facultative anaerobic	Extracellular
Yersinia pestis (plague)	Gram −	Facultative anaerobic	Extracellular
Gastrointestinal Infections			
Inflammatory Gastrointestinal Infections			
Bacillus anthracis (gastrointestinal anthrax)	Gram +	Facultative anaerobic	Extracellular
Clostridium difficile	Gram +	Anaerobic	Extracellular
Escherichia coli O157:H7	Gram −	Facultative anaerobic	Extracellular
Vibrio cholerae	Gram −	Facultative anaerobic	Extracellular
Invasive Gastrointestinal Infections			
Brucella abortus (brucellosis, undulant fever, leading to sepsis, heart infection)	Gram −	Aerobic	Intracellular
Helicobacter pylori (gastritis and peptic ulcers)	Gram −	Microaerophilic	Extracellular
Listeria monocytogenes (leading to sepsis and meningitis)	Gram +	Aerobic	Intracellular
Salmonella typhi (typhoid fever)	Gram −	Anaerobic	Extracellular
Shigella sonnei	Gram −	Facultative anaerobic	Extracellular
Food Poisoning			
Bacillus cereus	Gram +	Facultative anaerobic	Extracellular
Clostridium botulinum	Gram +	Anaerobic	Extracellular
Clostridium perfringens	Gram +	Anaerobic	Extracellular
Staphylococcus aureus	Gram +	Facultative anaerobic	Extracellular
Sexually Transmitted Infections			
Chlamydia trachomatis (pelvic inflammatory disease)	Not stainable	Aerobic	Intracellular
Neisseria gonorrhoeae (urethritis)	Gram −	Aerobic	Facultative intracellular
Treponema pallidum (spirochete; syphilis)	Gram −	Aerobic	Extracellular
Skin and Wound Infections			
Bacillus anthracis (cutaneous anthrax)	Gram +	Facultative anaerobic	Extracellular
Borrelia burgdorferi (Lyme disease; spirochete)	Gram −	Aerobic	Extracellular

TABLE 9.4 Examples of Common Bacterial Infections—cont'd

Microorganism	Gram Stain	Respiratory Pathway	Intracellular or Extracellular
Clostridium tetani (tetanus)	Gram +	Anaerobic	Extracellular
Clostridium perfringens (gas gangrene)	Gram +	Anaerobic	Extracellular
Mycobacterium leprae (leprosy)	Gram + (weakly)	Aerobic	Extracellular
Pseudomonas aeruginosa	Gram –	Aerobic	Extracellular
Rickettsia prowazekii (rickettsia; typhus)	Gram –	Aerobic	Obligate intracellular
Staphylococcus aureus	Gram +	Facultative anaerobic	Extracellular
Streptococcus pyogenes (group A)	Gram +	Facultative anaerobic	Extracellular
Eye Infections			
Chlamydia trachomatis (conjunctivitis)	Not stainable	Aerobic	Obligate intracellular
Haemophilus aegyptius (pink eye)	Gram —	Facultative anaerobic	Extracellular
Zoonotic Infections			
Bacillus anthracis (anthrax)	Gram +	Facultative anaerobic	Extracellular
Brucella abortus (brucellosis, also called undulant fever)	Gram –	Aerobic	Intracellular
Borrelia burgdorferi (spirochete; Lyme disease)	Gram –	Aerobic	Extracellular
Listeria monocytogenes	Gram +	Aerobic	Intracellular
Rickettsia rickettsii (rickettsia; Rocky Mountain spotted fever)	Gram –	Aerobic	Obligate intracellular
Rickettsia prowazekii (rickettsia; typhus)	Gram –	Aerobic	Obligate intracellular
Yersinia pestis (plague)	Gram –	Facultative anaerobic	Extracellular
Nosocomial Infections			
Enterococcus faecalis	Gram +	Facultative anaerobic	Extracellular
Enterococcus faecium	Gram +	Facultative anaerobic	Extracellular
Escherichia coli (cystitis)	Gram –	Facultative anaerobic	Extracellular
Pseudomonas aeruginosa	Gram –	Obligate anaerobic	Extracellular
Staphylococcus aureus	Gram +	Facultative anaerobic	Extracellular
Staphylococcus epidermidis	Gram +	Facultative anaerobic	Extracellular

TABLE 9.5 Comparison of Exotoxin and Endotoxin

Exotoxin	Endotoxin
Gram-negative and gram-positive microorganisms	Gram-negative microorganisms
A secreted protein	An integral part of cell wall
Highly antigenic	Poorly antigenic
Can be converted to a toxoid (made harmless) and remains antigenic and can be used for a vaccine (e.g., diphtheria or tetanus).	Cannot be converted to a toxoid

(ROS). These cytokines can cause fever, activate platelets, and promote intravascular coagulation or increase capillary permeability sufficient to permit escape of large volumes of plasma into surrounding tissue contributing to hypotension and, in severe cases, cause septic shock and or multiple organ failure with increased risk for mortality[2] (see Chapter 26).

Viral Infection

Viral diseases are common afflictions of humans and range from the common cold to cancers and acquired immunodeficiency syndrome (AIDS). Examples of human diseases caused by specific viruses are listed in Table 9.6. Viruses are obligatory intracellular microbes consisting of nucleic acid protected from the environment by a protein shell, the capsid. The viral genome can be double-stranded deoxyribonucleic acid (dsDNA), single-stranded DNA (ssDNA), double-stranded ribonucleic acid RNA (dsRNA), or single-stranded RNA (ssRNA). Viral replication depends totally on their ability to infect a permissive host cell—a cell that cannot resist viral invasion and replication.

Viral pathogens directly destroy or damage cells as part of their replication in infected cells. Transmission is usually from one infected individual to an uninfected individual by aerosols of respiratory tract fluids, contact with infected blood, sexual contact, transmission from an animal reservoir (zoonotic infection), or through a vector, such as mosquitoes. The viral life cycle is completely intracellular and involves several steps:

1. *Attachment* to a specific receptor on the target cell. The specificity of the virus-receptor attachment dictates the range of host cells that a particular virus will infect and therefore the clinical symptoms that reflect the alteration of the function or destruction of the specific infected cells.
2. *Penetration* (entrance into the cell by endocytosis or membrane fusion).
3. *Uncoating* is the release of viral nucleic acid from the viral capsid by viral or host enzymes.

DID YOU KNOW?

Staphylococcus aureus *Infections*

Different strains of *Staphylococcus aureus* (gram-positive cocci) cause a variety of infections in different organ systems. The center photograph shows *S. aureus* in sputum from an individual with pneumonia. The particular infection may depend on the toxin produced: exfoliative toxin (scalded skin syndrome), enterotoxins A–G (food poisoning), or toxic shock syndrome toxin-1 *(TSST-1).*

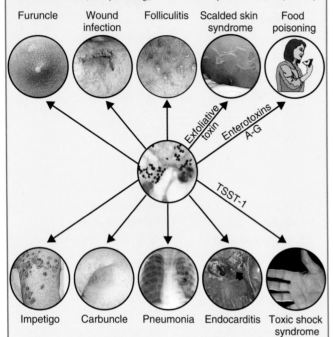

Furuncle   Wound infection   Folliculitis   Scalded skin syndrome   Food poisoning

Exfoliative toxin   Enterotoxins A–G

TSST-1

Impetigo   Carbuncle   Pneumonia   Endocarditis   Toxic shock syndrome

Toxic shock syndrome, carbuncle, impetigo, and wound infection photos: From Cohen J, Powderly WG: *Infectious diseases,* ed 3, St Louis, 2010, Mosby.
Folliculitis photo: From Goldman L, Ausiello D: *Cecil medicine,* ed 24, Philadelphia, 2012, Saunders.
Center photo and photos of food poisoning and endocarditis: From Kumar V et al: *Robbins and Cotran pathologic basis of disease,* ed 8, Philadelphia, 2010, Saunders.
Furuncle photo: From Long S et al: *Principles and practice of pediatric infectious diseases,* ed 4, Philadelphia, 2012, Saunders.
Scalded skin syndrome and pneumonia photos: From Mandell G et al: *Principles and practice of infectious diseases,* ed 7, Philadelphia, 2010, Churchill Livingstone.

4. *Replication* is the synthesis of viral proteins and messenger RNA (mRNA). The viruses inject their DNA or RNA into the host nucleus and use host resources for viral reproduction.
5. *Assembly* is the formation of new virions.
6. *Release* or shedding of new virions is by lysis or budding from the cell membrane. A select group of viruses (e.g., HIV, herpesviruses, influenza A, severe acute respiratory syndrome [SARS] coronavirus) bud from the surface of an infected cell, retaining a portion of the cell's plasma membrane (envelope) as added protection (Fig. 9.2).
   The effects of a virus on an infected cell vary greatly and often result in destruction of the cell.[3] These destructive processes can include cessation of DNA, RNA, and protein synthesis (e.g., herpesvirus); disruption of lysosomal membranes resulting in release of digestive lysosomal enzymes that can kill the cell (e.g., herpesvirus); fusion of host cells producing multinucleated giant cells (e.g., respiratory syncytial virus [RSV]); and alteration of the antigenic properties of the infected cell, causing the individual's immune system to attack the cell as if it were

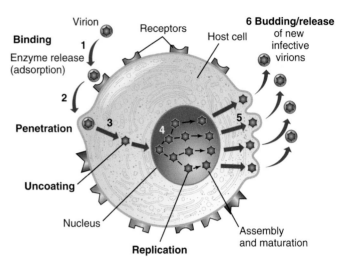

FIGURE 9.2 **Stages of Viral Infection of a Host Cell.** The virion (1) becomes attached to the cell's plasma membrane by absorption; (2) releases enzymes that weaken the membrane and allow it to penetrate the cell; (3) uncoats itself; (4) replicates; (5) matures forming new virions; and (6) escapes from the cell by budding or release from the plasma membrane. The virons can then spread to other host cells.

foreign (e.g., hepatitis B virus). Alternatively, there are viruses that cause transformation of host cells into cancerous cells resulting in uninhibited and unregulated growth (e.g., human papillomavirus [HPV]), or promote secondary bacterial infection in tissues damaged by viruses (e.g., RSV and influenza viruses).

Some viruses bypass intracellular defenses and hide within cells and away from normal inflammatory or immune responses in a process called *viral latency* (e.g., varicella zoster virus, HPV, and HIV). Varicella zoster virus (which causes chickenpox) will enter a latency phase and spread from mucosal and epidermal sites to remain dormant in the dorsal root ganglion. Later in life and in response to stimuli, such as stress, hormonal changes, or disease, the virus may exit latency and enter a productive cycle causing herpes zoster (shingles) or postherpetic neuralgia.

Viruses also can elude the immune system by making small changes to the genes that produce viral surface antigens, a process known as antigenic variation. The influenza A virus is a good example of how a virus uses this process to escape immune defenses. Influenza A virus has two surface glycoproteins known as hemagglutinin (HA) and neuraminidase (NA) antigens, which are the receptors for attachment to human target cells. Antibodies against these antigens are responsible for protection against influenza infection. Infections are seasonal, and vaccine protection gained from the previous year's infection does not totally protect against influenza in the following year because the HA and NA antigens undergo yearly change. Antigenic variation is usually relatively minor, known as antigenic drift, and results from the combination of two different strains of a virus to make a new virus. Individuals frequently have partial protection resulting from the previous year's infection or vaccination, which lessens the clinical effects or severity of the disease. A virus periodically undergoes a sudden major antigenic change known as antigenic shift (Fig. 9.3). Two or more different viruses combine to form a new strain having a mixture of surface antigens of the two or more original strains. For example, influenza A can infect birds and mammals, and shifts occur in animals coinfected by a human and an avian strain of influenza. The genome undergoes recombination, during which the human virus obtains a new HA or NA antigen. When an antigenic shift occurs, previous protection by vaccination may not

TABLE 9.6 Examples of Human Diseases Caused by Specific Viruses

Baltimore Classification	Family	Virus	Envelope	Main Route of Transmission	Disease
dsDNA	Adenoviruses	Adenovirus	No	Droplet contact	Acute febrile pharyngitis
	Herpesviruses	Herpes simplex virus type 1 (HSV-1)	Yes	Direct contact with saliva or lesions	Lesions in mouth, pharynx, conjunctivitis
		Herpes simplex virus type 2 (HSV-2)	Yes	Sexually, contact with lesions during birth	Sores on labia, meningitis in children
		Herpes simplex virus type 8 (HSV-8)	Yes	Sexually (?), body fluids	Kaposi sarcoma
		Epstein-Barr virus (EBV)	Yes	Saliva	Mononucleosis, Burkitt lymphoma
		Cytomegalovirus (CMV)	Yes	Body fluids, mother's milk, transplacental	Mononucleosis, congenital infection
		Varicella-zoster virus (VZV)	Yes	Droplet contact	Chickenpox, shingles
ssDNA	Papovaviruses	Human papillomavirus (HPV)	No	Direct contact	Warts, cervical carcinoma
dsRNA	Reoviruses	Rotavirus	No	Fecal–oral	Severe diarrhea
ssRNA+	Picornaviruses	Coxsackievirus	No	Fecal–oral, droplet contact	Nonspecific febrile illness, conjunctivitis, meningitis
		Hepatitis A virus	No	Fecal–oral	Acute hepatitis
		Poliovirus	No	Fecal–oral	Poliomyelitis
		Rhinovirus	No	Droplet contact	Common cold
	Flaviviruses	Hepatitis C virus	Yes	Blood, sexually	Acute or chronic hepatitis, hepatocellular carcinoma
		Yellow fever virus	Yes	Mosquito vector	Yellow fever
		Dengue virus	Yes	Mosquito vector	Dengue fever
		West Nile virus	Yes	Mosquito vector	Meningitis, encephalitis
	Togaviruses	Rubella virus	Yes	Droplet contact, transplacental	Acute or congenital rubella
	Coronaviruses	SARS	Yes	Droplets in aerosol or direct contact	Severe respiratory tract disease
	Caliciviruses	Norovirus	No	Fecal–oral	Gastroenteritis
ssRNA–	Orthomyxoviruses	Influenza virus	Yes	Droplet contact	Influenza
	Paramyxoviruses	Measles virus	Yes	Droplet contact	Measles
		Mumps virus	Yes	Droplet contact	Mumps
		Parainfluenza virus	Yes	Droplet contact	Croup, pneumonia, common cold
		Respiratory syncytial virus (RSV)	Yes	Droplet contact, hand-to-mouth	Pneumonia, influenza-like syndrome
	Rhabdoviruses	Rabies virus	Yes	Animal bite, droplet contact	Rabies
	Bunyaviruses	Hantavirus	Yes	Aerosolized animal fecal material	Viral hemorrhagic fever
	Filoviruses	Ebola virus	Yes	Direct contact with body fluids	Viral hemorrhagic fever
		Marburg virus	Yes	Direct contact with body fluids	Viral hemorrhagic fever
	Arenavirus	Lassa virus	Yes	Aerosolized animal fecal material	Viral hemorrhagic fever
ssRNA+ with RT	Retroviruses	HIV	Yes	Sexually, blood products	AIDS
dsDNA with RT	Hepadnaviruses	Hepatitis B virus	Yes	All body fluids	Acute or chronic hepatitis, hepatocellular carcinoma

AIDS, Acquired immunodeficiency syndrome; *DNA*, deoxyribonucleic acid; *ds*, double-stranded; *HIV*, human immunodeficiency virus; *RNA*, ribonucleic acid; *RT*, reverse transcriptase; *SARS*, severe acute respiratory syndrome; *ss*, single-stranded.

exist, resulting in a major pandemic (an epidemic that spreads over a large area, such as a continent or worldwide) and much more severe disease. Such an event occurred in 2009 with the emergence of H1N1 influenza ("swine flu"). These infections are monitored closely by such agencies as the Centers for Disease Control and Prevention (CDC) in Atlanta, Georgia, and the World Health Organization (WHO) in Geneva, Switzerland, with recommendations for prevention using the most current vaccines.

Generally, viruses rarely produce toxins or other destructive products that cause tissue damage, and the severity of clinical symptoms is secondary to the level of cytokines produced by the infected cells or in response to death of the cells. In most cases, the symptoms of viral infection (e.g., fever, aches, nausea) are generally mild, caused by the individual's own inflammatory response to infection, and usually resolve in a relatively short time. However, more severe local cellular effects may result from destruction of infected cells by lymphocytes. For example, the dermal and ocular lesions of herpes simplex virus infection result from T cell–mediated cytotoxicity of epithelial cells. Many viruses induce excessive production of proinflammatory cytokines and reactive oxygen species, all of which contribute to tissue damage. Severe systemic illness

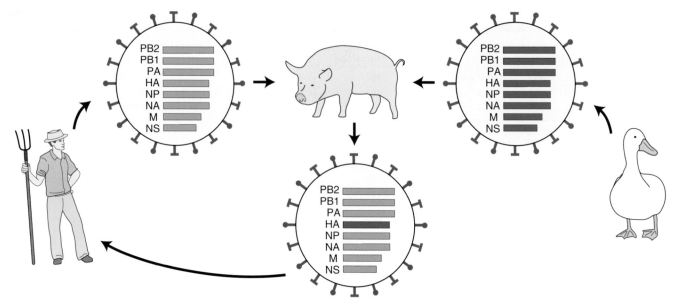

FIGURE 9.3 Antigenic Shifts in Influenza Virus. One theory proposes that antigenic shifts occur when a human influenza virus *(blue)* and an avian influenza virus *(red)* coinfect a species that is permissive for both. The eight single-stranded ribonucleic acid (ssRNA) strands are coexpressed in the same infected cell, resulting in mixing of the strands so that a hybrid virus can be produced. The hybrid virus indicated here contains all the genetic information of the original virus that infected humans but also contains a new hemagglutinin *(HA)*–containing stand from the avian virus. This virus expresses a new HA antigen and will be less susceptible to residual immunity that normally provides partial protection against yearly influenza infections.

also can occur in viral infection resulting in significant morbidity and mortality (e.g., influenza pneumonia, HIV).

Fungal Infection

Fungi are relatively large eukaryotic microorganisms with thick walls that have one of two basic structures: single-celled yeasts (spheres) or multicellular molds (filaments or hyphae) (Fig. 9.4). Some fungi can exist in either form and are called dimorphic fungi. They usually reproduce by simple division or budding. The cell walls of fungi are rigid and multilayered and composed of polysaccharides different from the peptidoglycans of bacteria. The lack of peptidoglycans allows fungi to resist the action of bacterial cell wall inhibitors, such as penicillin and cephalosporin. Molds are aerobic and yeasts are facultative anaerobes, which can adapt to anaerobic conditions.

Infections caused by fungi are called mycoses. Mycoses can be superficial, deep, or opportunistic. Superficial mycoses occur on or near skin or mucous membranes and usually produce mild and superficial disease. Fungi that invade the skin, hair, or nails are known as dermatophytes. The diseases they produce are called *tineas* (ringworm), for example, tinea capitis (scalp), tinea pedis (feet), and tinea cruris (groin). Chapter 43 discusses the various skin disorders caused by fungi.

Pathologic fungi cause disease by adapting to the host environment. Phagocytes and T lymphocytes are important in controlling fungi. Low white blood cell counts promote fungal infection, and infection control is particularly important for individuals who are immunosuppressed. Common pathologic fungi are summarized in Table 9.7.

By mechanisms similar to those described for bacteria, pathologic fungal infections damage tissue directly by secretion of enzymes and indirectly by initiation of an inflammatory response. Several toxins secreted by molds in the environment cause disease without fungal infection. Mycotoxins are produced by molds that grow on nuts, beans, and grains. Ingestion of these toxins affect muscle

coordination, causes tremors, and may be fatal. Other fungal toxins may cause cancer; aflatoxins produced by some *Aspergillus* species are especially carcinogenic.

C. albicans is the most common cause of fungal infections in humans. It is an opportunistic yeast that is a commensal inhabitant in the normal microbiome of many healthy individuals, residing in the skin, gastrointestinal tract, mouth, and vagina. *C. albicans* is normally under the control of local defense mechanisms, including members of the bacterial microbiome that produce antifungal agents. In healthy individuals antibiotic therapy can diminish the microbiome (e.g., diminished levels of *Lactobacillus* in the gastrointestinal or vaginal microbiome). *Candida* overgrowth may occur, resulting in localized infection, such as vaginitis or oropharyngeal infection (thrush).

In immunocompromised individuals, particularly those with diminished levels of neutrophils (neutropenia), disseminated infection may occur. *Candida* is the most common fungal infection in people with cancer (particularly acute leukemia and other hematologic cancers), transplantation (bone marrow and solid organ), and HIV/AIDS. Invasive candidiasis also may be secondary to indwelling catheters, intravenous lines, or peritoneal dialysis, which provides direct entrance into the bloodstream.

Disseminated candidiasis may involve deep infections of several internal organs, including abscesses in the kidney, brain, liver, and heart, and is characterized by persistent or recurrent fever, gram-negative shock-like symptoms (hypotension, tachycardia), and disseminated intravascular coagulation (DIC). The mortality rate among individuals with septic or disseminated candidiasis is about 30%.[4]

Parasitic Infection

Parasitic microorganisms establish a relationship in which the parasite benefits at the expense of the other species. Parasites range from a unicellular protozoan to large worms. Parasitic worms (helminths) include intestinal and tissue nematodes (e.g., hookworm, roundworm),

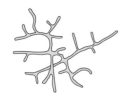

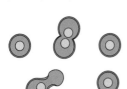

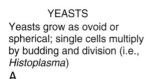

MOLDS
Filamentous fungi grow as multinucleate, branching hyphae, forming a mycelium (i.e., ringworm)

YEASTS
Yeasts grow as ovoid or spherical; single cells multiply by budding and division (i.e., *Histoplasma*)

A

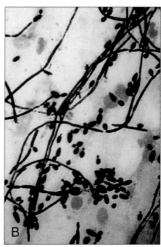

B

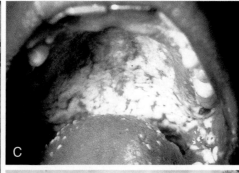

C

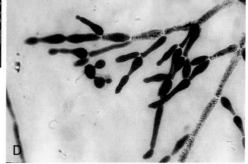

D

FIGURE 9.4 Morphology of Fungi. **A,** Fungi may occur in either mold or yeast forms, or they may be dimorphic. **B,** Photograph showing *Candida albicans* with both the mycelial and the yeast forms. **C,** Oral infection with *C. albicans* (candidiasis, i.e., thrush). **D,** Gram staining of sputum showing that clinical isolates of *C. albicans* present as chains of elongated budding yeasts (×1000). (**A, B,** from Goering R et al: *Mims' medical microbiology,* ed 5, London, 2013, Saunders. **C,** from McPherson R, Pincus M: *Henry's clinical diagnosis and management by laboratory methods,* ed 22, Philadelphia, 2012, Saunders; **D,** Courtesy of Dr. Stephen Raffanti.)

TABLE 9.7 Common Pathogenic Fungi

Primary Site of Infection	Fungus	Disease (Primary)	Symptoms
Superficial (no tissue invasion, little inflammation)	*Malassezia furfur*	Tinea versicolor, seborrheic dermatitis, dandruff	Red rash on body
Cutaneous (no tissue invasion, inflammatory response)	Dermatophytes	Tinea pedis (athlete's foot)	Scaling, fissures, pruritus
	Trichophyton mentagrophytes	Tinea cruris (jock itch)	Rash, pruritus
	Trichophyton rubrum	Tinea corporis (ringworm)	Lesion, raised border, scaling
	Microsporum canis		
	Candida albicans	Cutaneous candidiasis	Lesions in most areas of skin, mucous membranes, thrush, vaginal infection
Subcutaneous (tissue invasion)	*Sporothrix schenckii*	Sporotrichosis	Ulcers or abscesses on skin and other organ systems
Systemic (dimorphic; causes disease in healthy individuals)	*Stachybotrys chartarum,* or "black mold"	Black mold disease	Rash, headaches, nausea, pain
	Coccidioides immitis	Coccidioidomycosis	Valley fever, flulike symptoms
	Histoplasma capsulatum	Histoplasmosis	Lung, flu-like symptoms, disseminates to multiple organs, eye
	Blastomyces dermatitidis	Blastomycosis	Flulike symptoms, chest pains
Systemic (opportunistic)	*Aspergillus fumigatus, Aspergillus flavus*	Aspergillosis	Invasive to lungs and other organs
	Pneumocystis jiroveci	Pneumocystis pneumonia (PCP)	Pneumonia
	Cryptococcus neoformans	Cryptococcosis	Pneumonia-like illness, skin lesions, disseminates to brain, meningitis
	Candidia albicans	Systemic candidiasis	Sepsis, endocarditis, meningitis

TABLE 9.8   Examples of Human Diseases Caused by Parasites

Category	Subgroup	Species	Disease	Organs Affected/Symptoms
Protozoa	Ameboid	Entamoeba histolytica	Amebiasis	Dysentery, liver abscess
	Flagellate	Giardia lamblia	Giardiasis*	Diarrhea
		Trichomonas vaginalis	Trichomoniasis	Inflammation of reproductive organs
		Trypanosoma cruzi, Trypanosoma brucei	Chagas disease: African sleeping sickness	Generalized, blood and lymph nodes, progressing to cardiac and central nervous system
	Ciliate	Balantidium coli	Balantidiasis	Small intestines, invasion of colon, diarrhea
	Sporozoa (nonmotile)	Cryptosporidium parvum, Cryptosporidium hominis	Cryptosporidiosis*	Intestine, diarrhea
		Plasmodium spp.	Malaria	Blood, liver
		Toxoplasma gondii	Toxoplasmosis*	Intestine, eyes, blood, heart, liver
Helminths	Flukes (trematodes)	Fasciola hepatica	Fasciolosis	Liver destruction
		Schistosoma mansoni	Schistosomiasis	Blood, diarrhea, bladder, generalized symptoms
	Tapeworms (cestodes)	Taenia solium	Pork tapeworm	Encysts in muscle, brain, liver
	Roundworms (nematodes)	Ascaris lumbricoides	Ascariasis	Intestinal obstruction, bile duct obstruction
		Necator americanus (hookworm)	Hookworm disease	Intestinal parasite
		Trichinella spiralis	Trichinosis*	Intestine, diarrhea, muscle, CNS, death
		Wuchereria bancrofti	Filariasis, elephantiasis	Lymphatics
		Enterobius vermicularis (pinworm)	Pinworm infection	Intestines
		Onchocerca volvulus	Onchocerciasis	Blindness, dermatitis

*Most common in the United States.

flukes (e.g., liver fluke, lung fluke), and tapeworms. A protozoan is a eukaryotic, unicellular microorganism with a nucleus and cytoplasm. Pathogenic protozoa include malaria (Plasmodium), amebae (e.g., Entamoeba histolytica, which causes amoebic dysentery), and flagellates (e.g., Giardia lamblia, which causes diarrhea; Trypanosoma, which causes sleeping sickness). The most common parasitic infections in the United States include Toxoplasma gondii (a lifelong infection that may cause blindness, miscarriage, and central nervous system [CNS] abscesses) and Trichomonas vaginalis (a common sexually transmitted infection). Malaria is one of the most common infections worldwide and is caused by Plasmodium falciparum, a protozoan (unicellular) parasite. Important parasites of humans are listed in Table 9.8.

Many protozoan parasites are transmitted through vectors or ingested. Vectors include the tsetse fly (Trypanosoma cruzi, which causes Chagas disease, prevalent in South America; Trypanosoma brucei, which causes sleeping sickness, prevalent in Africa) and sand fleas (leishmaniasis). Water and food can be contaminated with protozoal parasites (e.g., E. histolytica, G. lamblia). Transmission of Plasmodium is through the bite of an infected female Anopheles mosquito, in which the parasite grows in the salivary gland.

The initial attachment to cells depends on the presence of the parasite in the bloodstream or gastrointestinal tract. Microorganisms in the bloodstream have surface proteins that allow them to attach to various receptors to infect macrophages, red blood cells, or organ cells such as the liver. For example, multiplication of Plasmodium occurs in erythrocytes and results in the release of additional parasites that infect other erythrocytes. Periodic (48-72 hours) lysis of the erythrocytes results in anemia and induction of cytokines (e.g., TNF-β, interferon-gamma [IFN-γ], IL-1) that provoke fever, chills, sweating, headache, muscle pains, and vomiting, Severe symptoms include anemia, pulmonary edema, and other complications causing death. Neurologic complications may result from infected red blood cells adhering to endothelium in capillaries of the brain. Most of the tissue damage caused by parasites is secondary to the release of enzymes that help invasion by destroying surrounding extracellular matrix and tissue.

ANTIBIOTIC/ANTIMICROBIAL RESISTANCE

Since the initiation of widespread use of penicillin during World War II, antibiotics have significantly prevented the spread of infections. Antibiotics are natural products of fungi, bacteria, and related microorganisms that affect the growth of other microorganisms. Some antibacterial antibiotics are bactericidal (kill the microorganism), whereas others are bacteriostatic (inhibit growth until the microorganism is destroyed by the individual's own protective mechanisms). The mechanisms of action of most antibiotics are (1) inhibition of the function or production of the cell wall/membrane, (2) prevention of protein synthesis, (3) blockage of DNA replication, or (4) interference with folic acid metabolism (Table 9.9). Because viruses use the enzymes of the host's cells, there has been far less success in developing antiviral antibiotics.

Immediately after antibiotics became widely used, antibiotic-resistant microorganisms were observed. Antibiotic-resistant infections develop yearly in > 2 million individuals, resulting in > 23,000 deaths. Antibiotic resistance to a single antibiotic has rapidly progressed to multiple-antibiotic resistance. The CDC released a lengthy document titled Antibiotic Resistance Threats in the United States, 2013, in which 18 pathogens were sorted into "Urgent Threats," "Serious Threats," and "Concerning Threats."[5] The most urgent threats are C. difficile, carbapenem (an "antibiotic of last resort" against penicillin-resistant organisms), resistant Enterobacteriaceae species (i.e., Klebsiella and E. coli), and drug-resistant N. gonorrhoeae.

Many other infections considered routine and easily treatable with penicillin are now resistant to almost all currently available antibiotics, including methicillin-resistant Staphylococcus aureus [MRSA] and Streptococcus pneumoniae, which causes pneumonia, meningitis, and acute otitis media (middle ear infection). Additionally, there are major increases in resistant Salmonella typhi (typhoid fever), Shigella (bloody diarrhea), Acinetobacter (pneumonia), Campylobacter (bloody diarrhea), Enterococcus (sepsis, wound infection, urinary tract infection), Pseudomonas aeruginosa (burn infection, sepsis), and M. tuberculosis (tuberculosis).[6] Antibiotic-resistant fungi (e.g., fluconazole-resistant C. albicans)

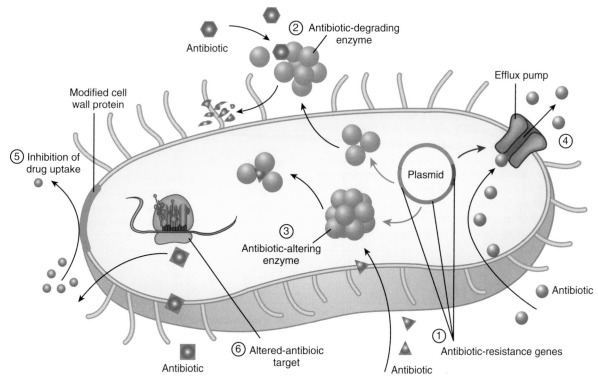

FIGURE 9.5 Mechanisms of Antibiotic Resistance. Mechanisms of antibiotic resistance include the following. **(1)** Resistance genes that are spread within the bacterial community by horizontal gene transfer to other generations of microbes. **(2)** Antibiotics are degraded by enzymes released from the microbe. **(3)** Antibiotics are altered by enzymes within the microbe. **(4)** Antibiotics are ejected from inside the microbe by efflux pumps in the cell membrane. **(5)** The cell wall can be modified to prevent antibiotic binding or uptake. **(6)** Modification of the cellular target of the antibiotic.

TABLE 9.9 Chemicals or Antimicrobials Identified That Prevent Growth of or Destroy Microorganisms	
Mechanism of Action	**Agents**
Inhibits synthesis of cell wall	Penicillins, cephalosporins, monobactams, carbapenems, vancomycin, bacitracin, cycloserine, fosfomycin
Cell membrane inhibitors	Amphotericin, ketoconazole, polymycin
Damages cytoplasmic membrane	Polymyxins, polyene antifungals, imidazoles
Alters metabolism of nucleic acid	Quinolones, rifampin, nitrofurans, nitroimidazoles
Inhibits protein synthesis	Aminoglycosides, tetracyclines, chloramphenicol, macrolides, clindamycin, spectinomycin
Inhibits folic acid synthesis (needed for protein synthesis)	Sulfonamides, trimethoprim
Alters energy metabolism	Trimethoprim, dapsone, isoniazid

Adapted from Visovsky CG et al: *Introduction to Clinical Pharmacology,* ed 9, St Louis, 2019, Elsevier.

have evolved and malarial parasites have recently developed broad drug resistance, including to chloroquine—the previous mainstay of the preventive and therapeutic arsenal of antimalarial drugs.

Microbes can use various mechanisms to resist or inactivate antibiotics (Fig. 9.5). The type of antibiotic affected by these resistance mechanisms is primarily determined by how the drug enters the microorganism or its mechanisms of action. For example, an enzyme called *beta-lactamase,* which is produced by most *S. aureus* species, prevents the action of penicillin on the microorganismal cell wall. Other antibiotics, such as fluoroquinolones and macrolides, are rendered ineffective by multiple resistance mechanisms.

Why have multiple antibiotic-resistant microorganisms emerged? Lack of compliance in completing the therapeutic regimen with antibiotics allows the selective resurgence of microorganisms that are more relatively resistant to the antibiotic. Overuse of antibiotics can lead to the destruction of the normal microbiome, allowing the selective overgrowth of antibiotic-resistant strains or pathogens that had previously been controlled. There also is concern that overuse of antibiotics to promote growth in animals used for food may result in ingestion of antibiotic-containing meat.

VACCINES AND PROTECTION AGAINST INFECTION

Active Immunization

Recovery from an infection generally results in the strongest resistance to a future infection with the same microbe. Vaccines are biologic preparations of antigens that, when administered, stimulate production of protective antibodies or cellular immunity against a specific pathogen without causing potentially life-threatening disease. The purpose of vaccination is to induce long-lasting protective immune responses under safe conditions. The primary immune response from vaccination is generally short lived; therefore booster injections are used to push the immune response through multiple secondary responses that result in large numbers of memory cells and sustained protective levels of antibody or T cells, or both. Many vaccines are used in the United States, and the CDC provides updated vaccine schedules, which are available at https://www.cdc.gov/vaccines/schedules/index.html.

Passive Immunotherapy

Passive immunotherapy is a form of countermeasure against pathogens in which preformed antibodies are given to the individual. Passive immunotherapy with human immunoglobulin has been approved for several infections, including hepatitis A and hepatitis B. Treatment of potential rabies infection after a bite combines passive and active immunization. Individuals who have been bitten receive a one-time injection with human rabies immunoglobulin, or, more recently, with monoclonal antibody to slow further viral proliferation, followed by multiple injections with a killed viral vaccine to induce greater protective immunity. More specific therapy with monoclonal antibodies is being evaluated for other infectious diseases. A monoclonal antibody against

RSV has been approved for therapy, and recently an experimental monoclonal antibody preparation is available for the treatment of Ebola virus infection. A vaccine also is available to control outbreaks of Ebola virus infections.[7]

In the past, vaccines and therapeutic antibodies were developed only for the most deadly pathogens. With the increase in antibiotic-resistant microorganisms, the development and widespread use of new vaccines and antibodies against these microorganisms must be considered.

> ✔ **QUICK CHECK 9.2**
> 1. How do antigenic changes in viral pathogens promote disease?
> 2. What are three mechanisms pathogens use to block the immune system?
> 3. What is the difference between an endotoxin and an exotoxin?
> 4. How do bacteria develop antibiotic resistance?

SUMMARY REVIEW

Microorganisms and Humans: a Dynamic Relationship

1. Infectious disease is a significant cause of morbidity and mortality in the United States and worldwide.
2. Pathogens have unique characteristics that influence their ability to overcome body defense mechanisms and cause disease.
3. The process of infection includes encounter and transmission, colonization, invasion, dissemination, and cellular or tissue damage by the pathogenic microorganisms.
4. There are four distinct stages of infection: incubation period, prodromal stage, invasion or acute illness stage, and convalescence.

Infectious Disease

1. Bacteria have virulence factors that promote their ability to cause infection and cell injury, including pili, flagella, capsules, enzymes, competition for iron, and toxins.
2. Bacteria produce exotoxins or endotoxins. Exotoxins are enzymes that can damage the plasma membranes of host cells or can inactivate enzymes critical to protein synthesis, and endotoxins activate the inflammatory response and produce fever.
3. Septicemia results from the proliferation of bacteria in blood. Toxins released by bloodborne bacteria cause the release of vasoactive enzymes that increase the permeability of blood vessels. Leakage from vessels causes hypotension that can result in septic shock.
4. Viruses are intracellular parasites. They enter host cells and use their metabolic processes to proliferate and cause disease.
5. Viruses that have invaded host cells may decrease protein synthesis; disrupt lysosomal membranes; form inclusion bodies, where synthesis of viral nucleic acids is occurring; fuse with host cells to produce giant cells; alter antigenic properties of the host cell; transform host cells into cancerous cells; and promote bacterial infection.

6. Viruses can elude the immune system by making small changes to the genes that produce viral surface antigens, a process known as *antigenic variation*.
7. Diseases caused by fungi are called *mycoses,* and fungi occur in two forms: yeasts (spheres) and molds (filaments or hyphae).
8. Dermatophytes are fungi that infect skin, hair, and nails with diseases, such as ringworm and athlete's foot.
9. *Candida albicans* is the most common cause of fungal infections in humans.
10. Parasitic microorganisms range from unicellular protozoa to large worms. Although less common in the United States, parasites and protozoa are common causes of infection worldwide.
11. Parasitic and protozoal infections are rarely transmitted from human to human. Infection mainly spreads through vectors (e.g., through mosquito bites) or through contaminated water or food (i.e., malaria, Chagas disease, sleeping sickness, and leishmaniasis).

Antibiotic/Antimicrobial Resistance

1. Pathogens can use various mechanisms to resist the effects of antibiotics, including transmission of resistance genes to new generations of bacteria, enzyme degradation of the antibiotic, ejection of the antibiotic from the pathogen, modification of the cell wall to prevent binding or uptake of the antibiotic, or modification of the target of the antibiotic.

Vaccines and Protection Against Infection

1. Vaccines are biologic preparations of antigens that, when administered, stimulate production of protective antibodies or cellular immunity against a specific pathogen.
2. Passive immunotherapy is the administration of preformed antibodies for protection against a specific pathogen, such as hepatitis A and B or rabies.

KEY TERMS

Antibiotic resistance, 206
Antigenic drift, 202
Antigenic shift, 202
Antigenic variation, 202

Antitoxin, 199
Bacteremia, 199
Biofilm, 198
Colonization, 197

Dermatophyte, 204
Dimorphic fungus (*pl.,* fungi), 204
Dissemination, 198

Encounter, 196
Endotoxin (lipopolysaccharide [LPS]), 199
Exotoxin, 199

REFERENCES

1. Uribe-Querol E, Rosales C: Control of phagocytosis by microbial pathogens, *Front Immunol* 8:1368, 2017.
2. Minasyan H: Sepsis and septic shock: pathogenesis and treatment perspectives, *J Crit Care* 40:229-242, 2017.
3. Almand EA, Moore MD, Jaykus L-A: Virus-bacteria interactions: an emerging topic in human infection, *Viruses* 9(3):E58, 2017.
4. Centers for Disease Control and Prevention (CDC): Invasive Candidiasis statistics, Atlanta GA, Author. Updated January 25, 2017, 2017. Available at: https://www.cdc.gov/fungal/diseases/candidiasis/invasive/statistics.html.
5. Centers for Disease Control and Prevention (CDC): Antibiotic resistance threats in the United States. Updated November 26, 2018, 2013.
   Available at: https://www.cdc.gov/drugresistance/threat-report-2013/index.html.
6. Nguyen L: Antibiotic resistance mechanisms in M. tuberculosis: an update, *Arch Toxicol* 90(7):1585-1604, 2016.
7. Espeland EM, et al: Safeguarding against Ebola: vaccines and therapeutics to be stockpiled for future outbreaks, *PLoS Negl Trop Dis* 12(4):e0006275, 2018.

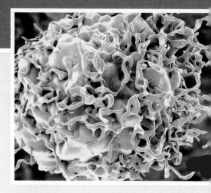

10

Stress and Disease

Lorey K. Takahashi, Kathryn L. McCance

CHAPTER OUTLINE

Stress is broadly defined as a perceived or anticipated threat that disrupts a person's well-being, or homeostasis, and exceeds the individual's capacity to meet the demands. The demands can be physical in nature (e.g., exposure cold temperatures, moving heavy equipment) or psychological (e.g., rush to meet exam deadlines, attempting to complete multiple job assignments). In everyday life, the term *stress* is commonly used to describe negative thoughts and uncontrolled feelings. Experiences that cannot be easily reconciled and threaten one's sense of security are considered stressful, and the random and constant external and internal challenges are called stressors.[1,2] Stressful events perceived as especially threatening, chaotic, and chronic are personal, such as loss of a family member, loss of job security, cancer diagnosis, physical abuse, social neglect, or feelings of social discrimination. The National Institute of Mental Health further defines *stress* in terms of how the brain responds to a demand by activating the neuroendocrine system (NES), the autonomic nervous system (ANS), and the immune system (IS). Importantly, chronic stress-induced activation of these physiologic systems has the potential to compromise recovery and predispose the individual to engage in a wide range of unhealthy coping strategies, such as foregoing sleep, eating high-calorie comfort foods, and withdrawing from physical activity. Continued engagement in these behavioral activities is linked to a number of serious illnesses, such as hypertension, depression, diabetes, and obesity. This chapter discusses the role played by the body and brain in relation to psychological and emotional stressors that promote the onset and progression of human diseases.

BACKGROUND AND GENERAL CONCEPTS OF STRESS

Traditional Overview of Stress

Walter B. Cannon used the term *stress* in both a physiologic and a psychological sense as early as 1914, and coined the term *fight-or-flight response* to describe the body's preparation to deal with threat. He applied the engineering concepts of stress and strain in a physiologic context and believed that emotional stimuli also were capable of causing stress. The physiologic reactions to stress included increased heart rate and blood supply of oxygen and glucose to muscles and the brain, elevated respiration, dilation of pupils, and inhibition of gastric secretions. It should be noted the "fight or flight" response involving the brain's perception of threat and rapid release of hormones is adaptive in protection from harm. Only when we overreact and cannot reconcile chronic threats will we become susceptible to the development of physical and mental disorders.

The concept of stress was further advanced by Hans Selye and discussed in terms of a chemical or physical change (i.e., physiologic stress, in response either to the external environment or within the body itself). Physiologic stress involves (1) enlargement of the adrenal gland, (2) decreased lymphocyte levels in blood from damage to lymphatic structures of the immune system, and (3) development of bleeding ulcers in the stomach and duodenal lining. Selye concluded that physiologic stress will impair the ability of the organism to resist future stressors and represented the hallmark pattern of a nonspecific stress response that was labeled general adaptation syndrome (GAS).

GAS involves three successive stages: the alarm, the resistance or adaptation, and the exhaustion stages. The alarm stage is the emergency reaction that prepares the body to fight or flee from threat. This stage involves the secretion of hormones and catecholamines to support physiologic/metabolic activity (Figs. 10.1 and 10.2) and boosts the immune system to thwart infection and disease. The ensuing resistance or adaptation stage requires continued mobilization of the body's resources to cope and overcome a sustained challenge. The exhaustion stage (currently described as allostatic overload; discussed later) occurs then the body's physiologic and immune systems no longer effectively cope with the stressor and marks the onset of diseases (diseases of adaptation). That is, when stress continues unabated and adaptation is not successful, body organs that are weak, such as the heart and kidney, may no longer function and lead to death.

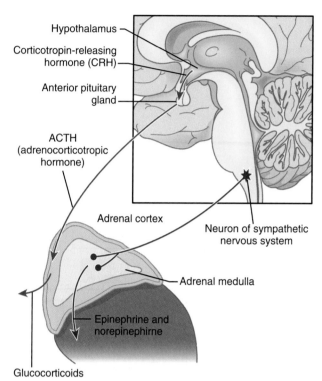

Hypothalamus

Corticotropin-releasing
hormone (CRH)

Anterior pituitary
gland

ACTH
(adrenocorticotropic
hormone)

Adrenal cortex

Neuron of sympathetic
nervous system

Adrenal medulla

Epinephrine and
norepinephirne

Glucocorticoids

FIGURE 10.1 The Alarm Reaction. The alarm reaction includes increased secretion of glucocorticoids (cortisol) by the adrenal cortex and increased secretion of epinephrine and small amounts of norepinephrine from the adrenal medulla. The response to the release of cortisol and sympathetic nerve activation is summarized in Fig. 10.2. *ACTH,* Adrenocorticotropic hormone. (Adapted from Thibodeau GA, Patton KT: *Anatomy & physiology,* ed 9, St Louis, 2016, Mosby.)

The Alarm Reaction; the Stress Response, Respectively

Although GAS is considered a cornerstone of stress research, studies in the mid-1950s began to show that psychological stressors were as effective as physical stressors in activating adrenal hormone secretion. For example, a dramatic increase in stress hormone secretion occurs when an animal is reexposed to a clicking sound previously paired with the aversive electric shock. Similarly, stress hormone secretion increases in human subjects confronted with psychological stressors, such as a stressful interview. A number of psychological factors, such as the degree of discomfort, unpleasantness, or suddenness of an unanticipated stimulus, are capable of activating the stress response.

Research from the 1970s confirmed a remarkable sensitivity of the central nervous system (CNS) and the endocrine system to emotional, psychological, and social influences. Psychological stressors can elicit a reactive or anticipatory stress response. For example, a routine medical examination involving no physical stressor may, nonetheless, elicit a reactive physiologic response, such as accelerated heart rate and dry mouth. Anticipatory responses can be generated by the fear of a potential encounter with a dangerous, unconditioned stimulus (e.g., a predator) or in conditioned situations when a person learns that a specific event is associated with an aversive outcome. A child with a history of parental abuse may show a physiologic stress response in anticipation of further abuse when that parent enters the room. Another well-known example of a conditioned emotional response is the recall of intense fear memories in posttraumatic stress disorder (PTSD). Military veterans and survivors of extreme natural disasters, car accidents, physical assaults, or rape show intense conditioned fear and debilitating responses that are triggered

by sounds, odors, visual images, or other stimuli associated with the traumatic event.

Modern Overview of Stress: Allostasis and Allostatic Overload

The emerging link between stress and disease became the basis of the concept of **allostasis**, introduced by Sterling and Eyer[3] (Fig. 10.3). This concept refers to "stability through change" and differs from the "fixed homeostasis model" in which physiologic regulation revolves around a narrow set point range. For example, after exposure to a challenging stressor, heighted physiologic secretion of stress hormones (e.g., cortisol) is expected to return to basal levels. By contrast, allostasis involves a dynamic adaptation with the brain continuously monitoring many parameters in anticipation of what the NES and the ANS system must do to meet future challenges. In other words, the body continuously adjusts its normal operating range (e.g., hormone secretion) in response to potential anticipated demands. Returning to initial basal hormone levels may not be the most adaptive strategy to cope with impending stressful encounters.

Physiologic and Behavioral Stress Responses

This active, ongoing maintenance of internal equilibrium increases allostatic load, an index of the cumulative wear and tear on the body caused by repeated activation of multiple physiologic systems over time in response to environmental demands. Chronic activation of regulatory systems has the potential to tax the body and brain and lead to the emergence of diseases and disorders. **Allostatic overload** is the term used to describe chronic overactivation of adaptive regulatory physiologic systems that may lead to pathophysiology and onset of disease. In short, frequent and longer exposures to stress accelerate the wear and tear on the body and brain (see Fig. 10.3).

Allostasis and allostatic overload are highly individualized. An event or situation considered normal in one person may be stressful to another as a result of genetic, environmental (or both), or experiential factors. The brain plays a key role in perceiving stress and determines when we have reached allostatic overload. Thus psychological or uncontrollable stress is increasingly recognized both as a precipitating factor for some diseases as well as a contributor that worsens symptoms in behavioral (e.g., anxiety), physiologic (e.g., chronic pain, asthma), or metabolic disorders (e.g., obesity, type 2 diabetes). In addition, stress disrupts the biologic process of sleep and growth and reproductive functions. In the United States, chronic exposure to toxic, allostatic overload is a contributing factor underlying early mortality (Table 10.1).

Examples of Stress-Related Diseases and Conditions

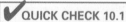

QUICK CHECK 10.1
1. How is stress related to unhealthy coping behaviors?
2. Briefly describe the three stages of GAS.
3. Define allostatic load and allostatic overload.

THE STRESS SYSTEMS

The perception or anticipation of a threat activates three major physiologic stress systems: the hypothalamic–pituitary–adrenal (HPA) axis; the sympathetic nervous system (SNS); and the immune system (IS). Acute activation of these stress-related systems modulates a broad range of mediators on the body and brain to protect and meet the physiologic and behavioral demands of the stressor to facilitate recovery (Fig. 10.4). For example, stress-induced activation of the SNS and the HPA axis triggers the release of hormones (e.g., epinephrine, cortisol),

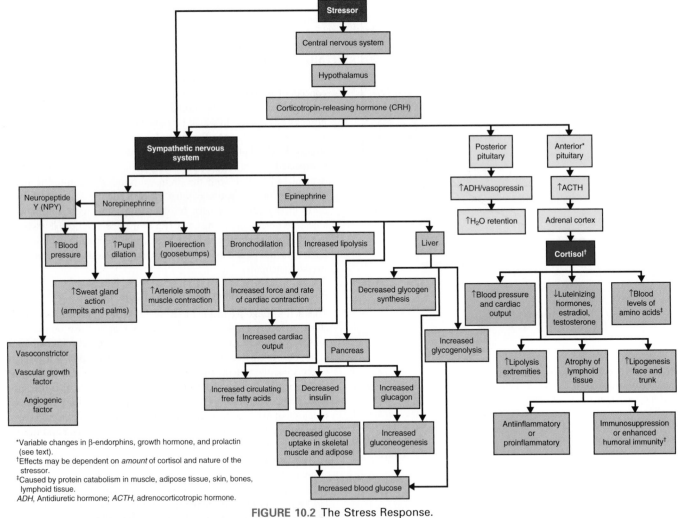

FIGURE 10.2 The Stress Response.

*Variable changes in β-endorphins, growth hormone, and prolactin (see text).

†Effects may be dependent on *amount* of cortisol and nature of the stressor.

‡Caused by protein catabolism in muscle, adipose tissue, skin, bones, lymphoid tissue.

ADH, Antidiuretic hormone; *ACTH,* adrenocorticotropic hormone.

FIGURE 10.3 Physiologic and Behavioral Stress Responses. Stress processes arise from bidirectional communication patterns between the brain and other physiologic systems (autonomic, immune, neural, and endocrine). Importantly, these bidirectional mechanisms are protective, promoting short-term adaptation (allostasis). Chronic stress mechanisms, however, can lead to long-term dysregulation and promote behavioral responses and physiologic responses that lead to stress-induced disorders/diseases (allostatic load), compromising health. (From McEwen BS: *Eur J Pharmacol* 583[2–3]:174–185, 2008.)

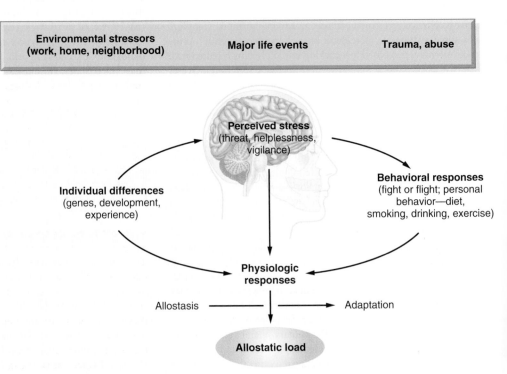

TABLE 10.1 Examples of Stress-Related Diseases and Conditions

Target Organ or System	Disease or Condition	Target Organ or System	Disease or Condition
Cardiovascular system	Coronary artery disease Hypertension Stroke Disturbances of heart rhythm	Gastrointestinal system	Ulcer Irritable bowel syndrome Diarrhea Nausea and vomiting Ulcerative colitis
Muscle	Tension headaches Muscle contraction backache	Genitourinary system	Diuresis Impotence Frigidity
Connective tissues	Rheumatoid arthritis (autoimmune disease) Related inflammatory diseases of connective tissue	Skin	Eczema Neurodermatitis Acne
Pulmonary system	Asthma (hypersensitivity reaction) Hay fever (hypersensitivity reactions)	Endocrine system	Type 2 diabetes mellitus Amenorrhea
Immune system	Immunosuppression or deficiency Autoimmune diseases	Central nervous system	Fatigue and lethargy Type A behavior Overeating Depression Insomnia

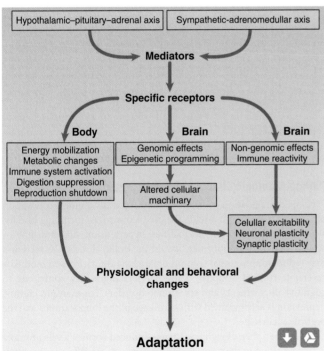

FIGURE 10.4 Adaptive Roles of Stress Systems. In response to stress, the hypothalamus activates the pituitary and adrenal cortex to secrete the glucocorticoid hormone cortisol. The hypothalamus also activates the sympathetic nervous system to release the catecholamines epinephrine and norepinephrine from the adrenal medulla and from nerve endings in the periphery. Together, the glucocorticoids and catecholamines prepare the body and brain for action and protect and keep the individual from harm with the accompanying activation of the immune system. See text for further details. (Adapted from Carlson NR, Birkett MA: *Physiology of behavior,* ed 12, New York, 2017, Pearson. Godoy LD, Rossignoli MT, Delfino-Pereira P, et al: A comprehensive overview on stress neurobiology: basic concepts and clinical implications, *Behav Neurosci* 12:127, 2018. DOI: 10.3389/fnbeh.2018.00127.)

which rapidly mobilizes resources necessary to prepare the body and brain for "fight or flight" responses to threat. In addition, both stress systems send signals to the immune system to release proinflammatory cytokines, such as interleukin-1 (IL-1), IL-6, and tumor necrosis factor-α (TNF-α). The release of these sympathetic, neuroendocrine, and immune factors has profound effects on immunity, behavior, and physiology.

Adaptive Roles of Stress Systems

Allostatic overload occurs when these protective physiologic regulatory systems are taxed by chronic, persistent exposure to threat and no longer able to adapt to the demands of the current and new stressors. Key physiologic changes involved in allostatic overload include exaggerated secretion of adrenal cortisol, catecholamines from the SNS, and proinflammatory cytokines that may initiate gene expression changes with widespread effects on neurobiologic structures and processes. Brain regions, including the hippocampus, amygdala, and prefrontal cortex, may undergo structural remodeling that alters connections between brain cells and consequently influences both the structure and function of brain circuits underlying adaptive behavioral, cognitive, and physiologic responses. Brain alterations may impact our ability to process information that promote beneficial coping strategies and instead increase the risk of developing mental illness and cognitive impairments.[1] Becoming "stressed out," or allostatic overload, may lead to sleep deprivation; elevated evening cortisol secretion; heightened insulin and blood glucose levels; increased blood pressure; reduced parasympathetic activity; increased levels of proinflammatory cytokines; and increased secretion of the hormone ghrelin (primarily by cells of the stomach and pancreas), which promotes appetite. To summarize, allostatic overload points to the damaging effects of chronic stress on mediating many disease processes.

Regulation of the Hypothalamic–Pituitary–Adrenal Axis

An essential feature of the stress hormone system is the regulation of the hypothalamic–pituitary–adrenal (HPA) axis (Fig. 10.5). Stress activates the hypothalamus to secrete corticotropin-releasing hormone (CRH), which binds to receptors on anterior pituitary cells, which, in

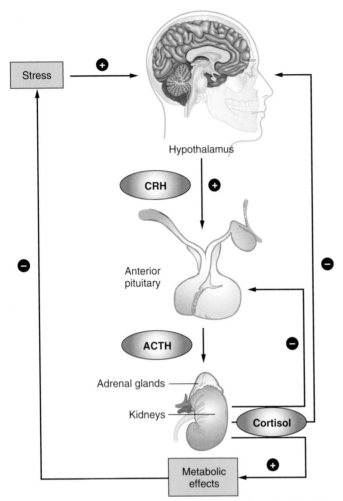

FIGURE 10.5 Hypothalamic–Pituitary–Adrenal (HPA) Axis. The response to stress begins in the brain. The hypothalamus is the control center in the brain for many hormones, including corticotropin-releasing hormone (CRH).

turn, produce **adrenocorticotropic hormone (ACTH)**. ACTH is then released into blood and transported to the adrenal glands located on the top of the kidneys. After binding to receptors on the cortex of the adrenal glands, the glucocorticoid (GC) hormone, primarily cortisol (cortisol is known outside the body as hydrocortisone), is released and reaches all tissues, including the brain.

Hypothalamic–Pituitary–Adrenal (HPA) Axis

A key aspect of the HPA axis is the negative feedback loops that inhibit further secretion of cortisol. Feedback loops between cortical and subcortical regions work together to return cortisol to allostatic levels that prevent cellular damage in the brain. Understanding the links between stress and HPA cortisol secretion are beginning to offer many insights into stress-related illnesses and health outcomes.

Notably, stressors can exert lasting effects on an organism's physiology and on the HPA axis through GC signaling that activates the mineralocorticoid receptor and the glucocorticoid receptor (GR). Stressor characteristics, including stressor duration, intensity, type, and context, has potential to alter the regulation of the HPA axis and secretion of GCs. Dysregulation of the HPA axis can be programmed in an age- and sex-dependent manner; these programming effects are linked with susceptibility to psychiatric and age-related diseases in both human studies and animal models. Furthermore, human and animal research

shows that stress and GCs may induce long-lasting alterations in epigenetic modifications and changes in DNA methylation.

Physiologic Effects of Cortisol

Cortisol reacts with numerous intracellular GRs (see Fig. 10.1) to exert diverse biologic actions. Cortisol regulates many functions including arousal, cognition, mood, sleep, metabolism, maintenance of cardiovascular tone, the immune and antiinflammatory responses, and growth and reproduction.

Cortisol plays a key role in mobilizing substances needed for cellular metabolism and stimulates gluconeogenesis or the formation of glucose from noncarbohydrate sources, such as amino acids or free fatty acids in the liver. In addition, cortisol enhances the elevation of blood glucose levels that is promoted by other hormones, such as epinephrine, glucagon, and growth hormone. Cortisol also inhibits the uptake and oxidation of glucose by many body cells. Overall, the cortisol-induced increase in carbohydrate metabolism serves to energize the body to cope with the stressor. The effects of cortisol are summarized in Table 10.2.

Cortisol has anabolic effects on protein metabolism by increasing the rate of protein synthesis and ribonucleic acid (RNA) in the liver and this effect is countered by cortisol's catabolic effect on protein stores in other tissues. Protein catabolism acts to increase levels of circulating amino acids; therefore chronic exposure to excess cortisol can severely deplete protein stores in muscle, bone, connective tissue, and skin.

Another important adaptive function of cortisol is to enhance immunity during acute stress. Cortisol exerts beneficial effects by inhibiting initial inflammatory effects, for example, vasodilation and increased capillary permeability. Cortisol also promotes resolution and repair by facilitating the actions of the GR, namely, the transcription of genetic material (through deoxyribonucleic acid [DNA] binding) within leukocytes. Because GCs are widely expressed, they influence virtually all immune cells. The adaptiveness or destructiveness of cortisol-induced effects may depend on the intensity, type, and duration of the stressor; the tissue involved; and the subsequent concentration and length of cortisol exposure.

Pathophysiologic Effects of Chronic Cortisol

Chronic dysregulation of the HPA axis, especially abnormal elevation of cortisol, is linked to a wide variety of disorders, including obesity, sleep deprivation, lipid abnormalities, hypertension, diabetes, atherosclerosis, and loss of bone density.[4] In the brain, chronic GC secretion may reduce hippocampal volume, enlarge the ventricles, and modulate reversible cortical atrophy.[4] These CNS changes may contribute to cognitive impairments and emotional disorders. For example, chronic depression is accompanied with shrinkage of the hippocampus and the prefrontal cortex.

In the periphery, heightened stress-induced cortisol levels promote gastric secretion in the stomach and intestines, potentially causing gastric ulcers, which may account for the gastrointestinal ulceration observed by Selye. Furthermore, GCs contribute to the development of metabolic syndrome and the pathogenesis of obesity by directly causing insulin resistance and influencing genetic variations that predispose to obesity[5,6] (see *Did You Know?* Chronic Stress-Induced Glucocorticoid Secretion Increases Inflammation and Insulin Resistance That Promotes Obesity and Health Issues).

The feedback mechanisms of the HPA axis sense and determine circulating glucocorticoid levels, whereas other tissues passively accept the actions of circulating glucocorticoids. Thus discrepancy in the glucocorticoid-sensing network between the HPA axis and peripheral tissues may produce peripheral tissue hyper- or hypocortisolism. High HPA axis reactivity to stress, in conjunction with increased peripheral

Chronic Stress-Induced Glucocorticoid Secretion Increases Inflammation and Insulin Resistance That Promotes Obesity and Health Issues

Chronic stress-induced HPA axis secretion of glucocorticoids (GCs) (i.e., cortisol) has diverse effects in the body and brain to promote obesity. In the brain, GCs stimulate food intake through direct actions on orexigenic neurons in the arcuate nucleus (ARC) of the hypothalamus, as well by stimulating the nucleus accumbens/ ventral tegmental (NAcc/VTA) pathways that reinforce the rewarding nature of food, especially high-calorie or "comfort foods," such as sweets, desserts, and chocolate cakes. In addition, continued secretion of GCs prevents the satiety or fullness effects of leptin and insulin by reducing the sensitivity of the brain to these hormones. In the periphery, GCs contribute to accumulation of visceral fat or white adipose tissue (WAT) by activating hormone-sensitive lipase (HSL), which enhances lipolysis and lipoprotein lipase (LPL) leading to fat storage. The increase in GRs in visceral fat and greater LPL activity serve to promote fat storage in adipose tissue. Diverse effects of GCs on the body and brain stimulate the motivation to seek and eat high caloric foods, which increase body fat and promote obesity (see figure below).

As individuals gain weight and become obese, the excessive amounts of adipose tissue begin to undergo apoptosis and activate macrophages in the traditional M1 inflammatory state. Here, tumor necrosis factor (TNF) is released, which recruits additional immune cells. When this low-grade inflammatory state continues, the fat tissues become resistant to insulin and open the pathway to developing type 2 diabetes and other health issues.

People who consume a healthy diet and engage in physical activity have small adipocytes accompanied by antiinflammatory immune cells (e.g., M2-type macrophages and CD4+ T-regulatory [Treg] cells) (see figure below). In contrast, positive energy balance and physical inactivity increases adipose tissue size with proinflammatory M1 macrophages that release proinflammatory adipokines (e.g., TNF, interleukin-6 [IL-6], C-reactive protein [CRP]). This low-grade inflammatory state accompanied by sedentary behavior increases the risk of developing insulin resistance, colon cancer, breast cancer, atherosclerosis, depression, and neurodegeneration (e.g., Parkinson disease, Alzheimer disease). Notably, regular engagement in physical activity has antiinflammatory effects that lessen the development of many of these health conditions.

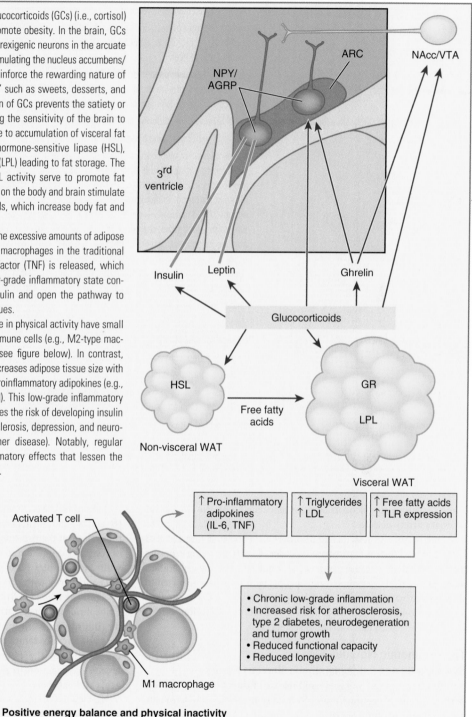

Data from: Gleeson M et al: *Nat Rev Immunol* 11(9):607-615, 2011; Odengaard JI, Chawala A: *F1000 Biol Rep* 4:13, 2012; Spencer SH, Tilbrook A: *Stress* 14(3):233-246, 2011.

TABLE 10.2   Physiologic Effects of Cortisol

Functions Affected	Physiologic Effects
Carbohydrate and lipid metabolism	Diminishes peripheral uptake and utilization of glucose; promotes gluconeogenesis in liver metabolism cells; enhances gluconeogenic response to other hormones; promotes lipolysis in adipose tissue
Protein metabolism	Increases protein synthesis in liver and decreases protein synthesis (including immunoglobulin synthesis) in muscle, lymphoid tissue, adipose tissue, skin, and bone; increases plasma level of amino acids; stimulates deamination in liver
Antiinflammatory effects (systemic effects)	High levels of cortisol used in drug therapy suppress inflammatory response and inhibit proinflammatory activity of many growth factors and cytokines; however, over time some individuals may develop tolerance to glucocorticoids, causing an increased susceptibility to both inflammatory and autoimmune diseases
Proinflammatory effects (possible local effects)	Cortisol levels released during stress response may increase proinflammatory effects
Lipid metabolism	Lipolysis in extremities and lipogenesis in face and trunk
Immune effects	*Treatment* levels of glucocorticoids are immunosuppressive; thus they are valuable agents used in numerous diseases/conditions; T-cell or innate immune system is particularly affected by these larger doses of glucocorticoids, with suppression of T-helper cell 1 (Th1) function or innate immunity; *stress* can cause a different pattern of immune response; these nontherapeutic levels can suppress innate (Th1) and increase adaptive (Th2) immunity—the so-called Th2 shift; several factors influence this complex physiology and include long-term adaptations, reproductive hormones (i.e., overall, androgens suppress and estrogens stimulate immune responses), defects of the hypothalamic–pituitary–adrenal axis, histamine-generated responses, and acute versus chronic stress; thus stress seems to cause a Th2 shift *systemically*, whereas *locally*, under certain conditions, it can induce proinflammatory activities and by these mechanisms may influence onset or course of infections, autoimmune/inflammatory, allergic, and neoplastic diseases
Digestive function	Promotes gastric secretion
Urinary function	Enhances excretion of calcium
Connective tissue function	Decreases proliferation of fibroblasts in connective tissue (thus delaying healing)
Muscle function	Maintains normal contractility and maximal work output for skeletal and cardiac muscle
Bone function	Decreases bone formation
Vascular system/myocardial function	Maintains normal blood pressure; permits increased responsiveness of arterioles to constrictive action of adrenergic stimulation; optimizes myocardial performance
Central nervous system function	Somehow modulates perceptual and emotional functioning; essential for normal arousal and initiation of daytime activity
Possible synergism with estrogen in pregnancy?	May suppress maternal immune system to prevent rejection of fetus

tissue sensitivity to glucocorticoids, is associated with the severity of coronary artery disease.

Notably, not all stress-related disorders are associated with elevated cortisol levels. Posttraumatic stress disorder (PTSD), involving exposure to a life-threatening trauma, induces a unique neurobiologic alteration in the HPA axis. For example, some people with PTSD are reported to show low urinary cortisol levels. The reduction in cortisol may reflect an adaptation of the body to protect itself from the deleterious effects of chronic, elevated glucocorticoid secretion.

The Autonomic Nervous System
Sympathetic and Parasympathetic Nervous Systems

Activation of the SNS induces rapid release of catecholamines (CAs), particularly norepinephrine, especially from sympathetic nerve terminals, and epinephrine, from the medulla of the adrenal gland. Sympathetic nerves also contain nonadrenergic mediators that amplify or antagonize the effects of adrenal catecholamines. CAs work in concert with the ANS to regulate the cardiovascular, pulmonary, hepatic, skeletal muscle, and immune systems.

The parasympathetic system balances the SNS and thus also influences adaptation or maladaptation to stressful events. The parasympathetic system generally opposes the sympathetic system, for example, the parasympathetic nervous system slows the heart rate. The parasympathetic system also has antiinflammatory effects.

CAs stimulate two major classes of receptors: α-adrenergic receptors (α_1 and α_2) and β-adrenergic receptors (β_1 and β_2). Table 14.7 summarizes the actions of the two subclasses of adrenergic receptors. (A discussion of receptors can be found in Chapters 1, 19, and 25.) Epinephrine binds with and activates both α and β receptors, whereas norepinephrine binds primarily with α receptors.

Epinephrine in the liver and skeletal muscles is rapidly metabolized. Epinephrine influences cardiac action by enhancing myocardial contractility (inotropic effect), increasing heart rate (chronotropic effect), and increasing venous return to the heart, ultimately increasing both cardiac output and blood pressure. Epinephrine dilates blood vessels to allow greater oxygenation to skeletal muscles and also mobilizes free fatty acids and cholesterol.

Catecholamines cannot cross the blood–brain barrier and are synthesized and secreted in the brain to promote arousal, increase vigilance, facilitate anxiety, and other emotional responses. The physiologic effects of the catecholamines on organs and tissues are summarized in Table 10.3.

Pathophysiologic Effects of Catecholamines

Catecholamine secretion increases proinflammatory cytokine production, which elevates heart rate and blood pressure and impairs wound healing. However, recent research indicates that chronic stress-induced increases in norepinephrine levels ultimately result in increased production of

TABLE 10.3   Physiologic Effects of Catecholamines*

Organ/Tissue	Process or Result
Brain	Increased blood flow; increased glucose metabolism
Cardiovascular system	Increased rate and force of contraction Peripheral vasoconstriction
Pulmonary system	Bronchodilation
Skeletal muscle	Increased glycogenolysis Increased contraction Increased dilation of muscle vasculature Decreased glucose uptake and utilization (decreases insulin release)
Liver	Increased glucose production Increased glycogenolysis
Adipose tissue	Increased lipolysis Decreased glucose uptake
Skin	Decreased blood flow
Gastrointestinal and genitourinary tracts	Decreased protein synthesis Decreased smooth muscle contraction Increased renin release Increased gastrointestinal sphincter tone
Lymphoid tissue	Acute as well as chronic stress inhibits several components of innate immunity, particularly decreasing natural killer cells
Macrophages	Inhibit and stimulate macrophage activity Depends on availability of type 1/proinflammatory cytokines, presence or absence of antigenic stressors, and peripheral corticotropin-releasing hormone (CRH)

*Some of these responses require glucocorticoids (e.g., cortisol) for maximal activity (see text for explanation).
Data from Elenkov IJ, Chrousos GP: *Ann N Y Acad Sci* 966:290–303, 2002; Granner DK: Hormones of the adrenal medulla. In Murray RK et al, editors: *Harper's biochemistry*, ed 25, New York, 2000, McGraw-Hill.

inflammatory leukocytes that adhere to vessel walls and promote the development of plaque.[7] Proteases released from these inflammatory leukocytes increase the risk of myocardial infarction and stroke by weakening the fibrous cap of the plaque, which can promote plaque rupture. In addition to a stress-induced increased risk of cardiovascular disease, the effects of stress on inflammatory cytokine secretion also influence depression, autoimmune disorders, and virally mediated cancers and may facilitate functional decline that leads to frailty, disability, and untimely death. Finally, stress-induced excessive levels of inflammatory cytokines during infection or inflammatory illness may activate a collection of nonspecific symptoms called the "sickness syndrome."

Role of the Immune System

The immune, nervous, and endocrine systems communicate through similar (and highly complex) pathways using hormones, neurotransmitters, neuropeptides, and immune cell products. Various components of immune system responses are affected by neuroendocrine-produced factors involved in the stress reaction. Several pathways regulate communication among these systems (Fig. 10.6).

Effects of Acute and Chronic Stress on the Immune System

Stress-induced secretion of HPA hormones and CAs by the sympathetic branch of the ANS directly influences the immune system. Immune cells have receptors for ACTH, CRH, endorphins, norepinephrine, growth hormone, steroids, and other products of the stress response. In addition, cholinergic, adrenergic, and peptidergic nerves innervate lymphoid organs, such as the thymus, spleen, lymph nodes, and bone marrow. Exposure to stress increases endogenous opiate secretion to enhance or suppress immune cell functions in a concentration-dependent manner (Table 10.4).

Lymphocytes also produce ACTH and endorphins in small amounts that influence the immune response in an autocrine (same cell stimulation) or paracrine (cell to cell) manner in ongoing immune and memory cytotoxic responses. The T-cell growth factor IL-2 can upregulate pituitary ACTH. Immune-derived cytokines have direct and indirect effects on HPA and adrenal cell functions. Thus the immune system has an adaptive role as a signal organ to alert other systems of internally threatening stimuli (e.g., infection, tissue damage, tumor cells). The release of immune inflammatory mediators (IL-6, TNF-β, interferon [IFN]) is triggered by bacterial or viral infections, cancer, tissue injury, and other stressors, which, in turn, initiate a stress response through the HPA pathway. Enhanced systemic production of these cytokines also induces other CNS and behavior changes during an acute infectious episode.

It is important to recognize that although inflammation is a normal response and considered beneficial, chronic stress accompanied by prolonged intrusive ruminations is related to maladaptive psychological functioning, which may lead to persistent immune dysregulation. Persistent stress and intrusive negative thoughts are associated with lower levels of natural killer (NK) cells and increased levels of proinflammatory cytokines, providing links among cognitive processing, the HPA hormone secretion, immune function, and disease. Chronic inflammatory processes characterized by prolonged secretion of proinflammatory cytokines include cardiovascular disease, osteoporosis, arthritis, type 2 diabetes mellitus, chronic obstructive pulmonary disease (COPD), and other diseases associated with aging. Prolonged severe stress may lead to enlargement of the adrenal gland with simultaneous involution of the thymus and lymph nodes. Chronic stress secretion of GCs impacts many immune cell functions, including decreased NK cell and T-cell cytotoxicity and impaired β-cell function. Thus prolonged secretion of

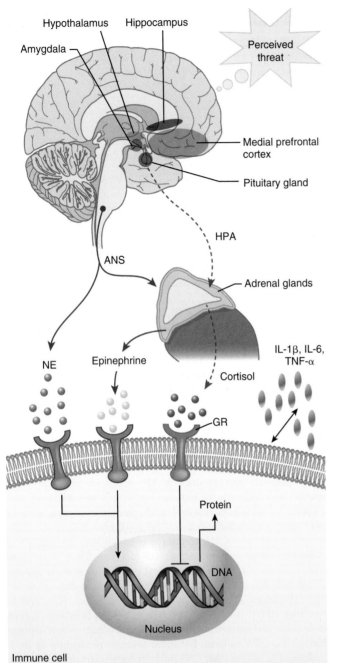

FIGURE 10.6 Neurophysiologic Pathways Linking Perceived Threat to Inflammation. Neurophysiologic pathways linking stress or threat-related neural activity in the amygdala, medial prefrontal cortex, and hippocampus with the hypothalamic–pituitary–adrenal (HPA) axis, the autonomic nervous system (ANS), and immune cells that increase inflammation. Threat perception activates the HPA axis, leading to increased release of the glucocorticoid hormone cortisol from the adrenal glands (broken lines). In addition, activation of the sympathetic arm of the ANS leads to increased release of the catecholamine epinephrine and norepinephrine (solid lines). Cortisol and catecholamines bind to receptors on immune cells to increase synthesis and release of cytokines, including interleukin-1β, interleukin-6, and tumor necrosis factor-α, which serve adaptive roles in protecting the body from disease. However, when chronic stress-induced cortisol secretion occurs, the glucocorticoid receptor (GR) becomes downregulated and limits the antiinflammatory effects of cortisol. In addition, the expression of proinflammatory genes are increasingly expressed that heighten the secretion of proinflammatory cytokines. Altogether these effects ultimately lead to elevated inflammation that increases the risk of disease. (From: O'Donovan A et al: *Neurosci Biobehav Rev* 37:96–108, 2013.)

cortisol may be an important mechanism underlying stress-related immune structure alterations, suppression of the immune response, and chronic inflammation.[6]

The elevation in inflammation levels also stems from chronic stimulation of the sympathetic nervous system and the gradual down-regulation of key antiinflammatory pathways, such as the HPA axis and the parasympathetic nervous system. Studies show that psychosocial stress-induced modulation of lymphoid and myeloid cells and chronic inflammation by cytokines, such as IL-6, are implicated in cancer progression, metastasis, and recurrence.

Stress-induced SNS release of CAs and activation of β-AR receptors are implicated in primary tumor growth and metastasis and colonization of tumors in distant tissues. In addition, stress-inducible inflammatory factors and genes, such as IL-6, are regulated by β2-AR signaling and are increased in circulation after stressor exposure. Circulating levels of IL-6, as well as gene polymorphisms of IL-6, are prognostic indicators of tumor progression, metastasis, and survival in human cancers. Importantly, peripheral immune cells, which are responsive to β-AR signaling and secrete IL-6 and other regulatory factors, reside within and around the tumor microenvironment and can promote or prevent malignant disease. Inflammatory cell recruitment into the primary tumor microenvironment may serve as a biomarker for early detection of disease progression or serve as a prognostic indicator of therapeutic success and resolution of disease.

A clear example of the adverse effects of chronic psychosocial stress is burnout, a syndrome associated with a number of negative consequences to workers' well-being and health. Work stress, especially burnout, is a significant predictor of adverse physical consequences, including hypercholesterolemia, type 2 diabetes, coronary heart disease, and hospitalization caused by a cardiovascular disorder, musculoskeletal pain, changes in pain experiences, prolonged fatigue, headaches, gastrointestinal issues, respiratory problems, severe injuries, and early mortality at age <45 years.

Potential mechanisms contributing to burnout include dysregulation of the HPA axis and ANS, which are accompanied by impaired immune function and inflammation. These interrelated stress systems, including burnout, increase the risk of adopting poor health choices (e.g., smoking, lack of physical activity and sleep, bad eating habits) that make the individual vulnerable to infectious disease, such as flu-like illnesses, the common cold, and gastroenteritis.

CHRONIC STRESS AT AN EARLY AGE INCREASES THE RISK OF DEVELOPING LONG-LASTING PATHOPHYSIOLOGIC ALTERATIONS LINKED TO POOR HEALTH AND TO DISEASE

Human brain development begins from the fetal period to the neonatal period, infancy, childhood, adolescence, and early adulthood. Throughout this developmental timespan, the brain is undergoing a host of critical changes, such as cell proliferation, cell migration, differentiation, and eventual synaptic maturation, and neuronal connections and functioning. These dynamic changes in the development of stress-responsive systems and brain structures, including the amygdala, hippocampus, and prefrontal cortex, can be significantly impacted by the effects of early stress to induce pathophysiologic alterations that are biologically embedded to increase the risk of later health and disease.

Many epidemiologic studies show that stress in women during pregnancy has the potential to adversely affect the early development of a child. Prenatal stress also increases the incidence of spontaneous abortions, fetal malformations, and preterm birth and impairs the intellectual, language, and emotional development of a child. Other

TABLE 10.4 Other Hormones That Influence the Stress Response

Hormone	Source	Action
β-Endorphins (endogenous opiates)	Pituitary and hypothalamus	• Activates endorphin (opiate) receptors on peripheral sensory nerves, leading to pain relief or analgesia • Hemorrhage increases levels to inhibit blood pressure or delay compensatory changes that would increase blood pressure
Growth hormone (GH, somatotropin)	Anterior pituitary gland	• Affects protein, lipid, and carbohydrate metabolism • Counters effects of insulin • Involved in tissue repair • May participate in growth and function of immune system • Levels increase after variety of stressful stimuli (cardiac catheterization, electroshock therapy, gastroscopy, surgery, fever, physical exercise) • Increased levels associated with psychologic stimuli (taking examinations, viewing violent or sexually arousing films, participating in certain psychological performance tests) • Prolonged stress (chronic stress) suppresses growth hormone
Prolactin	Anterior pituitary gland; numerous extrapituitary tissue sites	• Increases in response to many stressful stimuli (including such procedures as gastroscopy, proctoscopy, pelvic examination, and surgery); increased for in situ breast cancer • Requires more intense stimuli than those leading to increases in catecholamine or cortisol levels • Levels show little change after exercise
Oxytocin	Hypothalamus	• Promotes bonding and social attachment • In animals associated with reduced hypothalamic–pituitary–adrenal (HPA) activation levels and reduced anxiety
Testosterone	Leydig cells in testes	• Regulates male secondary sex characteristics and libido • Levels decrease after stressful stimuli (anesthesia, surgery, marathon running, mountain climbing) • Decreased by psychological stimuli; however, some data indicate that psychological stress associated with competition (e.g., pistol shooting) increases both testosterone and cortisol levels, especially in athletes older than 45 years of age • Markedly reduced in individuals with respiratory failure, burns, and congestive heart failure • Decreased levels occur during aging and are associated with lowered cortisol responsiveness to stress-induced inflammation
Estrogen	Ovaries	• Works in concert with oxytocin, exerting calming effect during stressful situations
Melatonin	Produced by pineal gland	• Increases during stress response; release is suppressed by light and increased in dark; receptors have been identified on lymphoid cells, possibly higher density of receptors on T cells than on B cells; suppression of lymphocyte function by trauma was reversed by melatonin
Somatostatin (SOM)	Produced by sensory nerve terminals found in and released from lymphoid cells and hypothalamus	• Natural killer (NK) cell function and immunoglobulin synthesis decreased by SOM; growth hormone secretion decreased by SOM
Vasoactive intestinal peptide (VIP)	Found in neurons of central nervous system (CNS) and in peripheral nerves	• VIP increases during stress; VIP-containing nerves are located in both primary and secondary lymphoid tissues, around blood vessels, and in gastrointestinal tract; VIP receptors are on both T and B cells; VIP may influence lymphocyte maturation; cytokine production by T cells is modified by VIP; B-cell and antibody production is influenced by VIP
Calcitonin gene–related peptide (CGRP)	Found in spinal cord motor neurons and in sensory neurons near dendritic cells of skin and in primary and secondary lymphoid tissues	• CGRP receptors are present on T and B lymphocytes; thus it is likely that CGRP can modulate immune function; CGRP may enhance acute inflammatory response because it is vasodilator; maturation of immune B lymphocytes is inhibited by CGRP; IL-1 is inhibited by CGRP, which is important for activation of T cells; it has been shown to interfere with lymphocyte activation
Neuropeptide Y (NPY)	Present in neurons of CNS and in neurons throughout body; colocalized in nerve terminals in lymphatic tissues with norepinephrine	• Lymphocytes have receptors for NPY and thus may modulate their function; several lines of evidence suggest that NPY is neurotransmitter and neurohormone involved in stress response; increased levels of NPY occur in plasma in response to severe or prolonged stress; may be responsible for stress-induced regional vasoconstriction (splanchnic, coronary, and cerebral); may also increase platelet aggregation. May be important in preventing depression.
Substance P (SP)	Produced by neuropeptide classified as tachykinin (increases heart rate subsequent to lowering blood pressure) found in brain, as well as nerves innervating secondary lymphoid tissues	• SP increases in response to stress; receptors for SP are found on membranes of both T and B cells, mononuclear phagocytic cells, and mast cells; proinflammatory activity induces release of histamine from mast cells during stress response; causes smooth muscle contraction, causes macrophages and T cells to release cytokines, and increases antibody production

studies reported increased propensity to acquire cardiovascular and metabolic disorders in later life. Prenatal stress is a predicator of low birth weight associated with a higher risk of depression during adolescence and adulthood.

Activation of the HPA axis and release of cortisol is suggested to be a major source mediating the negative effects of maternal stress on the fetus. High levels of stress-induced maternal cortisol secretion could cross the placental barrier and enter the fetus to alter brain development and the HPA axis.[8] Convincing data point to high maternal cortisol, a key biomarker of stress, during pregnancy with low birth weight. The consequences of cortisol-induced low birth weight have extended to disease risk in later life, including obesity, cardiovascular conditions (e.g., hypertension), and behavioral disorders attributed to altered brain structures. Thus exposure to elevated glucocorticoid secretion in early life dramatically compromises the well-being of the individual throughout life.

The fetus exposed to elevated levels of proinflammatory cytokines also is at risk of developing a range of neurodevelopmental disorders. Excessive exposure to proinflammatory cytokines has the potential to prenatally alter brain morphology, which compromises cognitive functioning in late life. An example is maternal obesity during gestation, which produces an inflammatory state linked to offspring neurodevelopmental alterations that predict insulin resistance, an elevated body mass index (BMI), and increased risk of attention-deficit/hyperactivity disorder.

The caregiving environment is believed to support and protect the child and buffer the potential effects of stress on altering the development of stress systems. However, allostatic overload or a chronic proinflammatory state induced by psychosocial stress in early life may result in a dysregulation of the HPA and ANS to predispose an individual to show increased hypervigilance to threat, poor emotional regulation, and increased health risk behaviors (e.g., poor dietary choices, risky behaviors). Childhood trauma involving physical, sexual, and emotional abuse or neglect is associated with psychiatric illnesses, including depression, anxiety, and PTSD and with health problems, such as rheumatoid arthritis, cardiovascular disease, metabolic syndrome, and cancer. A recent study reported that exposure to childhood trauma was associated with elevated baseline levels of peripheral C-reactive protein (CRP), TNF-α, and the cytokine IL-6 in adulthood.[9] CRP is a reliable marker of systemic inflammation, as well as a useful diagnostic marker for cardiovascular pathology. This chronic inflammatory state may be the culprit contributing to the development of mental disorders observed in adults exposed to childhood trauma.

A well-documented risk factor linked to chronic stress and poor health is low socioeconomic status (SES). Families with low SES are exposed to a host of stressors, such as financial unpredictability, household chaos and violence, noisy neighborhood, and disruption of family routines, all of which contribute to an increase in stress for both parents and children. Socioeconomically disadvantaged young children exhibit elevated levels of cortisol and mental illnesses, such as anxiety and depression.

These disorders likely originated from the effects of stress on brain development. Child maltreatment, a stressor likely to occur in low-SES families, provide support for the notion that both abuse and neglect have significant effects on brain structure and functional connectivity.[10] For example, people who suffered from maltreatment in childhood show greater amygdala reactivity to threat. In addition, functional connectivity is altered between brain areas (i.e., amygdala) responsible for threat detection and connective brain areas (prefrontal cortex) responsible for cognitive regulation of threat responses (see *Did You Know?* Early Life Stress Alters Brain Development).

Stress-induced developmental alterations in these neural circuits may sensitize the individual to thoughts or situations as threatening and increase the activation of stress systems and their negative consequences. Childhood poverty is linked with deficits in executive function through stress-related structural changes in the prefrontal cortex. Greater adolescent stress was associated with smaller prefrontal cortex volumes and poorer executive function. Stress-induced structural changes in the prefrontal cortex may impair working memory, executive function, attention, self-awareness, and inhibitory or impulse control. Overtime, the growing child may be less likely to develop cognitive, behavioral, and self-regulatory control of emotions that enable them to manage and adapt to stress (see *Did You Know?* Trauma's Effects Are Passed to Future Generations).

In children living in lower-SES households and from racial/ethnic minorities, there are neurobiologic alterations that increase the risk of age-related diseases widely linked to cardiometabolic morbidity

DID YOU KNOW?

Early Life Stress Alters Brain Development

A longitudinal study recently reported that exposure to stress in early life alters the maturation of adolescent's brains. By using magnetic resonance imaging (MRI) in children to assess how stress affects the natural pruning or culling of brain connections, different periods of development were found to be sensitive to different neurodevelopmental trajectories.

The researchers examined two life phases at ages 0 to 5 years and 14 to 17 years and collected data during the children's playtime sessions and interactions with parents, friends, and classmates, along with other factors. The amount of stress was compared with the synaptic pruning process in different areas of the brain responsible for functioning in social and emotional situations.

Researchers found that exposure to negative stressful experiences, such as illness or parental separation, occurring from age 0 to 5 years was associated with a faster maturation of the prefrontal cortex and amygdala during puberty. These parts of the brain are responsible for personality expression, decision making, moderating social behavior, and expressing emotions. The researchers suggest that although early-life stress accelerates brain maturation during adolescence, the rapidly maturing brain may compromise the normal effects of developmental plasticity, which may lead to subsequent mental and physical disorders.

In contrast, social or personal stress occurring at a later age exhibit a different developmental trajectory. From age 14 to 17 years, adolescents who were disliked by their peers showed reduced gray matter volume in different parts of the brain, including the prefrontal cortex and the hippocampus, which is responsible for memory. In addition, gray matter volume of the anterior cingulate was reduced and may be related to the higher incidence in antisocial traits reported at these ages. Callous, unemotional behavior occurring at this time may be linked to the subsequent development of psychopathy.

The study indicated that stressors can influence neurodevelopmental trajectories in different ways, depending on temporal developmental periods when the child is exposed to stress. The implication of these results is that temporal differences in stress-induced maturation of the brain may later affect different cognitive and mental health issues.

Data from: Tyborowska et al: *Sci Reports* 8:9201, 2018.

DID YOU KNOW?

Trauma's Effects Are Passed to Future Generations

Exposure to chronic, unpredictable stress in early life has a substantial, lasting effect on the physical and mental health of the developing child. Studies reported that early childhood adversity increases the risk of depression and cardiovascular-related disorders. Furthermore, children exposed to war trauma are especially at risk of developing depression, posttraumatic stress disorder, alcohol use disorders, and early mortality rates.

A recent study reported that the negative health effects of trauma can be passed from one generation to the next. This study traced the effects of war stress on women whose mothers were evacuated as children from Finland to Sweden during World War II. Women evacuated as children during the war were more than twice as likely to suffer from depression compared with female siblings or cousins who remained with their families. Of interest, however, is that the daughters of mothers who experienced evacuation to foster care during the war also required high rates of hospitalization, even though they were not exposed to early trauma. The elevated risk of mood disorders among daughters do not appear to be accounted for by maternal psychopathologic care because male offspring showed no significant intergenerational psychiatric effects.

The results showed a persistent effect of stress across generations, especially impacting females. Future work will be required to determine the underlying mechanisms linked to stress that were passed from the mother who experienced adversity in childhood to the affected daughter.

Data from: Betancourt et al: *JAMA Psychiatry* 75:5–6, 2018; Santavirta T et al: *JAMA Psychiatry* 75(1):21–27, 2018.

and mortality.[11] Chronic childhood adversity–induced activation of the HPA axis affects GC metabolism and immune function which predispose individuals to chronic inflammation, as indicated by elevations in IL-6, the proinflammatory CRP; fibrinogen; and other biomarkers associated with cardiometabolic disease. Of further interest, people living below the poverty level and have low education exhibit CRP levels nearly twice the value in those living above the poverty level.

Another consequence of childhood stress is an accelerated increase in BMI. Stress triggers the secretion of the neurohormone ghrelin, which increases appetite, food-seeking behavior, and food-associated reward. Children exposed to chronic stress also are deficient in leptin, a hormone involved in the regulation of energy balance. The imbalance in physiologic factors that normally regulate body weight likely contributes to the onset of obesity in children. Exposure to maternal stress also may increase the risk of childhood overweight/obesity, which may be caused by epigenetic modifications (i.e., DNA methylations cause changes in gene expression).

NEGATIVE EFFECTS OF STRESS ON TELOMERE LENGTH, AGING, AND DISEASE

Telomeres are DNA-based caps located at the end of chromosomes. These end-caps protect genetic information and degradation during cell division. Telomeric DNA naturally shortens with age during each replication. As telomeres shorten, cell senescence increases, and eventually cell apoptosis results.

Telomere shortening or attrition is linked to biologic aging and can be accelerated by a number of conditions associated with inflammation and oxidative stress. Shorter telomere length found in white blood cells reflects an increased risk of aging-related morbidity and mortality. Research showed that adults with telomeres in the shortest category had 25% greater early risk of death compared with those in the longest telomere category.[12] Shorter telomere lengths are found across a range of conditions in people with obesity, smoking, type 2 diabetes, and low SES.

Stress has a major influence on telomere shortening that can begin in utero by increasing early telomere damage, inflammation, and greater rate of leukocyte division. Maternal stress during pregnancy and childhood adversity are reported to impact telomere length during the periods of exposure as well as later in adulthood. Children who experienced cumulative exposures to violence (e.g., exposure to maternal domestic violence, frequent bullying, victimization or physical maltreatment by an adult) showed significantly more telomere erosion prior to puberty, even after adjusting for confounding factors. In adulthood, these individuals are at risk developing depression and metabolic disorders.

Childhood stress predicts elevated inflammation and individuals with early life stress experiences have heightened inflammatory response to psychosocial stress. Moreover, childhood adversity among older adults predicted both higher inflammatory markers and shorter telomere length in blood cells. Inflammation is also associated with increased proliferation of immune cells and, as a consequence, with more telomere erosion in those immune cells. These studies suggest a mediating effect of inflammation on telomere erosion. Another complementary mechanism is stress-induced cortisol elevation, which is associated with shorter telomere length in young children. Stress-induced secretion of cortisol may downregulate the activity of telomerase and increase oxidative stress, which, in turn, increases telomere attrition and susceptibility to develop age-related diseases.

COPING AND INTERVENTION STRATEGIES

Coping is the process of managing stressful challenges that impact the individual's resources.[13] Coping responses may be adaptive or maladaptive and the extent to which an individual responds to distress using effective positive coping strategies will determine the degree of successful moderation of the stress challenge (Fig. 10.7). Personality characteristics, such as academic achievement, motivation, optimism, and aggression are associated with differences in appraisal and response to stressors. These personality characteristics may facilitate or impede the efficacy of interventions for preventing disease and managing illness in a clinical setting.

Staying on the Good Side of the Stress Spectrum

Maladaptive coping responses to stressors, such as increased smoking, decreased exercise, and sleep, and poor diets provide an important pathway through which stressors influence the risk of disease. Constant disturbances of the sleep–wake cycle observed in many stressed people may exacerbate the pathophysiologic status of some individuals. Sleep deprivation and circadian disruption, even in young otherwise healthy individuals, have detrimental influences on respiratory and immune system function. Even partial sleep deprivation was associated with reduced NK-cell activity in healthy subjects. Altered immune functions also are found in people who cope by engaging in repressive behavior. For example, medical outpatients who exhibit repressive coping styles have lower monocyte counts, higher eosinophil counts, higher serum glucose levels, and more self-reported medication reactions.[14] School teachers who devote long hours without reward and are unable to

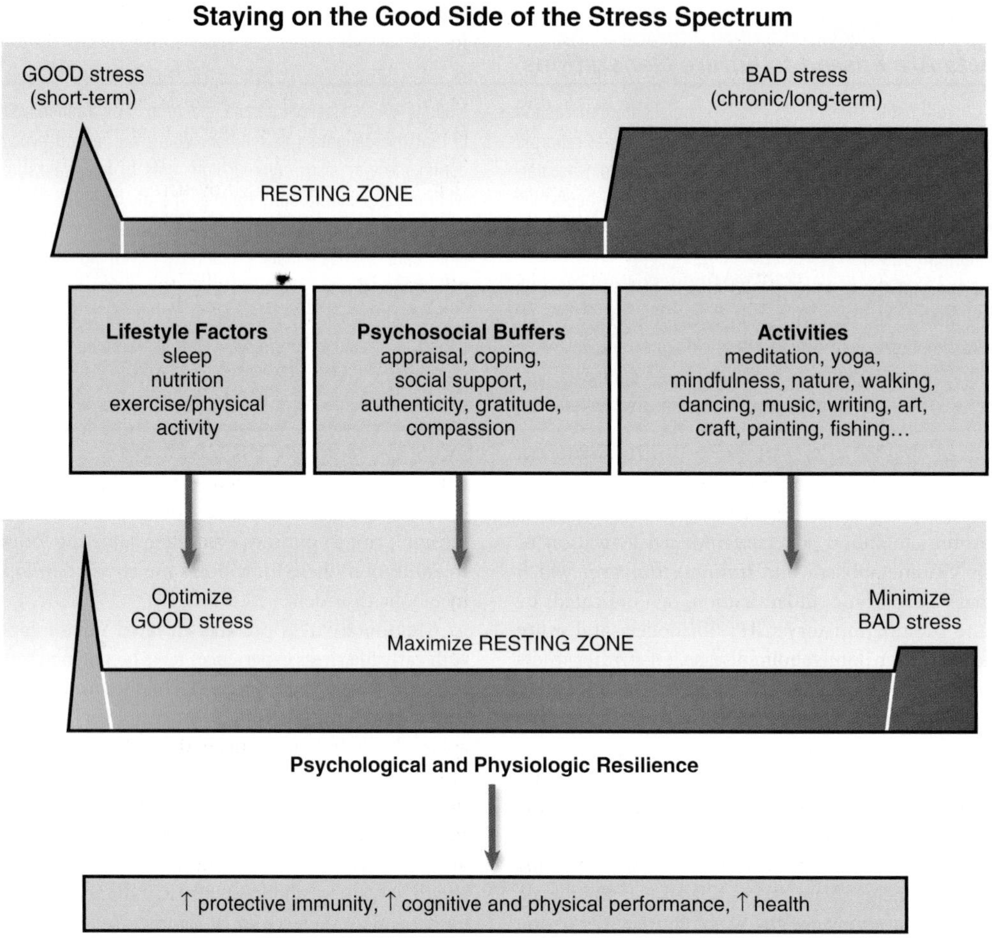

Staying on the Good Side of the Stress Spectrum

FIGURE 10.7 Staying on the Good Side of the Stress Spectrum. GOOD stress is shown on the left of the spectrum and involves a rapid biologic response to the stressor, followed by a rapid shutdown of the response upon cessation of the stressor. These responses support physiologic conditions that are likely to enhance protective immunity, cognitive and physical performance, and overall health. BAD stress, represented on the right of the spectrum, involves exposure to chronic or long-term biologic changes that are likely to result in dysregulation or suppression of immune function, a decrease in cognitive and physical performance, and an increased likelihood of disease. Short- and/or long-term stress is generally superimposed on a psychophysiologic RESTING ZONE of low/no stress that also represents a state of health maintenance/restoration. To maintain health, one needs to optimize GOOD stress, maximize the RESTING ZONE, and minimize BAD stress. Achieving psychological and physiologic resilience involves a multipronged approach. Sleep of good quality and duration that helps one feel rested in the morning, a moderate and healthy diet, and consistent and moderate exercise or physical activity are three LIFESTYLE FACTORS that are likely to enable one to stay on the "good" side of the stress spectrum. Effective appraisal and coping mechanisms, genuine gratitude, social support, and compassion toward others and oneself are likely to provide PSYCHOSOCIAL BUFFERS against bad stress and enable one to stay on the "good" side of the stress spectrum. Additionally, depending on individual preferences, ACTIVITIES, such as meditation, yoga, being in nature, exercise/physical activity, music, art, craft, dance, fishing, painting, also may reduce BAD stress, extend the RESTING ZONE, and optimize GOOD stress. Such personal activities are likely to involve different strokes for different folks and need not always be meditative or reflective in nature. (Adapted from Dhabhar FS, McEwen BS: Bidirectional effects of stress on immune function: possible explanations for salubrious as well as harmful effects. In Ader R, editor: *Psychoneuroimmunology*, vol IV, San Diego, 2007, Elsevier.)

disengage from work-related tasks also are found to have lower innate immune responses.

Coping strategies are especially beneficial when they are problem focused and receive social support. Effective interventions may result in greater stress resilience and improved psychological and physiologic outcomes. For example, women with recurrent metastatic breast cancer who attended weekly group counseling in conjunction with routine medical treatment lived an average of 19 months longer compared with control subjects, suggesting a positive influence of group support on these women.

It should be noted that social support for chronically ill individuals also affects the health of caregivers. Significant effects of stress manifested as depression, anxiety, and fatigue are found in those caring for a family member with cancer, Alzheimer disease, or burn trauma. Individuals offering chronic caregiving support have elevated levels of stress hormones and dysregulation of their immune system, which persists even after the end of the caregiving period. These stress-induced caregiver responses likely result from the unpredictable and uncontrollable nature of long-term caregiving support. However, caregivers who are offered enhanced social support appear to show improvement in behavior and in biomarkers of immune dysregulation.

Social support also can be beneficial for adults with limited education on how to care for themselves and for children who require caregiving attention. Child care requires teaching adults how to engage the young when the prefrontal cortex is developing in learning problem-solving skills, planning, and emotional self-regulation. The positive interactions between the caregiver and the child offer a way to alleviate any potential negative health effects of stress on adult and child family members.

Effects of Exercise

Coping behaviors, such as regular physical activity, can significantly enhance mental well-being and lessen symptoms of depression and anxiety as effectively as psychotherapy.[15] The beneficial effects of exercise are found at all age groups—from adolescents to the elderly. Stress-induced imbalances in brain neurotransmitters are noted in people with depression, which is associated with negative emotions, such as increased anger, confusion, fatigue, tension, and reduced vigor. Animal and human studies further indicate that maternal exercise during pregnancy has the potential to strengthen the cardiac autonomic control of the fetus that could reduce the prevalence of age-related diseases and lead to an increase in quality of life and life span.

Impairments in serotonin neurotransmission are linked to depression, which can be treated with selective serotonin reuptake inhibitors (SSRIs) in some cases. This antidepressant drug increases the availability of brain serotonin by preventing its reuptake in the synapse. A study reported that blood levels of serotonin increased in aerobic exercise participants compared with those in a control group (performing only stretching). This increase in serotonin was correlated with a decrease in depression similar to the effects of antidepressant medications. Senior men participating in a 16-week aerobic exercise regimen exhibited levels of blood tryptophan similar to elevated brain serotonin levels, which may explain the antidepressant effects of exercise in older adults.

The positive effects of exercise on depression also may occur as a result of the ability of exercise to reduce inflammation. Thus physical exercise may be improving the neuroimmune status observed in depression by reducing inflammation.

Another major benefit of exercise is to reduce not only the occurrence of stress-induced mental disorders but also obesity, a major public health problem in the United States and across the world. Because people exposed to chronic stress often seek high-calorie comfort foods as a way to alleviate stress, they are at risk to develop obesity, which is a major contributor of the pathophysiology of diabetes, heart disease, metabolic disorders, liver disease, cancer, inflammatory disorders, mental illnesses, and premature death. Obesity leads to a chronic low-grade inflammatory state caused by the activation and dysregulated production of proinflammatory cytokines (e.g., IL-1, IL-6, IL-17, and TNF) from adipocytes (fat cells) in adipose tissue. Coping with stress and obesity through exercise has the potential to reduce adipose tissue, attenuated serum proinflammatory cytokine levels, and create an antiinflammatory environment. The interplay between obesity, inflammation, and depression may be mediated through diet and exercise through the loss of adipose tissue and the restoration of adaptive immune and behavioral functions.[15]

Finally, another positive effect of exercise, especially aerobic exercise, is to enhance cognitive and brain functions. Exercise increases brain metabolism and brain structure and synaptic proteins, such as

brain-derived neurotrophic factor (BDNF). Some, but not all, studies in older adults reported associations between BDNF levels and exercise-related changes in memory and hippocampal volumes. Because the role of stress is linked to the development of cognitive and mental disorders, such as anxiety and depression, the positive effects of aerobic exercise on improving cognitive functions may be related to brain functions that are not compromised by stress.

Mindfulness Therapy

One type of cognitive therapy that is gaining increasing attention for the treatment of stress-related disorders is mindfulness therapy, which involves the personal monitoring of current experiences with acceptance; it is thought to dampen psychological and physiologic stress reactions, thereby limiting the cumulative impact of allostatic load or stress on health. Mindfulness therapy, such as mindfulness-based stress reduction (MBSR), is effective in coping with various medical conditions, including chronic pain and depression, and attenuating the negative perception of stress. MBSR facilitates a positive affect in individuals with HIV infection compared with a control group of participants over a 6-month follow-up period. Mindfulness training in adults with attention-deficit/hyperactivity disorder also improves neurocognitive deficits, such as attention deficit, and enhances emotional regulation and quality of life.

Mindfulness is believed to improve health by modulating the HPA secretion of cortisol, a primary product of the neuroendocrine stress system, with pervasive effects throughout the body and brain. As discussed earlier, chronic stress-induced secretion of cortisol is involved in a wide range of mental and physiologic health functions. A major role of mindfulness appears to return the allostatic load of cortisol to an allostatic state.[16] The neural mechanisms or stress systems linked to mindfulness training interventions appear to involve the top-down prefrontal cortical regions that modulate connected neural sites, such as the amygdala and the subgenual anterior cingulate cortex, which are activated by stress and contribute to stress reactions. In stressed adults, mindfulness was found to increase the resting state of the stress-regulatory region of the dorsolateral prefrontal cortex and decreases stress-related regions between the amygdala and the subgenual anterior cingulate cortex. These brain changes were linked to a reduction in stress biomarkers (i.e., cortisol, circulating IL-6) at a 4-month follow-up time point.

Although the majority of mindfulness interventions have focused on adults, recent research has begun to examine the beneficial effects of mindfulness on at-risk children and adolescents. These studies involving low-income urban children at risk of ongoing stresses found that school-based structured mindfulness interventions decreased negative coping behavior, anxiety, school-related PTSD symptoms, depression, and self-harm and resulted in a flatter cortisol curve. Students participating in a mindfulness curriculum also showed improvement in their sleep and self-esteem, greater well-being, and reduction in hostility. These outcomes of mindfulness classes appear effective in mitigating the toxic effects of stress in youth. The intervention of mindfulness beginning at a young age has the potential to teach valuable coping skills in at-risk children that may lower their long-term burden of disease in adulthood.

In summary, the current understanding of the role of stress in modulating the complex interplay between the brain and the body is beginning to offer promising avenues of effective interventions for health and disease. Alterations in biomarkers of stress systems (e.g., cortisol, NE, proinflammatory cytokines) are revealing insights into potential targets to address their causal basis in disease and mental disorders. However, treatments for many stress-related diseases will likely continue to be a major challenge. The young exposed to stress may have already undergone neuroanatomic, physiologic, and cognitive changes that are different from those in people exposed to stress in adulthood. The specific biologic changes induced by the length of stress exposure, the nature of the stressor, the age, sex, and genetic makeup of individual are a few of a number of factors that complicate the treatment of this disease. The dynamic nature of stress on the individual and the subsequent occurrence of chronic diseases may require early stress reduction interventions that prevent or reduce the toxic effects of stress on the body and the brain.

✔ **QUICK CHECK 10.2**
1. Define the HPA axis.
2. Define ANS.
3. How does the immune system participate in stress-related diseases?
4. Why do stress-related diseases occur?
5. What is coping, and why are some intervention activities effective in reducing stress-related diseases?

SUMMARY REVIEW

Background and General Concepts of Stress

1. Stress is broadly defined as a perceived or anticipated threat that activates stress-related systems in the body and the brain (the stress response).
2. The term *fight-or-flight response* was coined by Walter Cannon to describe how the brain's perception of threat and rapid physiologic responses prepares the body to deal with threat.
3. Cannon's view was further developed by Hans Selye in 1946 by demonstrating that internal or external stressors could result in adrenal gland enlargement, immune alterations (increased leukocytes), and gastrointestinal manifestations (ulcers). These global physiologic responses, characterized by Selye, were labeled general adaptation syndrome (GAS).
4. GAS occurs in three stages: the alarm stage; the stage of resistance or adaptation; and the stage of exhaustion. The latter stage is now referred to as *allostatic overload*. Diseases of adaptation develop if the stage of resistance or adaptation does not restore homeostasis. Although important, this approach is now thought to be greatly oversimplified.
5. Stress research continued into the mid-1950s to show that psychological stressors are as effective as physical stressors in activating adrenal gland hormone secretion. Psychological stressors can be anticipatory and triggered by expectations of an upcoming stressor or can be reactive to a stressor. Both of these psychological stressors are capable of eliciting a physiologic stress response.
6. The emerging link between stress and disease became the basis for the concept of allostasis (stability through change; monitoring the environment for adaptive response). This allostasis concept differs from a "fixed homeostasis model" (i.e., stress-induced heightened physiologic responses eventually returning to a narrow step point range) by involving a dynamic adaptation of the brain to constantly adjust its physiologic operating range to meet future anticipated demands. In other words, returning stress-induced hormone levels to prestress levels may not be the most adaptive strategy to cope with impending stressful encounters.
7. Chronic activation of regulatory stress systems has the potential to tax the body and the brain and lead to the emergence of diseases and disorders. In allostatic overload, chronic overactivation of adaptive regulatory physiologic systems may lead to pathophysiology and onset of disease.

The Stress Systems

1. The perception or anticipation of threat activates three major physiologic stress systems: (1) the hypothalamic–pituitary–adrenal (HPA) axis, (2) the sympathetic nervous system (SNS), and (3) the immune system (IS). Acute stress-induced activation of these stress systems modulates a broad range of mediators in the body and the brain to protect and meet the physiologic and behavioral demands of the stressor to facilitate recovery.

2. Key physiologic changes involved in allostatic overload include exaggerated or chronic secretion of adrenal cortisol, catecholamines from the SNS, and proinflammatory cytokines that may initiate gene expression changes with widespread effects on the body, and neurobiologic structures and processes.

3. Becoming "stressed out" by allostatic overload may lead to sleep deprivation, heightened insulin and blood glucose levels, increased blood pressure, and reduced parasympathetic activity. These physiologic consequences are often linked to insomnia, chronic pain and fatigue syndromes, obesity, metabolic syndrome, essential hypertension, type 2 diabetes, atherosclerosis and its cardiovascular consequences, osteoporosis, and autoimmune inflammatory and allergic disorders.

4. Activation of the HPA system involves sequential secretion of corticotropin-releasing hormone from the hypothalamus, which stimulates receptors in the anterior pituitary to secrete adrenocorticotropic hormone (ACTH), which, in turn, stimulates the adrenal cortex to secrete the glucocorticoid cortisol.

5. Cortisol secretion induced by stress binds to glucocorticoid receptors to activate diverse biologic actions throughout the body and the brain. The many adaptive functions include, but are not limited to, arousal, cognition, mood, metabolism, maintenance of cardiovascular tone, and effects on the immune system.

6. Cortisol's main effects involve metabolic processing by mobilizes glucose, amino acids, lipids, and fatty acids and delivers them to the bloodstream. As an example, anabolic effects of cortisol increase the rate of protein synthesis in the liver, whereas the catabolic effects of cortisol increase levels of amino acids, ultimately depleting protein stores in muscle, bone, skin, and connective tissue.

7. Chronic dysregulation of the HPA axis, especially abnormal elevated levels of cortisol, is linked to a wide variety of disorders, including obesity, metabolic syndrome, sleep deprivation, lipid abnormalities, coronary heart disease, diabetes, atherosclerosis, and loss of bone density. In the brain, chronic glucocorticoid secretion may lead to cognitive impairments and emotional disorders. For example, chronic depression is accompanied by shrinkage of the hippocampus and the prefrontal cortex.

8. Activation of the autonomic nervous system (ANS) consists of sympathetic stimulation of the adrenal medulla and nerve endings to rapidly secrete catecholamines (norepinephrine, epinephrine).

9. Epinephrine exerts its chief effects on the cardiovascular system by increasing cardiac output and blood flow to the heart, brain, and skeletal muscles by dilating vessels that supply these organs. It also dilates the airways, thereby increasing delivery of oxygen to the bloodstream.

10. The parasympathetic nervous system balances or restrains the sympathetic system, resulting in slowed heart rates and antiinflammatory effects. During prolonged stress (allostatic overload), the

parasympathetic system becomes less effective in opposing the sympathetic system.

11. Stress-induced secretion of HPA hormones and catecholamines (CAs) directly influences the immune system, which plays an adaptive role as a signal organ to alert other systems from internally threatening stimuli (e.g., infection, tissue damage, tumor cells). The release of immune inflammatory mediators (interleukin-6 [IL-6], tumor necrosis factor-β [TNF-β], interferon [IFN]) to protect the body is triggered by bacterial or viral infections, cancer, tissue injury, and other stressors.

12. Although inflammation is a normal response and considered beneficial, chronic stress accompanied by prolonged, intrusive, negative thoughts is related to maladaptive psychological functioning which may lead to persistent immune dysregulation. Chronic stress is linked to inflammatory processes and prolonged secretion of proinflammatory cytokines that promote cardiovascular disease, osteoporosis, arthritis, type 2 diabetes mellitus, chronic obstructive pulmonary disease (COPD), and other diseases associated with aging.

13. A clear example of the adverse effects of chronic psychosocial stress is burnout, a syndrome associated with a number of negative impact on workers' well-being and health. Mechanisms contributing to burnout likely include dysregulation of the HPA axis and the ANS, which are accompanied by impaired immune function and inflammation.

Chronic Stress at an Early Age Increases the Risk of Developing Long-Lasting Pathophysiologic Alterations Linked to Poor Health and to Disease

1. Children exposed to prenatal or postnatal stressors increase the risk of developing long-lasting pathophysiologic alterations linked to poor health and to disease.

2. High levels of stress-induced maternal cortisol secretion could cross the placental barrier and enter the fetus to cause low birth weight and increase the risk of disease in later life, including obesity, cardiovascular conditions (e.g., hypertension), and behavioral disorders (e.g., depression and attention-deficit/hyperactivity disorder).

3. Early exposure to psychosocial stressors (e.g., parental, sexual, or emotional abuse, low socioeconomic status [SES] or poverty) are linked to the development of dysregulated HPA and ANS leading to a chronic proinflammatory state that increases the risk of disease.

4. Early life stressors may impair brain systems that govern executive functions involved in attention, self-awareness, impulse control behavior that regulate emotions, and adaptive coping behavior.

Negative Effects of Stress on Telomere Length, Aging, and Disease

1. Telomeres are deoxyribonucleic acid (DNA)–based caps located at the end of chromosomes to protect genetic information and degradation during cell division.

2. Telomere shortening or attrition is linked to biologic aging and can be accelerated by a number of conditions associated with inflammation and oxidative stress. Shorter telomere length found in white blood cells reflects an increased risk of aging-related morbidity and

mortality and is associated with a range of conditions in people with obesity, smoking, type 2 diabetes, and low SES.

3. Stress has a major role on telomere shortening that can begin in utero by increasing early telomere damage, inflammation, and greater rate of leukocyte division.

4. Studies showed that childhood stress predicts telomere erosion and heightened inflammatory response to psychosocial stress and elevated risk of developing depression and metabolic disorders.

Coping and Intervention Strategies

1. Coping styles affect the ability of a person to handle stress. Personality characteristics, such as academic achievement, motivation, and optimism, increase likelihood of successfully dealing with stress. In addition, people who engage in coping strategies that receive social support develop greater stress resilience and improved psychological and physiologic outcomes.

2. Maladaptive coping responses to stress, such as increased smoking, decreased exercise and sleep, and poor diets, are likely to alter adaptive immune functions and increase susceptibility to disease.

3. Engagement in exercise as a means of coping with stress has beneficial effects at all ages. Exercise has the potential to rebalance neurotransmitter effects that were altered by stress. Exercise also may improve the neuroimmune status (i.e., inflammation) by inhibiting the secretion of proinflammatory cytokines. Exercise increases brain metabolism that improves cognitive functions that could be compromised by chronic exposure to stress.

4. Another major benefit of exercise is to reduce obesity, a major contributor of the pathophysiology of diabetes, heart disease, metabolic disorders, liver disease, cancer, inflammatory disorders, mental illnesses, and premature death. Coping with stress and obesity by exercising reduces adipose tissue, attenuates serum proinflammatory cytokine levels, and creates an antiinflammatory environment.

5. Mindfulness therapy is increasingly used to reduce the chronic impact of allostatic load on health. This therapy involves monitoring current experiences with acceptance and is effective in coping with various medical conditions, including chronic pain, depression, and attenuating the negative perception of stress.

6. Mindfulness appears to improve health by modulating the stress-induced secretion of cortisol by the HPA and by dampening brain regions activated by stress that play a role in the generation of stress reactions.

7. In young children exposed to constant uncontrolled environmental or psychosocial stressors, school-based, structured mindfulness interventions appear effective in mitigating the toxic effects of stress by decreasing negative coping behavior, anxiety and depression, self-harm, and flatten the elevated cortisol curve. Children receiving mindfulness interventions show improvement in their sleep, self-esteem, well-being, and reduction in hostility. Mindfulness teaches valuable coping skills that potentially reduce the likelihood of at-risk children developing chronic diseases in adulthood.

▌ KEY TERMS

Adaptation stage, 210

Adrenocorticotropic hormone (ACTH), 214, 224

Alarm stage, 210

Allostasis, 211

Allostatic overload, 211

Anticipatory response, 211

Catecholamine (CA), 216

Coping, 221

Corticotropin-releasing hormone (CRH), 213

Cortisol, 214

Diseases of adaptation, 210

Epinephrine, 216

Exhaustion stage, 210

General adaptation syndrome (GAS), 210

Homeostasis, 210

Hypothalamic–pituitary–adrenal (HPA) axis, 213

Physiologic stress, 210

Posttraumatic stress disorder (PTSD), 216

Reactive physiologic response, 211

Resistance or adaptation stage, 210

Stressor, 210

REFERENCES

1. McEwen BS: Brain on stress: how the social environment gets under the skin, *Proc Natl Acad Sci USA* 109:17180-17185, 2012.
2. Nicolaides NC, et al: Circadian endocrine rhythms: the hypothalamic-pituitary-adrenal axis and its actions, *Ann N Y Acad Sci* 1318:71-80, 2014.
3. Sterling P, Eyer J: Allostasis: a new paradigm to explain arousal pathology. In Fisher S, Reason J, editors: *Handbook of life stress, cognition, and health*, New York, 1988, John Wiley and Son, pp 629-649.
4. McEwen BS: Neurobiological and systemic effects of chronic stress, *Chronic Stress* 1:1–11, 2017.
5. Jonker MF, et al: The effect of urban green on small-area (healthy) life expectancy, *J Epidemiol Community Health* 68(10):999-1002, 2014.
6. Kiecolt-Glaser JK, et al: Psychoneuroimmunology: psychological influences on immune function and health, *J Consult Clin Psychol* 70(3):537-547, 2002.
7. Coutinho AE, Chapman KE: The anti-inflammatory and immunosuppressive effects of glucocorticoids, recent developments and mechanistic insights, *Mol Cell Endocrinol* 335(1):2-13, 2011.
8. Reynolds RM: Glucocorticoid excess and the developmental origins of disease: two decades of testing the hypothesis—2012 Curt Richter award winner, *Psychoneuroendocrinology* 38:1-11, 2013.
9. Baumeister D, et al: Childhood trauma and adulthood inflammation: a meta-analysis of peripheral C-reactive protein, interleukin-6 and tumour necrosis factor-α, *Mol Psychiatry* 21:642-649, 2016.
10. Teicher MH, et al: The effects of childhood maltreatment on brain structure, function and connectivity, *Nat Rev Neurosci* 17:652-666, 2016.
11. Danese A, McEwen BS: Adverse childhood experiences, allostasis, allostatic load, and age-related disease, *Physiol Behav* 106:29-39, 2012.
12. Weischer M, et al: Short telomere length, myocardial infarction, ischemic heart disease, and early death, *Arterioscler Thromb Vasc Biol* 32:822-829, 2012.
13. Folkman S, Lazarus RS: The relationship between coping and emotion: implications for theory and research, *Soc Sci Med* 26(3):309-317, 1988.
14. Frolkis VV: Stress-age syndrome, *Mech Ageing Dev* 69(1-2):93-107, 1993.
15. Mikkelsen K, et al: Exercise and mental health, *Maturitas* 106:48-56, 2017.
16. Creswell JD, Lindsay EK: How does mindfulness training affect health? A mindfulness stress buffering account, *Curr Dir Psychol Sci* 23(6):401-407, 2014.

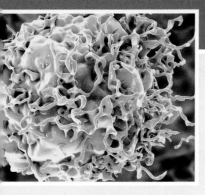

Cancer Biology

Kathryn L. McCance, Neal S. Rote

CHAPTER OUTLINE

Cancer is a leading cause of suffering and death in the developed world. Over the past 35 years, intensive research has led to a significantly enhanced understanding of this complex and frightening disease. It is now understood that cancer is a collection of more than 100 different diseases, each caused by a specific and often unique age-related accumulation of genetic and epigenetic alterations. Environment, heredity, and behavior interact to modify the risk of developing cancer and the response to treatment. Improvements in treatment strategies and supportive care, coupled with new, often individualized therapies based on advances of the basic pathophysiology of malignancy, have contributed to an increasing number of effective options for these diverse, often lethal disorders collectively called cancer.

CANCER TERMINOLOGY AND CHARACTERISTICS

The National Cancer Institute (NCI) of the National Institutes of Health (NIH) defines cancer as "diseases in which abnormal cells divide without control and are able to invade other tissues."[1] The term cancer comes from the Latin translation of the Greek word for crab, *karkinoma,* which the physician Hippocrates used to describe the appendage-like projections extending from tumors into adjacent tissue. The word tumor originally referred to any swelling that is caused by inflammation but is now generally reserved for describing a new growth, or neoplasm.

Tumor Classification and Nomenclature

The careful evaluation of each cancer is important for many reasons. Different cancers will have different causes, different rates and patterns of progression, and different responses to treatment. The classification starts with knowing the tissue and organ of origin, the extent of distribution to other sites, and the microscopic appearance of the lesion. Increasingly, it also includes a detailed description of the critical genetic changes in the cancer.

Benign and Malignant

Tumors can be benign or malignant (cancerous). Benign tumors are usually encapsulated with connective tissue and contain fairly well-differentiated cells and well-organized stroma (Fig. 11.1). They retain recognizable normal tissue structure and do not invade beyond their capsule, nor do they spread to regional lymph nodes or distant locations. Mitotic cells are very rarely present during microscopic analysis. Benign tumors are generally named according to the tissues from which they arise with the suffix "-oma," which indicates a tumor or mass. For example, a benign tumor of the smooth muscle of the uterus is a *leiomyoma,* and a benign tumor of fat cells is a *lipoma.* Benign tumors can become extremely large and, depending on their location in the body, can cause morbidity or be life-threatening. For example, a benign meningioma at the base of the skull may cause symptoms by compressing adjacent normal brain tissue.

Some tumors initially described as benign can progress to cancer and then are referred to as malignant tumors, which are distinguished from benign tumors by more rapid growth rates and specific microscopic alterations, including loss of differentiation and absence of normal tissue organization (Fig. 11.2). One of the microscopic hallmarks of cancer cells is anaplasia, the loss of cellular differentiation. Malignant

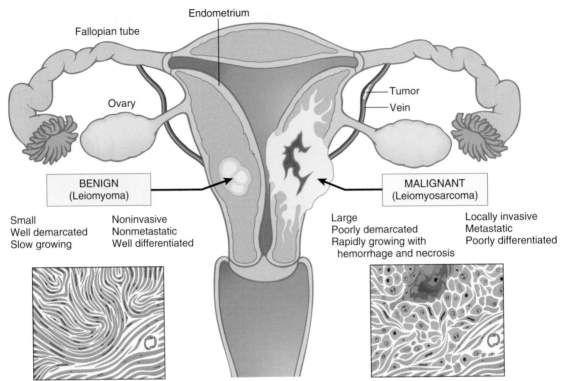

FIGURE 11.1 Comparison of a Benign Tumor and a Malignant Tumor of the Same Origin. (From Kumar V et al: *Robbins and Cotran pathologic basis of disease,* ed 9, Philadelphia, 2015, Saunders.)

cells are also **pleomorphic,** with marked variability of size and shape. They often have large darkly stained nuclei, and mitotic cells are common. Malignant tumors may have a substantial amount of stroma, but it is disorganized, with loss of normal tissue structure. Malignant tumors lack a capsule and grow to invade nearby blood vessels, lymphatics, and surrounding structures. The most important and most deadly characteristic of malignant tumors is their ability to spread far beyond the tissue of origin, a process known as *metastasis.*

Unlike benign tumors, which are named related to the tissue of origin, cancers generally are named according to the cell type from which they originate. Cancers arising in epithelial tissue are called **carcinomas,** and if they arise from or form ductal or glandular structures are named **adenocarcinomas.** Hence a malignant tumor arising from breast glandular tissue is a **mammary adenocarcinoma,** whereas an example of a benign breast tumor is a fibroadenoma. Cancers arising from mesenchymal tissue (including connective tissue, muscle, and bone) usually have the suffix **sarcoma.** For example, malignant cancers of skeletal muscle are known as *rhabdomyosarcomas.* Cancers of lymphatic tissue are called **lymphomas,** whereas cancers of blood-forming cells are called **leukemias.** However, many cancers, such as Hodgkin disease and Ewing sarcoma, are named for historical reasons that do not follow this nomenclature convention.

Carcinoma in situ

Carcinoma in situ (CIS) refers to preinvasive epithelial tumors of glandular or squamous cell origin. Cancers develop incrementally, as they accumulate specific genetic lesions. Careful surveillance for cancer often detects abnormal growths in epithelial tissues that have atypical cells and an increased proliferation rate compared with normal surrounding tissues. These early-stage cancers are localized to the epithelium and have not penetrated the local basement membrane or invaded the surrounding stroma. Based on these characteristics, they are not

malignant. CIS occurs in a number of sites, including the cervix, skin, oral cavity, esophagus, and bronchus. In glandular epithelium, in situ lesions occur in the stomach, endometrium, breast, and large bowel. In the breast, ductal carcinoma in situ (DCIS) fills the mammary ducts but has not progressed to local tissue invasion. DCIS lesions are readily treatable, although the optimal therapeutic approach is controversial. CIS lesions can have one of the following three fates: (1) they can remain stable for a long time, (2) they can progress to invasive and metastatic cancers, or (3) they can regress and disappear. CIS can vary from low-grade to high-grade dysplasia, with the high-grade lesions having the highest likelihood of becoming invasive cancers. The time that such preinvasive lesions remain in situ before becoming invasive is unknown. Some carcinomas of the cervix appear as preinvasive lesions in situ for several years before they progress to invasive carcinoma and metastatic tumors (Fig. 11.3). Knowing how to best treat low-grade CIS lesions is challenging, because the proportion that progress to cancer versus the proportion that will never cause clinical problems is usually not known. Although most persons prefer removal of any CIS as opposed to "watchful waiting," this topic continues to be a source of great debate.

✔ **QUICK CHECK 11.1**
1. What is cancer?
2. Identify the major differences between benign and malignant tumors.
3. What is carcinoma in situ?

THE BIOLOGY OF CANCER CELLS

In two seminal publications, Douglas Hanahan and Robert Weinberg[2,3] described what they considered the hallmarks of cancer. Both articles stimulated considerable discussion and, especially, debate. The original publication contained six hallmarks, but with time and new research

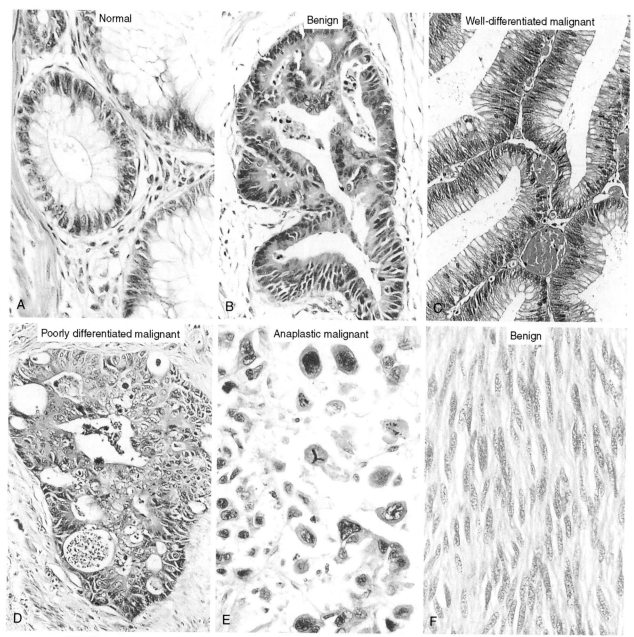

FIGURE 11.2 Loss of Cellular and Tissue Differentiation During the Development of Cancer.
The cells of a benign neoplasm **(B)** resemble those of the normal colonic epithelium **(A)**, in that they are columnar and have an orderly arrangement. Loss of some degree of differentiation is evident because the neoplastic cells do not show much mucin vacuolization (the large, clear cytoplasmic vacuoles seen in **A**). Cells of the well-differentiated malignant neoplasm **(C)** of the colon have a haphazard arrangement. In addition, although gland lumina are formed, they are architecturally abnormal and irregular. Nuclei vary in shape and size, especially compared with those illustrated in **(A)**. Cells in the poorly differentiated malignant neoplasm **(D)** have an even more haphazard arrangement, with very poor formation of gland lumina. The nuclei show greater variation in shape and size compared with those in the well-differentiated malignant neoplasm **(C)**. Cells in anaplastic malignant neoplasms **(E)** bear no relation to the normal epithelium, and no recognizable gland formation can be seen. Tremendous variation is found in the size of cells and their nuclei, with very intense staining (hyperchromatic nuclei). Not knowing the site of origin makes it impossible to classify this tumor by microscopic appearance alone. Well-differentiated tumors often resemble their cell of origin, as shown in the example of a benign tumor of smooth muscles **(F)**. (From Stevens A, Lowe J: *Pathology,* ed 2, London, 2000, Mosby.)

| NORMAL EPITHELIUM | LOW-GRADE INTRAEPITHELIAL NEOPLASIA | HIGH-GRADE INTRAEPITHELIAL NEOPLASIA | INVASIVE CARCINOMA |

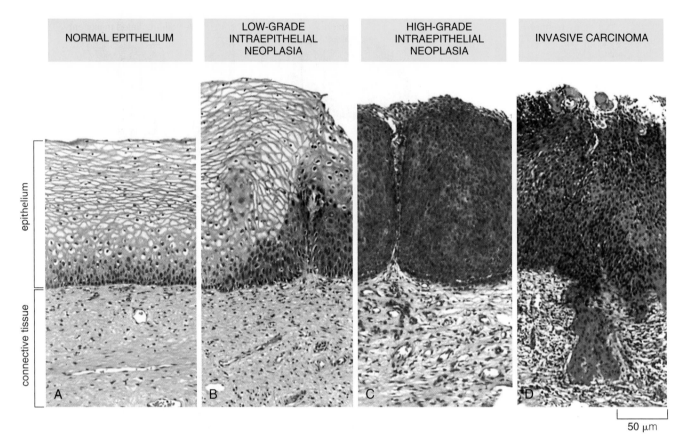

50 μm

FIGURE 11.3 Progression From Normal to Neoplasm in the Uterine Cervix. A sequence of cellular and tissue changes, progressing from low-grade to high-grade intraepithelial neoplasms (also called *carcinoma in situ*) and then to invasive cancer, often is seen in the development of cancer. In this example of the early stages of cervical neoplastic changes, the presence of anaplastic cells and loss of normal tissue architecture signify the development of cancer. The high rate of cell division and the presence of local mutagens and inflammatory mediators all contribute to the accumulation of genetic abnormalities that lead to cancer. (From Alberts B et al: *Molecular biology of the cell*, ed 5, New York, 2008, Garland.)

findings, increased to eight hallmarks and two traits that enable cancer progression. Their analysis remains the leading overview of why a cell is malignant. The following discussion is organized in the context of those 10 hallmarks/enablers (Fig. 11.4). Two fundamental concepts are the foundation for understanding the biology of cancer. Cancer is a complex disease, and the microenvironment of a tumor is a heterogeneous mixture of cells, both cancerous and benign. These concepts affect every stage of cancer development and evolve during that development. Tumor initiation, the process that produces the initial cancer cells, is dependent on mutational and epigenetic changes and characteristics of the microenvironment. Tumor promotion, the process during which the population of cancer cells expands with diversity of cancer cell phenotypes, is dependent on additional genetic mutations and epigenetic changes and a changing tumor microenvironment. Tumor progression, the process leading to spread of the tumor to adjacent and distal sites (metastasis), is governed by further genetic mutations, epigenetic aberrations, and changing microenvironments at the primary tumor and at sites of metastasis.

The fraction of individuals who develop cancer increases dramatically with age. Genetic changes may occur by both mutational and epigenetic mechanisms. Mutation generally means an alteration in the DNA sequence affecting expression or function of a gene (Fig. 11.5). Mutations include small-scale changes in DNA, such as point mutations—the alteration of one or a few nucleotide base pairs (see Chapter 2). This

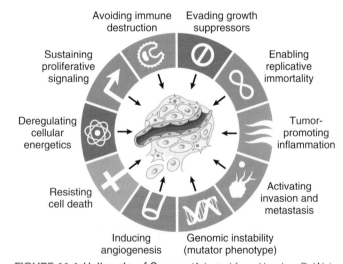

FIGURE 11.4 Hallmarks of Cancer. (Adapted from Hanahan D, Weinberg RA: *Cell* 144:646, 2011. In Kumar V et al: *Robbins and Cotran pathologic basis of disease*, ed 9, Philadelphia, 2015, Saunders.)

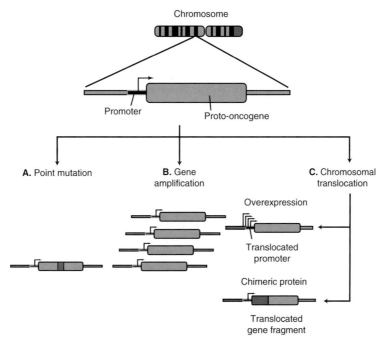

FIGURE 11.5 Oncogene Activation Mechanisms. Cellular genes may become cancerous oncogenes as a result of **(A)** point mutations that alter one or a few nucleotide base pairs, causing the production of a protein that is activated as a result of the altered sequence (e.g., RAS); **(B)** amplification of the cellular gene, resulting in higher levels of protein expression (e.g., MYCN in neuroblastoma); or **(C)** chromosomal transloca-tions that either (1) lead to the juxtaposition of a strong promoter, causing increased protein expression (MYC in Burkitt lymphoma), or (2) produce a novel fusion protein that is derived from gene fragments normally present on different chromosomes (BCR-ABL in chronic myeloid leukemia). (Adapted from Haber DA: *Molecular genetics of cancer* (WebMD). In ACP medicine, Danbury, Conn, 2004, WebMD.)

type of mutation can have profound effects on the activity of resultant proteins. Chromosome translocations are large changes in chromosome structure in which a piece of one chromosome is translocated to another chromosome. Gene amplification is the result of repeated duplication of a region of a chromosome, so that instead of the normal two copies of a gene, tens or even hundreds of copies are present. Gene expression also may be altered indirectly by epigenetic effects including DNA methylation, histone acetylation, or altered expression of non–coding RNA (see Chapter 3). Some mutations, referred to as driver mutations, "drive" the progression of cancer. There may be as many as 140 different driver mutations, although some are more critical than others, and each cancer only has a relatively small number of these. Not all mutations in cancer contribute to the malignant phenotype. Some are just random events and are referred to as passenger mutations; they are just along for the ride. After a critical number of driver mutations have occurred, the cell becomes cancerous. The cancer cell has a selective advantage over its neighbors; its progeny can accumulate faster than its nonmutant neighbors. This is referred to as clonal proliferation or clonal expansion (Fig. 11.6). As a clone with mutations proliferates, it may become an early-stage tumor, for example, a carcinoma in situ or a benign colonic polyp. The increasingly rapid cell division and impaired DNA repair mechanisms of cancer cells result in a continuing accumulation of mutations throughout the progression to the most aggressive metastatic lesion. Thus malignant transformation, the process by which a normal cell becomes a cancer cell, is directed by progressive accumulation of genetic and epigenetic changes that alter the basic nature of the cell and drive it to malignancy. The process of tumor development is a form of darwinian evolution; cells with a heritable change that confers a survival advantage out-compete their neighbors. Each cancer cell may

develop its own set of mutations resulting in a genomically heterogeneous mixture of cells with subsets that have accumulated more and more mutations that increase the cell's malignant potential. Thus many cancer cells that do not accumulate a critical set of mutations lose the competi-tion and die during this process.

The processes occurring during the development of cancer are, in many ways, analogous to wound healing. The initial proliferation of cancer cells and enlargement of the tumor elicit the synthesis of pro-inflammatory mediators by the cancer cells and adjacent nonmalignant cells. As with wound healing, mediators recruit inflammatory/immune cells (primarily T lymphocytes and macrophages, but also B cells and neutrophils) and cells normally associated with tissue repair (fibroblasts, adipocytes, mesenchymal stem cells, endothelial cells, and pericytes). These cells form the stroma (tumor microenvironment) that surrounds and infiltrates the tumor (Fig. 11.7).[4] In some conditions, stromal cells may make up 90% of the tumor mass. Extensive paracrine signaling among the stromal and cancer cells affects both populations; cancer cells increase proliferation and become more heterogeneous during tumor growth, and several populations of stromal cells undergo evolution to phenotypes that promote cancer progression and metastatic potential. Cancer heterogeneity or diversity arises from ongoing proliferation and mutation. Tumor-associated endothelial cells, fibroblasts, and inflammatory cells develop different and distinct gene expression profiles with unique cell surface molecules and patterns of secreted molecules. During this process there is often a great deal of cancer cell death, but the surviving cells are more aggressive and many take on a metastatic phenotype. Because continuing somatic mutations may be random, cancer cells in different regions of the tumor may be genetically diverse. Additionally, a population of cancer stem cells may arise, the origin of

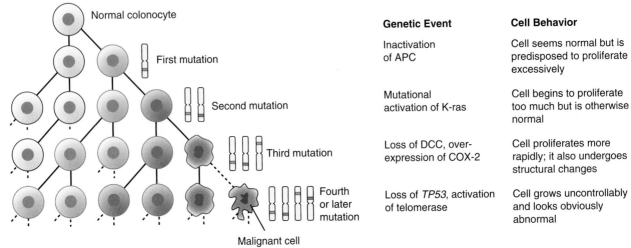

FIGURE 11.6 Clonal Proliferation Model of Neoplastic Progression in the Colon. During clonal proliferation, progressively altered populations of colon cells (colonocytes) arise over time. As genetic and epigenetic changes occur, different subclones (indicated by the different-colored cells) coexist for a time. Clones that grow the fastest out-compete other clones, producing even more malignant, and abnormal-appearing, growths. The sequential accumulation of mutations has been well studied in the progression from a normal colon cell to a benign intestinal polyp to a malignant colon cancer. One of the earliest mutations in colon cancer is loss of the tumor-suppressor gene *APC*. Additional mutations (often in the oncogene *RAS*), activation of COX-2, and loss of the tumor suppressors *DCC* and *TP53* occur as the lesion progresses from a benign polyp to an invasive carcinoma. *APC*, Adenomatous polyposis coli; *COX-2*, cyclooxygenase-2; DCC, deleted in colon cancer; TP53, p53 gene. (Modified from Mendelsohn I et al: *The molecular basis of cancer*, ed 2, Philadelphia, 2001, Saunders; and Kumar V et al: *Basic pathology*, ed 6, Philadelphia, 1997, Saunders.)

which is still unclear. Many of the hallmarks of cancer are consequences of cancer-stromal interactions (discussed later in the chapter).

Several of the hallmarks/enablers are primarily genomic alterations that initiate and maintain development of cancer. These will be discussed first and include sustained proliferative signaling, evading growth suppression, genomic instability, and replicative immortality (see Fig. 11.4). Other hallmarks/enablers are secondary to genomic change and include inducing angiogenesis and reprogramming energy metabolism. A third group, tumor resistance to destruction by the host's protective mechanisms, includes resistance to apoptotic cell death, tumor-promoting inflammation, and avoiding immune destruction. The last hallmark is the culmination of the previous nine: activating invasion and metastasis.

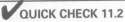

QUICK CHECK 11.2
1. Describe the differences between point mutations, chromosomal transloca- tions, and gene amplification in the process of cancer.
2. Define driver and passenger mutations in cancer development.
3. Why is the tumor microenvironment important to cancer progression?

Sustained Proliferative Signaling

The first and foremost hallmark of cancer is uncontrolled cellular proliferation. Normal cells generally only enter proliferative phases in response to growth factors that bind to specific receptors on the cell surface. The cytoplasmic components of the receptors are associated with signaling molecules that undergo activation and in turn activate intracellular signaling pathways leading to induction/activation of regulatory factors affecting DNA synthesis, entrance into the cell cycle, and changes in expression of other genes related to cell metabolism for optimal growth (Fig. 11.8). One example is initiation of proliferation by epidermal growth factor (EGF). EGF binds and cross-links two EGF

receptors on the cell surface. The cytoplasmic portions of the receptors are tyrosine kinases that attach phosphorus to tyrosine in neighboring proteins, including each other (autophosphorylation). Phosphorylation allows the receptor to attach to bridging protein, which links the EGF receptors to plasma membrane–associated inactive RAS. RAS is an acronym for "rat sarcoma," where it was found originally. Inactive RAS is associated with guanine diphosphate (GDP). Association between the EGF receptor and inactive RAS modifies the binding of GDP, which is replaced with guanine triphosphate (GTP). GTP activates RAS, which is a GTPase that converts GTP to GDP, during which it can activate signaling pathways such as the mitogen-activated protein kinase (MAPK) pathway and the phosphatidylinositol-3-kinase (PI3K) pathway. These signaling pathways phosphorylate other cytoplasmic proteins and affect activity and nuclear localization of transcription factors, such as myelocytomatosis viral oncogene homolog (MYC), that govern the transcription of cell cycle regulators, such as cyclins, and entrance into cellular proliferation. Proliferation can be discontinued through this pathway by decreased levels of growth factors in the environment or inactivation of signaling pathway components.

The genes that encode components of receptor-mediated pathways designed to regulate normal cellular proliferation are collectively called proto-oncogenes. Cancerous cells characteristically express mutated or overexpressed proto-oncogenes, which are called oncogenes. Oncogenes are independent of normal regulatory mechanisms; thus the cell is driven into a state of unregulated expression of proliferation signals and uncontrolled cell growth. Oncogenes can affect any portion of the growth factor pathways, such as described for EGF. For instance, most growth factors originate from neighboring cells, but some cancers acquire the ability to secrete growth factors that stimulate their own growth, a process known as autocrine stimulation. As described later in this chapter, noncancerous stromal cells within a tumor are frequently modified to benefit the cancer. In some instances, stromal cells produce

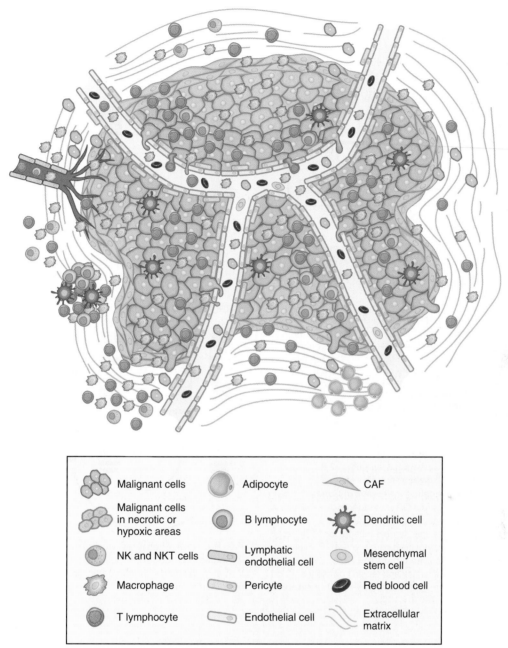

Malignant cells	Adipocyte	CAF
Malignant cells in necrotic or hypoxic areas	B lymphocyte	Dendritic cell
NK and NKT cells	Lymphatic endothelial cell	Mesenchymal stem cell
Macrophage	Pericyte	Red blood cell
T lymphocyte	Endothelial cell	Extracellular matrix

FIGURE 11.7 Cancers Live in a Complex Microenvironment. Cancer cells express tumor-specific antigens that ideally can be recognized by cells of the immune system and the inflammatory systems (natural killer cells, antitumor M1 macrophages, T-cytotoxic cells) and destroyed by apoptosis or undergo growth suppression by cytokines. However, successful cancers produce a variety of cytokines and chemokines that are chemoattractants for stromal cells that infiltrate the tumor and undergo change to pro-tumor phenotypes. These include tumor-associated M2 macrophages (TAMs), cancer-associated fibroblasts (CAFs), mesenchymal stem cells (MSCs), and immune suppressor cells of T-cell origin (T-regulatory cells) and myeloid origin (myeloid-derived suppressor cells). Through multiple receptor-mediated interactions between other stromal cells and the cancer cells, the stromal cells, and also the cancer cells, collectively produce a battery of additional cytokines, chemokines, growth factors, and proteases and secrete components of the extracellular matrix (ECM). The stromal reaction promotes tumor progression, including new blood vessel growth (angiogenesis), tumor cell proliferation and differentiation, suppression of immune rejection and tumor cell apoptosis, invasion, and commitment to metastasis. (From Balkwill FR, Capasso M, Hagemann T: *J Cell Sci* 125:5591-5596, 2012.)

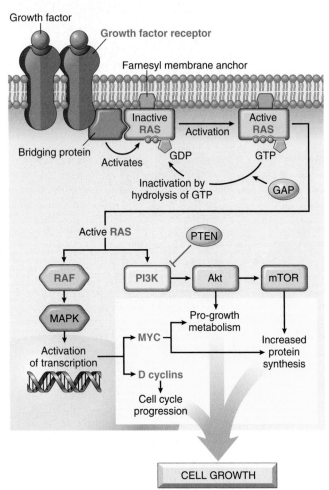

FIGURE 11.8 Growth Factor Signaling Pathways in Cancer. Growth factor receptors, RAS, PI3K, MYC, and D cyclins are oncoproteins that are activated by mutations in various cancers. GAPs apply brakes to RAS activation, and PTEN serves the same function for PI3K. *GAP*, GTPase-activating protein; *GDP*, guanosine diphosphate; *GTP*, guanosine triphosphate; *MAPK*, mitogen-activated protein kinase; *PI3K*, phosphoinositidyl-3-kinase; *PTEN*, phosphatase and tensin homologue. (From Kumar V et al: *Robbins and Cotran pathologic basis of disease*, ed 9, Philadelphia, 2015, Saunders.)

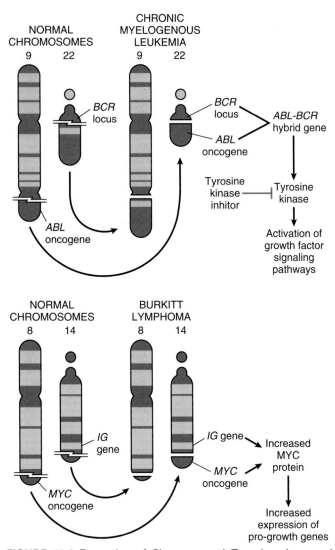

FIGURE 11.9 Examples of Chromosomal Translocations and Associated Oncogenes. See text for further explanation. (From Kumar V et al: *Robbins and Cotran pathologic basis of disease*, ed 9, Philadelphia, 2015, Saunders.)

excessive growth factors that drive the proliferation of cancer cells. Other cancers increase the expression of growth factor receptors; for example, in breast cancer, production of the **human epidermal growth factor receptor 2 (HER2),** also known as the epidermal growth factor receptor gene (ERBB2), is up-regulated and is hyperresponsive to low levels of EGF. Some breast and lung cancers are treated by inhibitors of HER2 and other EGF receptors that block this pathway.

Oncogenes may lead to constant activation of the signal cascade from the cell surface receptor to the nucleus. Up to a third of all cancers have an activating mutation in the RAS gene resulting in a continuous cell growth signal even when growth factors are missing (see Fig. 11.8). Other mutations in the EGF receptor pathway include excessive proliferation signaling by hyperactivation of the PI3 kinase.

Several types of genetic events can activate oncogenes. A point mutation that is frequently observed in lung cancer results in continuous activation of the EGF **receptor tyrosine kinase.** A point mutation in the *RAS* gene converts it from a regulated proto-oncogene to an unregulated oncogene. Activating point mutations in *RAS* are found

in many cancers, especially pancreatic and colorectal cancer. Specialized tests, such as direct DNA sequencing, can detect such point mutations in clinical samples.

Translocations can activate oncogenes by one of two distinct mechanisms (Fig. 11.9). First, a translocation can cause excess and inappropriate production of a proliferation factor. One of the best examples is the t(8;14) translocation found in many Burkitt lymphomas; t(8;14) designates a chromosome that has a piece of chromosome 8 fused to a piece of chromosome 14 (see Chapter 23). Burkitt lymphoma is an aggressive cancer of B lymphocytes. The **MYC proto-oncogene** found on chromosome 8 is normally activated at low levels in proliferating lymphocytes and is inactivated in mature lymphocytes. If the t(8;14) translocation occurs, the *MYC* gene is aberrantly placed under the control of a B-cell immunoglobulin gene *(IG)* present on chromosome 14. The *IG* gene is very active in maturing B lymphocytes. The t(8;14) translocation alters the control of *MYC;* its normal low level expression is switched to high levels, as directed by an *IG* gene promoter. Hyperproduction of **MYC protein** drives proliferation and blocks differentiation.

Second, chromosome translocations can lead to production of novel proteins with growth-promoting properties. In chronic myeloid leukemia (CML) a specific chromosome translocation is almost always present (see Fig. 11.9). This translocation, t(9;22), was first identified in association with CML in Philadelphia in 1960 and is often referred to as the Philadelphia chromosome. Translocation fuses two chromosomes in the middle of two different genes: *BCR* (break point cluster region gene) on chromosome 9 and *ABL* (Abelson gene) on chromosome 22. The result is production of a BCR-ABL fusion protein containing the first half of BCR and the second half of ABL (a nonreceptor tyrosine kinase). BCR-ABL is an unregulated protein tyrosine kinase that promotes growth of myeloid cells. Imatinib, a drug that specifically targets this tyrosine kinase, represents the first successful chemotherapy targeted against the product of a specific oncogenic mutation. Imatinib and related tyrosine kinase inhibitors (TKIs) are highly effective in the treatment of CML and, because of their specificity, lack the toxic side effects noted with nonspecific anticancer drugs. However, imatinib is not effective in cancers that do not have the t(9;22) translocation or related mutations. In modern personalized cancer therapy, knowledge of the specific genetic alteration can dictate the optimal drugs for the individual.

Oncogenes also may be activated by gene amplification (Fig. 11.10). Gene amplification results in increased expression of an oncogene, or in some cases drug resistance genes. The N-*MYC* oncogene, a member of the *MYC* family, is amplified in 25% of childhood neuroblastomas and confers a poor prognosis. The HER2 gene (*ERBB2*) is amplified in 20% of breast cancers.

Evading Growth Suppressors

Uncontrolled cancer cell proliferation also is related to inactivation of tumor-suppressor genes. Tumor-suppressor genes normally regulate the cell cycle, inhibit proliferation resulting from growth signals, stop cell division when cells are damaged, and prevent mutations. Hence they also have been referred to as anti-oncogenes. Whereas oncogenes are activated in cancers, tumor suppressors must be inactivated to allow cancer to occur (Table 11.1 and Fig. 11.11). A single genetic event can activate an oncogene because it can act in a dominant manner in the cell. However, we have two copies of each tumor-suppressor gene, one from each parent. Both copies must be inactivated; therefore two mutations are necessary.

A prototypical tumor-suppressor gene is the retinoblastoma *(RB) gene*. The *RB* gene resides on chromosome 13, in a region referred to as q14 (13q14). Normal cells receive diverse "antigrowth" signals from their normal environment. Contact with other cells, with basement membranes, and with some soluble factors normally signals cells to stop proliferating. Tumor-suppressor genes, such as *RB*, monitor

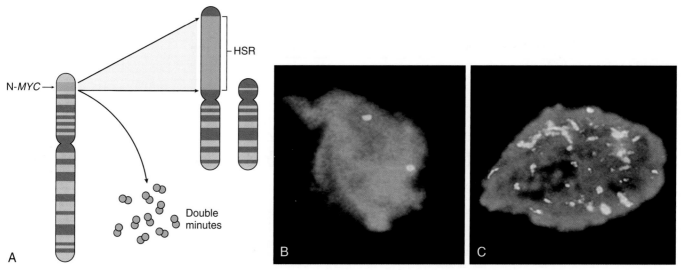

FIGURE 11.10 N-*MYC* Gene Amplification in Neuroblastoma. A, The N-MYC gene is present on chromosome 2, becomes amplified, and is seen either as extra chromosomal double minutes or as a chromosomal homologous staining region. The N-*MYC* gene is detected in human neuroblastoma cells using a technique called *FISH* (fluorescent in situ hybridization). B, A single pair of N-*MYC* genes is detected in normal cells and in low-grade neuroblastoma. C, Multiple amplified copies of the N-*MYC* gene are detected in some cases of neuroblastoma. Amplification of the N-*MYC* gene is strongly associated with a poor prognosis in childhood neuroblastoma. *HSR,* homologous staining region. (A from Kumar V et al: *Robbins and Cotran pathologic basis of disease,* ed 9, Philadelphia, 2015, Saunders. B and C courtesy Arthur R. Brothman, PhD, FACMG, University of Utah School of Medicine, Salt Lake City, Utah.)

TABLE 11.1 **Comparison of Cancer Gene Types**

Gene Type	Normal Function	Mutation Effect
Caretaker	DNA and chromosome stability	Chromosome instability and increased rates of mutation
Dominant oncogenes*	Encode proteins that promote growth (e.g., growth factors)	Overexpression or amplification causes gain of function
Tumor suppressors (recessive oncogenes)	Encode proteins that inhibit proliferation and prevent or repair mutations	Requires loss of function of both alleles to increase cancer risk

*Nonmutant state referred to as *proto-oncogene.*

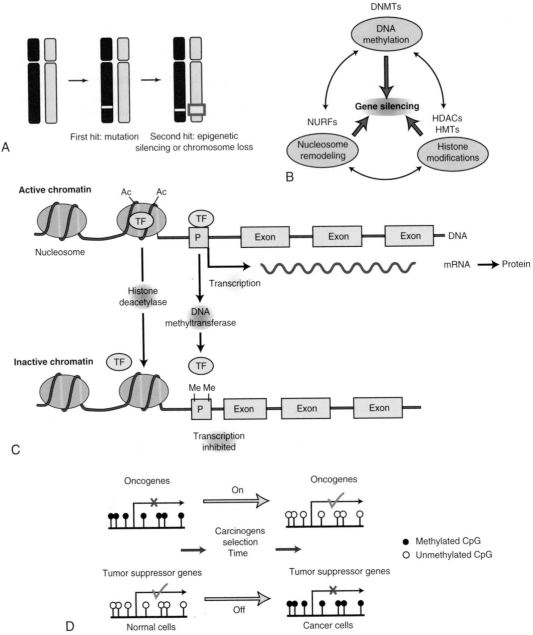

FIGURE 11.11 Silencing Tumor-Suppressor Genes. Tumor-suppressor genes can be deactivated by a variety of mechanisms. **A,** In this example, the first hit is a point mutation in a tumor-suppressor gene (white box), followed by either epigenetic silencing or chromosome loss of the second allele (red box). **B,** Genes can normally be silenced by a variety of interacting processes including DNA methylation, histone modification, nucleosome remodeling, and microRNA changes (not shown). A number of cellular enzymes contribute to these modifications, including DNA methyltransferases *(DNMTs)*, histone deacetylases *(HDACs)*, histone methyltransferases *(HMTs)*, and complex nucleosome remodeling factors *(NURFs)*. Gene silencing is essential for normal development and differentiation. **C,** Histone modification and promoter methylation regulate gene expression. Genes are transcribed when chromatin is modified by addition of acetyl *(Ac)* groups to specific lysine groups in histones. Gene expression can be turned off when specific acetyl groups are removed (by HDACs) or when the CpG-rich promoter regions of genes are modified by direct DNA methylation (by DNA methyltransferase). In addition, small endogenous RNA molecules (microRNAs, or miRNA) can bind to mRNA and reduce gene expression. **D,** Changes in promoter methylation turn cancer genes off and on. Oncogenes can be turned on by promoter hypomethylation, and tumor-suppressor genes can be turned off by promoter hypermethylation. Each of these changes can produce selective growth and survival advantages for the cancer cell. *Me,* Methylation; *mRNA,* messenger ribonucleic acid; *RNA,* ribonucleic acid; *TF,* transcription factor. (B adapted from Jones PA, Baylin SB: *Cell* 128:683-692, 2007; **C** from Gluckman PD et al: *N Engl J Med* 359[1]:66, 2008; **D** from Shames DS et al: *Curr Mol Med* 7:85-102, 2007.)

antigrowth cellular signals and block activation of the growth/division phase in the cell cycle; thus mutations in *RB* lead to persistent cell growth. Anti-proliferative activity of *RB* depends on the degree of protein phosphorylation. Low levels of phosphorylation (hypophosphorylation) result in *RB* binding to and inhibiting transcription factors that regulate genes controlling passage through the cell cycle. Growth factor–regulated kinases increase phosphorylation (hyperphosphorylation) and inactivation of *RB*. A variety of genetic mutations in cancers also inactivate *RB*, resulting in unregulated and continuous cellular proliferation. RB is mutated in childhood retinoblastoma, and in many lung, breast, and bone cancers as well. Most individuals with *RB* mutations have a subtle mutation, such as a point mutation, in one allele. The *RB* gene in the other chromosome may be inactivated through loss of the 13q14 region or epigenetic mechanisms.

Another classic tumor-suppressor gene is **tumor protein p53 *(TP53)***. The protein p53 has been called the *guardian of the genome*. TP53 monitors intracellular signals related to stress and activates **caretaker genes**—genes that are responsible for the maintenance of genomic integrity (Fig. 11.12). Many types of cellular stress (e.g., anoxia, oncogene expression, nuclear damage) produce intracellular signals (e.g., levels of nucleotides and glucose, degree of oxygenation, DNA damage, and other indicators of cellular abnormalities) detectable by p53. Normally p53 is in an inactive complex with inhibitor molecules. Stress activates kinases that phosphorylate p53 into an active suppressor of cell division and activator of caretaker genes. Caretaker genes encode proteins involved in repairing damaged DNA, such as occurs with errors in DNA replication, mutations caused by ultraviolet or ionizing radiation, and mutations caused by chemicals and drugs. The p53 protein also

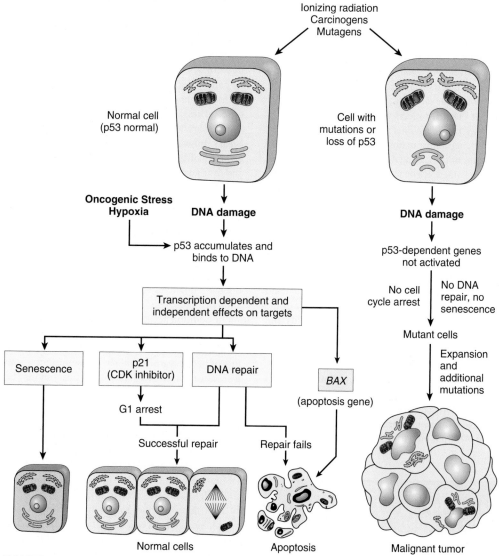

FIGURE 11.12 The Role of p53 in Maintaining the Integrity of the Genome. Activation of normal p53 by DNA-damaging agents or by hypoxia leads to cell cycle arrest in G₁ by up-regulation of the cell cycle inhibitor p21 and induction of DNA repair transcriptional up-regulation of the cyclin-dependent kinase inhibitor *CDKN1A* (encoding the cyclin-dependent kinase inhibitor p21) and the *GADD45* genes. Successful repair of DNA allows cells to proceed with the cell cycle. If DNA repair fails, *p53* triggers either apoptosis or senescence. In cells with loss or mutation of the *p53* gene, DNA damage does not induce cell cycle arrest or DNA repair, and genetically damaged cells proliferate, giving rise eventually to malignant neoplasms. (From Kumar V et al: *Robbins and Cotran pathologic basis of disease,* ed 9, Philadelphia, 2015, Saunders.)

controls initiation of cellular senescence (cease dividing) or apoptosis, and suppresses cell division until DNA repair is complete or other effects of stress are corrected. If not corrected, the cell enters senescence or apoptosis, thus preventing further DNA damage and mutations. Loss of function of *TP53* or caretaker genes leads to increased mutation rates and cancer.

Because inactivation of tumor-suppressor genes requires at least two mutations (one in each allele), a single germ cell mutation (sperm or egg) results in the transmission of cancer-causing genes from one generation to the next, producing families with a high risk for specific cancers. These inherited mutations that predispose to cancer are almost invariably in tumor-suppressor genes because only a single additional mutation in any other cell (somatic cell mutation) is needed to inactivate completely the tumor-suppressor gene (Table 11.2).

An example of increased risk for cancer that can be inherited is the familial form of retinoblastoma. A mutation in one *RB* allele is inherited so that only one additional mutation in the normal allele will lead to cancer (see Table 11.2). Approximately half of children with retinoblastoma have the inheritable form and most will develop tumors in both eyes (bilateral retinoblastoma). Also, Li-Fraumeni syndrome is a very rare inheritable loss-of-function mutation in *TP53* in one allele resulting in a 25-fold increase of developing malignancy at an early age (<50 years of age). These malignancies may include breast cancer, brain tumors, acute leukemia, soft tissue sarcomas, bone sarcoma, and adrenal cortical carcinoma. Other familial cancers with inheritable mutations in tumor-suppressor genes include Wilms tumor, a childhood cancer of the kidney (*WT1* gene); neurofibromatosis (*NF1* gene*)*; and familial polyposis coli or adenomas of the colon (*APC* gene). Characterization of cancer-causing genes and other genetic factors helps identify individuals prone to developing cancer and contributes to our understanding of sporadic cancers. Individuals known to carry mutations in tumor-suppressor genes are offered targeted cancer screening to facilitate early cancer detection and therapy.

Genomic Instability

Genomic instability refers to an increased tendency of alterations—mutability—in the genome during the life cycle of cells. Inherited and acquired mutations in caretaker genes that protect the integrity of the genome and DNA repair increase the level of genomic instability and risk for developing cancer. Acquired mutations in "guardians of the genome," such as *TP53*, that detect DNA damage and activate repair mechanisms result in an increasing accumulation of mutations. Xeroderma pigmentosum is a defect in the repair of DNA pyrimidine dimers created by ultraviolet (UV) light that increases the risk for skin cancers. Hereditary nonpolyposis colorectal cancer results from an inherited defect in repairing DNA base pair mismatches that occur occasionally during DNA replication. Affected individuals have an increased rate of small insertions and deletions in DNA, leading to a high rate of colon and other cancers. Some inherited mutations threaten the integrity of entire chromosomes. Bloom syndrome, caused by mutations in a DNA helicase, presents with an increased risk of several forms of cancer, and those with Fanconi aplastic anemia, caused by loss of function for repairing DNA double-strand breaks, have a particularly increased risk of acute myelogenous leukemia. These examples are autosomal recessive disorders in which affected individuals demonstrate marked chromosomal instability.

Genomic instability also may result from increased epigenetic silencing or modulation of gene function (see Chapter 3). Many cancers have increased methylation of DNA in the promoter region of tumor-suppressor genes. They also have associated changes in the modification of histones in the chromatin, often correlated with methylation of DNA. These changes alter the promoter regions of genes, leading to their silencing or altered gene expression.

Changes in gene regulation can affect not just single genes, but also entire intracellular signaling networks. Gene expression networks can be regulated by changes in microRNAs (miRNAs, or miRs) and other non–coding RNAs (ncRNAs). miRs regulate diverse signaling pathways; the miRs that stimulate cancer development and progression are termed oncomirs. miRs decrease the stability and expression of other genes by pairing with mRNA.

Mutations in *BRCA1* and *BRCA2* (breast cancer 1 and 2, early onset genes) are currently of clinical importance. Both are tumor-suppressors and caretaker genes that repair double-stranded DNA breaks. Inherited mutations in either gene greatly increase the risk for a variety of tumors, especially breast cancer in both women and men, and ovarian or prostate cancers. Approximately 12% of women generally will develop breast cancer within their lifetime, a recent large study found that about 72% of women with a high-risk *BRCA1* mutation and about 69% with a harmful *BRCA2* mutation will develop breast cancer by age 80.[5,6] Ovarian cancer occurs in approximately 1.3% of the general population, but about 44% of women with an inherited harmful mutation in *BRCA1* and about 17% with a mutation in *BRCA2* will develop ovarian cancer by age 80.[5,6] At-risk women are currently offered enhanced screening, prophylactic (risk reducing) surgery, and chemoprevention.

In addition to specific gene mutations and abnormal epigenetic silencing, chromosome instability also appears to be increased in malignant cells, resulting in a high rate of chromosome loss, as well as loss of heterozygosity and chromosome amplification. The underlying mechanism of this instability is not clear but may be caused by malfunctions in the cellular machinery that regulates chromosome segregation at mitosis.

Enabling Replication Immortality

A hallmark of cancer cells is their immortality; they seem to have an unlimited life span and will continue to divide for years under appropriate laboratory conditions. One of the most commonly used laboratory cell lines, HeLa cells, was derived from a cervical cancer specimen obtained in 1951 that continues to grow and divide in laboratories around the world. Most normal cells are not immortal and can divide only a limited number of times (known as the *Hayflick limit*) before they either enter senescence (cease dividing) or enter crisis (apoptosis) and die. One major block to unlimited cell division (i.e., immortality) is the size of a specialized structure called the *telomere*. Telomeres are protective ends, or caps, of repeating hexanucleotides (six nucleotide units) on each chromosome and are placed and maintained by a specialized enzyme called telomerase (Fig. 11.13). Telomerase is usually active only in germ cells (in ovaries and testes) and in stem cells. All other cells of the body lack telomerase activity. Therefore when non–germ cells begin to

TABLE 11.2 Some Familial Cancer Syndromes Caused by Loss of Tumor-Suppressor Gene Function	
Syndrome	Gene
Retinoblastoma	*RB1*
Li-Fraumeni syndrome	*p53 (TP53)*
Familial melanoma	*p16$^{INK\alpha}$ (CDKN2A)*
Neurofibromatosis	*Neurofibromin (NF1)*
Familial adenomatous polyps	*APC*
Breast cancer	*BRCA1*

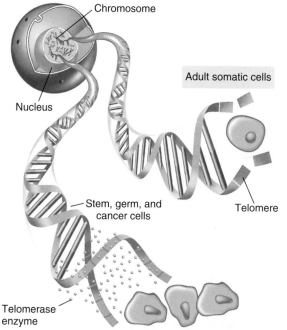

FIGURE 11.13 Control of Immortality: Telomeres and Telomerase. Normal adult somatic cells cannot divide indefinitely because the ends of their chromosomes are capped by telomeres. In the absence of the telomerase enzyme, telomeres become progressively shorter with each division until, when they are critically short, they signal to the cell to stop dividing. In germ cells, adult stem cells, and cancer cells the telomerase gene is "switched on," producing an enzyme that rebuilds the telomeres. Thus, like germ cells, the cancer cell becomes immortal and able to divide indefinitely without losing its telomeres.

proliferate abnormally their telomere caps shorten with each cell division. Short telomeres normally signal the cell to cease cell division. If the telomeres become critically small, the chromosomes become unstable and fragment, and the cells die.

Cancer cells are very heterogeneous, and many cells die as the cancer develops. When they reach a critical age, most cancer cells activate telomerase to restore and maintain their telomeres, thereby allowing continuous division. The trigger for reexpression of telomerase activity remains unclear, but seems to require expression of specific oncogenes, such as *RAS* or *MYC,* and loss of function of certain tumor-suppressor molecules, such as p53 and *RB.* Telomerase activity is restored in about 90% of cancers. The remaining cancers appear to recruit or originate from stem cells, becoming cancer stem cells that maintain levels of telomerase activity characteristically found in somatic stem cells. Because telomerase is specifically activated in cancer cells, and potentially in cancer stem cells, it is an attractive therapeutic target.

✔ **QUICK CHECK 11.3**
1. What are the heritable changes in cells that contribute to cancer development?
2. Define oncogene, proto-oncogene, and tumor-suppressor gene.
3. Biologically, why do tumor-suppressor genes have to be inactivated to cause cancer?
4. Define epigenetics and epigenetic silencing.
5. Distinguish between mutations in somatic cells versus in germ cells.
6. Define telomeres, telomerase, and senescence and describe their effects on cancer.

Cellular Adaptations
Inducing Angiogenesis

A major component of wound healing is the process of establishing new blood vessels within the tissue undergoing repair (called neovascularization or angiogenesis). Access to a blood supply also is obligatory for the growth and spread of cancer. Without a blood supply to deliver oxygen and nutrients, growth of a tumor is limited to about a millimeter in diameter.

Angiogenic factors and angiogenic inhibitors normally control development of new vessels. In cancerous tumors several mechanisms increase and maintain secretion of angiogenic factors by the cancer cells, as well as prevent release of angiogenic inhibitors. Hypoxia-inducible factor-1α (HIF-1α), an oxygen-sensitive transcription factor, is a major regulator of angiogenesis in normal tissue; HIF-1α is stabilized under hypoxic conditions and induces expression of pro-angiogenic factors, such as vascular endothelial growth factor (VEGF) and basic fibroblast growth factor (bFGF). Inactivation of tumor-suppressor genes (e.g., *p53*) or increased expression of oncogenes (e.g., *HER2*) leads to increased expression of HIF-1α–regulated angiogenic factors and increased vascularization. Increased expression of HIF-1α also is related to increased resistance to chemotherapy, increased tumor cell glycolysis, increased metastasis, and a poor prognosis. These effects may likely occur through an autocrine mechanism by which VEGF activates tumor-associated VEGF receptors. The use of angiogenic inhibitors targeting VEGF signaling can inhibit angiogenesis and diminish tumor growth.

Other routes of angiogenic factor induction include mutations in cancer oncogenes (e.g., *RAS, MYC*) that increase transcription of VEGF by cancer cells. Most cells in the tumor microenvironment also secrete VEGF, including tumor-infiltrating monocytes, endothelial cells, adipocytes, and cancer-associated fibroblasts. Angiogenesis inhibitors, such as thrombospondin-1 (TSP-1), normally bind to cellular surface receptors on inflammatory cells and negatively regulate angiogenesis in wound healing and tissue remodeling. The expression of angiogenesis inhibitors is under the control of p53, which is suppressed in cancer cells, thus diminishing the control of stromal inflammatory cell secretion of angiogenic factors.

Cancer cells and stromal cells may increase production of matrix metalloproteinases (MMPs) (e.g., MMP-9) (Fig. 11.14). MMPs are zinc-dependent proteases that digest the surrounding extracellular matrix (ECM). The ECM contains stored latent (inactive) forms of some angiogenic factors (e.g., bFGF, transforming growth factor-beta [TGF-β]). MMPs activate the stored forms into functional angiogenic factors.

The vessels formed within tumors differ from those in healthy tissue. They originate from endothelial sprouting from existing capillaries and irregular branching, rather than regular branching seen in healthy tissue. The interendothelial cell contact is less tight so the vessels are more porous and prone to hemorrhage, as well as allowing passage of tumor cells into the vascular system.

Reprogramming Energy Metabolism

Cancer cells live in a distinct environment from normal cells and have different nutritional requirements from nonproliferating cells. The successful cancer cell divides rapidly, with the consequent requirement for the building blocks to construct new cells. Nonmalignant cells in the presence of adequate oxygen normally generate adenosine triphosphate (ATP) by mitochondrial oxidative phosphorylation (OXPHOS), generating 36 ATP molecules from each glucose molecule that is broken down to water and carbon dioxide. In the absence of sufficient oxygen (hypoxia) normal cells perform glycolysis or the breakdown

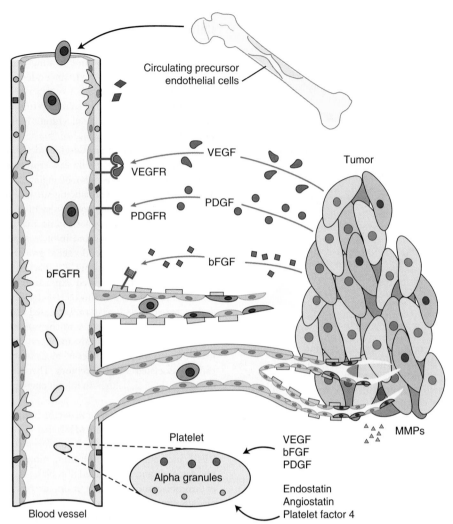

FIGURE 11.14 Tumor-Induced Angiogenesis. Malignant tumors secrete angiogenic factors and tissue-remodeling matrix metalloproteinases (MMPs) that actively induce the formation of new blood vessels. New blood vessels are formed from both local endothelial cells and circulating precursor cells recruited from the bone marrow. Circulating platelets can also release regulatory proteins into the tumor. *bFGF* and *bFGFR*, Basic fibroblast growth factor and its receptor, respectively; *MMPs*, matrix metalloproteinases; *PDGF* and *PDGFR*, platelet-derived growth factor and its receptor, respectively; *VEGF* and *VEGFR*, vascular endothelial growth factor and its receptor, respectively. (Adapted from Folkman J: *Nat Rev Drug Discov* 6[4]:273-286, 2007.)

of glucose by enzymes (anaerobic glycolysis), generating only two ATP molecules per molecule of glucose, with lactic acid and pyruvate as by-products.

Energy metabolism in cancer cells has received renewed attention and is deemed as important as other hallmark characteristics, such as sustained angiogenesis. In the 1920s, the emerging distinction between normal cells and cancer cells was first reported by Otto Warburg, termed the *Warburg effect*. The **Warburg effect** suggests that even in the presence of sufficient oxygen, cancer cells prefer to produce ATP through glycolysis instead of OXPHOS.[7] Thus the Warburg Effect is the use of glycolysis under normal oxygen conditions, hence the name **aerobic glycolysis.** Although aerobic glycolysis was postulated to arise from cancer-specific mitochondrial dysfunction, it is now apparent that this is instead a highly regulated and beneficial adaptation for cancer cells. The shift from OXPHOS to glycolysis allows lactate and other products of glycolysis to be used for the more efficient production of lipids, nucleosides, amino acids, and other molecular

building blocks needed for rapid cell growth. Recent work, however, challenges the Warburg Effect because mitochondrial OXPHOS still contributes in overall ATP generation under normal conditions for certain cancer cells and reduces significantly in hypoxic environments. Perhaps more significantly, the Warburg Effect does not focus on the metabolic interactions between cancer cells and other components of the microenvironment.[8,9] Ongoing investigations involve glucose, amino acids, and possibly lactate dehydrogenase and their importance in cancer metabolism.[10-12]

A new model, the **reverse Warburg effect,** may play a role in certain cancers.[9] Cancer cells may continue using the OXPHOS to generate large amounts of ATP. However, they also may manipulate the cancer-associated fibroblasts (CAFs), perhaps by inducing oxidative stress, to undergo aerobic glycolysis and secrete metabolites (e.g., lactate, pyruvate) that the cancer cells can use in the citric acid cycle (Krebs cycle) to feed OXPHOS and produce ATP. A secondary consequence would be induction of autophagy in the CAFs, resulting in consumption of the CAFs and release of materials needed by the cancer cell in the synthesis of new organelles.

Oncogenes can drive metabolic reprogramming, which enables cancer cells to:

- sustain deregulated proliferation,
- withstand challenges associated with oxygen and nutrient limitations,
- maintain a dedifferentiated state with associated alterations in gene expression, and
- corrupt the surrounding microenvironment to assist tumor growth and dissemination.[11]

Most studies have focused on glucose and glutamine, but a variety of other nutrients are used by cancer cells including sulfur-containing amino acids cysteine and methionine, essential fatty acids, choline, trace minerals, and vitamins.[11] A recent finding is that the mammalian/mechanistic target of rapamycin complex 1 (mTORC1) is a major nutrient sensor and regulator of cellular metabolic processes (Fig. 11.15).

Clinically the high glucose utilization of a cancer can be exploited for its detection. ^{18}F-Fluorodeoxyglucose (FDG) is incorporated into cells in the same way as glucose, with two key differences. Because it is missing a key hydroxyl group, it cannot be broken down by glycolysis, and thus FDG accumulates in cells. Because it is tagged with ^{18}F, it can be imaged by a positron emission tomography (PET) scan. Small metastatic tumor masses that are consuming huge amounts of glucose can readily be detected with this imaging method (Fig. 11.16).

Resistance to Destruction
Resisting Apoptotic Cell Death

Programmed cell death (apoptosis) is a mechanism by which individual cells can self-destruct under conditions of tissue remodeling or as a protection against aberrant cell growth that may lead to malignancy. Two pathways may trigger apoptosis (see Fig. 4.28). The intrinsic pathway (mitochondrial pathway) monitors cellular stress. Cellular stress may include DNA damage, genomic instability, aberrant proliferation, loss of adhesion to extracellular matrix or to adjacent cells, and other causes and characteristics of abnormal cellular physiology. The extrinsic pathway is activated through a plasma membrane receptor complex linked to intracellular activators of apoptosis (known as the *death receptor*).

Apoptotic pathways are dysregulated in most cancers. Most commonly, loss-of-function mutations to the *TP53* gene suppress activation of apoptosis during DNA damage. The balance between pro- and anti-apoptotic molecules also can be affected by overexpression of anti-apoptotic molecules or diminished expression of anti-apoptotic molecules resulting from mutations. Other mechanisms of providing resistance to apoptosis include down-regulation of caspases or production of caspase inhibitors. By whatever mechanism, or combination of mechanisms, successful cancers suppressed apoptotic pathways and increased resistance to cell death.

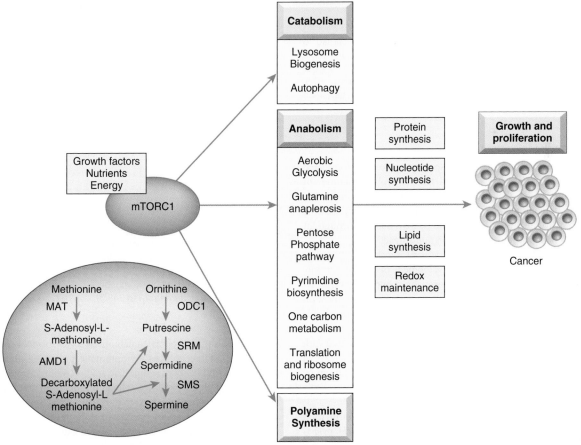

FIGURE 11.15 mTORC1: A Master Regulator of Metabolic Processes. The mTORC1 (mammalian target of rapamycin complex 1) signaling network is a sensor of intracellular energy and extracellular stimuli (e.g., nutrients, growth factors). It induces changes in intermediary metabolism to meet cellular homeostasis. mTORC1 promotes many anabolic processes, represses catabolic processes, and induces polyamine synthesis, thereby sustaining cell growth and proliferation. (Data from Gomes AP, Schild T, Blenis J: *Dev Cell* 42[2]:112-114, 2017.)

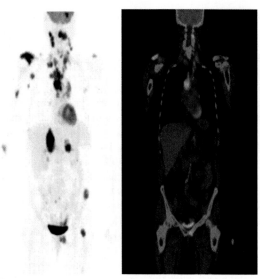

FIGURE 11.16 Intense Glucose Requirement of Cancer Aids in Diagnosis. A non–small cell lung cancer (NSCLC) lesion was surgically removed from this 54-year-old woman, and these images were obtained 5 years later. The positron emission tomography (PET) scan, using ^{18}F-deoxyglucose, shows metastatic lesions in the brain, right shoulder, and mediastinal and cervical lymph nodes, in addition to the liver, left pelvis, and proximal femur. *(Left)* PET whole-body image. *(Right)* Representative coronal image from the whole-body FDG-PET/CT–fused image of the same patient. The fused image consists of the CT image with the metabolic information superimposed in color. The pattern of distribution most likely is from the primary tumor to the large mediastinal lymph nodes, and then by lymphatic spread to cervical lymph nodes. Blood-borne dissemination produced the bone, brain, and liver metastases. Normally only the heart, brain, and bladder show a strong signal on PET scans. *CT,* Computed tomography; *FDG,* fluorodeoxyglucose. (Images courtesy John Hoffman, MD, Huntsman Cancer Institute, Salt Lake City, Utah.)

Tumor-Promoting Inflammation

Historically an immune/inflammatory response to cancer was considered a detrimental condition that successful tumors evolved methods of evading. We now realize that the relationship between a cancer and the inflammatory system is much more complex. The inflammatory response may contribute to the onset of cancer and be manipulated throughout the process to benefit tumor progression and spread.

Chronic inflammation has been recognized for close to 150 years as being an important factor in the development of cancer. Chronic inflammations may result from many causes, for example, solar irradiation, asbestos exposure (mesothelioma), pancreatitis, and infection (Table 11.3). Additionally, some organs appear to be more susceptible to the oncogenic effects of chronic inflammation (e.g., the gastrointestinal [GI] tract, prostate, thyroid gland). Individuals who have suffered with ulcerative colitis for 11 years or more have up to a 30-fold increase in the risk of developing colon cancer. Chronic viral hepatitis caused by hepatitis B virus (HBV) or hepatitis C virus (HCV) infection markedly increases the risk of liver cancer.

A specific example is the association between gastric inflammation induced by infection with the bacterium *Helicobacter pylori (H. pylori)* and the risk for gastric cancer. *H. pylori* is a bacterium that infects more than half of the world's population. Chronic infection with *H. pylori* is an important cause of peptic ulcer disease and is strongly associated with gastric carcinoma, a leading cause of cancer deaths worldwide. It also is associated with a less common cancer, gastric mucosa–associated lymphoid tissue (MALT) lymphomas. *H. pylori* infection is often acquired

TABLE 11.3 Chronic Inflammatory Conditions and Infectious Agents Associated With Neoplasms

Inflammatory Condition	Associated Neoplasm(s)
Asbestosis, silicosis	Mesothelioma, lung carcinoma
Bronchitis	Lung carcinoma
Cystitis, bladder inflammation	Bladder carcinoma
Gingivitis, lichen planus	Oral squamous cell carcinoma
Inflammatory bowel disease, Crohn disease, chronic ulcerative colitis	Colorectal carcinoma
Lichen sclerosus	Vulvar squamous cell carcinoma
Chronic pancreatitis, hereditary pancreatitis	Pancreatic carcinoma
Reflux esophagitis, Barrett esophagus	Esophageal carcinoma
Sialadenitis	Salivary gland carcinoma
Sjögren syndrome, Hashimoto thyroiditis	MALT lymphoma
Skin inflammation	Melanoma
Infectious Agent (Nonviral)	**Associated Neoplasm(s)**
Helicobacter pylori	Gastric adenocarcinoma, MALT lymphoma
Chronic bacterial cholecystitis	Gallbladder cancer
Schistosomiasis	Bladder, liver, rectal carcinoma; follicular lymphoma of spleen
Liver flukes	Cholangiocarcinoma
Infectious Agent (Viral)	**Associated Neoplasm(s)**
HIV-1	Non-Hodgkin lymphoma, squamous cell carcinomas, Kaposi sarcoma
Hepatitis B and hepatitis C	Hepatocellular carcinoma
Epstein-Barr virus	B-cell non-Hodgkin lymphoma, Burkitt lymphoma, nasopharyngeal carcinoma
KSHV/HHV8 and immunodeficiency	Kaposi sarcoma
HPV-16, -18, -31, others	Cervical, anogenital
HTLV-1	Adult T-cell leukemia/lymphoma

MALT, Mucosa-associated lymphoid tissue; *HIV-1,* human immunodeficiency virus type 1; *KSHV(HHV8),* Kaposi sarcoma herpesvirus/human herpes virus 8: *HPV,* human papillomavirus; *HTLV-1,* human T-cell lymphotropic virus type 1.
From Kuper H et al: *J Intern Med* 248(3):171-183, 2000.

in childhood and disproportionately affects lower socioeconomic classes. Although most infections are asymptomatic, prolonged chronic inflammation can lead to increased gastric acid secretion, atrophic gastritis, and duodenal ulcers, or benign cellular proliferation that can in a small fraction of individuals progress to dysplastic changes and finally gastric adenocarcinoma. *H. pylori* infection can both directly and indirectly produce genetic and epigenetic changes in cells of infected stomachs, including mutations in *TP53* and alterations in the methylation of specific genes. Eradication of *H. pylori* from infected individuals before the development of dysplasia may prevent the development of cancer. However, there is no expert consensus on the value of population screening and treatment strategies. The MALT lymphomas associated with chronic *H. pylori* infections may depend on chronic inflammation and antigenic stimulation associated with infections, and therefore treatment with antibiotics may be useful even in cases of early lymphoma.

Once cells with malignant phenotypes have developed, additional complex interactions occur between the tumor and the surrounding stroma and cells of the immune and inflammatory systems. Cancers disrupt the environment, initiate or enhance inflammation, and in turn recruit local and distant cells (macrophages, lymphocytes, and other cellular components of inflammation). The acute inflammatory response is initially designed to eliminate infection, but evolves to initiate and direct the healing process (see Chapter 6). Successful tumors appear capable of manipulating cells of the inflammatory response from a rejection response towards the phenotypes associated with wound healing and tissue regeneration; a process that includes induction in the damaged tissue of cellular proliferation, neovascularization, and local immune suppression. These activities benefit cancer progression, as well as increase resistance to chemotherapeutic agents.

One of the key cells that promote tumor survival is the tumor-associated macrophage (TAM). Tumors commonly produce cytokines and chemokines that are chemotactic factors for monocytes/macrophages (e.g., colony-stimulating factor-1 [CSF1; also known as *macrophage colony–stimulating factor* or *M-CSF*], the chemokine ligand 2 [CCL2; also known as *monocyte chemotactic protein-1* or *MCP-1*]). Levels of CCL2 in human breast cancer and cancers of the esophagus are related to the degree of macrophage infiltration and progression of the tumor. Most tumors have large numbers of TAMs, whose presence frequently correlates with a worse prognosis. Thus monocytes are attracted from the blood and into the tumor, where they mature into macrophages. Monocytes have the capacity to differentiate into several macrophage phenotypes, depending on the conditions in the microenvironment. The classic proinflammatory macrophage (M1) is the primary macrophage in the acute inflammatory response and is responsible for removal and destruction of infectious agents. During healing, however, a different phenotype (M2) produces antiinflammatory mediators to suppress ongoing inflammation and induce cellular proliferation, angiogenesis, and wound healing. TAMs appear to phenotypically mimic the M2 phenotype.

TAMs have diminished cytotoxic response, and develop the capacity to block T-cytotoxic cell and natural killer (NK)-cell functions and produce cytokines that are advantageous for tumor growth and spread. TAMs secrete cellular growth factors (e.g., TGF-β and fibroblast growth factor-2 [FGF-2]) that favor tumor cell proliferation, angiogenesis, and tissue remodeling, similar to their activities in wound healing. They also secrete angiogenesis factors (e.g., VEGF) that induce neovascularization and matrix metalloproteinases (MMPs) that degrade intercellular matrix. The overall effect is increased tumor growth, invasion of the blood vessels, increased oxygen to the tumor, and invasion through the degraded matrix into the local tissue.

Cancer-associated fibroblasts (CAFs) synthesize the extracellular matrix that surrounds and permeates the tumor. Cytokines and growth factors stored in the matrix as well as growth factors, metalloproteases, proteoglycans, and other molecules secreted by CAFs contribute greatly to cancer progression, local spread, and metastasis.[13]

Evading Immune Destruction

Many cancers express cell surface antigens that are not generally found on normal cells from the same tissue. Tumor-associated antigens include products of oncogenes, antigens from oncogenic viruses, oncofetal antigens (expressed in embryonic tissues and tumors), and altered glycoproteins and glycolipids. Viral and tumor antigens are processed by the tumor cell and presented on the cell surface by major histocompatibility complex (MHC) class I molecules and are targets of CD8+ T-cytotoxic cells (Tcyto) (see Chapter 7). NK cells recognize altered

cell surface glycoproteins and glycolipids. Thus cancer cells should be recognized as foreign and destroyed by the immune system. In the laboratory, T lymphocytes and NK cells recognize and kill cancer cells. This observation gave rise to two concepts—*immune surveillance* and *immunotherapy*. The immune surveillance hypothesis predicts that most developing malignancies are suppressed by an efficient immune response against tumor-associated antigens. The rationale for immunotherapy predicts that the immune system could be used to target tumor-associated antigens and destroy tumors clinically. Immunotherapy could be either active, by immunization with tumor antigens to elicit or enhance the immune response against a particular cancer, or passive, by injecting the person with cancer with antibodies or lymphocytes directed against the tumor antigens. However, the interactions between cancer and the immune system are more complex than originally envisioned and both hypotheses remain controversial.

What is the role of the immune system in protecting against cancer? The most clearly documented effective immune response is prophylactic and directed against oncogenic viruses. Several viruses have been associated with human cancer; human papillomavirus (HPV), Epstein-Barr virus (EBV; also known as HHV4), Kaposi sarcoma herpesvirus (KSHV; also known as HHV8), and hepatitis B and C viruses (HBV, HCV) are associated with about 15% of all human cancers worldwide[14] (see Table 11.3). Cancer of the cervix and hepatocellular carcinoma account for approximately 80% of virus-linked cancer cases.

Virtually all cervical cancer is caused by infection with specific types of HPV, which infects basal skin cells and commonly causes warts. There are more than 120 HPV types, but only about 40 can infect human mucosal tissue, and only a few (HPV-16, -18, -31, and -45) are associated with the highest risk for developing cervical, anogenital, and penile cancer. Most HPV infection is handled effectively and rapidly by the immune system and does not cause cancer. Cancer is more common in people with prolonged infection with HPV (a decade or more), during which the viral DNA becomes integrated into the genomic DNA of the infected basal cell of the cervix and directs the persistent production of viral oncogenes. Early oncogenic HPV infection is readily detected by the Papanicolaou (Pap) test, an examination of cervical epithelial scrapings. Early detection of atypical cells in a Pap test alerts health care providers to the possibility of cervical carcinoma in situ, which can be effectively treated. The Pap test is probably the most effective cancer-screening test developed to date. For women age 30 to 65 years old, additional testing for HPV infection of cervical cells (HPV test) should be added. Vaccines protecting against the common oncogenic HPV types (HPV-16 and HPV-18 [types that cause 70% of cervical cancers] and HPV-6 and HPV-11 [types that cause 90% of genital warts]) were approved for clinical use beginning in 2006; if these vaccines are administered to young women and men before an initial HPV infection, this is likely to prevent many cases of cervical cancer.

Chronic hepatitis B infections are common in parts of Asia and Sub-Saharan Africa and confer up to a 200-fold increased risk of developing liver cancer. Chronic hepatitis C infections have become increasingly recognized in Western countries. Up to 80% of liver cancer cases worldwide are associated with chronic hepatitis caused either by HBV or by HCV. The initial infection with hepatitis B or C is not associated with cancer; instead, it is acquisition of a chronic viral hepatitis that markedly increases cancer risk. In both cases, it appears that a lifetime of chronic liver inflammation predisposes to the development of hepatocellular carcinoma. Widespread use of the HBV vaccine is expected to significantly decrease the incidence of chronic hepatitis B and hence hepatocellular carcinoma. Unfortunately, a vaccine for HCV is not yet available.

For most other human tumor viruses, immunoprophylaxis is not yet available. EBV and HHV8 are members of the Herpesviridae family.

More than 90% of adults have been infected with EBV, usually as children and without symptoms. EBV infection during adolescence may cause infectious mononucleosis. The virus infects B lymphocytes and stimulates their limited proliferation and usually becomes latent throughout the individual's life. If the individual is immunosuppressed because of human immunodeficiency virus (HIV) infection or because of drugs given for an organ transplant, persistent EBV infection can lead to the development of B-cell lymphomas. EBV infection also is associated with Burkitt lymphoma in areas of endemic malaria and with nasopharyngeal carcinoma, a cancer endemic in Chinese populations in Southeast Asia. HHV8 is linked to the development of Kaposi sarcoma, a cancer that was once seen primarily in older men but now occurs in a markedly more virulent form in immunosuppressed individuals, especially those with acquired immunodeficiency syndrome (AIDS). HHV8 also has been linked to several rare lymphomas. Human T-cell lymphotropic virus type 1 (HTLV-1) is an oncogenic retrovirus linked to the development of adult T-cell leukemia and lymphoma (ATLL). HTLV is transmitted vertically (that is, inherited by children from infected parents) and horizontally (e.g., by breast-feeding, sexual intercourse, blood transfusions, and exposure to infected needles). Infection with HTLV may be asymptomatic, and only a small fraction of infected individuals develop ATLL, often many years after acquiring the virus.

Thus immunization has proven beneficial in preventing viral-induced cancers. The immune surveillance hypothesis, however, would predict that components of the immune system, especially T cells, monitor the body and destroy most evolving tumors, even those not caused by viruses. If the immune surveillance hypothesis is correct, compromise of the immune system by immunosuppressive drugs or development of genetic or acquired immune deficiencies would result in increased incidences of all types of cancer. However, defective immune responses generally only increase the risk for lymphoid cancers, many of which are associated with viral infections. For instance, individuals taking chronic powerful immunosuppressive drugs, such as those given for kidney, heart, or liver transplant, have a much higher risk of developing viral-associated cancers, with a 10-fold increased risk of non-Hodgkin lymphoma (caused by EBV) and up to a 1000-fold increased risk of Kaposi sarcoma (caused by HHV8). The same immunosuppressed individuals, however, have only a slight increase in the risk of common cancers such as lung and colon cancer (and this could well be because of increased inflammation at those sites), and no increase in the risk of breast or prostate cancer.

However, many tumors have an abundance of tumor-infiltrating lymphocytes (TILs). Although the immune cells frequently found in tumors were once thought to be futile attempts at an antitumor response, instead it appears that cancers actively recruit an immune and stromal response to assist in remodeling of tissues, formation of new blood vessels, and promotion of metastasis. NK cells are generally in low amounts in tumors. The predominant TILs are T-regulatory (Treg) cells. Treg cells are CD4+ cells that differentiate under the control of specific cytokines, primarily TGF-β. The role of Treg cells during wound healing is to control or limit the immune response to protect the host's own tissues against autoimmune reactions. Their role in tumors is manipulated to prevent a destructive antitumor immune response and provide cytokines that facilitate tumor cell proliferation and spread. Treg cells and TAMs, as well as other stromal cells, produce very high levels of TGF-β and interleukin-10 (IL-10). IL-10 is an immunosuppressive cytokine, which generally decreases T-helper cell 1 (Th1) and Th2 activity, suppresses antigen recognition and cell proliferation by Th cells, and suppresses the capacity of CD8+ T-cytotoxic (Tcyto) cells to recognize, proliferate, and kill tumor cells. The goal of current immunotherapy regimens is to reverse this relationship and facilitate T-cell–mediated cancer cell death (discussed later in this chapter).

The release of immunosuppressive factors into the tumor micro-environment also increases resistance of the tumor to chemotherapy and radiotherapy. Increased levels of Treg cells in blood and lymph nodes and infiltrating the tumor correlate with poor outcomes in breast and GI tumors. In advanced non–small cell lung cancer, an elevated ratio of Treg to Tcyto cells is related to a poor response to platinum-based chemotherapy. Immunosuppressive cytokines additionally lower the cancer cell's sensitivity to immune-mediated death (Fig. 11.17). With increasing heterogeneity of cells within the tumor, subpopulations of antigen-negative cancer cell variants may selectively outgrow more immune-sensitive cells. Variants may suppress the production of particular antigens or suppress levels of antigen-presenting MHC class I. Other cytokines appear to increase the cancer cells' resistance to apoptosis. For example, the Th2 cytokine IL-4 increases the resistance of thyroid cancer to chemotherapy; IL-6 produced by Th cells, adipocytes, and fibroblasts activates survival pathways in breast cancer leading to resistance to radiotherapy; and adipocytes enhance the transcription of the anti-apoptotic factor Bcl-2 in leukemia cells.

Activating Invasion and Metastasis

Metastasis is the spread of cancer cells from the site of the original tumor to distant tissues and organs through the body. Metastasis is a defining characteristic of cancer and is the major cause of death from

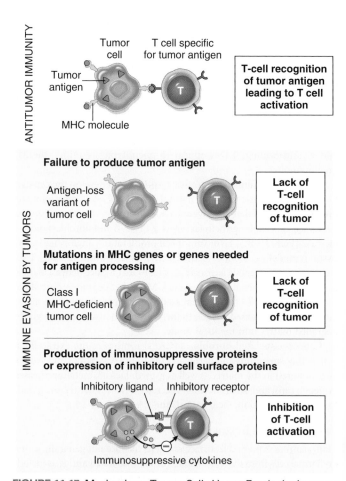

FIGURE 11.17 Mechanisms Tumor Cells Use to Evade the Immune System. Tumors may evade the immune response by losing expression of antigens or major histocompatibility complex (MHC) molecules or by producing immunosuppressive cytokines or ligands for inhibitory receptors on T cells. (From Kumar V et al: *Robbins and Cotran pathologic basis of disease,* ed 9, Philadelphia, 2015, Saunders.)

cancer. Cancer that has not metastasized can often be cured by a combination of surgery, chemotherapy, and radiation. These same therapies are frequently ineffective against cancer that has metastasized. For example, in appropriately treated women with localized low-stage breast cancer, the 5-year survival rate is often greater than 90%. Tragically, less than 30% of women with metastatic breast cancer are still alive 5 years after diagnosis. A growing body of basic and clinical research is defining the biologic principles of metastasis, with the hope that this improved understanding will lead to novel diagnostic approaches and better therapies to prevent and treat metastatic cancers.

How do cancer cells develop the ability to metastasize? Metastasis is a highly inefficient process. Cancer cells must surmount multiple physical and physiologic barriers in order to spread, survive, and proliferate in distant locations, and the destination must be receptive to the growth of the cancer. Changes in the tumor microenvironment initiate the metastatic process and may include stromal cell adaptation to increase tumor mass and intratumor hypoxia. As this diversity increases within the changing tumor microenvironment, some cancer cells evolve with multiple new abilities that can facilitate metastasis. The model for transition to metastatic cancer cells is called epithelial-mesenchymal transition.

Epithelial-mesenchymal transition (EMT) is a process that occurs normally in embryonic development, as well as wound healing and tissue repair. Generally, cells that have transitioned into a mesenchymal-like phenotype have suppressed expression of adhesion molecules with a loss of polarity, increased migratory capacity, elevated resistance to apoptosis, and demonstrated the potential to redifferentiate into other cell types. The transition to a mesenchymal-like phenotype is, in most cases, driven by cytokines and chemokines produced within the tumor microenvironment. IL-8 is an effective driver of carcinoma cells into EMT.

A degree of cellular "dedifferentiation" is necessary to produce the phenotype that can separate from the primary tumor and flourish in a potentially hostile secondary site. This results from a programmed transition of the still partially epithelial-like carcinoma to a more undifferentiated mesenchymal-like phenotype (Fig. 11.18). A similar process occurs with tumors of endothelial origin (endothelial-mesenchymal transition). The degree of dedifferentiation may be variable, but most cells undergoing EMT acquire stem cell traits that facilitate initial growth in a new microenvironment. The EMT is not a stable transition; after taking residence in the metastatic site, the tumor tends to regain some characteristics of the primary tumor, thus reverting to some extent to its epithelial origins. Because metastasis requires successful completion of each and every step, there may be many opportunities to interrupt this potentially lethal pathway.

Invasion, or local spread, is a prerequisite for metastasis. In its earliest stages, *local invasion* may occur by direct tumor extension. Eventually, however, cells migrate away from the primary tumor and invade the surrounding tissues (see Fig. 11.18). Invasion is a multistep process within EMT that includes diminished cell-to-cell adhesion, digestion of the surrounding extracellular matrix, and increased motility of individual cancer cells. TGF-β induces changes in expression of E-cadherin (an integral component of tight junctions) and of β_4-integrin in mammary gland tumor cells. The loss of E-cadherin in particular allows cells to detach from extracellular matrix and migrate more readily.

Recruitment of TAMs and other cell types is critical for invasion. Cells are normally attached to the extracellular matrix (ECM). TAMs and other stromal cells secrete proteases and protease activators, such as the MMPs and plasminogen activators, which promote digestion of connective tissue capsules and other structural barriers. Degradation of the surrounding ECM creates pathways through which cells can move, while releasing bioactive peptides as digestion products that further stimulate tumor growth and mobility.

Normal cells, when separated from their ECM, undergo anoikis, a form of apoptosis. Tumor cells adapted to a hypoxic environment have already been selected for resistance to apoptosis, often by loss of normal cell death pathways. The process of EMT frequently increases resistance to apoptosis.

To transition from local to distant metastasis, the cancer cells must also be able to invade local blood and lymphatic vessels, a task facilitated by stimulation of neoangiogenesis and lymphangiogenesis by factors such as VEGF. After release from the ECM and digestion of basement membranes, mobile cancer cells gain access to the circulation, perhaps facilitated by the leaky newly made vessels and attraction of the cells because of chemoattractants coming from these new vessels. Once in the circulation, metastatic cells must be able to withstand the physiologic stresses of travel in the blood and lymphatic circulation, including high shear rates and exposure to immune cells. One mechanism is for tumor cells to bind to blood platelets, giving them a protective coat of non-malignant blood cells that both shields the tumor cells and creates a small tumor embolus, or cancer clot, that can promote cancer cell survival in distant locations (see Fig. 11.18).

The neovascularization or natural formation of new blood vessels of a cancer offers malignant cells direct access into the venous blood and draining lymphatic vessels. The venous and lymphatic drainage networks associated with the primary tumor frequently determine the *pattern* of metastasis. Single cells, clumps, and even tumor fragments can disseminate by these routes. Anatomic patterns of lymphatic and venous blood flow help determine how colon cancers spread to the liver, liver cancers spread through the portal vein to the lungs, lung cancers spread through the systemic circulation to the brain, and breast cancer spreads through the lymphatics to axillary lymph nodes. Cancers often spread first to regional lymph nodes through the lymphatics and then to distant organs through the bloodstream.

There also is a major yet poorly understood selectivity of different cancers for different sites. Metastatic breast cancer often spreads through the bloodstream to bones but rarely to kidney or spleen, whereas lymphomas often spread to the spleen but uncommonly spread to bone. In a key study, different types of cancer cells were injected into the carotid artery of mice.[15] In spite of identical blood flow–mediated distribution of the cancer cells, each cell type produced cancers in very different parts of the brain. This tissue selectivity is likely caused by specific interactions between the cancer cells and specific receptors on the small blood vessels in different organs. Experimental metastasis studies in mice are beginning to reveal additional molecular reasons for this tissue specificity.

A cancer's ability to establish a metastatic lesion in a new location requires that the cancer *survive* in the specific environment and be capable of forming complex and heterogeneous tumors. In some cases, these tumor-initiating cells are very rare. Human cancers transplanted into special immune-deficient mice will grow and can metastasize. Experiments have been performed to determine how few cancer cells are capable of establishing a tumor; only 1 in 10,000 human colon cancer cells are able to reform a complex and heterogeneous colon cancer in mice; however, in human melanomas 1 in 4 cells can initiate a complex tumor in the appropriate mouse model. Thus the number of potentially metastatic cells may vary greatly with the particular cancer.

However, metastasis does not universally result in proliferation at a new site. Some cancer cells survive at a new site but do not proliferate to form a clinically relevant metastatic site. These cancer cells appear to exist in a state of *dormancy*. Cellular dormancy is cellular quiescence (quietness or inactivity), a stable, nonproliferative state that is reversible. Cells may remain quiescent for years before initiating proliferation. About two-thirds of breast cancer deaths occur after a 5-year disease-free interval. In other conditions, solitary tumor cells

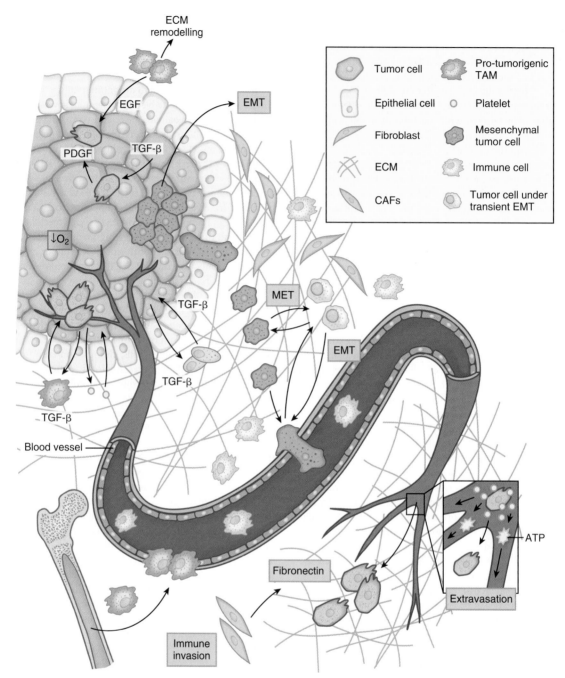

FIGURE 11.18 Epithelial-Mesenchymal Transition and Metastasis. The microenvironment supports metastatic dissemination and colonization at secondary sites. Stromal cells (e.g., mesenchymal stem cells [MSCs]), possibly facilitated by a relative decrease in oxygen levels in the tumor, contribute to the epithelial-to-mesenchymal transition (EMT) through which tumor cells develop a metastatic phenotype characterized by suppression of adhesion molecules and reduced adherence to adjacent cells and extracellular matrix, increased local invasion, and access to the blood and lymphatic circulations. One major mediator of this process is TGF-β, which is secreted by the tumor stroma. Intravascularization of tumor cells into the circulation is facilitated by protumorigenic TAMs, and CAFs tend to cluster at the leading edge of the invading cancer cells and secrete matrix metalloproteinases that promote digestion and remodeling of the surrounding ECM. Survival in the circulation is promoted by association with platelets and clotting factors that shield the cancer cells from cytotoxic immune cells (T-cytotoxic cells and NK cells). At a metastatic site, cancer cells adhere to local vascular endothelium, undergo extravascularization facilitated by the effects of ATP on the endothelium, and undergo mesenchymal-to-epithelial transition (MET). *ATP,* Adenosine triphosphate; *CAF,* cancer-associated fibroblast; *ECM,* extracellular matrix; *NK,* natural killer cell; *PDGF,* platelet-derived growth factor; *TAM,* tumor-associated macrophage; *TGF-β,* tumor growth factor-beta; *Treg,* T-regulatory cell; *VEGF,* vascular endothelial cell growth factor. (Adapted from Peinado H, Olmeda D, Cano A: *Nat Rev Cancer* 7[6]:415-428, 2007; Quail DF, Joyce JA: *Nat Med* 19[11]:1423-1437, 2013.)

can be detected in the blood years after a complete clinical remission in individuals, and many people with detectable micrometastases will not develop clinically obvious metastases. Cancer cell dormancy may be extremely common, even without a history of clinical cancer. Studies of deceased individuals without any history of cancer suggest that most individuals have dormant cancer cells that never adjusted to form a malignant tumor.

The causes of dormancy and, more importantly, escape from dormancy, and the development of a malignant cancer are unknown. Dormancy may result from features of the cell or the environmental niche, or both. Individuals with clinical cancers may shed disseminated tumor cells very early from premetastatic lesions. These early cells may have developed inadequately to a metastatic phenotype and thus cannot recruit cells into a supportive stroma or initiated angiogenesis. Another consideration is the niche itself. It is not clear whether a developing cancer secretes factors that enter the bloodstream and prepare potential metastatic niches. If so, early disseminated cancer cells may encounter nonsupportive niches that foster dormancy. A clear understanding of dormancy is needed because existing cancer therapies do not address this condition.

QUICK CHECK 11.4

1. Why is the stroma important for cancer growth and invasion?
2. Identify cancers that are the result of chronic inflammation.
3. Why does inflammation fuel cancer development/invasion?
4. Identify common viruses that can cause cancer.
5. How do cancers protect themselves from cell death?
6. What is the clinical significance of tumor cell dormancy?

CLINICAL MANIFESTATIONS OF CANCER

The clinical manifestations of cancer are numerous and depend on the localization and type of tumor, and some are apparent before actual diagnosis of a malignancy. Generally, the variety and intensity of symptoms will increase as the malignancy progresses.

Paraneoplastic Syndromes

Paraneoplastic syndromes are symptom complexes that are triggered by a cancer but are not caused by direct local effects of the tumor mass. They are most commonly caused by biologic substances released from the tumor (e.g., hormones, cytokines) or by an immune response triggered by the tumor. For example, a small fraction of carcinoid tumors release substances, including serotonin, into the bloodstream that cause flushing, diarrhea, wheezing, and rapid heartbeat. A number of cancers trigger an antibody response that attacks the nervous system, causing a variety of neurologic disorders that can precede other symptoms of cancer by months.

Although infrequent, paraneoplastic syndromes are significant because they may be the earliest symptom of an unknown cancer and, in affected individuals, can be serious, often irreversible, and sometimes life-threatening. Table 11.4 presents the classifications of paraneoplastic syndromes. Other clinical manifestations of cancer are summarized in Box 11.1. Factors predisposing individuals with cancer to infection are contained in Table 11.5.

Molecular Mechanisms of Cachexia

Cachexia is a multiorgan, energy wasting syndrome or type of energy balance disorder where energy intake is decreased and energy expenditure

---

BOX 11.1   Common Side Effects of Cancer and Cancer Therapy

Anemia: Commonly associated with malignancy, with 20% of persons diagnosed with cancer have hemoglobin concentrations less than 9 g/dl (normal value = 15 g/dl). Mechanisms of anemia include chronic bleeding (resulting in iron deficiency), severe malnutrition, cytotoxic chemotherapy, and malignancy in blood-forming organs. Chronic bleeding and iron deficiency can accompany colorectal or genitourinary malignancy. Iron also is malabsorbed in individuals with gastric, pancreatic, or upper intestinal cancer.

Bone density loss: Osteoporosis, or the less severe osteopenia, may occur secondary to hormone treatment, such as that used for breast cancer and prostate cancer, or in individuals treated with steroids.

Cachexia: A syndrome that has many symptoms, including anorexia, early satiety (filling), weight loss, anemia, asthenia (marked weakness), taste alterations, and altered protein, lipid, and carbohydrate metabolism. It is the most severe form of malnutrition associated with cancer and results in wasting, emaciation, and diminished quality of life. Cytokines and metabolites from the tumor may contribute to cachexia.

Cardiac and pulmonary damage: Chemotherapy and localized radiation can damage the heart and lungs, resulting in an increased risk of heart failure and decreased pulmonary function.

Fatigue: Severe fatigue is the most frequently reported and persistent symptom of cancer and cancer treatment, particularly chemotherapy. Suggested causes include sleep disturbances, chronic inflammation, anemia, depression, level of activity, nutritional status, and other environmental and physical factors.

Gastrointestinal (GI) tract: The rapidly proliferating cells of the GI tract are particularly sensitive to radiation and chemotherapy, which leads to oral ulcers (stomatitis), malabsorption, and diarrhea, in addition to an increased risk of infection from the individual's own microbiome.

Hair loss (alopecia) and skin: Some chemotherapy generally affects hair follicles, whereas radiation is more localized. The condition usually is temporary, although hair may regrow with a different texture initially. Decreased renewal rates of the epidermal layers in the skin may lead to skin breakdown and dryness, altering the normal barrier protection against infection. Radiation therapy may cause skin erythema (redness) and contribute to breakdown.

Infection: The most significant cause of complications and death in people with malignant disease is infection. Immune suppression, lymphopenia, and granulocytopenia may result from the underlying cancer or secondary to treatment, increasing the risk of serious microbial (e.g., bacterial and fungal) infections. The prevalence of hospital-acquired (nosocomial) infections increases because of indwelling medical devices, inadequate wound care, and the introduction of microorganisms from visitors and other individuals.

Infertility: Male or female infertility may result secondary to the cancer, surgical treatment, or treatment with chemotherapy or radiation. Many infertility clinics will freeze sperm, eggs, or embryos before the imitation of therapy.

Leukopenia and thrombocytopenia: Causes can include many chemotherapeutic drugs and radiation therapy because they are toxic to the bone marrow, often causing granulocytopenia and thrombocytopenia. Thrombocytopenia is a major cause of hemorrhage in people with cancer and often is treated with platelet transfusions.

Lymphedema: Accumulation of fluid in the tissues results from damage to the lymphatic system from lymphoid cancer or metastatic disease, surgery, or radiation treatment.

Pain: Pain may occur during the early stages of malignant disease but intensifies with disease progression. Direct pressure, obstruction, invasion of a sensitive structure, stretching of visceral surfaces, tissue destruction, infection, and inflammation all can cause pain. Chronic pain may result from nerve damage secondary to surgery, chemotherapy, or radiation.

TABLE 11.4 Paraneoplastic Syndromes

Clinical Syndromes	Major Forms of Underlying Cancer	Causal Mechanism
Endocrinopathies		
Cushing syndrome	Small cell carcinoma of the lung Pancreatic carcinoma Neural tumors	ACTH or ACTH-like substance
Syndrome of inappropriate antidiuretic hormone (SIADH) secretion	Small cell carcinoma of the lung Intracranial neoplasms	Antidiuretic hormone or atrial natriuretic hormones
Hypercalcemia	Squamous cell carcinoma of the lung Breast carcinoma Renal carcinoma Adult T-cell leukemia/lymphoma Ovarian carcinoma	PTHRP, TGF-α, TNF, IL-1
Hypoglycemia	Fibrosarcoma Other mesenchymal sarcomas Hepatocellular carcinoma	Insulin or insulin-like substance
Carcinoid syndrome	Bronchial adenoma (carcinoid) Pancreatic carcinoma Gastric carcinoma	Serotonin, bradykinin
Polycythemia	Renal carcinoma Cerebellar hemangioma Hepatocellular carcinoma	Erythropoietin
Nerve and Muscle Syndromes		
Myasthenia	Bronchogenic carcinoma	Immunologic
Disorders of the central and peripheral nervous systems	Breast carcinoma	Unknown
Dermatologic Disorders		
Acanthosis nigricans	Gastric carcinoma Lung carcinoma Uterine carcinoma	Immunologic; secretion of epidermal growth factor
Dermatomyositis	Bronchogenic carcinoma Breast carcinoma	Immunologic
Osseous, Articular, and Soft Tissue Changes		
Hypertrophic osteoarthropathy and clubbing of the fingers	Bronchogenic carcinoma	Unknown
Vascular and Hematologic Changes		
Venous thrombosis (Trousseau phenomenon)	Pancreatic carcinoma Bronchogenic carcinoma Other cancers	Tumor products (mucins that activate clotting)
Nonbacterial thrombotic endocarditis	Advanced cancers	Hypercoagulability
Anemia	Thymic neoplasms	Unknown
Others		
Nephrotic syndrome	Various cancers	Tumor antigens, immune complexes

ACTH, Adrenocorticotropic hormone; *IL,* interleukin; *PTHRP,* parathyroid hormone–related protein; *TGF,* transforming growth factor; *TNF,* tumor necrosis factor.
From Kumar V et al: *Pathologic basis of disease,* ed 7, Philadelphia, 2005, Saunders.

is increased (Fig. 11.19). A growing consensus indicates that the definition of cachexia involves two common factors: (1) weight loss mainly from loss of skeletal muscle and (2) body fat and inflammation.[16] It is often irreversible, affects 50% to 80% of people with cancer, causes substantial weight loss, and may account for up to 20% of cancer deaths.[16] Cachexia is dependent on the individual's response to tumor progression, with activation of the inflammatory response and energetic inefficiency involving the mitochondria.[16] Energy intake and expenditure depends on the tumor type and its growth phase. Because individuals who are being administered total parenteral nutrition still lose weight, increased resting energy expenditure may be the cause of the wasting syndrome. Investigators are studying the role of both mitochondria and sarcoplasmic reticulum (SR) in muscle function and the relationship to cachexia. Muscle weakness and fatigue are related to loss of myofibrillar proteins in muscle cells. Abnormalities in protein and amino acid metabolism are noted in cachectic muscle (Fig. 11.20). Contributing further to muscle wasting are an increase in apoptosis and an impaired capacity for regeneration. Many signaling pathways are involved in protein

TABLE 11.5 Factors Predisposing Individuals With Cancer to Infection

Factor	Basis
Age	Many common malignancies occur mostly in older age. Immunologic functions decline with age. General debility reduces immunocompetence. Immobility predisposes to infection. Far-advanced cancer often results in immobility and general debility that worsen with age. Elderly persons are predisposed to nutritional inadequacies. Malnutrition impairs immunocompetence.
Tumor	Nutritional derangements can result. Sites and circumstances favorable to the growth of microorganisms (obstruction, serous or blood effusion, ulceration) can be created. Far-advanced disease predisposes individuals to debility and immobility. Humoral or cellular immune defects may result. Metastasis to bone marrow may cause leukopenia or other defects in immunity.
Leukemias	Inadequate granulocyte production (impaired phagocytosis) results. Thrombocytopenia (bleeding) can occur. Late effect: chronic lung disease from *Pneumocystis carinii* pneumonia can develop during therapy.
Lymphomas and other mononuclear phagocyte malignancies	Humoral and cellular immune defects (anergy, altered immunoglobulin production) result. Late effect: splenectomy in children can cause increased susceptibility to infection.
Surgical treatment	Invasive procedure interrupts first lines of defense. Radical nature of surgery (removal of large blocks of tissue in lengthy procedures) causes hemorrhage, decreased tissue perfusion, creation of dead spaces, tissue necrosis, and devitalization of tissues. Procedure may be "dirty" surgery (bowel, infected, or contaminated areas). Surgery patients often are older and at poor risk. Long preoperative hospitalization often precedes surgery. Patients may have received previous adrenocorticosteroid therapy. Patients may have infections at sites remote from the operative area. Nutritional derangements (especially important in head and neck surgery) may result. Lymph node dissection may predispose patients to local infection and impair containment to area. Gynecologic surgery may result in fistulae. Lung surgery may cause bronchopleural fistulae. Debility and immobility may result.

Data from Donovan MI, Girton SF: *Cancer care nursing,* ed 2, New York, 1984; Appleton-Century-Crofts; and Murphy GP et al: *Clinical oncology,* ed 2, New York, 1994, American Cancer Society.

turnover leading to the wasting process and are activated by inflammatory mediators including cytokines, myostatin, and tumor-derived factors. In addition to muscle wasting, miRNAs may be involved in stimulating the breakdown of adipose tissue. In cancer cachexia, skeletal muscle loss includes major loss of white adipose tissue (WAT). The WAT loss is thought to be caused by (1) increased lipolysis, (2) decreased activity of lipoprotein lipase (LPL), and (3) decreased new or de novo lipogenesis in adipose tissue. New data show that WAT cells undergo a "browning" process during cancer cachexia where they change to beige cells called *BAT-like cells*. Browning is associated with increased thermogenesis. Tumor-derived compounds, such as IL-6 (which also may be released by immune cells) and parathyroid hormone–related protein (PTHRP), may be the drivers of thermogenesis.

An unusual and frustrating component of cancer care is the person's early satiety, or a sense of being full after only a few mouthfuls of food. Brain mediators are involved in the regulation of food intake and include appetite, satiation, taste, and smell of food. Therefore the brain is an important organ in anorexia and consequently altered energy balance. Both the orexigenic (appetite-stimulating) and anorexigenic (appetite-suppressing) brain pathways are profoundly altered. (Cytokines are discussed in detail in Chapters 6 and 7.)

DIAGNOSIS AND STAGING OF CANCER

Histologic Staging

Cancer can be discovered in many ways: after screening tests, from routine exams, and after investigation of symptoms. The symptoms a cancer produces are as diverse as the types of cancer. The location of the cancer can determine symptoms by physical pressure, obstruction, and loss of normal function, or a cancer can cause problems far away from its source by pressing on nerves or secreting bioactive compounds. Whatever the initial complaint, once the diagnosis is suspected and a tumor has been identified, it is essential that tumor tissue be obtained

to establish a definitive diagnosis and correctly classify the disease. Various methods of obtaining tissue are described in Table 11.6.

DID YOU KNOW?

Liquid Biopsy

As part of the precision medicine movement and patient-tailored therapies is liquid biopsy. A liquid biopsy is from cancer-derived components that circulate in the bloodstream and consists of the detection and isolation of circulating tumor cells, circulating tumor DNA, and exosomes. Circulating cell-free DNA fragments released from apoptotic or necrotic cancer cells are called circulating tumor DNA (ctDNA), and exosomes (EXOs) are membrane-encapsulated subcellular structures containing proteins and nucleic acids released by the tumor cells (see Fig. 12.17). A liquid biopsy will avoid traditional biopsies and surgical procedures that are invasive. Research and development is ongoing to perfect the liquid biopsy.

Data from Palmirotta R et al: Liquid biopsy of cancer: a multimodal diagnostic tool in clinical oncology, *Ther Adv Med Oncol* 10: 1758835918794630, 2018).

Once tissue is obtained, it is examined microscopically by the pathologist for the histologic hallmarks of cancer detailed in the beginning of this chapter. The classification of the cancer can be further facilitated by a variety of clinically available tests, including immunohistochemical stains, flow cytometry, electron microscopy, chromosome analysis, and genetic studies.

If the diagnosis of cancer is established, it is critical to determine if the cancer has spread, known as the *stage of the cancer.* Cancer staging initially involves determining the size of the tumor, the degree to which it has invaded locally, and the extent to which it has spread (metastasized) (Fig. 11.21). Specific molecular tests increasingly are used in staging. Diverse schemes are used for staging different tumors. In general, a

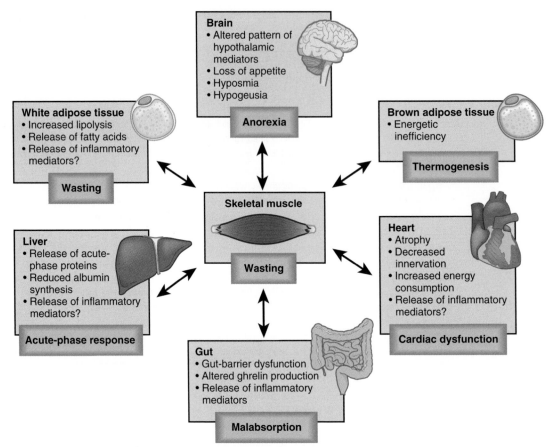

FIGURE 11.19 Cachexia: A Multiorgan Syndrome. Loss of skeletal muscle and of adipose tissue are major contributors to cachexia. But many other organs have a role in cachexia syndrome, and the wasting that occurs in muscle may depend on alterations in these other organs or tissues. Changes in hypothalamic function and activation of brown adipose tissue, in addition to alterations in liver and heart function, also are involved in the syndrome. Recent data suggests that the conversion of white adipose tissue to brown adipose tissue is triggered both by humoral inflammatory mediators, such as interleukin-6 (IL-6), and by tumor-derived compounds, such as parathyroid hormone–related protein (PTHRP). Some studies support a role for gut microbiota in cancer cachexia and the possibility of a relationship between the gut microbiota and skeletal muscle. (From Argilés JM et al: *Nat Rev Cancer* 14[11]:754-762, 2014; Bindels LB, Delzenne NM: *Int J Biochem Cell Biol* 45:2186-2190, 2013; Bindels LB et al: *PLOS One* 7[6]:e37971, 2012; Varian BJ et al: *Oncotarget* 7[11]:11803-11816, 2016.)

TABLE 11.6	**Obtaining Tissue—The Biopsy**	
Procedure	**Purpose**	**Example**
Excisional biopsy	Complete removal, usually with a margin of normal tissue	Full resection (e.g., mastectomy, partial colectomy)
Incisional biopsy	Removal of a portion of the lesion	Lymph node biopsy, muscle mass biopsy
Core needle biopsy	Often performed with direct vision or guided by ultrasound or computed tomography (CT)	Needle biopsy of prostate or liver mass
Fine-needle aspirate	Obtains dissociated cells for cytologic study but does not preserve the tissue structure	Thyroid, breast mass
Exfoliative cytology	Cells shed from the surface (e.g., from the cervix, sputum [lung], or urine)	Brushings from lung or colon endoscopy

four-stage system is used, with carcinoma in situ regarded as a special case. Cancer confined to the organ of origin is stage 1; cancer that is invasive locally is stage 2; cancer that has spread to regional structures, such as lymph nodes, is stage 3; and cancer that has spread to distant sites (e.g., a liver cancer that has spread to a lung or a prostate cancer that has spread to bone) is stage 4. One common scheme for standardizing staging is the World Health Organization's TNM system: *T* indicates tumor spread, *N* indicates node involvement, and *M* indicates the presence of distant metastasis (see Fig. 11.21). The prognosis generally worsens with increasing tumor size, lymph node involvement, and metastasis. Staging also may alter the choice of therapy; more aggressive therapy is delivered to more invasive disease.

Tumor Markers

During surveillance or diagnosis of cancer, as well as following therapy, specific biochemical markers of tumors have proven to be helpful. These **tumor markers** are substances produced by both benign and malignant cells that are either present in or on tumor cells or found in blood, spinal fluid, or urine. Some tumor markers have been known for many decades. Tumor markers include hormones, enzymes, genes, antigens, and antibodies (Table 11.7). If the tumor marker itself has biologic

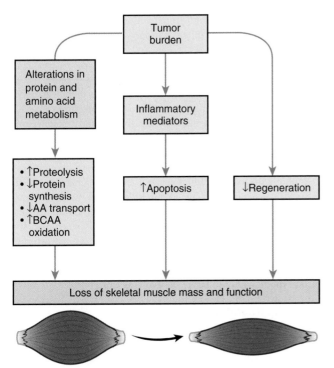

FIGURE 11.20 Wasting of Skeletal Muscle. Inflammation plays a major role in muscle wasting and is linked to alterations in protein and amino acid metabolism, activation of muscle cell apoptosis, and decreased regeneration *BCAA*, Branched-chain amino acids. (Adapted from Argilés JM et al: *Nat Rev Cancer* 14[11]:754-762, 2014.)

TABLE 11.7 Examples of Tumor Markers in Body Fluids		
Marker Name	Nature	Type of Tumor
Adrenocorticotropic hormone (ACTH)	Peptide hormone	Pituitary adenomas
Alpha fetoprotein (AFP)	70-kDa protein	Hepatic, germ cell
Beta-2 microglobulin (β2M)	11-kDa protein	Multiple myeloma, CLL
Beta-human chorionic gonadotropin (β-hCG)	Glycopeptide hormone β-chain	Germ cell, choriocarcinoma
CA15-3/CA27.29	Large MW glycoproteins	Breast
CA-125	Large MW glycoprotein	Ovary
CA19-9	201-dDa glycoprotein	Pancreas, gallbladder, bile duct, gastric
Calcitonin	3.4 kDa polypeptide hormone	Thyroid
Carcinoembryonic antigen (CEA)	200-kDa glycoprotein	GI, pancreas, lung, breast, etc.
Catecholamines	Epinephrine and precursors	Pheochromocytoma (adrenal medulla)
CD20		Non-Hodgkin lymphoma
Chromogranin A (CgA)	33-36 kDa glycosylated phosphoprotein	Neuroendocrine
	48-kDa protein	
Homovanillic acid/ vanillylmandelic acid (HVA/VMA)	Catecholamine metabolites	Neuroblastoma
Prostate-specific antigen (PSA)	33-kDa glycoprotein	Prostate
Urinary Bence Jones protein	Ig light chain	Multiple myeloma

CLL, Chronic lymphocytic leukemia, *GI*, gastrointestinal; *Ig*, immunoglobulin; *kDa*, kilodalton(s), *MW*, molecular weight.

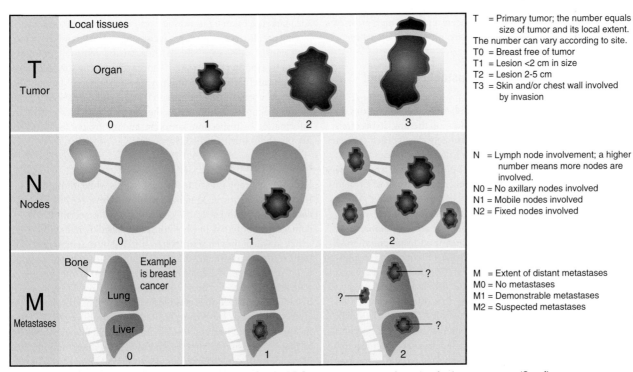

FIGURE 11.21 Tumor Staging by the TNM System. Example of staging for breast cancer. (See figure for explanation of the abbreviations.)

activity, then it can cause symptoms, such as those described in Table 11.7. For example, the adrenal medulla normally secretes the catecholamine epinephrine (adrenaline). Benign tumors of the adrenal medulla (pheochromocytoma) can produce catecholamines (e.g., adrenaline) in vast excess, leading to rapid pulse rate, high blood pressure, diaphoresis (i.e., sweating), and tremors. Detection of elevated blood or urine levels of catecholamines helps confirm the diagnosis, and treatment of the disease relieves the symptoms. Tumor markers can be used in three ways:

1. to screen and identify individuals at high risk for cancer;
2. to help diagnose the specific type of tumor in individuals with clinical manifestations relating to their tumor, as in adrenal tumors or enlarged liver or prostate; and
3. to follow the clinical course of a tumor.

To date, no tumor marker has proven satisfactory to screen populations of healthy individuals for cancer. Testing large populations will always detect a few normal individuals with test results at the high end of the normal distribution (the "false positives"), which can lead to expensive and invasive additional tests and unnecessary concern. Similarly, some individuals with disease will have test results in the normal range ("false negatives"). More importantly, some nonmalignant conditions also can produce tumor markers. The presence of an elevated tumor marker therefore may suggest a specific diagnosis, but it is not used alone as a definitive diagnostic test. For instance, prostate tumors secrete *prostate specific antigen (PSA)* into the blood. But enthusiasm has waned for routine testing for PSA levels, and now the US Preventive Services Task Force (USPSTF) recommends that clinicians inform men ages 55 to 69 years about the potential benefits and harms of PSA screening for prostate cancer.[17] Screening offers a small potential benefit of reducing the chance of dying of prostate cancer. Many men, however, will experience potential harms of screening, including false-positive results that require additional workup, overdiagnosis and overtreatment, and treatment complications such as incontinence and impotence. Falling levels of PSA after radiation or surgical therapy may indicate successful treatment for prostate cancer, and a later rise may indicate a recurrence. Identification of ideal sensitive and specific tumor markers that are elevated early in the course of common cancers remains a high priority because the early detection of cancer often improves the treatment outcome.

Classification of Tumors: Immunohistochemical and Genetic Analysis

Because knowledge about the cellular and molecular alterations in individual cancers can influence the choices of therapy, it becomes increasingly important for clinicians to accurately classify each cancer. The classification, and hence the treatment decisions, of cancers was originally based on gross and light microscopic appearance and is now commonly accompanied by immunohistochemical analysis of protein expression. Increasingly, this is supplemented by a more extensive genetic analysis of the tumors. The range of genetic analysis is expanding rapidly. In a research setting and increasingly in clinical settings, global gene expression and mutation analysis can be measured using polymerase chain reaction (PCR), microarray, or advanced DNA sequencing technology. These analyses can be used to classify tumors more precisely and may predict the most effective therapy. This detailed analysis of each tumor is a form of personalized medicine that offers therapy based on a very detailed knowledge of the characteristics of each individual's specific cancer. This enhanced molecular characterization subdivides cancers into therapeutically and prognostically relevant smaller groups. As an example, breast cancers can now be subclassified into over four types (luminal A, luminal B, basal-like, and others) based on their expression of specific markers, such as estrogen receptor, *HER2/Neu*,

and other specific genes and proteins. Each subtype has a different response to therapy and a different prognosis.

TREATMENT OF CANCER

Until late in the last century the mainstays of cancer therapy have been surgery, chemotherapy, and radiation therapy. These approaches have been highly successful for certain types of cancer, but have many limitations. Immunotherapy has been the holy grail of cancer therapists, but successes have been few. Cancer therapy is now in a process of rapid evolution. Armed with a more clear understanding that cancer is in fact multiple diseases that share general hallmarks/enablers and that the specific mechanisms underlying each hallmark may vary considerably among cancers (e.g., the large variety of oncogenes that may be used to differentiate cancers), modern cancer therapy is reaching a stage where complete genetic analysis of an individual cancer may determine the appropriate combination of therapies. Thus effective therapy may include a combination of reagents targeting several hallmarks and under constant modification to target the evolving cancer cells.

Classic Approaches
Surgery

Surgery plays many roles in the care of individuals with cancer. The multiple approaches to obtaining tissue for diagnosis have been discussed. Surgery is often the definitive treatment of cancers that do not spread beyond the limits of surgical excision. It also is indicated for the relief of symptoms, for instance, those caused by tumor mass obstruction. In selected high-risk diseases, surgery plays a role in the prevention of cancer. For example, individuals with familial adenomatous polyposis because of germline mutations of the *APC* gene have close to a 100% lifetime risk of colon cancer, so a prophylactic colectomy is indicated. Similarly, women with *BRCA1/2* mutations have a markedly increased risk of breast and ovarian cancer, and often choose prophylactic mastectomy or bilateral salpingo-oophorectomy (removal of ovaries and fallopian tubes), or both.

Key principles apply specifically to cancer surgery, including obtaining adequate surgical margins during a resection to prevent local recurrences, placing needle tracks and biopsy incision scars (that may be contaminated with cancer cells) carefully so they can be removed in subsequent incisions, avoiding the spread of cancer cells during surgical procedures through careful technique, and paying attention to obtaining adequate tissue specimens during biopsies so that the pathologist can be confident of the diagnosis. Additionally, the surgeon provides critical staging information by inspection, sampling, and removal of local and regional lymph nodes during procedures.

Radiation Therapy

Radiation therapy is used to kill cancer cells while minimizing damage to normal structures. Ionizing radiation damages cells by imparting enough energy to cause molecular damage, especially to DNA. The damage may be lethal, in which the cell is killed by radiation; potentially lethal, in which the cell is so severely affected by radiation that modifications in its environment will cause it to die; or sublethal, in which the cell can subsequently repair itself. Cellular compartments with rapidly renewing cells are, in general, more radiosensitive. Effective cell killing by radiation also requires good local delivery of oxygen, something not always present in large cancers. Radiation produces slow changes in most cancers and irreversible changes in normal tissues as well. Because of these irreversible changes, each tissue has a maximum lifetime dose of radiation it can tolerate. Radiation is well suited to treat localized disease in areas that are hard to reach surgically, for example, in the brain and pelvis. A number of radiation delivery methods are available, with external beam being the most common. Radiation sources, such as small ^{125}I-labeled capsules (also called *seeds*), can also be temporarily placed into body cavities, a delivery method termed brachytherapy. Brachytherapy is useful in the treatment of cervical, prostate, and head and neck cancers.

Chemotherapy

The era of modern chemotherapy began with the observation in World War II that mustard gas exposure caused suppression of the bone marrow. Related compounds, such as nitrogen mustard and cyclophosphamide, were then tested and produced clinical responses in hematologic malignancies, including lymphomas. Also in the late 1940s, based on the remarkable clinical observation that the vitamin folic acid could *increase* leukemia growth, antifolate drugs were developed (leading ultimately to methotrexate) that produced remissions in previously untreatable leukemia.

All chemotherapeutic agents take advantage of specific vulnerabilities in target cancer cells. Antimetabolites, such as methotrexate and L-asparaginase, block normal growth pathways in all cells, but leukemia and other cancer cells are exquisitely sensitive to folic acid and asparagine deprivation, whereas nonmalignant cells are far less sensitive. Similarly, some cancer cells are highly sensitive to DNA-damaging agents, such as cyclophosphamide and anthracyclines, because of the oncogenic mutations that accelerate the cell cycle and DNA synthesis. Cellular checkpoints prevent normal cells treated with microtubule-directed drugs, such as vincristine and the taxanes, from undergoing mitosis, whereas cancer cells treated with these agents lack normal checkpoints, continue through mitosis, and undergo mitotic catastrophe (see Chapter 1).

Single chemotherapeutic agents often shrink cancers, but these drugs given alone rarely, if ever, provide a cure. Hence chemotherapy drugs are usually given in combinations designed to attack a cancer from many different weaknesses at the same time and to limit the dose and therefore the toxicity of any single agent. Cancers contain a very large number of cells, and commonly a small fraction of those cells may be resistant to a particular drug. However, those cells are likely to be sensitive to the second or third drug in a chemotherapy cocktail. Scheduling of drug administration is also very important, with many studies showing cancers are more likely to develop drug resistance if there are significant delays between planned courses of chemotherapy.

Chemotherapy can be used for several distinct purposes. Induction chemotherapy seeks to cause shrinkage or disappearance of tumors. In Hodgkin lymphoma, for example, chemotherapy alone can be used in some cases to cure the disease. In other settings, chemotherapy may shrink the tumor and improve symptoms without ultimately providing a cure. Adjuvant chemotherapy is given after surgical excision of a cancer with the goal of eliminating micrometastases. Neoadjuvant chemotherapy is given before localized (surgical or radiation) treatment of a cancer. As with induction chemotherapy, the effectiveness, or lack thereof, of neoadjuvant therapy can be measured (for example, with follow-up scans). Neoadjuvant therapy can shrink a cancer so that surgery may spare more normal tissue. For example, in the bone cancer osteogenic sarcoma, neoadjuvant therapy often converts a large tumor mass into a much smaller mass, allowing the surgeon to perform a limb-sparing excision rather than an amputation.

A major complication of chemotherapy is death of rapidly dividing cells that are not cancerous, such as those of the bone marrow. Hematopoietic growth factors also have been used to counter the effects of chemotherapy on bone marrow cells.

Immunotherapy

The expression of unique antigens on cancer cells that can be targeted by T cells has driven the quest for effective therapies to initiate an immune response, boost a currently inadequate immune response, or convert a tumor-protective immune response to a destructive one.[18] Since the 1950s this quest has been characterized by promises and frustrations.

Tumor cell vaccines were one of the first attempts at immunotherapy for cancer and have been extremely effective in protecting individuals against infective agents. Several cancer cell vaccines continue to be tested, but so far none have been effective enough to be licensed.[19]

An immunotherapy approach approved by the Food and Drug Administration (FDA) is using sipuleucel-T for the treatment of metastatic prostate cancer that is resistant to conventional therapy. Dendritic cells are obtained from an individual with prostate cancer and incubated with a protein resulting from the fusion of prostatic acid phosphatase, a cancer antigen found in 95% of prostate cancers, and granulocyte-macrophage colony–stimulating factor (GM-CSF), an immune cell–stimulating cytokine. The dendritic cells process and present the antigen and are infused back into the patient. In clinical trials treatment with sipuleucel-T extended the lives of patients by 4.1 months. These results may not seem spectacular, but were meaningful in this group of individuals with very advanced and terminal disease. Other vaccine approaches against B-cell lymphoma and melanoma have shown promising results.

Passive immunotherapy using lymphocytes against cancer cell antigens has been attempted, with limited success, since the early 1970s. In recent years, passive administration of tumor-targeting lymphocytes (adoptive cell therapy [ACT]) has developed more promise as a result of various pretreatment ex vivo techniques that improve treatment efficacy. A major source of an individual's lymphocytes is those that have infiltrated the tumor (tumor-infiltrating lymphocytes [TILs]). The efficacy of these cells is increased by depleting the Treg cells within the population or by engineering the T-cell receptor for greater specificity against the tumor. Cancers have developed many mechanisms for escaping the cell killing effects of T-cytotoxic cells (Tc cells). Recognition of cancer-associated antigens by the Tc may be completely suppressed. Several approaches have been designed to bypass suppression of the T-cell receptor (TCR), which controls the specificity and function of Tc. One approach is the engineering of T cells with *chimeric* (sequences derived from two different genes; artificial) antigen receptors, or CAR T cells. CAR T therapies then use the individuals' own cells to create more specific cancer fighting cells (Fig. 11.22).

A family of monoclonal antibodies are currently approved for use against cancer. One group is called immune checkpoint inhibitors. These antibodies are directed against co-stimulatory molecules involved in repressing T-cell immune responses (see Chapter 7). By blocking inhibitory signals, T-cytotoxic cells may retain tumor-killing capacity.

Targeted Disruption of Cancer

As discussed previously, cancers appear to share a variety of hallmarks that contribute to the malignant phenotype. Recent molecular and genetic analyses of groups of cancer can classify an individual's cancer by the spectrum of mutations underlying the cancer phenotype. However, each of the therapeutic approaches described previously generally treats specific vulnerabilities of the cancer rather than a variety of contributing factors. That approach is not successful in most invasive cancers because some cancer cells may undergo further mutation leading to therapeutic resistance.

Exceptions include targeted drugs, used in combination with conventional chemotherapy, against very specific characteristics of selected cancers. For example, imatinib is a competitive inhibitor of tyrosine kinases, primarily the BCR-ABL tyrosine kinase (Table 11.8). It is highly effective in treating CML but ineffective in virtually all other cancers. Monoclonal antibodies against the CD20 antigen expressed on some B-cell lymphomas, the epidermal growth factor (EGF) receptor on colon cancers and head and neck cancers, and the HER2 EGF receptor on

TABLE 11.8 Examples of Molecular-Era Anticancer Drugs

Drug (Trade Name)	Type of Drug	Molecular Target	Disease
Imatinib (Gleevec)	Small molecule TKI	BCR-ABL tyrosine kinase, FGF receptor tyrosine kinase	Chronic myeloid leukemia (CML), gastrointestinal stromal tumor (GIST)
Erlotinib (Tarceva)	Small molecule TKI	EGF receptor tyrosine kinase	Subset of lung cancer
Trastuzumab (Herceptin)	Monoclonal antibody	HER2 receptor tyrosine kinase	HER2-positive breast cancer
Bevacizumab (Avastin)	Monoclonal antibody	VEGF receptor	Advanced colorectal cancer
Rituximab (Rituxan)	Monoclonal antibody	CD20 antigen on B lymphocytes	B-cell malignancies

EGF, Endothelial growth factor; *FGF,* fibroblast growth factor; *HER2,* human epidermal growth factor receptor 2; *TKI,* tyrosine kinase inhibitor; *VEGF,* vascular endothelial growth factor.

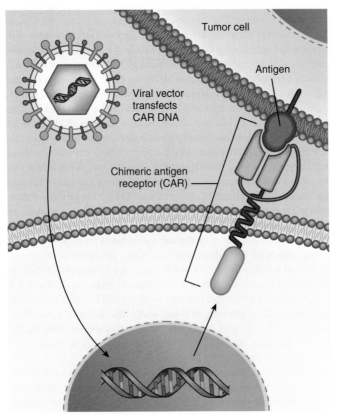

FIGURE 11.22 CAR T-Cell Immunotherapy. A person's T cells are extracted from blood and modified with a viral vector to express an artificial or a chimeric antigen receptor (CAR) for a particular cancer-associated antigen. T cells are then reinfused into the individual. The engineered cells recognize and kill cancerous cells. Side effects of the CAR T therapies can be mild to moderate, although some people may experience life-threatening reactions (e.g., cytokine release syndromes [CRS] and macrophage activation syndromes [MAS]). (Adapted from Brower V: *The CAR T-cell race.* Available at http://www.the-scientist.com/?articles.view/articleNo/42462/title/The-CAR-T-Cell-Race/. Accessed February 5, 2018.)

breast cancer are relatively successful.[20] These drugs are so tightly targeted they have much less toxicity than conventional chemotherapies that have targets in virtually all cells.

Tumor growth and progression are dependent on a variety of mutations leading to expression of oncogenes, inactivation of tumor-suppressor molecules, and interactions with inflammatory cells in the tumor microenvironment. These interactions foster angiogenesis, resistance to apoptosis and immune-mediated cancer cell death, altered tumor cell metabolism, and metastasis. A more efficacious therapeutic approach therefore may be a combination of drugs highly targeted to cancer hallmarks.[21]

More than 25 drugs are listed at the National Cancer Institute as cancer-targeting agents that inactivate oncogenes, block angiogenesis, and affect cancer cell metabolism. Monoclonal antibodies are available that induce apoptosis in tumor-infiltrating cells such as TAM, Treg cells, and tumor endothelium. Additionally, specific antagonists may neutralize the effects of cytokines, chemokines, and other tumor-enhancing mediators produced in the tumor microenvironment. These are usually in the form of monoclonal antibodies, which are available against TNF-α, VEGF, HER-2, and other ligands and their receptors. Such highly specific targeting would minimize secondary toxic effects. Information on the prevention of cancer by altering and eliminating high-risk lifestyle behaviors is contained in Chapter 12.

> ✔ **QUICK CHECK 11.5**
> 1. Describe the major clinical manifestations of cancer.
> 2. How is cancer diagnosed?
> 3. What are the most common treatments for cancer?

SUMMARY REVIEW

Cancer Terminology and Characteristics

1. Cancer is a disease in which abnormal cells divide uncontrollably and invade other tissues. A tumor is a new growth, or neoplasm.
2. Benign tumors are usually encapsulated and well differentiated with well-organized stroma and do not spread to distant locations. They are named for the tissues from which they arise. Benign tumors are noncancerous.
3. Malignant tumors are cancerous. Compared with benign tumors, malignant tumors have more rapid growth rates, specific microscopic alterations (anaplasia, or loss of differentiation, and pleomorphism, or variability in size and shape), absence of normal tissue organization, and no capsule. They invade blood vessels and lymphatics and have distant metastases. The stroma is disorganized with loss of normal tissue structure.

4. Cancers are named for the cell type from which they originate. Carcinomas arise from epithelial tissue, lymphomas are cancers of lymphatic tissue, and leukemias are cancers of blood-forming cells.

5. Carcinoma in situ (CIS) refers to noninvasive epithelial tumors of glandular or squamous cell origin. These early–stage cancers are localized to the epithelium and have not penetrated the local basement membrane.

The Biology of Cancer Cells

1. Cancer is a complex disease and the microenvironment of a tumor is a heterogenous mixture of cells, both cancerous and benign.

2. Tumor initiation is dependent on mutational and epigenetic changes and characteristics of the microenvironment. Tumor progression is governed further by more genetic mutations, epigenetic alterations, and changing microenvironment.

3. Genetic changes include small and large DNA mutations that alter genes, chromosomes, and non–coding RNAs, as well as epigenetic changes because of altered chemical modifications of DNA and histones.

4. Driver mutations "drive" the progression of cancer. Passenger mutations are random events that do not contribute to the malignant phenotype. After a critical number of driver mutations, the cell becomes cancerous.

5. Mutations activate growth-promotion pathways, block anti-growth signals, prevent apoptosis, stimulate telomerase and new blood vessel growth, and allow tissue invasion and distant metastasis.

6. The processes that occur during the development of cancer are analogous to wound healing. The proliferation of cancer cells and enlargement of the tumor elicit synthesis of proinflammatory mediators by the cancer cells and adjacent nonmalignant cells.

7. Like wound healing, mediators recruit inflammatory/immune cells and cells normally associated with tissue repair. These cells form the stroma (tumor microenvironment) that surrounds and infiltrates the tumor.

8. Cancer heterogeneity or diversity arises from ongoing proliferation and mutation.

9. Hallmarks of cancer that are primarily genomic alterations include sustained proliferative signaling, evading growth suppression, genomic instability, and replicative immortality. Other hallmarks secondary to genomic change include induction of angiogenesis, reprogramming energy metabolism, resistance to destruction, and activating invasion and metastasis.

10. Normal cells only enter proliferative phases in response to growth factors. Cancerous cells characteristically express mutated or over-expressed proto-oncogenes, referred to as oncogenes, which are independent of normal regulatory mechanisms and signal uncontrolled sustained proliferation.

11. Some oncogenes, such as RAS, result from point mutations. Other oncogenes can result from genetic translocations. Translocation can cause excess and inappropriate production of a proliferation factor, such as with Burkitt lymphoma. Translocations can also lead to production of novel proteins with growth-promoting properties, as is seen with the Philadelphia chromosome in chronic myeloid leukemias (CML).

12. Tumor-suppressor genes normally regulate cell cycle, but they must be inactivated in cancer cells by mutations to each allele, one from each parent.

13. A common mutation in cancer cells is inactivation of the tumor-suppressor gene tumor protein p53 (TP53), which activates caretaker genes, ones responsible for maintaining genomic integrity. Caretaker genes control expression of many genes that repair DNA damage,

suppress cellular proliferation during genomic repair, and initiate apoptosis. Inactivation of p53 results in increased mutation rates and cancer.

14. In rare families, a germ cell mutation (an inheritable mutation on a sperm or egg cell) in a tumor-suppressor gene, such as TP53 or the retinoblastoma gene (RB), may lead to a greatly increased risk for developing particular cancers.

15. Genomic instability refers to an increased tendency of alterations/mutations in the genome during the life cycle of cells. Genomic instability may result from increased epigenetic silencing or modulation of gene function.

16. Changes in gene regulation can affect entire networks of signaling, not just single genes. Gene expression networks can be regulated by changes in microRNAs (miRNAs or miRs) and other non–coding RNAs (ncRNAs).

17. Cancer cells are immortal. When they reach a critical age, cancer cells activate telomerase to restore and maintain their telomeres, thereby allowing cancer cells to divide repeatedly or become immortal.

18. Like many normal adult tissues, cancers can contain rare stem cells that provide a source of immortal cells. To fully eradicate a cancer, it may be necessary to target the cancer stem cell.

19. Access to the vascular system is essential for tumor growth. Cancerous tumors maintain secretion of angiogenic factors and prevent the release of angiogenic inhibitors, which stimulates new blood vessel growth (called neovascularization or angiogenesis).

20. The vessels formed within tumors originate from endothelial sprouting from existing capillaries and irregular branching, rather than regular branching seen in healthy tissue. The vessels are also more porous and prone to hemorrhage and allow passage of tumor cells into the vascular system.

21. Cancer cells are able to reprogram energy metabolism. The successful cancer cell divides rapidly, with the consequent requirement for the building blocks of new cells, such as ATP. Many cancer genes encourage aerobic glycolysis instead of oxidative phosphorylation, which allows for a more efficient production of molecular building blocks needed for rapid growth.

22. Oncogenes can drive metabolic reprogramming, enabling cancer cells to (1) maintain deregulated proliferation, (2) withstand challenges associated with oxygen and nutrient limitations, (3) maintain a dedifferentiated state with associated alterations in gene expression, and (4) corrupt the surrounding microenvironment to assist tumor growth and dissemination.

23. In cancer, defects in the intrinsic or extrinsic cell death pathways, or both, provide resistance to apoptotic cell death.

24. Some conditions of chronic inflammation increase the risk of developing cancer. A prime example is the association between gastric cancer and infection with Helicobacter pylori.

25. The inflammatory response may contribute to the onset of cancer and be manipulated throughout the process to benefit tumor progression and spread.

26. One of the key cells that promote tumor survival is the tumor-associated macrophage (TAM). Most tumors have large numbers of TAMs, whose presence may correlate with a worse prognosis. Cancer-associated fibroblasts contribute greatly to cancer progression, local spread, and metastasis.

27. Unique antigens and other markers on tumor cells can be recognized by T cells and NK cells of the immune system, leading to destruction of the tumor cell.

28. The immune surveillance hypothesis predicts that most developing malignancies are suppressed by an efficient immune response against tumor-associated antigens. Therefore the rationale for

immunotherapy predicts that the immune system could be used to target tumor-associated antigens and destroy tumors clinically.

29. The role of the immune system in protecting against cancer has been clearly documented against oncogenic viruses. Antibodies induced by vaccines against oncogenic viruses, such as human papillomavirus (HPV) and hepatitis B virus (HBV), protect against initial infection and development of cervical and liver tumors, respectively.

30. Cancer cells can evade rejection by the immune system by production of immunosuppressive factors, induction of immunosuppressive T-regulator cells, evolution of tumor-antigen negative variants, or suppressed expression of antigen-presenting MHC class I molecules.

31. Metastasis is the spread of cancer cells from the site of the original tumor to distant tissues and organs through the body and is the major cause of death from cancer.

32. Metastasis is a complex process that requires cells to have many new abilities, including the ability to invade, survive, and proliferate in a new environment.

33. Carcinomas undergo a process of epithelial-mesenchymal transition (EMT) during which many epithelial-like characteristics are lost (e.g., polarity, adhesion to basement membrane), resulting in increased migratory capacity, increased resistance to apoptosis, and a dedifferentiated stem cell–like state that favors growth in foreign microenvironments and establishment of metastatic disease.

34. Invasion, or local spread, consists of loss of cell-to-cell contact, degradation of the extracellular matrix (ECM), and increased motility of individual cancer cells. Stromal cells, particularly tumor-associated macrophages (TAMs), are essential to this process.

35. Some cancers appear to selectively home to particular metastatic sites, which may be a result of interactions between the cancer cells and specific receptors on the small blood vessels in different organs.

Clinical Manifestations of Cancer

1. Paraneoplastic syndromes are rare symptom complexes, often caused by biologically active substances released from a tumor or by an immune response triggered by a tumor, that manifest as symptoms not directly caused by the local effects of the cancer.

2. Common side effects of cancer and cancer therapy include anemia, bone density loss, cachexia, cardiac and pulmonary damage, fatigue, gastrointestinal issues, hair loss and skin conditions, infection, infertility, leukopenia and thrombocytopenia, lymphedema, and pain.

3. Anemia associated with cancer usually occurs because of malnutrition, chronic bleeding and resultant iron deficiency, chemotherapy, radiation, and malignancies in the blood-forming organs.

4. Cachexia is a multiorgan energy wasting syndrome where energy intake is decreased and energy expenditure is increased. Two factors are most significant: muscle loss and inflammation. Cachexia has many clinical manifestations including anorexia, early satiety (filling), weight loss, anemia, asthenia (marked weakness), taste alterations, and altered protein, lipid, and carbohydrate metabolism. Muscle wasting involves many protein signaling pathways and inflammatory mediators. Profoundly altered are both appetite-stimulating and appetite-suppressing brain pathways.

5. Fatigue is the most frequently reported symptom of cancer and cancer treatment.

6. The gastrointestinal tract relies on rapidly growing cells to provide an absorptive surface for nutrients. Both chemotherapy and radiation therapy may cause decreased cell turnover, thereby leading to oral ulcers (stomatitis), malabsorption, and diarrhea.

7. Alopecia (hair loss) results from chemotherapy effects on hair follicles. Alopecia is usually temporary, although hair may initially regrow with a different texture. Not all chemotherapeutic agents cause alopecia. Decreased renewal rates of the epidermal layers in the skin may lead to skin breakdown and dryness, altering the normal barrier protection against infection.

8. Infection is the most significant cause of complications and death. Immune suppression, lymphopenia, and granulocytopenia may result from the underlying cancer or secondary to treatment increasing the risk of serious microbial infections.

9. Leukopenia and thrombocytopenia are usually a result of chemotherapy (which is toxic to bone marrow) or radiation (which kills circulating leukocytes). Thrombocytopenia is a major cause of hemorrhage in people with cancer.

10. Pain is generally associated with the late stages of cancer. It can be caused by pressure, obstruction, invasion of a structure sensitive to pain, stretching, tissue destruction, and inflammation.

Diagnosis and Staging of Cancer

1. The diagnosis of cancer requires a biopsy and examination of tumor tissue by a pathologist. Cancer classification is established by a variety of tests.

2. Tumor staging involves the size of the tumor, the degree to which it has locally invaded, and the extent to which it has spread. A standard scheme for staging is the T (tumor spread), N (node involvement), and M (metastasis) system.

3. Tumor markers are substances (i.e., hormones, enzymes, genes, antigens, antibodies) found in cancer cells and in blood, spinal fluid, or urine. They are used to screen and identify individuals at high risk for cancer, to help diagnose specific types of tumors, and to follow the clinical course of cancer. To date, no tumor marker has proven satisfactory to screen populations of healthy individuals for cancer.

4. The classification, and hence the treatment decisions, of cancers was originally based on gross and light microscopic appearance, and is now commonly accompanied by immunohistochemical analysis of protein expression. Increasingly, this is supplemented by a more extensive molecular analysis of the tumors.

5. Cancer is treated routinely with surgery, radiation therapy, chemotherapy, and combinations of these modalities. However, cancer therapy is rapidly evolving, and genetic anaolysis may help determine appropriate therapies.

6. Surgical therapy is used for nonmetastatic disease (in which cure is possible by removing the tumor) and as a palliative measure to alleviate symptoms.

7. Ionizing radiation causes cell damage; therefore the goal of radiation therapy is to damage the tumor without causing excessive toxicity or damage to nondiseased structures.

8. The theoretic basis of chemotherapy is the vulnerability of tumor cells in various stages of the cell cycle. Modern chemotherapy uses combinations of drugs with different targets and different toxicities.

9. Induction chemotherapy seeks to cause shrinkage or disappearance of tumors. Adjuvant chemotherapy is given after surgical excision of a cancer with the goal of eliminating micrometastases. Neoadjuvant chemotherapy is given before localized (surgical or radiation) treatment of a cancer to shrink a cancer so that surgery may spare more normal tissue.

10. Immunotherapy attempts to modify the immune system from a cancer-protective state to a destructive condition.

11. Future treatment of tumors will, most likely, use a careful histologic and genetic analysis of individual cancers that prescribes a combination of tumor-targeting drugs to simultaneously disrupt multiple hallmarks of that particular cancer.

KEY TERMS

REFERENCES

1. National Cancer Institute (NCI): Fact sheet: what is cancer? Available at: www.cancer.gov/cancertopics/cancerlibrary/what-is-cancer. (Accessed November 30, 2014).
2. Hanahan D, Weinberg RA: Hallmarks of cancer, *Cell* 100(1):57-70, 2000.
3. Hanahan D, Weinberg RA: Hallmarks of cancer: the next generation, *Cell* 144(5):646-674, 2011.
4. Hanahan D, Coussens LM: Accessories to the crime: functions of cells recruited to the tumor microenvironment, *Cancer Cell* 21(3):309-322, 2012.
5. Kuchenbaecker KB, et al: Risks of breast, ovarian, and contralateral breast cancer for BRCA1 and BRCA2 mutation carriers, *J Am Med Assoc* 317(23):2402-2416, 2017.
6. National Cancer Institute (NCI): Fact Sheet: BRCA1 and BRCA2: cancer risk and genetic testing. Available at: www.cancer.gov/cancertopics/factsheet/Risk/BRCA. (Accessed November 30, 2018).

7. Martin D, Sabater B: The cancer Warburg effect may be a testable example of the minimum entropy production rate principle, *Phys Biol* 14(2):024001, 2017.
8. Das R, et al: Microenvironment-dependent growth of preneoplastic and malignant plasma cells in humanized mice, *Nat Med* 22:1351-1357, 2016.
9. Fu Y, et al: The reverse Warburg effect is likely to be an Achilles' heel of cancer that can be exploited for cancer therapy, *Oncotarget* 8(34):57813-57825, 2017.
10. Flores A: Increased lactate dehydrogenase activity is dispensable in squamous carcinoma cells of origin, *Nat Commun* 10(1):91, 2019.
11. Pavlova NN, Thompson CB: The emerging hallmarks of cancer metabolism, *Cell Metab* 23(1):27-47, 2016.
12. Tsun ZY, Possemato R: Amino acid management in cancer, *Semin Cell Dev Biol* 43:22-32, 2015.
13. Kalluri R: The biology and function of fibroblasts in cancer, *Nat Rev Cancer* 16(9):583-598, 2016.
14. McLaughlin-Drubin ME, Munger K: Viruses associated with human cancer, *Biochim Biophys Acta* 1782(3):127-150, 2008.

15. Fidler IJ, et al: The biology of melanoma brain metastasis, *Cancer Metastasis Rev* 18(3):387-400, 1999.
16. Argilés JM, et al: Cancer cachexia: understanding the molecular basis, *Nat Rev Cancer* 14(11):754-762, 2014.
17. US Preventive Services Task Force (USPSTF): Prostate cancer screening draft recommendations, 2017. Available at: https://www.uspreventiveservicestaskforce.org. (Accessed February 3, 2018).
18. Schumacher TN, Hacohen N: Neoantigens encoded in the cancer genome, *Curr Opin Immunol* 41(4):98-103, 2016.
19. Romero P, et al: The human vaccines project: a roadmap for cancer vaccine development, *Sci Transl Med* 8(334):1-7, 2016.
20. Sliwkowski MX, Mellman I: Antibody therapeutics in cancer, *Science* 341(6151):1192-1198, 2013.
21. Hanahan D: Rethinking the war on cancer, *Lancet* 383(9916):558-563, 2014.

12

Cancer Epidemiology

Kathryn L. McCance, Lois E. Brenneman

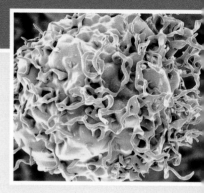

EVOLVE WEBSITE

CHAPTER OUTLINE

Cancer develops from a complex interaction of predisposing factors that include genetics and epigenetics, environmental-lifestyle factors, altered metabolism and biologic processes, and exposure to carcinogens (cancer-causing substances).[1-3] Many forms of cancer are preventable, particularly where predisposing factors include high-risk activities and exposure to known carcinogens (Fig. 12.1). Research has identified a number of factors known to promote cancer and influence mortality and morbidity in persons who develop cancer. Known risk factors include the following[4-6]:

- Lifestyle choices, such as smoking, alcohol intake, and diet
- Lack of physical exercise and obesity
- Certain infections and predisposing sexual practices
- Environmental factors, including exposure to sunlight, natural and medical ionizing radiation, and/or air, water and soil carcinogens
- Occupational carcinogen exposure
- Certain prescribed and illicit medications
- Socioeconomic factors that affect exposures, risk, and detection and treatment

Estimates of environmental factors and their risk of cancer vary. The International Agency for Research on Cancer (IARC) has identified more than 100 chemicals, occupations, physical agents, biologic agents, and other agents as human carcinogens.[4] Table 12.1 lists risk factors classified by cancer site within the body.

GENETICS, EPIGENETICS, AND TISSUE

Cancers are caused by environmental-lifestyle and genetic factors (Fig. 12.2). *Patterns* of cancer incidence around the world are primarily influenced by environmental and lifestyle factors. At the cellular level, cancer is *driven* by genetic and epigenetic alterations. Interacting factors that influence risk include immune and inflammatory systems, alterations in detoxifying enzymes, deoxyribonucleic acid (DNA) repair genes, and hormonal and metabolic factors (see Chapter 11). Inflammation, especially chronic inflammation, has a significant role in cancer development as do hormonal factors and abnormal glucose or lipid metabolism.

Cancer development and spread is influenced by the tissue microenvironment or stroma (surrounding supportive tissue) (see Chapter 11). Stromal tissue contains infiltrating immune cells, which can promote chronic inflammation. Chronic inflammation can *precede* and possibly *initiate* cancer changes (e.g., as noted in inflammation-induced colon cancer). Inflammation also can be caused by numerous environmental factors. Environmental factors are significant for lung and respiratory tract cancers where environmental proinflammatory factors include inhaled tobacco smoke, asbestos fibers, air pollutants from automotive exhaust, and industrial sources.[7-8] When malignant transformation develops, tumor cells continually interact with the surrounding stromal cells and, importantly, the infiltrated immune and inflammatory cells (see Chapter 11). Such interactions can influence the degree to which tumors grow in size or spread, or both

---

✔ QUICK CHECK 12.1

1. Discuss what is meant by "environment is the main cause of cancer."
2. What is the role of the microenvironment in cancer development and progression?

Text continued on p. 264

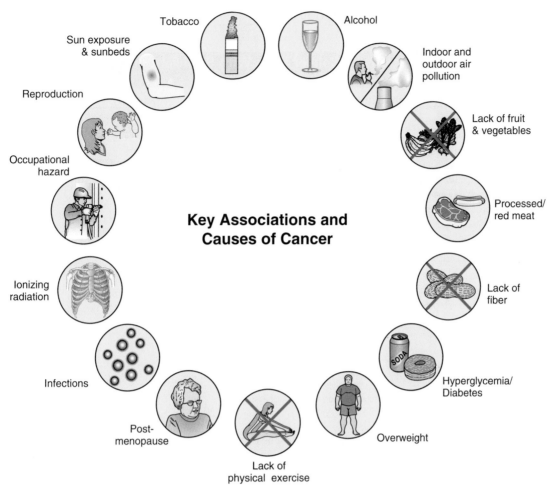

FIGURE 12.1 Key Associations and Causes of Cancer. Tobacco, diet and alcohol, obesity, pollution, lack of physical activity, hormones, infections, ionizing radiation, occupational hazards, reproductive factors, and ultraviolet light are key factors for cancer. Although diet is key and known to affect cancer risk, determining specific dietary factors has been very difficult and is emerging.

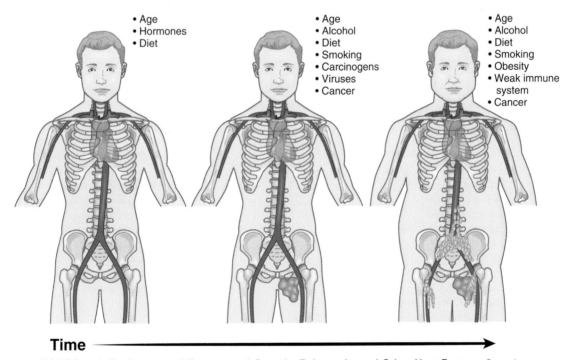

Time

FIGURE 12.2 Environmental Factors and Genetic, Epigenetic, and Other Host Factors. Over time a person's internal genetic makeup persistently interacts with external or environmental factors. Environmental factors (e.g., diet, smoking, alcohol use, hormones, certain viruses, chemical carcinogens) collectively interact with internal epigenetic factors and genetic mutations to destabilize normal biologic factors including immune factors for balancing growth and maturation. (Adapted from NCI: *Understanding cancer series: cancer: inside and outside factors*, Washington, DC, National Cancer Institute, National Institutes of Health, 2007.)

TABLE 12.1   List of Classifications by Cancer Sites With Sufficient or Limited Evidence in Humans*

Cancer Site	Carcinogenic Agents With Sufficient Evidence in Humans	Agents With Limited Evidence in Humans
Lip, Oral Cavity, and Pharynx		
Lip		Solar radiation
Oral cavity	Alcoholic beverages Betel quid with tobacco Betel quid without tobacco Human papillomavirus type 16 Tobacco, smokeless Tobacco smoking	
Salivary gland	X-radiation, γ-radiation	Radioiodines, including iodine-131
Tonsil	Human papillomavirus type 16	
Pharynx	Alcoholic beverages Betel quid with tobacco Human papillomavirus type 16 Tobacco smoking	Asbestos (all forms) Mate drinking, hot Printing presses Tobacco smoke, secondhand
Nasopharynx	Epstein-Barr virus Formaldehyde Salted fish, Chinese style Wood dust	
Digestive tract, upper	Acetaldehyde associated with consumption of alcoholic beverages	
Digestive Organs		
Esophagus	Acetaldehyde associated with consumption of alcoholic beverages Alcoholic beverages Betel quid with tobacco Betel quid without tobacco Tobacco, smokeless Tobacco smoking X-radiation, γ-radiation	Dry cleaning Mate drinking, hot Pickled vegetables (traditional Asian) Rubber production industry Tetrachloroethylene
Stomach	*Helicobacter pylori* Rubber production industry Tobacco smoking X-radiation, γ-radiation	Asbestos (all forms) Epstein-Barr virus Lead compounds, inorganic Nitrate or nitrite (ingested) under conditions that result in endogenous nitrosation Pickled vegetables (traditional Asian) Salted fish (Chinese style)
Colon and rectum	Alcoholic beverages Tobacco smoking X-radiation, γ-radiation	Asbestos (all forms) *Schistosoma japonicum*
Anus	Human immunodeficiency virus type 1 Human papillomavirus type 16	Human papillomavirus types 18, 33
Liver and bile duct	Aflatoxins Alcoholic beverages *Clonorchis sinensis* Estrogen-progestogen contraceptives Hepatitis B virus Hepatitis C virus *Opisthorchis viverrini* Plutonium Thorium-232 and its decay products Tobacco smoking (in smokers and in smokers' children) Vinyl chloride	Androgenic (anabolic) steroids Arsenic and inorganic arsenic compounds Betel quid without tobacco Human immunodeficiency virus type 1 Polychlorinated biphenyls *Schistosoma japonicum* Trichloroethylene X-radiation, γ-radiation
Gallbladder	Thorium-232 and its decay products	

TABLE 12.1 **List of Classifications by Cancer Sites With Sufficient or Limited Evidence in Humans*—cont'd**

Cancer Site	Carcinogenic Agents With Sufficient Evidence in Humans	Agents With Limited Evidence in Humans
Pancreas	Tobacco, smokeless Tobacco smoking	Alcoholic beverages Thorium-232 and its decay products X-radiation, γ-radiation
Digestive tract, unspecified		Radioiodines, including iodine-131
Respiratory Organs		
Nasal cavity and paranasal sinus	Isopropyl alcohol production Leather dust Nickel compounds Radium-226 and its decay products Radium-228 and its decay products Tobacco smoking Wood dust	Carpentry and joinery Chromium (VI) compounds Formaldehyde Textile manufacturing
Larynx	Acid mists, strong inorganic Alcoholic beverages Asbestos (all forms) Tobacco smoking	Human papillomavirus type 16 Mate drinking, hot Rubber production industry Sulfur mustard Tobacco smoke, secondhand
Lung	Aluminum production Arsenic and inorganic arsenic compounds Beryllium and beryllium products Bis(chloromethyl) ether; chloromethyl methyl ether (technical grade) Cadmium and cadmium compounds Chromium (VI) compounds Coal, indoor emissions from household combustion Coal gasification Coal-tar pitch Coke production Hematite mining (underground) Iron and steel founding MOPP (vincristine-prednisone-nitrogen mustard-procarbazine mixture) Nickel compounds Painting Plutonium Radon-222 and its decay products Rubber production industry Silica dust, crystalline Soot Sulfur mustard Tobacco smoke, secondhand Tobacco smoking X-radiation, γ-radiation	Acid mists, strong inorganic Art glass, glass containers, and pressed ware (manufacture of) Biomass fuel (primarily wood), indoor emissions from household combustion of Bitumens, oxidized, and their emissions during roofing Bitumens, hard, and their emissions during mastic asphalt work Carbon electrode manufacture α-Chlorinated toluenes and benzyl chloride (combined exposure) Cobalt metal with tungsten carbide Creosotes Engine exhaust, diesel Frying, emissions from high-temperature Insecticides, nonarsenical (occupational exposures in spraying and application) Printing processes 2,3,7,8-Tetrachlorodibenzo-*para*-dioxin Welding fumes
Bone, Skin, Mesothelium, Endothelium, and Soft Tissue		
Bone	Plutonium Radium-224 and its decay products Radium-226 and its decay products Radium-228 and its decay products X-radiation, γ-radiation	Radioiodines, including iodine-131
Skin (melanoma)	Solar radiation Ultraviolet-emitting tanning devices	

Continued

TABLE 12.1   List of Classifications by Cancer Sites With Sufficient or Limited Evidence in Humans*—cont'd

Cancer Site	Carcinogenic Agents With Sufficient Evidence in Humans	Agents With Limited Evidence in Humans
Skin (other malignant neoplasms)	Arsenic and inorganic arsenic compounds Azathioprine Coal-tar distillation Coal-tar pitch Cyclosporine Methoxypsoralen plus ultraviolet A Mineral oils, untreated or mildly treated Shale oils Solar radiation Soot X-radiation, γ-radiation	Creosotes Human immunodeficiency virus type 1 Human papillomavirus types 5 and 8 (in individuals with epidermodysplasia verruciformis) Nitrogen mustard Petroleum refining (occupational exposures) Ultraviolet-emitting tanning devices Merkel cell polyomavirus (MCV)
Mesothelium (pleura and peritoneum)	Asbestos (all forms) Erionite Painting	
Endothelium (Kaposi sarcoma)	Human immunodeficiency virus type 1 Kaposi sarcoma herpesvirus	
Soft tissue		Polychlorophenols or their sodium salts (combined exposures) Radioiodines, including iodine-131 2,3,7,8-Tetrachlorodibenzo-*para*-dioxin
Breast and Female Genital Organs		
Breast	Alcoholic beverages Diethylstilbestrol Estrogen-progestogen contraceptives Estrogen-progestogen menopausal therapy X-radiation, γ-radiation	Estrogen menopausal therapy Ethylene oxide Shift work that involves circadian disruption Tobacco smoking
Vulva	Human papillomavirus 16	Human immunodeficiency virus type 1
Vagina	Diethylstilbestrol (exposure in utero) Human papillomavirus 16	Human immunodeficiency virus type 1
Uterine cervix	Diethylstilbestrol (exposure in utero) Estrogen-progestogen contraceptives Human immunodeficiency virus type 1 Human papillomavirus types 16, 18, 31, 33, 35, 39, 45, 51, 52, 56, 58, 59 Tobacco smoking	Human papillomavirus types 26, 53, 66, 67, 68, 70, 73, 82 Tetrachloroethylene
Endometrium	Estrogen menopausal therapy Estrogen-progestogen menopausal therapy Tamoxifen	Diethylstilbestrol
Ovary	Asbestos (all forms) Estrogen menopausal therapy Tobacco smoking	Talc-based body powder (perineal use) X-radiation, γ-radiation
Male Genital Organs		
Penis	Human papillomavirus type 16	Human immunodeficiency virus type 1 Human papillomavirus type 18
Prostrate		Androgenic (anabolic) steroids Arsenic and inorganic arsenic compounds Cadmium and cadmium compounds Rubber production industry Thorium-232 and its decay products X-radiation, γ-radiation
Testis		Diethylstilbestrol exposure in utero
Urinary Tract		
Kidney	Tobacco smoking X-radiation, γ-radiation	Arsenic and inorganic arsenic compounds Cadmium and cadmium compounds Printing processes

TABLE 12.1 List of Classifications by Cancer Sites With Sufficient or Limited Evidence in Humans*—cont'd

Cancer Site	Carcinogenic Agents With Sufficient Evidence in Humans	Agents With Limited Evidence in Humans
Renal pelvis and ureter	Aristolochic acids, plants containing phenacetin Phenacetin, analgesic mixtures containing Tobacco smoking	Aristolochic acids
Urinary bladder	Aluminum production 4-Aminobiphenyl Arsenic and inorganic arsenic compounds Auramine production Benzidine Chlornaphazine Cyclophosphamide Magenta production 2-Naphthylamine Painting Rubber production industry *Schistosoma haematobium* Tobacco smoking *ortho*-Toluidine X-radiation, γ-radiation	4-Chloro-*ortho*-toluidine Coal-tar pitch Coffee Dry cleaning Engine exhaust, diesel Hairdressers and barbers (occupational exposure) Printing processes Soot Textile manufacturing
Eye, Brain, and Central Nervous System		
Eye	Human immunodeficiency virus type 1 Ultraviolet-emitting tanning devices Welding	Solar radiation
Brain and central nervous system	X-radiation, γ-radiation	Radiofrequency electromagnetic fields (including from wireless phones)
Endocrine Glands		
Thyroid	Radioiodines, including iodine-131 X-radiation, γ-radiation	
Lymphoid, Hematopoietic, and Related Tissue		
Leukemia and/or lymphoma	Azathioprine Benzene Busulfan 1,3-Butadiene Chlorambucil Cyclophosphamide Cyclosporine Epstein-Barr virus Etoposide with cisplatin and bleomycin Fission products, including strontium-90 Formaldehyde *Helicobacter pylori* Hepatitis C virus Human immunodeficiency virus type 1 Human T-cell lymphotropic virus type 1 Kaposi sarcoma herpesvirus Melphalan MOPP (vincristine-prednisone-nitrogen mustard-procarbazine mixture) Phosphorus-32 Rubber production industry Semustine (methyl-CCNU) Thiotepa Thorium-23 and its decay products Tobacco smoking Treosulfan X-radiation, γ-radiation	Bis(chloroethyl)nitrosourea Chloramphenicol Ethylene oxide Etoposide Hepatitis B virus Magnetic fields, extremely low frequency (childhood leukemia) Mitoxantrone Nitrogen mustard Painting (childhood leukemia from maternal exposure) Petroleum refining (occupational exposures) Polychlorophenols or their sodium salts (combined exposures) Radioiodines, including iodine-131 Radon-222 and its decay products Styrene Teniposide Tetrachloroethylene Trichloroethylene 2,3,7,8-Tetrachlorodibenzo-*para*-dioxin Tobacco smoking (childhood leukemia in smokers' children) Malaria (caused by infection with *Plasmodium falciparum* in holoendemic areas)

Continued

TABLE 12.1   List of Classifications by Cancer Sites With Sufficient or Limited Evidence in Humans*—cont'd

Cancer Site	Carcinogenic Agents With Sufficient Evidence in Humans	Agents With Limited Evidence in Humans
Multiple or Unspecific Sites		
Multiple sites (unspecified)	Cyclosporine Fission products, including strontium-90 X-radiation, γ-radiation (exposure in utero)	Chlorophenoxy herbicides Plutonium
All cancer sites (combined)	2,3,7,8-Tetrachlorodibenzo-*para*-dioxin	

***NOTE:** This table does not include factors not covered in the IARC Monographs, notably genetic traits, reproductive status, and some nutritional factors.

Adapted from Cogliano VJ et al: *J Natl Cancer Inst* 103:1-13, 2011. Available at http://jnci.oxfordjournals.org/content/early/2011/12/11/jnci.djr483.short?rss=1.

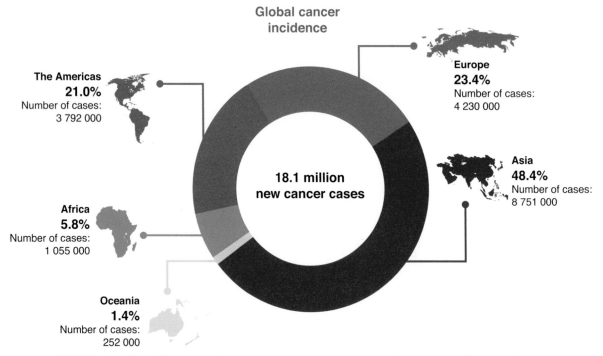

FIGURE 12.3 Global Cancer Incidence. New global cancer data from Globocan 2018 (From Bray F et al: *Ca Cancer J Clin* 68(6):394-424, 2018.)

Incidence and Mortality Trends

According to a report by GLOBOCAN, an estimated 18.1 million new cancer cases (17 million excluding nonmelanoma skin cancer) and 9.6 million cancer deaths (9.5 million excluding nonmelanoma skin cancer) were reported worldwide in 2018[9] (Fig. 12.3). In both sexes combined, lung cancer is the most commonly diagnosed cancer (11.6% of the total cases) and the leading cause of cancer death (18.4% of the total cancer deaths), followed closely by female breast cancer (11.6%), prostate cancer (7.1%), colorectal cancer (6.1%); colorectal cancer (9.2%), stomach cancer (8.2%), and liver cancer (8.2%) for mortality.[9] In males, lung cancer is the most frequent cancer and leading cause of cancer death followed by prostate and colorectal cancer (for incidence) and liver and stomach (for mortality). Among females, breast cancer is the most commonly diagnosed cancer and the leading cause of cancer death, followed by colorectal and lung cancer (for incidence), and lung cancer and colorectal cancer (for mortality). Cervical cancer ranks fourth for both incidence and mortality.[9] Worldwide, cancer is an important cause of morbidity and mortality despite the level of human development.[9] Variations in the magnitude and profile of the disease between and within world regions shows the extraordinary diversity of cancer.

IN UTERO AND EARLY LIFE CONDITIONS

It is widely accepted that a long latency period precedes the onset of adult cancers. Accumulating data suggest early life events influence later susceptibility to certain chronic diseases (Fig. 12.4). Developmental plasticity is the degree to which an organism's development is contingent on external cues from its environment. *Plasticity* refers to the ability of genes to organize physiologically or structurally in response to environmental conditions during fetal development. Specifically, the *developmental origins hypothesis* postulates that nutrition and other environmental factors affect cellular pathways during gestation, enabling a single genotype to produce a broad range of adult phenotypes. Maternal nutrition, as well as environment factors, are proposed as significant biologic influences. Persistent epigenetic adaptations, occurring early in

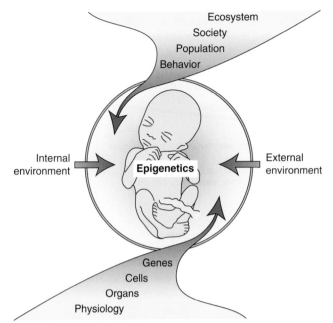

FIGURE 12.4 Fetal Vulnerability to External and Internal Environments. The fetus is particularly vulnerable to changes in the external and internal environments, which can have immediate and lifelong consequences. Such environmentally induced changes can occur at multiple levels, including molecular and behavioral. Ultimately these alterations may be epigenetic, inducing mitotically heritable alterations in gene expression without changing the DNA. (Adapted from Crews E, McLachlan JA: *Endocrinology* 147[6 suppl]:S4-S10, 2006.)

development, are believed to be associated with increased susceptibility to cancer and other adult-onset chronic diseases. Throughout in utero development, the placenta, as a regulator of the intrauterine environment, plays a major role in controlling growth and development. The Dutch Famine Birth Cohort is a well-known study of the effects of prenatal undernutrition in humans. Undernutrition in utero is linked to increased heart disease, metabolic disorders, and possibly breast cancer decades later. Early undernutrition in pregnancy is particularly important. Research suggests that undernutrition during the first trimester of pregnancy results in increased vulnerability to disease outcome in adulthood.

One of the best examples of early life events that trigger future cancer is the in utero exposure to diethylstilbestrol (DES), a synthetic estrogen. This medication was prescribed between 1938 and 1971 as a treatment for threatened miscarriage, premature birth, and abnormal bleeding. It became clear by the 1950s that DES altered the development of the reproductive system in the fetus; and, importantly, it did *not* prevent miscarriage. DES exposure in utero increases the risk of female reproductive tract cancer throughout a woman's childbearing years. More recent studies have revealed that daughters of women who took DES during pregnancy may have a slight increased risk of breast cancer before age 40.

Research from animal studies suggests a relationship between DES exposure and an increased rate of both a rare form of testicular cancer and prostate cancer. Whether DES-exposed sons will have increased rates of testicular or prostate cancer is unclear; more research is needed as the cohort of men age. Meta-analysis suggests that testicular cancer, hypospadias, and cryptorchidism are all positively associated with prenatal exposure to DES.

Newbold and colleagues have demonstrated that DES-related reproductive cancers in mice also occurred in the grandsons and grand-daughters of animals treated with DES.[10] In summary, fetal programming

TABLE 12.2   Differences Between Multigenerational and Transgenerational Phenotypes

Phenotype	Exposure	Definition
Multigenerational	Direct	Simultaneous exposure of multiple generations to an environmental factor
Transgenerational	Initial germline exposure (ancestral)	Transgenerational phenotype is transmitted to future generations via germline inheritance

TABLE 12.3   Somatic Versus Germ Cell Inheritance

Cell Type	Biologic Response
Somatic cells	Critical for adult-onset disease in exposed individual; not transmitted to future generations as transgenerational effect
Germ cells	Allows transmission between generations; promotes transgenerational phenotype

influences developmental origins of health and disease. It also may help explain epigenetic transgenerational effects (Tables 12.2 and 12.3).

QUICK CHECK 12.2
1. Define developmental plasticity.
2. Discuss how epigenetic processes can be modified by environmental factors.
3. Define the developmental basis of health and disease.

ENVIRONMENTAL-LIFESTYLE FACTORS

Tobacco Use

Smoking is carcinogenic and remains the most important cause of preventable death. Smoking causes cancer, heart disease, stroke, lung diseases, diabetes, and chronic obstructive pulmonary disease (COPD) that includes emphysema and chronic bronchitis. Smoking also increases risk for tuberculosis, certain eye diseases, and problems of the immune system, including rheumatoid arthritis and erectile dysfunction in males.[11] More than 16 million Americans are living with a disease caused by smoking.[11] In the United States, cigarette smoking accounts for more than 480,000 deaths each year, including more than 41,000 deaths resulting from secondhand smoke.[11] Worldwide, tobacco use causes more than 7 million deaths per year. [11] On average, smokers die 10 years earlier than nonsmokers.[11]

Smoking tobacco causes cancer in over 15 organ sites, but smoking affects nearly every organ of the body[12,13] (Fig. 12.5). Exposure to secondhand smoke causes cancer in nonsmokers, a fact that has particular significance for parents who smoke. The risks associated with smoking are greatest in persons who begin to smoke when young and continue throughout life; however, tobacco smoking is pandemic and affects all ages. Thousands of young people start smoking cigarettes every day.[11] Although the incidence of smoking is lower in women, the disease risks have risen sharply. The risks are now equal to those in men for lung cancer, chronic obstructive pulmonary disease, and cardiovascular disease.

Secondhand smoke, also called environmental tobacco smoke (ETS), is the combination of *sidestream smoke* (smoke from the burning end of a cigarette, cigar, or pipe) and *mainstream smoke* (smoke exhaled

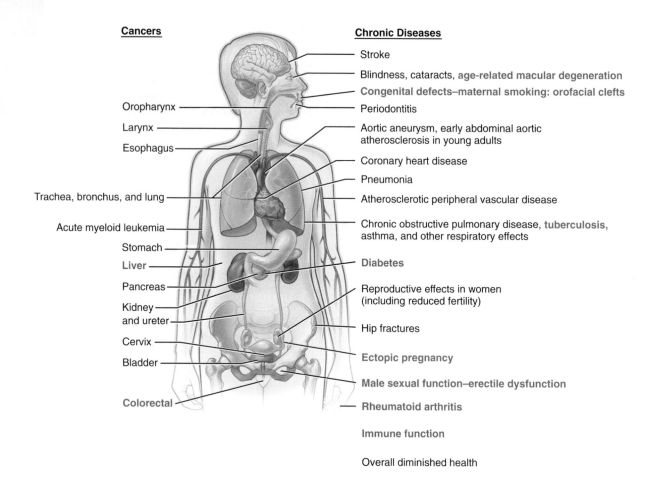

Cancers

- Oropharynx
- Larynx
- Esophagus
- Trachea, bronchus, and lung
- Acute myeloid leukemia
- Stomach
- Liver
- Pancreas
- Kidney and ureter
- Cervix
- Bladder
- Colorectal

Chronic Diseases

- Stroke
- Blindness, cataracts, age-related macular degeneration
- Congenital defects–maternal smoking: orofacial clefts
- Periodontitis
- Aortic aneurysm, early abdominal aortic atherosclerosis in young adults
- Coronary heart disease
- Pneumonia
- Atherosclerotic peripheral vascular disease
- Chronic obstructive pulmonary disease, tuberculosis, asthma, and other respiratory effects
- Diabetes
- Reproductive effects in women (including reduced fertility)
- Hip fractures
- Ectopic pregnancy
- Male sexual function–erectile dysfunction
- Rheumatoid arthritis
- Immune function
- Overall diminished health

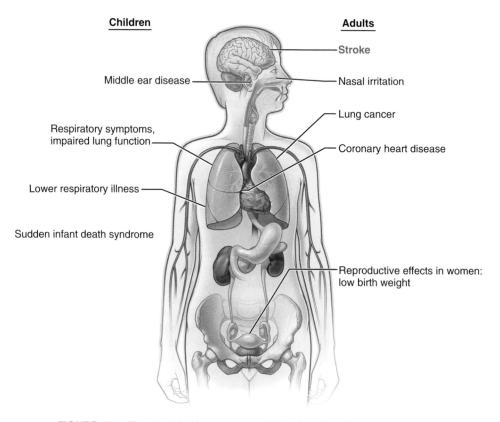

Children

- Middle ear disease
- Respiratory symptoms, impaired lung function
- Lower respiratory illness
- Sudden infant death syndrome

Adults

- Stroke
- Nasal irritation
- Lung cancer
- Coronary heart disease
- Reproductive effects in women: low birth weight

FIGURE 12.5 The Health Consequences Linked to Smoking. NOTE: The conditions in red are new diseases that have been causally linked to smoking. See text for discussion. Stroke is a new disease causally linked to secondhand smoke. (Reproduced from the World Cancer Research Fund/American Institute for Cancer Research. Diet, Nutrition, Physical Activity and Cancer: a Global Perspective. Continuous Update Project Expert Report 2018. Available at dietandcancerreport.org.)

directly by the smoker). More than 7000 chemicals have been identified in mainstream tobacco smoke; hundreds are toxic and about 70 can cause cancer.[13] During 2011 through 2012, about 58 million nonsmokers in the United States were exposed to secondhand smoke.[14] Nonsmokers who live with smokers are at risk for lung cancer, as well as numerous noncancerous conditions. It is a known risk factor for stroke. Secondhand smoke also is associated with decreased survival for nonsmokers with cancer. Other diseases related to secondhand smoke include age-related macular degeneration, tuberculosis, ectopic pregnancy, and diabetes mellitus. Secondhand smoke exposure increases inflammation, impairs immunity, and is a cause of rheumatoid arthritis. Additionally, another 100,000 babies were smoking-related fatalities who died of sudden infant death syndrome (SIDS), complications related to low birth weight, or other conditions arising as a direct result of parental smoking, especially if the mother is a smoker.[13]

Smoking tobacco is linked to numerous types of cancer, including the following:
- Cancers of the lung, upper aerodigestive tract (oral cavity, pharynx, larynx, nasal cavity, paranasal sinuses, esophagus), and stomach.
- Cancers of the lower urinary tract (renal pelvis, penis, and bladder)
- Cancers of the kidney, pancreas, cervix, and uterus
- Myeloid leukemia

Newly identified cancer risks attributable to smoking include liver and colorectal cancers. Smoking causes even more deaths from respiratory, vascular, and other diseases than do cancers discussed in later chapters.

Non-cigarette tobacco use also is hazardous. Cigar or pipe smoking is strongly related to cancers of the oral cavity, oropharynx, hypopharynx, larynx, esophagus, and lung. Cigar smokers who inhale are prone to develop coronary heart disease and chronic obstructive pulmonary disease (COPD). Pipe smokers have an increased risk of cancers of the lung, lip, throat, esophagus, larynx, pancreas, and colon and rectum. Smokeless tobacco is associated with oral cavity, esophageal, and pancreatic cancers.

Electronic cigarettes (e-cigarettes) come in many shapes and sizes, have a battery, a heating element, and a place to hold liquid. They produce an aerosol by heating liquid that usually contains nicotine, flavorings, and other chemicals. Use of e-cigarettes is sometimes called *vaping*. E-cigarettes can contain harmful and potentially harmful substances including nicotine, ultrafine particles that can be inhaled deeply in the lungs, flavoring (diacetyl), volatile organic compounds, cancer-causing chemicals, and heavy metals (tin, nickel, and lead).[15]

Cigarette smoke induces an inflammatory response and causes an increase in reactive oxygen species (ROS), causing oxidative stress. Oxidative stress can alter many cellular proteins. Cigarette smoking has both proinflammatory and immunosuppressive effects (impairs immune protection). Investigators are studying the genetic and epigenetic effects of both secondhand smoke and smoking (both maternal and paternal) during pregnancy on prenatal exposure and subsequent chronic diseases.

Diet

The influence of diet on cancer development is complicated. Cancer risks in older adults may depend as much on diet in early life as on current eating practices. Researchers targeting diet and disease associations face a variety of challenges, including accurate measurement of specific nutrients, food types, and dietary patterns. Convincing and probable judgments related to diet and nutrition, physical activity, and weight risk factors and the prevention of cancer are presented in Fig. 12.6. Much evidence exists that nutritional factors are related to cancer development (Fig. 12.7). Research is ongoing to understand the complexity of genomics, epigenomics, transcription factors (transcriptomics), proteomics, and metabolic factors (metabolomics) and the way that modifying any one of these factors influences cancer risk. **Nutrigenomics**

is the study of the effects of nutrition on the phenotypic variability of individuals based on genomic differences (see Fig. 12.7).

Nutrition, Obesity, Alcohol Consumption, and Physical Activity: Impacts on Cancer

Diet, weight, and activity level all influence risks for cancer development; they particularly impact specific types of cancers (Fig. 12.9). Everyday *choices* matter and impact the risk of developing cancer.

Nutrition

The implementation of dietary patterns and specific dietary recommendations are becoming more widespread. One pattern receiving much attention is the Mediterranean diet (MD). The MD has been reported to reduce mortality rates for chronic diseases, including cancer, cardiovascular diseases, and neurodegenerative diseases.[16] Culture and geographic location play a significant role in diet and health. For example, differences in the incidence of colorectal cancer with various geographic regions include variations in diet, particularly the consumption of red or processed meat; fiber; and alcohol. With geographic migration, risks and cancer patterns change, particularly when migrating individuals or stationary cultures adopt the so-called Western diet. Japan has seen a rapid increase in the incidence of colorectal cancer with the westernization of its diet. Fig. 12.8 shows cell functions thought to be influenced by diet, weight, and activity level.

Gene expression is influenced by epigenetic processes, such as DNA methylation or acetylation (addition of an acetyl group) (see Chapters 3 and 11). Dietary sources of methyl groups, including folate, methionine, betaine, serine, and choline, are primary potential donors as modulators of DNA methylation (Fig. 12.10). The European Prospective Investigation into Cancer and Nutrition (EPIC) found individuals with high plasma concentrations of methionine, choline, and betaine may be at reduced risk of colorectal cancer.[17] Other examples of epigenetic changes and diet are presented in Box 12.1.

BOX 12.1 Examples of Epigenetic Changes and Diet

- B vitamins (B_2, B_6, B_{12}) are modulators of DNA methylation
- Periconceptual maternal supplementation with 400 mcg of folic acid per day was associated with methylation in the offspring
- From the Waterland study, methylation effects were similar in all tissues examined. These data suggest that the methylation mechanism may alter stem cells early in embryogenesis before tissue differentiation and persist throughout life
- Severe folate deficiency, which increases the risk of hepatocellular cancer, induces hypomethylation of the *p53* tumor suppressor gene
- There is strong evidence for the epigenetic effects of organosulfur compounds from garlic and of isothiocyanates from cruciferous vegetables
- Sulforaphane from cruciferous vegetables can act as a histone deacetylase inhibitor to maintain DNA stability or modify transcription
- The potential role of dietary polyphenols, such as curcumin, resveratrol, genistein, epigallocatechin gallate (EGCG), and indole-3-carbinol, may promote antiproliferation and proapoptosis through epigenetic regulation of microRNAs (miRNAs).
- Natural agents in cancer therapies are being investigated in clinical trials

Data from World Cancer Research Fund/American Institute from Cancer Research: *Food, nutrition, physical activity, and the prevention of cancer: a global perspective*, Washington, DC, 2007, AICR and World Cancer Research Fund/American Institute for Cancer Research; *Diet, Nutrition, Physical Activity and Cancer: a Global Perspective*, Continuous Update Project Report 2018, available at dietandcancerreport.org.

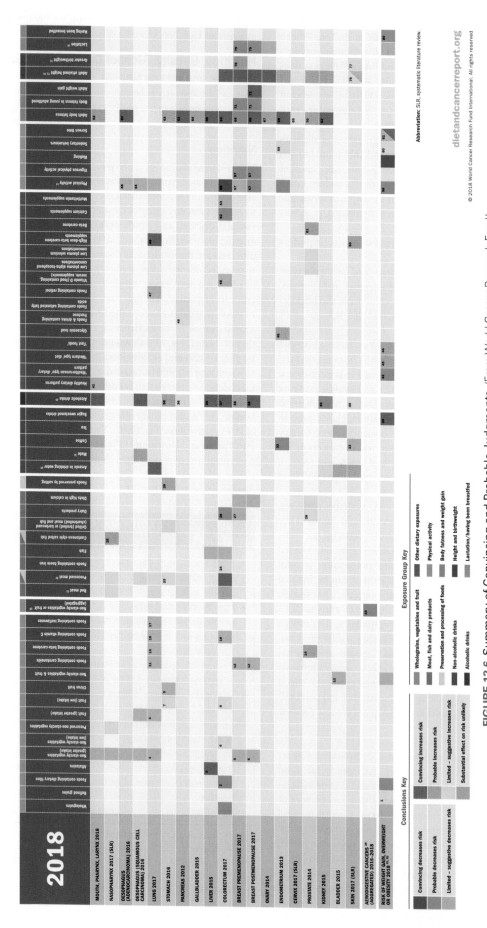

FIGURE 12.6 Summary of Convincing and Probable Judgments. (From World Cancer Research Fund/American Institute for Cancer Research: *Diet, nutrition, physical activity and cancer: a global perspective*, Continuous Update Project Expert Report 2018.)

dietandcancerreport.org

Abbreviation: SLR, systematic literature review.

Bioactive components have a profound effect on differentiation, and a major area of investigation is the differentiation of cancer stem cells. Cancer stem cells utilize several developmental mechanisms for self-renewal, and these mechanisms appear to be fundamental to the initiation and recurrence of tumors. Even if chemotherapy or radiation eliminates cancer cells, it is only when the cancer stem cells are destroyed that a full recovery is achievable. Repopulation with radioresistant or chemoresistant stem cells may significantly contribute to therapy resistance. Evidence from both drug and bioactive food constituents shows modifications in cancer stem cell self-renewal capabilities; for

example, retinoic acid may promote differentiation (versus a stem cell–like state) of breast cancer stem cells. Adequate consumption of specific food compounds, including vitamin A and D, genistein, green tea, epigallocatechin, sulforaphane, theanine, curcumin, choline, and possibly many others, may suppress cancer stem renewal.[18]

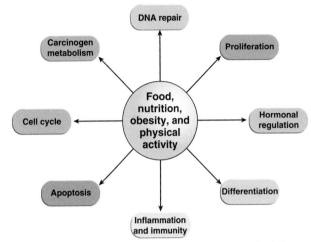

FIGURE 12.7 Basis for the Study of Food, Nutrition, Obesity, Physical Activity, and the Cancer Process. The genetic message in the DNA code is translated to RNA, and then into protein synthesis, and so determines metabolic processes. Research methods, called "-omics," address these different stages. (Adapted from World Cancer Research Fund/American Institute for Cancer Research: *Food, nutrition, physical activity, and the prevention of cancer: a global perspective,* Washington, DC, 2007, AICR.)

FIGURE 12.8 Food, Nutrition, Obesity, Physical Activity, and Cellular Processes Linked to Cancer. Food, nutrition, and physical activity can influence fundamental processes shown here, which may promote or inhibit cancer development and progression. (Reproduced from the World Cancer Research Fund/American Institute for Cancer Research. Diet, Nutrition, Physical Activity and Cancer: a Global Perspective. Continuous Update Project Expert Report 2018. Available at dietandcancerreport.org.)

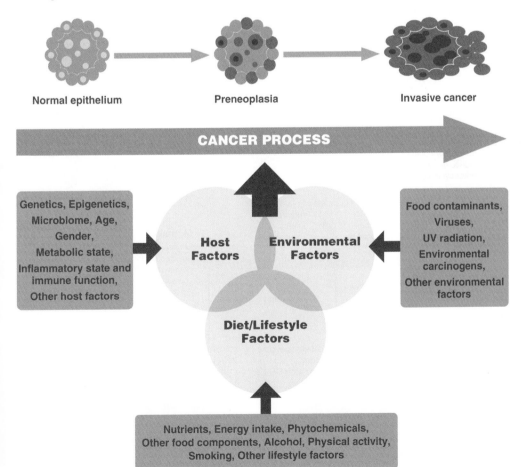

FIGURE 12.9 Diet, Nutrition, Physical Activity and Other Environmental Exposures Affect the Cancer Process. It can take many years for a normal cell to transform into invasive cancer cells. Carcinogenesis involves a complex interaction of diet, nutrition, physical activity, and other lifestyle and environmental factors with host factors that are related to inheritance, prior experience, and epigenetic changes. With time, the accumulated genetic damage and impairment of function, for example, DNA repair processes with aging, can all lead to carcinogenesis. Thus critical to this process are everyday lifestyle choices and exposures. (Adapted from World Cancer Research Fund/American Institute for Cancer Research Diet: *Nutrition, physical activity and cancer: a global perspective continuous update project expert report 2018.*)

Bioactive Food Substances in Epigenetics

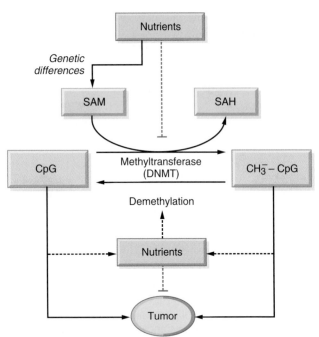

FIGURE 12.10 Dietary Factors, DNA Methylation, and Cancer. Certain dietary factors may supply methyl groups ($+CH_3$) that can be donated through *S*-adenosylmethionine *(SAM)* to many acceptors in the cell (DNA, proteins, lipids, and metabolites). Donation and removal (demethylation) are affected by numerous enzymes, including DNA methyltransferase *(DNMT)*. Increased DNMT activity occurs in many tumor cells. Hypermethylation can inhibit or silence tumor-suppressor genes (see Chapter 11, and DNA methylation inhibitors as anticancer agents can block DNMT, thus reactivating tumor-suppressor genes. DNA hypomethylation can reactivate and mutate genes, including cancer-causing oncogenes. *SAH, S*-Adenosylhomocysteine; *CH_3,* methyl group; *CpG site,* cytosine (C) lies next to guanine (G).

A variety of food constituents may influence DNA repair (Fig. 12.11). Observational studies suggest that malnutrition can reduce DNA repair from damage. In vivo studies have demonstrated that healthy adults consuming kiwi fruits, cooked carrots, or supplemental coenzyme Q_{10} improved their DNA repair.[19] Consumption of lycopene-rich vegetable juice was associated with significantly decreased damage to the DNA of lung epithelial cells in healthy adults.[20]

Humans are constantly exposed to a variety of compounds termed xenobiotics (the Greek word *xenos* means "foreign"; *bios* means "life") that include toxic, mutagenic, and carcinogenic chemicals. Many of these chemicals are found in the human diet and in drugs. Most xenobiotics are transported in the blood by lipoproteins and penetrate lipid membranes (see Chapter 4). The body has two main defense systems for counteracting these effects: (1) detoxification enzymes and (2) antioxidant systems (see Chapter 4). Once introduced into the body, xenobiotics are metabolized and detoxified, mainly in the liver. When a compound is absorbed through the gastrointestinal (GI) tract, it enters the hepatic circulation through the portal vein. The liver metabolizes the compound through several biochemical processes. This process of hepatic action is known as *first pass effect,* and it applies to both dietary and pharmaceutical xenobiotics. Drugs that are ingested orally, but not parenterally, are usually subject to first pass effect. The metabolic processes occurring in the liver prevent many potentially carcinogenic agents from entering the body after they are ingested from dietary sources. Although the liver is the main site of detoxification, this process occurs to a lesser extent at other sites (i.e., extrahepatic detoxification). Many foods enhance the efficiency and degree of detoxification of xenobiotics and thus serve a protective role in metabolizing carcinogens. Isothiocyanates from cruciferous vegetables, for example, induce detoxification enzymes. Foods can modify carcinogen metabolism and may modify carcinogenesis.

Certain enzymes (glutathione-*S*-transferases) are "enzyme housekeepers." These compounds are involved in the metabolism of environmental carcinogens and reactive oxygen species. Individuals who lack these enzymes may be at higher risk for cancers because of a decreased capacity to metabolize activated carcinogens into less toxic forms; for example,

FIGURE 12.11 Cell Cycle and Nutrition Regulation. Nutrition may influence the regulation of the normal cell cycle, which ensures correct DNA replication. G_0 represents the resting phase, G_1 the growth and preparation of the chromosome for replication, S the synthesis of DNA, G_2 the preparation of the cell for division, and M mitosis. (Adapted from World Cancer Research Fund/American Institute for Cancer Research: *Food, nutrition, physical activity, and the prevention of cancer: a global perspective,* Washington, DC, 2007, AICR.)

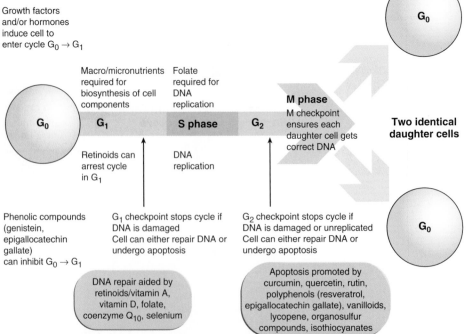

the fungi that produce aflatoxins grow on certain crops, such as peanuts and some grains. Aflatoxins are known carcinogens, activated by enzymes in the liver. They produce DNA adducts or a segment of DNA that is bound to a carcinogen. Such adducts can trigger the formation of a cancer cell. Individuals lacking protective enzymes are at higher risk for developing colon cancer. Diets high in isothiocyanates (from cruciferous vegetables) may decrease this risk. Individuals who consume diets high in red meat or processed meat have an increased risk of developing colorectal cancer, particularly if they carry certain genetic polymorphisms. Processed meats are meats preserved by smoking, curing, or salting. EPIC, which included 478,040 people from 10 countries, reported that the most convincing data are from meats that contain nitrites, nitrates, or other preservatives. Such products include bacon, sausages, bratwursts, frankfurters, and other nitrite-containing meats. The resulting *N*-nitroso compounds increase nitrogenous residues in the colon that can cause DNA damage.

Metabolic reactions that impact cancer development include procarcinogenic processes, as well as protective reactions. Some reactions activate dietary compounds to form potential carcinogens. Other metabolic processes inactivate ingested carcinogenic components, thus preventing DNA damage. Red meat has been the subject of considerable scrutiny. A high intake of red meat may result in the synthesis of higher levels of heme iron, a substance known to activate oxidative stress and inflammation in the colon. Additionally, meat may have certain thermoresistant oncogenic bovine viruses (e.g., polyoma-papilloma) or single-stranded DNA viruses. Cooking meats at high temperatures (pan frying or grilling) may pose additional hazards because it results in the formation of heterocyclic amines (HCAs) and polycyclic aromatic hydrocarbons (PAHs), both identified as carcinogens in laboratory animals. Fig. 12.12 illustrates the potential role of epigenetic modulation and environmental factors in cancer development. Future research is needed to define robust biomarkers of cancer risk.

Obesity

Obesity in most developed countries and urban areas of many developing countries has been increasing rapidly over the past 20 years. Obesity in the United States is epidemic. It has more than tripled since the 1970s, and recent data show that nearly 1 in 5 school-age children and young people (6 to 19 years of age) in the United States are obese.[21] Worldwide data from 2016 show that 1.9 billion adults, 18 years and older, were overweight. Of these, over 650 million were obese.[22] Globally accepted criteria for overweight status and obesity are based on the

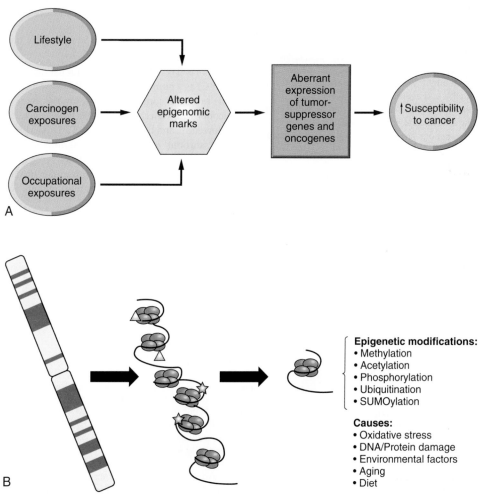

FIGURE 12.12 Epigenetic Modulation and Modifications. **A,** Overview of the potential role of epigenetic modulation by dietary and other environmental factors in cancer development. **B,** Epigenetic modulation model according to current knowledge. The different types of chemical modifications, such as methylation or acetylation, of promoter regions and/or other regulatory DNA sequences outside the gene can have a severe impact on gene transcription and translation and a resultant high modulation of gene expression and product (protein) functionality. (**B,** Adapted from Nowsheen S, et al.: *Cancer Letters* 342(3):213-222, 2014.)

body mass index (BMI). Widely accepted BMI standards are published by the World Health Organization (WHO) (Table 12.4) and is supported by numerous panels and federal agencies.

Obesity constitutes a startling setback to major improvements in other areas of health during the past century. Numerous health conditions are linked to obesity and physical inactivity. The long-term costs of obesity for both the individual and the society underlie the urgency to accelerate progress in obesity prevention

Obesity impacts energy balance, cancer risk, cancer recurrence, and survival. Research has significantly clarified the relationship between obesity and cancer risk. Evidence exists that being overweight or obese is linked to an increased risk of developing 11 cancers: liver, advanced prostate, ovarian, gallbladder, kidney, colorectal, esophageal (adenocarcinoma), postmenopausal breast, pancreatic, endometrial, and stomach (cardia) (Fig. 12.13).

The mechanisms of obesity-associated cancer risks are evolving; mechanisms may vary by the type of tumor and the distribution of body fat. Emerging data point to three main factors impacting obesity and cancer: (1) the insulin–insulin-like growth factor 1 (IGF-1) axis, (2) sex hormones, and (3) adipokines, or adipocyte-derived cytokines. Obesity-related metabolic changes include insulin resistance, hyperglycemia, dyslipidemia, hypoxia, and chronic inflammation. Because tumor growth is regulated by interactions between tumor cells and their tissue microenvironment, stromal compartments rich in adipose tissue can promote the development of tumor cells. Excess adipose tissue can enhance proinflammatory mediators, which attract macrophages and cancer-associated fibroblasts. All of these cells are tumor-promoting cell types. Additionally, the associated insulin resistance and hypoxia can trigger compensatory angiogenesis, thus providing an energy reservoir for any embedded cancer cells. During cancer progression, the cancer-associated adipocytes (CAAs) undergo both structural and functional alterations. Such changes create an environment favorable to increased invasiveness and aggression of cancer cells (see Fig. 12.13).

Increasing BMI is related to less favorable outcomes for recurrence, survival, and comorbidities (e.g., cardiovascular disease, diabetes, wound healing). The development of obesity and diabetes mellitus in aging survivors of childhood cancer and other endocrine disturbances is documented.

Alcohol Consumption

Alcohol is classified by the International Agency for Research on Cancer (IARC) as a human carcinogen. Excessive alcohol plays a contributory role in several common cancers. Overall, there are strong data linking alcohol with cancers of the mouth, pharynx, larynx, esophagus, liver, colorectum, and breast[23,24] (Table 12.5). The evidence does not support any "safe limit" of intake. The deleterious effects come from the ethanol content and are not affected by the type of drink consumed.

The mechanisms involved in alcohol-related carcinogenesis are from acetaldehyde, the first metabolite of ethanol oxidation. Other effects

TABLE 12.4 WHO Classification of Body Mass Index (BMI)

BMI (kg/m²)*	WHO Classification	Other Descriptions
<18.5	Underweight	Thin
18.5-24.9	Normal range	"Healthy," "normal," or "acceptable" weight
25-29.9	Preobese	Overweight
30-34.9	Obese class I	Obesity
35-39.9	Obese class II	—*
>40	Obese class III	Morbidly overweight

*The cutoffs are somewhat arbitrary, although they are derived from epidemiologic studies of BMI and overall mortality. It is important to understand that within each category of BMI there can be substantial individual variation in total and visceral adiposity and in related metabolic factors. These variations are also true for the normal range BMI.

WHO, World Health Organization.

Data available at http://apps.who.int/bmi/index.jsp?introPage=intro_3.html.

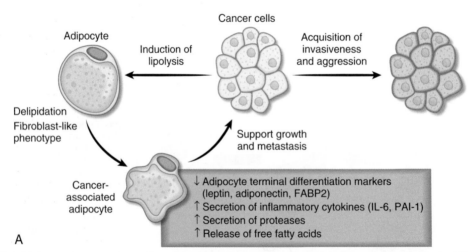

A

FIGURE 12.13 Structural and Functional Changes in Adipocytes and Interaction With the Microenvironment Contribute to Cancer Progression and Metastases: a Working Model. A, Signaling interactions occur between cancer cells and cancer-associated adipocytes. This interaction within the tumor microenvironment creates a place or *niche* permissive for cancer growth. Cancer cells stimulate the breakdown of lipids in adipocytes, leading to *delipidation* and the emergence of a fibroblast-like phenotype in adipocytes. The continuing alterations are associated with functional changes in the cells and include increased secretion of inflammatory mediators (cytokines) and proteases, and increased release of free fatty acids. All of these changes can support tumor growth and invasiveness.

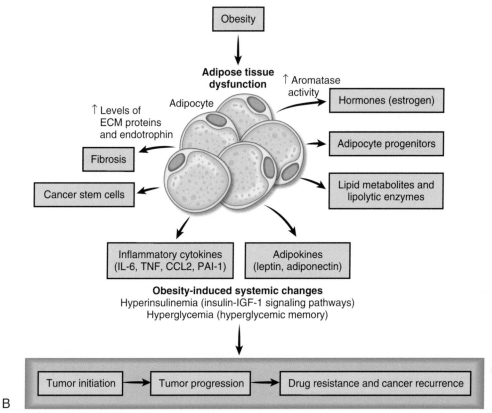

FIGURE 12.13, cont'd B, Obesity leads to excessive levels of proinflammatory cytokines, sex hormones, lipid metabolites, and altered adipokines. The altered adipose tissue becomes a source of various extracellular matrix proteins, cancer stem cells, and cancer-associated adipokines. Collectively these alterations contribute to tumor initiation, growth, and recurrence. The systemic metabolic changes of obesity—hyperinsulinemia and hyperglycemia—can further contribute to a tumor-permissive environment. *CCL2,* chemokine ligand 2; *ECM,* extracellular matrix; *FABP2,* fatty acid–binding protein 2; *IGF,* insulin-like growth factor; *IL,* interleukin; *TNF,* tumor necrosis factor. (Adapted from Park J et al: *Nat Rev Endocrinol* 10[8]:455-465, 2014.)

TABLE 12.5	**Alcoholic Drinks and Risk of Cancer***			
	DECREASES RISK		**INCREASES RISK**	
	Exposure	Cancer Site	Exposure	Cancer Site
Convincing			Alcoholic drinks	Mouth, pharynx and larynx, esophagus Colorectum (men)[†] Breast (premenopause and postmenopause)
Probable			Alcoholic drinks	Liver[‡] Colorectum (women)[‡]
Limited—suggestive				
Substantial effect on risk unlikely	Alcoholic drinks (adverse effect): kidney[§]			

*In the judgment of the Panel (WCRF/AICR), the factors listed modify the risk of cancer. Judgments are graded according to the strength of the evidence.

[†]The judgments for men and women are different because there are fewer data for women. Increased risk is only apparent above a threshold of 30 g/day of ethanol for both sexes.

[‡]Cirrhosis is an essential precursor of liver cancer caused by alcohol. The International Agency for Research on Cancer has graded alcohol as a class 1 carcinogen for liver cancer. Alcohol alone only causes cirrhosis in the presence of other factors.

[§]The evidence was sufficient to judge that alcoholic drinks are unlikely to have an adverse effect on the risk of kidney cancer; it was inadequate to draw a conclusion regarding the protective effect.

Adapted from World Cancer Research Fund/American Institute for Cancer Research (WCRF/AICR): *Second expert report: food, nutrition, physical activity, and the prevention of cancer: a global perspective,* London, 2007, Author.

result from the induction of cytochrome P-450 2E1 (genetic variant CYP2E1) leading to the generation of ROS and oxidative stress. Other factors include an increase in pro-carcinogens (e.g., nitrosamines), modulation of cellular regeneration (cell cycle), and commonly associated nutritional deficiencies (retinol, retinyl esters, folic acid, other vitamins). Such changes predispose the individual to enzyme and metabolic dysfunction, as well as structural abnormalities (e.g., altered mucosal integrity). Variations in several genes can increase the risk of alcohol-related carcinogenesis, and recent data suggest that the *ADHIB* gene (*ARG47His* variant) was associated with a decreased risk of esophageal cancer.[25]

Physical Activity

Regular exercise is reported to decrease the risk of breast cancer, colon cancer (men), and endometrial cancer independent of weight changes. Data are showing the vital importance of regular exercise in the primary and secondary prevention of several chronic diseases, including cardiovascular disease, hypertension, diabetes, cancer, obesity, depression, osteoporosis, and premature death. Annual deaths attributable to physical inactivity are reported between 3.2 million and 5.3 million deaths per year.[26,27] Several biologic mechanisms for physical activity and protection against cancer have been proposed including:

- Decreasing insulin and insulin-like growth factor (IGF) levels
- Decreasing obesity
- Increasing free radical scavenger systems
- Altering inflammatory mediators
- Decreasing levels of circulating sex hormones and metabolic hormones
- Improving immune function
- Decreasing oncogenes
- Enhancing cytochrome P-450, thus modifying carcinogen activation
- Increasing gut motility
- Increasing release of myokines or proteins from contracting muscles and their antitumor effects (see *Did You Know? Exercise and Anticancer Effects of Myokines*)

Many questions remain unanswered concerning the ideal frequency, intensity, and duration of exercise. According to the U.S. Department of Health and Human Services, significant health benefits are achieved when adults engage in at least 150 minutes (2 hours and 30 minutes) of moderate-intensity aerobic physical activity, 75 minutes (1 hour and 15 minutes) of vigorous intensity aerobic physical activity, or an equivalent combination of moderate- and vigorous-intensity activity every week.[28] The guidelines recommend at least 60 minutes of physical activity everyday (mostly moderate- or vigorous-intensity aerobic) for children and adolescents.[28] Being physically active after a cancer diagnosis is linked to improvement of cancer-specific outcomes for several cancer types. A Cochrane review found that aerobic exercise was beneficial for adults with cancer-related fatigue both during and after cancer treatment.[29] Another Cochrane review found exercise in children with cancer was associated with improved body composition, flexibility, and cardiorespiratory fitness.[30]

Air Pollution

The U.S. Environmental Protection Agency, WHO, the Institute for Health Metrics and Evaluation (IHME), and others report that long-term exposure to air pollution increases mortality and morbidity, and shortens life expectancy from cardiovascular disease, respiratory disease, and lung cancer.[31] State of Global Air 2018 presents the latest review of worldwide air pollution exposures and health impacts.[32] Air pollution is the leading environmental cause of death worldwide.[33] Globally 1 in 3 persons face a double burden—that is, exposure to household indoor pollution from burning (coal, charcoal, wood, dung, or other biomass) and outdoor air pollution.[33] Long-term exposure to outdoor and indoor air pollution contributed to 6.1 million premature deaths from stroke, heart attack, lung cancer, and chronic lung disease.[33]

Outdoor air pollution is a complex mixture of many known carcinogens; its relationship to lung cancer has been studied for more than 50 years. Past reviews of outdoor and household air pollution indicated that both were associated with increased rates of lung cancer. The most significant association involves exposures to increased levels of particles called particulate matter (see Chapter 4). Particulate matter (PM), also known as *particle pollution*, is a mixture of extremely small particles and liquid droplets. Particle pollution consists of a complex mix of acids (nitrates and sulfates), organic chemicals, metals, and soil or dust particles. IARC recently concluded that exposure to outdoor air pollution and to PM in outdoor air is carcinogenic to humans (IARC Group 1) and causes lung cancer.[34,35] The IARC's evaluation came from long-term epidemiologic studies involving residential exposure to air pollution. Specifically, the research has focused on lung cancer risks associated with exposure to $PM_{2.5}$ *particles* (aerodynamic diameter ≤2.5 µm) and PM_{10} particles (≤10 µm, or inhalable particles) (see Fig. 12.14). *Primary particles* are emitted directly from a source, for example, construction

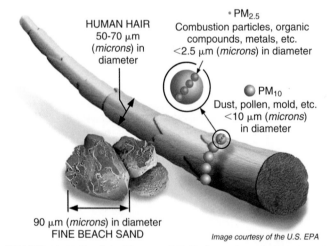

HUMAN HAIR
50-70 µm
(*microns*) in
diameter

• $PM_{2.5}$
Combustion particles, organic
compounds, metals, etc.
<2.5 µm (*microns*) in diameter

● PM_{10}
Dust, pollen, mold, etc.
<10 µm (*microns*)
in diameter

90 µm (*microns*) in diameter
FINE BEACH SAND

Image courtesy of the U.S. EPA

FIGURE 12.14 Particle Sizes and Pollution. (From Environmental Protection Agency: *Particulate matter updated March 18, 2013*, Washington, DC, 2013, Author.)

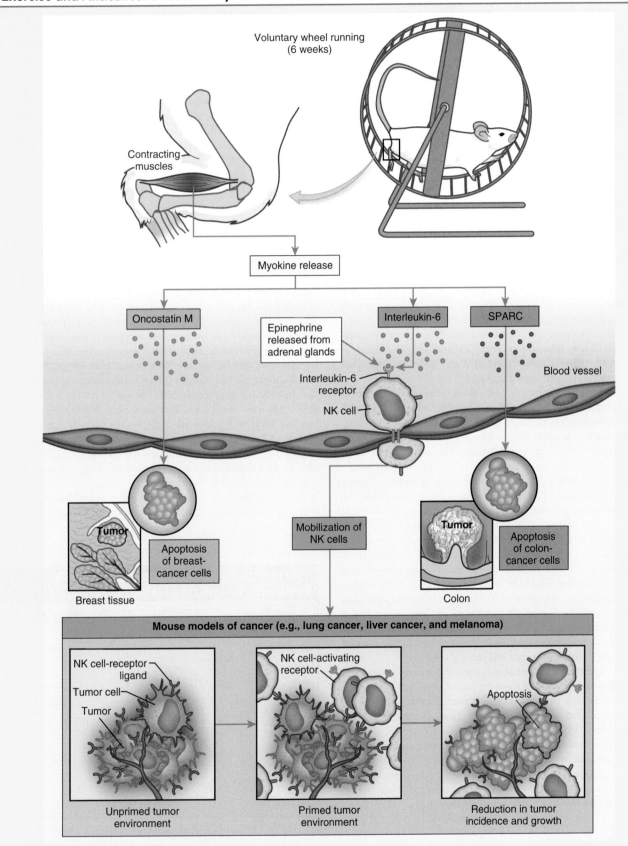

Exercise and contracting muscle fibers release myokines into the bloodstream, which can induce apoptosis in breast and colon cancer cells. In mouse models, investigators Pedersen and colleagues showed antitumor effects from myokine IL-6, which is elevated after exercise. IL-6 and epinephrine released from the adrenal gland move into the bloodstream and result in increased mobilization of natural killer (NK) lymphocytes, which migrate into tumors and destroy tumor cells.

Adapted from Lucia A, Ramirez M: *NEJM* 375(9):892894, 2016; Pedersen L, et al: *Cell Metab* 23:554-562, 2016.

sites, unpaved roads, fields, smokestacks, or fires. *Secondary particles* are emitted from power plants, industries, and automobiles. Worldwide exposure to $PM_{2.5}$ contributed to 4.1 million deaths from heart disease and stroke, lung cancer, chronic lung disease, and respiratory infections in 2016.[32]

The mechanisms of adverse effects of PM include (1) oxidative stress, (2) ROS generation, (3) DNA oxidative damage, (4) mutagenicity, (5) stimulation of proinflammatory factors, and (6) induction of senescence. Fine or ultrafine particles are easily absorbed by the lungs and phagocytosed by macrophages and neutrophils that release tissue-damaging inflammatory mediators. Insoluble particles cause pulmonary inflammation, which leads to oxidative stress and oxidation of DNA, proliferative response, and tissue remodeling progressing to fibrosis and tumor development.

Ozone, another component of outdoor air pollution, levels are rising around the world and contributed to 234,000 deaths from chronic lung disease.[32] Ozone levels remain high in both higher income and lower/middle income regions of the world.[32]

Studies of occupational exposure to diesel exhaust indicate an increased risk of lung cancer.[36] *Acute* exposure to diesel exhaust that contains particles is linked to lung, throat, and eye irritations; asthma attacks; and myocardial ischemia.[37] In 2012, the IARC classified diesel exhaust as a carcinogen. WHO has found that diesel exhaust is carcinogenic and causes lung cancer. Diesel exhaust is under study to understand other sites of potential cancer (e.g., bladder, larynx, colon) and if it has a role in cardiovascular disease.

Living close to certain industries is a recognized cancer risk factor. Overall, fine particle pollution also has been linked to other health problems including (1) premature death in people with heart or lung disease, (2) nonfatal heart attacks, (3) irregular heartbeat, (4) aggravated asthma, (5) decreased lung function, and (6) respiratory symptoms, including irritation of the airways, coughing, and shortness of breath. Other effects of particle pollution include reduced visibility (haze); environmental damage in lakes and streams, coastal waters, and river basins; depletion of nutrients in soil; and damage to forests and food crops.[38]

Indoor pollution is generally considered worse than outdoor pollution, partly because of cigarette smoke. Environmental tobacco smoke (ETS; passive smoking) can cause the formation of reactive oxygen free radicals and thus DNA damage. The IARC has classified ETS as a human carcinogen. Exposures from heating and cooking combustion sources (e.g., oil vapors, volatile toxicants) are risk factors for lung cancer. Some regions in China have shown high levels of lung cancer in women who spend much of their time indoors. Domestic coal use and ETS increase the risk of lung cancer in women and men.

Another significant indoor air pollutant is radon gas. **Radon** is a natural radioactive gas derived from the radioactive decay of uranium that is found in rock and soil. It can become trapped in houses and form carcinogenic radioactive decay products. Houses with radon hazards can be identified by testing and then can be modified by adding a mitigation system to prevent further radon contamination. Exposure levels are greater in underground mines as compared to houses. Most of the lung cancers associated with radon are bronchogenic; however, small cell carcinoma occurs with greater frequency in underground miners. According to the Environmental Protection Agency (EPA), radon is the leading cause of lung cancer in nonsmokers.

Ionizing Radiation

Much of the knowledge of the effects of ionizing radiation on human cancer has stemmed from observations of the Hiroshima and Nagasaki atomic bomb exposures, particularly from the Life Span Study conducted on this population. These data provide the best estimate of human

cancer risk over the dose range from 20 to 250 centigray (cGy). This range includes low linear energy transfer (LET) radiation, such as from x-rays or γ-rays. Other evidence is derived from groups exposed to ionizing radiation (IR) for medical reasons or various occupational exposures, for example, underground miners exposed to radon gas and other occupational exposures (Table 12.6). The atomic bomb exposures in Japan caused acute leukemias in both adults and children and increased frequencies of thyroid and breast carcinomas. Other cancers added to the list include lung, stomach, colon, esophageal, urinary tract cancers, and multiple myeloma. At Nagasaki and Hiroshima, the leukemia incidence in individuals 15 years or younger reached its peak 6 to 7 years after the explosions and has declined steadily since 1952. Those 45 years or older at the time of exposure had a latent period of 20 years before developing acute leukemia.

Age at the time of radiation exposure is one of the main factors in radiation-induced cancer.[39] Radiation exposures at early ages are the most radiosensitive; the initial damage from the exposure has a longer latent period to induce cancer. With time, sensitivity to radiation decreases until maturity, but it increases again at older ages.[39] From the Life Span Study cohort of the Japanese atomic bomb survivors, the excess relative risks (ERRs) for radiation-induced cancers as a function of age at exposure, were examined.[40] The ERR for cancer induction was higher during childhood and then decreased at exposure ages of 30 to 40 years of age.[40] The ERR of developing solid tumors increased upward again for exposure ages higher than 40 years of age.[40] Other investigators found among the Oak Ridge Y-12 uranium-processing plant workers that radiation doses received after the age of 45 showed a stronger association with cancer mortality than those received at younger ages.[41] In terms of carcinogenic events, radiation sensitivity increases with age among adults after age 40 to 45 years.[39] All together these findings suggest that this bimodal distribution reflects that radiation risks after early ages are related to *initiation* of cancer processes, whereas radiation risks after exposure at later ages are mostly associated with the *promotion* of preexisting premalignant cells.[40] Promotion is used here to mean the process by which an initiated cell clonally expands. Importantly, with

TABLE 12.6   Cancer Associated With Exposure to Ionizing Radiation

Cancer Type	AB	AS	PM	TC	TH	RP	UM	RD
Leukemia	X	X			X			X
Thyroid	X			X				
Breast	X		X					
Lung	X	X			X		X	
Bone						X		
Stomach	X	X						
Esophagus	X	X						
Lymphoma	X	X						X
Brain			X				X	
Liver				X				
Skin				X			X	X

AB, Atomic bomb survivors; *AS,* ankylosing spondylitis patients; *PM,* postpartum mastitis patients; *TC,* tinea capitis patients; *TH,* individuals receiving Thorotrast; *RD,* radiologists; *RP,* radium dial painters; *UM,* underground miners.
Data from Jones JA et al: Ionizing radiation as a carcinogen. In McQueen E, editor: *CA comprehensive toxicology,* ed 2, St Louis, 2010, Elsevier.

aging and life expectancy increasing it is not just radiosensitivity but also the increasing medical imaging procedures with age and the cumulative effective doses from these procedures.[42] Proposed mechanisms of age-related cellular changes after radiation exposure include oxidative stress, telomere attrition, compromise of DNA repair, and the inflammatory response.[39]

Human exposure to ionizing radiation includes emissions from the environment (e.g., radon), medical treatment exposures (x-rays, CT scans, radioisotopes), and other radioactive sources (Fig. 12.15). Health risks involve not only neoplastic diseases but also cardiovascular disease, including stroke, following high-dose medical exposure and lower doses in atomic bomb (A-bomb) survivors (BEIR VII).[43] Late effects of radiation in A-bomb survivors show persistent elevations of inflammatory markers, implying immunologic damage may be the cause of later-occurring cardiovascular effects.[44] For the first time, investigators using a model of umbilical vein endothelial cells demonstrated that low doses (0.05 Gy) of x-rays induce DNA damage and apoptosis in endothelial cells.[45] Cardiac and blood vessel damage may manifest years after completion of radiation therapy.[46] Chronic inflammation is increasingly implicated in radiation-induced late tissue injury.[47]

Other risks from IR include somatic mutations and tissue alterations that may contribute to other diseases, such as respiratory diseases, birth defects, and eye maladies. Animal studies suggest that inherited mutations may affect the incidence of diseases in future generations. The human embryo and fetus are particularly sensitive to IR; the health consequences of exposure even at low doses can be severe.[48] The consequences include growth retardation, malformations, impaired brain function, and cancer.[48] Mutations, if not repaired, are cumulative.[49] An important summary point in BEIR VII is the concern regarding high-dose diagnostic medical exposure, particularly computed tomography (CT) scans (see *Did You Know?* Increasing Use of Computed Tomography Scans and Risks). In

2009, the National Council on Radiation Protection and Measurements (NCRP)[50] reported Americans were exposed to more than seven times as much ionizing radiation from medical procedures as compared with levels of exposure for the 1980s. The increased exposure is mainly because of the rapid increase in the use of CT imaging.[51] The increase in CT imaging is largely driven by technologic improvements, which have led to increased applications, increased patient demand, increased physician utilization, and defensive medical practices.[52]

Radiation-induced damage depends not only on dose, fractionation, and mechanism of the radiation delivery but also on the inherent repair mechanisms of the organism. Bystander effects and radioprotective substances also are compelling considerations.[49]

Radiation-Induced Cancer

IR is a potent mutagen and carcinogen. It can penetrate cells and tissues, depositing random energy within tissues in the form of ionizations (e.g., excitation or removal of an electron from the target atom.) Such ionization can lead to irreversible or indirect damage secondary to the formation of water-based free radicals (radiolysis). The *general* characteristics of IR-induced carcinogenesis are well established. The past two decades have focused on *specific* cellular and molecular mechanisms, which impact cancer development. Considerations include dose-response relationships for chromosome aberrations, cell transformation, and both genetic and epigenetic expression. Other important areas of investigation include alternative targets, mutations in somatic cells, *nontargeted effects*, or the biologic effects that occur in nonirradiated cells, and effects on the microenvironment.

Ionizing radiation is a potent DNA-damaging agent causing cross-linking, nucleotide base damage, and single- or double-strand DNA breaks and disrupted cellular regulation processes leading to carcinogenesis. The double-strand break (DSB) (Fig. 12.16) is considered

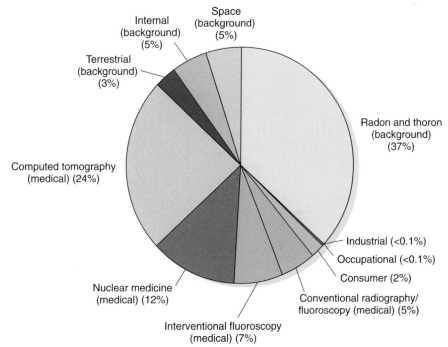

FIGURE 12.15 Pie Chart Showing Sources of Exposure to Ionizing Radiation. Percent contribution of various sources of exposure to the total collective effective dose (1,870,000 person-Sv) and the total effective dose per individual in the U.S. population (6.2 mSv) for 2006. Percent values have been rounded to the nearest 1%, except those <1%. *Sv,* Sievert. (From NCRP: *2009 Ionizing radiation exposure of the population of the United States,* NCRP Report No. 160, Bethesda, MD, 2009, Author.)

DID YOU KNOW?

Increasing Use of Computed Tomography Scans and Risks

A review article in the *New England Journal of Medicine* on computed tomography (CT) and radiation exposure has received much media attention. The article was written by radiology researchers at Columbia University. In short, the numbers of CT scans have greatly increased in the United States. This increase has occurred both as a diagnostic treatment for individuals with symptoms and as a diagnostic modality for individuals without symptoms (heart, lung, colon, and whole-body screening). Faster scanning times are partly responsible for increased CT use in pediatric populations. Typical doses are larger from CT scans than for a conventional examination (e.g., 50 times more radiation to the stomach than an x-ray). Based on data correlations from Japanese survivors of atomic bombs, the authors estimated that 1.5% to 2.0% of cancers in the United States might be attributable to CT radiation. The authors note that CT scans are sometimes ordered excessively and repeated unnecessarily because of defensive medicine. They also include three ways to reduce radiation exposure from CT: (1) reduce radiation doses in individual studies (i.e., use modern scanners), (2) substitute ultrasonography with magnetic resonance imaging (MRI) for CT whenever possible, and (3) order CT scans only when absolutely necessary. The NCRP estimates that 67 million CT scans (compared with 3 million in 1980), 18 million nuclear medicine procedures, 17 million interventional fluoroscopy procedures, and 18 million nuclear medicine procedures were performed in the United States in 2006.

Median Effective Radiation Dose for Each Type of CT Study

Anatomic Area, Study Type	Median (mSv)	Range (mSv)	Dose Equivalent (No. of Chest X-rays)
Head and Neck			
Routine head	2	0.3-6	30
Routine neck	4	0.7-9	55
Suspected stroke	14	4-56	199
Chest			
Chest, no contrast	8	2-24	117
Chest, with contrast	8	2-19	119
Suspected pulmonary embolus	10	2-30	137
Coronary angiogram	22	7-39	309
Abdomen-Pelvis			
Routine abdomen-pelvis, no contrast	15	3-43	220
Routine abdomen-pelvis, with contrast	16	4-45	234
Multiphase abdomen-pelvis	31	6-90	442
Suspected aneurysm or dissection	24	4-68	347

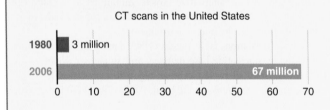

CT scans in the United States

1980   3 million
2006   67 million

0   10   20   30   40   50   60   70

Data from Brenner DJ, Hall E: *N Engl J Med* 357:2277, 2007; Brett AS: *J Watch* 28(1):3, 2008; Food and Drug Administration Public Health Notification: *Reducing radiation risk from computed tomography for pediatric and small adult patients,* Silver Spring, Md, 2001; Food and Drug Administration: *What are the radiation risks from CT?* Silver Spring, MD, 2017, Author.

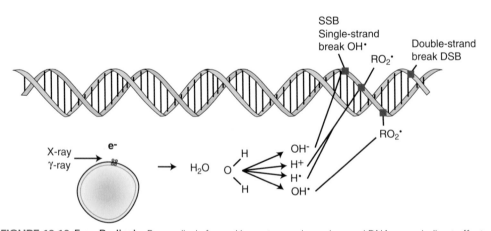

FIGURE 12.16 Free Radicals. Free radicals formed by water nearby and around DNA cause indirect effects. These free radicals have a short life as single free radicals. Oxygen can modify the reaction, enabling longer lifetimes of oxidative free radicals.

the hallmark lesion associated with IR. Importantly, DSBs are mostly commonly repaired by the *nonhomologous end joining (NHEJ) pathway.* This pathway is efficient for joining broken ends of DNA, however, errors can occur and the ability to repair may decline with age. Irradiated human cells that are unable to execute the NHEJ pathway are extremely vulnerable to large-scale mutations and chromosomal aberrations.[53]

Although evidence suggests that interindividual differences in radiation responses may be attributed to certain genes, IR can activate oncogenes, resulting in uncontrolled cell growth (see Chapter 11).

Tumor-suppressor genes also are sensitive to IR. Several tumor-suppressor genes have been identified that are deactivated by IR, and that promotes carcinogenesis. Recent research has shown that cells can detect and respond epigenetically, altering gene expression, after low doses of radiation.[54] Gene expression can change as a function of radiation dose and radiation type.[54]

Nontargeted Effects

Nontargeted effects (NTEs) are the biologic effects (e.g., genomic instability and bystander effects) that occur in cells not directly traversed by a radiation particle, but in the vicinity of a cell that has been exposed to IR or has received signals (cell-to-cell communication) from irradiated cells. These cells can participate in the final damage response. A long-held assumption is that cellular alterations—mutations and malignant transformation—occur only in cells directly irradiated. It is now known that cells not directly exposed to radiation but that instead are the progeny of cells irradiated many cell divisions previously may express a high level of gene mutations, cell lethality, and chromosomal aberration. These deleterious effects, stemming from previous generations of irradiated cells, are called genomic instability. Investigators are studying genomic instability as it may contribute to secondary cancers. The directly irradiated cells also can lead to genetic effects in so-called bystander cells, biologic effects known as the bystander effects. Bystander cells, or innocent cells, received no direct radiation exposure. In vivo studies in mice have found that localized radiation to the head led to induced bystander effects in the lead-shielded distant spleen tissue.[55] Bystander-related tumor induction (medulloblastoma) in shielded cerebellum of radiosensitive Patched-1 (Ptch1) heterozygous mice was demonstrated after x-ray exposure of the remainder of their bodies.[56] The bystander effect has been demonstrated in three-dimensional human tissues and in other whole animal organisms.[57] Both DSBs and apoptotic cell death were induced by bystander effects, supporting a signaling role between the irradiated cells (the targeted cells) and nonirradiated cells (the nontargeted or bystander cells) (Fig. 12.17). Numerous intercellular and intracellular signaling pathways are implicated in the bystander response, and these effects have been shown to be transmitted to cell descendants. Emerging data are showing the importance of exosomes mediating microRNA transfer and the cellular communication between the directly irradiated cells and the nonirradiated cells (see Chapter 1 and Fig. 12.18). Importantly, exosome communication is being studied as promoting a favorable inflammatory microenvironment that promotes cancer cell metastasis.[58] These bystander effects, demonstrated in vivo, reflect an ongoing inflammatory response (oxidative stress response) to the initial radiation-induced injury (Box 12.2). One hypothesis is that the stress response is caused by elevated ROS, which induce the subsequent genomic instability. Therapeutic interference with specific signaling pathways may result in genome stabilization.

BOX 12.2   A Paradigm Shift? Responses to Ionizing Radiation Mediated by Inflammatory Mechanisms

Many observations have not been supportive of the conventional paradigm of biologic responses to ionizing radiation (IR). The conventional paradigm is that the consequences of exposure to IR have been attributed solely to mutational DNA damage or cell death induced in irradiated cells at the time of exposure. The challenges to this paradigm come from three types of published data: (1) abscopal, or "out-of-field," effects, where radiation treatment to one local area of the body results in an antitumor effect distant to the radiation site; (2) detection of plasma factors in vivo (clastogenic [or capable of chromosome damage] factors) that can affect the survival and function of irradiated cells; and (3) effects in nonirradiated cells that are in the vicinity of irradiated cells (bystander effects) or in the descendants of irradiated cells several generations after the initial radiation exposure (genomic instability). These nontargeted effects are different than the targeted effects that arise in cells upon immediate deposition of energy at the time of radiation exposure. The nontargeted effects arise as a result of intracellular signaling and appear to represent a genotype-dependent balance (and various epigenetic influences) of toxic factors and cellular responses that may involve both oxidative stress and inflammatory type processes (see Fig. 12.17).

Data from Azzam E, Jay-Gerin JP: *Cancer Lett* 327(1-2):48-60, 2012; and Mukherjee D et al: *J Pathol* 232(3):289-299, 2014.

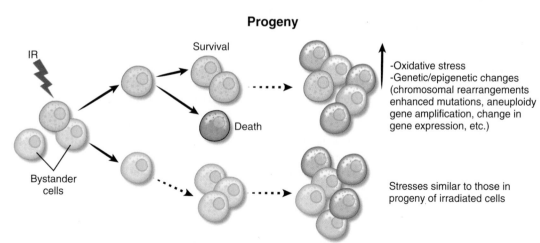

Progeny

- Oxidative stress
- Genetic/epigenetic changes (chromosomal rearrangements enhanced mutations, aneuploidy gene amplification, change in gene expression, etc.)

Stresses similar to those in progeny of irradiated cells

FIGURE 12.17 Radiation: Targeted and Nontargeted or Bystander Effects. Signaling from cells exposed to irradiation causes stressful effects, including oxidative stress, to those cells not directly irradiated (called *bystander cells*) and their progeny. These induced effects may be similar to those reported in the progeny of irradiated cells. (Adapted from Azzam EI et al: Ionizing radiation-induced metabolic oxidative stress and prolonged cell injury, *Cancer Lett* 327[1-2]:48-60, 2012.)

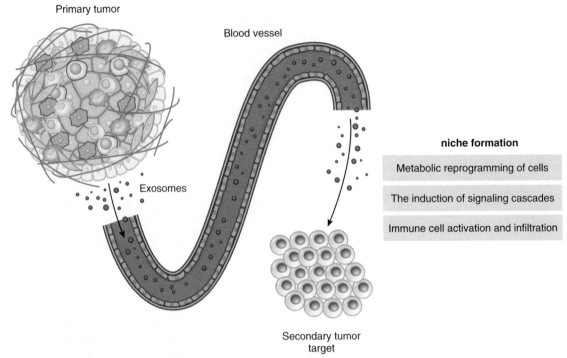

Primary tumor

Blood vessel

niche formation

Metabolic reprogramming of cells

The induction of signaling cascades

Immune cell activation and infiltration

Exosomes

Secondary tumor
target

FIGURE 12.18 Exosomes in Cancer. Exosomes are vesicles that carry cargo. Tumor-derived exosomes can be released into extracellular sites. These vesicles carry oncoproteins and nucleic acids that induce different signaling pathways and activation of different immune cells. This communication can promote a cancer-favorable inflammatory microenvironment that promotes cancer metastasis.*ESCRT*, endosomal sorting complex required for transport; *MVBs*, mutivesicular bodies. (Adapted from Rajagopal C, Harikumar KB: *Front Oncol* 8:66, 2018.)

Acute, Latent, and Microenvironmental Effects

IR causes both acute and persistent effects. Acute exposure to IR can cause damage to several organ systems, especially those with highly proliferative cells, such as the hematopoietic system, the skin, and the gastrointestinal system. Investigators have postulated that radiation's carcinogenic potential persists as a direct result of nontargeted radiation effects, which are known to alter cell signaling and induce changes in the microenvironment. Investigators report the brain's innate immune system is very vulnerable to cranial irradiation. The radiation alters the microenvironment and induces the recruitment of macrophages, which infiltrate the region. With improvement in cancer survival, the long-term risks of a second cancer developing from treatment become increasingly important.

Radiation-induced cancer in humans has latent periods, usually 5 to 10 years, but latency can span decades. British investigators have reported that for solid tumors, radiation-related excess risk begins to appear about 5 years after exposure in therapeutically irradiated groups. For leukemia, it appears within 5 years of exposure.[59] Using U.S. Surveillance Epidemiology and End Results (SEER) data, the estimated excess of secondary cancers that could be related to radiotherapy is about 8%. Data from the United Kingdom, which included diagnostic procedures but excluded therapeutic irradiation, yielded an estimation of 15%.[59,60]

Low Dose and Dose Rate

Recent events, including the 2011 Fukushima nuclear accident, terrorist attacks, and exposure to radiation from medical procedures, have increased the need to identify risks from exposure to low-level ionizing radiation. Risk estimates for human exposures to low-dose ionizing radiation are constantly debated. Determining risks from low doses of radiation is statistically difficult because it requires such large populations. Simulation models may provide reasonable approximations; theoretic models are still used to estimate response curves (Box 12.3).

Ultraviolet Radiation

Ultraviolet radiation, called UV radiation, comes from sunlight. Other sources of UV radiation include electric lights, black lights, and tanning lamps. UV radiation is divided into three major wavelengths: UVA, UVB, and UVC radiation. Most of the UV radiation received on earth is UVA; some is UVB.[61] UVA radiation is weaker than UVB but penetrates deeper into the skin and is more constant throughout the year regardless of weather conditions. UVB primarily affects the outer layer of the skin; and UVC radiation effects do not increase health risks as much as UVB radiation. UV radiation also can be important to health and produces vitamin D, necessary for the absorption of calcium and phosphorus from food, which is important for bone development. The WHO recommends 5 to 15 minutes of sun exposure two to three times a week. Overexposure, however, can result in acute and chronic health effects, particularly to the skin, the eyes, and the immune system.

There are three main types of skin cancer:
- Melanoma: cancer that forms in melanocytes (i.e., pigment cells)
- Basal cell carcinoma (BCC): cancer in the lower part of the epidermis or outer layer of the skin
- Squamous cell carcinoma (SCC): cancer in the flat cells that form the surface of the skin

Melanoma, the most lethal form of skin cancer, can occur at many site; however, certain sites are more common. In men it is often found on the skin on the head, the neck, between the shoulders, and the hips. In women, melanoma is more commonly found on the skin on

BOX 12.3 Theoretical Models to Understand Low-Dose Radiation

Several models include the linear no-threshold (LNT) relationship, in which any dose, including very low doses, has the potential to cause mutations (see **A**). Another model, the linear-quadratic relationship, proposes there is a risk mathematical term that is directly proportional to the dose (linear term) and another term proportional to the square of the dose (quadratic term) (see **B**). The threshold model proposes a threshold dose below which radiation may not cause cancer in humans (see **C**). Proponents of this model argue that such thresholds are derived, for example, from the ability to repair damage caused by lower doses of radiation. There is some evidence that low doses may actually produce a higher level of risk per unit of dose, which is called the *supralinear hypothesis* (see **D**). **E,** Stochastic or random probability is a major model for understanding low-dose radiation. Currently, the shape of the response curve for the low-dose region is really unknown.

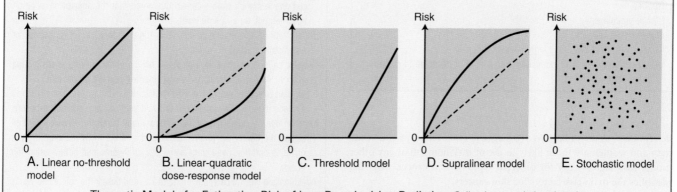

Theoretic Models for Estimating Risk of Low-Dose Ionizing Radiation. Collective population dose is expressed as a person-rem (roentgen equivalent, man). Estimating a collective dose then enables an application of a "constant risk factor" to obtain a statistical estimate of the number of additional cancers (above background radiation) from that exposure. These computations apply to low doses–low dose rates only (**A**). Many propose the best fit is the linear no-threshold (LNT) model (**B**). The most common alternative to the LNT model is the linear-quadratic model. The quadratic term is the square of the dose. The linear term is equal to zero (**C**). The threshold model is a threshold below which there is *no* increase in cancer risk. Proponents of this model argue that because some toxic chemicals/materials exhibit such thresholds, radiation must also have a threshold. Their arguments are related to repair of the radiation damage caused by lower doses of radiation (**D**). Some evidence exists that low levels of radiation produce a higher level of risk per unit dose, which is called the supralinear model. The stochastic model describes effects that are random and the events cannot be predicted (**E**). (Adapted from Makhijani A et al: *Science for the vulnerable: setting radiation and multiple exposure environmental health standards to protect those at most risk,* Takoma Park, MD, 2006, Institute for Energy and Environmental Research.)

the lower legs, between the shoulders, and the hips. Although rare in people with dark skin, in this population the melanoma is usually found under the fingernails or toenails or on the palms of the hands and soles of the feet. Based on some evidence, *intermittent acute* sun exposure causing sunburn is associated with an increased risk of melanoma. Melanomas on sun-exposed skin are heterogeneous (distinctly different biologically) tumors.

Basal cell carcinoma commonly occurs on the head and neck. Squamous cell carcinoma is found more commonly in men who work outdoors but can occur in anyone. SCC typically occurs on sun-exposed areas of the skin, including the nose, ears, lower lip, and dorsa of the hand. SCCs are composed of keratinizing cells and are more aggressive than BCC, however, the incidence of invasive SCC is low.

The incidence of basal cell carcinoma and squamous cell carcinoma is strongly correlated with lifetime sunlight exposure (i.e., photocarcinogenesis). Specific patterns of sunlight exposure, intermittent or chronic, confer different host effects. Intense intermittent recreational sun exposure has been associated with melanoma and BCC. Chronic occupational sun exposure has been associated with SCC. Tanning bed exposure is associated with an increased risk of BCC. The risk is higher in females and increases proportionately with increased use of indoor tanning facilities. (Other occupational factors are discussed in Chapter 43.) Depending on the time of day and skin type, acute sun exposure may result in sunburn. From epidemiologic studies,

sunburn is defined as a burn or pain or blistering, or a combination of these, which lasts for 2 or more days. Cumulative sun exposure is the additive effects of intermittent sun exposure, chronic sun exposure, or both. Other skin cancer risk factors include ionizing radiation, chronic arsenic ingestion, immunosuppression, and genetic factors. These skin cancers have a higher incidence among people with a light or fair skin tone, but they can occur in anyone, including those who do not usually burn from exposure to sunlight. The pathogenesis of non-melanoma skin cancers involves specific gene mutations, epigenetic alterations, oxidative stress, inflammation, and reduced immune surveillance (see Chapter 43 for a more complete discussion of skin cancers).

In the United States, skin cancer is the most common malignancy diagnosed. In 2019, an estimated number of new cases of melanoma of the skin was 96,480 and estimated deaths were 7230.[62] The actual numbers of non-melanoma skin cancers is unknown because they are not reported to cancer registries. Melanoma accounts for substantial morbidity and the majority of skin cancer deaths. Because mortality rates have not risen as rapidly as incidence rates, controversy exists as to whether the incidence rate is a true increase or is a result of overdiagnosis. The U.S. Preventive Services Task Force (USPSTF) concludes that the current evidence is insufficient for early detection of skin cancer, and the balance of benefit and harm of visual skin examination by a clinician to screen for skin cancer in asymptomatic adults cannot be

BOX 12.4   Common Risk Factors for Skin Cancers

Lighter natural skin color
Family history of skin cancer
A personal history of skin cancer
Exposure to sun through work and play
History of sunburns, especially early in life
History of indoor tanning
Skin that burns, reddens easily, or becomes painful in the sun
Freckles
Blue or green eyes
Blonde or red hair
Certain types of moles and a large number of moles
Higher coffee intake was associated with a modest decrease in melanoma (large cohort study)

BOX 12.5   Cell Phone Radiation and Children's Health: What Parents Need to Know

Use text messaging when possible and use cell phones in speaker mode or with the use of hands-free kits
When talking on the cell phone, try holding it an inch or more away from the head
Make only short or essential calls on cell phones
Avoid carrying your phone against the body, such as in a pocket, sock, or bra; cell phone manufacturers cannot guarantee that the amount of radiation absorbed will be at a safe level
Do not talk on the phone or text while driving; this increases the risk of automobile crashes
Exercise caution when using a phone or texting while walking or performing other activities; "distracted walking" injuries also are on the rise
If you plan to watch a movie on your device, download it first, then switch to airplane mode while watching it to avoid unnecessary radiation exposure
Keep an eye on signal strength (i.e., how many bars); the weaker your cell signal, the harder the phone has to work and the more radiation it gives off; it is better to wait until there is a stronger signal before using the device
Avoid making calls in cars, elevators, trains, and buses; the cell phone works harder to get a signal through metal so the power level increases
Remember that cell phones are not toys or teething items

Data from American Academy of Pediatrics, June 13, 2016. Available at http://www.healthychildren.org.

determined.[63] A major harm is overdiagnosis and overtreatment. White men and women are more likely to die of melanoma than any other group. Risk factors vary for different types of skin cancer. Box 12.4 identifies the main risk factors for skin cancers.

Electromagnetic Radiation

Electromagnetic radiation (EM or EMR) is energy in the form of magnetic and electric waves. Health risks associated with EM are very controversial and have been a concern for many decades, since at least the 1950s. Long-term low-level exposures of EM have been difficult to study. Recent research emphasis has involved low-intensity fields, intermediate radiofrequency (RF); and higher-frequency radiation from devices such as phones, broadcast antennas, Wi-Fi, security monitors, and others. Exposure to electric and magnetic fields is widespread. Electric fields are shielded or weakened by walls and other objects, but magnetic fields are not. Electromagnetic fields (EMFs) are, for example, generated by RF sources coupled with the body. The result induces electric and magnetic fields with associated currents inside tissue. The most common sources of radiofrequency electromagnetic radiation (RF-EMR) are wireless telecommunication devices and equipment including cell phones, smart meters, and portable wireless devices (laptop computers, and tablets).

The impact of EMR on human health has not been fully assessed. In addition, with competing priorities (convenience, financial interest, and health necessity), a consensus of the risk/benefit ratio of EMR exposure may be difficult to achieve. Safety standards vary significantly (up to 1000-fold) among countries. The National Institute of Environmental Health Sciences Electric and Magnetic Fields Working Group have recommended that low-frequency EMFs be classified as possible carcinogens. Low levels of low-frequency EMF and cancer led to the classification of EMF by the IARC as a possible cause of cancer.

The most extensively studied exposure is from use of wireless telephones (mobile and cordless); other exposures include occupational settings and sources from the general environment. Recent studies from the National Toxicology Program (NTP) showed *high* exposure to radiofrequency radiation (RFR) in rodents resulted in tumors in tissues surrounding the nerves in the hearts (schwannomas) of male rats, but not female rats or mice. The report included statistically significant increases in the number of rats and mice with tumors found in other organs at one or more of the exposure levels studied, including the brain, prostate gland, pituitary gland, adrenal gland, liver, and pancreas. The researchers in this report concluded that these findings were equivocal findings and will be reviewed further in 2018.[64] The mechanisms included genotoxicity, effects on immune function, gene and protein expression, DNA repair mechanisms, cell signaling, oxidative stress, decreased melatonin, and apoptosis. Long-term exposure to elevated magnetic fields may lead to increased free radical concentrations, which are associated with aging, cancers, and neurodegenerative diseases.

A main concern is for children since the effects of exposure may be compounded because of increased vulnerability to radiation and their longer use of cell phones into adulthood. In response to the NTP study discussed earlier, the American Academy of Pediatrics issued specific recommendations to reduce wireless cell phone exposure (Box 12.5). Chapter 13 discusses cancer in children.

✓ QUICK CHECK 12.3

1. What are the cancers associated with cigarette smoking?
2. What are some dietary components that may cause or offer protection from cancer?
3. What are the possible pathophysiologic mechanisms of obesity-associated cancer risk?
4. How does ionizing radiation contribute to carcinogenesis? UV radiation?
5. Discuss the most recent findings of the National Toxicology Program and exposure to cell phone radiofrequency energy.

Infection, Sexual and Reproductive Behavior

Infections with certain viruses, bacteria, and parasites are an important contributor to cancer worldwide. About 15% of new cancer cases have been attributed to carcinogenic infections. Infection and cancer rates vary widely by region and level of socioeconomic development; the higher the development, the lower the attributable fraction (AF) for infection. The most notable infections implicated in new cancer cases include *Helicobacter pylori (H. pylori)*, human papillomavirus (HPV), hepatitis B virus (HBV), hepatitis C virus (HCV), and

Epstein–Barr virus (EBV). *H. pylori* is the cause of about 75% of stomach cancers. Hepatitis B and hepatitis C infect the liver; together they account for the large majority of liver cancer cases (see Chapter 38). EBV is linked to nasopharyngeal carcinoma, Hodgkin lymphoma, diffuse large B-cell lymphoma (DLBCL), Burkitt lymphoma, EBV-associated malignant B-cell lymphoma, other lymphomas, and gastric adenocarcinoma.

(HPV is the most common sexually transmitted virus in the United States. HPV is very common worldwide and accounts for more than half of the total infection-attributable cancers in women worldwide. Most sexually active women and men will be infected with HPV at some point in their lives, and some are infected repeatedly. HPVs are a group of more than 200 related viruses and at least 13 are cancer causing. *Low-risk HPVs* are not associated with cancer but can cause skin warts, called *condylomata acuminata. High-risk,* or oncogenic, *HPVs* can cause cancer. HPV types 16 and 18 are responsible for the majority of cancers. Most high-risk HPV infections cause cytologic abnormalities or abnormal cell changes that disappear unexpectedly. According to the National Cancer Institute, most infections will be suppressed by an individual's immune system.[65] Persistence of infection with high-risk HPV is a precursor to the development of cervical intraepithelial neoplasia (CIN) (see Fig. 35.19), lesions, and invasive cervical cancers. HPV infection has been identified as a definite carcinogen for several types of cancer: cervical, penis, vulvar, vaginal, anal, and some oropharyngeal cancers (OPCs). The OPCs most commonly include the base of the tongue, tonsils, and pharynx. More than half of the OPCs in the United States are linked to HPV-16. The incidence of HPV-associated oropharyngeal cancer has increased during the past 20 years, especially among men. Persistent chronic inflammation-related HPV infection might drive oropharyngeal carcinogenesis. Factors that may increase the risk of developing cancer following a high-risk HPV infection include smoking, decreased immunity, having many children (cervical cancer), long-term oral contraceptive use (cervical cancer), poor oral hygiene (oropharyngeal cancer), and chronic inflammation. Although the main mode of HPV transmission is sexual contact, HPV has been found in virginal women before first intercourse.[66] One hypothesis for the virginal women is that as newborns they were exposed to cervical HPV infection from the mother. The possible modes of transmission in children, however, are controversial.

Current guidelines recommend that women should have a Pap test every 3 years beginning at age 21 to 29. Women 30 to 65 years of age may receive Pap testing with HPV screening every 5 years (preferred) or Pap testing alone every 3 years. After age 65, Pap testing and HPV screening are no longer recommended for women with previous normal testing results since the risk of new malignancy is low. Women who had a hysterectomy with removal of the uterine cervix for a noncancerous condition do not need Pap smears or HPV testing the rest of their lives. At this time, although the HPV vaccine does reduce the risk for cervical cancer, it does not change the frequency or need for Pap and HPV testing (see *Did You Know?* Human Papillomavirus Vaccine).

Other Viruses and Microorganisms

The relationship between viruses, bacteria, and cancer is discussed in Chapter 11 and appropriate chapters in Part Two. Human herpesvirus type 8 is linked to Kaposi sarcoma, and human T-cell lymphotropic virus type 1 is linked to leukemia and lymphoma. Other microorganisms involved in carcinogenesis include parasites such as *Opisthorchis viverrini* (bile duct cancer) and *Schistosoma haematobium* (bladder cancer). Their specific roles in carcinogenesis are thought to be related to functioning as cofactors or as direct carcinogens, or both.

Chemical and Occupational Hazards as Carcinogens

An estimated 100,000 synthetic chemicals are used in the United States.[67] Of those, only about 7% have been tested for their health effects[68]; another 1000 chemicals are added each year.[67] Exposure to chemicals occurs every day. Chemicals are present in air, soil, food, water, household products, toys, personal care products, workplaces, and homes. The number of known carcinogens in experimental animals is large. It is suspected that most of these chemical carcinogens are potentially carcinogenic in humans, but documentation is lacking. Table 12.1 provides a summary of a limited number of chemicals according to sufficient or limited evidence by IARC in humans by cancer site. A simplified overview of the Occupational Safety and Health Administration (OSHA) carcinogenic factors is presented in Table 12.7.

TABLE 12.7	Overview of OSHA-Relevant Carcinogenic Factors	
Group	**Example**
Chemicals	
Gases	Vinyl chloride
	Formaldehyde
Liquids, volatile	Trichloroethylene
	Tetrachloroethylene
	Methylchloride
	Styrene
	Benzene
	Xylene
Liquids, nonvolatile	Metalworking fluids
	Mineral oils
	Hair dyes
Solids, dust	Silica
	Wood dust
	Talc containing asbestiform fibers

Continued

TABLE 12.7 Overview of OSHA-Relevant Carcinogenic Factors—cont'd

Group	Example
Solids, fibers	Asbestos Man-made mineral fibers, for example, ceramic fibers
Solids	Lead Nickel compounds Chromium VI compounds Arsenic Beryllium Cadmium Carbon black Bitumen
Fumes, smoke	Welding fumes Diesel emissions Coal tar fumes Bitumen fumes Fire, combustion emissions PAHs Tobacco smoke
Mixtures	Solvents
Pesticides Halogenated organic compounds	DDT Ethylene dibromide
Others	Amitrole
Pharmaceuticals Antineoplastic drugs	MOPP (Mustargen, oncovin, procarbazine, and prednisone, a combination chemotherapy regimen used to treat Hodgkin disease) and other combined chemotherapies, including alkylating agents
Anesthetics	There is evidence from in vitro experiments that isoflurane increases cancer cells' potential to grow and migrate
Emerging Factors Air pollution and fine particulate matter	Emissions from motor vehicles, industrial processes, power generation, and other sources polluting the ambient air
Endocrine-disrupting compounds	Certain pesticides Certain flame retardants
Biologic Factors Bacteria	*Helicobacter pylori*
Viruses	Hepatitis B Hepatitis C
Mycotoxin-producing fungi	Bulk handling of agricultural foodstuffs (nuts, grain, maize, coffee), animal-feed production, brewing/malting, waste management, composting, food production, working with indoor molds, horticulture
Aspergillus flavus, A. parasiticus	Aflatoxin (A1)
Penicillium griseofulvum	Griseofulvin (IARC group 2B)
A. ochraceus, A. carbonarius, P. verrucosum	Ochratoxin A (group 2B)
A. versicolor, Emericella nidulans, Chaetomium spp., A. flavus, A. parasiticus	Sterigmatocystin (group 2B)
Fusarium spp.	Fumonisin B1 (group 2B)
Physical Factors Ionizing radiation	Radon X-rays
Ultraviolet radiation (UVR)	Solar radiation Artificial UVR
Ergonomics	Sedentary work

TABLE 12.7 Overview of OSHA-Relevant Carcinogenic Factors—cont'd

Group	Example
Other	
Work organization	Shift work that involves circadian disruption
	Static work
	Prolonged sitting and standing
Lifestyle factors	Stress-related obesity, smoking, drinking, drug consumption
Combinations of Various Factors	
Chemicals and radiation	Methoxsalen and UVA radiation
	Some chemicals, called *promoters*, can increase the cancer-causing ability of UVR. Conversely, UVR can act as a promoter and increase the cancer-causing ability of some chemicals, particularly coal tar and pitch.
Work organization and chemicals	Shift work and solvents

DDT, Dichlorodiphenyltrichloroethane; *IARC*, International Agency for Research on Cancer; *OSHA*, Occupational Safety and Health Administration; *PSHs*, polycyclic aromatic hydrocarbons; *UVA*, ultraviolet A.

Data from European Agency for Safety and Health at Work: *Exposure to carcinogens and work-related cancer: a review of assessment methods European Risk Observatory Report*, Luxembourg, 2014, European Agency for Safety and Health at Work Eu-OSHA. Available at http://europa.eu.OSHA, Occupational Safety and Health Administration

DID YOU KNOW?

Human Papillomavirus Vaccine

Every year in the United States:

- Nearly 1 in 4 adults in the U.S. have at least one strain of the human papillomavirus (HPV)
- About 12,000 women are diagnosed with HPV-related cervical cancer
- Almost 4000 women die from this disease
- About 1900 men get HPV-related penile or anal cancer

Vaccines are available in the United States to vaccinate for two, four, or nine strains of high-risk (HPV):

- Vaccines are recommended for females and males beginning at age 11 years and up to age 26, depending on sex and risk factors
- The Centers for Disease Control and Prevention (CDC) now recommends children ages 11 to 12 years receive two doses of HPV vaccine rather than the previously recommended three doses; the second dose should be given 6 to 12 months after the first dose

- Vaccines are highly effective in preventing high-risk HPV types associated with cervical cancer; they have been proven safe and effective by the CDC with ongoing safety monitoring
- Vaccines are not recommended for pregnant women because their safety is not yet established, but preliminary reports suggest that HPV vaccination in pregnancy may decrease vertical transmission during vaginal birth
- Vaccinated women still need cervical cancer screening at regular intervals
- The three-injection vaccine series is covered by most insurance plans, Medicaid, and the Vaccines for Children (VFC) program if individuals meet eligibility requirements, including age and financial need

For more information, visit the Centers for Disease Control and Prevention (CDC) STD website at http://www.cdc/std/default.htm.

Data from Centers for Disease Control and Prevention (CDC): *Human papillomavirus (HPV)*, Atlanta, GA, 2017, U.S. Department of Health and Human Services. Available at https://www.cdc.gov/mmwr/volumes/65/wr/mm6549a5.html, updated January 25, 2017; Centers for Disease Control and Prevention (CDC): *Multi-routine, & non-routine vaccine VISs*, Atlanta, GA, 2016, U.S. Department of Health and Human Services. Available at http://www.cdc.gov/vaccines/hcp/vis/index.html.

Chemical carcinogenesis involves genotoxic mechanisms and nongenotoxic mechanisms (Fig. 12.19). Genotoxic mechanisms create genetic damage and nongenotoxic mechanisms (inflammation, immunosuppression, ROS, receptor activation, epigenetic silencing) alter signal transduction.

A substantial percentage of cancers of the upper respiratory passages, lung, bladder, and peritoneum are attributed to occupational factors, however, fewer studies of nonsmokers exist. Millions of U.S. workers are exposed to substances tested as carcinogens in animal studies and some are found carcinogenic in human studies.[69] It has been estimated that 3% to 6% of all cancers worldwide are caused by workplace exposures to carcinogens. Textile industry workers are exposed to different kinds of chemicals (dyes, solvents, fiber dusts, others) continuously with known carcinogenic properties.[70] One notable occupational factor is asbestos, a heat-resistant, fibrous silicate mineral woven into fabrics and fire-resistant and insulating compounds, such as brake linings. Chrysotile asbestos, more than any other form, accounts for a majority of asbestos in buildings in the United States. Asbestos increases the risk

of mesothelioma and lung cancer. It may be implicated in other cancers, as well. Noncancerous disorders related to asbestos exposures include pleural plaques, diffuse pleural thickening, and pulmonary fibrosis. These asbestos-related disorders (ARDs) represent a significant occupational and public health concern. Asbestos was commonly used in homes and buildings built before the 1970s to insulate ceiling tiles, flooring, and pipe covers. In Western Europe, because of the long latency of disease onset, the epidemic of mesothelioma in building workers born after 1940 did not become apparent until the 1990s. Building materials containing asbestos have been banned in most developed countries, but such materials are still used in many developing countries, where the incidence of cases of ARDs is rising. No exposure to asbestos is without risk.

Carcinoma of the bladder has been linked with the manufacture of dyes, rubber, paint, and aromatic amines, especially β-naphthylamine and benzidine. Benzol inhalation is linked to leukemia in shoemakers and in workers employed in the rubber cement, explosives, and dye-manufacture industries. Other notable occupational hazards

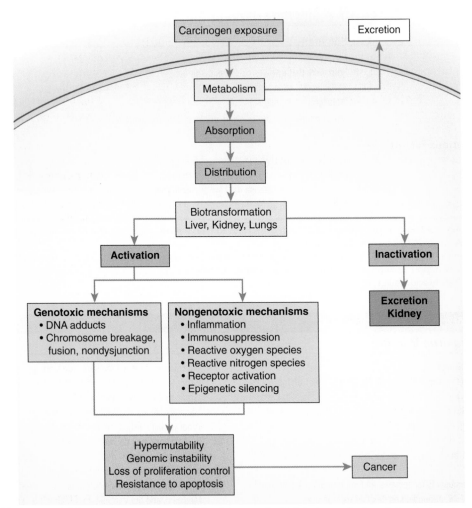

FIGURE 12.19 Mechanisms of Chemical Carcinogenesis. Cellular internalization of chemical carcinogens results in metabolic products that are either excreted or retained by the cell. Within the cell, carcinogens or their metabolic products can directly or indirectly affect the regulation and expression of genes involved in cell cycle control, DNA repair, cell differentiation, or apoptosis. Some chemical carcinogens act by *genotoxic* mechanisms, such as DNA adducts, chromosomal breakage, fusion, deletion, missegregation, and nondisjunction. Other carcinogens act by *nongenotoxic* mechanisms, such as induction of inflammation, immunosuppression, formation of reactive oxygen species (oxidative stress), activation of receptors, and epigenetic mechanisms, such as silencing. Both genotoxic and nongenotoxic mechanisms can alter signal transduction pathways that result in many features of cancer cells (Adapted from Luch A: *Nat Rev Cancer* 5:113-125, 2005.)

include heavy metals (high-nickel alloy, chromium VI compounds, inorganic arsenic), silica, polycyclic aromatic hydrocarbons, sulfuric acid, and chloromethyl ether. Disentangling data related to lung cancer, air pollution, and occupational risks is complex, especially in combination with other risk factors, such as active and passive smoking, other environmental factors, and genetic polymorphisms at multiple loci.

✔ **QUICK CHECK 12.4**

1. Identify the high-risk types of human papillomavirus (HPV) that are carcinogenic.
2. What components of air pollution are considered most important for carcinogenesis?
3. Describe the genotoxic and nongenotoxic mechanisms of chemical carcinogenesis.

▌ S U M M A R Y   R E V I E W

Genetics, Epigenetics, and Tissue

1. Cancer arises from a complicated and interacting web of multiple etiologies. Avoiding high-risk behaviors and exposure to individual carcinogens will prevent many types of cancers.
2. Risk factors for cancer include lifestyle behaviors (smoking, alcohol intake, diet), lack of physical exercise and obesity, certain

infections, environmental factors (exposure to sunlight or ionizing radiation), occupational exposure to carcinogens, and certain medications.

3. Cancers are caused by environmental-lifestyle factors and genetic/epigenetic factors. Interacting factors are weaker immune systems, variations in detoxifying enzymes or DNA repair genes, differences

in hormone levels, and metabolic factors. Altogether the biologic environment is modified by metabolic and hormonal factors, inflammation, and disordered glucose and lipid metabolism.

4. Cancer-causing factors are influenced by the surrounding microenvironment or stroma. Once malignant phenotypes have developed, complex interactions occur between the tumor, the surrounding stroma, and the cells of the immune and inflammatory systems.

5. Globally cancer is reported to become a major cause of morbidity and mortality in the coming decades.

6. In the United States, cancer incidence rates decreased for men and stayed about the same for women from 2003 to 2012. During this same time period, cancer incidence rates increased in children 0 to 19 years of age.

7. Overall, cancer death rates have continued to decline in men, women, and children. However, deaths caused by liver cancer increased at the highest rate of all reported cancer sites, and liver cancer incidence rates increased sharply.

In Utero and Early Life Conditions

1. Emerging data suggest early life events influence later susceptibility to chronic diseases.

2. Developmental plasticity is the degree to which an organism's development is contingent on its environment. Plasticity refers to the ability of genes to organize physiologically or structurally in response to environmental conditions during fetal development.

3. The developmental origins' hypothesis suggests that nutrition and other environmental factors affect cellular pathways during gestation, enabling a single genotype to produce a broad range of adult phenotypes. Maternal nutrition, as well as environment factors, are proposed as significant biological influences.

4. Undernutrition in utero is linked to increased heart disease, metabolic disorders, and possibly breast cancer decades later. Early versus late undernutrition in pregnancy indicated that the first trimester of pregnancy is particularly vulnerable to disease outcome in adulthood.

Environmental-Lifestyle Factors
Tobacco Use

1. Cigarette smoking is carcinogenic and the most important cause of cancer. Tobacco smoking causes cancer in more than 15 organ sites, and exposure to secondhand smoke and parental smoking causes cancer in children and in other nonsmokers. The risk is greatest in those who begin to smoke when young and continue throughout life. Smoking is, however, pandemic affecting all ages.

2. Worldwide, tobacco use causes more than 7 million deaths per year.

3. Environmental tobacco smoke (i.e., secondhand smoke) is a cause of stroke; increases the risk of death in people with cancer and cancer survivors as well as those with macular degeneration, tuberculosis, ectopic pregnancy, and diabetes mellitus. Secondhand smoke exposure increases inflammation, impairs immunity, and is a cause of rheumatoid arthritis.

4. Smoking tobacco is linked to cancers of the lung, upper aerodigestive tract, stomach, lower urinary tract, kidney, pancreas, cervix, uterus, and myeloid leukemia. Recently added to the list are liver cancer and colorectal cancer. Smoking causes even more deaths from respiratory, vascular, and other diseases than from cancer.

5. Cigar or pipe smoking is related to cancers of the oral cavity, oropharynx, hypopharynx, larynx, esophagus, and lung. Pipe smokers have an increased risk of cancers of lung, lip, throat, esophagus, larynx, pancreas, and colon and rectum.

6. Electronic cigarettes can contain harmful and potentially cancer-causing substances.

Diet

1. The influence of diet on cancer development is complicated. Cancer risks in older adults may depend as much on diet in early life as on current eating practices.

2. Nutrigenomics is the study of the effects of nutrition on the phenotypic variability of individuals based on genomic differences.

3. Nutrition, Obesity, Alcohol Consumption, and Physical Activity: Impacts on CancerDiet, weight, and activity level all influence risks for cancer development.

4. The implementation of dietary patterns, for example, the Mediterranean dietary pattern, and the promoting of specific dietary recommendations, is becoming more widespread.

5. The importance of diet has been illustrated by data showing changes in cancer risk among migrants in low-risk countries compared with those in high-risk countries. With geographic migration, risks and cancer patterns change, particularly with the adoption of the Western diet.

6. Bioactive components have a profound effect on differentiation, potentially including differentiation of cancer stem cells. Intake of specific food compounds may suppress cancer stem renewal.

7. A variety of food compounds may influence DNA repair.

8. Xenobiotics are toxic, mutagenic, and carcinogenic chemicals that humans are constantly exposed to. The body has defense systems for counteracting these effects. Many foods enhance the efficiency and degree of detoxification of xenobiotics and thus serve a protective role in metabolizing carcinogens.

9. Diets high in red meat or processed meat may lead to increased risks of development colorectal cancer. Means containing nitrites, nitrates, or other preservatives can leave residues in the colon that cause DNA damage.

10. Obesity has been increasing in developed countries and in urban areas of developing countries. Obesity in the United States is epidemic. Obesity impacts energy balance, cancer risk, cancer recurrence, and survival.

11. Obesity is a risk factor for 11 cancers: liver, advanced prostate, ovarian, gallbladder, kidney, colorectal, esophageal, breast (postmenopausal), pancreatic, endometrial, and stomach.

12. The mechanisms of obesity-associated cancer risks are evolving and vary by type of tumor and distribution of body fat. Emerging data point to are three main factors: (1) insulin-insulin-like growth factor (IGF-1) axis, (2) sex hormones, and (3) adipokines.

13. Metabolic changes in adipose tissue from obesity result in several alterations and include insulin resistance, hyperglycemia, dyslipidemia, hypoxia, and chronic inflammation. Tumor growth is regulated by interactions between tumor cells and their tissue microenvironment, so stromal compartments that are rich in adipose tissue can promote the development of tumor cells.

14. Alcohol is classified as a human carcinogen. Strong data link alcohol with cancers of the mouth, pharynx, larynx, esophagus, liver, colorectum, and breast.

15. Evidence does not show any safe limit of alcohol and the health effects are from ethanol regardless of the type of drink.

16. Alcohol-related carcinogenesis involves acetaldehyde, reactive oxygen species (ROS), pro-carcinogen activation, cellular regeneration, nutritional deficiencies, and enzyme and metabolic dysfunction.

17. Physical activity, independent of weight changes, reduces the risk for breast cancer, colon cancer (in men), and endometrial cancer.

18. Biologic mechanisms for the protective effects of physical activity include decreasing insulin and IGF levels, decreasing obesity, increasing free radical scavenger systems, altering inflammatory mediators, decreasing levels of circulating sex hormones and metabolic

hormones, improving immune function, decreasing oncogenes, enhancing cytochrome P-450 activity (thus modifying carcinogen activation), increasing gut motility, and increasing release of myokines (proteins from contracting muscles with antitumor effects).

19. Many unanswered questions remain regarding frequency of exercise, intensity, and duration.

20. Recent data encourage 150 minutes of moderate-intensity aerobic or 75 minutes of vigorous-intensity aerobic physical activity each week for adults. Children and adolescents should get at least 60 minutes of physical activity daily.

Air Pollution

1. Air pollution, indoor and outdoor, is the leading environmental cause of death worldwide. Long-term exposure to air pollution increases mortality and morbidity, and shortens life expectancy from cardiovascular, respiratory disease, and lung cancer.

2. There is a significant association between increased rates of lung cancer and exposure to particulate matter, a mixture of small particles and liquid droplets. Primary particles are emitted directly from a source, for example, construction sites, unpaved roads, fields, or smokestacks. Secondary particles are emitted from power plants, industries, and automobiles.

3. Diesel exhaust is carcinogenic and causes lung cancer. Acute exposure to diesel exhaust that contains particles is linked to lung, throat, and eye irritations; asthma attacks; and myocardial ischemia.

4. The mechanisms of adverse effects of particulate matter include (1) oxidative stress, (2) ROS generation, (3) DNA oxidative damage, (4) mutagenicity, (5) stimulation of proinflammatory factors, and (6) induction of senescence.

5. Fine particle pollution also is linked to (1) premature death in people with heart or lung disease, (2) nonfatal heart attacks, (3) irregular heartbeat, (4) aggravated asthma, (5) decreased lung function, and (6) respiratory symptoms.

6. Indoor air pollution is generally considered worse than outdoor pollution. Sources of indoor air pollution include tobacco smoke, heating and cooking combustion sources, radon, and coal use.

Ionizing Radiation (IR)

1. Much of the knowledge of the effects of ionizing radiation on human cancer has come from Hiroshima and Nagasaki atomic bomb exposures, particularly the Life Span Study. Other evidence is from exposure to radiation for medical reasons, underground miners, and other occupational exposures. Human exposure includes emissions from the environment, x-rays, CT scans, radioisotopes, and other radioactive sources.

2. Atomic bomb exposures in Japan caused acute leukemias and increased frequencies of thyroid, breast, lung, stomach, colon, esophageal, and urinary tract cancers and multiple myeloma.

3. Excess relative risks (ERRs) for radiation-induced cancers at a given age are much higher for individuals exposed during childhood, and decreased at the ages of 30-40 years. The ERR of developing solid tumors increased again for exposure ages higher than 40 years.

4. The bimodal age distribution reflects that radiation exposure in early ages is related to initiation of cancer processes, whereas exposure in later ages is associated with promotion of pre-existing premalignant cells.

5. Other health risks from radiation include cardiovascular effects and somatic mutations that may contribute to other diseases. These effects may manifest years after radiation exposure.

6. There is concern about the increased IR exposure from medical procedures, particularly CT scans.

7. IR is a potent mutagen and carcinogen; it can penetrate cells and tissues and deposit energy in tissues at random in the form of ionizations.

8. IR affects DNA by causing cross-linking, nucleotide base damage, and single- and double-strand DNA breaks. Disrupted cellular regulation processes can lead to carcinogenesis. The double-strand break is considered the hallmark lesion associated with IR.

9. It is now known that radiation may induce genomic instability to the progeny of the directly irradiated cells over many generations of cell divisions and can affect so-called innocent bystander cells. Investigators are studying genomic instability as it may contribute to secondary cancers.

10. The risks from low-dose radiation are constantly debated. Determining risks from low doses of radiation are statistically difficult because they require such large populations.

Ultraviolet Radiation (UVR)

1. Ultraviolet (UV) radiation comes from sunlight, electric lights, black lights, and tanning lamps. Most of the UV radiation received on earth is UVA and some UVB. UVA radiation is weaker than UVB, but UVA penetrates deeper into the skin and is more constant throughout the year despite the weather.

2. The incidence of basal cell carcinoma (BCC) and squamous cell carcinoma (SCC) is strongly correlated with lifetime sunlight exposure. Intense intermittent recreational sun exposure has been associated with melanoma and BCC. Chronic occupational sun exposure has been associated with SCC. Tanning bed use has been associated with an increased risk of BCC, especially in women.

3. Skin cancer risk factors include cumulative sun exposure (the additive effects of intermittent sun exposure, chronic sun exposure, or both), ionizing radiation, chronic arsenic ingestion, immunosuppression, and genetic factors.

4. The pathogenesis of nonmelanoma skin cancers involves specific gene mutations, epigenetic alterations, oxidative stress, inflammation, and reduced immune surveillance.

Electromagnetic Radiation (EMR)

1. EMR is energy in the form of magnetic and electric waves. Health risks associated with EMR are controversial. Exposure to electric and magnetic fields is widespread. Wireless telecommunication devices (e.g., cell phones, wireless laptops, smart meters) are the most common source of radiofrequency electromagnetic radiation (RF-EMR).

2. of the impact of EMR has not been fully assessed. Competing priorities (convenience, financial interest, and health necessity) may make a consensus on the risk/benefit ratio difficult to achieve.

3. Low-frequency electromagnetic fields (EMFs) have been classified as possible carcinogens.

4. The most extensively studied exposure is from use of wireless telephones.

5. Children are a main concern since the effects of exposure may be compounded because of increased vulnerability to radiation and their longer use of cell phones into adulthood.

Infection, Sexual and Reproductive Behavior

1. Infection with certain viruses, bacteria, and parasites are an important contributor to cancer worldwide. The most notable infections implicated in new cancer cases include Epstein-Barr virus (EBV), *Helicobacter pylori*, hepatitis B and C viruses (HBV and HCV), and human papillomavirus (HPV).

2. *H. pylori* is the cause of about 75% of stomach cancers. EBV is linked to nasopharyngeal carcinoma, Hodgkin lymphoma, diffuse

large B-cell lymphoma, Burkitt lymphoma, EBV-associated malignant B-cell lymphoma, other lymphomas, and gastric adenocarcinoma. HBV and HCV infect the liver and together account for the large majority of liver cancer cases.

3. HPV is the most common sexually transmitted virus in the United States. HPV accounts for more than half of the total infection-attributable cancers in women worldwide. HPV types 16 and 18 are responsible for the majority of cancers. Persistence of infection with high-risk HPV is a prerequisite for the development of cervical intraepithelial neoplasia, lesions, and invasive cancer.

4. HPV infection has been identified as a definite carcinogen for several types of cancer: cervical, penis, vulvar, vaginal, anal, and some oropharyngeal (including the base of the tongue, tonsils, and pharynx).

5. The incidence of HPV-associated oropharyngeal cancer has increased during the past 20 years, especially among men.

6. Biologic factors that may interact with HPV infection to increase cancer risk include smoking, decreased immunity, having many children, long-term oral contraceptive use, poor oral hygiene, and chronic inflammation.

7. HPV may be transmitted by genital contact (oral, touching, or sexual intercourse). The possible modes of transmission in children are controversial, however it is thought that newborn babies can be exposed to cervical HPV infection from the mother.

8. Although the HPV vaccine reduces the risk for cervical cancer, women should still get Pap tests and HPV screening at regular intervals.

Other Viruses and Microorganisms

1. Human herpes virus type 8 is linked to Kaposi sarcoma, and human T-cell lymphotropic virus type 1 is linked to leukemia and lymphoma.

2. Microorganisms involved in carcinogenesis include parasites such as *Opisthorchis viverrini* (bile duct cancer) and *Schistosoma haematobium* (bladder cancer).

Chemicals and Occupational Hazards as Carcinogens

1. An estimated 100,000 synthetic chemicals are used in the United States. Only 7% have been fully tested for their impact on health and another 1000 are added each year.

2. Exposure to chemicals occurs from air, soil, food, water, personal care products, toys, household products, medications, workplaces, and homes

3. A large number of chemicals are known carcinogens in experimental animals, and it is suspected that most of these are potentially carcinogenic in humans.

4. Chemical carcinogenesis involves genotoxic mechanisms (create genetic damage) and nongenotoxic mechanisms (alter signal transduction).

5. A substantial percentage of cancers of the upper respiratory passages, lung, bladder, and peritoneum are attributed to occupational factors. Notable occupational hazards include dyes, rubber, paint, aromatic amines, benzol, heavy metals, silica, polycyclic aromatic hydrocarbons, sulfuric acid, and chloromethyl ether. Asbestos is linked to an epidemic of mesothelioma and asbestos usage has been banned in most developed countries.

KEY TERMS

Asbestos, 285
Basal cell carcinoma (BCC), 280
Bystander effect, 279
Carcinogen, 258
Developmental plasticity, 264
Electromagnetic field (EMF), 282

Electromagnetic radiation (EM, EMR), 282
Electronic cigarette (e-cigarette), 267
Environmental tobacco smoke (ETS), 265
Genomic instability, 279

Melanoma, 280
Myokine, 274
Nontargeted effect (NTE), 274
Nutrigenomics, 267
Particulate matter (PM), 274
Radiofrequency electromagnetic radiation (RF-EMR), 282

Radon, 276
Squamous cell carcinoma (SCC), 280
UV radiation, 280
Xenobiotics, 270

REFERENCES

1. Clapp RW, et al: Environmental and occupational causes of cancer: a call to act on what we know, *Biomed Pharmacother* 61(10):631-639, 2007.

2. Clapp RW, et al: Environmental and occupational causes of cancer; new evidence 2005-2007, *Rev Environ Health* 23(1):1-37, 2008.

3. World Health Organization (WHO): World cancer report 2014, Geneva, Switzerland, 2014, Agency for Research on Cancer, World Health Organization.

4. Cogliano VJ, et al: Preventable exposures associated with human cancers, *J Natl Cancer Inst* 103(24):1827-1839, 2011.

5. Institute of Medicine (IOM): *Rebuilding the unity of health and the environment: a new vision of environmental health for the 21st century. Workshop summary*, Washington, DC, 2001, National Academy Press.

6. National Toxicology Program: *Report on carcinogens*, ed 12, Washington, DC, 2011, U.S. Department of Health and Human Services.

7. International Agency for Research on Cancer (IARC): Special report: policy—a review of human carcinogens—part C: metals, arsenic, dusts, and fibres, 2012. Available at http://monographs.iarc.fr/ENG/Monographs/vol100C/index.php. Accessed July 2012.

8. Straif K, et al: A review of human carcinogens—part C: metals, arsenic, dusts, and fibres, *Lancet Oncol* 10(5):453-454, 2009.

9. Bray F, et al: Global cancer statistics 2018: globocan estimates of incidence and mortality worldwide for 36 cancers in 185 countries, *CA Cancer J Clin* 68(6):394-424, 2018.

10. Newbold RR, et al: Adverse effects of the model environmental estrogen diethylstilbestrol are transmitted to subsequent generations, *Endocrinology* 147(6 Suppl):S11-S17, 2006.

11. Centers for Disease Control and Prevention (CDC): Smoking and tobacco use fast facts, Atlanta, GA, 2019, Office on Smoking and Health, National Center for Chronic Disease Prevention and Health Promotion.

12. Lushniak BD: A historic moment: the 50th anniversary of the first Surgeon General's Report on smoking and health, *Public Health Rep* 129(1):5-6, 2014.

13. Office of the Surgeon General: The health consequences of smoking—50 years of progress. A report of the Surgeon General executive summary, Rockville, MD, 2014, U.S. Department of Health and Human Services.

14. Centers for Disease Control and Prevention (CDC): Vital signs: disparities in nonsmokers' exposure to secondhand smoke—United States, 1999–2012, *MMWR Morb Mortal Wkly Rep* 64(4):103-108, 2015.

15. Centers for Disease Control and Prevention (CDC): Electronic cigarettes. Centers for Disease Control and Prevention, Office of Smoking and Health, U.S. Department of Health & Human Services, updated April 18, 2018. Accessed May 22, 2018.

16. Carruba G, et al: Nutrition, aging and cancer: lessons from dietary intervention studies, *Immun Ageing* 13:13, 2016.

17. Nitter M, et al: Plasma methionine, choline, betaine, and dimethylglycine, in relation to colorectal cancer risk in the European Prospective Investigation into Cancer and Nutrition (EPIC), *Ann Oncol* 25(8):1609-1615, 2014.

18. Kim YS, et al: Cancer stem cells: potential target for bioactive food components, *J Nutr Biochem* 23:691-698, 2012.

19. World Cancer Research Fund/American Institute for Cancer Research (WCRF/AICR): Second expert report: food, nutrition, physical activity, and the prevention of cancer: a global perspective, London, 2007, Author.

20. Arab L, et al: Lycopene and the lung, *Exp Biol Med (Maywood)* 227:894-899, 2002.

21. Hales CM, et al: Prevalence of obesity among adults and youth: United States, 2015-2016, *NCHS Data Brief* 288:1-8, 2017.

22. World Health Organization (WHO): Obesity and overweight, Geneva, 2018, Author.

23. American Cancer Society (ACS): *Alcohol and cancer*, Atlanta, GA, 2016, Author.

24. World Cancer Research Fund/American Institute for Cancer Research (SCRF/AICR): *Recommendations for cancer prevention*, Washington DC, 2016, American Institute for Cancer Research.

25. Mao N, et al: Association between alcohol dehydrogenase-2 gene polymorphism and esophageal cancer risk: a meta-analysis, *World J Surg Oncol* 14(1):191, 2016.

26. Lee IM, et al: Annual deaths attributable to physical inactivity: whither the missing 2 million? *Lancet* 381(9871):992-993, 2013.

27. World Health Organization (WHO): *Noncommunicable diseases*, Geneva, 2016, WHO Media Center.

28. U.S. Department of Health and Human Services (USDHHS): 2008 physical activity guidelines for Americans summary last updated 5/28/18, Washington, DC, 2018, Office of Disease Prevention and Health Promotion, Office of the Assistant Secretary for Health, Office of the Secretary, U.S. Department of Health and Human Services.

29. Cramp F, Byron-Daniel J: Exercise for the management of cancer-related fatigue in adults, *Cochrane Database Syst Rev* (11):CD006145, 2012.

30. Braam KI, et al: Physical exercise training interventions for children and young adults during and after treatment for childhood cancer, *Cochrane Database Syst Rev* (4):CD008796, 2013.

31. Cohen AJ, et al: Estimates and 25-year trends of the global burden of disease attributable to ambient air pollution: an analysis of data from the Global Burden of Diseases Study 2015, *Lancet* 389(10082):1907-1918, 2017.

32. Health Effects Institute: *State of global air 2018. Special report*, Boston, MA, 2018, Author.

33. GBD 2016 Risk Factors Collaborators: Global, regional, and national comparative risk assessment of 84 behavioural, environmental and occupational, and metabolic risks or clusters of risks, 1990-2016: a systematic analysis for the Global Burden of Disease Study 2016, *Lancet* 390(10100):1345-1422, 2017. Available at: https://www.ncbi.nlm.nih.gov/pubmed/28919119.

34. International Agency for Research on Cancer (IARC): Outdoor air pollution, *IARC Monogr Eval Carcinog Risks Hum* 109:2013. Lyon, France.

35. Loomis D, et al: The carcinogenicity of outdoor air pollution, *Lancet Oncol* 14:1262-1263, 2013.

36. Vineis P, et al: Outdoor air pollution and lung cancer: recent epidemiologic evidence, *Int J Cancer* 111(1):647-652, 2004.

37. Pruitt RC, et al: Chronic fine and course particulate exposure, mortality, and coronary heart disease in the Nurses' Health Study, *Environ Health Perspect* 117(11):1697-1701, 2009.

38. Environmental Protection Agency (EPA): *Particulate matter*, updated March 18, 2013, Washington, DC, 2013, Author.

39. Hernandez L, et al: Aging and radiation: bad companions, *Aging Cell* 14(2):153-161, 2015.

40. Shuryak I, et al: Cancer risks after radiation exposure in middle age, *J Natl Cancer Inst* 102(21):1606-1609, 2010.

41. Richardson DB, Wing S: Greater sensitivity to ionizing radiation at older age: follow-up of workers at Oak Ridge National Laboratory through 1990, *Int J Epidemiol* 28:428-436, 1999.

42. Fazel R, et al: Exposure to low-dose ionizing radiation from medical imaging procedures, *N Engl J Med* 361:849-857, 2009.

43. Preston DL, et al: Studies of mortality of atomic bomb survivors. Report 13: solid cancer and noncancer disease mortality: 1950–1997, *Radiat Res* 160:381-407, 2003.

44. Hoel DG: Ionizing radiation and cardiovascular disease, *Ann N Y Acad Sci* 1076:309-317, 2006.

45. Rombouts C, et al: Differential response to acute low dose radiation in primary and immortalized endothelial cells, *Int J Radiat Biol* 89(10):841-850, 2013.

46. Yusuf SW, et al: Radiation-induced heart disease: a clinical update, *Cardiol Res Pract* 2011:317659, 2011.

47. Mathias D, et al: Low-dose irradiation affects expression of inflammatory markers in the heart of ApoE mice, *PLoS ONE* 10(3):e0119661, 2015.

48. Centers for Disease Control and Prevention (CDC): *Radiation and pregnancy: a fact sheet for clinicians*, Atlanta GA, 2014, Centers for Disease Control and Prevention, National Center for Environmental Health (NCEH)/Agency for Toxic Substances and Disease Registry (ATSDR), National Center for Injury Prevention and Control (NCIPC).

49. Prasad KN, et al: Health risks of low dose ionizing radiation in humans: a review, *Exp Biol Med* 229(5):378-382, 2004.

50. National Council on Radiation Protection and Measurement (NCRP): 1929–2009 medical radiation exposure of the U.S. population greatly increased since the early 1980s, March 2009. Available at http://NCRPonline%2Corg.

51. Brenner DJ, Hall EJ: Computed tomography—an increasing source of radiation exposure, *N Engl J Med* 357(22):2277-2284, 2007.

52. Smith-Bendman R, et al: Use of diagnostic imaging studies and associated radiation exposure for patients enrolled in large integrated health care system, 1996-2010, *J Am Med Assoc* 307(22):2400-2409, 2012.

53. Little JB: Cellular radiation effects and the bystander response, *Mutat Res* 597:113-118, 2006.

54. Jones JA, et al: Ionizing radiation as a carcinogen. In McQueen CA, editor: *Comprehensive toxicology*, ed 2, St Louis, 2010, Elsevier.

55. Koturbash I, et al: In vivo bystander effects: cranial x-irradiation leads to elevated DNA damage, altered cellular proliferation and apoptosis, and increased p53 levels in shielded spleen, *Int J Radiat Oncol Biol Phys* 70(2):554-562, 2008.

56. Mancuso M, et al: Oncogenic bystander radiation effects in *Patched* heterozygous mouse cerebellum, *Proc Natl Acad Sci* 105(34):12445-12450, 2008.

57. Bertucci A, et al: Microbeam irradiation of the *C. elegans* nematode, *J Radiat Res* 50:A49-A54, 2009.

58. Rajagopal C, Harikumar KB: The origins and functions of exosomes in cancer, *Front Oncol* 8:66, 2018.

59. Parkin DM, Darby SC: Cancers in 2010 attributable to ionising radiation exposure in the UK, *BJ Cancer* 105:S57-S65, 2011.

60. Barrington de Gonzalez A, et al: Proportion of second cancers attributable to radiotherapy treatment in adults: a prospective cohort study in the US SEER cancer registries, *Lancet Oncol* 12(4):353-360, 2011.

61. Centers for Disease Control and Treatment (CDC): *Radiation and your health*, Atlanta, GA, 2014, Author. Available at www.cdc.gov/nceh/radiation/. Accessed August 17, 2014.

62. American Cancer Society (ACS): *Cancer facts & figures 2018*, Atlanta, GA, 2018, Author.

63. U.S. Preventive Services Task Force (USPSTF): Screening for skin cancer: US Preventive Services Task Force recommendation statement, *J Am Med Assoc* 316(4):429-435, 2016.

64. National Institute of Environmental Health Sciences: High exposure to radiofrequency radiation linked to tumor activity in male rats, News Release, February 2, 2018.

65. National Cancer Institute (NCI): Pap and HPV testing, National Cancer Institute, National Institutes of Health updated 09/09/2014. Available at www.cancer.gov/cancertopics/factsheet/detection/Pap-HPV-testing. Accessed September 16, 2014.

66. Smith EM, et al: Evidence for vertical transmission of HPV from mothers to infants, *Infect Dis Obstet Gynecol* 2010:326369, 2010. Available at: http://dx.doi.org/10.1155/2010/326369.

67. Agency for Toxic Substances and Disease Registry (ATSDR): *Chemicals, cancer, and you*, Atlanta, GA, Agency for Toxic Substances and Disease Registry, Division of Health Assessment and Consultation, U.S. Department of Health and Human Services. Available at www.atsdr.cdc.gov/.../Chemicals,%20Cancer,%20 and%20You%20FS.pdf. Accessed September 18, 2014.

68. Gray J: *State of the evidence 2008: the connection between breast cancer and the environment*, San Francisco, 2008, Breast Cancer Fund.

69. National Institute for Occupational Safety and Health (NIOSH): *Hazard evaluations, and field studies*, Atlanta, GA, 2015, Occupational Cancer National Institute for Occupational Safety and Health Division of Surveillance, CDC.

70. Singh Z, Chadha P: Textile industry and occupational cancer, *J Occu Med Toxicol* 11:39, 2016.

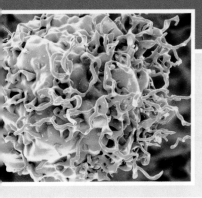

13

Cancer in Children and Adolescents

Lauri A. Linder

CHAPTER OUTLINE

Although cancer in children and adolescents is rare, it is the leading cause of death resulting from disease for this age group.[1] Survival rates among children and adolescents with cancer have dramatically improved since the 1960s. Today, over 80% of children and adolescents diagnosed with cancer will become long-term survivors of their disease. Factors leading to improved cure rates include combination chemotherapy, multimodal treatment for children with solid tumors, and multisite clinical trials.

INCIDENCE, ETIOLOGY, AND TYPES OF CHILDHOOD CANCER

Approximately 15,590 children and adolescents 19 years of age and younger were estimated to have cancer in the United States in 2018.[2] The overall incidence of childhood and adolescent cancer is 18.2 per 100,000 (Fig. 13.1).[3] Childhood cancer demonstrates a bimodal distribution, with peaks among children < 5 years of age and adolescents 15 to 19 years of age. In the United States, childhood cancer is also slightly more common in boys than in girls. The male/female ratio for childhood cancers is 1.2 : 1.0.[3]

In 2015, the cancer-related death rates among children and adolescents, from birth to age 19 years, were 2.5 per 100,000 for males and 2.1 per 100,000 for females.[3] By comparison, the cancer-related mortality rate in adults was 158.5 per 100,000 in 2015.[4]

Childhood cancers differ from those in adults. The most common types of cancer among adults include prostate, breast, lung, and colon cancers. In contrast, children are more likely to develop leukemias, brain tumors, and sarcomas. Although many adult cancers have associated lifestyle factors that could theoretically be avoided, such as smoking and exposure to the sun, very few environmental factors have been linked to cancer in children. More data are emerging to indicate that the developing child may be affected by epigenetic modifications resulting from parental exposures before conception, exposures in utero, and nutrition during early life.[5,6]

Most childhood cancers originate from the mesodermal germ layer. This layer develops into connective tissue, bone, cartilage, muscle, blood, blood vessels, gonads, kidney, and the lymphatic system (Fig. 13.2). As a result, the most common childhood cancers include leukemias, sarcomas, and embryonic tumors.

Childhood cancers are often diagnosed during peak times of physical growth and maturation. This accounts for the bimodal distribution in their incidence, with peak incidences among children age < 6 years and then again during adolescence. In general, childhood cancers are fast growing, resulting in a relatively short latency period—that is, the time from the initial exposure to the onset of symptoms. Cancer also is more common in white children relative to other racial groups (Table 13.1).

The distribution of cancer types changes during childhood and adolescence. Leukemia is the most frequent type of childhood cancer. Its peak incidence is among children 2 to 5 years of age. Tumors involving the brain and the central nervous system (CNS) are the second leading type of childhood cancer. The peak incidence of these tumors is among children age < 15 years; however, the incidence of specific subtypes of brain and CNS tumors varies across childhood and adolescence.

Lymphomas, both Hodgkin and non-Hodgkin types, are the third most common type of childhood cancer. Lymphoma is rare in children age < 5 years. It occurs most frequently in children and adolescents 10 years of age and older.

Embryonal tumors begin during intrauterine life. These tumors contain abnormal cells that appear to be immature embryonic tissue; they are unable to mature or differentiate into fully developed cells. Embryonal tumors are most often diagnosed early in life, usually before the child is 5 years of age. They are rare in older children, adolescents, and adults. The names of these tumors often include the root term *blast* (e.g., neuroblastoma, retinoblastoma), which indicates the embryonal stage of development.

Rhabdomyosarcoma is the most common soft tissue sarcoma of childhood. This tumor has a bimodal age distribution. Two-thirds of cases occur in children age < 6 years, and one-third occur in children

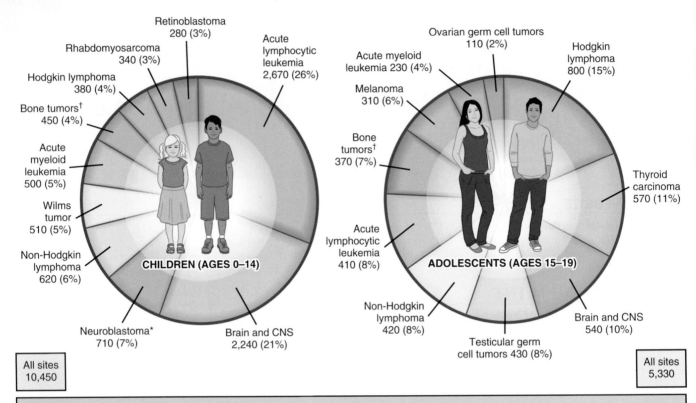

FIGURE 13.1 Estimated Cases for Childhood and Adolescent Cancers, United States, 2014. (Data from American Cancer Society, Atlanta, GA, 2014.)

TABLE 13.1   Childhood Age-Adjusted Cancer Incidence Rates for Children Younger Than 19 Years of Age by Primary Site, Race, and Ethnicity, United States*

Cancer Site	Non-Hispanic White	Non-Hispanic Black	Asian/Pacific Islander	Hispanic
All cancer sites combined	20.8	14.7	14.8	18.6
Brain and other nervous systems	5.9	3.7	3.4	4.5
Leukemia	5.5	3.8	4.3	6.5
Lymphoma	3.1	2.4	2.1	2.7
Other	6.5	4.1	4.3	5.3

*Rates are per 100,000 persons and are age-adjusted to the 2000 U.S. standard population (19 age groups—Census P25-1130).
Data modified from Ward E et al: *CA Cancer J Clin, 64*:83–103, 2014.

and adolescents 10 years of age and older. The two most common types of bone tumors are osteosarcoma and Ewing's sarcoma. These cancers are more likely to occur in adolescents age ≥ 15 years (Table 13.2).

Although sarcomas, leukemias, and lymphomas are cancers observed in childhood, they also occur in adults. Most adult cancers develop from epithelial tissue and are therefore carcinomas. Because carcinomas most often result from environmental exposures to carcinogens, they rarely occur in children. A long period (up to decades) of exposure is required until the development of carcinoma. The incidence of carcinomas increases between ages 15 and 19 years. Carcinoma is the most common cancer tissue type observed after adolescence.[3]

Etiology

The causes of cancer in children are largely unknown. A few environmental factors can predispose a child to cancer; however, there are no established causal factors for most childhood cancers. A number of host factors, many of which are genetic risk factors or congenital conditions, have been implicated in the development of childhood cancer (Table 13.3).

Most children who are diagnosed with cancer do not have known predisposing environmental or host factors. Because of their relatively short latency period, most childhood cancers do not lend themselves to early cancer warning signs. The American Cancer Society's seven

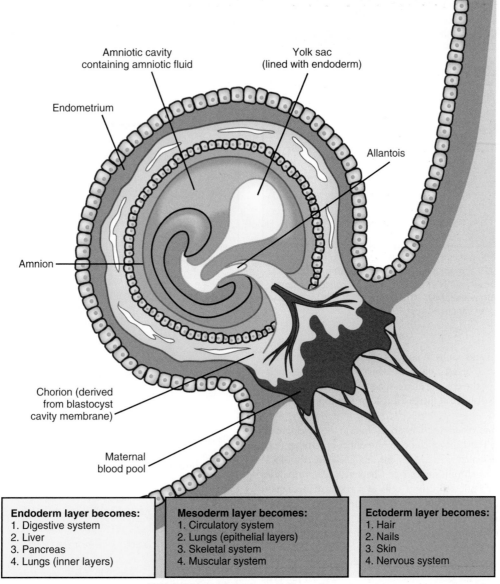

Amniotic cavity
containing amniotic fluid

Yolk sac
(lined with endoderm)

Endometrium

Allantois

Amnion

Chorion (derived
from blastocyst
cavity membrane)

Maternal
blood pool

Endoderm layer becomes:	Mesoderm layer becomes:	Ectoderm layer becomes:
1. Digestive system	1. Circulatory system	1. Hair
2. Liver	2. Lungs (epithelial layers)	2. Nails
3. Pancreas	3. Skeletal system	3. Skin
4. Lungs (inner layers)	4. Muscular system	4. Nervous system

FIGURE 13.2 Mesodermal Germ Layer.

warning signs are less relevant for children. These warning signs describe manifestations of environmentally caused carcinomas that are much more common among adults. Efforts to establish early population-based screening strategies for childhood cancers have not been effective. Children with a family history of cancer and who are known to have mutations associated with cancer, such as those involving the *TP53* gene, however, will receive additional screening.[7]

A multiple causation model is important for interpreting the results of epidemiologic studies. For example, laboratory and epidemiologic studies may indicate that exposure to a certain chemical or to ionizing radiation can cause leukemia, but not all children who are exposed will develop leukemia. More studies are needed to determine other host and environmental factors that interact with these exposures to cause the disease.

Genetic and Genomic Factors

Acquired or inherited mutations in individual genes may contribute to the development of cancer in children and adolescents. Mutations in > 150 oncogenes and tumor-suppressor genes have been associated

with the subsequent development of both childhood and adult cancers (Table 13.4). In general, children who develop cancer have a greater frequency of germline cancer predisposition genes compared with children who do not develop cancer.[8] Genes associated with childhood cancers also tend to differ from those associated with adult cancers.[9]

Fanconi anemia and Bloom syndrome are two autosomal recessive conditions that result in impaired deoxyribonucleic acid (DNA) repair and are risk factors for the development of acute leukemia. Retinoblastoma, a malignant embryonic tumor of the eye, occurs either as an inherited defect in the *RB1* gene or as an acquired mutation (see Chapter 18).

Leukemia is not an inherited genetic condition; however, siblings of children with leukemia have a two to four times increased risk for the development of leukemia compared with siblings of healthy children. The occurrence of leukemia in monozygous twins is estimated to be as high as 25%.

Li-Fraumeni syndrome (LFS) is an autosomal dominant disorder involving the *TP53* tumor-suppressor gene. Individuals with a mutation in the *TP53* gene have a significantly increased risk of cancer developing in childhood or adulthood compared with the general

TABLE 13.2 Childhood Age-Adjusted Invasive Cancer Incidence Rates by Primary Site and Age, United States*

Site	Birth to 14 Years	Birth to 19 Years
All sites	16.9	19.2
Leukemia (all types)	4.7	4.3
Acute lymphocytic leukemia	3.5	3.1
Brain and other nervous system	3.8	3.5
Soft tissue	1.1	1.1
Kidney and renal	0.9	0.8
Bones and joints	0.8	1.1
Non-Hodgkin lymphoma	1.1	1.4
Hodgkin lymphoma	0.6	1.4

*Rates are per 100,000 persons and are age-adjusted to the 2000 U.S. standard population (19 age groups—Census P25-1130).
Data modified from Howlader N et al: editors: *SEER cancer statistics review, 1975-2015*, Bethesda, MD, 2018, National Cancer Institute. Available at: https://seer.cancer.gov/csr/1975_2015.

TABLE 13.3 Congenital Factors Associated With Childhood Cancer

Syndrome	Associated Childhood Cancer
Chromosome Alterations	
Down syndrome	Acute leukemia
13q syndrome	Retinoblastoma
Chromosome Instability	
Ataxia-telangiectasia	Lymphoma
Bloom syndrome	Acute leukemia, lymphoma, Wilms tumor
Fanconi anemia	Acute myelogenous leukemia, myelodysplastic syndrome, hepatic tumors
Hereditary Syndromes	
Beckwith-Wiedemann syndrome	Wilms tumor, sarcoma, brain tumors, neuroblastoma, hepatoblastoma
Neurofibromatosis type I	Brain tumor, sarcomas, neuroblastomas, Wilms tumor, nonlymphocytic leukemia
Neurofibromatosis type II	Meningioma (malignant or benign), acoustic neuroma/schwannoma, gliomas, ependymomas
Tuberous sclerosis	Glial tumors
Li-Fraumeni syndrome	Sarcoma, adrenocortical carcinoma
Von Hippel-Lindau disease	Cerebellar hemangioblastoma, retinal angioma, renal cell carcinoma, pheochromocytomas
Ataxia-telangiectasia	Leukemia, lymphoma, brain tumors
Gorlin syndrome	Medulloblastoma, skin tumors
Immunodeficiency Disorders	
Congenital	
Agammaglobulinemia	Lymphoma, leukemia, brain tumors
Immunoglobulin A (IgA) deficiency	Lymphoma, leukemia, brain tumors
Wiskott-Aldrich syndrome	Leukemia, lymphoma
Acquired	
Aplastic anemia	Leukemia
Human immunodeficiency virus/Acquired immunodeficiency syndrome (HIV/AIDS)	Non-Hodgkin lymphoma, leiomyosarcoma
Organ transplantation	Leukemia, lymphoma
Congenital Malformation Syndromes	
Aniridia, hemihypertrophy, hamartoma, genitourinary anomalies	Wilms tumor
Cryptorchidism	Testicular tumor
Gonadal dysgenesis	Gonadoblastoma
Family Susceptibility	
Twin or sibling with leukemia	Leukemia

population. Children and adults in families affected by LFS are at risk for soft tissue sarcoma, breast cancer, leukemia, osteosarcoma, melanoma, and cancers of the colon, pancreas, adrenal cortex, and brain. Individuals with LFS also are at increased risk for developing multiple primary cancers.

Chromosomal abnormalities also may contribute to the development of childhood cancer. These may include abnormalities in number (e.g., aneuploidy) or in the structure (e.g., deletions, amplifications, translocations, and fragility) of chromosomes (see Chapter 2). Abnormalities may occur within the affected cancer cells as a result of malignant transformation. They also may be present as the consequence of a congenital syndrome.

A chromosomal translocation results from the rearrangement of two nonhomologous chromosomes. Translocations may result in the creation of a fusion gene, in which the two previously separate gene regions unite. Two fusion genes associated with acute lymphocytic leukemia (ALL) in children are the *BCR-ABL* gene, resulting from a translocation between chromosomes 9 and 22; and the *TEL-AML1* gene, resulting from a translocation between chromosomes 12 and 21.

Several syndromes associated with specific congenital malformations are associated with a higher incidence of cancer development. One of the more recognized syndromes is trisomy 21 (Down syndrome). Children with Down syndrome have a 10 to 20 times greater risk of developing leukemia compared with unaffected children. The age distribution for developing ALL among children with Down syndrome is similar to that of children without Down syndrome.

Wilms tumor, a malignant tumor of the kidney, is associated with a number of congenital anomalies, including genitourinary anomalies, aniridia (congenital absence of the iris), hemihypertrophy (muscular overgrowth of half of the body or face), and intellectual disabilities. Identifiable malformations and congenital predisposition syndromes are present in approximately 17% of children diagnosed with Wilms tumor.[10] These children with known predisposition syndromes are likely to receive additional early cancer screening.

Children with some congenital anomalies not associated with a known chromosomal syndrome also have an increased risk of developing childhood cancer. Children with ventricular septal defects have a 10 times greater risk of developing hepatoblastoma compared with healthy

TABLE 13.4   Selected Oncogenes and Tumor-Suppressor Genes Associated With Childhood Cancer

Gene	Associated Pediatric Tumor
Oncogenes	
ABL	Acute lymphoblastic leukemia
MYCN	Neuroblastoma
MYB	Neural tumors, leukemia, lymphoma, rhabdomyosarcoma, Wilms tumor, neuroblastoma
EGFR/erbB	Glioblastomas
NRAS	Neuroblastoma, leukemia, rhabdomyosarcoma
KRAS	Leukemia
ATM	Lymphoma, leukemia
Tumor-Suppressor Genes	
RB1	Retinoblastoma, sarcoma
WT1, WT2	Wilms tumor, leukemia
NF-1	Sarcoma, primitive neuroectodermal tumor, juvenile chronic myelocytic leukemia
NF-2	Brain tumors, melanoma, meningiomas
TP53	Sarcoma, leukemia, brain tumors, lymphoma
DCC	Ewing sarcoma, rhabdomyosarcoma, neuroblastoma
CDKN2A	Melanoma, acute lymphoblastic leukemia, Ewing sarcoma
CDC2L1	Non-Hodgkin lymphoma, neuroblastoma

Data from Beamer LC et al: *Nurs Clin North Am* 48(4):585–626, 2013; OMIM® Online Mendelian Inheritance in Man® An online catalog of human genes and genetic disorders. Available at: www.http://omim.org. Accessed June 24, 2018.

BOX 13.1   Factors That May Contribute to the Development of Childhood and Adolescent Cancers

- Genetic, genomic, and epigenetic factors
- Diet
- Immune function
- Occupational exposure
- Ionizing radiation
- Hormonal variations
- Viral illnesses
- Individual characteristics, such as the biologic, social, and physical environments

children, and children with CNS birth defects have a 10 to 20 times increased risk of developing some types of brain tumors.[11]

Environmental Factors

Finding the cause of any disease is typically a long, slow process that occurs over many years. No single factor determines whether cancer will develop in an individual, even if a specific environmental exposure explains a high proportion of the occurrence of a specific cancer (Box 13.1).

Prenatal Exposure

Prenatal exposure to some drugs and to ionizing radiation has been linked to childhood cancers. The most well-described drug is

TABLE 13.5   Drugs That May Increase Risk of Childhood Cancer

Drug Class	Uses	Cancer Risk
Anabolic androgenic steroids	Stimulate bone growth and appetite; induce puberty; increase muscle mass and physical strength	Hepatocellular carcinoma, Brain tumors
Epipodophyllotoxin and anthracycline chemotherapy agents	Cancer treatment	Leukemia
Immunosuppressive agents	Prevent organ rejection following transplantation surgery	Lymphoma

diethylstilbestrol (DES), which was prescribed by physicians to prevent recurrent spontaneous abortion. In 1971, DES was identified as a transplacental chemical carcinogen because adenocarcinomas of the vagina occurred in a small percentage of the daughters of women who took DES. No other studies have identified other drugs taken by pregnant women that may cause cancer in their children.

Current evidence suggests that an increased risk of childhood leukemia is associated with low levels of exposure to antenatal x-rays.[12,13] An association between antenatal x-ray exposure and childhood brain tumors has not been identified. Other current areas of research include exploring epigenetic modifications resulting from prenatal exposures and their role in future cancer development.

Childhood Exposure

Childhood exposures to ionizing radiation, drugs, electromagnetic fields, or viruses have been associated with the risk of cancer. Retrospective research has shown a significant correlation between radiation-induced malignancies and either radiotherapy (cancer treatment) or radiation exposure from diagnostic imaging[14] (see *Did You Know?* Radiation Risks and Pediatric Computed Tomography [CT]: Data from the National Cancer Institute). In contrast, some exposures may be protective against childhood cancer. Current research suggests that early exposure to common infections may help "prime" the immune system, thereby protecting the child against acute lymphoblastic leukemia.[15] Drug and environmental agents that are known to cause cancer in adults also are risks for exposure during childhood. A few drugs may increase cancer risk during childhood (Table 13.5).

The relationship between childhood cancer and other environmental factors (e.g., electromagnetic fields, small appliances, radon) has been the focus of many epidemiologic studies. To date, exposures to high-dose and high-dose rate ionizing radiation have been established as risk factors for childhood leukemia.[16] Multiple other possible environmental risk factors for childhood cancer have been explored. Results of these studies have been mixed, and no definitive causal pathway for childhood cancer has been determined (see *Did You Know?* Magnetic Fields and Development of Pediatric Cancer).

The strongest association between viruses and the development of cancer in children has been seen in cases of the Epstein-Barr virus (EBV) infection, which is linked to Burkitt lymphoma, nasopharyngeal carcinoma, and Hodgkin disease. Children with acquired immunodeficiency syndrome (AIDS) have an increased risk of developing non-Hodgkin lymphoma and Kaposi sarcoma. The use of highly active antiretroviral therapy (HAART) in the developed world has dramatically reduced the incidence of AIDS-related malignancies.

DID YOU KNOW?

Radiation Risks and Pediatric Computed Tomography (CT): Data From the National Cancer Institute

Computed tomography (CT) is the largest contributor to medical radiation exposure in the U.S. population. CT exposures represent only about 12% of diagnostic radiologic procedures in large hospitals; however it accounts for almost 49% of the U.S. population's collective radiation dose from all medical x-ray examinations. Concern about the risk of cancer in children associated with radiation exposure from CT is increasing. Epidemiologic studies have shown that children are more sensitive to radiation compared with adults. They also have a longer life expectancy compared with adults, and this increases the window of opportunity to express radiation damage. Children also may receive a higher radiation dose than necessary if the CT setting is not adjusted for their smaller size. The absolute cancer risks associated with CT, however, are very small. Lifetime risks of cancer because of CT exposures have been estimated by using projection models based on atomic bomb survivors. These risks are about 1 case of cancer for every 1000 people scanned, with a maximal incidence of about 1 case of cancer for every 500 people. The benefits of properly performed and clinically justified CT examinations should always outweigh the risks for an individual child. Minimizing radiation exposure from pediatric CT, whenever possible, will reduce the projected number of CT-related cancers.

Data from National Cancer Institute, National Institutes of Health: *NCI radiation risks and pediatric computed tomography (CT): a guide for health care workers,* Bethesda, MD, 2012, National Cancer Institute. Available at: https://www.cancer.gov/about-cancer/causes-prevention/risk/radiation/pediatric-ct-scans. Accessed June 20, 2018.

DID YOU KNOW?

Magnetic Fields and Development of Pediatric Cancer

Several recent reports have suggested an association between environmental sources and the development of cancer in children. The presence of low-frequency magnetic fields has been a concern for many years as a cause of childhood leukemia. The World Health Organization (WHO) identified a better understanding of health risks, including cancer, and exposure to low-frequency magnetic fields as a research priority in 2007. A recent meta-analysis evaluated nine case-control studies, representing eight different countries, conducted between 1997 and 2013 and involving 11,699 cases of children with leukemia and 13,194 controls. This meta-analysis identified an increased risk of childhood leukemia associated with high levels of magnetic field exposure ($\geq 0.4\ \mu T$). For additional perspective, < 1% of the children in these studies experienced this level of exposure. The WHO has estimated that only about 1% to 4% of children worldwide live in conditions that exceed $0.4\ \mu T$. Ongoing research is needed because environmental factors may require many years of exposure to cause disease. Additionally, an association between an environmental factor and childhood cancer does not establish causality. Research is needed to better understand the relationships between environmental factors and other factors associated with childhood cancers. Research also is needed to identify potential mechanisms by which environmental factors may contribute to the development of childhood cancer.

Data from: National Cancer Institute: *Electromagnetic fields and cancer.* Available at: https://www.cancer.gov/about-cancer/causes-prevention/risk/radiation/electromagnetic-fields-fact-sheet. Accessed June 24, 2018; World Health Organization: *Fact sheet: electromagnetic fields and public health: exposure to extremely low frequency fields.* Available at: www.who.int/peh-emf/publications/facts/fs322/en/. Accessed June 24, 2018; Zhao L et al: *Leuk Res* 38(3):269–274, 2014.

✔ **QUICK CHECK 13.1**

1. What are the main types of childhood cancer?
2. What are the overall incidences of childhood and adolescent cancers?
3. How does the etiology of childhood cancer differ from that of adult cancer?

PROGNOSIS

Greater than 80% of children diagnosed with cancer are cured. Factors leading to these improved cure rates include the use of combination chemotherapy, multimodal treatment, advances in biotherapy, and improvements in nursing and supportive care. Research centers for comprehensive childhood cancer treatment and cooperative study groups also have facilitated refinements in treatment protocols and data sharing, leading to improved survival rates.

Survival rates for children younger than 15 years of age have increased at a rate of 1.5% per year, which is similar to increases in survival rates for adults older than 50 years of age. Adolescents and young adults ages 15 and 24 years, however, have experienced increases in survival of < 0.5% per year.[3] A partial explanation for the relative lack of progress in similar cure rates among the adolescent population as in the younger pediatric population is the lack of participation in clinical trials. Between 1997 and 2005, the percentage of 15- to 19-year-olds with cancer participating in clinical trials was estimated at 10% to 15%. This value is approximately one-fourth the clinical trial rate of participation by children younger than 15 years of age. Several factors are likely to contribute to this lower participation. If adolescents are treated in adult

cancer centers, a clinical trial may not be available. Some clinical trials that are available to adults may not be open to adolescents younger than 18 years of age even if their disease biology is similar to that of adult disease,[17] and fewer trials are available for young adolescents. The National Cancer Institute (NCI) and pediatric and adult cooperative groups sponsored by the NCI have launched a national initiative to increase the numbers of adolescents and young adults participating in clinical trials.

Childhood cancer survivors have a greater risk of developing a second cancer later in life. This risk may be associated with a variety of factors, including specific types of chemotherapy, as well as radiation to certain areas of the body. Genetic factors and the type of the primary cancer also influence the risk of a second cancer. For example, children with a history of familial retinoblastoma are at increased risk of osteosarcoma developing later in life.

Because childhood cancer should be viewed as a chronic disease instead of a fatal illness, treatment includes attention to quality of life and symptom management. Even children whose cancers cannot be cured can experience improved quality of life with palliative care. Children and adolescents whose cancers are regarded as cured still face residual and late effects of their treatment. These late effects are more significant in children than in adults because children receive their treatment at a time when they are still physically immature and growing. Many late effects of cancer treatment need further study. These include physical impairments, reproductive dysfunction, soft tissue and bone atrophy, learning disabilities, secondary cancers, and psychological sequelae.

More must be learned about the genetic and genomic factors associated with childhood malignancies and about the genetic and genomic consequences of treatment. A referral to genetic services is appropriate for families of children whose cancer is known to be transmitted genetically (e.g., retinoblastoma, LFS).

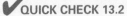

> **QUICK CHECK 13.2**
> 1. What are the most common childhood cancers, and how do they differ from adult cancers?
> 2. Why are carcinomas less likely to develop in children?
> 3. Compare the different etiologic factors associated with childhood cancers.

SUMMARY REVIEW

Incidence and Types of Childhood Cancers
1. Childhood cancer is a rare disease, but it remains the second leading cause of death in children.
2. Leukemia is the most common type of childhood cancer. Tumors involving the brain or central nervous system are the second most common type of childhood cancer.

Etiology
1. Most carcinomas are caused by cumulative exposure to carcinogens in the environment. Because children have not lived long enough for the consequence of these exposures to manifest, carcinomas are extremely rare in children.
2. Children with immunodeficiencies are at an increased risk of cancer because of an ineffective immune system.
3. Children with Down syndrome have an increased risk for the development of leukemia.
4. Risk factors that may be associated with the development of childhood cancer include inherited and acquired genetic and genomic changes, nutrition and diet, immune function, occupational exposure, hormonal variations, and viral illnesses, as well as other individual characteristics, such as biologic, social, or physical environments.

Prognosis
1. Childhood cancer survivors have a greater risk of developing a second cancer during their lifetime compared with the general population.
2. Reasons for improved survival among children and adolescents with cancer include research aimed at identifying less toxic treatments with fewer long-term side effects.

KEY TERMS

Embryonal tumor, 291
Li-Fraumeni syndrome (LFS), 293

Mesodermal germ layer, 291

Multiple causation model, 293

Wilms tumor, 294

REFERENCES

1. Heron M: Deaths: leading causes for 2015, *Natl Vital Stat Rep* 66(5):1-96, 2017. Available at: https://www.cdc.gov/nchs/data/nvsr/nvsr66/nvsr66_05.pdf. (Accessed 15 April 2018).
2. Siegel RL, Miller KD, Jemal A: Cancer statistics, 2018, *CA Cancer J Clin* 68(1):7-30, 2018.
3. Noone AM, et al, editors: *SEER cancer statistics review, 1975-2015*, Bethesda, MD, 2018, National Cancer Institute. Available at: http://seer.cancer.gov/csr/1975_2015/.
4. Murphy SL, et al: Deaths: final data for 2015, *Natl Vital Stat Rep* 66(6):7-75, 2017. Available at: https://www.cdc.gov/nchs/data/nvsr/nvsr66/nvsr66_06.pdf. (Accessed 20 April 2018).
5. Ghantous A, et al: Characterizing the epigenome as a key component of the fetal exposome in evaluating in utero exposures and childhood cancer risk, *Mutagenesis* 30:733-742, 2015.
6. Timms JA, et al: DNA methylation as a potent mediator of environmental risks in the development of childhood acute lymphoblastic leukemia, *Epigenomics* 8(4):519-536, 2016.
7. Kratz CP, et al: Cancer screening recommendations for individuals with Li-Fraumeni syndrome, *Clin Cancer Res* 23(11):e38-e45, 2017.
8. Zhang J, et al: Germline mutations in predisposition genes in pediatric cancer, *N Engl J Med* 373(24):2336-2346, 2015.
9. Ma X, et al: Pan-cancer genome and transcriptome analyses of 1,699 paediatric leukemias and solid tumors, *Nature* 555(7696):371-376, 2018.
10. Dumoucel S, et al: Malformations, genetic abnormalities, and Wilms tumor, *Pediatr Blood Cancer* 61(1):140-144, 2014.
11. Schraw JM, et al: Abstract LB-161, presented at the American Association for Cancer Research Annual Meeting, April 14-18, 2018, Chicago, IL.
12. Rajaraman P, et al: Early life exposure to diagnostic radiation and ultrasound scans and risk of childhood cancer: case-control study, *BMJ* 342:d472, 2011.
13. Wakeford R: The risk of childhood leukaemia following exposure to ionising radiation, *J Radiol Prot* 33(1):1-25, 2013.
14. Miglioretti DL, et al: Pediatric computed tomography and associated radiation exposure and estimated cancer risk, *JAMA Pediatr* 167(8):700-707, 2013.
15. Greaves M: A causal mechanism for acute lymphoblastic leukemia, *Nat Rev Cancer* 18(8):471-484, 2018.
16. Hsu WL, et al: The incidence of leukemia, lymphoma, and multiple myeloma among atomic bomb survivors: 1950-2001, *Radiat Res* 179(3):361-382, 2013.
17. Davis LE, et al: Clinical trial enrollment of adolescents and young adults with cancer, *Cancer* 123(18):3434-3440, 2017.

14

Structure and Function of the Neurologic System

Sue E. Huether

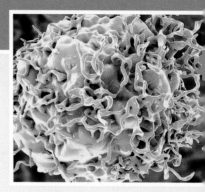

EVOLVE WEBSITE

CHAPTER OUTLINE

The human nervous system is a remarkable structure responsible for decision making, for the body's ability to interact with the environment, and for the regulation and control of activities involving our internal organs. It is a network composed of complex structures that transmit electrical and chemical signals between the brain and the body's many organs and tissues. This chapter provides a basic overview of the structure and function of the nervous system and supports the understanding of nervous system pathophysiology in the following chapters.

OVERVIEW AND ORGANIZATION OF THE NERVOUS SYSTEM

Although the nervous system functions as a unified whole, structures and functions have been divided here to facilitate understanding. Structurally, the nervous system is divided into the central nervous system and the peripheral nervous system. The central nervous system (CNS) consists of the brain and spinal cord, enclosed within the protective cranial vault and vertebrae, respectively. The peripheral nervous system (PNS) is composed of the cranial nerves and the spinal nerves and their ganglia. Peripheral nerve pathways are differentiated into afferent pathways (ascending pathways), which carry sensory impulses toward the CNS, and efferent pathways (descending pathways), which innervate skeletal muscle or effector organs by transmitting motor impulses away from the CNS (Fig. 14.1).

Functionally, the PNS can be divided into the somatic nervous system and the autonomic nervous system. The somatic nervous system consists of pathways that regulate voluntary motor control (e.g., skeletal muscle). The autonomic nervous system (ANS) is involved in regulation of the body's internal environment (viscera) through involuntary control of organ systems. The ANS is further divided into sympathetic and parasympathetic divisions. Organs innervated by specific components of the nervous system are called effector organs.

CELLS OF THE NERVOUS SYSTEM

Two basic types of cells constitute nervous tissue: neurons and supporting nonneuronal neuroglial cells. The neuron is the primary cell of the nervous system. It is an electrically excitable cell and transmits and receives information. Neuroglial cells provide structural support, protection, and nutrition for the neurons and facilitate neurotransmission. Neuroglial cells include astrocytes, microglia, and oligodendrocytes in the CNS; and Schwann (neurilemma) and satellite cells (a type of Schwann cell) in the PNS.

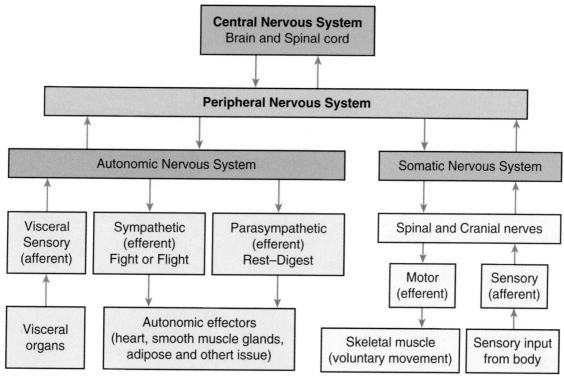

FIGURE 14.1 Organization of the Nervous System.

Neurons

Working alone or in units, neurons detect environmental changes and initiate body responses to maintain a dynamic steady state. Neuronal size and structure vary markedly, and each neuron is adapted to perform specialized functions. The cellular constituents of neurons include microtubules (transport substances within the cell), neurofibrils (very thin supportive fibers that extend throughout the neuron), microfilaments (thought to be involved in transport of cellular products), and Nissl substances (endoplasmic reticulum and ribosomes) involved in protein synthesis.

A neuron (Fig. 14.2) has three components: a cell body (soma), the dendrites (thin branching fibers of the cell), and the axons. Cell bodies for most neurons, even those extending axons into peripheral nerves, are located within the CNS. Those in the PNS usually are found in groups called ganglia (or plexuses—a group of relay nerves). The dendrites are extensions that carry nerve impulses *toward* the cell body. Axons are long, conductive projections that carry nerve impulses *away* from the cell body. The axon hillock is the cone-shaped process where the axon leaves the cell body. The first part of the axon hillock has the lowest threshold for stimulation, so action potentials begin there. A typical neuron has only one axon, which may be wrapped with a myelin sheath—a membrane made of a lipid material called myelin. In the CNS, myelin is produced by oligodendrocytes. In the PNS, myelin is produced by Schwann cells. The myelin sheaths are interrupted at regular intervals by the nodes of Ranvier. Nutrient exchange is not possible through the myelin sheath, although it can occur at the nodes of Ranvier. Axons can branch at the nodes of Ranvier, forming axon collaterals. Axons end with telodendria, branches that terminate with synaptic knobs, which are used in neurotransmission.

Where there is myelin, the velocity of nerve impulses increases. Myelin acts as an insulator that allows an action potential to leap between segments rather than flowing along the entire length of the membrane, yielding the increased velocity. This mechanism is referred to as saltatory conduction. Disorders of the myelin sheath (demyelinating diseases), such as multiple sclerosis and Guillain-Barré syndrome, demonstrate the important role myelin plays in nerve conduction (see Chapter 16). Conduction velocities depend not only on the myelin coating but also on the diameter of the axon. Larger axons transmit impulses at a faster rate.

Neurons are structurally classified on the basis of the number of processes (projections) extending from the cell body (see Fig. 14.2, *A*). There are four basic types of cell configuration: (1) unipolar, (2) pseudounipolar, (3) bipolar, and (4) multipolar. Unipolar neurons have one process, an axon, which branches shortly after leaving the cell body. One example is found in the retina. Pseudounipolar neurons (some call them *unipolar*) have one axon process and one dendrite process, but the dendrite and axon are fused to each other near the cell body and the axon then extends into the CNS. This configuration is typical of sensory neurons in both cranial and spinal nerves. Bipolar neurons have two distinct processes (one axon and one dendrite) arising directly from the cell body. This type of neuron connects the rod and cone cells of the retina. Multipolar neurons are the most common and have multiple processes capable of extensive branching. A motor neuron is typically multipolar.

Functionally, there are three types of neurons (their direction of transmission and typical configuration are noted in parentheses): (1) sensory (afferent, mostly pseudounipolar), (2) associational (interneurons, multipolar), and (3) motor (efferent, multipolar). Sensory neurons carry impulses from peripheral sensory receptors to the CNS. Associational neurons (interneurons) transmit impulses from neuron to neuron—that is, sensory to motor neurons. They are located solely within the CNS. Motor neurons transmit impulses away from the CNS to an effector (i.e., skeletal muscle or organs). In skeletal muscle the end processes form a neuromuscular (myoneural) junction (see Fig. 14.14 and the Spinal Cord section later in the chapter).

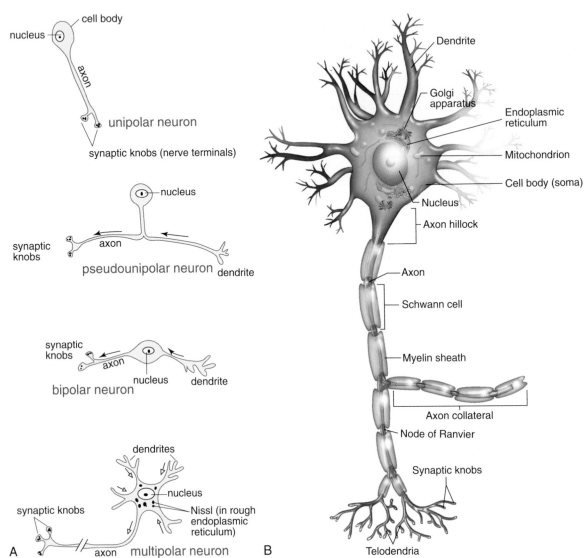

FIGURE 14.2 Neuron Structure. A, Structural classifications of neurons based on the number of processes: unipolar, pseudopolar, bipolar, and multipolar. **B,** Typical multipolar neuron: PNS neuron with multiple extensions from the cell body. *PNS,* Peripheral nervous system. (**A,** from Watson C, Kirkcaldie M, Paxinos G: *The brain,* London, 2011, Academic Press; **B,** modified from Patton KT, Thibodeau GA, Douglas MM: *Essentials of anatomy & physiology,* St Louis, 2012, Mosby.)

Neuroglia

Neuroglia ("nerve glue") are the general classification of nonneuronal cells that support the neurons of the nervous system. They comprise approximately 50% of the total brain and spinal cord volume. Neuroglia are present in both the CNS and PNS. Astrocytes, oligodendroglia (oligodendrocytes), ependymal cells, and microglia are found in the CNS; Schwann cells, nonmyelinating Schwann cells, and satellite glial cells are found in the PNS (Fig. 14.3). The different types of neuroglia serve different functions (Table 14.1).

Nerve Injury and Regeneration

Mature nerve cells do not divide, and injury can cause permanent loss of function. When an axon is severed, Wallerian degeneration occurs in the distal axon, the portion cut off from the cell body: (1) a characteristic swelling appears within the portion of the axon distal to the cut; (2) the neurofilaments hypertrophy; (3) the myelin sheath shrinks

and disintegrates; and (4) the axon degenerates and disappears. The myelin sheaths re-form into Schwann cells that align in a column between the severed part of the axon and the effector organ.

At the proximal end of the injured axon, similar changes occur but only back to the next node of Ranvier. The cell body responds to trauma by swelling and dying by chromatolysis (dispersing the Nissl substance) or apoptosis. During the repair process, the cell increases protein synthesis and mitochondrial activity. Approximately 7 to 14 days after the injury, new terminal sprouts project from the proximal segment and may enter the remaining Schwann cell pathway. (Fig. 14.4 contains a more detailed representation of these events.)

This process, however, is limited to myelinated fibers and generally occurs only in the PNS. The regeneration of axonal constituents in the CNS is limited by an increased incidence of scar formation and the different nature of myelin formed by the oligodendrocyte. Nerve regeneration depends on many factors, such as location of the injury, the type of injury, the presence of inflammatory responses, and the

CENTRAL NERVOUS SYSTEM NEUROGLIA

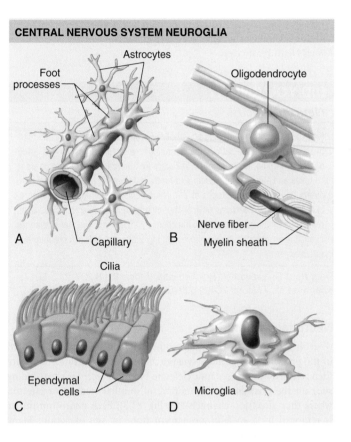

PERIPHERAL NERVOUS SYSTEM NEUROGLIA

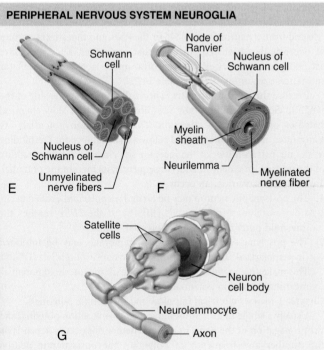

FIGURE 14.3 Types of Neuroglial Cells. Neuroglia of the central nervous system (CNS): **A,** Astrocytes attached to the outside of a capillary blood vessel in the brain. **B,** An oligodendrocyte with processes that wrap around nerve fibers in the CNS to form myelin sheaths. **C,** Ciliated ependymal cells forming a sheet that usually lines fluid cavities in the brain. **D,** A phagocytic microglial cell. Neuroglia of the peripheral nervous system (PNS): **E,** A Schwann cell supporting a bundle of nerve fibers in the PNS. **F,** Another type of Schwann cell encircling a peripheral nerve fiber to form a thick myelin sheath. **G,** Satellite cells, another type of Schwann cell, surround and support cell bodies of neurons in the PNS. (From Patton KT, et al: *Essentials of anatomy & physiology*, St Louis, 2012, Mosby.)

Cell Type	Primary Functions
TABLE 14.1 Support Cells of the Nervous System	
Central Nervous System	
Astrocytes	Form specialized contacts between neuronal surfaces and blood vessels
	Provide rapid transport for nutrients and metabolites
	Thought to form an essential component of blood–brain barrier
	Appear to be scar-forming cells of CNS, which may be foci for seizures
	Appear to work with neurons in processing information and memory storage
Oligodendroglia (oligodendrocytes)	Formation of myelin sheath in CNS
Microglia	Responsible for clearing cellular debris (phagocytic properties) and the key immune cell in the CNS
Ependymal cells	Serve as a lining for ventricles and choroid plexuses involved in production of cerebrospinal fluid
Peripheral Nervous System	
Schwann cells	Formation of myelin sheath in PNS
	Direct axonal regrowth and functional recovery in PNS
Nonmyelinating Schwann cells	Provide neuronal metabolic support and regeneration in PNS
Satellite glial cells	Surround sensory, sympathetic, and parasympathetic nerve cell bodies and ganglia to provide protection and promote cellular communication (similar to astrocytes in CNS)

CNS, Central nervous system; *PNS,* peripheral nervous system.

process of scarring. The closer the injury to the cell body of the nerve, the greater are the chances that the nerve cell will die and not regenerate. A crushing injury allows for fuller recovery compared with a cut injury. Crushed nerves sometimes recover fully, whereas cut nerves form connective tissue scars that block or slow regenerating axonal branches. Peripheral nerves injured close to the spinal cord recover poorly and slowly because of the long distance between the cell body and the peripheral termination of the axon.[1]

> **✓ QUICK CHECK 14.1**
> 1. How do the functions of the somatic and autonomic nervous systems differ?
> 2. What are the three components of a neuron?
> 3. How does myelin affect nerve impulse transmission?
> 4. Describe the process through which injured axons are repaired.

THE NERVE IMPULSE

Neurons generate and conduct electrical and chemical impulses by selectively changing the electrical potential of the plasma membrane and influencing other nearby neurons by releasing chemicals (neurotransmitters). An unexcited neuron maintains a resting membrane potential. When the membrane potential is sufficiently raised, an action potential is generated, and the nerve impulse then flows to all parts of the neuron. The action potential response occurs

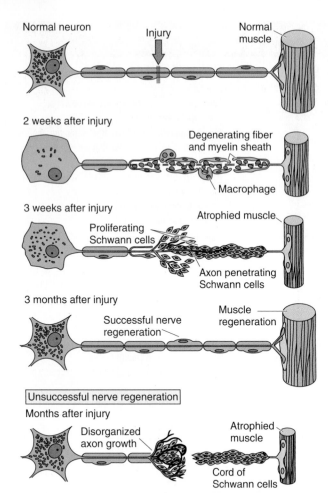

FIGURE 14.4 Peripheral Nerve Regeneration Following Injury. Schwann cells detach from the axons, proliferate, and, with recruited macrophages, help clear cellular and myelin debris. A damaged motor axon can regrow to its distal connection only if the neurilemma remains intact (to form a guiding tunnel) and if scar tissue does not block its pathway. (From Gartner LP: *Textbook of histology*, ed 4, Philadelphia, 2017, Elsevier.)

only when the stimulus is strong enough; if it is too weak, the membrane remains unexcited. This property is termed the *all-or-none response* (see Chapter 1 for a discussion of electrical impulse conduction).

Synapses

Neurons are not physically continuous with one another. The region between adjacent neurons is called a synapse (Fig. 14.5). The neurons that conduct a nerve impulse are named according to whether they relay impulses toward (presynaptic neurons) or away from (postsynaptic neurons) the synapse. The synapse is composed of a bulbous end of the presynaptic neuron (synaptic knob) that is separated from the postsynaptic neuron by a gap called the synaptic cleft. Impulses are transmitted across the synapse by chemical and electrical conduction (Only chemical conduction is discussed here. Chapter 1 contains information on electrical conduction [see Fig. 1.30]. When an impulse originates in a presynaptic neuron, the impulse reaches the vesicles, where chemicals (neurotransmitters) are stored in the synaptic bouton. Once released from the vesicles, the neurotransmitters diffuse across the synaptic cleft and bind to specific neurotransmitter (protein) receptor sites on the plasma membrane of the postsynaptic neuron, relaying the impulse (see Fig. 14.5).

Brain synapses can change in strength and number throughout life and this is known as synaptic plasticity or neuroplasticity (see *Did You Know? Neuroplasticity*).

Neurotransmitters

Neurotransmitters are chemicals synthesized in the neuron and localized in the presynaptic terminal (synaptic bouton). Neurotransmitters are then released into the synaptic cleft and bind to a receptor site (binding site) on the postsynaptic membrane of another neuron or effector, where they affect ion channels (see Fig. 14.5). Each neurotransmitter is removed by a specific mechanism from its site of action. Many substances are neurotransmitters, including norepinephrine, acetylcholine, dopamine, histamine, and serotonin. Many of these transmitters have more than one function. Neuromodulators are chemical messengers released from a neuron in the CNS or the PNS, and this affects a group of neurons that have receptors for that messenger. They may have excitatory or inhibitory effects. Neurotransmitter and neuromodulator substances are summarized in Table 14.2.

Because the neurotransmitter is normally stored on one side of the synaptic cleft and the receptor sites are on the other side, chemical synapses operate in one direction. Therefore action potentials are transmitted along a multineuronal pathway in one direction. The binding of the neurotransmitter at the receptor site changes the permeability of the postsynaptic neuron and, consequently, its membrane potential. Two possible scenarios can occur:

1. The postsynaptic neuron may be excited (depolarized), called excitatory postsynaptic potentials (EPSPs). If the EPSP reaches the threshold potential, an action potential is initiated.
2. The postsynaptic neuron's plasma membrane may be inhibited (hyperpolarized), called inhibitory postsynaptic potentials (IPSPs). This makes the membrane less likely to reach the threshold potential, meaning the action potential is inhibited.

Chapter 1 reviews electrical impulses and membrane potentials.

Usually a single EPSP cannot induce a neuron's action potential and the propagation of the nerve impulse. Whether this occurs depends on the number and frequency of potentials the postsynaptic neuron receives—a concept known as summation. Temporal summation (time relationship) refers to the effects of successive, rapid impulses received from a single neuron at the same synapse. Spatial summation (spacing effect) is the combined effects of impulses from a number of neurons onto a single neuron at the same time. Facilitation refers to the effect of EPSP on the plasma membrane potential. The plasma membrane is *facilitated* when summation brings the membrane closer to the threshold potential and decreases the stimulus required to induce an action potential. The effect that a chemical neurotransmitter has on the plasma

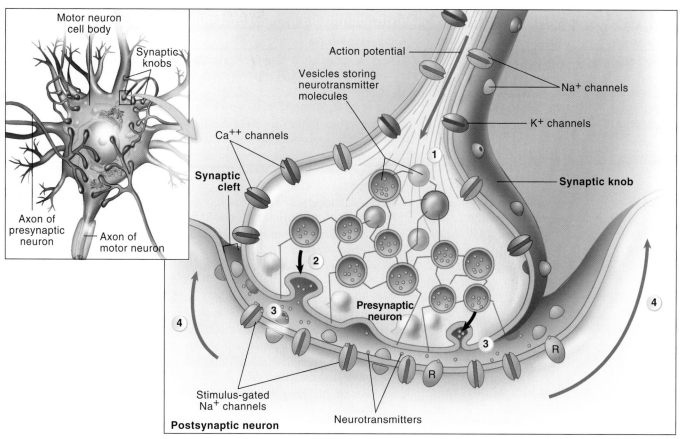

FIGURE 14.5 Neuronal Transmission and Synaptic Cleft. Details illustrate the synaptic knob of a presynaptic neuron, the plasma membrane of a postsynaptic neuron, and a synaptic cleft. At step **1**, the action potential arrives at the synaptic knob. At step **2**, the rapid exocytosis of neurotransmitter molecules from vesicles in the knob occurs. At step **3**, neurotransmitter diffuses into the synaptic cleft and binds to receptor molecules (*R*) in the plasma membrane of the postsynaptic neuron. The postsynaptic receptors directly or indirectly trigger the opening of stimulus gated ion channels, initiating a local potential in the postsynaptic neuron. At step **4**, the local potential may move toward the axon, where an action potential may begin. (Adapted from Patton KT: *Anatomy & physiology*, ed 10, St Louis, 2019, Mosby.)

membrane potential depends on the balance of these effects. The mechanisms of convergence (many neurons firing and converging on one neuron), divergence (one neuron firing and diverging on many neurons), summation, and facilitation allow for the integrative processes of the nervous system.

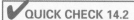

QUICK CHECK 14.2
1. Explain the process of the chemical conduction of impulses.
2. What are neurotransmitters? Give two examples.
3. Compare summation and facilitation of nerve impulses.

CENTRAL NERVOUS SYSTEM

Brain

The brain is a functionally integrated circuit of millions of neurons with different genomes, structures, molecular composition, networks, and connections. It weighs approximately 3 lb and receives 15% to 20% of the total cardiac output. The brain enables a person to reason, function intellectually, express personality and mood, and perceive and interact with the environment.

The cerebrum is the largest part of the brain and contains both gray matter and white matter. The three primary embryonic vesicles

(structural divisions) of the brain are (1) the forebrain (prosencephalon), (2) the midbrain (mesencephalon), and (3) the hindbrain (rhombencephalon). These three vesicles then develop further into the secondary vesicles and their structures which are summarized in Table 14.3 and Fig. 14.6. The midbrain, medulla, and pons comprise the brainstem, which connects the hemispheres of the brain, cerebellum, and spinal cord. A collection of nerve cell bodies (nuclei) within the brainstem makes up the reticular formation (Fig. 14.7). The reticular formation is a large network of diffuse nuclei that connect the brainstem to the cortex and control vital reflexes, such as cardiovascular function and respiration. It is essential for maintaining wakefulness and attention and therefore is referred to as the reticular activating system (see Fig. 14.7). Some nuclei within the reticular formation support specific motor movements, such as balance and posture.

Divisions of the brain are associated with different functions, but attributing specific functions to definite regions of the brain is not entirely accurate. However, for clinical considerations functional specificity is very useful for localizing pathologic conditions in various nervous system regions. Fig. 14.8, *C*, illustrates these regions and describes some of the areas. The mapping of brain networks is also helpful in discovering how varying parts of the brain are interconnected when performing a specific function (Box 14.1).

TABLE 14.2 Substances That Are Neurotransmitters or Neuromodulators

Substance	Effect	Clinical Example
Acetylcholine	Excitatory or inhibitory	Alzheimer disease (a type of dementia) is associated with a decrease in acetylcholine-secreting neurons. Myasthenia gravis (weakness of skeletal muscles) results from a reduction in acetylcholine receptors.
Norepinephrine	Excitatory or inhibitory	Cocaine and amphetamines,* resulting in overstimulation of postsynaptic neurons.
Serotonin	Generally inhibitory	Involved with mood, anxiety, and sleep induction. Levels of serotonin are elevated in schizophrenia (delusions, hallucinations, withdrawal).
Dopamine	Generally excitatory	Parkinson disease (depression of voluntary motor control) results from destruction of dopamine-secreting neurons. Drugs used to increase dopamine production induce vomiting and schizophrenia.
Histamine	Excitatory (H1 and H2 receptors) and inhibitory (H3 receptors)	No clear indication of histamine-associated pathologic conditions. Histamine is involved with arousal and attention and links to other brain transmitter systems.
Gamma-aminobutyric acid (GABA)	Majority of postsynaptic inhibition in brain	Drugs that increase GABA function have been used to treat epilepsy by inhibiting excessive discharge of neurons.
Glycine	Most postsynaptic inhibition in spinal cord	Glycine receptors are inhibited by strychnine.
Glutamate and aspartate	Excitatory	Drugs that block glutamate or aspartate, such as riluzole, used to treat amyotrophic lateral sclerosis. These drugs might prevent overexcitation from seizures and neural degeneration.
Endorphins and enkephalins	Generally inhibitory	Morphine and heroin bind to endorphin and enkephalin receptors on presynaptic neurons and reduce pain by blocking release of neurotransmitter.
Substance P	Generally excitatory	Substance P is a neurotransmitter in pain transmission pathways. Blocking release of substance P by morphine reduces pain.
Vasoactive intestinal peptide	Generally excitatory	Stimulates secretion, vasodilation, and smooth muscle relaxation (vasodilation, sphincter relaxation).

*Increase the release and block the reuptake of norepinephrine.
From Daroff RB et al: *Bradley's neurology in clinical practice*, ed 6, Philadelphia, 2012, Saunders.
ANS, Autonomic nervous system; *CNS,* central nervous system; *GI,* gastrointestinal; *PNS,* peripheral nervous system.

TABLE 14.3 Divisions of the Central Nervous System

Primary Brain Vesicles	Secondary Vesicles	Structures in Secondary Vesicles
Forebrain (prosencephalon)	Telencephalon	Cerebral hemispheres Cerebral cortex Basal ganglia
	Diencephalon	Epithalamus Thalamus Hypothalamus Subthalamus
Midbrain (mesencephalon)	Mesencephalon	Corpora quadrigemina (tectum—superior and inferior colliculi) Cerebral peduncles
Hindbrain (rhombencephalon)	Metencephalon	Cerebellum Pons
	Myelencephalon	Medulla oblongata
Spinal cord	Spinal cord	Spinal cord

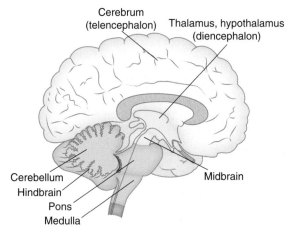

FIGURE 14.6 Structural Divisions of the Brain. (From Standring S: *Gray's anatomy: the anatomical basis of clinical practice*, ed 40, Philadelphia, 2008, Elsevier.)

Forebrain

Telencephalon. The telencephalon (cerebral hemispheres) consists of the cerebral cortex (the largest portion of the brain) and the basal ganglia (composed of several *nuclei*). The surface of the cerebral cortex is covered with convolutions called *gyri* (see Fig. 14.8), which greatly increase the cortical surface area and the number of neurons. Grooves between adjacent gyrus are termed sulci; deeper grooves are fissures. The cerebral cortex contains an outer layer of cell bodies of neurons (gray matter). The cerebral cortex is located in the frontal, parietal, temporal, and occipital lobes. White matter lies beneath the cerebral cortex and is composed of myelinated nerve fibers.

Lobes. The two cerebral hemispheres are separated by a deep groove known as the longitudinal fissure (see Fig. 14.9, *B*). The surface of each hemisphere is divided into lobes named after the region of the skull under which each lobe lies: frontal, parietal, occipital, and temporal lobes.

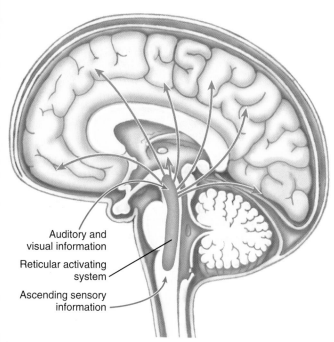

Auditory and
visual information

Reticular activating
system

Ascending sensory
information

FIGURE 14.7 Reticular Activating System (RAS). The RAS consists of nuclei in the brainstem reticular formation plus fibers that conduct sensory information to the nuclei and fibers that conduct from the nuclei to widespread areas of the cerebral cortex. Functioning of the reticular activating system is essential for consciousness.

BOX 14.1 Brain Networks

The architecture and integrated function of neural nodes, networks, and interconnected pathways within the brain are being mapped in the advancing field of human connectomics. Imaging techniques are combined with mathematical and computational models to produce visual representations of brain networks.

The figure below provides an illustration of brain connectivity showing interconnecting cortical pathways using diffusion tensor imaging tracking technology (the imaging of diffusion of water in tissue). Such mapping of the brain contributes to an understanding of the commonalities and individual differences of the normally functioning brain and changes associated with aging and disease (i.e., degenerative brain disease, epilepsy, schizophrenia, and brain tumors).

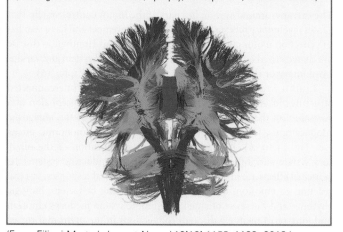

(From Filippi M et al: *Lancet Neurol* 12[12]:1189–1199, 2013.)

The posterior margin of the frontal lobe is on the central sulcus (fissure of Rolando), and it borders inferiorly on the lateral sulcus (Sylvian fissure, lateral fissure) (see Fig. 14.8, *A*). The prefrontal area is responsible for goal-oriented behavior (e.g., ability to concentrate), short-term or recall memory, the elaboration of thought, and inhibition of the limbic areas of the CNS. The premotor area (see Fig. 14.8, *C*) is involved in programming motor movements. This area contains the cell bodies that form part of the basal ganglia system. The frontal eye fields, which are involved in controlling eye movements, are located on the middle frontal gyrus.

The primary motor area is located along the precentral gyrus forming the primary voluntary motor area. It has a specific correspondence between a body region and an area in the brain (somatotopic organization) that is often referred to as a *homunculus* (little man) (see Fig. 14.9). Electrical stimulation of specific areas of this cortex causes specific muscles of the body to move. The axons traveling from the cell bodies in and on either side of this gyrus project fibers (axons) that form the pyramidal system. This system includes the corticobulbar tract that synapses in the brainstem and provides voluntary control of muscles in the head and neck, and the corticospinal tracts that descend into the spinal cord and provide voluntary control of muscles throughout the body (Fig. 14.15 later in the chapter). The Broca speech area is on the inferior frontal gyrus. It is usually on the left hemisphere and is responsible for the motor aspects of speech. Damage to this area, commonly as a result of a cerebrovascular accident (stroke), results in the inability to form words or at least some difficulty in forming words (expressive aphasia) (see Chapter 16).

The parietal lobe lies within the borders of the central, parietooccipital, and lateral sulci. This lobe contains the major area for somatic sensory input, located primarily along the postcentral gyrus (see Fig. 14.8), which is adjacent to the primary motor area. Communication between the motor and sensory areas (and among other regions in the cortex) is provided by association fibers. Much of this region is involved in sensory association (storage, analysis, and interpretation of stimuli). Fig. 14.9 shows the distribution of functions associated with both the primary motor area and the primary sensory area of the cerebral cortex.

The occipital lobe lies caudal to the parietooccipital sulcus and is superior to the cerebellum. The primary visual cortex is located in this region and receives input from the retinas. Much of the remainder of this lobe is involved in visual association. The temporal lobe lies inferior to the lateral fissure and is composed of the superior, middle, and inferior temporal gyri. The primary auditory cortex and its related association area lie deep within the lateral sulcus on the superior temporal gyrus. The Wernicke area, along with adjacent portions of the parietal lobe, constitutes a *sensory speech area*. This area is responsible for reception and interpretation of speech, and dysfunction may result in receptive aphasia or dysphasia. The temporal lobe also is involved in memory consolidation and smell.

Another lobe, the insula (insular lobe), lies hidden from view in the lateral sulci between the temporal and frontal lobes of each hemisphere. The insula processes sensory and emotional information and routes the information to other areas of the brain. Lying directly beneath the longitudinal fissure is a mass of white matter pathways called the corpus callosum (transverse or commissural fibers). This structure connects the two cerebral hemispheres through sensory and motor contralateral projection of axons and is essential in coordinating activities between hemispheres (see Fig. 14.8, *B*).

Basal ganglia. Inside the cerebrum are numerous tracts (white matter) and nuclei (gray matter). The major subcortical nuclei are called the basal ganglia (basal nuclei) system. The basal ganglia system is a group of nuclei that includes the caudate nucleus, putamen, and

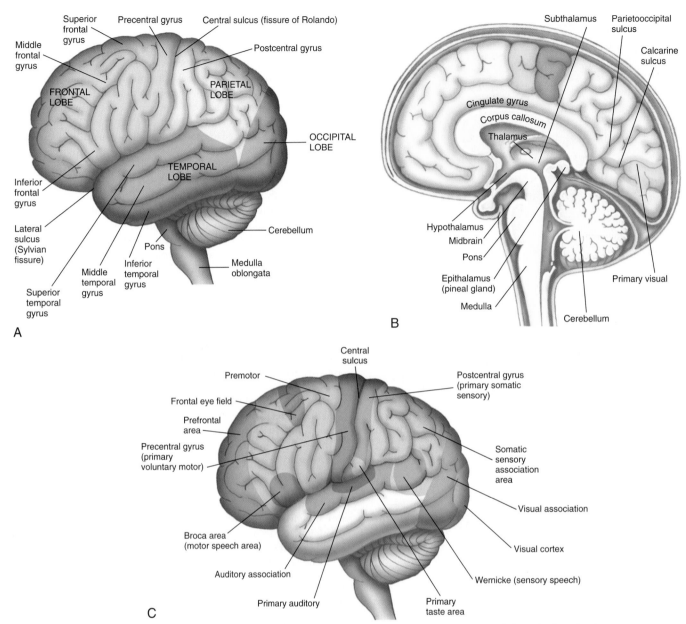

FIGURE 14.8 The Cerebral Hemispheres. A, Left hemisphere of cerebrum, lateral view. **B,** Functional areas of the cerebral cortex, midsagittal view. **C,** Functional areas of the cerebral cortex, lateral view.

globus pallidus (Fig. 14.10). The putamen and the globus pallidus together are called the lentiform nucleus (because they are shaped like a lentil). The caudate nucleus, putamen, and nucleus accumbens together are called the striatum. Functionally, the substantia nigra is a component of the basal ganglia. It synthesizes dopamine, a neurotransmitter and precursor of norepinephrine. The nuclei of the basal ganglia are important for voluntary movement and cognitive and emotional functions (i.e., the nucleus accumbens has pleasure and reward functions).

The internal capsule is a thick layer of white matter in which axons of afferent (sensory) and efferent (motor) pathways pass to and from the cerebral cortex through the center of the cerebral hemispheres and between the caudate and lentiform nuclei (see Fig. 14.10, *B*).

The basal ganglia plus their direct and indirect interconnections with the thalamus, premotor cortex, red nucleus, reticular formation, and spinal cord have been considered part of the extrapyramidal system.

The extrapyramidal system is a part of the motor control system that causes involuntary reflexes and coordinated movement and has a stabilizing effect on motor control. Parkinson disease and Huntington disease are characterized by disruption of the extrapyramidal system and various involuntary or exaggerated motor movements (see Chapter 16).

Limbic system. The limbic system is a group of interconnected structures located between the telencephalon and diencephalon and surrounding the corpus callosum. It is composed of the amygdala, hippocampus, fornix, hypothalamus, and related autonomic nuclei (see Fig. 14.10, *A*). It is an extension or modification of the olfactory system and influences the autonomic and endocrine systems. Its principal effects are involved in primitive behavioral responses, visceral reaction to emotion, motivation, mood, feeding behaviors, biologic rhythms, and the sense of smell. The limbic system mediates emotion and long-term memory through connections in the prefrontal cortex (limbic cortex).

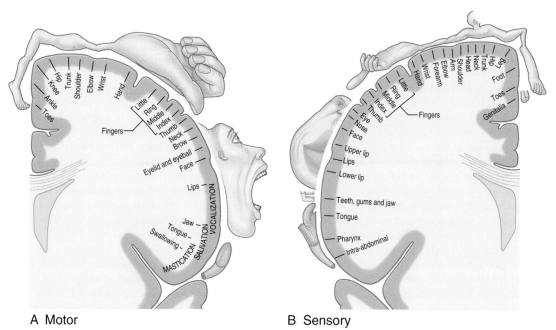

A Motor   B Sensory

FIGURE 14.9 Primary Somatic Sensory (A) and Motor (B) Areas of the Cortex. A, The motor homunculus shows proportional somatotopic representation in the main motor area. **B,** The sensory homunculus shows proportional somatotopic representation in the somaesthetic cortex. (From Standring S et al: *Gray's anatomy*, ed 40, Edinburgh, Churchill Livingstone, 2008.)

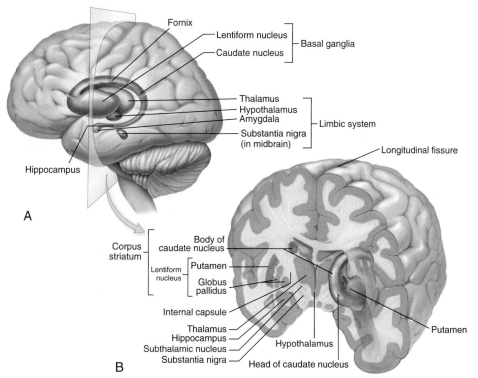

FIGURE 14.10 Basal Ganglia. A, The basal ganglia seen through the cortex of the left cerebral hemisphere. **B,** The basal ganglia seen in a frontal (coronal) section of the brain. The nucleus accumbens is not visible in this figure; it lies between the caudate nucleus and putamen. (From Patton KT, Thibodeau GA: *Anatomy & physiology*, ed 9, St Louis, 2016, Mosby.)

Diencephalon. The diencephalon (interbrain), surrounded by the cerebrum and sitting on top of the brainstem, has four divisions: epithalamus, thalamus, hypothalamus, and subthalamus (see Table 14.3 and Fig. 14.8). The epithalamus forms the roof of the third ventricle (a brain cavity) and composes the most superior portion of the diencephalon. The diencephalon controls vital functions and visceral activities and is closely associated with those of the limbic system.

The thalamus borders and surrounds the third ventricle. It is a major integrating center for afferent impulses to the cerebral cortex. Various sensations are perceived at this level, but cortical processing is required for interpretation. The thalamus serves also as a relay center for information from the basal ganglia and cerebellum to the appropriate motor area.

The hypothalamus forms the base of the diencephalon. The hypothalamus functions to (1) maintain a constant internal environment and (2) implement behavioral patterns. Integrative centers control ANS function, regulate body temperature and endocrine function, and adjust emotional expression. The hypothalamus exerts its influence through the endocrine system, as well as through neural pathways (Box 14.2). The subthalamus flanks the hypothalamus laterally. It serves as an important basal ganglia center for motor activities.

Midbrain

Mesencephalon. The midbrain (mesencephalon) is composed of three structures: the corpora quadrigemina (located on the tectum, the ceiling of the midbrain), which is composed of the two pairs of superior colliculi and two pairs of inferior colliculi; the tegmentum (the floor of the midbrain), which is composed of the red nucleus, substantia nigra, and the basis pedunculi. The tegmentum and basis pedunculi are collectively called the cerebral peduncles.

The superior colliculi are involved with voluntary and involuntary visual motor movements (e.g., the ability of the eyes to track moving objects in the visual field). The inferior colliculi accomplish similar motor activities but involve movements affecting the auditory system (e.g., positioning the head to improve hearing). The red nucleus receives ascending sensory information from the cerebellum and projects a minor motor pathway, the rubrospinal tract, to the cervical spinal cord. The basis pedunculi are made up of efferent fibers of the corticospinal, corticobulbar, and corticopontocerebellar tracts.

Other notable structures of this region are the nuclei of the third and fourth cranial nerves. The cerebral aqueduct (aqueduct of Sylvius), which carries cerebrospinal fluid (CSF), also traverses this structure. Obstruction of this aqueduct is often the cause of hydrocephalus.

Hindbrain

Metencephalon. The major structures of the metencephalon are the cerebellum and the pons. The cerebellum (see Fig. 14.8) is composed

of gray matter and white matter, and its cortical surface is convoluted, similar to the surface of the cerebrum. It also is divided by a central fissure into right and left lobes connected by the vermis.

The cerebellum is responsible for reflexive, involuntary fine-tuning of motor control and for maintaining balance and posture through extensive neural connections with the medulla (through the inferior cerebellar peduncle) and with the midbrain (through the superior cerebellar peduncle). The two hemispheres are connected to the pons by the middle cerebellar peduncles. These connections allow extensive sampling of visual, vestibular, and proprioceptive data from other regions of the CNS and periphery.

The pons (bridge) is easily recognized by its bulging appearance below the midbrain and above the medulla. Primarily it transmits information from the cerebellum to the brainstem and between the two cerebellar hemispheres. The nuclei of the fifth through eighth cranial nerves are located in this structure.

Myelencephalon. The myelencephalon usually is called the *medulla oblongata* and forms the lowest portion of the brainstem. Reflex activities, such as heart rate, respiration, blood pressure, coughing, sneezing, swallowing, and vomiting, are controlled in this area. The nuclei of cranial nerves IX through XII are located in this region.

A major portion of the descending motor pathways (i.e., corticospinal tracts) cross to the other side, or decussate, at the medulla (see Fig. 14.15 later in the chapter). These pathways, together with other areas of decussation in the CNS, are the basis for the phenomenon of contralateral control, when cerebral impulses control function on the opposite side of the body. Sleep–wake rhythms also are processed by neural influences from lower brain centers and are associated with a complex group of diffuse structures and functions (see Chapter 15), including the reticular activating system (cells that receive collateral signals from the afferent sensory pathways and project the signals to the higher brain centers, thus controlling CNS activity) (see Fig. 14.7).

> **QUICK CHECK 14.3**
> 1. Name the three major divisions of the brain and their component parts.
> 2. Describe the limbic system's functions.
> 3. What are the two major functions of the hypothalamus?

Spinal Cord

The spinal cord is the portion of the CNS that lies within the vertebral canal and is surrounded and protected by the vertebral column. The spinal cord has many functions, including connection of the brain and the body through a long nerve cable, somatic and autonomic reflexes, motor pattern control, and sensory and motor modulation. The spinal cord originates in the medulla oblongata and ends at the level of the first or second lumbar vertebra in adults (Fig. 14.11). The end of the spinal cord, the conus medullaris, is cone shaped. Spinal nerves continue from the end of the spinal cord and form a nerve bundle called the cauda equina. The filament anchor from the conus medullaris to the coccyx is the filum terminale. The coverings of the spinal cord are illustrated in Fig. 14.11, C.

Grossly the spinal cord is divided into vertebral sections (8 cervical, 12 thoracic, 5 lumbar, 5 sacral, and 1 coccygeal) that correspond to paired nerves (see Fig. 14.11, A). A cross section of the spinal cord (Fig. 14.12) is characterized by a butterfly-shaped inner core of gray matter (containing nerve cell bodies). The central canal is filled with cerebrospinal fluid and lies in the center of this region and extends through the spinal cord from its origin in the fourth ventricle. The gray matter of the spinal cord is divided into three regions and displays specific

---

BOX 14.2 Functions of the Hypothalamus

- Visceral and somatic responses
- Affectual responses
- Hormone synthesis
- Sympathetic and parasympathetic activity
- Temperature regulation
- Fluid balance
- Appetite and feeding responses
- Physical expression of emotions
- Sexual behavior
- Pleasure-punishment centers
- Level of arousal or wakefulness

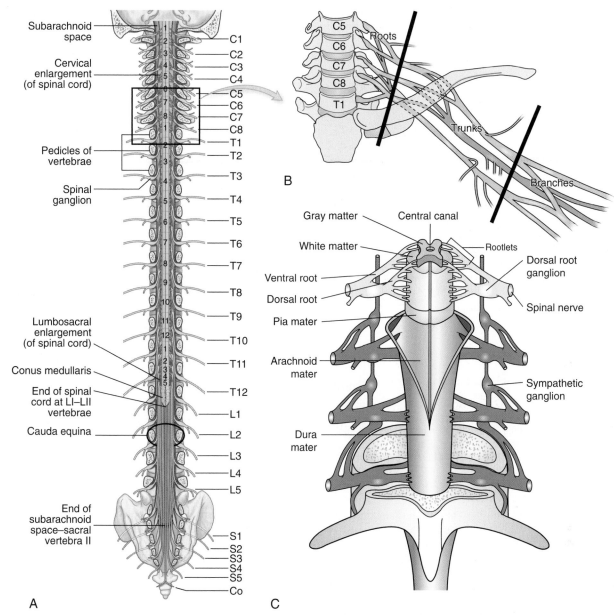

FIGURE 14.11 Vertebral Canal, Spinal Cord, and Spinal Nerves. A, Spinal cord and nerve root; cranial through sacral nerve distributions. **B,** Enlarged schematic of the brachial plexus is shown. The general schematic of a spinal nerve can be compared to a tree, with roots, trunks, and branches. **C,** Coverings of the spinal cord. The dura mater is shown in purple. Note how it extends to cover the spinal nerve roots and nerves. The arachnoid mater is highlighted in pink and the pia mater in orange. (**A,** Drake R et al: *Gray's anatomy for students,* ed 3, London, 2015, Churchill Livingstone. **B,** from Chung KC et al: *Practical management of pediatric and adult brachial plexus palsies,* London, 2012, Saunders. **C,** from Patton KT, Thibodeau GA: *Structure and function of the body,* ed 15, St Louis, 2016, Mosby.)

functional characteristics. These regions include the posterior horn, or dorsal horn (composed primarily of interneurons and axons from sensory neurons whose cell bodies lie in the dorsal root ganglion). At the tip of the posterior horn is the substantia gelatinosa, a structure involved in pain transmission (see Chapter 15). The lateral horn contains cell bodies involved with the ANS. The anterior horn, or ventral horn, contains the nerve cell bodies for efferent pathways that leave the spinal cord by way of spinal nerves.

Surrounding gray matter is white matter, which forms ascending and descending pathways called spinal tracts. Spinal tracts are named to denote their beginning and ending points. For example, the

spinothalamic tract (see Fig. 14.12) carries sensory nerve impulses from the spinal cord to the thalamus in the diencephalon. Numerous spinal tracts are grouped into columns according to their location within white matter. These include the anterior columns, lateral columns, and posterior (dorsal) columns (see Fig. 14.12).

Neural circuits in the spinal cord, when activated, display specific sets of motor responses. Reflex arcs form basic units that respond to stimuli and provide protective circuitry for motor output. Structures needed for a reflex are a receptor, an afferent (sensory) neuron, an efferent (motor) neuron, and an effector muscle or gland. A simple reflex arc may contain only two neurons (Fig. 14.13). Interneurons are

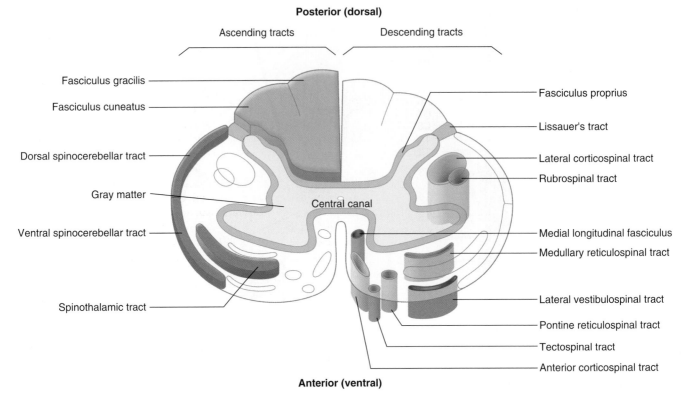

FIGURE 14.12 The Spinal Cord. All ascending *(sensory)* and descending *(motor)* tracts are present bilaterally. In this figure, ascending tracts are emphasized on the left side and descending tracts are emphasized on the right side. The location of the Lissauer tract and the fasciculus proprius (which contain both ascending and descending fibers) are also shown. (From Crossman AR, Neary D: *Neuroanatomy: an illustrated colour text,* ed 4, London, 2015, Churchill Livingstone.)

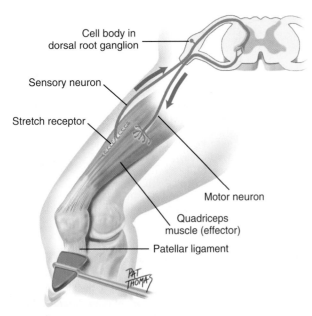

FIGURE 14.13 Cross-Section of Spinal Cord Showing Simple Reflex Arc. (From Jarvis C: *Physical examination & health assessment,* ed 7, St Louis, 2016, Saunders.)

usually present and provide a link between sensory and motor neurons. The motor effects of reflex arcs generally occur before the event is perceived in the brain's higher centers. Much internal environmental regulation is mediated by reflex activity involving the ANS.

Afferent pathways transmit sensory information from peripheral receptors toward the cerebrum. The pathways terminate in the cerebral or cerebellar cortex, or both. Efferent pathways primarily relay information away from the cerebrum to the brainstem or spinal cord. **Upper motor neurons** are completely contained within the CNS. Their primary roles are controlling fine motor movement and influencing/modifying spinal reflex arcs and circuits. Generally upper motor neurons form synapses with interneurons, which then form synapses with lower motor neurons that project into the periphery. **Lower motor neurons** directly influence muscles. Their cell bodies lie in the gray matter of the brainstem and of the spinal cord, but their processes extend out of the CNS and into the PNS. Destruction of upper motor neurons usually results in initial paralysis followed within days or weeks by partial recovery, whereas destruction of the *lower motor neurons* leads to paralysis unless peripheral nerve damage is followed by nerve regeneration and recovery (see Fig. 14.4). Differences in injury to upper and lower motor neurons are presented in Chapter 16.

Muscle activity (i.e., stimulation and contraction) is regulated by nerve impulses. Motor neurons innervate one or more muscle cells, forming **motor units**, which consist of a neuron and the skeletal muscles it stimulates. The junction between the axon of the motor neuron and the plasma membrane of the muscle cell is called the neuromuscular (myoneural) junction (Fig. 14.14). (Injury to motor neurons is discussed in Chapter 16.)

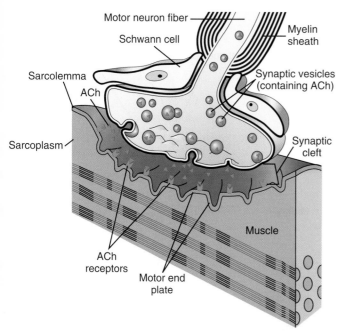

FIGURE 14.14 Normal Neuromuscular Junction. This figure shows how the distal end of a motor neuron fiber forms a synapse, or "chemical junction," with an adjacent muscle fiber. Neurotransmitters (specifically, acetylcholine [ACh]) are released from the neuron's synaptic vesicles and diffuse across the synaptic cleft. There they stimulate receptors in the motor end-plate region of the sarcolemma. (From Damjanov I: *Pathology for the health professions*, ed 4, St Louis, 2012, Saunders.)

Motor Pathways

Clinically relevant motor pathways are the lateral corticospinal (connects motor cortex with anterior horn cells in the spinal cord) and pyramidal tracts (connects the motor cortex with the medullary pyramids and descend to synapse with lower motor neurons of several cranial nerves in the brain stem or spinal cord); and the extrapyramidal reticulospinal, vestibulospinal, and rubrospinal tracts. The corticospinal and corticobulbar pathways are essentially the same tract and consist of a two-neuron chain (Fig. 14.15). The cell bodies (upper motor neurons) originate in and around the precentral gyrus; pass through the corona radiata (connects motor and sensory pathways) of the cerebrum, the internal capsule, middle three-fifths of the cerebral pedunculus, pons, and pyramid; and decussate (cross contralaterally) in the medulla oblongata and form the lateral corticospinal tract of the spinal cord (see Figs. 14.12 and 14.15, *A*) and thus control the opposite side of the body. The corticobulbar tract axons synapse on motor cranial nuclei within the brainstem that control muscles of the face, head, and neck. The lateral corticospinal tract axons leave the tract to go to specific interneurons or motor neurons in the anterior horn. The lateral corticospinal tract has the same somatotopic organization as the body (see Figs. 14.9 and 14.15, *A*). These lower motor neurons project through nerves to specific muscles. These tracts are involved in precise motor movements. The reticulospinal tract arises in the reticular formation of the medulla or pons (see Fig. 14.12) and modulates motor movement by inhibiting and exciting spinal activity. The vestibulospinal tract arises from a vestibular nucleus in the pons and causes the extensor muscles of the body to rapidly contract, most dramatically witnessed when a person starts to fall backward. The rubrospinal tract originates in the red nucleus, decussates, and terminates in the cervical spinal cord. It is important for muscle movement and fine muscle control in the upper extremities.

Sensory Pathways

The three clinically important spinal afferent pathways are the posterior column, anterior spinothalamic tract, and lateral spinothalamic tract (see Figs. 14.12 and 14.15, *B*). The posterior (dorsal) column (fasciculus gracilis and fasciculus cuneatus) carries fine-touch sensation, two-point discrimination, and proprioceptive information (i.e., epicritic information). The posterior column is formed by a three-neuron chain. The first neuron of the chain is the primary afferent neuron. It also is the sensory neuron of the reflex arc. After entering the spinal cord, it sends its axon ipsilaterally (on the same side) up the spinal cord to a specific part of the posterior column and synapses in the three posterior column nuclei in the medulla oblongata. For example, a basketball player who is > 6 feet tall has primary afferent neurons that could be 6 feet long, running from the great toe up to the medulla oblongata. The axon of the second-order neuron crosses contralaterally in the medial lemniscus and ascends in the medulla and pons to synapse with a specific nucleus of the thalamus. The third-order neuron, originating in the thalamus, continues the tract into the internal capsule, corona radiata, and postcentral gyrus (see Figs. 14.8, and 14.15, *B*).

The anterior and lateral spinothalamic tracts are responsible for vague touch sensation and for pain and temperature perception, respectively (see Figs. 14.12 and 14.15). These modalities are referred to as protopathic. These tracts also form a three-neuron chain. However their primary afferent neurons synapse in the posterior horn of the spinal cord is not just at the level they enter the intervertebral foramen but in a number of spinal segments above and below their point of entry. This is an example of divergence. The axons of the second-order neurons in the posterior horn cross to the contralateral side in the spinal cord in the lateral column, ascend to the same thalamic nucleus as the posterior column pathway, and continue with the posterior column pathway to the postcentral gyrus.

Protective Structures
Cranium

The cranium is composed of eight bones. The cranial vault encloses and protects the brain and its associated structures. The galea aponeurotica, which is a thick, fibrous band of tissue overlying the cranium between the frontal and occipital muscles, affords added protection to the skull. The subgaleal space has venous connections with the dural sinuses. If there is increased intracranial pressure, blood can be shunted to the space, thus reducing pressure in the intracranial cavity. The subgaleal space is also a common site for wound drains after intracranial surgery.

The floor of the cranial vault is irregular and contains many foramina (openings) for cranial nerves, blood vessels, and the spinal cord to exit. The cranial floor is divided into three fossae (depressions). The frontal lobes lie in the anterior fossa, the temporal lobes and base of the diencephalon lie in the middle fossa (temporal fossa), and the cerebellum lies in the posterior fossa. These terms are commonly used anatomic landmarks to describe the location of intracranial lesions.

Meninges

Surrounding the brain and spinal cord are three protective membranes: the dura mater, the arachnoid, and the pia mater. Collectively they are called the meninges (Fig. 14.16, *C*). The dura mater (meaning literally "hard mother") is composed of two layers, with the venous sinuses formed between them. The outermost layer forms the periosteum (endosteal layer) of the skull. The inner dura (meningeal layer) is responsible for forming rigid membranes that support and separate various brain structures.

One of these membranes, the falx cerebri, dips between the two cerebral hemispheres along the longitudinal fissure. The falx cerebri is

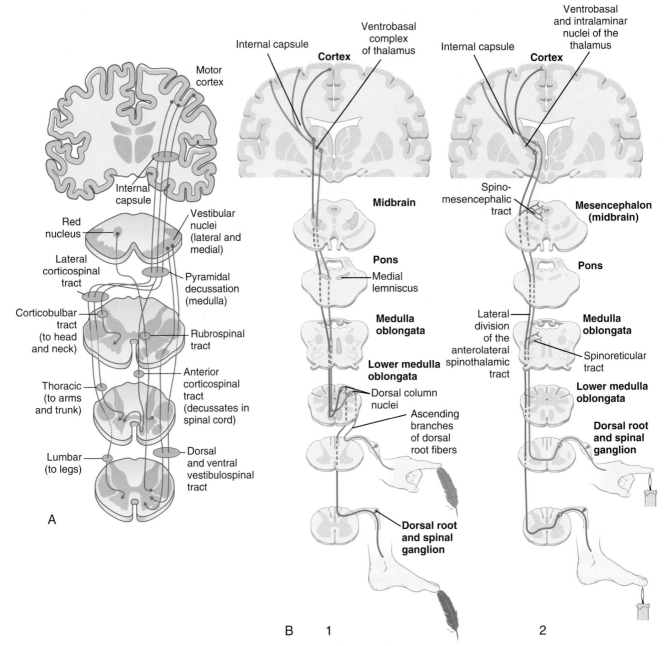

FIGURE 14.15 Examples of Somatic Motor and Sensory Pathways. A, Motor tracts. The pyramidal pathway through the lateral corticospinal tract and the extrapyramidal pathways through the rubrospinal, reticulospinal, and vestibulospinal tracts. **B,** Sensory tracts. 1, The dorsal column-medial lemniscal pathway for transmitting critical types of tactile signals: touch/proprioception. Note the lateral corticospinal tract decussation, the point where it crosses to the other side, is in the lower medulla. 2, Anterior and lateral divisions of the anterolateral spinothalamic sensory tract: pain/temperature. Note the decussation is in the spinal cord. (**A,** from Compston A et al: *McAlpine's multiple sclerosis,* ed 4, London, 2006, Churchill Livingstone. **B,** from Hall JE: *Guyton and Hall textbook of medical physiology,* ed 13, Philadelphia, 2016, Saunders.)

anchored anteriorly to the base of the brain at the crista galli of the ethmoid bone. The tentorium cerebelli, a common landmark, is a membrane that separates the cerebellum below from the cerebral structures above. Internal to the dura mater is the location of the arachnoid, a spongy, web-like structure that loosely follows the contours of the cerebral structures.

The subdural space lies between the dura and arachnoid. Many small bridging veins that have little support traverse the subdural space. Their disruption results in a subdural hematoma (see Chapter 17). The

subarachnoid space lies between the arachnoid and the pia mater and contains CSF (see Fig. 14.16,C). Unlike the dura mater and the arachnoid, the delicate pia mater adheres to the contours of the brain and spinal cord. It provides support for blood vessels serving brain tissue. The choroid plexuses, which are structures that produce CSF, arise from the pial membrane.

The spinal cord is anchored to the vertebrae by extension of the meninges (see Fig. 14.11, C). The meninges continue beyond the end of the spinal cord (at vertebrae levels L1 and L2) to the lower portion

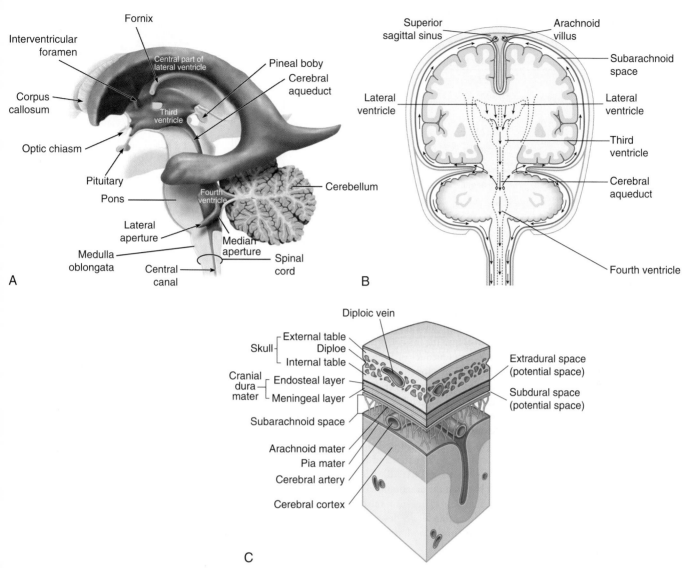

FIGURE 14.16 Flow of Cerebrospinal Fluid (CSF) and Meninges of the Brain. A, Ventricles highlighted in blue within a translucent brain in a left lateral view. **B,** Flow of cerebral spinal fluid. The fluid produced by filtration of blood by the choroid plexus of each ventricle flows inferiorly through the lateral ventricles, interventricular foramen, third ventricle, cerebral aqueduct, fourth ventricle, and subarachnoid space to the blood. **C,** Meninges of the brain in relation to CSF and venous blood flow. (**A, B,** from Waugh A, Grant A: *Ross and Wilson anatomy and physiology in health and illness,* ed 12, London, 2012, Churchill Livingstone. **C,** from Drake R, et al: *Gray's anatomy for students,* ed 3, London, 2015, Churchill Livingstone.)

of the sacrum. CSF contained within the subarachnoid space also circulates inferiorly to about the second sacral vertebra.

The meninges form potential and real spaces important to understanding functional and pathologic mechanisms. For example, between the dura mater and skull lies a potential space termed the extradural space (also called the epidural space) (see Fig. 14.16, *C*). The arterial supply to the meninges consists of blood vessels that lie within grooves in the skull. A skull fracture can severe one of these vessels and produce an epidural hematoma.

Cerebrospinal Fluid and the Ventricular System

Cerebrospinal fluid (CSF) is a clear, colorless fluid similar to blood plasma and interstitial fluid. The intracranial and spinal cord structures float in CSF and are thereby partially protected from jolts and blows. The buoyant properties of the CSF also prevent the brain from tugging

on meninges, nerve roots, and blood vessels. (Constituents of CSF are listed in Table 14.4.) Between 125 and 150 mL of CSF is circulating within the ventricles (small cavities) and subarachnoid space at any given time. Approximately 600 mL of CSF is produced daily.

Ependymal cells in the choroid plexuses of the lateral, third, and fourth ventricles produce the major portion of CSF. (Ventricles are illustrated in Fig. 14.16, *A*.) These plexuses are characterized by a rich network of blood vessels supplied by the pia mater and lie close to the ependymal cells. The tight junctions of the choroid blood vessel provide a limiting barrier between CSF and blood, which functions similarly to the blood–brain barrier (see the Blood–Brain Barrier section).

CSF exerts pressure within the brain and the spinal cord. When a person is supine, CSF pressure is about 80 to 180 mm of water pressure, or approximately 5 to 14 mm of mercury pressure, but doubles when the person moves to the upright position. CSF flow results from

TABLE 14.4 Composition of Cerebrospinal Fluid

Constituent	Normal Value
Sodium (Na^+)	148 mM
Potassium (K^+)	2.9 mM
Chloride (Cl^-)	125 mM
Bicarbonate (HCO_3^-)	22.9 mM
Glucose (fasting)	50-75 mg/dL (60% of serum glucose)
pH	7.3
Protein	15-45 mg/dL
Albumin	80%
Globulin	6-10%
Blood cells	
White (lymphocyte)	0-6/mm³
Red	0

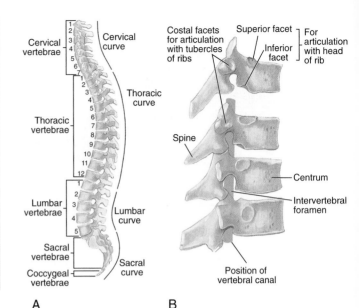

FIGURE 14.17 Vertebral Column. A, The normal curves and regions of the vertebral column. The vertebrae in each region are numbered. **B,** Lateral view of several vertebrae showing how they articulate. (From Solomon E: *Introduction to human anatomy and physiology,* ed 4, St Louis, 2016, Saunders.)

the pressure gradient between the arterial system and the CSF-filled cavities. Beginning in the lateral ventricles, the CSF flows through the interventricular foramen (foramen of Monro) into the third ventricle and then passes through the cerebral aqueduct (aqueduct of Sylvius) into the fourth ventricle (see Fig. 14.16, *B*). From the fourth ventricle the CSF may pass through either the paired lateral apertures (foramen of Luschka) or the median aperture (foramen of Magendie) before communicating with the subarachnoid spaces of the brain and spinal cord. CSF does not, however, accumulate. Instead, it is reabsorbed into the venous circulation through the arachnoid villi. The arachnoid villi protrude from the arachnoid space, through the dura mater, and lie within the blood flow of the venous sinuses (see Fig. 14.16, *B*). CSF is reabsorbed through a pressure gradient between the arachnoid villi and the cerebral venous sinuses. The villi function as one-way valves directing CSF outflow into the blood but preventing blood flow into the subarachnoid space. Thus CSF is formed from blood, and after circulating throughout the CNS, it returns to blood.

Vertebral Column

The vertebral column (Fig. 14.17) is composed of 33 vertebrae: 7 cervical, 12 thoracic, 5 lumbar, 5 fused sacral, and 4 fused coccygeal. Between each interspace (except for the fused sacral and coccygeal vertebrae) is an intervertebral disk (Fig. 14.18). At the center of the intervertebral disk is the nucleus pulposus, a pulpy mass of elastic fibers. The intervertebral disk absorbs shocks, preventing damage to the vertebrae. The intervertebral disk is also a common source of back problems. If too much stress is applied to the vertebral column, the disk contents may rupture and protrude into the spinal canal, causing compression of the spinal cord or nerve roots.

✓ QUICK CHECK 14.4
1. What information is conveyed in the ascending and descending spinal tracts?
2. Contrast the functions of upper and lower motor neurons.
3. Name the protective structures of the central nervous system, and briefly describe each one.

BLOOD SUPPLY

Blood Supply to the Brain

The brain receives approximately 20% of the cardiac output, or 800 to 1000 mL of blood flow per minute. Cerebral blood flow is autoregulated

to maintain a stable flow during fluctuating perfusion pressures. Carbon dioxide is a primary regulator for blood flow within the CNS. It is a potent vasodilator, and its effects ensure an adequate blood supply.

The brain derives its arterial supply from two systems: the internal carotid arteries and the vertebral arteries (Fig. 14.19). The internal carotid arteries supply a proportionately greater amount of blood flow. They originate at the common carotid arteries, enter the cranium through the base of the skull, and pass through the cavernous sinus. After forming some small branches, these arteries divide into the anterior and middle cerebral arteries (Fig. 14.20). The vertebral arteries originate at the subclavian arteries and pass through the transverse foramina of the cervical vertebrae, entering the cranium through the foramen magnum. They join at the junction of the pons and medulla to form the basilar artery (see Fig. 14.20). The basilar artery divides at the level of the midbrain to form paired posterior cerebral arteries.

The circle of Willis (see Fig. 14.20, *B*) provides an alternative route for blood flow when one of the contributing arteries is obstructed (collateral blood flow). The circle of Willis is formed by the posterior cerebral arteries, posterior communicating arteries, internal carotid arteries, anterior cerebral arteries, and anterior communicating artery. The anterior cerebral, middle cerebral, and posterior cerebral arteries leave the circle of Willis and extend to various brain structures, serving their associated brain territories. The border zone is the area between the major arterial territories (Table 14.5 and Fig. 14.21 describe the structures served, the functional relationships, and the pathologic considerations related to occlusion of cerebral arteries).

Cerebral venous drainage does not parallel its arterial supply, whereas the venous drainage of the brainstem and cerebellum does parallel the arterial supply of these structures. The cerebral veins are classified as superficial and deep veins. The veins drain into venous plexuses and dural sinuses (formed between the dural layers) and eventually join the internal jugular veins at the base of the skull (Fig. 14.22). Adequacy of venous outflow can significantly affect intracranial pressure. For example, when individuals with a head injury turn or let their heads fall to the side, the action partially occludes venous return, and intracranial pressure can increase because of decreased flow through the jugular veins.

Blood–Brain Barrier

The **blood–brain barrier (BBB)** describes cellular structures that selectively inhibit certain potentially harmful substances in blood from entering the interstitial spaces of the brain or CSF, thus allowing neurons to function normally. Endothelial cells in brain capillaries with their intracellular tight junctions are the site of the BBB. Supporting cells include astrocytes, pericytes (Fig. 14.23), and microglia.[2] Some substances, including glucose, lipid soluble molecules, electrolytes, and chemicals, can cross into and out of the brain facilitated by transport molecules. This has substantial implications for drug therapy because certain types of antibiotics and chemotherapeutic drugs show a greater propensity than others for crossing this barrier. Breakdown of the BBB can contribute to invasion of the brain by toxic molecules or pathogens promoting neuroinflammation and neurodegeneration.

Blood Supply to the Spinal Cord

The spinal cord derives its blood supply from branches off the vertebral arteries and from branches from various regions of the aorta. The **anterior spinal artery** and the paired **posterior spinal arteries** branch from the vertebral artery at the base of the cranium and descend alongside the spinal cord. Arterial branches from vessels exterior to the spinal cord follow the spinal nerve through the intervertebral foramina, pass through the dura, and divide into the anterior and posterior radicular arteries (Fig. 14.24).

The radicular arteries eventually connect to the spinal arteries. Branches from the radicular and spinal arteries form plexuses whose branches penetrate the spinal cord, supplying the deeper tissues. Venous drainage parallels the arterial supply closely and drains into venous sinuses located between the dura and periosteum of the vertebrae.

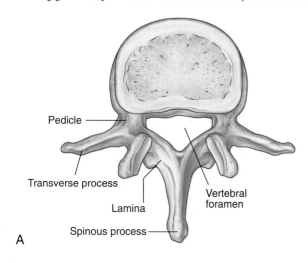

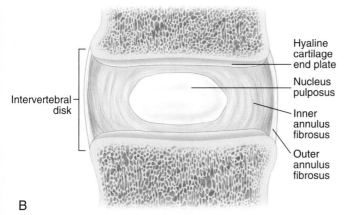

FIGURE 14.18 Intervertebral Disk. **A,** The normal curves and regions of the vertebral column. The vertebrae in each region are numbered. **B,** Lateral view of several vertebrae showing how they articulate. (**A,** from Drake R, Vogl AW, Mitchell AWM: *Gray's anatomy for students,* ed 3, London, 2015, Churchill Livingstone. **B,** from Lawry GV, et al: *Fam's musculoskeletal examination and joint injection techniques,* ed 2, Philadelphia, 2010, Mosby.)

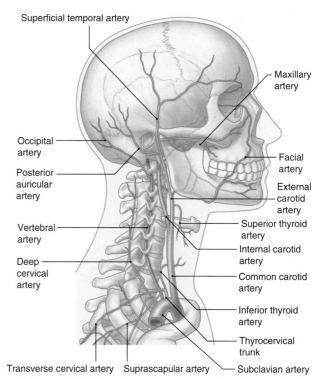

FIGURE 14.19 Major Arteries of the Head and Neck. (From Moses KP, et al: *Atlas of clinical gross anatomy,* ed 2, Philadelphia, 2013, Saunders.)

TABLE 14.5	Arterial Systems Supplying the Brain	
Arterial Origin	**Structures Served**	**Conditions Caused by Occlusion**
Anterior cerebral artery	Basal ganglia; corpus callosum; medial surface of cerebral hemispheres; superior surface of frontal and parietal lobes	Hemiplegia on contralateral side of body, greater in lower than in upper extremities
Middle cerebral artery	Frontal lobe; parietal lobe; temporal lobe (primarily cortical surfaces)	Aphasia in dominant hemisphere and contralateral hemiplegia (see Chapter 16)
Posterior cerebral artery	Part of diencephalon (thalamus, hypothalamus) and temporal lobe; occipital lobe	Visual loss; sensory loss; contralateral hemiplegia if cerebral peduncle affected

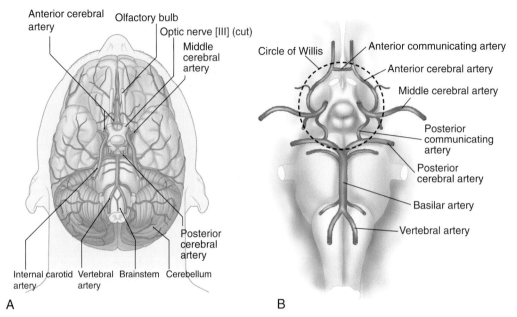

A   B

FIGURE 14.20 **Arteries at the Base of the Brain.** The arteries that compose the circle of Willis are the two anterior cerebral arteries, joined to each other by the anterior communicating artery and two short segments of the internal carotids, off of which the posterior communicating arteries connect to the posterior cerebral arteries. (**A,** from Moses KP, et al: *Atlas of clinical gross anatomy,* ed 2, Philadelphia, 2013, Saunders. **B,** from Hagen-Ansert S: *Textbook of diagnostic sonography,* ed 7, St Louis, 2012, Mosby.)

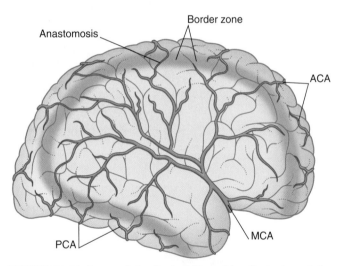

FIGURE 14.21 **Areas of the Brain Affected by Occlusion of the Anterior, Middle, and Posterior Cerebral Artery Branches.** *ACA,* Gray area affected by occlusion of branches of anterior cerebral artery; *MCA,* pink area affected by occlusion of branches of middle cerebral artery; *PCA,* orange area affected by occlusion of branches of posterior cerebral artery. Occlusions can occur in the cortical or deep areas of the border zone. (From Fitzgerald MJT et al: *Clinical neuroanatomy and neuroscience,* ed 6, Philadelphia, 2012, Saunders.)

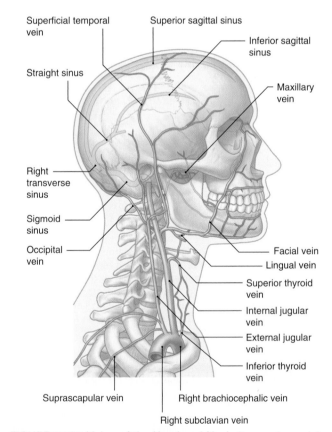

FIGURE 14.22 **Veins of the Head and Neck.** Deep veins and dural sinuses are projected on the skull. Note two superficial veins in the face are tributaries that send blood through emissary veins in the skull foramen into deep veins inside the skull terminating in the internal jugular vein. (From Moses KP, et al: *Atlas of clinical gross anatomy,* ed 2, Philadelphia, 2013, Saunders.)

✔**QUICK CHECK 14.5**
1. Describe the circle of Willis and explain its role in supplying blood to the brain.
2. What is the source of the spinal cord's blood supply?

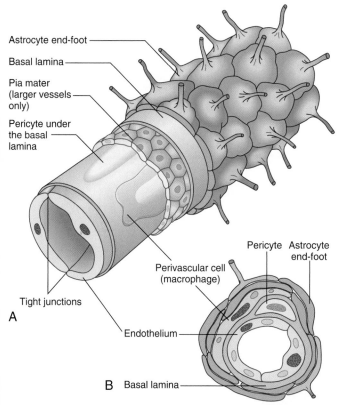

Astrocyte end-foot

Basal lamina

Pia mater (larger vessels only)

Pericyte under the basal lamina

Tight junctions

A

Perivascular cell (macrophage)

Pericyte   Astrocyte end-foot

Endothelium

B Basal lamina

FIGURE 14.23 Blood–Brain Barrier. A, Cellular structure of brain capillary. Endothelial cell membranes with tight junctions create a physical barrier between capillary blood and the brain, restricting movement of bacteria or neurotoxic substances. The pia mater is present only in larger vessels. **B,** Cross-section. (From Standring S: *Gray's anatomy*, ed 41, London, 2016, Elsevier.)

PERIPHERAL NERVOUS SYSTEM

The **peripheral nervous system (PNS)** includes the nerves outside the central nervous system (see Fig. 14.1). The somatic nervous system is the part of the PNS that controls voluntary muscle movement (efferent nerves) and sensory information (afferent nerves). The spinal nerves originate in the spinal cord. The cranial nerves originate in the brain and pass out of the skull. A peripheral nerve is composed of individual axons/dendrites, with most wrapped in a myelin sheath. These individual fibers are arranged in bundles called *fascicles* (Fig. 14.25, *B*). The coverings provide structural support, a blood supply, and interstitial compartments necessary for the delivery of essential electrolytes to support nerve impulse conduction.

The 31 pairs of **spinal nerves** derive their names from the vertebral level from which they exit: 8 cervical, 12 thoracic, 5 lumbar, 5 sacral and 1 coccygeal. The first cervical nerve exits above the first cervical vertebra, and the rest of the spinal nerves exit below their corresponding vertebrae. From the thoracic region (and inferiorly), nerves correspond to the vertebral level above their exit (see Fig. 14.11).

Spinal nerves contain both sensory and motor neurons and are called **mixed nerves**. Their structure can be compared to that of a tree (see Fig. 14.11, *B*). They arise as rootlets that combine into *roots* lateral to anterior and posterior horns of the spinal cord. These two spinal nerve roots converge in the region of the intervertebral foramen to form the spinal nerve *trunk*. Shortly after converging, the spinal nerve divides into anterior and posterior rami (*branches*). The anterior rami (except the thoracic) initially form **plexuses** (networks of nerve fibers), which then branch into the peripheral nerves. Instead of forming plexuses, the thoracic nerves pass through the intercostal spaces and innervate regions of the thorax.

The main spinal nerve plexuses innervate the skin and the underlying muscles of the limbs. The **brachial plexus**, for example, is formed by the last four cervical nerves (C5 to C8) and the first thoracic nerve (T1) (see Fig. 14.11). The brachial plexus innervates the nerves of the arm, wrist, and hand.

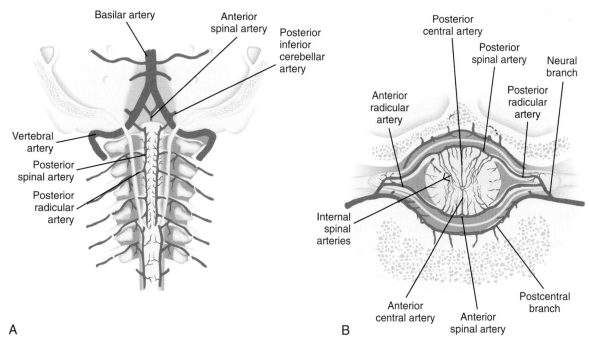

Basilar artery

Anterior spinal artery

Posterior inferior cerebellar artery

Vertebral artery

Posterior spinal artery

Posterior radicular artery

Posterior central artery

Posterior spinal artery

Neural branch

Posterior radicular artery

Anterior radicular artery

Internal spinal arteries

Anterior central artery

Anterior spinal artery

Postcentral branch

A

B

FIGURE 14.24 Arteries of the Spinal Cord. A, Arteries of cervical cord exposed from the rear. **B,** Arteries of spinal cord diagrammatically shown in horizontal section. (Redrawn from Rudy EB, editor: *Advanced neurological and neurosurgical nursing*, St Louis, 1984, Mosby.)

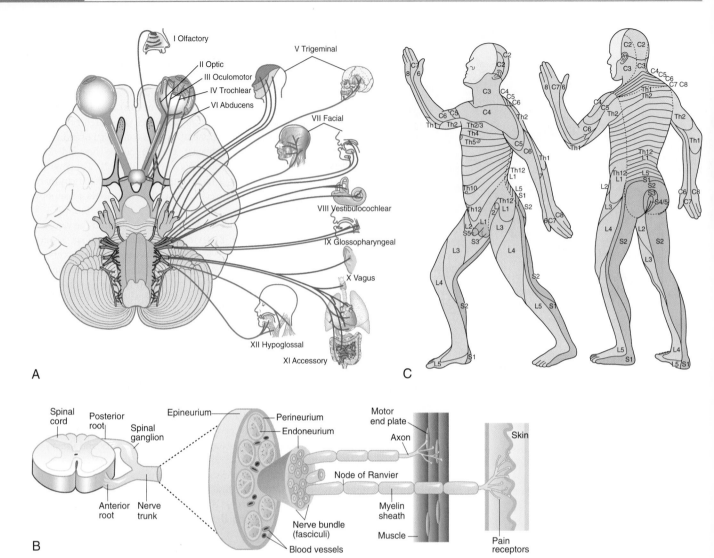

FIGURE 14.25 Cranial and Peripheral Nerves and Skin Dermatomes. A, Ventral surface of the brain showing attachment of the cranial nerves. The red lines indicate motor function, and the blue lines indicate sensory function. **B,** Peripheral nerve trunk and coverings. **C,** Dermatome map, anterolateral view (left) and posterolateral view (right). (**A,** from Applegate E: *The anatomy and physiology learning system,* ed 4, St Louis, 2011, Saunders. **C,** from Salvo SG: *Mosby's pathology for massage therapists,* ed 3, St Louis, 2014, Mosby.)

The posterior rami of each spinal nerve, with their many processes, are distributed to a specific area in the body. Sensory signals thus arise from specific sites associated with a specific spinal cord segment. Specific areas of cutaneous (skin) innervation at these spinal cord segments are called **dermatomes** (Fig. 14.25, *C*).

Like spinal nerves, **cranial nerves** are categorized as peripheral nerves. Most of these are mixed nerves (like the spinal nerves), although some are purely sensory or purely motor. Cranial nerves connect to nuclei in the brain and brainstem (see Fig. 14.25, *A*). Table 14.6 describes the cranial nerves and how to test them.

AUTONOMIC NERVOUS SYSTEM

The **autonomic nervous system (ANS)** coordinates and maintains a steady state among body organs and regulates cardiac muscle, smooth muscle, and the glands of the body.[3] This system is considered an involuntary system because one generally cannot *will* these functions to happen. Components of the ANS are located in both the CNS and the PNS, but the ANS is considered to be part of the efferent division

of the PNS. The ANS is separated both structurally and functionally into two divisions: (1) the sympathetic nervous system and (2) the parasympathetic nervous system (Fig. 14.26). The effects of these two divisions is usually antagonistic, which means one stimulates an effector and one inhibits an effector. In this way an effector, such as the heart or the blood vessels, can be precisely controlled. Many neurons of the ANS travel in the spinal nerves and certain cranial nerves. The widespread activity of this system indicates that its components are distributed all over the body. The peripheral autonomic nerves carry mainly efferent fibers and that will be the emphasis here. The *visceral* or *enteric autonomic nervous system* is a neural system that controls sensory and motor function of the gastrointestinal tract and operates independently of the brain and spinal cord.

The CNS has cardiovascular and respiratory centers in the reticular formation, and both the sympathetic and the parasympathetic areas in the hypothalamus. CNS pathways interconnect all these areas and project to autonomic areas in the brain stem and spinal cord. Both divisions of the ANS are composed of autonomic nerves, ganglia, and plexuses. These structures, in turn, are made up of efferent (motor) autonomic

TABLE 14.6   The Cranial Nerves

Number and Name	Function	How Tested
I. Olfactory	Purely sensory; carries impulses for sense of smell	Person is asked to sniff aromatic substances, such as oil of cloves and vanilla, and to identify them
II. Optic	Purely sensory; carries impulses for vision	Vision and visual field tested with an eye chart and by testing point at which person first sees an object (finger) moving into visual field; inside of eye is viewed with ophthalmoscope to observe blood vessels of eye interior
III. Oculomotor	Contains motor fibers to inferior oblique and to superior, inferior, and medial rectus extraocular muscles that direct eyeball; levator muscles of eyelid; smooth muscles of iris and ciliary body; and proprioception (sensory) to brain from extraocular muscles	Pupils examined for size, shape, and equality; pupillary reflex tested with a penlight (pupils should constrict when illuminated); ability to follow moving objects
IV. Trochlear	Proprioceptor and motor fibers for superior oblique muscle of eye (extraocular muscle)	Tested in common with cranial nerve III relative to ability to follow moving objects
V. Trigeminal	Both motor and sensory for face; conducts sensory impulses from mouth, nose, surface of eye, and dura mater; also contains motor fibers that stimulate chewing muscles	Sensations of pain, touch, and temperature tested with safety pin and hot and cold objects; corneal reflex tested with a wisp of cotton; motor branch tested by asking subject to clench teeth, open mouth against resistance, and move jaw from side to side
VI. Abducens	Contains motor fibers to lateral rectus muscle and proprioceptor fibers from same muscle to brain	Tested in common with cranial nerve III relative to ability to move each eye laterally
VII. Facial	Mixed: (1) supplies motor fibers to muscles of facial expression and to lacrimal and salivary glands and (2) carries sensory fibers from taste buds of anterior part of tongue	Anterior two-thirds of tongue tested for ability to taste sweet (sugar), salty, sour (vinegar), and bitter (quinine) substances; symmetry of face checked; subject asked to close eyes, smile, whistle, and so on; tearing tested with ammonia fumes
VIII. Vestibulocochlear (acoustic)	Purely sensory; vestibular branch transmits impulses for sense of equilibrium; cochlear branch transmits impulses for sense of hearing	Hearing checked by air and bone conduction by use of a tuning fork; vestibular tests: Bárány and caloric tests
IX. Glossopharyngeal	Mixed: (1) motor fibers serve pharynx (throat) and salivary glands, and (2) sensory fibers carry impulses from pharynx, posterior tongue (taste buds), and pressure receptors of carotid artery	Gag and swallow reflexes checked; subject asked to speak and cough; posterior one-third of tongue may be tested for taste
X. Vagus	Fibers carry sensory and motor impulses for pharynx; a large part of this nerve is parasympathetic motor fibers, which supply smooth muscles of abdominal organs; receives sensory impulses from viscera	Same as for cranial nerve IX (IX and X are tested in common) because they both serve muscles of throat
XI. Spinal accessory	Provides sensory and motor fibers for sternocleidomastoid and trapezius muscles and muscles of soft palate, pharynx, and larynx	Sternocleidomastoid and trapezius muscles checked for strength by asking subject to rotate head and shrug shoulders against resistance
XII. Hypoglossal	Carries motor fibers to muscles of tongue and sensory impulses from tongue to brain	Subject asked to stick out tongue, and any position abnormalities are noted

neurons that conduct impulses away from the brainstem or spinal cord and down to the autonomic effectors. The efferent component of the ANS is a two-neuron system. **Preganglionic neurons** (myelinated) conduct impulses from the brainstem or spinal cord to an autonomic ganglion, where they synapse with a postganglionic neuron. **Postganglionic neurons** (unmyelinated) conduct impulses away from the ganglion to the effector (Fig. 14.27). This arrangement contrasts with the efferent somatic nervous system, where a single motor neuron travels from the CNS to the innervated structure without passing through the ganglia (see Fig. 14.27, *D*).

Anatomy of the Sympathetic Nervous System

The **sympathetic nervous system** mobilizes energy stores in times of need (e.g., in the "fight or flight" or stress response) (see Chapter 10

and Fig. 10.2). The sympathetic division is innervated by cell bodies located from the first thoracic (T1) through the second lumbar (L2) regions of the spinal cord and therefore is called the **thoracolumbar division** (see Fig. 14.26). The preganglionic axons of the sympathetic division form synapses shortly after leaving the spinal cord in the **sympathetic (paravertebral) ganglia**. These preganglionic axons travel in several different ways: (1) directly synapsing with postganglionic neurons in the sympathetic chain ganglion at their level; (2) by traveling up the sympathetic chain ganglia; (3) by traveling down the sympathetic chain ganglion before forming synapses with a higher or lower postganglionic neuron; or (4) by traveling through the sympathetic chain ganglion to synapse with collateral ganglia (i.e., the **splanchnic nerves**, which lead to **collateral ganglia** on the front of the aorta). The collateral ganglia are named according to the branches

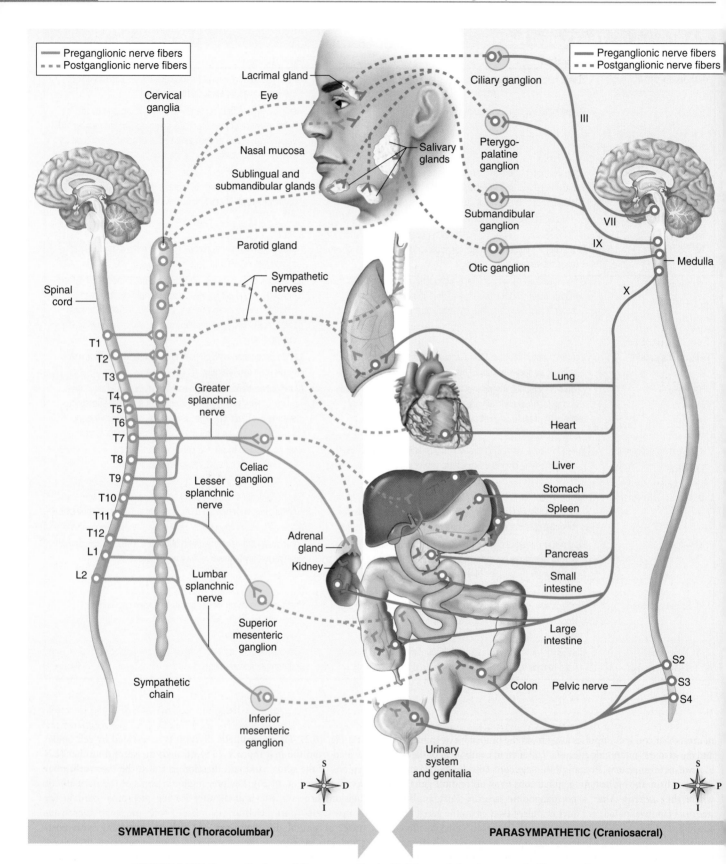

SYMPATHETIC (Thoracolumbar)

PARASYMPATHETIC (Craniosacral)

FIGURE 14.26 Sympathetic and Parasympathetic Divisions of the Autonomic Nervous System.
Preganglionic neuron cell bodies are located in the brainstem and sacral cord segments (parasympathetic or "craniosacral" division) and thoracic and upper lumbar cord segments (sympathetic or "thoracolumbar" division). The axons of these neurons synapse with postganglionic neurons, which innervate smooth muscle, cardiac muscle, and glands of the body. The postganglionic neuron cell bodies may be located in distinct autonomic ganglia *(represented by circles)* or very near the wall of the innervated visceral organ. Note that sympathetic fibers provide the only innervation to peripheral effectors (sweat glands, arrector pili muscles, adipose tissue, and blood vessels). (From Patton KA: *Anatomy & physiology*, ed 10, St Louis, 2019, Elsevier.)

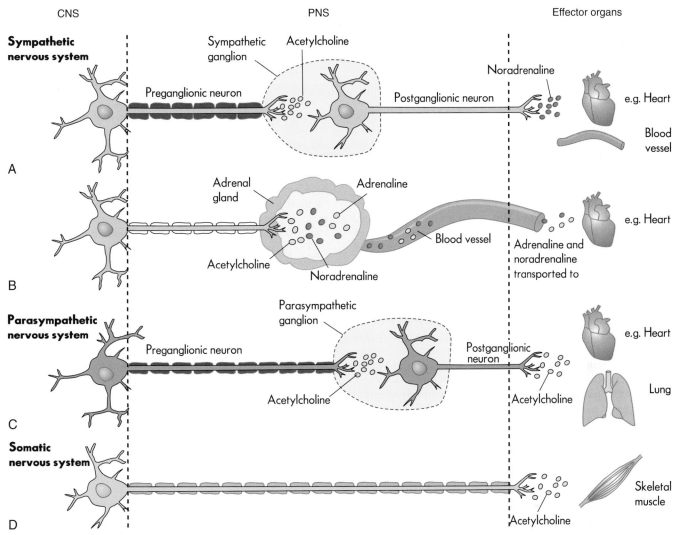

FIGURE 14.27 Comparison of Neurotransmitters and Receptors Between the Sympathetic and Parasympathetic Nervous Systems. Although not part of the autonomic nervous system, the somatic nervous system is included because of its similarity for comparison. In each case, the cell body of the first neuron is located in the central nervous system. (From Craft J, et al: *Understanding pathophysiology*, Australian adaptation, ed 2, Marrickville, Australia, 2015, Elsevier Australia.)

of the aorta nearest them, namely the celiac, superior mesenteric, and inferior mesenteric ganglia (see Fig. 14.26). Postganglionic neurons leave the collateral ganglia and innervate the viscera below the diaphragm.

Preganglionic sympathetic neurons that innervate the adrenal medulla also travel in the splanchnic nerves and *do not* synapse before reaching the gland (see Figs. 14.26 and 14.27, *B*). The secretory cells in the adrenal medulla are considered modified postganglionic neurons. Because preganglionic sympathetic fibers are all myelinated, travel to the adrenal medulla is quick, and innervation causes the rapid release of epinephrine and norepinephrine, which are mediators of the fight-or-flight response (see Chapter 10).

Anatomy of the Parasympathetic Nervous System

The parasympathetic nervous system conserves and restores energy when a person is at rest. The nerve cell bodies of this division are located in the cranial nerve nuclei and in the sacral region of the spinal cord and therefore constitute the craniosacral division. Unlike the sympathetic branch, the preganglionic fibers in the parasympathetic division are

longer and travel close to the organs they innervate before forming synapses with the relatively short postganglionic neurons (see Fig. 14.26). Parasympathetic nerves arising from nuclei in the brainstem travel to the viscera of the head, thorax, and abdomen within cranial nerves—including the oculomotor (III), facial (VII), glossopharyngeal (IX), and vagus (X) nerves.

Preganglionic parasympathetic nerves that originate from the sacral region of the spinal cord run either separately or together with some spinal nerves. The preganglionic axons unite to form the pelvic splanchnic nerve, which innervates the viscera of the pelvic cavity. These preganglionic axons synapse with postganglionic neurons in terminal ganglia located close to the organs they innervate.

Similar to the spinal nerves, the autonomic nerves also form plexuses. These are networks of nerves that have both parasympathetic and sympathetic neurons. They are usually located near the organs they innervate. Examples include the celiac (solar) plexus (contains the celiac ganglia and innervates many abdominal and pelvic organs), the cardiac plexus (innervates the heart), and Meissner and Auerbach plexuses (innervate the gastrointestinal tract).

Neurotransmitters and Neuroreceptors

Sympathetic preganglionic fibers and parasympathetic preganglionic and postganglionic fibers release acetylcholine—the same neurotransmitter released by somatic efferent neurons (see Fig. 14.27). These fibers are characterized by cholinergic transmission. Most postganglionic sympathetic fibers release norepinephrine (noradrenaline) and thus are considered to function by adrenergic transmission. A few postganglionic sympathetic fibers, such as those that innervate the sweat glands, release acetylcholine.

The action of catecholamines (adrenalin, noradrenaline) varies with the type of neuroreceptor stimulated. It should be remembered that catecholamines also are released by the adrenal medulla gland that physiologically and biochemically resembles the sympathetic nervous system. Two types of adrenergic receptors exist, α and β. Cells of the effector organs may have one or both types of adrenergic receptors. α-Adrenergic receptors have been further subdivided according to the action produced. α_1-Adrenergic activity is associated mostly with excitation or stimulation; α_2-adrenergic activity is associated with relaxation or inhibition. Most of the α-adrenergic receptors on effector organs belong to the α_1 class. β-Adrenergic receptors are classified as β_1-adrenergic receptors (which facilitate increased heart rate and contractility and cause the release of renin from the kidney) and β_2-adrenergic receptors (which facilitate all remaining effects attributed to β receptors).[4] Norepinephrine stimulates all α_1 and β_1 receptors and only certain β_2 receptors. The primary response from norepinephrine, however, is stimulation of α_1-adrenergic receptors that cause vasoconstriction. Epinephrine strongly stimulates all four types of receptors and induces general vasodilation because of the predominance of β receptors in muscle vasculatures. (Table 14.7 summarizes the effects of neuroreceptors on their effector organs.)

Functions of the Autonomic Nervous System

Many body organs are innervated by both the sympathetic and parasympathetic nervous systems. The two divisions often cause opposite responses; for example, sympathetic stimulation of the stomach causes decreased peristalsis, whereas parasympathetic stimulation of the intestine increases peristalsis. In general, sympathetic stimulation promotes responses for the protection of the individual. For example, sympathetic activity increases blood glucose levels and temperature and increases heart rate and blood pressure. In emergency situations, a generalized and widespread discharge of the sympathetic system occurs and is known as the "fight or flight" reflex or acute stress response (see Chapter 10).

This is accomplished by an increased firing frequency of sympathetic fibers and by activation of sympathetic fibers normally silent and at rest (fibers to the sweat glands, pilomotor muscles, and the adrenal medulla, as well as vasodilator fibers to muscle). Regulation of vasomotor tone is considered the single most important function of the sympathetic nervous system. (Fig. 14.28 illustrates some of the most important functions of the sympathetic nervous system.)

Increased parasympathetic activity promotes rest and tranquility and is characterized by reduced heart rate and enhanced visceral functions concerned with digestion. Stimulation of the vagus nerve (cranial nerve X) in the gastrointestinal tract increases peristalsis and secretion, as well as the relaxation of sphincters. Activation of parasympathetic fibers in the head, provided by cranial nerves III, VII, and IX, causes constriction of the pupil, tear secretion, and increased salivary secretion. Stimulation of the sacral division of the parasympathetic system contracts the urinary bladder and facilitates the process of penile erection.

The parasympathetic system lacks the generalized and widespread response of the sympathetic system. Specific parasympathetic fibers are activated to regulate particular functions. Although the actions of the parasympathetic and sympathetic systems are usually antagonistic, there are exceptions. Peripheral vascular resistance, for example, is increased dramatically by sympathetic activation but is not altered appreciably by activity of the parasympathetic system. Most blood vessels involved in the control of blood pressure are innervated by sympathetic nerves. To decrease blood pressure, therefore, it is more important to block or paralyze the continuous (tonic) discharge of the sympathetic system than to promote parasympathetic activity.

The CNS mechanisms involved in the aging process are extremely complex, and many questions have yet to be answered. *Geriatric Considerations: Aging & the Nervous System* contains a summary of the structural, cellular, cerebrovascular, and functional changes that occur in the nervous system with aging.

✔ QUICK CHECK 14.6

1. What are ganglia? Give two examples in the PNS.
2. What are the cranial nerves? Give three examples.
3. Describe the anatomy and function of the PNS.
4. What are the structural and functional divisions of the ANS?
5. Compare cholinergic and adrenergic transmission.
6. What are the functions of the ANS?

TABLE 14.7 Actions of Autonomic Nervous System Neuroreceptors

Effector Organ or Tissue	Adrenergic Receptors	Adrenergic Effects	Cholinergic Effects
Eye, iris			
Radial muscle	α_1	Dilation	—
Sphincter muscle	—	—	Constriction
Eye, ciliary muscle	β_2	Relaxation for far vision	Contraction for near vision
Lacrimal glands	α_1	Secretion	Secretion
Nasopharyngeal glands	—	—	Secretion
Salivary glands	α_1	Secretion of potassium and water	Secretion of potassium and water
	β	Secretion of amylase	—
Heart			
Sinoatrial (SA) node	β_1, β_2	Increase heart rate	Decrease heart rate; vagus arrest

TABLE 14.7   Actions of Autonomic Nervous System Neuroreceptors—cont'd

Effector Organ or Tissue	Adrenergic Receptors	Adrenergic Effects	Cholinergic Effects
Atrial	β_1, β_2	Increase contractility and conduction velocity	Decrease contractility; shorten action potential duration
Atrioventricular (AV) junction	β_1, β_2	Increase automaticity and propagation velocity	Decrease automaticity and propagation velocity
Purkinje system	β_1, β_2	Increase automaticity and propagation velocity	—
Ventricles	β_1, β_2	Increase contractility	Slight decrease in contraction
Arterioles			
Coronary	α_1, α_2, β_2	Constriction, dilation	Dilation
Skin and mucosa	α_1, α_2	Constriction	Dilation
Skeletal muscle	α, β_2	Dilation, constriction	Dilation
Cerebral	α_1	Constriction (slight)	Dilation
Pulmonary	α_1, β_2	Constriction, dilation	Dilation
Mesenteric	α_1	Constriction	Dilation
Renal	α_1, β_1, β_2	Constriction, dilation	Dilation
Salivary glands	α_1, α_2	Constriction	Dilation
Veins, systemic	α_1, α_2, β_2	Constriction, dilation	—
Lung			
Bronchial muscle	α_2	Relaxation	Contraction
Bronchial glands	α_1, β_2	Decrease secretion; increase secretion	Stimulation
Stomach			
Motility	α_1, α_2, β_1, β_2	Decrease (usually)	Increase
Sphincters	α_1	Contraction (usually)	Relaxation (usually)
Secretion	α_2	Inhibition	Stimulation
Liver	α_1, β_2	Glycogenolysis and gluconeogenesis	—
Gallbladder and ducts	β_2	Relaxation	Contraction
Pancreas			
Acini	α	Decrease secretion	Secretion
Islet cells	α_2, β_2	Decrease secretion; increase secretion	—
Intestine			
Motility and tone	α_1, α_2, β_1, β_2	Decrease	Increase
Sphincters	α_1	Contraction	Relaxation (usually)
Secretion	α_2	Inhibition	Stimulation
Adrenal medulla	—	Secretion of epinephrine and norepinephrine	
Kidney			
Renin secretion	α_1, β_1	Decrease; increase	—
Ureter			
Motility and tone	β_1	Increase	Increase (?)
Urinary bladder			
Detrusor	β_2	Relaxation	Contraction
Trigone and sphincter	α_1	Contraction	Relaxation
Sex organs, male	α_1	Ejaculation	Erection
Skin			
Pilomotor muscles	α_1	Contraction	—
Sweat glands	α_1	Localized secretion	—
Fat cells	α_2, β_1, β_2, β_3	Inhibition of lipolysis; stimulation of lipolysis	—
Pineal gland	β	Melatonin synthesis	—

Modified from Brunton LL et al, editors: *Goodman & Gilman's the pharmacological basis of therapeutics,* ed 12, New York, 2010, McGraw-Hill; Yagiela JA et al: *Pharmacology and therapeutics for dentistry,* ed 6, St Louis, 2011, Mosby.

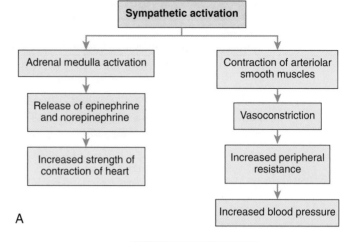

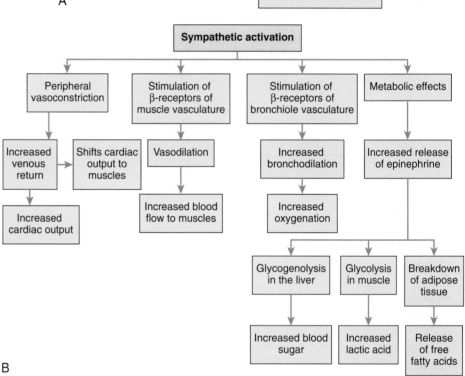

FIGURE 14.28 Examples of Important Functions of the Sympathetic Nervous System. **A,** Regulation of vasomotor tone. **B,** Regulation of strenuous muscular exercise ("fight-or-flight" or stress response). (See also Chapter 10 and Fig. 10.2 for more detail on the stress response.)

GERIATRIC CONSIDERATIONS

Aging and the Nervous System

Structural Changes With Aging

Decreased brain weight and size, particularly frontal regions
Increase in ventricular volume
Fibrosis and thickening of the meninges
Narrowing of gyri and widening of sulci
Increase in size of ventricles

Cellular Changes With Aging

Decrease in number of neurons not consistently related to changes in mental function
Decreased myelin
Lipofuscin deposition (a pigment resulting from cellular autodigestion)
Decreased number of dendritic processes and synaptic connections
Intracellular neurofibrillary tangles; significant accumulation in cortex associated with Alzheimer dementia
Imbalance in amount and distribution of neurotransmitters
Decrease in glucose metabolism

Cerebrovascular Changes With Aging

Arterial atherosclerosis (may cause infarcts and scars)
Increased permeability of blood–brain barrier
Decreased vascular density

Functional Changes With Aging

Decreased tendon reflexes
Progressive deficit in taste and smell
Decreased vibratory sense
Decrease in accommodation and color vision
Decrease in neuromuscular control with change in gait and posture
Sleep disturbances
Memory impairments
Cognitive alterations associated with chronic disease
Functional changes and nervous system aging have significant individual variation

Data from Chételat G et al: *Neuroimage* 76:167–177, 2013; Fjell AM, Walhovd KB: *Rev Neurosci* 21(3):187–221, 2010; Fjell AM et al: *Prog Neurobiol* 117:20–40, 2014; Xekardaki A et al: *Adv Exp Med Biol* 821:11–17, 2015.

SUMMARY REVIEW

Overview and Organization of the Nervous System

1. The divisions of the nervous system have been categorized as either structural (central nervous system [CNS] and peripheral nervous system [PNS]) or functional (somatic nervous system and autonomic nervous system [ANS]).
2. The CNS is contained within the brain and spinal cord.
3. The PNS is composed of cranial and spinal nerves, which carry impulses toward the CNS (afferent—sensory) and away from the CNS (efferent—motor) to and from target organs or skeletal muscle.

Cells of the Nervous System

1. The neuron and neuroglial cells (nonnerve cells) constitute nervous tissue. The neuron is specialized to transmit and receive electrical and chemical impulses, whereas the neuroglial cell provides supportive and maintenance functions.
2. The neuron is composed of a cell body, dendrite(s), and an axon. A myelin sheath around selected axons forms insulation that allows faster nerve impulse conduction.
3. The neuron is further divided into unipolar, pseudounipolar, bipolar, and multipolar categories, according to its structure and particular mechanics of impulse transmission.

The Nerve Impulse

1. The region between adjacent neurons is the synapse, and the region between the neuron and muscle is the neuromuscular junction.
2. Neurotransmitters are responsible for chemical conduction across the synapse, and the nerve impulse is regulated predominantly by a balance of inhibitory postsynaptic potentials (IPSPs) and excitatory postsynaptic potentials (EPSPs), temporal and spatial summation, and convergence and divergence.

The Central Nervous System

1. The cerebrum is the largest part of the brain and contains gray matter and white matter. The cerebral cortex is the outer layer of the brain and contains only gray matter arranged in folds; composed mostly of cell bodies.
2. The brain is contained within the cranial vault and is divided into three distinct regions: (1) forebrain, (2) hindbrain, and (3) midbrain.
3. The forebrain includes the *telencephalon* (the two cerebral hemispheres) and allows conscious perception of internal and external stimuli, thought and memory processes, and voluntary control of skeletal muscles. The deep portion of the forebrain is termed the *diencephalon* and processes incoming sensory data. The center for voluntary control of skeletal muscle movements is located along the precentral gyrus in the frontal lobe, whereas the center for perception is along the postcentral gyrus in the parietal lobe. The Broca area (inferior frontal gyrus – motor function) and the Wernicke area (superior temporal gyrus – sensory function) are major speech centers.
4. The midbrain is primarily a relay center for motor and sensory tracts, as well as a center for auditory and visual reflexes.
5. The hindbrain allows sampling and comparison of sensory data, which are received from the periphery and motor impulses of the cerebral hemispheres, for the purpose of coordination and refinement of skeletal muscle movement.
6. The spinal cord contains most of the nerve fibers that connect the brain with the periphery. The corticospinal tracts are descending pyramidal (motor) pathways from the motor cortex. The rubrospinal and reticulospinal tracts are descending extrapyramidal tracts that coordinate movement. The anterior, posterior, and lateral spinothalamic tracts carry sensory information to the brainstem and thalamus, where information is relayed to the sensory cortex. Reflex arcs are sensory and motor circuits completed in the spinal cord and influenced by the higher centers in the brain.
7. The CNS is protected by the bony cranium, meninges (dura mater, arachnoid, membrane, and pia mater), cerebrospinal fluid (CSF), and vertebral column. CSF is formed from blood components in the choroid plexuses of the ventricles and is reabsorbed in the arachnoid villi (located in the dural venous sinuses) after circulating through the brain and subarachnoid space.
8. The paired carotid and vertebral arteries supply blood to the brain and connect to form the circle of Willis. The major branches projecting from the circle of Willis are the anterior, middle, and posterior cerebral arteries. Drainage of blood from the brain is accomplished through the venous sinuses and jugular veins.
9. The blood–brain barrier is provided by tight junctions between the cells of brain capillary endothelial cells and surrounding supporting cells.
10. Blood supply to the spinal cord originates from the vertebral arteries and branches arising from the aorta.

The Peripheral Nervous System

1. The cranial and spinal nerves constitute the PNS. The PNS relays information from the CNS to muscle and effector organs through cranial and spinal nerve tracts arranged in fascicles (multiple fascicles bound together form the peripheral nerve).

The Autonomic Nervous System

1. The ANS is responsible for maintaining a steady state in the internal environment. Two opposing systems make up the ANS: (1) the sympathetic nervous system (thoracolumbar division) responds to stress by mobilizing energy stores and prepares the body to defend itself, and (2) the parasympathetic nervous system (craniosacral division) conserves energy and the body's resources. Both systems function, more or less, at the same time. The enteric autonomic nervous system controls the function of the gastrointestinal tract.

KEY TERMS

Acetylcholine, 322
Adrenergic transmission, 322
Afferent (sensory) neuron, 309
Afferent pathway (ascending pathway), 298
α-Adrenergic receptor, 322
Anterior column, 309

Anterior fossa, 311
Anterior horn (ventral horn), 309
Anterior spinal artery, 315
Anterior spinothalamic tract, 311
Arachnoid, 312
Arachnoid villi, 314

Association fiber, 305
Associational neuron (interneuron), 299
Astrocyte, 300
Autonomic nervous system (ANS), 298, 298
Axon, 299

Axon hillock, 299
Basal ganglia (basal nuclei) system, 305
Basilar artery, 314
Basis pedunculi, 308
β-Adrenergic receptor, 322
Bipolar neuron, 299

REFERENCES

1. Sulaiman W, Gordon T: Neurobiology of peripheral nerve injury, regeneration, and functional recovery: from bench top research to bedside application, *Ochsner J* 13(1):100-108, 2013.

2. Daneman R, Prat A: The blood-brain barrier, *Cold Spring Harb Perspect Biol* 7(1):a020412, 2015.
3. Karemaker JM: An introduction into autonomic nervous function, *Physiol Meas* 38(5):R89-R118, 2017.

4. Siegel R, et al: *Basic neurochemistry: molecular, cellular, and medical aspects*, ed 8, Philadelphia, 2012, Academic Press.

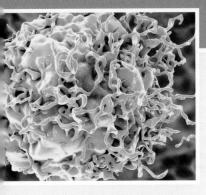

15

Pain, Temperature, Sleep, and Sensory Function

George W. Rodway, Sue E. Huether

EVOLVE WEBSITE

http://evolve.elsevier.com/Huether/
Student Review Questions
Audio Key Points

Case Studies
Animations
Quick Check Answers

Alterations in sensory function may involve dysfunctions of the general or the special senses. Dysfunctions of the general senses include chronic pain, abnormal temperature regulation, and tactile or proprioceptive dysfunction. Like pain, variations in temperature can signal disease. Fever is a common manifestation of dysfunction and is often the first symptom observed in an infectious or inflammatory condition.

Sleep is a normal cyclic process that restores the body's energy and maintains normal functioning. Sleep deprivation causes a wide range of clinical manifestations. Dysfunctions of the special senses include visual, auditory, vestibular, olfactory, and gustatory (taste) disorders.

PAIN

Pain is a complex experience. It is comprised of dynamic interactions between physical, cognitive, spiritual, emotional, and environmental factors and cannot be characterized as only a response to injury. McCaffery defined pain as "whatever the experiencing person says it is, existing whenever he says it does."[1] The International Association for the Study of Pain and the American Pain Society defined pain as "an unpleasant sensory and emotional experience associated with actual or potential tissue damage or described in terms of such damage."[2] A more recent proposal for the definition of pain is "pain is a mutually recognizable somatic experience that reflects a person's apprehension of threat to their bodily or existential integrity."[3] Acute pain is protective and promotes withdrawal from painful stimuli, allows the injured part to heal, and teaches avoidance of painful stimuli.

Neuroanatomy of Pain

Three parts of the nervous system are responsible for the sensation, perception and response to pain:
1. The *afferent pathways,* which begin in the peripheral nervous system (PNS), travel to the spinal gate in the dorsal horn and then ascend to areas in the diencephalon (thalamus, epithalamus, and hypothalamus) and cortex.
2. The *interpretive centers* located in the subcortical and cortical networks, brainstem, midbrain, diencephalon, and cerebral cortex.
3. The *efferent pathways* that descend from the central nervous system (CNS) back to the dorsal horn of the spinal cord.

The processing of potentially harmful (noxious) stimuli through a normally functioning nervous system is called **nociception**. **Nociceptors**, or pain receptors, are free nerve endings in the afferent peripheral nervous system. When they are stimulated, they cause **nociceptive pain**. The cell bodies of nociceptors are located in the dorsal root ganglia (DRG) for the body and in the trigeminal ganglion for the face. Nociceptors have a peripheral and central axonal branch that innervates their target organ and the spinal cord, respectively. Nociceptors are unevenly distributed throughout the body, so the relative sensitivity to pain differs according to their location (Table 15.1). Nociceptors respond to different types of noxious stimuli: mechanical (pressure or mechanical distortion), thermal (extreme temperatures), or chemical (acids or chemicals of inflammation, such as bradykinin, histamine, leukotrienes, or prostaglandins). Nociception involves four phases: transduction, transmission, perception, and modulation.[4]

Pain transduction begins when nociceptors are activated by a noxious stimulus, causing ion channels (sodium, potassium, calcium) on nociceptors to open, creating electrical impulses that travel through axons of

TABLE 15.1 Stimuli That Activate Nociceptors (Pain Receptors)

Location of Receptor	Provoking Stimuli
Skin	Pricking, cutting, crushing, burning, freezing
Gastrointestinal tract	Engorged or inflamed mucosa, distention or spasm of smooth muscle, traction on mesenteric attachment
Skeletal muscle	Ischemia, injuries of connective tissue sheaths, necrosis, hemorrhage, prolonged contraction, injection of irritating solutions
Joints	Synovial membrane inflammation
Arteries	Piercing, inflammation
Head	Traction, inflammation, or displacement of arteries, meningeal structures, and sinuses; prolonged muscle contraction
Heart	Ischemia and inflammation
Bone	Periosteal injury: fractures, tumor, inflammation

two primary types of nociceptors that are transmitted to the spinal cord, brainstem, thalamus, and cortex (see Fig. 14.15).[5] The two primary types of nociceptors are: **A-delta (Aδ) fibers** and **C fibers**. Aδ fibers are larger myelinated fibers that rapidly transmit sharp, well-localized "fast" pain sensations, such as intense heat or a pinprick to the skin. Activation of these fibers causes a spinal reflex withdrawal of the affected body part from the stimulus, before a pain sensation is perceived. C fibers are the most numerous, are smaller and unmyelinated, and are located in muscle, tendons, body organs, and in the skin. They slowly transmit dull, aching, or burning sensations that are poorly localized and often constant.

Pain transmission is the conduction of pain impulses along the Aδ and C fibers (primary-order neurons) into the dorsal horn of the spinal cord (Fig. 15.1). Here they form synapses with excitatory or inhibitory interneurons (second-order neurons) in the substantia gelatinosa of the dorsal horn. The impulses then synapse with projection neurons (third-order neurons), cross the midline of the spinal cord, and ascend to the brain through two lateral spinothalamic tracts. The anterior spinal thalamic tract carries fast impulses for acute sharp pain. The lateral spinothalamic tract carries slow impulses for dull or chronic pain. The fast sharp pain is perceived first, followed by dull, throbbing pain. These tracts connect to the reticular formation, hypothalamus, thalamus (the major relay station of sensory information), and limbic system. The impulses are then projected to the somatosensory cortex for interpretation of the location and intensity of the pain (see Fig. 15.1), and to other areas of the brain for an integrated response to pain.

Pain perception is the conscious awareness of pain, which occurs primarily in the reticular and limbic systems and the cerebral cortex. Interpretation of pain is influenced by many factors, including genetics, cultural preferences, sex roles, age, level of health, and life experience, including past pain experiences. Three systems interact to produce the

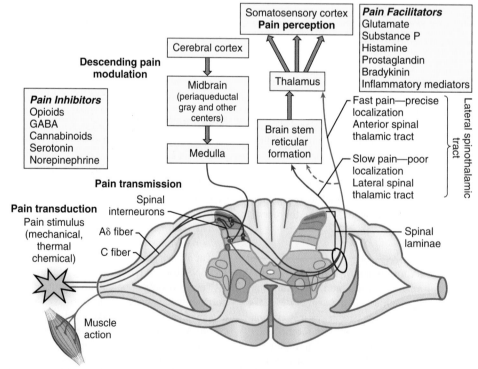

FIGURE 15.1 Transmission of Pain Sensations. The Aδ and C fibers synapse in the laminae of the dorsal horn, cross over to the contralateral spinothalamic tract, and then ascend to synapse in the midbrain through the neospinothalamic and paleospinothalamic tracts. Impulses are then conducted to the sensory cortex. Descending pain inhibition is initiated in the cerebral cortex or from the midbrain and medulla.

perception of pain.[6] The **sensory-discriminative system** is mediated by the somatosensory cortex and is responsible for identifying the presence, character, location, and intensity of pain. The **affective-motivational system** determines an individual's conditioned avoidance behaviors and emotional responses to pain. It is mediated through the reticular formation, limbic system, and brainstem. The **cognitive-evaluative system** overlies the individual's learned behavior concerning the experience of pain and therefore can modulate perception of pain. It is mediated through the cerebral cortex. The integration of these three systems is referred to as the "pain matrix"[7] or networks of cerebral connectivity.

Pain threshold and tolerance are subjective phenomena that influence an individual's perception of pain. They can be influenced by genetics, sex, cultural perceptions, expectations, role socialization, physical and mental health, and age (Table 15.2).

Pain threshold is defined as the lowest intensity of pain that a person can recognize.[2] Intense pain at one location may increase the threshold in another location. For example, a person with severe pain in one knee is more likely to experience less intense chronic back pain (this is called **perceptual dominance**). Because of perceptual dominance, pain at one site may mask other painful areas. Stress, excessive physical exertion, acupuncture, sexual activity, and other factors can increase the levels of circulating neuromodulators, thereby raising the pain threshold.

Pain tolerance is defined as the greatest intensity of pain that a person can endure.[2] It varies greatly among people and in the same person over time because of the body's ability to respond differently to noxious stimuli. Pain tolerance generally *decreases* with repeated exposure to pain, fatigue, anger, boredom, apprehension, and sleep deprivation and may *increase* with alcohol consumption, persistent use of opioid medications, hypnosis, distracting activities, and strong beliefs or faith.

Pain Modulation

Pain modulation involves many different mechanisms that increase or decrease the transmission of pain signals throughout the nervous system. Depending on the mechanism, modulation can occur before, during, or after pain is perceived.[8]

Neurotransmitters of Pain Modulation

A wide variety of neurotransmitters act to modulate control over transmission of pain impulses in the periphery, spinal cord, and brain. The peripheral triggering mechanisms that initiate release of excitatory neurotransmitters include tissue injury (prostaglandins, histamine, bradykinin) and chronic inflammatory lesions (lymphokines). Glutamate, aspartate, substance P, and calcitonin are common excitatory neurotransmitters in the brain and spinal cord. These substances sensitize nociceptors by reducing the activation threshold, leading to increased responsiveness of nociceptors.

Inhibitory neurotransmitters in the CNS include gamma-aminobutyric acid (GABA) and glycine. Norepinephrine and 5-hydroxytryptamine (serotonin) contribute to pain inhibition in the CNS but can excite peripheral nerves.

Endogenous opioids are a family of morphine-like neuropeptides that inhibit transmission of pain impulses in the periphery, spinal cord, and brain by binding with specific opioid receptors (mu [μ], kappa [κ], and delta [δ]) on neurons. They inhibit ion channels, preventing the release of excitatory neurotransmitters, such as substance P and glutamate, in the dorsal horn. In the midbrain they influence descending inhibitory pathways[9] (Fig. 15.2). In peripheral inflamed tissue, opioids are produced and released from immune cells and activate opioid receptors on sensory nerve terminals.[10] Opioid receptors are widely distributed throughout the body and are responsible for general sensations of well-being and modulation of many physiologic processes, including control of respiratory and cardiovascular functions, stress and immune responses, gastrointestinal function, reproduction, and neuroendocrine control.[11,12]

Enkephalins are the most prevalent of the natural opioids and bind to δ opioid receptors. **Endorphins** (endogenous morphine) are produced in the brain. The best studied endorphin is β-endorphin, which binds to μ receptors and is purported to produce the greatest sense of exhilaration as well as substantial natural pain relief. **Dynorphins** are the most potent of the endogenous opioids, binding strongly with κ receptors to impede pain signals. Paradoxically, they play a role in neuropathic pain and in mood disorders and drug addiction. **Endomorphins** bind with μ receptors and have potent analgesic effects. **Nociceptin/orphanin FQ** is an opioid that *induces* pain or hyperalgesia but does not interact with opioid receptors. The nociceptin receptor is widely distributed throughout the PNS and CNS and is also associated with inflammation, immune regulation, mood, and emotion.

Synthetic and natural opiates have pharmacologic actions similar to morphine and bind as direct agonists to the opioid receptors. Morphine has a 50 times higher affinity for μ receptors in comparison with other opioids. Naloxone is the only clinically used opioid receptor antagonist, with a higher affinity for the μ receptors than for the other receptors.

TABLE 15.2	**Pain Perception in Infants, Children, and Elderly Persons**		
	Infants	**Children**	**Elderly Persons**
Pain threshold	Painful neonatal experiences increase pain sensitivity (lower threshold); pain may be increased with future procedures	Lower or same as adults	Individual responses may vary but pain threshold may be elevated
Physiologic symptoms	Increased heart rate, blood pressure, and respiratory rate; flushing or pallor, sweating, and decreased oxygen saturation	Same as infants; nausea and vomiting	Same as infants and children; nausea and vomiting; may be decreased in individuals with cognitive impairment
Behavioral responses	Changes in facial expression, crying, and body movements, with lowered brows drawn together; vertical bulge and furrows in forehead between brows; broadened nasal root; tightly closed eyes; angular, square-shaped mouth, chin quiver; withdrawal of affected limbs, rigidity, flailing	Individual responses vary	Individual responses vary and may be influenced by presence of painful chronic diseases and decline in renal, intestinal, hepatic, cardiovascular, and neurologic function; individuals with cognitive impairment may demonstrate changes in behavior (e.g., combative or withdrawn, increased confusion)

Data from Anand KJS: *Acta Paediatr* 106(9):1438-1444, 2017; Lautenbacher S et al: *Neurosci Biobehav Rev* 75:104-113, 2017; Tracy B, Sean Morrison R: *Clin Ther* 35(11):1659-1668, 2013; Walker SM: *Paediatr Anaesth* 24(1):39-48, 2014.

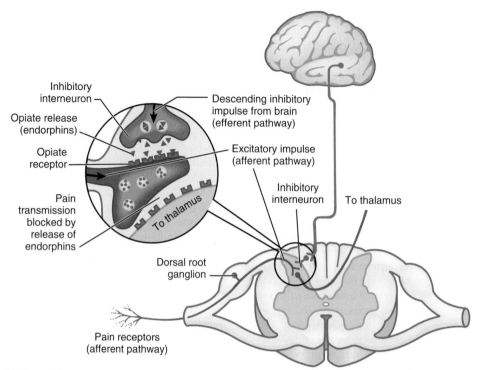

FIGURE 15.2 Descending Pathway and Endorphin Response. In this figure, a descending inhibitory impulse is transmitted from the brain to an inhibitory interneuron in the dorsal horn, stimulating the release of endorphin. The endorphin activates a mu opioid receptor and results in inhibition of pain transmission to ascending pathways.

Endocannabinoids are synthesized from phospholipids and are classified as eicosanoids. They activate cannabinoid CB$_1$ (primarily in the CNS) and CB$_2$ receptors (primarily in immune tissue [e.g., the spleen]) to modulate pain and other functions, including memory, appetite, immune function, sleep, stress response, thermoregulation, and addiction. CB$_1$ receptors decrease pain transmission by inhibiting release of excitatory neurotransmitters in the spinal dorsal horn, periaqueductal gray (PAG; the gray matter surrounding the cerebral aqueduct), thalamus, rostral ventromedial medulla (RVM), and amygdala. Cannabis (marijuana) produces a resin containing cannabinoids. Cannabinoids are analgesic in humans, but their use is limited by their psychoactive and addictive properties. Work is in progress to develop cannabinoid receptor agonists that do not have addictive side effects.[13,14]

Pathways of Modulation

Descending inhibitory and facilitatory pathways and nuclei inhibit or facilitate pain. Inhibitory pathways can activate opioid receptors and inhibit release of excitatory neurotransmitters, facilitate release of inhibitory neurotransmitters, or stimulate inhibitory interneurons. Afferent stimulation of particularly the ventromedial medulla and PAG in the midbrain stimulates efferent pathways, which inhibit ascending pain signals at the dorsal horn. The RVM stimulates descending pathways that facilitate or inhibit pain in the dorsal horn.

Segmental pain inhibition occurs when A-beta (Aβ) fibers (large myelinated fibers that transmit touch and vibration sensations) are stimulated and the impulses arrive at the same spinal level or segment as impulses from Aδ or C fibers. They stimulate an inhibitory interneuron and decrease pain transmission. An example is rubbing an area that has been injured to relieve pain.

Diffuse noxious inhibitory control (DNIC) is an inhibitory pain system that involves a spinal-medullary-spinal pathway. Pain is relieved when two noxious or painful stimuli occur at the same time from different sites (pain inhibiting pain). This also is known as heterosegmental pain inhibition or conditioned pain modulation and is the basis for pain relief with acupuncture, deep massage, or intense cold or heat.[15]

Expectancy-related cortical activation (placebo effect [beneficial expectations] or nocibo effect [adverse expectations]) can exert control over analgesic systems to attenuate or intensify pain.[16] In other words, cognitive expectations can cause real, measurable physiologic effects that share some of the same descending pain pathways as the pain modulatory systems.

Clinical Descriptions of Pain

Pain can be described in a variety of ways. Because of the complex nature of pain, however, many terms overlap, and more than one description is often used. The broad categories of pain are summarized in Box 15.1. Some of the most common clinical pain presentations are summarized here.

Acute pain (nociceptive pain) is a normal protective mechanism that alerts the individual to a condition or experience that is immediately harmful to the body and mobilizes the individual to take prompt action to relieve it. Acute pain is transient, usually lasting seconds to days, sometimes up to 3 months. It begins suddenly and is relieved after the chemical mediators (usually related to inflammation) that stimulate pain receptors are removed. Stimulation of the autonomic nervous system results in physical manifestations, including increased heart rate, hypertension, diaphoresis, and dilated pupils. Anxiety related to the pain experience, including its cause, treatment, and prognosis, is common, as is the hope of recovery and expectation of limited duration.

Acute pain arises from cutaneous, deep somatic, or visceral structures and can be classified as (1) somatic, (2) visceral, or (3) referred. Somatic pain arises from the skin (i.e., from an abrasion or a laceration), joints (pain from arthritis or injured tendons), and muscles (strain from

BOX 15.1   Categories of Pain

I. Neurophysiologic Pain
  A. Nociceptive pain
    1. Somatic (e.g., skin, muscle, bone)
    2. Visceral (e.g., intestine, liver, stomach)
    3. Referred
  B. Neuropathic (non-nociceptive)
    1. Central pain (lesion in brain or spinal cord)
    2. Peripheral pain (lesion in peripheral nervous system)
II. Neurogenic Pain
  A. Neuralgia (pain in the distribution of a nerve)
  B. Constant
    1. Sympathetically independent
    2. Sympathetically dependent
III. Temporal Pain (time related, duration)
  A. Acute pain
    1. Somatic
    2. Visceral
    3. Referred
  B. Chronic (pain lasting longer than 3 months)
IV. Pain Location
  A. Abdominal pain
  B. Chest pain
  C. Headache
  D. Low back pain
  E. Orofacial pain
  F. Pelvic pain
V. Etiologic Pain
  A. Cancer pain
  B. Dental pain
  C. Inflammatory pain
  D. Ischemic pain
  E. Vascular pain

Adapted from Mersky H: Taxonomy and classification of chronic pain syndromes. In Benzon HT et al, editors: *Practical management of pain*, ed 5, pp 13-18, St Louis, 2014, Mosby.

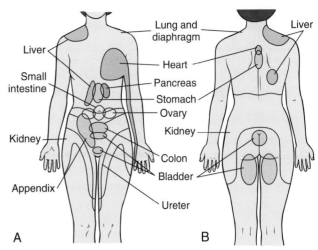

FIGURE 15.3 Sites of Referred Pain. A, Anterior view. B, Posterior view.

Chronic or persistent pain has been defined as lasting for more than 3 to 6 months in adults and is pain lasting well beyond the expected normal healing time. It varies with the type of injury and among individuals.[17] Chronic or persistent pain serves no purpose and is poorly understood and causes suffering. It often appears to be out of proportion to any observable tissue injury. It may be ongoing (e.g., low back pain) or intermittent (e.g., migraine headaches). Changes in the PNS and CNS that cause dysregulation of nociception and pain modulation processes (peripheral and central sensitization) are thought to lead to chronic pain (see the discussion of neuropathic pain later in this section).

Neuroimaging studies have demonstrated brain changes in individuals with chronic pain, which may lead to cognitive deficits and decreased ability to cope with pain.[18] These negative manifestations of chronic pain are thought to be due, in part, to the stress of coping with continuous pain and may be reversible when pain is controlled. Because it is not yet possible to predict when acute pain will develop into chronic pain, early treatment of acute pain is encouraged.

Physiologic responses to intermittent chronic pain are similar to those for acute pain, whereas persistent pain allows for physiologic adaptation, producing a normal heart rate and blood pressure. This leads many to mistakenly conclude that people with chronic pain are malingering because they do not appear to be in pain. As chronic pain progresses, certain behavioral and psychologic changes often emerge, including depression, difficulty eating and sleeping, preoccupation with the pain, and avoidance of pain-provoking stimuli.[19] The desire to relieve pain and the need to hide it become conflicting drives for those with chronic pain, who fear being labeled complainers.[20] Chronic pain is perceived as meaningless and is often associated with a sense of hopelessness as more time elapses and no relief seems possible. Some of the chronic pain syndromes are listed in Table 15.3. Comparison of acute and chronic pain is summarized in Table 15.4. Chronic pain associated with specific organ systems is discussed in later chapters. Neuropathic pain is presented next.

Neuropathic pain is chronic pain initiated or caused by a primary lesion or dysfunction in the nervous system and leads to long-term changes in pain pathway structures (neuroplasticity) and abnormal processing of sensory information.[21] There is amplification of pain without stimulation by injury or inflammation. Neuropathic pain is often described as burning, shooting, shocklike, or tingling. It is characterized by increased sensitivity to painful or nonpainful stimuli with

overuse or muscle injury). It is either sharp and well localized (especially fast pain carried by Aδ fibers) or dull, aching, throbbing, and poorly localized, as seen in polymodal C fiber transmissions. Visceral pain is transmitted by C fibers and refers to pain in internal organs and the lining of body cavities; it tends to be poorly localized with an aching, gnawing, throbbing, or intermittent cramping quality. It is carried by sympathetic fibers and is associated with nausea and vomiting, hypotension and, in some cases, shock. Visceral pain often radiates (spreads away from the actual site of the pain) or is referred. Examples of conditions that cause visceral pain include gallstones, pancreatitis, kidney stones, bowel obstruction, appendicitis, and bladder infection. Referred pain is felt in an area removed or distant from its point of origin—the area of referred pain is supplied by the same spinal segment as the actual site of pain. Referred pain can be acute or chronic. Impulses from many cutaneous and visceral neurons converge on the same ascending neuron, and the brain cannot distinguish between the different sources of pain. Because the skin has more receptors, the painful sensation is experienced at the referred site instead of at the site of origin. Referred pain can be acute or chronic. For example, the pain of pancreatitis may be felt in the right shoulder or scapula, or pain from the heart may be referred to the left shoulder or arm. Fig. 15.3 illustrates common areas of referred pain and their associated sites of origin.

TABLE 15.3	Common Chronic Pain Syndromes
Condition	Description
Persistent low back pain	Most common chronic pain condition Results from poor muscle tone, inactivity, muscle strain, or sudden, vigorous exercise
Myofascial pain syndromes	Pain results from muscle spasm, tenderness, stiffness, or injury to muscle and fascia with peripheral and central sensitization Examples include myositis, fibrositis, myalgia, fibromyalgia, and muscle strain Trigger points—small hypersensitive regions in muscle or connective tissues that, when stimulated, produce pain in a specific area As disorder progresses, pain becomes increasingly generalized
Chronic postoperative pain	Persistent pain that can occur with disruption or cutting of sensory nerves; examples include post-thoracotomy, postmastectomy; risk factors may include preexisting pain and genetic susceptibility
Cancer pain	Attributed to advance of disease, treatment, or coexisting disease entities
Deafferentation pain	Pain because of alteration of sensory input into central nervous system is caused by damage to peripheral nerves Common types include severe burning pain triggered by various stimuli, such as cold, light touch, or sound, and complex regional pain syndromes (occur after peripheral nerve injury and are characterized by continuous, severe, burning pain associated with vasomotor changes and muscle wasting)
Hyperalgesia	Increased sensitivity and decreased pain threshold to tactile and painful stimuli Pain is diffuse, modified by fatigue and emotion, and mixed with other sensations May result from chronic irritation of central nervous system areas
Hemiagnosia	Loss of ability to identify source of pain on one side of body Painful stimuli on that side produce discomfort, anxiety, moaning, agitation, and distress but no attempt to withdraw from stimulus Associated with stroke
Phantom limb pain	Pain experienced in amputated limb after stump has completely healed; may be immediate or occur months later; associated with preamputation pain, acute postoperative pain Exact cause is unknown, thought to originate in brain; can be influenced by emotions/sympathetic stimulation
Complex regional pain syndrome	Chronic pain is usually associated with limb injury, surgery, or fractures Characterized by autonomic and neuroinflammatory features and pain out of proportion to expected pain

TABLE 15.4	Comparison of Acute and Chronic Pain	
Characteristic	Acute Pain	Chronic Pain
Experience	An event	A situation; state of existence
Source	External agent or internal disease, injury, or inflammation	Unknown; if known, treatment is prolonged or ineffective
Onset	Usually sudden	May be sudden or develop insidiously
Duration	Transient (up to 3 months); usually of short duration Resolves with treatment and healing	Prolonged (months to years); lasts beyond expected normal healing time
Pain identification	Painful and nonpainful areas generally well identified	Painful and nonpainful areas less easily differentiated; change in sensations becomes more difficult to evaluate
Clinical signs	Typical response pattern with more visible signs Anxiety and emotional distress common	Response patterns vary; fewer overt signs (adaptation) Can interfere with sleep, productivity, and quality of life
Significance	Significant (informs person something is wrong); protective	Person looks for significance and meaning; serves no useful purpose
Pattern	Self-limiting or readily corrected	Continuous or intermittent; intensity may vary or remain constant
Course	Suffering usually decreases over time	Suffering usually increases over time
Actions	Leads to actions to relieve pain	Leads to actions to modify pain experience
Prognosis	Likelihood of eventual complete relief	Complete relief usually not possible

hyperalgesia, allodynia (the induction of pain by normally nonpainful stimuli), and the development of spontaneous pain.[22] Neuropathic pain is classified as either peripheral or central and is associated with central and peripheral sensitization. Peripheral neuropathic pain is caused by peripheral nerve lesions. Peripheral sensitization is an increase in the sensitivity and excitability of primary sensory neurons and cells in the DRG. Examples include nerve entrapment, diabetic neuropathy, and chronic pancreatitis.

Central neuropathic pain is caused by a lesion or dysfunction in the brain or spinal cord. A progressive repeated stimulation of group C neurons (known as *wind-up*) in the dorsal horn leads to central sensitization, an increased sensitivity of central pain signaling neurons. This results in pathologic changes in the CNS that cause chronic pain. Examples include brain or spinal cord trauma, tumors, vascular lesions, multiple sclerosis, Parkinson disease, postherpetic neuralgia, and phantom limb pain.

The following mechanisms have been implicated in the cause of neuropathic pain:[21]

- Changes in sensitivity of neurons—lower threshold with peripheral and central sensitization
- Spontaneous impulses from regenerating peripheral nerves
- Alterations in the DRG and spinothalamic tract in response to peripheral nerve injury (i.e., deafferentation pain—loss of pain-related afferent information to the brain)
- Loss of pain inhibition and stimulation of pain facilitation by excitatory neurotransmitters in the dorsal horn (e.g., release of glutamate)
- Loss of descending inhibitory pain modulation
- Hyperexcitable spinal interneurons stimulated by Aβ fibers (non-painful stimulation of pain)
- Release of nociceptive inflammatory cytokines, chemokines, and growth factors by activated glial cells
- Structural and functional alterations in brain processing neural networks

Because of the complexity of the causes of neuropathic pain syndromes, they are difficult to treat. Multimodal therapy is often needed, including nondrug treatment.[23]

> ✔ **QUICK CHECK 15.1**
> 1. What is the difference between Aδ and C fibers?
> 2. Give two examples of pain excitatory and inhibitory neurotransmitters.
> 3. How do Aβ fibers inhibit pain and cause pain?
> 4. What are two differences between nociceptive pain and neuropathic pain?

TEMPERATURE REGULATION

Human **thermoregulation** is achieved through precise balancing of heat production, heat conservation, and heat loss The normal range of body temperature is considered to be 36.2° to 37.7° C (96.2° to 99.4° F) overall, but a person's individual body parts will vary in temperature. Body temperature rarely exceeds 41° C (105.8° F). The extremities are generally cooler than the trunk, and the temperature at the core of the body (as measured by rectal temperature) is generally 0.5° C higher than the surface temperature (as measured by oral temperature). Internal temperature varies in response to activity, environmental temperature, and daily fluctuation (circadian rhythm). Oral temperatures fluctuate within 0.2° to 0.5° C during a 24-hour period. Women tend to have wider fluctuations that follow the menstrual cycle, with a sharp rise in temperature just before ovulation. The daily fluctuating temperature in both sexes peaks around 6 PM and is at its lowest during sleep. Maintenance of body temperature within the normal range is necessary for life.

Control of Body Temperature

Temperature regulation (thermoregulation) is mediated primarily by the hypothalamus and endocrine system. Peripheral thermoreceptors in the skin, liver, and skeletal muscle (unmyelinated C fibers and thinly myelinated Aδ fibers) and central thermoreceptors in the hypothalamus, spinal cord, viscera, and great veins provide the hypothalamus with information about body temperatures. If these temperatures are low or high, the hypothalamus triggers heat production and heat conservation or heat loss mechanisms.[24]

Body heat is produced by the chemical reactions of metabolism and skeletal muscle tone and contraction. The heat-producing mechanism (chemical or nonshivering thermogenesis) begins with hypothalamic thyrotropin releasing hormone (TRH); it stimulates the anterior pituitary to release thyroid-stimulating hormone (TSH), which acts on the thyroid gland and stimulates the release of thyroxine. Thyroxine then acts on the adrenal medulla, causing the release of epinephrine into the bloodstream. Epinephrine causes cutaneous vasoconstriction, stimulates glycolysis, and increases metabolic rate, thus increasing body heat. Norepinephrine and thyroxine activate brown fat thermogenesis where energy is released as heat (nonshivering thermogenesis) instead of as adenosine triphosphate (ATP). Heat is distributed by the circulatory system.

The hypothalamus also triggers heat conservation by stimulating the sympathetic nervous system and results in increased skeletal muscle tone, initiating the shivering response and producing vasoconstriction. Sympathetic stimulation also constricts peripheral blood vessels. Centrally warmed blood is shunted away from the periphery to the core of the body, where heat can be retained. This involuntary mechanism takes advantage of the insulating layers of the skin and subcutaneous fat to protect the core temperature. The hypothalamus relays information to the cerebral cortex about cold, and voluntary responses result. Individuals typically bundle up, keep moving, or curl up in a ball. These types of voluntary physical activities respectively provide insulation, increase skeletal muscle activity, and decrease the amount of skin surface available for heat loss through radiation, convection, and conduction.

The hypothalamus responds to warmer core and peripheral temperatures by reversing the same mechanisms resulting in heat loss. Heat loss is achieved through (1) radiation, (2) conduction, (3) convection, (4) vasodilation, (5) evaporation (sweating), (6) decreased muscle tone, (7) increased respiration, (8) voluntary measures, and (9) adaptation to warmer climates (i.e., increasing or decreasing the volume of sweat). Table 15.5 summarizes further information about heat production and loss.

Temperature Regulation in Infants and Elderly Persons

Infants (particularly low birth weight infants) and elderly persons require special attention to maintenance of body temperature. Term infants produce sufficient body heat, primarily through metabolism of brown fat, but cannot conserve heat produced because of their small body size, greater ratio of body surface to body weight, and inability to shiver. Infants also have little subcutaneous fat and thus are not as well insulated as adults. Children also have a greater ratio of body surface to body weight, lower sweating rate, higher peripheral blood flow in the heat, and a greater extent of vasoconstriction in the cold than adults. They can acclimatize to changes in environmental temperatures, but do so at a lower rate than adults.

Elderly persons respond poorly to environmental temperature extremes because of their slowed blood circulation, structural and functional skin changes, overall decreased heat-producing activities, and the presence of disease (i.e., congestive heart failure, chronic lung disease, diabetes mellitus, or peripheral vascular disease). Cold stress in older adults also decreases coronary perfusion.[25] In addition, elderly persons have a decreased shivering response (delayed onset and decreased effectiveness), slowed metabolic rate, decreased vasoconstrictor response, diminished or absent ability to sweat, decreased peripheral sensation, desynchronized circadian rhythm, decreased perception of heat and cold, decreased thirst, decreased nutritional reserves, decreased brown adipose tissue, and decreased shivering response.[26]

Pathogenesis of Fever

Fever (febrile response) is a temporary resetting of the hypothalamic thermostat to a higher level in response to exogenous or endogenous pyrogens. **Exogenous pyrogens** (endotoxins produced by pathogens; see Chapter 9) stimulate the release of **endogenous pyrogens** from phagocytic cells, including tumor necrosis factor-alpha (TNF-α), interleukin-1 (IL-1), interleukin-6 (IL-6), and interferon (IFN). These

TABLE 15.5　Mechanisms of Heat Production and Heat Loss

Condition	Description
Heat Production	
Chemical reactions of metabolism	Occur during ingestion and metabolism of food and while maintaining body at rest (basal metabolism); occur in body core (e.g., liver)
Skeletal muscle contraction	Gradual increase in muscle tone or rapid muscle oscillations (shivering)
Nonshivering thermogenesis	Epinephrine is released and produces rapid, transient increase in heat production by raising basal metabolic rate; quick, brief effect that counters heat lost through conduction and convection; involves brown adipose tissue, which decreases markedly in older adults; thyroid hormone increases metabolism
Heat Loss	
Radiation	Heat loss through electromagnetic waves emanating from surfaces with temperature higher than surrounding air
Conduction	Heat loss by direct molecule-to-molecule transfer from one surface to another, so that warmer surface loses heat to cooler surface
Convection	Transfer of heat through currents of gases or liquids; exchanges warmer air at body's surface with cooler air in surrounding space
Vasodilation	Diverts core-warmed blood to surface of body, with heat transferred by conduction to skin surface and from there to surrounding environment; occurs in response to autonomic stimulation under control of hypothalamus
Evaporation	Body water evaporates from surface of skin and linings of mucous membranes; major source of heat reduction connected with increased sweating in warmer surroundings
Decreased muscle tone	Exhausted feeling caused by moderately reduced muscle tone and curtailed voluntary muscle activity
Increased respiration	Air is exchanged with environment through normal process; minimal effect
Voluntary mechanisms	"Stretching out" and "slowing down" in response to high body temperatures; increasing body surface area available for heat loss; dressing in light-colored, loose-fitting garments
Adaptation to warmer climates	Gradual process beginning with lassitude, weakness, and faintness; proceeding through increased sweating, lowered sodium content, decreased heart rate, and increased stroke volume and extracellular fluid volume; and terminating in improved warm weather functioning and decreased symptoms of heat intolerance (work output, endurance, and coordination increase; subjective feelings of discomfort decrease)

pyrogens raise the thermal set point by inducing the hypothalamic synthesis of prostaglandin E_2 (PGE_2). This produces an integrated response that raises body temperature through an increase in heat production and conservation (Fig. 15.4). The individual feels colder, dresses more warmly, decreases body surface area by curling up, and may go to bed in an effort to get warm. Body temperature is maintained at the new level until the fever "breaks," when the set point begins to return to normal with decreased heat production and increased heat reduction mechanisms. The individual feels very warm, dons cooler clothes, throws off the covers, and stretches out. Once the body has returned to a normal temperature the individual feels more comfortable and the hypothalamus adjusts thermoregulatory mechanisms to maintain the new temperature.

Fever of unknown origin (FUO) is a body temperature of greater than 38.3° C (101° F) for longer than 3 weeks' duration that remains undiagnosed after 3 days of hospital investigation, 3 outpatient visits, or 1 week of ambulatory investigation. The clinical categories of FUO include infectious, rheumatic/inflammatory, neoplastic, HIV-associated, and miscellaneous disorders.[27]

Benefits of Fever

Moderate fever helps the body respond to infectious processes through several mechanisms[28,29]:

1. Raising of body temperature kills many microorganisms and adversely affects their growth and replication.
2. Higher body temperatures decrease serum levels of iron, zinc, and copper—minerals needed for bacterial replication.
3. Increased temperature causes lysosomal breakdown and autodestruction of cells, preventing viral replication in infected cells.
4. Heat increases lymphocytic transformation tend motility of polymorphonuclear neutrophils, facilitating the immune response.

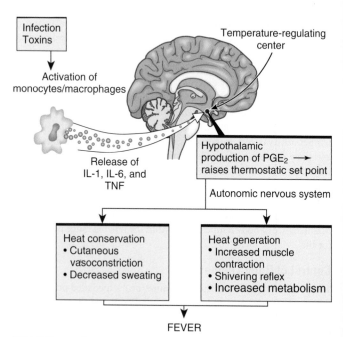

FIGURE 15.4 Production of Fever. When monocytes/macrophages are activated, they secrete cytokines such as interleukin-1 (IL-1), interleukin-6 (IL-6), and tumor necrosis factor (TNF), which reach the hypothalamic temperature-regulating center. These cytokines promote the synthesis and secretion of prostaglandin E_2 (PGE_2) in the anterior hypothalamus. PGE_2 increases the thermostatic set point, and the autonomic nervous system is stimulated, resulting in shivering, muscle contraction, peripheral vasoconstriction, and increased metabolism mediated by thyroid hormone. (From Lewis SM et al: *Medical-surgical nursing: assessment and management of clinical problems*, ed 9, St Louis, 2014, Mosby.)

5. Phagocytosis is enhanced, and production of antiviral interferon is augmented.

Suppression of fever with antipyrogenic medications can be effective but should be used with caution.[30,31] Infection and fever responses in elderly persons and children may vary from those in normal adults. Box 15.2 lists the principal features associated with fever at these extremes of age.[32]

Disorders of Temperature Regulation

Hyperthermia

Hyperthermia is elevation of the body temperature without an increase in the hypothalamic set point. Hyperthermia can produce nerve damage, coagulation of cell proteins, and death. At 41° C (105.8° F), nerve damage produces convulsions in the adult. Death results at 43° C (109.4° F). Hyperthermia may be therapeutic, accidental, or associated with stroke or head trauma. Prevention of hyperthermia in stroke and head trauma assists in limiting brain injury.[33]

Therapeutic hyperthermia is a form of local, regional, or whole-body hyperthermia used to destroy pathologic microorganisms or tumor cells by facilitating the host's natural immune process or tumor blood flow.[34] The forms of accidental hyperthermia are summarized as follows[35]:

1. Heat cramps—severe, spasmodic cramps in the abdomen and extremities that follow prolonged sweating and associated sodium loss. Usually occur in those not accustomed to heat or those performing strenuous work in very warm climates. Fever, rapid pulse rate, and increased blood pressure accompany the cramps.
2. Heat exhaustion—results from prolonged high core or environmental temperatures, which cause profound vasodilation and profuse sweating, leading to dehydration, decreased plasma volumes, hypotension, decreased cardiac output, and tachycardia. Symptoms include weakness, dizziness, confusion, nausea, and fainting.
3. Heat stroke—a potentially lethal result of an overstressed thermoregulatory center. Heat stroke can be caused by exertion, by overexposure to environmental heat, or from impaired physiologic mechanisms for heat loss. With very high core temperatures (>40° C [104° F]), the regulatory center ceases to function and the body's heat loss mechanisms fail. Symptoms include high core temperature, absence of sweating, rapid pulse rate, confusion, agitation, and coma. Complications include cerebral edema, degeneration of the CNS, swollen dendrites, renal tubular necrosis, and hepatic failure with delirium, coma, and eventually death if treatment is not undertaken.[36]
4. Malignant hyperthermia—a potentially lethal hypermetabolic complication of a rare inherited muscle disorder that may be triggered by inhaled anesthetics and depolarizing muscle relaxants.[37] The syndrome involves altered calcium function in muscle cells with hypermetabolism, uncoordinated muscle contractions, increased muscle work, increased oxygen consumption, and a raised level of lactic acid production. Acidosis develops, and body temperature rises, with resulting tachycardia and cardiac dysrhythmias, hypotension, decreased cardiac output, and cardiac arrest. Signs resemble those of coma—unconsciousness, absent reflexes, fixed pupils, apnea, and occasionally a flat electroencephalogram. Oliguria and anuria are common. It is most common in children and adolescents.

Hypothermia

Hypothermia (core body temperature less than 35° C [95° F]) produces depression of the CNS and respiratory system, vasoconstriction, alterations in microcirculation and coagulation, and ischemic tissue damage. Hypothermia may be accidental or therapeutic (Box 15.3). Most tissues can tolerate low temperatures in controlled situations, such as surgery. However, in severe hypothermia, ice crystals form on the inside of the cell, causing cells to rupture and die. Tissue hypothermia slows cell metabolism, increases the blood viscosity, slows microcirculatory blood flow, facilitates blood coagulation, and stimulates profound vasoconstriction (also see Frostbite, Chapter 43).

Trauma and Temperature

Major body trauma can affect temperature regulation through various mechanisms. Damage to the CNS, inflammation, increased intracranial pressure, or intracranial bleeding typically produces a body temperature of greater than 39° C (102.2° F). This sustained noninfectious fever, often referred to as a central fever, appears with or without bradycardia. A central fever does not induce sweating and is very resistant to antipyretic therapy.[38] Other traumatic mechanisms that produce temperature alterations include accidental injuries, hemorrhagic shock, major surgery, and thermal burns. The severity and type of alteration (hyperthermia or hypothermia) vary with the severity of the cause and the body system affected.

> ✔ **QUICK CHECK 15.2**
> 1. Why is temperature regulation important?
> 2. What are the principal heat production methods? Heat loss methods?
> 3. How does the hypothalamus alter its set point to change body temperature?
> 4. Compare and contrast hyperthermia and hypothermia and their effects on the body.

SLEEP

Sleep is an active multiphase process that provides restorative functions and promotes memory consolidation. Complex neural circuits, interacting hormones, and neurotransmitters involving the hypothalamus, thalamus, brainstem, and cortex control the timing of the sleep-wake cycle and coordinate this cycle with circadian rhythms (24-hour rhythm cycles).[39] Normal sleep has two primary phases that can be documented by electroencephalogram (EEG), a test that detects electrical activity in your brain: rapid eye movement (REM) sleep (20% to 25% of sleep time) and slow-wave (non-REM) sleep. Non-REM sleep is further divided into three stages (N1, N2, N3) from light to deep sleep. REM cycles do not typically start to occur until about 90 minutes into sleep. Four to six cycles of REM and non-REM sleep occur each night in an adult.[40]

The hypothalamus is a major sleep center, and the hypocretins (orexins), acetylcholine, and glutamate are neuropeptides secreted by the hypothalamus that promote wakefulness. Prostaglandin D₂, adenosine, melatonin, serotonin, ʟ-tryptophan, gamma-aminobutyric acid (GABA), and growth factors promote sleep. The pontine reticular formation is primarily responsible for generating REM sleep, and projections from the thalamocortical network produce non-REM sleep.[41]

BOX 15.2 Effects of Fever at the Extremes of Age

Elderly Persons
Show decreased fever response to infection; therefore benefits of fever are reduced.
High morbidity and mortality result from lack of beneficial aspects.

Children
Develop higher temperatures than adults for relatively minor infections.
Febrile seizures before age 5 years are not uncommon.

BOX 15.3   Defining Characteristics of Hypothermia

Accidental Hypothermia

The unintentional decrease in core temperature to less than 35° C (95° F) results from sudden immersion in cold water, prolonged exposure to cold environments, diseases that diminish the ability to generate heat, or altered thermoregulatory mechanisms. It is most common among young and elderly persons.

Factors That Increase Risk

1. Hypothyroidism
2. Hypopituitarism
3. Malnutrition
4. Parkinson disease
5. Rheumatoid arthritis
6. Chronic increased vasodilation
7. Failure of thermoregulatory control resulting from cerebral injury, ketoacidosis, uremia, sepsis, and drug overdose

Response Mechanisms

1. Peripheral vasoconstriction—shunts blood away from cooler skin to core to decrease heat loss and produces peripheral tissue ischemia
2. Intermittent reperfusion of extremities (Lewis phenomenon) helps preserve peripheral oxygenation until core temperature drops dramatically
3. Hypothalamic center induces shivering; thinking becomes sluggish, and coordination is depressed

4. Stupor; heart rate and respiratory rate decline; cardiac output diminishes; metabolic rate falls; acidosis; eventual ventricular fibrillation and asystole occur at 30° C (86° F) and lower

Treatment

1. Most changes are reversible with rewarming
2. Core temperature greater than 30° C (86° F)—active rewarming (external)
3. Core temperature less than 30° C (86° F) or with severe cardiovascular problems—active core rewarming (internal)

Therapeutic Hypothermia (Targeted Temperature Management)

Used to slow metabolism and preserve ischemic tissue during surgery (e.g., limb reimplantation) and after cardiac arrest. Studies are in progress to evaluate outcomes of hypothermia for management of neurologic injury.

Effects and Cautions

1. Stresses the heart, leading to ventricular fibrillation and cardiac arrest (may be desired outcome in open heart surgery when heart must be stopped)
2. Exhausts liver glycogen stores by prolonged shivering
3. Surface cooling may cause burns, frostbite, and fat necrosis
4. Immunosuppression with increased infection risk
5. Slows drug metabolism

From Carwell M: *Crit Care Nurs Q* 41(2):102-108, 2018; Kraft J, Karpenko A, Rincon F: *Curr Neurol Neurosci Rep* 16(2):18, 2016.

Rapid eye movement (REM) sleep is initiated by *REM-on* and *REM-off* neurons in the pons and mesencephalon. REM sleep occurs about every 90 minutes beginning 1 to 2 hours after non-REM sleep begins. This sleep is known as *paradoxical sleep* because the EEG pattern is similar to that of the normal awake pattern and the brain is very active with dreaming. REM and non-REM sleep alternate throughout the night, with lengthening intervals of REM sleep and fewer intervals of deeper stages of non-REM sleep toward morning. The changes associated with REM sleep include increased parasympathetic activity and variable sympathetic activity associated with rapid eye movement; muscle relaxation; loss of temperature regulation; altered heart rate, blood pressure, and respiration; penile erection in men and clitoral engorgement in women; release of steroids; and many memorable and often bizarre, dreams. Respiratory control appears largely independent of metabolic requirements and oxygen variation. Loss of normal voluntary muscle control in the tongue and upper pharynx may produce respiratory obstruction which, in turn, can precipitate apneic events. Cerebral blood flow increases. REM sleep is associated with memory consolidation.[42]

Non-REM sleep accounts for 75% to 80% of sleep time in adults and is initiated when inhibitory signals are released from the hypothalamus. Sympathetic tone is decreased, and parasympathetic activity is increased during non-REM sleep, creating a state of reduced activity. The basal metabolic rate falls by 10% to 15%; temperature decreases 0.5° to 1° C (0.9° to 1.8° F); heart rate, respiration, blood pressure, and muscle tone decrease; and knee jerk reflexes are absent. Pupils are constricted. During the various stages, cerebral blood flow to the brain decreases and growth hormone is released, with corticosteroid and catecholamine levels depressed. Box 15.4 summarizes sleep characteristics in infants and elderly persons.

Sleep Disorders

Because classification of sleep disorders is complex, a system has been established by the American Academy of Sleep Medicine and includes six classifications: (1) insomnia, (2) sleep-related breathing disorders, (3) central disorders of hypersomnolence, (4) circadian rhythm sleep-wake disorders, (5) parasomnias, (6) sleep-related movement disorders.[43] The most common disorders are summarized here.

Common Dyssomnias

Insomnia is the inability to fall or stay asleep; it is accompanied by fatigue, malaise, and difficulty with performance during wakefulness and may be mild, moderate, or severe. It may be transient, lasting a few days or months (primary insomnia), and related to travel across time zones or caused by acute stress, or very commonly inadequate "sleep hygiene." Sleep hygiene simply refers to behavioral and environmental practices that are intended to promote better-quality sleep (e.g., avoiding all-nighters and caffeine late in the evening). Chronic insomnia can be idiopathic, start at an early age, and be associated with drug or alcohol abuse, chronic pain disorders, chronic depression, the use of certain drugs, obesity, aging, genetics, and environmental factors that result in hyperarousal.[44]

Obstructive sleep apnea syndrome (OSAS) is the most commonly diagnosed sleep disorder and occurs in all age groups. However, the incidence of OSAS increases with age beyond 60 years. Major risk factors include obesity, male sex, older age, and postmenopausal status (not on hormone therapy) in women, and increased size of tonsillar and adenoid tissue.[45] A lack of daytime sleepiness often lessens awareness of a potential sleep disorder, and many persons are never properly diagnosed and treated.[46] OSAS results from partial or total upper airway obstruction to airflow recurring during sleep with excessive loud snoring, gasping, and multiple apneic episodes that last 10 seconds or longer. *Central sleep apnea* is the temporary absence or diminution of ventilatory effort during sleep with decreased sensitivity to carbon dioxide and oxygen tensions, and decreased airway dilator muscle activation. *Obesity hypoventilation syndrome* may be related to leptin resistance because leptin also is a respiratory stimulant. The periodic breathing eventually

BOX 15.4 Sleep Characteristics of Infants, Children, and Elderly Persons

Infants

- Infants sleep 10 to 16 hours per day: 50% REM (active) sleep, 25% non-REM (inactive) sleep.
- Infant sleep cycles are 50 to 60 minutes in length; 10 to 45 minutes of REM sleep accompanied by movement of the arms, legs, and facial muscles followed by about 20 minutes of non-REM sleep.
- At 1 year, REM and non-REM sleep cycles are about equal in length and infants sleep through the night with about two naps per day.

Children

- Children assume an adult sleep pattern between 3 and 5 years and sleep about 9 to 10 hours per night.
- Inadequate sleep in adolescents is associated with obesity, depression, and poor academic performance.

Elderly Persons

- Total sleep time is decreased with a longer time to fall asleep and poorer-quality sleep.
- Total time in slow-wave and final phase of non-REM sleep decreases by 15% to 30%.
- Increases in stage 1 and 2 non-REM sleep, attributable to an increased number of spontaneous arousals.
- Elderly individuals tend to go to sleep earlier in the evening and wake earlier in the morning because of a phase advance in their normal circadian sleep cycle.
- Alterations in sleep patterns occur about 10 years later in women than in men.
- Sleep disorders are more likely in the elderly and increase risks of morbidity, mortality, and changes in cognitive function.

From Gulia KK, Kumar VM: *Psychogeriatrics* 18(3):155-165, 2018; Owens J; *Pediatrics* 134(3):e921-e932, 2014; Scullin MK, Bliwise DL: *Perspect Psychol Sci* 10(1):97-137, 2015.
REM, rapid eye movement; non-REM, non-rapid eye movement

produces arousal, which interrupts the sleep cycle, reducing total sleep time and producing sleep and REM deprivation. Sleep apnea produces hypercapnia and low oxygen saturation and if left untreated, eventually leads to polycythemia, pulmonary hypertension, systemic hypertension, stroke, right-sided congestive heart failure, dysrhythmias, liver congestion, cyanosis, and peripheral edema.

Hypersomnia (excessive daytime sleepiness) is associated with OSAS. Individuals may fall asleep while driving a car, working, or even while conversing, with significant safety concerns.[47] Sleep deprivation also can result in impaired mood and cognitive function characterized by impairments of attention, episodic memory, working memory, and executive functions (i.e., decision-making ability).

Polysomnography is needed to diagnose OSAS, in addition to the history and physical examination. Treatments include use of nasal continuous positive airway pressure (CPAP) and dental devices, surgery of the upper airway and jaw in selected individuals, and management of obesity.[48] Adenotonsillar hypertrophy is the major cause of obstructive sleep apnea in children, and obesity increases the risk. Adenotonsillectomy is the treatment of choice.[49]

Narcolepsy is a primary hypersomnia with disruption in sleep-wake cycles characterized by hallucinations, sleep paralysis and, rarely, cataplexy (brief spells of muscle weakness). Narcolepsy is usually sporadic or can occur in families. Type I narcolepsy (narcolepsy with cataplexy) is associated with immune-mediated destruction of hypocretin (orexin)-secreting cells in the hypothalamus. Orexins stimulate wakefulness. Type II narcolepsy (narcolepsy without cataplexy) is associated with normal levels of orexins (hypocretins) and the cause is unknown.[50]

Circadian rhythm sleep disorders are common disorders of the 24-hour sleep-wake schedule (circadian rhythm sleep disorders). They can result from extrinsic causes, such as rapid time zone changes (or jet-lag syndrome), alternating the sleep schedule (rotating work shifts) involving 3 hours or more in sleep time, or changing the total sleep time from day to day. Intrinsic causes include *advanced sleep phase disorder* (early morning waking–early evening sleeping) resulting in sleep loss if social requirements are for late sleeping, or *delayed sleep phase disorder* (late morning waking–late night to early morning sleeping) with loss of sleep because of required early morning rising (common in adolescents). These changes desynchronize the circadian rhythm, which can depress the degree of vigilance, performance of psychomotor tasks, and arousal. A circadian rhythm sleep disorder known as shift work sleep disorder affects many shift workers who rotate or swing long shifts (such as nurses), particularly between the hours of 2200 (10 PM) and 0600 (6 AM). Our sleep-wake cycle is driven by circadian rhythms, and the disruption of this circadian influence may cause problems in the short term, such as cognitive deficits and difficulty concentrating. However, long-term health consequences of shift work sleep disorder may be quite serious and include depression/anxiety, increased risk for cardiovascular disease, and increased all-cause mortality. Sleep cycle phenotype also has a genetic basis and influences the timing and cycles of sleep and can affect advances or delays in sleep-wake times.[51,52]

Common Parasomnias

Parasomnias are unusual behaviors occurring during non-REM stage 3 (slow-wave) sleep (non-REM parasomnias).[53] These behaviors include sleepwalking, having night terrors, rearranging furniture, eating food, exhibiting sleep sex or violent behavior, and having restless legs syndrome. REM sleep behavior disorder (RBD) is manifested by loss of REM paralysis, leading to potentially injurious dream enactment. Nonmotor symptoms are nonspecific and include olfactory dysfunction, abnormal color vision, autonomic dysfunction, excessive daytime sleepiness, depression, and cognitive impairment. RBD is a common prodromal manifestation of Parkinson disease.[54]

Two dysfunctions of sleep (somnambulism and night terrors) are common in children and may be related to CNS immaturity. Somnambulism (sleepwalking) is a non-REM parasomnia disorder primarily of childhood and appears to resolve within a few years. Sleepwalking is therefore not associated with dreaming, and the child has no memory of the event on awakening. Sleepwalking in adults is often associated with sleep-disordered breathing. Night terrors are characterized by sudden apparent arousals in which the child expresses intense fear or emotion. However, the child is not awake and can be difficult to arouse. Once awakened, the child has no memory of the night terror event. Night terrors are not associated with dreams. Although this problem occurs most often in children, adults also may experience it with corresponding daytime anxiety.

Restless Leg Syndrome

Restless legs syndrome (RLS)/Willis Ekbom disease is a common sensorimotor disorder associated with unpleasant sensations (prickling, tingling, crawling) and nonvolitional periodic leg movements that occurs at rest and is worse in the evening or at night. There is a compelling urge to move the legs for relief, with a significant effect on sleep and quality of life. The disorder is more common in women, during pregnancy, the elderly, and individuals with iron deficiency. RLS has a familial tendency and is associated with a circadian fluctuation of dopamine in the substantia nigra. Iron is a cofactor in dopamine production, and some individuals respond to iron administration as well as dopamine agonists. Diagnostic and treatment guidelines have been established to assist with disease management.[55]

✓ **QUICK CHECK 15.3**
1. Describe REM and non-REM sleep.
2. What is the major difference between the dyssomnias and parasomnias?

THE SPECIAL SENSES

Vision

The eyes are complex sense organs responsible for vision. Within a protective casing, each eye has receptors, a lens system for focusing light on the receptors, and a system of nerves for conducting impulses from the receptors to the brain. Visual dysfunction may be caused by abnormal ocular movements or alterations in visual acuity, refraction, color vision, or accommodation. Visual dysfunction also may be the secondary effect of another neurologic disorder.

The Eye

The wall of the eye consists of three layers: (1) sclera, (2) choroid, and (3) retina (Fig. 15.5). The sclera is the thick, white, outermost layer. It becomes transparent at the cornea—the portion of the sclera in the central anterior region that allows light to enter the eye. The choroid is the deeply pigmented middle layer that prevents light from scattering inside the eye. The iris, part of the choroid, has a round opening, the pupil, through which light passes. Smooth muscle fibers control the size of the pupil so that it adjusts to bright light or dim light and to close or distant vision.

The retina is the innermost layer of the eye and contains millions of rods and cones—special photoreceptors that convert light energy into nerve impulses. Rods mediate peripheral and dim light vision and are densest at the periphery. Cones are color and detail receptors, and densest in the center of the retina. There are no photoreceptors where the optic nerve leaves the eyeball; this creates the optic disc, or blind spot. Lateral to each optic disc is the macula lutea, the area of most distinct vision, and in the center is the fovea centralis, a tiny area that contains only cones and provides the greatest visual acuity (see Fig. 15.5).

Nerve impulses pass through the optic nerves (second cranial nerve) to the optic chiasm (see Fig. 15.8). The nerves from the inner (nasal) halves of the retinas cross to the opposite side and join fibers from the outer (temporal) halves of the retinas to form the optic tracts (see Fig. 15.8). The fibers of the optic tracts synapse in the dorsal lateral geniculate nucleus and pass by way of the optic radiation (or geniculocalcarine tract) to the primary visual cortex in the occipital lobe of the brain. Some fibers terminate in the suprachiasmatic nucleus (SCN) of the hypothalamus (located above the optic chiasm) and are involved in circadian regulation of the sleep-wake cycle. Light entering the eye is focused on the retina by the lens—a flexible, biconvex, crystal-like structure. The flexibility of the lens allows a change in curvature with contraction of the ciliary muscles, called *accommodation*, and allows the eye to focus on objects at different distances. The lens divides the anterior chamber into (1) the aqueous chamber and (2) the vitreous chamber. Aqueous humor fills the aqueous chamber and helps maintain pressure inside the eye, as well as provide nutrients to the lens and cornea. Aqueous humor is secreted by the ciliary processes and reabsorbed into the canal of Schlemm. If drainage is blocked, intraocular pressure increases, causing glaucoma. The vitreous chamber is filled with a gel-like substance called vitreous humor that cannot regenerate. Vitreous humor helps prevent the eyeball from collapsing inward.

The central retinal artery provides blood to the inner retinal surface, and the choroid supplies nutrients to the outer surface of the retina. Six extrinsic eye muscles allow gross eye movements and permit eyes to follow a moving object (Fig. 15.6).

Visual Dysfunction

Alterations in ocular movements. Abnormal ocular movements result from oculomotor, trochlear, or abducens cranial nerve dysfunction (see Table 14.6). The three types of eye movement disorders are (1) strabismus, (2) nystagmus, and (3) paralysis of individual extraocular muscles.

In strabismus, one eye deviates from the other when the person is looking at an object. This is caused by a weak or hypertonic muscle in one eye. The deviation may be upward, downward, inward (entropia), or outward (extropia). Strabismus in children requires early intervention to prevent amblyopia (reduced vision in the affected eye caused by cerebral blockage of the visual stimuli). The primary symptom of strabismus is diplopia (double vision). Causes include neuromuscular disorders of the eye muscle, diseases involving the cerebral hemispheres, or thyroid disease.

Nystagmus is an involuntary unilateral or bilateral rhythmic movement of the eyes. It may be present at rest or when the eye moves. Pendular nystagmus is characterized by a regular back and forth movement of the eyes. In jerk nystagmus, one phase of the eye movement is faster than the other. Nystagmus may be caused by imbalanced reflex activity of the inner ear, vestibular nuclei, cerebellum, medial longitudinal fascicle, or nuclei of the oculomotor, trochlear, and abducens cranial nerves (see Table 14.6 and Fig. 14.25). Drugs, retinal disease, diseases involving the cervical cord, stroke syndromes, brain tumors, and brain trauma also may produce nystagmus.

Paralysis of specific extraocular muscles may cause limited abduction, abnormal closure of the eyelid, ptosis (drooping of the eyelid), or diplopia

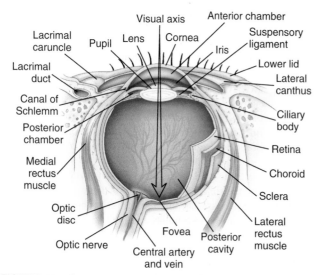

FIGURE 15.5 Internal Anatomy of the Eye. (Adapted from Patton KT, Thibodeau GA: *Structure & function of the human body,* ed 13, St Louis, 2008, Mosby.)

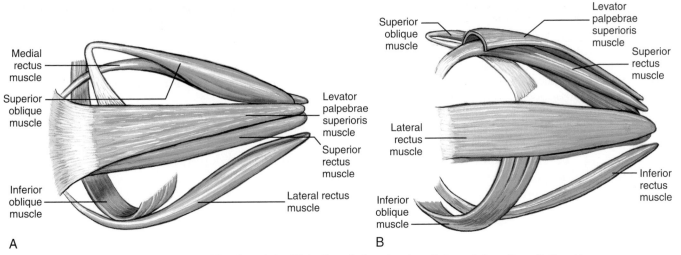

FIGURE 15.6 Extrinsic Muscles of the Right Eye. **A,** Superior view. **B,** Lateral view. (From Dutton JJ: *Atlas of clinical and surgical orbital anatomy,* ed 2, Philadelphia, 2011, Saunders.)

TABLE 15.6   Changes in the Eye Caused by Aging

Structure	Change	Consequence
Cornea	Thicker and less curved	Increase in astigmatism
Formation of gray ring at edge of cornea (arcus senilis)	Not detrimental to vision	
Anterior chamber	Decrease in size and volume caused by thickening of lens	Occasionally exerts pressure on Schlemm canal and may lead to increased intraocular pressure and glaucoma
Lens	Increase in opacity	Decrease in refraction with increased light scattering (blurring) and decreased color vision (green and blue); can lead to cataracts
Ciliary muscles	Reduction in pupil diameter, atrophy of radial dilation muscles	Persistent constriction (senile miosis); decrease in critical flicker frequency*
Retina	Reduction in number of rods at periphery, loss of rods and associated nerve cells	Increase in minimum amount of light necessary to see an object

*The rate at which consecutive visual stimuli can be presented and still be perceived as separate.

(double vision) as a result of unopposed muscle activity. Trauma or pressure in the area of the cranial nerves or diseases such as diabetes mellitus and myasthenia gravis also paralyze specific extraocular muscles.

Alterations in visual acuity. Visual acuity is the ability to see objects in sharp detail. With advancing age, the lens of the eye becomes less flexible and adjusts slowly, and there is altered refraction of light by the cornea and lens. Thus visual acuity declines with age. Table 15.6 contains a summary of changes in the eye caused by aging. Specific causes of visual acuity changes are (1) amblyopia, (2) scotoma (blind spot in visual field), (3) cataracts, (4) papilledema, (5) dark adaptation, (6) glaucoma, (7) retinal detachment, and (8) macular degeneration (Table 15.7).

A cataract is a cloudy or opaque area in the ocular lens and leads to visual loss when located on the visual axis (see Fig. 15.5). It is the leading cause of blindness in the world. The incidence of cataracts increases with age as lens proteins break down, leading to opacification. Cataracts develop because of alterations of metabolism and transport of nutrients within the lens. Although the most common form of cataract is degenerative, cataracts also may occur congenitally or as a result of infection, radiation, trauma, drugs, or diabetes mellitus. Cataracts cause decreased visual acuity, blurred vision, glare, and decreased color

perception. Cataracts are treated by removal of the entire lens and replacement with an intraocular artificial lens.

Glaucomas are the second leading cause of blindness and are characterized by intraocular pressures greater than 12 to 20 mm Hg with death of retinal ganglion cells and their axons and irreversible loss of vision.[56] There are three primary types of glaucoma:

1. *Open angle.* This type of glaucoma is characterized by outflow obstruction of aqueous humor at the trabecular meshwork or canal of Schlemm even though there is adequate space for drainage; often this is an inherited disease and is a leading cause of blindness with few preliminary symptoms.

2. *Angle closure* or *narrow angle.* In this type of glaucoma there is displacement of the iris toward the cornea with obstruction of the trabecular meshwork and obstruction of outflow of aqueous humor from the anterior chamber; it may occur acutely with a sudden rise in intraocular pressure, causing pain and visual disturbances.

3. *Congenital closure.* This is a rare disease associated with congenital malformations and other genetic anomalies.

Angle closure glaucoma is a medical emergency. Both medical and surgical therapies are available to control intraocular pressure for all types of glaucoma.

TABLE 15.7   Causes of Visual Acuity Changes

Disorder	Description
Amblyopia	Reduced or dimmed vision; cause unknown
	Associated with strabismus
	Accompanies such diseases as diabetes mellitus, renal failure, and malaria and use of drugs such as alcohol and tobacco
Scotoma	Circumscribed defect of central field of vision
	Often associated with retrobulbar neuritis and multiple sclerosis, compression of optic nerve by tumor, inflammation of optic nerve, pernicious anemia, methyl alcohol poisoning, and use of tobacco
Cataract	Cloudy or opaque area in ocular lens—the leading cause of blindness
	Incidence increases with age because most commonly a result of degeneration; other causes are congenital
Papilledema	Edema and inflammation of optic nerve where it enters eyeball
	Caused by obstruction of venous return from retina by one of three main sources: increased intracranial pressure, retrobulbar neuritis, or changes in retinal blood vessels
Dark adaptation	With age, eye does not adapt as readily to dark
	Also, changes in quantity and quality of rhodopsin are causative; vitamin A deficiencies can produce this at any age
Glaucoma	Increased intraocular pressures (>12-20 mm Hg)
	Loss of acuity results from pressure on optic nerve, which blocks flow of nutrients to optic nerve fibers, leading to their death; second leading cause of blindness
Retinal detachment	Tear or break in retina with accumulation of fluid and separation from underlying tissue; seen as floaters, flashes of light, or a curtain over visual field; risks include extreme myopia, diabetic retinopathy, sickle cell disease

Age-related macular degeneration (AMD) is a severe and irreversible loss of vision and a major cause of blindness in older individuals. Hypertension, cigarette smoking, diabetes mellitus, and a family history of AMD are risk factors. The degeneration usually occurs after the age of 60 years. There are two forms: atrophic (dry, nonexudative) and neovascular (wet, exudative). The atrophic form is more common and is slowly progressive with inflammation and accumulation of lipofuscin (a lysosomal pigmented residue) and drusen (waste products from photoreceptors) in the retina and may include limited night vision and difficulty reading. The neovascular form includes accumulation of drusen and lipofuscin, abnormal choroidal blood vessel growth, leakage of blood or serum, retinal detachment, fibrovascular scarring, loss of photoreceptors, and more severe and rapid loss of central vision. Treatment includes anti–vascular endothelial growth factor (anti-VEGF) injection for wet macular degeneration and antioxidant vitamins for dry macular degeneration. Daily high doses of vitamins C and E, beta-carotene, and the minerals zinc and copper—called the AREDS formulation—can help slow the progression to advanced AMD.[57]

Alterations in accommodation. Accommodation refers to changes in the shape of the lens and allows for a change of focus from distant to near images. Accommodation is mediated through the oculomotor nerve. Pressure, inflammation, age, and disease of the oculomotor nerve may alter accommodation, causing diplopia, blurred vision, and headache.

Loss of accommodation with advancing age is termed presbyopia, a condition in which the ocular lens becomes larger, firmer, and less elastic. The major symptom is reduced near vision, causing the individual to hold reading material at arm's length. Treatment includes corrective forward, contact, and intraocular lenses or laser refractive surgery for monovision.[58]

Alterations in refraction. Alterations in refraction are the most common visual problem. Causes include irregularities of the corneal curvature, the focusing power of the lens, and the length of the eye. The major symptoms of refraction alterations are blurred vision and headache. Three types of refraction alterations are as follows (Fig. 15.7):

Myopia—nearsightedness: Light rays are focused in front of the retina when the person is looking at a distant object.

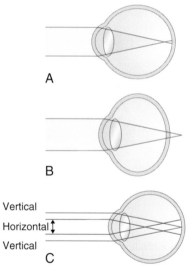

FIGURE 15.7 Alterations in Refraction. **A,** Myopic eye. Parallel rays of light are brought to a focus in front of the retina. **B,** Hyperopic eye. Parallel rays of light come to a focus behind the retina in the unaccommodative eye. **C,** Simple myopic astigmatism. The vertical bundle of rays is focused on the retina; the horizontal rays are focused in front of the retina. (From Stein HA et al: *The ophthalmic assistant: a text for allied and associated ophthalmic personnel,* ed 9, Philadelphia, 2013, Saunders.)

Hyperopia—farsightedness: Light rays are focused behind the retina when a person is looking at a near object.

Astigmatism—unequal curvature of the cornea: Light rays are bent unevenly and do not come to a single focus on the retina. Astigmatism may coexist with myopia, hyperopia, or presbyopia.

Alterations in color vision. Normal sensitivity to color diminishes with age because of the progressive yellowing of the lens that occurs with aging. All colors become less intense, although color discrimination for blue and green is greatly affected. Color vision deteriorates more rapidly for individuals with diabetes mellitus than for the general population.

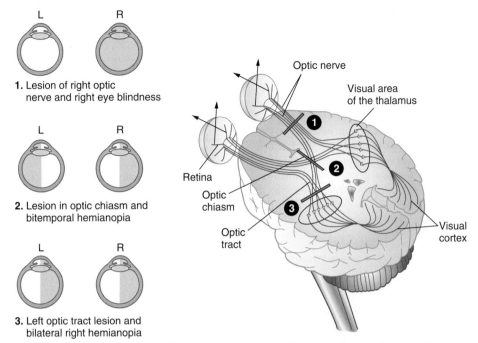

1. Lesion of right optic nerve and right eye blindness

2. Lesion in optic chiasm and bitemporal hemianopia

3. Left optic tract lesion and bilateral right hemianopia

FIGURE 15.8 Visual Pathways and Defects. (Modified from Thompson JM et al: *Mosby's clinical nursing*, ed 5, St Louis, 2002, Mosby.)

Abnormal color vision also may be caused by color blindness and is an X-linked genetic trait.[59] Congenital color blindness affects 6% to 8% of the male population and about 0.5% of the female population. Although many forms of color blindness exist, most commonly the affected individual cannot distinguish red from green. In the most severe form (achromatopsia) individuals see only shades of gray, black, and white. Acquired color vision deficiency occurs with ocular, neurologic, or systemic disease.

Neurologic disorders causing visual dysfunction. Vision may be disrupted at many points along the visual pathway, causing various defects in the visual field. Visual changes may cause defects or blindness in the entire visual field or in half of a visual field (hemianopia). Fig. 15.8 illustrates the many areas along the visual pathway that may be damaged and the associated visual changes. Injury to the optic nerve causes same-side blindness. Injury to the optic chiasm (the X-shaped crossing of the optic nerves) can cause various defects, depending on the location of the injury.

External Eye Structure and Disorders

Protective external eye structures include the eyelids (palpebrae), conjunctivae, and lacrimal apparatus. The eyelids control the amount of light reaching the eyes, and the conjunctiva lines the eyelids. Tears released from the lacrimal apparatus bathe the surface of the eye and prevent friction, maintain hydration, and wash out foreign bodies and other irritants (Fig. 15.9).

Infection and inflammatory responses are the most common conditions affecting the supporting structures of the eyes. Blepharitis is an inflammation of the eyelids caused by *Staphylococcus* or seborrheic dermatitis. A hordeolum (stye) is an infection (usually staphylococcal) of the sebaceous glands of the eyelids, usually centered near an eyelash. A chalazion is a noninfectious lipogranuloma of the meibomian (oil-secreting) gland that often occurs in association with a hordeolum and appears as a deep nodule within the eyelid. These conditions present with redness, swelling, and tenderness and are treated symptomatically. Entropion is a common eyelid malposition in which the lid margin

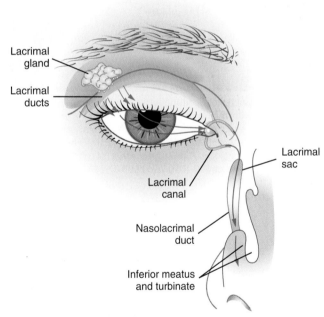

FIGURE 15.9 Lacrimal Apparatus. Fluid produced by lacrimal glands (tears) streams across the eye surface, enters the canals, and then passes through the nasolacrimal duct to enter the nose. (From Applegate E: *The anatomy and physiology learning system*, ed 4, St Louis, 2011, Saunders.)

turns inward against the eyeball. There are both surgical and nonsurgical treatments to reposition the lid margin.

Conjunctivitis is an inflammation of the conjunctiva (mucous membrane covering the front part of the eyeball) caused by viruses (most common), bacteria, allergies, or chemical irritants.[60]

Acute bacterial conjunctivitis (pinkeye) is highly contagious and often caused by *Staphylococcus, Haemophilus, Streptococcus pneumoniae,* and *Moraxella catarrhalis,* although other bacteria may be involved (Fig. 15.10). In children younger than 6 years, *Haemophilus* infection often leads to otitis media (conjunctivitis-otitis syndrome). Preventing the spread of the microorganism with meticulous hand washing and use of separate towels is important. The disease also is treated with antibiotics.

Viral conjunctivitis is caused by an adenovirus. It, too, is contagious, with symptoms of watering, redness, and photophobia. Allergic conjunctivitis is associated with a variety of antigens, including pollens. Chronic conjunctivitis results from any persistent conjunctivitis. Trachoma (chlamydial conjunctivitis) is caused by *Chlamydia trachomatis* and often is associated with poor hygiene and leads to corneal scarring. It is the leading cause of preventable blindness in the world.

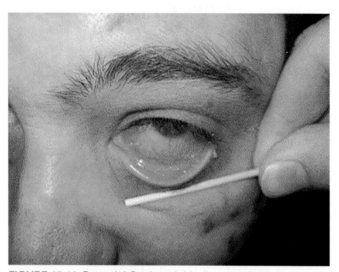

FIGURE 15.10 Bacterial Conjunctivitis. Staphylococcal conjunctivitis of the left eye with mild erythema and inflammatory edema of the eyelids. Purulent exudate can be seen at the lateral canthus. (From Durkin SR et al: Recurrent staphylococcal conjunctivitis associated with facial impetigo contagiosa, *Am J Ophthalmol* 141(1):189-190, 2006. Available at https://doi.org/10.1016/j.ajo.2005.07.079.)

Keratitis is an infection of the cornea caused by bacteria or viruses. Bacterial infections can cause corneal ulceration, and type 1 herpes simplex virus can involve both the cornea and the conjunctiva. *Acanthamoeba* keratitis can occur from contact lens wear because of poor hygiene. Severe ulcerations with residual scarring require corneal transplantation.

Hearing
The Normal Ear

The ear is divided into three areas: (1) the external ear, involved only with hearing; (2) the middle ear, involved only with hearing; and (3) the inner ear, involved with both hearing and equilibrium.

The external ear is composed of the pinna (auricle), which is the visible portion of the ear, and the external auditory canal, a tube that leads to the middle ear (Fig. 15.11). The external auditory canal is surrounded by the bones of the cranium. The opening (meatus) of the canal is just above the mastoid process. The air-filled sinuses, called mastoid air cells, of the mastoid process promote conductivity of sound between the external and the middle ear. The tympanic membrane separates the external ear from the middle ear. Sound waves entering the external auditory canal hit the tympanic membrane (eardrum) and cause it to vibrate.

The middle ear is composed of the tympanic cavity, a small chamber in the temporal bone. Three ossicles (small bones known as the malleus [hammer], incus [anvil], and stapes [stirrup]) transmit the vibration of the tympanic membrane to the inner ear. When the tympanic membrane moves, the malleus moves with it and transfers the vibration to the incus, which passes it on to the stapes. The stapes presses against the oval window, a small membrane of the inner ear. The movement of the oval window promotes movement of the round window and sets the fluids of the inner ear in motion (Fig. 15.12).

The eustachian (pharyngotympanic) tube connects the middle ear with the thorax. Normally flat and closed, the eustachian tube opens briefly when a person swallows or yawns, and it equalizes the pressure in the middle ear with atmospheric pressure. Equalized pressure permits the tympanic membrane to vibrate freely. Through the eustachian tube the mucosa of the middle ear is continuous with the mucosal lining of the throat.

The inner ear is a system of osseous labyrinths (bony, mazelike chambers) filled with a fluid, the perilymph. The bony labyrinth is

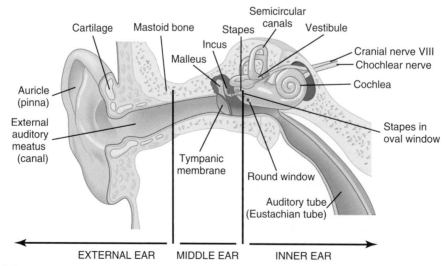

FIGURE 15.11 External, Middle, and Inner ears. (Anatomic structures are not drawn to scale.) (From Applegate E: *The anatomy and physiology learning system,* ed 4, St Louis, 2011, Saunders.)

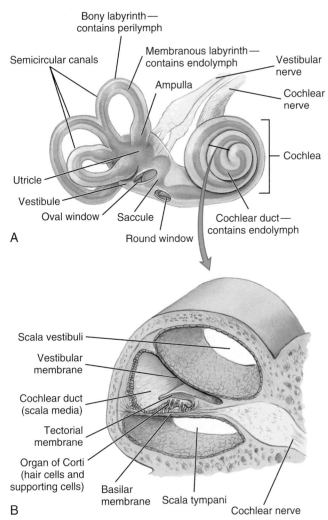

Scala vestibuli
Vestibular membrane
Cochlear duct (scala media)
Tectorial membrane
Organ of Corti (hair cells and supporting cells)
Basilar membrane
Scala tympani
Cochlear nerve

B

Bony labyrinth— contains perilymph
Semicircular canals
Membranous labyrinth— contains endolymph
Ampulla
Vestibular nerve
Cochlear nerve
Cochlea
Utricle
Vestibule
Oval window
Saccule
Round window
Cochlear duct— contains endolymph

A

FIGURE 15.12 The Inner Ear. A, The bony labyrinth *(tan)* is the hard outer wall of the entire inner ear and includes the semicircular canals, vestibule, and cochlea. Within the bony labyrinth is the membranous labyrinth *(purple),* which is surrounded by perilymph and filled with endolymph. Each ampulla in the vestibule contains a crista ampullaris that detects changes in head position and sends sensory impulses through the vestibular nerve to the brain. **B,** Section of the membranous cochlea. Hair cells in the organ of Corti detect sound and send the information through the cochlear nerve. The vestibular and cochlear nerves join to form the eighth cranial nerve. (From Applegate E: *The anatomy and physiology learning system,* ed 4, St Louis, 2011, Saunders.)

divided into the cochlea, the vestibule, and the semicircular canals (see Fig. 15.12). Suspended in the perilymph is the endolymph-filled membranous labyrinth that basically follows the shape of the bony labyrinth.

Within the cochlea is the organ of Corti, which contains hair cells (hearing receptors). Sound waves that reach the cochlea through vibrations of the tympanic membrane, ossicles, and oval window set the cochlear fluids into motion. Receptor cells on the basilar membrane are stimulated when their hairs are bent or pulled by fluid movement. Once stimulated, hair cells transmit impulses along the cochlear nerve (a division of the vestibulocochlear nerve) to the auditory cortex of the temporal lobe in the brain (see Fig. 15.12 and view an animation at https://www.youtube.com/watch?v=46aNGGNPm7s). This is where interpretation of the sound occurs.

The semicircular canals and vestibule of the inner ear contain equilibrium receptors. In the semicircular canals the dynamic equilibrium receptors respond to changes in direction of movement. Within each semicircular canal is the crista ampullaris, a receptor region composed of a tuft of hair cells covered by a gelatinous cupula. When the head is rotated, the endolymph in the canal lags behind and moves in the direction opposite to the head's movement. The hair cells are stimulated, and impulses are transmitted through the vestibular nerve (a division of the vestibulocochlear nerve) to the cerebellum.

The vestibule in the inner ear contains maculae—receptors essential to the body's sense of static equilibrium. As the head moves, otoliths (small pieces of calcium salts) move in a gel-like material in response to changes in the pull of gravity. The otoliths pull on the gel, which in turn pulls on the hair cells in the maculae. Nerve impulses in the hair cells are triggered and transmitted to the brain (see Fig. 15.12). Thus the ear not only permits the hearing of a large range of sounds but also assists with maintaining balance through the sensitive equilibrium receptors (see animation at https://www.youtube.com/watch?v=YMIMvBa8XGs).

Auditory Dysfunction

Between 5% and 10% of the general population have impaired hearing, and it is the most common sensory defect. The major categories of auditory dysfunction are conductive hearing loss, sensorineural hearing loss, mixed hearing loss, and functional hearing loss. Hearing loss may range from mild to profound. Auditory changes caused by aging are common and incremental (see the box *Geriatric Considerations: Aging & Changes in Hearing*).

Conductive hearing loss. A conductive hearing loss occurs when a change in the outer or middle ear impairs conduction of sound from the outer to the inner ear. Conditions that commonly cause a conductive hearing loss include impacted cerumen, foreign bodies lodged in the ear canal, benign tumors of the middle ear, carcinoma of the external auditory canal or middle ear, eustachian tube dysfunction, otitis media, acute viral otitis media, chronic suppurative otitis media, cholesteatoma (accumulation of keratinized epithelium), and otosclerosis.

Symptoms of conductive hearing loss include diminished hearing and soft speaking voice. The voice is soft because often the individual hears his or her voice, conducted by bone, as loud.

Sensorineural hearing loss. A sensorineural hearing loss is caused by impairment of the organ of Corti or its central connections. The loss may occur gradually or suddenly. Conditions causing sensorineural loss include congenital and hereditary factors, noise exposure, aging, Ménière disease, ototoxicity, systemic disease (syphilis, Paget disease, collagen diseases, diabetes mellitus), neoplasms, and autoimmune processes.[61] Congenital and neonatal sensorineural hearing loss may be caused by maternal rubella, ototoxic drugs, prematurity, traumatic delivery, erythroblastosis fetalis, bacterial meningitis, and congenital hereditary malfunction. Diagnosis often is made when delayed speech development is noted. Sudden onset bilateral sensorineural hearing loss is a medical emergency.

Presbycusis is the most common form of sensorineural hearing loss in elderly people. Its cause may be atrophy of the basal end of the organ of Corti, loss of auditory receptors, changes in vascularity, or stiffening of the basilar membranes. Drug ototoxicities (drugs that cause destruction of auditory function) have been observed after exposure to various chemicals; for example, antibiotics such as streptomycin, neomycin, gentamicin, and vancomycin; diuretics such as ethacrynic acid and furosemide; and chemicals such as salicylate, quinine, carbon monoxide, nitrogen mustard, arsenic, mercury, gold, tobacco, and alcohol. In most instances, the drugs and chemicals listed initially cause tinnitus (ringing in the ear), followed by a progressive high-tone sensorineural hearing loss that is permanent.

GERIATRIC CONSIDERATIONS
Aging & Changes in Hearing*

Changes in Structure	Changes in Function
Cochlear hair cell degeneration	Inability to hear high-frequency sounds (presbycusis, sensorineural loss); interferes with understanding speech; hearing may be lost in both ears at different times
Loss of auditory neurons in spiral ganglia of organ of Corti	Inability to hear high-frequency sounds (presbycusis, sensorineural loss); interferes with understanding speech; hearing may be lost in both ears at different times
Degeneration of basilar (cochlear) conductive membrane of cochlea	Inability to hear at all frequencies but more pronounced at higher frequencies (cochlear conductive loss)
Decreased vascularity of cochlea	Equal loss of hearing at all frequencies (strial loss); inability to disseminate localization of sound
Loss of cortical auditory neurons	Equal loss of hearing at all frequencies (strial loss); inability to disseminate localization of sound

*Hearing loss affects about 33% of older people. Hearing loss is associated with declining cognitive function, changes in perception, comprehension, and memory, but causal mechanisms are not clearly known.
Data from Frisina RD: *Ann N Y Acad Sci* 1170:708-717, 2009; Jayakody DMP et al: *Front Neurosci* 12:125, 2018; Roth TN: *Handb Clin Neurol* 129:357-373, 2015.

Mixed and functional hearing loss. A mixed hearing loss is caused by a combination of conductive and sensorineural losses. With functional hearing loss, which is rare, the individual does not respond to voice and appears not to hear. It is thought to be caused by emotional or psychologic factors.

Ménière disease. Ménière disease (endolymphatic hydrops is an episodic chronic disorder of the middle ear with an unknown etiology that can be unilateral or bilateral. There is excessive endolymph and pressure in the membranous labyrinth that disrupts both vestibular and hearing functions. There are four symptoms: recurring episodes of vertigo (often accompanied by severe nausea and vomiting), hearing loss, ringing in the ears (tinnitus), and a feeling of fullness in the ear. Treatment is symptomatic with medical management or surgical management when medications fail.[62]

Ear Infections

Otitis externa. Otitis externa is the most common inflammation of the outer ear and may be acute or chronic, infectious or noninfectious. The most common origins of acute infections are bacterial microorganisms including *Pseudomonas, Staphylococcus aureus*, and, less commonly, *Escherichia coli*. Fungal infections are less common. Infection usually follows prolonged exposure to moisture (swimmer's ear). The earliest symptoms are inflammation with pruritus, swelling, and clear drainage, progressing to purulent drainage with obstruction of the canal. Tenderness and pain with earlobe retraction accompany inflammation. Acidifying solutions are used for early treatment and prevention. Topical antimicrobials usually provide effective treatment for later stages of disease.[63] Chronic infections are more often related to allergy or skin disorders.

Otitis media. Otitis media is a common infection of infants and children. Most children have one episode by 3 years of age. The most common pathogens are *Streptococcus pneumoniae, Haemophilus influenzae*, and *Moraxella catarrhalis*. Predisposing factors include allergy, sinusitis, submucosal cleft palate, adenoidal hypertrophy, eustachian tube dysfunction, and immune deficiency. Breast-feeding is a protective factor. Recurrent acute otitis media may be genetically determined.[64]

Acute otitis media (AOM) is associated with ear pain, fever, irritability, inflamed tympanic membrane, and fluid in the middle ear. The appearance of the tympanic membrane progresses from erythema to opaqueness with bulging as fluid accumulates. There is an increasing prevalence of AOM caused by penicillin-resistant microorganisms. Otitis media with effusion (OME) is the presence of fluid in the middle ear without symptoms of acute infection (Fig. 15.13).

Treatment includes symptom management, particularly of pain, with watchful waiting, antimicrobial therapy for severe illness, and placement of tympanostomy tubes when there is persistent bilateral effusion and significant hearing loss. Complications include mastoiditis, brain abscess, meningitis, and chronic otitis media with hearing loss. Persistent middle ear effusions may affect speech, language, and cognitive abilities. Multivalent vaccines for influenza result in modest prevention of acute otitis media.[65]

Olfaction and Taste

Olfaction (smell) is a function of cranial nerve I and part of cranial nerve V. Taste (gustation) is a function of multiple nerves in the tongue, soft palate, uvula, pharynx, and upper esophagus innervated by cranial nerves VII and IX. Both of these cranial nerves are influenced by hormones within the sensory cells. Dysfunctions of smell and taste may occur separately or jointly. The strong relationship between smell and taste creates the sensation of flavor. If either sensation is impaired, the perception of flavor is altered. Olfactory structures are illustrated in Fig. 15.14.

Olfactory cells, located in the olfactory epithelium, are the receptor cells for smell. Seven different primary classes of olfactory stimulants have been identified: (1) camphoraceous, (2) musky, (3) floral, (4) peppermint, (5) ethereal, (6) pungent, and (7) putrid. The primary sensations of taste are (1) sour, (2) salty, (3) sweet, (4) bitter, and (5) umami (savory taste of glutamate). Taste buds (fungiform, foliate, and circumvallate) sensitive to each of the primary sensations are located in specific areas of the tongue: sweet near the tip, salty on frontal sides, sour on the posterior sides, bitter on the very back, and umami overall surface of tongue.

Sensitivity to odors declines steadily with aging. (See the box *Geriatric Considerations: Aging & Changes in Olfaction and Taste* for a summary of changes in olfaction and taste with aging.)

Olfactory and Taste Dysfunctions

Olfactory dysfunctions include the following:
1. Hyposmia—impaired sense of smell
2. Anosmia—complete loss of sense of smell
3. Olfactory hallucinations—smelling odors that are not really present
4. Parosmia—abnormal or perverted sense of smell

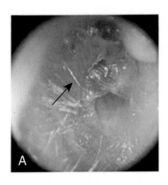
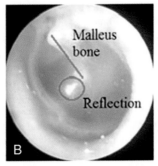
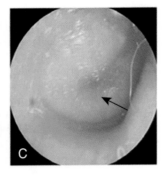

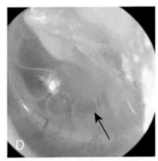
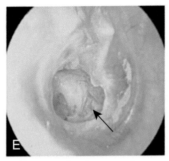

FIGURE 15.13 Otitis Media. A, Obstructing wax or foreign bodies in external ear canal *(see arrow)* precluding visualization of the TM to establish an OM diagnosis. **B,** A normal TM (n-TM) showing a semitransparent pearly white TM, triangular shaped light reflex, and malleus bone clearly visible (red ring and line, respectively). **C,** Acute otitis media showing a bulging TM with red color *(see arrow)*. **D,** Otitis media with effusion *(see arrow)* showing a retracted TM and fluid in the middle ear *(see arrow)*. **E,** Chronic suppurative otitis media showing a TM perforation *(see arrow)*. *TM,* tympanic membrane. (From Myburgh HC et al: Otitis media diagnosis for developing countries using tympanic membrane image-analysis, *EBioMedicine* 5:156–160, 2016. Available at https://www.sciencedirect.com/science/article/pii/S2352396416300500.)

GERIATRIC CONSIDERATIONS

Aging & Changes in Olfaction and Taste

- Decline in sensitivity to odors, usually after age 80, occurs.
- Loss of olfaction may diminish appetite, taste, and food selection and may affect nutrition.
- Inability to smell toxic fumes or gases can pose a safety hazard.
- Decline in taste sensitivity is more gradual than decline in sense of smell.
- Higher concentrations of flavors required to stimulate taste.
- Taste may be influenced by decreased salivary secretion.

The sense of taste can be impaired by injury. Altered taste may be attributed to impaired smell associated with injury near the hippocampus.

Hypogeusia is a decrease in taste sensation, whereas **ageusia** is an absence of the sense of taste. These disorders result from cranial nerve injuries and can be specific to the area of the tongue innervated. **Dysgeusia** is a perversion of taste in which substances possess an unpleasant flavor (i.e., metallic). Alterations in taste may compromise adequate nutrition or cause anorexia.[66]

✔ **QUICK CHECK 15.4**
1. List the major structures of the eye.
2. Visual disorders fall into several categories; name them.
3. How does fluid accumulate in the middle ear during otitis media?
4. What factors are involved in the sensation of flavor?

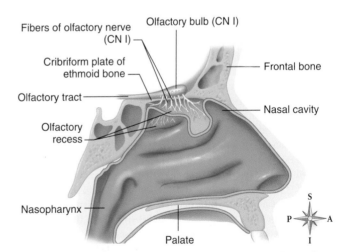

FIGURE 15.14 Olfaction. Midsagittal section of the nasal area shows the location of major olfactory sensory structures. (From Patton KT, Thibodeau GA, Douglas MM: *Essentials of anatomy & physiology,* St Louis, 2012, Mosby.)

SOMATOSENSORY FUNCTION

Touch

The sensation of **touch** involves four afferent fiber types that mediate tactile sensation, and there may be an additional sensory nerve that transmits pleasurable touch.[67] Receptors sensitive to touch are present in the skin with high densities in the fingers and lips. Meissner and pacinian corpuscles sense movement across the skin and vibration, respectively. Merkel disks sense sustained light touch, and Ruffini endings respond to deep sustained pressure, stretch, and joint position. Specific sensory input is carried to the higher levels of the CNS by the dorsal column of the spinal cord and the anterior spinothalamic tract.

The cutaneous senses develop before birth, but structural growth continues into early adulthood. Then a gradual decline occurs, with loss in tactile discrimination with advancing age.[68] Abnormal tactile perception may be caused by alterations at any level of the nervous system, from the receptor to the cerebral cortex. Factors that interrupt or impair reception, transmission, perception, or interpretation of touch—including trauma, tumor, infection, metabolic changes, vascular changes, and degenerative diseases—may cause tactile dysfunction. In addition, most tactile sensations evoke affective responses that determine whether the sensation is unpleasant, pleasant, or neutral.

Proprioception

Proprioception is the awareness of the position of the body and its parts. It depends on impulses from the inner ear and from receptors in joints and ligaments. Sensory data are transmitted to higher centers, primarily through the dorsal columns and the spinocerebellar tracts, with some data passing through the medial lemnisci and thalamic radiations to the cortex. These stimuli are necessary for the coordination of movements, the grading of muscular contraction, and the maintenance of equilibrium.

As with tactile dysfunction, any factor that interrupts or impairs the reception, transmission, perception, or interpretation of proprioceptive stimuli also alters proprioception and increases the risk for falls and injury. A progressive loss of proprioception has been reported in elderly persons with an increased risk for falls and injury.[69] Two common causes are vestibular dysfunction and neuropathy.

Specific vestibular dysfunctions are vestibular nystagmus and vertigo. Vestibular nystagmus is the constant, involuntary movement of the eyeball and develops when the semicircular canal system is overstimulated. Vertigo is the sensation of spinning that occurs with inflammation of the semicircular canals in the ear. The individual may feel either that he or she is moving in space or that the world is revolving. Vertigo often causes loss of balance, and nystagmus may occur. Ménière disease can cause loss of proprioception during an acute attack, so that standing or walking is impossible.

Peripheral neuropathies also can cause proprioceptive dysfunction. They may be caused by several conditions and commonly are associated with renal disease and diabetes mellitus. Although the exact sequence of events is unknown, neuropathies cause a diminished or absent sense of body position or position of body parts. Gait changes often occur.

✔ **QUICK CHECK 15.5**
1. How are different touch receptors distributed over the body?
2. What are two causes of alterations in proprioception?

■ SUMMARY REVIEW

Pain

1. Pain (nociception) is a complex, sensory experience involving emotion, cognition, and motivation. Acute pain is protective, promoting withdrawal from painful stimuli.
2. Three portions of the nervous system are responsible for the sensation, perception, and response to pain: (1) the afferent pathways, (2) the interpretive centers in the central nervous system, and (3) the efferent pathways.
3. Nociception involves four phases: transduction, transmission, perception, and modulation.
4. Pain transduction begins when nociceptors (pain receptors) are activated by noxious stimulants. There are two types of nociceptors: mylinated Aδ fibers transmit sharp, "fast" pain; smaller, unmyelinated C fibers more slowly transmit dull, less localized pain.
5. Pain transmission is the conduction of pain impulses along the nociceptors into the spinal cord and eventually to the brain.
6. Pain perception is the conscious awareness of pain. It occurs with the integration of three systems. The sensory-discriminative system (mediated by the somatosensory cortex) identifies the location and intensity of pain. The affective-motivational system (mediated by the reticular formation, limbic system, and brain stem) controls emotional and affective responses to pain. The cognitive-evaluative system (mediated by the cortex) coordinates the meaning an experience of pain.
7. Pain threshold is the lowest intensity of pain that a person can recognize. Pain tolerance is the greatest level of pain that an individual is prepared to tolerate. Both are subjective and influenced by many factors.
8. Pain modulation increases or decreases the transmission of pain signals throughout the nervous system. Neuromodulators of pain include substances that (1) stimulate pain nociceptors (e.g.,

prostaglandins, bradykinins, lymphokines, substance P, glutamate) and (2) suppress pain (e.g., GABA, endogenous opioids, endocannabinoids). Some substances excite peripheral nerves but inhibit central nerves (e.g., serotonin, norepinephrine).

9. Endogenous opioids inhibit pain transmission and include enkephalins, endorphins, dynorphins, and endomorphins. They are produced in the central nervous system and by immune cells.
10. Descending inhibitory and facilitatory pathways and nuclei inhibit or facilitate pain. Efferent pathways from the ventromedial medulla and periaqueductal gray inhibit pain impulses at the dorsal horn. The rostroventromedial medulla (RVM) stimulates efferent pathways that facilitate or inhibit pain in the dorsal horn
11. Segmental pain inhibition occurs when impulses from Aβ fibers (touch and vibration sensations) arrive at the same spinal level as impulses from Aδ or C fibers.
12. Diffuse noxious inhibitory control occurs when pain signals from two different sites are transmitted simultaneously and inhibit pain through a spinal-medullary-spinal pathway.
13. Because of the complex nature of pain, classifications of pain often overlap, and more than one description is often used.
14. Acute pain is a signal to the person of a harmful stimulus and may be (1) somatic (skin, joints, muscles), (2) visceral (inner organs, body cavities), or (3) referred (present in an area distant from its origin). The area of referred pain is supplied by the same spinal segment as the actual site of pain.
15. Chronic pain is pain lasting well beyond the expected normal healing time and may be ongoing (e.g., low back pain) or intermittent (e.g., migraine headaches). Psychologic, behavioral, and physiologic responses to chronic pain include depression, sleep disorders, preoccupation with pain, lifestyle changes, and physiologic adaptation.

16. Neuropathic pain is increased sensitivity to painful or nonpainful stimuli and results from abnormal processing of pain information in the peripheral or central nervous system.

Temperature Regulation

1. Temperature regulation (thermoregulation) is achieved through precise balancing of heat production, heat conservation, and heat loss. Body temperature is maintained in a range around 37° C (98.6° F).
2. Temperature regulation is mediated by the hypothalamus and endocrine system through peripheral thermoreceptors in the skin, liver, and skeletal muscle and central thermoreceptors in the hypothalamus, spinal cord, viscera, and great veins.
3. Heat is produced through chemical reactions of metabolism and skeletal muscle contraction. Heat is distributed by the circulatory system.
4. Heat is lost through radiation, conduction, convection, vasodilation, decreased muscle tone, evaporation of sweat, increased respiration, voluntary mechanisms, and adaptation to warmer climates.
5. Infants do not conserve heat well because of their greater body surface/mass ratio and decreased amounts of subcutaneous fat. Elderly persons have poor responses to environmental temperature extremes as a result of slowed blood circulation, structural and functional changes in the skin, and overall decrease in heat-producing activities.
6. Fever involves the "resetting of the hypothalamic thermostat" to a higher level. When the fever breaks, the set point returns to normal. Fever is triggered by the release of exogenous pyrogens from bacteria or the release of endogenous pyrogens (cytokines) from phagocytic cells.
7. Fever of unknown origin is a body temperature greater than 38.3° C (101° F) for longer than 3 weeks that remains undiagnosed after 3 days of investigation.
8. Fever production aids responses to infectious processes. Higher temperatures kill many microorganisms, promote immune responses, and decrease serum levels of iron, zinc, and copper, which are needed for bacterial replication.
9. Hyperthermia (marked warming of core temperature) can produce nerve damage, coagulation of cell proteins, and death. Therapeutic hyperthermia may be used to promote natural immune processes or promote tumor blood flow. Forms of accidental hyperthermia include heat cramps, heat exhaustion, heat stroke, and malignant hyperthermia. Heat stroke and malignant hyperthermia are potentially lethal.
10. Hypothermia (marked cooling of core temperature) slows the rate of cell metabolism, increases the viscosity of the blood, slows blood flow through the microcirculation, facilitates blood coagulation, and stimulates profound vasoconstriction. Hypothermia may be accidental or therapeutic.
11. 11. Major body trauma can affect temperature regulation by damaging the CNS or causing inflammation, increased intracranial pressure, or intracranial bleeding. It results in a sustained, noninfectious fever called central fever.

Sleep

1. Sleep is an active process that provides restorative functions and promotes memory consolidation. Sleep is divided into rapid eye movement (REM) and non-REM stages, each of which has its own series of stages. While asleep, an individual progresses through REM and non-REM (slow wave) sleep multiple times in a predictable cycle.

2. REM sleep is controlled by mechanisms in the pons and mesencephalon. It is known as paradoxical sleep because the EEG pattern is similar to that of an awake person. The brain is very active with dreaming.
3. Non-REM sleep is controlled by release of inhibitory signals from the hypothalamus and accounts for 75% to 80% of sleep time. The body is in a state of reduced activity.
4. The sleep patterns of the newborn and young child vary from those of the adult in total sleep time, cycle length, and percentage of time spent in each sleep cycle. Elderly persons experience a total decrease in sleep time.
5. The restorative, reparative, and growth processes occur during slow-wave (non-REM) sleep. Sleep deprivation can cause profound changes in personality and functioning.
6. Sleep disorders include (1) dyssomnias, which are disorders of initiating or maintaining sleep (i.e., insomnia, obstructive sleep apnea syndrome, hypersomnia, or disorders of the sleep-wake schedule) and (2) parasomnias, which are unusual behaviors during sleep (i.e., sleepwalking or night terrors and restless legs syndrome).

The Special Senses

1. The special senses include vision, hearing, olfaction, and taste.
2. The eyes are responsible for vision. The wall of the eye has three layers: sclera, choroid, and retina. The retina contains millions of baroreceptors known as rods and cones that receive light through the lens and then convey signals to the optic nerve and subsequently to the visual cortex of the brain.
3. The eye is filled with vitreous and aqueous humor, which prevent it from collapsing.
4. The major alterations in ocular movement include strabismus, nystagmus, and paralysis of the extraocular muscles.
5. Alterations in visual acuity (the ability to see objects in sharp detail) can be caused by amblyopia, scotoma, cataracts, papilledema, dark adaptation, glaucoma, retinal detachment, and macular degeneration. Visual acuity decreases with age due to structural eye changes.
6. A cataract is a cloudy or opaque area in the ocular lens and leads to visual loss when located on the visual axis. Cataracts are the leading cause of blindness in the world.
7. Glaucomas are characterized by intraocular pressures with death of retinal ganglion cells and their axons.
8. Age-related macular degeneration is irreversible loss of vision with atrophic (dry) or neovascular (wet) forms.
9. Alterations in accommodation (changes in lens shape that changes focus from distant to near images) develop with increased intraocular pressure, inflammation, age, and disease of the oculomotor nerve. Presbyopia is loss of accommodation caused by loss of elasticity of the lens with aging.
10. Alterations in refraction, including myopia, hyperopia, and astigmatism, are the most common visual disorders.
11. Alterations in color vision can be related to yellowing of the lens with aging and color blindness, an inherited trait.
12. Trauma or disease of the optic nerve pathways can cause defects or blindness in the entire visual field or in half of the visual field (hemianopia).
13. The eyelids, conjunctivae, and lacrimal apparatus protect the eye externally. Infections are the most common disorders; they include blepharitis, conjunctivitis, chalazion, and hordeolum.
14. Blepharitis is an inflammation of the eyelid; a hordeolum (stye) is an infection of the eyelid's sebaceous gland; and a chalazion is an infection of the eyelid's meibomian gland.
15. Conjunctivitis is an inflammation of the conjunctiva, and can be acute or chronic, bacterial, viral, or allergic. Redness, edema, pain,

and lacrimation are common symptoms. Trachoma (chlamydial conjunctivitis) is the leading cause of preventable blindness in the world and is associated with poor hygiene.

16. Keratitis is a bacterial or viral infection of the cornea that can lead to corneal ulceration.

17. The ears are responsible for hearing. The ear is composed of external, middle, and inner structures.

18. The external ear structures are the pinna, auditory canal, and tympanic membrane. The external ear is only involved in hearing.

19. The middle ear is composed of the tympanic cavity (containing three bones: the malleus, the incus, and the stapes), oval window, eustachian tube, and fluid. These transmit sound vibrations to the inner ear. The middle ear is only involved in hearing.

20. The inner ear is involved in both hearing and equilibrium. It includes the bony and membranous labyrinths that transmit sound waves through the cochlea and to the cochlear nerve and ultimately to the brain. The semicircular canals and vestibule help maintain balance through the equilibrium receptors.

21. Impaired hearing is the most common sensory defect, occurring in 5% to 10% of the general population.

22. Hearing loss can be classified as conductive, sensorineural, mixed, or functional.

23. Conductive hearing loss occurs when sound waves cannot be conducted through the middle ear.

24. Sensorineural hearing loss develops with impairment of the organ of Corti or its central connections. Presbycusis is the most common form of sensorineural hearing loss in elderly people.

25. A combination of conductive and sensorineural loss is a mixed hearing loss. Loss of hearing with no known organic cause is a functional hearing loss.

26. Ménière disease is a disorder of the middle ear that affects hearing and balance.

27. Otitis externa is an infection of the outer ear associated with prolonged exposure to moisture.

28. Otitis media is an infection of the middle ear that is common in children. Accumulation of fluid (effusion) behind the tympanic membrane is a common finding.

29. Olfaction (smell) is a function of cranial nerve I and part of cranial nerve V. Taste (gustation) is a function of multiple nerves in the tongue, soft palate, uvula, pharynx, and upper esophagus innervated by cranial nerves VII and IX

30. The perception of flavor is altered if olfaction or taste dysfunctions occur. Sensitivity to odor and taste decreases with aging.

31. Hyposmia is an impaired sense of smell, and anosmia is the complete loss of the sense of smell.

32. Hypogeusia is a decrease in taste sensation, and ageusia is the absence of the sense of taste.

Somatosensory Function

1. The sensation of touch is a function of receptors present in the skin, and the sensory response is conducted to the brain through the dorsal column and anterior spinothalamic tract.

2. Alterations in touch can result from alterations at any level of the nervous system.

3. Proprioception is the awareness of the position and location of the body and its parts. Proprioceptors are located in the inner ear, joints, and ligaments. Proprioceptive stimuli are necessary for balance, coordinated movement, and grading of muscular contraction.

4. Disorders of proprioception can occur at any level of the nervous system and result in impaired balance and lack of coordinated movement. Vestibular nystagmus is the constant, involuntary movement of the eyeball and develops when the semicircular canal system is overstimulated. Vertigo is the sensation of spinning that occurs with inflammation of the semicircular canals in the ear.

KEY TERMS

A-beta (Aβ) fiber, 330
Accidental hyperthermia, 335
Accommodation, 340
Acute bacterial conjunctivitis (pinkeye), 342
Acute otitis media (AOM), 344
Acute pain, 330
A-delta (Aδ) fiber, 328
Affective-motivational system, 329
Age-related macular degeneration (AMD), 340
Ageusia, 345
Allergic conjunctivitis, 342
Allodynia, 332
Amblyopia, 338
Anosmia, 344
Aqueous humor, 338
Astigmatism, 340
Blepharitis, 341
Cannabinoid, 330
Cannabis, 330
Cataract, 339
Central fever, 335
Central neuropathic pain, 332
Central sensitization, 332

C fiber, 328
Chalazion, 341
Choroid, 338
Chronic conjunctivitis, 342
Chronic pain, 331
Circadian rhythm sleep disorder, 337
Cochlea, 343
Cognitive-evaluative system, 329
Color blindness, 341
Conductive hearing loss, 343
Cone, 338
Conjunctivitis, 341
Cornea, 338
Crista ampullaris, 343
Descending inhibitory pathway, 330
Diffuse noxious inhibitory control (DNIC), 330
Diplopia, 338
Dynorphin, 329
Dysgeusia, 345
Endocannabinoid, 330
Endogenous opioid, 329
Endogenous pyrogen, 333
Endomorphin, 329

Endorphin, 329
Enkephalin, 329
Entropion, 341
Equilibrium receptor, 343
Eustachian (pharyngotympanic) tube, 342
Excitatory neurotransmitter, 329
Exogenous pyrogen, 333
Expectancy-related cortical activation, 330
External auditory canal, 342
Facilitatory pathway, 330
Fever, 333
Fever of unknown origin (FUO), 334
Fovea centralis, 338
Functional hearing loss, 344
Glaucoma, 339
Hair cell, 343
Heat cramp, 335
Heat exhaustion, 335
Heat stroke, 335
Heterosegmental pain inhibition or conditioned pain modulation, 330
Hordeolum (stye), 341

Hyperopia, 340
Hypersomnia, 337
Hyperthermia, 335
Hypogeusia, 345
Hyposmia, 344
Hypothermia, 335
Incus (anvil), 342
Inhibitory neurotransmitter, 329
Insomnia, 336
Iris, 338
Jerk nystagmus, 338
Keratitis, 342
Lens, 338
Macula lutea, 338
Maculae, 343
Malignant hyperthermia, 335
Malleus (hammer), 342
Mastoid air cell, 342
Mastoid process, 342
Meissner corpuscle, 345
Ménière disease (endolymphatic hydrops), 344
Merkel disk, 346
Mixed hearing loss, 344
Myopia, 340
Narcolepsy, 337

REFERENCES

1. McCaffery M: *Nursing practice theories related to cognition, bodily pain and nonenvironment interactions*, Los Angeles, CA, 1968, University of California at Los Angeles Students' Store.
2. International Association for the Study of Pain (IASP): IASP pain terminology, pain terms, last updated December 14, 2017. Available at: https://www.iasp-pain.org/Education/Content.aspx?ItemNumber=1698#Pain. (Accessed 2 May 2019).
3. Cohen M, Quintner J, van Rysewyk S: Reconsidering the International Association for the Study of Pain definition of pain, *Pain Rep* 3(2):e634, 2018.
4. Ellison DL: Physiology of pain, *Crit Care Nurs Clin North Am* 29(4):397-406, 2017.
5. Yam MF, et al: General pathways of pain sensation and the major neurotransmitters involved in pain regulation, *Int J Mol Sci* 19(8):2164, 2018.
6. Casey KL: Forebrain mechanisms of nociception and pain: analysis through imaging, *Proc Natl Acad Sci USA* 96(14):7668-7674, 1999.
7. Garcia-Larrea L, Peyron R: Pain matrices and neuropathic pain matrices: a review, *Pain* 154(Suppl 1):S29-S43, 2013.
8. Kirkpatrick DR, et al: Therapeutic basis of clinical pain modulation, *Clin Transl Sci* 8(6):848-856, 2015.
9. Lau BK, Vaughan CW: Descending modulation of pain: the GABA disinhibition hypothesis of analgesia, *Curr Opin Neurobiol* 29C:159-164, 2014.
10. Ninkovic J, Roy S: Role of the mu-opioid receptor in opioid modulation of immune function, *Amino Acids* 45(1):9-24, 2013.
11. Bodnar RJ: Endogenous opiates and behavior, *Peptides* 31(12):2325-2359, 2010, 2009.
12. Busch-Dienstfertig M, Stein C: Opioid receptors and opioid peptide-producing leukocytes in inflammatory pain—basic and therapeutic aspects, *Brain Behav Immun* 24(5):683-694, 2010.
13. Donvito G, et al: The endogenous cannabinoid system: a budding source of targets for treating inflammatory and neuropathic pain, *Neuropsychopharmacology* 43(1):52-79, 2018.
14. Starowicz K, Finn DP: Cannabinoids and pain: sites and mechanisms of action, *Adv Pharmacol* 80:437-475, 2017.
15. van Wijk G, Veldhuijzen DS: Perspective on diffuse noxious inhibitory controls as a model of endogenous pain modulation in clinical pain syndromes, *J Pain* 11(5):408-419, 2010.
16. Colloca L, Grillon C: Understanding placebo and nocebo responses for pain management, *Curr Pain Headache Rep* 18(6):419, 2014.

17. Crofford LJ: Chronic pain: where the body meets the brain, *Trans Am Clin Climatol Assoc* 126:167-183, 2015.
18. Martucci KT, Mackey SC: Imaging pain, *Anesthesiol Clin* 34(2):255-269, 2016.
19. Garland EL: Pain processing in the human nervous system: a selective review of nociceptive and biobehavioral pathways, *Prim Care* 39(3):561-571, 2012.
20. Miles A, et al: Managing constraint: the experience of people with chronic pain, *Soc Sci Med* 61(2):431-441, 2005.
21. Colloca L, et al: Neuropathic pain, *Nat Rev Dis Primers* 3:17002, 2017.
22. Bennett GJ: What is spontaneous pain and who has it?, *J Pain* 13(10):921-929, 2012.
23. Bonakdar RA: Integrative pain management, *Med Clin North Am* 101(5):987-1004, 2017.
24. Romanovsky AA: The thermoregulation system and how it works, *Handb Clin Neurol* 156:3-43, 2018.
25. Gao Z, et al: Altered coronary vascular control during cold stress in healthy older adults, *Am J Physiol Heart Circ Physiol* 302(1):H312-H318, 2012.
26. Székely M, Garai J: Thermoregulation and age, *Handb Clin Neurol* 156:377-395, 2018.
27. Cunha BA, Lortholary O, Cunha CB: Fever of unknown origin: a clinical approach, *Am J Med* 128(10):1138.e1-1138.e15, 2015.
28. Barone JE: Fever: fact and fiction, *J Trauma* 67(2):406-409, 2009.
29. Cannon JG: Perspective on fever: the basic science and conventional medicine, *Complement Ther Med* 21(Suppl 1):S54-S60, 2013.
30. Purssell E, While AE: Does the use of antipyretics in children who have acute infections prolong febrile illness? A systematic review and meta-analysis, *J Pediatr* 163(3):822-827, 2013.
31. Wing R, et al: Fever in the pediatric patient, *Emerg Med Clin North Am* 31(4):1073-1096, 2013.
32. Roghmann MC, et al: The relationship between age and fever magnitude, *Am J Med Sci* 322(2):68-70, 2001.
33. Wang H, et al: Brain temperature and its fundamental properties: a review for clinical neuroscientists, *Front Neurosci* 8:307, 2014.
34. Habash RWY: Therapeutic hyperthermia, *Handb Clin Neurol* 157:853-868, 2018.
35. Gomez CR: Disorders of body temperature, *Handb Clin Neurol* 120:947-957, 2014.
36. Al Mahri S, Bouchama A: Heatstroke, *Handb Clin Neurol* 157:531-545, 2018.
37. Bandschapp O, Girard T: Malignant hyperthermia, *Swiss Med Wkly* 142:w13652, 2012.

38. Zawadzka M, Szmuda M, Mazurkiewicz-Bełdzińska M: Thermoregulation disorders of central origin—how to diagnose and treat, *Anaesthesiol Intensive Ther* 49(3):227-234, 2017.
39. Potter GD, et al: Circadian rhythm and sleep disruption: causes, metabolic consequences, and countermeasures, *Endocr Rev* 37(6):584-608, 2016.
40. Iber C, et al: *The AASM manual for the scoring of sleep and associated events*, Westchester, IL, 2007, American Academy of Sleep Medicine.
41. España RA, Scammell TE: Sleep neurobiology from a clinical perspective, *Sleep* 34(7):845-858, 2011.
42. Peever J, Fuller PM: The biology of REM sleep, *Curr Biol* 27(22):R1237-R1248, 2017.
43. American Academy of Sleep Medicine: *International classification of sleep disorders, third edition: diagnostic and coding manual*, Westchester, IL, 2014, Author.
44. Buysse DJ: Insomnia, *J Am Med Assoc* 309(7):706-716, 2013.
45. Veasey SC, Rosen IM: Obstructive sleep apnea in adults, *N Engl J Med* 380(15):1442-1449, 2019.
46. Berry RB: *Fundamentals of sleep medicine*, Philadelphia, 2012, Elsevier.
47. Rosenberg RP: Clinical assessment of excessive daytime sleepiness in the diagnosis of sleep disorders, *J Clin Psychiatry* 76(12):e1602, 2015.
48. Ferguson MS, Magill JC, Kotecha BT: Narrative review of contemporary treatment options in the care of patients with obstructive sleep apnea, *Ther Adv Respir Dis* 11(11):411-423, 2017.
49. Brockbank JC: Update on pathophysiology and treatment of childhood obstructive sleep apnea syndrome, *Paediatr Respir Rev* 24:21-23, 2017.
50. Golden EC, Lipford MC: Narcolepsy: diagnosis and management, *Cleve Clin J Med* 85(12):959-969, 2018.
51. Jagannath A, et al: The genetics of circadian rhythms, sleep and health, *Hum Mol Genet* 26(R2):R128-R138, 2017.
52. Pavlova M: Circadian rhythm sleep-wake disorders, *Continuum (Minneap Minn)* 23(4, Sleep Neurology):1051-1063, 2017.
53. Fleetham JA, Fleming JA: Parasomnias, *CMAJ* 186(8):E273-E280, 2014.
54. Fraigne JJ, et al: REM sleep at its core—circuits, neurotransmitters, and pathophysiology, *Front Neurol* 6:123, 2015.
55. Allen RP: Restless legs syndrome/Willis Ekbom disease: evaluation and treatment, *Int Rev Psychiatry* 26(2):248-262, 2014.
56. Weinreb RN, Aung T, Medeiros FA: The pathophysiology and treatment of glaucoma: a review, *J Am Med Assoc* 311(18):1901-1911, 2014.

57. Chew EY, et al: Long-term effects of vitamins C, E, beta-carotene and zinc on age related macular degeneration, AREDS Report No. 35, *Ophthalmology* 120(8):1604-1611, 2013.
58. Liu HH, Hu Y, Cui HP: Femtosecond laser in refractive and cataract surgeries, *Int J Ophthalmol* 8(2):419-426, 2015.
59. Simunovic MP: Colour vision deficiency, *Eye (Lond)* 24(5):747-755, 2010.
60. Alfonso SA, Fawley JD, Alexa Lu X: Conjunctivitis, *Prim Care* 42(3):325-345, 2015.
61. Lasak JM, et al: Hearing loss: diagnosis and management, *Prim Care* 41(1):19-31, 2014.

62. Nevoux J, et al: International consensus (ICON) on treatment of Ménière's disease, *Eur Ann Otorhinolaryngol Head Neck Dis* 135(1S):S29-S32, 2018.
63. Hajioff D, MacKeith S: Otitis externa, *BMJ Clin Evid* 2015:2015. pii 0510.
64. Rye MS, et al: Genetic susceptibility to otitis media in childhood, *Laryngoscope* 122(3):665-675, 2012.
65. Norhayati MN, Ho JJ, Azman MY: Influenza vaccines for preventing acute otitis media in infants and children, *Cochrane Database Syst Rev* (10):CD010089, 2017.

66. Visvanathan R, Chapman IM: Undernutrition and anorexia in the older person, *Gastroenterol Clin North Am* 38(3):393-409, 2009.
67. McGlone F, Reilly D: The cutaneous sensory system, *Neurosci Biobehav Rev* 34(2):148-159, 2010.
68. Norman JF, et al: Aging and curvature discrimination from static and dynamic touch, *PLoS ONE* 8(7):e68577, 2013.
69. Sohn J, Kim S: Falls study: proprioception, postural stability, and slips, *Biomed Mater Eng* 26(Suppl 1):S693-S703, 2015.

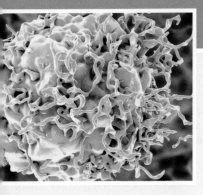

16

Alterations in Cognitive Systems, Cerebral Hemodynamics, and Motor Function

Barbara J. Boss, Sue E. Huether

EVOLVE WEBSITE

CHAPTER OUTLINE

Intellectual and behavioral functions are achieved by integrated processes of cognitive systems, sensory systems, and motor systems. The purpose of this chapter is to present the concepts and processes of alterations in these systems as an approach to understanding the manifestations of neurologic dysfunction that can occur with disease or injury. Some specific diseases also are presented here (i.e., Parkinson disease, Huntington disease, and amyotrophic lateral sclerosis) because they best fit here. (Specific disorders of the central and peripheral nervous system are presented in Chapter 17. Alterations in sensory function were presented in Chapter 15.)

The neural systems essential to cognitive function are (1) attentional systems that provide arousal and maintenance of attention over time; (2) memory and language systems by which information is remembered and communicated; and (3) affective or emotive systems that mediate mood, emotion, and intention. These core systems are fundamental to the processes of abstract thinking and reasoning. The products of abstraction and reasoning are organized and made operational through executive attentional networks. The normal functioning of these networks manifests through the motor network in a behavioral array viewed by others as appropriate to human activity and successful living.

ALTERATIONS IN COGNITIVE SYSTEMS

Consciousness is a state of awareness both of oneself and of the environment, and a set of responses to that environment. Consciousness has two distinct components: arousal (state of awakeness or alertness) and awareness (content of thought). **Arousal** is mediated by the reticular activating system, which regulates aspects of attention and information processing and maintains consciousness. Awareness encompasses all cognitive functions and is mediated by attentional systems, memory systems, language systems, and executive systems.

Alterations in Arousal

Alterations in level of arousal may be caused by structural, metabolic, or psychogenic (functional) disorders.

PATHOPHYSIOLOGY Structural alterations in arousal are divided according to the primary location of the pathologic condition. Causes include infection, vascular alterations, neoplasms, traumatic injury, congenital alterations, degenerative changes, polygenic traits, and metabolic disorders.

Supratentorial disorders (above the tentorium cerebelli) produce changes in arousal by either diffuse or localized dysfunction. Diffuse dysfunction may be caused by disease processes affecting the cerebral cortex or the underlying subcortical white matter (e.g., encephalitis). Disorders outside the brain but within the cranial vault (extracerebral) that can produce diffuse dysfunction include neoplasms, closed-head trauma with subsequent subdural bleeding, and accumulation of pus in the subdural space. Localized dysfunction occurs when masses develop within the brain substance (intracerebral). The sources of these masses include bleeding, infarcts, emboli, and tumors. Such localized destructive processes directly impair function of the thalamic or hypothalamic activating systems or secondarily compress these structures in a process of herniation.

Infratentorial disorders (below the tentorium cerebelli) produce a decline in arousal by (1) direct destruction or compression of the reticular activating system and its pathways (e.g., demyelinating disorders or accumulations of blood or pus and growth of tumors) or (2) the brainstem (midbrain, pons, medulla) may be destroyed either by direct invasion or by indirect impairment of its blood supply.

Metabolic disorders produce a decline in arousal by alterations in delivery of energy substrates as occurs with hypoxia, electrolyte disturbances, or hypoglycemia. Metabolic disorders caused by liver or renal failure cause alterations in neuronal excitability because of failure to metabolize or eliminate drugs and toxins. All the systemic diseases that eventually produce nervous system dysfunction are part of this metabolic category.

Psychogenic alterations in arousal (unresponsiveness), although uncommon, may signal general psychiatric disorders. Despite apparent unconsciousness, the person actually is physiologically awake, and the neurologic examination reflects normal responses.

CLINICAL MANIFESTATIONS AND EVALUATION Five patterns of neurologic function are critical to the evaluation of consciousness: (1) level of consciousness, (2) pattern of breathing, (3) pupillary reaction, (4) oculomotor responses, and (5) motor responses. Patterns of clinical manifestations help in determining the extent of brain dysfunction and serve as indexes for identifying increasing or decreasing central nervous system (CNS) function. Distinctions are made between

metabolic and structurally induced manifestations (Table 16.1). The types of manifestations suggest the mechanism of the altered arousal state (Table 16.2).

Level of consciousness is the most critical clinical index of nervous system function, with changes indicating either improvement or deterioration of the individual's condition. A person who is alert and oriented to self, others, place, and time is considered to be functioning at the highest level of consciousness, which implies full use of all the person's cognitive capacities. From this normal alert state, levels of consciousness diminish in stages from confusion and disorientation (can occur simultaneously) to coma, each of which is clinically defined (Table 16.3).

Patterns of breathing help evaluate the level of brain dysfunction and coma (Fig. 16.1). Rate, rhythm, and pattern should be evaluated. Breathing patterns can be categorized as hemispheric or brainstem patterns (Table 16.4).

With normal breathing, a neural center in the forebrain (cerebrum) produces a rhythmic pattern. When consciousness decreases, lower brainstem centers regulate the breathing pattern by responding only to changes in arterial carbon dioxide ($Paco_2$) levels. This pattern is called *posthyperventilation apnea. Cheyne-Stokes respiration* is an abnormal rhythm of ventilation with alternating periods of tachypnea and apnea with a crescendo-decrescendo pattern. Increases in $Paco_2$ levels lead to tachypnea. The $Paco_2$ level then decreases to below normal, and breathing stops (apnea) until the carbon dioxide reaccumulates and again stimulates tachypnea (see Fig. 16.1). In cases of opiate or sedative drug overdose, the respiratory center is depressed, so the rate of breathing gradually decreases until respiratory failure occurs.

Pupillary changes indicate the presence and level of brainstem dysfunction because brainstem areas that control arousal are adjacent to areas that control the pupils (Fig. 16.2). For example, severe ischemia and hypoxia usually produce dilated, fixed pupils. Hypothermia may cause fixed pupils.

Some drugs affect the pupils and must be considered in evaluating individuals in comatose states. Large doses of atropine and scopolamine (drugs that block parasympathetic stimulation) fully dilate and fix the pupils. Doses of sedatives in sufficient amounts to produce coma cause the pupils to become midposition or

TABLE 16.1	**Clinical Manifestations of Metabolic and Structural Causes of Altered Arousal**	
Manifestations	**Metabolically Induced**	**Structurally Induced**
Blink to threat (cranial nerves II, VII)	Equal	Asymmetric
Optic discs (cranial nerve II)	Flat, good pulsation	Papilledema
Extraocular movement (cranial nerves III, IV, VI)	Roving eye movements; normal doll's eyes and calorics	Gaze paresis, nerve palsy
Pupils (cranial nerves II, III)	Equal and reactive; may be dilated (e.g., atropine), pinpoint (e.g., opiates), or midposition and fixed (e.g., glutethimide [Doriden])	Asymmetric or nonreactive; may be midposition (midbrain injury), pinpoint (pons injury), large (tectal injury)
Corneal reflex (cranial nerves V, VII)	Symmetric response	Asymmetric response
Grimace to pain (cranial nerve VII)	Symmetric response	Asymmetric response
Motor function movement	Symmetric	Asymmetric
Muscle tone	Symmetric	Paratonic (rigid), spastic, flaccid, especially if asymmetric
Posture	Symmetric	Decorticate, especially if symmetric; decerebrate, especially if asymmetric (see Fig. 16.6)
Deep tendon reflexes	Symmetric	Asymmetric
Babinski sign	Absent or symmetric response	Present
Sensation	Symmetric	Asymmetric

TABLE 16.2 Differential Characteristics of States Causing Altered Arousal

Mechanism	Manifestations
Supratentorial mass lesions compressing or displacing diencephalon or brainstem	Initiating signs usually of focal cerebral dysfunction: vomiting, headache, hemiparesis, ocular signs, seizures, coma Signs of dysfunction progress rostral to caudal Neurologic signs at any given time point to one anatomic area (e.g., diencephalon, mesencephalon, medulla) Motor signs often asymmetric
Infratentorial mass of destruction causing coma	History of preceding brainstem dysfunction or sudden onset of coma Localizing brainstem signs precede or accompany onset of coma and always include oculovestibular abnormality Cranial nerve palsies usually manifest "bizarre" respiratory patterns that appear at onset
Metabolic coma Exogenous toxins (drugs) Endogenous toxins (organ system failure)	Confusion and stupor commonly precede motor signs Motor signs usually are symmetric Pupillary reactions usually are preserved Asterixis, myoclonus, tremor, and seizures are common Acid–base imbalance with hyperventilation or hypoventilation is common
Psychiatric unresponsiveness	Lids close actively; pupils reactive or dilated (cycloplegics) Oculocephalic reflexes are unpredictable; oculovestibular reflexes are physiologic (nystagmus is present) Motor tone is inconsistent or normal Eupnea or hyperventilation is usual No pathologic reflexes are present Electroencephalogram (EEG) is normal

TABLE 16.3 Levels of Altered Consciousness

State	Definition
Confusion	Loss of ability to think rapidly and clearly; impaired judgment and decision making
Disorientation	Beginning loss of consciousness; the person may exhibit restlessness, anxiety, and irritation; disorientation to time occurs first, followed by disorientation to place and familiar others (family members) and impaired memory; recognition of self is lost last
Lethargy	Limited spontaneous movement or speech; easy arousal with normal speech or touch; may or may not be oriented to time, place, or person
Obtundation	Mild to moderate reduction in arousal (awakeness) with limited response to environment; falls asleep unless stimulated verbally or tactilely; answers questions with minimal response
Stupor	Condition of deep sleep or unresponsiveness from which person may be aroused or caused to open eyes only by vigorous and repeated stimulation; response is often withdrawal or grabbing at stimulus
Light coma	Associated with purposeful movement on stimulation
Coma	Associated with nonpurposeful movement only on stimulation
Deep coma	Associated with unresponsiveness or no response to any stimulus

moderately dilated, unequal, and commonly fixed to light. Opiates cause pinpoint pupils. Severe barbiturate intoxication may produce fixed pupils.

Oculomotor responses are resting, spontaneous, and reflexive eye movements. They change at various levels of brain dysfunction in comatose individuals. Persons with metabolically induced coma, except with barbiturate-hypnotic and phenytoin poisoning, generally retain ocular reflexes even when other signs of brainstem damage are present. Destructive or compressive injury to the brainstem causes specific abnormalities of the oculocephalic and oculovestibular reflexes (Figs. 16.3 and 16.4). Injuries that involve an oculomotor nucleus or nerve (cranial nerve III) cause the involved eye to deviate outward, producing a resting dysconjugate lateral position of the eye.

Assessment of motor responses helps evaluate the level of brain dysfunction and determine the most severely damaged side of the brain. The patterns of response may be (1) purposeful; (2) inappropriate, generalized motor movement; or (3) not present. Motor signs indicating loss of cortical inhibition that are commonly associated with decreased consciousness include primitive reflexes and rigidity (paratonia) (Fig. 16.5). Primitive reflexes include grasping, reflex sucking, snout reflex, and palmomental reflex, all of which are normal in the newborn but disappear in infancy. Abnormal flexor and extensor responses in the upper and lower extremities are defined in Table 16.5 and illustrated in Fig. 16.6.

Vomiting, yawning, and hiccups are complex reflex-like motor responses that are integrated by neural mechanisms in the lower brainstem. These responses may be produced by compression or diseases involving tissues of the medulla oblongata (e.g., infection, tumors, infarction). They also may occur when there is benign stimuli to the vagal nerve (i.e., from the gut, liver, and kidney). Most CNS disorders produce nausea and vomiting. Vomiting without nausea indicates direct involvement of the central neural mechanism (or pyloric obstruction; see Chapters 38 and 39). Vomiting often accompanies CNS injuries that (1) involve the vestibular nuclei (cranial nerve VIII) or its immediate projections, particularly when double vision (diplopia) also is present; (2) impinge directly on the floor of the fourth ventricle; or (3) produce brainstem compression secondary to increased intracranial pressure.

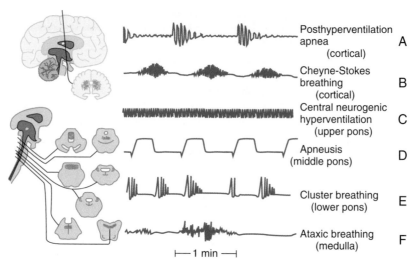

FIGURE 16.1 Abnormal Respiratory Patterns With Corresponding Level of Central Nervous System Activity. **A,** Posthyperventilation apnea is seen with bilateral cerebral dysfunction. **B,** Cheyne-Stokes respiration is seen with metabolic injury and lesions in the forebrain and diencephalon. **C,** Central neurogenic hyperventilation is most commonly seen with metabolic encephalopathies (lesion of midbrain, pons or medulla). **D,** Apneustic breathing (inspiratory pauses) is seen in patients with bilateral pontine lesions. **E,** Cluster breathing and ataxic breathing are seen in lesions at the pontine medullary junction. **F,** Ataxic breathing occurs when the medullary ventral respiratory nuclei are injured. (From Urden LD et al: *Critical care nursing: diagnosis and management,* ed 6, St Louis, 2010, Mosby.)

TABLE 16.4	**Patterns of Breathing**	
Breathing Pattern	**Description**	**Location of Injury**
Hemispheric Breathing Patterns		
Normal	After a period of hyperventilation that lowers arterial carbon dioxide pressure (Pa_{CO_2}), individual continues to breathe regularly but with reduced depth.	Response of nervous system to an external stressor—not associated with injury to CNS
Posthyperventilation apnea	Respirations stop after hyperventilation has lowered the concentration of carbon dioxide in the blood (P_{CO_2}) level below normal. Rhythmic breathing returns when P_{CO_2} level returns to normal.	Associated with diffuse bilateral metabolic or structural disease of cerebrum
Cheyne-Stokes respirations	Breathing pattern has a smooth increase (crescendo) in rate and depth of breathing (hyperpnea), which peaks and is followed by a gradual smooth decrease (decrescendo) in rate and depth of breathing to point of apnea, when cycle repeats itself. Hyperpneic phase lasts longer than apneic phase.	Bilateral dysfunction of deep cerebral or diencephalic structures; seen with supratentorial injury and metabolically induced coma states
Brainstem Breathing Patterns		
Central neurogenic hyperventilation	A sustained, deep, rapid, but regular pattern (hyperpnea) occurs, with a decreased Pa_{CO_2} and a corresponding increase in pH and the partial pressure of oxygen in the arterial blood (Pa_{O_2}).	May result from CNS damage or disease that involves midbrain and upper pons; seen after increased intracranial pressure and blunt head trauma
Apneusis	A prolonged inspiratory cramp (a pause at full inspiration) occurs; a common variant of this is a brief end-inspiratory pause of 2 or 3 sec, often alternating with an end-expiratory pause.	Indicates damage to respiratory control mechanism located at pontine level; most commonly associated with pontine infarction but documented with hypoglycemia, anoxia, and meningitis
Cluster breathing	A cluster of breaths has a disordered sequence with irregular pauses between breaths.	Dysfunction in lower pontine and high medullary areas
Ataxic breathing	Completely irregular breathing occurs, with random shallow and deep breaths and irregular pauses. Rate is often slow.	Originates from a primary dysfunction of medullary neurons controlling breathing
Gasping breathing pattern (agonal gasps)	A pattern of deep "all-or-none" breaths is accompanied by a slow respiratory rate.	Indicative of a failing medullary respiratory center

CNS, Central nervous system.

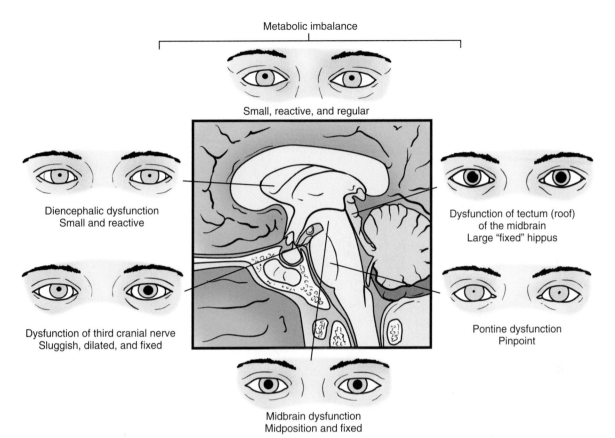

FIGURE 16.2 Appearance of Pupils at Different Levels of Consciousness.

QUICK CHECK 16.1
1. Why are structural as well as metabolic factors capable of producing coma?
2. Why is level of consciousness the most critical index of central nervous system function?
3. How do changes in $Paco_2$ cause Cheyne-Stokes respirations in coma?
4. What level of brain injury is associated with oculomotor changes?

BOX 16.1   Criteria for Brain Death

1. Completion of all appropriate diagnostic and therapeutic procedures with no possibility of brain function recovery
2. Unresponsive coma (no motor or reflex movements)
3. No spontaneous respiration (apnea)
4. No brainstem functions (ocular responses to head turning or caloric stimulation; dilated, fixed pupils; no gag or corneal reflex [see Figs. 16.3 and 16.4])
5. Isoelectric (flat) electroencephalogram (EEG) (electrocerebral silence)
6. Persistence of these signs for an appropriate observation period

Summarized from Wijdicks EF et al: *Neurology* 74(23):1911-1918, 2010.

Outcomes of Alterations in Arousal

Outcomes of alterations in arousal fall into two categories: *extent of disability (morbidity)* and *mortality*. Outcomes depend on the cause and extent of brain damage and the duration of coma. Some individuals may recover consciousness and an original level of function, some may have permanent disability, and some may never regain consciousness and experience neurologic death. Two forms of neurologic death—brain death and cerebral death—result from severe pathologic conditions and are associated with irreversible coma. Other possible outcomes are a vegetative state, a minimally conscious state, or locked-in syndrome. The extent of disability has four subcategories: recovery of consciousness, residual cognitive function, psychologic function, and vocational function.

Brain death (total brain death) occurs when the brain is damaged so completely that it can never recover (irreversible) and cannot maintain the body's internal homeostasis. State laws define brain death as irreversible cessation of function of the entire brain, including the brainstem and cerebellum. On postmortem examination, the brain is autolyzing (self-digesting) or already autolyzed. Brain death has occurred when there is no evidence of brain function for an extended period.[1] The abnormality of brain function must result from structural or known

metabolic disease and must *not* be caused by a depressant drug, alcohol poisoning, or hypothermia. An isoelectric, or flat, electroencephalogram (EEG) (electrocerebral silence) for 6 to 12 hours in a person who is not hypothermic and has not ingested depressant drugs indicates brain death. The clinical criteria used to determine brain death are noted in Box 16.1. A task force for determination of brain death in children recommended the same criteria as for adults, but with a longer observation period.[2]

Cerebral death, or irreversible coma, is death of the cerebral hemispheres exclusive of the brainstem and cerebellum. Brain damage is permanent, and the individual is forever unable to respond behaviorally in any significant way to the environment. The brainstem may continue to maintain internal homeostasis (i.e., body temperature, cardiovascular functions, respirations, and metabolic functions). The survivor of cerebral death may remain in a coma or emerge into a persistent vegetative state (VS) or a minimally conscious state. In coma, the eyes are usually closed

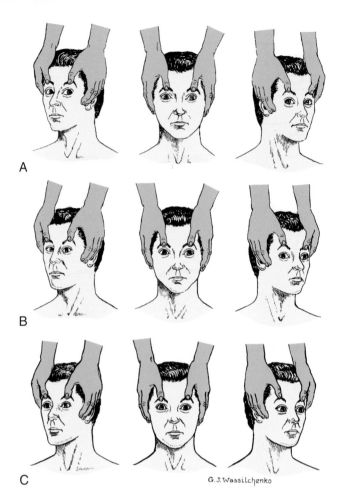

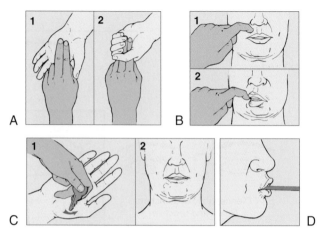

FIGURE 16.5 Pathologic Reflexes. A, Grasp reflex. **B,** Snout reflex. **C,** Palmomental reflex. **D,** Suck reflex.

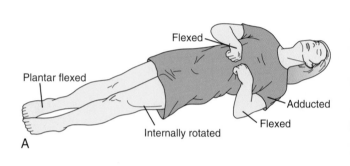

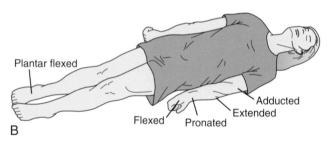

FIGURE 16.6 Decorticate and Decerebrate Posture/Responses. A, Decorticate posture/response. Flexion of arms, wrists, and fingers with adduction in upper extremities. Extension, internal rotation, and plantar flexion in lower extremities. Both sides. **B,** Decerebrate posture/response. All four extremities in rigid extension, with hyperpronation of forearms and plantar extension of feet. (From deWit SC, Kumagai CK: *Medical-surgical nursing,* ed 2, St Louis, 2013, Saunders.)

FIGURE 16.3 Test for Oculocephalic Reflex Response (Doll Eyes Phenomenon). A, Normal response—eyes turn together to side opposite from turn of head. **B,** Abnormal response—eyes do not turn in conjugate manner. **C,** Absent response—eyes move in direction of head movement (brainstem injury). (From Rudy EB: *Advanced neurological and neurosurgical nursing,* St Louis, 1984, Mosby.)

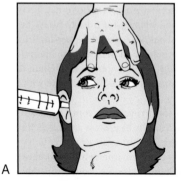
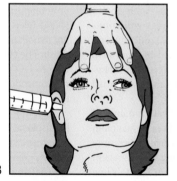
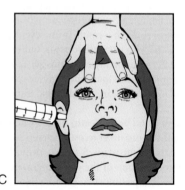

FIGURE 16.4 Test for Oculovestibular Reflex (Caloric Ice Water Test). A, Ice water is injected into the ear canal. Normal response—conjugate eye movements. **B,** Abnormal response—dysconjugate or asymmetric eye movements. **C,** Absent response—no eye movements.

TABLE 16.5	**Abnormal Motor Responses With Decreased Responsiveness**	
Motor Response	**Description**	**Location of Injury**
Decorticate posturing/rigidity: upper extremity flexion, lower extremity extension	Slowly developing flexion of arm, wrist, and fingers with adduction in the upper extremity and extension, internal rotation, and plantar flexion of lower extremity	Hemispheric damage above midbrain releasing medullary and pontine reticulospinal systems
Decerebrate posturing/rigidity: upper and lower extremity extensor responses	Opisthotonos (hyperextension of vertebral column) with clenching of teeth; extension, abduction, and hyperpronation of arms; and extension of lower extremities	Associated with severe damage involving midbrain or upper pons
	In acute brain injury, shivering and hyperpnea may accompany unelicited recurrent decerebrate spasms	Acute brain injury often causes limb extension regardless of location
Extensor responses in upper extremities accompanied by flexion in lower extremities		Pons
Flaccid state with little or no motor response to stimuli		Lower pons and upper medulla

with no eye opening. The person does not follow commands, speak, or have voluntary movement.

A **persistent vegetative state** is complete unawareness of the self or surrounding environment and complete loss of cognitive function. The individual does not speak any comprehensible words or follow commands. Sleep-wake cycles are present, eyes open spontaneously, and blood pressure and breathing are maintained without support. Brainstem reflexes (pupillary, oculocephalic, chewing, swallowing) are intact, but cerebral function is lost. There is bowel and bladder incontinence. Recovery is unlikely if the state persists for 12 months. In a **minimally conscious state (MCS, minimally preserved consciousness)** individuals may follow simple commands, manipulate or reach for objects, gesture or give yes/no responses, have intelligible speech, and have movements such as blinking or smiling. Individuals may remain permanently in this state or progress to minimal ability to understand and communicate.[3]

With **locked-in syndrome** there is complete paralysis of voluntary muscles with the exception of eye movement. Content of thought and level of arousal are intact, but the efferent pathways are disrupted. The injury is at the base of the pons with the reticular formation intact and often is caused by basilar artery occlusion.[4] Thus the individual cannot communicate through speech or body movement but is fully conscious, with intact cognitive function. Vertical eye movement and blinking are a means of communication.

Alterations in Awareness

Awareness (content of thought) encompasses all cognitive functions, including awareness of self, environment, and affective states (i.e., moods). Awareness is mediated by all of the core networks under the guidance of executive attention networks, including selective attention and memory. Executive attention networks involve abstract reasoning, planning, decision making, judgment, error correction, and self-control. Each attentional function is a network of interconnected brain areas and not localized to a single brain area.

Selective attention (orienting, focusing) refers to the ability to select specific information to be processed from available, competing environmental and internal stimuli, and to focus on that stimulus (i.e., to concentrate on a specific task without being distracted).[5] *Selective visual attention* is the ability to select objects from multiple visual stimuli and process them to complete a task (i.e., selecting a square red object from among various objects when sorting objects according to configuration and color). *Selective auditory* or *hearing attention* is the ability to select or filter specific sounds and process them to complete a task (i.e., listening to a person's verbal directions and blocking out background music or traffic noise). Multiple areas of the brain are involved in selective attention including cortical areas, thalamic nuclei, and the limbic system.

Selective attention deficits can be temporary, permanent, or progressive. Disorders associated with selective attention deficits include seizure activity, parietal lobe contusions, subdural hematomas, stroke, gliomas or metastatic tumor, late Alzheimer dementia, frontotemporal dementia, and psychotic disorders.

Memory is the recording, retention, and retrieval of information. **Working memory (short-term memory)** is remembering temporary information long enough to make a decision or complete a task (seconds to a few minutes). For example, remembering the first sentences in a paragraph in order to understand the concepts included by the end of the paragraph. **Long-term memory** can last indefinitely and last a lifetime. **Amnesia** is the loss of memory and can be mild or severe. Two types of amnesia are retrograde amnesia and anterograde amnesia. The person experiencing **retrograde amnesia** has difficulty retrieving or recalling past personal history memories (i.e., place of birth or high school graduation) or past factual memories (i.e., current address or phone number). **Anterograde amnesia** is the inability to form new personal or factual memories (i.e., where a car is parked or recognize a person one has met in the preceding minutes) but memories of the distant past are retained and retrieved. **Global amnesia** is a combination of anterograde and retrograde amnesia. Such individuals may not be able to recall where they are, how they arrived there, where or when they were born, or recognize family and friends. **Image processing** is a higher level of memory function and includes the ability to integrate sensory data and language to form concepts, assign meaning, and make abstractions. Alterations in image processing include an inability to form concepts and generalizations or to reason. Thinking is very concrete. For example, a person will not understand the abstract phrase "walking on eggs shells" and may look at his or her feet for the eggshells. These memory disorders may be temporary (e.g., after a seizure) or permanent (e.g., after severe head injury or in Alzheimer disease). There may be only the memory disorder, or the memory disorder may be associated with other cognitive disorders, including an inability to make decisions or sustain attention. Table 16.6 contains the clinical manifestations of alterations in attention and memory.

Executive attention deficits include the inability to maintain sustained attention and a working memory deficit. Sustained attention deficit is an inability to set goals and recognize when an object meets a goal. A working memory deficit is an inability to remember instructions and information needed to guide behavior. Executive attention

TABLE 16.6   Clinical Manifestations of Alterations in Attention and Memory

Deficit	Clinical Signs	Symptoms
Attention		
Selective attention (orienting)	Inability to focus attention; decreased eye, head, and body movements associated with focusing on stimuli; decreased search and scanning; faulty orientation to stimuli, causing safety problems	Person reports inability to focus attention, failure to perceive objects and other stimuli (history of injuries, falls, safety problems); can exhibit neglect syndrome (i.e., unilateral neglect with failure to groom or recognize one side of the body)
Memory		
Antegrade amnesia (inability to form new memories)	*Left hemisphere:* disorientation to time, situation, place, name, person (verbal identification); impaired language memory (e.g., names of objects); impaired semantic memory *Right hemisphere:* disorientation to self, person (visual), place (visual); impaired episodic memory (personal history); impaired emotional memory *Either or both hemispheres:* confusion; behavioral change	Person reports disorientation, confusion, "not listening," "not remembering"; reports by others of person being disoriented, not able to remember, not able to learn new information
Retrograde amnesia (loss of past memories)	*Left hemisphere:* inability to retrieve personal history, past medical history; unaware of recent current events *Right hemisphere:* inability to recognize persons, places, objects, music, and so on from past	Person reports remote memory problems; others report that person cannot recall formerly known information
Image processing	Inability to categorize (identify similarities and differences) or sort; inability to form concepts; inability to analyze relationships; misinterpretations; inability to interpret proverbs Inability to perform deductive reasoning (convergent reasoning); inability to perform inductive reasoning (divergent reasoning); inability to abstract; concrete reasoning demonstrated; delusions	Reports by others of frequent misinterpretation of data, failure to conceptualize or generalize information Reports by others of predominantly concrete thinking; lack of understanding of everyday situations, healthcare regimens, and such; delusional thinking
Executive Attention Deficits		
Vigilance	Failure to stay alert and orient to stimuli	Person reports decreased alertness or ability to orient
Detection	Lack of initiative (anergy); lack of ambition; lack of motivation; flat affect; no awareness of feelings; appears depressed, apathetic, and emotionless; fails to appreciate deficit; disinterested in appearance; lacks concern about childish or crude behavior	Reports by others of laziness or apathy, flat affect, or lack of emotional expression; failure to exhibit or be aware of feelings
Mild	Responds to immediate environment but no new ideas; grooming and social graces are lacking	Reports by others of lack of ambition, motivation, or initiative; failure to carry out adult tasks; lack of social graces and new ideas
Severe	Motionless; lack of response to even internal cues; does not respond to physical needs; does not interact with surroundings Inability to use feedback regarding behavior; failure to recognize omissions and errors in self-care, speech, writing, and arithmetic; impaired cue utilization; overestimation of performance Failure to shift response set; failure to change behavior when conditions change; cue utilization may be impaired	Reports by others of failure to groom or toilet self, unawareness of surroundings and own physical needs Reports by others of not changing behavior when requested; unawareness of limitations; does not recognize and correct errors in dressing, grooming, toileting, eating, and such; fails to recognize speech and arithmetic errors; careless speech Reports by others of failure to use feedback; inability to incorporate feedback (does not correct when feedback is given)
Working memory (recent or short-term memory)	Inability to set goals or form goals; indecisiveness Failure to make plans; inability to produce a complete line of reasoning; inability to make up a story; appears impulsive Failure to initiate behavior; failure to maintain behavior; failure to discontinue behavior; slowness to alternate response for the next step; motor perseveration	Reports by others of failure to set goals, indecisiveness Reports by others of failure to plan, impulsiveness, "does not think things through" Reports by others of not knowing where to begin, inability to carry out sequential acts (maintain a behavior), inability to cease a behavior

deficits may be temporary, progressive, or permanent. ADHD is a common disorder of childhood that can continue through adulthood (Box 16.2).

PATHOPHYSIOLOGY Very generally, the primary pathophysiologic mechanisms that operate in disorders of awareness are (1) direct destruction caused by ischemia and hypoxia or indirect destruction resulting from compression and (2) the effects of toxins and chemicals or metabolic disorders. Disorders of selective attention, at least as they relate to visual orienting behavior, are produced by disease that involves portions of the midbrain. For example, disease affecting the superior colliculus (associated with retinal signals) manifests as a slowness in orienting attention. Parietal lobe disease may produce *unilateral neglect syndrome* or lack of awareness of one side of the body or lack of response to stimuli on one side of the body. It can occur after a stroke. An individual may groom or dress on only one side or eat food from only

BOX 16.2   Attention-Deficit/Hyperactivity Disorder

Initially attention-deficit/hyperactivity disorder (ADHD) was viewed as a neurodevelopmental disorder of childhood. It is now recognized that 50% to 75% of persons diagnosed in childhood have continuing symptoms into adulthood. Often the diagnosis is first made in adolescence or young adulthood, when behavioral control and self-organization are expected of the person. The ability to function at work, at home, and in social situations is often impaired because of inattentiveness, hyperactivity, impulsivity, and problems with executive function. Continued treatment, including medications for symptomatic adults, is supported. The multifactorial patterns of inheritance and gene–environment interactions are under investigation, as are the pathogenesis and pathophysiology of this complex disorder. Findings from structural and functional neuroimaging suggest the involvement of developmentally abnormal brain networks related to cognition, attention, emotion, and sensorimotor functions. Hopefully new findings will lead to improved prevention, diagnosis, treatment options, and functional outcomes.

Data from Bonvicini C, Faraone SV, Scassellati C: *Mol Psychiatry* 21(7):872-884, 2016; Gallo EF, Posner J: *Lancet Psychiatry* 3(6):555-567, 2016; Leahy LG: *Arch Psychiatr Nurs* 32(6), 2018.

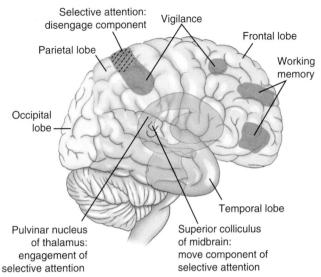

FIGURE 16.7 Right Cortical, Subcortical, and Brainstem Areas of the Brain Mediating Cognitive Function. (From Boss GJ, Wilkerson R: Communication: language and pragmatics. In Hoeman SP, editor: *Rehabilitation nursing; prevention, intervention & outcomes*, ed 4, p 508, St Louis, 2008, Mosby.)

one side of the plate. **Sensory inattentiveness** is a form of neglect. The person is able to recognize individual sensory input from the dysfunctional side when asked but ignores the sensory input from the dysfunctional side when stimulated from both sides (**extinction**). The entire complex of denial of dysfunction, loss of recognition of one's own body parts, and extinction sometimes is referred to as *hemineglect* or **neglect syndrome**.

A disorder in vigilance may be produced by disease in the prefrontal areas. Dysfunction in the right anterior cingulate gyrus (part of the "emotional" limbic system) and basal ganglia (coordination of fluid movement) may cause detection problems (i.e., being able to choose among objects without making an error). Problems with working memory may be produced with left lateral frontal lobe injury. Anterograde amnesia originates from pathologic conditions in the hippocampus and related temporal lobe structures; the diencephalic region, including the thalamus; and the basal forebrain. Retrograde amnesia and higher-level memory deficits originate from pathologic conditions in the widely distributed association areas of the cerebral cortex (see Fig. 14.8, *C*). Executive attention deficits are associated with alterations in the frontal and prefrontal cortex (cognitive functions) including the anterior cingulate gyrus, supplementary motor area, and portions of the basal ganglia.

CLINICAL MANIFESTATIONS   Clinical manifestations of selective attention deficits, memory deficits, and executive attention function deficits are presented in Table 16.6.

EVALUATION AND TREATMENT   Immediate medical management is directed at diagnosing the cause and treating reversible factors. Rehabilitative measures generally focus on compensatory or restorative activities and recently have been greatly facilitated by computer technology and other electronic devices.

QUICK CHECK 16.2
1. Why is irreversible coma different from brain death?
2. What is the difference between anterograde and retrograde amnesia?
3. What is an example of neglect syndrome?

Data-Processing Deficits

Data-processing deficits are problems associated with recognizing and processing sensory information. These deficits include agnosia, aphasia, and acute confusional states.

Agnosia

Agnosia is a defect of pattern recognition—a failure to recognize the form and nature of objects. Agnosia can be tactile, visual, or auditory, but generally only one sense is affected. For example, an individual may be unable to identify a safety pin by touching it with a hand but is able to name it when looking at it. Agnosia may be as minimal as a finger agnosia (failure to identify by name the fingers of one's hand) or more extensive, such as a color agnosia (an inability to name and distinguish colors, for example describing a brown dog as pink). Although agnosia is associated most commonly with cerebrovascular accidents, it may arise from any pathologic process that injures specific areas of the brain.

Aphasia

Aphasia is impairment of comprehension or production of language with impaired communication. The terms *aphasia* and *dysphasia* are often used interchangeably; the term *aphasia* is used here. Comprehension or use of symbols, in either written or verbal language, is disturbed or lost. Aphasia results from dysfunction in the left cerebral hemisphere, including the inferior frontal gyrus and superior temporal gyrus, and the subcortical and cortical connecting networks (Fig. 16.7). Aphasias usually are associated with a cerebrovascular accident involving the middle cerebral artery or one of its many branches. Language disorders, however, may arise from a variety of injuries and diseases including vascular, neoplastic, traumatic, degenerative, metabolic, or infectious causes. Most language disorders result from acute processes or a chronic residual deficit of the acute process.

Aphasias have been classified anatomically (i.e., Wernicke [sensory speech area] or Broca area [motor speech area] aphasias) or functionally as disorders of fluency (quality and content of speech). *Expressive aphasia*, also known as Broca, motor, or nonfluent aphasia, involves loss of the ability to produce spoken or written language, with slow or difficult speech. Verbal comprehension is usually present. Expressive aphasia is differentiated from *dysarthria,* in which words cannot be articulated clearly as a result of cranial nerve damage or muscle impairment. *Receptive aphasia,* also known as Wernicke, sensory, or fluent aphasia, involves an inability to understand written or spoken language. Speech is fluent, flowing at a normal rate, but words and phrases have no meaning. *Anomic aphasia* is a sensory aphasia distinguished by difficulty finding words and naming a person or object. Circumlocution, or describing an object as a way of trying to name something, is common in anomic aphasia. Auditory comprehension is present in *conductive aphasia,* but there is impaired verbatim repetition. Naming also can be impaired. The person recognizes the errors and tries to correct them. Speech is fluent, but words and sounds may be transposed. Damage is in the left hemisphere to networks that connect the Broca and Wernicke areas. *Transcortical aphasias* are rare and can be motor, sensory, or mixed. They involve areas of the brain that connect into the language centers. *Global aphasia* is the most severe aphasia and involves both expressive and receptive aphasia. The individual is nonfluent or mute; cannot read or write; and has impaired comprehension, naming, reading, and writing. Global aphasia is usually associated with a cerebrovascular accident involving the middle cerebral artery. Table 16.7 compares types of aphasias, and Table 16.8 illustrates some of the language disturbances. Pure aphasias are rare and are often mixed, making diagnosis difficult. All types of aphasia usually improve with speech rehabilitation.

Acute Confusional States and Delirium

Acute confusional states (ACSs) (also may be known as *delirium* or *acute organic brain syndromes* or *acute brain failure*) are transient disorders of cognitive function, consciousness, or perception and may have either a sudden or a gradual onset. Delirium can be considered as a type of acute confusional state, but for this discussion acute confusional states and delirium are considered to be synonymous. There are many medical conditions associated with delirium, and they are summarized in Box 16.3. Acute confusional states arise from disruption of widely distributed brain networks rather than in a discrete area of the brain. Most metabolic disturbances (i.e., hypoglycemia, thyroid disorders, liver or kidney disease) that produce delirium interfere with neuronal metabolism or synaptic transmission. Several neurotransmitters are involved, including decreased acetylcholine and excess dopamine. Many drugs and toxins also interfere with neurotransmission function at the synapse. The types of delirium include hyperactive and hypoactive states. Some individuals fluxuate between the two states and have mixed delirium.

BOX 16.3 Conditions Causing Acute Confusional States/Delirium

Drug intoxication
Alcohol or drug withdrawal
Metabolic disorders (e.g., hypoglycemia, thyroid storm)
Brain trauma or surgery or tumors
Meningoencephalitis
Postanesthesia
Febrile illnesses or heat stroke
Electrolyte imbalance, dehydration
Heart, kidney, or liver failure
Sepsis and proinflammatory cytokines

PATHOPHYSIOLOGY AND CLINICAL MANIFESTATIONS Delirium (hyperactive confusional state) is an acute disturbance in attention and awareness, associated with autonomic nervous system overactivity and typically develops over 2 to 3 days.[6] It commonly occurs in critical care units, after surgery, during withdrawal from CNS depressants (i.e., alcohol or narcotic agents), and in hospitalized elderly.[7] Risk factors include medications (i.e., narcotics, benzodiazepines, anticholinergic medications), acute infection or sepsis, surgery, electrolyte disturbances, hypoxia, and metabolic disorders (liver or kidney disease, hypoglycemia, and thyroid disorders).

Delirium initially manifests as restlessness, irritability, difficulty in concentrating, insomnia, tremulousness, and poor appetite. Some persons experience seizures. Unpleasant, even terrifying dreams or hallucinations may occur. In a fully developed delirium state, the individual is completely inattentive and perceptions are grossly altered, with extensive misperception and misinterpretation. The person appears distressed and often perplexed; conversation is incoherent. Frank tremor and high levels of restless movement are common. The individual cannot sleep, is flushed, and has dilated pupils, a rapid pulse rate (tachycardia), elevated temperature, and profuse sweating (diaphoresis). Delirium usually abates suddenly or gradually in 2 to 3 days, although occasionally delirium states persist for weeks.

Excited delirium syndrome (ExDS), also known as *agitated delirium,* is a type of hyperactive delirium that can lead to sudden death. Its symptoms include altered mental status, combativeness, aggressiveness, tolerance to significant pain, rapid breathing, sweating, severe agitation, elevated temperature, noncompliance or poor awareness to direction from police or medical personnel, inability to become fatigued, unusual or superhuman strength, and inappropriate clothing for the current environment.

Hypoactive delirium (hypoactive confusional state) is associated with right-sided frontal-basal ganglion disruption (an area of the brain associated with coordinated movement and alertness).It may occur in individuals who have fevers or metabolic disorders (i.e., chronic liver or kidney failure), or who are under the influence of CNS depressants. The individual exhibits decreases in alertness, attention span, accurate perception, interpretation of the environment, and reaction to the environment. Forgetfulness and apathy are prominent, speech may be slow, and the individual dozes frequently with little spontaneous movement.

EVALUATION AND TREATMENT The initial goals are to (1) establish that the individual is confused and (2) determine the cause of the confusion (organic or functional) (Table 16.9). The next step is to differentiate whether the confusion is delirium or an underlying dementia; the syndromes can overlap. Individuals with dementia are at increased risk for developing delirium. Table 16.10 contains a comparison of the features differentiating delirium and dementia. A complete history, physical examination, laboratory tests (electrocardiogram and blood, urine, cerebrospinal fluid, and radiologic studies), and review of medications are needed. Several assessment scales are available to guide evaluation (such as the Nursing Delirium Screening Scale and Confusion Assessment Method).[8,9] Once the cause is established, treatment is directed at controlling the primary disorder with supportive measures used as appropriate. Delirium is preventable in some individuals.[10]

✔QUICK CHECK 16.3

1. What are two types of dysphasia?
2. How does dysphasia differ from dysarthria?
3. What are some causes of delirium?

TABLE 16.7   Major Types of Aphasia

Type	Expression	Verbal Comprehension	Repetition	Reading Comprehension	Writing	Location of Lesion	Cause of Lesion
Expressive							
Broca, nonfluent or motor aphasia	Cannot find words, difficulty writing	Relatively intact	Impaired	Variable	Impaired	Left posteroinferior frontal lobe (Broca area)	Occlusion of one or several branches of left middle cerebral artery supplying inferior frontal gyrus
Transcortical motor, nonfluent aphasia	Halting speech	Intact	Intact	Impaired	Impaired	Anterior superior frontal lobe	Occlusion at the border zone between two arterial territories
Receptive							
Wernicke, receptive fluent or sensory aphasia	Meaningless verbal language, inappropriate words or unable to monitor language for correctness so errors are not recognized Intonation, accent, cadence, rhythm, and articulation normal	Impaired; disturbance in understanding all language	Impaired	Impaired	Impaired	Left posterosuperior temporal lobe (Wernicke area)	Occlusion of inferior division of left middle cerebral artery
Conductive dysphasia	Difficulty repeating words, phrases spoken to them; naming is impaired	Intact	Severely impaired	Variable	Variable	Inferior and posterior temporal lobe; parietotemporal junction	Occlusion in distributions of left middle cerebral artery
Anomic aphasia	Hesitancy, difficulty recalling names, objects, or numbers	Intact	Impaired	Variable	Intact except for anomia	Left temporoparietal zones; arcuate fasciculus	Diffuse left hemisphere brain disease
Transcortical sensory, fluent aphasia	Repeats words and phrases spoken to them	Poor	Intact	Impaired	Impaired	Posterior temporal lobe	Occlusion at the border zone between two cerebral arterial territories
Other							
Transcortical mixed motor and sensory, nonfluent	Repeats words and phrases spoken to them	Impaired	Intact	Impaired	Impaired	Left cerebral hemisphere; spares the perisylvian cortex	Occlusion at the border zone between two cerebral arterial territories
Global or nonfluent; summation of motor and sensory aphasia	Mute	Impaired	Impaired	Impaired	Impaired	Large areas of the left cortex and subcortical regions	Occlusion of left middle cerebral artery of left internal carotid artery, tumors, other mass lesions, hemorrhage, embolic occlusion of ascending parietal or posterior temporal branch of middle cerebral artery

Dementia

Dementia is an acquired deterioration and a progressive failure of many cerebral functions that includes impairment of intellectual processes with a decrease in orienting, memory, language, judgment, and decision making. Because of declining intellectual ability, the individual may exhibit alterations in behavior, for example, agitation, wandering, and aggression.

PATHOPHYSIOLOGY   Mechanisms leading to dementia include neuron degeneration, compression of brain tissue, atherosclerosis of cerebral vessels, brain trauma, infection, and neuroinflammation. Genetic predisposition is associated with neurodegenerative diseases, including Alzheimer, Huntington, and Parkinson diseases. CNS infections, including the human immunodeficiency virus (HIV) and slow-growing viruses associated with Creutzfeldt-Jakob disease, also lead to nerve cell degeneration and brain atrophy.

CLINICAL MANIFESTATIONS   The onset of dementia is generally slow, and symptoms are usually irreversible. Clinical manifestations of the major dementias are presented in Table 16.11.

EVALUATION AND TREATMENT   Establishing the cause for dementia may be complicated, but individuals with clinical manifestations of dementia should be evaluated with laboratory and neuropsychological testing to identify underlying conditions that may be treatable. Unfortunately, no specific cure exists for most progressive dementias. Therapy is directed at maintaining and maximizing use of the remaining capacities, restoring functions if possible, and accommodating to lost abilities. Helping the family understand the process and to learn ways to assist the individual are essential.

Alzheimer Disease

Alzheimer disease (AD) (dementia of Alzheimer type [DAT], senile disease complex) is the leading cause of severe cognitive dysfunction in older persons. The three forms of AD are nonhereditary sporadic or late-onset AD (70% to 90%), early-onset familial AD (FAD), and early-onset AD (very rare). In 2019, an estimated 5.8 million Americans had AD; about two-thirds were women.[11]

PATHOPHYSIOLOGY   The exact cause of AD is unknown, but both early onset and late onset have genetic associations. Early-onset FAD has been linked to three genes with mutations on chromosome 21 (abnormal amyloid precursor protein 14 *[APP14]*, abnormal presenilin 1 *[PSEN1]*, and abnormal presenilin 2 *[PSEN2]*). Late-onset AD may be related to the involvement of chromosome 19 with the apolipoprotein E gene-allele 4 *(APOE4)*. Sporadic late-onset AD is the most common, and does not have a specific genetic association; however, the cellular pathology is the same as that for gene-associated early- and late-onset AD.[12] DNA methylation is a potential epigenetic marker for AD.[13]

Pathologic alterations in the brain include the accumulation of extracellular neuritic plaques containing a core of amyloid beta protein and intraneuronal neurofibrillary tangles of tau protein. Neuritic plaques disrupt nerve impulse transmission and cause death of neurons (Fig. 16.8). They are more concentrated in the cerebral cortex and

TABLE 16.8   Examples of Aphasia

Disorder	Example
Wernicke/Fluent/Sensory Aphasia	
Verbal paraphasia	*Question:* What did the car do?
	Patient: The car would spit sweetly down the road.
	(The car sped swiftly down the road.)
Wernicke/Fluent/Sensory Aphasia	
Literal paraphasia	*Request:* Say, "Persistence is essential to success."
	Patient: Mesastence is instans to success.
Wernicke/Fluent/Sensory Aphasia	
Neologism	*Question:* What do you call this? (Pointing to a plant.)
	Patient: It's a logper.
Anomic dysphasia (circumlocution example)	*Question:* What do you call this? (Pointing to a plant.)
	Patient: Something that grows.
	Patient: It's…
	Or
	Question: What did you do this morning?
	Patient: Reading.
	Question: Were you reading a book or newspaper?
	Patient: One of those.
Broca or Motor Aphasia	
Telegraphic style	*Question:* Where is your daughter?
	Patient: New Orleans … home … Monday.

From Boss BJ: *J Neurosurg Nurs* 16(3):151-160, 1984.

TABLE 16.9   Differences Between Organic and Functional Confusion

Factor	Organic Confusion	Functional Confusion
Memory impairment	Recent more impaired than remote	No consistent difference between recent and remote
Disorientation		
Time	Within own lifetime or reasonably near future	May not be related to person's lifetime
Place	Familiar place or one where person might easily be found	Bizarre or unfamiliar places
Person	Sense of identity usually preserved	Sense of identity diminished
	Misidentification of others as familiar	Misidentification of others based on delusion system
Hallucinations	Visual, vivid	Auditory more frequent
	Animals and insects common	Bizarre and symbolic
Illusions	Common	Not prominent
Delusions	Concern everyday occurrences and people	Bizarre and symbolic
Confused	Spotty confusion	More consistent
	Clear intervals mixed with confused episodes	No tendency to become worse at night
	Worse at night	

From Morris M, Rhodes M: *Am J Nurs* 72(9):1632, 1972.

TABLE 16.10   Comparison of Delirium and Dementia

Feature	Delirium	Dementia
Age	Usually older	Usually older
Onset	Acute—common during hospitalization	Usually insidious and progressive; acute in some cases of strokes/trauma
Associated conditions	Urinary tract infection, thyroid disorders, hypoxia, hypoglycemia, toxicity, fluid-electrolyte imbalance, renal insufficiency, trauma, postsurgical anesthesia	May have no other conditions Brain trauma
Course	Fluctuating/reversible with treatment	Chronic slow decline—more stable
Duration	Hours to days and months in some cases	Months to years
Attention	Inability to focus or sustain attention	Intact early; often impaired late
Sleep-wake cycle	Disrupted	Disturbances are common
Alertness	Impaired	There may be fluctuations
Orientation	Impaired	Intact early; impaired late
Behavior	Agitated, withdrawn/depressed	Intact early
Speech	Incoherent, disorganized	Word-finding problems or aphasia
Thoughts	Disorganized, delusions	Impoverished
Perceptions	Hallucinations/illusions	Usually intact early

Adapted from Fong TG et al: *Lancet Neurol* 14(8):823-832, 2015.

TABLE 16.11   Clinical Manifestations of the Major Degenerative Dementias

Disease	Mental Status	Neurobehavior	Neurologic Examination
Alzheimer disease	Memory loss, disorientation to place and time, loss of facial recognition	Initially normal; progressive cognitive, language, abstraction, and judgment impairment	Initially normal
Creutzfeldt-Jakob disease	Variable, frontal/executive, focal cortical, memory	Depression, anxiety, decreased cognitive function and memory loss	Myoclonus, rigidity, parkinsonism
Dementia with Lewy body (Lewy body dementia)	Initially affects concentration and attention, then memory or cognition loss but unpredictable levels of ability, attention, or alertness; delirium prone	Visual hallucinations, depression, sleep disorder, delusions, transient loss of consciousness	Parkinsonism Changes in walking or movement may present first
Frontotemporal disorders/ degeneration/ dementia	Primary progressive aphasia variant Language loss with talking less and speech becoming hesitant or loss of understanding of language, may precede memory loss; spares drawing	Behavioral variant frontotemporal dementia Loss of empathy (emotional blunting), apathy, increased inappropriate or decline in personal or social conduct, loss of judgment and reasoning, hyperorality, euphoria, depression	Caused by corticobasal degeneration and progressive supranuclear palsy variants
Huntington disease	Subtle decline in decision making, planning, organizing and recognizing emotion of others several years prior to motor symptoms	Apathy, loss of interest early; impaired cognition, judgment, and memory can occur as prodromal manifestations; loss of smell recognition; decline of finger tapping speed.	Chorea, bradykinesia, dystonia
Vascular dementia	Frontal/executive, cognitive slowing; memory can be intact	Often but not always sudden, usually within 3 months of a stroke; variable; apathy, falls, focal weakness, delusions, anxiety	Usually motor slowing, spasticity; can be normal or may have symptom improvement with stroke recovery

Data from Bott NT et al: *Neurodegener Dis Manag* 4(6):439-454, 2014; Darrow MD: *Prim Care* 42(2):195-204, 2015; Hugo J, Ganguli M: *Clin Geriatr Med* 30(3):421-442, 2014; Nordberg A: *Nat Rev Neurol* 11(2):69-70, 2015.

hippocampus (an area of the brain associated with memory). Loss of synapses, acetylcholine, and other neurotransmitters contributes to the decline of memory and attention and the loss of other cognitive functions associated with AD. The loss of neurons results in brain atrophy with widening of sulci and shrinkage of gyri (see Fig. 16.8).

CLINICAL MANIFESTATIONS   AD has a long preclinical and prodromal course. Pathophysiologic changes can occur decades before the appearance of the clinical dementia syndrome. The disease progresses from mild short-term memory deficits and culminates in total loss of cognitive and executive functions. Initial clinical manifestations are insidious and often are attributed to forgetfulness, emotional upset, or other illness. The individual becomes progressively more forgetful over time, particularly in relation to recent events. Memory loss increases as the disorder advances. The person becomes disoriented and confused and loses the ability to concentrate. Abstraction, problem solving, and

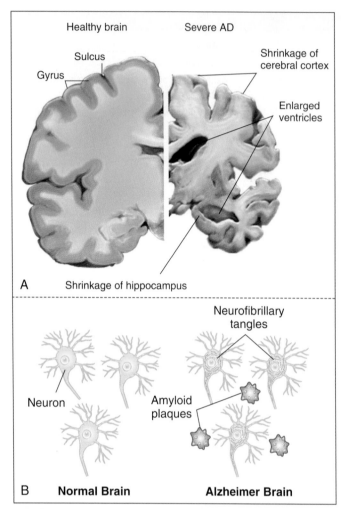

A, Comparison of Normal and Alzheimer Brain. The brain decreases in volume and weight, the sulci widen, and the gyri thin, especially in the temporal and frontal lobes. The ventricles enlarge to fill the space. B, Common pathologic findings in Alzheimer disease. (A from National Institute on Aging Scientific Images: *Brain images.* Available at https://www.nia.nih.gov/health/alzheimers-disease-fact-sheet#changes.)

FIGURE 16.8 Common Pathologic Findings in Alzheimer Disease.

judgment gradually deteriorate with failure in mathematic calculation ability, language, and visuospatial orientation. The mental status changes induce behavioral changes, including irritability, agitation, and restlessness. Mood changes also result from the deterioration in cognition. The person may become anxious, depressed, hostile, emotionally labile, and prone to mood swings. Motor changes may occur if the posterior frontal lobes are involved, causing rigidity and flexion posturing. Weight loss can be significant. Great variability in age of onset, intensity and sequence of symptoms, and location and extent of brain abnormalities is common. Stages for the progression of AD are summarized in Table 16.12.

EVALUATION AND TREATMENT   The diagnosis of AD is made by ruling out other causes. Clinical criteria have been developed to assist diagnosis.[14] The clinical history, including mental status examinations (mini–mental status examination, clock drawing; and geriatric depression scale); laboratory tests; brain imaging of structure, blood flow, and metabolism; and the course of the illness (which may span 5 years or more), is used to assess progression of the disease. Efforts are in progress to identify imaging and biochemical markers for risk assessment and early diagnosis and progression of Alzheimer type and other neurodegenerative causes of dementia[15] (see *Did You Know?* Biomarkers and Neurodegenerative Dementia).

DID YOU KNOW?

Biomarkers and Neurodegenerative Dementia

Neurodegenerative disease processes that lead to dementia begin many years before clinical manifestations are evident for Alzheimer disease, Huntington disease, and Parkinson disease. Efforts are under way to identify neuroimaging techniques to visualize Aβ deposits and neurodegenerative lesions. Predictive biomarkers for tau protein, amyloid β peptides, and apolipoprotein E4 in the brain, spinal fluid, and blood will guide a more comprehensive understanding of the etiology and biologic pathways that mediate neurodegeneration. Identification and profiling of such images and molecules will promote early identification of risk factors, enhance preventive and protective measures, provide alerts for progression from mild to advanced stages, and accelerate development of presymptomatic and personalized treatment for these diseases.

Data from Zetterberg H et al: *Mol Brain* March 28, 12(1):26, 2019; Hampel H et al: *Nat Rev Neurol* 14(11):639-652, 2018; Mahalingam S, Chen MK: *Semin Neurol* 39(2):188-199, 2019.

TABLE 16.12 **Progression of Alzheimer Disease**

Stage	Mild Cognitive Impairment	Early Stage	Middle Stage	Late Stage	End Stage
Cognitive	Mild memory loss	Measurable short-term memory loss; difficulty with word finding; other cognition problems compared with previous behavior	Moderate to severe cognitive problems: impaired reasoning, judgment, and problem solving; disorientation to time, place, and person; difficulty planning and organizing; progressive memory loss	Little cognitive ability; language not clear	No significant cognitive function; loss of orientation to self
Functional	Possibly depression (vs. apathy); mild anxiety	Mild IADL problems	IADL-dependent; some ADL problems	ADL-dependent; incontinent	Nonambulatory/bedbound; unable to eat related to failure to sense hunger or thirst, difficulty swallowing

ADL, (Basic) activities of daily living; *IADL,* instrumental activities of daily living (independent performance of activities).
Adapted from National Conference of Gerontological Nurse Practitioners and the National Gerontological Nursing Association: *Counseling Points* 1(1):6, 2008; Peña-Casanova J et al: *Arch Med Res* 43(8):686-693, 2012.

Treatment is directed at using devices to compensate for the impaired cognitive function, such as memory aids; maintaining unimpaired cognitive functions; and maintaining or improving the general state of hygiene, nutrition, and health. Cholinesterase inhibitors have shown a modest effect on cognitive function in mild to moderate AD. Memantine, an *N*-methyl-D-aspartate (NMDA) receptor antagonist, blocks glutamate activity and may slow progression of disease in moderate to severe AD. Treatments, beginning in the preclinical stage, are being developed to prevent, modify, or halt disease pathology.[16]

Vascular Dementia

Vascular dementia is the second most common cause of dementia after AD. It is a consequence of cerebrovascular disease. Vascular dementia is associated with large artery disease, cardioembolism, small vessel disease of the brain, and stroke, all of which can cause hypoperfusion in the brain. It is more common in men. Risk factors include diabetes, hypercholesterolemia, hypertension, and smoking. Treatment is directed at preventing these risk factors.[17]

Frontotemporal Dementia

Frontotemporal dementia (FTD), previously known as Pick disease, is a rare disease. There is a familial association with an age of onset less than 60 years. The majority of cases involve mutations of genes encoding tau protein. There is degeneration of the frontal and anterior frontal lobes. Three distinct clinical syndromes are presented in frontotemporal degeneration, depending on the site of atrophy: (1) behavioral variant of frontotemporal dementia (changes in personality and judgment), (2) progressive nonfluent aphasia (problems with language and writing skills), and (3) semantic dementia (problems forming words and sentences).[18] There is no specific treatment.

Seizure Disorders

Seizure disorders represent a manifestation of disease and not a specific disease entity. A seizure is a sudden, transient disruption in brain electrical function caused by abnormal excessive discharges of cortical neurons. Epilepsy is a disease of the brain with recurrence of unpredictable seizures. The term convulsion is sometimes applied to seizures and refers to the tonic-clonic (jerky, contract-relax) movement associated with some seizures. (Seizures in children are presented in Chapter 18.)

Conditions Associated With Seizure Disorders

Any disorder that alters the neuronal environment may cause seizure activity. Conditions that may produce a seizure are metabolic disorders, congenital malformations, genetic predisposition, perinatal injury, postnatal trauma, myoclonic syndromes (sudden involuntary jerking of muscles), infection, brain tumor, vascular disease, and drug or alcohol abuse. The onset of seizures also may indicate the presence of an ongoing primary neurologic disease. Metabolic and structural causes of recurrent seizures in adults are summarized in Table 16.13. The cause of seizures is often unknown.

The threshold for seizures may be lowered by hypoglycemia, fatigue or lack of sleep, emotional or physical stress, fever, large amounts of water ingestion, constipation, use of antipsychotic drugs (i.e., chlorpromazine and clozapine) especially when combined with alcohol, withdrawal from depressant drugs (including alcohol), or hyperventilation (respiratory alkalosis). Some environmental stimuli, such as blinking lights, a poorly adjusted television screen, loud noises, certain music, certain odors, or merely being startled, have been known to initiate a seizure. Women may have increased seizure activity immediately before or during menses.

TABLE 16.13 Structural/Metabolic Causes of Recurrent Seizures in Adults	
Age at Onset	**Probable Cause**
Young adults (18 to 35 yr)	Alcohol or drug withdrawal (e.g., barbiturates, benzodiazepines) Brain tumor Idiopathic Illicit drug use (e.g., cocaine, amphetamine) Posttraumatic brain injury Perinatal insults
Older adults (>35 yr)	Alcohol or drug withdrawal (e.g., barbiturates, benzodiazepines) Brain tumor Cerebrovascular disease (e.g., stroke, aneurysm, arteriovenous malformations, infection) CNS degenerative diseases (e.g., Alzheimer disease, multiple sclerosis) Idiopathic Metabolic disorders (e.g., uremia, hepatic failure, electrolyte abnormalities, hypoglycemia) Posttraumatic brain injury

CNS, Central nervous system.
Data from Daroff RB et al: *Bradley's neurology in clinical practice,* ed 6, Saunders, 2012, Philadelphia.

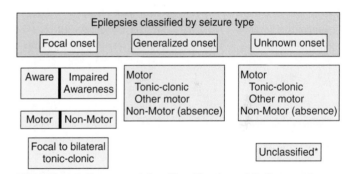

FIGURE 16.9 Framework for Classification of Epilepsy. *Due to inadequate information or inability to place in other categories.

Types of Seizure

Seizures are classified in different ways: by clinical manifestations, site of origin, EEG correlates, or response to therapy. Types of seizures and clinical manifestations are presented in Table 16.14. Terms used to describe seizure activity are defined in Table 16.15. The International League Against Epilepsy also has developed a framework to assist with classifying epilepsy (Fig. 16.9).[19]

PATHOPHYSIOLOGY Epilepsy is the result of the interaction of complex genetic mutations with environmental effects. These effects cause abnormalities in synaptic transmission, an imbalance in the brain's excitatory and inhibitory neurotransmitters, the development of abnormal nerve connections, or loss of nerves after injury.[20] A group of neurons may exhibit a sudden, depolarization shift, triggering a discharge of action potentials and function as an epileptogenic focus. These epileptogenic neurons are hypersensitive and are more easily activated by triggers, such as hyperthermia, hypoxia, hypoglycemia, hyponatremia, repeated sensory stimulation, and certain sleep phases. Epileptogenic neurons fire more frequently and with greater amplitude. When the

TABLE 16.14   Types of Seizures and Clinical Manifestations

Type	Clinical Manifestations
Focal seizures (previously partial seizures)	Seizures originating in one area of the brain; an aura is common **Motor** Tonic: stiffening of body muscles with falling; loss of consciousness; can occur in sleep; more common in infants and children Atonic: sudden, brief loss of muscle tone with falling (drop attacks); usually no loss of consciousness Myoclonic: sudden brief shock-like jerks or twitches of the arms and/or legs; may drop things; no impairment of consciousness; frequently occurs shortly after awakening Tonic-clonic: Abrupt loss of consciousness, body stiffening (tonic) and then shaking (clonic); may begin with sudden cry, sometimes loss of bladder control or biting of tongue; usually lasts about 2 minutes, followed by a period of confusion, agitation, and fatigue; headaches and soreness are common afterwards Hypermotor: bimanual or bipedal motor activity such a kicking and thrashing, clapping and rubbing of both hands, hugging, sometimes with sexual automatisms and autonomic changes with or without preserved awareness **Nonmotor** Sensory: numbness, tingling or burning sensation, flashing lights, auditory experiences Cognitive: aphasia, hallucination, memory or attention impairment Emotional or affective: fear, agitation, anger, crying, laughing, paranoia Autonomic: blushing, pallor, increased or decreased heart-rate, hyper- or hypoventilation nausea
Without loss of awareness	Recall, responsiveness, and consciousness are intact
Impaired awareness (also known as complex focal seizure)	Loss of consciousness or awareness; vague or dreamlike state
Awareness unknown	Unable to determine awareness
Focal to bilateral tonic-clonic seizure	Begins in one part of brain (focal seizure) and spreads to both sides of brain followed by generalized tonic-clonic seizure; loss of consciousness
Generalized seizures	Seizures originating in both sides of the brain simultaneously; can include tonic, atonic, clonic, myoclonic, myoclonic-atonic, clonic-tonic-clonic activity (see above descriptions)
Epileptic spasms (formerly known as infantile spasms)	Episodes of sudden flexion or extension involving neck, trunk, and extremities; clinical manifestations range from subtle head nods to violent body contractions (jackknife seizures); onset between 3 and 12 months of age; may occur after infancy, may be idiopathic, genetic, result of metabolic disease, or in response to CNS insult; spasms occur in clusters of 5 to 150 times per day; EEG shows large-amplitude, chaotic, and disorganized pattern called "hypsarrhythmia"
Epilepsy syndromes (examples)	Seizure disorder that displays a group of signs and symptoms that occur collectively and characterize or indicate a particular condition; usually associated with genetic or developmental cause
Neonatal seizures	Wide variety of abnormal clinical activity, including rhythmic eye movements, chewing, and swimming movements; common in neonatal seizures; there are 5 main types of neonatal seizures: (1) subtle seizures (50%), (2) tonic seizures (5%), (3) clonic seizures (25%), (4) myoclonic seizures (20%), (5) nonparoxysmal repetitive behaviors
Lennox-Gastaut syndrome	Epileptic syndrome with onset in early childhood, 1 to 5 years of age; includes various generalized seizures (tonic-clonic, atonic [drop attacks], akinetic, absence, and myoclonic); EEG has characteristic "slow spike and wave" pattern; results in mental retardation and delayed psychomotor developments
Juvenile myoclonic epilepsy	Generalized epilepsy syndrome with onset in adolescence; multifocal myoclonus; seizures often occur early in morning, aggravated by lack of sleep or after excessive alcohol intake; occasional generalized convulsions; requires long-term medication treatment
Unclassified Epileptic Seizures	Etiology remains unknown; seizures do not have distinct clinical and EEG features
Simple febrile seizures	Common in children younger than 5 to 6 years of age; brief (less than a few minutes) generalized convulsions associated with high fever; important to exclude meningitis as cause of seizures; usually do not develop epilepsy
Pseudoseizures	Nonepileptic phenomena that look like epileptic seizures; diagnosis often requires video-EEG monitoring to capture spells, and determine that EEG is normal during clinical events; frequently occurs in setting of child abuse
Status Epilepticus	Continuing or recurring seizure activity in which recovery from seizure activity is incomplete; unrelenting seizure activity can last 30 min or more; other forms can evolve into status epilepticus; medical emergency that requires immediate intervention

CNS, Central nervous system; *EEG*, electroencephalogram.
Data from: Fisher RS et al: Operational classification of seizure types by the International League Against Epilepsy: Position Paper of the ILAE Commission for Classification and Terminology. *Epilepsia* 58(4):522-530, 2017. Available at https://www.ilae.org/news-and-media/news-about-ilae/new-ilae-seizure-classification. Accessed July 7, 2019.

TABLE 16.15 Terminology Applied to Phases of a Seizure Disorder

Term	Definition
Preictal Phase	
Prodroma	Early clinical manifestation (such as malaise, headache, a sense of depression or alterations in smell, taste, hearing or vision) that may occur a few days to hours before onset of a seizure
Aura	A partial seizure experienced as a peculiar sensation preceding onset of generalized seizure that may take the form of gustatory, visual, or auditory experience or a feeling of dizziness, numbness, or just "a funny feeling"
Ictal Phase	The event of the seizure
Tonic Phase	A state of muscle contraction in which there is excessive muscle tone
Clonic Phase	A state of alternating contraction and relaxation of muscles
Postictal Phase	Time period immediately following cessation of seizure activity

BOX 16.4 Cerebral Hemodynamics

Cerebral blood flow (CBF) to the brain is normally maintained at a rate that matches the local metabolic needs of the brain.

Cerebral perfusion pressure (CPP) (70-90 mm Hg) is the pressure required to perfuse the cells of the brain.

Cerebral blood volume (CBV) is the amount of blood in the intracranial vault at a given time.

Cerebral blood oxygenation is measured by oxygen saturation in the internal jugular vein.

Intracranial pressure (ICP) normally is 1 to 15 mm Hg, or 60 to 180 cm H_2O.

intensity of firing reaches a threshold point, the excitation spreads across the brain. Excitation of the subcortical, thalamic, and brainstem areas corresponds to the tonic phase (muscle contraction with increased muscle tone) and is associated with loss of consciousness. The clonic phase (alternating contraction and relaxation of muscles) begins when inhibitory neurons in the cortex, anterior thalamus, and basal ganglia react to the cortical excitation. The seizure discharge is interrupted, producing intermittent muscle contractions that gradually decrease and finally cease. The epileptogenic neurons are then exhausted.

During seizure activity, oxygen is consumed at a high rate—about 60% greater than normal. Although cerebral blood flow also increases, oxygen is rapidly depleted, along with glucose, and lactate accumulates in brain tissue. Thus continued severe seizure activity has the potential for progressive brain injury and irreversible damage. In addition, if a seizure focus in the brain is active for a prolonged period, a mirror focus may develop in contralateral normal tissue and cause more widespread seizure activity across the brain.

CLINICAL MANIFESTATIONS   The clinical manifestations associated with seizure depend on its type (see Table 16.14). Two types of symptoms signal the preictal phase of a generalized tonic-clonic seizure: prodroma, early manifestations occurring hours to days before a seizure and may include anxiety, depression, or inability to think clearly; and an aura, unusual sensory experiences or a partial seizure that immediately precedes the onset of a generalized tonic-clonic seizure. Both symptoms may become familiar to the person experiencing recurrent generalized seizures and may enable the person to prevent injuries during the seizure. The ictus is the episode of the epileptic seizure with tonic-clonic activity. Relaxation of urinary and bowel sphincters may occur, leading to bladder and bowel incontinence. Airway maintenance needs to be ensured. The postictal state follows an epileptic seizure and can include signs of headache, confusion, dysphasia, memory loss, and paralysis that may last hours or a day or two. Deep sleep also is common. Status epilepticus in adults is a state of continuous seizures lasting more than 5 minutes, or rapidly recurring seizures before the person has fully regained consciousness from the preceding seizure, or a single seizure lasting more than 30 minutes.

EVALUATION AND TREATMENT   The health history, a physical examination, and laboratory tests of blood and urine (concentrations of blood glucose, serum calcium, blood urea nitrogen, and urine sodium; and creatinine clearance time) can identify systemic diseases known to promote seizures. Brain imaging and cerebrospinal fluid (CSF) examination help identify neurologic diseases associated with seizures. The EEG is used to assess the type of seizure and determine its focus in brain tissue.

Treatment for a seizure disorder is to first correct or control its cause if possible. If this is not possible, the major means of management is the judicious administration of antiseizure medications. Dietary treatments (e.g., ketogenic and Atkins diet) are effective for some individuals.[21] Surgical interventions can improve seizure control and quality of life in people with drug-resistant epilepsy.

✓ QUICK CHECK 16.4
1. What are some major difference between delirium and dementia?
2. What is an eliptogenic focus?
3. What is epilepsy?

ALTERATIONS IN CEREBRAL HEMODYNAMICS

An injured brain reacts with structural, chemical, and pathophysiologic changes. Primary brain injury is the original trauma, and secondary brain injury is a consequence of alterations in cerebral blood flow, intracranial pressure, and oxygen delivery. Target values for relevant cerebral blood flow parameters are summarized in Box 16.4).

Alterations in cerebral blood flow (CBF) are related to three injury states: inadequate cerebral perfusion, normal cerebral perfusion but with an elevated intracranial pressure, and excessive cerebral blood volume (CBV). Treatments for these injury states are directed at improving or maintaining cerebral perfusion pressure (CPP), as well as controlling intracranial pressure. (The pathophysiology specific to primary and secondary traumatic brain injury is discussed in Chapter 17.)

Increased Intracranial Pressure

Increased intracranial pressure (IICP) may result from an increase in intracranial content as occurs with tumor growth, cerebral edema, excess CSF, or hemorrhage. An increase in intracranial content necessitates an equal reduction in volume of the other cranial contents to maintain cerebral perfusion. The most readily displaced content is CSF. If intracranial pressure remains high after CSF displacement out of the cranial vault, CBV and CBF are altered.

There are four progressive stages of IICP. In *stage 1 of intracranial hypertension*, vasoconstriction and external compression of the venous system occur in an attempt to further decrease the intracranial pressure. Thus during the first stage of intracranial hypertension, intracranial pressure (ICP) may not change because of the effective compensatory

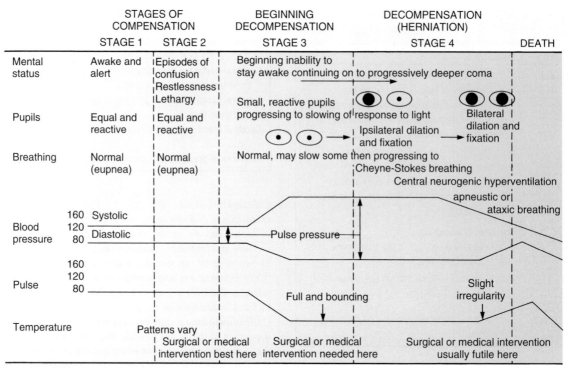

	STAGES OF COMPENSATION		BEGINNING DECOMPENSATION	DECOMPENSATION (HERNIATION)	
	STAGE 1	STAGE 2	STAGE 3	STAGE 4	DEATH
Mental status	Awake and alert	Episodes of confusion Restlessness Lethargy	Beginning inability to stay awake continuing on to progressively deeper coma		
Pupils	Equal and reactive	Equal and reactive	Small, reactive pupils progressing to slowing of response to light → Ipsilateral dilation and fixation	Bilateral dilation and fixation	
Breathing	Normal (eupnea)	Normal (eupnea)	Normal, may slow some then progressing to Cheyne-Stokes breathing Central neurogenic hyperventilation apneustic or ataxic breathing		
Blood pressure	160 Systolic 120 80 Diastolic		Pulse pressure		
Pulse	160 120 80		Full and bounding	Slight irregularity	
Temperature	Patterns vary				
	Surgical or medical intervention best here		Surgical or medical intervention needed here	Surgical or medical intervention usually futile here	

FIGURE 16.10 Clinical Correlates of Compensated and Uncompensated Stages of Intracranial Hypertension. (From Beare PG, Myers JL: *Principles and practice of adult health nursing,* ed 3, St Louis, 1998, Mosby.)

mechanisms, and there may no detectable symptoms (Fig. 16.10). Small increases in volume, however, cause an increase in pressure, and the pressure may take longer to return to baseline. This pressure change can be detected with ICP monitoring.

In *stage 2 of intracranial hypertension,* there is continued expansion of intracranial contents. The resulting increase in ICP may exceed the ability of the brain's compensatory mechanisms to adjust. The pressure begins to compromise neuronal oxygenation. Systemic arterial vasoconstriction occurs in an attempt to elevate the systemic blood pressure sufficiently to overcome the IICP and maintain perfusion. Clinical manifestations at this stage usually are subtle and transient, including episodes of confusion, restlessness, drowsiness, and slight pupillary and breathing changes (see Fig. 16.10). Interventions at this stage reduce ICP and promote better clinical outcomes.

In *stage 3 of intracranial hypertension,* ICP begins to approach arterial pressure. The brain tissues begin to experience hypoxia and hypercapnia, and the individual's condition rapidly deteriorates. Clinical manifestations include decreasing levels of arousal or central neurogenic hyperventilation, widened pulse pressure, bradycardia, and small, sluggish pupils (see Fig. 16.10).

Dramatic sustained rises in ICP are not seen until all compensatory mechanisms have been exhausted. Then dramatic rises in ICP occur over a very short period. **Autoregulation** is the compensatory alteration in the diameter of the intracranial blood vessels designed to maintain a constant blood flow during changes in cerebral perfusion pressure. Autoregulation is lost with progressively increased ICP. Accumulating carbon dioxide may still cause vasodilation locally, but without autoregulation this vasodilation causes the blood pressure in the vessels to drop and the blood volume to increase. The brain volume is thus further increased, and ICP continues to rise. Small increases in volume cause dramatic increases in ICP, and the pressure takes much longer to return to baseline. As the ICP begins to approach systemic blood pressure, cerebral perfusion pressure falls and cerebral perfusion slows

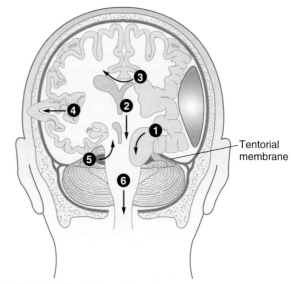

FIGURE 16.11 Brain Herniation Syndromes. Herniations can occur both above and below the tentorial membrane. Supratentorial: **1,** uncal (transtentorial); **2,** central; **3,** cingulate; **4,** transcalvarial (external herniation through an opening in the skull). Infratentorial: **5,** upward herniation of cerebellum; **6,** cerebellar tonsillar move down through foramen magnum.

dramatically. The brain tissues experience severe hypoxia, hypercapnia, and acidosis.

In *stage 4 of intracranial hypertension,* brain tissue shifts (herniates) from the compartment of greater pressure to a compartment of lesser pressure. IICP in one compartment of the cranial vault is not evenly distributed throughout the other vault compartments (see Figs. 16.10 and 16.11). With this shift in brain tissue, the herniating brain tissue's blood supply is compromised, causing further ischemia and hypoxia in the herniating tissues. The volume of content within the lower-pressure compartment increases, exerting pressure on the brain tissue that normally occupies that compartment, and thus impairs its blood supply. For example, herniation into the brainstem impairs the vital cardiovascular and respiratory regulatory centers and can cause death. The herniation process markedly and rapidly increases ICP. Mean systolic arterial pressure soon equals ICP, and CBF ceases at this point. The types of herniation syndromes are outlined in Box 16.5.

Cerebral Edema

Cerebral edema is an increase in the fluid content of brain tissue (Fig. 16.12). The result is increased extracellular or intracellular tissue volume. It occurs after brain insult from trauma, infection, hemorrhage, tumor growth, ischemia, infarction, or hypoxia. The harmful effects of cerebral edema are caused by distortion of blood vessels, displacement of brain tissues, increase in ICP, and eventual herniation of brain tissue to a different brain compartment.

There are three types of cerebral edema: (1) vasogenic edema, (2) cytotoxic (metabolic) edema, and (3) interstitial/hydrocephalic edema.[22] There is often overlap among the three types of edema. Vasogenic edema is clinically the most important and common type. It is caused by increased permeability of the capillaries that comprise the blood–brain

barrier. Consequently, plasma proteins leak into the extracellular spaces, drawing water to them, and increasing the water content of the brain interstitial spaces. Vasogenic edema begins in the area of injury (brain trauma, tumors, inflammation) and spreads, with fluid accumulating in the white matter at the site of injury. Edema promotes more edema because of ischemia from the increasing ICP.

Clinical manifestations of vasogenic edema include focal neurologic deficits, disturbances of consciousness, and a severe increase in ICP. Vasogenic edema resolves by slow diffusion of fluid back into the bloodstream.

In cytotoxic edema (cellular brain edema), the accumulation of fluid is in the cells of the brain (neuronal, glial, and endothelial cells) rather than in the interstitial spaces. The blood–brain barrier is intact. Accumulation of toxic factors directly causes failure of the active transport systems. The cells lose their potassium and gain larger amounts of sodium. Water follows by osmosis into the cells, so that the cells swell. Cytotoxic edema occurs principally in the gray matter and may contribute to vasogenic edema. It occurs with head injury, hypoxia, and arterial infarction.

Interstitial/hydrocephalic edema is most often seen with noncommunicating hydrocephalus. The edema is caused by the movement of CSF from the lining of the ventricles into the extracellular spaces of the brain tissues (transependymal edema). The brain fluid volume increases predominantly around the ventricles, with increased hydrostatic pressure within the white matter. The size of the white matter is reduced because of the rapid disappearance of myelin lipids.

Treatment of cerebral edema is directed at decreasing IICP. Treatment can include the use of oxygen, osmotherapy (e.g., mannitol), diuretics, the placement of a CSF drain tube, and maintenance of systemic blood pressure with fluid management. Steroids (dexamethasone) may be used to treat edema associated with brain tumors.

Hydrocephalus

The term hydrocephalus refers to various conditions characterized by excess fluid in the cerebral ventricles, subarachnoid space, or both. Hydrocephalus occurs because of interference with CSF flow caused by increased fluid production, obstruction within the ventricular system, or defective reabsorption of the fluid. A tumor of the choroid plexus may, in rare instances, cause overproduction of CSF. The types of hydrocephalus are reviewed in Table 16.16.

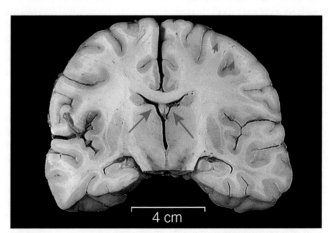

FIGURE 16.12 Brain Edema. This coronal section of the cerebrum demonstrates marked compression in the lateral ventricles *(long arrows)* and flattening of gyri *(short arrows)* from extensive bilateral cerebral edema. Edema increases intracranial pressure, leading to herniation. (From Klatt EC: *Robbins and Cotran atlas of pathology,* ed 2, Philadelphia, 2010, Saunders.)

BOX 16.5   Brain Herniation Syndrome

Supratentorial Herniation

1. *Uncal herniation.* Occurs when the uncus or hippocampal gyrus, or both, shifts from the middle fossa through the tentorial notch into the posterior fossa, compressing the ipsilateral third cranial nerve, the contralateral third cranial nerve, and the mesencephalon. Uncal herniation generally is caused by an expanding mass in the lateral region of the middle fossa. The classic manifestations of uncal herniation are a decreasing level of consciousness, pupils that become sluggish before fixing and dilating (first the ipsilateral, then the contralateral pupil), Cheyne-Stokes respirations (which later shift to central neurogenic hyperventilation), and the appearance of decorticate and then decerebrate posturing.
2. *Central herniation.* Occurs when there is a straight downward shift of the diencephalon through the tentorial notch. It may be caused by injuries or masses located around the outer perimeter of the frontal, parietal, or occipital lobes; extracerebral injuries around the central apex (top) of the cranium; bilaterally positioned injuries or masses; and unilateral cingulate gyrus herniation. The individual rapidly becomes unconscious; moves from Cheyne-Stokes respirations to apnea; develops small, reactive pupils and then dilated, fixed pupils; and passes from decortication to decerebration.
3. *Cingulate gyrus herniation.* Occurs when the cingulate gyrus shifts under the falx cerebri. Little is known about its clinical manifestations.
4. *Transcalvarial.* The brain shifts through a skull fracture or a surgical opening in the skull. This type of external herniation may occur during a craniectomy—surgery in which a flap of skull is removed. This type of herniation prevents the piece of skull from being replaced.

Infratentorial Herniation

1. The most common syndrome is *cerebellar tonsillar herniation.* The cerebellar tonsil shifts through the foramen magnum because of increased pressure within the posterior fossa. The clinical manifestations are an arched, stiff neck, paresthesias in the shoulder area, decreased consciousness, respiratory abnormalities, and pulse rate variations. Occasionally the force produces an *upward transtentorial herniation* of a cerebellar tonsil or the lower brainstem. There is increased intracranial pressure (ICP) but no specific set of clinical manifestations associated with infratentorial herniation.

TABLE 16.16 Types of Hydrocephalus

Type	Mechanism	Cause
Noncommunicating	Obstruction of CSF flow between ventricles Aqueduct stenosis Arnold-Chiari malformation (brain extension through foramen magnum) Compression by tumor	Congenital abnormality
Communicating	Impaired absorption of CSF within subarachnoid space Compression of subarachnoid space by a tumor High venous pressure in sagittal sinus Head injury Congenital malformation	Infection with inflammatory adhesions
	Increased CSF secretion by choroid plexus	Secreting tumor

CSF, Cerebrospinal fluid.

QUICK CHECK 16.5
1. What are the four stages of increased intracranial pressure?
2. How does supratentorial herniation differ from infratentorial herniation?
3. What is the major difference between vasogenic and cytotoxic cerebral edema?
4. How is communicating hydrocephalus different from noncommunicating hydrocephalus?

Hydrocephalus may develop from infancy through adulthood. Communicating hydrocephalus is defective resorption of CSF from the cerebral subarachnoid space and is found more often in adults. Noncommunicating hydrocephalus (internal hydrocephalus, intraventricular hydrocephalus) is obstruction within the ventricular system and is seen more often in children (see Fig. 18.7). Congenital hydrocephalus is ventricular enlargement before birth and is rare.

PATHOPHYSIOLOGY The obstruction of CSF flow associated with hydrocephalus produces increased pressure and dilation of the ventricles proximal to the obstruction. The increased pressure and dilation cause atrophy of the cerebral cortex and degeneration of the white matter tracts. Selective preservation of gray matter occurs.

CLINICAL MANIFESTATIONS Most cases of hydrocephalus develop gradually and insidiously over time. Acute hydrocephalus presents with signs of rapidly developing IICP. The person quickly deteriorates into a deep coma if not promptly treated. Normal-pressure hydrocephalus (dilation of the ventricles without increased pressure) develops slowly and occurs more commonly in the elderly. The individual or family members may notice declining memory and cognitive function. The triad symptoms of an unsteady, broad-based gait with a history of falling, incontinence, and dementia is common.[23]

EVALUATION AND TREATMENT The diagnosis is based on the physical examination and imaging procedures. Hydrocephalus can be treated by surgery to resect cysts, neoplasms, or hematomas or by ventricular bypass into the normal intracranial channel or into an extracranial compartment using a shunting procedure. Excision or coagulation of the choroid plexus is a treatment option to reduce formation of CSF or when a papilloma (a benign tumor) is present. In normal-pressure hydrocephalus, reduction in CSF is achieved through diuresis or placement of a ventriculoperitoneal shunt.

ALTERATIONS IN NEUROMOTOR FUNCTION

Movements are complex patterns of activity controlled by the cerebral cortex, the pyramidal system, the extrapyramidal system, and the motor neurons in muscles (motor units). Dysfunction in any of these areas can cause motor dysfunction. General neuromotor dysfunctions are associated with changes in muscle tone, movement, and complex motor performance.

Alterations in Muscle Tone

Normal muscle tone involves a slight resistance to passive movement. Throughout the range of motion, the resistance is smooth, constant, and even. The alterations of muscle tone and their characteristics and causes are summarized in Table 16.17.

Hypotonia

Hypotonia is decreased muscle tone. With passive muscle movement there is little or no resistance. Normally there is some resistance or tone to relaxed muscles. Causes include cerebellar damage and pure pyramidal tract damage (a rare occurrence). Hypotonia manifests with minimal weakness and normal or slightly exaggerated reflexes. Cerebellar damage contributes to ataxia (loss of control of body movements) and intention tremor. A pure pyramidal tract injury produces hypotonia and weakness. Hypotonia also occurs when nerve impulses needed for muscle tone are lost, such as in spinal cord injury or cerebrovascular accident.

Individuals with hypotonia tire easily or are weak. They may have difficulty rising from a sitting position, sitting down without using arm support, and walking up and down stairs. They may have an inability to stand on their toes. Because of their weakness, accidents during ambulatory and self-care activities are common. The joints become hyperflexible, so persons with hypotonia may be able to assume positions that require extreme joint mobility. The joints may appear loose. The muscle mass atrophies because of decreased input entering the motor unit, and muscles appear flabby and flat. Muscle cells are gradually replaced by connective tissue and fat. Fasciculations (muscle twitches) may be present in some cases.

Hypertonia

Hypertonia is increased muscle tone. With passive movement of a muscle there is resistance to stretch. Hypertonia is caused by upper motor neuron damage with loss of inhibitory control (see the section Upper Motor Neuron Syndromes). The four types of hypertonia are spasticity (usually corticospinal in origin) (Figs. 16.13 and 16.15), paratonia (gegenhalten), dystonia (Fig. 16.14), and rigidity (usually extrapyramidal in origin). Four types of rigidity are described: plastic or lead-pipe, cogwheel, gamma (independent of stretch reflex pathways), and alpha (dependent on stretch reflex pathways) (see Table 16.17).

Individuals with hypertonia tire easily or are weak. Passive movement and active movement are affected equally, except in paratonia, in which more active than passive movement is possible. As a result of hypertonia and weakness, accidents occur during ambulatory and self-care activities.

The muscles may atrophy because of decreased use. However, hypertrophy occasionally occurs as a result of the overstimulation of muscle fibers. Overstimulation occurs when the motor unit reflex arc remains intact and functioning but is not inhibited by higher centers.

TABLE 16.17 Alterations in Muscle Tone

Alterations	Characteristics	Cause
Hypotonia	Passive movement of a muscle mass with little or no resistance Muscles may be moved rapidly without resistance	Thought to be caused by decreased muscle spindle activity as a result of decreased excitability of neurons (e.g., muscular dystrophy, cerebral palsy)
Flaccidity	Associated with limp, atrophied muscles, and paralysis	Occurs typically when nerve impulses necessary for muscle tone are lost
Hypertonia	Increased muscle resistance to passive movement May be associated with paralysis May be accompanied by muscle hypertrophy	Results when lower motor unit reflex arc continues to function but is not mediated or regulated by higher centers (e.g., stroke, brain tumors, multiple sclerosis)
Spasticity	A gradual increase in tone causing increased resistance until tone suddenly diminishes, which results in clasp-knife phenomenon; increased deep tendon reflexes (hyperreflexia); clonus (spread of reflexes)	Exact mechanism unclear; appears to arise from an increased excitability of alpha motor neurons to any input because of absence of descending inhibition of pyramidal systems (e.g., multiple sclerosis, brain trauma, cerebral palsy)
Paratonia (gegenhalten)	Resistance to passive movement, which varies in direct proportion to force applied	Exact mechanism unclear; associated with frontal lobe injury (e.g., progressive Alzheimer dementia)
Dystonia	Sustained involuntary muscle contraction with twisting movement	Produced by slow muscular contraction; lack of reciprocal inhibition of muscle (e.g., neuroleptic drug side effects, meningitis)
Rigidity	Muscle resistance to passive movement of a rigid limb that is uniform in both flexion and extension throughout the motion	Occurs as a result of constant, involuntary contraction of muscle—usually involves extrapyramidal tracts (e.g., Parkinson disease)
Plastic or lead-pipe rigidity	Increased muscular tone relatively independent of degree of force used in passive movement; does not vary throughout the passive movement	Associated with basal ganglion damage (e.g., Parkinson disease)
Cogwheel rigidity	Uniform resistance may be interrupted by a series of brief jerks, resulting in movements much like a ratchet, "cogwheel" phenomenon	Associated with basal ganglion damage
Gamma rigidity	Characterized by extensor posturing (decerebrate rigidity)	Loss of excitation of extensor inhibitory areas by cerebral cortex decreasing inhibition of alpha and gamma motor neurons
Alpha rigidity	Impaired relaxation characterized by extensor rigidity of skeletal muscle after contraction	Loss of cerebellum input to lateral vestibular nuclei

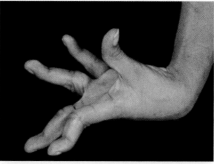

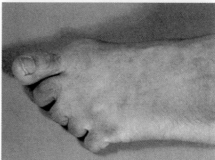

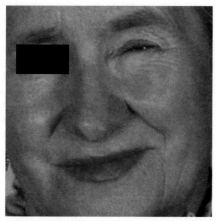

FIGURE 16.13 Paroxysm of Left-Sided Hemifacial Spasm. (From Perkin GD: *Mosby's color atlas and text of neurology*, ed 2, London, 2002, Mosby.)

FIGURE 16.14 Dystonic Posturing of the Hand and Foot. (From Perkin GD: *Mosby's color atlas and text of neurology*, ed 2, London, 2002, Mosby.)

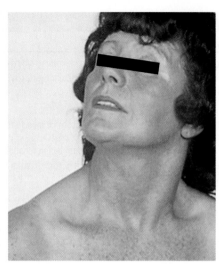

FIGURE 16.15 Spasmodic Torticollis. A characteristic head posture related to spasticity. (From Perkin GD: *Mosby's color atlas and text of neurology,* ed 2, London, 2002, Mosby.)

This causes continual muscle contraction, resulting in enlargement of the muscle mass and the development of firm muscles.

Alterations in Muscle Movement

Movement requires a change in the contractile state of muscles. Abnormal movements occur when CNS dysfunction alters muscle innervation. The neurotransmitter *dopamine* has a role in several movement disorders. Some movement disorders (e.g., the akinesias) result from too little dopaminergic activity, whereas others (e.g., chorea, ballism, tardive dyskinesia) result from too much dopaminergic activity. Still others are not primarily related to dopamine function. Movement disorders are not necessarily associated with muscle mass, strength, or tone but are neurologic dysfunctions that result in insufficient or excessive movement or involuntary movement. Movement disorders can be idiopathic or associated with specific diseases of the CNS, such as Parkinson disease and Huntington disease.

Hyperkinesia is excessive, purposeless movement. Within this category are a number of specific dysfunctions, including tremors (Table 16.18). Also included under the general category of hyperkinesias are *dyskinesias* and abnormal involuntary movements. Huntington disease symptoms are the hallmark of hyperkinesia (see the section Huntington Disease).

Paroxysmal dyskinesias are rare abnormal, episodic, involuntary movements that occur as spasms. The type of dyskinesia varies depending on the specific disorder. These involuntary movements include dystonia (uncontrollable twisting, repetitive movement resulting in abnormal posture), chorea (abnormal jerky movements), athetosis (writhing movements), and ballism (flailing limb movements), or a combination of these.

Tardive dyskinesia is the involuntary movement of the face, lip, tongue, trunk, and extremities. Although the condition occurs occasionally in individuals with Parkinson disease, it usually occurs as a side effect of prolonged antipsychotic drug therapy. The most common symptom of tardive dyskinesia is rapid, repetitive, stereotypic movements, such as continual chewing with intermittent protrusions of the tongue, lip smacking, and facial grimacing. The symptoms also are called *extrapyramidal symptoms* because the extrapyramidal system controls involuntary reflexes and coordination of movement and posture.

Other movement disorders in this category are (1) complex repetitive movements, including automatism (unconscious behavior), stereotypy (ritualistic behavior such as rocking), complex tics such as Tourette syndrome (see *Did You Know?* Tourette Syndrome), compulsions, perseverations, and mannerisms; (2) excessive reactions to certain stimuli; and (3) paroxysmal excessive activity, including cataplexy (a sudden and uncontrollable muscle weakness or paralysis often triggered by a strong emotion, such as excitement or laughter) and excessive startle reaction.

Huntington Disease

Huntington disease (HD), also known as *Huntington chorea,* is a relatively rare, hereditary, degenerative hyperkinetic movement disorder. The onset of HD is usually between 35 and 44 years of age, when the trait may already have been passed to the person's children. The disorder has a prevalence rate of approximately 3 to 7 per 100,000 people of European ancestry, but it occurs in all races.[24]

PATHOPHYSIOLOGY   HD is inherited from one or both parents who have the autosomal dominant trait with high penetrance. The genetic defect of HD is on chromosome 4. There is an abnormally long polyglutamine tract in the huntingtin (htt) protein that is toxic to neurons. The age of symptom onset is related to the length of the repeat sequences and mechanisms of toxicity. Repeat lengths greater than 60 cause the juvenile form of the disease.[25] Fathers, but not mothers, with high normal alleles do not develop HD but are at risk of transmitting potentially penetrant HD alleles (≥36) to their offspring, who can develop HD.[26]

The principal pathologic feature of HD is severe degeneration of the basal ganglia, particularly the caudate nucleus, with progression to involve other parts of the brain. Tangles of huntingtin protein collect in the brain cells. Depletion of gamma-aminobutyric acid (GABA), an inhibitory neurotransmitter, is the principal biochemical alteration in Huntington disease. It alters the integration of motor and mental function.

CLINICAL MANIFESTATIONS   Symptoms of HD progress slowly over 15 to 20 years. Symptoms are extrapyramidal and include involuntary hyperkinetic movements, such as chorea, athetosis, and ballism (Table

TABLE 16.18 Types of Hyperkinesia and Tremor

Type	Characteristics	Causes
Hyperkinesia		
Chorea*	Nonrepetitive muscular contractions, usually of extremities or face; random pattern of irregular, involuntary rapid contractions of groups of muscles; disappears with sleep, decreases with resting; increases with emotional stress and attempted voluntary movement	Associated with excess concentration of or supersensitivity to dopamine within basal ganglia
Athetosis*	Disorder of distal muscle postural fixation; slow, sinuous, irregular movements most obvious in distal extremities, more rhythmic than choreiform movements and always much slower; movements accompany characteristic hand posture; slowly fluctuating grimaces	Occurs most commonly as result of injury to putamen of basal ganglion; exact pathophysiologic mechanism is not known
Ballism	Disorder of proximal muscle postural fixation with wild flinging movement of limbs; movement is severe and stereotyped, usually lateral; does not lessen with sleep; ballism is most common on one side of body, a condition termed *hemiballism*	Results from injury to subthalamic nucleus (one of nuclei that comprise basal ganglia); thought to be caused by reduced inhibitory influence in nucleus, a release phenomenon; hemiballism results from injury to contralateral subthalamic nucleus
Hyperactivity	State of prolonged, generalized, increased activity that is largely involuntary but may be subject to some voluntary control; not highly stereotyped but rather manifests as continuous changes in total body posture or in excessive performance of some simple activity, such as pacing under inappropriate circumstances	May be caused by frontal and reticular activating system injury
Wandering	Tendency to wander without regard for environment	"Release phenomenon" associated with bilateral injury to globus pallidus or putamen
Akathisia	Special type of hyperactivity; mild compulsion to move (usually more localized to legs); severe, frenzied motion possible; movements are partly voluntary and may be transiently suppressed; carrying out movement brings sense of relief; frequent complication of antipsychotic drugs	Dopaminergic transmission may be involved
Tremor at Rest		
Parkinsonian tremor	Rhythmic, oscillating movement affecting one or more body parts Regular, rhythmic, slower flexion-extension contraction; involves principally metacarpophalangeal and wrist joints; alternating movements between thumb and index finger described as "pill rolling"; disappears during voluntary movement	Caused by regular contraction of opposing groups of muscles Loss of inhibitory influence of dopamine in the basal ganglia, causing instability of basal ganglial feedback circuit within cerebral cortex
Postural Tremor		
Asterixis (tremor of hepatic encephalopathy)	Irregular flapping movement of hands accentuated by outstretching arms	Exact mechanisms responsible unknown; thought to be related to accumulation of products normally detoxified by liver (e.g., ammonia)
Metabolic	Rapid, rhythmic tremor affecting fingers, lips, and tongue; accentuated by extending body part; enhanced physiologic tremor	Occurs in conditions associated with disturbed metabolism or toxicity, as in thyrotoxicosis (hyperthyroidism), alcoholism, and chronic use of barbiturates, amphetamines, lithium, or amitriptyline (Elavil); exact mechanism responsible unknown
Essential (familial)	Tremor of fingers, hands, and feet; absent at rest but accentuated by extension of body part, prolonged muscular activity, and stress	Not associated with any other neurologic abnormalities; cause unknown
Intention Tremor		
Cerebellar	Tremor initiated by movement, maximal toward end of movement	Occurs in disease of dentate nucleus (one of deep cerebellar nuclei responsible for efferent output) and superior cerebellar peduncle (stalklike structure connected to pons); caused by errors in feedback from periphery and errors in preprogramming goal-directed movement
Rubral	Rhythmic tremor of limbs that originates proximally by movement	Results from lesions involving dentatorubrothalamic tract (a spinothalamic tract connecting red nucleus in reticular formation and dentate nucleus in cerebellum)
Myoclonus	Series of shocklike, nonpatterned contractions of portion of a muscle, entire muscle, or group of muscles that cause throwing movements of a limb; usually appear at random but frequently triggered by sudden startle; do not disappear during sleep	Associated with an irritable nervous system and spontaneous discharge of neurons; structures associated with myoclonus include cerebral cortex, cerebellum, reticular formation, and spinal cord

*Choreoathetosis involves both chorea and athetosis; precise pathophysiology is unknown.

16.18). Chorea, the most common type of jerky abnormal movement, begins in the face and arms, eventually affecting the entire body. There is emotional lability and progressive dysfunction of intellectual and thought processes that may precede motor symptoms. Any one of these features may mark the onset of the disease. Cognitive deficits include slow thinking, loss of working memory, and reduced capacity to plan, organize, and sequence. Restlessness, disinhibition, and irritability are common. Apathy, depression, and anxiety can be disabling.

EVALUATION AND TREATMENT   The diagnosis of HD is based on the family history and clinical presentation of the disorder. Genetic testing confirms the diagnosis. Neuroradiologic abnormalities can be demonstrated up to 15 years before clinical symptoms. No known treatment is effective in halting the degeneration or progression of symptoms, and the disease is fatal. Symptomatic drug therapies are available.[27,28]

Hypokinesia

Hypokinesia (decreased movement) is loss of voluntary movement despite preserved consciousness and normal peripheral nerve and muscle function. Types of hypokinesia include akinesia, bradykinesia, and loss of associated movement. Parkinson disease symptoms are the hallmark of hypokinesia.

Akinesia is a decrease in voluntary and associated movements. It is related to dysfunction of the extrapyramidal system and caused by either a deficiency of dopamine or a defect of the postsynaptic dopamine receptors, which occurs in parkinsonism.

Bradykinesia is slowness of voluntary movements. All voluntary movements become slow, labored, and deliberate, with difficulty in (1) initiating movements, (2) continuing movements smoothly, and (3) performing synchronous (at the same time) and consecutive tasks. Both akinesia and bradykinesia involve a delay in the time it takes to start to perform a movement.

Loss of associated movement accompanies hypokinesia. The normal, habitually associated movements that provide skill, grace, and balance to voluntary movements are lost. Decreased associated movements accompanying emotional expression cause an expressionless face, a statue-like posture, absence of speech inflection, and absence of spontaneous gestures. Decreased associated movements accompanying locomotion cause reduction in arm and shoulder movements, hip swinging, and rotary motion of the cervical spine.

Parkinson Disease

Parkinson disease (PD) is a complex motor disorder accompanied by systemic nonmotor and neurologic symptoms. Etiologic classification of parkinsonism includes primary parkinsonism (hereditary and sporadic) and secondary parkinsonism. Primary PD begins after the age of 40 years, with the incidence increasing after 60 years. It is more prevalent in males and a leading cause of neurologic disability in individuals older than 60 years. Approximately 60,000 new cases are diagnosed in the United States each year.[29] The familial form represents about 10% of PD; however, the majority of cases are sporadic or idiopathic. Secondary parkinsonism is parkinsonism caused by disorders other than PD (i.e., head trauma, infection, neoplasm, atherosclerosis, toxins, drug intoxication). Drug-induced parkinsonism, caused by neuroleptics, antiemetics, and antihypertensives, is the most common secondary form and usually is reversible.

PATHOPHYSIOLOGY   The pathogenesis of primary PD is unknown. Several gene mutations have been identified that influence nerve function in PD. Gene–environment interactions are probable causes of neurodegeneration in PD. The primary pathology is degeneration of the basal ganglia (see Fig. 14.10) with accumulation of dysfunctional or misfolded

α-synuclein protein and loss of dopamine-producing neurons in the substantia nigra and dorsal striatum. The resulting depletion of dopamine, an inhibitory neurotransmitter, and relative excess of cholinergic (excitatory) activity in the feedback circuit are manifested by hypertonia (tremor and rigidity) and hypokinesia, producing a syndrome of abnormal movement called parkinsonism (Parkinson syndrome, parkinsonian syndrome, paralysis agitans) (Fig. 16.16). Neuroimaging shows degeneration of dopaminergic neurons preceding the onset of motor symptoms by as long as 3 to 6 years.[30] Collections of α-synuclein protein form *Lewy bodies* resulting in neurodegeneration and dementia after years of the disease.[31] Loss of cholinergic subcortical input into the cortex is associated with nonmotor symptoms of PD.[32]

CLINICAL MANIFESTATIONS   The classic manifestations of PD are resting tremor, rigidity, bradykinesia/akinesia, postural disturbance, dysarthria, and dysphagia. They may develop alone or in combination, but as the disease progresses, all are usually present. There is no true paralysis. The symptoms are always bilateral but usually involve one side early in the illness. Because the onset is insidious, the beginning of symptoms is difficult to document. Early in the disease, reflex status, sensory status, and mental status usually are normal. Loss of smell can be an early nonmotor symptom. Postural abnormalities (flexed, forward leaning), difficulty walking, and weakness develop as neurodegeneration progresses (Fig. 16.17). Speech may be slurred.

Disorders of equilibrium result from postural abnormalities. The person with Parkinson disease cannot make the appropriate postural adjustment to tilting or falling and falls like a post when starting to tilt. The short, accelerating steps of the individual with Parkinson disease are an attempt to maintain an upright position while walking. Individuals are also unable to right themselves when changing from a reclining or crouching position to a standing position and when rolling over from a supine to a lateral or prone position.

Nonmotor symptoms are common. Sleep disorders and excessive daytime sleepiness are commonly experienced. Sensory disturbances (pain and impaired smell and vision), urinary urgency, difficulty

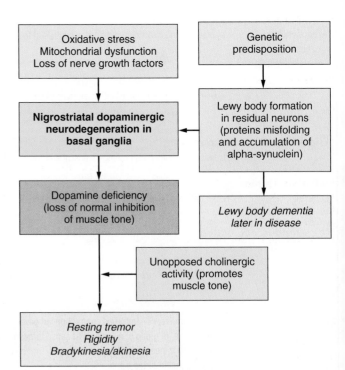

FIGURE 16.16 Pathophysiology of Parkinson Disease.

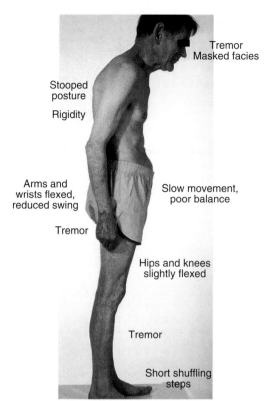

FIGURE 16.17 Stooped Posture of Parkinson Disease. (From Perkin DG: *Mosby's color atlas and text of neurology,* ed 2, London, 2002, Mosby.)

concentrating, depression, and hallucinations are some of the nonmotor symptoms of PD. Autonomic-neuroendocrine changes also contribute to nonmotor symptoms and include inappropriate diaphoresis, orthostatic hypotension, drooling, gastric retention, constipation, and urinary retention.

Progressive dementia is more common in persons older than 70 years. Mental status may be further compromised by the side effects of the medication taken to control symptoms.

EVALUATION AND TREATMENT   The diagnosis of PD is based on the history and clinical features of the disease. Causes of secondary parkinsonism are first excluded. Specific gene panels and imaging studies are evolving for early diagnosis.[33,34]

Treatment of PD is symptomatic, with drug therapy to decrease dyskinesia. Because of troublesome side effects and loss of effectiveness, however, drug therapy may not be started until the symptoms become incapacitating. Deep brain stimulation (i.e., subthalamic neurostimulation) is replacing surgery to treat persons unresponsive to drug therapy. Implants of stem cells and fetal cells, as well as gene therapy, are strategies for future treatments.[35,36] Dysphagia and general immobility are special problems of the individual with PD, requiring interdisciplinary efforts to improve nutrition and functional status.

Upper and Lower Motor Neuron Syndromes
Upper Motor Neuron Syndromes

Upper motor neuron syndromes are the result of injury to motor pathways that descend from the motor cortex (Figs. 16.18 and 16.19). The nerves travel in the pyramidal (corticospinal) tracts and synapse on lower motor neurons in the brainstem or anterior spinal cord. Upper motor neuron injury may be in the cerebral cortex, the subcortical white matter, the internal capsule, the brainstem, or the spinal cord but

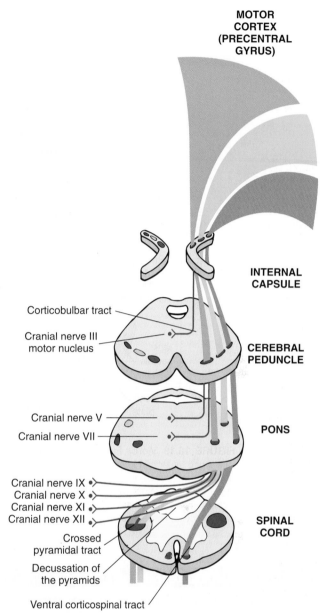

FIGURE 16.18 Structures of the Upper Motor Neuron, or Pyramidal, System. Pyramidal system fibers are shown to originate primarily in cells in the precentral gyrus of the motor cortex; to converge at the internal capsule; to descend to form the central third of the cerebral peduncle; to descend further through the pons, where small fibers supply cranial nerve motor nuclei along the way; to form pyramids at the medulla, where most of the fibers decussate (cross over); and then to continue to descend in the lateral column of white matter of the spinal cord. A few fibers descend without crossing at the level of the medulla (i.e., the ventral (anterior) corticospinal tract).

above the anterior horn cell. Injury may be caused by trauma, a stroke, or tumors (these are discussed in Chapter 17). The injury causes upper motor neuron signs and symptoms that are summarized in Table 16.19.

Paresis (weakness) is partial paralysis with incomplete loss of muscle power. Paralysis is loss of motor function so that a muscle group is unable to overcome gravity. Different terms are used to describe the location of the paralysis (Box 16.6). Upper motor neuron paresis (weakness) or paralysis is also known as *spastic paresis/paralysis.* Upper motor neuron injury initially causes flaccid paralysis. However, within

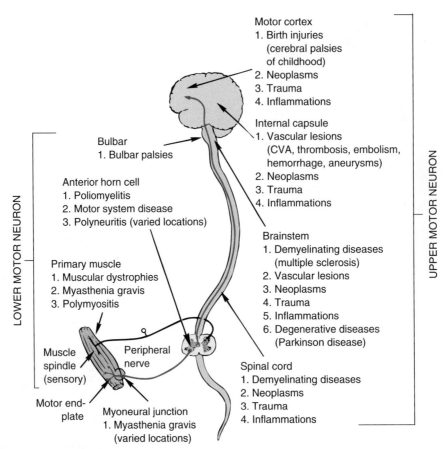

FIGURE 16.19 Motor Function Syndromes. Disturbances in motor function are classified pathologically along upper and lower motor neuron structures. It should be noted that the same pathologic condition occurs at more than one site in an upper motor neuron *(top right)*. A few pathologic conditions involve both upper and lower motor neuron structures, as in amyotrophic lateral sclerosis, for example. Other lesion sites include myoneural junction and primary muscle, making it possible to classify conditions as neuromuscular and muscular, respectively.

BOX 16.6 Location of Paresis/Paralysis

Hemiparesis/hemiplegia is paresis/paralysis of the upper and lower extremities on one side.

Diplegia is paralysis of corresponding parts of both sides of the body as a result of cerebral hemisphere injuries.

Paraparesis/paraplegia is weakness/paralysis of the lower extremities as a result of lower spinal cord injury.

Quadriparesis/quadriplegia is paresis/paralysis of all four extremities as a result of upper spinal cord injury.

---

a few weeks there is a gradual return of motor function that is overactive. Upper motor neuron paresis/paralysis involves a series of motor dysfunctions resulting from interruption of the pyramidal system. The clinical manifestations reflect muscle overactivity and include excessive, regularly occurring movements, such as clonus (rhythmic contractions) and spasms. They are the result of loss of descending inhibitory control. There is great variation, depending on the suddenness of onset and the age of the individual.

If the pyramidal system is interrupted above the level of the pons, the hand and arm muscles are greatly affected. Paralysis rarely involves all the muscles on one side of the body, even when the hemiplegia results from complete damage to the internal capsule. Bilateral movements, such as those of the eye, jaw, and larynx, as well as those of the trunk, are affected only slightly, if at all. Predominantly the limbs are affected.

Paralysis associated with an upper motor neuron syndrome rarely remains flaccid for a prolonged time. After a few days or weeks, a gradual return of spinal reflexes marks the end of spinal shock (see Chapter 17). Hypertonia and hyperreflexia occur particularly in antigravity muscles (e.g., the soleus muscles of the leg, the hamstrings of the leg, the gluteus maximus, the quadriceps femoris, and spinal erector muscles of the back).

Spasticity is common, although rigidity occasionally occurs. Most often, passive range-of-motion movements cause "clasp-knife" rigidity, probably by activating the stretch receptors in the muscle spindles and the Golgi tendon organ. (Muscle function is discussed in Chapter 40.) With pyramidal motor syndrome, the flexors of the arms and the extensors of the legs are predominantly affected.

Lower Motor Neuron Syndromes

Alpha motor neurons are the large motor neurons with their cell bodies in the anterior horn of the spinal cord and the motor nuclei of the brainstem. These lower motor neurons bring nerve impulses from upper motor neurons to skeletal muscles through the anterior spinal roots or cranial nerves and cause muscle contraction (Fig. 16.20). Damage to alpha motor neurons can occur in the anterior horn cell, nerve root,

TABLE 16.19 Upper and Lower Motor Neuron Syndromes Signs and Symptoms

Upper Motor Neuron (Pyramidal Cells—Motor Cortex)	Lower Motor Neuron (Cranial Nerve Nuclei—Brainstem; Ventral Horn—Spinal Cord)
Muscle groups are affected	Individual muscles may be affected
Mild weakness (paresis)	Mild weakness (paresis)
Spastic paralysis	Flaccid paralysis
Minimal disuse muscle atrophy	Marked muscle atrophy
No fasciculations	Fasciculations
Hyperreflexia, increased muscle stretch reflexes (clasp-knife spasticity; resistance to passive flexion that releases abruptly to allow easy flexion)	Hyporeflexia, decreased muscle stretch reflexes
Clonus may be present	Clonus not present
Hypertonia, spasticity	Hypotonia, flaccidity
Pathologic reflexes (Babinski and Hoffmann signs, loss of abdominal reflexes)	No Babinski sign
Often initial impairment of only skilled movements	Asymmetric and may involve one limb only in beginning to become generalized as disease progresses

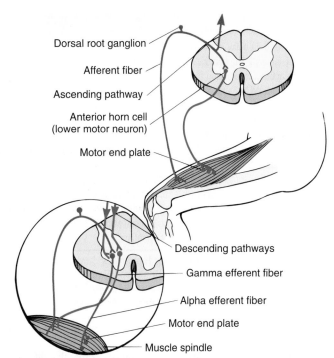

FIGURE 16.20 Structures Composing Lower Motor Neuron, Including Motor (Efferent) and Sensory (Afferent) Elements. *(Top)* Anterior horn cell (alpha motor neuron with cell body in anterior gray column of spinal cord), axon terminates in motor end plate as it innervates extrafusal muscle fibers in quadriceps muscle. *(Detailed enlargement)* Sensory and motor elements of gamma loop system. Gamma efferent fibers shown innervating the muscle spindle (sensory receptor of skeletal muscle). Contraction of muscle spindle fibers stretches the central portion of the spindle and causes the gamma afferent spindle fiber to transmit impulse centrally to the cord. Muscle spindle gamma afferent fibers in turn synapse on the anterior horn cell, and impulses are transmitted by way of alpha efferent fibers to skeletal (extrafusal) muscle, causing it to contract. Muscle spindle discharge is interrupted by active contraction of skeletal muscle fibers.

Labels in figure: Dorsal root ganglion; Afferent fiber; Ascending pathway; Anterior horn cell (lower motor neuron); Motor end plate; Descending pathways; Gamma efferent fiber; Alpha efferent fiber; Motor end plate; Muscle spindle

nerve plexus, or peripheral nerve. The damage causes **lower motor neuron syndromes** and impairs both voluntary and involuntary movement in the muscles innervated by the involved nerves (see Table 16.19 and Fig. 16.19). The degree of paralysis or paresis is proportional to the number of lower motor neurons affected. If only some of the motor units that supply a muscle are affected, only partial paralysis or paresis results. If all motor units are affected, complete paralysis results. Other clinical manifestations also are proportional to the degree of dysfunction, but the precise manifestations depend on the location of the dysfunction in the motor unit and in the CNS.

Small motor (gamma) neurons maintain muscle tone, protect the muscle from injury, and are needed for normal motor movement. Gamma neurons depend on input from the muscle spindle in skeletal muscle (see Fig. 16.20). Dysfunction in this motor system (the gamma loop) impairs tone and reduces tendon reflexes, causing hyporeflexia. The muscles become susceptible to damage from hyperextensibility. Generally, the large and small motor neuron systems are equally affected. Therefore the muscle has reduced tone or hypotonia and is accompanied by hyporeflexia or areflexia (loss of tendon reflexes) and **flaccid paresis/paralysis**.

Denervated muscles (i.e., muscles that have lost their nervous system input) atrophy over weeks to months, mostly from disuse, and demonstrate **fasciculations** (muscle rippling or quivering under the skin). Occasionally, denervated muscles cramp. **Fibrillation** is isolated contraction of a single muscle fiber because of metabolic changes in denervated muscle and is not clinically visible.

Motor Neuron Diseases

Motor neuron diseases result from progressive degeneration of upper or lower motor neurons in the spinal cord, brainstem, or cortex. The pathologic processes that give rise to motor neuron diseases can be sporadic or inherited. Sporadic inflammatory processes (virally induced, postinfectious, or postvaccination) may injure or destroy anterior horn

cells or cranial nerve cell bodies (e.g., polio, Guillain-Barré syndrome (see Chapter 17), or amyotrophic lateral sclerosis [see the next section]). Some inflammatory processes are mild and can be followed by rapid cellular recovery (e.g., facial nerve [Bell] palsy) (Box 16.7).

Damage to one or more of the cranial nerve nuclei is called *cranial nerve palsy*. It may be caused by vascular occlusion, tumor, aneurysm, tuberculosis, or hemorrhage. A group of rare degenerative disorders principally cause progressive lower motor neuron atrophy. **Spinal muscular atrophy (SMA)** is an inherited autosomal recessive degenerative disease of the anterior horn cells of the spinal cord. SMA causes weakness and atrophy of skeletal muscles. A **bulbar palsy** involves the cranial nerves in the motor nuclei of the medulla (cranial nerves IX [glossopharyngeal], X [vagus], XI [accessory], and XII [hypoglossal]). The term *bulb* was so named because the medulla was originally called the bulb. **Progressive bulbar palsy** involves degeneration of the glossopharyngeal, vagus, and hypoglossal cranial nerves. The clinical manifestations of bulbar palsies include paresis or paralysis of the jaw, face, pharynx, and tongue musculature. All these manifestations become progressively worse, leading to aspiration, malnutrition, possible dehydration, and an inability to communicate verbally.

Amyotrophic Lateral Sclerosis

Amyotrophic lateral sclerosis ([ALS], sporadic motor neuron disease, sporadic motor system disease, motor neuron disease [MND], Lou

---

BOX 16.7   Facial Nerve (Bell) Palsy

Facial nerve (Bell) palsy is an acute unilateral lower motor neuron paralysis of cranial nerve VII. The etiology remains unknown. There is usually an inflammatory reaction compressing the facial nerve, particularly in the narrowest segment, followed by demyelinating neural change. The most distressing signs are unilateral facial weakness and the inability to smile or whistle. Facial palsy may be caused by reactivation of herpesviruses in cranial nerve VII (facial), geniculate ganglia, or an autoimmune response. The signs usually have an acute onset (within 72 hours). Herpes simplex type 1 has been detected in up to 78% of cases and herpes zoster in 30% of cases. Severe pain with facial palsy and a vesicular rash in the ear or mouth suggest herpes zoster infection. Ramsay Hunt syndrome (herpes zoster oticus) is rare, but complete recovery is less than 50%. Recovery from facial palsy is usually complete. Both disorders may be treated with combination antivirals and oral steroids. Treatment should be individualized according to severity of symptoms.

Data from Baugh RF et al: *Otolaryngol Head Neck Surg* 149(3 Suppl):S1-S27, 2013; De Ru JA, Van Benthem PP: *Evid Based Med* 19(1):15, 2014; Eviston TJ et al: *J Neurol Neurosurg Psychiatry* 86(12):1356-1361, 2015; Glass GE, Tzafetta K: *Fam Pract* 31(6):631-642, 2014.

Gehrig disease) is a worldwide neurodegenerative disorder that diffusely involves lower and upper motor neurons, resulting in progressive muscle weakness. *Amyotrophic* (without muscle nutrition or progressive muscle wasting) refers to the predominant lower motor neuron component of the syndrome. *Lateral sclerosis,* scarring of the pyramidal (corticospinal) tract in the lateral column of the spinal cord, refers to the upper motor neuron component of the syndrome.

ALS may begin at any time from the fourth decade of life; its peak occurrence is between 60 and 69 years, with about 1 to 2.6 cases per 100,000 population in the United States. The prevalence is higher in males.[37] Most cases of ALS are sporadic. A subset (about 5% to 10%) of persons has a familial form with genetic mutations that contribute to the neurotoxicity affecting motor neurons. Gene and environmental interactions are being evaluated as a cause of ALS.[38] ALS is fatal from respiratory failure, usually within 3 years of diagnosis. A small percentage of individuals live 5 to 10 years or longer.

PATHOPHYSIOLOGY   The cause of ALS is unknown. The principal pathologic feature of ALS is degeneration of lower and upper motor neurons. There is a decrease in large motor neurons in the spinal cord, brainstem, and cerebral cortex (premotor and motor areas), with ongoing degeneration in the remaining motor neurons. Death of the motor neuron results in axonal degeneration and secondary demyelination with glial proliferation and sclerosis (scarring). Widespread neural degeneration of nonmotor neurons in the spinal cord and motor cortices, as well as in the premotor, sensory, and temporal cortices, has been found, including areas that involve cognition.

Lower motor neuron degeneration denervates motor units. Adjacent, still viable lower motor neurons attempt to compensate by distal intramuscular sprouting, reinnervation, and enlargement of motor units.

CLINICAL MANIFESTATIONS   The initial symptoms of the disease are heterogeneous and may be related to lower or upper motor neuron dysfunction or both. About 60% of individuals have a spinal form of the disease, with focal muscle weakness beginning in the arms and legs and progressing to muscle atrophy, spasticity, and loss of manual dexterity and gait. No associated mental, sensory, or autonomic symptoms are present. ALS with progressive bulbar palsy presents with difficulty speaking and swallowing. Peripheral muscle weakness and atrophy

usually occur within 1 to 2 years, including the muscles of ventilation. These individuals have an improved response to treatment with noninvasive ventilation.[39]

The lower motor neuron syndrome consists of weakness of individual muscles, progressing to flaccid paralysis, associated with hypotonia, and primary muscle atrophy (i.e., atrophy caused by denervation). Frontotemporal dementia may occur concurrently.[40]

EVALUATION AND TREATMENT   Diagnosis of the syndrome is based predominantly on the history and physical examination with no evidence of other neuromuscular disorders. Genetic testing is available. Electromyography and muscle biopsy results verify lower motor neuron degeneration and denervation. Imaging studies and CSF biomarkers can assist in making the diagnosis. There is no curative treatment. Riluzole (Rilutek), an antiglutamate and edaravone (Radicava) a free-radical scavenger, are the only drugs approved by the U.S. Food and Drug Administration for treatment of ALS, and they prolong life for months. Supportive and rehabilitative management are directed toward preventing complications of malnutrition and immobility. Psychologic support of the affected individual and the family is extremely important.

ALTERATIONS IN COMPLEX MOTOR PERFORMANCE

The alterations in complex motor performance include disorders of posture (stance), disorders of gait, and disorders of expression.

Disorders of Posture (Stance)

An inequality of tone in muscle groups, because of a loss of normal postural reflexes, results in a posturing of limbs. Equilibrium and balance are disrupted. Many reflex systems govern tone and posture, but the most important factor in posture control is the stretch reflex, in which extensor (antigravity) muscle stretching causes increased extensor tone and inhibited flexor tone. Four types of disorders of posture are (1) dystonic posture, (2) decorticate posture, (3) decerebrate posture/response, and (4) basal ganglion posture.

Dystonia is the maintenance of an abnormal posture through muscular contractions. When muscular contractions are sustained for several seconds, they are called dystonic movements. When contractions last for longer periods, they are called dystonic postures. Dystonic postures may last for weeks, causing permanent, fixed contractures. Dystonia has been associated with basal ganglia abnormality, but the exact pathophysiologic mechanisms are unknown. One dystonic posture is decorticate posture/response (striatal posture or upper motor neuron dysfunction posture), which may be unilateral or bilateral.

Decorticate posture/response (also referred to as antigravity posture or hemiplegic posture) is characterized by upper extremities flexed at the elbows and held close to the body and by lower extremities that are externally rotated and extended (see Fig. 16.6). Decorticate posture/response is thought to occur when the brainstem is not inhibited by the cerebral cortex motor area. Upper motor neuron posture is more commonly described as the arm flexed at the elbow with a wrist drop, the leg inadequately bent at the knee, the hip excessively circumabducted, and the presence of footdrop.

Decerebrate posture/response refers to increased tone in extensor muscles and trunk muscles, with active tonic neck reflexes. When the head is in a neutral position, all four limbs are rigidly extended (see Fig. 16.6). The decerebrate posture is caused by severe injury to the brain and brainstem, resulting in overstimulation of the postural righting and vestibular reflexes.

Basal ganglion posture refers to a stooped, hyperflexed posture with a narrow-based, short-stepped gait. Basal ganglion dysfunction accounts for this posture. This posture abnormality results from the loss of normal postural reflexes and not from defects in proprioceptive, labyrinthine, or visual function. Dysfunctional equilibrium results when the individual loses stability and cannot make the appropriate postural adjustment to tilting or loss of balance, falling instead. Dysfunctional righting is the inability to right oneself when changing from a lying or crouching to a standing position or when rolling from the supine to the lateral or prone position. Dysfunctional postural fixation is the involuntary flexion of the head and neck, causing the person difficulty in maintaining an upright trunk position while standing or walking.

Disorders of Gait

Four predominant types of gait associated with neurologic disorders are (1) upper motor neuron dysfunction gait (spastic gait), (2) cerebellar (ataxic) gait, (3) basal ganglion gait, and (4) frontal lobe ataxic gait. As with posture, equilibrium and balance are affected with gait disturbances.[41]

Several upper motor neuron gaits exist. Injury to the pyramidal (cortospinal) system with loss of accompanying inhibitory control accounts for these gaits (e.g., stroke, cerebral palsy, multiple sclerosis, spinal cord tumor). With mild forms, the individual may have footdrop with fatigue and hip and leg pain. A spastic gait, which is associated with unilateral injury, manifests by a shuffling gait with the leg extended and held stiff, causing a scraping over the floor surface. The leg swings improperly around the body rather than being appropriately lifted and placed. The foot may drag on the ground, and the person tends to fall to the affected side. A scissors gait is associated with bilateral injury and spasticity. The legs are adducted so they touch each other. As the person walks, the legs are swung around the body but then cross in front of each other because of adduction.

A cerebellar (ataxic) gait is wide-based with the feet apart and often turned outward or inward for greater stability. The pelvis is held stiff, and the individual staggers when walking. Cerebellar dysfunction with loss of coordination accounts for this particular gait.

A basal ganglion gait is a broad-based gait in which the person walks with small steps and a decreased arm swing. The head and body are flexed and the arms semiflexed and abducted, whereas the legs are flexed and rigid in more advanced states. The basal ganglia modulate and coordinate motor function; dysfunction accounts for this gait. It is associated with Parkinson disease.

A frontal lobe ataxic gait is associated with start hesitation, gait ignition failure, a wide-based gait, body sway and falls, loss of control of truncal motion, shuffling, and freezing. The gait is associated with bilateral frontal lobe damage or degeneration. Power and coordination of the legs is normal when tested in the seated or lying position. The pattern may change as the frontal disease progresses. The slowness of walking, lack of heel-shin or upper limb ataxia, dysarthria, or nystagmus distinguishes the wide stance from cerebellar gait ataxia.[42]

Gait disorders are often accompanied by balance, coordination, and sensory dysfunction that further alter mobility and increase risk for falls. Assessment and intervention strategies are important for prevention of injury.

Disorders of Expression

Disorders of expression involve the motor aspects of communication and include (1) hypermimesis, (2) hypomimesis, and (3) apraxia/dyspraxia. Hypermimesis commonly manifests as pathologic laughter or crying. Pathologic laughter is associated with right hemisphere injury, and pathologic crying is associated with left hemisphere injury. The exact pathophysiology is not known. Hypomimesis manifests as aprosody—the loss of emotional language. Receptive aprosody involves an inability to understand emotion in speech and facial expression. Expressive aprosody involves the inability to express emotion in speech and facial expression. Aprosody is associated with right hemisphere damage.

Apraxia/dyspraxia is a disorder of learned skilled movements with difficulty planning and executing coordinated motor movements. The term is often used interchangeably with dyspraxia. It can be developmental, beginning at birth (developmental apraxia), or associated with vascular disorders (common in stroke), trauma, tumors, degenerative disorders, infections, or metabolic disorders. People with apraxia have difficulty performing tasks requiring motor skills, including speaking, writing, using tools or utensils, playing sports, following instructions, and focusing.[43]

True apraxias occur when the connecting pathways between the left and right cortical areas are interrupted. Apraxias may result from any pathologic process that disrupts the cortical areas necessary for the conceptualization and execution of a complex motor act or the communication pathways within the left hemisphere or between the hemispheres.[43,44]

EXTRAPYRAMIDAL MOTOR SYNDROMES

Because the extrapyramidal system encompasses all the motor pathways except the pyramidal system, two types of motor dysfunction make up the extrapyramidal motor syndromes: (1) the basal ganglia motor syndromes and (2) the cerebellar motor syndromes. Unlike pyramidal motor syndromes, both extrapyramidal motor syndromes result in movement or posture disturbance without significant paralysis, along with other distinctive symptoms (Table 16.20).

Basal ganglia motor syndromes are caused by an imbalance of dopaminergic and cholinergic activity in the corpus striatum. A relative excess of cholinergic activity produces hypokinesia (decreased movement) and hypertonia. A relative excess of dopaminergic activity produces hyperkinesia and hypotonia. Symptoms associated with Parkinson and

TABLE 16.20 Pyramidal Versus Extrapyramidal Motor Syndrome

Manifestations	Pyramidal Motor Syndrome	Extrapyramidal Motor Syndrome
Unilateral movement	Paralysis of voluntary movement	Little or no paralysis of voluntary movement
Tendon reflexes	Increased tendon reflexes	Normal or slightly increased tendon reflexes
Babinski sign	Present	Absent
Involuntary movements	Absence of involuntary movements	Presence of tremor, chorea, athetosis, or dystonia
Muscle tone	Spasticity in muscles (e.g., clasp-knife phenomenon) Hypertonia present in flexors of arms and extensors of legs	Plastic rigidity (equal throughout movement) or intermittent—cogwheel rigidity (generalized but predominantly in flexors of limbs and trunk) Hypotonia, weakness and gait disturbances in cerebellar disease

Huntington diseases are exemplary of disorders of the basal ganglia. Cerebellar motor syndromes are associated with ataxia and other symptoms affecting coordinated movement and balance. Cerebellar disorders primarily influence the same side of the body, so that damage to the right cerebellum generally causes symptoms on the right side of the body.

✓ QUICK CHECK 16.6

1. What are three symptoms of upper motor neuron disease?
2. What are three symptoms of lower motor neuron disease?
3. How does decerebrate posture differ from decorticate posture?
4. What motor symptoms would be characteristic of extrapyramidal diseases?

SUMMARY REVIEW

Alterations in Cognitive Systems

1. The neural systems essential to cognitive function are: (1) attentional systems that provide arousal and maintenance of attention over time; (2) memory and language systems by which information is remembered and communicated; and (3) affective or emotive systems that mediate mood, emotion, and intention.

2. Consciousness is a state of awareness of oneself and the environment, and a set of responses to that environment.

3. Consciousness has two components: arousal (state of awakeness or alertness) and awareness (content of thought).

4. An altered level of arousal occurs by pathologies that alter localized or diffuse brain structure and metabolic disorders that alter delivery of energy substrates. The five patterns of neurologic function critical to the evaluation of consciousness are level of consciousness, pattern of breathing, pupillary reaction, oculomotor responses, and motor responses.

5. Level of consciousness is the most critical index of nervous system function. From a normal alert state, consciousness can diminish in stages through confusion, disorientation, lethargy, obtundation, stupor, and coma.

6. Breathing pattern, rate, and rhythm help evaluate brain dysfunction and coma.

7. Pupillary changes reflect changes in level of brainstem function, drug action, and response to hypoxia and ischemia.

8. Oculomotor responses are resting, spontaneous, and reflexive eye movements and reflect alterations in brainstem function.

9. Level of brain function manifests by changes in generalized motor responses or no responses. The most severely damaged side of the brain can be determined by assessing motor response.

10. Loss of cortical inhibition associated with decreased consciousness produces abnormal flexor and extensor movements.

11. Brain death results from irreversible brain damage, with an inability to maintain internal homeostasis.

12. Cerebral death or irreversible coma represents permanent brain damage, with an ability to maintain cardiac, respiratory, and other vital functions.

13. A persistent vegetative state is complete unawareness of the self or surrounding environment and complete loss of cognitive function. Brainstem reflexes (pupillary, oculocephalic, chewing, swallowing) are intact but cerebral function is lost.

14. Locked-in syndrome is complete paralysis of voluntary muscles, with the exception of eye movement, with retention of consciousness.

15. Alterations in awareness include alterations in executive attention (abstract reasoning, planning, decision making, judgment, error correction, and self-control) and memory.

16. With a deficit in selective attention, mediated by midbrain, thalamus, and parietal lobe structures, the individual cannot focus on selective stimuli and thus neglects those stimuli.

17. In amnesia, some past memories are lost (retrograde amnesia) and new memories cannot be stored (anterograde amnesia). Global amnesia is a combination of anterograde and retrograde amnesia.

18. Frontal areas mediate vigilance, detection, and working (short-term) memory.

19. With vigilance deficits, the person cannot maintain sustained concentration.

20. With detection deficits, the person is unmotivated and unable to set goals and plan.

21. Data-processing deficits are problems associated with recognizing and processing sensory information, and include agnosias, dysphasias, acute confusional states, and dementias.

22. Agnosias are defects of pattern recognition and may be tactile, visual, or auditory.

23. Aphasia (dysphasia) is an impairment of comprehension or production of language. Aphasia may be expressive or receptive.

24. Acute confusional states are characterized chiefly by transient disorders of awareness.

25. Delirium can be hyperactive (excited delirium syndrome) with intense autonomic nervous system activation, or hypoactive with frontal basal ganglia disruption.

26. Dementia is a slowly progressive deterioration in cerebral function with loss of intellectual processes and memory.

27. Alzheimer disease is a chronic irreversible dementia that is related to altered production or failure to clear amyloid from the brain with plaque formation and formation of neurofibrillary tangles.

28. Vascular dementia is a consequence of cerebrovascular disease, and treatment is directed at preventing the risk factors of diabetes, hypercholesterolaemia, hypertension, and smoking.

29. Frontotemporal dementias are rare early-onset degenerative diseases similar to Alzheimer disease.

30. Seizures represent a sudden, chaotic discharge of cerebral neurons with transient alterations in brain function. Seizures may be generalized or focal and can result from metabolic disorders, congenital malformations, genetic predisposition, perinatal injury, postnatal trauma, myoclonic syndromes, infection, brain tumor, vascular disease, and drug or alcohol abuse.

Alterations in Cerebral Hemodynamics

1. Alterations in cerebral blood flow are related to inadequate cerebral perfusion, normal cerebral perfusion but with an elevated intracranial pressure, and excessive cerebral blood volume.

2. Increased intracranial pressure (IICP) may result from edema, excess cerebrospinal fluid, hemorrhage, or tumor growth. When intracranial pressure approaches arterial pressure, hypoxia and hypercapnia produce brain damage.

3. The herniation process rapidly increases ICP. Types of supratentorial herniation include (1) uncal (uncus and/or hippocampal gyrus shift from the middle fossa through the tentorial notch into the posterior fossa), (2) central (downward shift of the diencephalon through the tentorial notch), (3) cingulate gyrus (cingulate gyrus shifts under the falx cerebri), and (4) transcalvarial (brain shifts through a skull fracture or a surgical opening in the skull).

4. The most common infratentorial herniation is a shift of the cerebellar tonsils through the foramen magnum.

5. Cerebral edema is an increase in the fluid content of the brain resulting from trauma, infection, hemorrhage, tumor growth, ischemia, infarction, or hypoxia. The three types of cerebral edema are vasogenic, cytotoxic, and interstitial.

6. Hydrocephalus comprises a variety of disorders characterized by an excess of fluid within the ventricles, subarachnoid space, or both. Hydrocephalus occurs because of interference with cerebrospinal fluid flow caused by increased fluid production, obstruction within the ventricular system, or defective reabsorption of the fluid.

Alterations in Neuromotor Function

1. General neuromotor dysfunctions are associated with changes in muscle tone, movement, and complex motor performance.

2. Normal muscle tone involves a slight resistance that is smooth, constant, and even to passive movement. Hypotonia and hypertonia are the main categories of altered tone.

3. Hypotonia is decreased muscle tone. It is associated with pyramidal tract or cerebellar injury. Muscles are flaccid and weak with atrophy.

4. Hypertonia is increased muscle tone. The four types of hypertonia are spasticity, paratonia, dystonia, and rigidity.

5. Alterations in muscle movements occur when CNS dysfunction alters muscle innervation. Movement disorders are not necessarily associated with muscle mass, strength, or tone but are neurologic dysfunctions that result in insufficient or excessive movement or involuntary movement. Movement disorders can be idiopathic or associated with specific diseases of the central nervous system, such as Parkinson disease and Huntington disease.

6. Hyperkinesia is excessive purposeless movement, including chorea, athetosis, ballism, akathisia, tremor, and myoclonus. Paroxysmal dyskinesias are rare abnormal, episodic, involuntary movements that occur as spasms.

7. Huntington disease is a rare, hereditary movement disorder involving severe degeneration of the basal ganglia and cerebral cortex that commonly manifests between 25 and 45 years of age. An excess of dopaminergic activity causes involuntary hyperkinetic movements, such as chorea (jerky, abnormal movement), athetosis (slow, sinuous, irregular movements), and ballism (violent flailing movement of the limbs).

8. Hypokinesia is loss of voluntary movement despite preserved consciousness and normal peripheral nerve and muscle function. Akinesia is a decrease in voluntary movements; bradykinesia is a slowness of voluntary movements.

9. Parkinson disease is a degenerative disorder of the basal ganglia with loss of dopamine-secreting neurons. Dopamine depletion and excess cholinergic activity cause tremor, rigidity, and akinesia.

Progressive dementia may be associated with an advanced stage of the Parkinson disease.

10. Upper motor neuron syndromes are the result of injury to motor pathways that descend from the motor cortex. Injury may occur in the cerebral cortex, the subcortical white matter, the internal capsule, the brainstem, or the spinal cord. Upper motor neuron syndromes are characterized by paresis (partial paralysis), paralysis, hypertonia, and hyperreflexia.

11. Lower motor neuron syndromes involve damage to the alpha motor neurons—the large motor neurons in the anterior horn of the spinal cord and the motor nuclei of the brainstem. Lower motor neuron syndromes manifest by impaired voluntary and involuntary movements and flaccid paresis or paralysis.

12. Motor neuron diseases result from progressive degeneration of upper or lower motor neurons in the spinal cord, brainstem, or cortex (e.g., polio, Gullian-Barré syndrome, or amyotrophic lateral sclerosis).

13. Amyotrophic lateral sclerosis involves degeneration of both upper and lower motor neurons with progressive muscle weakness and atrophy. No associated mental, sensory, or autonomic symptoms are present.

Alterations in Complex Motor Performance

1. Alterations in complex motor performance include disorders of posture (stance), disorders of gait, and disorders of expression.

2. Inequality of tone in muscle groups results in abnormal posturing of the limbs. Disorders of posture include dystonic posture, decerebrate posture/response, basal ganglion posture, and senile posture.

3. Disorders of gait associated with neurologic disorders include upper motor neuron dysfunction gait (spastic gait), cerebellar (ataxic) gait, basal ganglion gait, and frontal lobe ataxic gait.

4. Disorders of expression include hypermimesis (pathologic laughter or crying), hypomimesis (loss of emotional language/communication), and apraxia/dyspraxia. Apraxia is an impairment of the conceptualization or execution of a complex motor act.

Extrapyramidal Motor Syndromes

1. Extrapyramidal motor syndromes include basal ganglia and cerebellar motor syndromes.

2. Basal ganglia disorders are caused by an imbalance of dopaminergic and cholinergic activity. A relative excess of cholinergic activity produces hypokinesia and hypertonia; a relative excess of dopaminergic activity produces hyperkinesia and hypotonia.

3. Cerebellar motor syndromes are associated with ataxia and other symptoms affecting coordinated movement and balance, usually on the same side of the body as the side of the cerebellar lesion.

KEY TERMS

Acute confusional state (ACS), 360
Acute hydrocephalus, 370
Agnosia, 359
Akinesia, 374
Alzheimer disease (AD) (dementia of Alzheimer type [DAT], senile disease complex), 362
Amnesia, 357
Amyotrophic lateral sclerosis ([ALS] sporadic motor

neuron disease, sporadic motor system disease, motor neuron disease [MND], Lou Gehrig disease), 377
Anterograde amnesia, 357
Aphasia, 359
Apraxia/dyspraxia, 379
Arousal, 351
Aura, 367
Autoregulation, 368
Awareness (content of thought), 357

Basal ganglia motor syndrome, 379
Basal ganglion gait, 379
Basal ganglion posture, 378
Bradykinesia, 374
Brain death (total brain death), 355
Bulbar palsy, 377
Cerebellar (ataxic) gait, 379
Cerebellar motor syndrome, 380
Cerebral death (irreversible coma), 355

Cerebral edema, 369
Cerebral perfusion pressure (CPP), 367
Clonic phase, 367
Communicating hydrocephalus, 370
Congenital hydrocephalus, 370
Consciousness, 351
Convulsion, 365
Cytotoxic edema, 369
Decerebrate posture/response, 378

REFERENCES

1. Wijdicks EF, et al: Evidence-based guideline update: determining brain death in adults: report of the Quality Standards Subcommittee of the American Academy of Neurology, *Neurology* 74(23):1911-1918, 2010.
2. Nakagawa TA, et al: Guidelines for the determination of brain death in infants and children: an update of the 1987 task force recommendations, *Crit Care Med* 39(9):2139-2155, 2011.
3. Hodelín-Tablada R: Minimally conscious state: evolution of concept, diagnosis and treatment, *MEDICC Rev* 18(4):43-46, 2016.
4. Golubović V, et al: Two different manifestations of locked-in syndrome, *Coll Antropol* 37(1):313-316, 2013.
5. Carrasco M: Visual attention: the past 25 years, *Vision Res* 51(13):1484-1525, 2011.
6. Zaal IJ, Slooter AJ: Delirium in critically ill patients: epidemiology, pathophysiology, diagnosis and management, *Drugs* 72(11):1457-1471, 2012.
7. Marcantonio ER: Delirium in hospitalized older adults, *N Engl J Med* 377(15):1456-1466, 2017.
8. Gaudreau JD, et al: Fast, systematic, and continuous delirium assessment in hospitalized patients: the nursing delirium screening scale, *J Pain Symptom Manage* 29(4):368-375, 2005.
9. Confusion Assessment Method. Available at https://www.mnhospitals.org/Portals/0/Documents/ptsafety/LEAPT%20Delirium/Confusion%20Assessment%20Method%20-%20CAM.pdf. (Accessed 5 July 2019).
10. Ghaeli P, et al: Preventive intervention to prevent delirium in patients hospitalized in intensive care unit, *Iran J Psychiatry* 13(2):142-147, 2018.
11. Alzheimer's Association: Alzheimers disease facts and figures, 2019. Available at: https://www.alz.org/media/Documents/alzheimers-facts-and-figures-2019-r.pdf.
12. Loy CT, et al: Genetics of dementia, *Lancet* 383(9919):828-840, 2014.

13. Qazi TJ, et al: Epigenetics in Alzheimer's disease: perspective of DNA methylation, *Mol Neurobiol* 55(2):1026-1044, 2018.
14. Cummings JL, et al: International Work Group criteria for the diagnosis of Alzheimer disease, *Med Clin North Am* 97(3):363-368, 2013.
15. Aisen PS, et al: On the path to 2025: understanding the Alzheimer's disease continuum, *Alzheimers Res Ther* 9(1):60, 2017.
16. Epperly T, Dunay MA, Boice JL: Alzheimer disease: pharmacologic and nonpharmacologic therapies for cognitive and functional symptoms, *Am Fam Physician* 95(12):771-778, 2017.
17. Tariq S, Barber PA: Dementia risk and prevention by targeting modifiable vascular risk factors, *J Neurochem* 144(5):565-581, 2018.
18. Olney NT, Spina S, Miller BL: Frontotemporal dementia, *Neurol Clin* 35(2):339-374, 2017.
19. Fisher RS, et al: Operational classification of seizure types by the International League Against Epilepsy: Position Paper of the ILAE Commission for Classification and Terminology, *Epilepsia* 58(4):522-530, 2017. Available at https://www.ilae.org/news-and-media/news-about-ilae/new-ilae-seizure-classification.
20. Stafstrom CE, Carmant L: Seizures and epilepsy: an overview for neuroscientists, *Cold Spring Harb Perspect Med* 5(6):2015.
21. Nei M, et al: Ketogenic diet in adolescents and adults with epilepsy, *Seizure* 23(6):439-442, 2014.
22. Michinaga S, Koyama Y: Pathogenesis of brain edema and investigation into anti-edema drugs, *Int J Mol Sci* 16(5):9949-9975, 2015.
23. Williams MA, Malm J: Diagnosis and treatment of idiopathic normal pressure hydrocephalus, *Continuum (Minneap Minn)* 22(2 Dementia):579-599, 2016.
24. Agostinho LA, et al: A systematic review of the intergenerational aspects and the diverse genetic profiles of Huntington's disease, *Genet Mol Res* 12(2):1974-1981, 2013.
25. Labbadia J, Morimoto RI: Huntington's disease: underlying molecular mechanisms and emerging

concepts, *Trends Biochem Sci* 38(8):378-385, 2013.
26. Ross CA, Tabrizi SJ: Huntington's disease: from molecular pathogenesis to clinical treatment, *Lancet Neurol* 10(1):83-98, 2011.
27. National Institutes of Health and Human Services (DHHS), Genetic and Rare Diseases Information Center: Huntington disease. Available at: https://rarediseases.info.nih.gov/diseases/6677/huntington-disease. (Accessed 13 November 2018).
28. Pagan F, Torres-Yaghi Y, Altshuler M: The diagnosis and natural history of Huntington disease, *Handb Clin Neurol* 144:63-67, 2017.
29. Parkinson Disease Foundation, 2018. Available at: http://www.parkinson.org/Understanding-Parkinsons/Causes-and-Statistics/Statistics.
30. Gaig C, Tolosa E: When does Parkinson's disease begin?, *Mov Disord* 24(Suppl 2):S656-S664, 2009.
31. Gomperts SN: Lewy body dementias: dementia with lewy bodies and Parkinson disease dementia, *Continuum (Minneap Minn)* 22(2 Dementia):435-463, 2016.
32. Schaeffer E, Berg D: Dopaminergic therapies for non-motor symptoms in Parkinson's disease, *CNS Drugs* 31(7):551-570, 2017.
33. Barber TR, et al: Neuroimaging in pre-motor Parkinson's disease, *Neuroimage Clin* 15:215-227, 2017.
34. Miller DB, O'Callaghan JP: Biomarkers of Parkinson's disease: present and future, *Metabolism* 64(3 Suppl 1):S40-S46, 2015.
35. Elkouzi A, et al: Emerging therapies in Parkinson disease—repurposed drugs and new approaches, *Nat Rev Neurol* 15(4):204-223, 2019.
36. Parmar M: Towards stem cell based therapies for Parkinson's disease, *Development* 145(1):2018.
37. Talbott EO, Malek AM, Lacomis D: The epidemiology of amyotrophic lateral sclerosis, *Handb Clin Neurol* 138:225-238, 2016.

38. Martin S, Al Khleifat A, Al-Chalabi A: What causes amyotrophic lateral sclerosis?, *F1000Res* 6:371, 2017.
39. Khamankar N, et al: Associative increases in amyotrophic lateral sclerosis survival duration with non-invasive ventilation initiation and usage protocols, *Front Neurol* 9:578, 2018.
40. Wen X, et al: Pathogenic determinants and mechanisms of ALS/FTD linked to hexanucleotide repeat expansions in the C9orf72 gene, *Neurosci Lett* 636:16-26, 2017.
41. Vachranukunkiet T, Esquenazi A: Pathophysiology of gait disturbance in neurologic disorders and clinical presentations, *Phys Med Rehabil Clin N Am* 24(2):233-246, 2013.
42. Thompson PD: Frontal lobe ataxia, *Handb Clin Neurol* 103:619-622, 2012.
43. Foundas AL: Apraxia: neural mechanisms and functional recovery, *Handb Clin Neurol* 110:335-345, 2013.
44. Zadikoff C, Lang AE: Apraxia in movement disorders, *Brain* 128(Pt 7):1480-1497, 2005.

Disorders of the Central and Peripheral Nervous Systems and Neuromuscular Junction

Barbara J. Boss, Sue E. Huether

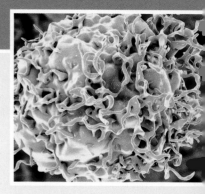

EVOLVE WEBSITE

CHAPTER OUTLINE

Alterations in central nervous system (CNS) function are caused by traumatic injury, vascular disorders, tumor growth, infectious and inflammatory processes, and metabolic derangements, including nutritional deficiencies and drugs or chemicals. Alterations in peripheral nervous system function involve the nerve roots, a nerve plexus, the peripheral nerves, or the neuromuscular junction.

CENTRAL NERVOUS SYSTEM DISORDERS

Traumatic Brain and Spinal Cord Injury

Traumatic Brain Injury

Traumatic brain injury (TBI) is an alteration in brain function or other evidence of brain pathology caused by an external force. The most common causes are falls for children and older adults followed by unintentional blunt trauma and motor vehicle accidents. Males have the highest incidence in every age group. The incidence of TBI is highest among American Indian/Alaska Natives and African Americans and in lower- and median-income families.[1] In recent years, individuals with TBI have shown improved survival. Advancements have been made in enhanced safety measures (e.g., passive seat restraints, air bags, protective head gear), reduced transport time to hospitals or trauma centers, improved on-scene medical management, imaging of brain injury, prevention and management of secondary brain injury, and a better understanding of all degrees of brain injury severity.

TBI can be classified as primary or secondary. Primary brain injury is caused by a direct impact. The injury can be a focal brain injury, affecting only one area of the brain, or a diffuse brain injury (diffuse axonal injury [DAI]), which involves more than one area of the brain.

Both types of injury can be associated with the same initiating event. Focal brain injury and DAI each account for about half of all injuries. Focal brain injury accounts for more than two-thirds of head injury deaths. More severely disabled survivors, including those surviving in an unresponsive state or reduced level of consciousness, have DAI. Secondary injury is an indirect consequence of the primary injury. It includes systemic and brain tissue responses with a cascade of cellular and molecular cerebral events (Table 17.1). TBI can be mild, moderate, or severe. The Glasgow Coma Scale (GCS) is used to grade severity of injury (Table 17.2). Most TBIs are mild. The hallmark of a severe TBI is loss of consciousness for 6 hours or more.[2]

Primary brain injury

Focal brain injury. Focal brain injury can be caused by closed (blunt) trauma or open (penetrating) trauma. Closed injury is more common and involves either the head striking a hard surface (e.g., motor vehicle accidents or falls), a rapidly moving object striking the head (e.g., a baseball or falling objects), or by blast waves. The dura remains intact, and brain tissues are not exposed to the environment. Focal brain injuries include contusions, subdural hematomas, epidural hematomas, and intracerebral hemorrhage. Blunt trauma may result in both focal brain injuries and DAIs, and they can occur at the same time (see Table 17.1). Open injury occurs with penetrating trauma or skull fracture. A break in the dura results in exposure of the cranial contents to the environment.

Closed brain injuries are specific, grossly observable brain lesions that occur in a precise location; most blunt trauma injuries are mild. Injury to the cranial vault, vessels, and supporting structures can produce more severe damage, including contusions and epidural, subdural, and

TABLE 17.1   Classification of Brain Injuries

Type of Injury	Mechanism
Primary Brain Injury	
Focal Brain Injury	Localized injury from impact
Closed injury	Blunt trauma
Coup	Injury is directly below site of forceful impact
Contrecoup	Injury is on opposite side of brain from site of forceful impact
Epidural (extradural) hematoma	Vehicular accidents, minor falls, sporting accidents
Subdural hematoma	Forceful impact: vehicular accidents or falls, especially in elderly persons or persons with chronic alcohol abuse
Subarachnoid hemorrhage	Bleeding caused by forceful impact, usually vehicular accidents or long distance falls
Open injury	Penetrating trauma: missiles (bullets) or sharp projectiles (knives, ice picks, axes, screwdrivers)
Compound fracture	Objects strike head with great force or head strikes object forcefully; temporal blows, occipital blows, upward impact of cervical vertebrae (basilar skull fracture)
Diffuse Axonal Injury (can occur with focal injury)	Traumatic shearing forces; tearing of axons from twisting and rotational forces with injury over widespread brain areas; moving head strikes hard, unyielding surface or moving object strikes stationary head; torsional head motion without impact
Secondary Brain Injury	
Systemic processes	Hypotension, hypoxia, anemia, hypercapnia, and hypocapnia
Intracerebral processes	Inflammation, cerebral edema, increased intracranial pressure (IICP), brain herniation, decreased cerebral perfusion pressure, ischemia
Cellular processes	Release of excitatory neurotransmitters (glutamate); failure of cell ion pumps, mitochondrial failure; disruption of blood brain barrier

TABLE 17.2   Glasgow Coma Scale (GCS)*

Score[†]	Best Eye Response Score (4)	Best Verbal Response Score (5)	Best Motor Response Score (6)
1	No eye opening	No verbal response	No motor response
2	Eye opening to pain	Incomprehensible sounds	Extension to pain
3	Eye opening to verbal command	Inappropriate words	Flexion to pain
4	Eyes open spontaneously	Confused	Withdrawal from pain
5	NA	Oriented	Localizing pain
6	NA	NA	Obeys commands

*The GCS is scored between 3 and 15, with 3 being the worst and 15 the best. It is composed of the sum of three parameters: Best Eye Response (E), Best Verbal Response (V), and Best Motor Response (M). Mild Brain Injury = 13 or higher; Moderate Brain Injury = 9 to 12; Severe Brain Injury = 8 or lower.
[†]It is important to break the scoring report into its components, for example, E3V3M5 = GCS 11. A total score is meaningless without this information. Age affects the GCS. Elderly individuals with a traumatic brain injury (TBI) have higher (better) GCS scores than younger individuals with a TBI of similar anatomic severity.
Data from Teasdale G, Jennett B: *Lancet* 2:81-84, 1974; Salottolo K et al: *J Am Med Assoc Surg* 149(7):727-734, 2014.

because of the concentration of force. Brain edema forms around and in damaged neural tissues, contributing to increasing intracranial pressure (see Chapter 16). Multiple hemorrhages, edema, infarction, and necrosis can occur within the contused areas. The tissue has a pulpy quality. The maximal effects of these injuries peak 18 to 36 hours after severe head injury.

Contusions occur most commonly in the frontal lobes, the temporal lobes, and at the frontotemporal junction. Injuries in these areas cause changes in attention, memory, intellectual function, affect, emotion, and behavior. Less commonly, contusions occur in the parietal and occipital lobes. Focal cerebral contusions are usually superficial, involving just the brain gyri. Hemorrhagic contusions may coalesce into a large confluent intracranial hematoma.

A contusion may be evidenced by immediate loss of consciousness (generally accepted to last no longer than 5 minutes), loss of reflexes (individual falls to the ground), transient cessation of respiration, brief period of bradycardia, and decrease in blood pressure (lasting 30 seconds to a few minutes). Vital signs may stabilize to normal values in a few seconds; reflexes then return, and the person regains consciousness over minutes to days. With more severe injury, residual deficits may persist, and some persons never regain a full level of consciousness.

Evaluation is based on the results of the health history, level of consciousness according to the GCS (see Table 17.2), outcomes of imaging studies, and assessment of vital parameters (e.g., intracranial pressure [ICP] and electroencephalogram [EEG]). Large contusions and lacerations with hemorrhage may be surgically excised. Treatment is otherwise directed at controlling intracranial pressure, neuroprotection, and managing symptoms.

An epidural (extradural) hematoma is bleeding between the dura mater and the skull. It represents 1% to 2% of major head injuries and occurs in all age groups, but most commonly in those 20 to 40 years old. The temporal fossa is the most common site of epidural hematoma caused by injury, commonly to the middle meningeal artery and less commonly to the meningeal vein or dural sinus (see Fig. 17.2). Both sites of hematoma can result in brain herniation (see Fig. 16.11).

intracerebral hematomas. The injury may be a coup injury (injury at site of impact) or a contrecoup injury (injury from brain rebounding and hitting the opposite side of skull) (Fig. 17.1). Compression of the skull at the point of impact produces contusions or brain bruising from blood leaking from an injured vessel. The severity of contusion varies with the amount of energy transmitted by the skull to underlying brain tissue. The smaller the area of impact, the more severe the injury

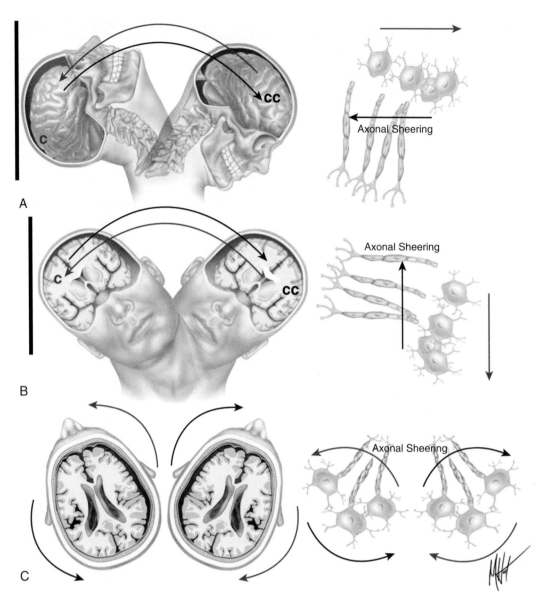

FIGURE 17.1 Coup and Contrecoup Focal Injury With Acceleration/Deceleration Axonal Shearing. **A,** Sagittal force causing coup *(c)* and contrecoup injury *(cc)*. **B,** Lateral force causing coup *(c)* and contrecoup *(cc)* injury. **C,** Axial or rotational injury with shearing of axons, particularly at base of brain. Acceleration/deceleration axonal shearing injury occurs throughout the brain (red and blue directional arrows in all three images). (Borrowed from Pascual JM, Preito R: Surgical management of severe closed head injury in adults. In Quinones-Hinojosa A, editor: *Schmidek and Sweet operative neurosurgical techniques,* ed 6, vol 2, pp 1513-1538, Philadelphia, 2012, Saunders. Originally redrawn from Adams JH: Brain damage in fatal nonmissile head injury in man. In Braakman R, editor: *Handbook of clinical neurology, head injury,* vol 13, pp 43-63, Amsterdam, 1990, Elsevier Science Publishers BV; Gennarelli TA et al: *Ann Neurol* 12:564-574, 1982.)

Individuals with temporal epidural hematomas lose consciousness at injury. If a vein is bleeding (a slower bleed), one-third of those affected then become lucid for a few minutes to a few days. As the hematoma accumulates, a headache of increasing severity, vomiting, drowsiness, confusion, and seizure occur. The expanding hematoma causes temporal lobe herniation, and the level of consciousness is rapidly lost, with ipsilateral pupillary dilation and contralateral hemiparesis. Imaging usually is needed to diagnose epidural hematoma. The prognosis is good if intervention is initiated before bilateral dilation of the pupils occurs. Epidural hematomas are medical emergencies requiring evaluation, monitoring, and surgical evacuation of the hematoma.[3]

A subdural hematoma is bleeding between the dura mater and the arachnoid membrane covering the brain and is caused by tearing of veins.[4] It is the most common cause of a traumatic intracranial mass lesion, occurring in about 10% to 20% of individuals. Nontraumatic subdural hematoma can rarely develop in association with anticoagulant therapy or vascular malformations. *Acute subdural hematomas* develop rapidly, commonly within hours, and usually are located at the top of the skull. *Subacute subdural hematomas* develop more slowly, often over 48 hours to 2 weeks. *Chronic subdural hematomas* develop over weeks to months. These subdural hematomas act like expanding masses, increasing ICP that eventually compresses the bleeding vessels (see Fig. 17.2). Brain herniation can result. With a chronic subdural hematoma,

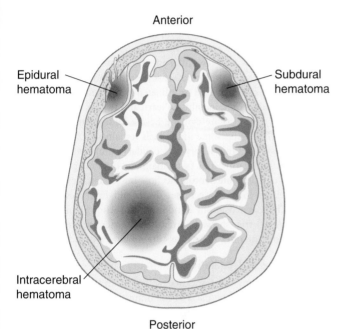

Anterior

Epidural hematoma

Subdural hematoma

Intracerebral hematoma

Posterior

FIGURE 17.2 Brain Hematomas.

the existing subdural space gradually fills with blood. A vascular membrane forms around the hematoma in approximately 2 weeks. Further enlargement may take place.

In acute, rapidly developing subdural hematomas, the expanding clots directly compress the brain. As the ICP rises, bleeding veins are compressed. Thus bleeding can be self-limiting, although cerebral compression and displacement of brain tissue can cause temporal lobe herniation.

An acute subdural hematoma classically begins with headache, drowsiness, restlessness or agitation, slowed cognition, and confusion. These symptoms worsen over time and progress to loss of consciousness, respiratory pattern changes, and pupillary dilation (i.e., the symptoms of temporal lobe herniation). Homonymous hemianopia (loss of vision in either the right or the left field [see Fig. 15.8]), dysconjugate gaze, and gaze palsies also may occur. Severity of injury is measured using the GCS, ICP monitoring, and brain imaging. Generally, clinical deterioration, a clot thickness greater than 10 mm, or a midline shift greater than 5 mm are suggested as critical parameters for surgery to remove the clot.[5]

Of those individuals affected by chronic subdural hematomas, 80% have chronic headaches and tenderness over the hematoma on palpation. Most persons appear to have a progressive dementia with generalized rigidity (paratonia). Chronic subdural hematomas require clot evacuation.

Intracerebral hematomas (bleeding within the brain) occur in 2% to 3% of persons with head injuries. The hematomas may be single or multiple and are associated with contusions. Although most commonly located in the frontal and temporal lobes, they may occur in the hemispheric deep white matter. Penetrating injury or shearing forces traumatize small blood vessels. The intracerebral hematoma then acts as an expanding mass, increasing the ICP, compressing brain tissues, and causing edema (see Fig. 17.2). Delayed intracerebral hematomas may appear 3 to 10 days after the head injury. Intracerebral hematomas also can occur with nontraumatic brain injury, such as hemorrhagic stroke.

Intracerebral hematomas cause a decreasing level of consciousness. Coma or a confusional state from other injuries, however, can make the cause of this increasing unresponsiveness difficult to detect. Contralateral hemiplegia also may develop and, as the ICP rises, temporal lobe

herniation may occur. In delayed intracerebral hematoma, the presentation is similar to that of a hypertensive brain hemorrhage—sudden, rapidly progressive decreased level of consciousness with pupillary dilation, breathing pattern changes, hemiplegia, and bilateral positive Babinski reflexes (stroking the lateral side of the sole of the foot causes extension of the big toe—moves up—with fanning of the other toes).

The history and physical examination help establish the diagnosis, and imaging confirms it. Surgical evacuation of a hematoma is performed, considering clinical signs and symptoms, size and location of the hematoma, and associated comorbid conditions. Otherwise, treatment is directed at reducing the ICP and allowing the hematoma to reabsorb slowly.

Open brain injury (trauma that penetrates the dura mater) produces both focal and diffuse injuries and includes compound skull fractures and missile injuries (e.g., bullets, rocks, shell fragments, knives, and blunt instruments). A compound skull fracture opens a communication between the cranial contents and the environment and should be investigated whenever lacerations of the scalp, tympanic membrane, sinuses, eye, or mucous membranes are present. Such fractures may involve the cranial vault or the base of the skull (basilar skull fracture). Cranial nerve damage and spinal fluid leak may occur with a basilar skull fracture.

The mechanisms of open brain trauma are crush injury (laceration and crushing of whatever the missile touches) and stretch injury (blood vessels and nerves damaged without direct contact as a result of stretching). The tangential injury is to the coverings and the brain (scalp and brain lacerations) and may also include skull fractures and meningeal or cerebral lacerations from projectiles and debris driven into the brain substance.

Most persons lose consciousness with open brain injury. The depth and duration of the coma are related to the location of injury, extent of damage, and amount of bleeding. Open brain injury often requires débridement of the traumatized tissues to prevent infection and to remove blood clots, thereby reducing ICP. The ICP also is managed with dehydrating agents, osmotic diuretics, or a combination of these drugs. Broad-spectrum antibiotics are administered to prevent infection.

A compound fracture may be diagnosed through physical examination, skull X-ray films, or both. Basilar skull fracture is determined on the basis of clinical findings, such as spinal fluid leaking from the ear or nose. Skull X-rays often do not demonstrate the fracture, although intracranial air or air in the sinuses on imaging is indirect evidence of a basilar skull fracture. Bed rest and close observation for meningitis and other complications are prescribed for a basilar skull fracture.

Diffuse brain injury. Diffuse brain injury (diffuse axonal injury [DAI]) involves widespread areas of the brain and occurs with all severities of brain injury. DAI is defined clinically as coma lasting 6 or more hours after TBI. In mild DAI, coma lasts 6 to 24 hours. In moderate DAI, coma lasts longer than 24 hours but without abnormal posturing. In severe cases of DAI, coma duration is longer than 24 hours, with signs of brainstem impairment. Mechanical effects from high levels of acceleration and deceleration injury, such as whiplash, or rotational forces cause shearing of delicate axonal fibers and white matter tracts that project to or from the cerebral cortex (see Fig. 17.1). The most severe axonal injuries are located more peripheral to the brainstem, causing extensive cognitive and affective impairments, as seen in survivors of TBI from motor vehicle crashes. Axonal damage reduces the speed of information processing and responding and causes behavioral, cognitive, and physical changes.[6]

Pathophysiologically, axonal damage can be seen only with an electron microscope and involves numerous axons, either alone or in conjunction with actual tissue tears. Advanced imaging techniques assist in defining areas of injury. Areas where axons and small blood vessels are torn appear as small hemorrhages. More damaged axons are visible 12 hours to several days after the initial injury. The severity of diffuse injury correlates with how much shearing force was applied to the brainstem. DAI is not associated with intracranial hypertension immediately after injury; however, acute brain swelling, caused by vasodilation, increased intravascular blood flow within the brain, and increased cerebral blood volume, is seen often and can result in hypoxic-ischemic injury and death. DAI may induce long-term neurodegenerative processes. These changes may continue for years after injury, with the development of chronic traumatic encephalopathy and Alzheimer disease–like pathologic changes.[7]

Secondary brain injury. Secondary brain injury is an indirect result of primary brain injury, including trauma and stroke syndromes. Both systemic and cerebral processes are contributing factors. Systemic processes include hypotension, hypoxia, anemia, hypercapnia, and hypocapnia. Cerebral contributions include inflammation, cerebral edema, increased intracranial pressure (IICP), decreased cerebral perfusion pressure, cerebral ischemia, and brain herniation. Cellular and molecular brain damage from the effects of primary injury develops hours to days later and causes disruption of the blood–brain barrier and neuronal death. Mechanisms include oxidative stress, excitotoxicity (excessive stimulation by excitatory neurotransmitters, such as glutamate), and mitochondrial failure.

The management of secondary brain injury is related to prevention of hypoxia and maintenance of cerebral perfusion pressure. Management includes removal of hematomas and treatment of hypotension, hypoxemia, anemia, intracranial pressure, fluid and electrolyte balance, body temperature, and ventilation. The development of neuroprotective agents is in progress but is difficult because of the complexity of multiple interacting secondary injury cascades.[8] Nutrition management has emerged as critically important in the care of individuals with severe brain injury.[9] Long-term recovery and mortality can be influenced by systemic complications, such as pneumonia, fever, infections, and immobility, that contribute to further brain injury and delays in repair and recovery.

Categories of traumatic brain injury. Several categories of TBI exist and are presented here as mild, moderate, and severe. The terms *concussion* and *traumatic brain injury* are often used interchangeably. The severity of TBI commonly considers the duration of loss of consciousness, the GCS score, posttraumatic amnesia, and brain imaging results.[10]

Mild traumatic brain injury (mild concussion) is characterized by immediate but transitory clinical manifestations. There may be no loss of consciousness, or loss of consciousness may last less than 30 minutes. Most blunt trauma injuries cause mild concussion. The GCS score is 13 to 15. The initial confusional state lasts for 1 to several minutes, possibly with amnesia for events preceding the trauma (retrograde amnesia). Persons may experience headache, nausea, vomiting, impaired ability to concentrate, and difficulty sleeping for up to a few days. A blood test to evaluate for the presence of mild TBI in adults is available to determine if there is a need for a computed tomography (CT) scan.[11]

Moderate traumatic brain injury (moderate concussion) is any loss of consciousness lasting more than 30 minutes and up to 6 hours. The GCS score is 9 to 12. A basal skull fracture may be present, but there is no brainstem injury; however, there is transitory decerebration or decortication (see Fig. 16.6). The person is confused and experiences posttraumatic amnesia that lasts for more than 24 hours. There often are permanent deficits in selective attention, vigilance, detection, working memory, data processing, vision or perception, and language, as well as mood and affect changes ranging from mild to severe. Brain imaging is abnormal.

Severe traumatic brain injury (severe concussion) is loss of consciousness lasting more than 6 hours. The GCS is 3 to 8. Frequently there are associated signs of brainstem damage, including changes in pupillary reaction, cardiac and respiratory symptoms, decorticate or decerebrate posturing (see Fig. 16.6), and abnormal reflexes. Brain imaging is abnormal. IICP appears 4 to 6 days after injury. Pulmonary complications occur frequently, with profound sensorimotor and cognitive system deficits. Severely compromised coordinated movements and verbal and written communication, inability to learn and reason, and inability to modulate behavior also are evident. Severe injury causes permanent neurologic deficits, and some individuals remain in a vegetative state or die as a result of brain injury or secondary complications.

The goal of treating TBI is to maintain cerebral perfusion and oxygenation and promote neuroprotection. Implementation of management guidelines for TBI decreases death and improves neurologic outcome. The Corticosteroid Randomization After Significant Head Injury (CRASH) trial showed corticosteroids increase mortality with acute TBI; consequently, these drugs are no longer used.[12]

Complications of Traumatic Brain Injury

Many complications are associated with TBI and are related to the severity of injury and the parts of the brain that are affected. Altered states of consciousness can range from confusion to deep coma (see Table 16.3). Cognitive deficits; hydrocephalus; sensory-motor disorders, including pain, paresis, and paralysis; and loss of coordination may be present. Three of the most common posttraumatic brain syndromes are summarized below.

Postconcussion syndrome, including headache, dizziness, fatigue, nervousness or anxiety, irritability, insomnia, depression, inability to concentrate, and forgetfulness, may last for weeks to months after a mild concussion. Treatment entails reassurance and symptomatic relief in addition to 24 hours of close observation after the concussion in the event bleeding or swelling in the brain occurs. Symptoms requiring further evaluation and treatment include drowsiness or confusion, nausea or vomiting, severe headache, memory deficit, seizures, drainage of cerebrospinal fluid from the ear or nose, weakness or loss of feeling in the extremities, asymmetry of the pupils, and double vision. Guidelines for the management of pediatric and adult concussion are available.[13-15] Guidelines have been published for the management of sports-related concussion.[16]

Posttraumatic seizures (epilepsy) occur in about 10% to 20% of TBIs, with the highest risk among open brain injuries. Seizures can occur early, within days, and up to 2 to 5 years or longer after the trauma. Causal mechanisms are poorly understood. Seizure prevention using drugs, such as phenytoin, is initiated for moderate to severe TBI at the time of injury. Studies are ongoing to test drugs that prevent the development of posttraumatic seizures.[17]

Chronic traumatic encephalopathy (CTE) (previously called *dementia pugilistica*) is a progressive dementing disease that develops with repeated brain injury associated with sporting events, blast injuries in soldiers, or work-related head trauma. Hyperphosphorylated tau neurofibrillary tangles are present in the brain, and research is in progress to discover the mechanistic link between neurotrauma and CTE. CTE is associated with violent behaviors, loss of control, depression, suicide, memory loss, cognitive change, and change in motor function. It is diagnosed from history and clinical evaluation and at autopsy.[18]

✔ **QUICK CHECK 17.1**

1. How is a concussion different from a contusion?
2. How does focal brain injury differ from diffuse brain injury?
3. Why is head motion the principal causative mechanism of diffuse brain injury?

TABLE 17.3   Spinal Cord Injuries

Injury	Description
Cord concussion	Results in temporary disruption of cord-mediated functions
Cord contusion	Bruising of neural tissue causes swelling and temporary loss of cord-mediated functions
Cord compression	Pressure on cord causes ischemia to tissues; must be relieved (decompressed) to prevent permanent damage to spinal cord
Laceration	Tearing of neural tissues of spinal cord; may be reversible if only slight damage sustained by neural tissues; may result in permanent loss of cord-mediated functions if spinal tracts are disrupted
Transection	Severing of spinal cord causes permanent loss of function
Complete	All tracts in spinal cord are completely disrupted; all cord-mediated functions below transection are completely and permanently lost
Incomplete	Some tracts in spinal cord remain intact, together with functions mediated by these tracts; has potential for recovery although function is temporarily lost
Preserved sensation only	Some demonstrable sensation below level of injury
Preserved motor nonfunctional	Preserved motor function without useful purpose; sensory function may or may not be preserved
Preserved motor functional	Preserved voluntary motor function that is functionally useful
Hemorrhage	Bleeding into neural tissue as a result of blood vessel damage; usually no major loss of function
Damage or obstruction of spinal blood supply	Causes local ischemia

Spinal Cord and Vertebral Injury

Each year 17,700 persons experience serious spinal cord injury. Male sex and ages 16 to 30 years are strong risk factors. Motor vehicle crashes are the leading cause of injury, followed by falls and then violence, other events, and sports activities.[19] Elderly people are particularly at risk for trauma that results in serious spinal cord injury because of preexisting degenerative vertebral disorders.

PATHOPHYSIOLOGY   Primary spinal cord injury occurs with the initial mechanical trauma and immediate tissue destruction. Injuries to the cord are summarized in Table 17.3. Primary spinal cord injury occurs if an injured spine is not adequately immobilized immediately following injury. Primary spinal cord injury also may occur in the absence of vertebral fracture or dislocation and is related to longitudinal stretching of the cord with or without flexion or extension of the vertebral column, or both. The stretching causes altered axon transport, edema, myelin degeneration, and retrograde or Wallerian neural degeneration (see Chapter 14).

Secondary spinal cord injury is a complex pathophysiologic cascade of vascular, cellular, and biochemical events that begins within a few minutes after injury and continues for weeks. Secondary injury includes hemorrhages, inflammation, edema, and ischemia. Hemorrhages develop in the central gray matter, and edema develops in the white matter, impairing the microcirculation of the cord. The hemorrhages and edema are followed by vasospasm and vascular occlusion, reduced perfusion, and development of ischemic areas, which are maximal at the level of injury and two cord segments above and below it. Cord swelling increases the individual's degree of dysfunction, making it difficult to distinguish functions permanently lost from those temporarily impaired. In the cervical region at C1-C4, cord swelling may be life-threatening because cardiovascular and respiratory control functions can be lost. Excitotoxicity (excessive stimulation by excitatory neurotransmitters, such as glutamate), intracellular calcium overload, oxidative damage, and cell death occur similarly to those previously described for TBI. Spared neurons continue to be chronically injured, with death of oligodendrocytes and myelin degeneration, axonal disruption, glial scarring, cystic cavitation, and release of inhibitory mediators. The process presents a physical and chemical barrier to regeneration.[20]

Vertebral injuries result from acceleration, deceleration, or deformation forces occurring at impact. These forces cause vertebral fractures, dislocations, and penetration of bone fragments that can cause compression to the tissues, pull or exert traction (tension) on the tissues, or cause shearing of tissues so they slide into one another (Figs. 17.3 to 17.6). Vertebral injuries can be classified as (1) simple fracture—a single break usually affecting transverse or spinous processes; (2) compressed (wedged) vertebral fracture—vertebral body compressed anteriorly; (3) comminuted (burst) fracture—vertebral body shattered into several fragments; and (4) dislocation.

The vertebrae fracture readily with both direct and indirect trauma. When the supporting ligaments are torn, the vertebrae move out of alignment, and dislocations occur. A horizontal force moves the vertebrae straight forward; if the individual is in a flexed position at the time of injury, the vertebrae are then angulated. Flexion and extension injuries may result in dislocations. (Bone, ligament, and joint injuries are presented in Table 17.4.)

Vertebral injuries in adults occur most often at vertebrae C1 to C2 (cervical), C4 to C7 (cervical), and T10 (thoracic) to L2 (lumbar) (see Fig. 14.11), the most mobile portions of the vertebral column. The spinal cord also occupies most of the vertebral canal in the cervical and lumbar regions, so it can be easily injured in these locations.

CLINICAL MANIFESTATIONS   Spinal shock is the temporary loss of spinal cord functions below the lesion. Spinal shock develops immediately after injury because of loss of continuous tonic discharge from the brain or brainstem and inhibition of central descending impulses that control and modulate spinal cord neurons. It is caused by cord hemorrhage, edema, or anatomic transection. Normal activity of spinal cord cells at and below the level of injury ceases, with complete loss of reflex function, flaccid paralysis, absence of sensation, loss of bladder and rectal control, transient drop in blood pressure, bradycardia, and poor venous circulation. The condition also results in disturbed thermal control because the sympathetic nervous system is damaged. The hypothalamus cannot regulate body heat through vasoconstriction and increased metabolism; therefore the individual assumes the temperature of the air (poikilothermia). Spinal shock generally lasts 2 to 3 days. It terminates with the reappearance of reflex activity, hyperreflexia, spasticity, and reflex emptying of the bladder, all of which may take weeks to months. Table 17.5 summarizes the clinical manifestations of spinal cord injury.

Neurogenic shock, also called *vasogenic shock,* occurs with cervical or upper thoracic cord injury above T6 and may be seen in addition to spinal shock. Neurogenic shock is caused by the absence of sympathetic activity through loss of supraspinal control and unopposed parasympathetic tone mediated by the intact vagus nerve. Symptoms include vasodilation, hypotension, bradycardia, and failure of body temperature regulation. Neurogenic shock may be complicated by hypovolemic or cardiogenic shock if there is concurrent heart failure or blood loss (see Chapter 26).

Loss of motor and sensory function depends on the extent and level of injury. Paralysis of the lower half of the body with both legs involved is termed *paraplegia.* Paralysis involving all four extremities

is termed *quadriplegia* (tetraplegia). In complete quadriplegia, the level of injury is above C6 and all upper extremity function is lost. In incomplete quadriplegia, function at or above C6 is preserved, leaving the shoulder, upper arm, and some forearm muscle control intact. The initial clinical manifestations associated with acute spinal cord injury are related to spinal shock described above and include (1) rapid development of flaccid paralysis below the level of injury, (2) loss of sensations in the lower extremities and possibly lower trunk (depending on the level of injury), and (3) loss of spinal and autonomic reflexes below the level of injury. The duration of this areflexic state is highly variable. In most persons, reflex activity

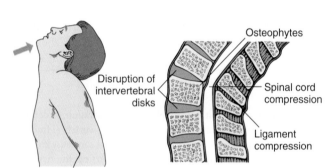

FIGURE 17.3 Hyperextension Injuries of the Spine. Hyperextension injuries of the spine can result in fracture or nonfracture injuries with spinal cord damage.

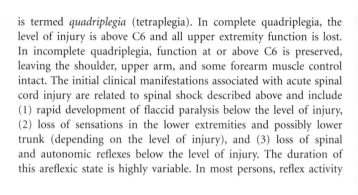

FIGURE 17.5 Axial Compression Injuries of the Spine. In axial compression injuries of the spine, the spinal cord is contused directly by retropulsion of bone or disk material into the spinal canal.

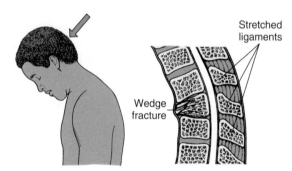

FIGURE 17.4 Flexion Injury of the Spine. Hyperflexion produces translation (subluxation) of vertebrae that compromises the central canal and compresses spinal cord parenchyma or vascular structures.

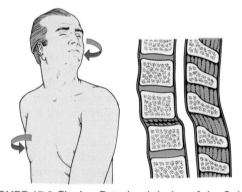

FIGURE 17.6 Flexion-Rotation Injuries of the Spine.

TABLE 17.4	Mechanisms of Vertebral Injury Involving Bone, Ligaments, and Joints		
Mechanism of Injury	Location of Vertebral Injury	Forces of Injury	Location of Injury
Hyperextension	Fracture and dislocation of posterior elements, such as spinous processes, transverse processes, laminae, pedicles, or posterior ligaments	Results from forces of acceleration/deceleration and sudden reduction in anteroposterior diameter of spinal cord	Cervical area
Hyperflexion	Fracture or dislocation of vertebral bodies, disks, or ligaments	Results from sudden and excessive force that propels neck forward or causes an exaggerated lateral movement of neck to one side	Cervical area
Vertical compression (axial loading)	Shattering fractures	Results from a force applied along an axis from top of cranium through vertebral bodies	T12 to L2
Rotational forces (flexion-rotation)	Rupture support ligaments in addition to producing fractures	Add shearing force to acceleration forces	Cervical area

returns in about a week. Return of spinal neuron excitability occurs slowly. Depending on the degree of damage, either of the following can occur: (1) motor, sensory, reflex, and autonomic functions return to normal; or (2) autonomic neural activity in the isolated segment develops. Spasticity is common, with hyperreflexia, clonus, and painful muscle spasms. Sometimes after several months, episodes of autonomic hyperreflexia occur.

Autonomic hyperreflexia (dysreflexia) is a syndrome of sudden, massive reflex sympathetic discharge associated with spinal cord injury at level T6 or above. It occurs because descending inhibition is blocked (Fig. 17.7). It may occur after spinal shock resolves and be a recurrent complication. Characteristics include paroxysmal hypertension (up to 300 mm Hg, systolic), a pounding headache, blurred vision, sweating above the level of the lesion, with flushing of the skin, nasal congestion, nausea, piloerection caused by pilomotor spasm, and bradycardia (30 to 40 beats/min). The symptoms may develop singly or in combination. The condition can cause serious complications (stroke, seizures, myocardial ischemia, and death) and requires immediate treatment.

In autonomic hyperreflexia, sensory receptors below the level of the cord lesion are stimulated. The intact autonomic nervous system reflexively responds with an arteriolar spasm that increases blood pressure. Baroreceptors in the cerebral vessels, the carotid sinus, and the aorta sense the hypertension and stimulate the parasympathetic system. The heart rate decreases, but the visceral and peripheral vessels do not dilate because efferent impulses cannot pass through the cord.

The most common cause is a distended bladder or rectum; however, any sensory stimulation (i.e., skin or pain receptors) can elicit autonomic hyperreflexia. Intravenous fluids may be required to maintain blood pressure. Drug therapy may be required to lower blood pressure and reduce complications. Bladder, bowel, and skin care management are important preventive strategies. Education of the individual and family regarding triggers and acute management is important, as is wearing a medic alert tag.[21]

EVALUATION AND TREATMENT Diagnosis of spinal cord injury is based on physical examination and imaging studies. Neurogenic shock must be differentiated from other kinds of shock (i.e., hypovolemic shock). For a suspected or confirmed vertebral fracture or dislocation, regardless of the presence or absence of spinal cord injury, the immediate intervention is immobilization of the spine to prevent further injury. Decompression and surgical fixation may be necessary. Blood pressure control, lung function, nutrition, skin integrity,

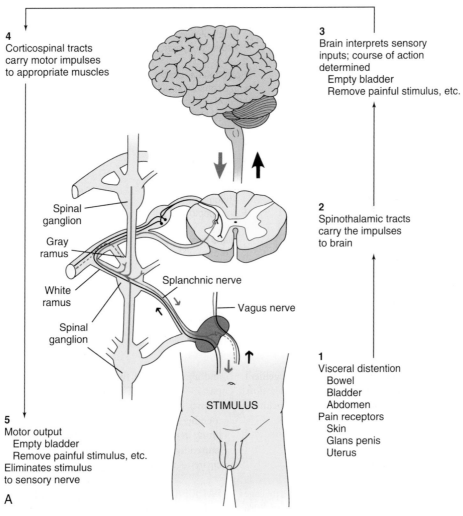

4
Corticospinal tracts carry motor impulses to appropriate muscles

3
Brain interprets sensory inputs; course of action determined
  Empty bladder
  Remove painful stimulus, etc.

Spinal ganglion

Gray ramus

White ramus

Spinal ganglion

Splanchnic nerve

Vagus nerve

STIMULUS

2
Spinothalamic tracts carry the impulses to brain

1
Visceral distention
  Bowel
  Bladder
  Abdomen
Pain receptors
  Skin
  Glans penis
  Uterus

5
Motor output
  Empty bladder
  Remove painful stimulus, etc.
Eliminates stimulus to sensory nerve

A

FIGURE 17.7 Autonomic Hyperreflexia. A, Normal response pathway.   *Continued*

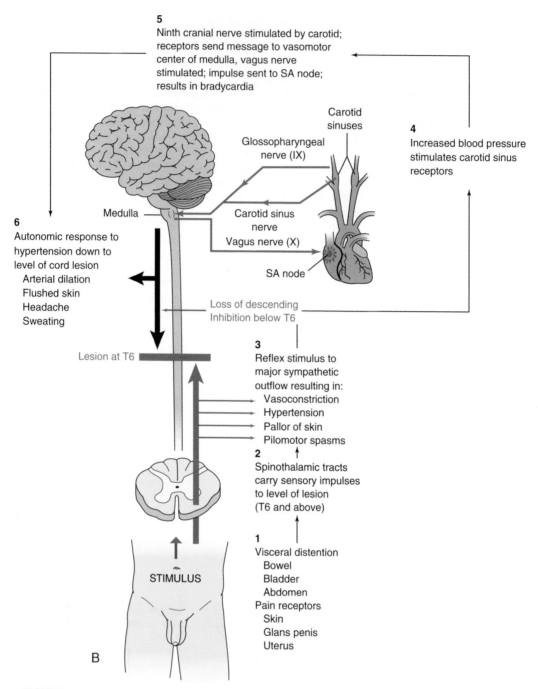

5
Ninth cranial nerve stimulated by carotid; receptors send message to vasomotor center of medulla, vagus nerve stimulated; impulse sent to SA node; results in bradycardia

Carotid sinuses

Glossopharyngeal nerve (IX)

4
Increased blood pressure stimulates carotid sinus receptors

Medulla

Carotid sinus nerve
Vagus nerve (X)

SA node

6
Autonomic response to hypertension down to level of cord lesion
    Arterial dilation
    Flushed skin
    Headache
    Sweating

Loss of descending Inhibition below T6

Lesion at T6

3
Reflex stimulus to major sympathetic outflow resulting in:
    Vasoconstriction
    Hypertension
    Pallor of skin
    Pilomotor spasms

2
Spinothalamic tracts carry sensory impulses to level of lesion (T6 and above)

1
Visceral distention
    Bowel
    Bladder
    Abdomen
Pain receptors
    Skin
    Glans penis
    Uterus

STIMULUS

B

FIGURE 17.7, cont'd B, Autonomic hyperreflexia pathway. *SA,* Sinoatrial. (Modified from Rudy EB: Advanced neurological and neurosurgical nursing, St Louis, 1984, Mosby.)

prevention of pressure ulcers, and bladder and bowel management must be addressed. Plans for rehabilitation need early consideration. Both neuroprotective and neuroregenerative strategies are under clinical investigation.[22,23]

Degenerative Disorders of the Spine
Low Back Pain

Low back pain (LBP) affects the area between the lower rib cage and gluteal muscles and often radiates into the thighs. About 80% of the population experiences LBP at some time during their lives,

and about 25% of the adult population has experienced LBP in the past 3 months.[24] The burdens of disability include psychological, financial, occupational, and social effects on the person and family members. Risk factors include occupations that require repetitious lifting in the forward bent-and-twisted position, exposure to vibrations caused by vehicles or industrial machinery, obesity, osteoporosis, and cigarette smoking.

PATHOPHYSIOLOGY   Most cases of LBP are idiopathic or nonspecific, and no precise diagnosis is possible. Acute LBP is often associated with muscle or ligament strain and is more common in individuals younger

TABLE 17.5	**Clinical Manifestations of Spinal Cord Injury**
Stage	**Manifestations**

Spinal Shock Stage
Complete spinal cord
  transection
	Loss of motor function
	  1. Quadriplegia with injuries of cervical spinal cord
	  2. Paraplegia with injuries of thoracic spinal cord
	Muscle flaccidity
	Loss of all reflexes below level of injury
	Loss of pain, temperature, touch, pressure, and proprioception below level of injury
	Pain at site of injury caused by zone of hyperesthesia above injury
	Atonic bladder and bowel
	Paralytic ileus with abdominal distention
	Loss of vasomotor tone in lower body parts; low and unstable blood pressure
	Loss of perspiration below level of injury
	Loss or extreme depression of genital reflexes, such as penile erection and bulbocavernous reflex
	Dry and pale skin; possible ulceration over bony prominences
	Respiratory impairment

Partial spinal cord
  transection
	Asymmetric flaccid motor paralysis below level of injury
	Asymmetric reflex loss
	Preservation of some sensation below level of injury
	Vasomotor instability less severe than that seen with complete cord transection
	Bowel and bladder impairment less severe than that seen with complete cord transection
	Preservation of ability to perspire in some portions of body below level of injury
	Brown-Séquard syndrome (associated with penetrating injuries, hyperextension and flexion, locked facets, and compression fractures)
	  1. Ipsilateral paralysis or paresis below level of injury
	  2. Ipsilateral loss of touch, pressure, vibration, and position sense below level of injury
	  3. Contralateral loss of pain and temperature sensations below level of injury
	Cauda equina syndrome (compression of nerve roots below L1 caused by fracture and dislocation of spine or large posterocentral
	  intervertebral disk herniation)
	  1. Lower extremity motor deficits
	  2. Variable sensorimotor dysfunction
	  3. Variable reflex dysfunction
	  4. Variable bladder, bowel, and sexual dysfunction

Heightened Reflex Activity Stage	Emergence of Babinski reflexes Hyperactive ankle and knee reflexes Reflex urinary incontinence and defecation Episodes of hypertension Defective heat-induced sweating Development of extensor reflexes, first in muscles of hip and thigh, later in leg

than 50 years of age without a history of cancer. The interspinous bursae can be a source of pain, particularly in the lumbar vertebrae. The ligaments of the spine are supplied with pain receptors, and all of these ligaments are vulnerable to traumatic tears (sprains) and fracture. Diskogenic pain also may be related to inflammation and nerve sprouting within the disk[25] (Fig. 17.8, *A*).

Common causes of chronic LBP include degenerative disk disease, spondylolysis (vertebral stress fracture), spondylolisthesis (vertebra slides forward or slips in relation to a vertebra below), spinal osteochondrosis (abnormal bone growth), spinal stenosis, and lumbar disk herniation (see Fig. 17.8, *B* and *C*). Other causes include tension caused by tumors or disk prolapse, bursitis, synovitis, spinal immobility, inflammation caused by infection (as in osteomyelitis), and pain referred from viscera or the posterior peritoneum. Systemic causes of LBP include bone diseases, such as osteoporosis or osteomalacia, and hyperparathyroidism. Anatomically, LBP must originate from innervated structures, but deep pain is widely referred and varies. The nucleus pulposus has no intrinsic innervation, but when extruded or herniated through a prolapsed disk,

it irritates the spinal nerve and causes pain referred to the segmental area (see Fig. 17.8, *C*).

CLINICAL MANIFESTATIONS Some individuals with acute LBP have pain along the distribution of a lumbar nerve root (radicular pain), most commonly involving the sciatic nerve (sciatica). Sciatica is often accompanied by neurosensory and motor deficits, such as tingling, numbness, and weakness in various parts of the leg and foot. Chronic LBP may be associated with progressive motor or sensory deficits, cauda equina syndrome (new-onset bowel or bladder incontinence or urinary retention, loss of anal sphincter tone, and saddle anesthesia), a history of cancer metastasis to bone, and suspected spinal infection.

EVALUATION AND TREATMENT Diagnosis of LBP is based on the history and physical examination. Imaging and nerve conduction studies are obtained with severe neurologic deficit or serious underlying disease. Diagnosis and treatment guidelines are available to plan therapy.[26] Most

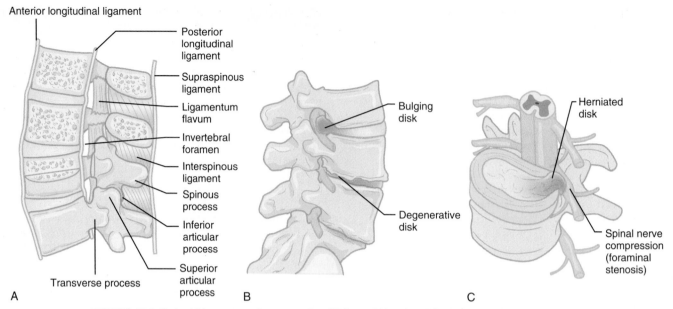

FIGURE 17.8 Spinal Ligaments, Degenerating Disk, and Herniated Disk. **A,** Ligaments of the spine. **B,** Bulging disk with spinal nerve compression and degenerative disk showing collapse of vertebral body. **C,** Herniated disk with spinal nerve compression.

individuals with acute LBP benefit from a nonspecific short-term treatment regimen of rest, analgesic medications, exercises, physical therapy, and education. Surgical treatments, specifically diskectomy and spinal fusions, are used for individuals not responding to medical management or for emergency management of cauda equina syndrome. Individuals with chronic LBP may benefit from antiinflammatory and muscle relaxant medications, exercise programs, massage, topical heat, spinal manipulation, acupuncture, cognitive-behavioral therapies, and interdisciplinary care. There is scant evidence for efficacy of opioids for chronic LBP, but a high risk for addiction. The complexity of causes contributes to the difficulty in defining pathogenesis and clearly defining the most effective therapies.

Degenerative Joint Disease

Degenerative disk disease. Degenerative disk disease (DDD) is common in individuals 30 years of age and older. It is, in part, a process of normal aging as a response to continuous vertical compression of the spine (axial loading). DDD includes a genetic component, involving genes that code for spinal cartilage. The combination of environmental interactions and genetic predisposition increases susceptibility to lumbar disk disease by disrupting normal building and maintenance of cartilage, with inflammation and physical compression of the intervertebral disk tissue.[27] The annulus (outer fibrous ring) can tear, and the disk can herniate, pinching nerves or placing strain on the spine. The pathologic findings in DDD include disk protrusion, spondylolysis and/or subluxation (spondylolisthesis), degeneration of vertebrae, and spinal stenosis. Lumbar disk disease commonly affects adults at some point in their lives. However, only a small percentage of people with degenerative disk disease have any functional incapacity because of pain.

Spondylolysis. Spondylolysis is a structural defect (degeneration, fracture, or developmental defect) in the pars interarticularis of the vertebral arch (the joining of the vertebral body to the posterior structures). The lumbar spine at L5 is affected most often. Mechanical pressure may cause an anterior or posterior displacement of the deficient vertebra (spondylolisthesis). Heredity plays a significant role, and spondylolysis is associated with an increased incidence of other congenital spinal defects. Symptoms include lower back and lower limb pain.

Spondylolisthesis. Spondylolisthesis, an osseous defect of the pars interarticularis, allows a vertebra to slide anteriorly in relation to the vertebra below. This commonly occurs at L5-S1. Spondylolisthesis is graded from 1 to 4 based on the percentage of slip that occurs. Grades 1 and 2 have symptoms of pain in the lower back and buttocks, muscle spasms in the lower back and legs, and tightened hamstrings. Conservative management includes exercise, rest, and back bracing. Vertebral slippage in grades 3 and 4 usually requires surgical intervention.

Spinal stenosis. Spinal stenosis is a narrowing of the spinal canal that causes pressure on the spinal nerves or cord. It can be congenital or acquired (more common) and is associated with trauma or arthritis. Spinal stenosis is categorized by the area of the spine affected: cervical, thoracic, or lumbar. Acquired conditions include a bulging disk, facet hypertrophy, or a thick, ossified posterior longitudinal ligament. Symptoms are related to the area of the spine affected and can produce pain; numbness; and tingling in the neck, hands, arms, or legs, with weakness and difficulty walking. Surgical decompression is recommended for those with chronic symptoms and those who do not respond to medical management.

Herniated Intervertebral Disk

Herniation of an intervertebral disk is a displacement of the nucleus pulposus or annulus fibrosus beyond the intervertebral disk space (see Fig. 17.8, *C*). Rupture of an intervertebral disk usually is caused by trauma, degenerative disk disease, or both. Risk factors are weight-bearing sports, light weight lifting, and certain work activities, such as repeated lifting. Men are affected more often than women, with the highest incidence in the 30- to 50-year age group. Most commonly affected are the lumbosacral disks L4-L5 and L5-S1. Disk herniation occasionally occurs in the cervical area, usually at C5-C6 and C6-C7.

Herniations at the thoracic level are extremely rare. The herniation may occur immediately, within a few hours, or months to years after injury.

PATHOPHYSIOLOGY   In a herniated disk, the ligament and posterior capsule of the disk are usually torn, allowing the nucleus pulposus to extrude and compress the nerve root. The vascular supply may be compromised and cause inflammatory changes in the nerve root (radiculitis). Occasionally, the injury tears the entire disk loose, causing the disk capsule and nucleus pulposus to protrude onto the nerve root or compress the spinal cord.

CLINICAL MANIFESTATIONS   The location and size of the herniation into the spinal canal, together with the amount of space in the canal, determine the clinical manifestations associated with the injury (Fig. 17.9). Compression or inflammation, or both, of a spinal nerve resulting from disk herniation follows a dermatomal distribution called radiculopathy (Fig. 17.10). A herniated disk in the lumbosacral area is associated with pain that radiates along the sciatic nerve course over the buttock and into the calf or ankle. The pain occurs with straining, including coughing and sneezing, and usually on straight leg raising. Other clinical manifestations include limited range of motion of the lumbar spine; tenderness on palpation in the sciatic notch and along the sciatic nerve; impaired pain, temperature, and touch sensations in the L4-L5 or L5-S1

dermatomes of the leg and foot; decreased or absent ankle jerk reflex; and mild weakness of the foot. More rarely, there is development of cauda equine syndrome (see Table 17.5).

With the herniation of a lower cervical disk, paresthesias (sensation of tingling, numbness, or burning) and pain are present in the upper arm, forearm, and hand along the affected nerve root distribution. Neck motion and straining, including coughing and sneezing, may increase neck and nerve root pain. Neck range of motion is diminished. Slight weakness and atrophy of biceps or triceps muscles may occur; the biceps or triceps reflex may decrease. Occasionally, signs of both corticospinal and sensory tract impairments appear, including motor weakness of the lower extremities, sensory disturbances in the lower extremities, and presence of a Babinski reflex.

EVALUATION AND TREATMENT   Diagnosis of a herniated intervertebral disk is made through the history and physical examination, imaging, electromyography, and nerve conduction studies. Evidenced-based practice guidelines have been published to guide treatment options.[28] Most herniated disks heal spontaneously over time and do not require surgery. Diskectomy is indicated if there is evidence of severe compression (weakness or decreased deep tendon, bladder, or bowel reflexes) or if a conservative approach is unsuccessful. Cauda equina syndrome rarely develops and requires emergency surgical evaluation and long-term follow-up.[29]

Cerebrovascular Disorders

Cerebrovascular disease (CVD) is any abnormality of the brain caused by a pathologic process in the blood vessels. CVD is the most frequently occurring neurologic disorder and frequently requires hospitalization. Included in this category are lesions of the vessel wall, occlusion of the vessel lumen by thrombus or embolus, rupture of the vessel, and alteration in blood quality, such as increased blood viscosity.

The brain abnormalities induced by cerebrovascular disease are either (1) ischemia with or without infarction (death of brain tissues) or (2) hemorrhage. The common clinical manifestation of CVD is a cerebrovascular accident or stroke. The symptoms occur suddenly and are focal (i.e., slurred speech, difficulty swallowing, limb weakness, or paralysis). In its mildest form, a cerebrovascular accident is so minimal that it is almost unnoticed. In its most severe form, hemiplegia, coma, and death result.

Cerebrovascular Accidents (Stroke Syndromes)

Cerebrovascular accidents (CVAs, stroke syndromes) are the leading cause of disability; they are the third leading cause of death in women and the fifth leading cause of death in men in the United States. Of all strokes, 87% are ischemic and 13% are hemorrhagic (intracerebral 10% and subarachnoid 3%). About 25% of strokes are recurrent strokes. Although hemorrhagic strokes are less common, they account for about 40% of stroke-related deaths. About 75% of CVAs occur among those older than 65 years. The incidence is greater in African Americans than in other ethnic groups. Persons with both hypertension and type 2 diabetes mellitus have an increase in stroke incidence and an increase in stroke mortality.[30] CVAs are classified pathophysiologically as ischemic or hemorrhagic. If there is no identifiable cause of an ischemic stroke, it is classified as *undetermined* or *cryptogenic*. Risk factors for stroke are summarized in Box 17.1.

Ischemic stroke. Ischemic stroke occurs when there is obstruction to arterial blood flow to the brain from thrombus formation, an embolus, or hypoperfusion related to decreased blood volume or heart failure. The inadequate blood supply results in ischemia (inadequate cellular oxygen) and can progress to infarction (death of tissue).

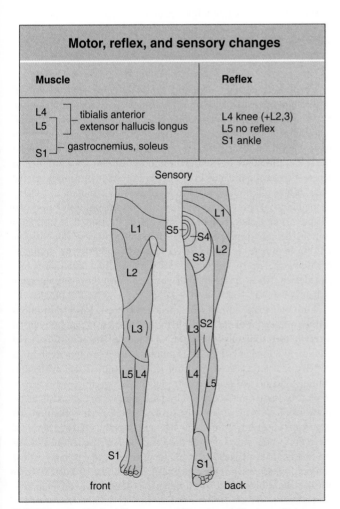

Motor, reflex, and sensory changes

Muscle		Reflex
L4 ⎤	tibialis anterior	L4 knee (+L2,3)
L5 ⎦	extensor hallucis longus	L5 no reflex
S1 ⎦	gastrocnemius, soleus	S1 ankle

Sensory

front   back

FIGURE 17.9 Clinical Features of Herniated Nucleus Pulposus.

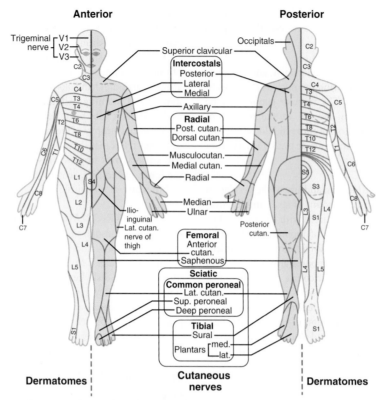

FIGURE 17.10 Sensory Nerve Distribution of Skin Dermatomes. (Redrawn from Patton HD et al, editors: *Introduction to basic neurology*, Philadelphia, 1976, WB Saunders. Borrowed from Canale ST, Beaty JH: *Campbell's operative orthopaedics*, ed 12, St Louis, 2013, Mosby.)

BOX 17.1   Risk Factors for Stroke

- Poorly controlled or uncontrolled arterial hypertension
- Smoking, which increases the risk of stroke by 2 to 4 times
- Insulin resistance and diabetes mellitus
- Atrial fibrillation
- Polycythemia (excess red blood cells) and thrombocythemia (excess platelets)
- High total cholesterol or low high-density lipoprotein (HDL) cholesterol, elevated lipoprotein-a
- Congestive heart disease and peripheral vascular disease
- Hyperhomocysteinemia
- Sickle cell disease
- Postmenopausal hormone therapy
- High sodium intake >2300 mg; low potassium intake <4700 mg
- Obesity
- Sleep apnea
- Depression
- *Chlamydia pneumoniae* infection
- Physical inactivity
- Family history of ischemic stroke

Thrombotic strokes (cerebral thromboses) arise from arterial obstruction caused by thrombus formation in arteries supplying the brain or intracranial vessels. Conditions causing increased coagulation (e.g., dehydration) or inadequate cerebral perfusion (e.g., hypotension or prolonged vasoconstriction from malignant hypertension) increase the risk of thrombosis. Cerebral thrombosis develops most often from atherosclerosis and inflammatory disease processes that damage arterial walls. It may take as long as 20 to 30 years for obstruction to develop at the branches and curvatures found in the cerebral circulation (see Chapter 26 for a discussion of atherogenesis). The smooth stenotic area can degenerate, forming an ulcerated area of the vessel wall. Platelets and fibrin adhere to the damaged wall, and a clot forms, gradually occluding the artery. Thrombotic strokes also occur when parts of a clot detach, travel upstream, and obstruct blood flow, causing acute ischemia.

Embolic stroke involves fragments that break from a thrombus formed outside the brain, usually in the heart, aorta, or common carotid artery. Other sources of embolism include fat, air, tumor, bacterial clumps, and foreign bodies. The embolus usually involves small brain vessels and obstructs at a bifurcation or other point of narrowing, thus causing ischemia. An embolus may plug the lumen entirely and remain in place or shatter into fragments and become part of the vessel's blood flow. Risk factors for an embolic stroke include atrial fibrillation, left ventricular aneurysm or thrombus, left atrial thrombus, recent myocardial infarction, endocarditis, rheumatic valve disease, mechanical valvular prostheses, atrioseptal defects, patent foramen ovale, and primary cardiac tumors. In persons who experience an embolic stroke, a recurrent stroke usually follows because the source of emboli continues to exist. Embolization is usually in the distribution of the middle cerebral artery (see Fig. 14.21). Ischemic strokes in children are associated with congenital heart

Transient ischemic attacks (TIAs) are episodes of neurologic dysfunction lasting no more than 1 hour and resulting from temporary obstruction of brain blood flow. The clinical manifestations of a TIA may include weakness, numbness, sudden confusion, loss of balance, or a sudden severe headache. The use of brain imaging modalities often reveals a brain infarction. About 12% of individuals experiencing a TIA will have a stroke.[30]

disease, cerebral arteriovenous malformations, and sickle cell disease (see Chapter 18).

Lacunar strokes (lacunar infarcts or small vessel disease) are usually caused by occlusion of a single, deep perforating artery that supplies a small penetrating vessel causing ischemic lesions (0.5 to 15 mm) deep in the brain (i.e., thalamus or basal ganglia) but not in the cortex. The small area of brain infarction is called a *lacune*. Because of the location and small area of infarction, they may manifest as pure motor or sensory deficits.[31] Lacunar strokes are associated with untreated high blood pressure.

Hypoperfusion, or hemodynamic stroke, is associated with *systemic* hypoperfusion caused by cardiac failure, pulmonary embolism, or bleeding that results in inadequate blood supply to the brain. Stroke may occur more readily if there is carotid artery occlusion. Symptoms are usually bilateral and diffuse.

PATHOPHYSIOLOGY Cerebral infarction results when an area of the brain loses its blood supply because of vascular occlusion. Causes include (1) acute vascular occlusion (e.g., embolus or thrombi), (2) gradual vessel occlusion (e.g., atheroma), and (3) partial occlusion of stenotic vessels. Cerebral thrombi and cerebral emboli most commonly produce occlusion, but atherosclerosis and hypertension are the dominant underlying processes.

There is a central core of irreversible ischemia and necrosis within a cerebral infarction. The central core is surrounded by a zone or rim of borderline hypoxic tissue known as the penumbra or ischemic penumbra. Hypoxia in the penumbra is not severe enough to result in structural damage. Prompt restoration of perfusion in the penumbra by injection of thrombolytic agents promotes perfusion and may prevent necrosis and loss of neurologic function. The window of opportunity for protecting the penumbra is about 3 hours.

Cerebral infarctions are ischemic or hemorrhagic. In *ischemic infarcts,* the affected area becomes pale and softens 6 to 12 hours after the occlusion. Necrosis, swelling around the insult, and mushy disintegration appear by 48 to 72 hours after infarction. There is infiltration of macrophages and phagocytosis of necrotic tissue. The necrosis resolves by about the second week, ultimately leaving a cavity surrounded by glial scarring.

Hemorrhagic transformation of an ischemic stroke is bleeding that occurs into the infarcted area through leaking vessels. Hemorrhagic transformation may be exacerbated by thrombolytic therapy and occurs more commonly with massive ischemic infarction. Guidelines are available for treatment.[32]

CLINICAL MANIFESTATIONS Clinical manifestations of thrombotic and embolic stroke vary, depending on the artery obstructed. Different sites of obstruction create different occlusion syndromes and are summarized in Table 17.6.[33] Contralateral sensory and motor manifestations occur on the opposite side of the body from the location of the brain lesion because motor tracts originate in the cortex and most cross over in the medulla. Sensory tracts originate in the periphery and cross over in the spinal cord. Ipsilateral manifestations occur on the same side as the brain lesion but are rare in stroke syndromes.

EVALUATION AND TREATMENT Imaging is used to diagnose stroke. Treatment of ischemic stroke is focused on (1) restoring brain perfusion in a time frame that does not contribute to reperfusion injury, (2) counteracting ischemic pathways, (3) lowering cerebral metabolic demand so that the susceptible brain tissue is protected against impaired perfusion, (4) preventing recurrent ischemic events, and (5) promoting tissue restoration. Intravenous thrombolysis, using tissue-type plasminogen activator (tPA), is given within 3 and up to 4.5 hours of onset of

TABLE 17.6 Signs and Symptoms of Stroke Involving Major Cerebral Vessels

Cerebral Vessel	Signs and Symptoms
Anterior cerebral artery (ACA)	Contralateral leg more than arm weakness (hemiparesis) and minimal numbness; akinetic mutism (inability to move or speak) if bilateral vessel involvement
Middle cerebral artery (MCA)	Contralateral upper limb more than leg weakness (hemiparesis) and numbness, ipsilateral hemianopsia and aphasia if stroke in dominant hemisphere
Posterior cerebral artery (PCA)	Contralateral weakness and dizziness, hemianopsia and ataxia
Basilar artery	Difficulty breathing, ataxia (impaired balance and coordination), nystagmus (involuntary, rapid eye movement), vomiting, coma
Cerebellar artery	Ataxia, vertigo, headache, nausea and vomiting, slurred speech

symptoms. Other strategies include endovascular intraarterial thrombolysis, thrombectomy, and placement of removable stents.[34] Supportive management is given to control cerebral edema and increased intracranial pressure and to provide neuroprotection. Arresting the disease process and preventing recurrent stroke by control of risk factors is critical, and antiplatelet therapy may be instituted. Separate guidelines are available for the assessment and management of acute ischemic stroke[35] and for the prevention of stroke risk in women.[36] Rehabilitation is indicated for ischemic strokes, and recovery of function is often possible.

Hemorrhagic stroke. Hemorrhagic stroke occurs within the brain tissue (intracerebral, the most common) or in the subarachnoid or subdural spaces. The primary cause of intracerebral hemorrhagic stroke is chronic hypertension. Other causes include tumors, coagulation disorders, trauma, or illicit drug use, particularly cocaine. Hypertensive causes of hemorrhagic stroke involve primarily smaller arteries and arterioles that have been damaged by chronic hypertension. Microaneurysms in these smaller vessels may precipitate the bleeding. Prevention or control of hypertension reduces the incidence of hemorrhagic stroke.

Subarachnoid hemorrhage (hematoma) is associated with ruptured aneurysms or arteriovenous malformations or brain trauma. *Subdural hemorrhage* (hematoma) is usually associated with brain trauma (see the Traumatic Brain Injury section).

PATHOPHYSIOLOGY A mass of blood is formed when there is bleeding into the brain tissue. The most common sites for hypertensive hemorrhages are in the deeper parts of the brain: the basal ganglia, the thalamus, the pons, and the caudate nucleus. Adjacent brain tissue is deformed, compressed, and displaced. This causes ischemia, edema, IICP, and necrosis. Rupture or seepage of blood into the ventricular system often occurs and is associated with higher mortality. Maximal cerebral edema develops in approximately 72 hours and takes about 2 weeks to subside. Most persons survive an initial ischemic stroke unless there is massive cerebral edema, which is nearly always fatal. The cerebral hemorrhage resolves through reabsorption. A cavity forms, surrounded by a dense scar after reabsorption of the blood.

CLINICAL MANIFESTATIONS The clinical manifestations of hemorrhagic stroke are similar to those for ischemic stroke and depend on the location and size of the bleeding. Symptoms can occur suddenly and with activity. Once a deep unresponsive state occurs, the person rarely survives. The immediate prognosis is grave; however, if the person survives, recovery of function is often possible.

It is difficult to differentiate ischemic from hemorrhagic stroke based on symptoms. Individuals experiencing intracranial hemorrhage from a ruptured or leaking aneurysm have one of three sets of symptoms: (1) onset of an excruciating generalized headache with an almost immediate lapse into an unresponsive state; (2) headache but with consciousness maintained and there may be seizures, nausea, and vomiting; and (3) sudden lapse into unconsciousness. If the hemorrhage is confined to the subarachnoid space, there may be no local signs. If bleeding spreads into the brain tissue, hemiparesis/paralysis, dysphasia, or homonymous hemianopia (visual field loss on the same side of both eyes) may be present. Warning signs of an impending aneurysm rupture include headache, transient unilateral weakness, transient numbness and tingling, and transient speech disturbance. However, such warning signs are often absent.

EVALUATION AND TREATMENT The neurologic exam and brain imaging are important to stroke diagnosis. Treatment of intracranial bleeding, regardless of the cause, focuses on stopping or reducing the bleeding; controlling blood pressure, edema, and IICP; preventing rebleeding; and preventing vasospasm. Surgical treatments, including endovascular approaches, are options for ruptured aneurysms, vascular malformations, and subarachnoid hemorrhage.[37]

Intracranial aneurysm. An intracranial aneurysm is a dilation or ballooning of a cerebral vessel from a weakness in the vessel wall. Risk factors include arteriosclerosis, congenital abnormality, cocaine use, trauma, smoking, or family history. The size may vary from 2 mm to 2 or 3 cm. Most aneurysms are located at bifurcations in or near the circle of Willis, in the vertebrobasilar arteries, or within the carotid system, where there is higher wall shear stress (frictional force of blood against the endothelium of a blood vessel) and flow turbulence (see Figs. 14.20 and 14.21. Aneurysms may be single but, in some instances, more than one is present. In these instances, the aneurysms may be unilateral or bilateral. The peak incidence of rupture occurs in persons 50 to 59 years of age, with the incidence in postmenopausal women slightly higher than that in men.

PATHOPHYSIOLOGY No single pathologic mechanism exists.[38] Aneurysms rupture through thin areas of blood vessels, often at bifurcation sites. There is hemorrhage into the subarachnoid space that spreads rapidly, producing localized changes in the cerebral cortex and focal irritation of nerves and arteries. Bleeding ceases when a fibrin-platelet plug forms at the point of rupture and as a result of compression. Blood undergoes reabsorption through arachnoid villi, usually within 3 weeks.

Aneurysms may be classified on the basis of their shape. *Saccular aneurysms (berry aneurysms)* occur frequently (in approximately 2% of the population) and can result from congenital abnormalities in the tunica media (middle layer) of the arterial wall and wall weakening related to atherosclerosis and hypertension. The sac gradually grows over time. A saccular aneurysm may be (1) round with a narrow stalk connecting it to the parent artery, (2) broad-based without a stalk, or (3) cylindrical (Figs. 17.11 and 17.12). The highest incidence of rupturing or bleeding (subarachnoid hemorrhage) is among persons 20 to 50 years of age.

Fusiform aneurysms (giant aneurysms) are less common, occur as a result of diffuse arteriosclerotic changes, and are found most commonly in the basilar arteries or terminal portions of the internal carotid arteries (see Fig. 17.11). They act as space-occupying lesions.

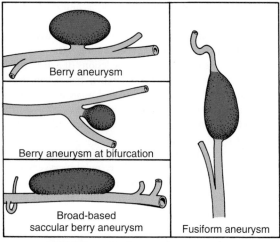

FIGURE 17.11 Types of Aneurysms.

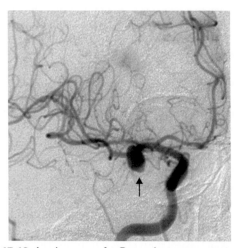

FIGURE 17.12 Angiogram of a Berry Aneurysm. In this contrast-enhanced lateral view, a portion of the cerebral arterial circulation can be seen as a berry aneurysm *(arrow)* involving the middle cerebral artery of the circle of Willis at the base of the brain. (From Klatt EC: *Robbins and Cotran atlas of pathology,* ed 3, Philadelphia, 2015, Saunders.)

CINICAL MANIFESTATIONS Aneurysms often are asymptomatic, and their presence is unknown until discovered incidentally or at autopsy. Clinical manifestations include sudden severe headache or dizziness and cranial nerve compression, but the signs vary, depending on the location and size of the aneurysm. Cranial nerves III, IV, V, and VI (see Table 14.6) are affected most often. Unfortunately, the most common first indication of the presence of an aneurysm is an acute subarachnoid hemorrhage, intracerebral hemorrhage, or combined subarachnoid-intracerebral hemorrhage (see the Hemorrhagic Stroke section).

EVALUATION AND TREATMENT Diagnosis before a bleeding episode is made through arteriography. After a subarachnoid or intracerebral hemorrhage, a tentative diagnosis of an aneurysm is based on clinical manifestations, history, and imaging. Treatments for intracranial aneurysm are both medical (i.e., control of hypertension and vasospasm) and surgical (i.e., external ventricular drain placement, microvascular clipping, or placement of endovascular coils).[39]

Subarachnoid hemorrhage. Subarachnoid hemorrhage (SAH) is the escape of blood from a defective or injured vessel into the subarachnoid space. Individuals at risk for a subarachnoid hemorrhage are those with intracranial aneurysm, intracranial arteriovenous malformation (see the next section), hypertension, a family history of SAH, and those who have sustained head injuries. Subarachnoid hemorrhages often recur, especially from a ruptured intracranial aneurysm.

PATHOPHYSIOLOGY When a vessel is leaking, blood oozes into the subarachnoid space. When a vessel tears, blood under pressure is pumped into the subarachnoid space. Autoregulation of blood flow is impaired, and there is a compensatory increase in systolic blood pressure.[40] The expanding hematoma acts like a space-occupying lesion and expands intracranial volume. There is compression and displacement of brain tissue with increased intracranial pressure, decreased perfusion pressure and cerebral blood flow, blood–brain barrier breakdown, brain edema, inflammation, and cell death. Secondary brain injury can occur as described for traumatic brain injury. In addition, the escaped blood coats nerve roots, clogs arachnoid granulations impairing CSF reabsorption, and obstructs foramina (passages) within the ventricular system impairing CSF circulation. Ultimately, granulation tissue is formed. There may be meningeal scarring with impairment of CSF reabsorption and secondary hydrocephalus. Mortality in SAH is about 50% at 1 month.

Delayed cerebral ischemia is a syndrome of progressive neurologic deterioration (i.e., development of hemiparesis or aphasia) associated with cerebral artery vasospasm. It occurs in 3 to 14 days after a subarachnoid hemorrhage in about 50% of cases. There is vasospasm related to the release of vasoactive substances during the hemorrhage; loss of autoregulation of blood flow, and neuron electrical activity (cortical spreading depolarization) that affects adjacent areas of the brain. Vasospasm with microthrombosis causes decreased cerebral perfusion with extension of ischemic injury and increased risk of death.[41]

CLINICAL MANIFESTATIONS Early manifestations associated with leaking vessels are episodic and include headache, changes in mental status or level of consciousness, nausea or vomiting, and focal neurologic defects (weakness or paralysis, loss of sensation, aphasia). A ruptured vessel causes a sudden, throbbing, "explosive" headache, accompanied by nausea and vomiting, visual disturbances, motor deficits, and loss of consciousness related to a dramatic rise in ICP. Meningeal irritation and inflammation often occur, causing neck stiffness (nuchal rigidity), photophobia, blurred vision, irritability, restlessness, and low-grade fever. A positive **Kernig sign** (straightening the knee with the hip and knee in a flexed position produces pain in the back and neck regions) and a positive **Brudzinski sign** (passive flexion of the neck produces neck pain and increased rigidity) may appear. No localizing signs are present if the bleeding is confined completely to the subarachnoid space. However, they may develop if there is delayed cerebral ischemia.

The Hunt and Hess SAH grading system is commonly used and is based on the description of the clinical manifestations[42] (Table 17.7). Rebleeding is a significant risk with a high mortality (up to 70%). The period of greatest risk is during the first 72 hours and up to 2 weeks after the initial episode of bleeding. Rebleeding is manifested by a sudden increase in blood pressure and ICP, along with a deteriorating neurologic status.

Seizures occur in 25% of persons with an SAH, and hydrocephalus after a bleeding episode occurs in 20% of cases. Hypothalamic dysfunction, manifested by salt wasting, hyponatremia, and electrocardiograph (ECG) changes, is common.

EVALUATION AND TREATMENT The diagnosis of an SAH is based on the clinical presentation, imaging, and cerebrospinal fluid evaluation. Treatment is directed at controlling intracranial pressure,

TABLE 17.7 Subarachnoid Hemorrhage Classification Scale

Category	Description
Grade I	Neurologic status intact; mild headache, slight nuchal rigidity
Grade II	Neurologic deficit evidenced by cranial nerve involvement; moderate to severe headache with more pronounced meningeal signs (e.g., photophobia, nuchal rigidity)
Grade III	Drowsiness and confusion with or without focal neurologic deficits; pronounced meningeal signs
Grade IV	Stuporous with pronounced neurologic deficits (e.g., hemiparesis, dysphasia); nuchal rigidity
Grade V	Deep coma state with decerebrate posturing and other brainstem functioning

From Tateshima S, Duckwiler G: Vascular diseases of the nervous system. In Daroff RB et al, editors: *Bradley's neurology in clinical practice*, Philadelphia, 2012, Saunders.

improving cerebral perfusion pressure, preventing ischemia and hypoxia of neural tissues, and avoiding rebleeding episodes. Surgical intervention is common. Treatment guidelines are available to direct therapy.[39]

Vascular malformation. Vascular malformations are rare congenital vascular lesions. An **arteriovenous malformation (AVM)** is a mass of dilated vessels between the arterial and venous systems (arteriovenous fistula) without an intervening capillary bed. AVMs may occur in any part of the brain and vary in size from a few millimeters to large malformations. They occur equally in males and females and, occasionally, in families. Although AVMs are usually present at birth, symptoms exhibit a delayed age of onset and commonly occur before 30 years of age.

PATHOPHYSIOLOGY AVMs have abnormal blood vessel structure with abnormally thin walls.[43] There is direct shunting of arterial blood into the venous vasculature without the dissipation of the arterial blood pressure. One or several arteries may feed the AVM. Over time, they become tortuous and dilated, with an increased risk for rupture. With moderate to large AVMs, sufficient blood is shunted into the malformation to deprive surrounding tissue of adequate blood perfusion.

CLINICAL MANIFESTATIONS Twenty percent of persons with an AVM have a characteristic chronic, nondescript headache, although some experience migraine. About 50% of persons experience seizures. The other 50% experience an intracerebral, subarachnoid, or subdural hemorrhage with progressive neurologic deficits. Bleeding from an AVM into the subarachnoid space causes symptoms identical to those associated with a ruptured aneurysm. If bleeding is into the brain tissue, focal signs that develop resemble a stroke that is progressing in severity. Ten percent of persons experience hemiparesis or other focal signs. At times, noncommunicating hydrocephalus (see Chapter 16) develops with a large AVM that extends into the ventricular lining. Some AVMs never cause symptoms.

EVALUATION AND TREATMENT A systolic bruit over the carotid artery in the neck, the mastoid process, or the eyeball in a young person is almost always diagnostic of an AVM. Confirming diagnosis is made by imaging. Treatment options include direct surgical excision, endovascular embolization, or radiotherapy.[44]

Primary Headache Syndromes

Headache is a common neurologic disorder and is usually a benign symptom.[45] However, it can be associated with serious disease, such as brain tumor, meningitis, or cerebrovascular disease. The headache syndromes discussed here are the chronic, recurring type not associated with structural abnormalities or systemic disease and include migraine, cluster, and tension headaches. Characteristics of the major types of headache syndromes are summarized in Table 17.8.

Migraine

Migraine is an episodic neurologic disorder characterized by a headache lasting 4 to 72 hours. It is diagnosed when any two of these features occur: unilateral head pain, throbbing pain, pain worsens with activity, moderate or severe pain intensity; *and* at least one of these features: nausea and/or vomiting, or photophobia and phonophobia.[46] Migraine is broadly classified as (1) *migraine with aura* with visual, sensory, or motor symptoms; (2) *migraine without aura* (most common); and (3) *chronic migraine.*

Migraine occurs in 18% of women, 6% of men and 10% of children in the United States. It is more common in those 25 to 55 years of age.[47] There often is a family history of migraine. In susceptible women, migraine occurs most frequently before and during menstruation and is decreased during pregnancy and menopause. The cyclic withdrawal of estrogen and progesterone may trigger attacks of migraine.[48]

Migraine is caused by a combination of multiple genetic and environmental factors. Migraine may be precipitated by triggers that decrease the threshold for a migraine. Triggers can be genetic or associated with fatigue, oversleeping, missed meals, overexertion, weather change, stress or relaxation from stress, hormonal changes (menstrual periods), excess afferent stimulation (bright lights, strong smells), and chemicals (alcohol or nitrates).

The pathophysiologic basis for migraine is complex and not clearly established. There is no identifiable pathology, but there are associated changes in brain metabolism and blood flow. Current theories include neurologic, vascular, hormonal, and neurotransmitter components. Migraine aura is associated with cortical spreading depression (CSD). CSD is a spontaneous self-propagating wave of glial and neuronal depolarization, resulting in hyperactivity, that starts in the occipital region and spreads across the cortex. CSD initiates the release of excitatory neurotransmitters that activate the trigeminal vascular system (afferent projections from cranial nerve V), stimulating vasodilation of dural blood vessels, activation of inflammation, peripheral and central sensitization of pain receptors (hypersensitivity to pain), and activation of areas of the brainstem and forebrain that modulate pain. Release of inflammatory mediators with sterile meningeal inflammation, edema of blood vessels, and release of neurotransmitters may be important components of migraine pain.[49] The clinical phases of a migraine attack are as follows:

1. *Premonitory phase:* Up to one-third of persons have premonitory symptoms hours to days before the onset of the aura or headache. These symptoms may include fatigue, irritability, loss of concentration, stiff neck, and food cravings.
2. *Migraine aura:* Up to one-third of persons have aura symptoms at least some of the time that may last up to 1 hour. Symptoms can be visual, sensory, or motor.
3. *Headache phase:* Throbbing pain usually begins on one side and spreads to include the entire head. Headache may be accompanied by fatigue, nausea, and vomiting or dizziness. There may be hypersensitivity to anything touching the head. Symptoms may last from 4 to 72 hours (usually about a day).
4. *Recovery phase:* Irritability, fatigue, or depression may take hours or days to resolve.

The diagnosis of migraine is made from the medical history and physical examination. The differential diagnosis is confirmed by imaging and EEG. The management of migraine includes avoidance of triggers (e.g., darkening the room, applying ice). Sleeping can provide some relief with the onset of acute migraine. Pharmacologic management for the treatment and prevention of migraine is available.[50] A transcutaneous electrical stimulation device providing trigeminal neurostimulation has been approved by the Food and Drug Administration for the prevention of migraine.[51]

Chronic migraines usually begin as episodic migraines that increase in frequency over time. Chronic migraine occurs at least 15 days in a

TABLE 17.8   Characteristics of Common Headaches

| | MIGRAINE | | Cluster Headache/ | |
	Without Aura	With Aura (25%-30%)	Proximal Hemicrania	Tension-Type Headache
Age of onset	Childhood, adolescence, or young adulthood	Childhood, adolescence, or young adulthood	Young adulthood, middle age	Young adulthood, middle age
Sex	Higher in females	Higher in females	Male	Not sex specific
Family history of headaches	Yes	Yes	No	Yes
Onset and evolution	Slow to rapid	Slow to rapid	Rapid	Slow to rapid
Time course	Episodic	Episodic	Clusters in time	Episodic, may become constant
Quality	Usually throbbing	Usually throbbing	Steady	Steady
Location	Variable, unilateral to bilateral	Variable, unilateral to bilateral	Orbit, temple, cheek	Variable
Associated features	Prodrome, vomiting	Aura: visual, sensory, language, and motor disturbance Prodrome, vomiting	Lacrimation, rhinorrhea, Horner syndrome	None

month (can occur daily or on a near-daily basis) for more than 3 months. Chronic migraines are associated with overuse of analgesic migraine medications (sometimes called *rebound headaches*), obesity, and caffeine overuse. Treatment is similar to that for episodic migraine.

Cluster Headache

Cluster headaches are one of a group of disorders referred to as *trigeminal autonomic cephalalgias* (headaches involving the autonomic division of the trigeminal nerve). They occur in one side of the head (proximal hemicranias) primarily in men between 20 and 50 years of age. The pain may alternate sides with each headache episode and is severe, stabbing, and throbbing. These uncommon headaches occur in clusters (up to 8 attacks per day) and last for minutes to hours for a period of days, followed by a long period of spontaneous remission. Cluster headache has an episodic and a chronic form with extreme pain intensity and short duration. If the cluster of attacks occurs more frequently without sustained spontaneous remission, the condition is classified as *chronic cluster headaches* (10% to 20% of cases) (see Table 17.8). Triggers are similar to those that cause migraine headache.

Trigeminal activation occurs, but the mechanism is unclear. The pathogenic mechanism for pain is related to the release of vasoactive substances and the formation of neurogenic inflammation. Autonomic dysfunction is characterized by sympathetic underactivity and parasympathetic activation. There is unilateral trigeminal distribution of severe pain with ipsilateral autonomic manifestations, including tearing and ptosis of the eye on the affected side, and congestion of the nasal mucosa. Prophylactic drugs are used to treat cluster headache, and avoidance of triggers also is important. Acute attacks are managed with oxygen inhalation, sumatriptan or inhaled ergotamine administration, and nerve stimulation. New drugs are under investigation.[52]

Tension-Type Headache

Tension-type headache (TTH) is the most common type of recurrent headache. The average age of onset is during the second decade of life. It is a mild to moderate bilateral headache with a sensation of a tight band or pressure around the head with gradual onset of pain. The headache occurs in episodes and may last for several hours or several days. It is not aggravated by physical activity. Chronic tension-type headache (CTTH) evolves from episodic tension-type headache and represents headache that occurs at least 15 days per month for at least 3 months.

Both central and peripheral mechanisms operate in causing tension headache. It is not a vascular headache. The central pain mechanism is associated with chronic tension headache and a peripheral mechanism with episodic tension headache. The central mechanism probably involves hypersensitivity of pain fibers from the trigeminal nerve that leads to central sensitization (see Chapter 15). The peripheral sensitization of myofascial sensory nerves may contribute to muscular hypersensitivity and the development of CTTH. Headache sufferers have more localized pain and tenderness of pericranial muscles. Many individuals have both tension-type and migraine headaches.

Mild tension-type headaches are treated with ice, and more severe forms are treated with aspirin or nonsteroidal antiinflammatory drugs. CTTHs are best managed with a tricyclic antidepressant and behavioral and relaxation therapy. Some individuals benefit from injection of botulinum toxin A. Long-term use of analgesics or other drugs, such as muscle relaxants, antihistamines, tranquilizers, caffeine, and ergot alkaloids, should be avoided.[53]

Infection and Inflammation of the Central Nervous System

The central nervous system (CNS) may be infected by bacteria, viruses, fungi, parasites, and mycobacteria. The invading organisms enter the nervous system either by spreading through arterial blood vessels or by directly invading the nervous tissue from another site of infection. Neurologic infections produce disease by several mechanisms: direct neuronal or glial infection, mass lesion formation, inflammation with subsequent edema, interruption of cerebrospinal fluid (CSF) pathways, neuronal or vascular damage, and secretion of neurotoxins. An immune process may initiate an inflammatory reaction.

Meningitis

Meningitis is inflammation of the brain or spinal cord. Infectious meningitis may be caused by bacteria, viruses, fungi, parasites, or toxins. The infection may be acute, subacute, or chronic, with the pathophysiology, clinical manifestations, and treatment differing for each type of microorganism.

Bacterial meningitis. Bacterial meningitis is primarily an infection of the pia mater and arachnoid villi, the subarachnoid space, the ventricular system, and the CSF. Meningococci (*Neisseria meningitidis*) and pneumococci (*Streptococcus pneumoniae*) are the most common pathogens in adults.[54]

With pneumococcal meningitis, young persons and those more than 40 years of age are mostly affected with outbreaks in dormitories or military bases. Predisposing conditions are otitis or sinusitis (25%), immunocompromised status (16%), and pneumonia (12%). The disease is spread by respiratory droplets and contact with contaminated saliva or respiratory tract secretions (kissing, coughing, sneezing, or sharing utensils, food, and drink). Carriers of the meningococcal bacteria do not develop meningitis but may pass it on to others.

Meningococci and pneumococci are inhaled and attach to epithelial cells in the nasopharynx, where they cross the mucosal barrier, enter the bloodstream, travel to cerebral blood vessels, cross the blood–brain barrier, and infect the meninges. With bacterial infection, large numbers of neutrophils are recruited to the subarachnoid space. Release of cytotoxic inflammatory agents and bacterial toxins alter the blood–brain barrier, causing cerebral edema and damaging brain tissue. The inflammatory exudate thickens the CSF and interferes with normal CSF flow around the brain and spinal cord, possibly obstructing arachnoid villi and producing hydrocephalus. Meningeal cells become edematous, and the combined exudate and edematous cells increase ICP. Engorged blood vessels and thrombi can disrupt blood flow, causing further injury.

The clinical manifestations of bacterial meningitis can be grouped into infectious signs, meningeal signs, and neurologic signs. The clinical manifestations of systemic infection include fever, tachycardia, and chills. The clinical manifestations of meningeal irritation are a severe throbbing headache, severe photophobia, nuchal rigidity, and positive Kernig and Brudzinski signs. The neurologic signs include a decrease in consciousness, cranial nerve palsies, focal neurologic deficits (e.g., hemiparesis/hemiplegia and ataxia), and seizures. Often there is projectile vomiting. As the ICP increases, papilledema develops and delirium may progress to unconsciousness and death. With meningococcal meningitis, a petechial or purpuric rash covers the skin and mucous membranes. A rare complication is acute infectious purpura fulminans. This is a rapidly progressive syndrome of hemorrhagic infarction of the skin and disseminated intravascular coagulation that can lead to multiple organ failure, ischemic necrosis of digits and limbs with amputation required, and death. It is caused by bacterial endotoxin and inflammatory cytokines.

Rapid diagnosis, antibiotic administration, and supportive treatment are important to prevent morbidity and mortality from bacterial meningitis. Diagnosis is based on physical examination, blood cultures, and the results of nasopharyngeal smear and antigen tests. CSF analysis and cultures are required for differential diagnosis. Serious complications, including septic shock, disseminated intravascular coagulation, purpura fulminans, limb damage, and multiple organ failure, require intensive multidisciplinary care. Vaccinations are available to prevent meningococcal, pneumococcal, and *Haemophilus influenzae* meningitis.[55]

Viral meningitis. Viral meningitis (aseptic meningitis) is thought to be limited to the meninges. An identifiable bacterium cannot be found in the CSF. The most common viruses are enteroviral viruses (echovirus, coxsackievirus, and nonparalytic poliomyelitis), arboviruses, and herpes simplex type 2. Viruses enter the nervous system by crossing the blood–brain barrier, by direct spread along peripheral nerves, or through the choroid plexus epithelium (Fig. 17.13). Recognition of viral antigens by immune cells activates the inflammatory response. The clinical manifestations of viral meningitis are similar to those of bacterial meningitis but milder. Viral meningitis is managed pharmacologically with antiviral drugs and steroids.

Fungal meningitis. Fungal meningitis is a chronic, much less common condition than bacterial or viral meningitis. The infection most often occurs in persons with impaired immune responses or alterations in normal body flora. It develops insidiously, usually over days or weeks. Fungi in the nervous system usually produce a granulomatous reaction, forming granulomata or gelatinous masses in the meninges at the base of the brain. Fungi also may extend along the perivascular sites in the subarachnoid space and into the brain tissue, producing arteritis with thrombosis, infarction, and communicating hydrocephalus. Meningeal fibrosis develops later in the inflammatory process. Cranial nerve dysfunction, caused by compression, often results from the granulomata and fibrosis. The first manifestations are often those of dementia (see Chapter 16) or communicating hydrocephalus (see Chapter 16). The individual is characteristically afebrile. Antifungal treatments are microorganism specific and effective.

Encephalitis

Encephalitis is an acute inflammation of the brain, usually of viral origin. The most common forms are caused by bites of mosquitos, ticks, or flies. Herpes simplex type 1 is the most common sporadic cause of encephalitis. Viruses infect specific cell types in the CNS, as shown in Fig. 17.13. Referred to as infectious viral encephalitides, encephalitis may occur as a complication of systemic viral diseases such as poliomyelitis, rabies, or mononucleosis, or it may arise after recovery from viral infections such as rubella, varicella, rubeola, or yellow fever. Encephalitis also may follow vaccination with a live attenuated virus vaccine if the vaccine has an encephalitis component (e.g., measles, mumps, and rubella). Typhus, trichinosis, malaria, and schistosomiasis also are associated with encephalitis.[56]

With the exception of California viral encephalitis, which is endemic, the arthropod-borne encephalitides occur in epidemics, varying in geographic and seasonal incidence (*Did You Know?* West Nile Virus). Eastern equine encephalitis is the most serious but least common of the encephalitides.

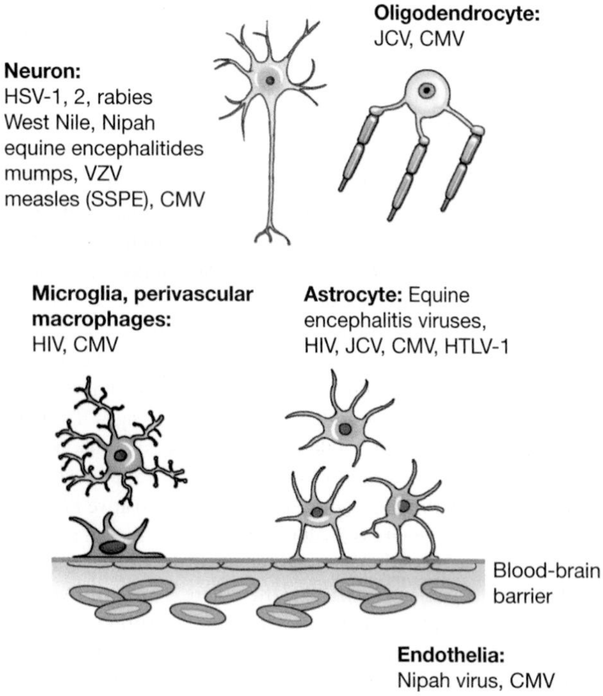

Neuron:
HSV-1, 2, rabies
West Nile, Nipah
equine encephalitides
mumps, VZV
measles (SSPE), CMV

Oligodendrocyte:
JCV, CMV

Microglia, perivascular macrophages:
HIV, CMV

Astrocyte: Equine encephalitis viruses, HIV, JCV, CMV, HTLV-1

Blood-brain barrier

Endothelia:
Nipah virus, CMV

FIGURE 17.13 Viral Infection in the Central Nervous System. Viruses infect specific cell types within the central nervous system (CNS), depending on the particular properties of the virus together with individual cell membrane proteins expressed on permissive cell types. Normally the brain is protected from circulating pathogens and toxins by the blood–brain barrier. *CMV,* Cytomegalovirus; *HIV,* human immunodeficiency virus; *HSV,* herpes simplex virus; *HTLV-1,* human T-cell lymphotropic virus (causes T-cell leukemia); *JCV,* John Cunningham virus (a polyomavirus causing progressive multifocal leukoencephalopathy); *SSPE,* subacute sclerosing panencephalitis; *VZV,* varicella-zoster virus. (Adapted from Power C, Noorbakhsh G: Central nervous system viral infections: clinical aspects and pathogenic mechanisms. In Gilman S, editor: *Neurobiology of disease,* p 488, Burlington, MA, 2007, Elsevier.)

DID YOU KNOW?

West Nile Virus

West Nile virus (WNV), a *Flavivirus* transmitted predominantly by the *Culex* mosquito, is the most common cause of epidemic meningoencephalitis in North America and the leading cause of arboviral encephalitis in the United States. Humans and horses, as well as other mammals, are incidental hosts. Birds and mosquitoes are life cycle hosts, and the greatest amount of virus is carried by mosquitos in early fall. WNV also can be transmitted through blood transfusions and organ transplants. Health experts think that transmission from mother to unborn child and through breast milk is possible.

The human incubation period is 2 to 14 days. Most individuals develop no symptoms. About 20% of those infected have mild symptoms that last 4 to 6 days and generally include fever, headache, skin rash, and lymphadenopathy. Less than 1% of affected persons develop severe illness, including WN encephalitis, marked by headache, disorientation, stupor, coma, seizures, and movement disorders, including tremor, ataxia, extrapyramidal signs, and paralysis. WN meningitis is characterized by meningeal signs of severe headache, high fever, and nuchal rigidity. Myelitis and polyradiculitis also may be present. Abnormalities in the thalamus, basal ganglia, and cerebellum are often seen on magnetic resonance imaging in people with severe infection. Identifiable risk factors are very young or advanced age, immunocompromise, and pregnancy.

A preliminary diagnosis is made if IgM for the virus is found in serum or cerebrospinal fluid. A rapid test became available in 2007. Plaque reduction neutralization assay (PRNA) is the confirmatory test. Treatment is supportive care. No West Nile vaccine has been developed for humans. Environmental control and prevention of mosquito bites is the best protection. Since 2003, all blood banks use blood-screening tests for WNV. There is a vaccine for horses, but there is not an approved vaccine for humans.

Data from Centers for Disease Control and Prevention (CDC): *West Nile virus,* updated August 7, 2018, available at: https://www.cdc.gov/westnile/; Ronca SE, Murray KO, Nolan MS: *Emerg Infect Dis* 25(2):325-327, 2019.

PATHOPHYSIOLOGY Viruses gain access to the CNS through the bloodstream, olfactory bulb, or choroid plexus, or from peripheral nerves. Meningeal involvement is present in all encephalitides. The various encephalitides may cause widespread nerve cell degeneration. Edema, necrosis with or without hemorrhage, and IICP develop.

CINICAL MANIFESTATIONS Encephalitis ranges from a mild infectious disease to a life-threatening disorder. Mild symptoms include malaise, headache, body aches, nausea, and vomiting. Dramatic clinical manifestations include fever, difficulty with word finding, seizure activity, cranial nerve palsies, paresis and paralysis, involuntary movement, abnormal reflexes, and delirium or confusion progressing to unconsciousness. Signs of marked ICP may be present.

EVALUATION AND TREATMENT Diagnosis is made by the history and clinical presentation, aided by CSF examination and culture, serologic studies, white blood cell count, CT scan, or magnetic resonance imaging (MRI). Empirical treatment is specific to the type of virus and may include antiviral agents, antibiotics, and steroids. Herpes encephalitis is treated with antiviral agents, such as acyclovir. Measures to control the ICP are paramount.

Brain or Spinal Cord Abscess

Abscesses are localized collections of pus within the parenchyma of the brain or spinal cord and are rare. Immunosuppressed persons are particularly at risk.

Brain abscesses are classified as epidural, subdural, or intracerebral. *Epidural brain abscesses (empyemas)* are associated with osteomyelitis in a cranial bone. *Subdural brain abscesses* (empyemas) arise from a sinus infection or a vascular source. *Intracerebral brain abscesses* arise from a vascular source. Spinal cord abscesses are very rare and classified as epidural or intramedullary (within the spinal cord). Epidural spinal abscesses usually originate as osteomyelitis in a vertebra; the infection then spreads into the epidural space. (Osteomyelitis is discussed in Chapter 41.)

PATHOPHYSIOLOGY Microorganisms gain entrance to the CNS by direct extension or distribution along the wall of a vein. Infective emboli carry organisms from distant sites. Illegal drug users who share needles are at risk, as are immunosuppressed persons. For example, *Toxoplasma gondii* is producing an ever-increasing number of CNS abscesses in persons with acquired immunodeficiency syndrome (AIDS).[57] Streptococci, staphylococci, and *Bacteroides sp.*, often combined with anaerobes, are the most common bacteria that cause abscesses; however, yeast and fungi also may be involved.

Brain abscesses progress from localized inflammation to a necrotic core with the formation of a connective tissue capsule, usually within 14 days or longer.[58] Existing abscesses also tend to spread and form daughter abscesses.

CINICAL MANIFESTATIONS Early manifestations include low-grade fever, headache (most common symptom), nausea and vomiting, neck pain and stiffness, confusion, drowsiness, sensory deficits, and communication deficits. Later manifestations are associated with an expanding mass and include decreased attention span, memory deficits, decreased visual acuity and narrowed visual fields, papilledema, ocular palsy, ataxia, dementia, and seizures. The development of symptoms may be very insidious, often making an abscess difficult to diagnose.

Extradural brain abscesses are associated with localized pain, purulent drainage from the nasal passages or auditory canal, fever, localized tenderness, and neck stiffness. Clinical manifestations of spinal cord abscesses have four stages: (1) spinal aching; (2) severe root pain, accompanied by spasms of the back muscles and limited vertebral movement; (3) weakness caused by progressive cord compression; and (4) paralysis.

EVALUATION AND TREATMENT The diagnosis is suggested by clinical features and confirmed by imaging studies. Antibiotics and surgical aspiration or excision are usually indicated. The ICP may have to be managed. Spinal cord abscesses are treated with surgical decompression or aspiration, antibiotic therapy, and supportive therapy.

Neurologic Complications of Acquired Immunodeficiency Syndrome

The most common neurologic complication associated with AIDS is human immunodeficiency virus–associated neurocognitive disorder (HAND), a range of disorders that includes mild neurocognitive disorder and HIV-associated dementia, which is rare. Combined antiretroviral therapy (cART) with more efficient CNS drug penetration has reduced the prevalence and improved survival for individuals with HAND. Milder forms of the disease may persist because of longer life and the ability of the virus to survive within brain tissue in some individuals.

The onset of clinical manifestations includes neurocognitive impairment, behavioral disturbance, and motor abnormalities. Specific manifestations can include an organic psychosis with agitation, inappropriate behavior, and hallucinosis. Motor signs can include difficulty speaking, progressive loss of balance, gait disturbances, or paralysis. Diagnosis is difficult during early stages of manifestations. CSF analysis and imaging help establish the diagnosis. HIV antiretroviral treatment improves survival for individuals with severe HAND but does not reverse the impairment.[59]

Demyelinating Disorders

Demyelinating disorders are the result of damage to the myelin nerve sheath and affect neural transmission. They can occur in either the central (i.e., multiple sclerosis) or the peripheral (i.e., Guillain-Barré syndrome) nervous system. Contributing factors include genetics, infections, autoimmune reactions, environmental toxins, and unknown factors.

Multiple Sclerosis

Multiple sclerosis (MS) is a chronic immune-mediated inflammatory disease involving degeneration of CNS myelin, scarring (sclerosis or plaque formation), and loss of axons. The etiology of MS is unknown. The onset of MS is usually between 20 and 40 years of age and is more common in women. Men may have a more severe progressive course. The prevalence rate is higher in northern latitudes. Inconclusive risk factors that may be involved include environmental factors, such as smoking; vitamin D deficiency; obesity; infection, including Epstein-Barr virus infection; and genetic factors.[60]

PATHOPHYSIOLOGY MS is a diffuse and progressive CNS autoimmune inflammatory disease that affects white and gray matter throughout the brain and spinal cord. There are multiple focal areas of myelin loss within the CNS called *plaques*. The plaques form when autoreactive T and B cells cross the blood–brain barrier and attack myelin, triggering release of inflammatory mediators and loss of oligodendrocytes (myelin-producing cells). Activation of glia cells (brain macrophages) contributes to inflammation and injury. Loss of myelin disrupts nerve conduction, with subsequent death of neurons and brain atrophy. Normal-appearing white matter can be microscopically very abnormal, and gray matter lesions and atrophy have been documented during later stages of the disease process.[61] These degenerative processes begin before symptom onset and can progress throughout a person's life (Fig. 17.14). *Spinal*

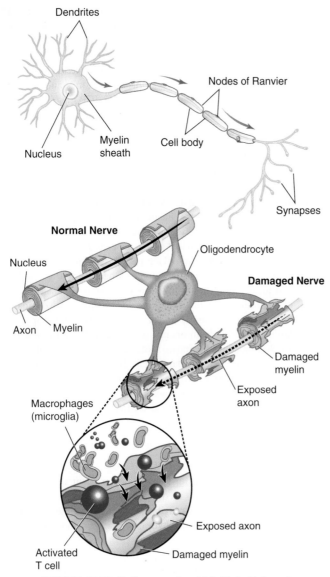

FIGURE 17.14 Pathogenesis of Multiple Sclerosis.

MS can occur concurrently with or independently of brain lesions. The multifocal, multistage features of MS lesions produce symptoms that are multiple and variable.

CINICAL MANIFESTATIONS The most common initial symptoms of MS are paresthesias of the face, trunk, or limbs; weakness; impaired gait; or urinary incontinence, indicating diffuse CNS involvement. Visual impairment is associated with optic neuritis. Cerebellar and corticospinal involvement presents as nystagmus, ataxia, and weakness, with all four limbs involved. Intention tremor and slurred speech may also occur.

The onset, duration, and severity of symptoms are different for each person. Disease exacerbations (also known as *relapses* or *flares*) are the temporary occurrence or worsening of symptoms. The symptoms may be mild or serious, may last for several days or weeks, and may be followed by progressive symptoms, including include paresthesias, difficulty speaking, ataxia, or visual changes. The mechanism of these exacerbations is related to delayed or blocked conduction caused by inflammation and demyelination. Various events can occur immediately before the exacerbation of symptoms and are regarded as precipitating

factors or triggers, including trauma, emotional stress, and pregnancy. Painful sensory events, spastic paralysis, and bowel and bladder incontinence are common with spinal involvement.[62] Recovery from symptoms during remissions is caused by down-regulation of inflammation and the restoration of axonal function, either by remyelination, the resolution of inflammation, or the restoration of conduction to demyelinated axons.

The subtypes of MS are based on the clinical course and are summarized in Table 17.9. A *clinically isolated syndrome* of neurologic symptoms that lasts 24 hours or less may initially occur. It can be related to inflammation and demyelination but may never progress to develop into multiple sclerosis. Most persons present with a remitting-relapsing course and without treatment transition to the progressive types with insidious neurologic decline that occurs over years. Early cognitive changes are common and may include poor judgment, apathy, emotional lability, and depression.

EVALUATION AND TREATMENT There is no single test available to diagnose or rule out MS. Diagnostic criteria include the history, clinical examination in combination with MRI (most sensitive test), CSF findings, and evoked potentials.[63] Persistently elevated levels of CSF immunoglobulin G (IgG) are found in about two-thirds of individuals with MS, and oligoclonal IgG bands on electrophoresis are found in more than 90% of individuals with MS. Evoked potential studies aid diagnosis by detecting decreased conduction velocity in visual, auditory, and somatosensory pathways. MRI is the most sensitive available method of detecting demyelinated plaques and monitoring disease.

The treatment goal in MS is prevention of exacerbations, prevention of permanent neurologic damage, and control of symptoms. Disease-modifying drugs are initiated with diagnosis and include corticosteroids, immunosuppressants, and immune system modulators.[64] Continuous monitoring is important because of the increased risk for infection when taking these drugs. Plasma exchange may be used in persons who do not respond to steroids. Drugs are also available for symptom control. The long-term benefit of these drugs is under investigation.[65] Supportive care includes participation in a regular exercise program, cessation of smoking, and avoidance of overwork, extreme fatigue, and heat exposure. The administration of vitamin D to prevent disease progression is being evaluated, but a recent report found no therapeutic effect.[66] Stem cell therapy is under investigation.[67]

Guillain-Barré Syndrome

Guillain-Barré syndrome is a rare demyelinating disorder caused by a humoral and cell-mediated immunologic reaction directed at the peripheral nerves. It usually occurs after a respiratory tract or gastrointestinal infection. The clinical manifestations can vary from tingling and weakness to paralysis of the legs or complete quadriplegia, respiratory insufficiency, and autonomic nervous system instability. Intravenous immunoglobulin or plasmapheresis is used during the acute phase and followed by aggressive rehabilitation.[68] Recovery occurs within weeks to months or up to 2 years. About 30% of individuals have residual weakness.

✔ **QUICK CHECK 17.3**
1. What are two differences between the symptoms of migraine and cluster headaches?
2. How can bacterial meningitis lead to an amputation?
3. How are macrophages involved in the neurologic complications of HIV infection.
4. What are the autoimmune mechanisms that cause MS lesions?

TABLE 17.9   Types of Multiple Sclerosis

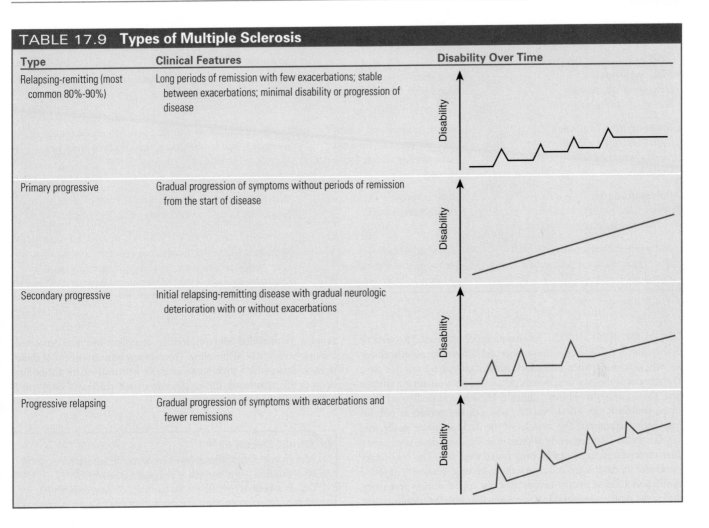

Type	Clinical Features	Disability Over Time
Relapsing-remitting (most common 80%-90%)	Long periods of remission with few exacerbations; stable between exacerbations; minimal disability or progression of disease	
Primary progressive	Gradual progression of symptoms without periods of remission from the start of disease	
Secondary progressive	Initial relapsing-remitting disease with gradual neurologic deterioration with or without exacerbations	
Progressive relapsing	Gradual progression of symptoms with exacerbations and fewer remissions	

PERIPHERAL NERVOUS SYSTEM AND NEUROMUSCULAR JUNCTION DISORDERS

Peripheral Nervous System Disorders

The peripheral nervous system is composed of motor anterior horn cells fibers, sensory dorsal root ganglia fibers, and peripheral autonomic ganglia and their axons. Acute or chronic disease processes, inflammation, or trauma may injure these peripheral nerves and cause a neuropathy. Mononeuropathies affect a single nerve. Multiple mononeuropathies (multiplex) involve two or more individual nerves. Polyneuropathy is generalized involvement of peripheral nerves that is usually bilateral and symmetrical and can involve motor, sensory, and autonomic nerves simultaneously. Autonomic neuropathies involve the autonomic nervous system. Examples of peripheral neuropathies are summarized in Table 17.10. Neuropathic pain is reviewed in Chapter 15.

Neuromuscular Junction Disorders

Transmission of the nerve impulse at the neuromuscular junction requires the release of adequate amounts of neurotransmitter from the presynaptic terminals of the axon and effective binding of the released transmitter to the receptors on the membranes of muscle cells (see Fig. 14.14). Botulism food poisoning results from the botulinum neurotoxin released from *Clostridium botulinum*. The toxin inhibits the release of acetylcholine at the myoneural junction and causes flaccid paralysis. Myasthenia gravis is the most prevalent of the neuromuscular junction disorders and is presented next.

Myasthenia Gravis

Myasthenia gravis (MG) is an acquired chronic autoimmune disease mediated by antibodies against the acetylcholine receptor (AChR) at the postsynaptic membrane of the neuromuscular junction. The disease is rare and more common in women. Thymic tumors, pathologic changes in the thymus, and other autoimmune diseases are associated with the disorder. (Autoimmune mechanisms are discussed in Chapter 8.) Ocular myasthenia is more common in males, involves weakness of the eye muscles and eyelids, and may include swallowing difficulties and slurred speech.

PATHOPHYSIOLOGY   MG results from a defect in nerve impulse transmission at the neuromuscular junction. The postsynaptic AChRs on the muscle cell's plasma membrane are no longer recognized as "self" and elicit T-cell–dependent formation of IgG autoantibodies. The autoantibodies fix onto AChR sites, blocking the binding of acetylcholine. Eventually the antibody action destroys receptor sites. This loss of AChR sites causes diminished transmission of the nerve impulse across the neuromuscular junction and decreased muscle depolarization. Symptomatic individuals without anti-AChR antibodies may have antibodies against muscle-specific kinase (MuSK), an enzyme required for maintenance of the neuromuscular junction, with similar symptoms. Why this autosensitization occurs is unknown. Thymomas occur in about half of MG cases. It is thought they are associated with loss of self-tolerance, but the actual mechanism is unknown.[69]

TABLE 17.10	**Types of Peripheral Neuropathies**	
Type	**Cause**	**Example**
Mononeuropathy Motor: weakness, paralysis Sensory: numbness, pain	Trauma, compression, infection, inflammation, tumor	Sciatica, carpel tunnel syndrome, radial nerve palsy, facial palsy
Mononeuritis Multiplex Motor: weakness, paralysis Sensory: numbness, pain Patchy distribution involving two or more nerves	Metabolic (hyperglycemia, toxins), connective tissue (autoimmune mechanisms) or vascular (hypoxemia) disorders	Usually associated with systemic disease: diabetes mellitus, vasculitis, lupus erythematosus; radiculopathies (spinal nerve roots), and nerve plexus injury
Polyneuropathy Affects sensory, motor and autonomic nerves simultaneously in a symmetric distribution	Systemic metabolic, toxic, autoimmune and infectious diseases	Hyperglycemia, uremia, alcoholism, chemotherapy, Guillain-Barré syndrome, human immunodeficiency virus (HIV) infection
Autonomic Neuropathy Affects sympathetic and parasympathetic nerve fibers	Usually associated with systemic disease: i.e., diabetes mellitus, vasculitis, lupus erythematosus	Alterations in heart rate, blood pressure (dizziness, fainting), bladder function (incontinence or urinary retention). gastrointestinal function (diarrhea or constipation) or thermal regulation

CINICAL MANIFESTATIONS MG has an insidious onset. The variable distribution of AChR sites or the number and different forms of antibodies may determine when and which muscle groups are affected first. The muscles of the eyes, face, mouth, throat, and neck usually are affected first. There can be drooling and difficulty chewing and swallowing food. These problems can affect nutrition and put the person at risk for respiratory aspiration. The muscles of the neck, shoulder girdle, and hip flexors are less frequently affected, but muscle fatigue is common after exercise and there can be progressive weakness. The respiratory muscles of the diaphragm and chest wall can become weak, with impaired ventilation. Clinical manifestations may first appear during pregnancy, during the postpartum period, or in conjunction with the administration of certain anesthetic agents. The progression of MG varies; it appears first as a mild case that spontaneously remits, with a series of relapses and symptom-free intervals ranging from weeks to months. Over time, the disease can progress. Myasthenic crisis can develop as the disease progresses; this occurs when severe muscle weakness causes extreme quadriparesis or quadriplegia, respiratory insufficiency with shortness of breath, and extreme difficulty in swallowing. The individual in myasthenic crisis is in danger of respiratory arrest.

Cholinergic crisis may arise from anticholinesterase drug toxicity with increased intestinal motility, episodes of diarrhea and complaints of intestinal cramping, bradycardia, pupillary constriction, increased salivation, and diaphoresis. These symptoms are caused by the smooth muscle hyperactivity secondary to excessive accumulation of acetylcholine at the neuromuscular junctions and excessive parasympathetic-like activity. As in myasthenic crisis, the individual is in danger of respiratory arrest.

EVALUATION AND TREATMENT The diagnosis of MG is made on the basis of a response to edrophonium chloride (Tensilon, an acetyl-cholinesterase inhibitor), results of electromyographic (EMG) studies, and detection of antibodies. With the intravenous administration of the drug, immediate demonstrable improvement in muscle strength usually persists for several minutes. Imaging helps to determine whether a thymoma is present. Current treatments for MG have improved the prognosis, including in those who have ocular myasthenia.

Anticholinesterase drugs, steroids, and immunosuppressant drugs (e.g., azathioprine and cyclosporine) are used to treat MG and prevent myasthenic crisis. For individuals with cholinergic crisis, anticholinergic drugs are withheld until blood levels are nontoxic; in addition, ventilatory support is provided and respiratory complications are prevented. Plasmapheresis may be lifesaving. Thymectomy is the treatment of choice in individuals with a thymoma and those with anti-AChR antibodies, because this terminates the production of self-reactive T cells and B cells that produce the antibodies.[70]

QUICK CHECK 17.4
1. What symptoms would differentiate a mononeuropathy from a polyneuropathy?
2. What would be a manifestation of an autonomic neuropathy?
3. Why do antibodies contribute to the weakness of myasthenia gravis?

TUMORS OF THE CENTRAL NERVOUS SYSTEM

CNS tumors include both brain and spinal cord tumors. Primary CNS tumors had an estimated 23,880 new cases and 16,830 deaths in the United States in 2018.[71] The incidence of CNS tumors increases to age 70 years and then decreases. CNS tumors are the second most common group of tumors occurring in children. Approximately 70% to 75% of all intracranial tumors in children are located infratentorially (see Chapter 18), and in adults 70% are located supratentorially. Peripheral nerve tumors are rare in children and common in adults. Carcinogenesis is discussed in Chapter 11, pituitary tumors are discussed in Chapter 20, and cerebral tumors in children are discussed in Chapter 18.

Brain Tumors

Tumors within the cranium can be either primary or metastatic. *Primary brain tumors* originate from brain substance, including neuroglia, neurons, cells of blood vessels, and connective tissue. *Extracerebral tumors* originate outside substances of the brain and include meningiomas, acoustic nerve tumors, and tumors of the pituitary and pineal glands. *Metastatic (secondary) brain tumors* are the most prevalent and arise in organ systems outside the brain and spread to the brain. Sites of intracranial tumors are illustrated in Fig. 17.15.

Local effects of cranial tumors are caused by the destructive action of the tumor itself on a particular site in the brain and by compression, causing decreased cerebral blood flow. Generalized effects result from IICP caused by growth of the tumor, obstruction of the ventricular system, hemorrhages in and around the tumor, or cerebral edema

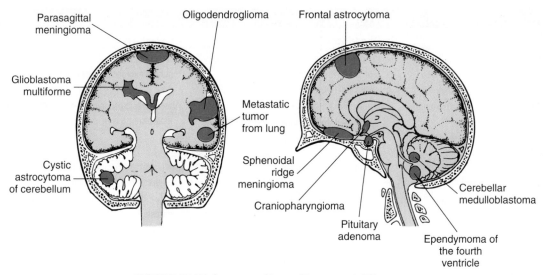

FIGURE 17.15 Common Sites of Intracranial Tumors.

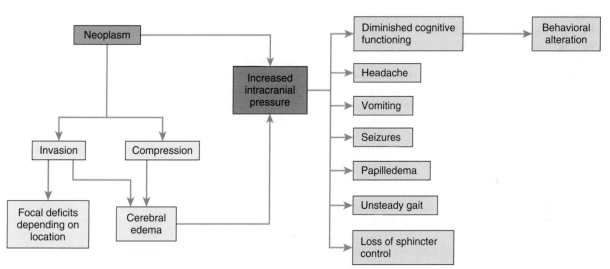

FIGURE 17.16 Origin of Clinical Manifestations Associated With an Intracranial Neoplasm.

(Fig. 17.16). Manifestations include headache, seizures, visual disturbances, unstable gait, and cranial nerve dysfunction.

Intracranial brain tumors do not metastasize as readily as tumors in other organs because there are no lymphatic channels within the brain substance. If metastasis does occur, it is usually through seeding of cerebral blood or CSF during cranial surgery or through artificial shunts.

Primary Brain (Intracerebral) Tumors

Primary brain (intracerebral) tumors, also called gliomas (cells that support brain neurons), include astrocytomas, oligodendrogliomas, glioblastoma multiforme, and ependymomas. They account for about 2% of all cancers in the United States. The etiology for primary brain tumors is not clearly known. Ionizing radiation is the only known environmental risk factor.

Surgical or radiosurgical excision, surgical decompression, chemotherapy, radiotherapy, and hyperthermia are treatment options for these tumors. Supportive treatment is directed at reducing edema. New treatment options are emerging. (Cancer treatment is discussed in Chapter 11.)

Astrocytoma. Astrocytomas are the most common glioma (about 75% of all tumors of the brain and spinal cord).[71] The World Health Organization (WHO) divides astrocytomas into four grades based on histopathologic features, cellular density, atypia, mitotic activity, microvascular proliferation, and necrosis (Table 17.11). Grades I and II are generally benign or slow growing and most common in children. They can progress to a higher grade. Grades III and IV are faster-growing malignant tumors. They may occur anywhere in the brain or spinal cord and are generally located in the cerebrum, hypothalamus, or pons. Low-grade astrocytomas tend to be located laterally or supratentorially in adults and in a midline or near-midline position in children.

Headache (caused by pressure on blood vessels and meninges) and subtle neurobehavioral changes may be early signs. Other neurologic symptoms evolve slowly, and IICP occurs late in the tumor's course. Onset of a focal seizure disorder between the second and sixth decades of life suggests an astrocytoma. Low-grade astrocytomas are treated with surgery or by external radiation. About 50% of persons survive 5 years when surgery is followed by radiation therapy (RT).[71,72]

Grades III and IV astrocytomas are found predominantly in the frontal lobes and cerebral hemispheres, although they may occur in the

TABLE 17.11 Grades of Astrocytomas

Grade*	Type	Description	Characteristics
I	Pilocytic astrocytoma	Common in children and young adults and people with neurofibromatosis type 1; common in cerebellum	Least malignant, well differentiated; grows slowly; near-normal microscopic appearance, noninfiltrating
II	Diffuse, low-grade astrocytoma (fibrillary, gemistocytic, protoplasmic) Oligodendroglioma	Common in young adults; more common in cerebrum but can occur in any part of brain	Abnormal microscopic appearance; grows slowly; infiltrates to adjacent tissue; may recur at higher grade
III	Anaplastic (malignant) astrocytoma Anaplastic oligodendroglioma	Common in young adults	Malignant; many cells undergoing mitosis; infiltrates adjacent tissue; frequently recurs at higher grade
IV	Glioblastoma (glioblastoma multiforme)	Common in older adults, particularly men Predominant in cerebral hemispheres	Poorly differentiated; increased number of cells undergoing mitosis; bizarre microscopic appearance; widely infiltrates; neovascularization; central necrosis.

*World Health Organization grading system for central nervous system tumors.
Data from American Brain Tumor Association: *About brain tumors: a primer for patients and care givers,* Chicago IL, 2015, Author, available at: http://www.abta.org/secure/about-brain-tumors-a-primer.pdf.

brainstem, cerebellum, and spinal cord. Men are twice as likely to have astrocytomas as women; in the 15- to 34-year-old age group they are the third most common brain cancer, whereas in the 35- to 54-year-old age group they are the fourth most common.

A Grade IV astrocytoma, known as **glioblastoma multiforme (GBM)**, is the most lethal and common type of primary brain tumor. They are highly vascular and extensively irregular and infiltrative, making them difficult to remove surgically. Fifty percent of glioblastomas are bilateral or at least occupy more than one lobe at the time of death. The typical clinical presentation for a glioblastoma multiforme is that of diffuse, nonspecific clinical signs, such as headache, irritability, and "personality changes," that progress to more clear-cut manifestations of increased intracranial pressure, including headache on position change, papilledema, vomiting, or seizure activity. Symptoms may progress to include definite focal signs, such as hemiparesis, dysphasia, dyspraxia, cranial nerve palsies, and visual field deficits.

Higher-grade astrocytomas are treated surgically and with radiotherapy and chemotherapy. Recurrence is common, and survival time is less than 5 years for grade III and IV tumors. Bevacizumab is an antiangiogenic monoclonal antibody that has been approved for the treatment of recurrent GBM in the USA and Canada.[73]

Oligodendroglioma. Oligodendrogliomas constitute about 2% of all brain tumors and 10% to 15% of all gliomas. They are typically slow-growing, low-grade tumors (grade II). Most oligodendrogliomas are macroscopically indistinguishable from other gliomas and may be a mixed type of oligodendroglioma and astrocytoma. Most are found in the frontal and temporal lobes, often in the deep white matter, but they can be found in other parts of the brain and spinal cord. Malignant degeneration occurs in approximately one-third of affected persons. These tumors are known as *anaplastic oligodendrogliomas* (grade III).

More than 50% of individuals experience a focal or generalized seizure as the first clinical manifestation. Only half of those with an oligodendroglioma have IICP at the time of diagnosis and surgery, and only one-third develop focal manifestations. Treatment includes surgery, radiotherapy, and chemotherapy or combination therapy.[74]

Ependymoma. Ependymomas are nonencapsulated gliomas that arise from ependymal cells. They are rare in adults, usually occurring in the spinal cord.[75] However, in children ependymomas are typically located in the brain. They constitute about 1.9% of all primary brain tumors in adults, about 4% in children, and 5.7% in adolescents. Approximately 70% of these tumors occur in the fourth ventricle, with others found in the third and lateral ventricles and posterior portion of the spinal cord. Approximately 40% of infratentorial (cerebellum) ependymomas occur in children younger than 10 years. Cerebral (supratentorial) ependymomas occur at all ages.

Fourth ventricle ependymomas present with difficulty in balance, unsteady gait, uncoordinated muscle movement, and difficulty with fine motor movement. The clinical manifestations of a lateral and third ventricle ependymoma that involves the cerebral hemispheres are seizures, visual changes, and hemiparesis. Blockage of the CSF pathway produces hydrocephalus and presents with headache, nausea, and vomiting.

The interval between first manifestations and surgery may be as short as 4 weeks or as long as 7 or 8 years. Ependymomas are treated with radiotherapy, radiosurgery, and chemotherapy. Overall, about 84% of persons survive 5 years.[76]

Primary Extracerebral Tumors

Meningioma. Meningiomas constitute about a third of all intracranial tumors, and only 1% are malignant. Most occur in adults age 65 years or older.[77] These tumors usually originate from the arachnoidal (meningeal) cells in the dura mater and rarely from arachnoid cells of the choroid plexus of the ventricles. Meningiomas are located most commonly in the olfactory grooves, on the wings of the sphenoid bone (at the base of the skull), in the tuberculum sellae (next to the sella turcica), on the superior surface of the cerebellum, and in the cerebellopontine angle and spinal cord. Rarely, they can involve the optic nerve sheath, with loss of visual acuity. The cause of meningiomas is unknown.

A meningioma is sharply circumscribed and adapts to the shape it occupies. It may extend to the dural surface and erode the cranial bones or produce an osteoblastic reaction. Meningiomas are slow growing, and clinical manifestations occur when they reach a certain size and begin to press on the brain tissue. Focal seizures are often the first manifestation, and IICP is less common than with gliomas.

There is a 20% recurrence rate, even with complete surgical excision. If only partial resection is possible, the tumor recurs. Radiation therapies also are used to slow growth.

Nerve sheath tumors. Neurofibromas (benign nerve sheath tumors) are a group of autosomal dominant disorders of the nervous system. They include neurofibromatosis type 1, previously known as von Recklinghausen disease, and neurofibromatosis type 2. The two types are also known as *peripheral* and *central neurofibromatosis,* respectively.

Neurofibromatosis type 1 (NF1) is the most prevalent with an incidence of about 1 in 3500 people. *Neurofibromin 1 (NF1)* is a gene that encodes the protein neurofibromin, a tumor suppressor (prevents cells from growing and dividing too rapidly), primarily in adult neurons. Mutations of *NF1* cause multiple cutaneous neurofibromas, cutaneous macular lesions (café-au-lait spots and freckles). Less commonly, there are bone and soft tissue tumors. Inactivation of the *NF1* gene results in loss of function of neurofibromin in Schwann cells (produce the myelin sheath around axons) and promotes tumorigenesis (neurofibromas). Cognitive and learning disabilities are present in about 50% of affected individuals.[78]

Neurofibromatosis type 2 (NF2) is rare and occurs in about 1 in 40,000 to 60,000 people. The *neurofibromin 2 (NF2)* gene product is neurofibromin 2 or merlin, a tumor-suppressor protein that inhibits cell growth. Mutations promote development of CNS tumors, particularly schwannomas, although other tumor types can occur (meningiomas, ependymomas, astrocytomas, and neurofibromas). Schwannomas of the vestibular nerves present with hearing loss and deafness. Other symptoms may include loss of balance and dizziness. Schwannomas also may develop in other cranial, spinal, and peripheral nerves. In these cases, cutaneous signs are less prominent.

Genetic testing is available for the management of families susceptible to neurofibromas, and prenatal diagnosis is possible. Diagnosis is based on clinical manifestations and neuroimaging studies, and diagnostic criteria have been established for NF1.[79] Surgery is the major treatment. Individuals with NF2 have extensive morbidity and reduced life expectancy, particularly with early age of onset. Genetically tailored drugs are likely to provide personalized therapy for both of these devastating conditions.

Metastatic brain tumors. Metastatic brain tumors from systemic cancers are 10 times more common than primary brain tumors, and about 20% to 40% of persons with cancer have metastasis to the brain.[80] Common primary sites include the lung, breast, and skin (e.g., melanomas). Metastasis to the brain is thought to be through vascular channels (see Chapter 11).

Metastatic brain tumors produce signs resembling those of glioblastomas, although several unusual syndromes do exist. Carcinomatous (metastatic cancer) encephalopathy causes headache, nervousness, depression, trembling, confusion, forgetfulness, and gait disorder. In carcinomatosis of the cerebellum, headache, dizziness, and ataxia are found. Carcinomatosis of the craniospinal meninges (also called *carcinomatous meningitis*) manifests with headache, confusion, and symptoms of cranial or spinal nerve root dysfunction. Metastatic brain tumors carry a poor prognosis. Treatment is guided by the pathology of the original tumor; the number, size, and location of the brain metastasis; and prior cancer treatments. With the development of new drugs that cross the blood–brain barrier, chemotherapy and immunotherapy are increasingly recommended.[81] Survival time is about 1 year.

Spinal Cord Tumors

Primary spinal cord tumors are rare and represent about 2% of CNS tumors. They may be extramedullary extradural, intradural

extramedullary, or intradural intramedullary. Intramedullary tumors, originate within the neural tissues of the spinal cord. Extramedullary tumors originate from tissues outside the spinal cord. Intramedullary tumors are primarily gliomas (astrocytomas and ependymomas). Gliomas are difficult to resect completely, and radiotherapy is required. Spinal ependymomas may be completely resected and are more common in adults. Extramedullary tumors are either peripheral nerve sheath tumors (neurofibromas or schwannomas) or meningiomas. Neurofibromas are generally found in the thoracic and lumbar region, whereas meningiomas are more evenly distributed through the spine. Complete resection of these tumors can be curative.

Metastatic spinal cord tumors are usually carcinomas (i.e., from breast, lung, or prostate cancer), lymphomas, or myelomas. Their location is often extradural, the cancer having proliferated to the spine through direct extension from tumors of the vertebral structures or from extraspinal sources extending through the interventricular foramen or bloodstream.

PATHOPHYSIOLOGY   Intramedullary spinal cord tumors produce dysfunction by both invasion and compression. Extramedullary spinal cord tumors produce dysfunction by compressing adjacent tissue, not by direct invasion. Metastases from spinal cord tumors occur from direct extension or seeding through the CSF or bloodstream.

CINICAL MANIFESTATIONS   An acute onset of clinical manifestations suggests a vascular occlusion of vessels supplying the spinal cord, whereas gradual and progressive symptoms suggest compression. The compressive syndrome (sensorimotor syndrome) involves both the anterior and the posterior spinal tracts, and motor function and sensory function are affected as the tumor grows. Pain is usually a presenting symptom.

The irritative syndrome (radicular syndrome) combines the clinical manifestations of a cord compression with radicular pain that occurs in the sensory root distribution and indicates root irritation. The segmental manifestations include segmental sensory changes, such as paresthesias and impaired pain and touch perception; motor disturbances, including cramps, atrophy, fasciculations, and decreased or absent deep tendon reflexes; and continuous spinal pain.

EVALUATION AND TREATMENT   The diagnosis of a spinal cord tumor is made through imaging techniques, CT-guided needle biopsy, or open biopsy. Involvement of specific cord segments is established. Any metastases also are identified. Treatment varies, depending on the nature of the tumor and the person's clinical status, but surgery is essential for all spinal cord tumors.[82]

✔ QUICK CHECK 17.3
1. What is the difference between a primary and a metastatic brain tumor?
2. What is an astrocytoma?
3. What are some common signs and symptoms of compressive and irritative spinal cord tumor syndromes?

SUMMARY REVIEW

Central Nervous System Disorders

1. Traumatic brain injury (TBI) is an alteration in brain function caused by an external force. The most common causes of TBI are falls, unintentional blunt trauma, and motor vehicle accidents. TBI is classified as primary or secondary.

2. Primary brain injury is caused by direct impact and involves neural injury, primary glial injury, and vascular responses. Primary brain injuries can be focal (involving only one area of the brain) or diffuse (involving more than one area of the brain).

3. Causes of focal brain injury include closed (blunt) trauma or open (penetrating) trauma.

4. Closed trauma is more common and involves the head striking a surface or an object striking the head. These injuries include contusion, extradural hematoma, subdural hematoma, and intracerebral hematoma. Injury may be caused by coup or contrecoup injury or both.

5. Open brain injury involves a skull fracture with exposure of the cranial vault to the environment, and may result from compound skull fractures and missile injuries. Open brain injury can produce both focal and diffuse injuries.

6. Diffuse brain injury (diffuse axonal injury) results from shearing forces that result in axonal damage. Diffuse brain injury is seen clinically as coma lasting 6 or more hours following TBI.

7. Secondary brain injury develops from systemic and intracranial responses to primary brain trauma that result in further brain injury and neuronal death.

8. Categories of TBI are mild, moderate, and severe and are based on the Glasgow Coma Scale (GCS), duration of loss of consciousness, posttraumatic amnesia, and brain imaging results.

9. Complications of TBI include postconcussion syndrome, posttraumatic seizures, and chronic traumatic encephalopathy.

10. Spinal cord and vertebral injury involves damage to neural tissues by compressing tissue, pulling or exerting tension on tissue, or shearing tissues so that they slide into one another. Vertebral fracture occurs with direct or indirect trauma.

11. Spinal cord injury involves primary and secondary injury similar to the processes of traumatic brain injury.

12. Spinal cord injury may cause spinal shock with temporary cessation of all motor, sensory, reflex, and autonomic functions below the lesion. Spinal shock generally lasts 2 to 3 days.

13. Neurogenic shock (vasogenic shock) is caused by loss of sympathetic nerve activity and occurs with cervical or upper thoracic cord injury (above T6) and can occur concurrently with spinal shock. Symptoms include vasodilation, hypotension, bradycardia, and loss of temperature control.

14. Loss of motor and sensory function depends on the extent and level of injury. Paralysis of the lower half of the body with both legs involved is called paraplegia. Paralysis involving all four extremities is called quadriplegia.

15. Return of spinal neuron excitability occurs slowly. Spasticity and hyperreflexia are common.

16. Autonomic hyperreflexia (dysreflexia) is a syndrome of sudden, massive reflex sympathetic discharge associated with spinal cord injury at level T6 or above. Flexor spasms are accompanied by severe hypertension, a pounding headache, blurred vision, profuse sweating, nasal congestion, nausea, piloerection, and bradycardia. Autonomic hyperreflexia requires emergency medical management.

17. Degenerative disorders of the spine include low back pain, degenerative joint disease, and herniated intervertebral disk.

18. Low back pain is pain between the lower rib cage and gluteal muscles and often radiates into the thigh. Common causes of chronic low back pain include degenerative disk disease, spondylolysis, spondylolisthesis, spinal osteochondrosis, spinal stenosis, and lumbar disk herniation. Other causes are tension, inflammation, referred pain, and bone diseases.

19. Degenerative joint disease includes degenerative disk disease, spondylolysis, spondylolisthesis, and spinal stenosis.

20. Degenerative disk disease is an alteration in intervertebral disk tissue and can be related to normal aging, inflammation, and compression.

21. Spondylolysis is a structural defect of the spine with displacement of the vertebra.

22. Spondylolisthesis involves forward slippage of the vertebra and can include a crack or fracture of the pars interarticularis, usually at the L5-S1 vertebrae.

23. Spinal stenosis is a narrowing of the spinal canal that causes pressure on the spinal nerves or cord.

24. Herniation of an intervertebral disk is a protrusion of part of the nucleus pulposus. Herniation most commonly affects the lumbosacral disks (L5-S1 and L4-L5). The extruded pulposus compresses the nerve root, causing pain that radiates along the sciatic nerve course.

25. Cerebrovascular disease is the most frequently occurring neurologic disorder and is any abnormality of the brain caused by a pathologic process in the blood vessels The brain abnormalities seen with cerebrovascular disease are either ischemia (with or without infarction) or hemorrhage.

26. Cerebrovascular accidents (stroke syndromes) are a common clinical manifestation of cerebrovascular disease. Strokes are classified pathophysiologically as ischemic or hemorrhagic (intracranial hemorrhage).

27. Ischemic stroke occurs when there is obstruction to arterial blood flow to the brain from thrombus formation (thrombotic stroke), an embolus (embolic stroke), or hypoperfusion related to decreased blood volume or heart failure (hemodynamic stroke). The inadequate blood supply results in ischemia and can progress to infarction.

28. Transient ischemic attacks (TIAs) are temporary decreases in brain blood flow with an increased risk of stroke.

29. Lacunar strokes are caused by ischemia from occlusion of a small vessel deep in the brain.

30. Hemorrhagic strokes occur within brain tissue (intracerebral) or in the subarachnoid or subdural space. The primary cause of intracerebral hemorrhagic stroke is chronic hypertension.

31. Intracranial aneurysms result from defects in the vascular wall and are classified on the basis of form and shape. They are often asymptomatic, but the signs vary depending on the location and size of the aneurysm. They are a cause of subarachnoid hemorrhage.

32. A subarachnoid hemorrhage occurs when blood escapes from defective or injured vasculature into the subarachnoid space. When a vessel tears, blood under pressure is pumped into the subarachnoid space. The blood produces an inflammatory reaction in these tissues and increased intracranial pressure.

33. An arteriovenous malformation (AVM) is a mass of dilated blood vessels. Although usually present at birth, symptoms are delayed and usually occur before age 30.

34. Headache is a common neurologic disorder and is usually a benign symptom. Chronic recurring headaches include migraine, cluster, and tension headaches.

35. Migraine headache is an episodic headache lasting 4 to 72 hours that can be associated with triggers, and may have an aura associated with a cortical spreading depression that alters cortical blood flow. Pain is related to overactivity in the trigeminal vascular system.

36. Cluster headaches are a group of disorders known as trigeminal autonomic cephalalgias and occur primarily in men. They occur in clusters over a period of days with extreme pain intensity and short duration, and are associated with trigeminal nerve activation.

37. Tension-type headache is the most common recurrent headache. Episodic-type headaches involve a peripheral pain mechanism, and the chronic type involves a central pain mechanism and may be related to hypersensitivity of pain fibers from the trigeminal nerve.

38. Infection and inflammation of the CNS can be caused by bacteria, viruses, fungi, parasites, and mycobacteria.

39. Meningitis is inflammation of the brain or spinal cord and is classified as bacterial (i.e., meningococci), aseptic (viral or nonpurulent), or fungal. Bacterial meningitis primarily is an infection of the pia mater, the arachnoid, and the fluid of the subarachnoid space. Viral (aseptic) meningitis is thought to be limited to the meninges. Fungal meningitis is a chronic, less common type of meningitis.

40. Encephalitis is an acute inflammation of the brain, usually of viral origin. The most common forms are caused by bites of mosquitos, ticks, or flies and by and herpes simplex type 1. Meningeal involvement appears in all encephalitides. Herpes encephalitis is treated with antiviral agents.

41. Brain or spinal cord abscesses often originate from infections outside the CNS. Microorganisms gain access to the CNS from adjacent sites or spread along the wall of a vein. Brain abscesses progress from localized inflammation to a necrotic core with the formation of a connective tissue capsule, usually within 14 days or longer.

42. The common neurologic complication of AIDS is HIV-associated neurocognitive disorder, a range of disorders that includes mild neurocognitive disorder and HIV-associated dementia. The onset of clinical manifestations includes neurocognitive impairment, behavioral disturbance, and motor abnormalities.

43. Demyelinating disorders are the result of damage to the myelin nerve sheath that can occur in either the central (i.e., multiple sclerosis) or the peripheral (i.e., Guillain-Barré syndrome) nervous system.

44. Multiple sclerosis (MS) is a chronic immune-mediated inflammatory demyelinating disorder with scarring (sclerosis) and loss of axons. The pathogenesis is unknown. Demyelination is associated with plaque formation.

45. Guillain-Barré syndrome is a rare demyelinating disorder caused by a humoral and cell-mediated immunologic reaction directed at the peripheral nerves usually following an infection.

Peripheral Nervous System and Neuromuscular Junction Disorders

1. Injury to peripheral nerves by disease processes, inflammation, or trauma can cause a neuropathy. Neuropathies can be mononeuropathies (affecting a single nerve), multiple mononeuropathies (involving two or more individual nerves), polyneuropathy (generalized involvement of peripheral nerves), or autonomic neuropathies (involving the nervous system).

2. The most prevalent neuromuscular junction disorder is myasthenia gravis, which is a disorder of voluntary muscles characterized by muscle weakness and fatigability. It is considered an autoimmune disease and is associated with an increased incidence of other autoimmune diseases.

3. Myasthenia gravis results from a defect in nerve impulse transmission at the neuromuscular junction. Antibody action destroys the receptor sites, causing decreased transmission of the nerve impulse across the neuromuscular junction.

Tumors of the Central Nervous System

1. Tumors within the cranium can be primary intracerebral, primary extracerebral, or metastatic (secondary).

2. Primary intracerebral tumors originate from brain substance and include astrocytomas, oligodendrogliomas, glioblastoma multiforme, and ependymomas.

3. Extracerebral tumors originate outside of the substances of the brain and include meningiomas and nerve sheath tumors.

4. Metastatic tumors arise in organ systems outside the brain and spread to the brain. Common primary sites include lung, breast, skin, kidney, and colorectal areas.

5. Brain tumors cause local and generalized manifestations. Manifestations include headache, seizures, visual disturbances, unstable gain, and cranial nerve dysfunction.

6. Spinal cord tumors are classified as intramedullary tumors (within the neural tissues) or extramedullary tumors (outside the spinal cord). Metastatic spinal cord tumors are usually carcinomas, lymphomas, or myelomas.

7. Intramedullary spinal cord tumors produce dysfunction by both invasion and compression. Extramedullary spinal cord tumors produce dysfunction by compression of adjacent tissue, not by direct invasion.

KEY TERMS

REFERENCES

1. Centers for Disease Control and Prevention (CDC), National Center for Injury Prevention and Control: Traumatic brain injury in the United States: get the facts; updated April 27, 2017. Available at: https://www.cdc.gov/traumaticbraininjury/get_the_facts.html.

2. Edwards P, et al: Final results of MRC CRASH, a randomised placebo-controlled trial of intravenous corticosteroid in adults with head injury—outcomes at 6 months, *Lancet* 365(9475):1957-1959, 2005.

3. Zakaria Z, et al: Extradural haematoma—to evacuate or not? Revisiting treatment guidelines, *Clin Neurol Neurosurg* 115(8):1201-1205, 2013.

4. Vega RA, Valadka AB: Natural history of acute subdural hematoma, *Neurosurg Clin North Am* 28(2):247-255, 2017.

5. Karibe H, et al: Surgical management of traumatic acute subdural hematoma in adults: a review, *Neurol Med Chir (Tokyo)* 54(11):887-894, 2014.

6. Vieira RC, et al: Diffuse axonal injury: epidemiology, outcome and associated risk factors, *Front Neurol* 7:178, 2016.

7. McKee AC, Daneshvar DH: The neuropathology of traumatic brain injury, *Handb Clin Neurol* 127:45-66, 2015.

8. Desai M, Jain A: Neuroprotection in traumatic brain injury, *J Neurosurg Sci* 62(5):563-573, 2018.

9. Curtis L, Epstein P: Nutritional treatment for acute and chronic traumatic brain injury patients, *J Neurosurg Sci* 58(3):151-160, 2014.

10. Centers for Disease Control and Prevention (CDC): Traumatic brain injury and concussion, severe TBI; Last reviewed April 2, 2019. Available at: https://www.cdc.gov/traumaticbraininjury/severe.html.

11. Voelker R: Taking a closer look at the biomarker test for mild traumatic brain injury, *J Am Med Assoc* 319(20):2066-2067, 2018.

12. Hoshide R, et al: Do corticosteroids play a role in the management of traumatic brain injury?, *Surg Neurol Int* 7:84, 2016.

13. Centers for Disease Control and Prevention (CDC): Traumatic brain injury and concussion: Updated mild traumatic brain injury guideline for adults; Last reviewed March 6, 2019. Available at: https://www.cdc.gov/traumaticbraininjury/mtbi_guideline.html.

14. Brain Trauma Foundation: Guidelines for the acute medical management of severe traumatic brain injury in infants, children, and adolescents—second edition, *Pediatr Crit Care Med* 13(1):S1-S82, 2012. Available at: https://www.cns.org/sites/default/files/guideline-pdf/guidelines_pediatric2_0.pdf.

15. Ontario Neurotrauma Foundation: Guidelines for diagnosing and managing pediatric concussion, ed 1, Toronto, 2014, Author. Available at: http://onf.org/system/attachments/266/original/GUIDELINES_for_Diagnosing_and_Managing_Pediatric_Concussion_Recommendations_for_HCPs__v1.1.pdf.

16. McCrory P, et al: Consensus statement on concussion in sport—the 5(th) International Conference on Concussion in Sport held in Berlin, October 2016, *Br J Sports Med* 51(11):838-847, 2017. Available at: https://bjsm.bmj.com/content/early/2017/04/26/bjsports-2017-097699.

17. Saletti PG, et al: In search of antiepileptogenic treatments for post-traumatic epilepsy, *Neurobiol Dis* 123:86-99, 2019.

18. Willis MD, Robertson NP: Chronic traumatic encephalopathy: identifying those at risk and understanding pathogenesis, *J Neurol* 264(6):1298-1300, 2017.

19. National Spinal Cord Injury Statistical Center: Spinal cord injury facts and figures at a glance. Available at: https://www.nscisc.uab.edu/Public/Facts%20and%20Figures%20-%202018.pdf. (Accessed 18 July 2018).

20. Ahuja CS, et al: Traumatic spinal cord injury-repair and regeneration, *Neurosurgery* 80(3S):S9-S22, 2017.

21. Hou S, Rabchevsky AG: Autonomic consequences of spinal cord injury, *Compr Physiol* 4(4):1419-1453, 2014.

22. Hachem LD, Ahuja CS, Fehlings MG: Assessment and management of acute spinal cord injury: from point of injury to rehabilitation, *J Spinal Cord Med* 40(6):665-675, 2017.

23. Kim YH, Ha KY, Kim SI: Spinal cord injury and related clinical trials, *Clin Orthop Surg* 9(1):1-9, 2017.

24. National Institute of Neurological Disorders and Stroke: Low back pain fact sheet; Last updated July 6, 2018. Available at: https://www.ninds.nih.gov/Disorders/Patient-Caregiver-Education/Fact-Sheets/Low-Back-Pain-Fact-Sheet.

25. Ito K, Creemers L: Mechanisms of intervertebral disk degeneration/injury and pain: a review, *Global Spine J* 3(3):145-152, 2013.

26. U.S. Department of Veterans Affairs: BA/DoD clinical practice guidelines: diagnosis and treatment of low back pain (LBP) (2017). Available at: https://www.healthquality.va.gov/guidelines/pain/lbp/.

27. Dowdell J, et al: Intervertebral disk degeneration and repair, *Neurosurgery* 80(3S):S46-S54, 2017.

28. Kreiner DS, et al: An evidence-based clinical guideline for the diagnosis and treatment of lumbar disc herniation with radiculopathy, *Spine J* 14(1):180-191, 2014.

29. Korse NS, et al: The long term outcome of micturition, defecation and sexual function after spinal surgery for cauda equina syndrome, *PLoS ONE* 12(4):e0175987, 2017.

30. Benjamin EJ, et al: Heart disease and stroke statistics-2018 update: a report from the American Heart Association, *Circulation* 137(12):e67-e492, 2018.

31. Wardlaw JM, et al: Lacunar stroke is associated with diffuse blood-brain barrier dysfunction, *Ann Neurol* 65(2):194-202, 2009.

32. Yaghi S, et al: Treatment and outcome of hemorrhagic transformation after intravenous alteplase in acute ischemic stroke: a scientific statement for healthcare professionals from the American Heart Association/American Stroke Association, *Stroke* 48(12):e343-e361, 2017.

33. Pare JR, Kahn JH: Basic neuroanatomy and stroke syndromes, *Emerg Med Clin North Am* 30(3):601-615, 2012.

34. Rangel-Castilla L, et al: Endovascular intracranial treatment of acute ischemic strokes, *J Cardiovasc Surg (Torino)* 57(1):36-47, 2016.

35. Powers WJ, et al: 2018 guidelines for the early management of patients with acute ischemic stroke: a guideline for healthcare professionals from the American Heart Association/American Stroke Association, *Stroke* 49(3):e46-e110, 2018. Available at: http://stroke.ahajournals.org/content/early/2018/01/23/STR.0000000000000158.

36. Bushnell C, et al: Guidelines for the prevention of stroke in women: a statement for healthcare professionals from the American Heart Association/American Stroke Association, *Stroke* 45(5):1545-1588, 2014. Available at: http://stroke.ahajournals.org/content/early/2014/02/06/01.str.0000442009.06663.48.

37. Burns JD, Fisher JL, Cervantes-Arslanian AM: Recent advances in the acute management of intracerebral hemorrhage, *Neurosurg Clin N Am* 29(2):263-272, 2018.

38. Sadasivan C, et al: Physical factors effecting cerebral aneurysm pathophysiology, *Ann Biomed Eng* 41(7):1347-1365, 2013.

39. Grasso G, Alafaci C, Macdonald RL: Management of aneurysmal subarachnoid hemorrhage: state of the art and future perspectives, *Surg Neurol Int* 8:11, 2017.

40. Budohoski KP, et al: Clinical relevance of cerebral autoregulation following subarachnoid haemorrhage, *Nat Rev Neurol* 9(3):152-163, 2013.

41. Foreman B: The pathophysiology of delayed cerebral ischemia, *J Clin Neurophysiol* 33(3):174-182, 2016.

42. Cavanaugh SJ, Gordon VL: Grading scales used in the management of aneurismal subarachnoid hemorrhage: a critical review, *J Neurosci Nurs* 34:288-295, 2002.

43. Novakovic RL, et al: The diagnosis and management of brain arteriovenous malformations, *Neurol Clin* 31(3):749-763, 2013.

44. Narayanan M, Atwal GS, Nakaji P: Multimodality management of cerebral arteriovenous malformations, *Handb Clin Neurol* 143:85-96, 2017.

45. Onderwater GLJ, et al: Primary headaches, *Handb Clin Neurol* 146:267-284, 2017.

46. International Headache Society (IHS): HIS classification ICHD-II 1. *The international classification of headache disorders. In:* Migraine, ed 3. Available at: http://ihs-classification.org/en/02_klassifikation/02_teil1/01.00.00_migraine.html. (Accessed 19 July 2018).

47. Migraine Research Foundation: Migraine fact sheet. Available at: www.migraineresearchfoundation.org/fact-sheet.html. (Accessed 19 July 2018).

48. Pavlović JM: Evaluation and management of migraine in midlife women, *Menopause* 25(8):927-929, 2018.

49. Dodick DW: A phase-by-phase review of migraine pathophysiology, *Headache* 58(Suppl 1):4-16, 2018.

50. Grimsrud KW, Halker Singh RB: Emerging treatments in episodic migraine, *Curr Pain Headache Rep* 22(9):61, 2018.

51. U.S. Food and Drug Administration (US FDA): FDA news release: FDA allows marketing of first medical device to prevent migraine headaches; March 11 2014. Available at: www.fda.gov/newsevents/newsroom/pressannouncements/ucm388765.htm.

52. Doesborg P, Haan J: Cluster headache: new targets and options for treatment, *F1000 Res* 7:339, 2018.

53. Barbanti P, et al: Treatment of tension-type headache: from old myths to modern concepts, *Neurol Sci* 35(Suppl 1):17-21, 2014.

54. Centers for Disease Control and Prevention (CDC): Meningitis, chapter 2: epidemiology of meningitis caused by *Neisseria meningitidis*, *Streptococcus pneumoniae*, and *Haemophilus influenza*; Last updated March 15, 2012. Available at: https://www.cdc.gov/meningitis/lab-manual/chpt02-epi.html.

55. Centers for Disease Control and Prevention (CDC): Vaccines and immunization; Last updated April 23,

2018. Available at: https://www.cdc.gov/vaccines/index.html.

56. Rust RS: Human arboviral encephalitis, *Semin Pediatr Neurol* 19(3):130-151, 2012.

57. Wang ZD, et al: Prevalence and burden of Toxoplasma gondii infection in HIV-infected people: a systematic review and meta-analysis, *Lancet HIV* 4(4):e177-e188, 2017.

58. Alvis Miranda H, et al: Brain abscess: current management, *J Neurosci Rural Pract* 4(Suppl 1):S67-S81, 2013.

59. Eggers C, et al: HIV-1-associated neurocognitive disorder: epidemiology, pathogenesis, diagnosis, and treatment, *J Neurol* 264(8):1715-1727, 2017.

60. Tarlinton RE, et al: The interaction between viral and environmental risk factors in the pathogenesis of multiple sclerosis, *Int J Mol Sci* 20(2):2019.

61. Mallucci G, et al: The role of immune cells, glia and neurons in white and gray matter pathology in multiple sclerosis, *Prog Neurobiol* 127-128:1-22, 2015.

62. Ciccarelli O, et al: Spinal cord involvement in multiple sclerosis and neuromyelitis optica spectrum disorders, *Lancet Neurol* 18(2):185-197, 2019.

63. Thompson AJ, et al: Diagnosis of multiple sclerosis: 2017 revisions of the McDonald criteria, *Lancet Neurol* 17(2):162-173, 2018.

64. Dargahi N, et al: Multiple sclerosis: immunopathology and treatment update, *Brain Sci* 7(7):2017.

65. Wingerchuk DM, Carter JL: Multiple sclerosis: current and emerging disease-modifying therapies and treatment strategies, *Mayo Clin Proc* 89(2):225-240, 2014.

66. Zheng C, et al: The efficacy of vitamin D in multiple sclerosis: a meta-analysis, *Mult Scler Relat Disord* 23:56-61, 2018.

67. National Institutes of Health (NIH), Northwestern University: *Stem cell therapy for patients with multiple sclerosis failing alternate approved therapy—a randomized study. In* Clinical Trials.gov. [Verified July 2018.] Available from: http://clinicaltrials.gov/ct2/show/NCT00273364.

68. Verboon C, van Doorn PA, Jacobs BC: Treatment dilemmas in Guillain-Barré syndrome, *J Neurol Neurosurg Psychiatry* 88(4):346-352, 2017.

69. Cacho-Díaz B, et al: Myasthenia gravis as a prognostic marker in patients with thymoma, *J Thorac Dis* 10(5):2842-2848, 2018.

70. Kim H, et al: Factors predicting remission in thymectomized patients with acetylcholine receptor antibody-positive myasthenia gravis, *Muscle Nerve* 58(6):796-800, 2018.

71. American Cancer Society (ACS): Cancer facts & figures 2018, Atlanta, 2018, Author. Available at: https://www.cancer.org/content/dam/cancer-org/research/cancer-facts-and-statistics/annual-cancer-facts-and-figures/2018/cancer-facts-and-figures-2018.pdf. (Accessed July 2018).

72. Grier JT, Batchelor T: Low grade gliomas in adults, *Oncologist* 11:681-693, 2006.

73. Polivka J, Jr, et al: Advances in experimental targeted therapy and immunotherapy for patients with glioblastoma multiforme, *Anticancer Res* 37(1):21-33, 2017.

74. Simonetti G, et al: Clinical management of grade III oligodendroglioma, *Cancer Manag Res* 7:213-223, 2015.

75. Gerstner ER, Pajtler KW: Ependymoma, *Semin Neurol* 38(1):104-111, 2018.

76. Collaborative Ependymoma Research Network: Ependymoma statistics; Revised August 2016. Available at: http://www.cern-foundation.org/education/ependymoma-basics/ependymoma-statistics.

77. Cancer Net: Meningioma guide; July, 2017. Available at: https://www.cancer.net/cancer-types/meningioma/introduction.

78. Vogel AC, Gutmann DH, Morris SM: Neurodevelopmental disorders in children with neurofibromatosis type 1, *Dev Med Child Neurol* 59(11):1112-1116, 2017.

79. DeBella K, et al: Use of the National Institutes of Health criteria for diagnosis of neurofibromatosis 1 in children, *Pediatrics* 105(3 Pt 1):608-614, 2000.

80. Ostrom QT, Wright CH, Barnholtz-Sloan JS: Brain metastases: epidemiology, *Handb Clin Neurol* 149:27-42, 2018.

81. Kotecha R, et al: Recent advances in managing brain metastasis, *F1000Res* 7:2018.

82. Tredway TL: Minimally invasive approaches for the treatment of intramedullary spinal tumors, *Neurosurg Clin North Am* 25(2):327-336, 2014.

18

Alterations of Neurologic Function in Children

Russell J. Butterfield, Sue E. Huether

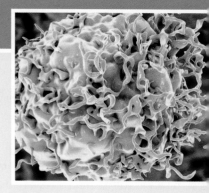

EVOLVE WEBSITE

http://evolve.elsevier.com/Huether/
Student Review Questions
Audio Key Points

Case Studies
Animations
Quick Check Answers

CHAPTER OUTLINE

Neurologic disorders in children can occur from infancy through adolescence and include congenital malformations, genetic defects in metabolism, brain injuries, infection, tumors, and other disorders that affect neurologic function.

DEVELOPMENT OF THE NERVOUS SYSTEM IN CHILDREN

The nervous system develops from the embryonic ectoderm through a complex, sequential process that begins on about day 40 of gestation from the formation of the neural tube. By about day 175, the brain has developed into all of its parts (Fig. 18.1). The brain continues the formation of network connections and synapses from birth to many years postnatally. Many different events happen simultaneously, and critical periods must pass uninterrupted if the vulnerable fetus is to develop normally. Genetic and environmental factors (e.g., nutrition, hormones, oxygen levels, toxins, alcohol, drugs, maternal infections, maternal disease) can have a significant effect on neural development[1,2] (see *Did You Know?* Alcohol-Related Neurodevelopmental Disorder [ARND]).

The growth and development of the brain occur rapidly from the third month of gestation through the first year of life, reflecting the proliferation of neurons and glial cells. Although basically all of the neurons that an individual will ever have are present at birth, development of skills, such as walking, talking, and thinking, depends on these cells making correct connections with other cells and on myelination of the axons making those connections. The head is the fastest-growing body

DID YOU KNOW?
Alcohol-Related Neurodevelopmental Disorder

Alcohol-related neurodevelopment disorder (ARND) is a type of alcohol spectrum disorder with long-lasting neurobehavioral and cognitive deficiencies as a result of fetal alcohol exposure. It is among the most common causes of mental deficits that persist throughout adulthood. ARND is 100% preventable, and there is no known amount of alcohol that is safe to consume while pregnant. The prevalence of ARND has been reported as 1.1% to 5%. Alcohol crosses the placenta and the blood–brain barrier and exerts teratogenic effects on the developing brain throughout fetal development. Alcohol exposure during the first trimester can lead to fetal brain volume reduction and can be related to apoptosis, neurodegeneration, and suppression of neurogenesis. Diagnosis of ARND includes prenatal and/or postnatal growth retardation, facial dysmorphology, central nervous system dysfunction, and neurobehavioral disabilities. Screening, education, and prevention programs are critical for promoting alcohol-free pregnancies.

Data from May PA et al: *J Am Med Assoc* 319(5):474-482, 2018; Hoyme HE et al: *Pediatrics* 138(2):pii: e20154256, 2016; Nakhoul MR et al: *J Alcohol Drug Depend* 5(1):pii: 257, 2017.

part during infancy. One-half of postnatal brain growth is achieved by the first year and is 90% complete by age 6 years. The cortex thickens with maturation, and the sulci deepen as a result of rapid expansion of the surface area of the brain. Cerebral blood flow and oxygen consumption during these years are about twice those of the adult brain.

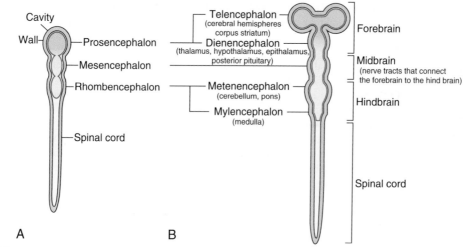

FIGURE 18.1 Development of the Brain and Spinal Cord. A, The anterior part of the neural tube enlarges to form the three primary vesicles of the brain. The narrow posterior part forms the spinal cord. **B,** Primary and secondary vesicles develop into various parts of the brain.

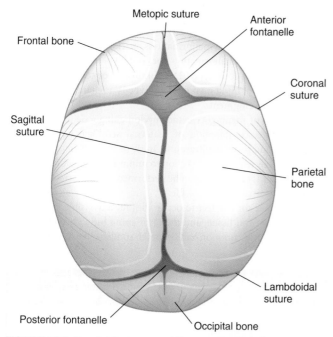

FIGURE 18.2 Cranial Sutures and Fontanelles in Infancy. Fibrous union of the suture lines and interlocking of the serrated edges occurs by 6 months; solid union requires approximately 12 years. (Head growth charts are available from the Centers for Disease Control and Prevention at www.cdc.gov/nchs/data/series/sr_11/sr11_246.pdf.)

TABLE 18.1	Reflexes of Infancy	
Reflex	**Age of Appearance**	**Age at Which Reflex Should No Longer Be Obtainable**
Moro	Birth	3 months
Stepping	Birth	6 weeks
Sucking	Birth	4 months awake 7 months asleep
Rooting	Birth	4 months awake 7 months asleep
Palmar grasp	Birth	6 months
Plantar grasp	Birth	10 months
Tonic neck	2 months	5 months
Neck righting	4 to 6 months	24 months
Landau	3 months	24 months
Parachute reaction	9 months	Persists indefinitely

The bones of the infant's skull are separated at the suture lines, forming two **fontanelles**, or "soft spots": one diamond-shaped anterior fontanelle and one triangular-shaped posterior fontanelle. The sutures allow for expansion of the rapidly growing brain. The posterior fontanelle may be open until 2 to 3 months of age; the anterior fontanelle normally does not fully close until 18 months of age (Fig. 18.2). Head growth almost always reflects brain growth. Monitoring the fontanelles and careful measurement and plotting of the head circumference on standardized growth charts are essential elements of the pediatric examination

Because of the immaturity of much of the human forebrain at birth, neurologic examination of the infant detects mostly reflex responses that require an intact spinal cord and brainstem. Absence of expected reflex responses at the appropriate age indicates general depression of central or peripheral motor functions. Asymmetric responses may indicate lesions in the motor cortex or peripheral nerves or may occur with fractures of bones after traumatic delivery or postnatal injury. As cerebral cortical function matures, the neonatal reflexes disappear in a predictable order as voluntary motor functions supersede them (Table 18.1). Abnormal persistence of these reflexes is seen in infants with developmental delays or with central motor lesions.

> ✓ **QUICK CHECK 18.1**
> 1. When does development of the brain begin?
> 2. What is a major function of the fontanelles?
> 3. Why do many of the reflexes of infancy disappear by 1 year of age?

STRUCTURAL MALFORMATIONS

Central nervous system (CNS) malformations are responsible for 75% of fetal deaths and 40% of deaths during the first year of life. CNS malformations account for 33% of all apparent congenital malformations, and 90% of CNS malformations are defects of neural tube closure.

Defects of Neural Tube Closure

Neural tube defects (NTDs) are an arrest of the normal development of the brain and spinal cord during the first month of embryonic development. They occur in about 4000 pregnancies in the United States each year, although there are significant regional prevalence variations.[3] Fetal death often occurs in the more severe forms, thereby reducing the actual prevalence of neural defects at birth.

The cause of neural tube defects is believed to be multifactorial (a combination of genes and environment). No single gene has been found to cause neural tube defects.[4] Folic acid deficiency during preconception and early stages of pregnancy increases the risk for neural tube defects, and supplementation (400 mcg of folic acid per day) ensures adequate folate status. Other risk factors include a previous NTD pregnancy, maternal diabetes or obesity, use of anticonvulsant drugs (particularly valproic acid), and maternal hyperthermia.[5,6]

Defects of neural tube closure are divided into two categories: (1) anterior midline defects (ventral induction) and (2) posterior defects (dorsal induction). Anterior midline defects may cause brain and face abnormalities, with the most extreme form being cyclopia, in which the child has a single midline orbit and eye with a protruding noselike proboscis above the orbit. Spina bifida (split spine) is the most common neural tube defect. Vertebrae fail to close in spina bifida, and the defect includes anencephaly (an, "without"; enkephalos, "brain"), encephalocele, meningocele, myelomeningocele, and spina bifida occulta. Disorders of embryonic neural development are summarized in Fig. 18.3.

Anencephaly is an anomaly in which the soft, bony component of the skull and part of the brain are missing. This disorder occurs in approximately 1206 pregnancies in the United States each year.[7] These infants are stillborn or die within a few days after birth. The pathologic mechanism is unknown. Diagnosis is often made prenatally by using ultrasound or evaluating the maternal serum alpha fetoprotein (AFP).

Encephalocele refers to a herniation or protrusion of the brain and meninges through a defect in the skull, resulting in a saclike structure. The incidence is approximately 1 in 12,200 live births (340 babies) in the United States each year.[8]

Meningocele is a saclike cyst of meninges filled with spinal fluid and is a mild form of spina bifida (Fig. 18.4). It develops during the first 4 weeks of pregnancy when the neural tube fails to close completely. The cystic dilation of meninges protrudes through the vertebral defect but does not involve the spinal cord or nerve roots and may produce no neurologic deficit or symptoms. Meningoceles occur with equal frequency in the cervical, thoracic, and lumbar spine areas.

Myelomeningocele (meningomyelocele; spina bifida cystica) is a hernial protrusion of a saclike cyst (containing meninges, spinal fluid, and a portion of the spinal cord with its nerves) through a defect in the posterior arch of a vertebra. It is most commonly located in the lumbar and lumbosacral regions, the last regions of the neural tube to close. Myelomeningocele is one of the most common developmental anomalies of the nervous system, with an incidence rate ranging from 0.5 to 1 per 1000 pregnancies.[9]

Meningocele and myelomeningoceles are evident at birth as a pronounced skin defect on the infant's back (see Fig. 18.4). The bony prominences of the unfused neural arches can be palpated at the lateral border of the defect. The defect usually is covered by a transparent membrane that may have neural tissue attached to its inner surface. This membrane may be intact at birth or may leak cerebrospinal fluid (CSF), thereby increasing the risks of infection and neuronal damage.

The spinal cord and nerve roots are malformed below the level of the lesion, resulting in loss of motor, sensory, reflex, and autonomic

functions. A brief neurologic examination concentrating on motor function in the legs, reflexes, and sphincter tone is usually sufficient to determine the level above which spinal cord and nerve root function is preserved (Table 18.2). This is useful to predict if the child will ambulate, require bladder catheterization, or be at high risk for developing scoliosis (see Chapter 42).

Hydrocephalus occurs in 85% of infants with myelomeningocele.[10] Seizures also occur in 30% of those with myelodysplasia. Visual and perceptual problems, including ocular palsies, astigmatism, and visuoperceptual deficits, are common. Motor and sensory functions below the level of the lesions are altered. Often these problems worsen as the child grows and the cord ascends within the vertebral canal, pulling primary scar tissue and tethering the cord.[11] Several musculoskeletal deformities are related to this diagnosis, as are spinal deformities.

Myelomeningoceles are almost always associated with the Chiari II malformation (Arnold-Chiari malformation).[10] This is a complex malformation of the brainstem and cerebellum in which the cerebellar tonsils are displaced downward into the cervical spinal canal. The upper medulla and lower pons are elongated and thin, and the medulla is also displaced downward and sometimes has a "kink" (Fig. 18.5). The Chiari II malformation is associated with hydrocephalus from pressure that blocks the flow of cerebrospinal fluid; syringomyelia, an abnormality causing cysts at multiple levels within the spinal cord; and cognitive and motor deficits.

Other types of Chiari malformations are not associated with spina bifida. Type I Chiari malformation does not involve the brainstem and may be asymptomatic. In type III, the brainstem or cerebellum extends into a high cervical myelomeningocele. Type IV is characterized by lack of cerebellar development.

Most cases of meningocele and myelomeningocele are diagnosed prenatally by a combination of maternal serologic testing (alpha fetoprotein) and prenatal ultrasound. In these cases, the fetus is usually delivered by elective cesarean section to minimize trauma during labor. Surgical repair is critical and can be performed by in utero fetal surgery or during the first 72 hours of life.[12,13]

It is possible for a defect to occur without any visible exposure of meninges or neural tissue, and the term spina bifida occulta is then used. The defect is common and occurs to some degree in 10% to 25%

TABLE 18.2 Functional Alterations in Myelomeningocele Related to Level of Lesion

Level of Lesion	Functional Implications
Thoracic	Flaccid paralysis of lower extremities; variable weakness in abdominal trunk musculature; high thoracic level may mean respiratory compromise; absence of bowel and bladder control
High lumbar	Voluntary hip flexion and adduction; flaccid paralysis of knees, ankles, and feet; may walk with extensive braces and crutches; absence of bowel and bladder control
Mid lumbar	Strong hip flexion and adduction; fair knee extension; flaccid paralysis of ankles and feet; absence of bowel and bladder control
Low lumbar	Strong hip flexion, extension, and adduction and knee extension; weak ankle and toe mobility; may have limited bowel and bladder function
Sacral	Normal function of lower extremities; normal bowel and bladder function

Modified from Sandler AD: *Pediatr Clin North Am* 57(4):879-892, 2010.

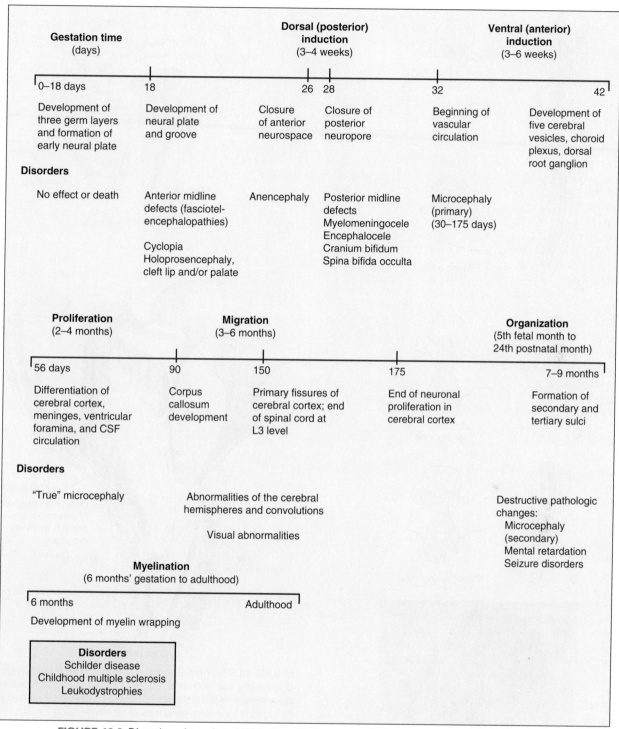

FIGURE 18.3 Disorders Associated With Specific Stages of Embryonic Development. *CSF,* Cerebrospinal fluid.

of infants. Spina bifida occulta usually causes no neurologic dysfunction because the spinal cord and spinal nerves are normal. A sacral dimple on examination of a newborn infant can be associated with spina bifida occulta and can be evaluated with ultrasound. Tethered cord syndrome may develop after surgical correction for myelomeningocele. The cord becomes abnormally attached or tethered as a result of scar tissue as the cord transcends the vertebral canal with growth.[14] The cord can be untethered surgically.

Craniosynostosis

Skull malformations range from minor, insignificant defects to major defects that are incompatible with life. Craniosynostosis (craniostenosis) is the premature closure of one or more of the cranial sutures (sagittal, coronal, lambdoid, metopic) during the first 18 to 20 months of the infant's life. The incidence of craniosynostosis is about 4 per 10,000 live births.[15] Males are affected twice as often as females. Fusion of a cranial suture prevents growth of the skull perpendicular to the

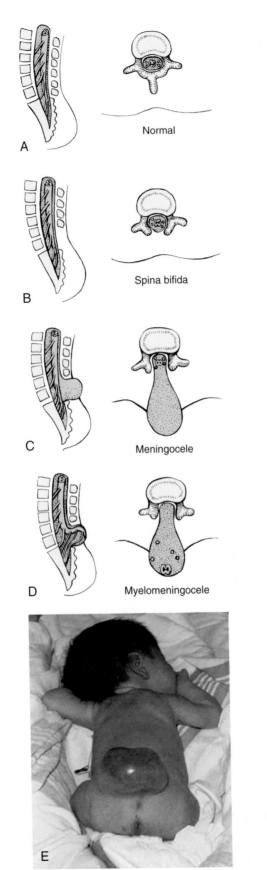

FIGURE 18.4 Normal Spine, Spina Bifida, Meningocele, Myelo-meningocele. Myelomeningocele with an intact sac. (From Hock-enberry MJ, Wilson D: *Wong's nursing care of infants and children,* ed 10, St Louis, 2015, Mosby.)

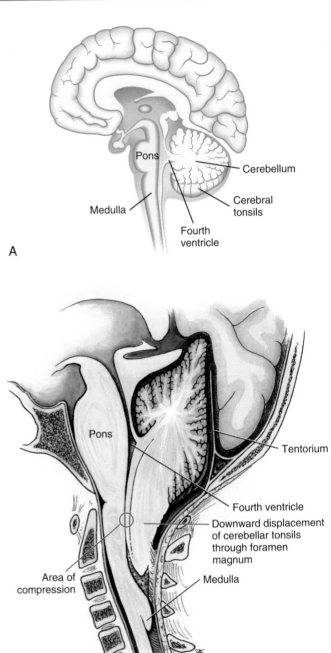

FIGURE 18.5 Normal Brain and Arnold-Chiari II Malformation. A, Diagram of a normal brain. **B**, Diagram of an Arnold-Chiari II malformation, showing downward displacement of the cerebellar tonsils and medulla through the foramen magnum causing, compression and obstruction of cerebrospinal fluid flow. (**B** modified from Barrow Neurological Institute of St Joseph's Hospital and Medical Center. Reprinted with permission.)

suture line, resulting in an asymmetric shape of the skull. The general term *plagiocephaly*, meaning "misshapen skull," is used to describe deformities that result from craniosynostosis or from asymmetric head posture (positional). When a single coronal suture fuses prematurely, the head is flattened on that side in front. When the sagittal suture fuses prematurely, the head is elongated in the anteroposterior direction (known as scaphocephaly).[16] Single suture craniosynostosis is usually only a cosmetic issue. Rarely, when multiple sutures fuse prematurely, brain growth may be restricted and surgical repair may prevent neurologic dysfunction (Fig. 18.6). *Syndromic craniosynostosis*

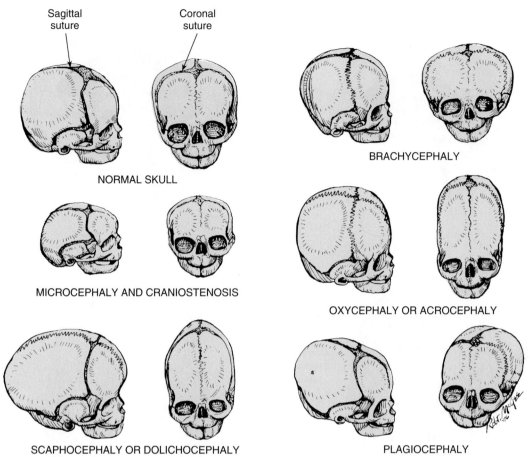

Sagittal suture   Coronal suture

NORMAL SKULL

BRACHYCEPHALY

MICROCEPHALY AND CRANIOSTENOSIS

OXYCEPHALY OR ACROCEPHALY

SCAPHOCEPHALY OR DOLICHOCEPHALY

PLAGIOCEPHALY

FIGURE 18.6 Normal and Abnormal Head Configurations. *Normal skull:* The bones are separated by membranous seams until the sutures gradually close. *Microcephaly and craniostenosis:* In microcephaly, the head circumference is more than 2 standard deviations below the mean for age, gender, race, and gestation, reflecting a small brain. Craniosynostosis is premature closure of the sutures. *Scaphocephaly or dolichocephaly* (frequency 56%): Premature closure of the sagittal suture, resulting in restricted lateral growth. *Brachycephaly:* Premature closure of the coronal suture, resulting in excessive lateral growth. *Oxycephaly or acrocephaly* (frequency 5.8% to 12%): Premature closure of all coronal and sagittal sutures, resulting in accelerated upward growth and a small head circumference. *Plagiocephaly* (frequency 13%): Unilateral premature closure of the coronal suture, resulting in asymmetric growth. (From Hockenberry MJ, Wilson D: *Wong's nursing care of infants and children,* ed 10, St Louis, 2015, Mosby.)

involves deformities in other systems (i.e., the heart, limbs, and CNS).

Malformations of Brain Development

Reduced proliferation or accelerated apoptosis (programmed cell death) of brain cells causes congenital microcephaly (microencephaly—small brain). Increased proliferation of brain cells causes megalencephaly (macrencephaly—abnormally large brain). Both disorders are rare. Diagnosis is made by clinical history, family history, and brain imaging.[17,18]

Microcephaly is a defect in brain growth as a whole (see Fig. 18.6). Cranial size is significantly below average for the infant's age, gender, race, and gestation. The small size of the skull reflects a small brain (microencephaly), which is caused by reduced proliferation or accelerated apoptosis. *True (primary) microcephaly* is usually caused by an autosomal recessive genetic or chromosomal defect. *Secondary (acquired) microcephaly* is associated with various causes, such as intrauterine infection (including emergence of the Zika virus); trauma; metabolic disorders; maternal anorexia experienced during the third trimester of pregnancy; in utero exposure to alcohol, toxins, or certain medications; and the

presence of other genetic syndromes. Children with microcephaly are usually developmentally delayed.

Cortical dysplasias are defects in brain development and related to failure of embryonic neurons to migrate to the right places in the brain. These disorders may range from a small area of abnormal tissue to an entire brain that is smooth and without the normal configuration of gyri and sulci, known as *lissencephaly,* or a brain that has too many small gyri (folds), known as *polymicrogyria.* There is a specific genetic defect for some of these disorders; others are multifactorial or acquired (e.g., intrauterine trauma or infection). Cortical dysplasias increase the risk for seizures that are difficult to control and cause developmental delay and motor dysfunction. Genetic testing assesses risk in other family members and guides therapy.[19,20]

Congenital hydrocephalus is present at birth and characterized by increased CSF pressure and enlargement of the ventricles. The overall incidence of hydrocephalus is approximately 1 to 3 per 1000 live births.[21] The incidence of hydrocephalus that is not associated with myelomeningocele is approximately 0.5 to 1 per 1000 live births.[21] Hydrocephalus may be caused by blockage within the ventricular system where the CSF flows, an imbalance in the production of CSF, or a reduced

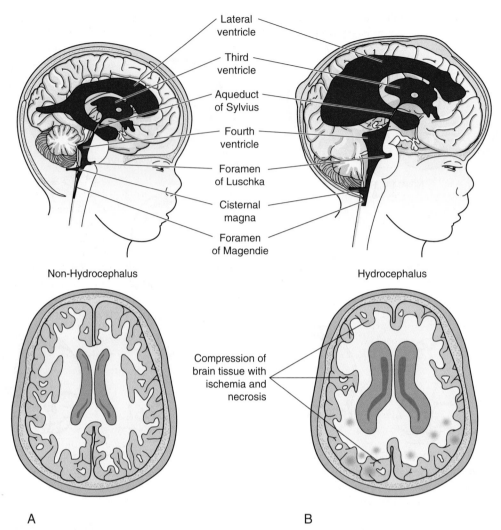

FIGURE 18.7 Hydrocephalus—Blockage in the Flow of Cerebrospinal Fluid. **A,** Patent cerebrospinal fluid circulation. **B,** Enlarged lateral and third ventricles caused by obstruction of circulation (e.g., stenosis of aqueduct of Sylvius).

reabsorption of CSF.[22] The increased pressure within the ventricular system dilates the ventricles and pushes and compresses the brain tissue against the skull cavity (Fig. 18.7) When hydrocephalus develops before fusion of the cranial sutures, the skull can expand to accommodate this additional space-occupying volume and preserve neuronal function. (Types of hydrocephalus are discussed in Chapter 16.)

Congenital hydrocephalus may cause fetal death in utero, or the increased head circumference may require cesarean delivery of the infant. Symptoms depend directly on the cause and rate of hydrocephalus development. When there is separation of the cranial sutures, a resonant note sounds when the skull is tapped, a manifestation called the **Macewen sign,** or **"cracked pot" sign.** The eyes may assume a staring expression, with sclera visible above the cornea, called *sunsetting.* Treatment outcomes are variable. Cognitive impairment in children with hydrocephalus is often related to associated brain malformations or episodes of shunt failure or infection. Approximately 40% to 65% of children with uncomplicated congenital hydrocephalus complete schooling and are employed when treated successfully with shunting or endoscopic third ventriculostomy and choroid plexus cauterization.[23-25]

The **Dandy-Walker malformation (DWM)** is a congenital defect of the cerebellum characterized by a large posterior fossa cyst that communicates with the fourth ventricle, cerebellar hypoplasia, and macrocephaly. DWM is commonly associated with hydrocephalus caused by compression of the aqueduct of Sylvius. Other causes of obstructions within the ventricular system that can result in hydrocephalus include brain tumors, cysts, trauma, arteriovenous malformations, blood clots, infections, and the Chiari malformations.

> ✔ **QUICK CHECK 18.2**
> 1. List two defects of neural tube closure.
> 2. Why do motor and sensory functions worsen with growth in a child with a neural tube defect?
> 3. What food source or dietary supplement helps prevent neural tube defects?

ALTERATIONS IN FUNCTION: ENCEPHALOPATHIES

Encephalopathy, meaning brain pathology, is a general category that includes a number of syndromes and diseases (see Chapter 17). These disorders may be acute or chronic, as well as static or progressive.

Static (Nonprogressive) Encephalopathies

Static or **nonprogressive encephalopathy** describes a neurologic condition caused by a fixed lesion without active and ongoing disease. Causes include brain malformations or brain injury that may occur during gestation or birth, or at any time during childhood. The degree of neurologic impairment is directly related to the extent of the injury or malformation. Anoxia, trauma, and infections are the most common causes of injury to the nervous system in the perinatal period. Infections, metabolic disturbances (acquired or genetic), trauma, toxins, and vascular disease may injure the nervous system in the postnatal period.[26]

Cerebral palsy is a disorder of movement, muscle tone, or posture that is caused by injury or abnormal development in the immature brain, before, during, or after birth up to 1 year of age. Cerebral palsy is one of the most common crippling disorders of childhood, affecting nearly 500,000 children in the United States alone. Although the exact incidence is unknown, studies suggest that the prevalence is approximately 1 in 323 children in the United States.[27]

Risk factors include prenatal or perinatal cerebral hypoxia, hemorrhage, infection, genetic abnormalities, or low birth weight. Cerebral palsy can be classified on the basis of neurologic signs and motor symptoms, with the major types being spasticity, dystonia, ataxia, or a combination of these symptoms (mixed). Diplegia, hemiplegia, or tetraplegia may be present.

Pyramidal/spastic cerebral palsy is the most common. It results from damage to corticospinal pathways (upper motor neurons) and is associated with increased muscle tone, persistent primitive reflexes, hyperactive deep tendon reflexes, clonus, rigidity of the extremities, scoliosis, and contractures. Extrapyramidal/nonspastic cerebral palsy is less common and is caused by damage to cells in the basal ganglia or cerebellum and includes two subtypes: dystonic and ataxic. Dystonic (dyskinetic) cerebral palsy is associated injury to the basal ganglia with extreme difficulty in fine motor coordination and purposeful movements. Movements are stiff, uncontrolled, and abrupt. Ataxic cerebral palsy is caused by damage to the cerebellum, with alterations in coordination and movement. There is a broad-based gait in an attempt to maintain balance, and tremor is common with intentional movements. A child may have symptoms of each of these cerebral palsy types, which leads to a mixed disorder.[28]

Children with cerebral palsy often have associated neurologic disorders, such as seizures and intellectual impairment ranging from mild to severe. Other complications include visual impairment, communication disorders, respiratory problems, bowel and bladder problems, and orthopedic disabilities.[29]

Inherited Metabolic Disorders of the Central Nervous System

A large number of inherited metabolic disorders have been identified, typically leading to diffuse brain dysfunction. Early diagnosis and treatment is vital if these infants are to survive without severe neurologic problems. Newborn metabolic screening for 28 metabolic conditions (in most states) has led to most of these children being identified before symptoms develop. Inborn errors of metabolism are present at birth, and most cause disturbances of the nervous system, although they may not manifest until childhood or even adulthood. Defects in amino acid and lipid metabolism are among the most common and are presented here.

Defects in Amino Acid Metabolism

Defects in amino acid metabolism are caused by genetic defects resulting in lack of a normal protein and absence of enzymatic activity. The defects include (1) those in which the transport of an amino acid is impaired; (2) those involving an enzyme or cofactor deficiency; and (3) those encompassing certain chemical components, such as branched-chain or sulfur-containing amino acids.

Phenylketonuria. Phenylketonuria (PKU) is an example of an inborn error of metabolism characterized by phenylalanine hydroxylase deficiency and the inability of the body to convert the essential amino acid phenylalanine to tyrosine (Fig. 18.8). PKU is an autosomal recessive inborn error of metabolism characterized by mutations of the phenylalanine hydroxylase *(PAH)* gene. PKU has an incidence of 1 per 10,000 to 15,000 live births in the United States.[30]

Most natural food proteins contain about 15% phenylalanine, an essential amino acid. Phenylalanine hydroxylase controls the conversion of this essential amino acid to tyrosine in the liver. The body uses tyrosine in the biosynthesis of proteins, melanin, thyroxine, and the catecholamines in the brain and adrenal medulla. Phenylalanine hydroxylase deficiency causes an accumulation of phenylalanine in the serum. Elevated phenylalanine levels result in developmental abnormalities of the cerebral cortical layers, defective myelination, and cystic degeneration of the gray and white matter. Unfortunately, brain damage occurs before the metabolites can be detected in the urine, and damage continues as long as phenylalanine levels remain high. Nonselective newborn screening is used to detect PKU in the United States and in more than 30 other countries. Treatment, consisting of reduction of dietary phenylalanine (PKU diet), is effective and allows for normal development. Mutations in the *PAH* gene are by far the most common cause of PKU, although there are other types of PKU as well. In one such variation, there is impaired synthesis of cofactors (e.g., tetrahydrobiopterin [BH_4]), which contributes to elevated levels of phenylalanine. Individuals with impaired synthesis of BH_4 have a positive response when sapropterin, a synthetic form of tetrahydrobiopterin, is included in their treatment.[31]

Defects in Lipid Metabolism

Disorders of lipid metabolism are termed lysosomal storage diseases because each disorder in this group can be traced to a missing lysosomal enzyme. Lysosomal storage disorders include more than 50 known

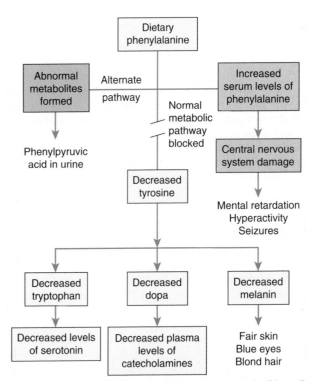

FIGURE 18.8 Metabolic Error and Consequences in Phenylketonuria. (From Hockenberry MJ, Wilson D: *Wong's nursing care of infants and children,* ed 10, St Louis, 2015, Mosby.)

genetic disorders. The incidence of lysosomal storage disorders is approximately 1 in 5000 live births.[32] These disorders cause an excessive accumulation of a particular cell product, occurring in the brain, liver, spleen, bone, and lung, and thus involving several organ systems. Generally these disorders are not included in newborn screening. Some of these disorders may be treated with enzyme replacement therapy.[33] Perhaps the best known of the lysosomal storage disorders is Tay-Sachs disease (GM_2 gangliosidosis), an autosomal recessive disorder caused by deficiency of the lysosomal enzyme hexosaminidase A (HexA), an enzyme that degrades GM_2 gangliosides (fatty acids) within nerve cell lysosomes. Most individuals diagnosed are of Jewish ancestry, although sporadic cases appear in the non-Jewish population. Onset of this disease usually occurs when the infant is 4 to 6 months old. Symptoms of Tay-Sachs include an exaggerated startle response to loud noise, seizures, developmental regression, dementia, and blindness. Death from this disease is almost universal and occurs by 5 years of age. Screening for carriers of the gene defect concomitant with counseling to prevent disease transmission is possible.[34]

✔ QUICK CHECK 18.3
1. List three types of cerebral palsy.
2. Why does failure to metabolize phenylalanine result in such widespread and devastating effects on development?

Intoxications of the Central Nervous System

Drug-induced encephalopathies must always be considered a possibility in the child with unexplained neurologic changes. Such encephalopathies may result from accidental ingestion, therapeutic overdose, intentional overdose, or ingestion of environmental toxins. Approximately 45.2% of all poison exposures in 2017 occurred in children younger than 6 years of age, with the highest incidence being 1- and 2-year-old children. The most commonly ingested poisons in children are cosmetics and personal care products, cleaning substances, and over-the-counter analgesics and other medications.[35]

Lead poisoning results in high blood levels of lead. If lead poisoning is untreated, lead encephalopathy results and is responsible for serious and irreversible neurologic damage. Those at greatest risk are children ages 2 to 3 years and children prone to the practice of pica—the habitual, purposeful, and compulsive ingestion of nonfood substances, such as clay, soil, and paint chips or paint dust. Lead intoxication also may occur from chronic exposure to lead in cosmetics, inhalation of gasoline vapors, and ingestion of airborne lead.[36] Fetal neurotoxicity occurs with maternal lead exposure, particularly during the first trimester.[37] Details related to lead intoxication are described in Chapter 4.

Infections of the Central Nervous System

Meningitis is an infection of the meninges and subarachnoid space of the brain and spinal cord. Encephalitis is inflammation within the brain. In many infections of the meninges, encephalitis also is present and the term meningoencephalitis is used. The origin of such inflammation and acute encephalopathy can be caused by bacteria, viruses, or other microorganisms. Aseptic meningitis has no evidence of bacterial infection but may be associated with viral infection, systemic disease, or drugs.

Bacterial Meningitis

Acute bacterial meningitis is one of the most serious infections to which infants and children are susceptible. The introduction of conjugate vaccines against Haemophilus influenzae type B, Streptococcus pneumoniae, and Neisseria meningitidis (meningococcus) has decreased the incidence of bacterial meningitis.[38] Vaccines for serogroup B N. meningitidis are now available.[39]

Group B Streptococcus causes lethal meningitis and sepsis in neonates and is transmitted to the child from the mother's birth canal. S. pneumoniae is the most common microorganism in children 1 to 23 months of age. Staphylococcal or streptococcal meningitis can occur in children of any age but shows a predilection for children who have had neurosurgery, skull fracture, or a complication of systemic bacterial infection. Infections that originate in the middle ear, sinuses, or mastoid cells also may lead to S. pneumoniae infection in children. Children with sickle cell disease or who have had a splenectomy are particularly at high risk for infection.

Escherichia coli and group B beta-hemolytic streptococci are the most common causes of meningitis in the newborn period. The second most common microorganism causing bacterial meningitis, particularly in children younger than 4 years, is Neisseria meningitidis (meningococcus) and it has the potential to occur in epidemics. Approximately 2% to 5% of healthy children are carriers of N. meningitidis. As the incidence of N. meningitidis infection increases in adolescence and with crowded environments, such as in dormitories and among military personnel, it is recommended that all individuals 11 to 12 years of age receive two immunizations against this pathogen. Teens and young adults (16- through 23-year-olds) also may be vaccinated with a serogroup B meningococcal vaccine.[40]

Pathogens enter the nervous system by direct extension from a contiguous source (e.g., paranasal sinuses or mastoid cells) or, more commonly, by hematogenous spread (e.g., infective endocarditis, pneumonia, neurosurgical procedures, severe burns). Pathogens then cross the blood–brain barrier, enter the CSF, and multiply. Bacterial toxins increase cerebrovascular permeability, causing alterations in blood flow and edema. Increased intracranial pressure (IICP) may be increased further by obstruction to the CSF circulation. Herniation of the brainstem causes death.

Acute bacterial meningitis often is preceded by an upper respiratory tract or a gastrointestinal infection. Inflammation leads to the general symptoms of fever, headache, vomiting, and irritability and the CNS symptoms of photophobia, nuchal and spinal rigidity, decreased level of consciousness, and seizures. Irritation of the meninges and spinal roots causes pain and resistance to neck flexion (nuchal rigidity), a positive Kernig sign (resistance to knee extension in the supine position with the hips and knees flexed against the body), and a positive Brudzinski sign (flexion of the knees and hips when the neck is flexed forward rapidly). With severe meningeal irritation the child may demonstrate opisthotonic posturing (rigid arching of the back with the head extended). Infants may have bulging fontanelles. Meningococcal meningitis can produce a characteristic petechial rash.

Viral meningitis may result from a direct infection caused by a virus, or it may be secondary to disease, such as measles, mumps, herpes, or leukemia. The hallmark of viral meningitis, or aseptic meningitis, is a mononuclear response in the CSF and the presence of normal glucose levels as well. The clinical manifestations are similar to those in bacterial meningitis, although usually milder.

Viral encephalitis in children is similar to viral encephalitis in adults (see Chapter 17, and Fig. 17.13) and can be difficult to distinguish from viral meningitis. Viruses can directly invade the brain, causing inflammation; or postinfectious encephalitis can develop as a result of an autoimmune response.[41] (Encephalopathy resulting from infection with the human immunodeficiency virus [HIV] is discussed in Chapters 8 and 17.)

CEREBROVASCULAR DISEASE IN CHILDREN

Perinatal Stroke

Perinatal arterial ischemic stroke is estimated at 1 in 4000 live births and is a leading cause of perinatal brain injury, cerebral palsy, and lifelong disability. Although a cause for perinatal stroke is usually not found, clotting abnormalities may make the child prone to further vascular events.

Childhood Stroke

Childhood stroke occurs in 1.3 to 1.6 per 100,000 children per year and may be divided into two categories: ischemic and hemorrhagic.[42,43]

Ischemic (occlusive) stroke is rare in children and may result from embolism, sinovenous thrombosis, or congenital or iatrogenic narrowing of vessels, leading to decreased flow of blood and oxygen to areas of the brain. Children with arterial ischemic stroke do not have the typical adult risk factors of atherosclerosis and hypertension. Approximately 40% of children with acute ischemic stroke have no identifiable risk factors.[44] Sickle cell disease, cerebral arteriopathies, and cardiac anomalies are the common disorders associated with arterial ischemic stroke.[45]

Hemorrhagic stroke is most commonly caused by bleeding from congenital cerebral arteriovenous malformations and is rare in children younger than 19 years. Intraventricular hemorrhage associated with premature birth is related to immature blood vessels and unstable blood pressure. There is a high risk of developing posthemorrhagic hydrocephalus in very-low-birthweight (<1000 gm) preterm infants.[46]

The clinical presentation of stroke varies according to the vessels involved and the age of the individual. Symptoms include hemiplegia, weakness, seizures, headaches, high fever, nuchal rigidity, hemianopia, sensory changes, facial palsy, and temporary aphasia. Obtaining a thorough history of evolving symptoms and risk factors is important for diagnosis. Laboratory studies may be indicated. Neuroimaging studies assist in determining the extent of the disease. Surgery is an option for treatment, and anticoagulants and antithrombotics may be used in selected cases.

Moyamoya disease is a rare, chronic, progressive vascular stenosis of the circle of Willis. There is obstruction of arterial flow to the brain and the development of small basal arterial collateral vessels that vascularize the hypoperfused brain distal to the occluded vessels.[47] Moyamoya means a *puff of smoke* in Japanese and represents the appearance of these small vessels. The cause is unknown.

Epilepsy and Seizure Disorders in Children

The incidence of epilepsy varies greatly with age, geographic location, and study design. Approximately 470,000 children in the United States had epilepsy in 2015.[48]

Seizures are the abnormal discharge of electrical activity within the brain. When a sufficient number of neurons become overexcited, they discharge abnormally, which sometimes results in clinical manifestations (seizures) with alterations in motor function, sensation, autonomic function, behavior, and consciousness. The manifestations depend on the site and spread of abnormal electrical activity within the brain. If a child has more than one unprovoked seizure within 24 hours, that child is said to have **epilepsy**, although there are a few exceptions—one example being febrile seizures. Seizures may result from diseases that are primarily neurologic (CNS) or are systemic and affect CNS function secondarily (such as diabetes). Seizures can be caused by structural abnormalities of the brain, hypoxia, intracranial hemorrhage, CNS infection, traumatic injury, electrolyte imbalance, or inborn metabolic disturbances. Febrile seizures are benign and the most common type of childhood seizure. Seizures are sometimes clearly familial. Often the cause of epilepsy is unknown and presumed to have a genetic basis. (Table 16.14 summarizes the major types of seizures.)

CHILDHOOD TUMORS

Brain Tumors

Brain tumors are the most common solid tumor, the second most common primary neoplasm in children (after leukemia), and can be benign or malignant.[49] They are the leading cause of cancer-related death in children, and the 5-year survival is about 74%, varying significantly by tumor type. Primary brain tumors arise from brain tissue and do not metastasize outside the brain. The cause of brain tumors is unknown, although genetic, environmental, and immune factors have been investigated. Exposure to radiation therapy has been the only environmental factor consistently related to the development of brain tumors.[50]

Brain tumors can arise from any CNS cell, and tumors are classified by cell type. The most common tumors are embryonal tumors, including medulloblastoma, atypical medulloblastoma, atypical teratoid rhabdoid tumors, CNS primitive neuroectodermal tumors, and high-grade gliomas, including glioblastomas, diffuse pontine gliomas, and other malignant astrocytomas. Other tumor types are less common, including low-grade astrocytomas (especially pilocytic astrocytomas), neuronal and mixed neuronal-glial tumors, and ependymal tumors (ependymomas). Brain tumors in children are often located in the posterior fossa (Fig. 18.9). The types and characteristics of the more common childhood brain tumors are summarized in Table 18.3.

Signs and symptoms of brain tumors in children vary from generalized and vague to localized and related specifically to an anatomic area. Signs of IICP may occur, including headache, vomiting, lethargy, and irritability. If a young child complains of repeated and worsening headache, a thorough investigation should take place because headache is an uncommon complaint in young children. Headache caused by IICP usually is worse in the morning and gradually improves during the day, when the child is upright and venous drainage is enhanced. The frequency of headache and other symptoms increases as the tumor grows. Irritability or possible apathy and increased somnolence also may result. Like headache, vomiting occurs more commonly in the morning. Often it is *not* preceded by nausea and may become projectile, differing from a gastrointestinal disturbance in that the child may be ready to eat immediately after vomiting. Other signs and symptoms include increased head circumference with bulging fontanelles in the child younger than 2 years, cranial nerve palsies, and papilledema (Box 18.1).

Localized findings relate to the degree of disturbance in physiologic functioning in the area where the tumor is located. Children with infratentorial tumors (posterior fossa) exhibit localized signs of impaired coordination and balance, including ataxia, gait difficulties, truncal ataxia, and loss of balance. Supratentorial tumors of the cerebral hemispheres are more common in neonates and adolescents and are usually gliomas.[51]

Most pediatric brain tumors require surgical resection. Aggressive radiation and chemotherapy are required for high-grade tumors. Advances are being made in areas of immunotherapy and targeted molecular therapy.[52]

Embryonal Tumors

Neuroblastoma

Neuroblastoma is an embryonal tumor originating from neural crest tissues of the sympathetic nervous system outside the CNS. It is the most common cancer in infants less than 1 year of age. Although it accounts for only about 6% of pediatric malignancies (about 800 new cases per year), neuroblastoma causes about 15% of cancer deaths in children.[53]

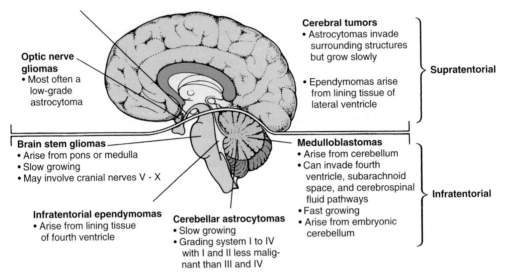

Craniopharyngiomas
- Located adjacent to the sella turcica (structure containing the pituitary gland), often considered to lie supratentorial
- Considered to have benign properties but is life threatening because of its location near vital structures

Optic nerve gliomas
- Most often a low-grade astrocytoma

Cerebral tumors
- Astrocytomas invade surrounding structures but grow slowly
- Ependymomas arise from lining tissue of lateral ventricle

Supratentorial

Brain stem gliomas
- Arise from pons or medulla
- Slow growing
- May involve cranial nerves V - X

Medulloblastomas
- Arise from cerebellum
- Can invade fourth ventricle, subarachnoid space, and cerebrospinal fluid pathways
- Fast growing
- Arise from embryonic cerebellum

Infratentorial

Infratentorial ependymomas
- Arise from lining tissue of fourth ventricle

Cerebellar astrocytomas
- Slow growing
- Grading system I to IV with I and II less malignant than III and IV

FIGURE 18.9 Location of Brain Tumors in Children. (From Ostrom QT et al: *Neuro Oncol* 19(suppl_5):v1-v88, 2017.)

TABLE 18.3	More Common Brain Tumors in Children	
Type	**Characteristics**	**Treatment**
Astrocytoma	Arises from astrocytes, often in cerebellum or lateral cerebral hemisphere Slow growing, solid or cystic Often very large before diagnosed Varies in degree of malignancy	*Cerebellar astrocytoma* Surgery; possibly curative Radiation and chemotherapy not proved successful but may delay recurrence *Cerebral astrocytoma* Surgery if resection is possible Radiation useful for all grades of astrocytoma Chemotherapy beneficial in higher grade tumors, but further study required
Medulloblastoma (neuroectodermal tumor)	Often located in cerebellum, extending into fourth ventricle and spinal fluid pathway Can extend outside central nervous system Rapidly growing malignant tumor	Treatment is age and tumor type dependent Surgery, primarily as partial resection to relieve increased intracranial pressure and "debulk" tumor Radiation as primary treatment; may include spinal radiation Chemotherapy showing some promise in conjunction with craniospinal radiation Targeted therapies for molecular subgroups are in development
Ependymoma	Arises from ependymal cells lining ventricles Circumscribed, solid, nodular tumors	Tumor possibly indolent for many years Surgery rarely curative; risk of resecting an infratentorial tumor too great Radiation for palliation (current controversy over whether local or craniospinal radiation is best) Chemotherapy used for recurrent disease but with disappointing results Targeted therapies for molecular subgroups are in development
Brainstem glioma	Arises from pons Numerous cell types Compresses cranial nerves V through X	Surgery, resection occasionally possible Radiation, primarily palliative treatment Chemotherapy not yet proven beneficial New protocols and agents being studied

More than with any other cancer, neuroblastoma has been associated with spontaneous remission, commonly in infants. Prognosis is worse for children older than 2 years of age with disseminated disease. Although familial tendency has been noted in individual cases, a nonfamilial or sporadic pattern is found in most children with neuroblastoma. Familial cases of neuroblastoma are considered to have an autosomal dominant pattern of inheritance (mechanisms of inheritance are discussed in Chapter 2).

The most common location of neuroblastoma is in the retroperitoneal region, most often in the adrenal medulla. The tumor is evident as an abdominal mass and may cause anorexia, bowel and bladder alteration, and sometimes spinal cord compression. The second most common location of neuroblastoma is the mediastinum (15% of cases), where the tumor may cause dyspnea or infection related to airway obstruction. Rarely, neuroblastoma may arise from the cervical sympathetic ganglion.

BOX 18.1   Clinical Manifestations of Brain Tumors

Headache
Recurrent and progressive
In frontal or occipital area
Worse on arising; pain lessens during the day
Intensified by lowering head and straining, such as when defecating, coughing, sneezing

Vomiting
With or without nausea or feeding
Progressively more projectile
More severe in morning
Relieved by moving and changing position

Neuromuscular Changes
Incoordination or clumsiness
Loss of balance (use of wide-based stance, falling, tripping, banging into objects)
Poor fine motor control
Weakness
Hyporeflexia or hyperreflexia
Positive Babinski sign
Spasticity
Paralysis

Behavioral Changes
Irritability
Decreased appetite

Failure to thrive
Fatigue (frequent naps)
Lethargy
Coma
Bizarre behavior (staring, automatic movements)

Cranial Nerve Neuropathy
Cranial nerve involvement varies according to tumor location. The most common signs are:
Head tilt
Visual defects (nystagmus, diplopia, strabismus, episodic "graying out" of vision, and visual field defects)

Vital Sign Disturbances
Decreased pulse and respiratory rates
Increased blood pressure
Decreased pulse pressure
Hypothermia or hyperthermia

Other Signs
Seizures
Cranial enlargement*
Tense, bulging fontanelle at rest*
Separating suture*
Nuchal rigidity
Papilledema (edema of optic nerve)

*Present only in infants and young children.
From Hockenberry MN: *Wong's essentials of pediatric nursing,* ed 7, St Louis, 2007, Mosby.

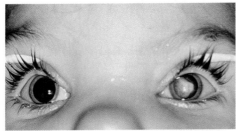

FIGURE 18.10 **Retinoblastoma.** The tumor occupies a large portion of the inside of the eye globe. (From Damjanov I: *Pathology for the health professions,* ed 3, St Louis, 2006, Saunders. Courtesy Dr. Walter Richardson and Dr. Jamsheed Khan, Kansas City, Kan.)

A number of systemic signs and symptoms are characteristic of neuroblastoma, including weight loss, irritability, fatigue, and fever. Intractable diarrhea occurs in some children and is caused by tumor secretion of a hormone called *vasoactive intestinal polypeptide (VIP).* Most children with neuroblastoma have increased amounts of catecholamines and associated metabolites in their urine. High levels of urinary catecholamines and serum ferritin are associated with a poor prognosis.

Retinoblastoma

Retinoblastoma is a rare congenital eye tumor of young children that originates in the retina of one or both eyes (Fig. 18.10). Two forms of retinoblastoma are exhibited: inherited and acquired. The inherited form of the disease generally is diagnosed during the first year of life. The acquired disease most commonly is diagnosed in children 2 to 3 years of age and involves unilateral disease.[54]

Approximately 40% of retinoblastomas are inherited as an autosomal dominant trait with incomplete penetrance (see Fig. 2.22). The remaining 60% are acquired. The "two-hit" hypothesis explains the occurrence of both hereditary and acquired forms of the disease.[55] This hypothesis predicts that two separate transforming events or "hits" must occur in a normal retinoblast cell to cause the cancer. Further, it proposes that in the inherited form, the first hit or mutation occurs in the germ cell (inherited from either parent), and the mutation is contained in every cell of the child's body. Only a second, random mutation in a retinoblast cell is needed to transform that cell into cancer. Multiple tumors are observed in the inherited form because these second mutations are likely to occur in several of the approximately 1 million to 2 million retinoblast cells. In contrast, the acquired form of retinoblastoma requires two *independent* hits or mutations to occur in the same somatic cell (after the egg is fertilized) for the transformation to cancer. This is much less likely to happen. Fig. 18.11 illustrates the "two-hit" model for these two patterns of mutation.

The primary sign of retinoblastoma is leukocoria, a white pupillary reflex (white reflex) also called *cat's eye reflex,* which is caused by the mass behind the lens (see Fig. 18.10). This easy to identify sign can be missed. Other signs and symptoms include strabismus; a red, painful eye; and limited vision.

Because retinoblastoma is a treatable tumor, dual priorities are saving the child's life and restoring useful vision. The prognosis for most children with retinoblastoma is excellent, with a greater than 90% long-term survival.

> ✔ **QUICK CHECK 18.4**
> 1. Why are the principal symptoms of brain tumors in children related to brainstem function?
> 2. Why is the "two-hit" hypothesis more likely to apply in the inherited form of retinoblastoma?

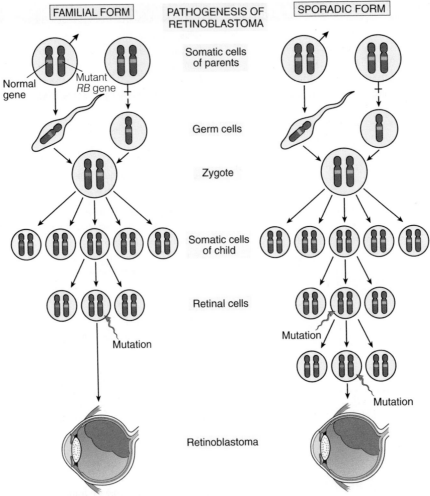

FIGURE 18.11 The Two-Mutation Model of Retinoblastoma Development. In inherited retinoblastoma, the first mutation is transmitted through the germline of an affected parent. The second mutation occurs somatically in a retinal cell, leading to development of the tumor. In sporadic retinoblastoma, development of a tumor requires two somatic mutations.

SUMMARY REVIEW

Development of the Nervous System in Children

1. Growth and development of the brain occur most rapidly during fetal development and during the first year of life.
2. The bones of the skull are joined by sutures, and the wide, membranous junctions of the sutures (known as *fontanelles*) allow for brain growth and close by 18 months of age.
3. At birth, the forebrain is immature, so neurologic examination is primarily of reflex responses that require an intact spinal cord and brainstem.

Structural Malformations

1. Neural tube defects (NTDs) are an arrest of the normal development of the brain and spinal cord during the first month of embryonic development. Risk factors include folic acid deficiency, previous NTD pregnancy, maternal diabetes or obesity, use of anticonvulsants, and maternal hyperthermia.
2. Spina bifida (failure of vertebral closure) is the most common NTD and includes anencephaly (absence of part of the skull and brain), encephalocele (herniation of the meninges and brain through a skull defect), meningocele (a saclike meningeal cyst of spinal fluid

that protrudes through a vertebral defect), myelomeningocele (like a meningocele that also contains a portion of the spinal cord with its nerves), and spina bifida occulta.
3. Premature closure of the cranial sutures causes craniosynostosis, resulting in an asymmetric skull shape. If multiple sutures fuse prematurely, brain growth may be restricted.
4. Microcephaly is a defect in brain cell proliferation that leads to a small brain, small skull, and usually developmental delays.
5. Cortical dysplasias are defects in brain development that result in abnormal arrangements of brain tissue.
6. Congenital hydrocephalus, characterized by increased cerebrospinal fluid (CSF) pressure, results from overproduction, impaired absorption, or blockage of circulation of CSF. Dandy-Walker deformity, which is commonly associated with hydrocephalus, is caused by cystic dilation of the fourth ventricle and aqueductal compression.

Alterations in Function: Encephalopathies

1. Static (nonprogressive) encephalopathies are disorders of the brain caused by a fixed lesion without active and ongoing disease. They

can occur during gestation, birth, or childhood and can be caused by endogenous or exogenous factors.

2. Cerebral palsy can be caused by prenatal or perinatal cerebral hypoxia or perinatal trauma, with symptoms of motor dysfunction (including increased muscle tone, increased reflexes, and loss of fine motor coordination), mental retardation, seizure disorders, or developmental disabilities.

3. Inherited metabolic disorders that damage the nervous system include defects in amino acid metabolism (phenylketonuria) and lipid metabolism (Tay-Sachs disease) and result in abnormal behavior, seizures, and deficient psychomotor development.

4. Seizure disorders are abnormal discharges of electrical activity within the brain. They are associated with numerous nervous system disorders and more often are a generalized rather than a partial type of seizure.

5. Accidental ingestion, therapeutic overdose, intentional overdose, or ingestion of environmental toxins, such as in lead poisoning, can cause serious neurologic damage.

6. Bacterial meningitis is commonly caused by *Neisseria meningitidis* or *Streptococcus pneumoniae* and may result from respiratory tract or gastrointestinal infections; symptoms include fever, headaches, photophobia, seizures, rigidity, and stupor.

7. Viral meningitis may result from direct infection or be secondary to a systemic viral infection (e.g., measles, mumps, herpes, or leukemia).

Cerebrovascular Disease in Children

1. Perinatal arterial ischemic stroke is a leading cause of perinatal brain injury, cerebral palsy, and lifelong disability.

2. Ischemic (occlusive) stroke is rare in children but can occur from embolism, sickle cell disease, cerebral arteriopathies, and cardiac anomalies.

3. Hemorrhagic stroke can occur in association with immature blood vessel associated with prematurity or cerebral arteriovenous malformations.

4. Moyamoya is a rare, progressive vascular stenosis of the circle of Willis that obstructs arterial blood flow to the brain.

5. Seizures are abnormal discharges of electrical activity within the brain. More than one unprovoked seizure within 24 hours indicates epilepsy.

6. Seizures can be caused by structural abnormalities of the brain, hypoxia, intracranial hemorrhage, CNS infection, traumatic injury, electrolyte imbalance, or inborn metabolic disturbances.

7. Febrile seizures are benign and the most common type of childhood seizure.

Childhood Brain Tumors

1. Brain tumors are the second most common type of childhood cancer and are the leading cause of cancer related death in children

2. Symptoms of brain tumors may be generalized or localized. The most common general symptoms are the result of increased intracranial pressure and include headache, irritability, vomiting, somnolence, and bulging of fontanelles.

3. Localized findings relate to the degree of disturbance in physiologic functioning in the area where the tumor is located. Localized signs of infratentorial tumors in the cerebellum include impaired coordination and balance.

4. Neuroblastoma is an embryonal tumor of the sympathetic nervous system and can be located anywhere there is sympathetic nervous tissue. Symptoms include weight loss, irritability, fatigue, fever, and intractable diarrhea. Neuroblastoma has been associated with spontaneous remission in infants.

5. Retinoblastoma is a congenital eye tumor that has two forms: inherited and acquired.

KEY TERMS

Acute bacterial meningitis, 422
Anencephaly, 416
Aseptic meningitis, 422
Ataxic cerebral palsy, 421
Cerebral palsy, 421
Chiari II malformation (Arnold-Chiari malformation), 416
Congenital hydrocephalus, 419
Cortical dysplasias, 419
Craniosynostosis, 417
Cyclopia, 416
Dandy-Walker malformation (DWM), 420

Dystonic (dyskinetic) cerebral palsy, 421
Encephalitis, 422
Encephalocele, 416
Encephalopathy, 420
Epilepsy, 423
Extrapyramidal/nonspastic cerebral palsy, 421
Fontanelle, 415
Hemorrhagic stroke, 423
Ischemic (occlusive) stroke, 423
Lead poisoning, 422
Lysosomal storage disease, 421

Macewen sign ("cracked pot" sign), 420
Meningitis, 422
Meningocele, 416
Microcephaly, 419
Moyamoya disease, 423
Myelomeningocele (meningomyelocele, spina bifida cystica), 416
Neural tube defect (NTD), 416
Neuroblastoma, 423
Phenylketonuria (PKU), 421
Pica, 422

Pyramidal/spastic cerebral palsy, 421
Retinoblastoma, 425
Seizure, 423
Spina bifida (split spine), 416
Spina bifida occulta, 416
Static encephalopathy (nonprogressive encephalopathy), 420
Tay-Sachs disease (GM_2 gangliosidosis), 422
Tethered cord syndrome, 417
Viral encephalitis, 422
Viral meningitis, 422

REFERENCES

1. Beard JL: Why iron deficiency is important in infant development, *J Nutr* 138(12):2534-2536, 2008.
2. Todorich B, et al: Oligodendrocytes and myelination: the role of iron, *Glia* 57(5):467-478, 2009.
3. Centers for Disease Control and Prevention (CDCP): Birth defects and folic acids. Updated September 15, 2017. Available at: https://www.cdc.gov/healthcommunication/toolstemplates/entertainmented/tips/BirthDefects.html.

4. Copp AJ, et al: Neural tube defects: recent advances, unsolved questions, and controversies, *Lancet Neurol* 12(8):799-810, 2013.
5. Centers for Disease Control and Prevention (CDC): CDC grand rounds: additional opportunities to prevent neural tube defects with folic acid fortification, *MMWR Morb Mortal Wkly Rep* 59(31):980-984, 2010.
6. Meador KJ: Comment: valproate dose effects differ across congenital malformations, *Neurology* 81(11):1002, 2013.
7. Centers for Disease Control and Prevention (CDC): Facts about anecephaly. Last reviewed November 21,

2017. Available at: www.cdc.gov/ncbddd/birthdefects/Anencephaly.html.
8. Centers for Disease Control and Prevention (CDC): Facts about encephalocele. Last reviewed November 21, 2017. Available at: www.cdc.gov/ncbddd/birthdefects/Encephalocele.html.
9. Behrman R, et al: *Nelson' textbook of pediatrics*, ed 17, Philadelphia, 2004, Saunders.
10. Tamburrini G, et al: Myelomeningocele: the management of the associated hydrocephalus, *Childs Nerv Syst* 29(9):1569-1579, 2013.
11. Adzick NS: Fetal myelomeningocele: natural history, pathophysiology, and in-utero intervention,

Semin Fetal Neonatal Med 15(1):9-14, 2009.

12. Adzick NS: MOMS investigators: a randomized trial of prenatal versus postnatal repair of myelomeningocele, *N Engl J Med* 364(11):993-1004, 2011.

13. Adzick NS: Fetal surgery for spina bifida: past, present, future, *Semin Pediatr Surg* 22(1):10-17, 2013.

14. Moldenhauer JS: In utero repair of spina bifida, *Am J Perinatol* 31(7):595-604, 2014.

15. Centers for Disease Control and Prevention (CDCP): Facts about craniosynostosis. Last reviewed November 21, 2017. Available at: https://www.cdc.gov/ncbddd/birthdefects/craniosynostosis.html.

16. Ciurea AV, et al: Actual concepts in scaphocephaly: (an experience of 98 cases), *J Med Life* 4(4):424-431, 2011.

17. Alvarado-Socarras JL, et al: Congenital microcephaly: a diagnostic challenge during Zika epidemics, *Travel Med Infect Dis* 2018. S1477-8939(18)30013-30019.

18. Pavone P, et al: Clinical review on megalencephaly: a large brain as a possible sign of cerebral impairment, *Medicine (Baltimore)* 96(26):e6814, 2017.

19. Barkovich JA, et al: A developmental and genetic classification for malformations of cortical development: update, *Brain* 135(Pt 5):1348-1369, 2012, 2012.

20. Romero DM, Bahi-Buisson N, Francis F: Genetics and mechanisms leading to human cortical malformations, *Semin Cell Dev Biol* 76:33-75, 2018.

21. Garton HJ, Piatt JH, Jr: Hydrocephalus, *Pediatr Clin North Am* 51:305-325, 2004.

22. McAllister JP, Jr: Pathophysiology of congenital and neonatal hydrocephalus, *Semin Fetal Neonatal Med* 17(5):285-294, 2012.

23. Constantini S, et al: Neuroendoscopy in the youngest age group, *World Neurosurg* 79(2 Suppl):S23, e1-e11, 2013.

24. Kahle KT, et al: Hydrocephalus in children, *Lancet* 387(10020):788-799, 2016.

25. Paulsen AH, Lundar T, Lindegaard KF: Pediatric hydrocephalus: 40-year outcomes in 128 hydrocephalic patients treated with shunts during childhood. Assessment of surgical outcome, work participation, and health-related quality of life, *J Neurosurg Pediatr* 16(6):633-641, 2015.

26. Marret S, et al: Pathophysiology of cerebral palsy, *Handb Clin Neurol* 111:169-176, 2013.

27. Centers for Disease Control and Prevention (CDCP): Data and statistics for cerebral palsy. Page last reviewed March 9, 2018. Available at: https://www.cdc.gov/ncbddd/cp/data.html.

28. Krigger KW: Cerebral palsy: an overview, *Am Fam Physician* 73(1):91-100, 2006.

29. Pruitt DW, Tsai T: Common medical comorbidities associated with cerebral palsy, *Phys Med Rehabil Clin North Am* 20(3):453-467, 2009.

30. National Institutes of Health, Genetics Home Reference: Phenylketonuria. Available at: https://ghr.nlm.nih.gov/condition/phenylketonuria#resources. (Accessed 21 May 2019).

31. Somaraju UR, Merrin M: Sapropterin dihydrochloride for phenylketonuria, *Cochrane Database Syst Rev* (3):CD008005, 2015.

32. Platt FM: Sphingolipid lysosomal storage disorders, *Nature* 510(7503):68-75, 2014.

33. Ortolano S, et al: Treatment of lysosomal storage diseases: recent patents and future strategies, *Recent Pat Endocr Metab Immune Drug Discov* 8(1):9, 2014.

34. Patterson MC: Gangliosidoses, *Handb Clin Neurol* 113:1707-1708, 2013.

35. National Poison Control Center: Poison Statistics National Data 2017. Available at: https://www.poison.org/poison-statistics-national. (Accessed 22 May 2019).

36. Advisory Committee on Childhood Lead Poisoning Prevention: Interpreting and managing blood lead levels <10 µg/dL in children and reducing childhood exposures to lead: recommendations of CDC's Advisory Committee on Childhood Lead Poisoning Prevention, *MMWR Recommend Rep* 56(RR-8):1-14, 2007. Available at: www.cdc.gov/mmwr/preview/mmwrhtml/rr5608a1.htm.

37. Liu J, et al: Lead exposure at each stage of pregnancy and neurobehavioral development of neonates, *Neurotoxicology* 44:1-7, 2014.

38. McIntyre PB, et al: Effect of vaccines on bacterial meningitis worldwide, *Lancet* 380(9854):1703-1711, 2012.

39. Beeslaar J, et al: Clinical data supporting a 2-dose schedule of MenB-FHbp, a bivalent meningococcal serogroup B vaccine, in adolescents and young adults, *Vaccine* 36(28):4004-4013, 2018.

40. Centers for Disease Control and Prevention (CDCP): Vaccines and preventable diseases: meningococcal: who needs to be vaccinated?

Page last reviewed July 26, 2019. Available at: https://www.cdc.gov/vaccines/vpd/mening/index.html.

41. Weingarten L, et al: Encephalitis, *Pediatr Emerg Care* 29(2):235-241, 2013.

42. Kirton A, deVeber G: Paediatric stroke: pressing issues and promising directions, *Lancet Neurol* 14(1):92-102, 2015.

43. Mallick AA, O'Callaghan FJ: The epidemiology of childhood stroke, *Eur J Paediatr Neurol* 14(3):197-205, 2010.

44. Lopez-Vicente M, et al: Diagnosis and management of pediatric arterial ischemic stroke, *J Stroke Cerebrovasc Dis* 19(3):175-183, 2010.

45. Felling RJ, et al: Pediatric arterial ischemic stroke: epidemiology, risk factors, and management, *Blood Cells Mol Dis* 67:23-33, 2017.

46. Ellenbogen JR, Waqar M, Pettorini B: Management of post-haemorrhagic hydrocephalus in premature infants, *J Clin Neurosci* 31:30-34, 2016.

47. Kronenburg A, et al: Recent advances in moyamoya disease: pathophysiology and treatment, *Curr Neurol Neurosci Rep* 14(1):423, 2014.

48. Zack MM, Kobau R: National and state estimates of the numbers of adults and children with active epilepsy—United States, *MMWR Morb Mortal Wkly Rpt* 66:821-825, 2015.

49. Central Brain Tumor Registry of the United States: 2018 CBTRUS fact sheet. Available at: http://www.cbtrus.org/factsheet/factsheet.html.

50. American Cancer Society (ACS): Risk factors for brain and spinal cord tumors in children. Accessed August 6, 2019. Available at: https://www.cancer.org/cancer/brain-spinal-cord-tumors-children/causes-risks-prevention/risk-factors.html.

51. Jacques G, Cormac O: Central nervous system tumors, *Handb Clin Neurol* 112:931-958, 2013.

52. Segal D, Karajannis MA: Pediatric brain tumors: an update, *Curr Probl Pediatr Adolesc Health Care* 46(7):242-250, 2016.

53. American Cancer Society (ACS): What are the key statistics about neuroblastoma? Last revised January 9, 2019. Available at: http://www.cancer.org/cancer/neuroblastoma/detailedguide/neuroblastoma-key-statistics.

54. Rodriguez-Galindo C, et al: Retinoblastoma, *Pediatr Clin North Am* 62(1):201-223, 2015.

55. Knudson AG, Jr: Mutation and cancer: a statistical study of retinoblastoma, *Proc Natl Acad Sci USA* 68(4):820-823, 1971.

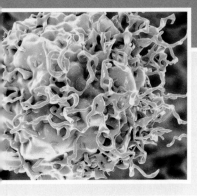

19

Mechanisms of Hormonal Regulation

Valentina L. Brashers, Sue E. Huether

EVOLVE WEBSITE

CHAPTER OUTLINE

The endocrine system is composed of various glands located throughout the body (Fig. 19.1). These glands can synthesize and release special chemical messengers called *hormones.* The endocrine, nervous, and immune systems work together to regulate responses to the internal and external environments. The endocrine system has five general functions: (1) differentiation of the reproductive and central nervous systems in the developing fetus; (2) stimulation of sequential growth and development during childhood and adolescence; (3) coordination of the male and female reproductive systems, which makes sexual reproduction possible; (4) maintenance of an optimal internal environment throughout life; and (5) initiation of corrective and adaptive responses when emergency demands occur. Hormones convey specific regulatory information among cells and organs and are integrated with the nervous system to maintain communication and control. The mechanisms of communication and control occur within a cell *(autocrine)*, between local cells *(paracrine)*, and between cells located remotely from each other *(endocrine).*

MECHANISMS OF HORMONAL REGULATION

Endocrine glands respond to specific signals by synthesizing and releasing hormones into the circulation, which then trigger intracellular responses. All hormones share certain general characteristics:

1. Hormones have specific rates and rhythms of secretion. Three basic patterns of secretion are (a) diurnal patterns, (b) pulsatile and cyclic patterns, and (c) patterns that depend on levels of circulating substrates (e.g., calcium, sodium, potassium, or the hormones themselves).
2. Hormones operate within feedback systems, either negative or positive, to maintain an optimal internal environment.

3. Hormones affect only target cells with specific receptors for the hormone and then act on these cells to initiate specific cell functions or activities.
4. Steroid hormones are either excreted directly by the kidneys or metabolized by the liver, which inactivates them and renders the hormone more water soluble for renal excretion. Peptide hormones are catabolized by circulating enzymes and eliminated in the feces or urine.

Hormones may be classified according to structure, gland of origin, effects, or chemical composition. (Table 19.1 categorizes known hormones based on structure.) The secretion and mechanisms of action of hormones represent an extremely complex system of integrated responses. The endocrine and nervous systems work together to regulate responses to the internal and external environments.

Regulation of Hormone Release

Hormones are released either to respond to an altered cellular environment or to maintain the level of another hormone or substance. One or more of the following mechanisms regulates hormone release: (1) chemical factors (such as blood glucose or calcium levels), (2) endocrine factors (a hormone from one endocrine gland controlling another endocrine gland), and (3) neural control. For example, insulin is secreted by the chemical stimulation of increased plasma glucose levels, cortisol from the adrenal cortex is an endocrine factor that regulates and stimulates insulin secretion, and direct stimulation of the insulin-secreting cells of the pancreas by the autonomic nervous system is a form of neural control.

Feedback systems provide precise monitoring and control of the cellular environment. Both negative- and positive-feedback systems are important for maintaining hormone levels within physiologic ranges.

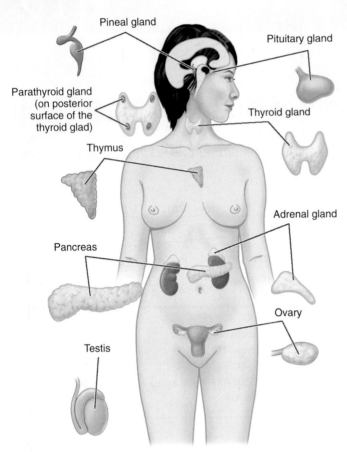

FIGURE 19.1 Major Endocrine Glands. (From Applegate E: *The anatomy and physiology learning system*, ed 4, St Louis, 2011, Saunders.)

TABLE 19.1 Structural Categories of Hormones	
Structural Category	**Examples**
Water Soluble	
Peptides	Growth hormone
	Insulin
	Leptin
	Parathyroid hormone
	Prolactin
Glycoproteins	Follicle-stimulating hormone
	Luteinizing hormone
	Thyroid-stimulating hormone
Polypeptides	Adrenocorticotropic hormone
	Antidiuretic hormone
	Calcitonin
	Endorphins
	Glucagon
	Hypothalamic hormones
	Lipotropins
	Melanocyte-stimulating hormone
	Oxytocin
	Somatostatin
	Thymosin
	Thyrotropin-releasing hormone
Amines	Epinephrine
	Norepinephrine
Lipid Soluble	
Thyroxine (an amine but lipid soluble)	Both thyroxine (T_4) and triiodothyronine (T_3)
Steroids (cholesterol is a precursor for all steroids)	Estrogens
	Glucocorticoids (cortisol)
	Mineralocorticoids (aldosterone)
	Progestins (progesterone)
	Testosterone
Derivatives of arachidonic acid (autocrine or paracrine action)	Leukotrienes
	Prostacyclins
	Prostaglandins
	Thromboxanes

Positive feedback occurs when a neural, chemical, or endocrine response increases the synthesis and secretion of a hormone. Negative feedback occurs when a changing chemical, neural, or endocrine response to a stimulus decreases the synthesis and secretion of a hormone. Fig. 19.2 illustrates both positive and negative feedback within the hypothalamus-pituitary axis and the thyroid gland. Positive feedback occurs when thyrotropin-releasing hormone (TRH) is released from the hypothalamus in response to low thyroid hormone levels. TRH stimulates the secretion of thyroid-stimulating hormone (TSH), which then stimulates the synthesis and secretion of the thyroid hormones thyroxine (T_4) and triiodothyronine (T_3). Negative feedback occurs when increasing levels of T_4 and T_3 feedback on the pituitary and hypothalamus to inhibit TRH and TSH synthesis and decrease the synthesis and production of thyroid hormones. The lack of positive or negative feedback on hormonal release often results in pathologic changes in hormone production (see Chapter 20).

Hormone Transport

Once hormones are released into the circulatory system, they are distributed throughout the body. The protein (peptide) hormones (see Table 19.1) are water soluble and generally circulate in free (unbound) forms. Water-soluble hormones generally have a half-life of seconds to minutes because they are catabolized by circulating enzymes. For example, insulin has a half-life of 3 to 5 minutes and is catabolized by insulinases. Lipid-soluble hormones (see Table 19.1), such as cortisol and adrenal androgens, are transported bound to a water-soluble carrier or transport protein and can remain in the blood for hours to days. Only free hormones (those not bound to a carrier protein) can signal a target

cell. Because there is equilibrium between the concentrations of free hormones and hormones bound to plasma proteins, a significant change in the concentration of binding (carrier) proteins can affect the concentration of free hormones in the plasma. For example, malnutrition and liver disease can lower the serum levels of the carrier protein albumin, causing a decrease in the lipid-soluble hormones thyroxine, cortisol, and aldosterone. (Mechanisms of hormone binding are discussed in Chapter 1.) Free hormone levels can be measured using a variety of measurement techniques, including radioimmunoassay (RIA), enzyme-linked immunosorbent assay (ELISA), or bioassay.

Hormone Receptors

Although a hormone is distributed throughout the body, only those cells with appropriate receptors for that hormone, termed target cells, are affected. Hormone receptors of the target cell have two main functions: (1) to recognize and bind specifically and with high affinity to their particular hormones and (2) to initiate a signal to appropriate intracellular effectors.

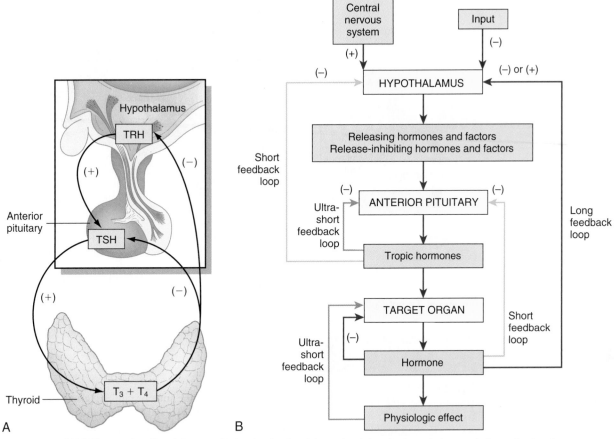

FIGURE 19.2 Feedback Loops. Endocrine feedback loops involving the hypothalamus-pituitary gland and end organs; in this example, the thyroid gland is illustrated (endocrine regulation). *TRH,* Thyroid-releasing hormone; *TSH,* thyroid-stimulating hormone; *T₃,* triiodothyronine; *T₄,* tetraiodothyronine (thyroxine).

The sensitivity of the target cell to a particular hormone is related to the total number of receptors per cell or the affinity of the receptors for the hormone: the more receptors or the higher the affinity of the receptors, the more sensitive the cell to the stimulating effects of the hormone. Low concentrations of hormone increase the number or affinity of receptors per cell; this is called up-regulation. High concentrations of hormone decrease the number or affinity of receptors; this is called down-regulation (Fig. 19.3). Thus the cell can adjust its sensitivity to the concentration of the signaling hormone. The receptors on the plasma membrane are continuously synthesized and degraded, so that changes in receptor concentration or affinity may occur within hours. Various physiochemical conditions can affect both the receptor number and the affinity of the hormone for its receptor. Some of these physiochemical conditions are the fluidity and structure of the plasma membrane, pH, temperature, ion concentration, diet, and the presence of other chemicals (e.g., drugs). Finally, mutations may affect receptor number or structure.

Types of Hormone Receptors

Hormone receptors may be located in the plasma membrane or in the intracellular compartment of the target cell (Fig. 19.4). Water-soluble (peptide) hormones, which include the protein hormones and the catecholamines, have a high molecular weight and cannot diffuse across the cell membrane. They interact or bind with receptors located in or on the cell membrane. Lipid-soluble hormones diffuse freely across the plasma and nuclear membranes and bind with cytosolic or nuclear

Up-Regulation

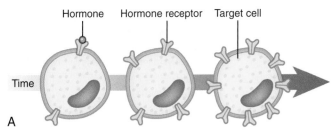

Down-Regulation

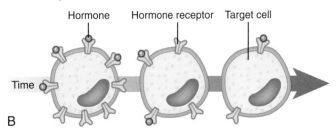

FIGURE 19.3 Regulation of Target Cell Sensitivity. A, Low hormone level and up-regulation, or an increase in the number of receptors. **B,** High hormone level and down-regulation, or a decrease in the number of receptors.

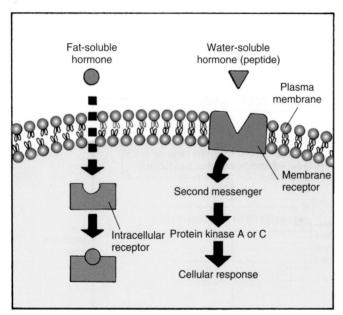

FIGURE 19.4 Hormone Binding at Target Cell.

TABLE 19.2   Second Messengers Identified for Specific Hormones

Second Messenger	Associated Hormones
Cyclic AMP	Adrenocorticotropic hormone (ACTH)
	Luteinizing hormone (LH)
	Human chorionic gonadotropin (hCG)
	Follicle-stimulating hormone (FSH)
	Thyroid-stimulating hormone (TSH)
	Antidiuretic hormone (ADH)
	Thyrotropin-releasing hormone (TRH)
	Parathyroid hormone (PTH)
	Glucagon
Cyclic GMP	Atrial natriuretic peptide
Calcium and IP$_3$	Angiotensin II
	Gonadotropin-releasing hormone (GnRH)
	Antidiuretic hormone (ADH)
	Luteinizing hormone–releasing hormone (LHRH)
Tyrosine kinases	Insulin
	Growth hormone
	Leptin
	Prolactin

AMP, Adenosine monophosphate; *GMP,* guanosine monophosphate; *IP$_3$,* inositol triphosphate.

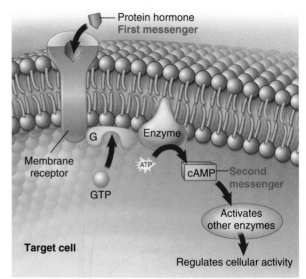

FIGURE 19.5 Mechanism of First and Second Messenger Action. The hormone acts as a "first messenger," delivering its message via the bloodstream to a membrane receptor in the target cell much like a key fits into a lock. The "second messenger" causes the cell to respond and perform its specialized function. (From Patton KT, Thibodeau GA: *Structure & function of the body,* ed 15, St Louis, 2016, Mosby.)

receptor, although receptors for some lipid-soluble hormones are located in or near the plasma membrane.[1]

Water-soluble hormone binding with plasma membrane receptors initiates a complex cascade of intracellular effects. In this cascade, the hormone is termed the **first messenger.** The hormone-receptor interaction initiates a signal that generates a small molecule inside the cell, called the **second messenger.** The second messenger conveys the signal from the receptor to the cytoplasm and nucleus of the cell and mediates the effect of the hormone on the target cell. Second messengers include cyclic adenosine monophosphate (cAMP), cyclic guanosine monophosphate (cGMP), calcium, inositol triphosphate (IP$_3$), and the tyrosine kinase system (Table 19.2). The second messenger cAMP increases when

first messengers from the anterior pituitary gland, such as adrenocorticotropic hormone (ACTH) and TSH, bind to a cell membrane receptor. Increased levels of intracellular cAMP activate protein kinases, leading to activation or deactivation of intracellular enzymes (Fig. 19.5). cGMP also functions as a second messenger following receptor binding of first messengers, such as atrial natriuretic peptide and nitric oxide. The second messenger IP$_3$ is increased in response to angiotensin II and antidiuretic hormone (ADH) receptor binding and triggers a release of intracellular calcium. This leads to the formation of the calcium-calmodulin complex, which mediates the effects of calcium on intracellular activities that are crucial for cell metabolism and growth. Finally, some hormone first messengers, such as insulin, growth hormone, and prolactin, bind to surface receptors that directly activate second messengers of the tyrosine kinase family. These tyrosine kinases include the Janus family of tyrosine kinases (JAK) and signal transducers and activators of transcription (STAT). They regulate a wide range of intracellular processes that contribute to cellular metabolism and growth.

Receptors for lipid-soluble hormones are in the cytosol and nucleus and directly modulate gene expression without complex second messengers (Fig. 19.6). With the exception of thyroid hormones, the lipid-soluble hormones are synthesized from cholesterol (giving rise to the term "steroid") (see Table 19.1). Because these are relatively small, lipophilic, hydrophobic molecules, lipid-soluble hormones can cross the lipid plasma membrane by simple diffusion (see Chapter 1). The effects of lipid-soluble hormones on cytosol and nuclear receptors can take hours to days, however, activation of receptors for lipid-soluble hormones in the plasma membrane are associated with rapid responses (seconds to minutes) as shown in Fig. 19.6.

✔ **QUICK CHECK 19.1**
1. What are hormones? By what mechanisms do they function?
2. What is meant by negative-feedback regulation of hormone release?
3. How do first messengers differ from second messengers?
4. Where are the receptors located for lipid-soluble hormones?

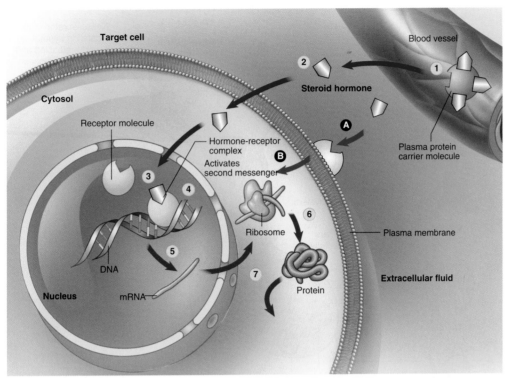

FIGURE 19.6 Steroid Hormone Mechanism. Lipid-soluble steroid hormone molecules detach from the carrier protein (**1**) and pass through the plasma membrane (**2**). Hormone molecules then diffuse into the nucleus, where they bind to a receptor to form a hormone-receptor complex (**3**). This complex then binds to a specific site on a deoxyribonucleic acid *(DNA)* molecule (**4**), triggering transcription of the genetic information encoded there (**5**). The resulting messenger ribonucleic acid *(mRNA)* molecule moves to the cytosol, where it associates with a ribosome, initiating synthesis of a new protein (**6**). This new protein—usually an enzyme or channel protein—produces specific effects on the target cell (**7**). The classic genomic action is typically slow *(red arrows)*. Steroids also may exact rapid effects *(green arrows)* by binding to receptors on the plasma membrane (**A**) and activating an intercellular second messenger (**B**). (From Patton KT, Thibodeau GA: *Anatomy & physiology,* ed 9, St Louis, 2016, Mosby.)

STRUCTURE AND FUNCTION OF THE ENDOCRINE GLANDS

Hypothalamic–Pituitary System

The hypothalamic–pituitary axis (HPA) forms the structural and functional basis for central integration of the neurologic and endocrine systems, creating what is called the *neuroendocrine system.* The HPA produces several hormones that affect a number of diverse body functions (Fig. 19.7), including thyroid, adrenal, and reproductive functions.

The **hypothalamus** is located at the base of the brain. It is connected to the pituitary gland by the pituitary stalk (Fig. 19.8). The hypothalamus is connected to the anterior pituitary through hypophysial portal blood vessels (Fig. 19.9) and to the posterior pituitary via a nerve tract referred to as the *hypothalamohypophysial tract* (Fig. 19.10). These connections are vital to the functioning of the hypothalamic–pituitary system. The hypothalamus contains special neurosecretory cells that synthesize and secrete the hypothalamic-releasing hormones that regulate the release of hormones from the anterior pituitary. In addition, these cells synthesize the hormones ADH (also called *vasopressin*) and oxytocin, which are released from the posterior pituitary gland. These hormones are summarized in Table 19.3.

The **pituitary gland** is located in the sella turcica (a saddle-shaped depression of the sphenoid bone at the base of the skull). It weighs approximately 0.5 g, except during pregnancy, when its weight increases by about 30%. It is composed of two distinctly different lobes: (1)

the anterior pituitary, or adenohypophysis; and (2) the posterior pituitary, or neurohypophysis (see Fig. 19.7). These two lobes differ in their embryonic origins, cell types, and functional relationship to the hypothalamus.

The Anterior Pituitary

The **anterior pituitary** (adenohypophysis) is composed of three regions: (1) the pars distalis, (2) the pars tuberalis, and (3) the pars intermedia. The **pars distalis** is the major component of the anterior pituitary and is the source of the anterior pituitary hormones. The **pars tuberalis** is a thin layer of cells on the anterior and lateral portions of the pituitary stalk. The **pars intermedia** lies between the two and secretes melanocyte-stimulating hormone in the fetus. In the adult, the distinct pars intermedia disappears and the individual cells are distributed diffusely throughout the pars distalis and pars nervosa (neural lobe) of the posterior pituitary.

The anterior pituitary is composed of two main cell types: (1) the **chromophobes,** which appear to be nonsecretory; and (2) the **chromophils,** which are the secretory cells of the adenohypophysis. The chromophils are subdivided into seven secretory cell types, and each cell type secretes a specific hormone or hormones. In general, the anterior pituitary hormones are regulated by (1) secretion of hypothalamic releasing factors, (2) feedback effects of the hormones secreted by target glands, and (3) direct effects of other mediating neurotransmitters.

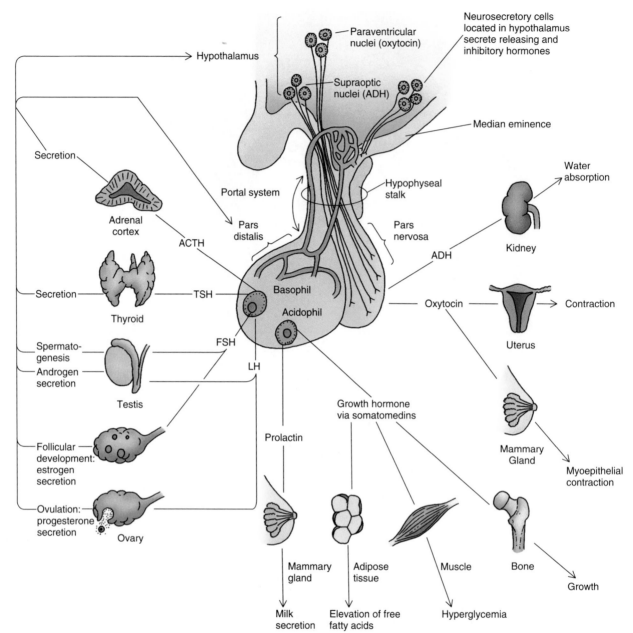

FIGURE 19.7 The Hypothalamic-Pituitary Axis and Its Target Organs. *ACTH,* adrenocorticotropic hormone; *ADH,* antidiuretic hormone; *FSH,* follicle-stimulating hormone; *LH,* luteinizing hormone; *TSH,* thyroid-stimulating hormone. (From Gartner LP, Hiatt JL: *Color textbook of histology,* ed 3, Philadelphia, 2007, Saunders.)

The anterior pituitary secretes tropic hormones that affect the physiologic function of specific target organs (see Fig. 19.7 and Table 19.4). Melanocyte-stimulating hormone (MSH) promotes the pituitary secretion of melanin, which darkens skin color. The glycoprotein hormones follicle-stimulating hormone (FSH) and luteinizing hormone (LH) influence reproductive function and are discussed in Chapter 34. Adrenocorticotropic hormone (ACTH) regulates the release of cortisol from the adrenal cortex. Thyroid-stimulating hormone (TSH) regulates the activity of the thyroid gland. The roles of ACTH and TSH are discussed later in this chapter. Growth hormone (GH) and prolactin are called the somatotropic hormones and have diverse effects on body tissues. GH secretion is controlled by two hormones from the hypothalamus: growth hormone–releasing hormone (GHRH), which increases GH secretion; and somatostatin, which inhibits GH secretion.

GH is essential to normal tissue growth and maturation and also impacts aging, sleep, nutritional status, stress, and reproductive hormones.

Many of the anabolic functions of GH are mediated, at least in part, by the insulin-like growth factors (IGFs), also known as the *somatomedins.* There are two primary forms of IGF, IGF-1 and IGF-2, of which IGF-1 is the most biologically active. They both circulate bound to a group of IGF-binding proteins (IGFBPs) modulating their availability. IGF-1 binds to IGF-1 receptors, mediating the anabolic effects of GH. IGF-1 also binds to insulin receptors, providing an insulin-like effect on skeletal muscle. IGF-2 has important effects on fetal growth. Because of the anabolic effects of GH and IGF-1, they can be used to treat growth disorders, increase muscle mass, and potentially slow the aging process; but there are concerns about their safety (see *Did You Know?* Growth Hormone and Insulin-like Growth Factor in Aging).

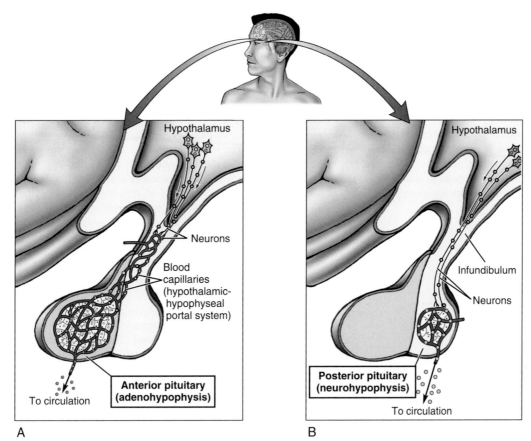

FIGURE 19.8 Pituitary Gland. The pituitary gland sits within the sella turcica of the sphenoid bone of the skull. **A,** Relationship of the hypothalamus to the anterior pituitary gland. **B,** Relationship of the hypothalamus to the posterior pituitary gland. (From Herlihy B: *The human body in health and illness,* ed 5, St Louis, 2015, Saunders.)

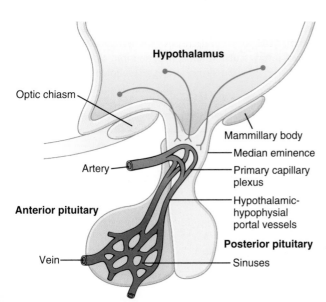

FIGURE 19.9 Hypophysial Portal System. (From Hall JE: *Guyton and Hall textbook of medical physiology,* ed 13, Philadelphia, 2016, Saunders.)

DID YOU KNOW?

Growth Hormone and Insulin-Like Growth Factor in Aging

The aging process is associated with many hormonal and metabolic changes. The amounts of growth hormone (GH) and insulin-like growth factor (IGF) decline with aging, a process that has been called the "somatopause." Clinical findings related to somatotropic hormone changes with aging include increased visceral fat, decreased lean body mass, decreased bone density, and changes in reproductive and cognitive function. The underlying mechanisms of aging and its relationship to GH and IGF are complex. For example, these hormones not only promote bone and muscle growth, but they also may be factors in determining overall life span and ability to respond to physiologic stress. GH and IGF effects on inflammation and immunity also are important in the aging process. Although many studies suggest that a deficiency of these hormones leads to an acceleration of the aging process, there are other studies suggesting that lower lifetime levels of these hormones may confer longevity by providing protection from cancer and other age-related diseases. As these hormones are used to treat a wider range of disorders and for different age groups, more information about their safety is emerging and newer formulations, such as biosimilar recombinant human growth hormone (rhGH), are being tested.

Data from Ashpole NM et al: *Exp Gerontol* 68:76-81, 2015; Balasubramanian P, Longo VD: *Growth Horm IGF Res* 28:66-68, 2016; Borras Perez MV et al: *Drug Des, Devel Ther* 11:1497-1503, 2017; Di Bona D et al: *Curr Vasc Pharmacol* 12:674-681, 2014; Junnila RK et al: *Nat Rev Endocrinol* 9(6):366-376, 2013; Li Z et al: *Oncotarget* 7(49):81862-81869, 2016.

Prolactin primarily functions to induce milk production during pregnancy and lactation. It has immune stimulatory effects and modulates immune and inflammatory responses with both physiologic and pathologic reactions. Its synthesis is stimulated by vasoactive intestinal polypeptide, serotonin, and growth factors. Release of prolactin is inhibited by dopamine.

The Posterior Pituitary

The embryonic posterior pituitary (neurohypophysis) is derived from the hypothalamus and is comprised of three parts: (1) the median eminence, located at the base of the hypothalamus; (2) the pituitary stalk; and (3) the infundibular process, also known as the *pars nervosa* or *neural lobe*. The median eminence is composed largely of the nerve endings of axons from the ventral hypothalamus. It often is designated as part of the posterior pituitary and contains at least 10 biologically active hypothalamic releasing hormones, as well as the neurotransmitters dopamine, norepinephrine, serotonin, acetylcholine, and histamine. The pituitary stalk contains the axons of neurons that originate in the supraoptic and paraventricular nuclei of the hypothalamus and connects the pituitary gland to the brain. Axons originating in the hypothalamus terminate in the pars nervosa, which secretes the hormones of the posterior pituitary (see Fig. 19.10).

The posterior pituitary secretes two polypeptide hormones: (1) antidiuretic hormone (ADH), also called *arginine vasopressin*; and (2) oxytocin. These hormones differ by only two amino acids. They are synthesized—along with their binding proteins, the neurophysins—in the supraoptic and paraventricular nuclei of the hypothalamus (see Fig. 19.10). They are packaged in secretory vesicles and are moved down the axons of the pituitary stalk to the pars nervosa for storage. The release of ADH and oxytocin is mediated by cholinergic and adrenergic neurotransmitters. The major stimulus to both ADH and oxytocin release is glutamate, whereas the major inhibitory input is through gamma-aminobutyric acid (GABA). Before release into the circulatory system, ADH and oxytocin are split from the neurophysins and are secreted in unbound form.

Antidiuretic hormone. The major homeostatic function of the posterior pituitary is the control of plasma osmolality as regulated by antidiuretic hormone (ADH) (see Chapter 5). At physiologic levels, ADH increases the permeability of the distal renal tubules and collecting ducts (see Chapter 31). This increased permeability leads to increased water reabsorption into the blood, thus concentrating the urine and reducing serum osmolality. The secretion of ADH is regulated primarily by the osmoreceptors of the hypothalamus, located near or in the supraoptic nuclei. As plasma osmolality increases, these osmoreceptors are stimulated, the rate of ADH secretion increases, thirst is stimulated increasing water intake, and more water is reabsorbed by the kidney. The plasma is diluted back to its set-point osmolality. ADH has no direct effect on electrolyte levels, but by increasing water reabsorption, serum electrolyte concentrations may decrease because of a dilutional effect.[2]

ADH secretion also is stimulated by decreased intravascular volume, as monitored by baroreceptors in the left atrium, in the carotid arteries, and in the aortic arches. Stress, trauma, pain, exercise, nausea, nicotine, exposure to heat, and drugs such as morphine also increase ADH secretion. ADH secretion decreases with decreased plasma osmolality, increased intravascular volume, hypertension, alcohol ingestion, and an increase in estrogen, progesterone, or angiotensin II levels.

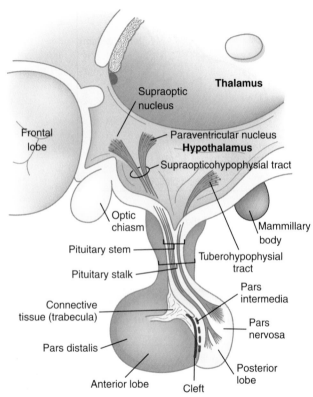

FIGURE 19.10 Nerve Tracts From Hypothalamus to Posterior Lobe of Pituitary Gland.

TABLE 19.3	**Hypothalamic Hormones**	
	Hormone	**Action**
Target the anterior pituitary	Thyrotropin-releasing hormone (TRH)	Stimulates release of thyroid-stimulating hormone (TSH); modulates prolactin secretion
	Gonadotropin-releasing hormone (GnRH)	Stimulates release of follicle-stimulating hormone (FSH) and luteinizing hormone (LH)
	Somatostatin	Inhibits release of growth hormone (GH) and TSH
	Growth hormone–releasing hormone (GHRH)	Stimulates release of GH
	Corticotropin-releasing hormone (CRH)	Stimulates release of adrenocorticotropic hormone (ACTH) and β-endorphin
	Substance P	Inhibits synthesis and release of adrenocorticotropic hormone (ACTH); stimulates secretion of GH, FSH, LH, and prolactin
	Prolactin-inhibiting factor (PIF, dopamine)	Inhibits synthesis and secretion of prolactin
	Prolactin-releasing factor (PRF)	Stimulates secretion of prolactin
Travel to posterior pituitary for release	Antidiuretic hormone (ADH)	Increases water reabsorption through the renal collecting ducts to reduce plasma osmolarity
	Oxytocin	Stimulates contraction of the uterus and milk ejection in lactating women

TABLE 19.4 Tropic Hormones of the Anterior Pituitary and Their Functions

Hormone	Target Organs	Functions
Adrenocorticotropic hormone (ACTH)	Adrenal gland (cortex)	Increased steroidogenesis (cortisol and androgenic hormones); synthesis of adrenal proteins contributing to maintenance of adrenal gland
Melanocyte-stimulating hormone (MSH)	Anterior pituitary	Promotes secretion of melanin and lipotropin by anterior pituitary; makes skin darker
Somatotropic Hormones		
Growth hormone (GH)	Muscle, bone, liver	Regulates metabolic processes related to growth and adaptation to physical and emotional stressors, muscle growth, increased protein synthesis, increased liver glycogenolysis, increased fat mobilization
	Liver	Induces formation of somatomedins, or insulin-like growth factors (IGFs) that have actions similar to insulin
Prolactin	Breast	Milk production
Glycoprotein Hormones		
Thyroid-stimulating hormone (TSH)	Thyroid gland	Increased production and secretion of thyroid hormone
		Increased iodide uptake; promotes hypertrophy and hyperplasia of thymocytes
Luteinizing hormone (LH)	*In women:* granulosa cells	Ovulation, progesterone production
	In men: Leydig cells	Testicular growth, testosterone production
Follicle-stimulating hormone (FSH)	*In women:* granulosa cells	Follicle maturation, estrogen production
	In men: Sertoli cells	Spermatogenesis
β-Lipotropin	Adipose cells	Fat breakdown and release of fatty acids
β-Endorphins	Adipose cells; brain opioid receptors	Analgesia; may regulate body temperature, food and water intake

Physiologic levels of ADH do not significantly impact vessel tone. However, ADH was originally named *vasopressin* because, at extremely high levels, it causes vasoconstriction and a resulting increase in arterial blood pressure. For example, high doses of ADH (given as the drug vasopressin) may be administered to achieve hemostasis during hemorrhage and to raise blood pressure in shock states.

Oxytocin. Oxytocin is responsible for contraction of the uterus and milk ejection in lactating women and may affect sperm motility in men. In both genders, oxytocin has an antidiuretic effect similar to that of ADH. In women, oxytocin is secreted in response to suckling and mechanical distention of the female reproductive tract. Oxytocin binds to its receptors on myoepithelial cells in the mammary tissues and causes contraction of those cells, which increases intramammary pressure and milk expression ("let-down" reflex). Oxytocin acts on the uterus near the end of labor to enhance the effectiveness of contractions, promote delivery of the placenta, and stimulate postpartum uterine contractions, thereby preventing excessive bleeding. The function of this hormone is discussed in detail in Chapter 34.

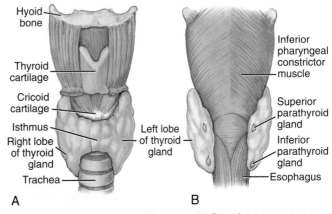

FIGURE 19.11 Thyroid and Parathyroid Glands. A, Anterior view. **B,** Posterior view. (From Fehrenbach MJ, et al: *Illustrated anatomy of the head and neck,* ed 4, St Louis, 2012, Saunders.)

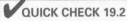

QUICK CHECK 19.2
1. What is the relationship between the hypothalamus and the pituitary?
2. What is the action of antidiuretic hormone (ADH)?

Pineal Gland

The pineal gland is located near the center of the brain and is composed of photoreceptive cells that secrete melatonin. It is innervated by noradrenergic sympathetic nerve terminals controlled by pathways within the hypothalamus. Melatonin release is stimulated by exposure to dark and inhibited by light exposure. It is synthesized from tryptophan, which is first converted to serotonin and then to melatonin. Melatonin regulates circadian rhythms and reproductive systems, including the secretion of the gonadotropin-releasing hormones and the onset of puberty. It also plays an important role in immune regulation and is postulated to impact the aging process. Further effects of melatonin include increasing nitric oxide release from blood vessels, removing toxic oxygen free radicals, and decreasing insulin secretion. Melatonin has been used therapeutically in humans to help with sleep disturbances, jet lag, and psychological and inflammatory disorders. Its utility for numerous other disorders is being explored.

Thyroid and Parathyroid Glands

The thyroid gland, located in the neck just below the larynx, produces hormones that control the rates of metabolic processes throughout the body. The four parathyroid glands are near the posterior side of the thyroid and function to control serum calcium levels (Fig. 19.11).

Thyroid Gland

Two lobes of the thyroid gland lie on either side of the trachea, inferior to the thyroid cartilage and joined by a small band of tissue termed the isthmus. The pyramidal lobe is superior to the isthmus (see Fig. 19.11). The normal thyroid gland is not visible on inspection, but it may be palpated on swallowing, which causes it to be displaced upward.

The thyroid gland consists of follicles that contain follicular cells surrounding a viscous substance called *colloid* (Fig. 19.12). The follicular cells synthesize and secrete the thyroid hormones. Neurons terminate on blood vessels within the thyroid gland and on the follicular cells themselves, so neurotransmitters (acetylcholine, catecholamines) may directly affect the secretory activity of follicular cells and thyroid blood flow. Approximately a 2-month supply of thyroid hormone is stored in the gland.

Also found in the thyroid are parafollicular cells, or C cells (see Fig. 19.12). C cells secrete various polypeptides, including calcitonin. At high levels, calcitonin, also called *thyrocalcitonin,* lowers serum calcium levels by inhibiting bone-resorbing osteoclasts. However, in humans the metabolic consequences of calcitonin deficiency or excess do not appear to be significant. (Bone resorption is explained in Chapter 40.) Calcitonin can be used therapeutically to treat a number of bone disorders, including osteogenesis imperfecta, osteoporosis, and Paget bone disease, among others. Parafollicular cells can give rise to medullary thyroid carcinoma.

Regulation of thyroid hormone secretion. Thyroid hormone (TH) is regulated through a negative-feedback loop involving the hypothalamus, the anterior pituitary, and the thyroid gland (see Fig. 19.2). This loop is initiated by thyrotropin-releasing hormone (TRH), which is synthesized and stored within the hypothalamus. TRH is released into the hypothalamic-pituitary portal system and circulates to the anterior pituitary, where it stimulates the release of TSH.

TSH is a glycoprotein synthesized and stored within the anterior pituitary. When TSH is secreted by the anterior pituitary, it circulates to bind with receptors on the plasma membrane of the thyroid follicular cells. The primary effect of TSH on the thyroid gland is to cause an immediate release of stored TH and an increase in TH synthesis. TSH also increases growth of the thyroid gland by stimulating thymocyte hyperplasia and hypertrophy. As TH levels rise, there is a negative-feedback effect on the HPA to inhibit TRH and TSH release, which

then results in decreased TH synthesis and secretion. TH synthesis is also controlled by serum iodide levels and by circulating selenium-dependent enzymes, called *deiodinases,* which inactivate the precursor molecule thyroxine.

Synthesis of thyroid hormone. Thyroid hormone synthesis is summarized in these steps:

1. Uniodinated thyroglobulin (a large glycoprotein) is produced by the endoplasmic reticulum of the thyroid follicular cells.
2. Tyrosine (an amino acid) is incorporated into the thyroglobulin of follicular cells as it is synthesized.
3. Iodide (the inorganic form of iodine) is actively transferred from the blood into the colloid by carrier proteins located in the outer membrane of the follicular cells. This active transport system is called the *iodide trap* and is very efficient at accumulating the trace amounts of iodide from the blood.
4. Iodide is oxidized and quickly attaches to tyrosine within the thyroglobulin molecule.
5. Coupling of iodinated tyrosine forms thyroid hormones. Triiodothyronine (T_3) is formed from the coupling of monoiodotyrosine (one iodine atom and tyrosine) and diiodotyrosine (two iodine atoms and tyrosine). Tetraiodothyronine (T_4), commonly known as thyroxine, is formed from the coupling of two diiodotyrosines.
6. Thyroid hormones are stored attached to thyroglobulin within the colloid until they are released into the circulation.

The thyroid gland normally produces 90% T_4 and 10% T_3. Once released into the circulation, T_3 and T_4 are primarily transported bound to thyroxine-binding globulin (TBG), though some TH is transported by thyroxine-binding prealbumin (transthyretin), albumin, or lipoproteins. The bound form serves as a reservoir, whereas the unbound (free) form is active. In the body tissues, most of the T_4 is converted to T_3, which acts on the target cell.

Actions of thyroid hormone. TH has a significant effect on the growth, maturation, and function of cells and tissues throughout the body. TH binds to intracellular receptor complexes and then influences the genetic expression of specific proteins. TH is essential for normal growth and neurologic development in the fetus and infant and affects metabolic, neurologic, cardiovascular, and respiratory functioning across the life span. In addition, TH is required for the metabolism and function of blood cells, as well as normal muscle functioning and the integrity of skin, nails, and hair. Similar to some steroid hormones, TH also

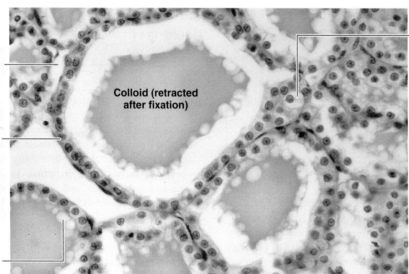

Blood vessels are found around the follicles.

Follicular epithelium In the inactive follicle, the follicular epithelium is simple low cuboidal, or squamous. During their active secretory phase, the cells become columnar.

Area of colloid resorption

Colloid (retracted after fixation)

A C cell can be distinguished from surrounding follicular cells by its pale cytoplasm.
   Two more effective identification approaches are:
1. Immunocytochemistry, using an antibody to calcitonin.
2. Electron microscopy, to visualize calcitonin-containing cytoplasmic granules.

FIGURE 19.12 Thyroid Follicle Cells.

affects cell metabolism by altering protein, fat, and glucose metabolism and, as a result, increasing heat production and oxygen consumption. Additionally, TH has permissive effects throughout the body by optimizing the actions of other hormones and neurotransmitters.[3]

Parathyroid Glands

Normally two pairs of small parathyroid glands are present behind the upper and lower poles of the thyroid gland (see Fig. 19.11). However, their number may range from two to six.

The parathyroid glands produce **parathyroid hormone (PTH),** which is the single most important factor in the regulation of the serum calcium concentration. A decrease in serum calcium stimulates PTH secretion, which acts to increase the serum calcium concentration and decrease the level of serum phosphate (Fig. 19.13). PTH acts directly on the bone to release calcium by stimulating osteoclast activity. PTH also acts on the kidney to increase calcium reabsorption while phosphate reabsorption is decreased. The resultant increase in the serum calcium concentration inhibits PTH secretion. **1,25-Dihydroxy-vitamin D$_3$** (the active form of vitamin D) is activated by the kidney and works as a cofactor with PTH to promote calcium and phosphate absorption in the gut and enhance bone mineralization. Vitamin D also plays an important role in metabolic processes and controlling inflammation. It has been found to be deficient in the majority of individuals in the United States (see *Did You Know?* Vitamin D).

Phosphate and magnesium concentrations also affect PTH secretion. An increase in the serum phosphate level decreases the serum calcium level by causing calcium-phosphate precipitation into soft tissue and bone, which indirectly stimulates PTH secretion. Hypomagnesemia in persons with normal calcium levels acts as a mild stimulant to PTH secretion; however, in persons with hypocalcemia, hypomagnesemia decreases PTH secretion.

✔ **QUICK CHECK 19.3**

1. How does the anterior pituitary regulate the thyroid gland?
2. What form of thyroid hormone is biologically active?
3. What two organs are the sites of action of parathyroid hormone (PTH)?

DID YOU KNOW?

Vitamin D

Vitamin D is essential for bone health and is widely used for the prevention and treatment of postmenopausal osteoporosis and renal osteodystrophy. More recently, vitamin D deficiency has been found to affect more than 75% of all Americans, and more than 90% of Americans with pigmented skin. Inadequate serum levels of vitamin D have been linked to numerous disorders, including infections, cancer, heart disease, dementia, diabetes, chronic pain syndromes, and autoimmune disorders, but cause and effect has never been established. In fact, recent reviews have found that there is still inadequate evidence that vitamin D supplementation reduces the risk for any of these nonskeletal conditions. However, many health organizations recommend an increased intake of vitamin D–containing foods (seafood, vitamin D–fortified juices, and milk products), increased exposure to sunlight, and supplementation with vitamin D. The Institute of Medicine currently recommends 400 to 800 units of vitamin D per day for children and adults and 400 units for infants up to 12 months of age.

Data from LeFevre ML, LeFevre NM: *Am Fam Physician* 97(4):254-260, 2018; Mihos CG et al: *Cardiol Rev* 25(4):189-196, 2017; Mondul AM et al: *Epidemiol Rev* 39(1):28-48, 2017; National Institutes of Health, Office of Dietary Supplements: *Vitamin D.* Updated November 9, 2018. Available at https://ods.od.nih.gov/factsheets/VitaminD-HealthProfessional/; Pilz S et al: *Anticancer Res.* 38(2):1145-1151, 2018.

Endocrine Pancreas

The **pancreas** is both an endocrine gland that produces hormones and an exocrine gland that produces digestive enzymes. (The exocrine function of the pancreas is discussed in Chapter 37.) The pancreas is located behind the stomach, between the spleen and the duodenum, and houses the **islets of Langerhans.** The islets of Langerhans have four types of hormone-secreting cells: **alpha cells,** which secrete glucagon; **beta cells,** which secrete insulin and amylin; **delta cells,** which secrete gastrin and somatostatin; and **F (or PP) cells,** which secrete pancreatic polypeptide. These hormones regulate carbohydrate, fat, and protein

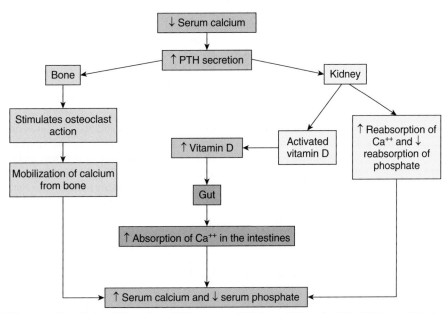

FIGURE 19.13 The Role of Parathyroid Hormone (PTH) and Vitamin D in Calcium Metabolism.

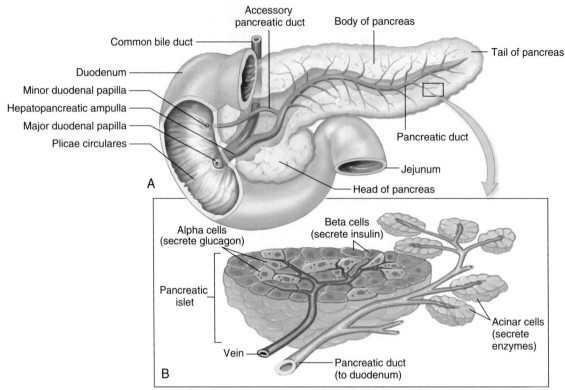

FIGURE 19.14 The Pancreas. A, Pancreas dissected to show main and accessory ducts. The main duct may join the common bile duct, as shown here, to enter the duodenum by a single opening at the major duodenal papilla, or the two ducts may have separate openings. The accessory pancreatic duct is usually present and has a separate opening into the duodenum. **B,** Exocrine glandular cells (around small pancreatic ducts) and endocrine glandular cells of the pancreatic islets (adjacent to blood capillaries). Exocrine pancreatic cells secrete pancreatic juice, alpha endocrine cells secrete glucagon, and beta cells secrete insulin. (From Patton KT, Thibodeau GA: *Structure & function of the body,* ed 15, St Louis, 2016, Mosby.)

metabolism. (The pancreas is illustrated in Fig. 19.14.) Nerves from both the sympathetic and the parasympathetic divisions of the autonomic nervous system innervate the pancreatic islets.

Insulin

The beta cells of the pancreas synthesize insulin from the precursor proinsulin, which is formed from a larger precursor molecule, preproinsulin. Proinsulin is composed of A peptide and B peptide connected by a C peptide and two disulfide bonds. C peptide is cleaved by proteolytic enzymes, leaving the bonded A and B peptides as the insulin molecule. Insulin circulates freely in the plasma and is not bound to a carrier. C peptide level can be measured in the blood and used as an indirect measurement of serum insulin synthesis.

Secretion of insulin is regulated by chemical, hormonal, and neural control. The primary stimulus for insulin secretion is an increase in blood levels of glucose. Insulin secretion also is stimulated by the parasympathetic nervous system usually before eating a meal. Other factors stimulating insulin secretion include some amino acids (leucine, arginine, and lysine) and gastrointestinal hormones (glucagon, gastrin, cholecystokinin, secretin). Insulin secretion diminishes in response to low blood levels of glucose (hypoglycemia), high levels of insulin (through negative feedback to the beta cells), and sympathetic stimulation of the beta cells in the islets.

At the target cell, insulin signaling is initiated when insulin binds and activates its cell surface receptor. These receptors are found on cells throughout the body.[4] The sensitivity of the insulin receptor is a key component in maintaining normal cellular function. Insulin sensitivity is affected by age, weight, abdominal fat, and physical activity. Insulin resistance has been implicated in numerous diseases, including hypertension, heart disease, and type 2 diabetes mellitus. Adipocytes release a number of hormones and cytokines that are altered in obesity and have an important impact on insulin sensitivity (see Chapter 21). The most effective measures shown to improve insulin sensitivity in humans are weight loss and exercise.

Insulin promotes cellular glucose uptake through glucose transporters (GLUT). An intracellular cascade of phosphorylation events, protein–protein interactions, and second-messenger generation then occurs, resulting in diverse metabolic events (see details in Fig. 19.15). Insulin is an anabolic hormone that promotes glucose uptake primarily in liver, muscle, and adipose tissue. It also increases the synthesis of proteins, carbohydrates, lipids, and nucleic acids. It functions mainly in the liver, muscle, and adipose tissue. The net effect of insulin in these tissues is to stimulate protein and fat synthesis and decrease the blood glucose level. The brain, red blood cells, kidney, and lens of the eye do not require insulin for glucose transport. Insulin also facilitates the intracellular transport of potassium (K$^+$), phosphate, and magnesium.

Amylin

Amylin (or islet amyloid polypeptide) is a peptide hormone co-secreted with insulin by beta cells in response to nutrient stimuli. It regulates blood glucose concentration by delaying gastric emptying and suppressing glucagon secretion after meals. Amylin also has a satiety effect, which reduces food intake. Through these mechanisms, amylin works with insulin to prevent hyperglycemia.

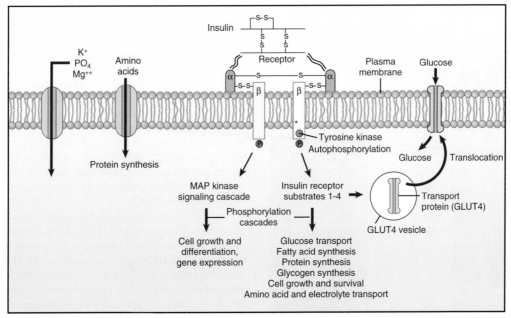

FIGURE 19.15 Insulin Action on Cells. Binding of insulin to its receptor causes autophosphorylation of the receptor, which then itself acts as a tyrosine kinase that phosphorylates insulin receptor substrates 1-4 *(IRS-1-4)*. Numerous target enzymes, such as protein kinase B and mitogen-activated protein (MAP) kinase, are activated, and these enzymes have a multitude of effects on cell function. The glucose transporter *(GLUT4)* is recruited to the plasma membrane, where it facilitates glucose entry into the cell. The transport of amino acids, potassium, magnesium, and phosphate into the cell is also facilitated. The synthesis of various enzymes is induced or suppressed, and cell growth is regulated by signal molecules that modulate gene expression. (Redrawn from Levy MN et al, editors: *Berne & Levy principles of physiology*, ed 4, St Louis, 2006, Mosby.)

Glucagon

Glucagon is antagonistic to the effects of insulin. Glucagon release is stimulated by low glucose levels and sympathetic stimulation and is inhibited by high glucose levels. It is produced by the alpha cells of the pancreas and by cells lining the gastrointestinal tract. Glucagon acts primarily in the liver and increases the blood glucose concentration by stimulating glycogenolysis and gluconeogenesis in muscle and lipolysis in adipose tissue.

Pancreatic Somatostatin

Somatostatin is produced by delta cells of the pancreas in response to food intake and is essential in carbohydrate, fat, and protein metabolism. It is different from hypothalamic somatostatin, which inhibits the release of growth hormone and TSH. Pancreatic somatostatin is involved in regulating alpha-cell and beta-cell function within the islets by inhibiting secretion of insulin, glucagon, and pancreatic polypeptide.

Gastrin, Ghrelin, and Pancreatic Polypeptide

Pancreatic gastrin stimulates the secretion of gastric acid. It is postulated that fetal pancreatic gastrin secretion is necessary for adequate islet cell development. Ghrelin stimulates GH secretion, controls appetite, and plays a role in obesity and the regulation of insulin sensitivity. Pancreatic polypeptide is released by F cells in response to hypoglycemia and protein-rich meals. It inhibits gallbladder contraction and exocrine pancreas secretion and is frequently increased in individuals with pancreatic tumors or diabetes mellitus.

Adrenal Glands

The adrenal glands are paired, pyramid-shaped organs behind the peritoneum and close to the upper pole of each kidney. Each gland is surrounded by a capsule, embedded in fat, and well supplied with blood

from the aorta and phrenic and renal arteries. Venous return from the left adrenal gland is to the renal vein and from the right adrenal gland is to the inferior vena cava.

Each adrenal gland consists of two separate portions—an outer cortex and an inner medulla. These two portions have different embryonic origins, structures, and hormonal functions. The adrenal cortex and medulla function like two separate but interrelated glands (Fig. 19.16).

Adrenal Cortex

The adrenal cortex accounts for 80% of the weight of the adult gland. The cortex is histologically subdivided into the following three zones:
1. The zona glomerulosa, the outer layer, constitutes about 15% of the cortex and primarily produces the mineralocorticoid aldosterone.
2. The zona fasciculata, the middle layer, constitutes 78% of the cortex and secretes the glucocorticoids cortisol, cortisone, and corticosterone.
3. The zona reticularis, the inner layer, constitutes 7% of the cortex and secretes mineralocorticoids (aldosterone), adrenal androgens and estrogens, and glucocorticoids.

The cells of the adrenal cortex are stimulated by ACTH from the pituitary gland. All hormones of the adrenal cortex are synthesized from cholesterol. The best-known pathway of steroidogenesis involves the conversion of cholesterol to pregnenolone, which is then converted to the major corticosteroids.

Glucocorticoids

Functions of the glucocorticoids. The glucocorticoids are steroid hormones that have metabolic, neurologic, antiinflammatory, and growth-suppressing effects. These functions (Fig. 19.17) have direct effects on carbohydrate metabolism. These hormones increase the blood glucose concentration by promoting gluconeogenesis in the liver and by decreasing uptake of glucose into muscle cells, adipose cells, and

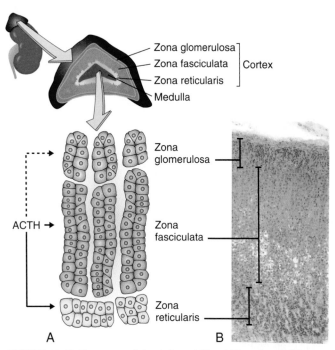

FIGURE 19.16 Structure of the Adrenal Gland Showing Cell Layers (Zonae) of the Cortex. **A,** Adrenal glands. Each gland consists of a cortex and a medulla. The cortex has three layers: zona glomerulosa, zona fasciculata, and zona reticularis. **B,** A portion of the medulla is visible at the lower right in the photomicrograph (×35) and at the bottom of the drawing. (**A** from Damjanov I: *Pathophysiology,* Philadelphia, 2008, Saunders; **B** from Kierszenbaum A: *Histology and cell biology,* St Louis, 2002, Mosby.)

lymphatic cells. In extrahepatic tissues, the glucocorticoids stimulate protein catabolism and inhibit amino acid uptake and protein synthesis.

The glucocorticoids act at several sites to suppress immune and inflammatory reactions. Adaptive immunity is affected by a glucocorticoid-mediated inhibitory effect on the proliferation of T lymphocytes, which results in a decrease in cellular immunity (see Chapter 7). Glucocorticoids affect innate immunity and inflammation through several pathways, including decreased function of macrophages and natural killer cells, suppression of inflammatory cytokines, and decreased release of proteolytic enzymes. Psychological and physiologic stress increases glucocorticoid production, which provides a pathway for the well-described decrease in immunity seen in both acute and chronic stress conditions (see Chapter 10). Use of glucocorticoids for the treatment of disease also leads to suppression of innate and adaptive immunity and the challenging complications of infection and poor wound healing (see Chapter 9).

Glucocorticoids appear to potentiate the effects of catecholamines, including sensitizing the arterioles to the vasoconstrictive effects of norepinephrine, thus increasing the blood pressure. Thyroid hormone and growth hormone effects on adipose tissue are also potentiated by glucocorticoids. Other effects of glucocorticoids include inhibition of bone formation, inhibition of ADH secretion, and stimulation of gastric acid secretion. A metabolite of cortisol may act like a barbiturate and depress nerve cell function in the brain, accounting for the noted effects on mood, such as anxiety and depression, associated with steroid level fluctuation in disease or stress.

Cortisol. The most potent naturally occurring glucocorticoid is cortisol. It is the main secretory product of the adrenal cortex and is needed to maintain life and protect the body from stress (see Fig. 10.2). Cortisol circulates in bound form attached to albumin but is primarily

bound to the plasma protein transcortin. A smaller amount circulates in free form and diffuses into cells with specific intracellular receptors for cortisol. Cortisol secretion is regulated primarily by the hypothalamus and the anterior pituitary gland (Fig. 19.18). Corticotropin-releasing hormone (CRH) is produced by several nuclei in the hypothalamus and stored in the median eminence. Once released, CRH travels through the portal vessels to stimulate the production of ACTH, which is the main regulator of cortisol secretion.

Three factors appear to be primarily involved in regulating the secretion of ACTH: (1) negative-feedback effects of high circulating levels of cortisol; (2) diurnal rhythms, with peak levels during sleep; and (3) psychological and physiologic stress increases ACTH secretion, leading to increased cortisol levels. (Neurologic mechanisms regulating sleep are discussed in Chapter 15.)

Once ACTH is secreted, it binds to specific plasma membrane receptors on the cells of the adrenal cortex and on other extra-adrenal tissues. Because both adrenal and extra-adrenal tissues have ACTH receptors, a number of effects result from stimulation by ACTH. In addition to increasing adrenocortical secretion of cortisol, ACTH maintains the size and synthetic functions of the adrenal cortex through activation of crucial enzymes and storage of cholesterol for metabolism into steroid hormones. Extra-adrenal effects of ACTH include stimulation of melanocytes and activation of tissue lipase. ACTH is rapidly inactivated in the circulation, and the liver and kidneys remove the deactivated hormone.

Mineralocorticoids: aldosterone. Mineralocorticoid steroids directly affect ion transport by epithelial cells, causing sodium retention and potassium and hydrogen loss. Aldosterone is the most potent naturally occurring mineralocorticoid and conserves sodium by increasing the activity of the sodium pump of epithelial cells. (The sodium pump is described in Chapter 1.)

Aldosterone synthesis and secretion is regulated primarily by the renin-angiotensin system (described in Chapter 31). The renin-angiotensin system is activated by sodium and water depletion, increased potassium levels, and a diminished effective blood volume. Angiotensin II is the primary stimulant of aldosterone synthesis and secretion; however, sodium and potassium levels also may directly affect aldosterone secretion.

Aldosterone maintains extracellular volume by acting on distal nephron epithelial cells to increase reabsorption of sodium and excretion of potassium and hydrogen. This renal effect takes 90 minutes to 6 hours. Fluid and electrolyte regulation is addressed in more detail in Chapter 5. Other effects of aldosterone include enhancement of cardiac muscle contraction, stimulation of ectopic ventricular activity through secondary cardiac pacemakers in the ventricles, stiffening of blood vessels with increased vascular resistance, and decrease in fibrinolysis.

Adrenal estrogens and androgens. The healthy adrenal cortex secretes minimal amounts of estrogen and androgens. ACTH appears to be the major regulator. Some of the weakly androgenic substances secreted by the cortex (dehydroepiandrosterone [DHEA], androstene-dione) are converted by peripheral tissues to stronger androgens, such as testosterone, thus accounting for some androgenic effects initiated by the adrenal cortex. Peripheral conversion of adrenal androgens to estrogens is enhanced in aging or obese persons, as well as in those with liver disease or hyperthyroidism. The biologic effects and metabolism of the adrenal sex steroids do not vary from those produced by the gonads (see Chapter 34).

Adrenal Medulla

The chromaffin cells (pheochromocytes) of the adrenal medulla secrete and store the catecholamines epinephrine (adrenaline) and norepinephrine (noradrenaline). Both are synthesized from the amino acid phenylalanine (Fig. 19.19). The adrenal medulla, together with the sympathetic division of the autonomic nervous system, is embryonically

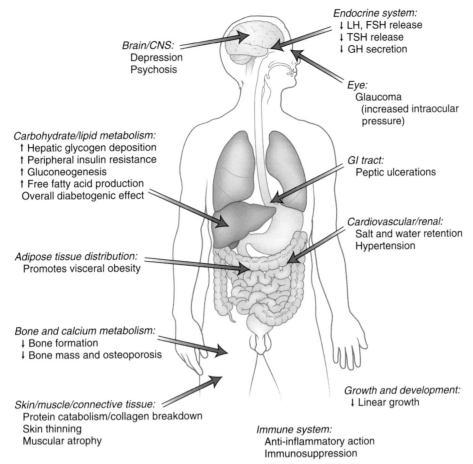

FIGURE 19.17 Effects of Glucocorticoids on the Body. (From Stewart PM, Krone NP: The adrenal cortex. In Melmed S et al, editors: *Williams textbook of endocrinology,* ed 12, Philadelphia, 2011, Saunders.)

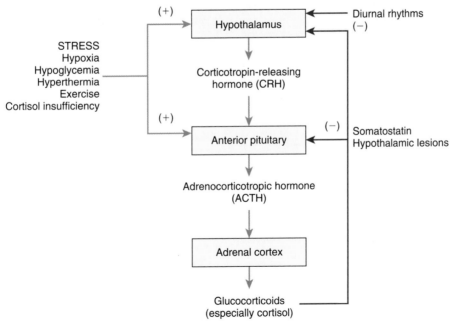

FIGURE 19.18 Feedback Control of Glucocorticoid Synthesis and Secretion.

derived from neural crest cells. Only 30% of circulating epinephrine comes from the adrenal medulla (the other 70% is released from nerve terminals), and the medulla is only a minor source of norepinephrine. The adrenal medulla functions as a sympathetic ganglion without postganglionic processes. Sympathetic cholinergic preganglion fibers terminate on the chromaffin cells and secrete catecholamines directly into the bloodstream. The catecholamines acting in the blood are therefore hormones and not neurotransmitters.

Physiologic stress to the body (e.g., traumatic injury, hypoxia, hypoglycemia, and many others) triggers the exocytosis of the storage granules from chromaffin cells, with release of epinephrine and norepinephrine into the bloodstream. Once released, the catecholamines remain in the plasma for only seconds to minutes. The catecholamines exert their biologic effects after binding to plasma membrane receptors (α_1, α_2, β_1, β_2, and β_3) in target cells. This binding activates the adenylyl cyclase system (an intracellular second messenger system). Catecholamines have diverse effects on the entire body. Their release and the body's response have been characterized as the "fight or flight" response (stress response) (see Figs. 10.2 and 10.3 and Tables 10.3 and 10.4). Metabolic effects of catecholamines promote hyperglycemia through a variety of mechanisms, including interference with the usual glucose regulatory feedback mechanisms. Catecholamines are rapidly removed from the plasma by neuron absorption for storage in new cytoplasmic granules, or metabolically inactivated and excreted in the urine. Catecholamines also directly inhibit secretion by decreasing the formation of the enzyme tyrosine hydroxylase (the rate-limiting step).

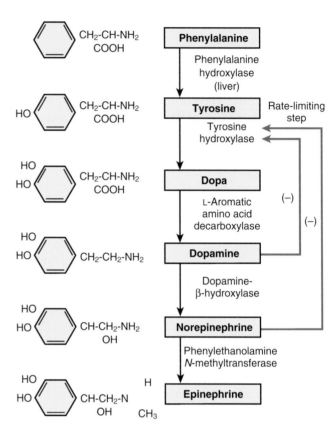

FIGURE 19.19 Synthesis of Catecholamines.

> ✔ **QUICK CHECK 19.4**
> 1. What are the islets of Langerhans? Where are they located?
> 2. Compare and contrast the actions of pancreatic alpha, beta, delta, and F cells.
> 3. What is the most potent naturally occurring glucocorticoid, and how is its secretion related to that of adrenocorticotropic hormone (ACTH)?
> 4. How does aldosterone influence fluid and electrolyte balance?
> 5. What are catecholamines?

GERIATRIC CONSIDERATIONS

Aging and Its Effects on Specific Endocrine Glands

General Endocrine Changes With Aging
Aging has many effects on the neuroendocrine system. There are complex changes within the hypothalamic/pituitary axis, and altered biologic activity of hormones, altered circulating levels of hormones, altered secretory response of the endocrine glands, altered metabolism of hormones, and loss of circadian control of hormone secretion are among the findings.

Pituitary
Posterior: Decrease in size; reduced antidiuretic hormone (ADH) secretion.
Anterior: Increased fibrosis and moderate increase in size of gland; decline in growth hormone release.

Thyroid
Glandular atrophy, fibrosis, nodularity, and increased inflammatory infiltrates; decreased T_4 secretion and turnover, decline in T_3 (especially in men), diminished thyroid-stimulating hormone (TSH) secretion; reduced response of plasma TSH concentration to thyroid-releasing hormone (TRH) administration (especially in men).

Growth Hormone and Insulin-Like Growth Factors
The amounts of growth hormone (GH) and insulin-like growth factors (IGF) decline with aging, which contributes to decreases in muscle size and function, reduced fat and bone mass, and changes in reproductive and cognitive function. Increased visceral fat, decreased lean body mass, and decreased bone density are common in older adults.

Pancreas
It is common for older individuals to have glucose intolerance or diabetes, and these disorders frequently are undiagnosed in aging adults. Mechanisms include decreased insulin receptor activity and decreased beta-cell secretion of insulin.

Adrenal
Decreased dihydroepandrosterone (DHEA) levels lead to decreased synthesis of androgen-derived estrogen and testosterone; decreased metabolic clearance of glucocorticoids and cortisol causes decreased cortisol secretion; there also are decreased levels of aldosterone. Circadian patterns of adrenocorticotropic hormone (ACTH) and cortisol secretion may change with aging.

Gonads
Postmenopausal women have decreased estrogen and progesterone, increased follicle-stimulating hormone, and relative increases in androgen levels; these changes have numerous physiologic and pathophysiologic consequences (see Chapter 34); in men there is a gradual decrease in serum testosterone levels, leading to decreased sexual activity, decreased muscle strength, and decreased bone mineralization.

SUMMARY REVIEW

Mechanisms of Hormonal Regulation

1. The endocrine system has five general functions: (1) differentiation of the reproductive and central nervous systems in the developing fetus; (2) stimulation of sequential growth and development during childhood and adolescence; (3) coordination of the male and female reproductive systems, which makes sexual reproduction possible; (4) maintenance of an optimal internal environment throughout life; and (5) initiation of corrective and adaptive responses when emergency demands occur.

2. Hormones are chemical messengers synthesized by endocrine glands and, when released, trigger intracellular responses.

3. Hormones have specific rates and rhythms of secretion: diurnal, pulsatile/cyclic, and patterns dependent on other circulating substances.

4. Hormones have specific negative- and positive-feedback mechanisms. Positive feedback occurs when a neural, chemical, or endocrine response increases the synthesis and secretion of a hormone. Negative feedback occurs when a changing chemical, neural, or endocrine response to a stimulus decreases the synthesis and secretion of a hormone.

5. Water-soluble hormones circulate throughout the body in unbound form, whereas lipid-soluble hormones (e.g., steroid and thyroid hormones) circulate throughout the body bound to carrier proteins. Only unbound hormones can signal a target cell.

6. Hormones affect only target cells with appropriate receptors and then act on these cells to initiate specific cell functions or activities.

7. Hormone receptors on target cells have two main functions: (1) to recognize and bind specifically and with high affinity to their particular hormones; and (2) to initiate a signal to appropriate intracellular effectors.

8. Receptors for hormones may be located on the plasma membrane or in the intracellular compartment of a target cell.

9. Water-soluble hormones (i.e., protein hormones and catecholamines) act as first messengers, binding to receptors in the cell's plasma membrane. The signals initiated by hormone-receptor binding are then transmitted into the cell by the action of second messengers (e.g., cAMP, cGMP, or tyrosine kinase) and mediate the action of the hormone on the target cell (i.e., protein synthesis or cellular growth).

10. Lipid-soluble hormones (including steroid and thyroid hormones) cross the plasma membrane by diffusion. These hormones diffuse directly into the cell nucleus and bind to nuclear receptors. Rapid responses of steroid hormones may be mediated by plasma membrane receptors.

Structure and Function of the Endocrine Glands

1. The hypothalamic-pituitary axis (HPA) forms the structural and functional basis for the neuroendocrine system.

2. The hypothalamus is connected to the pituitary gland by the pituitary stalk. The hypothalamus regulates anterior pituitary function by secreting releasing or inhibiting hormones and factors into the portal circulation.

3. Hypothalamic hormones include prolactin-releasing factor (PRF), which stimulates secretion of prolactin; prolactin-inhibiting factor (PIF, dopamine), which inhibits prolactin secretion; thyrotropin-releasing hormone (TRH), which affects release of thyroid hormones; growth hormone–releasing hormone (GHRH), which stimulates the release of growth hormone (GH); somatostatin, which inhibits the release of GH and thyroid-stimulating hormone (TSH); gonadotropin-releasing hormone (GnRH), which facilitates the release of follicle-stimulating hormone (FSH) and luteinizing hormone (LH); corticotropin-releasing hormone (CRH), which facilitates the release of adrenocorticotropic hormone (ACTH) and endorphins; and substance P, which inhibits ACTH release and stimulates the release of a variety of other hormones.

4. The pituitary gland consists of anterior and posterior portions that have different functional relationships to the hypothalamus.

5. Hormones of the anterior pituitary are regulated by (1) secretion of hypothalamic-releasing factors, (2) feedback effects from hormones secreted by target organs, and (3) mediating effects of neurotransmitters.

6. Hormones of the anterior pituitary include ACTH, melanocyte-stimulating hormone (MSH), somatotropic hormones (GH, prolactin), and glycoprotein hormones—FSH, LH, and TSH.

7. The posterior pituitary secretes antidiuretic hormone (ADH), which also is called vasopressin, and oxytocin.

8. ADH controls serum osmolality, increases permeability of the renal tubules to water, and causes vasoconstriction when administered pharmacologically in high doses.

9. Oxytocin causes uterine contraction and lactation in women and may have a role in sperm motility in men. In both men and women, oxytocin has an antidiuretic effect similar to that of ADH.

10. The pineal gland secretes melatonin, which regulates circadian rhythms and reproduction.

11. The two-lobed thyroid gland contains follicles, which secrete some of the thyroid hormones, and C cells, which secrete calcitonin.

12. Regulation of thyroid hormone (TH) involves a negative-feedback loop initiated by TRH and involving the hypothalamus, anterior pituitary, thyroid gland, and numerous biochemical variables.

13. TSH, which is synthesized and stored in the anterior pituitary, stimulates secretion of TH by activating intracellular processes, including uptake of iodine necessary for the synthesis of TH in the thyroid gland.

14. Synthesis of TH depends on the glycoprotein thyroglobulin, which contains a precursor of TH, tyrosine. Tyrosine then combines with iodine to form precursor molecules of the thyroid hormones thyroxine (T_4) and triiodothyronine (T_3). These hormones are then stored within thyroid colloid until released into the circulation.

15. When released into the circulation, T_3 and T_4 are bound by carrier proteins in the plasma, which store these hormones and provide a buffer for rapid changes in hormone levels. The free form is the active form.

16. Thyroid hormones alter protein synthesis and have a wide range of metabolic effects on proteins, carbohydrates, lipids, vitamins, and other hormones and neurotransmitters. TH also affects heat production and cardiac function.

17. The paired parathyroid glands are located behind the upper and lower poles of the thyroid. These glands secrete parathyroid hormone (PTH), an important regulator of serum calcium and phosphate levels.

18. PTH secretion increases levels of ionized calcium and decreases levels of phosphate in the plasma. In the kidney, PTH increases reabsorption of calcium and decreases reabsorption of phosphorus.

19. The endocrine pancreas contains the islets of Langerhans, which consist of alpha cells, beta cells, delta cells, and F cells. These cells secrete hormones that regulate carbohydrate, fat, and protein metabolism in the body.

20. Alpha cells produce glucagon, which is secreted inversely to blood glucose concentrations and helps increase blood glucose.

21. Beta cells synthesize insulin and secrete amylin. Insulin is a hormone that regulates blood glucose concentrations and overall body metabolism of fat, protein, and carbohydrates. Amylin suppresses glucagon secretion and has a satiety effect.
22. Delta cells secrete somatostatin, which inhibits glucagon and insulin secretion.
23. F cells secrete pancreatic polypeptide, which inhibits gallbladder contraction and exocrine pancreatic secretion.
24. The paired adrenal glands are situated above the kidneys. Each gland consists of an outer adrenal cortex, which secretes steroid hormones, and an inner adrenal medulla, which secretes catecholamines.
25. The steroid hormones secreted by the adrenal cortex are synthesized from cholesterol. These hormones include glucocorticoids, mineralocorticoids, and adrenal androgens and estrogens.
26. Glucocorticoids directly affect carbohydrate metabolism by increasing blood glucose concentration through gluconeogenesis in the liver and by decreasing uptake of glucose. Glucocorticoids also inhibit immune and inflammatory responses, suppress growth, and promote protein catabolism.
27. The most potent naturally occurring glucocorticoid is cortisol, which is necessary for the maintenance of life and for protection from stress. Secretion of cortisol is regulated by the hypothalamus and anterior pituitary.
28. Cortisol secretion is related to secretion of ACTH, which is stimulated by corticotropin-releasing hormone (CRH). ACTH binds with receptors of the adrenal cortex, which activates intracellular mechanisms and leads to cortisol release.
29. Mineralocorticoids are steroid hormones that directly affect ion transport epithelial cells, causing sodium retention and potassium and hydrogen loss.
30. Aldosterone is the most potent of the naturally occurring mineralocorticoids. Its primary role is conserving sodium by increasing the activity of the sodium pump of epithelial cells.
31. Aldosterone secretion is regulated primarily by the renin-angiotensin system and by sodium and potassium levels.
32. The principal site of aldosterone action is the kidney, where it causes sodium reabsorption and potassium and hydrogen excretion.
33. Androgens and estrogens secreted by the adrenal cortex act in the same way as those secreted by the gonads.
34. The adrenal medulla secretes the catecholamines epinephrine and norepinephrine. Physiologic stress to the body triggers their release.
35. Catecholamines bind with various target cells and are taken up by neurons or excreted in the urine. Catecholamines cause a range of metabolic effects (e.g., hyperglycemia) characterized as the "fight or flight" response.

Geriatric Considerations: Aging and Its Effects on Specific Endocrine Gland

1. Altered biologic activity, circulating levels, and metabolism of hormones occurs with aging.
2. The pituitary has reduced ADH and GH secretion. The thyroid has reduced T4, T3, and TSH secretion.
3. Reductions in GH and IGF with aging contributes to decreases in muscle size and function, reduced fat and bone mass, and changes in reproductive and cognitive function.
4. The adrenal gland shows decreased levels of estrogen and testosterone, cortisol, and aldosterone.

KEY TERMS

Adrenal cortex, 441
Adrenal gland, 441
Adrenal medulla, 442
Adrenocorticotropic hormone (ACTH), 434
Aldosterone, 442
Alpha cell, 439
Amylin, 440
Anterior pituitary, 433
Antidiuretic hormone (ADH), 436
Beta cell, 439
C cell, 438
Calcitonin, 438
Chromophil, 433
Chromophobe, 433
Corticotropin-releasing hormone (CRH), 442
Cortisol, 442
Delta cell, 439

1,25-Dihydroxy-vitamin D3, 439
Down-regulation, 431
F (or PP) cell, 439
First messenger, 432
Follicle, 438
Follicle-stimulating hormone (FSH), 434
Gastrin, 441
Ghrelin, 441
Glucagon, 441
Glucocorticoid, 441
Growth hormone (GH), 434
Hormone, 429
Hormone receptor, 430
Hypothalamus, 433
Insulin, 440
Islet of Langerhans, 439
Isthmus, 438
Luteinizing hormone (LH), 434

Median eminence, 436
Melanocyte-stimulating hormone (MSH), 434
Melatonin, 437
Mineralocorticoid, 442
Negative feedback, 430
Oxytocin, 436
Pancreas, 439
Pancreatic polypeptide, 441
Parathyroid hormone (PTH), 439
Pars distalis, 433
Pars intermedia, 433
Pars nervosa, 436
Pars tuberalis, 433
Pituitary gland, 433
Pituitary stalk, 436
Positive feedback, 430
Posterior pituitary (neurohypophysis), 436

Prolactin, 434
Pyramidal lobe, 438
Second messenger, 432
Somatostatin, 441
Target cell, 430
Thyroid gland, 438
Thyroid hormone (TH), 438
Thyroid-stimulating hormone (TSH), 430, 434
Thyrotropin-releasing hormone (TRH), 438
Thyroxine-binding globulin (TBG), 438
Tropic hormone, 434
Up-regulation, 431
Zona fasciculata, 441
Zona glomerulosa, 441
Zona reticularis, 441

REFERENCES

1. Schwartz N, et al: Rapid steroid hormone actions via membrane receptors, *Biochim Biophys Acta* 1863(9):2289-2298, 2016.
2. Bankir L, Bichet DG, Morgenthaler NG: Vasopressin: physiology, assessment and osmosensation, *J Intern Med* 282(4):284-297, 2017.
3. Little AG: Local regulation of thyroid hormone signaling, *Vitam Horm* 106:1-17, 2018.
4. Tokarz VL, MacDonald PE, Klip A: The cell biology of systemic insulin function, *J Cell Biol* 217(7):2273-2289, 2018.

20

Alterations of Hormonal Regulation

Valentina L. Brashers, Sue E. Huether

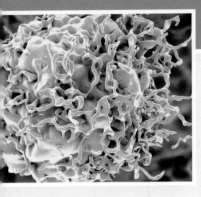

EVOLVE WEBSITE

http://evolve.elsevier.com/Huether/
Student Review Questions
Audio Key Points

Case Studies
Animations
Quick Check Answers

CHAPTER OUTLINE

Functions of the endocrine system involve complex interactions between hormones and most body systems that maintain dynamic steady states and influence tissue growth and reproductive capabilities. Endocrine system dysfunction is usually caused by hypersecretion or hyposecretion of the various hormones, leading to abnormal hormone concentrations in the blood. Dysfunction also may result from abnormal cell receptor function or from altered intracellular response to the hormone–receptor complex.

MECHANISMS OF HORMONAL ALTERATIONS

Significantly elevated or significantly depressed hormone levels may result from two primary mechanisms: (1) inappropriate amounts of hormone delivered to the target cell, or (2) inappropriate responses by the target cell (Table 20.1). Inappropriate amounts of hormone can result from disorders of endocrine glands, causing them to synthesize too little or too much hormone, failure of feedback systems designed to control hormone release, dysfunctional or ectopically produced hormones (hormones produced from nonendocrine sources), or defects in delivery of the hormone in the bloodstream.

Target cells may not respond appropriately to hormonal stimulation for a number of reasons. Target cells may have too many or too few cell surface receptors. Those receptors may be abnormal and insensitive, or they may be blocked or stimulated by antibodies. There also may be intracellular disorders that cause a failure of the target cell to respond to receptor stimulation. For example, there may be inadequate synthesis of second messengers, such as cyclic adenosine monophosphate (cAMP), or the cell may respond abnormally to the second messenger if levels of intracellular enzymes or proteins are altered. (Second messengers for various hormones are listed in Table 19.2.)

ALTERATIONS OF THE HYPOTHALAMIC–PITUITARY SYSTEM

The most common cause of apparent hypothalamic dysfunction is interruption of the pituitary stalk. Such interruptions prevent hypothalamic hormones from reaching the pituitary gland. Damage to the pituitary stalk can be caused by destructive lesions, rupture after head injury, surgical transection, or tumor. Without hypothalamic hormones, the pituitary releases inadequate amounts of follicle-stimulating hormone (FSH), luteinizing hormone (LH), adrenocorticotropic hormone (ACTH), thyroid stimulating hormone (TSH), and growth hormone (GH) (Fig. 20.1). The control of prolactin is predominantly inhibitory by hypothalamic dopamine. It does not have endocrine target tissue and therefore lacks a regulatory feedback pathway. The effects of these changes in pituitary hormones are discussed later in this chapter.

Diseases of the Posterior Pituitary

Diseases of the posterior pituitary cause either increased or decreased secretion of antidiuretic hormone (ADH, arginine vasopressin). An

TABLE 20.1 Mechanisms of Hormone Alterations

Inappropriate Amounts of Hormone Delivered to Target Cell	Inappropriate Response by Target Cell
Inadequate Hormone Synthesis	**Cell Surface Receptor–Associated Disorders**
1. Inadequate quantity of hormone precursors	1. Decrease in the number of receptors
2. Secretory cell unable to convert precursors to active hormone	2. Impaired receptor function
	3. Presence of antibodies against specific receptors
Failure of Feedback Systems	
1. Do not recognize positive feedback, leading to inadequate hormone synthesis	
2. Do not recognize negative feedback, leading to excessive hormone synthesis	
Dysfunctional or Ectopic Hormones	**Intracellular Disorders**
1. Inadequate biologically free hormone	1. Inadequate synthesis of a second messenger
2. Hormone degraded at an altered rate	2. Intracellular enzymes or proteins are altered
3. Circulating inhibitors	
4. Ectopic production of hormones	
Dysfunctional Delivery System	
1. Inadequate blood supply	
2. Inadequate carrier proteins	

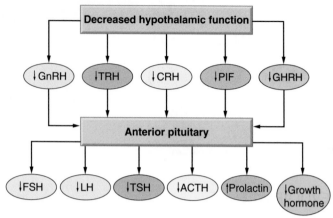

FIGURE 20.1 Loss of Hypothalamic Hormones. *ACTH,* Adrenocorticotropic hormone; *CRH,* corticotropin-releasing hormone; *FSH,* follicle-stimulating hormone; *GHRH,* growth hormone–releasing hormone; *GnRH,* gonadotropin-releasing hormone; *LH,* luteinizing hormone; *PIF,* prolactin inhibitory factor (probably dopamine); *TRH,* thyrotropin-releasing hormone; *TSH,* thyroid-stimulating hormone.

excess amount of this hormone results in water retention, whereas deficiencies in the amount or response to ADH result in water loss These complex pathophysiologic states not only have significant clinical effects on the modulation of body fluids and electrolytes but also affect cognitive and emotional responses to stress.

Syndrome of Inappropriate Antidiuretic Hormone Secretion

The syndrome of inappropriate ADH secretion (SIADH) is characterized by high levels of ADH in the absence of normal physiologic stimuli for its release.[1] A common cause of SIADH is the ectopic production of ADH by tumors, such as cancers of the lung, stomach, pancreas, bladder, prostate, and endometrium; lymphomas; and sarcomas. Pulmonary disorders associated with SIADH include pneumonia (e.g., tuberculosis), asthma, cystic fibrosis, and respiratory failure requiring mechanical ventilation. Central nervous system disorders that may cause SIADH include encephalitis, meningitis, intracranial hemorrhage, tumors, and trauma.

Iatrogenic causes of SIADH include surgery and medications. Any surgery can result in increased ADH secretion for as long as 5 to 7 days after surgery. The precise mechanism is uncertain but is likely related to fluid and volume changes after surgery, the amount and type of intravenous fluids given, and the use of narcotic analgesics. Medications are an important cause of SIADH, especially in the elderly. These include narcotics, general anesthetics, antidepressants, antipsychotics, chemotherapeutic agents, and nonsteroidal antiinflammatory drugs.

PATHOPHYSIOLOGY The cardinal features of SIADH are the result of enhanced renal free water retention. ADH induces the insertion of a water channel protein, called *aquaporin-2,* into the tubular luminal membrane, which increases water reabsorption by the kidneys. (Renal function is discussed in Chapter 31.) This results in an expansion of extracellular fluid volume that leads to dilutional hyponatremia (low serum sodium concentration) and hypoosmolarity. Urine is inappropriately concentrated with respect to serum osmolarity because water is reabsorbed that normally would be excreted.

CLINICAL MANIFESTATIONS The symptoms of SIADH result from hyponatremia (see Chapter 5) and are determined by its severity and rapidity of onset. Thirst, impaired taste, anorexia, dyspnea on exertion, fatigue, and dulled sensorium occur when the serum sodium level decreases rapidly. Gastrointestinal symptoms, including vomiting and abdominal cramps, occur with a drop in sodium concentration from 130 to 120 mEq/L. There is weight gain from water retention, but peripheral edema is absent. Serum sodium levels below 115 mEq/L cause confusion, lethargy, muscle twitching, and convulsions; severe and sometimes irreversible neurologic damage may occur. Symptoms usually resolve with correction of hyponatremia.

EVALUATION AND TREATMENT A diagnosis of SIADH is based on these findings: (1) serum hypoosmolality and hyponatremia, (2) urine hyperosmolarity (i.e., urine osmolality is greater than expected for the concomitant serum osmolality), and (3) the absence of conditions that can alter volume status (e.g., adrenal or thyroid dysfunction, congestive heart failure, or renal insufficiency).

The treatment of SIADH involves the correction of any underlying causal problems, fluid restriction with careful monitoring of sodium status and neurologic symptoms, and administration of vasopressin receptor antagonists (vaptans). In severe SIADH, emergency correction of severe hyponatremia by careful administration of hypertonic saline may be required. Resolution usually occurs within 3 days. If hyponatremia is corrected too rapidly, a severe neurologic syndrome called *central pontine myelinolysis* can ensue. Demeclocycline, which causes the renal tubules to develop resistance to ADH, and vasopressin (ADH) receptor antagonists may be used to treat resistant or chronic SIADH.

Diabetes Insipidus

Diabetes insipidus (DI) is characterized by insufficient ADH activity, leading to the loss of too much free water into the urine. The two major forms of DI are:

1. *Neurogenic* or *central DI.* Caused by the insufficient secretion of ADH, it occurs when any organic lesion of the hypothalamus, pituitary stalk, or posterior pituitary interferes with ADH synthesis, transport, or release. Causative lesions include primary brain tumors, traumatic brain injury, hypophysectomy, aneurysms, thrombosis, infections, and immunologic disorders. It can also be caused by hereditary disorders that affect ADH genes or result in structural changes in the pituitary gland.
2. *Nephrogenic DI.* Caused by inadequate response of the renal tubules to ADH. Acquired nephrogenic DI is caused by disorders and drugs that damage the renal tubules. These disorders include pyelonephritis, amyloidosis, destructive uropathies, and polycystic kidney disease. Drugs that may induce a reversible form of nephrogenic DI include lithium carbonate, colchicine, amphotericin B, loop diuretics, general anesthetics, and demeclocycline. There are several genetic causes of nephrogenic DI, including a mutation in the gene that codes for aquaporin-2, which is one of the four water transport channels in the renal tubule.[2]

A rare form of DI, called *gestational DI,* is associated with pregnancy in which the level of the vasopressin-degrading enzyme vasopressinase is increased, resulting in ADH deficiency. Clinical manifestations are usually mild and do not require treatment.

PATHOPHYSIOLOGY Individuals with DI have a partial to total inability to concentrate urine. Insufficient ADH activity causes excretion of large volumes of dilute urine, leading to increased plasma osmolality. In conscious individuals, the thirst mechanism is stimulated and induces polydipsia. Dehydration develops rapidly without ongoing fluid replacement. If the individual with DI cannot conserve as much water as is lost in the urine, serum hypernatremia and hyperosmolality occur. Concentrations of other serum electrolytes generally are not affected.

CLINICAL MANIFESTATIONS The clinical manifestations of DI include polyuria, nocturia, continuous thirst, and polydipsia. The urine output is varied but can increase from the normal output of 1 to 2 L/day to as much as 8 to 12 L/day. Individuals with long-standing DI develop a large bladder capacity and hydronephrosis (see Chapter 32). Neurogenic DI usually has an abrupt onset, whereas nephrogenic DI usually has a more gradual onset. Table 20.2 compares the signs and symptoms of DI and SIADH.

EVALUATION AND TREATMENT DI is diagnosed by the findings of a low urine osmolality with associated elevated serum sodium and osmolality. The diagnosis of DI is generally confirmed through water deprivation testing in which urine output is maintained despite dehydration. An evaluation for underlying reversible central or renal causes should be undertaken.

Dipsogenic or *primary polydipsia* may be confused with DI. It is usually the result of a psychiatric condition that causes the chronic ingestion of extremely large quantities of fluid, which washes out the renal concentration gradient, resulting in partial resistance to ADH.

Treatment of neurogenic DI is based on the extent of the ADH deficiency. Fluid replacement using oral or intravenous routes is usually adequate. Some individuals require ADH replacement with the synthetic vasopressin analog desmopressin (DDAVP). Management of nephrogenic DI requires treatment of any reversible underlying disorders, discontinuation of etiologic medications, and correction of associated electrolyte disorders. Drugs that potentiate the action of otherwise insufficient

TABLE 20.2 Signs and Symptoms of Diabetes Insipidus and Syndrome of Inappropriate Antidiuretic Hormone Secretion

Signs and Symptoms	Diabetes Insipidus	Syndrome of Inappropriate Antidiuretic Hormone Secretion
Urine output	High	Low
Urine osmolality	Low	High
Urine specific gravity	Low	High
Serum sodium	High	Low
Serum osmolality	High	Low
Symptoms	Polyuria, thirst, weight loss, high urine output, signs of dehydration	Water retention, weight gain, low urine output, nausea, vomiting, mental changes

amounts of endogenous ADH, such as thiazide diuretics, chlorpropamide, carbamazepine, and clofibrate, may be used in individuals with incomplete ADH deficiency. New treatments aimed at reversing aquaporin-2 dysfunction are being developed.

Diseases of the Anterior Pituitary
Hypopituitarism

Hypopituitarism is characterized by the absence of one or more anterior pituitary hormones or the complete failure of all anterior pituitary hormone functions.[3] The most common causes of hypopituitarism are pituitary infarction or space-occupying lesions. Pituitary infarction may occur when there is significant blood loss or hypovolemic shock. This also may occur in women during the postpartum period (Sheehan syndrome). Space-occupying lesions include pituitary adenomas or aneurysms, which can enlarge and compress the pituitary gland. Other causes of hypopituitarism include traumatic brain injury, removal or destruction of the gland, infections (e.g., meningitis, syphilis, tuberculosis), autoimmune hypophysitis, and certain drugs (e.g., bexarotene, carbamazepine, ipilimumab). A rare congenital form of hypopituitarism results from an early mutation of the prophet of pituitary transcription factor *(PROP-1)* gene, which affects embryonic pituitary development.

PATHOPHYSIOLOGY The pituitary gland is highly vascular and relies heavily on portal blood flow from the hypothalamus. It is therefore vulnerable to ischemia and infarction. Infarction results in tissue necrosis and edema with swelling of the gland. Over time, fibrosis of pituitary tissue occurs, and the symptoms of hypopituitarism develop. Adenomas and aneurysms may compress otherwise normal secreting pituitary cells and lead to compromised hormonal output. These lesions further impede blood supply because of enlargement of the pituitary within the fixed compartment of the sella turcica.

CLINICAL MANIFESTATIONS The signs and symptoms of hypofunction of the anterior pituitary are variable and depend on which hormones are affected. In panhypopituitarism, all hormones are deficient and the individual suffers from multiple complications.

ACTH deficiency with associated loss of cortisol is a potentially life-threatening disorder. Symptoms of cortisol insufficiency include nausea, vomiting, anorexia, fatigue, and weakness. Hypoglycemia results from increased insulin sensitivity, decreased glycogen reserves, and decreased gluconeogenesis associated with hypocortisolism. ACTH deficiency also is associated with changes in aldosterone secretion, with resulting decreases in the glomerular filtration rate and urine output.

TSH deficiency causes cold intolerance, skin dryness, lethargy, and decreased metabolic rate. The symptoms usually are less severe than those of primary hypothyroidism.

The onset of FSH and LH deficiencies in women of reproductive age is associated with amenorrhea and atrophy of the vagina, uterus, and breasts. In postpubertal males, the testicles atrophy and facial hair growth is diminished. Both men and women experience decreased body hair and diminished libido.

GH deficiency in children is manifested by growth failure and a condition known as *hypopituitary dwarfism* (Fig. 20.2). Symptoms of chronic adult GH deficiency syndrome include increased body fat, decreased strength and lean body mass, osteoporosis, reduced sweating, dry skin, and psychological problems, including depression, social withdrawal, fatigue, loss of motivation, and a diminished feeling of well-being. Dyslipidemias and atherosclerotic cardiovascular disease may occur.

EVALUATION AND TREATMENT The diagnostic evaluation of suspected pituitary disease includes simultaneous measurements of the levels of tropic hormones from the pituitary and target endocrine glands. Imaging of the pituitary (magnetic resonance imaging [MRI] or computed tomography [CT] scans) is critical to assess for anatomic lesions, such as tumors.

Management of hypopituitarism requires correction of the underlying disorder as quickly as possible. Replacement of target gland hormones that are deficient is essential (such as cortisol, thyroid hormone, GH,

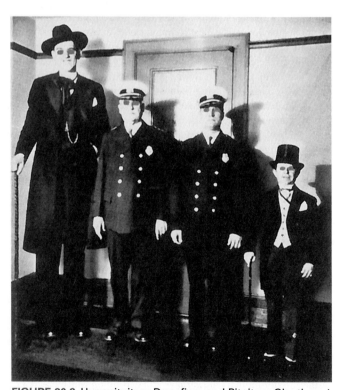

FIGURE 20.2 Hypopituitary Dwarfism and Pituitary Giantism. A pituitary giant and dwarf contrasted with normal-size men. Excessive secretion of growth hormone by the anterior lobe of the pituitary gland during the early years of life produces giants of this type, whereas deficient secretion of this substance produces well-formed dwarfs. (From Patton KT, Thibodeau GA: *Anatomy & physiology,* ed 8, St Louis, 2013, Mosby.)

and sex-specific steroid hormones). In cases of acute circulatory collapse, immediate therapy with glucocorticoids and intravenous fluids is critical.

Hyperpituitarism: Primary Adenoma

Pituitary adenomas usually are benign, slow-growing tumors that arise from cells of the anterior pituitary. The cause of pituitary adenomas is not known, and most occur sporadically. Altered gene expression is commonly detected, and familial pituitary adenomas occur as part of syndromes affecting other organs, such as multiple endocrine neoplasia type 1. About 50% are microscopic (microadenomas) found incidentally, are hormonally silent, and do not pose significant hazards to the individual. Larger adenomas (macroadenomas) are associated with morbidity and mortality attributable to alterations in hormone secretion or to invasion or impingement of surrounding structures.[4]

PATHOPHYSIOLOGY Local expansion of the adenoma may impinge on the optic chiasma and cause various visual disturbances. If the tumor is locally aggressive, invasion of the cavernous sinuses may occur, resulting in compromise of cranial nerve function. Extension to the hypothalamus disturbs control of wakefulness, thirst, appetite, and temperature.

Hormonal effects of adenomas include hypersecretion from the adenoma itself and hyposecretion from surrounding pituitary cells. The adenomatous tissue secretes the hormone of the cell type from which it arose, without regard to regulatory feedback mechanisms (autonomous function). Because of the pressure exerted by the tumor in the unexpandable bony sella turcica, hyposecretion from those cells that are most sensitive to pressure is common (FSH-and LH-secreting cells).

CLINICAL MANIFESTATIONS The clinical manifestations of pituitary adenomas are related to tumor growth and hormone hypersecretion or hyposecretion. Increased tumor size causes headache, fatigue, neck pain or stiffness, and seizures. Visual changes include visual field impairments (often beginning in one eye and progressing to the other) and temporary blindness. If the tumor infiltrates other cranial nerves, neuromuscular function is affected.

Pituitary adenomas are most often associated with increased secretion of growth hormone and prolactin. Gonadotropic hyposecretion results in menstrual irregularity in women, decreased libido, and receding secondary sex characteristics in both men and women. If the tumor exerts sufficient pressure, thyroid and adrenal hypofunction may occur because of lack of TSH and ACTH, resulting in the symptoms of hypothyroidism and hypocortisolism, respectively.

EVALUATION AND TREATMENT Diagnosis of pituitary adenoma involves physical and laboratory evaluations, including pertinent hormone assays and radiographic examination of the skull (MRI [preferred] or contrast-enhanced CT). The goal of treatment is to protect the individual from the effects of tumor growth and to control hormone hypersecretion while minimizing damage to appropriately secreting portions of the pituitary. Depending on tumor size and type, individuals may be treated by administration of specific medications to suppress tumor growth, transsphenoidal tumor resection, or radiation therapy, including stereotactic treatments.

> ✔ **QUICK CHECK 20.1**
> 1. What are the major causes of inappropriate amounts of hormone being delivered to the target cell?
> 2. Why do individuals with the syndrome of inappropriate antidiuretic hormone (SIADH) secrete concentrated urine?
> 3. Why may individuals with a pituitary adenoma develop visual disturbances?

Hypersecretion of Growth Hormone: Acromegaly

Acromegaly results from continuous exposure to high levels of GH and insulin-like growth factor 1 (IGF-1). It almost always is caused by a GH-secreting pituitary adenoma.[5] Acromegaly is usually diagnosed in adults in the 40- to 59-year-old age group, although it is often present for years before diagnosis. It is a slowly progressive disease and, if untreated, is associated with a decreased life expectancy. Deaths from acromegaly are caused by heart disease secondary to hypertension and coronary artery disease, stroke, diabetes mellitus, or malignancy (colon or lung cancers).

PATHOPHYSIOLOGY With a GH-secreting adenoma, only slight elevations of GH and IGF-1 can stimulate growth. In children and adolescents whose epiphyseal plates have not yet closed, the effect of increased GH levels is termed giantism (see Fig. 20.2). Skeletal growth is excessive, with some individuals becoming 8 or 9 feet tall. In the adult, epiphyseal closure has occurred, and increased amounts of GH and IGF-1 cause connective tissue proliferation and increased cytoplasmic matrix, as well as bony proliferation that results in the characteristic appearance of acromegaly (Fig. 20.3).

GH also has significant effects on glucose, lipid, and protein metabolism. Hyperglycemia results from adipocyte inflammation and GH inhibition of peripheral glucose uptake and increased hepatic glucose production, followed by compensatory hyperinsulinism and, finally, insulin resistance. Diabetes mellitus occurs when the pancreas cannot secrete enough insulin to offset the effects of GH. Excessive levels of GH and IGF-1 also affect the cardiovascular system, and hypertension, cardiomegaly, and left ventricular heart failure are seen in one-third to one-half of individuals with acromegaly. GH also acts on the renal tubules to increase phosphate reabsorption, leading to mild hyperphosphatemia. Approximately 20% of GH-secreting tumors also secrete prolactin. Because the adenoma becomes increasingly a space-occupying lesion, hypopituitarism may occur because of compression of surrounding hormone-secreting cells.

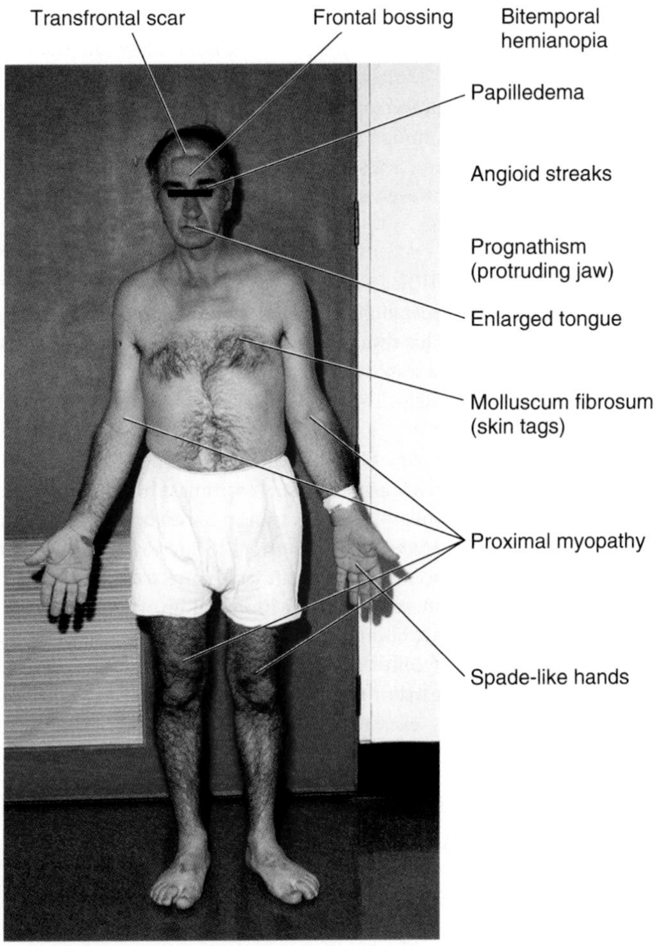

CLINICAL MANIFESTATIONS With connective tissue proliferation, individuals with acromegaly have an enlarged tongue, interstitial edema, enlarged and overactive sebaceous and sweat glands (leading to increased body odor), and coarse skin and body hair. Bony proliferation involves periosteal vertebral growth and enlargement of the bones of the face, hands, and feet (see Fig. 20.3). The lower jaw and forehead also protrude.

Increased IGF-1 levels cause ribs to elongate at the bone–cartilage junction, leading to a barrel-chested appearance, and increased proliferation of cartilage in joints, which causes backache and arthralgias. With bony and soft tissue overgrowth, nerve entrapment occurs, leading to peripheral nerve damage manifested by weakness, muscular atrophy, footdrop, and sensory changes in the hands.

Symptoms of diabetes mellitus, such as polyuria and polydipsia, may occur. Acromegaly-associated hypertension is usually asymptomatic until heart failure symptoms develop. Increased tumor size results in central nervous system symptoms of headache, seizure activity, visual disturbances, and papilledema. If compression hypopituitarism occurs, gonadotropin secretion may be affected, causing amenorrhea in women and sexual dysfunction in men. Increased prolactin results in hypogonadism.

EVALUATION AND TREATMENT Diagnosis is confirmed by clinical features of the disease, MRI scans, and elevated levels of GH and IGF-1. The goals of treatment are to normalize or reduce GH secretion and relieve or prevent complications related to tumor expansion. The treatment of choice is transsphenoidal surgical removal of the GH-secreting adenoma. Radiation therapy may be effective when rapid control of GH levels is not essential, when the individual is not a good surgical candidate, or when hyperfunction persists after subtotal resection. Somatostatin analogs (e.g., octreotide or lanreotide) normalize IGF-1 and GH levels. Dopaminergic agonists may be helpful, especially if the tumor also secretes prolactin. Cardiovascular, metabolic, and symptoms of tumor compression often improve with treatment. Skeletal abnormalities are irreversible.

Prolactinoma

Pituitary tumors that secrete prolactin, prolactinomas, are the most common hormonally active pituitary tumors. Other conditions, such as renal failure, polycystic ovarian disease, primary hypothyroidism, breast stimulation, or even the stress of venipuncture, can increase prolactin levels. Prolactin is under tonic inhibitory hypothalamic control through the secretion of dopamine. Thus medications that block the effects of dopamine can increase prolactin levels. These include some antipsychotics, metoclopramide, tricyclic antidepressants, and methyldopa. Estrogens can increase prolactin concentration by stimulating hyperplasia of prolactin-secreting cells. Any process that interferes with the delivery of dopamine from the hypothalamus to the lactotrophs (pituitary stalk tumor, pituitary stalk transection, or compressive pituitary tumor) also results in hyperprolactinemia. Because thyrotropin-releasing hormone (TRH) stimulates prolactin secretion, prolactin may be elevated in individuals with primary hypothyroidism.

FIGURE 20.3 Acromegaly. (From Talley NJ, O'Connor S: *Clinical examination*, ed 7, Australia, 2014, Churchill Livingstone.)

Labels on figure:
- Transfrontal scar
- Frontal bossing
- Bitemporal hemianopia
- Papilledema
- Angioid streaks
- Prognathism (protruding jaw)
- Enlarged tongue
- Molluscum fibrosum (skin tags)
- Proximal myopathy
- Spade-like hands

PATHOPHYSIOLOGY The hallmark of a prolactinoma is sustained increases in the levels of serum prolactin, which has multiple effects on female and male reproductive organs. Pathologic elevations of prolactin suppress LH and FSH, resulting in estrogen and progesterone deficiency in women and low testosterone levels in men.

Hypopituitarism may occur because of the compression of surrounding hormone-secreting cells. Central nervous system symptoms may develop because of growth and pressure of the adenoma within the sella turcica. These complications are especially common with what are called macro (>1 cm in diameter) or giant (>4 cm in diameter) prolactinomas.

CLINICAL MANIFESTATIONS Women with hyperprolactinemia generally present with galactorrhea (nonpuerperal milk production) and menstrual disturbances, including amenorrhea. Estrogen deficiency also may cause hirsutism, and fractures may occur because of osteopenia or osteoporosis. Hyperprolactinemia in men causes gynecomastia, hypogonadism, and erectile dysfunction, although they often are not diagnosed until they develop symptoms related to the increasing size of the adenoma (i.e., headache or visual impairment).

EVALUATION AND TREATMENT The diagnostic evaluation of hyperprolactinemia includes a careful history to exclude medications that may cause elevations in prolactin concentration. Screening for hypothyroidism is mandatory. MRI scanning of the pituitary is indicated to determine the size and location of an adenoma.

Dopaminergic agonists (cabergoline) are the treatment of choice for prolactinomas. Decreases in tumor size and restoration of fertility in previously anovulatory women are common. In individuals resistant or intolerant to these medications, transsphenoidal surgery and radiotherapy are options. New chemotherapeutic and targeted molecular therapies are being explored in selected cases.

ALTERATIONS OF THYROID FUNCTION

Disorders of thyroid function develop as a result of primary dysfunction or disease of the thyroid gland or, secondarily, as a result of pituitary or hypothalamic alterations. Primary thyroid disorders result in either increased or decreased thyroid hormone (TH) levels. These disorders also cause secondary feedback effects on pituitary TSH. For example, when there are primary elevations in the TH level, the TSH level will secondarily decrease because of negative feedback. When the TH level is decreased because of a condition affecting the thyroid gland, the TSH level will be elevated. Central (secondary) thyroid disorders are related to disorders of pituitary gland TSH production. When there is excessive TSH production, the TH level is elevated secondary to the primary elevation of the TSH concentration. The reverse is true with inadequate TSH production.

The majority of primary thyroid diseases are idiopathic and caused by autoimmune mechanisms that affect the gland. Although the exact genetic and environmental influences are not known, some individuals experience a predominantly cellular autoimmune response (some antithyroid autoantibodies also are involved) with resultant destruction of the thyroid gland, leading to hypothyroidism. Others experience a predominantly antibody-mediated autoimmune response that stimulates the gland, leading to hyperthyroidism. The most common autoimmune hypothyroid condition is called *Hashimoto thyroiditis*,[6] and the most common autoimmune hyperthyroid condition is called *Graves disease*[7] (Fig. 20.4).

Thyrotoxicosis/Hyperthyroidism
PATHOPHYSIOLOGY Thyrotoxicosis is a condition that results from any cause of increased TH levels and can result from dysfunction of

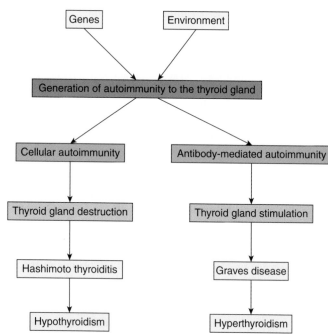

FIGURE 20.4 Autoimmune Mechanisms in Primary Thyroid Disease.

the pituitary, the thyroid gland, ectopic thyroid tissue, or the ingestion of excessive amounts of TH medication. Hyperthyroidism is a form of thyrotoxicosis in which excess amounts of TH are secreted from the thyroid gland[8] (Fig. 20.5). *Primary hyperthyroidism* results from thyroid gland dysfunction and is most commonly caused by Graves disease, toxic multinodular goiter, and solitary toxic adenoma. *Central (secondary) hyperthyroidism* is less common and is caused by TSH-secreting pituitary adenomas. Each condition is associated with a specific pathophysiology and manifestations; however, all forms of thyrotoxicosis share some common characteristics.

CLINICAL MANIFESTATIONS The clinical features of thyrotoxicosis are attributable to the metabolic effects of increased circulating levels of thyroid hormones. This results in an increased metabolic rate, with heat intolerance and increased tissue sensitivity to stimulation by the sympathetic nervous system. The major manifestations are summarized in Fig. 20.6.

Elevated serum thyroxine (T_4) and triiodothyronine (T_3) levels and suppressed serum TSH levels are diagnostic for primary hyperthyroidism. By contrast, central (secondary) hyperthyroidism caused by TSH-secreting pituitary tumors is characterized by normal to increased TSH levels despite elevated TH concentrations. Treatment is directed at controlling excessive TH production, secretion, or action and involves antithyroid drug therapy, radioactive iodine therapy (absorbed only by thyroid tissue, causing death of cells), or surgical removal of nodules or part of the thyroid gland. A major complication of all forms of treatment for hyperthyroidism is excessive ablation of the gland, leading to hypothyroidism.

Hyperthyroid Conditions
Graves disease. Graves disease is the underlying cause of 50% to 80% of cases of hyperthyroidism with a prevalence of approximately 3% of women and 0.5% of men in the United States.[9] Although the exact cause of Graves disease is not known, genetic factors interacting with environmental triggers play an important role in the pathogenesis. Graves disease is classified as an autoimmune disease and results from a form of type II hypersensitivity (see Chapter 8) in which there is

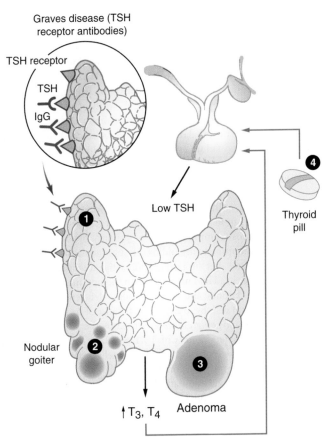

Graves disease (TSH receptor antibodies)

TSH receptor

TSH

IgG

1

Low TSH

Nodular goiter

2

3

Adenoma

4

Thyroid pill

$\uparrow T_3, T_4$

FIGURE 20.5 Common Causes of Hyperthyroidism. Hyperthyroidism may have several causes, among them: **1,** Graves disease; **2,** toxic multinodular goiter; **3,** follicular adenoma; **4,** thyroid medication. (Adapted from Damjanov I: *Pathology for the health professions,* ed 4, St Louis, 2012, Saunders.)

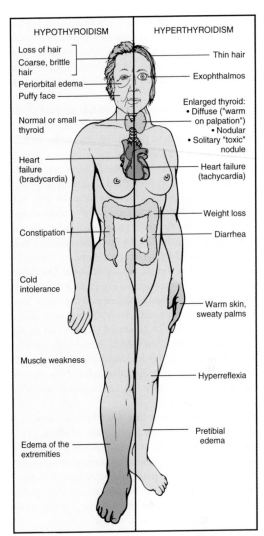

HYPOTHYROIDISM | HYPERTHYROIDISM

Loss of hair
Coarse, brittle hair
Periorbital edema
Puffy face

Normal or small thyroid

Heart failure (bradycardia)

Constipation

Cold intolerance

Muscle weakness

Edema of the extremities

Thin hair

Exophthalmos

Enlarged thyroid:
• Diffuse ("warm on palpation")
• Nodular
• Solitary "toxic" nodule

Heart failure (tachycardia)

Weight loss

Diarrhea

Warm skin, sweaty palms

Hyperreflexia

Pretibial edema

FIGURE 20.6 Clinical Manifestations of Hyperthyroidism and Hypothyroidism. (From Damjanov I: *Pathology for the health professions,* ed 4, St Louis, 2012, Saunders.)

stimulation of the thyroid by autoantibodies directed against the TSH receptor. These autoantibodies, called *thyroid-stimulating immunoglobulins* (TSIs; also called *thyroid-stimulating antibodies* [TSAbs] or *thyroid receptor antibodies* [TRAbs]), override the normal regulatory mechanisms. TSI stimulation of TSH receptors in the gland results in hyperplasia of the gland (goiter) and increased synthesis of TH, especially of triiodo-L-thyronine (T_3). Increased levels of TH result in the classic signs and symptoms of hyperthyroidism illustrated in Fig. 20.6. TSH production by the pituitary is inhibited through the usual negative feedback loop.

Autoimmunity also contributes to the two major distinguishing clinical manifestations of Graves disease (ophthalmopathy and dermopathy [pretibial myxedema]) (Fig. 20.7). Two categories of ophthalmopathy associated with Graves disease are (1) functional abnormalities resulting from hyperactivity of the sympathetic division of the autonomic nervous system (lag of the globe on upward gaze and of the upper lid on downward gaze) and (2) infiltrative changes involving the orbital contents with enlargement of the ocular muscles. These changes affect more than half of individuals with Graves disease. Orbital connective tissue accumulation, inflammation, and edema of the orbital contents result in exophthalmos (protrusion of the eyeball), periorbital edema, and extraocular muscle weakness leading to diplopia (double vision). The individual may experience irritation, pain, lacrimation, photophobia, blurred vision, decreased visual acuity, papilledema, visual field impairment, exposure keratosis, and corneal ulceration.

A small number of individuals with Graves disease who have very high levels of TSI experience pretibial myxedema (Graves dermopathy), characterized by subcutaneous swelling on the anterior portions of the legs and by indurated and erythematous skin. Graves dermopathy

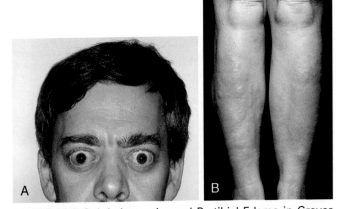

A B

FIGURE 20.7 Ophthalmopathy and Pretibial Edema in Graves Disease. A, Exophthalmos (large and protruding eyeballs, often in association with a large goiter). **B,** Pretibial myxedema associated with Graves disease; note lumpy and swollen appearance from accumulation of connective tissue and pinkish purple discoloration. (**A** from Belchetz P, Hammond P: *Mosby's color atlas and text of diabetes and endocrinology,* Edinburgh, 2003, Mosby; **B** from Habif T: *Clinical dermatology,* ed 5, St Louis, 2009, Mosby.)

is associated with TSI stimulation of fibroblasts and T lymphocytes, causing excessive amounts of hyaluronic acid production in the dermis and subcutaneous tissue. These manifestations occasionally appear on the hands, giving the appearance of clubbing of the fingers (thyroid acropachy). Fig. 20.8 provides an overview of the pathophysiology of Graves disease.

Hyperthyroidism resulting from nodular thyroid disease. The thyroid gland normally enlarges in response to the increased demand for TH that occurs in puberty, pregnancy, and iodine-deficient states, as well as in individuals with immunologic, viral, or genetic disorders. When the condition resulting in increased TH resolves, TSH secretion normally subsides and the thyroid gland returns to its original size.

Irreversible changes can occur in some follicular cells so that these cells form nodules that function autonomously and produce excessive amounts of TH. Toxic multinodular goiter occurs when there are several hyperfunctioning nodules leading to hyperthyroidism. Unlike Graves disease, there is absence of an autoimmune stimulus. If only one nodule is hyperfunctioning, it is termed toxic adenoma. The classic clinical manifestations of hyperthyroidism (see Fig. 20.6) usually develop slowly, and exophthalmos and pretibial myxedema do not occur. Nodules may be palpable on physical examination, and there is increased uptake of radioactive iodine. There is an increased incidence of malignancy in toxic nodular goiter, so most individuals should undergo a fine-needle aspiration biopsy of suspicious nodules before treatment. Treatment consists of a combination of radioactive iodine (may increase risk of solid cancer-related death, including breast cancer death[9a]), surgery, and antithyroid medications.

Thyrotoxic crisis. Thyrotoxic crisis (thyroid storm) is a rare but dangerous worsening of the thyrotoxic state in which TH levels rise dramatically and death can occur within 48 hours without treatment. The condition may develop spontaneously but usually occurs in individuals who have undiagnosed or partially treated Graves disease and who are subjected to physiologic stress, such as infection, pulmonary or cardiovascular disorders, trauma, seizures, surgery (especially thyroid surgery), obstetric complications, or dialysis.

The systemic manifestations of thyrotoxic crisis include hyperthermia; tachycardia, especially atrial tachydysrhythmias; heart failure; agitation or delirium; and nausea, vomiting, or diarrhea contributing to fluid volume depletion. Treatment includes drugs that block TH synthesis (i.e., propylthiouracil or methimazole), beta blockers, glucocorticoids, iodine, and supportive care.

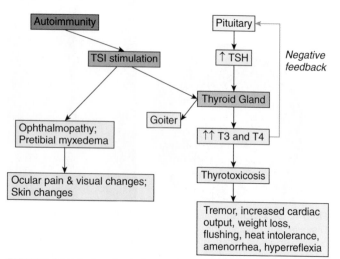

FIGURE 20.8 Pathophysiology of Graves Disease. *TSI,* Thyroid-stimulating immunoglobulins (antibodies); *TSH,* thyroid-stimulating hormone; *T₃,* triiodothyronine; *T₄,* tetraiodothyronine.

Hypothyroidism

Hypothyroidism results from deficient production of TH by the thyroid gland. Hypothyroidism is the most common disorder of thyroid function, affecting approximately 3.7% of the U.S. population, and occurs more commonly in women.[10] It may be primary or central. Primary hypothyroidism accounts for the majority of all cases. Central (secondary) hypothyroidism is much less common and is related to either pituitary or hypothalamic failure. Subclinical hypothyroidism is a mild thyroid failure estimated to occur in 4% to 8% of U.S. adults.[11] It is defined as an elevation in TSH levels with normal levels of circulating TH.

PATHOPHYSIOLOGY In *primary hypothyroidism,* loss of thyroid function leads to decreased production of TH and increased secretion of TSH and TRH. The most common causes of primary hypothyroidism in adults include autoimmune thyroiditis (Hashimoto disease), iatrogenic loss of thyroid tissue after surgical or radioactive treatment for hyperthyroidism or after head and neck radiation therapy, medications (e.g., lithium and amiodarone), and endemic iodine deficiency. Infants and children may present with hypothyroidism because of congenital defects. *Central (secondary) hypothyroidism* is caused by the pituitary's failure to synthesize adequate amounts of TSH or a lack of TRH. Pituitary tumors that compress surrounding pituitary cells or the consequences of their treatment are the most common causes of central hypothyroidism. Other causes include traumatic brain injury, subarachnoid hemorrhage, or pituitary infarction. Hypothalamic dysfunction results in low levels of TH, TSH, and TRH.

CLINICAL MANIFESTATIONS Hypothyroidism generally affects all body systems and occurs insidiously over months or years. Decreased TH levels lower energy metabolism and heat production. The individual develops a low basal metabolic rate, cold intolerance, lethargy, and slightly lowered basal body temperature (see Fig. 20.6). The decrease in the level of TH leads to excessive TSH production, which stimulates thyroid tissue and causes goiter.

The characteristic sign of severe or long-standing hypothyroidism is myxedema, which results from the altered composition of the dermis and other tissues. The connective tissue fibers are separated by large amounts of protein and mucopolysaccharide. This complex binds water, producing nonpitting, boggy edema, especially around the eyes, hands, and feet and in the supraclavicular fossae (Fig. 20.9). The tongue and laryngeal and pharyngeal mucous membranes thicken, producing thick, slurred speech and hoarseness. Myxedema coma, a medical emergency, is a diminished level of consciousness associated with severe hypothyroidism. Signs and symptoms include hypothermia without shivering, hypoventilation, hypotension, hypoglycemia, and lactic acidosis. Older individuals with comorbid conditions, such as pulmonary or urinary infections, congestive heart failure, or cerebrovascular accident, and with moderate or untreated hypothyroidism are particularly at risk for developing myxedema coma. It also may occur after overuse of narcotics or sedatives or after an acute illness in hypothyroid individuals. Symptoms of hypothyroidism in older adults should not be attributed to normal aging changes.

EVALUATION AND TREATMENT The diagnosis of primary hypothyroidism is made by documentation of the clinical symptoms of hypothyroidism and measurement of increased levels of TSH and decreased levels of TH (total T₃ and both total and free T₄). Central hypothyroidism is diagnosed by finding low TH and low serum TSH levels. Hormone replacement therapy with the hormone levothyroxine is the treatment of choice for both primary and central thyroid disorders.

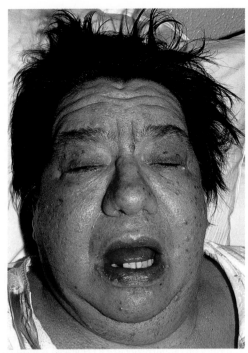

FIGURE 20.9 Myxedema. Note edema around eyes and facial puffiness. The hair is dry. (From Bolognia JL et al: *Dermatology,* ed 3, St Louis, 2012, Mosby.)

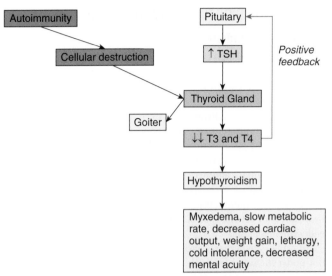

FIGURE 20.10 Pathophysiology of Hashimoto Thyroiditis. *TSH,* Thyroid-stimulating hormone; *T₃,* triiodothyronine; *T₄,* tetraiodothyronine.

Hypothyroid Conditions

Hashimoto disease. The most common cause of primary hypothyroidism in the U.S. is autoimmune thyroiditis (Hashimoto disease), which results in gradual, inflammatory destruction of thyroid tissue. This disorder is linked with several genetic risk factors and is often associated with other autoimmune conditions. Infiltration of the thyroid with autoreactive T lymphocytes, antithyroid antibodies (antithyroid peroxidase and antithyroglobulin antibodies), and natural killer cells induces inflammation, glandular apoptosis, and tissue destruction (Fig. 20.10).

Uncommon causes of hypothyroidism. Other, less common causes of hypothyroidism are subacute thyroiditis and postpartum thyroiditis. Subacute thyroiditis (de Quervain thyroiditis) is a rare nonbacterial inflammation of the thyroid gland often preceded by a viral infection. It is accompanied by fever, tenderness, and enlargement of the thyroid gland and transient hypothyroidism before the gland recovers normal activity. Symptoms may last for 2 to 4 months, and nonsteroidal antiinflammatory drugs or corticosteroids usually resolve symptoms. Postpartum thyroiditis generally occurs up to 6 months after birthing with a course similar to that seen in subacute thyroiditis. Iatrogenic hypothyroidism results from ablation of the thyroid gland during treatment for hyperthyroid conditions.

Congenital hypothyroidism. Hypothyroidism in infants occurs when thyroid tissue is absent (thyroid dysgenesis) or with hereditary defects in TH synthesis. Thyroid dysgenesis occurs more often in female infants, with permanent abnormalities in 1 of every 4000 live births. The affected fetus is dependent on maternal thyroxine for the first 20 weeks of gestation, then becomes deficient in TH. TH is essential for fetal growth and for the development of brain tissue, so the infant will suffer developmental and cognitive disabilities if left untreated. Hypothyroidism may not be evident at birth. Symptoms may include high birth weight, hypothermia, delay in passing meconium, and neonatal jaundice. Cord blood can be examined in the first days of life for measurement of T₄ and TSH levels. The probability of normal growth and intellectual function is high if treatment with levothyroxine is started before the child is 3 or 4 months old. The earlier thyroid hormone replacement is initiated, the better the child's outcome.

Without early screening, hypothyroidism may not be evident until after 4 months of age. Symptoms include difficulty eating, hoarse cry, and protruding tongue caused by myxedema of oral tissues and vocal cords; hypotonic muscles of the abdomen with constipation, abdominal protrusion, and umbilical hernia; subnormal temperature; lethargy; excessive sleeping; slow pulse rate; and cold, mottled skin. Skeletal growth is stunted because of impaired protein synthesis, poor absorption of nutrients, and lack of bone mineralization. The child will be dwarfed with short limbs, if not treated. Dentition is often delayed. Cognitive disability varies with the severity of hypothyroidism and the length of delay before treatment is initiated.

Thyroid Carcinoma

Thyroid carcinoma is the most common endocrine malignancy and is the sixth most common cancer in the U.S in women.[12] Exposure to ionizing radiation, especially during childhood, is the most consistent causal factor. Papillary and follicular thyroid carcinomas are the most frequent, and medullary and anaplastic thyroid carcinomas are less common.

The cancer is typically discovered as a small thyroid nodule or metastatic tumor in the lungs, brain, or bone. Changes in voice and swallowing and difficulty breathing are related to tumor growth impinging on the trachea or esophagus. The diagnosis of thyroid cancer is generally made by ultrasonography and then by fine-needle aspiration of a thyroid nodule. Most individuals with thyroid carcinoma have normal T₃ and T₄ levels and are therefore euthyroid.

Treatment may include partial or total thyroidectomy, TSH suppression therapy (levothyroxine), radioactive iodine therapy (in iodine-concentrating tumors), postoperative radiation therapy, and chemotherapy (especially in anaplastic carcinoma).[13] New insights into the molecular pathogenesis of thyroid carcinoma are leading to new therapies.

> ✔ **QUICK CHECK 20.2**
> 1. Compare the clinical manifestations of hyperthyroidism and hypothyroidism.
> 2. What is Graves disease?
> 3. What is Hashimoto disease?
> 4. How does thyroid carcinoma present clinically?

ALTERATIONS OF PARATHYROID FUNCTION

Hyperparathyroidism

Hyperparathyroidism is characterized by greater than normal secretion of parathyroid hormone (PTH) with associated hypercalcemia. Hyperparathyroidism is classified as primary, secondary, or tertiary.

PATHOPHYSIOLOGY Primary hyperparathyroidism is characterized by inappropriate excess secretion of PTH by one or more of the parathyroid glands.[14] It is one of the most common endocrine disorders. Approximately 80% to 85% of cases are caused by parathyroid adenomas, another 10% to 15% result from parathyroid hyperplasia, and approximately 1% of cases are caused by parathyroid carcinoma. In addition, primary hyperparathyroidism may be caused by a variety of genetic causes, especially the genes that cause multiple endocrine neoplasia.

In primary hyperparathyroidism, PTH secretion is increased and is not under the usual feedback control mechanisms. The calcium level in the blood rises because of increased bone resorption and gastrointestinal absorption of calcium but fails to inhibit PTH secretion by the parathyroid gland. Some individuals with primary hyperparathyroidism maintain normal levels of calcium despite elevated levels of PTH and are diagnosed only when they develop osteoporosis.

Secondary hyperparathyroidism is a compensatory response of the parathyroid glands to chronic hypocalcemia, which is commonly associated with decreased activation of vitamin D in individuals with renal failure (see Chapter 32). Secretion of PTH is elevated, but PTH cannot achieve normal calcium levels because of insufficient levels of activated vitamin D. Other causes of secondary hyperparathyroidism include a dietary deficiency of vitamin D or calcium; decreased intestinal absorption of vitamin D or calcium; and ingestion of drugs, such as phenytoin, phenobarbital, and laxatives, which either accelerate the metabolism of vitamin D or decrease intestinal absorption of calcium.

Tertiary hyperparathyroidism can develop after any long-standing period of hypocalcemia, such as is seen with chronic dialysis, renal transplantation, or gastrointestinal malabsorption. Parathyroid chief cell hyperplasia leads to is excessive secretion of PTH and may cause hypercalcemia.

CLINICAL MANIFESTATIONS Hypercalcemia and hypophosphatemia are the hallmarks of primary hyperparathyroidism. Hypercalcemia and hypophosphatemia may be asymptomatic, or affected individuals may present with symptoms related to the muscular, nervous, and gastrointestinal systems, including fatigue, headache, depression, anorexia, and nausea and vomiting. Excessive osteoclastic and osteocytic activity causes bone resorption, resulting in osteoporosis, pathologic fractures, kyphosis of the dorsal spine, and compression fractures of the vertebral bodies. (Bone resorption is discussed in Chapter 40.)

Hypercalcemia means that the renal tubules must filter large amounts of calcium, leading to hypercalciuria and production of an abnormally alkaline urine. PTH hypersecretion enhances renal phosphate excretion and results in hypophosphatemia and hyperphosphaturia (see Chapter 5). The combination of these three variables—hypercalciuria, alkaline urine, and hyperphosphaturia—predisposes the individual to the formation of calcium stones, particularly in the renal pelvis or renal collecting ducts. These stones may be associated with infections and impaired renal function. Chronic hypercalcemia also is associated with mild insulin resistance, necessitating increased insulin secretion to maintain normal glucose levels.

Secondary hyperparathyroidism caused by renal disease presents clinically not only with the complications of bone resorption but also with the symptoms of hypocalcemia and hyperphosphatemia, such as muscle spasms and cardiovascular complications (see Chapter 5)

EVALUATION AND TREATMENT The diagnosis of primary hyperparathyroidism is suggested by the concurrent findings of elevated PTH levels and an increased ionized calcium concentration. Imaging procedures are used to localize adenomas before surgery. Observation of asymptomatic individuals with mild hypercalcemia is recommended; these individuals are advised to avoid dehydration and limit dietary calcium intake. Definitive treatment of more severe primary hyperparathyroidism involves surgical removal of the solitary adenoma or, in the case of hyperplasia, complete removal of three and partial removal of the fourth hyperplastic parathyroid glands.

If the serum calcium concentration is low despite elevated levels of PTH, secondary hyperparathyroidism is likely. Evaluation for renal function may indicate chronic renal disease. Treatment for secondary hyperparathyroidism in chronic renal disease requires calcium replacement, dietary phosphate restriction and phosphate binders, and vitamin D replacement. Treatment also may include calcimimetics, which work to increase parathyroid calcium receptor sensitivity, thus lowering PTH levels.

Hypoparathyroidism

Hypoparathyroidism (abnormally low PTH levels) is most commonly caused by damage to the parathyroid glands during thyroid surgery. This occurs because of the anatomic proximity of the parathyroid glands to the thyroid (see Fig. 19.11). Hypomagnesemia is another cause of low PTH levels. Hypoparathyroidism also is associated with genetic syndromes, including familial hypoparathyroidism and DiGeorge syndrome (see Chapter 8). There is an inherited condition called *pseudohypoparathyroidism* that causes a defect in tissue responsiveness to PTH. Pseudohypoparathyroidism is associated with hypocalcemia despite normal to elevated levels of PTH.

PATHOPHYSIOLOGY No matter the cause, the absence of PTH impairs resorption of calcium from bone and the renal tubules, leading to hypocalcemia. Deficient PTH also stimulates increased renal reabsorption of phosphate, leading to hyperphosphatemia. Hyperphosphatemia further lowers the calcium concentration by inhibiting the activation of vitamin D, thereby lowering the gastrointestinal absorption of calcium.

Hypomagnesemia inhibits PTH secretion. Hypomagnesemia may be related to chronic alcoholism, malnutrition, malabsorption, increased renal clearance of magnesium caused by the use of aminoglycoside antibiotics or certain chemotherapeutic agents, or prolonged magnesium-deficient parenteral nutritional therapy. When serum magnesium levels return to normal, however, PTH secretion returns to normal.

CLINICAL MANIFESTATIONS Symptoms associated with hypoparathyroidism are primarily those of hypocalcemia (see Chapter 5). Hypocalcemia causes muscle spasms, which can progress to tetany, dry skin, and loss of body and scalp hair. Irreversible complications include hypoplasia of developing teeth, horizontal ridges on the nails, cataracts, basal ganglia calcifications (which may be associated with a parkinsonian syndrome), and bone deformities, including brachydactyly and bowing of the long bones.

EVALUATION AND TREATMENT A low PTH level, along with a low serum calcium concentration and a high phosphorus level in the absence of renal failure, intestinal disorders, or nutritional deficiencies, suggests hypoparathyroidism. Measurement of the serum magnesium level and urinary calcium excretion also can help in diagnosis. Treatment is directed toward alleviation of the hypocalcemia. In acute states, this involves parenteral administration of calcium, which corrects the serum calcium concentration within minutes. Chronic maintenance of the serum calcium level is achieved with pharmacologic doses of cholecalciferol (vitamin D_3) and oral calcium. PTH hormone replacement with recombinant human parathyroid hormone (rhPTH) is safe and effective.

✓ **QUICK CHECK 20.3**
1. How does excessive parathyroid hormone (PTH) affect bones?
2. What are the results of a lack of circulating PTH?

DYSFUNCTION OF THE ENDOCRINE PANCREAS: DIABETES MELLITUS

Diabetes mellitus is a group of metabolic diseases characterized by hyperglycemia resulting from defects in insulin secretion, insulin action, or both. In 2015, an estimated 30.3 million people (9.4%) in the U.S. had diabetes, and another 7.2 million were estimated to be undiagnosed.[15] The American Diabetes Association (ADA)[16] classifies four categories of diabetes mellitus[17]:

1. Type 1 diabetes (caused by autoimmune beta-cell destruction, usually leading to absolute insulin deficiency)[17]
2. Type 2 diabetes (caused by progressive loss of beta-cell insulin secretion, frequently with a background of insulin resistance)[18]
3. Gestational diabetes mellitus (GDM) (diabetes diagnosed in the second or third trimester of pregnancy that was not clearly overt diabetes prior to gestation)
4. Specific types of diabetes mellitus due to other causes

Specific types of diabetes include monogenic diabetes syndromes (e.g., neonatal diabetes and maturity-onset diabetes of the young [MODY]), disease of the exocrine pancreas (e.g., cystic fibrosis), and drug- or chemical-induced diabetes (e.g., glucocorticoid use in the treatment of human immunodeficiency virus [HIV] infection and/or acquired immunodeficiency syndrome [AIDS] or after organ transplantation).

The diagnosis of diabetes mellitus is based on glycosylated hemoglobin (HbA$_{1C}$) levels; fasting plasma glucose (FPG) levels; oral glucose tolerance testing (OGTT); or random glucose levels in an individual with symptoms[16] (Box 20.1). **Glycosylated hemoglobin** refers to the permanent attachment of glucose to hemoglobin molecules and reflects the average plasma glucose exposure over the life of a red blood cell (approximately 120 days). It provides a more accurate measure for monitoring long-term control of blood glucose levels.

The ADA classification "categories at increased risk for diabetes" (or prediabetes) describes nondiabetic elevations of the HbA$_{1C}$, FPG, or 2-hour plasma glucose value during an OGTT[16] (see Box 20.1). The Centers for Disease Control and Prevention (CDC) estimates that 84.1 million U.S. adults (34%) aged 18 years or older have prediabetes.[15] This classification includes impaired glucose tolerance (IGT), which results from diminished insulin secretion; and impaired fasting glucose (IFG), which is caused by enhanced hepatic glucose output. Individuals with IGT and IFG are at increased risk of cardiovascular disease and premature death and carry up to a 50% 5-year risk of developing diabetes, particularly type 2 diabetes. Thus prevention of diabetes with lifestyle interventions is essential.

Types of Diabetes Mellitus
Type 1 Diabetes Mellitus

Type 1 diabetes mellitus accounts for 5% to 10% of diabetes cases and is the most common pediatric chronic disease. It currently affects approximately 1.25 million U.S. children, and the incidence is increasing.[15] Between 10% and 13% of individuals with newly diagnosed type

---

BOX 20.1   Diagnostic Criteria for Diabetes Mellitus

1. HbA$_{1C}$ (as measured in a DCCT-referenced assay) ≥6.5%
   OR
2. FPG ≥126 mg/dl (7 mmol/L); fasting is defined as no caloric intake for at least 8 hr
   OR
3. 2-hr plasma glucose ≥200 mg/dl (11.1 mmol/L) during OGTT
   OR
4. In an individual with classic symptoms of hyperglycemia or hyperglycemic crisis, a random plasma glucose ≥200 mg/dl (11.1 mmol/L)

In the absence of unequivocal hyperglycemia, criteria 1 through 3 diagnosis requires two abnormal test results from the same sample or in two separate test samples

Categories of Increased Risk for Diabetes
1. FPG 100 to 125 mg/dl
2. 2-hr PG 140 to 199 mg/dl during OGTT
3. HbA$_{1C}$ 5.7% to 6.4%

DCCT, Diabetes Control and Complications Trial; *FPG,* fasting plasma glucose; *HbA$_{1C}$,* hemoglobin A$_{1C}$ or glycosylated hemoglobin; *OGTT,* oral glucose tolerance testing; *PG,* plasma glucose.
Data from American Diabetes Association: Classification and diagnosis of diabetes: standards of medical care in diabetes—2019, *Diabetes Care* 42(Suppl 1):S13-S28, 2019. Available at http://care.diabetesjournals.org/content/42/Supplement_1/.

---

1 diabetes have a first-degree relative (parent or sibling) with type 1 diabetes, and there is a 50% concordance rate in twins. Diagnosis is rare during the first 9 months of life and peaks at 12 years of age (see Table 20.3).

PATHOPHYSIOLOGY   Two distinct types of type 1 diabetes have been identified: idiopathic and autoimmune. *Idiopathic type 1 diabetes mellitus* is far less common than autoimmune diabetes, has a strong genetic component, and occurs mostly in people of Asian or African descent. Affected individuals have no evidence of beta-cell autoimmunity and have varying degrees of insulin deficiency.

Autoimmune type 1 diabetes mellitus is a slowly progressive disease that destroys beta cells of the pancreas. There are strong genetic associations with histocompatibility leukocyte antigen (HLA) class II alleles *HLA-DQ* and *HLA-DR*. Environmental factors that have been implicated include exposure to certain drugs, foods, and viruses. These gene-environment interactions result in the formation of autoantigens that are expressed on the surface of pancreatic beta cells and circulate in the bloodstream and lymphatics (Fig. 20.11). Cellular immunity (T-cytotoxic cells and macrophages) and humoral immunity (autoantibodies against islet cells, insulin, glutamic acid decarboxylase [GAD], and other cytoplasmic proteins) are stimulated, resulting in beta-cell destruction and apoptosis. Over time, 80% to 90% of the insulin-secreting beta cells of the islet of Langerhans are destroyed, insulin synthesis declines, and hyperglycemia develops.

Insulin normally suppresses secretion of glucagon, and thus hypoinsulinemia leads to a marked increase in glucagon secretion. In addition to the decline in insulin secretion, there is decreased secretion of amylin (another beta-cell hormone), which also leads to an increase in glucagon. **Glucagon,** a hormone produced by the alpha cells of the islets, acts in the liver to increase the blood glucose level by stimulating glycogenolysis and gluconeogenesis.. Thus both a lack of insulin and a relative excess of glucagon contribute to hyperglycemia in type 1 diabetes.

TABLE 20.3 Epidemiology and Etiology of Diabetes Mellitus in the United States

	Type 1 Diabetes: Primary Beta-Cell Defect or Failure	Type 2 Diabetes: Insulin Resistance With Inadequate Insulin Secretion
Incidence		
Frequency	5-10% of all cases of diabetes mellitus Prevalence rate is 0.17%	Accounts for most cases (≈90-95%) Prevalence rate for adults is 9.3%
Change in incidences	Incidence is increasing	Incidence in adults more than tripled in the past 3 decades.
Characteristics		
Age at onset	Peak onset at age 11-13 yr (slightly earlier for girls than for boys); rare in children younger than 9 mos and adults older than 30 yrs	Risk of developing diabetes increases after age 40 yr
Sex	Similar in males and females	Similar in males and females
Racial distribution	Rates for whites 1.5-2 times higher than for other ethnic groups	Risk is highest for African Americans and Native Americans
Weight	Generally normal or underweight	Obesity is common and is a frequent contributing factor to precipitate type 2 diabetes among those susceptible
Etiology		
Common theory	*Autoimmune:* genetic and environmental factors, resulting in gradual process of autoimmune destruction in genetically susceptible individuals *Nonautoimmune:* Unknown	Genetic susceptibility (polygenic) combined with environmental determinants; defects in beta-cell function combined with insulin resistance Associated with long-duration obesity
Presence of antibody	Autoantibodies to insulin and to glutamic acid decarboxylase (GAD_{65})	Autoantibodies not present
Insulin resistance	Insulin resistance at diagnosis is unusual, but may occur as individual ages and gains weight	Insulin resistance is virtually universal and multifactorial in origin
Insulin secretion	Severe insulin deficiency or no insulin secretion at all	Typically increased at time of diagnosis, but progressively declines over course of illness

Data from American Diabetes Association: *Diabetes Care* 40(Suppl 1): S11-S24, 2017. Available at: http://care.diabetesjournals.org/content/diacare/suppl/2016/12/15/40.Supplement_1.DC1/DC_40_S1_final.pdf); Centers for Disease Control: *National diabetes statistics report 2017.* Available at https://www.cdc.gov/diabetes/data/statistics/statistics-report.htm.

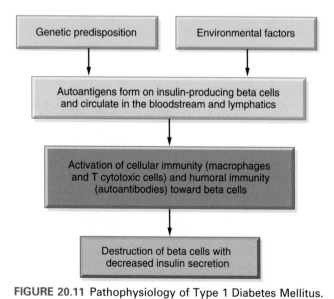

FIGURE 20.11 Pathophysiology of Type 1 Diabetes Mellitus.

BOX 20.2 Criteria for the Diagnosis of Metabolic Syndrome

Three of these five traits must be present:
1. Increased waist circumference as determined by population and country-specific definitions (>40 inches in men; >35 inches in women in the United States)
2. Plasma triglycerides ≥150 mg/dl
3. Plasma high-density lipoprotein (HDL) cholesterol <40 mg/dl (men) or <50 mg/dl (women)
4. Blood pressure: systolic ≥130 and or diastolic ≥85 mm Hg
5. Fasting plasma glucose ≥100 mg/dl
Drug treatment for these conditions is an alternative indicator.

From Alberti KG et al: *Circulation* 120(16):1640-1645, 2009.

The natural history of type 1 diabetes involves a long preclinical period before insulin deficiency and hyperglycemia develop. Glucose accumulates in the blood and appears in the urine as the renal threshold for glucose is exceeded, producing an osmotic diuresis and symptoms of polyuria and thirst (Table 20.4). Wide fluctuations in blood glucose levels occur. Insulin deficiency also causes protein and fat breakdown, resulting in weight loss. Excessive metabolism of fats and proteins leads to high levels of circulating ketones, causing a condition known as *diabetic ketoacidosis* (DKA) (see the Acute Complications of Diabetes section).

Although most individuals with type 1 diabetes are of normal or decreased weight, there are increasing numbers of individuals who have both type 1 diabetes and the clinical manifestations of metabolic syndrome, including obesity, dyslipidemia, and hypertension (Box 20.2). These individuals are at high risk for chronic complications of diabetes, including heart disease and stroke.

TABLE 20.4 Clinical Manifestations and Mechanisms for Type 1 Diabetes Mellitus

Manifestation	Rationale
Polydipsia	Because of elevated blood glucose levels, water is osmotically attracted from body cells, resulting in intracellular dehydration and stimulation of thirst in hypothalamus
Polyuria	Hyperglycemia acts as an osmotic diuretic; amount of glucose filtered by glomeruli of kidney exceeds that which can be reabsorbed by renal tubules; glycosuria results, accompanied by large amounts of water lost in urine
Polyphagia	Depletion of cellular stores of carbohydrates, fats, and protein results in cellular starvation and a corresponding increase in hunger
Weight loss	Weight loss occurs because of fluid loss in osmotic diuresis and loss of body tissue as fats and proteins are used for energy
Fatigue	Metabolic changes result in poor use of food products, contributing to lethargy and fatigue
Recurrent infections (e.g., boils, carbuncles, and bladder infection)	Growth of microorganisms is stimulated by increased glucose levels; tissue ischemia and neuropathy contribute to the risk of infection; diabetes also is associated with systemic immunocompromise.
Prolonged wound healing	Impaired blood supply hinders healing
Genital pruritus	Hyperglycemia and glycosuria favor fungal growth; candidal infections, resulting in pruritus, are a common presenting symptom in women
Visual changes	Blurred vision occurs as water balance in eye fluctuates because of elevated blood glucose levels; microvascular disease resulting in diabetic retinopathy may ensue
Paresthesias	Paresthesias are common manifestations of diabetic neuropathies
Cardiovascular symptoms (e.g., chest pain, extremity pain, and neurologic deficits)	Diabetes contributes to macrovascular disease with formation of atherosclerotic plaques that involve coronary, peripheral, and cerebral vessels

CLINICAL MANIFESTATIONS The common clinical manifestations of type 1 diabetes result from both insulin deficiency and hyperglycemia. These manifestations are described in Table 20.4. Acute complications also may include hypoglycemia and DKA, which are described later in this chapter. Chronic complications include renal, nervous system, cardiac, peripheral vascular, retinal, and bony tissue dysfunction.

EVALUATION AND TREATMENT The criteria for diagnosis of type 1 diabetes are the same as those for type 2 diabetes (see Box 20.1). To estimate the severity of beta-cell destruction, C-peptide, a component of proinsulin released during insulin production, can be measured in the serum as a surrogate for insulin levels. The zinc transporter 8 autoantibody (ZnT8Ab) test has been approved for diagnosis of type 1 diabetes and is the best way to distinguish between type 1 and type 2. diabetes. Other important aspects of evaluation include looking for evidence of acute and chronic complications of type 1 diabetes.

There are no approved treatments for preventing destruction of the beta cells. Currently, treatment regimens are designed to achieve optimal glucose level control (as measured by the HbA_{1C} value) without causing episodes of significant hypoglycemia. A comprehensive, individual-centered collaborative management plan is essential.[16] Management requires individual planning according to type of disease, age, and activity level, but all individuals require some combination of insulin therapy, meal planning, an exercise regimen, and glucose monitoring. There are several different types of insulin preparations available, and there are new technologies for more physiologic insulin delivery systems. Many different kinds of therapies are being tested to prevent the autoimmune destruction of beta cells, including immunosuppression with antirejection drugs and stem cell transplantation (see *Did You Know?* Immunotherapy for the Prevention and Treatment of Type 1 Diabetes).

DID YOU KNOW?

Immunotherapy for the Prevention and Treatment of Type 1 Diabetes

Many different kinds of immunologic approaches are being tested to prevent the autoimmune destruction of beta cells in type 1 diabetes. These treatments are aimed at preserving insulin synthesis early in the course of the disease. Though research in this area has been ongoing for over 30 years, with limited success, our knowledge of the disease mechanisms and immunologic features of type 1 diabetes has expanded significantly, and new approaches to immunotherapy are being developed. Some interventions being explored create generalized immunosuppression, including mycophenolate mofetil, monoclonal antibodies to B cells (rituximab), monoclonal antibodies to T cells (otelixizumab, teplizumab), interleukin-1 blockade, and cyclosporine. Unfortunately, these treatments cause many side effects. More focused immunologic therapies are "antigen specific," which means they suppress only the parts of the immune response that are attacking the beta cells. One approach that has shown promising (but mixed) results has been the use of vaccines to induce T-regulatory cells that suppress the immune attack on specific antigens. Another ambitious new approach to preserving beta-cell function is through the introduction of stem cells, which decrease autoimmune responses and may engraft and become insulin-producing beta cells. Clinical trials are needed to evaluate long-term remission.

Data from Aghazadeh Y, Nostro MC: *Curr Diab Rep* 17(6):37, 2017; Bone RN, Evans-Molina C: *Curr Diab Rep* 17(7):50, 2017; Desai T, Shea LD: *Nat Rev Drug Discov* 16(5):338-350, 2017; Nambam B, Bratina N, Schatz D: *Diabetes Technol Ther* 20(Suppl 1):S86-S93, 2018.

Type 2 Diabetes Mellitus

Type 2 diabetes mellitus (non–insulin-dependent diabetes mellitus) affects 9.3% of adults in the U.S.[15] Prevalence is highest among American Indians and Alaska Natives (16%) and lowest among non-Hispanic whites (7.6%). There also is an increased prevalence of type 2 diabetes in children, especially in obese children (see Table 20.3).

Genetic abnormalities combined with environmental influences result in the basic pathophysiologic mechanisms of type 2 diabetes, which are insulin resistance and decreased insulin secretion by beta cells (Fig. 20.12). The most well-recognized risk factors are family history, age, obesity, hypertension, poor diet, and physical inactivity. More than 60 genes have been identified that are associated with type 2 diabetes, including those that code for beta-cell mass, beta-cell function (ability to sense blood glucose levels, insulin synthesis, and insulin secretion), proinsulin and insulin molecular structures, insulin receptors, hepatic synthesis of glucose, glucagon synthesis, and cellular responsiveness to insulin stimulation.

There is increasing evidence that diet, including diet during pregnancy, influences the long-term risk of type 2 diabetes in children and adults. Diets high in fruits, vegetables, fiber, and nuts reduce risk; diets high in simple carbohydrates, saturated fats, and red meat are associated with an increased risk. Weight gain and a lack of exercise also contribute to the risk for type 2 diabetes. Current evidence also suggests that the intestinal microbiome has a significant effect on the risk of developing diabetes.

PATHOPHYSIOLOGY Insulin resistance is defined as a suboptimal response of insulin-sensitive tissues (especially liver, muscle, and adipose tissue) to insulin. Several mechanisms are involved in abnormalities of the insulin signaling pathway and contribute to insulin resistance. These include an abnormality of the insulin molecule, high amounts of insulin antagonists, down-regulation of the insulin receptor, and alteration of glucose transporter (GLUT) proteins.

Obesity is one of the most important contributors to insulin resistance and diabetes and acts through several important mechanisms:

1. Adipokines (cytokines produced by adipose tissue): Increased serum levels of leptin (leptin resistance) and decreased levels of adiponectin result in inflammation and decreased insulin sensitivity.
2. Free fatty acids (FFAs): Increased FFAs, along with intracellular deposits of triglycerides and cholesterol, lead to decreased tissue responses to insulin.

3. Inflammation: Adipocyte-associated mononuclear cells and inflammatory cytokines released from adipocytes induce insulin resistance and are cytotoxic to beta cells.
4. Mitochondrial dysfunction: Decreased insulin-induced mitochondrial activity leads to insulin resistance.
5. Hyperinsulinemia: Obesity is correlated with hyperinsulinemia and decreased insulin receptor density.

Compensatory hyperinsulinemia prevents the clinical appearance of diabetes for many years. Eventually, however, a decrease in beta-cell mass and a reduction in normal beta-cell function develops and leads to a relative deficiency of insulin activity.

The glucagon concentration is increased in type 2 diabetes because pancreatic alpha cells become less responsive to glucose inhibition, resulting in an increase in glucagon secretion. These abnormally high levels of glucagon increase the blood glucose level by stimulating glycogenolysis and gluconeogenesis. As was discussed under type 1 diabetes, type 2 diabetes also is associated with a deficiency in amylin, further increasing glucagon levels. Pramlintide, a synthetic analog of amylin, is used for treatment in type 2 diabetes.

Hormones released from the gastrointestinal (GI) tract play a role in insulin resistance, beta-cell function, and diabetes. Ghrelin is a peptide produced in the stomach and pancreatic islets that regulates food intake, energy balance, and hormonal secretion. Decreased levels of circulating ghrelin have been associated with insulin resistance and increased fasting insulin levels. The incretins are a class of peptides that are released from the GI tract in response to food intake and function to increase the secretion of insulin and have many other positive effects on metabolism. The most studied incretin is called *glucagon-like peptide 1* (GLP-1), and studies have demonstrated that beta-cell responsiveness to GLP-1 is reduced both in prediabetes and in type 2 diabetes. Incretin therapies include GLP-1 receptor agonists (GLP-1 RAs) and dipeptidyl peptidase IV (DPP-IV) inhibitors, which can help control postprandial glucose levels by promoting glucose-dependent insulin secretion.

The kidneys also influence the pathophysiology of type 2 diabetes. Renal reabsorption of glucose through the sodium-glucose cotransporter 2 (SGLT2) is an important controller of serum glucose levels, and medications aimed at blocking it have resulted in decreased measurements for blood glucose level, weight, and blood pressure (see *Did You Know?* Selective Sodium-Glucose Cotransporter 2 Inhibitors for Type 2 Diabetes Mellitus Therapy).

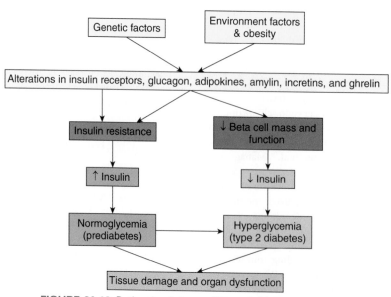

FIGURE 20.12 Pathophysiology of Type 2 Diabetes Mellitus.

DID YOU KNOW?

Selective Sodium-Glucose Cotransporter 2 Inhibitors for Type 2 Diabetes Mellitus Therapy

Under normal conditions, the kidneys act to filter, reabsorb, and return to the circulation almost all of the glucose in the blood. Filtered glucose is actively reabsorbed by specific transporters located on the apical membrane of proximal tubular cells. These transporters are termed *sodium-glucose cotransporter 1 and 2* (SGLT1 and SGLT2). Approximately 90% of glucose is reabsorbed in the proximal renal tubule by SGLT2. The remaining 10% is reabsorbed lower in the tubule by SGLT1. Glucose reabsorption by SGLT2 continues even when plasma glucose levels are abnormally elevated, and glucose begins to be excreted in the urine only once the renal threshold is exceeded (at about 180 to 200 mg/dl). Inhibition of SGLT2 prevents renal reabsorption of glucose and facilitates its excretion in the urine. With an increase in glucose excretion, individuals with type 2 diabetes experience weight loss and serum glucose levels fall independently of insulin levels or beta-cell function. Studies indicate that SGLT2 inhibitors provide protection against diabetic heart disease and may eventually be used as first-line medications for individuals with cardiac complications. SGLT2 inhibitors currently in use in the U.S. include canagliflozin, empagliflozin, dapagliflozin, and ipragliflozin, either as monotherapy or as adjunctive therapy. The FDA has issued warnings regarding adverse effects that include ketoacidosis, serious urinary tract infections, increased rates of toe amputation, and an increased risk of lowered bone density and fractures.

Data from Consoli A et al: *Expert Opin Drug Saf* 17(3):293-302, 2018; Faillie JL: *Pharmacol Res* 118:71-81, 2017; Kashiwagi A, Maegawa H: *J Diabetes Investig* 8(4):416-427, 2017; Li J et al: *Medicine (Baltimore)* 96(27):e7201, 2017; Garcia-Ropero A et al: *Expert Opin Drug Metab Toxicol* 14(12):1287-1302, 2018; Rieg T, Vallon V: *Diabetologia* 61(10):2019-2086, 2018.

As you have learned, many organs contribute to insulin resistance, chronic hyperglycemia, and the consequences of type 2 diabetes. These causes and consequences are summarized in Fig. 20.13, and the complications of type 2 diabetes will be discussed later in this chapter.

CLINICAL MANIFESTATIONS The clinical manifestations of type 2 diabetes are nonspecific. The individual with type 2 diabetes may show some classic symptoms of diabetes, such as polyuria and polydipsia, but more often will have nonspecific symptoms, such as fatigue, pruritus, recurrent infections, visual changes, or symptoms of neuropathy (paresthesias or weakness). The affected individual is often overweight, dyslipidemic, and hypertensive. In those whose diabetes has progressed without treatment, symptoms related to coronary artery, peripheral artery, cerebrovascular disease, and retinopathy may develop.

EVALUATION AND TREATMENT The diagnostic criteria for type 2 diabetes are the same as those for type 1 (see Box 20.1). The metabolic syndrome is a constellation of disorders (central obesity, dyslipidemia, prehypertension, and an elevated FBG) that together confer a high risk of developing type 2 diabetes and associated cardiovascular complications (see Box 20.2).

As with type 1 diabetes, the goal of treatment for individuals with type 2 diabetes (and metabolic syndrome) is the restoration of near-euglycemia (normal blood glucose) levels and correction of related metabolic disorders. Prevention and treatment of type 2 diabetes, especially in those individuals with prediabetes, hinges on diet and exercise.[16] Diet should match activity levels and include more complex carbohydrates (rather than simple sugars), foods low in fats, adequate protein, and fiber. Obesity management results in improved glucose

tolerance. Bariatric surgery improves glycemic control, decreases the risk of cardiovascular disease, and promotes weight loss in those morbidly obese.[16]

For individuals who require further intervention, oral hypoglycemic agents are indicated.[16] Currently, metformin is considered the primary pharmacologic choice for the treatment of type 2 diabetes. If the HbA$_{1C}$ target is not maintained over 3 months, a GLP-1 receptor agonist (incretin) may be added.[16] If treatment goals are still not met, a combination of drugs, including SGLT2 inhibitors, may be required (see *Did You Know? Selective Sodium-Glucose Cotransporter 2 Inhibitors for Type 2 Diabetes Mellitus Therapy*). Insulin therapy may be needed in the later stage of type 2 diabetes because of loss of beta-cell function, which is progressive over time.

Gestational Diabetes Mellitus and Specific Types of Diabetes Mellitus From Other Causes

As listed in Table 20.3, the ADA classification of diabetes mellitus not only includes the most common forms of diabetes (type 1 and type 2) but also encompasses GDM and specific types of diabetes mellitus from other causes.

Gestational diabetes mellitus (GDM) complicates approximately 7% of pregnancies and is defined as diabetes diagnosed in the second or third trimester of pregnancy that was not clearly overt diabetes prior to gestation.[16] An OGTT is used to confirm the diagnosis. However, this definition means that many women with previously undiagnosed type 1 or type 2 diabetes are diagnosed with GDM, and many of them have progressive disease after delivery. Therefore the ADA recommends that women with risk factors for diabetes be screened at their initial prenatal visit and that women diagnosed during pregnancy should continue to be monitored postpartum and at least every 3 years for persistent or recurrent diabetes.[16] Careful glucose control prenatally, during pregnancy, and after delivery is essential to the short- and long-term health of both mother and baby.

Specific types of diabetes from other causes include monogenic diabetes syndromes (e.g., MODY), disease of the exocrine pancreas (e.g., cystic fibrosis), and drug- or chemical-induced diabetes (e.g., with glucocorticoid use, in the treatment of HIV/AIDS, or after organ transplantation). Maturity-onset diabetes of youth (MODY) usually presents before 25 years of age and includes at least 13 genetic mutations that affect critical enzymes involved in beta-cell function but with little impact on insulin action.[16] The diagnosis of MODY should be considered in individuals who have atypical clinical presentations, who are diagnosed within the first 6 months of life (neonatal diabetes), and who have a strong family history of diabetes. Diagnosis includes genetic testing for the three most common forms of MODY. Management is similar to that used for type 2 diabetes. Diabetes also can result from pancreatic damage incurred through the effects of cystic fibrosis, medications, and immunosuppression after organ transplantation.

Acute Complications of Diabetes Mellitus

The major acute complications of diabetes mellitus are hypoglycemia, DKA, and hyperosmolar hyperglycemic nonketotic syndrome.[19] A comparison of these complications is summarized in Table 20.5).

Hypoglycemia in diabetes is sometimes called *insulin shock* or *insulin reaction*. Individuals with type 1 diabetes require insulin to manage their diabetes and are at more risk for hypoglycemia than those with type 2 diabetes because they have more severe deficits in their ability to control serum glucose levels. Significant drops in blood sugar most often occur when there is an unexpected change in caloric intake or exercise without appropriate modification of insulin dosing. Hypoglycemia sometimes occurs in type 2 diabetes during treatment with oral hypoglycemic medications. Symptoms include pallor, tremor, anxiety,

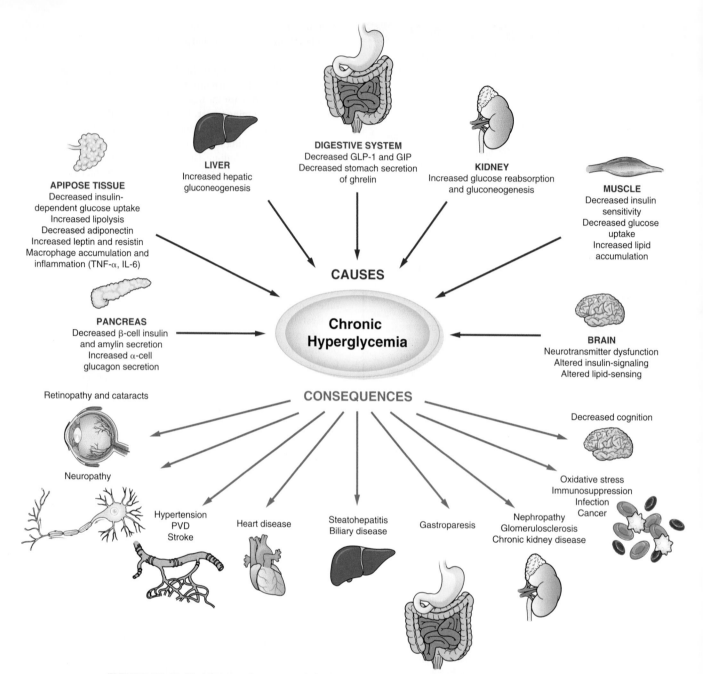

FIGURE 20.13 Multiorgan Causes and Common Consequences of Chronic Hyperglycemia in Type 2 Diabetes. *GLP-1,* Glucagon-like peptide 1; *GIP,* gastric inhibitory polypeptide; *IL,* interleukin; *PVD,* peripheral vascular disease; *TNF,* tumor necrosis factor.

tachycardia, palpitations, diaphoresis, headache, dizziness, irritability, fatigue, poor judgment, confusion, visual disturbances, hunger, seizures, and coma. Treatment requires immediate replacement of glucose either orally or intravenously. Glucagon for home use can be prescribed for individuals who are at high risk. Prevention is achieved with individualized management of medications and diet, monitoring of blood glucose levels, and education.

Diabetic ketoacidosis (DKA) is a serious complication related to a deficiency of insulin and an increase in the levels of insulin counterregulatory hormones (catecholamines, cortisol, glucagon, GH) (Fig. 20.14). DKA is much more common in type 1 diabetes because insulin is more deficient (see Table 20.5). It is characterized

by hyperglycemia, acidosis, and ketonuria. Insulin normally stimulates lipogenesis and inhibits lipolysis, thus preventing fat catabolism. With insulin deficiency, lipolysis is enhanced and there is an increase in the amount of nonesterified fatty acids delivered to the liver. The consequence is increased glyconeogenesis, contributing to hyperglycemia and the production of ketone bodies (acetoacetate, hydroxybutyrate, and acetone) by the mitochondria of the liver at a rate that exceeds peripheral use. Accumulation of ketone bodies causes a drop in pH, resulting in metabolic acidosis and transient hyperkalemia. Symptoms of DKA include Kussmaul respirations (hyperventilation in an attempt to compensate for the acidosis), postural dizziness, central nervous system depression, ketonuria, anorexia, nausea, abdominal pain, thirst, and

TABLE 20.5   Common Acute Complications of Diabetes Mellitus

Hypoglycemia in Persons With Diabetes Mellitus	Diabetic Ketoacidosis	Hyperglycemic Nonketotic Syndromes
Synonyms		
Insulin shock, insulin reaction	Diabetic coma syndrome	Hyperosmolar hyperglycemia nonketotic coma
Persons at Risk		
Individuals taking insulin Individuals with rapidly fluctuating blood glucose levels Individuals with type 2 diabetes taking oral hypoglycemic agents	Individuals with type 1 diabetes Individuals with undiagnosed diabetes	Older adults with type 2 diabetes, nondiabetic persons with predisposing factors, such as pancreatitis; individuals with undiagnosed diabetes
Predisposing Factors		
Excessive insulin or oral hypoglycemic agent intake, lack of sufficient food intake, excessive physical exercise, abrupt decline in insulin needs (e.g., renal failure, immediately postpartum), simultaneous use of insulin-potentiating agents or beta-blocking agents that mask symptoms	Stressful situation such as infection, accident, trauma, emotional stress; omission of insulin; medications that antagonize insulin	Infection, medications that antagonize insulin, comorbid condition
Typical Onset		
Rapid	Slow	Slowest
Presenting Symptoms		
Adrenergic reaction: pallor, sweating, tachycardia, palpitations, hunger, restlessness, anxiety, tremors Neurogenic reaction: fatigue, irritability, headache, loss of concentration, visual disturbances, dizziness, hunger, confusion, transient sensory or motor defects, convulsions, coma, death	Malaise, dry mouth, headache, polyuria, polydipsia, weight loss, nausea, vomiting, pruritus, abdominal pain, lethargy, shortness of breath, Kussmaul respirations, fruity or acetone odor to breath	Polyuria, polydipsia, hypovolemia, dehydration (parched lips, poor skin turgor), hypotension, tachycardia, hypoperfusion, weight loss, weakness, nausea, vomiting, abdominal pain, hypothermia, stupor, coma, seizures
Laboratory Analysis		
Serum glucose <30 mg/dl in newborn (first 2-3 days) and <55-60 mg/dl in adults	Glucose levels >250 mg/dl, reduction in bicarbonate concentration, increased anion gap, increased plasma levels of β-hydroxybutyrate, acetoacetate, and acetone	Glucose levels >600 mg/dl, lack of ketosis, serum osmolarity >320 mOsm/L, elevated blood urea nitrogen and creatinine levels

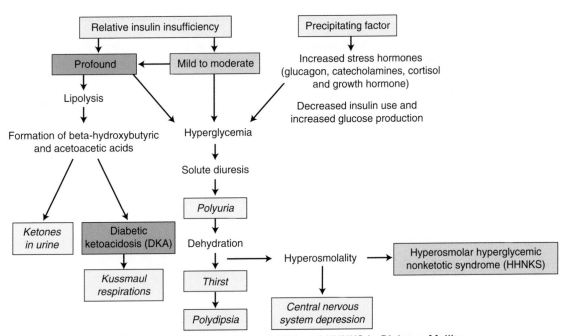

FIGURE 20.14 Pathophysiology of DKA and HHNKS in Diabetes Mellitus.

polyuria. DKA is managed with a combination of fluids, insulin, and electrolyte replacement.

Hyperosmolar hyperglycemic nonketotic syndrome (HHNKS) is an uncommon but significant complication of type 2 diabetes mellitus with a high overall mortality. It occurs more often in elderly individuals who have other comorbidities, including infections or cardiovascular or renal disease. HHNKS differs from DKA because type 2 diabetes is characterized by a lesser degree of insulin deficiency, which therefore prevents lipolysis and the production of ketones (see Fig. 20.14). However, hyperglycemia is usually more profound in HHNKS leading to more polyuria and fluid deficiency. Therefore the clinical features of HHNKS include a very high serum glucose concentration and osmolarity without metabolic acidosis. Clinical manifestations include severe dehydration; loss of electrolytes (especially potassium); and neurologic changes, such as stupor. Management includes fluid, insulin, and electrolyte replacement.

Chronic Complications of Diabetes Mellitus

A number of serious complications are associated with any type of poorly controlled diabetes mellitus. Most complications are associated with insulin resistance or deficit and chronic hyperglycemia. Insulin resistance or deficit renders cells unable to process glucose normally, so they resort to a number of alternative pathways for glucose metabolism, particularly through activation of the polyol pathway. This pathway results in the accumulation of sorbitol and glutathione, both of which contribute to chronic tissue damage. Hyperglycemia leads to a number of deleterious effects, including abnormalities in intracellular communication (e.g., protein kinase C pathways) and the attachment of glucose to proteins, lipids, and nucleic acids (glycation). Therefore glycation creates what are called *advanced glycation end products* (AGEs), which interfere with many crucial cellular processes. The cumulative effect of these abnormal processes leads to the microvascular (damage to capillaries; retinopathies, nephropathies, and neuropathies) and macrovascular (damage to larger vessels; coronary artery, peripheral vascular, and cerebral vascular disease) complications of chronic diabetes mellitus (Table 20.6).

Microvascular Disease

Diabetic microvascular complications are characterized by occlusion of capillaries, with associated ischemia of tissues. It is a leading cause of blindness, end-stage kidney failure, and various neuropathies. The frequency and severity of lesions appear to be proportional to the duration of the disease (more or less than 10 years) and the status of glycemic control. Hypoxia and ischemia accompany microvascular disease, especially in the eye, kidney, and nerves. Many individuals with type 2 diabetes will present with microvascular complications because of the long duration of asymptomatic hyperglycemia that generally precedes diagnosis. This underscores the need to screen for diabetes.

Diabetic retinopathy. Diabetic retinopathy is a leading cause of blindness worldwide and is a common complication of type 2 diabetes because of the likelihood of long-standing hyperglycemia before diagnosis. Most individuals with diabetes will eventually develop retinopathy and also are more likely to develop cataracts and glaucoma (see Chapter 15).

Diabetic retinopathy results from relative hypoxemia, damage to retinal blood vessels, red blood cell (RBC) aggregation, and hypertension[20] (Fig. 20.15). The three stages of retinopathy that lead to loss of vision are *nonproliferative* (stage I), characterized by an increase in retinal capillary permeability, vein dilation, microaneurysm formation, and superficial (flame-shaped) and deep (blot) hemorrhages; *preproliferative* (stage II), a progression of retinal ischemia, with areas of poor perfusion that culminate in infarcts; and *proliferative* (stage III), the result of neovascularization (angiogenesis) and fibrous tissue formation within the retina or optic disc. Traction of the new vessels on the vitreous humor may cause retinal detachment or hemorrhage into the vitreous humor, with severe blurring or loss of vision. Macular edema is the leading cause of blurred vision among persons with diabetes. Blurring of vision also can be a consequence of hyperglycemia and sorbitol accumulation in the lens. Dehydration of the lens, aqueous humor, and vitreous humor also reduces visual acuity.

Diabetic nephropathy. Diabetes is the most common cause of chronic kidney disease and end-stage kidney disease, and nearly half

TABLE 20.6	Chronic Complications of Diabetes Mellitus	
Complications	**Pathologic Mechanisms**	**Associated Symptoms**
Microvascular		
Retinopathy	Microaneurysms, exudates, hemorrhages, formation of new blood vessels scarring, retinal detachment. Macular edema may also occur.	Progresses from no visual changes to loss of visual acuity and blindness. Symptoms worsened by hyperosmolar lens edema and cataract formation.
Nephropathy	Glomerulosclerosis, glomerular perfusion and pressure changes, protein glycation	Microalbuminuria and hypertension slowly progressing to end-stage kidney failure
Neuropathy	Oxidative stress, poor perfusion and ischemia, loss of nerve growth factor	Sensorimotor polyneuropathy progressing to distal paresthesias in feet and hands, muscle wasting, Charcot joints, falls and injuries. Autonomic neuropathy progressing to postural hypotension, gastroparesis, urinary retention and erectile dysfunction.
Skin and foot lesions	Loss of sensation, poor perfusion, suppressed immunity, and increased risk of infection	Pressure ulcers and delayed wound healing; abscess formation; necrosis and gangrene of toes and feet; infection and osteomyelitis
Macrovascular		
Cardiovascular	Accelerated atherosclerosis	Hypertension, coronary artery disease, cardiomyopathy, and heart failure
Cerebrovascular	Same as above	Increased risk for ischemic and thrombotic stroke
Peripheral vascular	Same as above	Claudication, nonhealing ulcers, gangrene
Infection		
	Impaired immunity, tissue ischemia, recurrent trauma, delayed wound healing, urinary retention	Skin and wound infections, urinary tract infections, increased risk for sepsis

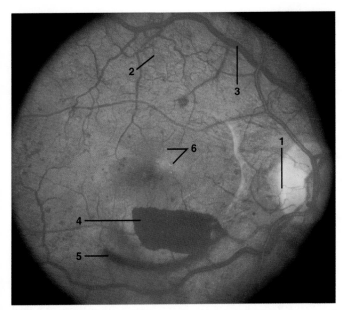

FIGURE 20.15 Diabetic Retinopathy. Neovascularization is present at the optic nerve *(1)* and along vascular pathways *(2)*. Retinal veins are engorged *(3)* and a preretinal boat-shaped hemorrhage *(4)* is present below the fovea. A more diffuse mild vitreous hemorrhage *(5)* is present below the preretinal hemorrhage. A few small, hard exudates are visible in the fovea *(6)*. (From Palay DA, Krachmer JH: *Primary care ophthalmology,* ed 2, St Louis, 2006, Mosby.)

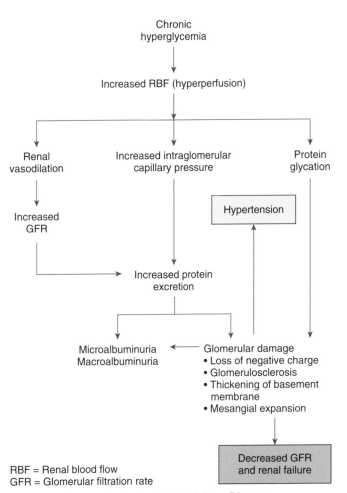

RBF = Renal blood flow
GFR = Glomerular filtration rate

FIGURE 20.16 Diabetic Kidney Disease.

of individuals with diabetes mellitus develop diabetic kidney disease.[21] Renal glomerular changes occur early in diabetes mellitus, occasionally preceding the overt manifestation of the disease. The glomeruli are injured by hyperglycemia with protein glycation (bonding of a glucose molecule to a protein), high renal blood flow (hyperfiltration), and intraglomerular hypertension exacerbated by systemic hypertension (Fig. 20.16). There is progressive glomerulosclerosis and decreased glomerular blood flow and glomerular filtration that can progress to renal failure.

Microalbuminuria is the first manifestation of diabetic kidney dysfunction and signals the onset of systemic diabetic complications. Before proteinuria, no clinical signs or symptoms of progressive glomerulosclerosis are likely to be evident. Later, hypoproteinemia, reduction in plasma oncotic pressure, fluid overload, anasarca (generalized body edema), and hypertension may occur. As renal function continues to deteriorate, individuals with type 1 diabetes may experience hypoglycemia (because of loss of renal insulin metabolism), which necessitates a decrease in insulin therapy. As the glomerular filtration rate drops below 10 ml/min, uremic signs, such as nausea, lethargy, acidosis, anemia, and uncontrolled hypertension, occur (see Chapter 32 for a discussion of renal failure). Early diagnosis and control of hypertension and hyperglycemia decreases the severity of nephropathy and delays the onset of end-stage kidney disease.

Diabetic neuropathies. Diabetic neuropathy is the most common complication of diabetes. The underlying pathologic mechanism includes metabolic and vascular factors related to chronic hyperglycemia with ischemia and demyelination contributing to neural changes and delayed conduction. Both somatic and peripheral nerve cells show diffuse or focal damage, resulting in polyneuropathy.[22] Loss of pain, temperature, and vibration sensation is more common than motor involvement and often involves the extremities first in the hands and feet. Motor neuropathies can affect muscle groups, particularly of the legs and feet, contributing to deformity and unstable balance. Peripheral neuropathy

can cause Charcot arthropathy, a progressive deterioration of weight-bearing joints, typically in the foot and ankle. Distal neuropathies combined with vascular complications, infection, or injury can lead to amputation (Fig. 20.17).

Autonomic neuropathies include delayed gastric emptying, diabetic diarrhea, altered bladder function (e.g., decreased sensation of bladder fullness, urge or overflow incontinence), impotence, orthostatic hypotension, and heart rate variability, with both tachycardia and bradycardia. Neuropathy may occur during periods of "good" glucose control and may be the initial clinical manifestation of type 2 diabetes. Chronic hyperglycemia also can cause cognitive dysfunction with alterations in learning and memory.

Macrovascular Disease

Macrovascular disease (lesions in large- and medium-sized arteries) increases morbidity and mortality and increases the risk for hypertension, accelerated atherosclerosis, cardiovascular disease, stroke, and peripheral vascular disease, particularly among individuals with type 2 diabetes mellitus. (Atherosclerosis is discussed in Chapter 26.) Children with poorly controlled diabetes have higher risk for macrovascular complications within 1 to 2 decades. The process tends to be more severe and accelerated in the presence of other risk factors, including obesity, hyperlipidemia, and smoking.

Cardiovascular disease. Cardiovascular disease is the primary cause of death of people with diabetes, with higher risk for women. Hypertension often coexists with diabetes mellitus. Diabetes also is associated with deleterious changes in serum lipids, including high

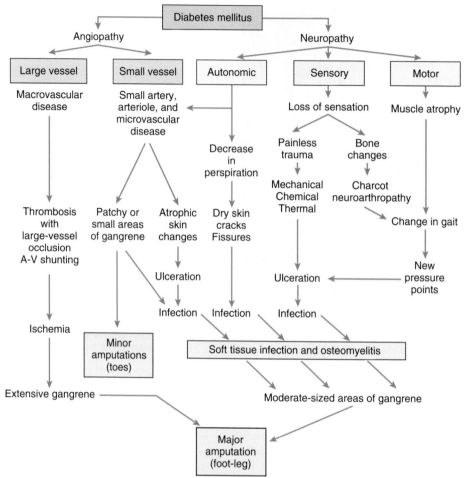

FIGURE 20.17 How Foot Lesions of Diabetes Lead to Amputation. (From Levin ME et al: *The diabetic foot*, ed 5, St Louis, 1993, Mosby.)

levels of low-density lipoproteins (LDLs), and low levels of high-density lipoproteins (HDLs). The combination of diabetes, hypertension dyslipidemia, and obesity (metabolic syndrome) greatly increases the risk for atherosclerotic cardiovascular disease, particularly coronary artery disease (CAD) and stroke. CAD results from vessel injury related to insulin resistance and hyperglycemia, leading to accelerated atherosclerosis (see Chapter 26). In general, the prevalence of CAD increases with the duration but not the severity of diabetes, and the onset can be silent.

The incidence of *congestive heart failure* is higher in individuals with diabetes, even without myocardial infarction. This may be related to cardiomyopathy and the presence of increased amounts of collagen in the ventricular wall and ventricular hypertrophy. There is reduced mechanical compliance of the heart during filling with diastolic and, eventually, systolic failure. (Heart disease is described in Chapter 26.)

Stroke. Stroke is twice as common in those with diabetes (particularly type 2 diabetes) as in the nondiabetic population. As in CAD, accelerated atherosclerosis of the cerebral vessels results from insulin resistance and hyperglycemia, especially when associated with hypertension and hyperlipidemia (see Chapter 17).

Peripheral vascular disease. Diabetes mellitus increases the incidence of peripheral vascular disease (PVD). Age, duration of diabetes, genetics, and additional risk factors (smoking, hyperlipidemia, hypertension) influence the development and management of PVD. PVD in those with diabetes is more diffuse and often involves arteries below

the knee. Occlusions of the small arteries and arterioles can lead to claudication (pain from reduced blood flow during exercise), ulcers, gangrene, and amputation. The lesions begin as ulcers and progress to osteomyelitis or gangrene, requiring amputation (see Fig. 20.17). Peripheral neuropathies and an increased risk for infection advance the disease.

Infection

The individual with diabetes is at an increased risk for infection throughout the body for several reasons:
1. *The senses.* Impaired vision caused by retinal changes and impaired touch caused by neuropathy lead to loss of protection, with injury and repeated trauma, open wounds, and soft tissue or osseous infection, particularly in the legs and feet.
2. *Hypoxia.* Once skin integrity is compromised, susceptibility to infection increases as a result of hypoxia. In addition, the glycosylated hemoglobin in the RBCs impedes the release of oxygen to tissues and contributes to delayed wound healing.
3. *Pathogens.* Some pathogens proliferate rapidly because of increased glucose in body fluids, which provides an excellent source of energy.
4. *Blood supply.* Decreased blood supply results from vascular changes and reduces the supply of white blood cells to the affected area.
5. *Suppressed immune response.* Chronic hyperglycemia impairs both innate and adaptive immune responses, including abnormal chemotaxis and vasoactive responses, and defective phagocytosis.

ALTERATIONS OF ADRENAL FUNCTION

Disorders of the Adrenal Cortex

Disorders of the adrenal cortex are related either to hyperfunction or to hypofunction. Hyperfunction that causes increased secretion of cortisol (hypercortisolism) leads to Cushing disease or Cushing syndrome. Hyperfunction that causes increased secretion of adrenal androgens or estrogens leads to virilization or feminization. Hyperfunction that causes increased levels of aldosterone leads to hyperaldosteronism, which may be primary or secondary. These syndromes often have overlapping features. Hypofunction of the adrenal cortex leads to Addison disease.

Hypercortical Function (Cushing Syndrome, Cushing Disease)

Cushing syndrome refers to the clinical manifestations resulting from chronic exposure to excess cortisol regardless of cause. Cushing disease refers to excess endogenous secretion of ACTH.[23] *ACTH-dependent hypercortisolism* (about 80% of cases) results from overproduction of pituitary ACTH by a pituitary adenoma (most common and can occur at any age) or by an ectopic secreting nonpituitary tumor, such as a small cell carcinoma of the lung (more common in older adults). *ACTH-independent hypercortisolism* is caused by cortisol secretion from a rare benign or malignant tumor of one or both adrenal glands (more common in children). A Cushing-like syndrome may develop as a side effect of long-term pharmacologic administration of glucocorticoids.

PATHOPHYSIOLOGY   With ACTH-dependent hypercortisolism, the excess ACTH stimulates excess production of cortisol and there is loss of feedback control of ACTH secretion. In individuals with ACTH-dependent hypercortisolism, secretion of both cortisol and adrenal androgens is increased, and cortisol-releasing hormone is inhibited. In contrast, ACTH-independent secreting tumors of the adrenal cortex generally secrete only cortisol. Elevated cortisol levels suppress CRH and ACTH levels. When the secretion of cortisol by the tumor exceeds normal cortisol levels, symptoms of hypercortisolism develop.

CLINICAL MANIFESTATIONS   Weight gain is the most common feature and results from the accumulation of adipose tissue in the trunk, facial, and cervical areas. These characteristic patterns of fat deposition have been respectively described as "truncal obesity," "moon face," and "buffalo hump" (Figs. 20.18 and 20.19).

Glucose intolerance occurs because of cortisol-induced insulin resistance and increased gluconeogenesis and glycogen storage by the liver. Overt diabetes mellitus develops in approximately 20% of individuals with hypercortisolism. Polyuria is a manifestation of hyperglycemia and resultant glycosuria.

Protein wasting is caused by the catabolic effects of cortisol on peripheral tissues. Muscle wasting leads to muscle weakness. In bone, loss of the protein matrix leads to osteoporosis, with pathologic fractures, vertebral compression fractures, bone and back pain, kyphosis, and reduced height. Cortisol interferes with the action of GH in long bones; thus children who present with short stature may be experiencing growth

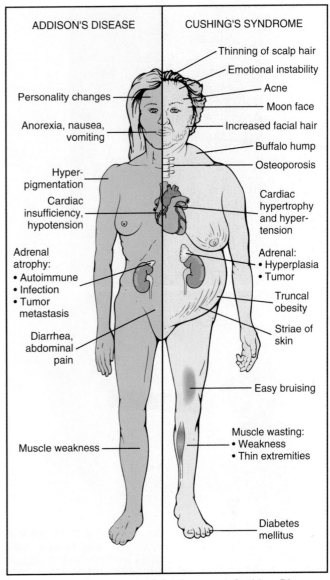

FIGURE 20.18 Symptoms of Addison and Cushing Diseases. (From Goodman CC, Kelly Snyder TE: *Differential diagnosis for physical therapists*, ed 5, Philadelphia, 2013, Saunders.)

retardation related to Cushing syndrome rather than GH deficiency. Bone disease may contribute to hypercalciuria and resulting renal stones.

In the skin, loss of collagen leads to thin, weakened integumentary tissues through which capillaries are more visible and are easily stretched by adipose deposits. Together, these changes account for the characteristic purple striae seen in the trunk area. Loss of collagenous support around small vessels makes them susceptible to rupture, leading to easy bruising, even with minor trauma. Thin, atrophied skin is also easily damaged, leading to skin breaks and ulcerations. Bronze or brownish hyperpigmentation of the skin, mucous membranes, and hair occurs when there are very high levels of ACTH.

With elevated cortisol levels, vascular sensitivity to catecholamines increases significantly, leading to vasoconstriction and hypertension. Mineralocorticoid effects promote hypokalemia and sodium and water retention with transient weight gain. Suppression of the immune system and increased susceptibility to infections also occur. Approximately 50% of individuals with Cushing syndrome experience irritability and depression, disturbed sleep, difficulty concentrating, memory loss, and,

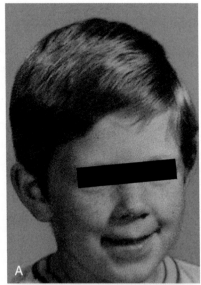
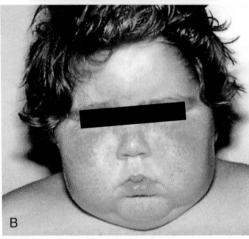

FIGURE 20.19 Cushing Syndrome. A, Individual before onset of Cushing syndrome. B, Individual 4 months later. Moon facies is clearly demonstrated. (From Zitelli BJ et al: *Zitelli and Davis' atlas of pediatric physical diagnosis,* ed 6, London, 2012, Saunders.)

rarely, schizophrenia-like psychosis. Females with ACTH-dependent hypercortisolism may experience symptoms of increased adrenal androgen levels (virilism), with increased hair growth (especially facial hair), acne, and oligomenorrhea. Rarely, unless an adrenal carcinoma is involved, do androgen levels become high enough to cause changes of the voice, recession of the hairline, and hypertrophy of the clitoris.

EVALUATION AND TREATMENT Routine laboratory examinations may reveal hyperglycemia, glycosuria, hypokalemia, and metabolic alkalosis. A variety of laboratory tests are used to confirm the diagnosis of hypercortisolism and to determine the underlying disorder. These include serum and urinary cortisol levels, serum ACTH levels, and dexamethasone suppression testing. Late-evening salivary cortisol levels are used as a screening. Tumors are diagnosed using imaging procedures.

Treatment is specific for the cause of hypercorticoadrenalism and includes surgery, medication, and radiation. Differentiation between pituitary ectopic and adrenal causes is essential for effective treatment. Without treatment, individuals with Cushing syndrome have a high risk for developing overwhelming infection and significant complications from generalized arteriosclerosis and hypertensive disease.

Congenital Adrenal Hyperplasia

Congenital adrenal hyperplasia results from an inherited deficiency of an enzyme that is critical in cortisol biosynthesis. Because cortisol is not produced efficiently, the concentration of ACTH increases and causes adrenal hyperplasia, which results in the overproduction of mineralocorticoids or androgens, or both. The most common form is a 21-hydroxylase deficiency, which involves both mineralocorticoid and cortisol synthesis. Affected female children are virilized, and infants of both sexes exhibit salt wasting. Prenatal diagnosis is available, and treatment guidelines have been developed. Disease management requires treatment with glucocorticoids and mineralocorticoids and management of sex steroid excess.

Hyperaldosteronism

Hyperaldosteronism is characterized by excessive adrenal secretion of aldosterone. Both primary and secondary forms of hyperaldosteronism can occur.

Primary hyperaldosteronism (Conn syndrome, primary aldosteronism) is caused by excessive secretion of aldosterone from an abnormality of the adrenal cortex, usually a single benign aldosterone-producing adrenal adenoma.[24] Bilateral adrenal nodular hyperplasia and adrenal carcinomas account for the remainder of cases.

Secondary hyperaldosteronism results from an extra-adrenal stimulus of aldosterone secretion, most often through the secretion of excess angiotensin II in response to decreased circulating blood volume (e.g., in dehydration, shock, or hypoalbuminemia) and decreased delivery of blood to the kidneys (e.g., renal artery stenosis, heart failure, or hepatic cirrhosis). Here, the activation of the renin-angiotensin system and subsequent aldosterone secretion may be seen as compensatory, although in some instances (e.g., congestive heart failure) the increased circulating volume further worsens the condition. Other causes of secondary hyperaldosteronism are Bartter syndrome, a renal tubular defect causing hypokalemia, and renin-secreting tumors of the kidney.

PATHOPHYSIOLOGY In *primary hyperaldosteronism,* pathophysiologic alterations are caused by excessive aldosterone secretion and the fluid and electrolyte imbalances that ensue. Hyperaldosteronism promotes (1) increased renal sodium and water reabsorption with corresponding hypervolemia (see Chapter 5) and hypertension and (2) renal excretion of hydrogen and potassium (see Chapter 5). The extracellular fluid volume overload, hypertension, and suppression of renin secretion are characteristic of primary disorders. Hypokalemic alkalosis, changes in myocardial conduction, and skeletal muscle weakness may be seen, particularly with severe potassium depletion.

In *secondary hyperaldosteronism,* renin secretion is stimulated by pressure-initiated cellular changes at the juxtaglomerular apparatus (see Chapter 31). This leads to an increase in angiotensin II and aldosterone with sodium and water retention and increased circulating blood volume.

CLINICAL MANIFESTATIONS Hypertension, hypokalemia, and hypervolemia are the hallmarks of primary hyperaldosteronism, and renin levels are suppressed. Hypertension is resistant to treatment and can lead to the development of left ventricular dilation and hypertrophy, vascular disease, and kidney disease. Edema is often absent.

EVALUATION AND TREATMENT Various clinical and laboratory evaluations are useful in assessing hyperaldosteronism:
1. Measurement of blood pressure: hypertension is usually present.
2. Serum and urinary electrolyte levels: hypernatremia and metabolic alkalosis may be present.

3. Plasma aldosterone-to-renin ratio and aldosterone suppression testing: an increased aldosterone-to-renin ratio is present in primary hyperaldosteronism.
4. Imaging techniques may be used to localize an aldosterone-secreting adenoma.

Treatment includes management of hypertension, hypervolemia, and hypokalemia, most often with aldosterone receptor antagonists, such as spironolactone, eplerenone, or angiotensin-converting enzyme (ACE) inhibitors. If an aldosterone-secreting adenoma is present, it must be surgically removed.

Hypersecretion of Adrenal Androgens and Estrogens

Hypersecretion of adrenal androgens and estrogens may be caused by adrenal tumors (adenomas or carcinomas), Cushing syndrome, or defects in steroid synthesis. The clinical syndrome that is manifested depends on the hormone secreted, the sex of the individual, and the age at which the hypersecretion is initiated. Hypersecretion of estrogens causes feminization, the development of female secondary sex characteristics. Hypersecretion of androgens causes virilization, the development of male secondary sex characteristics (Fig. 20.20).

The effects of an estrogen-secreting tumor are most evident in males and result in gynecomastia, testicular atrophy, and decreased libido. In female children, such tumors may lead to early development of secondary sex characteristics. The changes caused by an androgen-secreting tumor are more easily observed in females and include excessive face and body

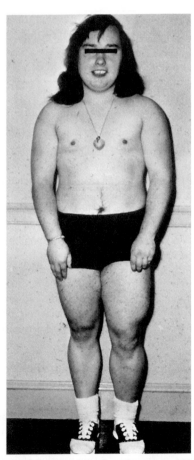

FIGURE 20.20 Virilization. Virilization of a young girl by an androgen-secreting tumor of the adrenal cortex. Masculine features include lack of breast development, increased muscle bulk, and hirsutism (excessive hair). (From Thibodeau GA, Patton KT: *The human body in health & disease,* ed 4, St Louis, 2010, Mosby.)

hair (hirsutism), clitoral enlargement, deepening of the voice, amenorrhea, acne, and breast atrophy. In children, virilizing tumors promote precocious sexual development and bone aging. Treatment of adrenal tumors usually involves surgical excision.

Adrenocortical Hypofunction

Hypocortisolism (low levels of cortisol secretion) develops either because of inadequate stimulation of the adrenal glands by ACTH or because of a primary inability of the adrenals to produce and secrete the adrenocortical hormones. Sometimes there is partial dysfunction of the adrenal cortex, so only synthesis of cortisol, aldosterone, or the adrenal androgens is affected.

Addison disease. Primary adrenal insufficiency is termed Addison disease. It is relatively rare, occurring most often in adults aged 30 to 60 years, although it may appear at any time. In the U.S., Addison disease is most commonly caused by autoimmune mechanisms that destroy adrenal cortical cells. Chronic infections that affect the adrenal gland, such as tuberculosis, account for the majority of cases of primary adrenal insufficiency in underdeveloped countries.

PATHOPHYSIOLOGY Addison disease is characterized by inadequate corticosteroid and mineralocorticoid synthesis and elevated levels of serum ACTH (loss of negative feedback). Idiopathic Addison disease (organ-specific autoimmune adrenalitis) causes adrenal atrophy and hypofunction and is an organ-specific autoimmune disease resulting from autoantibodies and autoreactive T cells that attach the adrenal cortical cells. It may occur in childhood (type 1) or adulthood (type 2) and is associated with other autoimmune diseases, especially Hashimoto thyroiditis, pernicious anemia, and idiopathic hypoparathyroidism. In some cases, Addison disease may be inherited as an autosomal recessive trait. (Mechanisms of inheritance are described in Chapter 2). The adrenal glands in idiopathic Addison disease are smaller than normal and may be misshapen.

CLINICAL MANIFESTATIONS The symptoms of Addison disease are the result of hypocortisolism and hypoaldosteronism and are often nonspecific. With mild to moderate hypocortisolism, symptoms begin with weakness and easy fatigability. Skin changes, including hyperpigmentation and vitiligo, may occur. As the condition progresses, anorexia, nausea, vomiting, and diarrhea may develop. Of greatest concern is the development of hypotension that can progress to complete vascular collapse and shock. This is known as *adrenal crisis,* or Addisonian crisis, and most often develops in individuals who have undiagnosed disease and experience a physiologic stress.

EVALUATION AND TREATMENT Serum and urine levels of cortisol are depressed with primary hypocortisolism, and ACTH levels are increased. Because of dehydration, blood urea nitrogen levels may increase. The serum glucose level is low. Eosinophil and lymphocyte counts often are elevated. Hyperkalemia is seen in Addison disease and may cause mild alkalosis (see Chapter 5). The ACTH stimulation test may be used to evaluate serum cortisol levels.

The treatment of Addison disease involves lifetime glucocorticoid and mineralocorticoid replacement therapy, together with dietary modifications and correction of any underlying disorders. The individual's diet should include at least 150 mEq of sodium per day; sodium intake should be increased if the individual experiences excessive sweating or diarrhea. With acute stressors (e.g., infection, surgery, or trauma), additional cortisol must be administered.

Secondary hypocortisolism. Secondary hypocortisolism commonly results from prolonged administration of exogenous glucocorticoids; they suppress ACTH secretion and cause adrenal atrophy, resulting in inadequate corticosteroidogenesis once the exogenous glucocorticoids are withdrawn. Decreased ACTH secretion also can result from pituitary infarction, pituitary tumors that compress ACTH-secreting cells, or hypophysectomy. In all instances of low ACTH levels, adrenal atrophy occurs and endogenous adrenal steroidogenesis is depressed. Clinical manifestations of secondary hypocortisolism are similar to those of Addison disease, although hyperpigmentation usually does not occur. The renin-angiotensin system usually is normal, so aldosterone and potassium levels also tend to be normal.

Tumors of the Adrenal Medulla

Hyperfunction of the adrenal medulla is caused by pheochromocytomas (chromaffin cell tumors) or sympathetic paragangliomas of the adrenal medulla. These are rare tumors, but 10% to 20% are malignant and may metastasize. Occurrence is usually sporadic, although nearly half are associated with genetic markers that may be inherited.

PATHOPHYSIOLOGY   Pheochromocytomas and sympathetic paragangliomas cause excessive production of norepinephrine, although large tumors secrete both epinephrine and norepinephrine. Approximately 5% of people with these tumors have no symptoms, apparently because the tumor is nonfunctioning. Such tumors can, however, release catecholamines, especially in response to a stressor, such as surgery.

CLINICAL MANIFESTATIONS   The clinical manifestations of a pheochromocytoma and sympathetic paragangliomas are related to the chronic effects of catecholamine secretion and include persistent hypertension, headache, pallor, diaphoresis, tachycardia, and palpitations. Hypertension results from increased peripheral vascular resistance and may be sustained or paroxysmal. An acute episode of hypertension related to hypersecretion of catecholamines may follow specific events, such as exercise, excessive ingestion of tyrosine-containing foods (aged cheese, red wine, beer, yogurt), ingestion of caffeine-containing foods, external pressure on the tumor, and induction of anesthesia. Hypertension unresponsive to drug therapy is often the first indication of a pheochromocytoma. Headaches appear because of sudden changes in catecholamine levels in the blood, affecting cerebral blood flow. Hypermetabolism and sweating are related to chronic activation of sympathetic receptors in adipocytes, hepatocytes, and other tissues. Glucose intolerance may occur because of catecholamine-induced inhibition of insulin release by the pancreas. These tumors tend to be extremely vascular and can rupture, causing massive and potentially fatal hemorrhage.

EVALUATION AND TREATMENT   Symptoms of pheochromocytoma can be insidious or intermittent and difficult to diagnose. A diagnosis is made when increased catecholamine production is found in the blood or urine. The site of the tumor is then determined using abdominal imaging techniques. Because of the possibility of metastasis, whole-body scanning may be done. Genetic testing can guide therapy.

Management of catecholamine excess is essential to prevent hypertensive emergencies and requires the use of α- and β-adrenergic blockers. The usual treatment of pheochromocytoma is surgical excision of the tumor. Medical therapy is continued to stabilize blood pressure before, during, or after surgery. Malignant pheochromocytoma is rarely curable and is usually managed by a combination of surgical debulking of the tumor combined with chemotherapy.

> **✔ QUICK CHECK 20.5**
> 1. What are the clinical manifestations of hyperaldosteronism?
> 2. What are the primary causes of hypocortisolism?
> 3. What are pheochromocytomas?

SUMMARY REVIEW

Mechanisms of Hormonal Alterations
1. Abnormalities in endocrine function may be caused by elevated or depressed hormone levels that result from (1) disorders within glands that cause them to synthesize abnormal amounts of hormone, (2) faulty feedback systems, (3) dysfunctional or ectopically produced hormones, or (4) defects in carrying the hormone in the bloodstream.
2. Target cells may fail to respond to hormones because of (1) cell surface receptor–associated disorders, or (2) intracellular disorders.

Alterations of the Hypothalamic–Pituitary System
1. Dysfunction in the action of hypothalamic hormones is most commonly related to interruption of the connection between the hypothalamus and pituitary—the pituitary stalk.
2. Disorders of the posterior pituitary include syndrome of inappropriate antidiuretic hormone secretion (SIADH) and diabetes insipidus. SIADH is characterized by abnormally high ADH secretion; diabetes insipidus is characterized by abnormally low ADH secretion.
3. In SIADH, high ADH levels cause retention of excess free water, leading to hyponatremia and hypoosmolality. SIADH is caused by ectopic production of ADH by tumors, surgical procedures, pulmonary disorders, and central nervous system disorders.
4. Diabetes insipidus may be neurogenic (caused by insufficient amounts of ADH) or nephrogenic (caused by an inadequate response to ADH). Low ADH results in excess free water loss leading to hypernatremia and hyperosmolality. Its principal clinical features are polyuria and polydipsia.
5. Diseases of the anterior pituitary include hypopituitarism, hyperpituitarism, acromegaly, and prolactinoma.
6. Hypopituitarism is characterized by the absence of anterior pituitary hormones or the complete failure of all anterior pituitary hormone functions. The most common causes of hypopituitarism are pituitary infarction or space-occupying lesions.
7. Hypopituitarism can affect any or all of the pituitary hormones and symptoms may range from mild to life-threatening, depending on the hormone affected. Adrenocorticotropic hormone (ACTH) deficiency is a potentially life-threatening disorder. Growth hormone (GH) deficiency causes increased body fat, decreased muscle mass, and psychologic problems in adults; and hypopituitary dwarfism in children.
8. Hyperpituitarism is caused by pituitary adenomas. These are usually benign, slow-growing tumors that arise from cells of the anterior pituitary.
9. Expansion of a pituitary adenoma causes both neurologic and secretory effects. Pressure from the expanding tumor causes hyposecretion of surrounding cells, dysfunction of the optic chiasma (leading to visual disturbances), dysfunction of the hypothalamus, and some cranial nerves.
10. Hypersecretion of GH in adults causes acromegaly and is most commonly the result of a pituitary adenoma. Prolonged, abnormally high levels of GH lead to proliferation of body and connective

tissue and slowly developing renal, thyroid, and reproductive dysfunction.

11. Excessive GH secretion in children with open epiphyseal plates causes giantism.

12. Prolactinomas, pituitary tumors that secrete prolactin, result in galactorrhea, hirsutism, amenorrhea, hypogonadism, and osteopenia.

Alterations of Thyroid Function

1. Alterations in thyroid function can be primary or secondary. Primary thyroid diseases are caused by dysfunction or disease of the thyroid gland, usually the result of autoimmunity, leading to either increased or decreased thyroid hormone (TH) levels. Secondary thyroid disorders are related to disorders of pituitary gland thyroid-stimulating hormone (TSH) function.

2. Thyrotoxicosis is a general condition resulting from elevated TH levels. Hyperthyroidism is defined as excessive secretion of TH from the thyroid gland. Common clinical manifestations include increased metabolic rate, heat intolerance, and weight loss.

3. Graves disease, the most common form of hyperthyroidism, is caused by an autoimmune mechanism that stimulates the TSH receptors on the thyroid gland. It is characterized by thyrotoxicosis and circulating thyroid-stimulating immunoglobulins. The two distinguishing clinical manifestations are ophthalmopathy and dermopathy (pretibial myxedema).

4. Toxic nodular goiter and toxic multinodular goiter occur when there are independently functioning follicular cells that form adenomas, which produce excessive TH.

5. Thyrotoxic crisis is a severe form of hyperthyroidism that is often associated with physiologic stress.

6. Hypothyroidism is caused by deficient production of TH by the thyroid gland. Primary hypothyroidism has increased levels of TSH and is caused by autoimmune thyroiditis, loss of thyroid tissue, medications, and iodine deficiency. Secondary hypothyroidism has decreased levels of TSH and is caused by hypothalamic or pituitary dysfunction.

7. Symptoms of hypothyroidism depend on the degree of TH deficiency. Common manifestations include decreased energy metabolism, cold intolerance, decreased heat production, lethargy, and myxedema.

8. Myxedema is a sign of hypothyroidism caused by alterations in connective tissue with water-binding proteins that lead to edema and thickened mucous membranes. Myxedema coma is a severe form of hypothyroidism that may be life-threatening without emergency medical treatment.

9. Autoimmune thyroiditis (Hashimoto disease) is the most common cause of primary hypothyroidism in the US, and involves autoimmune destruction of the thyroid gland and gradual loss of thyroid function.

10. Subacute thyroiditis is a nonbacterial inflammation of the thyroid gland that is often preceded by a viral infection.

11. Postpartum thyroiditis generally occurs up to 6 months after giving birth. Iatrogenic hypothyroidism results from ablation of the thyroid gland during treatment for hyperthyroid conditions.

12. Congenital hypothyroidism is the absence of thyroid tissue during fetal development or defects in hormone synthesis and, if untreated, can lead to severe physical and cognitive disorders.

13. Thyroid carcinoma is associated with exposure to ionizing radiation, especially in childhood.

Alterations of Parathyroid Function

1. Hyperparathyroidism, which may be primary, secondary, or tertiary, is characterized by greater than normal secretion of parathyroid hormone (PTH). Hyperparathyroidism leads to neuromuscular symptoms, bone damage, and renal stones.

2. Primary hyperparathyroidism is caused by an interruption of the normal mechanisms that regulate calcium and PTH levels. Hallmark manifestations include hypercalcemia and hypophosphatemia.

3. Secondary hyperparathyroidism is a compensatory response to hypocalcemia and often occurs with chronic renal failure and vitamin D deficiency.

4. Tertiary hyperparathyroidism develops after long-standing hypocalcemia, especially in individuals undergoing renal dialysis or transplantation.

5. Hypoparathyroidism, defined by abnormally low PTH levels, is caused by thyroid surgery, autoimmunity, or genetic mechanisms.

6. The lack of circulating PTH in hypoparathyroidism causes hypocalcemia, hyperphosphatemia, and decreased bone resorption.

Dysfunction of the Endocrine Pancreas: Diabetes Mellitus

1. Diabetes mellitus is a group of metabolic diseases characterized hyperglycemia resulting from defects in insulin secretion, insulin action, or both.

2. A diagnosis of diabetes mellitus is based on elevated plasma glucose concentrations and measurement of glycosylated hemoglobin. Classic signs and symptoms are often present as well.

3. Diabetes mellitus is classified as type 1, type 2, or gestational.

4. Type 1 diabetes mellitus is caused by autoimmune beta-cell destruction, usually leading to absolute insulin deficiency. It is characterized by loss of beta cells, presence of islet cell antibody, lack of insulin, excess of glucagon, and altered metabolism of fat, protein, and carbohydrates.

5. In type 1 diabetes mellitus, hyperglycemia causes polyuria and polydipsia resulting from osmotic diuresis. Hypoglycemia and diabetic ketoacidosis may be seen.

6. Type 2 diabetes mellitus is caused by progressive loss of beta-cell insulin secretion frequently on the background of insulin resistance. Genetic susceptibility is triggered by environmental factors. The most compelling environmental risk factor for type 2 diabetes is obesity.

7. In the obese, many factors, including metabolic syndrome, altered adipokines, increased fatty acids, inflammation, and hyperinsulinemia, contribute to the development of insulin resistance and hyperglycemia.

8. Early in the course of type 2 diabetes mellitus, hyperinsulinemia occurs in order to overcome underlying insulin resistance. Over time, however, the weight and number of beta cells decrease and insulin levels decline. There also are decreased levels of amylin, ghrelin, and incretins and glucagon concentration is increased. All contribute to chronic hyperglycemia.

9. Gestational diabetes is glucose intolerance diagnosed during the second or third trimester of pregnancy.

10. The category other specific types of diabetes include monogenetic forms of diabetes called maturity-onset diabetes of youth (MODY).

11. Acute complications of diabetes mellitus include hypoglycemia, diabetic ketoacidosis, and hyperosmolar hyperglycemic nonketotic syndrome.

12. Hypoglycemia in diabetes is a complication related to insulin treatment.

13. Diabetic ketoacidosis (DKA) develops when there is an absolute or relative deficiency of insulin and an increase in the insulin counterregulatory hormones of catecholamines—cortisol, glucagon, and growth hormone. DKA presents with hyperglycemia, acidosis, and ketonuria.

14. Hyperosmolar hyperglycemic nonketotic syndrome is pathophysiologically similar to DKA, although a lack of ketosis resulting acidosis indicates some level of insulin action. Severe dehydration and electrolyte imbalance are present.

15. Chronic complications of diabetes mellitus include microvascular disease (e.g., neuropathy, retinopathy, nephropathy), macrovascular disease (e.g., coronary artery disease, stroke, peripheral vascular disease), and infection.

16. Microvascular disease is characterized by obstruction of capillaries and decreased tissue perfusion.

17. Macrovascular disease associated with diabetes mellitus is most often related to the proliferation of atherosclerotic plaques in the arterial wall.

18. The incidence of coronary heart disease, peripheral vascular disease, and stroke is greater in those with diabetes than in nondiabetic individuals.

19. Individuals with diabetes are at risk for a variety of infections. Infection may be related to sensory impairment and resulting injury, hypoxia, increased proliferation of pathogens in elevated concentrations of glucose, decreased blood supply associated with vascular damage, and impaired immune protection.

Alterations of Adrenal Function

1. Disorders of the adrenal cortex are related to hyperfunction (secreting too much hormone) or hypofunction (secreting too little hormone).

2. Increased secretion of cortisol (hypercortisolism) is usually caused by Cushing disease (pituitary-dependent) and very rarely can be caused by ectopic production of ACTH. Complications include obesity, diabetes, protein wasting, immune suppression, and mental status changes.

3. Congenital adrenal hyperplasia is a genetic disorder with overproduction of mineralocorticoids or androgens, or both.

4. Excessive aldosterone secretion causes hyperaldosteronism, which may be primary or secondary. Primary hyperaldosteronism is caused by an abnormality of the adrenal cortex. Secondary hyperaldosteronism involves renin and angiotensin secretion in response to renal underperfusion.

5. Hyperaldosteronism promotes increased sodium reabsorption (with corresponding hypervolemia), increased extracellular volume (which is variable), hypokalemia related to renal reabsorption of sodium, and excretion of potassium.

6. Hypersecretion of adrenal androgens and estrogens can be a result of adrenal tumors, either adenomas or carcinomas; Cushing syndrome; or defects in steroid synthesis. Hypersecretion of estrogens causes feminization, the development of female secondary sexual characteristics. Hypersecretion of androgens causes virilization, the development of male secondary sexual characteristics.

7. Hypocortisolism, or low levels of cortisol, is caused secondarily by inadequate adrenal stimulation by ACTH or because of primary adrenal insufficiency, termed Addison disease.

8. Addison disease is characterized by elevated ACTH levels with inadequate corticosteroid and mineralocorticoid synthesis.

9. Manifestations of Addison disease are related to hypocortisolism and hypoaldosteronism. Symptoms include weakness, fatigability, hyperpigmentation, vitiligo, anorexia, vomiting, and diarrhea. The development of hypotension can progress to complete vascular collapse and shock, known as adrenal crisis, or Addisonian crisis.

10. Secondary hypocortisolism commonly results from prolonged administration of exogenous glucocorticoids that suppress ACTH secretion. Decreased ACTH secretion also can result from pituitary infarction, pituitary tumors, or hypophysectomy. In all instances of low ACTH levels, adrenal atrophy occurs and endogenous adrenal steroidogenesis is depressed.

11. Hyperfunction of the adrenal medulla is usually caused by a pheochromocytoma, a catecholamine-producing tumor. Symptoms of catecholamine excess include hypertension, palpitations, tachycardia, glucose intolerance, excessive sweating, and constipation.

KEY TERMS

Acromegaly, 451
Addison disease, 469
Amylin, 457
Central (secondary) thyroid disorders, 452
Congenital adrenal hyperplasia, 468
Cushing disease, 467
Cushing syndrome, 467
Cushing-like syndrome, 467
Diabetes insipidus (DI), 449
Diabetes mellitus, 457
Diabetic ketoacidosis (DKA), 462
Diabetic neuropathy, 465
Diabetic retinopathy, 464
Feminization, 469
Gestational diabetes mellitus (GDM), 461
Ghrelin, 460
Giantism, 451
Glucagon, 457
Glycosylated hemoglobin, 457

Hyperaldosteronism, 468
Hypercortisolism, 467
Hyperosmolar hyperglycemic nonketotic syndrome (HHNKS), 464
Hyperparathyroidism, 456
Hyperthyroidism, 452
Hypocortisolism, 469
Hypoglycemia, 461
Hypoparathyroidism, 456
Hypopituitarism, 449
Hypothyroidism, 454
Iatrogenic hypothyroidism, 455
Idiopathic Addison disease (organ-specific autoimmune adrenalitis), 469
Incretin, 460
Insulin resistance, 460
Macular edema, 464
Maturity-onset diabetes of youth (MODY), 461
Myxedema, 454

Myxedema coma, 454
Panhypopituitarism, 449
Pheochromocytoma (chromaffin cell tumor), 470
Pituitary adenoma, 450
Postpartum thyroiditis, 455
Pretibial myxedema (Graves dermopathy), 453
Primary adrenal insufficiency, 469
Primary hyperaldosteronism (Conn syndrome, primary aldosteronism), 468
Primary hyperparathyroidism, 456
Primary thyroid disorder, 452
Prolactinoma, 451
Secondary hyperaldosteronism, 468
Secondary hyperparathyroidism, 456
Secondary hypocortisolism, 469

Subacute thyroiditis (de Quervain thyroiditis), 455
Subclinical hypothyroidism, 454
Syndrome of inappropriate ADH secretion (SIADH), 448
Tertiary hyperparathyroidism, 456
Thyroid carcinoma, 455
Thyrotoxic crisis (thyroid storm), 454
Thyrotoxicosis, 452
Toxic adenoma, 454
Toxic multinodular goiter, 454
Type 1 diabetes mellitus, 457
Type 2 diabetes mellitus (non–insulin-dependent diabetes mellitus), 460
Virilization, 469

REFERENCES

1. Moritz ML: Syndrome of inappropriate antidiuresis, *Pediatr Clin North Am* 66(1):209-226, 2019.
2. Kavanagh C, Uy NS: Nephrogenic diabetes insipidus, *Pediatr Clin North Am* 66(1):227-234, 2019.
3. Higham CE, Johannsson G, Shalet SM: Hypopituitarism, *Lancet* 388(10058):2403-2415, 2016.
4. Molitch ME: Diagnosis and treatment of pituitary adenomas: a review, *JAMA* 317(5):516-524, 2017.
5. Dineen R, Stewart PM, Sherlock M: Acromegaly, *QJM* 110(7):411-420, 2017.
6. Caturegli P, De Remigis A, Rose NR: Hashimoto thyroiditis: clinical and diagnostic criteria, *Autoimmun Rev* 13(4-5):391-397, 2014.
7. Bartalena L: Graves' disease complications. In De Groot LJ, editor: *Endotext [Internet]*, South Dartmouth, MA, 2000, MDText.com. Available at: http://www.ncbi.nlm.nih.gov/books/NBK285551/. Last update February 20, 2018.
8. De Leo S, Lee SY, Braverman LE: Hyperthyroidism, *Lancet* 388(10047):906-918, 2016.
9. Burch HB, Cooper DS: Management of Graves disease: a review, *J Am Med Assoc* 314(23):2544-2554, 2015.
9a. Kitahara CM, et al: Association of radioactive iodine treatment with cancer mortality in patients with hyperthyroidism, *JAMA Intern Med* 179(8):1034-1042, 2019.
10. Aoki Y, et al: Serum TSH and total T4 in the United States population and their association with participant characteristics: National Health and Nutrition Examination Survey (NHANES 1999-2002), *Thyroid* 17(12):1211-1223, 2007.
11. Baumgardner C, Blum MR, Rodondi N: Subclnical hypothyroidism: summary of evidence in 2014, *Swiss Med Wkly* 144:w14058, 2014.
12. American Cancer Society (ACS): *Cancer facts and figures 2019*, Atlanta, Ga, 2019, Author.
13. Cabanillas ME, McFadden DG, Durante C: Thyroid cancer, *Lancet* 388(10061):2783-2795, 2016.
14. Duan K, Gomez Hernandez K, Mete O: Clinicopathological correlates of hyperparathyroidism, *J Clin Pathol* 68(10):771-787, 2015.
15. Centers for Disease Control and Prevention (CDC): National diabetes statistics report, 2017. Available at: https://www.cdc.gov/diabetes/data/statistics/statistics-report.html. Page last reviewed March 6, 2018.
16. American Diabetes Association: Standards of medical care in diabetes—2019: abridged for primary care providers, *Diabetes Care* 42(Suppl 1):S1-S194, 2018. Available at: http://clinical.diabetesjournals.org/content/diaclin/early/2018/12/16/cd18-0105.full.pdf.
17. Atkinson MA, et al: Type 1 diabetes, *Lancet* 383(9911):69-82, 2014.
18. Bellou V, et al: Risk factors for type 2 diabetes mellitus: an exposure-wide umbrella review of meta-analyses, *PLoS ONE* 13(3):e0194127, 2018.
19. Pasquel FJ, Umpierrez GE: Hyperosmolar hyperglycemic state: a historic review of the clinical presentation, diagnosis, and treatment, *Diabetes Care* 37(11):3124-3131, 2014.
20. Gardner TW, Davila JR: The neurovascular unit and the pathophysiologic basis of diabetic retinopathy, *Graefes Arch Clin Exp Ophthalmol* 255(1):1-6, 2017.
21. Mora-Fernández C, et al: Diabetic kidney disease: from physiology to therapeutics, *J Physiol* 592(18):3997-4012, 2014.
22. Juster-Switlyk K, Smith AG: Updates in diabetic peripheral neuropathy, *F1000Res* 5:2016.
23. Castinetti F, et al: Cushing's disease, *Orphanet J Rare Dis* 7:41, 2012.
24. Gyamlani G, et al: Primary aldosteronism: diagnosis and management, *Am J Med Sci* 352(4):391-398, 2016.

21

Obesity, Starvation, and Anorexia of Aging

Sue E. Huether

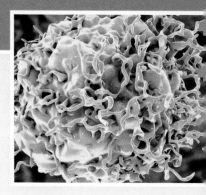

EVOLVE WEBSITE

CHAPTER OUTLINE

Obesity of one of the most common and costly chronic diseases in the world. The causes are complex, multifactorial, and associated with an increased risk of many comorbid diseases. Alternatively, starvation and anorexia of aging also are common conditions. The purpose of this chapter is to present an overview of the function of adipose tissue and the pathophysiology of obesity, starvation, and the anorexia of aging.

ADIPOSE TISSUE

Adipose tissue provides insulation and mechanical support, secretes hormonelike signaling molecules known as *adipokines,* and contributes to immune cell function. It is the body's major energy reserve to fuel other tissues. Adipocytes are fat-storing cells that store calories in the form of triglycerides (triglycerol), synthesize triglycerides from glucose, and mobilize energy in the form of free fatty acids (FFAs) and glycerol. Adipose tissue is classified according to color as white adipose tissue (WAT), brown adipose tissue (BAT), and beige adipose tissue (bAT). These tissue types are found in different locations and have different functions.[1] Most adipose tissue in the body is WAT.

White adipocytes, which are derived from connective tissue, are located in visceral (central) and subcutaneous (peripheral) stores of WAT. WAT also is found in muscle, providing mechanical protection and sliding of muscle bundles, as well as in bone marrow. WAT contains various cells, including macrophages, mast cells, neutrophils, fibroblasts, endothelial cells, blood vessels, nerves, and precursor adipocytes. White adipocytes contain a single triglyceride fat droplet or vacuole. A low nutritional state, stimulation of the beta adrenergic sympathetic nervous system and release of catecholamines (epinephrine and norepinephrine), activates lipolysis in WAT to release FFAs and glycerol into the circulation. FFAs and glycerol can then be used for energy metabolism.

Subcutaneous or peripheral adipose tissue is more likely to be stored by hyperplasia (adipogenesis), the formation of new fat cells from preadipocytes. These adipocytes are smaller and have a greater fat storage capacity. Subcutaneous fat has higher leptin production, lower adiponectin production, lower production of inflammatory cytokines, and lower association with insulin resistance. Expansion of subcutaneous fat is a healthier expansion of fat tissue and is associated with fewer complications of obesity.

Visceral adipose tissue is located in the abdomen and surrounding intra-abdominal organs. Visceral WAT is more likely to store fat by adipocyte hypertrophy. Visceral adipocytes store fat as triglycerides, primarily in the form of very-low-density lipoprotein (VLDL), derived from hepatic and dietary sources. Visceral fat is more hormonally active than subcutaneous fat and releases leptin and inflammatory mediators. Excess visceral fat is associated with impaired lipid and glucose metabolism, insulin resistance, metabolic syndrome, and an increased risk of cardiovascular disease and cancer.[2] Thus the complications of obesity are related to where fat is stored, not just the accumulation of fat stores.

Estrogen and estrogen receptors have a role in fat metabolism. They enhance the deposition of WAT in the subcutaneous tissue and inhibit it in visceral tissue. This may explain the higher incidence of peripheral obesity among premenopausal women and the increase in central obesity with menopause and in men.[3]

Bone marrow adipose tissue (MAT) is found in all bones, and it increases with obesity and age in long bones. With obesity, MAT releases adipokines that affect osteoblast and osteoclast function and alters hematopoiesis. In general, excessive MAT is associated with osteoporosis and fractures.[4]

Brown adipocytes form BAT and are derived from muscle tissue and have multiple lipid droplets. They are rich in mitochondria that contain iron, which gives them a brown color. Exposure to cold, activation of the sympathetic nervous system, catecholamines, and activation of triiodothyronine (T_3) stimulate BAT to generate heat rapidly through the oxidation of FFAs acids and glucose. This is known as *nonshivering thermogenesis;* it occurs at a rate 50-fold greater than in WAT and protects against obesity and metabolic syndrome.[5] Estrogen-related receptors also participate in nonshivering thermogenesis in BAT.[6]

Neonates generate body heat from BAT primarily located in the interscapular and perirenal regions. It traditionally was thought that BAT did not persist into adult life. However, positron emission tomography (PET) scanning has shown that adults also have BAT. It is most common in lean individuals, usually located in the neck, supraclavicular, axillary, paravertebral, and perirenal regions.[7] There also is an inverse relationship between the amount of BAT and both body mass index and age. Interindividual differences in BAT-mediated thermogenesis may explain some of the variability in obesity susceptibility and the increased prevalence of obesity with aging. Variation in BAT and bAT also may be factors in the natural regulation of weight reduction.

Located within WAT, particularly in subcutaneous fat stores, are beige, or "brite" (from "brown in white"), adipocytes that form bAT. Beige adipocytes are a subpopulation of white adipocytes that also contain multiple mitochondria but not in the numbers associated with BAT. Beige adipocytes emerge within WAT with chronic exposure to cold and exercise. This is known as the *beiging* or *browning* of WAT. They disappear with elevated ambient temperatures,[8] and with warm adaptation bAT reverts to WAT. Leptin and insulin together promote bAT, increasing energy expenditure and weight loss. bAT is diminished in obesity. Because the beiging (browning) of adipose tissue protects against obesity and metabolic syndrome, efforts are in progress to discover whether there is a therapeutic way to stimulate the synthesis and activity of BAT and bAT as an approach to preventing or treating obesity and diabetes mellitus.[9]

Adipose Tissue as an Endocrine Organ

Adipose tissue is also an endocrine organ, and adipocytes secrete adipokines. Adipokines are cell-signaling proteins that function like hormones, having autocrine, paracrine, and endocrine actions. Adipokines include all the biologically active substances synthesized by WAT. They are necessary for numerous functions in body tissues.[10] These substances function in the regulation of appetite, food intake and energy expenditure, lipid storage, insulin secretion and sensitivity, immune and inflammatory responses, coagulation, fibrinolysis, angiogenesis, fertility, vascular homeostasis, blood pressure regulation, and bone metabolism. Excess WAT causes dysregulation of the secretion and function of adipokines, contributing to the many complications of obesity.

Adipokines are important to understand because they are targets of both experimental and currently available drugs and weight loss programs used to treat obesity and its complications. Examples of adipokines are provided as a reference in Box 21.1 (a summary of adipokines and their role in caloric intake, energy metabolism, and obesity is presented later in this chapter). The regulation of food intake and energy balance is summarized next.

Regulation of Food Intake and Energy Balance

Regulation of food intake and energy balance is a complex process controlled by central and peripheral physiological signals.[11] Centrally, the arcuate nucleus (ARC) in the hypothalamus regulates food intake

---

BOX 21.1 Examples of Adipokines Secreted by Adipose Tissue

Adipokines

Increased in Obesity

Leptin (Leptin Resistance)
Inhibits appetite and stimulates energy expenditure
Satiety (hunger/appetite suppression) and regulation of eating behavior by hypothalamus
Sympathoactivation
Insulin sensitizing in liver and skeletal muscle
Modulating role in reproduction, angiogenesis, immune response, blood pressure control, and osteogenesis
Promotes inflammation (a harmful effect)

Angiopoietin-Related Protein 2 (a Vascular Endothelial Growth Factor)
Insulin resistance
Promotes inflammation

Angiotensinogen, Angiotensin Type 1 and Type 1 Receptors, Renin, and Angiotensin-Converting Enzyme
Vasoconstriction
Inflammation
Lipogenesis
Insulin resistance

Retinol-Binding Protein 4 (RBP4) (From Visceral White Adipose Tissue [WAT]; Role Not Clear)
Promotes insulin resistance in muscle
Promotes angiogenesis

Visfatin (From Visceral WAT)
Mimics insulin, binds to insulin receptors and promotes insulin sensitivity
Promotes adhesion of monocytes to endothelial cells and promotes plaque instability (harmful in cardiac disease)

Decreased in Obesity
Adiponectin
Insulin sensitizing
Antiinflammatory
Antiatherogenic

Apelin
Improves insulin sensitivity in muscle
Promotes vasodilation by blocking angiotensin
Promotes cardiac contractility

Proinflammatory Cytokines (Increased in Obesity)
Interleukin-6
Promotes insulin resistance
Inhibits adipogenesis
Decreases adiponectin secretion
Promotes inflammation

Monocyte Chemoattractant Protein 1
Attracts macrophages
Promotes insulin resistance
Promotes atherogenesis

Macrophage Products
Plasminogen activator inhibitor 1 (from visceral WAT)
Promotes clot formation (inhibits fibrinolysis) by inhibiting tissue plasminogen activator and urokinase (also released by endothelial cells)
Promotes insulin resistance
Prostaglandin E2 and leukotriene B4
Promotes inflammation
Tumor necrosis factor-alpha
Promotes insulin resistance
Promotes inflammation

Data from Giralt M, Cereijo R, Villarroya F: *Hand Exp Pharmacol* 233:265-282, 2016; Luo L, Liu M: *J Endocrinol* 231(3):R77-R99, 2016.

and energy metabolism by balancing the opposing effects of two sets of neurons. One set of neurons promotes appetite, stimulates eating, and decreases metabolism (anabolic). These are known as *orexigenic neurons*, which are stimulated by molecules called *orexins*. Another set of neurons suppresses appetite, inhibits eating, and increases metabolism. These are known as *anorexigenic neurons*, which are stimulated by molecules called *anorexins*. The hypothalamic orexin and anorexin signaling pathways are transmitted through the autonomic nervous and endocrine systems to regulate and balance appetite, food intake, energy metabolism, and body temperature. The hypothalamus also communicates with higher brain centers related to reward, pleasure, memory, and addictive behavior. These higher centers can override hypothalamic control of food intake and satiety, which increases consumption of highly palatable foods and results in increased fat stores.[12]

Peripherally, the gastrointestinal tract secretes a number of hormones (see Box 21.2) that also control hunger and satiety. In addition, adipokines can function as orexins or anorexins and provide peripheral signals for the control of food intake and energy expenditure. They are described in the Adipokines and Obesity section later in the chapter.

✔ **QUICK CHECK 21.1**
1. What are three functions of adipose tissue?
2. How do white adipocytes differ from brown and beige adipocytes?
3. What are adipokines?
4. What are orexins and anorexins?

OBESITY

Obesity is an increase in body adipose tissue and an endocrine and metabolic disorder that has become epidemic worldwide. **Obesity** is defined differently in adults and children. In adults, it is a body mass index (BMI) that exceeds 30 kg/m². In children, it is a BMI greater than or equal to the age- and sex-specific 95th percentile of the growth charts published in 2000 by the Centers for Disease Control and Prevention (CDC).[13] Obesity develops when caloric intake exceeds caloric expenditure in genetically susceptible individuals. Between 2015 and 2016, the incidence among U.S. adults was 39.8% and 18.5% among children and adolescents between ages 2 and 19 years. Children tend to become obese adults. Ethnic differences also are seen in the rates of obesity: Hispanics (47%), non-Hispanic blacks (46.8%), non-Hispanic whites (37.9%), and non-Hispanic Asians (12.7%).[14]

BOX 21.2   Gastrointestinal Hormones and Obesity

Ghrelin: Stomach (decreased in obesity, but increased after eating; role in obesity not clear)
  Stimulates hunger and controls gastric motility and acid secretion, stimulates growth hormone
Glucagon-like peptide 1 (GLP-1): Large intestine (decreased in obesity)
  Stimulates insulin secretion; inhibits glucagon release; slows gastric emptying to reduce postprandial hyperglycemia, increases satiety
Peptide YY: Small intestine (decreased in obesity)
  Reduces appetite, inhibits gastric motility, increases energy expenditure
Cholecystokinin: Small intestine (probably increased in obesity)
  Increases satiation; reduces food intake; stimulates gallbladder contraction; release of pancreatic enzymes and insulin; slows gastric emptying

---

Obesity is the fifth leading cause of death in the United States and accounts for high health care costs worldwide.[15] Three leading causes of death in the United States are associated with obesity: cardiovascular disease, type 2 diabetes mellitus, and cancer (liver, advanced prostate, ovarian, gallbladder, kidney, colorectal, esophageal, postmenopausal breast, pancreatic, endometrial, and stomach).[16] Obesity also is a risk factor for hypertension, stroke, hyperlipidemia, gallstones, nonalcoholic steatohepatitis (NASH), gastroesophageal reflux, hiatal hernia, osteoarthritis, infectious disease, asthma, obstructive sleep apnea, and chronic kidney disease. However, some studies have shown that mild obesity in older individuals is associated with lower mortality (the obesity paradox), but the mechanisms are not clear.[17] The causes and consequences of obesity are multiple and complex, and rapidly advancing research is underway on the causal mechanisms, complications, and treatment.

Genotype and gene–environment interactions are important predisposing factors (*Did You Know? Obesogens*). Single-gene defects (monogenic defects) are rare, and obesity is usually polygenic and associated with other phenotypes, such as endocrine disorders (i.e., diabetes mellitus and hypothyroidism) and mental retardation (i.e., Down and Prader-Willi syndromes).[18] Metabolic abnormalities that contribute to obesity include Cushing syndrome, Cushing disease, polycystic ovary syndrome, growth hormone deficiency, hypothyroidism, and hypothalamic injury. Contributing environmental factors include food intake (low nutrient, energy-dense foods), physical inactivity, obesogens, and socioeconomic status (both high and low income). Obesity also is associated with adverse social and psychological consequences, including depression and mood disorders.[19]

DID YOU KNOW?
Obesogens

Obesogens (also known as *endocrine-disrupting chemicals*) are exogenous chemicals that contribute to the development of obesity. These molecules stimulate adipogenesis and fat storage and also interfere with neuroendocrine control of appetite and satiety. Developmental exposure to environmental obesogens is proposed to contribute to the epidemic of obesity, in addition to a high caloric intake, a sedentary lifestyle, and genetic predisposition. In early life, these substances are included in the maternal diet (i.e., phytoestrogens) or are associated with exposure to pesticides (i.e., organophosphates), plastics (phthalates, bisphenol-A), personal care products, and household and other consumer products that can cross the placental barrier or be transmitted, or both, through breast milk. Epigenetic changes in gene regulation and expression effect adipocyte differentiation, adipogenesis, and lipid metabolism, resulting in obesity in later life. Animal studies indicate that these genetic changes can be transmitted through generations of families.

Data from Darbre PD: *Curr Obes Rep* 6(1):18-27, 2017; Janesick AS, Blumberg B: *Am J Obstet Gynecol* 214(5):559-565; 2016; Nappi F, et al: *Int J Environ Res Public Health* 13(8):765, 2016; Stel J, Legler J: *Endocrinology* 156(10):3466-3472, 2015.

PATHOPHYSIOLOGY   The pathophysiology of obesity is complex and involves the interaction of peripheral and central neuroendocrine pathways, numerous adipokines, hormones, and neurotransmitters[20] (Fig. 21.1). The adipocyte is the cellular basis of obesity. Excess fat is stored in mature white adipocytes when energy balance is positive (excess caloric intake in relation to energy expenditure). These adipocytes undergo hypertrophy and adipogenesis (hyperplasia), store triglycerol, and secrete adipokines. Adipokines circulate in the blood at concentrations that increase or decrease in relation to body fat mass and provide

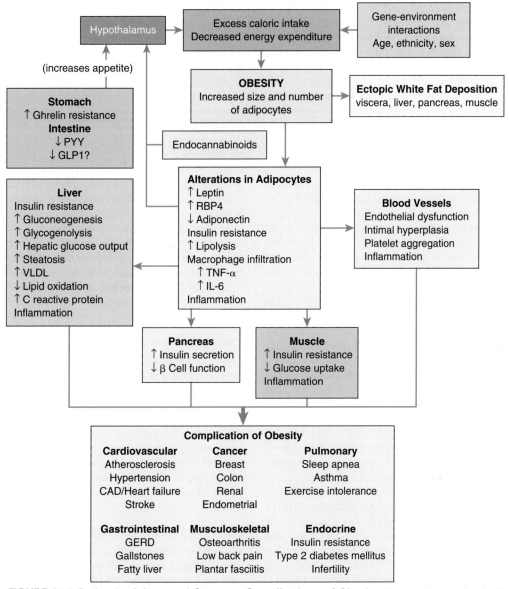

FIGURE 21.1 Pathophysiology and Common Complications of Obesity. See text for details. *Ang/ AT2,* Angiotensinogen/angiotensin 2; *CAD,* coronary artery disease; *FFA,* free fatty acids; *GERD,* gastro-esophageal reflux disease; *GLP1,* glucagon-like peptide 1; *IL-6,* interleukin-6; *PYY,* intestinal peptide YY; *RBP4,* retinol-binding protein 4; *TNF-α,* tumor necrosis factor-alpha; *VLDL,* very-low-density lipoprotein.

signals to the central nervous system for regulation of hunger, satiety, and energy balance, as described previously.[21] WAT accumulation causes dysfunction in the regulation and interaction of this signaling system and contributes to the complications and consequences of obesity.

Adipokines and Obesity

Leptin is a product of the obesity gene (*Ob* gene) and is expressed primarily by adipocytes. Leptin levels increase after eating and act on the hypothalamus to inhibit orexigenic neurons and stimulate anorexigenic neurons to suppress appetite and increase energy expenditure. At low leptin levels (i.e., during fasting), leptin stimulates food intake and reduces energy expenditure. This balance regulates body weight and energy expenditure within a fairly narrow range. Leptin levels increase as the number of adipocytes increases. However, high leptin levels are ineffective at decreasing appetite and energy expenditure, a condition associated with obesity and known as central *leptin resistance*.

Leptin resistance fails to inhibit orexigenic hypothalamic satiety signaling and promotes overeating and excessive weight gain. Leptin also regulates hepatic gluconeogenesis, insulin sensitivity, and glucose and lipid metabolism in liver, muscle, and adipose tissue. Peripheral leptin resistance (i.e., in muscle and adipose tissue) results in hyperglycemia, hyperinsulinemia, and hyperlipidemia and also stimulates macrophages and endothelial cells to produce proinflammatory mediators. The cause of leptin resistance is unknown. It may be related to a defect in leptin transport, an inability of leptin to cross the blood–brain barrier, an alteration in the permissive effect of leptin, or a defect in or suppression of the leptin receptor. The low-grade inflammation that accompanies obesity also is thought to contribute to leptin resistance. Chronic hyperleptinemia also stimulates the sympathetic nervous system, oxidative stress, chronic low-grade inflammation, and ventricular hypertrophy and contributes to the pathogenesis of hypertension, atherosclerosis, cardiovascular disease, and cancer associated with obesity.[22]

Adiponectin, which is produced primarily by visceral adipose tissue but also by cardiomyocytes and skeletal muscle, increases energy expenditure. It also has insulin-sensitizing and antiinflammatory properties. Plasma levels of adiponectin decrease with visceral obesity, and resistance to adiponectin action develops. Decreased adiponectin levels are associated with increased hepatic gluconeogenesis, insulin resistance, decreased skeletal muscle glucose uptake, and increased levels of inflammatory mediators, such as interleukin-6 (IL-6) and tumor necrosis factor-alpha (TNF-α). Adiponectin serves as an antiinflammatory and antiatherogenic plasma protein; it also has an important role in vascular remodeling, and it is cardioprotective. Decreased levels of adiponectin are associated with type 2 diabetes mellitus and an increased risk for coronary artery disease resulting from hyperlipidemia, hypertension, and factors that promote thrombosis and inflammation.[23]

Decreased beta cell function and insulin resistance are associated with obesity. The mechanisms are not clear, but an association exists between hyperlipidemia and increased fat storage, macrophages and inflammation, and alterations in adipokines. Leptin resistance and decreased adiponectin also contribute to insulin resistance. Insulin resistance results in hyperinsulinemia, hyperglycemia, and a predisposition to type 2 diabetes mellitus. **Retinol-binding protein 4** (binds vitamin A) is an adipokine produced both in the liver and by adipocytes. It is increased in visceral adiposity and contributes to inflammation and insulin resistance in the liver and muscles; it also is associated with hepatic steatosis (fatty liver) and cardiovascular disease.[24]

Endocannabinoids (i.e., anandamide) are arachidonic acid derivatives (unsaturated, essential fatty acids) expressed in both the brain and peripheral nerve tissues. They have effects on endocannabinoid (CB) receptors in orexigenic pathways. They increase appetite, enhance nutrient absorption, stimulate lipogenesis, and increase WAT accumulation by acting at both central (CB1 receptor) and peripheral sites (CB2 receptor). They also inhibit energy expenditure and thermogenesis. An increase in endocannabinoids is proposed to be associated with obesity.[25]

Angiotensinogen (AGT) is produced in the liver and by adipocytes and is increased in obesity. AGT is the precursor to angiotensin 1 (AGTI), which is then converted to angiotensin 2 (AGTII). The effects of AGTII include vasoconstriction, renal retention of sodium and water, and release of aldosterone. Increased AGTII from adipose tissue also promotes lipogenesis, oxidative stress, inflammation, and insulin resistance. All of these effects contribute to the complications associated with obesity.[26]

Gastrointestinal hormones also play a role in the complex pathophysiology of obesity (Box 21.2). The most significant ones are reviewed next.

Ghrelin is produced by the stomach gastric mucosa. It increases in response to fasting and chronic caloric restriction and decreases after food intake. Ghrelin stimulates food intake and fat storage and prevents life-threatening falls in blood glucose. Ghrelin is thought to have antilipolytic effects and stimulates lipogenesis in visceral WAT, leading to an increase in body weight and body fat mass. Ghrelin also stimulates the release of growth hormone (GH) from anterior pituitary cells, the release of gastric acid, gastrointestinal motility, and pancreatic secretion of insulin. It has satiety, vasodilatory, and cardioprotective effects. An elevation in FFAs and GH after eating normally decreases the release of ghrelin. However, obesity is associated with a decreased plasma level of ghrelin, and plasma ghrelin levels do not fall after eating. This is known as *ghrelin resistance*. The mechanisms for this response are not clear, and the role of ghrelin in obesity has yet to be clearly defined.[27]

Glucagon-like peptide 1 (GLP-1) is an anorexigenic hormone secreted by intestinal endocrine cells when nutrients enter the small intestine. GLP-1 stimulates pancreatic glucose-dependent insulin secretion, decreases blood glucose levels, delays gastric emptying, suppresses appetite, increases satiety, and increases energy expenditure. GLP-1 levels may be decreased in obese individuals, and a GLP-1 receptor analogue has been approved to treat both obesity and type 2 diabetes mellitus.[28]

Peptide YY (PYY) is released from intestinal endocrine cells in response to nutrients entering the intestine. PPY inhibits gastric motility and decreases appetite; it decreases with obesity.[21]

Cholecystokinin (CCK) is secreted by proximal small intestinal cells after food intake. Its actions include gallbladder contraction, release of pancreatic enzymes and insulin, satiation, and reduced food intake. CCK is reduced in obesity.[29]

Lipotoxicity

Chronic positive energy balance and obesity can overwhelm fat storage by adipocytes, resulting in altered lipid metabolism and insulin resistance. Normally, insulin can inhibit lipolysis by activation of insulin receptors in adipocytes. With obesity, adipocytes are resistant to insulin inhibition of lipolysis. With a chronic increased energy intake, the increase in adipocyte size and number in visceral WAT exceeds the supporting vascular supply, resulting in hypoxia and inflamed and fibrotic adipose tissues. Excess lipolysis and FFAs are distributed to nonadipose cells (e.g., kidney, liver, heart, skeletal muscle). When their utilization capacity is exceeded, cellular dysfunction or death occurs, and this is known as *lipotoxicity*.[30]

Obesity and Inflammation

Obesity produces a state of chronic, low-grade inflammation in WAT. Macrophages, lymphocytes, neutrophils, and mast cells infiltrate enlarged adipocytes and release inflammatory cytokines (e.g., TNF-α, and IL-6)[31] (see Box 21.1). The inflammatory state is supported by increased leptin, decreased adiponectin, and increased resistin (a hormone released by macrophages that promotes insulin resistance and inflammation). The inflammatory state, accelerated lipolysis, and lipotoxicity contribute to the development of insulin resistance, metabolic syndrome (see Chapter 20 and Box 20.2), and the complications of obesity, including type 2 diabetes mellitus, cardiovascular disease, kidney disease, NASH, and cancer.[32]

Obesity and the Gut Microbiome

Changes in the intestinal microbiome also are associated with obesity, although the mechanisms are not clear. Microbes (mostly bacteria) are found in high concentration in the lower gastrointestinal tract, and the bacterial composition is affected by genetics, diet, use of antibiotics and other medications, and energy balance. These bacteria have considerable variability among individuals and participate in the breakdown of complex carbohydrates, nutrient absorption, inflammatory responses, gut permeability, and bile acid metabolism. Gut microbial fermentation of dietary fiber produces short chain fatty acids (acetate, butyrate, and propionate), which function as energy sources and signaling molecules that affect the host's energy metabolism and inflammation. Gut microbiota transplanted from obese mice into germ-free mice or from an obese human twin have shown that the gut microbiota may have a causal role in the development of obesity and insulin resistance.[33] More studies are needed to determine how changes in the microbiota contribute to body weight regulation, metabolism, low-grade inflammation, and increased adiposity, and how manipulation of the gut microbiota can assist in preventing or treating obesity.

✔ **QUICK CHECK 21.2**
1. What are obesogens?
2. How do leptin and adiponectin contribute to the complications of obesity?
3. How does lipotoxicity damage peripheral organs (e.g., the heart and liver)?
4. Why is obesity associated with a proinflammatory state?

CLINICAL MANIFESTATIONS Obesity usually presents with two different forms or phenotypes of adipose tissue distribution: visceral and peripheral.[34] *Visceral obesity* (also known as intra-abdominal, central, or masculine obesity) occurs when the distribution of body fat is localized around the abdomen and upper body, resulting in an apple shape. Visceral obesity is associated with accelerated lipolysis and has an increased risk for chronic systemic inflammation, metabolic syndrome, obstructive sleep apnea syndrome, type 2 diabetes mellitus, cardiovascular complications, osteoarthritis, and cancer. Visceral venous blood drains into the portal vein, contributing to higher liver synthesis of plasma lipids and increasing the risk of NASH.[35]

Peripheral obesity (also known as subcutaneous, gluteal-femoral, or feminine obesity) occurs when the distribution of body fat is extraperitoneal and distributed around the thighs and buttocks and through the muscle, resulting in a pear shape; it is more common in premenopausal women. Peripheral and subcutaneous fat is less metabolically active and lipolytic and releases fewer adipokines (particularly adiponectin) than visceral fat. Risk factors are still present for the complications of obesity, but they are less severe than for visceral obesity.[1]

Normal-weight obesity (NWO) describes a phenotype of individuals who have a normal body weight and BMI but also a body fat percentage greater than 30%. These individuals are at risk for metabolic dysregulation, increases in inflammatory cytokines, insulin resistance, an increased risk of cardiovascular disease and other complications of obesity, and a higher mortality.[36] Another phenotype associated with obesity is metabolically healthy obesity (Box 21.3).

EVALUATION AND TREATMENT All children and adults should be screened for obesity. Several methods are available for estimating or measuring the amount of adipose tissue: anthropometric measurements including weight, height, and circumferences or various body diameters (i.e., waist-to-hip ratios and waist circumference); skinfold thickness (measured with skinfold calipers); ultrasound to measure peripheral body fat; and bioelectric impedance and underwater hydrostatic weighing to calculate total body fat. The only method for directly measuring total body fat is by dual energy x-ray absorptiometry (DXA) scanning, an enhanced type of x-ray imaging.

In clinical practice, anthropometric and body diameter measures are most commonly used to calculate the BMI because they are the easiest to measure and most cost-effective. Body mass indices have been established based on height, weight, age, sex, and ethnicity. Overweight

is defined as a BMI greater than 25 kg/m^2, and obesity is a BMI greater than 30 kg/m^2. BMI charts are available for children ages 2 to 20 years; these can be used for comparison during adulthood, because obese children generally become obese adults.

However, the BMI does not measure the amount and location of body fat. The waist circumference (more than 40 inches [102 cm] for men and more than 35 inches [88 cm] for women) adds information to assist with disease risk assessment in general practice. Obesity risk assessment is available from the American Association of Clinical Endocrinologists and the American College of Endocrinology.[37] No specific diagnostic criteria for obesity have been established.

Obesity is a chronic disease for which various treatment approaches have been used, including correction of metabolic abnormalities and individually tailored life style interventions, such as weight reduction diets and exercise programs. Additional treatments include psychotherapy, behavioral modification, self-motivation, and support systems.[38,39]

Several drugs have been approved for the pharmacologic management of obesity.[40] Currently, bariatric surgical procedures (i.e., the Roux-en-Y gastric bypass, adjustable gastric banding, and sleeve gastrectomy) offer the most significant reduction in weight, reduction in comorbidities, and decrease in insulin resistance for the treatment of obesity (see *Did You Know?* Outcomes of Bariatric Surgery). Efforts are continuing to identify the molecular and neuroendocrine causes of obesity. This will lead to more specific and personalized prevention and treatment strategies.

BOX 21.3 Metabolically Healthy Obesity

Metabolically healthy obesity (MHO, also known as the *obesity paradox*) describes a phenotype of about 10% to 30% of individuals who are obese but have no metabolic obesity–associated complications; specifically these individuals have high insulin sensitivity, an absence of metabolic syndrome, a high level of cardiorespiratory fitness, an adequate inflammatory profile (high adiponectin, and low C-reactive protein, tumor necrosis factor-alpha, and interleukin-6) and a decreased risk for morbidity and mortality. However, there is no standard definition for this phenotype, and complications related to pulmonary function and orthopedics, as well as other disorders, are often not described. MHO is more prevalent among those with an absence of visceral fat accumulation, among women, and among those who are more physically active. Research is in progress to better understand the genetics, body fat distribution patterns, metabolic pathways, adipocyte differentiation, lifestyle practices, age-related adverse outcomes, patterns of morbidity and mortality, and therapeutic options for these individuals.

Data from Goossens GH: *Obes Facts* 10(3):207-215, 2017; Neeland IJ, Poirier P, Després JP: Circulation 137(13):1391-1406, 2018.

DID YOU KNOW?
Outcomes of Bariatric Surgery

Bariatric surgery (BS), also known as *metabolic surgery*, results in significant and sustained weight loss, reduced fat mass, and control of obesity-related complications for individuals with severe obesity, including extremely obese children and adolescents, compared to other treatments. BS results in reduced insulin resistance, improved glycemic control, reduced levels of triglycerides, improved secretion of glucagon-like peptide 1 (GLP-1) with improved cardiovascular and liver function, resolution of metabolic syndrome and type 2 diabetes mellitus, and correction of sleep apnea. Improvements in cognitive function, including attention, executive function, and memory, have been documented. Depression and anxiety also have improved, but there may be lingering depression. Physical functioning improves but may be related to efficiency and not absolute improvement in cardiorespiratory or muscle function. More data is needed to understand the long-term complications, long-term survival, and microvascular and macrovascular events associated with BS. Changes in hypothalamic signaling also may occur, with increases in anorexigenic signals and decreases in orexigenic signals. However, more research is needed to understand these mechanisms of change in energy homeostasis and metabolism. Changes in the intestinal secretion of hormones and the microbiota also have been observed after BS, but the specific changes that may promote or inhibit weight loss have yet to be determined.

Data from Beamish AJ, Reinehr T: *Eur J Endocrinol* 176(4):D1-D15, 2017; Frikke-Schmidt H et al: *Obes Rev* 17(9):795-809, 2016; Jumbe S, Hamlet C, Meyrick J: *Curr Obes Rep* 2017 Mar;6(1):71-78, 2017; Kang JH, Le QA: *Medicine (Baltimore)* 96(46):e8632, 2017.

✔ QUICK CHECK 21.3

1. What is the difference between visceral (central) and peripheral (subcutaneous) obesity?
2. What factors contribute to the complications of obesity?
3. What are three treatment options for obesity?

STARVATION

Malnutrition is lack of nourishment from inadequate amounts of calories, protein, vitamins, or minerals and is caused by an improper diet, alterations in digestion or absorption, chronic disease, or a combination of these factors. Starvation is a reduction in energy intake that leads to weight loss. Short-term starvation and long-term starvation have different effects. Therapeutic short-term starvation is part of many weight reduction programs because it causes an initial rapid weight loss that reinforces the individual's motivation to diet. Therapeutic long-term starvation is used in medically controlled environments to facilitate rapid weight loss in morbidly obese individuals. Pathologic long-term starvation can be caused by poverty; chronic diseases of the cardiovascular, pulmonary, hepatic, and digestive systems; malabsorption syndromes; human immunodeficiency virus (HIV) infection; cancer; and anorexia nervosa.[41]

Short-term starvation, or extended fasting, consists of several days of total dietary abstinence or deprivation. The body responds with mechanisms to protect protein mass. For 4 to 6 hours after the last meal, the body is in a well-fed state and its energy requirements are supplied by glucose from recently ingested carbohydrates. Once all available energy has been absorbed from the intestine, glycogen in the liver is converted to glucose through glycogenolysis, the splitting of glycogen into glucose. This process peaks within 4 to 8 hours, and gluconeogenesis begins. Gluconeogenesis is the formation of glucose from noncarbohydrate molecules: lactate, pyruvate, amino acids, and the glycerol portion of fats from lipolysis. Like glycogenolysis, gluconeogenesis takes place within the liver. Both of these processes deplete stored nutrients and thus cannot meet the body's energy needs indefinitely. Lipolysis and proteins continue to be catabolized to a minimal degree, providing carbon for the synthesis of glucose.[42]

Long-term starvation begins after several days of dietary abstinence and eventually causes death from proteolysis. Absolute deprivation of food causes marasmus, or protein-energy malnutrition (loss of muscle mass, body fat depletion, and absence of edema). Protein deprivation in the presence of carbohydrate intake is called kwashiorkor (loss of muscle mass with sustained body fat). Marasmic kwashiorkor (edematous, severe childhood malnutrition) is a combination of chronic energy deficiency and chronic or acute protein deficiency and inadequate micronutrients.[43] These conditions are described in Chapter 39.

Anorexia nervosa is a psychological cause of long-term starvation. Cachexia (also known as cytokine-induced malnutrition) is physical wasting with loss of weight and muscle atrophy, fatigue, and weakness. Inflammatory mediators (i.e., TNF-α, interferon-γ, IL-1, and IL-6) and an increased catabolic response are associated with the cachexia.[44] Cancer, acquired immunodeficiency syndrome (AIDS), tuberculosis, and other major chronic progressive proinflammatory diseases contribute to cachexia. Anorexia and cachexia often occur together.

The major metabolic characteristic of long-term starvation is a decreased dependence on gluconeogenesis and an increased use of ketone bodies (products of lipid and pyruvate metabolism) as a cellular energy source. During long-term starvation, depressed insulin levels and increased levels of glucagon, cortisone, epinephrine, and growth hormones promote lipolysis in adipose tissue. Lipolysis liberates fatty acids, which supply energy to cardiac and skeletal muscle cells, and ketone bodies, which sustain brain tissue. Fatty acid, or ketone body, oxidation meets most of the energy needs of the cells. (Some glucose is still needed as fuel for brain tissue and red blood cells.) Once the supply of adipose tissue is depleted, proteolysis begins. The breakdown of muscle and visceral protein is the last process the body engages in to supply energy for life. Death results from severe alterations in electrolyte balance and loss of renal, pulmonary, and cardiac function.[45]

Adequate ingestion of appropriate nutrients is the obvious treatment for starvation. In medically induced starvation, the body is maintained in a ketotic state until the desired amount of adipose tissue has been lysed. Starvation imposed by chronic disease, long-term illness, malabsorption syndromes, and chronic eating disorders is treated with enteral or parenteral nutrition. Perioperative or critical care management of nutrition is necessary to prevent unnecessary starvation.[46] Care must be taken to prevent refeeding syndrome (Box 21.4) during the treatment of long-term starvation.

ANOREXIA OF AGING

Anorexia of aging is defined as a decrease in appetite or food intake in older adults. It can occur in illness-free individuals and with an adequate food supply. The resulting undernutrition leads to adverse outcomes and may affect up to 20% to 30% of elders.[47] The anorexia of aging results from multiple age-related changes, including reduced energy needs, waning hunger, diminished senses of smell and taste, decreased production of saliva, altered gastrointestinal satiety control mechanisms, and the presence of comorbidities. Centrally, aging is associated with decreased orexigenic signals (e.g., levels of ghrelin or ghrelin resistance and reduced hypothalamic receptors, or both) and increased anorexigenic signals (e.g., decreased levels of leptin, insulin, PPY, and CCK), which lead to loss of appetite and diminished food intake. Chronic low-grade inflammation with elevated cytokines also can contribute to delayed gastric emptying and decreased motility of the small intestine. Risk factors for the anorexia of aging include functional impairments and deficiencies (e.g., loss of vision, poor dentition, inability to prepare foods); medical and psychiatric conditions (e.g., malabsorption syndromes and depression); loneliness and grief; medications, including polypharmacy; social isolation; and abuse or neglect.[48] The consequences of anorexia of aging include malnutrition, physical frailty, mitochondrial dysfunction, reduced regenerative capacity,

---

BOX 21.4   Refeeding Syndrome

Refeeding syndrome is a life-threatening condition that occurs in severely malnourished individuals when parenteral or enteral nutritional therapy is initiated. During starvation, loss of body minerals causes the movement of phosphate, magnesium, and potassium ions out of the cells and into the plasma. When refeeding starts, an increase in insulin levels stimulates the movement of glucose and these ions back into the cells, and the plasma concentrations can decrease to dangerously low levels, causing hypophosphatemia, hypomagnesemia, hypokalemia, hyponatremia, hypocalcemia, and vitamin deficiency (particularly thiamin). Alterations usually occur within 72 hours after the start of nutritional therapy.

Hypophosphatemia contributes to alterations in red blood cell shape and function, contributing to tissue hypoxia and increased respiratory drive. Rapid expansion of the extracellular fluid volume also can occur with carbohydrate refeeding and may cause fluid overload. The consequences of these alterations include life-threatening dysrhythmias, congestive heart failure, muscle weakness (including respiratory muscles), and death. Individuals at greatest risk are those with starvation from any cause, including anorexia nervosa, chronic diseases, aging, morbid obesity with massive weight loss, and prolonged fasting. Refeeding syndrome is prevented by identifying at-risk individuals; slowly reinstituting feeding (about 20 kcal/kg/day for the first few days); and monitoring plasma levels of phosphate, potassium, magnesium, and calcium during the change from catabolic to anabolic metabolism.

Data from Aubry E et al: *Clin Exp Gastroenterol* 11:255-264, 2018; Crook MA: *Nutrition* 30(11-12):1448-1455, 2014.

increased oxidative stress, and imbalanced hormones. Currently no specific treatments exist for the anorexia of aging, although numerous supportive strategies are used (e.g., improved food access and appearance, dental and eye care, social stimulation). Mortality rates have been shown to be higher in those with anorexia of aging and unintentional weight loss.[49]

> ✔ **QUICK CHECK 21.3**
> 1. How are glucose levels maintained during short-term starvation?
> 2. What is the difference between marasmus and kwashiorkor?
> 3. What causes death in long-term starvation?
> 4. What factors contribute to the anorexia of aging?

▮ SUMMARY REVIEW

Adipose Tissue

1. Adipose tissue provides insulation and tissue support and is the body's major energy reserve, storing and releasing triglycerides and glycerol.
2. Adipose tissue is classified according to color: WAT, BAT, and bAT.
3. WAT contains macrophages, mast cells, neutrophils, fibroblasts, endothelial cells, blood vessels, nerves, and precursor adipocytes.
4. WAT is the largest fat depot and is located in visceral (central) and subcutaneous (peripheral) sites. It also is located in muscle and bone marrow.
5. White adipocytes store fat as a single lipid droplet or vacuole.
6. With a positive energy balance, WAT storage increases by adipocyte hypertrophy (more common in visceral fat) and adipogenesis (hyperplasia, more common in subcutaneous fat).
7. Estrogen enhances the deposition of subcutaneous fat compared to visceral fat.
8. BAT has multiple lipid droplets that are rich in mitochondria containing iron, which gives them a brown color. Exposure to cold, sympathetic activation and release of catecholamines, and activation of T_3 generates heat through free fatty acid oxidation (nonshivering thermogenesis).
9. Both neonates and adults have BAT, but not in the amounts of WAT.
10. bAT emerges within WAT with exposure to cold and exercise. This is known as the beiging of WAT.
11. BAT and bAT both protect against obesity and metabolic syndrome.
12. MAT is found in all bones. With obesity, MAT releases adipokines that affect osteoblast and osteoclast function. Excessive MAT is associated with osteoporosis and fractures.
13. Adipose tissue is an endocrine organ that secretes hormones, called *adipokines,* with autocrine, paracrine, and endocrine actions necessary for metabolic function and immune responses.
14. Regulation of food intake and energy balance are accomplished by balancing opposing sets of neurons in the arcuate nucleus: orexigenic neurons (promote appetite, stimulate eating, and decrease metabolism) and anorexigenic neurons (suppress appetite, inhibit eating, and increase metabolism). Peripherally, gastrointestinal hormones and adipokines also control food intake and energy expenditure.
15. Brain centers related to reward, pleasure, memory, and addictive behavior can override hypothalamic control of food intake and satiety, causing increased fat stores by increasing consumption of highly palatable foods.

Obesity

1. Obesity is an increase in body adipose tissue and an endocrine and metabolic disorder that develops when caloric intake exceeds energy expenditure. Obesity is defined as a BMI greater than 30 kg/m² in adults and a BMI greater than or equal to the age- and sex-specific 95th percentile of the 2000 CDC growth charts in children.
2. Obesity is an epidemic that has occurred worldwide in both adults and children. It is the fifth leading cause of death in the United States. Three leading causes of death in the U.S. are associated with obesity: cardiovascular disease, type 2 diabetes mellitus, and certain cancers. Obesity also increases the risk for numerous other systemic disorders.
3. Single-gene (rare) and polygenic disorders and metabolic disorders are associated with obesity, as are gene–environment interactions.
4. Adipokines and gastrointestinal hormones are altered with obesity and contribute to associated complications.
5. Leptin resistance occurs when leptin levels increase with obesity and promote overeating and excessive weight gain, hyperglycemia, hyperinsulinemia, and hyperlipidemia. It also stimulates macrophages and endothelial cells to produce proinflammatory mediators.
6. Adiponectin levels decrease with obesity, contributing to insulin resistance, inflammation, and hyperlipidemia.
7. Retinol-binding protein 4 levels are increased in visceral adiposity and promote insulin resistance and hepatic steatosis.
8. Endocannabinoids are increased in obesity and promote appetite, enhance nutrient absorption, stimulate lipogenesis, and inhibit energy expenditure.
9. Angiotensinogen and angiotensin 2 increase in obesity, promoting vasoconstriction, inflammation, lipogenesis, oxidative stress, and insulin resistance.
10. Gastrointestinal hormones (ghrelin, GLP-1, PYY, and CCK) also provide signals that control food intake and energy expenditure and are involved in the pathophysiology of obesity.
11. Ghrelin increases with obesity and stimulates food intake, promotes the release of growth hormone, and stimulates lipogenesis. It also has satiety, vasodilatory, cardioprotective, and antiproliferative effects; its role in obesity is not clear.
12. GLP-1 promotes insulin secretion, delays gastric emptying, suppresses appetite, increases satiety, increases energy expenditure, and is decreased with obesity.
13. PYY inhibits gastric motility, decreases appetite, and is decreased with obesity.
14. CCK is released after food intake and stimulates insulin secretion and satiation, decreases food intake, and is reduced in obesity.
15. Lipotoxicity occurs with excess adipocyte fat storage and lipolysis with distribution of free fatty acids to peripheral organs, resulting in cellular dysfunction and death.
16. Obesity is a state of chronic low-grade inflammation caused by expansion of adipocyte macrophages, neutrophils, lymphocytes, and mast cells, which release inflammatory mediators.
17. The chronic inflammation, alterations in adipokine action, and accelerated lipolysis related to excessive fat contribute to the complications of obesity, particularly insulin resistance, type 2 diabetes mellitus, cardiovascular disease, and cancer.
18. Changes in the intestinal microbiome also contribute to obesity, but the mechanisms need to be defined.
19. Obesity has two major phenotypes: visceral obesity (also known as intra-abdominal, central, or masculine obesity) and peripheral

obesity (also known as subcutaneous, gluteal-femoral, or feminine obesity). Visceral obesity has the greatest risk for accelerated lipolysis, chronic inflammation, insulin resistance, and associated complications.

20. Normal-weight obesity describes individuals with a normal body weight and BMI but with greater than 30% body fat. These individuals are at risk for metabolic dysregulation, increases in inflammatory cytokines, insulin resistance, increased risk for cardiovascular disease, and higher mortality.

21. Treatment of obesity may include correction of metabolic abnormalities and individually tailored lifestyle interventions (diets, exercise, behavioral modifications, self-motivation) and psychotherapy. The current most effective treatment for extreme obesity is bariatric surgery.

22. New drugs are being developed that target specific molecules and will provide a personalized approach to treatment.

Starvation

1. The body responds to short-term starvation (several days of total dietary abstinence or deprivation) with mechanisms to protect protein mass, using the processes of glycogenolysis and gluconeogenesis. Neither of these processes can meet the body's energy needs indefinitely because they deplete stored nutrients.

2. Long-term starvation (begins after several days of dietary abstinence) results in an initial decreased dependence on gluconeogenesis and an increased use of ketone bodies as a cellular energy source, followed by lipolysis in adipose tissue. In the absence of adequate nutrition, long-term starvation results in proteolysis, with death resulting from severe alterations in electrolyte balance and loss of renal, pulmonary, and cardiac function.

Anorexia of Aging

1. Anorexia of aging is a decrease in appetite or food intake in older adults that leads to undernutrition, resulting in a decline in function and an increased risk for morbidity and mortality.

2. Contributing factors related to aging include diminished sensory functions, poor dentition, decreased gastric emptying, decreased hunger and satiety, effects of medications, and social isolation and neglect.

KEY TERMS

Adipocyte, 474
Adipokine, 475
Adiponectin, 478
Adipose tissue, 474
Angiotensinogen (AGT), 478
Anorexia nervosa, 480
Beige adipocyte, 475
Brown adipocyte, 474

Cachexia, 480
Cholecystokinin (CCK), 478
Endocannabinoid, 478
Ghrelin, 478
Glucagon-like peptide 1 (GLP-1), 478
Kwashiorkor, 480
Leptin, 477

Leptin resistance, 477
Malnutrition, 480
Marasmus, 480
Metabolically healthy obesity, 479
Normal-weight obesity (NWO), 479
Obesity, 476

Obesogen, 476
Peptide YY (PYY), 478
Peripheral obesity, 479
Refeeding syndrome, 480
Retinol-binding protein 4, 478
Starvation, 480
Visceral obesity, 479
White adipocyte, 474

REFERENCES

1. Kwok KH, Lam KS, Xu A: Heterogeneity of white adipose tissue: molecular basis and clinical implications, *Exp Mol Med* 48:e215, 2016.
2. Lee MJ, Wu Y, Fried SK: Adipose tissue heterogeneity: implication of depot differences in adipose tissue for obesity complications, *Mol Aspects Med* 34(1):1-11, 2013.
3. Palmer BF, Clegg DJ: The sexual dimorphism of obesity, *Mol Cell Endocrinol* 402:113-119, 2015.
4. Suchacki KJ, Cawthorn WP: Molecular interaction of bone marrow adipose tissue with energy metabolism, *Curr Mol Biol Rep* 4(2):41-49, 2018.
5. Kiefer FW: Browning and thermogenic programing of adipose tissue, *Best Pract Res Clin Endocrinol Metab* 30(4):479-485, 2016.
6. Gantner ML, et al: Complementary roles of estrogen-related receptors in brown adipocyte thermogenic function, *Endocrinology* 157(12):4770-4781, 2016.
7. Virtanen KA: The rediscovery of BAT in adult humans using imaging, *Best Pract Res Clin Endocrinol Metab* 30(4):471-477, 2016.
8. Ikeda K, Maretich P, Kajimura S: The common and distinct features of brown and beige adipocytes, *Trends Endocrinol Metab* 29(3):191-200, 2018.
9. Mulya A, Kirwan JP: Brown and beige adipose tissue: therapy for obesity and its comorbidities?, *Endocrinol Metab Clin North Am* 45(3):605-621, 2016.
10. Booth A, et al: Adipose tissue: an endocrine organ playing a role in metabolic regulation, *Horm Mol Biol Clin Investig* 26(1):25-42, 2016.
11. Abdalla MM: Central and peripheral control of food intake, *Endocr Regul* 51(1):52-70, 2017.
12. Gadde KM, et al: Obesity: pathophysiology and management, *J Am Coll Cardiol* 71(1):69-84, 2018.

13. Centers for Disease Control and Prevention (CDC): Overweight and obesity, last reviewed April 1, 2019. Available at: https://www.cdc.gov/obesity. (Accessed 11 June 2019).
14. Hales CM, et al: *Prevalence of obesity among adults and youth: United States, 2015–2016, National Center for Health Statistics (NCHS) data brief, no 288,* Hyattsville MD, 2017, National Center for Health Statistics. Available at: https://www.cdc.gov/nchs/products/databriefs/db288.htm.
15. Smith KB, Smith MS: Obesity statistics, *Prim Care* 43(1):121-135, 2016.
16. Lauby-Secretan B, et al: Body fatness and cancer—viewpoint of the IARC Working Group, *N Engl J Med* 375:794-798, 2016.
17. Wang S, Ren J: Obesity paradox in aging: from prevalence to pathophysiology, *Prog Cardiovasc Dis* 61(2):182-189, 2018.
18. Albuquerque D, et al: Current review of genetics of human obesity: from molecular mechanisms to an evolutionary perspective, *Mol Genet Genomics* 290(4):1191-1221, 2015.
19. Jantaratnotai N, et al: The interface of depression and obesity, *Obes Res Clin Pract* 11(1):1-10, 2017.
20. Heymsfield SB, Wadden TA: Mechanisms, pathophysiology, and management of obesity, *N Engl J Med* 376(3):254-266, 2017.
21. Mishra AK, Dubey V, Ghosh AR: Obesity: an overview of possible role(s) of gut hormones, lipid sensing and gut microbiota, *Metabolism* 65(1):48-65, 2016.
22. Friedman J: The long road to leptin, *J Clin Invest* 126(12):4727-4734, 2016.
23. Wang ZV, Scherer PE: Adiponectin, the past two decades, *J Mol Cell Biol* 8(2):93-100, 2016.
24. Liu Y, et al: Retinol-binding protein 4 induces hepatic mitochondrial dysfunction and promotes hepatic steatosis, *J Clin Endocrinol Metab* 101(11):4338-4348, 2016.

25. Mazier W, et al: The endocannabinoid system: pivotal orchestrator of obesity and metabolic disease, *Trends Endocrinol Metab* 26(10):524-537, 2015.
26. Ramalingam L, et al: The renin angiotensin system, oxidative stress and mitochondrial function in obesity and insulin resistance, *Biochim Biophys Acta* 1863(5):1106-1114, 2016.
27. Cui H, López M, Rahmouni K: The cellular and molecular bases of leptin and ghrelin resistance in obesity, *Nat Rev Endocrinol* 13(6):338-351, 2017.
28. Burcelin R, Gourdy P: Harnessing glucagon-like peptide-1 receptor agonists for the pharmacological treatment of overweight and obesity, *Obes Rev* 18(1):86-98, 2016.
29. Miller LJ, Desai AJ: Metabolic actions of the type 1 cholecystokinin receptor: its potential as a therapeutic target, *Trends Endocrinol Metab* 27(9):609-619, 2016.
30. Ertunc ME, Hotamisligil GS: Lipid signaling and lipotoxicity in metaflammation: indications for metabolic disease pathogenesis and treatment, *J Lipid Res* 57(12):2099-2114, 2016.
31. Chatzigeorgiou A, Chavakis T: Immune cells and metabolism, *Handb Exp Pharmacol* 233:221-249, 2016.
32. Ellulu MS, et al: Obesity and inflammation: the linking mechanism and the complications, *Arch Med Sci* 13(4):851-863, 2017.
33. Komaroff AL: The microbiome and risk for obesity and diabetes, *J Am Med Assoc* 317(4):355-3356, 2017.
34. Goossens GH: The metabolic phenotype in obesity: fat mass, body fat distribution, and adipose tissue function, *Obes Facts* 10(3):207-215, 2017.
35. Lopes HF, et al: Visceral adiposity syndrome, *Diabetol Metab Syndr* 8:40, 2016.
36. Franco LP, Morais CC, Cominetti C: Normal-weight obesity syndrome: diagnosis, prevalence, and clinical implications, *Nutr Rev* 74(9):558-570, 2016.

37. Garvey WT, et al: American Association of Clinical Endocrinologists and American College of Endocrinology position statement on the 2014 advanced framework for a new diagnosis of obesity as a chronic disease, *Endocr Pract* 20:977-989, 2014.

38. Golden A: Current pharmacotherapies for obesity: a practical perspective, *J Am Assoc Nurse Pract* 29(S1):S 43-S52, 2017.

39. Tsai AG, et al: Treatment of obesity in primary care, *Med Clin North Am* 102(1):35-47, 2018.

40. Bray GA, et al: Management of obesity, *Lancet* 387(10031):1947-1956, 2016.

41. Jensen GL, Wheeler D: A new approach to defining and diagnosing malnutrition in adult critical illness, *Curr Opin Crit Care* 18(2):206-211, 2012.

42. Finn PF, Dice JF: Proteolytic and lipolytic responses to starvation, *Nutrition* 22(7-8):830-844, 2006.

43. Tierney EP, Sage RJ, Shwayder T: Kwashiorkor from a severe dietary restriction in an 8-month infant in suburban Detroit, Michigan: case report and review of the literature, *Int J Dermatol* 49(5):500-506, 2010.

44. Petruzzelli M, Wagner EF: Mechanisms of metabolic dysfunction in cancer-associated cachexia, *Genes Dev* 30(5):489-501, 2016.

45. Berkley JA, et al: Prognostic indicators of early and late death in children admitted to district hospital in Kenya: cohort study, *BMJ* 326(7385):361, 2003.

46. Reintam Blaser A, Berger MM: Early or late feeding after ICU admission?, *Nutrients* 9(12):E1278, 2017.

47. Sanford AM: Anorexia of aging and its role in frailty, *Curr Opin Clin Nutr Metab Care* 20(1):54-60, 2017.

48. Landi F, et al: Anorexia of aging: assessment and management, *Clin Geriatr Med* 33(3):315-323, 2017.

49. Wysokiński A, et al: Mechanisms of the anorexia of aging—a review, *Age (Dordr)* 37(4):9821, 2015.

22

Structure and Function of the Hematologic System

Sue E. Huether

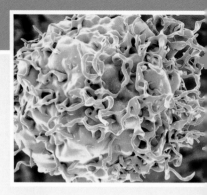

EVOLVE WEBSITE

http://evolve.elsevier.com/Huether/
Student Review Questions
Audio Key Points

Case Studies
Animations
Quick Check Answers

CHAPTER OUTLINE

All the body's tissues and organs require oxygen and nutrients to survive. These essential needs are provided by the blood that flows through miles of vessels throughout the human body. The red blood cells provide the oxygen, and the fluid portion of the blood carries the nutrients. The blood also cleans discarded waste from the tissues and transports cells (white blood cells) and other ingredients that are necessary for protecting the entire body from injury and infection.

COMPONENTS OF THE HEMATOLOGIC SYSTEM

Composition of Blood

Blood consists of various cells that circulate suspended in a solution of protein and inorganic materials (plasma), which is approximately 91% water and 9% dissolved substances (solutes). The blood volume amounts to about 6 quarts (5.5 L) in adults. The continuous movement of blood guarantees that critical components are available to all parts of the body to carry out their chief functions: (1) delivery of substances needed for cellular metabolism in the tissues, (2) removal of the wastes of cellular metabolism, (3) defense against invading microorganisms and injury, and (4) maintenance of acid–base balance.

Plasma and Plasma Proteins

In adults, plasma accounts for 50% to 55% of blood volume (Fig. 22.1). Plasma is a complex aqueous liquid containing a variety of organic and inorganic elements (Table 22.1). The concentration of these elements varies, depending on diet, metabolic demand, hormones, and vitamins. Plasma differs from serum in that serum is free of clotting proteins (e.g., fibrinogen). The clotting proteins may interfere with some diagnostic tests.

Plasma contains a large number of proteins (plasma proteins). These vary in structure and function and can be classified primarily into two major groups, albumin and globulins, plus a small amount of clotting proteins. Most plasma proteins are produced by the liver. The major exception is antibody, which is produced by plasma cells (B cells) in the lymph nodes and other lymphoid tissues (see Chapter 7).

Albumin (about 57% of total plasma protein) serves as a carrier molecule for both normal components of blood and drugs. Its most essential role is regulation of the passage of water and solutes through the capillaries. Albumin molecules are large and do not diffuse freely through the vascular endothelium, and thus they maintain the critical colloidal osmotic pressure (or oncotic pressure) that regulates the passage of fluids and electrolytes into the surrounding tissues (see Chapters 1 and 5). Water and solute particles tend to diffuse out of the arterial portions of the capillaries because blood pressure (hydrostatic pressure) is greater in arterial than in venous blood vessels. Water and solutes move from tissues into the venous portions of the capillaries, where the pressures are reversed, oncotic pressure being greater than intravascular pressure or hydrostatic pressure (see Fig. 5.1). In the case of decreased production of albumin (e.g., cirrhosis, other diffuse liver diseases, protein malnutrition) or excessive loss of albumin (e.g., certain kidney diseases), the reduced plasma oncotic pressure leads to excessive movement of water and solutes into the tissue and decreased blood volume.

Most of the remaining plasma proteins are globulins (about 38% of total plasma protein), which are often classified by their properties in

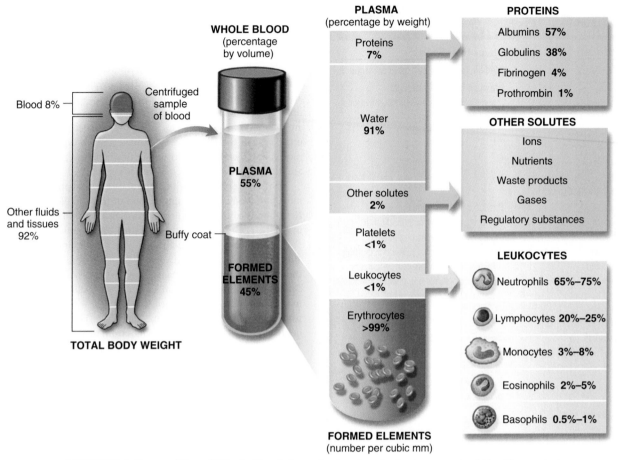

FIGURE 22.1 Composition of Whole Blood. Approximate values for the components of blood in a normal adult. (From Patton KT, Thibodeau GA: *The human body in health & disease*, ed 7, St Louis, 2018, Mosby.)

an electric field (serum electrophoresis). Under the normal conditions used to perform serum electrophoresis, albumin is the most rapidly moving protein. The globulins are classified by their movement relative to albumin: alpha globulins (those moving most closely to albumin) include high-density lipoproteins [HDLs], prothrombin, and proteins that transport hormones, beta globulins (includes low-density lipoproteins [LDLs]), and gamma globulins (those with the least movement). The gamma-globulin region consists primarily of antibodies (see Chapter 7).

Plasma proteins also can be classified by function: clotting, defense, transport, or regulation. The clotting factors or proteins promote coagulation and stop bleeding from damaged blood vessels. Fibrinogen is the most plentiful of the clotting factors and is the precursor of the fibrin clot (see Fig. 22.16). Proteins involved in defense, or protection, against infection include antibodies and complement proteins (see Chapters 6 and 7). Transport proteins specifically bind and carry a variety of inorganic and organic molecules, including iron (transferrin), copper (ceruloplasmin), lipids and steroid hormones (lipoproteins) (see Chapter 1), and vitamins (e.g., retinol-binding protein for vitamin A transport). Regulatory proteins include a variety of enzymatic inhibitors (e.g., α_1-antitrypsin) that protect the tissues from damage; precursor molecules (e.g., kininogen) that are converted into active biologic molecules when needed; and protein hormones (e.g., cytokines) that communicate between cells.

Plasma also contains several inorganic ions that regulate cell function, osmotic pressure, and blood pH. These include electrolytes; sodium,

potassium, calcium, chloride, and phosphate. (Electrolytes are described in Chapters 1 and 5.)

Cellular Components of the Blood

The cellular elements of the blood are broadly classified as red blood cells (erythrocytes), white blood cells (leukocytes), and platelets. The components of the blood are listed in Table 22.2.

Erythrocytes. Erythrocytes (red blood cells) are the most abundant cells of the blood, occupying approximately 48% of the blood volume in men and about 42% in women. There are 4.2 to 6.2 million erythrocytes/mm³ circulating in normal blood. Erythrocytes are primarily responsible for tissue oxygenation. Hemoglobin (Hb) carries the gases, and electrolytes regulate gas diffusion through the cell's plasma membrane. The mature erythrocyte lacks a nucleus and cytoplasmic organelles (e.g., mitochondria), so it cannot synthesize protein or carry out oxidative reactions. Because it cannot undergo mitotic division, the erythrocyte has a limited life span (approximately 100 to 120 days).

The erythrocyte's size and shape are ideally suited to its function as a gas carrier. It is a small disk with two unique properties: (1) a *biconcave* shape and (2) the capacity to be *reversibly deformed*. The flattened, biconcave shape provides a surface area/volume ratio that is optimal for gas diffusion into and out of the cell and for deformity. During its life span, the erythrocyte, which is 6 to 8 μm in diameter, repeatedly circulates through splenic sinusoids and capillaries that are only 2 μm in diameter. Reversible deformity enables the erythrocyte to assume a

TABLE 22.1 Organic and Inorganic Components of Arterial Plasma

Constituent	Major Functions
Water	Medium for carrying all other constituents
Electrolytes Na$^+$ K$^+$ Ca^{2+} Mg^{2+} Cl$^-$ HCO$_3^-$ Phosphate (mostly HPO$_4^-$)	Maintain H$_2$O in extracellular compartment; act as buffers; function in membrane excitability
Proteins Albumins Globulins Fibrinogen Transferrin Ferritin	Provide colloid osmotic pressure of plasma; act as buffers; bind other plasma constituents (e.g., lipids, hormones, vitamins, minerals); clotting factors; enzymes; enzyme precursors; antibodies (immunoglobulins); hormones; transporters
Gases CO$_2$ content O$_2$ N$_2$	 By-product of oxygenation, most CO$_2$ content is from HCO$_3^-$ and acts as buffer Oxygenation By-product of protein catabolism
Nutrients Glucose and other carbohydrates Total amino acids Total lipids Cholesterol Individual vitamins Individual trace elements Iron	Provide nutrition and substances for tissue repair
Waste Products Urea Creatinine (from creatine) Uric acid (from nucleic acids) Bilirubin (from heme)	 End product of protein catabolism End product from energy metabolism End product from protein metabolism End product of red blood cell destruction
Individual hormones	Functions specific to target tissue

BUN, Blood urea nitrogen; *Ca^{2+},* calcium; *Cl$^-$,* chloride; *CO$_2$,* carbon dioxide; *H$_2$O,* water; *HCO$_3^-$,* bicarbonate; *HPO$_4^-$,* phosphorus; *K$^+$,* potassium; *Mg^{2+},* magnesium; *N$_2$,* nitrogen; *Na$^+$,* sodium. Data from Vander AJ et al: *Human physiology: the mechanisms of body function,* New York, 2001, McGraw-Hill.

more compact torpedo-like shape, squeeze through the microcirculation (diapedesis), and return to normal (Fig. 22.2).

Leukocytes. Leukocytes (white blood cells) defend the body against organisms that cause infection and also remove debris, including dead or injured host cells of all kinds (Fig. 22.3). The leukocytes act primarily in the tissues but are transported in the circulation. The average adult has approximately 5000 to 10,000 leukocytes/mm^3 of blood.

Leukocytes are classified according to structure as either granulocytes or agranulocytes and according to function as either phagocytes or immunocytes. The granulocytes, which include neutrophils, basophils, and eosinophils, are all phagocytes. (Phagocytic action is described in Chapter 6.) Of the agranulocytes, the monocytes and macrophages are phagocytes, whereas the lymphocytes are immunocytes (cells that create immunity; see Chapter 7).

Granulocytes. The granulocytes have a nucleus with several lobes (polymorphonuclear) and many membrane-bound granules in their cytoplasm. These granules contain enzymes capable of killing microorganisms and catabolizing debris ingested during phagocytosis. The granules also contain powerful biochemical mediators with inflammatory and immune functions. These mediators, along with the digestive enzymes, are released from granulocytes in response to specific stimuli and affect other cells in the circulation. Granulocytes are capable of amoeboid movement, by which they migrate through vessel walls (diapedesis) and then to sites where their action is needed.

The neutrophil (polymorphonuclear neutrophil [PMN]) is the most numerous and best understood of the granulocytes (Fig. 22.4). Neutrophils constitute about 65% to 75% of the total leukocyte count in adults. The results vary by laboratory and populations studied.

Neutrophils are the chief phagocytes of early inflammation. Soon after bacterial invasion or tissue injury, neutrophils migrate out of the capillaries and into the damaged tissue, where they ingest and destroy contaminating microorganisms and debris. Neutrophils are sensitive to the environment in damaged tissue (e.g., low pH, enzymes released from damaged cells) and die in 1 or 2 days. The breakdown of dead neutrophils releases digestive enzymes from their cytoplasmic granules. These enzymes dissolve cellular debris and prepare the site for healing.

Eosinophils, which have large, coarse granules, constitute only about 2% to 5% of the normal leukocyte count in adults. Using a spectrum of pattern-recognition receptors, eosinophils are capable of amoeboid movement and phagocytosis. Unlike neutrophils, eosinophils ingest antigen-antibody complexes and are induced by immunoglobulin E (IgE)–mediated hypersensitivity reactions to attack parasites[1] (see Chapter 7). Eosinophil secondary granules contain toxic chemicals (e.g., major basic protein, eosinophil cationic protein, eosinophil peroxidase, eosinophil-derived neurotoxin) that are highly destructive to parasites and viruses. Eosinophil granules also contain a variety of enzymes (e.g., histaminase) that help control inflammatory processes. Eosinophils also release proinflammatory molecules, including leukotrienes, prostaglandins, platelet-activating factor (PAF), and a variety of cytokines (e.g., interleukin-1 [IL-1], IL-6, tumor necrosis factor-alpha [TNF-α], granulocyte-macrophage colony-stimulating factor [GM-CSF]) and chemokines (e.g., IL-8). Type I hypersensitivity allergic reactions and asthma are characterized by high eosinophil counts that may be involved in a dual role: regulation of inflammation and contribution to the destructive inflammatory processes observed in allergic reactions and the lungs of persons with asthma.

Basophils, which make up less than 1% of leukocytes, are structurally similar to the mast cells (see Fig. 22.4). Basophils contain cytoplasmic granules with histamine, chemotactic factors, proteolytic enzymes (e.g., elastase, lysophospholipase), and an anticoagulant (heparin). Stimulation of basophils also induces synthesis of vasoactive lipid molecules (e.g., leukotrienes) and cytokines, including IL-6, which affects differentiation of type 1 T-helper cells (Th1 cells) (focus on intracellular parasites) and type 2 T-helper cell (Th2 cells) (focus on extracellular parasites). Basophils also are a particularly rich source of the cytokine IL-4, which preferentially guides B-cell differentiation toward plasma cells that secrete IgE (see Chapter 7).

Agranulocytes. The agranulocytes—monocytes, macrophages, and lymphocytes—contain relatively fewer granules than granulocytes. Monocytes and macrophages make up the mononuclear phagocyte system (MPS) (see Chapter 6). Both monocytes and macrophages participate in the immune and inflammatory response, being powerful phagocytes. They also ingest dead or defective host cells, particularly blood cells.

TABLE 22.2 Cellular Components of the Blood

Cell	Structural Characteristics	Function	Life Span
Erythrocyte (red blood cell)	Nonnucleated cytoplasmic disk containing hemoglobin	Gas transport to and from tissue cells and lungs	80-120 days
Leukocyte (white blood cell)	Nucleated cell	Body defense mechanisms	See below
Neutrophil	Segmented polymorphonuclear granulocyte	Phagocytosis, particularly during early phase of inflammation	4 days
Eosinophil	Segmented polymorphonuclear granulocyte	Control of inflammation, phagocytosis, defense against parasites, allergic reactions	Unknown
Basophil	Segmented polymorphonuclear granulocyte	Mast cell–like functions, associated with allergic reactions	Unknown
Monocyte and macrophage	Large mononuclear phagocyte	Phagocytosis; mononuclear phagocyte system	Months or years
Lymphocyte	Mononuclear immunocyte	Humoral and cell-mediated immunity (see Chapter 7)	Days or years, depending on type
Natural killer cell	Large granular lymphocyte	Defense against some tumors and viruses (see Chapters 6 and 7)	Unknown
Platelet	Irregularly shaped cytoplasmic fragment (not a cell)	Hemostasis after vascular injury; normal coagulation and clot formation/retraction; release of growth factors	8-11 days

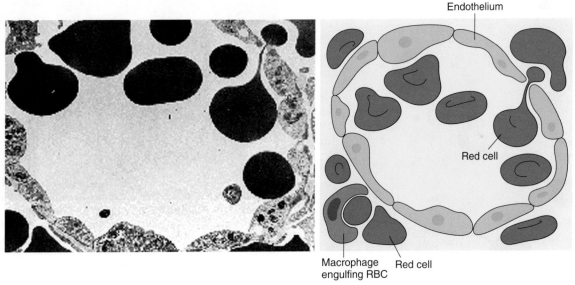

FIGURE 22.2 Red Cells Moving in the Spleen. Transmission electron micrograph and schematic of erythrocytes in the process of moving by diapedesis from the red pulp cords into the sinus lumen. They resume their normal shape after squeezing through. Note the degree of deformability required for red cells to pass through the wall of the sinus. (From Damjanov I, Linder J, editors: *Anderson's pathology*, ed 10, St Louis, 1996, Mosby. Schematic from Kumar V, Fausto N, Abbas A: *Robbins & Cotran pathologic basis of disease*, ed 7, St Louis, 2005, Saunders.)

Monocytes are immature macrophages (see Fig. 22.4). Monocytes are formed and released by the bone marrow into the bloodstream. As they mature, monocytes migrate into a variety of tissues (e.g., liver, spleen, lymph nodes, peritoneum, gastrointestinal tract) and fully mature into tissue macrophages to become part of the MPS. Other monocytes may mature into macrophages and migrate out of the vessels in response to infection or inflammation.

The mononuclear phagocyte system (MPS) (formerly called the reticuloendothelial system) consists of monocytes that differentiate without dividing and reside in the tissues for months or perhaps years. Cells of the MPS ingest and destroy (by phagocytosis) unwanted materials, such as foreign protein particles, circulating immune complexes,

microorganisms, debris from dead or injured cells, defective or injured erythrocytes, and dead neutrophils. Table 22.3 lists the various names given to macrophages localized in specific tissues.

Lymphocytes constitute about 20% to 25% of the total leukocyte count and are the primary cells of the immune response (see Fig. 22.4 and Chapter 6. Most lymphocytes transiently circulate in the blood and eventually reside in lymphoid tissues as mature T cells, B cells, or plasma cells.

Natural killer (NK) cells, which resemble lymphocytes, kill some types of tumor cells (in vitro) and some virus-infected cells without prior exposure (see Chapters 6 and 7). They develop in the bone marrow and circulate in the blood.

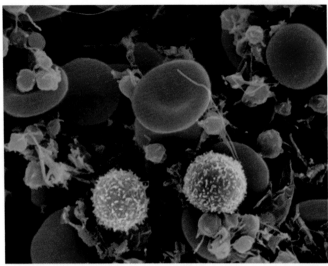

FIGURE 22.3 Blood Cells and Platelets. Leukocytes are spherical and have irregular surfaces with numerous extending pili. Leukocytes are the cotton candy–like cells *(yellow)*. Erythrocytes are flattened spheres with a depressed center *(red)*. Platelets are the smaller *(green)* cell fragments. (Copyright Dennis Kunkel Microscopy, Inc.)

TABLE 22.3 Mononuclear Phagocyte System

Name of Cell	Location
Monocytes/macrophages	Bone marrow and peripheral blood
Kupffer cells (inflammatory macrophages)	Liver
Alveolar macrophages	Lung
Histiocytes	Connective tissue
Macrophages	Bone marrow
Fixed and free macrophages	Spleen and lymph nodes
Pleural and peritoneal macrophages	Serous cavities
Microglial cells	Nervous system
Mesangial cells	Kidney
Osteoclasts	Bone
Langerhans cells	Skin
Dendritic cells	Lymphoid tissue

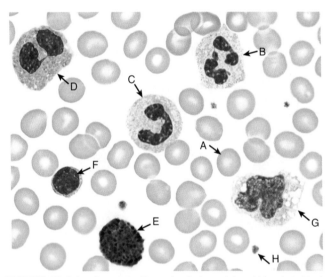

FIGURE 22.4 Leukocytes. Normal cells in peripheral blood. **A,** Erythrocyte (red blood cell). **B,** Neutrophil (segmented); **C,** Neutrophil (banded); **D,** Eosinophil; **E,** Basophil; **F,** Lymphocyte; **G,** Monocyte; **H,** Platelet. (From Keohane E, Smith L, Walenga J: *Rodak's hematology,* ed 5, St. Louis, 2016, Saunders).

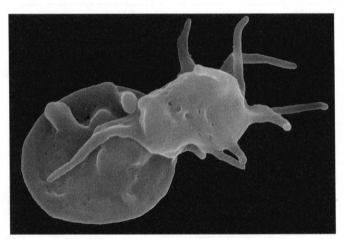

FIGURE 22.5 Colored Micrograph of Platelets. The platelet on the left is moderately activated, with a generally round shape and the beginning of formation of pseudopodia (footlike extensions from the membrane). The platelet on the right is fully activated, with extensive pseudopodia. (Copyright Dennis Kunkel Microscopy, Inc.)

Platelets. Platelets (thrombocytes) are not true cells, but rather irregularly shaped anuclear cytoplasmic fragments that are essential for blood coagulation and control of bleeding. They are formed in the bone marrow by fragmentation of very large cells (40 to 100 μm in diameter) known as megakaryocytes. They contain cytoplasmic granules and can release adhesive proteins and coagulation and growth factors when stimulated by injury to a blood vessel. Platelets can assume different shapes and form adhesive pseudopodia (long surface extensions) that increase their surface area and promote interconnectedness and adherence to collagen fibers in damaged vascular walls, plugging vascular openings to control bleeding (Fig. 22.5).

The normal platelet concentration is about 150,000 to 400,000 platelets/mm^3 of circulating blood, although the normal ranges may vary slightly from laboratory to laboratory. An additional one-third of the body's available platelets are in a reserve pool in the spleen. A platelet circulates for approximately 8 to 11 days, and is then removed by macrophages, mostly in the spleen.

> ✔ **QUICK CHECK 22.1**
> 1. What are the unique properties of the erythrocyte's shape?
> 2. Why are plasma proteins important to blood volume?
> 3. Which leukocytes are granulocytes?
> 4. Compare and contrast granulocytes, agranulocytes, phagocytes, and immunocytes.
> 5. What is the MPS?

Lymphoid Organs

The lymphoid system is closely integrated with the circulatory system. The lymphoid organs, some of which are merely aggregations of lymphoid tissue, are classified as primary or secondary. The **primary lymphoid** organs are the thymus and the bone marrow. The secondary lymphoid organs consist of the spleen, lymph nodes, tonsils, and Peyer patches in the ileum of the small intestine. All of the lymphoid organs link the hematologic and immune systems in that they are sites of residence, proliferation, differentiation, or function of lymphocytes and mononuclear phagocytes (monocytes and macrophages). The liver, which is primarily a digestive organ and is described in Chapter 37, synthesizes both coagulant and anticoagulant proteins.

Spleen

The spleen is the largest of the lymphoid organs. It serves as a site of fetal hematopoiesis, filters blood-borne antigens and cleanses the blood through the action of mononuclear phagocytes, initiates an immune response to blood-borne microorganisms, destroys aged erythrocytes, and serves as a reservoir for blood.

The spleen is a concave, encapsulated organ that weighs about 150 g and is about the size of a fist. Strands of connective tissue (trabeculae) extend throughout the spleen from the splenic capsule, dividing it into compartments that contain masses of lymphoid tissue called *splenic pulp* (white and red). The spleen is interlaced with many blood vessels, some of which can distend to store blood.

Arterial blood that enters the spleen first encounters the white splenic pulp, which consists of masses of lymphoid tissue containing macrophages and lymphocytes, primarily T lymphocytes in proximity to the arterioles (the periarterial lymphoid sheath) (Fig. 22.6). Cellular clumps (lymphoid follicles) are formed in the white pulp around the splenic arterioles. The lymphoid follicles consist primarily of B lymphocytes and are the chief sites of immune function within the spleen. Here blood-borne antigens encounter lymphocytes, initiating the immune response and the conversion of lymphoid follicles into germinal centers in the middle of the follicle where B cells proliferate and differentiate during the humoral immune response (see Chapter 7).

Some of the blood continues through the microcirculation and enters highly distensible storage areas, called *venous sinuses,* in the red pulp of the spleen. The venous sinuses (and the red pulp) can store more than 300 ml of blood. Sudden reductions in blood pressure cause the sympathetic nervous system to stimulate constriction of the sinuses and expel as much as 200 ml of blood into the venous circulation, helping restore blood volume or pressure in the circulation and increasing the hematocrit by as much as 4%.

The endothelial lining of the venous sinuses is discontinuous (having gaps between endothelial cells) and therefore extremely permeable so that blood cells are allowed to exit the circulation. The red pulp contains a system of loosely interconnected resident macrophages that provide the principal site of splenic filtration. Because of the slow circulation in the sinuses, the macrophages easily phagocytose old, damaged, or dead blood cells of all kinds (but chiefly erythrocytes), microorganisms, macromolecules, and particles of debris. Hemoglobin from phagocytosed erythrocytes is catabolized, and heme (iron) is stored in the cytoplasm of the macrophages or released back into the blood. Blood that filters through the red pulp then moves through the venous sinuses and into the portal circulation (blood flowing to the liver).

The spleen is not absolutely necessary for life or for adequate hematologic function. However, splenic absence as a result of any cause (atrophy, traumatic injury, or removal because of disease) has several secondary effects on the body. For example, leukocytosis (high levels of circulating leukocytes) often occurs after splenectomy, suggesting that the spleen exerts some control over the rate of proliferation of leukocyte stem cells in the bone marrow or their release into the bloodstream. Circulating levels of iron also may decrease, reflecting the spleen's role in the iron cycle (see the Iron Cycle section). The immune response to encapsulated bacteria (e.g., *Streptococcus pneumoniae* [pneumococcus], *Neisseria meningitidis* [meningococcus], and *Haemophilus influenzae*), which is primarily an IgM response, may be severely diminished, resulting in increased susceptibility to disseminated infections. Loss of the spleen results in an increase in morphologically defective blood cells in the circulation, confirming the spleen's role in removing old or damaged cells.

Lymph Nodes

Structurally lymph nodes are part of the lymphatic system. Lymphatic vessels collect interstitial fluid from the tissues and transport it, as lymph, through vessels of increasing size to the thoracic duct, which drains into the superior vena cava and returns the lymph to the circulation. Lymph nodes are distributed throughout the body and provide filtration of the lymph during its journey through the lymphatics. Each lymph node is enclosed in a fibrous capsule, branches of which (trabeculae) extend inward to partition the node into several compartments (Fig. 22.7). Reticular fibers of connective tissue divide the compartments into a meshwork throughout the lymph node. The node consists of outer (cortex) and inner (paracortex) cortical areas and an inner medulla.

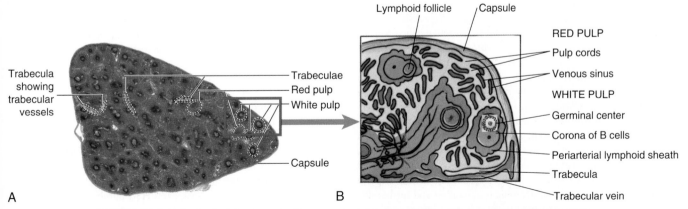

FIGURE 22.6 Splenic Architecture. A, Cross-section of the spleen. The spleen is enclosed in a capsule with the interior pulp divided into compartments by strands of connective tissue. The splenic pulp contains regions that are rich in lymphocytes (white pulp) and those containing erythrocytes (red pulp). **B**, Subcapsular splenic structures. (**A** from Telser AG, Young JK, Baldwin KM: *Elsevier's integrated histology,* St Louis, 2007, Mosby; **B** from Gartner LP, Hiatt JL: *Color textbook of histology,* ed 3, Philadelphia, 2007, Elsevier.)

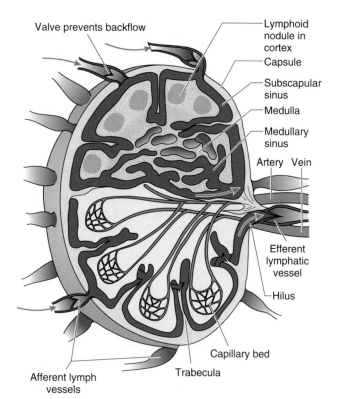

FIGURE 22.7 Cross-Section of Lymph Node. Several afferent valved lymphatics bring lymph to node. A single efferent lymphatic leaves the node at the hilus. *Note that the artery and vein also enter and leave at the hilus. Arrows show direction of lymph flow.* (Adapted from Gartner LP, Hiatt JL: *Color textbook of histology*, ed 3, Philadelphia, 2007, Saunders.)

Lymph enters through multiple small afferent lymphatic vessels into the subcapsular sinus, just beneath the capsule, and drains into the cortical sinuses to the medullary sinuses, from which the lymph is collected and leaves the node by way of the efferent lymphatic vessel. Blood flows into the lymph nodes through the lymphatic artery, which ends in groups of postcapillary venules distributed throughout the outer cortex. The blood is drained through the lymphatic vein.

Functionally, lymph nodes are part of the hematologic and immune systems and are the primary site for the first encounter between antigen and lymphocytes. Lymphocytes enter the lymph node from the blood through the postcapillary venules by means of diapedesis across the endothelial lining (see Fig. 22.2 for an example of diapedesis). Macrophages reside in the lymph node; help filter the lymph of debris, foreign substances, and microorganisms; and provide antigen-processing functions. The dendritic cells encounter and process antigens (see Chapter 7) and microorganisms in other tissues, enter the lymph node through the afferent lymph vessels, and migrate throughout the nodes. The reticular network provides adhesive surfaces for trapping large numbers of phagocytes and lymphocytes and facilitates their organization into follicles or primary nodules. The presence of antigen, either removed from the lymph by macrophages or presented on the surface of dendritic cells, results in the production of secondary nodules containing germinal centers. In the germinal centers lymphocytes, particularly B cells, respond to antigenic stimulation by undergoing proliferation and further differentiation into memory cells and plasma cells (see Chapter 7). Plasma cells migrate to the medullary cords. The B-lymphocyte proliferation in response to a great deal of antigen (e.g., during infection) may result in lymph node enlargement and tenderness (reactive lymph node), which can be palpable during a physical examination.

QUICK CHECK 22.2
1. Why is the spleen considered a hematologic organ? Why can humans live without it?
2. Why are lymph nodes considered part of the hematologic system?

DEVELOPMENT OF BLOOD CELLS

Bone Marrow

Bone marrow is confined to the cavities of bone and is the primary site of residence of hematopoietic stem cells (HSCs). Adults have two kinds of bone marrow: red marrow (active or hematopoietic marrow; also called myeloid tissue) and yellow marrow (inactive marrow). Bone cavities contain only red marrow at birth. The large quantity of fat in adult marrow is responsible for its yellow appearance. Not all bones contain active marrow. In adults, active marrow is found primarily in the flat bones of the pelvis (34%), vertebrae (28%), cranium and mandible (13%), and sternum and ribs (10%), and in the extreme proximal portions of the humerus and femur (4% to 8%). Stem cells for transplant are commonly harvested from the flat bones of the pelvis. Inactive marrow predominates in cavities of other bones. (Bones are discussed further in Chapter 40). The hematopoietic marrow consists of a variety of cellular and molecular microenvironments, called bone marrow niches.[2] Niches support the cells by direct cell-to-cell signaling and production of growth factors and cytokines important for retention, expansion, maintenance, and quiescence (inactive or dormant) of HSCs.

At least two populations of stem cells are found in bone marrow niches. Hematopoietic stem cells (HSCs) are progenitors of all hematologic cells.[3] Mesenchymal stem cells (MSCs) are stromal cells (connective tissue cells) that can differentiate into a variety of cells, including osteoblasts, adipocytes (store fat), chondrocytes (produce cartilage), sinusoidal endothelial cells, fibroblasts, and other stromal cells (connective tissue cells) that have a role in maintaining HSCs. Both populations of stem cells undergo continuous proliferation and self-renewal in the niches of the microenvironment of the bone marrow so that additional HSCs and MSCs are produced to replace those undergoing differentiation.

Hematopoietic marrow is vascularized by the primary arteries of the bones. Arterial vessels enter the bone, branch near the endosteum into smaller arterioles and capillaries, and drain into venous sinusoids. Hematopoietic marrow and yellow marrow fill the spaces surrounding the network of venous sinuses. Newly produced blood cells traverse narrow openings between endothelial cells (diapedesis) in the venous sinus walls and thus enter the circulation. Dormant or quiescent HSCs localize near small arterioles of the endosteal region until stimulated to proliferate.

Osteoblasts are derived from fibroblasts and are responsible for construction of bone. Osteoclasts are multinucleate cells of monocytic origin that remodel bone by resorption. Both cells are located near the endosteum (inner lining of compact bone) and can produce cytokines that affect proliferation and maintenance of hematopoietic cells.

Megakaryocytes and macrophages promote HSC migration and proliferation in the niches of the bone marrow. Megakaryocytes lie close to vascular sinuses and also produce platelets releasing them into the blood stream. Adipocytes suppress HSC numbers.

Cellular Differentiation

All humans originate from a single cell (the fertilized egg) that has the capacity to proliferate and eventually differentiate into the huge diversity of cells of the human body. After fertilization, the egg divides over a

5-day period to form a hollow ball (blastocyst) that implants on the uterus. Until about 3 days after fertilization, each cell (blastomere) is undifferentiated and retains the capacity to differentiate into any cell type. In the 5-day blastocyst, the outer layer of cells has undergone differentiation and commitment to become the placenta. Cells of the inner cell mass, however, continue to have unlimited differentiation potential (currently referred to as being *embryonic pluripotent stem cells*) and can grow into different kinds of tissue—blood, nerves, heart, bone, and so forth. After implantation, cells of the inner cell mass begin differentiation into other cell types. *Differentiation* is a multistep process and results in intermediate groups of stem cells with more limited, but still impressive, abilities to differentiate into many different types of cells. These are known as *multipotent stem cells* and include the HSCs.

Within the bone marrow niches each type of blood cell originates from HSCs that proliferate and differentiate under control of a variety of cytokines and growth factors. As with all stem cells, the HSCs are self-renewing (they have the ability to proliferate without further differentiation) so that a relatively constant population of stem cells is available. Some HSCs will continue differentiation into hematopoietic progenitor cells. Progenitor cells retain proliferative capacity but are *committed* to possible further differentiation into particular (unipotent) lineages of hematologic cells. The cell lineages include lymphoid lineages (T and B lymphocytes, NK cells) and myeloid lineages (monocytes, macrophages, neutrophils, basophils, eosinophils, megakaryocyte/platelets, and erythrocytes) (see Fig. 22.9).

Several cytokines participate in hematopoiesis, particularly colony-stimulating factors (CSFs or hematopoietic growth factors), which stimulate the proliferation of progenitor cells and their progeny and initiate the maturation events necessary to produce fully mature cells. Multiple cell types in hematopoietic organs, including endothelial cells, fibroblasts, granulocytes, monocytes, and lymphocytes, produce the necessary CSFs.

Hematopoiesis in the bone marrow occurs in two separate pools: the bone marrow stem cell pool—with eventual release of mature cells into the blood—and the circulating stem cell pool (Fig. 22.8). The bone marrow pool, the largest pool, contains cells that are proliferating and maturing in preparation for release into the circulation and mature cells that are stored for later release into the blood. The circulating stem cell pool contains multipotential and unipotential stem cells, partially committed progenitor cells, and mature functional cells.

Under certain conditions, the levels of circulating hematologic cells need to be rapidly replenished. Medullary hematopoiesis can be accelerated by any or all of three mechanisms: (1) conversion of yellow bone marrow, which does not produce blood cells, to red marrow, which does, by the actions of erythropoietin (a hormone produced primarily by the kidney that stimulates erythrocyte production); (2) faster proliferation of stem cells; and (3) faster differentiation of daughter cells (cells committed to differentiation).

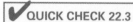

QUICK CHECK 22.3
1. Why is the stem cell system important to hematopoiesis?
2. What role do stromal cells play in hematopoiesis?

Hematopoiesis

Hematopoiesis is the production of blood cells. Blood cell production is constantly ongoing, occurring in the liver and spleen of the fetus and only in bone marrow (*medullary hematopoiesis*) after birth. This process involves the biochemical stimulation of populations

of relatively undifferentiated cells to undergo mitotic division (i.e., proliferation) and maturation (i.e., differentiation) into mature hematologic cells (Fig. 22.9). Although proliferation and differentiation are usually sequential, certain blood cells proliferate and differentiate simultaneously. Erythrocytes and neutrophils generally differentiate fully before entering the blood, but monocytes and lymphocytes continue to mature in the blood and in secondary lymphatic organs. The typical human requires about 100 billion new blood cells per day.

Hematopoiesis continues throughout life, increasing in response to a need to replenish aged or destroyed circulating cells or in response to infection. In general, long-term stimuli, such as chronic diseases, cause a greater increase in hematopoiesis than do acute conditions, such as hemorrhage. Various abnormalities in medullary hematopoiesis have been identified and are discussed in Chapter 23.

Extramedullary hematopoiesis is blood cell production in tissues other than bone marrow (e.g., liver and spleen). Extramedullary hematopoiesis, however, is usually a sign of disease and can occur in pernicious anemia, sickle cell anemia, thalassemia, hemolytic disease of the newborn (erythroblastosis fetalis), hereditary spherocytosis (abnormal sphere-shaped red blood cells [RBCs]), and certain leukemias.

Development of Erythrocytes

Erythropoiesis is the development of RBCs. In the confines of the bone marrow, progenitor cells proliferate and differentiate into large, nucleated proerythroblasts, which are committed to producing erythroid cells (Fig. 22.11). The proerythroblast differentiates through several intermediate forms of erythroblast (sometimes called normoblast) while progressively eliminating most intracellular structures (including the nucleus), synthesizing hemoglobin, and becoming more compact, eventually assuming the shape and characteristics of an erythrocyte. The last immature form is the reticulocyte. Except in newborns, only reticulocytes and erythrocytes are released into the bloodstream. The normal reticulocyte count is 1% of the total RBC count. Approximately 1% of the body's circulating erythrocyte mass normally is generated every 24 hours. Therefore the reticulocyte count is a useful clinical index of erythropoietic activity and indicates whether new red cells are being produced.

Regulation of erythropoiesis. In healthy humans, the total volume of circulating erythrocytes remains surprisingly constant. Most steps of erythropoiesis are primarily under the control of a feedback loop involving erythropoietin (EPO) and other cytokines. In conditions of tissue hypoxia, EPO is secreted primarily by the peritubular cells of the kidney (Fig. 22.10). Rising circulating levels of EPO cause a compensatory increase in erythrocyte production. The normal steady-state rate of production of 2.5 million erythrocytes per second can increase to 17 million per second under anemic or low-oxygen states, such as high-altitude environments or pulmonary disease. Thus the body responds to reduced oxygenation of blood in two ways: (1) by increasing the intake of oxygen through increased respiration and (2) by increasing the oxygen-carrying capacity of the blood through increased erythropoiesis.

Recombinant human erythropoietin (r-HuEPO) is used in individuals with anemia secondary to decreased EPO from chronic renal failure. An immediate effect of EPO administration is an increase in the blood reticulocyte count, followed by increasing levels of erythrocytes. The most significant side effect is increased blood pressure.

Hemoglobin synthesis. Erythrocytes form hemoglobin in the bone marrow. Hemoglobin (Hb), the oxygen-carrying protein of the erythrocyte, constitutes approximately 90% of the cell's dry weight. Hb-packed

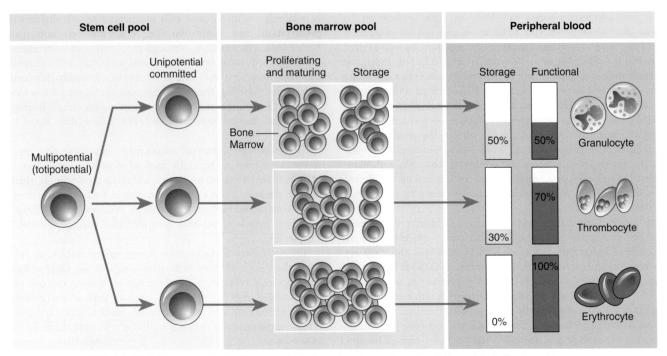

FIGURE 22.8 Hematopoiesis. Hematopoiesis from the stem cell pool; activity mainly in the bone marrow and in the peripheral blood.

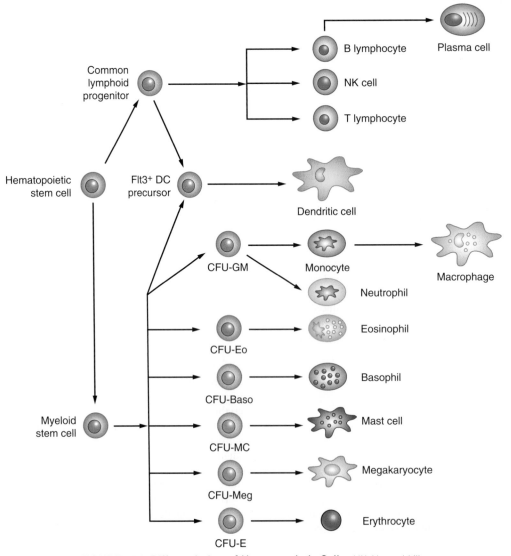

FIGURE 22.9 Differentiation of Hematopoietic Cells. *NK,* Natural killer.

blood cells take up oxygen in the lungs and exchange it for carbon dioxide in the tissues. Hb increases the oxygen-carrying capacity of blood by 100-fold. Each Hb molecule is composed of two pairs of polypeptide chains (the **globins**) and four colorful complexes of iron plus protoporphyrin (the hemes), which are responsible for the blood's ruby-red color (Fig. 22.12).

Several variants of Hb exist, and they differ only slightly in primary structure based on the use of different polypeptide chains: alpha, beta, gamma, delta, epsilon, or zeta.[4] Hb A, the most common type in adults, is composed of two α- and two β-polypeptide chains ($\alpha_2\beta_2$) (see Fig. 22.12). A normal variant, fetal Hb (Hb F), is a complex of two α- and two γ-polypeptide chains ($\alpha_2\gamma_2$) that binds oxygen with a much greater affinity than adult Hb.

Heme is a large, flat, iron-protoporphyrin disk that is synthesized in the mitochondria and can carry one molecule of oxygen (O_2). Thus, an individual Hb molecule with its four hemes can carry four oxygen molecules. If all four oxygen-binding sites are occupied by oxygen, the molecule is said to be saturated. Through a series of biochemical reactions, **protoporphyrin**, a complex four-ringed molecule, is produced and bound with ferrous iron. It is crucial that the iron be correctly charged; reduced ferrous iron (Fe^{2+}) can bind oxygen, whereas ferric iron (Fe^{3+}) cannot. Binding of O_2 to ferrous iron temporarily oxidizes Fe^{2+} to Fe^{3+} (**oxyhemoglobin**), but after the release of O_2 the body reduces the iron to Fe^{2+} and reactivates the Hb (**deoxyhemoglobin** [reduced hemoglobin]). Without reactivation, the Fe^{3+}-containing Kb (**methemoglobin**) cannot bind O_2. An excess of ferric iron occurs with certain drugs and chemicals, such as nitrates and sulfonamides, and reduces oxygen-carrying capacity.

Hb undergoes a conformational change when binding O_2. When one of the iron molecules binds O_2, the porphyrin ring changes shape, increasing the exposure of the three remaining iron atoms to O_2. This greatly increases the affinity for the oxygen-carrying capacity of Hb, as occurs in the lungs. When oxygen is unloaded from Hb, the oxygen-carrying capacity of hemoglobin is low, facilitating the transport of carbon dioxide back to the lungs.

Several other molecules can competitively bind to deoxyhemoglobin. Carbon monoxide (CO) directly competes with O_2 for binding to Fe^{2+} with an affinity that is about 200-fold greater than that of O_2. Thus even a small amount of CO can dramatically decrease the ability of Hb to bind and transport O_2. Hb also binds carbon dioxide (CO_2), but at

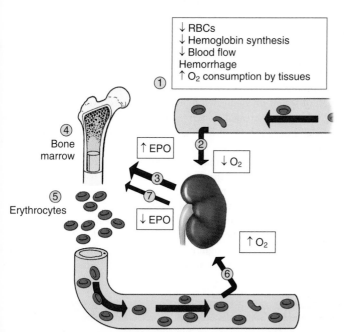

FIGURE 22.10 Role of Erythropoietin in Regulation of Erythropoiesis. (1) Decreased arterial oxygen levels result in decreased tissue oxygen (hypoxia) that (2) stimulates the kidney to increase production (3) of erythropoietin. Erythropoietin is carried to the bone marrow (4) and binds to erythropoietin receptors on proerythroblasts, resulting in increased red cell production (5). The increased release of red cells into the circulation frequently corrects the hypoxia in the tissues. Perception of normal oxygen levels by the kidney (6) causes diminished production (7) of erythropoietin (negative feedback) and a return to normal levels of erythrocyte production. *EPO,* Erythropoietin; *O₂,* oxygen in the blood and tissue; *RBCs,* red blood cells.

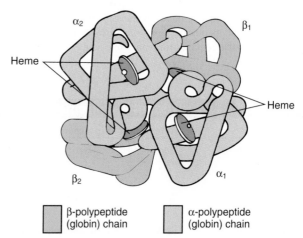

FIGURE 22.12 Molecular Structure of Hemoglobin. Molecule is spherical and contains a pair of α-polypeptide chains, a pair of β-polypeptide chains, and four heme groups.

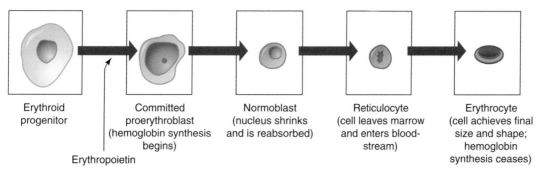

FIGURE 22.11 Erythrocyte Differentiation. Erythrocyte differentiation from large nucleated progenitor cells to small nonnucleated erythrocytes.

a binding site separate from where O_2 binds. In the lungs, CO_2 is released, allowing hemoglobin to bind O_2.

Nitric oxide (NO) produced by blood vessels is a major mediator of relaxation and dilation of the vessel walls. In the lungs, Hb can concurrently bind O_2 to the Fe^{2+} and NO to cysteine residues in the globins. As Hb transfers its O_2 to tissue, it may also shed small amounts of NO, contributing to dilation of the blood vessels and helping transfer of the O_2 into tissues. Erythrocytes may also play a role in the maintenance of vascular relaxation.

Nutritional requirements for erythropoiesis. Normal development of erythrocytes and synthesis of hemoglobin depend on an optimal biochemical state and adequate supplies of the necessary building blocks, including protein, vitamins, and minerals (Table 22.4). If these components are lacking for a prolonged time, erythrocyte production slows and anemia (insufficient numbers of functional erythrocytes) may result (see Chapter 23).

Erythropoiesis cannot proceed in the absence of vitamins, especially B_{12}, folate (folic acid), B_6, riboflavin, pantothenic acid, niacin, ascorbic acid, and vitamin E. Vitamin B_{12} is stored in the liver and used as needed in erythropoiesis. Decreased B_{12} or folate absorption may lead to pernicious (megaloblastic) anemia. Intrinsic factor is secreted by the stomach and promotes the absorption of vitamin B_{12} in the ileum. Folate is necessary for deoxyribonucleic acid (DNA) and ribonucleic acid (RNA) synthesis in precursor RBCs, and lack of folate results in an increase in abnormally large nucleated precursor RBCs (megaloblasts) with a reduced capacity to carry O_2. Folate is absorbed principally in the upper small intestine and is stored in the liver. Folate deficiency is more common than vitamin B_{12} deficiency and occurs more rapidly. Folate supplements are prescribed for pregnant women because pregnancy increases the demand for folate. Supplements may prevent anemia and can protect against neural tube defects because folate is also required for embryonic neural tube closure (see Chapter 18).

Normal destruction of senescent erythrocytes. Mature erythrocytes have cytoplasmic enzymes capable of glycolysis (anaerobic glucose metabolism) and production of small quantities of adenosine triphosphate (ATP). ATP provides the energy needed to maintain cell function and keep its plasma membrane pliable. Metabolic processes diminish as the erythrocyte ages, so less ATP is available to maintain plasma membrane function. The aged or senescent red cell becomes increasingly fragile and loses its reversible deformability, becoming susceptible to rupture while passing through narrowed regions of the microcirculation.

Additionally, the plasma membrane of senescent red cells undergoes phospholipid rearrangement, signaling macrophages to selectively remove and sequester the senescent red cells. If the spleen is dysfunctional or absent, macrophages in the liver (Kupffer cells) assume control of this process. During digestion of Hb in the macrophage, porphyrin reduces to unconjugated bilirubin, which is conjugated (made water soluble) and excreted from the liver into the intestine or into bile (Fig. 22.13). Bacteria in the intestinal lumen transform conjugated bilirubin into urobilinogen. Although a small portion is reabsorbed and excreted by the kidneys, most urobilinogen is excreted in feces. Conditions causing accelerated erythrocyte destruction increase the load of serum unconjugated bilirubin, increased liver conjugation of bilirubin, and increased urinary excretion of urobilinogen. Gallstones (cholelithiasis) can result from a chronically elevated rate of bilirubin excretion.

Iron cycle. Approximately 67% of total body iron is bound to heme in erythrocytes (Hb), and about 5% to 10% is bound to heme-containing myoglobin in muscle cells. Approximately 30% is stored in mononuclear phagocytes (i.e., macrophages) and hepatic parenchymal cells as either ferritin (iron bound to protein) or hemosiderin (intracellular bound iron). The remaining 3% (less than 1 mg) is lost daily in urine, sweat, bile, sloughing of epithelial cells from the skin and intestinal mucosa, and minor bleeding, as occurs with menstruation

TABLE 22.4 Nutritional Requirements for Erythropoiesis

Nutrient	Role in Erythropoiesis	Consequence of Deficiency*
Protein (amino acids)	Structural component of plasma membrane	Decreased strength, elasticity, and flexibility of membrane; hemolytic anemia
	Synthesis of hemoglobin	Decreased erythropoiesis and life span of erythrocytes
Cobalamin (vitamin B_{12})	Synthesis of DNA, maturation of erythrocytes, facilitator of folate metabolism;	Macrocytic (megaloblastic) anemia
Folate (folic acid)	Synthesis of DNA and RNA, maturation of erythrocytes	Macrocytic (megaloblastic) anemia
Vitamin B_6 (pyridoxine)	Heme synthesis	Microcytic-hypochromic anemia
Vitamin B_2 (riboflavin)	Oxidative reactions	Normocytic-normochromic anemia
Vitamin C (ascorbic acid)	Iron metabolism, acts as reducing agent to maintain iron in its ferrous (Fe^{2+}) form	Normocytic-normochromic anemia
Pantothenic acid	Heme synthesis	Unknown in humans†
Niacin	None, but needed for respiration in mature erythrocytes	Unknown in humans
Vitamin E	Heme synthesis (?);protection against oxidative damage in mature erythrocytes	Hemolytic anemia with increased cell membrane fragility; shortens life span of erythrocytes in individual with cystic fibrosis
Iron	Hemoglobin synthesis	Iron deficiency anemia
Copper	Optimal mobilization of iron from tissues to plasma	Microcytic-hypochromic anemia

*See Chapter 23.

†Although pantothenic acid is important for optimal synthesis of heme, experimentally induced deficiency failed to produce anemia or other hematopoietic disturbances.

DNA, Deoxyribonucleic acid; *RNA,* ribonucleic acid.

Data from Lee GR et al: *Wintrobe's clinical hematology,* ed 9, Philadelphia, 1993, Lea & Febiger; Harmening DM: *Clinical hematology and fundamentals of hemostasis,* ed 3, Philadelphia, 1997, FA Davis.

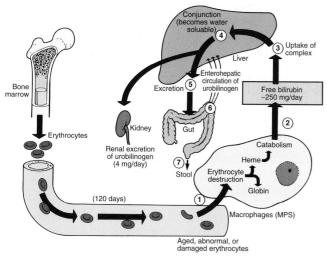

FIGURE 22.13 Metabolism of Bilirubin Released by Heme Breakdown. (1) Senescent red blood cells (RBCs) are consumed by macrophages. During digestion, (2) the porphyrin in the RBC reduces to bilirubin. (3) Bilirubin is taken up by the liver, where it is (4) conjugated by glucuronyl transferase and then is (5) excreted as bile. (6) Bacteria in the intestine transform conjugated bilirubin into urobilogen, (7) most of which is excreted in feces. *MPS,* Mononuclear phagocyte system.

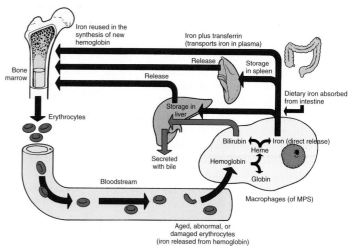

FIGURE 22.14 Iron Cycle. Iron released from gastrointestinal epithelial cells circulates in the bloodstream associated with its plasma carrier, transferrin. It is delivered to erythroblasts in bone marrow, where most of it is incorporated into hemoglobin. Mature erythrocytes circulate for approximately 120 days, after which they become senescent and are removed by the mononuclear phagocyte system *(MPS).* Macrophages of the MPS (mostly in the spleen) break down ingested erythrocytes and return iron to the bloodstream directly or after storing it as ferritin or hemosiderin.

in women. There is no excretory mechanism for iron. Unbound, or free, iron is toxic to human cells. Approximately 25 mg of iron is required daily for erythropoiesis; only 1 to 2 mg of iron is dietary, and the remainder is obtained from continual recycling of iron from erythrocytes through a process known as the **iron cycle.**[5] Pregnant women require more iron to meet the needs of the placenta and growing fetus.

The methemoglobin released from the breakdown of senescent or damaged erythrocytes is dissociated by the enzyme heme oxygenase, and the iron is released into the bloodstream, where it binds again to transferrin or is stored in the macrophage's cytoplasm as ferritin or hemosiderin (Fig. 22.14). Unavailable stores of iron are present in cytochromes, catalases, and peroxidase enzymes.

Ferritin is the major intracellular iron storage protein. **Apoferritin** is ferritin without attached iron. Apoferritin binds to free Fe^{2+} and stores it as Fe^{3+}, becoming ferritin. Excess accumulations of iron produce large intracellular iron storage complexes, known as **hemosiderin.** The iron within deposits of hemosiderin is poorly available because it is not water-soluble, but it is available when iron requirements increase. The most common cause of hemosiderin deposition is simple bruising. Hemosiderin in small amounts within iron-rich tissues (i.e., spleen, liver, bone marrow) is considered normal. Large aggregates or its presence in tissue, such as the lungs or subcutaneous tissue, suggests a pathologic condition known as hemosiderosis.

Iron from either dietary sources, release of iron stores, or erythrocyte catabolism is transported in the blood bound to **apotransferrin,** thus becoming **transferrin.** Transferrin is transported to the bone marrow, where it binds to transferrin receptors on erythroblasts. Transferrin receptors are on the plasma membrane of all nucleated cells, but at particularly high levels on erythroid precursors and rapidly proliferating cells (e.g., lymphocytes), and are thought to be the only route of cellular entry for transferrin-attached iron. Transferrin is recycled (transferrin cycle) by intracellular dissociation of iron from transferrin and secretion of the resultant apotransferrin to the bloodstream. The iron is transported to the erythroblast's mitochondria (the site of Hb production), where

the enzyme heme synthetase inserts Fe^{2+} into protoporphyrin to form heme. Heme then is bound to globin to form Hb. Iron not used in erythropoiesis is stored temporarily as ferritin or hemosiderin and later excreted or recycled.

The body's iron homeostasis is primarily controlled by the hormone hepcidin. **Hepcidin** is a protein synthesized in the liver and released into the plasma, where it is bound with high affinity to α_2-macroglobulin and with less affinity to albumin. Hepatocellular hepcidin production is regulated physiologically by the levels of iron in the body, rate of erythropoiesis, and percentage of oxygen saturation. Hepatocytes (liver cells) sense levels of circulating iron by means of receptors for transferrin. Excess iron is stored in hepatocytes and macrophages, and hepatocytes sense these levels by means of receptors for bone morphogenetic protein (BMP), which stimulates hepcidin activity.

Hepcidin regulates iron levels through its binding capacity to ferroportin, which is a transmembrane iron exporter found in the plasma membrane of cells that transport or store iron, including macrophages, hepatocytes, enterocytes (intestinal cells), and erythrocytes. The body's total iron balance is maintained through controlled absorption rather than excretion. Dietary iron (primarily as Fe^{2+}) is transported directly across the membranes of enterocytes in the duodenum and proximal jejunum and is carried in the plasma by transferrin. (Transport mechanisms are described in Chapter 1.) Hepcidin induces internalization and degradation of ferroportin, thus leading to increased intracellular iron stores, decreased dietary iron absorption, and decreased levels of circulating iron. Decreased production of hepcidin leads to release of stored iron and increased dietary absorption. Thus, if the body's iron stores are low or the demand for erythropoiesis increases, dietary iron is transported rapidly through the epithelial cell and into the plasma. If body stores are high and erythropoiesis is not increased, iron transport is stopped. Hepcidin production also can be induced by inflammation. During inflammation, increased levels of hepcidin lead to sequestering of iron as a result of down-regulation of ferroportin expression on macrophages and enterocytes and thus can cause anemia.

Development of Leukocytes

Myelopoiesis is the development of granulocytes (neutrophils, eosinophils, and basophils) and monocytes from the differentiation of myeloid progenitor cells in the bone marrow (the pathways of differentiation are shown in Fig. 22.9). The maturation of myeloid cells is under the direction of specific growth factors for each cell type. Granulocytes are released into the blood within 10 to14 days of development. They become two pools of cells—those functional cells that are circulating, and those stored around the walls of the blood vessels, often called the **marginating storage pool**. The marginating storage pool primarily consists of neutrophils that can rapidly move into tissues and mucous membranes when needed (i.e., during inflammation or infection). Monocytes are released into the blood and travel to various tissues to become tissue macrophages and dendritic cells within 1 or 2 days after release (see Table 22.3).

Lymphopoiesis (lymphocytopoiesis) is the generation of lymphocytes from lymphoid progenitor cells released into the bloodstream to undergo further maturation in the primary and secondary lymphoid organs (see Chapter 7). Lymphocytes can exist in the body from days to years and can increase in the presence of infection.

Development of Platelets

Thrombopoiesis is the development of platelets. Platelets (thrombocytes) are derived from stem cells and progenitor cells that differentiate into megakaryocytes (see Fig. 22.9). During thrombopoiesis, the megakaryocyte nucleus enlarges and becomes extremely polyploidy (up to 100-fold or more of the normal amount of DNA) without cellular division. Concurrently, the numbers of cytoplasmic organelles (e.g., internal membranes, granules) increase and the cell develops cellular surface elongations and branches that progressively fragment into platelets.[6] A single large (up to 100 μm) megakaryocyte may produce thousands of smaller platelets (2 to 3 μm). Like erythrocytes, platelets released from the bone marrow lack nuclei but contain granules that promote their stickiness.

About two-thirds of platelets enter the circulation, and the remainder resides in the splenic pool. **Thrombopoietin (TPO)**, a hormone growth factor, stimulates the production and differentiation of megakaryocytes and is the main regulator of the circulating platelet numbers.[7] TPO is primarily produced by the liver and induces platelet production in the bone marrow. Platelets express receptors for TPO and, when circulating platelet levels are normal, TPO is adsorbed onto the platelet surface and prevented from accessing the bone marrow and initiating further platelet production. When platelet levels are low, however, the amount of TPO exceeds the number of available platelet TPO receptors, and free TPO can enter the bone marrow. During inflammation IL-6 induces increased production of TPO, which increases production of newly formed platelets, which are more thrombogenic.

Platelets circulate in the bloodstream for about 10 days before beginning to lose their ability to carry out biochemical reactions. Senescent platelets are sequestered and destroyed in the spleen by macrophage phagocytosis.

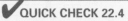

QUICK CHECK 22.4
1. Why is the reticulocyte count important?
2. Why is iron important to erythropoiesis?
3. What happens to aging erythrocytes?
4. What specific cells are involved in development of leukocytes?

MECHANISMS OF HEMOSTASIS

Hemostasis is the arrest of bleeding by formation of blood clots at sites of vascular injury. As a result of hemostasis, damaged blood vessels may maintain a relatively steady state of blood volume, pressure, and flow. Three equally important interactive components of hemostasis are the vasculature (endothelial cells and subendothelial matrix), platelets, and clotting factors.[8] The general sequence of events in hemostasis is (1) vascular injury leads to a transient arteriolar vasoconstriction to limit blood flow to the affected site; (2) damage to the endothelial cell lining of the vessel exposes prothrombogenic subendothelial connective tissue matrix, leading to platelet adherence and activation and formation of a *hemostatic plug* to prevent further bleeding (primary hemostasis); (3) tissue factor, produced by the endothelium, collaborates with secreted platelet factors and activated platelets to activate the clotting (coagulation) system to form fibrin clots and further prevent bleeding (secondary hemostasis); and (4) the fibrin/platelet clot contracts to form a more permanent plug, and regulatory pathways are activated (fibrinolysis) to limit the size of the plug and begin the healing process. The relative importance of the hemostatic mechanisms clearly varies with vessel size. Damage to large vessels cannot easily be controlled by hemostasis but requires vascular contraction and dramatically decreased blood flow into the damaged vessels (Table 22.5).

Function of Blood Vessels

The vessel walls consist of a layer of endothelial cells that adhere to an underlying subendothelial matrix of connective tissue. The matrix contains a variety of proteins, including collagen, fibronectin, and laminins. Endothelial cells adhere to the matrix and to each other through receptors that are expressed only on the intercellular and basal surfaces.

Under normal conditions the endothelium actively regulates blood flow and prevents spontaneous activation of platelets and the clotting system. Endothelial cells produce **nitric oxide (NO)**, also known as endothelium-derived vasorelaxant factor (EDRF),[9] and synthesize **prostacyclin (prostaglandin I$_2$ [PGI$_2$])**, both of which are vasodilators

---

TABLE 22.5 Types of Bleeding: Sources, Vessel Size, and Sealing Requirements			
Types and Sources of Bleeding	**Involved Vessel**	**Size**	**Sealing Requirements**
Pinpoint petechial hemorrhage (blood leakage from small vessels)	Capillary	Smallest	Generally direct sealing
	Venule		Mostly fused platelets
	Arteriole		Mostly fused platelets
Ecchymosis (large, soft tissue bleeding)	Vein		Vascular contraction, fused platelets, perivascular and intravascular hemostatic factor activation (see Fig. 20.16)
Rapidly expanding "blowout" hemorrhage	Artery	Largest	Greater vascular contraction, more fused platelets, greater perivascular and intravascular hemostatic factor activation

Modified from Harmening DM, editor: *Clinical hematology and fundamentals of hemostasis,* ed 3, Philadelphia, 1997, FA Davis.

that modulate blood flow and pressure and maintain platelets in an inactive state. Synergism between PGI_2 and NO is significant. PGI_2 production varies a great deal in response to stimuli, whereas NO is released continually to regulate vascular tone. Endothelium also produces adenosine diphosphatase, which degrades adenosine diphosphate (ADP), a potent activator of platelets.

The endothelial cell surface contains antithrombotic molecules, such as glycosaminoglycans (e.g., heparan sulfate), thrombomodulin, and plasminogen activators. These limit platelet activation and fibrin deposition. Although thrombomodulin and plasminogen activators help control hemostasis in normal vessels, their effects are magnified during vascular damage and clot formation.

As a result of damage to the vessels, the endothelial cell barrier is frequently compromised, the remaining endothelial cells are activated by products of tissue damage, and the underlying subendothelial matrix is exposed. Endothelial cells contain intracellular structures that contain von Willebrand factor (vWF, clotting factor VIII), which is released during vascular injury and activates platelets.

Function of Platelets

Platelets normally circulate freely, suspended in plasma, in an unactivated state. The roles of platelets are to (1) contribute to regulation of blood flow into a damaged site by induction of vasoconstriction (vasospasm); (2) initiate platelet–platelet interactions, resulting in formation of a platelet plug to stop further bleeding; (3) activate the coagulation (or clotting) cascade to stabilize the platelet plug; and (4) initiate repair processes, including clot retraction and clot dissolution (fibrinolysis) and release of growth factors.[10] The normal platelet count ranges from 150,000 to 400,000/mm³. Thrombocytopenia (abnormally low numbers of platelets) develops if the platelet count drops below 100,000/mm³, and an individual may experience longer than normal clotting times. Spontaneous major bleeding episodes do not generally occur unless the platelet count falls below 20,000/mm³.

Damage to the vessel initiates a process of platelet activation: (1) increased platelet *adhesion* to the damaged vascular wall; (2) *activation* leading to platelet degranulation, which stimulates changes in platelet shape and biochemistry; (3) *aggregation* as platelet–vascular wall and platelet-platelet adherence increases; and (4) activation of the clotting system and development of an immobilizing meshwork of platelets and fibrin (see *Did You Know?* Sticky Platelet Syndrome).

DID YOU KNOW?

Sticky Platelet Syndrome

Sticky platelet syndrome (SPS) is a pathologic inherited autosomal dominant procoagulant condition that causes thrombi in arteries, veins, or capillaries. The procoagulation is caused by an increase in platelet stickiness (aggregation) when stressful events cause the release of epinephrine and or adenosine diphosphate. The disease is relatively frequent but often remains clinically silent until a significant stressful event. SPS accounts for about 21% of unexplained arterial thrombotic episodes, including stroke. Pregnancy complications related to placental thrombi include fetal growth retardation and fetal loss, and less often venous thromboembolism. The first thrombotic event usually occurs in individuals less than 40 years of age and can occur in both men and women. Diagnosis is made by laboratory evaluation of platelet aggregation. Treatment is low-dose aspirin (acetylsalicylic acid) or clopidogrel if there is aspirin resistance.

Data from: Kubisz P et al: *Expert Rev Hematol* 9(1):21-35, 2016; Kubisz P, Holly P, Stasko J: *Semin Thromb Hemost* 45(1):61-68, 2019; Sokol J et al: *Semin Thromb Hemost* 43(1):8-13, 2017.

Adhesion

Normally platelets are generally observed "rolling" along the margins of vessels. At sites of vessel injury, however, platelets become adherent to the site of endothelial damage, where the subendothelial matrix is exposed and endothelial cells have released vWF and decreased their antithrombotic activities. Platelet adhesion is mostly mediated by the binding of platelet surface receptor glycoprotein Ib (GPIb) to vWF.

Activation

As a result of interactions with the endothelium or the subendothelial matrix, as well as exposure to inflammatory mediators produced by the endothelium and other cells, the platelets are activated. Activation results in reorganization of the platelet cytoskeleton, leading to dynamic changes in platelet shape from smooth spheres to those with spiny projections (increases surface area) (see Fig. 22.5) and degranulation (also called the platelet-release reaction) and resulting in the release of various potent biochemicals.

Platelets contain three types of granules: dense bodies, alpha granules, and lysosomes. The contents of the dense bodies and alpha granules are particularly important in hemostasis. The dense bodies contain ADP, serotonin, and calcium. ADP recruits and activates other platelets through specific receptors. During activation the platelet plasma membrane experiences several important changes, including becoming ruffled and sticky; undergoing cellular spreading to make tight contacts between neighboring platelets, causing the platelet plug to seal the injured endothelium; and externalizing the phospholipid phosphatidylserine, which provides a matrix for activation of clotting factors (Fig. 22.15). Serotonin is a vasoactive amine that functions like histamine and increases vasodilation and vascular permeability. Calcium is necessary for many of the adhesive interactions as well as for intracellular signaling mechanisms that control platelet activation.

Alpha granules contain a mixture of clotting factors (e.g., fibrinogen), growth and angiogenic factors (e.g., platelet-derived growth factor [PDGF]), and angiogenesis inhibitors (e.g., platelet factor 4). Platelet factor 4 also is a heparin-binding protein and enhances clot formation at the site of injury. Depending on the particular stimulus, platelets may selectively release promoters or inhibitors of angiogenesis. Many of these mediators either promote or inhibit platelet activity and the eventual process of clot formation. PDGF stimulates smooth muscle cells and promotes tissue repair.

Platelets also initiate production of the prostaglandin derivative thromboxane A_2 (TXA_2), which counters the effects of PGI_2 produced by endothelial cells. TXA_2 causes vasoconstriction and promotes the degranulation of platelets, whereas PGI_2 promotes vasodilation and inhibits platelet degranulation.

Aggregation

Platelet aggregation is stimulated primarily by TXA_2 and ADP, which induce functional fibrinogen receptors on the platelet. The glycoprotein IIb/IIIa (GPIIb/IIIa) complex (also called *integrin αIIbβ₃*) undergoes a conformational change during activation to become a calcium-dependent receptor for fibrinogen, allowing it to bind other matrix proteins (e.g., fibronectin, fibrinogen, thrombospondin). Although the GPIIb/IIIa complex is the most abundant fibrinogen receptor on the platelet, receptors for vWF and collagen also contribute to the process.

If blood vessel injury is minor, hemostasis is achieved temporarily by formation of the platelet plug within 3 to 5 minutes of injury. Platelet plugs seal the many minute ruptures that occur daily in the microcirculation, particularly in capillaries. With too few platelets, numerous small hemorrhagic areas called *purpuras* develop under the skin and throughout the tissues (see Chapter 23).

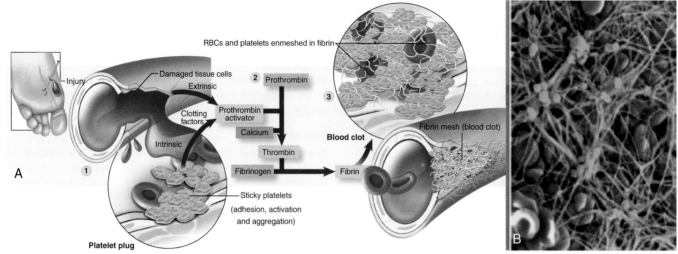

FIGURE 22.15 Blood-Clotting Mechanism. A, The complex clotting mechanism can be summarized into three basic steps: **(1)** release of clotting factors from both injured tissue cells and sticky platelets at the injury site (which form a temporary platelet plug); **(2)** series of chemical reactions that eventually result in the formation of thrombin that converts fibrinogen to fibrin, and **(3)** fibrin traps blood cells and platelets to form a clot. **B,** False color scanning electron micrograph showing a blood clot: fibrin fibers *(green),* platelets *(purple),* and erythrocytes *(red).* (Image courtesy of Y. Veklich & J. W. Weisel). An electron micrograph showing entrapped RBCs in a fibrin clot. (**A** from Patton KT, Thibodeau GA: *The human body in health & disease,* ed 7, St Louis, 2018, Mosby; **B** from Wei L et al: *Acta Biomaterialia* 60[15]:264-274, 2017.)

Function of Clotting Factors

A blood clot is a meshwork of protein strands that stabilizes the platelet plug and traps other cells, such as erythrocytes, phagocytes, and microorganisms (see Fig. 22.15). The strands are made of fibrin, which is produced by the clotting (coagulation) system. The clotting system was described in Chapter 6 and consists of a family of proteins that circulate in the blood in inactive forms. Initiation of the system results in sequential activation (cascade) of multiple members of the system until a fibrin clot is created.

The clotting system is usually presented as two pathways of initiation (intrinsic and extrinsic pathways) that join in a common pathway. The intrinsic pathway is activated when Hageman factor (factor XII) in plasma contacts negatively charged subendothelial substances exposed by vascular injury. The extrinsic pathway is activated when tissue thromboplastin, a substance released by damaged endothelial cells, reacts with clotting factors, particularly factor VII. Both pathways lead to the common pathway and activation of factor X, which proceeds to clot formation. As with the complement cascade, the clotting system is complex with a large number of alternative activators and inhibitors. There also is interaction between components of the intrinsic and extrinsic pathways so that an activated member of one pathway may activate a member of the other pathway (e.g., factor VIIa of the extrinsic pathway can directly activate factor IX of the intrinsic pathway).

Activated platelets are important participants in clotting. The phosphatidylserine-rich surface produced during platelet activation provides a matrix on which several important complexes of clotting factors are formed. These include the intrinsic pathway's *tenase complex* (factor X and activated factors VIII and IX) that activates factor X and the *prothrombinase complex* (prothrombin and activated factors X and V) that activates prothrombin into thrombin. Thrombin then converts fibrinogen into fibrin, which polymerizes into a fibrin clot (see Fig. 22.15). Thrombin has broad activity in the inflammatory response. In addition to producing fibrin, thrombin is an activator of other coagulation proteins (e.g., factors V, VIII, XI, XIII), platelets (e.g., aggregation, degranulation), endothelial cells (e.g., up-regulation of adhesion molecules for leukocytes, increased NO, PGI_2, PDGF), and monocytes (e.g., cytokine secretion and increased receptors for endothelial cells).

Control of Hemostatic Mechanisms

Under normal conditions, spontaneous activation of hemostasis is prevented by factors residing on the endothelial cell surface. These include thrombin inhibitors (e.g., antithrombin III), tissue factor inhibitors (e.g., tissue factor pathway inhibitor), and mechanisms for degrading activated clotting factors (e.g., protein C). Antithrombin III (AT-III) is a circulating inhibitor of plasma serine proteases. AT-III is produced by the liver and binds to heparin sulfate found naturally on the surface of endothelial cells, or with heparin administered clinically to prevent thrombosis. Heparin induces a change in AT-III that greatly enhances its capacity to inhibit thrombin and other activated clotting factors. Tissue factor pathway inhibitor (TFPI) is produced by endothelial cells and platelets; complexes to, and reversibly inhibits, factor Xa in the prothrombinase complex; and also inhibits other activated clotting factors.

Thrombomodulin is a thrombin-binding protein on the surface of endothelial cells. Protein C in the circulation binds to thrombomodulin in a thrombin-dependent manner and is converted to activated protein C. Activated protein C, in association with a cofactor (protein S), degrades factors Va and VIIIa. Deficiencies of AT-III, protein C, or protein S are important causes of hypercoagulation (increased clotting). Expression of thrombomodulin and the endothelial cell protein C receptor is down-regulated by cytokines and other products of inflammation (e.g., IL-1α, tumor necrosis factor-alpha [TNF-α], endotoxin), thereby enhancing clot formation.

Retraction and Lysis of Blood Clots

After a clot is formed, it retracts, or "solidifies." Fibrin strands shorten, becoming denser and stronger, which approximates the edges of the injured vessel wall and seals the site of injury. Retraction is facilitated by the large numbers of platelets trapped within the fibrin meshwork. The platelets contract and "pull" the fibrin threads closer together while releasing a factor that stabilizes the fibrin. Contraction expels serum from the fibrin meshwork. This process usually begins within a few minutes after a clot has formed, and most of the serum is expelled within 20 to 60 minutes.

Lysis (breakdown) of blood clots is carried out by the **fibrinolytic system** (Fig. 22.16). Another plasma protein, plasminogen, is converted to **plasmin** by several products of coagulation and inflammation, especially by the enzymatic action of **tissue plasminogen activator (t-PA)**. Endothelial cells express t-PA, which is activated maximally after binding to fibrin. Another activator of plasminogen is **urokinase-like plasminogen activator (u-PA)**. The u-PA binds to a specific cellular u-PA receptor (u-PAR), causing activation of plasminogen. This urokinase is the major activator of fibrinolysis in the *extravascular,* or tissue, compartment, whereas t-PA is largely involved in *intravascular* fibrinolysis. Several cancers appear to use membrane-bound u-PA to digest intercellular matrix and greatly facilitate tumor invasion and metastasis. Both t-PA and u-PA have been used clinically to treat diseases associated with a blood clot (e.g., pulmonary embolism, myocardial infarction, stroke).

Plasmin is an enzyme that dissolves clots (fibrinolysis) by degrading fibrin and fibrinogen into **fibrin degradation products (FDPs)**. A major FDP is D-dimer. Measurement of levels of circulating D-dimer (a small protein fragment of fibrin degradation) has been used for diagnosis because D-dimer can be elevated in cases of deep venous thrombosis (DVT) or pulmonary embolism (PE). Blood tests for evaluating the hematologic system are listed in Table 22.6.

> **QUICK CHECK 22.5**
> 1. Why are platelets necessary to stop bleeding?
> 2. Briefly describe the steps of platelet adhesion and aggregation.
> 3. How does plasminogen initiate fibrinolysis?

PEDIATRICS AND BLOOD

Blood cell counts tend to rise above adult levels at birth and then decline gradually throughout childhood. Table 22.7 lists normal ranges during infancy and childhood. The immediate rise in values is the result of accelerated hematopoiesis during fetal life and the increased numbers of cells that result from the trauma of birth and cutting of the umbilical cord.

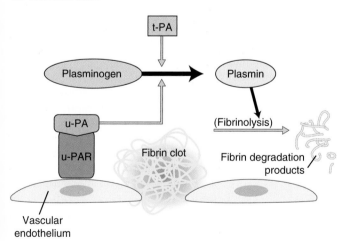

FIGURE 22.16 The Fibrinolytic System. Fibrinolysis is initiated by the binding of plasminogen to fibrin. Although tissue plasminogen activator *(t-PA)* initiates intravascular fibrinolysis, urokinase plasminogen activator *(u-PA)* is the major activator of fibrinolysis in tissue (extravascular). Plasmin digests the fibrin into smaller soluble pieces (fibrin degradation products). *u-PAR,* Urokinase-like plasminogen activator receptor.

Average blood volume in the full-term neonate is about 85 ml/kg of body weight. The premature infant has a slightly larger blood volume of 90 ml/kg of body weight. In both full-term and premature infants, blood volume decreases during the first few months. Thereafter the average blood volume is about 75 to 80 ml/kg, which is similar to that of older children and adults.

The hypoxic intrauterine environment stimulates erythropoietin production in the fetus and accelerates fetal erythropoiesis, producing polycythemia (excessive proliferation of erythrocyte precursors) in the newborn. After birth, the oxygen from the lungs saturates arterial blood, and more oxygen is delivered to the tissues. In response to the change from a placental to a pulmonary oxygen supply during the first few days of life, levels of erythropoietin and the rate of blood cell formation decrease. The active rate of fetal erythropoiesis is reflected by the large numbers of immature erythrocytes (reticulocytes) in the peripheral blood of full-term neonates. After birth, the number of reticulocytes decreases by 50% every 12 hours, so it is rare to find an elevated reticulocyte count after the first week of life. During this period of rapid growth, the rate of erythrocyte destruction is greater than that in later childhood and adulthood. In full-term infants, the normal erythrocyte life span is 60 to 80 days; in premature infants, it may be as short as 20 to 30 days; and in children and adolescents, it is the same as that in adults—100 to 120 days.

The postnatal fall in hemoglobin and hematocrit values is more marked in premature infants than it is in full-term infants. In preschool and school-aged children, hemoglobin, hematocrit, and RBC counts gradually rise. Metabolic processes within the erythrocytes of neonates differ significantly from those found in erythrocytes of normal adults. The relatively young population of erythrocytes in newborns consumes greater quantities of glucose than do erythrocytes in adults. Platelet counts in full-term neonates are comparable with those in adults and remain so throughout infancy and childhood.

White blood cells develop and mature during fetal life, including neutrophils, monocyte-macrophages, eosinophils, and lymphocytes, but the function of the cells at birth is weak because the cells are immature. At birth the lymphocyte count is high, and it continues to rise during the first year of life. Then it steadily declines until the lower value seen in adults is reached. The neutrophil count, like the lymphocyte count, is high at birth and rises during the first days of life. After 2 weeks, the neutrophil count falls to within or below the normal adult range. Although the exact age can vary by approximately 7 years of age, the neutrophil count is the same as that of an adult. The eosinophil count is higher in the first year of life and higher in children than in teenagers or adults. Monocyte counts also are high in the first year of life but then decrease to adult levels.

Newborn infants are at risk for impaired phagocytosis, bacterial infections, and delayed wound healing. Immature lymphocytes also increase the risk for viral infection, and there is a weak response to the production of antibodies and a poor response to foreign antigens. Protection against infectious disease is provided by passive IgG antibody transfer from the mother transplacentally and in breast milk. By 2 months of age the white blood cells have matured enough for the infant to begin receiving protection from infectious disease by vaccination. As the child ages, immunity is further enhanced by intercurrent infection and vaccinations, with the formation of antibodies and memory T cells that provide lifelong protection.[11]

AGING AND BLOOD

Blood composition changes little with age, although some components may be altered by iron deficiency. Values of total serum iron level, total iron-binding capacity, and intestinal iron absorption are all decreased

TABLE 22.6 Common Blood Tests for Evaluating Hematologic Function

Cell Type and Test	Property Evaluated by Test	Possible Hematologic Cause of Abnormal Findings*
Erythrocyte		
Red cell count	Number (in millions) of erythrocytes/µl of blood	Altered erythropoiesis, anemias, hemorrhage, Hodgkin disease, leukemia
Mean corpuscle volume (MCV)	Size of erythrocytes	Anemias, thalassemias
Mean corpuscle hemoglobin (MCH)	Amount of hemoglobin in each erythrocyte (by weight)	Anemias, hemoglobinopathy
Mean corpuscular hemoglobin concentration (MCHC)	Concentration of hemoglobin in each erythrocyte (percentage of erythrocyte occupied by hemoglobin)	Anemias, hereditary spherocytosis
Hemoglobin determination	Amount of hemoglobin (by weight)/dl of blood	Anemias
Hematocrit determination	Percentage of a given volume of blood that is occupied by erythrocytes	Hemorrhage, polycythemia, erythrocytosis, anemias, leukemia
Reticulocyte count	Number of reticulocytes/µl of blood (also expressed as percentage of reticulocytes in total red blood cell count)	Hyperactive or hypoactive bone marrow function
Erythrocyte osmotic fragility test	Cellular shape (biconcavity), structure of plasma membrane	Anemias, hemolytic disease caused by ABO or Rh incompatibility, Hodgkin disease, polycythemia vera, thalassemia major
Hemoglobin electrophoresis	Relative percentage of different types of hemoglobin in erythrocytes	Sickle cell disease, sickle cell trait, hemoglobin C disease, hemoglobin C trait, thalassemias
Sickle cell test	Presence of hemoglobin S in erythrocytes	Sickle cell trait, sickle cell anemia
Glucose-6-phosphate dehydrogenase (G6PD) deficiency test	Deficiency of G6PD in erythrocytes	Hemolytic anemia
Hemoglobin Metabolism		
Serum ferritin determination	Depletion of body iron (potential deficiency of heme synthesis)	Iron deficiency anemias
Total iron-binding capacity (TIBC)	Amount of iron in serum plus amount of transferrin available in serum ($\mu\gamma/\delta\gamma$)	Hemorrhage, iron deficiency anemia, hemochromatosis, hemosiderosis, iron overload, anemias, thalassemia
Transferrin saturation	Percentage of transferrin that is saturated with iron	Acute hemorrhage, hemochromatosis, hemosiderosis, sideroblastic anemia, iron deficiency anemia, iron overload, thalassemia
Porphyrin analysis (protoporphyrin analysis)	Concentration of protoporphyrin in erythrocytes (mcg/dl), an indicator of iron-deficient erythropoiesis	Megaloblastic anemia, congenital erythropoietic porphyria
Direct antiglobulin test (DAT)	Antibody binding to erythrocytes	Hemolytic disease of newborn, autoimmune hemolytic anemia, drug-induced hemolytic anemia, transfusion reaction
Antibody screen test (indirect Coombs test)	Detection of antibodies to erythrocyte antigens (other than ABO antigens)	Same as for DAT
Leukocytes: Differential White Cell Count (Absolute Number of a Type of Leukocyte/µl of Blood)		
Neutrophil count	Neutrophils/µl	Myeloproliferative disorders, hematopoietic disorders, hemolysis, infection
Lymphocyte count	Lymphocytes/µl	Infectious lymphocytosis, infectious mononucleosis, hematopoietic disorders, anemias, leukemia, lymphosarcoma, Hodgkin disease
Plasma cell count	Plasma cells/µl	Infectious mononucleosis, lymphocytosis, plasma cell leukemia
Monocyte count	Monocytes/µl	Hodgkin disease, infectious mononucleosis, monocytic leukemia, non-Hodgkin lymphoma, polycythemia vera
Eosinophil count	Eosinophils/µl	Hematopoietic disorders, parasitic infections, allergic reactions
Basophil count	Basophils/µL	Chronic myelogenous leukemia, hemolytic anemias, Hodgkin disease, polycythemia vera

TABLE 22.6   Common Blood Tests for Evaluating Hematologic Function—cont'd

Cell Type and Test	Property Evaluated by Test	Possible Hematologic Cause of Abnormal Findings*
Platelets and Clotting Factors		
Platelet count	Number of circulating platelets (in thousands)/µl of blood	Anemias, multiple myeloma, myelofibrosis, polycythemia vera, leukemia, disseminated intravascular coagulation (DIC), hemolytic disease of the newborn, transfusion reaction, lymphoproliferative disorders
Bleeding time	Duration of bleeding after a standardized superficial puncture wound of skin, integrity of platelet plug, measured in minutes following puncture	Leukemia, anemias, DIC, fibrinolytic activity, purpuras, hemorrhagic disease of the newborn, infectious mononucleosis, multiple myeloma, clotting factor deficiencies, thrombasthenia, thrombocytopenia, von Willebrand disease
Clot retraction test	Platelet number and function, fibrinogen quantity and use, measured in hours required for expression of serum from a clot incubated in a test tube	Acute leukemia, aplastic anemia, factor XIII deficiency, increased fibrinolytic activity, Hodgkin disease, hyperfibrinogenemia or hypofibrinogenemia, idiopathic thrombocytopenic purpura, multiple myeloma, polycythemia vera, secondary thrombocytopenia, thrombasthenia
Platelet adhesion studies	Ability of platelets to adhere to foreign surfaces	Anemia, macroglobulinemia, Bernard-Soulier syndrome, multiple myeloma, myeloid metaplasia, plasma cell dyscrasias, thrombasthenia, thrombocytopathy, von Willebrand disease
Platelet aggregation tests	Ability of platelets to adhere to one another	Afibrinogenemia, Bernard-Soulier syndrome, thrombasthenia, hemorrhagic thrombocythemia, myeloid metaplasia, plasma cell dyscrasias, platelet release defects, polycythemia vera, preleukemia, sideroblastic anemia, von Willebrand disease, Waldenström macroglobulinemia, hypercoagulability
Whole blood clotting time (Lee-White coagulation time)	Overall ability of blood to clot, as measured in minutes in a test tube	Afibrinogenemia, clotting factor deficiencies, excessive fibrinolysis, hemorrhagic disease of the newborn, hypofibrinogenemia, hypoprothrombinemia, leukemia
Circulating anticoagulants (immunoglobulin G [IgG] antibodies that inhibit coagulation)	Presence of antibodies that neutralize clotting factors and inhibit coagulation, as indicated by prolonged clotting time, prothrombin time, or partial thromboplastin time	Afibrinogenemia, presence of fibrin-fibrinogen degradation products, macroglobulinemia, multiple myeloma, DIC, plasma cell dyscrasias
Partial thromboplastin time (PTT)	Effectiveness of clotting factors (except factors VII and VIII), effectiveness of intrinsic pathway of coagulation cascade, as measured by a test tube (in seconds)	Presence of circulating anticoagulants, DIC, clotting factor deficiencies, excessive fibrinolysis, hemorrhagic disease of the newborn, hypofibrinogenemia and afibrinogenemia, prothrombin deficiency, von Willebrand disease, acute hemorrhage
Prothrombin time	Effectiveness of activity of prothrombin, fibrinogen, and factors V, VII, and X; effectiveness of vitamin K–dependent coagulation factors of extrinsic and common pathways of coagulation cascade as measured in a test tube (in seconds)	Hypofibrinogenemia, dysfibrinogenemia, and afibrinogenemia; presence of circulating anticoagulants; DIC; deficiency of factors V, VII, or X; presence of fibrin degradation products, increased fibrinolytic activity, hemolytic jaundice, hemorrhagic disease of the newborn; acute leukemia, polycythemia vera, prothrombin deficiency, multiple myeloma
Thrombin time	Quantity and activity of fibrinogen as measured in a test tube (in seconds)	Hypofibrinogenemia, dysfibrinogenemia, and afibrinogenemia; presence of circulating anticoagulants; hemorrhagic disease of the newborn, polycythemia vera; increase in fibrinogen-fibrin degradation products; increased fibrinolytic activity
Fibrinogen assay	Amount of fibrinogen available for fibrin formation	Acute leukemia, congenital hypofibrinogenemia or afibrinogenemia, DIC, increased fibrinolytic activity, severe hemorrhage
Fibrin-fibrinogen degradation products (fibrin-fibrinogen split products)	Fibrinogenic activity as measured by levels of fibrin-fibrinogen degradation products (in µL/ml of blood)	Transfusion reactions, DIC, internal hemorrhage in the newborn, deep vein thrombosis, pulmonary embolism

*See Chapter 23.

Data from Bick RL et al: *Hematology: clinical and laboratory practice*, St Louis, 1993, Mosby; Byrne CJ et al: *Laboratory tests: implications for nursing care*, Menlo Park, CA, 1986, Addison-Wesley.

TABLE 22.7 Mean Hematologic Differential Counts From Birth to Adulthood

Hematologic Differential	Newborn (Cord Blood)	2 Weeks of Age	3 Months of Age	6 Months to 6 Years of Age	7-12 Years of Age	Adult
Hemoglobin (g/dl)	16.8	16.5	12	12	13	13
Hematocrit (%)	55	50	36	37	38	40
Reticulocytes (%)	5	1	1	1	1	1
Leukocytes (WBCs/mm^3)	18,000	12,000	12,000	10,000	8000	8000
Neutrophils (%)	61	40	30	45	55	55
Lymphocytes (%)	31	48	63	48	38	35
Eosinophils (%)	2	3	2	2	2	2
Monocytes (%)	6	9	5	5	5	5
Platelets (10^3/mm^3)	290	252	150-400	150-400	150-400	150-400

WBCs, White blood cells.

somewhat in elderly persons. The erythrocyte life span is normal, although the erythrocytes are replenished more slowly after bleeding and their deformability decreases with advanced age.[12] Hemoglobin levels may be low, and the plasma membranes of erythrocytes become increasingly fragile, with portions being lost, presumably because of physical trauma inflicted during circulation.

Lymphocyte function decreases with age (see Chapter 7), causing changes in cellular immunity and some decline in T-cell function. The humoral immune system is less able to respond to antigenic challenge and to vaccination.

Platelet numbers tend to decrease in elderly persons, yet platelet adhesiveness increases. Fibrinogen levels and levels of factors V, VII, and IX and also vWF tend to be increased.[13] These changes could be considered a normal process of aging.

SUMMARY REVIEW

Components of the Hematologic System

1. Blood consists of a variety of components—about 91% water and 9% solutes. In adults, the total blood volume is approximately 5.5 L.
2. Plasma, a complex aqueous liquid, contains two major groups of plasma proteins: albumins and globulins.
3. The cellular elements of blood are the red blood cells (erythrocytes), white blood cells (leukocytes), and platelets.
4. Erythrocytes are the most abundant cells of the blood, occupying approximately 48% of the blood volume in men and approximately 42% in women. Erythrocytes are responsible for tissue oxygenation.
5. Leukocytes are fewer in number than erythrocytes and constitute approximately 5000 to 10,000 cells/mm^3 of blood. Leukocytes defend the body against infection and remove dead or injured host cells.
6. Leukocytes are classified as either granulocytes (neutrophils, eosinophils, basophils) or agranulocytes (monocytes/macrophages, lymphocytes, natural killer cells).
7. The mononuclear phagocyte system (MPS) is composed of monocytes in bone marrow and peripheral blood and macrophages in tissue. Cells of the MPS ingest and destroy unwanted materials, such as foreign protein particles, circulating immune complexes, microorganisms, debris from dead or injured cells, defective or injured erythrocytes, and dead neutrophils.
8. Platelets are irregularly shaped anuclear cytoplasmic fragments. Platelets are essential for blood coagulation and control of bleeding.
9. The lymphoid organs are sites of residence, proliferation, differentiation, or function of lymphocytes and mononuclear phagocytes.
10. The spleen is the largest lymphoid organ and functions as the site of fetal hematopoiesis, filters and cleanses the blood, and acts as a reservoir for lymphocytes and other blood cells.
11. The lymph nodes are the site of development or activity of large numbers of lymphocytes, monocytes, and macrophages.

Development of Blood Cells

1. Bone marrow consists of red (active or hematopoietic) marrow and yellow (inactive) marrow.
2. The hematopoietic marrow consists of a variety of cellular and molecular microenvironments called niches. Niches support the hematopoietic stem cells by direct cell-to-cell signaling and production of growth factors and cytokines important for retention, expansion, maintenance, and quiescence.
3. The bone marrow contains multiple populations of stem cells. Hematopoietic stem cells develop into blood cells. Mesenchymal stem cells develop into osteoblasts, adipocytes, chondrocytes, sinusoidal endothelial cells, fibroblasts, and other stromal cells.
4. Osteoblasts (responsible for construction of bone) and osteoclasts (remodel bone by resorption) produce cytokines that affect proliferation and maintenance of hematopoietic cells.
5. Specific hematopoietic growth factors (e.g., colony-stimulating factors) are necessary for the adequate production of myeloid, erythroid, lymphoid, and megakaryocytic lineages.
6. Hematopoiesis, or blood cell production, occurs in the liver and spleen of the fetus and in the bone marrow after birth.
7. Hematopoiesis involves two stages: mitotic division (i.e., proliferation) and maturation (i.e., differentiation). Each type of blood cell has parent cells called stem cells.
8. Hematopoiesis continues throughout life to replace blood cells that grow old and die, are killed by disease, or are lost through bleeding.
9. Regulation of erythropoiesis (development of red blood cells) is mediated by erythropoietin, which is secreted by the kidneys in response to tissue hypoxia. Erythropoietin causes a compensatory

increase in erythrocyte production if the oxygen content of the blood decreases because of anemia, high altitude, or pulmonary disease.

10. Hemoglobin, the oxygen-carrying protein of the erythrocyte, enables the blood to transport 100 times more oxygen than could be transported dissolved in plasma alone.

11. Erythropoiesis depends on the presence of vitamins (especially vitamin B_{12}, folate, vitamin B_6, riboflavin, pantothenic acid, niacin, ascorbic acid, and vitamin E).

12. The iron cycle reutilizes iron released from old or damaged erythrocytes. Iron binds to transferrin in the blood, is transported to macrophages, and is stored in the cytoplasm as ferritin.

13. Iron homeostasis is controlled by hepcidin, a small hormone produced by hepatocytes, which regulates ferroportin, the principal transporter of iron from stores in hepatocytes and macrophages and from intestinal cells that absorb dietary iron.

14. Myelopoiesis is the development of granulocytes (neutrophils, eosinophils, and basophils) and monocytes from the differentiation of myeloid progenitor cells in the bone marrow. Granulocytes are released into the blood and are either functioning cells that circulate in the blood or stored cells that are stored around the walls of blood vessels (marginating storage pool). Monocytes are released into the blood and travel to various tissues to become tissue macrophages and dendritic cells.

15. Lymphocytes, which are generated from lymphoid progenitor cells in a process called lymphopoiesis, are released into the bloodstream to undergo further maturation in the primary and secondary lymphoid organs

16. Platelets develop from megakaryocytes by a process called thrombopoiesis, which is controlled by thrombopoietin. During thrombopoiesis, megakaryocytes undergo mitosis but not cell division and the cytoplasm and plasma membrane fragment into platelets.

Mechanisms of Hemostasis

1. Hemostasis, or arrest of bleeding, involves (1) vasoconstriction (vasospasm), (2) formation of a platelet plug, (3) activation of the clotting cascade, (4) formation of a blood clot, and (5) clot retraction and clot dissolution.

2. The normal vascular endothelium prevents spontaneous clotting by producing factors such as nitric oxide (NO) and prostacyclin I_2 (PGI_2) that relax the vessels and prevent platelet activation.

3. Platelet activation involves three linked processes: (1) adhesion, (2) activation, and (3) aggregation.

4. A blood clot is a meshwork of protein strands that stabilizes the platelet plug. The strands are made of fibrin. Fibrin is the end product of the coagulation cascade.

5. Lysis of blood clots is the function of the fibrinolytic system. Plasmin, a proteolytic enzyme, splits fibrin and fibrinogen into fibrin degradation products that dissolve the clot.

Pediatrics and Blood

1. Blood cell counts tend to rise above adult levels at birth and then decline gradually throughout childhood. Platelet counts in full-term neonates are comparable with those in adults and remain so throughout infancy and childhood.

2. White blood cells develop during fetal life but the function of the cells at birth is weak as the cells are immature.

3. Newborn infants are at risk for impaired phagocytosis, bacterial infections, and delayed wound healing. Immature lymphocytes also increase risk for viral infection and there is a weak response to the production of antibodies and a poor response to foreign antigens.

Aging and Blood

1. Blood composition changes little with age. Erythrocyte replenishment may be delayed after bleeding, presumably because of iron deficiency.

2. Lymphocyte function appears to decrease with age. Particularly affected is a decrease in cellular immunity.

3. Platelet numbers decrease with age, but adhesiveness increases.

KEY TERMS

Agranulocyte, 486
Albumin, 484
Antithrombin III (AT-III), 498
Apoferritin, 495
Apotransferrin, 495
Basophil, 486
Blood clot, 498
Bone marrow (myeloid tissue), 490, 490
Bone marrow niche, 490
Clotting (coagulation) system, 498
Clotting factor, 485
Colony-stimulating factor (CSF, hematopoietic growth factor), 491
D-Dimer, 499
Deoxyhemoglobin, 493
Eosinophil, 486
Erythroblast (normoblast), 491
Erythrocyte, 485
Erythropoiesis, 491

Erythropoietin, 491
Fibrin degradation product (FDP), 499
Fibrinogen, 485
Fibrinolysis, 497
Fibrinolytic system, 499
Globin, 493
Globulin, 484
Glycoprotein IIb/IIIa (GPIIb/GPIIIa) complex, 497
Granulocyte, 486
Hematopoiesis, 491
Hematopoietic stem cells (HSCs), 490
Heme, 493
Hemoglobin (Hb), 491
Hemosiderin, 495
Hemostasis, 496
Hepcidin, 495
Immunocyte, 486
Iron cycle, 495
Leukocyte, 486

Lymph node, 489
Lymphocyte, 487
Lymphopoiesis (lymphocytopoiesis), 496
Macrophage, 487
Marginating storage pool, 496
Megakaryocyte, 488
Mesenchymal stem cell (MSC), 490
Methemoglobin, 493
Monocyte, 487
Mononuclear phagocyte system (MPS), 487
Myelopoiesis, 496
Natural killer (NK) cells, 487
Neutrophil (polymorphonuclear neutrophil [PMN]), 486
Nitric oxide (NO), 496
Oncotic pressure, 484
Osteoblast, 490
Osteoclast, 490
Oxyhemoglobin, 493

Phagocyte, 486
Plasma, 484
Plasma protein, 484
Plasmin, 499
Platelet adhesion, 497
Platelet aggregation, 497
Platelet (thrombocyte), 488
Platelet-release reaction, 497
Primary lymphoid organs, 488
Proerythroblast, 491
Prostacyclin (prostaglandin I_2 [PGI_2]), 496
Protein, 485
Protein C, 498
Protein S, 498
Protoporphyrin, 493
Reticulocyte, 491
Secondary lymphoid organ, 489
Serum, 484
Spleen, 489

REFERENCES

1. Weller PF, Spencer LA: Functions of tissue-resident eosinophils, *Nat Rev Immunol* 17(12):746-760, 2017.
2. Morrison SJ, Scadden DT: The bone marrow niche for haematopoietic stem cells, *Nature* 505(7483):327-334, 2014. Available from: https://www.ncbi.nlm.nih.gov/pmc/articles/PMC4514480/.
3. NIH Stem Cell Information Home Page: In *Stem Cell Information* [World Wide Web site], Bethesda, MD: National Institutes of Health, U.S. Department of Health and Human Services, 2016. (Cited August 10, 2019). Available at https://stemcells.nih.gov/info/basics.htm.
4. Thom CS, et al: Hemoglobin variants: biochemical properties and clinical correlates, *Cold Spring Harb Perspect Med* 3(3):a011858, 2013.
5. Kim A, Nemeth E: New insights into iron regulation and erythropoiesis, *Curr Opin Hematol* 22(3):199-205, 2015.
6. Machlus KR, et al: Interpreting the development dance of the megakaryocyte: a review of the cellular and molecular processes mediating platelet formation, *Br J Haematol* 165(2):227-236, 2014.
7. Hitchcock IS, Kaushansky K: Thrombopoietin from beginning to end, *Br J Haematol* 165(2):259-268, 2014.
8. Garmo C, Burns B. Physiology, clotting mechanism, *StatPearls [Internet]*, Treasure Island (FL), StatPearls Publishing, 2018 Jan-. Available from: http://www.ncbi.nlm.nih.gov/books/NBK507795. (Accessed 21 June 2018).
9. Ahmad A, et al: Role of nitric oxide in the cardiovascular and renal systems, *Int J Mol Sci* 19(9):2018.
10. Tomaiuolo M, Brass LF, Stalker TJ: Regulation of platelet activation and coagulation and its role in vascular injury and arterial thrombosis, *Interv Cardiol Clin* 6(1):1-12, 2017.
11. Simon AK, Hollander GA, McMichael A: Evolution of the immune system in humans from infancy to old age, *Proc Biol Sci* 282(1821):2015. 20143085.
12. de Haan G, Lazare SSL: Aging of hematopoietic stem cells, *Blood* 131(5):479-487, 2018.
13. Favaloro EJ, Franchini M, Lippi G: Aging hemostasis: changes to laboratory markers of hemostasis as we age—a narrative review, *Semin Thromb Hemost* 40(6):621-633, 2014.

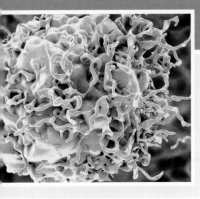

23

Alterations of Hematologic Function

Kathryn L. McCance

Alterations of erythrocyte function involve either insufficient or excessive numbers of erythrocytes in the circulation or normal numbers of cells with abnormal components. Anemias are conditions in which there are too few erythrocytes or an insufficient volume of erythrocytes in the blood. Polycythemias are conditions in which erythrocyte numbers or volume is excessive. All of these conditions have many causes and are pathophysiologic manifestations of a variety of disease states.

Many disorders involving leukocytes range from increased numbers of leukocytes (i.e., leukocytosis) in response to infections to proliferative disorders (such as leukemia). Many hematologic malignancies and nonhematologic malignancies metastasize to the bone marrow and affect leukocyte production. Thus a large portion of this chapter is devoted to malignant disease.

The primary role of clotting (hemostasis) is to stop bleeding through an interaction of endothelium lining the vessels, platelets, and clotting factors. A large number of disease states may increase or decrease clotting in any of the three main components of the clotting process.

ANEMIA

Classification and General Characteristics

Anemia is a reduction in the total number of erythrocytes in the circulating blood or a decrease in the quality or quantity of hemoglobin. Anemias commonly result from (1) impaired erythrocyte production, (2) blood loss (acute or chronic), (3) increased erythrocyte destruction, or (4) a combination of these three factors. Anemias are classified by their causes

(e.g., anemia of chronic disease) or by the changes that affect the size, shape, or substance of the erythrocyte. Total circulating red blood cell mass is affected by changes in plasma volume caused by dehydration (hemoconcentration) and fluid retention (hemodilution). The most common classification of anemias is based on the changes that affect the cell's size and hemoglobin content (Table 23.1). Terms used to identify anemias reflect these characteristics. Terms that end with *-cytic* refer to cell size, and those that end with *-chromic* refer to hemoglobin content. Additional terms describing erythrocytes found in some anemias are anisocytosis (assuming various sizes) and poikilocytosis (assuming various shapes).

CLINICAL MANIFESTATIONS The main alteration of anemia is a reduced oxygen-carrying capacity of the blood resulting in tissue hypoxia. Symptoms of anemia vary, depending on the body's ability to compensate for the reduced oxygen-carrying capacity. Anemia that is mild and starts gradually is usually easier to compensate and may cause problems for the individual only during physical exertion. As red cell reduction continues, symptoms become more pronounced and alterations in specific organs and compensation effects are more apparent. Compensation generally involves the cardiovascular, respiratory, and hematologic systems (Fig. 23.1).

A reduction in the number of blood cells in the blood causes a reduction in the consistency and volume of blood. Initial compensation for cellular loss is movement of interstitial fluid into the blood, causing an increase in plasma volume. This movement maintains an adequate

TABLE 23.1 Morphologic Classification of Anemias

Structure of Erythrocytes	Name and Mechanism of Anemia	Primary Cause
Macrocytic-normochromic anemia: large, abnormally shaped erythrocytes, normal hemoglobin concentrations	Pernicious anemia: lack of vitamin B₁₂; abnormal DNA and RNA synthesis in erythroblast; premature cell death	Congenital or acquired deficiency of intrinsic factor (IF); genetic disorder of DNA synthesis
	Folate deficiency anemia: lack of folate; premature cell death	Dietary folate deficiency
Microcytic-hypochromic anemia: small, abnormally shaped erythrocytes and reduced hemoglobin concentration	Iron deficiency anemia: lack of iron for hemoglobin; insufficient hemoglobin	Chronic blood loss, dietary iron deficiency, disruption of iron metabolism or iron cycle
	Sideroblastic anemia: dysfunctional iron uptake by erythroblasts and defective porphyrin and heme synthesis	Congenital dysfunction of iron metabolism in erythroblasts, acquired dysfunction of iron metabolism as result of drugs or toxins
	Thalassemia: impaired synthesis of α- or β-chain of hemoglobin A; phagocytosis of abnormal erythroblasts in marrow	Congenital genetic defect of globin synthesis
Normocytic-normochromic anemia: normal size, normal hemoglobin concentration	Aplastic anemia: insufficient erythropoiesis	Depressed stem cell proliferation
	Posthemorrhagic anemia: blood loss	Increased erythropoiesis; iron depletion
	Hemolytic anemia: premature destruction (lysis) of mature erythrocytes in circulation	Increased fragility of erythrocytes
	Sickle cell anemia: abnormal hemoglobin synthesis, abnormal cell shape with susceptibility to damage, lysis, and phagocytosis	Congenital dysfunction of hemoglobin synthesis
	Anemia of chronic inflammation; abnormally increased demand for new erythrocytes	Chronic infection or inflammation; malignancy

DNA, Deoxyribonucleic acid; *RNA,* ribonucleic acid.

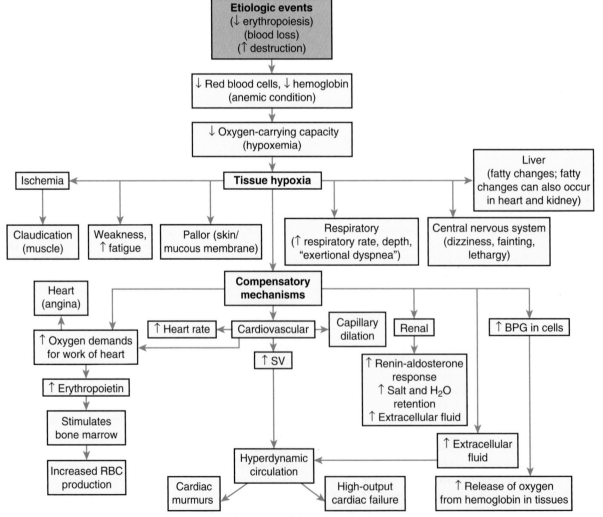

FIGURE 23.1 Progression and Manifestations of Anemia. *BPG,* Bisphosphoglycerate; *SV,* stroke volume.

blood volume, but the viscosity (thickness) of the blood decreases. The "thinner" blood flows faster and more turbulently than normal blood, causing a hyperdynamic circulatory state. This hyperdynamic state creates cardiovascular changes—increased stroke volume and heart rate. These changes may lead to cardiac dilation and heart valve insufficiency if the underlying anemic condition is not corrected.

Hypoxemia, reduced oxygen level in the blood, further contributes to cardiovascular dysfunction by causing dilation of arterioles, capillaries, and venules, thus increasing flow through them. Increased peripheral blood flow and venous return further contributes to an increase in heart rate and stroke volume in a continuing effort to meet normal oxygen demand and prevent cardiopulmonary congestion. These compensatory mechanisms may lead to heart failure.

Tissue hypoxia creates additional demands and effects on the pulmonary and hematologic systems. The rate and depth of breathing increase in an effort to increase oxygen availability accompanied by an increase in the release of oxygen from hemoglobin. All of these compensatory mechanisms may cause individuals to experience shortness of breath (dyspnea), a rapid and pounding heartbeat, dizziness, and fatigue. In mild chronic cases, these symptoms may be present only when there is an increased demand for oxygen (e.g., during physical exertion), but in severe cases, symptoms may be experienced even at rest.

Manifestations of anemia may be seen in other parts of the body. The skin, mucous membranes, lips, nail beds, and conjunctivae become either pale because of reduced hemoglobin concentration or yellowish (jaundiced) because of accumulation of end products of red cell destruction (hemolysis) if that is the cause of the anemia. Tissue hypoxia of the skin results in impaired healing and loss of elasticity, as well as thinning and early graying of the hair. Nervous system manifestations may occur in which the cause of anemia is a deficiency of vitamin B_{12}. Myelin degeneration occurs, causing a loss of nerve fibers in the spinal cord, resulting in paresthesias (numbness), gait disturbances, extreme weakness, spasticity, and reflex abnormalities. Decreased oxygen supply to the gastrointestinal (GI) tract often produces abdominal pain, nausea, vomiting, and anorexia. Low-grade fever (<101° F [38.3° C]) occurs in some anemic individuals and may result from the release of leukocyte pyrogens from ischemic tissues.

When the anemia is severe or acute in onset (e.g., hemorrhage), the initial compensatory mechanism is peripheral blood vessel constriction, diverting blood flow to essential vital organs. Decreased blood flow detected by the kidneys activates the renin-angiotensin response, causing salt and water retention in an attempt to increase blood volume. These situations are considered to be emergencies and require immediate intervention to correct the underlying problem that caused the acute blood loss; therefore long-term compensatory mechanisms do not develop.

Therapeutic interventions for slowly developing anemic conditions require treatment of the underlying condition and decrease of associated symptoms. Therapies include transfusion, dietary correction, and administration of supplemental vitamins or iron.

Anemias of Blood Loss
Acute Blood Loss

Posthemorrhagic anemia is a normocytic-normochromic anemia (NNA) caused by acute blood loss. Acute blood loss is mainly a loss of intravascular volume, and the effects depend on the rate of hemorrhage that can lead to cardiovascular collapse, shock, and death. A major cause of acute blood loss is trauma. Severe trauma is a rising global problem. An annual worldwide death rate from traumatic injury is more than 5.8 million or 1 in 10 mortalities.[1,2] The leading cause of potentially preventable death among injured individuals is uncontrolled posttraumatic bleeding. The pathophysiologic mechanisms of traumatic

injury are evolving (see *Did You Know?* Traumatic Injury, Bleeding, and Coagulopathy).

If acute blood loss is not severe, complete recovery is possible. Within 24 hours of blood loss, lost plasma is replaced by water and electrolytes from tissues and interstitial spaces into the vascular system. The hematocrit becomes lowered because of resulting hemodilution. A rapid elevation of circulating neutrophils and platelets occurs within a few hours from the shift of leukocytes into the circulation and a release of leukocytes from the bone marrow. The platelet count can rise significantly. Erythropoietin is stimulated from the reduction in tissue oxygenation and increases bone marrow production of erythrocytes. However, if blood loss is external, iron stores may be depleted and erythropoiesis may be impeded. Hemorrhage that is chronic (occult [i.e., bleeding ulcer or neoplasm]) produces less prominent adaptations, but an iron deficiency anemia (IDA) may develop. To restore blood volume, saline, dextran, albumin, or plasma is typically used, and with large blood losses it may be necessary to transfuse fresh whole blood (see *Did You Know?* Patient-Centered Blood Management).

DID YOU KNOW?

Patient-Centered Blood Management

Red blood cell transfusion is the main treatment to correct anemia; however, it is one of the top five overused procedures and carries its own risk and economic burdens. In an effort to improve patient outcomes, patient blood management (PBM) is a patient-centered and multidisciplinary approach to effectively manage anemia, reduce iatrogenic blood loss, and improve outcomes for those with anemia. Some hospitals are implementing PBM in practice.

Data from Meybohm P et al: *Perioper Med* 6:5, 2017.

Chronic Blood Loss

Anemia from chronic blood loss occurs if the loss is greater than the replacement capacity of the bone marrow. If iron stores are depleted, IDA can occur.

Anemias of Diminished Erythropoiesis

The anemias of diminished red cell production are many and varied and can be classified according to the underlying mechanism (Table 23.2). The most common anemias of diminished red cell production are the result of ineffective erythrocyte DNA synthesis mainly caused by nutritional deficiencies of vitamin B_{12} (cobalamin) or folate (folic acid). These anemias are also called macrocytic (megaloblastic) anemias.

Megaloblastic Anemias

The macrocytic (megaloblastic) anemias are characterized by unusually large stem cells (megaloblasts) in the marrow that mature into erythrocytes that are unusually large in size (macrocytic), thickness, and volume. These anemias are the result of ineffective erythrocyte deoxyribonucleic acid (DNA) synthesis, commonly caused by deficiencies of vitamin B_{12} (cobalamin) or folate (folic acid). Vitamin B_{12} is dependent on dietary B_{12} intake. Plants and vegetables contain little cobalamin and strictly vegetarian and macrobiotic diets do not provide adequate amounts. Another cause of megaloblastic anemia is pernicious anemia, caused by autoimmune destruction of parietal cells that make intrinsic factor (IF) (protein transporter necessary for vitamin B_{12} absorption in the intestine).

The defective erythrocytes in megaloblastic anemias die prematurely, which decreases their numbers in the circulation, causing anemia. Premature death of damaged erythrocytes, eryptosis, is a common mechanism of cellular loss in individuals with anemia secondary to

DID YOU KNOW?

Traumatic Injury, Bleeding, and Coagulopathy

Emerging is the understanding that persons with bleeding trauma are already showing signs of coagulopathy upon hospital admission. The presence of coagulopathy is related to an increase risk of multiple organ failure and death (see Chapter 26). Acute coagulopathy associated with traumatic injury is now recognized as a multifactorial condition caused by bleeding-induced shock, tissue-related thrombin-thrombomodulin-complex generation, and activation of the anticoagulant and fibrinolytic pathways (see Figure). The severity of the coagulopathy disorder is affected by preexisting and treatment factors that contribute to acidosis, hypothermia, hemodilution, hypoperfusion and coagulation factor consumption. Coagulopathy is modified by brain injury, age, genetic background, comorbidities, inflammation, medications (oral anticoagulants), and prehospital fluid administration. New terms for trauma-associated coagulopathic physiology include acute traumatic coagulopathy, early coagulation of trauma, acute coagulopathy of trauma-shock, trauma-induced coagulopathy, and trauma-associated coagulopathy. New guidelines recommend that individuals be transferred directly to trauma centers to improve outcomes.

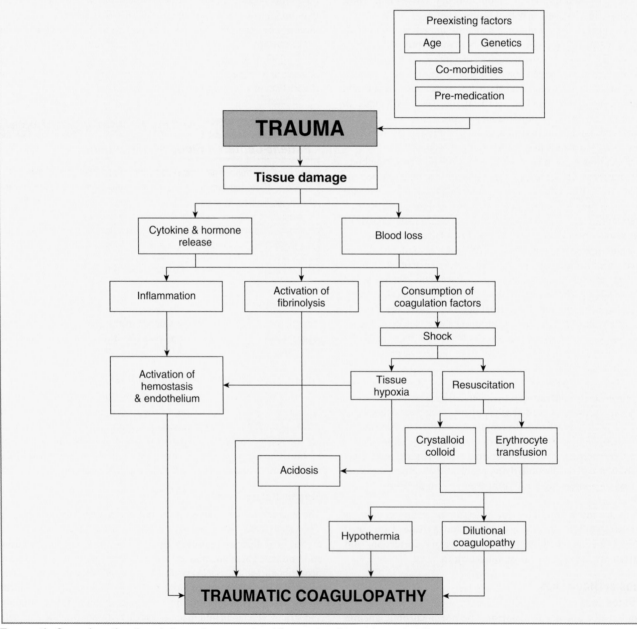

Traumatic Coagulopathy. Preexisting and trauma–related factors contribute to coagulopathy.
Box data from Firth D et al: *J Thromb Haemost* 8[9]:1919-1925, 2010; MacLeod JB et al: *J Trauma* 55[1]:39-44, 2003; Maegele M et al: *Injury* 38[3]:298-304, 2007; Rossaint R et al: *Crit Care* 20:100, 2016. Figure adapted from Rossaint R et al: *Crit Care* 20:100, 2016.

TABLE 23.2 Classification of Anemia According to Underlying Mechanism

Mechanism	Specific Examples
Blood Loss	
Acute blood loss	Trauma
Chronic blood loss	Gastrointestinal tract lesions, gynecologic disturbances*
Increased Red Cell Destruction (Hemolysis)	
Inherited Genetic Defects	
Red cell membrane disorders	Hereditary spherocytosis, hereditary elliptocytosis
Enzyme deficiencies	
Hexose monophosphate shunt enzyme deficiencies	G6PD deficiency, glutathione synthetase deficiency
Glycolytic enzyme deficiencies	Pyruvate kinase deficiency, hexokinase deficiency
Hemoglobin abnormalities	
Deficient globin synthesis	Thalassemia syndromes
Structurally abnormal globins (hemoglobinopathies)	Sickle cell disease, unstable hemoglobins
Acquired Genetic Defects	
Deficiency of phosphatidylinositol-linked glycoproteins	Paroxysmal nocturnal hemoglobinuria
Antibody-mediated destruction	Hemolytic disease of the newborn (Rh disease), transfusion reactions, drug-induced, autoimmune disorders
Mechanical trauma	
Microangiopathic hemolytic anemias	Hemolytic uremic syndrome, disseminated intravascular coagulation, thrombotic thrombocytopenia purpura
Cardiac traumatic hemolysis	Defective cardiac valves
Repetitive physical trauma	Bongo drumming, marathon running, karate chopping
Infections of red cells	Malaria, babesiosis
Toxic or chemical injury	Clostridial sepsis, snake venom, lead poisoning
Membrane lipid abnormalities	Abetalipoproteinemia, severe hepatocellular liver disease
Sequestration	Hypersplenism
Decreased Red Cell Production	
Inherited Genetic Defects	
Defects leading to stem cell depletion	Fanconi anemia, telomerase defects
Defects affecting erythroblast maturation	Thalassemia syndromes
Nutrition Deficiencies	
Deficiencies affecting DNA synthesis	B_{12} and folate deficiencies
Deficiencies affecting hemoglobin synthesis	Iron deficiency anemia
Erythropoietin deficiency	Renal failure, anemia of chronic disease
Immune-mediated injury of progenitors	Aplastic anemia, pure red cell aplasia
Inflammation-mediated iron sequestration	Anemia of chronic disease
Primary hematopoietic neoplasms	Acute leukemia, myelodysplasia, myeloproliferative disorders
Space-occupying marrow lesions	Metastatic neoplasms, granulomatous disease
Infections of red cell progenitors	Parvovirus B19 infection
Unknown mechanisms	Endocrine disorders, hepatocellular liver disease

*Most often cause of anemia is iron deficiency, not bleeding.
G6PD, Glucose-6-phosphate dehydrogenase.
From Kumar V, Abbas A, Aster JC: *Robbins & Cotran pathologic basis of disease*, ed 9, Philadelphia, 2015, Saunders.

deficiencies of iron, infections (e.g., malaria, mycoplasma), chronic diseases (e.g., diabetes, renal disease), genetic diseases (e.g., beta-thalassemia, glucose-6-phosphate dehydrogenase [G6PD] deficiency, sickle cell trait), and myelodysplastic syndrome.[3]

Defective DNA synthesis in megaloblastic anemias causes red cell growth and development to proceed at unequal rates. DNA synthesis and cell division are blocked or delayed. However, ribonucleic acid (RNA) replication and protein (hemoglobin) synthesis proceed normally.

Asynchronous development leads to an overproduction of hemoglobin during prolonged cellular division, creating a larger than normal erythrocyte with a disproportionately small nucleus. With each cell division, the disproportion between RNA and DNA becomes more apparent.

Pernicious anemia. Pernicious anemia (PA) is a type of megaloblastic anemia and is caused by vitamin B_{12} deficiency. The deficiency is often associated with the end stage of type A chronic atrophic

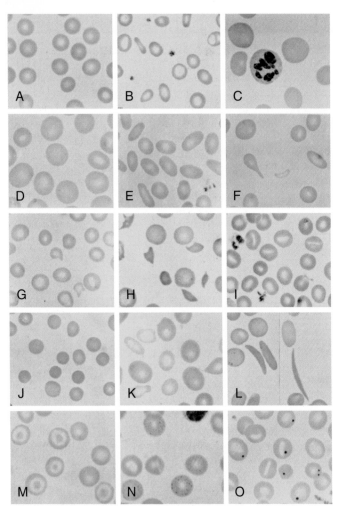

FIGURE 23.2 Appearance of Red Blood Cells in Various Disorders. A, Normal blood smear. **B,** Hypochromic-microcytic anemia (iron deficiency). **C,** Macrocytic anemia (pernicious anemia). **D,** Macrocytic anemia in pregnancy. **E,** Hereditary elliptocytosis. **F,** Myelofibrosis (teardrop). **G,** Hemolytic anemia associated with prosthetic heart valve. **H,** Microangiopathic anemia. **I,** Stomatocytes. **J,** Spherocytes (hereditary spherocytosis). **K,** Sideroblastic anemia; note the double population of red blood cells. **L,** Sickle cell anemia. **M,** Target cells (after splenectomy). **N,** Basophil stippling in case of unexplained anemia. **O,** Howell-Jolly bodies (after splenectomy). (From Wintrobe MM et al: *Clinical hematology,* ed 8, Philadelphia, 1981, Lea & Febiger.)

(autoimmune) gastritis (Fig. 23.2, *C*). Autoimmune gastritis impedes the production of IF, which is required for vitamin B_{12} uptake from the gut. *Pernicious* means highly injurious or destructive and reflects the fact that this condition was once fatal. It most commonly affects individuals older than age 30 who are of Northern European descent; however, it has now been recognized in all populations and ethnic groups.

PATHOPHYSIOLOGY   The main disorder in PA is the absence of IF. IF is secreted by gastric cells and forms a complex with vitamin B_{12} (B_{12}-IF) in the small intestine. B_{12} vitamin is essential for nuclear maturation and DNA synthesis in red blood cells. Deficiency of IF may be congenital or, more often, an autoimmune process directed against gastric parietal cells. Congenital IF deficiency is a genetic disorder with an autosomal recessive inheritance pattern. Although the autoimmune component may have a genetic component, the pattern of transmission has not been identified. PA also is frequently a component of autoimmune

polyendocrinopathy, which is a cluster of autoimmune diseases of endocrine organs. Autoimmune thyroiditis and type 1 diabetes mellitus, in particular, are associated with PA. Other causes include surgical removal of the stomach, resection of the ileum, and tapeworms. Associated conditions that increase demand for vitamin B_{12} include pregnancy, hyperthyroidism, chronic infection, and disseminated cancer. A history of infection with *Helicobacter pylori (H. pylori)* may cause an increase in antibodies that bind and damage the parietal cell. Environmental conditions may contribute to chronic gastritis, including excessive alcohol or hot tea ingestion and smoking.

The presence of PA with autoimmune gastritis (type A chronic gastritis) leads to gastric atrophy from destruction of parietal and zymogenic (relating to an enzyme) cells. Individuals with PA commonly have autoantibodies against the gastric H^+-K^+ ATPase, which is the major protein constituent of parietal cell membranes. Early in progression of disease, the gastric submucosa becomes infiltrated with inflammatory cells. These cells include autoreactive T cells, and it appears that these cells initiate gastric mucosal injury and trigger the formation of autoantibodies. The susceptibility to develop PA is linked to genetic variants involving the inflammasome, which suggests a relationship to innate immunity. Gastric mucosal atrophy, in which gastric parietal cells are destroyed, results in a deficiency of all secretions of the stomach—hydrochloric acid, pepsin, and IF. A direct correlation exists between the severity of the gastric lesion and the degree of malabsorption of vitamin B_{12}.

CLINICAL MANIFESTATIONS   PA develops slowly (over 20 to 30 years), so by the time an individual seeks treatment, it is usually severe. Early symptoms are often ignored because they are nonspecific and vague and include infections, mood swings, and GI, cardiac, or kidney ailments. When the hemoglobin level has decreased to 7 to 8 g/dl, the individual experiences classic symptoms of PA: weakness, fatigue, paresthesias of feet and fingers, difficulty walking, loss of appetite, abdominal pain, weight loss, and a sore tongue that is smooth and beefy red. The skin may become "lemon yellow" (sallow), caused by a combination of pallor and jaundice. Hepatomegaly, indicating right-sided heart failure, may be present in the elderly along with splenomegaly that is nonpalpable.

Neurologic manifestations result from nerve demyelination that may produce neuronal death. The posterior and lateral columns of the spinal cord also may be affected, causing a loss of position and vibration sense, ataxia, and spasticity. These complications pose a serious threat because they are not reversible, even with appropriate treatment. The cerebrum also may be involved with manifestations of affective disorders, most commonly of the depressive types. Low levels of vitamin B_{12} have been associated with neurocognitive disorders. An increased prevalence of serum vitamin B_{12} deficiency has been reported among individuals with Alzheimer disease.

EVALUATION AND TREATMENT   Diagnosis of PA is based on clinical manifestations and several test results, including blood tests, bone marrow aspiration, serologic studies, and gastric biopsy. The presence of circulating antibodies against parietal cells and IF also is useful in diagnosis. Gastric biopsy reveals total achlorhydria (absence of hydrochloric acid), which is diagnostic for PA.

Replacement of vitamin B_{12} (cobalamin) is the treatment of choice. Initial injections of vitamin B_{12} are administered weekly until the deficiency is corrected, followed by monthly injections for the remainder of the individual's life. The effectiveness of cobalamin replacement therapy is determined by a rising reticulocyte count. Blood counts return to normal within 5 to 6 weeks. PA cannot be cured, so maintenance therapy is lifelong. Conventional wisdom and practice assumed that oral preparations were ineffective because there was no IF to facilitate absorption of vitamin B_{12}. However, recent experience has shown that higher doses of orally administered vitamin B_{12} will be absorbed across the small bowel and that this treatment is beneficial.

Untreated PA is fatal, usually because of heart failure. With replacement therapy of vitamin B_{12}, mortality has decreased significantly. Death from PA is now rare, and relapses are often the result of noncompliance with therapy.

Folate deficiency anemia. A deficiency of folic acid results in a megaloblastic anemia having the same pathologic consequences as those caused by vitamin B_{12} deficiency. Folate (folic acid) is an essential vitamin required for RNA and DNA synthesis within the maturing erythrocyte. Folates are coenzymes required for the synthesis of thymine and purines (adenine and guanine) and the conversion of homocysteine to methionine. Deficient production of thymine, in particular, affects cells undergoing rapid division (e.g., bone marrow cells undergoing erythropoiesis). Humans are totally dependent on dietary intake to meet the daily requirement of 50 to 200 mg/day. Increased amounts are required for lactating and pregnant females. Folate is absorbed from the upper small intestine and does not require any other element (i.e., IF) to facilitate absorption. After absorption, folate circulates through the liver, where it is stored. Folate deficiency occurs more often than B_{12} deficiency, particularly in alcoholics and individuals with chronic malnourishment. It is estimated that at least 10% of North Americans are folate deficient, but the incidence has been decreasing in the United States since the fortification of foods with folate and the increased use of folate supplements.

Clinical manifestations are similar to the malnourished appearance of individuals with PA. Specific manifestations include cheilosis (scales and fissures of the mouth), stomatitis (inflammation of the mouth), and painful ulcerations of the buccal mucosa and tongue characteristic of burning mouth syndrome. *Burning mouth syndrome* may be secondary to a large number of disorders (e.g., extremely dry mouth, infection, autoimmune disease, nutritional deficiencies, and other conditions). Dysphagia, flatulence, and watery diarrhea also may be present, as well as histologic changes in the GI tract suggestive of those in sprue (chronic absorption disorder). Undiagnosed inflammatory bowel disease (e.g., Crohn disease, ulcerative colitis) may be the underlying cause of folate malabsorption in some individuals, and folate deficiency may suppress proliferation of the intestinal mucosa, leading to exacerbation of GI damage. Neurologic manifestations, if present, may be caused by thiamine deficiency, which often accompanies folate deficiency.

Evaluation of folate deficiency is based on blood tests, measurement of serum folate levels, and clinical manifestations. Treatment requires administration of oral folate preparations until adequate blood levels are obtained and manifestations are reduced or eliminated. Long-term therapy is not necessary if the appropriate dietary adjustments are made to maintain adequate intake. Manifestations of anemia disappear within 1 to 2 weeks after administration of folate.

Microcytic-Hypochromic Anemias

The microcytic-hypochromic anemias are characterized by abnormally small erythrocytes that contain unusually reduced amounts of hemoglobin (see Fig. 23.2, *B*). IDA is the most common nutritional disorder of the microcytic-hypochromic anemias.

Iron deficiency anemia. IDA is the most common nutritional disorder worldwide, occurring in both developed and developing countries. IDA is common in the United States, particularly in toddlers, adolescent girls, and women of childbearing age. Other populations at risk for IDA include those living in poverty, infants consuming cow's milk (decreased bioavailability of iron), older individuals ingesting restricted diets, and teenagers with poor diets (junk food). The

bioavailability of iron is particularly important because only 10% to 15% of ingested iron is absorbed.

Men typically ingest more iron than women, and premenopausal women, especially during pregnancy, have an increased requirement. Increased requirement is a major cause of iron deficiency in growing infants, children, and adolescents. The causes of IDA include (1) dietary deficiency, (2) impaired absorption, (3) increased requirement, (4) chronic blood loss, (5) impaired absorption (e.g., sprue, disorders of fat absorption), and (6) chronic diarrhea. Other causes for both sexes include use of medications that cause GI bleeding (e.g., aspirin or nonsteroidal antiinflammatory drugs [NSAIDS]), surgical procedures that decrease stomach acidity and other functions, and eating disorders. Excessive menstrual bleeding causes primary IDA in females, and males may experience bleeding as a result of ulcers, hiatal hernia, esophageal varices, cirrhosis, hemorrhoids, ulcerative colitis, or cancer. An occult bleeding source, such as colon cancer or other GI cancers or lesions, can lead to IDA; the astute clinician who understands the cause of IDA may be cancerous can save a life. An increased prevalence of iron deficiency has been observed in overweight children, adolescents, women, and those undergoing bariatric surgery.[4]

Children in developing countries are often affected by chronic parasite infestations that result in blood and iron loss that is greater than dietary intake, thus causing IDA. Treatment of helminth infections improves the anemia as well as appetite and growth. *H. pylori* infections are a frequent cause of iron-refractory or iron-dependent anemia of previously unknown origin in adults. *H. pylori* impairs iron uptake. IDA is associated with an increased absorption of other elements, for example, lead (Pb) and cadmium (Cd). Heavy exposure to Pb and Cd causes anemia, and treatment for iron deficiency is associated with a decrease in lead levels. Deficiencies in vitamins C, B_1, and B_6 enhance sensitivity toward Pb and Cd toxicity.

PATHOPHYSIOLOGY IDA is a hypochromic-microcytic anemia and occurs when iron stores are depleted. Although there is no intrinsic dysfunction in iron metabolism with inadequate dietary intake or excessive blood loss, both conditions deplete iron stores and reduce hemoglobin synthesis. With iron deficiency, various metabolic disorders lead to either insufficient iron delivery to bone marrow or impaired iron use within the marrow. Paradoxically, iron stores may be sufficient but delivery is inadequate to maintain heme synthesis, thus producing a functional or relative iron deficiency. Iron in the form of hemoglobin is in constant demand by the body. Iron is recyclable; therefore the body maintains a balance between iron that is contained in hemoglobin and iron that is in storage and available for future hemoglobin synthesis (see Chapter 22). Blood loss disrupts this balance by creating a need for more iron, thus depleting the iron stores more rapidly to replace the iron lost from bleeding. Iron contributes to immune function by regulating several immune mechanisms.

Acquired *hypoferremia* (deficiency of iron in the blood) may be part of the body's response to infection. Many pathogens require iron for survival; thus hypoferremia would hamper their growth. The precise benefits or detriments of iron deficiency and immunity, however, are still controversial.

IDA occurs when the demand for iron exceeds the supply and develops slowly through three overlapping stages. Stage I is characterized by decreased bone marrow iron stores; hemoglobin and serum iron remain normal. In stage II, iron transportation to bone marrow is diminished, resulting in iron-deficient erythropoiesis. Stage III begins when the small hemoglobin-deficient cells enter the circulation to replace the normal aged erythrocytes that have been removed from the circulation. The manifestations of IDA appear in stage III, when there is depletion of iron stores and diminished hemoglobin production.

CLINICAL MANIFESTATIONS Symptoms of IDA begin gradually, and individuals may not seek medical attention until hemoglobin levels have decreased to about 7 to 8 g/dl. Nonspecific early symptoms include fatigue, weakness, shortness of breath, and pale earlobes, palms, and conjunctivae (Fig. 23.3). As the condition progresses and becomes more severe, structural and functional changes occur in epithelial tissue (see Fig. 23.3). **Koilonychia** or *spoon-shaped* fingernails become brittle, thin, and coarsely ridged as a result of impaired capillary circulation (see Fig. 23.3, *B*) Other manifestations include cheilosis (scales and fissures of the mouth), stomatitis (inflammation of the mouth), and painful ulcerations of the buccal mucosa and tongue characteristic of burning (glossitis) (see Fig. 23.3, *C*). Burning mouth syndrome may be secondary to a large number of disorders (e.g., extremely dry mouth, infection, autoimmune disease, nutritional deficiencies, and other conditions). Difficulty in swallowing (dysphagia) is associated with an esophageal *web,* a thin, concentric extension of normal esophageal tissue consisting of mucosa and submucosa at the juncture between the hypopharynx and esophagus. Dysphagia is worsened by hyposalivation. Individuals with IDA also exhibit gastritis, neuromuscular changes, headache, irritability, tingling, numbness, and vasomotor disturbances. Alterations in gait are rare.

Iron deficiency in children is associated with numerous adverse manifestations, especially cognitive impairment. Cognitive impairment may be long-lasting and irreversible (see Chapter 24).

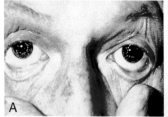
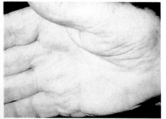
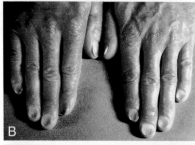
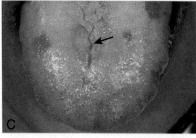

FIGURE 23.3 Manifestations of Iron Deficiency Anemia. A, Pallor and iron deficiency. Pallor of the skin, mucous membranes, and palmar creases in an individual with a hemoglobin level of 9 g/dl. Palmar creases become as pale as the surrounding skin when the hemoglobin level approaches 7 g/dl. **B,** Koilonychia. The nails are concave, ridged, and brittle. **C,** Glossitis. Tongue of individual with iron deficiency anemia has bald, fissured appearance caused by loss of papillae and flattening. (From Hoffbrand AV, Pettit JE, Vyas P: *Color atlas of clinical hematology,* ed 4, London, 2009, Mosby; **B** courtesy Dr. S.M. Knowles.)

EVALUATION AND TREATMENT Initial evaluation is based on symptoms and decreased levels of hemoglobin and hematocrit. Anemia appears only when iron stores are depleted and accompanied by lower than normal serum iron, ferritin, and transferrin saturation levels. Other blood tests may be done. A sensitive indicator of heme synthesis is the amount of free erythrocyte protoporphyrin (FEP) within erythrocytes. An initial step in treatment of IDA is to identify and eliminate sources of blood loss. Otherwise replacement therapy may be ineffective. Parenteral iron replacement is used in instances of uncontrolled blood loss, intolerance to oral iron replacement, intestinal malabsorption, or poor adherence to oral therapy.

Iron replacement therapy is required and very effective, and hematocrit levels should improve within 1 to 2 months of therapy. Serum ferritin level, however, is a more precise measurement of improvement. A rapid decrease in fatigue, lethargy, and other associated symptoms is generally seen within the first month of therapy. Replacement therapy may continue for many months. Menstruating females may need daily oral iron replacement therapy until menopause.

Anemia of Chronic Disease

Anemia of chronic disease (**ACD**, also called **anemia of inflammation** [**AI**]), is a mild to moderate anemia resulting from decreased erythropoiesis and impaired iron utilization in individuals with conditions of chronic systemic disease or inflammation (e.g., infections, cancer, and chronic inflammatory or autoimmune diseases). ACD is a common type of anemia in hospitalized individuals. Table 23.3 lists the possible causes of ACD. ACD also is commonly noted in the presence of congestive heart failure (CHF). The anemia develops after 1 to 2 months of disease activity. The initial severity is related to the underlying disorder, but, although persistent, it usually does not progress. Individuals may be asymptomatic, or the anemia may be a chance clinical finding. ACD shares features observed in individuals with chronic obstructive pulmonary disease (COPD); in persons with critical illnesses after acute events such as major surgery, severe trauma, myocardial infarction, and sepsis; and in the elderly. It shares some features with anemia noted in some cancers.

ACD is one of the most common conditions encountered in medicine and is possibly only secondary to IDA in overall incidence. In individuals older than age 65, anemia is present in 10% of those who live in the community and in more than 50% of those who reside in nursing homes, with two-thirds of cases being ACD or unexplained anemia.

TABLE 23.3 Underlying Causes of Anemia of Chronic Disease

Associated Diseases	Estimated Prevalence (%)
Infections: acute and chronic; viral infections including HIV infection, bacterial, parasitic, fungal	18-95
Cancer: hematologic, solid tumor	30-77
Autoimmune	8-71
Rheumatoid arthritis, systemic lupus	8-70
erythematosus and connective-tissue diseases, vasculitis, sarcoidosis, inflammatory bowel disease	25-30
Chronic rejection after solid-organ transplantation	
CKD and inflammation	

ACD, Anemia of chronic disease; *CKD,* chronic kidney disease.
Data from Weiss G, Goodnough LT: *N Engl J Med* 352(10):1011-1023, 2005.

The elderly may be predisposed to ACD related to age-associated hematopoietic changes with increased concentrations of inflammatory cytokines. These cytokines play a significant role in the development of ACD. The elderly with characteristics of ACD without an underlying malignancy or inflammatory condition are described as having primary defective iron utilization syndrome.

PATHOPHYSIOLOGY ACD results from a combination of (1) decreased erythrocyte life span, (2) suppressed production of erythropoietin, (3) ineffective bone marrow response to erythropoietin, and (4) altered iron metabolism and iron dynamics in macrophages. During chronic inflammation, a large variety of cytokines are released by lymphocytes, macrophages, and the affected tissue. Impaired iron metabolism is partially the result of iron sequestration. Fig. 23.4 includes the pathophysiology of ACD with normal and altered iron metabolism.

Erythrocyte destruction is the result of eryptosis (described earlier in this chapter). Most of the diseases responsible for ACD damage to erythrocytes results in macrophage activity. Normal iron transport by transferrin also may be decreased as a result of inflammation-related increases in the levels of circulating lactoferrin and apoferritin. Lactoferrin is a member of the transferrin family of nonheme, iron-binding glycoproteins and, under normal conditions, is present in the blood in only small amounts. During inflammation, neutrophils release lactoferrin to bind iron and reduce its availability for bacteria. However, the affinity of iron for lactoferrin is 260 times greater than that for transferrin. Lactoferrin-bound iron is removed by the mononuclear-phagocyte system and converted into ferritin, the storage form of iron. Apoferritin also has a higher affinity for iron and affects available iron in a similar manner.

The erythropoietic defect in ACD is failure to increase erythropoiesis in response to decreased numbers of erythrocytes. In part, decreased erythropoiesis results from diminished production of erythropoietin by the kidneys. In addition, the failure in erythropoiesis may reflect decreased responsiveness of erythroid progenitors to erythropoietin. Decreased availability of iron would diminish the rate of erythropoiesis. Proliferation of erythroid cells also is inhibited by proinflammatory cytokines. Loss of integrins may prevent adequate interaction with stromal cells and matrix proteins and inhibit erythropoiesis.

Platelet function may be defective in these individuals, which results in chronic bleeding and loss of erythrocytes. Anemia may arise from the direct action of bacterial toxins.

CLINICAL MANIFESTATIONS The anemia of ACD is usually in the mild to moderate range. With a significant drop in hemoglobin levels, clinical manifestations of IDA appear.

EVALUATION AND TREATMENT Initially, ACD is normocytic-normochromic, but with persistence it becomes hypochromic and microcytic. ACD is characterized by abnormal iron metabolism, low levels of circulating iron, and reduced levels of transferrin. The most significant finding of ACD is very high total body iron storage, although inadequate iron is released from the bone marrow for erythropoiesis. A first indication of ACD is often a failure to respond to conventional iron replacement therapy. Levels of erythropoietin are generally lower than expected for the degree of anemia. Individuals frequently present with low or normal total iron-binding capacity (TIBC), normal or high serum ferritin levels, and low concentrations of soluble

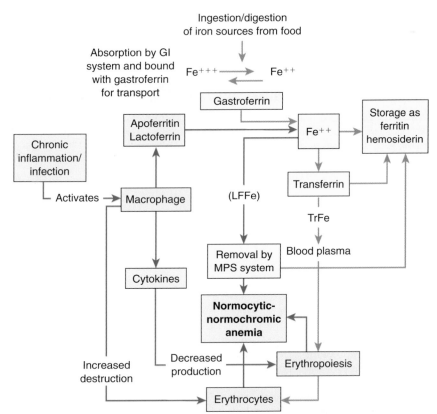

FIGURE 23.4 Pathophysiology of Anemia of Chronic Disease. Normal iron metabolism is indicated by the *blue arrows*. Abnormal mechanisms that are instrumental in the development of anemia of chronic inflammation are indicated by *red arrows*. (See discussion in text.) *GI,* Gastrointestinal.

transferrin receptor. It occasionally may be difficult to differentiate ACD from IDA.

Use of erythropoietin in treatment of ACD associated with arthritis, malignancies, and acquired immunodeficiency syndrome (AIDS) has met with limited success. Individuals with severe anemia secondary to chronic kidney disease (CKD) can be treated successfully with erythropoietin and treatments to increase iron stores.[5] However, the optimal degree of restoration of hemoglobin levels has not been determined; a return to normal levels increases the risk of hypertension, stroke, and death.[6] Transfusion of critically ill individuals may worsen the outcome and increase morbidity and mortality.[7] The principal treatment is easement of the underlying disorder. Individuals with ACD, but without evidence of inflammatory or infectious conditions, are screened for malignancies.

Aplastic and Hemolytic Anemia

Aplastic anemia (AA) is a hematopoietic failure or bone marrow aplasia with a reduction in the effective production of mature cells by the bone marrow, causing peripheral pancytopenia (anemia, neutropenia, and thrombocytopenia), which is a reduction or absence of all three blood cell types. Hemolytic anemia is premature accelerated destruction of erythrocytes, either episodically or continuously. These two types of anemia are discussed in Table 23.4.

✔**QUICK CHECK 23.1**

1. How do cell size and content determine classification of anemia?
2. Why is iron important to hemoglobin synthesis, and why is iron deficiency related to anemia?
3. Discuss the pathophysiology of iron deficiency anemia
4. Discuss the characteristics of anemia of chronic disease and why it is considered one of the most common conditions encountered in medicine.
5. How is anemia diagnosed?

MYELOPROLIFERATIVE RED CELL DISORDERS

Hematologic dysfunction results from an overproduction of cells, as well as a deficiency. One or more hematopoietic lines may be overproduced in the marrow in response to exogenous (e.g., exposure to radiation, drugs) or endogenous (e.g., physiologic compensatory response, immune disorder) signals. Excessive red cell production is classified as polycythemia (Table 23.5). Polycythemia exists in two forms: relative and absolute. Relative polycythemia results from hemoconcentration of the blood associated with dehydration that may be caused by decreased water intake, diarrhea, excessive vomiting, or increased use of diuretics. Its development is usually of minor consequence and resolves with fluid administration or treatment of underlying conditions.

Absolute polycythemia consists of two forms: primary and secondary. *Secondary polycythemia,* the most common of the two, is a physiologic response resulting from erythropoietin secretion caused by hypoxia. This hypoxia is noted in individuals living at higher altitudes (>10,000 ft), smokers with increased blood levels of carbon dioxide (CO), and individuals with COPD or heart failure, or both. Abnormal types of hemoglobin (e.g., San Diego, Chesapeake), which have a greater affinity for oxygen, also cause secondary polycythemia, as does inappropriate secretion of erythropoietin by certain tumors (e.g., renal cell carcinoma, hepatoma, and cerebellar hemangioblastomas).

Polycythemia Vera

Polycythemia vera (PV) (also known as *primary polycythemia*) is a slowly growing blood cancer in which the bone marrow makes too many red blood cells. It is a stem cell disorder with hyperplastic and neoplastic bone marrow alterations. PV is characterized by an abnormal uncontrolled proliferation of red blood cells (frequently with increased levels of white blood cells [leukocytosis] and platelets [thrombocytosis]). The increase in red cells (*polycythemia*) is responsible for most of the clinical symptoms, including an increase in blood volume and viscosity. PV is one of several disorders collectively known as *chronic*

TABLE 23.4   Normocytic-Normochromic Anemias

	Pathophysiology	Clinical Manifestations	Evaluation and Treatment
Aplastic	Rare; may result from infiltrative disorders of bone marrow, autoimmune diseases, renal failure, splenic dysfunction, vitamin B_{12} or folate deficiency, parvovirus infection, or exposure to radiation, drugs, and toxins; also may be congenital Common stem cell population may be altered so it cannot proliferate or differentiate, or stem cell environment is altered to inhibit erythropoiesis Outcome ranges from death to minimal manifestations	Classic cardiovascular and respiratory manifestations with thrombocytopenia, hemorrhage into tissues, leukopenia, and infection	Bone marrow biopsy determines whether anemia is caused by pure red cell aplasia or hypoplasia Treat underlying disorder or prevent further exposure to causative agent Blood transfusions, marrow transplant, and pharmacologic stimulation of bone marrow function
Hemolytic	Acquired: caused by infection, systemic disease, drugs or toxins, liver disease, kidney disease, abnormal immune responses Hereditary: caused by abnormalities of RBC membrane or cytoplasmic contents; present at birth Hemolysis: in blood vessels or lymphoid tissues that filter blood (e.g., spleen, liver) Erythrocytes: rigid, slowing their passage and making them vulnerable to phagocytosis Types: warm antibody disease (mediated by IgG antibody specific for erythrocyte antigens), cold antibody disease (mediated by IgM), and drug induced	Splenomegaly, jaundice, aplastic, hemolytic, or megaloblastic crises can develop with viral infection With severe disease, bones become deformed and pathologic fractures occur Cardiovascular and respiratory manifestations correspond with severity of anemia	

AIDS, Acquired immunodeficiency syndrome; *RBC,* red blood cell; *SLE,* systemic lupus erythematosus.

TABLE 23.5   Disorders Classified as Polycythemia

Type of Polycythemia	Mechanism of Increased Erythropoiesis	Cause of Associated Disorder
Primary polycythemia (polycythemia vera)	Excessive proliferation of erythroid precursors in marrow; JAK2 mutation, increased sensitivity of stem cell to erythropoietin	Possible mutation in erythropoietin receptor
Secondary polycythemia	Physiologic increase in erythropoietin secretion by kidneys in response to underlying systemic disorder	Tissue hypoxia caused by cardiopulmonary disorders (chronic obstructive pulmonary disease, congestive heart failure), decreased barometric pressure, cardiovascular malformations causing mixing of arterial and venous blood, methemoglobinemia, carboxyhemoglobinemia, smoking, obesity
	"Nonphysiologic"* increase in erythropoietin secretion	Renal disorders, cerebellar hemangioblastomas, hepatoma (liver tumor), ovarian carcinoma, uterine leiomyoma, pheochromocytoma, adrenocortical hypersecretion
Familial polycythemia	Genetically induced increase in erythroid precursors of marrow; Abnormal hemoglobin with increased oxygen affinity; Decreased 2,3-DPG; Increased sensitivity of stem cells to erythropoietin; Increased erythropoietin secretion	Genetic defect

2,3-DPG, 2,3-Diphosphoglycerate.
*Nonphysiologic means that there is no obvious physiologic explanation for hypersecretion of erythropoietin.

myeloproliferative disorders (CMPDs) (Box 23.1). These disorders include certain leukemias, essential thrombocytosis, and chronic bone marrow fibrosis. The disorders all result from abnormal regulation of the hematopoietic stem cells. Specifically, the common pathogenic feature is the presence of a mutation in the Janus kinase 2 gene (*JAK2* gene) resulting in an overproduction of blood cells. Normally, the *JAC2* gene makes a protein that helps the body produce blood cells (see Pathophysiology). Because of numerous characteristics (e.g., overproduction of different blood cells, marrow hypercellularity, or fibrosis) shared by these disorders and a lack of specific molecular markers, the diagnosis can be quite challenging. The major characteristics shared by these disorders include (1) involvement of a hematopoietic progenitor cell, (2) overproduction of one or more of the formed elements in blood in the absence of a defined stimulus, (3) dominance by a transformed progenitor cell, (4) hypercellular bone marrow or fibrosis, (5) chromosomal (cytogenetic) abnormalities, (6) predisposition to thrombus formation and hemorrhage, and (7) spontaneous transformation to leukemia.

PV is quite rare, with an estimated incidence of 2.3 per 100,000 individuals; peak incidence is between the ages of 60 and 80 years, with a median incidence of 55 to 60. However, PV has been observed in individuals younger than the age of 40. Males are twice as likely as females to develop PV. It is more common in whites of Eastern European Jewish ancestry. PV is rarely seen in children or in multiple members of a single family; however, an autosomal dominant form exists that causes increased secretion of erythropoietin.

PATHOPHYSIOLOGY   PV is a chronic neoplastic, nonmalignant condition characterized by overproduction of red blood cells (frequently with increased levels of white blood cells and platelets) and splenomegaly. Erythrocytosis is the essential component of PV. Proliferation of erythroid progenitors occurs in the bone marrow independent of the hormone erythropoietin, but the cells express a normal erythropoietin receptor. More than 95% of individuals with PV have an acquired mutation in the tyrosine kinase, Janus kinase 2 (JAK2). Normal JAK2 increases the activity of the erythropoietin receptor and is self-regulatory so that JAK2 activity diminishes over time. The mutation associated

with PV negates the self-regulatory activity of JAK2 so that the erythropoietin receptor is constantly active regardless of the level of erythropoietin. Overall, the mutated tyrosine kinases bypass normal controls, causing growth factor–independent proliferation and survival of marrow progenitors or precursor cells. The cause of the mutation is unknown.

CLINICAL MANIFESTATIONS   PV is uncommon and occurs insidiously. Clinical manifestations of PV are a result of the increased red cell mass and hematocrit. Usually there is an increase in blood volume. Together all of these factors cause abnormal blood flow that increases blood viscosity, creating a hypercoagulable state that results in clogging and occlusion of blood vessels. Tissue injury (ischemia) and death (infarction) is the outcome of blood vessel blockage. These outcomes are directly correlated with hematocrit levels. Increases in numbers of thrombocytes, as well as production of dysfunctional platelets, also contribute to this hypercoagulable condition.

Circulatory alterations caused by the thick, sticky blood give rise to other manifestations, such as plethora (ruddy, red color of the face, hands, feet, ears, and mucous membranes) and engorgement of retinal and cerebral veins. Other symptoms may include headache, drowsiness, delirium, mania, psychotic depression, chorea, and visual disturbances. Individuals frequently have an enlarged spleen with abdominal pain and discomfort. Death from cerebral thrombosis is approximately five times greater in individuals with PV.

Cardiovascular function, despite the vascular alterations, remains relatively normal. Cardiac workload and output remain constant; however, increased blood volume does increase blood pressure. Coronary blood flow may be affected, precipitating angina, although cardiovascular infarctions are uncommon. Other cardiovascular manifestations include Raynaud phenomenon and thromboangiitis obliterans.

A unique feature of PV, and helpful in diagnosis, is the development of intense, painful itching that appears to be intensified by heat or exposure to water *(aquagenic pruritus)* so that individuals avoid exposure to water, particularly warm water when bathing or showering. The intensity of itching is related to the concentration of mast cells in the skin and is generally not responsive to antihistamines or topical lotions.

BOX 23.1 World Health Organization (WHO) Classification of Myeloid Malignancies

1. Acute myeloid leukemia (AML) and related neoplasms*
2. Myeloproliferative neoplasms (MPN)
   2.1. Chronic myeloid leukemia, *BCR-ABL1* positive (CML)
   2.2. *BCR-ABL1*-negative MPN
      2.2.1. Polycythemia vera
      2.2.2. Primary myelofibrosis (PMF)
      2.2.3. Prefibrotic PMF
      2.2.4. Essential thrombocythemia (ET)
   2.3. Other MPN
      2.3.1. Chronic neutrophilic leukemia (CNL)
      2.3.2. Chronic eosinophilic leukemia, not otherwise specified (CEL-NOS)
      2.3.3. Mastocytosis
      2.3.4. Myeloproliferative neoplasm, unclassified (MPN-U)
3. Myelodysplastic syndromes (MDS)
   3.1. Refractory cytopenia† with unilineage dysplasia (RCUD)
      3.1.1. Refractory anemia (ring sideroblasts <15% of erythroid precursors)
      3.1.2. Refractory neutropenia
   3.2. Refractory anemia with ring sideroblasts (RARS; dysplasia limited to erythroid lineage and ring sideroblasts ≥15% of bone marrow erythroid precursors)
   3.3. Refractory cytopenia with multilineage dysphasia (RCMD; ring sideroblast count does not matter)
   3.4. Refractory anemia with excess blasts (RAEB)
      3.4.1. RAEB-1 (2%-4% circulating *or* 5%-9% marrow blasts)
      3.4.2. RAEB-2 (5%-19% circulating *or* 10%-19% marrow blasts *or* Auer rods present)
   3.5. MDS associated with isolated del(5q)
   3.6. MDS, unclassified
4. MDS/MPN
   4.1. Chronic myelomonocytic leukemia (CMML)
   4.2. Atypical chronic myeloid leukemia, *BCR-AB1* negative
   4.3. Juvenile myelomonocytic leukemia (JMML)
   4.4. MDS/MPN, unclassified
      4.4.1. Provisional entry: Refractory anemia with ring sideroblastic associated with marked thrombocytosis (RARS-T)
5. Myeloid and lymphoid neoplasms with eosinophilia and abnormalities of *PDGFRA,*‡ *PDGFRB,*‡ *FGFRI*‡
   5.1. Myeloid and lymphoid neoplasms with *PDGFRA* rearrangement
   5.2. Myeloid neoplasms with *PDGFRB* rearrangement
   5.3. Myeloid and lymphoid neoplasms with *FGFRI* abnormalities

*Acute myeloid leukemia-related precursor neoplasms include "therapy-related myelodysplastic syndrome" and "myeloid sarcoma."
†Either mono- or bi-cytopenia: hemoglobin <10 g/dl, absolute neutrophil count <1.8 × 10⁹/L, or platelet count <100 × 10⁹/L. However, higher blood counts do not exclude the diagnosis in the presence of unequivocal histologic/cytogenic evidence for myelodysplastic syndrome.
‡Genetic rearrangements involving platelet-derived growth factor receptor α/β *(PDFRA/PDFRB)* or fibroblast growth factor receptor 1 *(FGFR1).*
From Tefferi A, Barbui T: *Am J Hematol* 90(2):162-173, 2015.

EVALUATION AND TREATMENT   PV is frequently suspected because of clinical features, such as a thrombotic event, splenomegaly, or aquagenic pruritus. Blood and laboratory findings, characterized by an absolute increase in red blood cells and in total blood volume, confirm the diagnosis. Median hematocrit levels may range from 44.4% to 47.5%,

and red blood cell counts may range from 7×10^{12} to $7 \times 10^{13}/\mu L$. Erythrocytes appear normal, but anisocytosis may be present. There also may be moderate increases in white blood cells and platelets. A bone marrow examination may be done but is not very valuable unless performed in association with cytogenetic and molecular studies for relevant mutations in JAK2. The presence of a JAK2 mutation confirms the diagnosis.

Treatment of PV consists of reducing red cell proliferation and blood volume, controlling symptoms, and preventing clogging and clotting of the blood vessels. In low-risk individuals (e.g., those younger than age 60 or with no history of thrombosis and without risk factors for cardiovascular disease), the recommended therapy is phlebotomy (300 to 500 ml at a time to reduce erythrocytosis and blood volume) and low-dose aspirin. Frequent phlebotomies also reduce iron levels, a condition that impedes erythropoiesis.

Hydroxyurea, a nonalkylating myelosuppressive, is the drug of choice for myelosuppression because of a reduced incidence to cause leukemia and thrombosis. Radioactive phosphorus (^{32}P) also is used as an effective and easily tolerated intervention to suppress erythropoiesis. Its effects may last up to 18 months. Side effects of ^{32}P include suppression of hematopoiesis resulting in anemia, leukopenia, and thrombocytopenia. Acute leukemia is also a side effect, although most often it occurs only after 7 or more years of treatment, making its use in elderly persons more common. Interferon (IFN)-alpha has been used when other forms of treatment have failed. Newer drugs that inhibit the JAK2 pathway are being investigated.

Survival for 10 to 15 years is common. However, without proper treatment, 50% of individuals with PV die within 18 months of the onset of initial symptoms because of thrombosis or hemorrhage. A significant potential outcome of PV is the conversion to acute myeloid leukemia (AML), occurring spontaneously in 10% of affected individuals and generally being resistant to conventional therapy. Although PV is a chronic disorder, appropriate therapy results in remissions and prevention of significant pathologic outcomes.

Iron Overload

Iron overload can be primary, as in hereditary hemochromatosis (HH), or secondary. The secondary causes of iron overload include anemias with inefficient erythropoiesis (e.g., AA), dietary iron overload, or conditions that require repeated blood transfusions or iron dextran injections.

Hereditary Hemochromatosis

Hemochromatosis is caused by excessive iron absorption. Hereditary hemochromatosis (HH) is a common inherited, autosomal recessive disorder of iron metabolism and is characterized by increased GI iron absorption with subsequent tissue iron deposition. Excess iron is deposited first in the liver and pancreas, followed by the heart, joints, and endocrine glands. Excess iron causes tissue damage that can lead to diseases such as cirrhosis, diabetes, heart failure, arthropathies, and impotence.

HH is classified by type (1, 2, 3, and 4) depending on age of onset and other mostly genetic factors. Type 1 is the most common type, and type 4 (also called ferroportin disease) begins as adults. Men with type 1 or type 4 hemochromatosis usually develop symptoms between the ages of 40 and 60, and women develop them after menopause. Type 2 hemochromatosis is a juvenile-onset disorder. Iron accumulation begins early in life, and symptoms appear in childhood. Type 3 hemochromatosis is usually intermediate between types 1 and 2. Symptoms of type 3 hemochromatosis can begin before age 30.

PATHOPHYSIOLOGY   Mutations in several genes can cause HH. Type 1 hemochromatosis results from mutations in the *HFE* gene, and type

2 hemochromatosis results from mutations in either the *HJV* or *HAMP* gene. Mutations in the *FR2* gene cause type 3, and mutations in the *SLC40A1* gene cause type 4 hemochromatosis.[8] The proteins produced from these genes play the important roles of regulating absorption, transport, and storage of iron. With HH, regulation of dietary iron is abnormal, causing iron accumulation. HFE protein interacts with other proteins on the cell surface to detect the amount of iron in the body. HFE protein also regulates an important protein called **hepcidin**, which governs iron regulation.[9] Hepcidin is produced by the liver and determines how much iron is absorbed from the diet and then released from body storage sites. Mutations in any of the genes for HH impair the control of iron absorption during digestion and alter the distribution of iron to other body sites.[8] Eventually, iron accumulates in tissues and organs disrupting their normal function.

CLINICAL MANIFESTATIONS Clinical *HFE*-HH, more common in men than women, is characterized by excessive storage of iron in the liver, skin, pancreas, heart, joints, and testes. In untreated individuals, early symptoms may include abdominal pain, weakness, and weight loss. The risk of cirrhosis is significantly increased when the serum ferritin level is higher than 1000 ng/ml. Other findings include progressive increase in skin pigmentation; diabetes mellitus; CHF; and/or dysrhythmias, arthritis, and hypogonadism.[10] Many individuals are diagnosed as a result of serum iron studies as part of a health-screening panel.

EVALUATION AND TREATMENT Published practice guidelines for diagnosis and management of hemochromatosis are from the American Association for the Study of Liver Disease (AASLD) and the European Association for the Study of the Liver (EASL). Serum ferritin concentration is used to establish the disease status and prognosis (Fig. 23.5).

A specialized magnetic resonance imaging (MRI) technique approved by the U.S. Food and Drug Administration can estimate hepatic iron concentration. Therapeutic phlebotomy to remove excess iron is indicated in the presence of iron overload or evidence of end-organ damage (e.g., advanced cirrhosis, cardiac failure, skin pigment changes, or diabetes). Periodic phlebotomy is a simple, inexpensive, and effective treatment. Initially, phlebotomy may be needed weekly, but once therapeutic ferritin levels are reached, phlebotomy may be needed only every 2 to 3 months. Iron chelation therapy is not recommended unless an individual has

an elevated serum ferritin concentration with anemia, which renders phlebotomy impossible. Such circumstances are uncommon in individuals with *HFE*-HH. Individuals should be instructed to refrain from taking iron supplements and consuming raw fish or shellfish. Vaccination against hepatitis A and B is advised.

ALTERATIONS OF LEUKOCYTE FUNCTION

Leukocyte function (infection fighting) is affected if too many or too few white cells are present in the blood or if the cells that are present are structurally or functionally defective. **Quantitative leukocyte disorders** result from decreased production in the bone marrow or accelerated destruction of cells in the circulation. In addition, quantitative alterations occur in response to infections.

Qualitative leukocyte disorders consist of disruptions of leukocyte function. Phagocytic cells (granulocytes, monocytes, macrophages) may lose their ability to act as effective phagocytes, and the lymphocytes may lose their ability to respond to antigens. (Disruptions of inflammatory and immune processes caused by leukocyte disorders are described in Chapter 6.) Other leukocyte alterations include infectious mononucleosis and cancers of the blood—leukemia and multiple myeloma (MM).

Quantitative Alterations of Leukocytes

Leukocytosis is present when the count is higher than normal; **leukopenia** is present when the count is lower than normal. Leukocytosis and leukopenia may affect a specific type of white blood cell and may result from a variety of physiologic conditions and alterations.

Leukocytosis occurs as a normal protective response to physiologic stressors, such as invading microorganisms, strenuous exercise, emotional changes, temperature changes, anesthesia, surgery, pregnancy, and some drugs, hormones, and toxins. It also is caused by pathologic conditions, such as malignancies and hematologic disorders. Unlike leukocytosis, leukopenia is never normal and is defined as an absolute blood cell count less than 4000 cells/μl. Leukopenia is associated with a decrease in neutrophils, which increases risk for infection. When the neutrophil count falls to less than 1000/μl, the risk of infection increases drastically. With counts below 500/μl, the possibility for life-threatening infections is high. Leukopenia may be caused by radiation, anaphylactic shock,

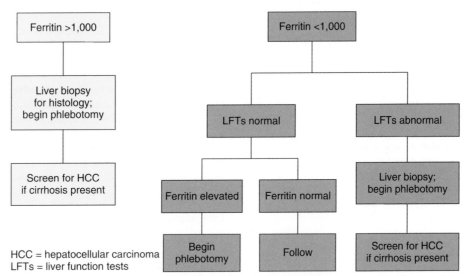

FIGURE 23.5 Ferritin Concentration to Help Direct Clinical Management. *HCC,* Hepatocellular carcinoma; *LFTs,* liver function tests. (From Adam MP et al: *HFE*-associated hereditary hemochromatosis, *GeneReviews* [Internet], Seattle WA, 2018, University of Washington, Seattle.)

autoimmune disease (e.g., systemic lupus erythematosus [SLE]), immune deficiencies (see Chapter 8), and certain drugs, such as glucocorticoids and chemotherapeutic agents.

Granulocytes and Monocytes

Increased numbers of circulating granulocytes (neutrophils, eosinophils, basophils) and monocytes are chiefly a physiologic response to infection. Increased numbers also occur as a result of myeloproliferative disorders that increase stem cell proliferation in the bone marrow.

Decreased numbers occur when infectious processes deplete the supply of circulating granulocytes and monocytes, drawing them out of the circulation and into infected tissues faster than they can be replaced. Decreases also can be caused by disorders that suppress marrow function, such as severe congenital neutropenia or immune-related neutropenia.

Granulocytosis—an increase in granulocytes (neutrophils, eosinophils, or basophils)—begins when stored blood cells are released. Neutrophilia is another term that may be used to describe *granulocytosis* because neutrophils are the most numerous of the granulocytes (Table 23.6). Neutrophilia occurs in the early stages of infection or inflammation and is established when the absolute count exceeds 7500/μl. Release and depletion of stored neutrophils stimulates granulopoiesis to replenish neutrophil reserves. Specific conditions associated with neutrophilia and other white blood cells are identified in Table 23.6.

When the demand for circulating mature neutrophils exceeds the supply, immature neutrophils (and other leukocytes) are released from the bone marrow. Premature release of the immature cells is responsible for the phenomenon known as a shift-to-the-left, or leukemoid reaction. This refers to the microscopic detection of disproportionate numbers of immature leukocytes in peripheral blood smears. Many diagrams present cellular differentiation and maturation progressing from left to right within the drawing, instead of vertically as shown in Fig. 22.8. The early release of immature white cells prevents the completion of the sequence and shifts the distribution of leukocytes in the blood toward those on the left side of the diagram. This phenomenon is also seen in the blood smear of individuals with leukemia, hence the term *leukemoid reaction.* As infection or inflammation diminishes, and granulopoiesis replenishes circulating granulocytes, a shift-to-the-right, or return to normal, occurs.

Neutropenia is a condition associated with a reduction in circulating neutrophils and exists clinically when the neutrophil count is less than 2000/μl. Reduction in neutrophils occurs in severe prolonged infections when production of granulocytes cannot keep up with demand. Severe neutropenia, granulocytopenia (less than 500/μl), or agranulocytosis (complete absence of granulocytes in blood) is usually secondary to arrested hematopoiesis in the bone marrow or massive cell destruction in the circulation. Chemotherapeutic agents used to treat hematologic and other malignancies cause bone marrow suppression. Several other drugs cause agranulocytosis, which occurs rarely but carries a high mortality of 10% to 50%. Clinical manifestations of agranulocytosis include severe infection (particularly of the respiratory system) leading to septicemia, general malaise, fever, tachycardia, and ulcers in the mouth and colon. If this condition remains untreated, sepsis caused by agranulocytosis results in death within 3 to 6 days. Other conditions associated with neutropenia are identified in Table 23.6.

Other causes of neutropenia, in the absence of infection, may be (1) decreased neutrophil production or ineffective granulopoiesis, (2) reduced neutrophil survival, and (3) abnormal neutrophil distribution and sequestration. Neutropenia also is classified as primary or secondary, and primary disorders are further identified as congenital or acquired. Primary acquired neutropenia is associated with multiple conditions. The megaloblastic anemias (vitamin B_{12} and folate deficiency), as well as starvation and anorexia nervosa, cause neutropenia because of an inadequate supply of vitamins and nutrients for protein production.

Congenital defects in neutrophil production include cyclic neutropenia, neutropenia with congenital immunodeficiencies, and multiple syndromes. Reduced neutrophil survival and abnormal distribution and sequestration are usually secondary to other disorders. Neutropenia occurs in a variety of immunologic disorders, particularly SLE, rheumatoid arthritis, Felty and Sjögren syndromes, splenomegaly, and drug-related causes.

Eosinophilia is an absolute increase (>450/μl) in the total number of circulating eosinophils. Allergic disorders (type 1) associated with asthma, hay fever, parasitic infections, and drug reactions often cause eosinophilia. Hypersensitivity reactions trigger the release of eosinophilic chemotaxic factor of anaphylaxis (ECF-A), and histamine from mast cells attracts eosinophils to the area. Mast cells release interleukin-5 (IL-5), which stimulates the bone marrow to produce more eosinophils into the blood. Areas with abundant mast cells, such as the respiratory and GI tracts, are commonly affected. Eosinophilia also may occur in dermatologic disorders, eosinophilia-myalgia syndrome, and parasitic invasion. Other conditions that cause eosinophilia are detailed in Table 23.6.

Eosinopenia, a decrease in the number of circulating eosinophils, generally is caused by migration of eosinophils into inflammatory sites. It also may be seen in Cushing syndrome and as a result of stress caused by surgery, shock, trauma, burns, or mental distress. Other conditions that cause eosinopenia are detailed in Table 23.6.

Basophilia, an increase in the number of circulating basophils, is rare and generally is a response to inflammation and immediate hypersensitivity reactions. Basophils contain histamine that is released during an allergic reaction. Increased numbers of basophils are seen in myeloproliferative disorders, such as chronic myeloid leukemia and myeloid metaplasia. Other conditions that are associated with basophilia are listed in Table 23.6.

Basopenia (also known as *basophilic leukopenia*) is a decrease in circulating numbers of basophils. It is seen in hyperthyroidism, acute infection, ovulation and pregnancy, and long-term therapy with steroids. Other conditions associated with basopenia are listed in Table 23.6.

Monocytosis is an increase in numbers of circulating monocytes (generally >800/μl). It is often transient and not related to a dysfunction of monocyte production. If present, it is usually associated with neutropenia during bacterial infections, particularly in the late stages or recovery stage, when monocytes are needed to phagocytize surviving microorganisms and debris. Increased monocytes also may indicate marrow recovery from agranulocytosis. Monocytosis is often seen in chronic infections such as tuberculosis (TB), brucellosis, listeriosis, and subacute bacterial endocarditis (SBE). Monocytosis has been found to correlate with the extent of myocardial damage after myocardial infarctions. Other conditions associated with monocytosis are identified in Table 23.6. Monocytopenia, a decrease in the number of circulating monocytes, is rare but has been identified with hairy cell leukemia and prednisone therapy.

Lymphocytes

Quantitative alterations of lymphocytes occur when lymphocytes are activated by antigenic stimuli, usually microorganisms (see Chapter 7). Lymphocytosis (absolute lymphocytosis) is an increase in the number or proportion of lymphocytes in the blood. It is rare in acute bacterial infections and is seen most commonly in acute viral infections, particularly those caused by the Epstein-Barr virus (EBV), a causative agent

TABLE 23.6   Other Conditions Associated With Neutrophils, Eosinophils, Basophils, Monocytes, and Lymphocytes

Condition	Cause	Example
Neutrophil		
Neutrophilia (granulocytosis)	Inflammation or tissue necrosis	Surgery, burns, MI, pneumonitis, rheumatic fever, rheumatoid arthritis
	Infection	Bacterial: gram-positive (staphylococci, streptococci, pneumococci), gram-negative (*Escherichia coli, Pseudomonas* species)
	Physiologic	Exercise, extreme heat or cold, third-trimester pregnancy, emotional distress
	Hematologic	Acute hemorrhage, hemolysis, myeloproliferative disorder, chronic granulocytic leukemia
	Drugs or chemicals	Epinephrine, steroids, heparin, histamine, endotoxin
	Metabolic	Diabetes (acidosis), eclampsia, gout, thyroid storm
	Neoplasm	Liver, GI tract, bone marrow
Neutropenia	Decreased marrow production	Radiation, chemotherapy, leukemia, aplastic anemia, abnormal granulopoiesis
	Increased destruction	Splenomegaly, hemodialysis, autoimmune disease
	Prolonged infection	Gram-negative (typhoid), viral (influenza, hepatitis B, measles, mumps, rubella), severe infections, protozoal infections (malaria)
Eosinophil		
Eosinophilia	Allergy	Asthma, hay fever, drug sensitivity
	Infection	Parasites (trichinosis, hookworm), chronic (fungal, leprosy, TB)
	Malignancy	CML, lung, stomach, ovary, Hodgkin disease
	Dermatosis	Pemphigus, exfoliative dermatitis (drug-induced)
	Drugs	Digitalis, heparin, streptomycin, tryptophan (eosinophilia-myalgia syndrome), penicillins, propranolol
Eosinopenia	Stress response	Trauma, shock, burns, surgery, mental distress
	Drugs	Steroids (Cushing syndrome)
Basophil		
Basophilia	Inflammation	Infection (measles, chickenpox), hypersensitivity reaction (immediate)
	Hematologic	Myeloproliferative disorders (CML, polycythemia vera, Hodgkin lymphoma, hemolytic anemia)
	Endocrine	Myxedema, antithyroid therapy
Basopenia	Physiologic	Pregnancy, ovulation, stress
	Endocrine	Graves disease
Monocyte		
Monocytosis	Infection	Bacterial (subacute bacterial endocarditis, TB), recovery phase of infection
	Hematologic	Myeloproliferative disorders, Hodgkin disease, agranulocytosis
	Physiologic	Normal newborn
Monocytopenia	Rare	
Lymphocyte		
Lymphocytosis	Physiologic	4 months to 4 years
	Acute infection	Infectious mononucleosis, CMV infection, pertussis, hepatitis, mycoplasma pneumonia, typhoid
	Chronic infection	Congenital syphilis, tertiary syphilis
	Endocrine	Thyrotoxicosis, adrenal insufficiency
	Malignancy	ALL, CLL, lymphosarcoma cell leukemia
Lymphocytopenia	Immunodeficiency syndrome	AIDS, agammaglobulinemia
	Lymphocyte destruction	Steroids (Cushing syndrome), radiation, chemotherapy
		Hodgkin lymphoma
		CHF, renal failure, TB, SLE, aplastic anemia

AIDS, Acquired immunodeficiency syndrome; *ALL,* acute lymphocytic leukemia; *CHF,* congestive (left) heart failure; *CLL,* chronic lymphocytic leukemia; *CML,* chronic myelogenous leukemia; *CMV,* cytomegalovirus; *GI,* gastrointestinal; *MI,* myocardial infarction; *SLE,* systemic lupus erythematosus; *TB,* tuberculosis.

in infectious mononucleosis. Other specific disorders associated with lymphocytosis are listed in Table 23.6.

Lymphocytopenia is a decrease in the number of circulating lymphocytes in the blood. It may be attributed to (1) abnormalities of lymphocyte production associated with neoplasias and immune deficiencies and (2) destruction by drugs, viruses, or radiation. It is also known to occur without any detectable cause. Conditions associated with lymphocytopenia are identified in Table 23.6. The lymphocytopenia associated with heart failure and other acute illnesses may be caused by elevated cortisol levels. Lymphocytopenia is a major problem in

AIDS. AIDS-related lymphocytopenia is caused by human immunodeficiency virus (HIV), which destroys T-helper lymphocytes. (For a detailed discussion of AIDS, see Chapter 9.)

Infectious Mononucleosis

Infectious mononucleosis (IM) is a benign, acute, self-limiting, lymphoproliferative clinical syndrome characterized by acute viral infection of B lymphocytes (B cells). It is associated with several human tumors, such as lymphomas and nasopharyngeal carcinoma. The most common cause is EBV. EBV is a ubiquitous herpesvirus and accounts for the majority of IM cases. Other viruses that cause symptoms resembling IM include cytomegalovirus (CMV), adenovirus, HIV, hepatitis A, influenza A and B, and rubella, as well as the bacteria *Toxoplasma gondii, Corynebacterium diphtheriae,* and *Coxiella burnetii.* The classic symptoms of IM are pharyngitis, lymphadenopathy, and fever. In individuals with immunodeficiency, the proliferation of infected B cells may be uncontrolled and can lead to the development of B-cell lymphomas.[11] Individuals who are coinfected with malaria or HIV are at increased risk of developing EBV-associated lymphomas, including Burkitt lymphoma (BL). EBV also is etiologically linked to subgroups of Hodgkin lymphoma (HL).

Approximately 50% to 85% of children are infected with EBV by age 4, and more than 90% of adults have indications of subclinical EBV infections. These early infections are usually asymptomatic and provide immunity to EBV; thus early EBV infections rarely develop into IM. IM may arise when the initial infection occurs during adolescence or later, but still only results in IM in 35% to 50% of these individuals. Symptomatic IM usually affects young adults between ages 15 and 35 years, with the peak incidences occurring between ages 15 and 24 years; males have a later peak (18 to 24 years) than females. The overall incidence rate for this age group is 6 to 8 cases per 1000 persons per year. Children from low socioeconomic environments are particularly susceptible to infections with EBV. IM is uncommon in individuals older than age 40; however, if it does occur, IM is more commonly caused by CMV.

Transmission of EBV is usually through saliva from close personal contact (e.g., kissing, hence the term *kissing disease*). The virus also may be secreted in other mucosal secretions of the genital, rectal, and respiratory tracts, as well as blood. The infection begins with widespread invasion of the B lymphocytes, which have receptors for EBV. The virus initially infects the oropharynx, nasopharynx, and salivary epithelial cells with later spread into lymphoid tissues and B cells. Once the virus enters the bloodstream, the infection spreads systemically.

PATHOPHYSIOLOGY In the immunocompetent individual, unaffected B cells produce antibodies (immunoglobulin G [IgG], IgA, IgM) against the virus. At the same time, there is a massive activation and proliferation of cytotoxic T cells (CD8) that are directed against EBV-infected cells (see Chapter 7). The immune response against EBV-infected cells is largely responsible for the cellular proliferation in the lymphoid tissue (lymph nodes, spleen, tonsils, and, occasionally, liver). Sore throat and fever are caused by inflammation at the site of initial viral entry and initial infection (the mouth and throat). Outcomes of EBV are presented in Fig. 23.6.

CLINICAL MANIFESTATIONS The incubation period for IM is approximately 30 to 50 days. Early flulike symptoms, such as headache, malaise, joint pain, and fatigue, may appear during the first 3 to 5 days, although some individuals are without symptoms. At the time of diagnosis, the individual commonly presents with the classic group of symptoms: fever, sore throat (pharyngitis), cervical lymph node enlargement, and fatigue. The pharyngitis is usually diffuse with a whitish or grayish green thick exudate. It can be painful, causing the individual

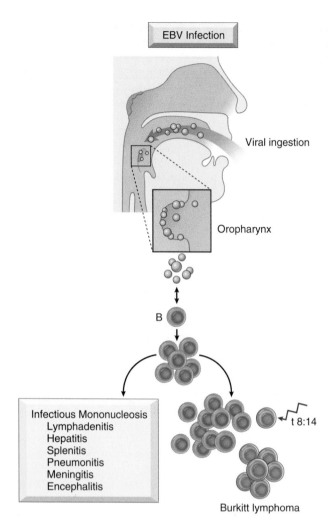

FIGURE 23.6 Outcomes of Epstein-Barr Virus (EBV). In individuals with normal immune function, infection is typically asymptomatic or leads to mononucleosis. With immunodeficiency, proliferation of B cells may be uncontrolled and progress to the development of B-cell neoplasms. Individuals without evidence of immunodeficiency can also develop EBV-positive neoplasms. In Burkitt lymphoma, the individual's susceptibility to EBV causes B cells to undergo genetic alterations (usually an 8;14 chromosomal translocation). EBV also is implicated in Hodgkin lymphoma, nasopharyngeal carcinoma, and other rare non-Hodgkin lymphomas. (From Kumar V, Abbas A, Aster JC: *Robbins & Cotran pathologic basis of disease,* ed 9, Philadelphia, 2015, Saunders.)

to seek treatment. Characteristics with progression may include a generalized lymphadenopathy, enlarged spleen, and appearance in the blood of atypical activated T lymphocytes (mononucleosis cells). IM is usually self-limiting, and recovery occurs in a few weeks. Fatigue, however, may last for 1 to 2 months after resolution of the infection.

Severe clinical complications are rare. With progression of IM, general lymph node enlargement may develop with enlargement of the spleen and liver. Splenomegaly is clinically evident 50% of the time and is demonstrated radiologically 100% of the time. Difficulty in detecting splenomegaly with physical examination contributes to the underestimation of actual enlargement. Splenic rupture is rare (only 0.1% to 0.5% of all cases) and can occur spontaneously as a result of mild trauma, arising primarily in men younger than 25 years of age and between days 4 and 21 after the onset of symptoms. It is the most common cause of death related to IM. Other causes of fatalities are hepatic failure, extensive bacterial infection, and viral myocarditis. Other organ systems are rarely involved, but such involvement may be present with characteristic manifestations, such as fulminant hepatitis with jaundice and anemia, encephalitis, meningitis, Guillain-Barré syndrome, and Bell palsy. Eye manifestations may include eyelid and periorbital edema, dry eyes, keratitis, uveitis, and conjunctivitis. Reye syndrome has been known to develop in children with EBV infection. Pulmonary and respiratory failure has been documented, but is more likely to occur in immunocompromised individuals. Approximately 3% to 10% of adults older than 40 years of age have never been infected with EBV and are susceptible to IM later in life. In these individuals, the classic symptoms are not generally present, making diagnosis more difficult.

EVALUATION AND TREATMENT Children commonly present with fever, sore throat, lymphadenitis, and manifestations discussed earlier. Young adults present with malaise, fatigue, and lymphadenopathy and often a fever of unknown origin. The blood of affected individuals contains an increased number of white blood cells with many atypical lymphocytes. The diagnosis of IM depends on the following specific findings: (1) an increase in the number of lymphocytes, commonly based on Hoagland criteria of at least 50% lymphocytes and at least 10% atypical lymphocytes in the blood, (2) a positive heterophile antibody (heterogeneous group of IgM antibodies that are agglutinins against nonhuman red blood cells [e.g., sheep, horse]) reaction (Monospot test), and (3) a rising titer of specific antibodies for EBV antigens. Use of the Monospot test is limited because other infections (e.g., CMV, adenovirus) and toxoplasmosis also produce heterophilic antibodies. Thus 5% to 15% of Monospot tests yield false-positive results. Heterophilic antibodies in the blood increase as the condition progresses, although some individuals and children younger than 4 years of age do not produce them. Diagnosis of EBV infection specifically may be increased with newer viral-specific tests that identify EBV-specific antibodies.

IM is usually self-limiting and medical intervention is rarely required. Treatment is supportive and consists of rest and alleviation of symptoms with analgesics and antipyretics. Aspirin is avoided with children because of its association with Reye syndrome. Streptococcal pharyngitis, which occurs in 20% to 30% of cases, is treated with penicillin or erythromycin, not ampicillin—ampicillin is known to cause a rash. Bed rest with avoidance of strenuous activity and contact sports is indicated. Steroids may be used but only with severe complications, such as impending airway obstruction or other organ involvement (central nervous system [CNS] manifestations, thrombocytopenic purpura, myocarditis, pericarditis) is evident. Acyclovir has been used in immunocompromised individuals but is not considered standard therapy. In the rare event of splenic rupture, the treatment has been removal of the spleen and continues to be the choice in hemodynamically unstable individuals. Current research, however, is suggesting that it may be better to repair the spleen to avoid overwhelming postsplenectomy infection (OPSI). Children are at greater risk then adults for OPSI.

> **QUICK CHECK 23.2**
> 1. What condition is manifested chiefly by an increase in the numbers of circulating granulocytes and monocytes?
> 2. What is the cause of infectious mononucleosis (IM)?
> 3. What are the classic symptoms of IM?

Lymphoid Neoplasm: Leukemias

Leukemia is a clonal malignant disorder of the bone marrow and usually, but not always, of the blood. The common pathologic feature of all forms of leukemia is an uncontrolled proliferation of malignant leukocytes, causing an overcrowding of bone marrow and decreased production and function of normal hematopoietic cells. Chromosomal abnormalities and translocations are common in the majority of leukemias. When genes become mutated, they create genomic aberrations that block cell maturation and activate pro–growth signaling pathways that prevent apoptotic cell death.

With time, the overall classification of leukemia has become increasingly complex with notable changes. These changes have created a blurring between the once discrete categories *lymphoma* and *leukemia*. Some cancers known as *lymphoma* have *leukemic* presentations, and evolution to leukemia is not unusual during the progression of incurable lymphoma. The World Health Organization (WHO) currently groups the lymphoid neoplasms into five broad categories, which are defined by the cell of origin:
1. Precursor B-cell neoplasms (immature B cells)
2. Peripheral B-cell neoplasms (mature B cells)
3. Precursor T-cell neoplasms (immature T cells)
4. Peripheral T-cell and NK (natural killer)-cell neoplasms (mature T cells and NK cells)
5. Hodgkin lymphoma (Reed-Sternberg [RS] cell and variants)

Most lymphoid neoplasm classifications relate to stages of cell differentiation of B-cell or T-cell differentiation (Fig. 23.7, *A*). Fig. 23.7, *B* provides a simple schematic overview of the main types of leukemia.

Acute leukemia is characterized by undifferentiated or immature cells, usually a blast cell. The onset of disease is abrupt and rapid. Without treatment, disease progression results in a short survival time. In chronic leukemia, the predominant cell is more differentiated but does not function normally, with a relatively slow progression. There are four general types of leukemia: acute lymphocytic (ALL), acute myelogenous (AML), chronic lymphocytic (CLL), and chronic myelogenous (CML).

Leukemia occurs with varying frequencies at different ages and is more common in adults than in children. It is estimated that more than 61,780 cases of leukemia were newly diagnosed in 2019, with males having a slightly higher incidence than females (Table 23.7). Estimated

TABLE 23.7 Estimated New Cases and Deaths From Leukemia in the United States—2014

Types of Leukemia	TOTAL NEW CASES (Proportion of New Cases) (%)	NEW CASES BY SEX		DEATHS BY SEX	
		Male	Female	Male	Female
All types	61,780 (100)	35,920	25,860	13,150	9,690
Acute lymphocytic leukemia	5,930 (12)	3,280	26,500	850	650
Chronic lymphocytic leukemia	20,720 (30)	12,880	7,840,	3,930	2,220
Acute myelogenous leukemia	21,450 (36)	11,650	9,800	6,290	4,630
Chronic myelogenous leukemia	8,990 (11)	5250	3,740	660	480
Other	4,690 (11)	2,860	1,830	3,130	2,220

Data from American Cancer Society: *Cancer facts and figures—2019,* Atlanta, 2019, The Society.

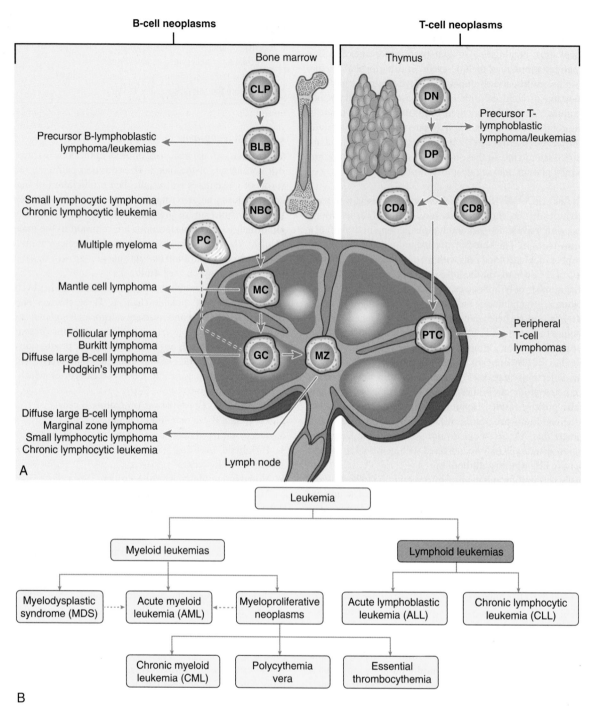

FIGURE 23.7 Origin of Lymphoid Neoplasms. A, Specific lymphoid tumors emerge from stages of B- and T-cell differentiation. **B,** Overview of main types of leukemia. Acute myeloid lymphoma *(AML)* may arise de novo or be preceded by myelodysplastic phase. Not all cases of myelodysplastic syndrome (MDS) evolve to AML *(dashed line)*. Some myelodysplastic neoplasms can transform into AML, although very rarely *(dotted line)*. *BLB,* Pre-B lymphoblast; *CLP,* common lymphoid precursor; *DN,* CD4/CD8 double-negative pro-T cell; *DP,* CD4/CD8 double-positive pre-T cell; *GC,* germinal-center B cell; *MC,* mantle B cell; *MZ,* marginal zone B cell; *NBC,* naïve B cell; *PTC,* peripheral T cell. **(A,** from Kumar V, Abbas A, Aster JC: *Robbins & Cotran pathologic basis of disease,* ed 9, Philadelphia, 2015, Saunders; **B,** from Khwaja A et al: Acute myeloid leukaemia, *Nat Rev Dis Pimers* 2:16010, 2016.)

deaths for 2019 was 22,840 individuals.[12] CLL and AML are the most common types in adults. CML is found mostly in adults (see Chapter 24 for leukemia in children).

Over the past 2 decades, the rates of induced remission and survival in most forms of leukemia have increased. Current survival rates range from 24% for AML to 81% for CLL, and as high as 91% for children and adolescents younger than 15 years of age with ALL.[13] Risk factors for the onset of leukemia include environmental factors, genetic factors, and other diseases (see Acute Leukemias and Chronic Leukemias sections for further discussion on risk factors).

PATHOPHYSIOLOGY All leukemias have certain pathophysiologic features in common. Most lymphoid neoplasms arise from B-cell and T-cell differentiation pathways (see Fig. 23.7, *A*). The hypothesis of origin for leukemias is "clonal disorders driven by genetically abnormal progenitor cells or stem-like cancer cells (SLCCs)." The majority (85% to 90%) of lymphoid neoplasms are of B-cell origin, followed by T-cell tumors and, rarely, NK-cell tumors. Abnormal immature white blood cells, called leukemic blasts, fill the bone marrow and can spill into the blood. Leukemic blasts literally "crowd out" the bone marrow and cause cellular proliferation of the other cell lines to decrease or cease. Normal granulocytic-monocytic, lymphocytic, erythrocytic, and megakaryocytic progenitor cells can cease to function, leading to pancytopenia (a reduction in all cellular components of the blood). Genetic translocations (mitotic errors) are observed in leukemic cells. The most common genetic abnormality is the reciprocal translocation between chromosomes 9 and 22—t(9;22) (q34;q11), the Philadelphia chromosome. The Philadelphia chromosome was first observed in persons with CML and is present in 95% of those with CML, 3% of individuals with AML, 25% to 30% of adults with ALL, and 2% to 10% of children with ALL.[14] This translocation results in the novel fusion of the *BCR1* gene region from chromosome 22 and the proto-oncogene *ABL1* from chromosome 9 (Fig. 23.8). The BCR-ABL1 joining results in the expression of a unique fused oncoprotein, BCR-ABL1. The ABL1 protein is involved in the signaling pathway that promotes cell proliferation. The BCR-ABL1 variant proves to be essential for transformation into leukemic cells. BCR-ABL1 appears to excessively activate intracellular pathways, leading to increased proliferation, decreased sensitivity to apoptosis, and premature release of immature cells into the circulation. In most leukemias and lymphomas a single major genetic abnormality, such as the t(9;22) translocation, does not lead to an aggressive malignancy. The initial event is usually followed by a series of secondary genetic changes. Therefore the original tumor becomes genetically unstable and diverse. In the majority of cases, leukemic cells are ejected into the blood, where they accumulate. These cells also may infiltrate and accumulate in the liver, spleen, lymph nodes, and other organs throughout the body. The presentation of large numbers of leukemic cells in the blood may be one of the most dramatic indicators of leukemia; however, leukemia is still a primary disruption of the bone marrow.

Acute leukemias. Acute leukemias include two types: acute lymphocytic leukemia (ALL) and acute myelogenous leukemia (AML). ALL is an aggressive, fast-growing leukemia with too many lymphoblasts or immature white blood cells found in blood and bone marrow. It also is called *acute lymphoblastic leukemia.* AML is an aggressive fast-growing leukemia with too many myeloblasts (i.e., immature white blood cells that are not lymphoblasts) found in the bone marrow and blood. It also is called *acute myeloblastic leukemia (AML)* and *acute nonlymphocytic leukemia (ANLL).* Acute leukemias are seen in both sexes and in all ages. AML is the more common acute leukemia in adults, with the median age at diagnosis around 70 years. There is a rise in the age-related incidence around 40 to 50 years of age, and a steep increase from 60 to 64 years of age. Mortality for all acute leukemias in the United States is about 7 per 100,000. In children younger than 15 years, leukemia accounts for one-third of all deaths from cancer. North America and Scandinavian countries have the highest mortality; Eastern European countries, Asia (except Japan), and Central America have the lowest mortality. The higher mortality in Japan is the result of the atomic bombs dropped in World War II. Blacks have consistently shown a lower mortality than whites. More than 5930 new cases of ALL and 21,450 cases of AML were estimated in 2019, with more than 1500 deaths from ALL and 10,920 deaths from AML.[12]

Increased risk for ALL has been linked to exposure to x-rays before birth, being exposed to ionizing radiation (postnatally), past treatment with chemotherapy, and certain genetic conditions. Leukemia has a statistically significant tendency to reappear in families. Increased risk in adults also has been linked to exposure to cigarette smoke. Large doses of ionizing radiation in particular result in an increased incidence of myelogenous leukemia. There is growing concern about the effect of low-dose radiation on subsequent risk of leukemia.[15] Infections with HIV or hepatitis C virus increase the risk for lymphoid neoplasms. It is now widely accepted that some types of leukemia are caused by infection with the human T-cell leukemia/lymphoma virus-1 (HTLV-1). AML is the most frequently reported secondary cancer after high doses

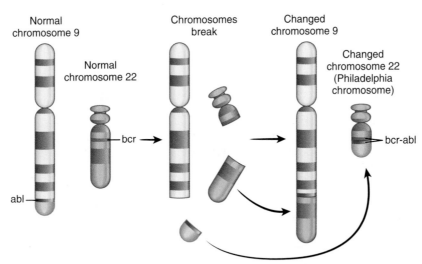

FIGURE 23.8 Philadelphia Chromosome. A piece of chromosome 9 and a piece of chromosome 22 break off and trade places. The *BCR-ABL* gene is formed on chromosome 22 where the piece of chromosome 9 attaches. The changed chromosome 22 is called the Philadelphia chromosome. (Adapted from National Cancer Institute: *Childhood acute lymphoblastic leukemia treatment,* Bethesda, MD, 2014, National Institutes of Health.)

of chemotherapy for HL, non-Hodgkin lymphoma (NHL), MM, ovarian cancer, and breast cancer. Acute leukemia also may develop secondary to certain acquired disorders, such as CML, CLL, HL, and others. Unlike other forms of leukemia, ALL develops at different rates in different geographic locations and the reason is unclear. People from developed countries and of higher socioeconomic categories have an increased incidence of ALL.

PATHOPHYSIOLOGY ALL presumably progresses from malignant transformation of B- or C-cell progenitor cells (like a stem cell) (Fig. 23.9). Most cases of ALL occur in children and often in the first decade (see Chapter 24). Although adults account for about 20% of all cases, their mortality rate is significantly higher. The significant difference between the incidence of ALL in adults and children may be because of differences in the biology of the disease.

B-cell ALL occurs mainly in children and is strongly associated with chromosomal aneuploidy of various types. Adult ALL is a mixture of cancers of precursor B- and T-cell origin. The identification of mutations found in ALL is ongoing and includes mutations that drive cell growth and mutations that increase tyrosine kinase activity.

AML is the most common adult leukemia. Genetic alterations in AML alter genes that encode transcription factors needed for normal myeloid differentiation; consequently, differentiation becomes arrested. These mutations affect the epigenome, suggesting that epigenetic alterations are key in AML. Mutations may lead to proliferation by activating growth factor signaling, as well as a decreased rate of apoptosis. Thus the bone marrow and peripheral blood are characterized by leukocytosis and a predominance of blast cells. With an increase in immature blasts, they displace normal myelocytic blood cells, megakaryocytes, and erythrocytes. This displacement can lead to complications of bleeding, anemia, and infection. Several hereditary conditions are known to increase the risk for AML (e.g., Down syndrome, Fanconi aplastic anemia, Bloom syndrome, and others).

CLINICAL MANIFESTATIONS Within days to a few weeks of the first symptoms is an abrupt stormy onset, which is more prevalent in ALL. The clinical manifestations of all varieties of acute leukemia are generally similar. Mechanisms associated with common manifestations are summarized in Table 23.8. Signs and symptoms related to bone marrow depression include fatigue caused by anemia, bleeding resulting from thrombocytopenia, and fever caused by infection. Bleeding may occur in the skin, gums, mucous membranes, and GI tract. Visible signs include petechiae and ecchymosis, as well as discoloration of the skin, gingival bleeding, hematuria, and midcycle or heavy menstrual bleeding.

Infection sites include the mouth, throat, respiratory tract, lower colon, urinary tract, and skin and may be caused by gram-negative bacilli (*Escherichia coli*), *Pseudomonas aeruginosa*, and *Klebsiella pneumoniae*. Fever is an early sign and is often accompanied by chills.

Anorexia is accompanied by weight loss, diminished sensitivity to sour and sweet tastes, wasting of muscle, and difficulty swallowing. Liver, spleen, and lymph node enlargement occurs more commonly in ALL than in AML. Liver and spleen enlargement commonly occur together. The leukemic individual often experiences abdominal pain and tenderness. Pain in the bones and joints is thought to result from leukemia infiltration with secondary stretching of the periosteum.

Neurologic manifestations are common and may be caused by either leukemic infiltration or cerebral bleeding. Headache, vomiting, papilledema, facial palsy, blurred vision, auditory disturbances, and meningeal irritation can occur if leukemic cells infiltrate the cerebral or spinal meninges.

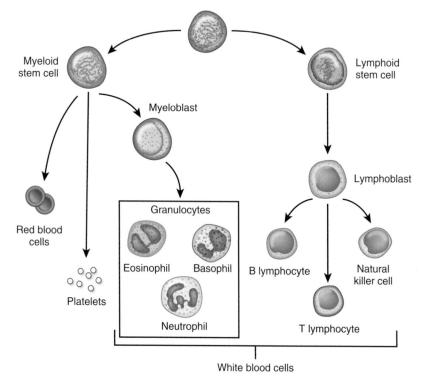

FIGURE 23.9 Leukemia Arises From Stem-Like Cells. A blood stem cell undergoes multiple steps to finally become a red blood cell, platelet, or white blood cell. (Modified from National Cancer Institute: Adult acute lymphoblastic leukemia treatment (PDQ), Bethesda, MD, 2014, Author. Available from http://www.cancer.gov/cancertopics/pdq/treatment/adultALL/HealthProfessional. Accessed January 9, 2015.)

TABLE 23.8   Clinical Manifestations and Related Pathophysiology in Leukemia

Clinical Manifestations	Laboratory Abnormalities	Cause	Comments
Anemia	Relative *proportion* of erythroblasts to total count (decreased in anemia) is key	Decreased stem cell input or ineffective erythropoiesis, or both	In acute leukemia, anemia is usually present from beginning, often first symptom noticed, and severe; mild form without symptoms is common in CML and CLL; hemorrhage common in acute forms, occasional in CML, but rare in CLL
Bleeding (purpura, petechiae, ecchymosis, hemorrhage)	Decreased and possibly abnormal platelets	Reduction in megakaryocytes leading to thrombocytopenia	Bleeding more common in acute than in chronic leukemia
Infection	Increased multisegmented neutrophils	Opportunistic organisms; decreased protection resulting from granulocytopenia or immune deficiency secondary to chemotherapy, corticosteroids, and disease process	Major sites of infection: oral cavity, throat, lower colon, urinary tract, lungs, and skin; prevention of infection focuses on restoring host defenses, decreasing invasive procedures, and reducing colonization of microorganisms
Weight loss	Decreased 24-hr urinary creatinine excretion; hypoalbuminemia	Condition can be attributed to pain, depression, chemotherapy, radiation therapy, loss of appetite, and alterations in taste	Severe weight loss may be related to excess production of TNF-α
Bone pain	Often no radiographic evidence of bone problems	Result of bone infiltration by leukemic cells or intramedullary infection	If combination drug regimens are ineffective, radiation therapy is used
Liver, spleen, and lymph node enlargement	Biopsy abnormal for liver and spleen	Leukemic cell infiltration	Lymph nodes also undergo leukemia proliferation in CLL
Elevated uric acid level	Normal excretion of uric acid is 300-500 mg/day; leukemic individual can excrete 50 times more	Increased catabolism of protein and nucleic acid; urate precipitation increased from dehydration caused by anorexia or fever and drug therapy	Hyperuricemia is present in both acute leukemia and CML; treatment focuses on increasing urine pH or decreasing acid production with drug allopurinol

CLL, Chronic lymphocytic leukemia; *CMA,* chronic myelocytic leukemia; *RBC,* red blood cell.

EVALUATION AND TREATMENT   Diagnosis is made through examination of blood cells and bone marrow. For ALL, diagnostic confusion with AML, hairy cell leukemia, and malignant lymphoma is not uncommon.[16] It is critical to obtain an accurate diagnosis because of the differences in treatment and prognosis of ALL and AML.[16] Also critical is that bone marrow aspirates should be done by an experienced oncologist, hematologist, hematopathologist, or general pathologist experienced in interpreting conventional and specially stained specimens.[16]

Chemotherapy, used in various combinations, is the treatment of choice for leukemia. Other types of treatment include radiation therapy, chemotherapy with stem cell transplant, and other drug therapy. Supportive measures include blood transfusions, antibiotics, antifungals, and antivirals. It is critical that stem cell transplants be done in hospitals with very experienced staff for both the procedure and the recovery phase.

Attainment of complete remission requires fairly aggressive treatment. Treatment is divided into two phases: remission induction (to attain remission) and postremission (to maintain remission). Historically, maintenance therapy for AML was administered for several years but it is not included in most current treatment clinical trials in the United States, except for promyelocytic leukemia.[16] Postremission therapy appears to be more effective when given immediately after remission is achieved.[16] Because only 5% of individuals with AML develop CNS disease, prophylactic treatment is not indicated.[16] Since the 1970s, 5-year survival rates for those with ALL have increased from 38% to 65% for adults and from 53% to 85% for children. The survival rate for AML is much lower. Factors influencing increased survival rate include the use of combined and multimodality treatment methods; improved supportive services, such as blood banking and nutritional support; and antimicrobial treatment. The presence of the Philadelphia chromosome (observed in about 5% of children with ALL, in 30% of adults with ALL, and occasionally in AML) is a poor prognostic indicator.

Myelosuppression is both a consequence of leukemia and a treatment for the disease. Hematologic support with blood products and granulocyte colony-stimulating factor (G-CSF) or granulocyte-macrophage colony-stimulating factor (GM-CSF) has effectively shortened the time of neutropenia and improved survival by reducing the risk for infection.

Chronic leukemias.   The two main types of chronic leukemia are (1) chronic myelogenous leukemia (CML) and (2) chronic lymphocytic leukemia (CLL). CML is also called *chronic granulocytic leukemia* and *chronic myeloid leukemia.* CML can occur, depending on the lineage of the malignant cells (e.g., chronic neutrophilic leukemia [CNL] or chronic eosinophilic leukemia [CEL]). CML is a slowly progressing disease with too many blood cells (not lymphocytes) made in the bone marrow. In adults, CLL is the most common leukemia in in the Western world. CLL is a slow-growing cancer in which too many immature lymphocytes are found, mostly in the blood and bone marrow. CLL and small lymphocytic lymphoma (SLL; also CLL/SLL) differ only in the amount of proliferation of peripheral blood lymphocytes. Unlike cells in acute leukemia, chronic leukemic cells are well differentiated and can be readily identified. CML is mostly a disease of adults but can occur in children or adolescents. The peak incidence is the fifth to sixth decades. Individuals with chronic leukemia have a longer life expectancy, usually extending several years from the time of diagnosis.

It is estimated there were 20,720 new cases of CLL and 3930 deaths in 2019, and 8990 new cases of CML and 1140 deaths in 2019.[12] CML is one of a group of diseases called myeloproliferative disorders—acquired abnormalities in signaling pathways that lead to growth factor–independent proliferation. The only known cause of CML is exposure to ionizing radiation, and the cause of CLL is unknown.

PATHOPHYSIOLOGY CML is clonal and thought to arise from a hematopoietic stem cell. The cells observed in CML are heterogeneous in differentiation, depending on the stage of the disease. During the chronic phase, the predominant cell is a long-lasting hematopoietic stem cell. The Philadelphia chromosome (see Fig. 23.8) is present in more than 95% of persons diagnosed with CML, and the presence of the BCR-ABL1 protein is responsible for initiation of CML (Fig. 23.10). CLL involves malignant transformation and progressive accumulation of B lymphocytes and rarely is of T-cell origin. CLL cells that accumulate

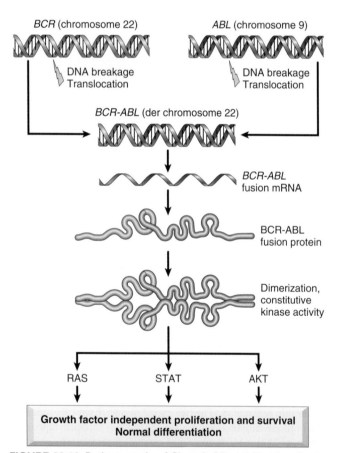

FIGURE 23.10 Pathogenesis of Chronic Myeloid Leukemia. The breakage and joining of *BCR* and *ABL* creates the chimeric fusion gene *BCR-ABL*. *BCR-ABL* genetically encodes an active BCR-ABL intracellular tyrosine kinase (an enzyme that controls intracellular "on-off" switches). The ABL kinase in turn induces signaling through the same pro-growth and pro-survival pathways that are activated by normal hematologic growth factors. Altogether the activation of many downstream pathways drives growth factor–independent proliferation and survival of bone marrow progenitors. *der chromosome* is a structurally rearranged chromosome. *AKT,* Serine/threonine kinases; *BCR-ABL,* breakpoint cluster region-Abelson; *RAS,* rat sarcoma; *STAT,* signal transducer and activator of transcription. (From Kumar V et al: *Robbins & Cotran pathologic basis of disease,* ed 9, St Louis, 2015, Elsevier.)

in the bone marrow do not interfere with normal blood cell production to the extent found in acute leukemias. This significant feature may explain the reduced severity in the beginning stage of disease. The major pathophysiologic deficit in CLL is the failure of B cells to mature into plasma cells that synthesize immunoglobulins, resulting in hypogammaglobulinemia (60% of individuals).

CLINICAL MANIFESTATIONS Chronic leukemia advances slowly and insidiously. Approximately 70% of individuals with CLL are asymptomatic at the time of diagnosis. When symptoms do appear, the most common finding is lymphadenopathy. The most significant effect of CLL is suppression of humoral immunity and increased infection with encapsulated bacteria. Frequently, the level of neutrophils is depressed, which adds to the risk of infection. Invasion of most organ cells is uncommon, but infiltration does occur in lymph nodes, liver, spleen, and salivary glands. CNS involvement is rare. Approximately 10% of individuals develop a more aggressive malignancy, usually a diffuse large B-cell lymphoma. In these individuals, extreme fatigue, weight loss, night sweats, low-grade fever, elevated levels of the enzyme lactic dehydrogenase, hypercalcemia, anemia, and thrombocytopenia are common.

Individuals with CML may progress through three phases of the disease: a chronic phase lasting 2 to 5 years, during which symptoms may not be apparent; an accelerated phase of 6 to 18 months, during which the primary symptoms develop; and a terminal blast phase ("blast crisis") with a survival of only 3 to 6 months. The accelerated phase is characterized by excessive proliferation and accumulation of malignant cells. Splenomegaly is prominent and becomes painful, but lymphadenopathy generally is not present. Liver enlargement also occurs, but liver function is rarely altered. Hyperuricemia is common and produces gouty arthritis. Infections, fever, and weight loss also are seen often. The terminal blast phase is characterized by rapid and progressive leukocytosis with an increase in basophils. In the later stages of the terminal phase, which then resembles AML, blast cells or promyelocytes predominate and the individual experiences a "blast crisis."

The acute effects of CML resemble those of acute leukemia but with more prominent and painful splenomegaly. Lymphadenopathy generally is found only in the acute phase of the disease. Hyperuricemia is usually present and produces gouty arthritis. Infections, fever, and weight loss are common findings with CML.

EVALUATION AND TREATMENT Diagnosis of chronic leukemia depends on laboratory analyses of peripheral blood and bone marrow. Diagnosis of CLL is based on detection of a monoclonal B-cell lymphocytosis in the blood. The cells must have the characteristic immunophenotype (CD5+, CD19+, CD20 [weak], CD23+) at levels in excess of 5000 cells/μl over a sustained period of time (usually 4 weeks). Confusion with other diseases may be avoided by determination of cell surface markers.

Treatment of CLL ranges from periodic observation with treatment of infection, hemorrhage, or immunologic complications. Because the disease mostly occurs in the elderly and the rate of progression is slow, it is often simply observed until the disease progresses. Randomized trials show no survival advantage for immediate versus delayed treatment of those individuals with early-stage disease.[17] For individuals with progressing CLL, treatment with conventional doses of chemotherapy is not curative; selected individuals treated with allogeneic stem cell transplantation have achieved prolonged disease-free survival.[18] Antileukemic therapy is frequently unnecessary in uncomplicated early disease.[18] From older clinical trials (1970s through the 1990s), the median survival for all individuals ranges from 8 to 12 years.[18] However, a large variation in survival exists, ranging from several months to a normal life expectancy. Treatment must be individualized based on the clinical behavior of the disease.[18] Complications of pancytopenia, including hemorrhage and infection, are a major cause of death. Typically, individuals with CLL survive 10 years or more. Those with certain risk factors, however, have a more aggressive disease, shortening survival to less than 3 years.

Current treatment modalities for CML do not cure the disease or prevent blastic transformation. Standard treatment consists of combined chemotherapy, biologic response modifiers, and allogenic stem cell transplantation. Stem cell transplantation use is limited by donor availability and high toxicity in older adults (older than 65 years). Imatinib mesylate (Gleevec), a tyrosine kinase inhibitor, led to changes in the management of CML. Other tyrosine kinase inhibitors have been developed; however, concerns about disease persistence and resistance still exist.[19] Gleevec produces a complete cytogenic response in more than 80% of newly diagnosed persons; however, it does not cure CML because it does not kill leukemia stem cells both in the laboratory and in vivo.

> ### ✔ QUICK CHECK 23.3
> 1. Why are those with leukemia at high risk for infections?
> 2. What is the significance of the Philadelphia chromosome, and how is it related to leukemia?

ALTERATIONS OF LYMPHOID FUNCTION

Lymphadenopathy

Lymphadenopathy is characterized by enlarged lymph nodes (Fig. 23.11). Lymph node enlargement occurs because of an increase in the size and number of its germinal centers caused by proliferation of lymphocytes and monocytes (immature phagocytes) or invasion by malignant cells. Normally, lymph nodes are not palpable or are barely palpable. Enlarged lymph nodes are characterized by being palpable and often also may be tender or painful to touch, although not in all situations.

Localized lymphadenopathy usually indicates drainage of an area associated with an inflammatory process or infection (reactive lymph node). *Generalized lymphadenopathy* occurs less often and is usually seen in the presence of infections, autoimmune diseases, or disseminated malignancy. Palpable nodes, however, do not always indicate serious disease and may indicate a minor trauma or infection. The location and size of the enlarged nodes are important factors in diagnosing the cause of the lymphadenopathy, as are the individual's age, sex, and geographic location. Generalized lymphadenopathy occurs with NHLs, CLL, histiocytosis, and disorders that produce lymphocytosis. In general, lymphadenopathy results from four types of conditions: (1) neoplastic disease, (2) immunologic or inflammatory conditions, (3) endocrine disorders, or (4) lipid storage diseases. Diseases of unknown cause, including autoimmune diseases and reactions to drugs, also may lead to generalized lymphadenopathy.

Malignant Lymphomas

Lymphomas consist of a diverse group of neoplasms that develop from the proliferation of malignant lymphocytes in the lymphoid system. The WHO publishes the Revised European American Lymphoma (REAL) classification based on the cell type from which the lymphoma probably originated. The basic groups include *HL* and *NHL*. Three major groups of lymphoid malignancies based on morphology and cell lineage include (1) B-cell neoplasms; (2) T-cell neoplasms, and NK-cell neoplasms. MM, which was previously classified independently, is included as a B-cell lymphoma. NHL can be further divided into cancers that have an *indolent*, slow-growing course, and those with an *aggressive*, fast-growing, course. Both HL and NHL occur in children and adults, and the overall treatment and prognosis depend on the stage and type of lymphoma.

Lymphoma is the most common blood cancer in the United States. Incidence rates of lymphoma differ with respect to age, sex, geographic location, and socioeconomic class. The estimated new cases of lymphoma include 8110 cases of HL and 74,200 cases of NHL.[12] It was estimated in 2019 that 19,970 will die from NHL and 1000 from HL. Since the early 1970s, the incidence of NHL has nearly doubled. The exact reason for this increase remains a mystery; however, a modest portion of the increase had been attributed to lymphomas developing in association with immune deficiencies, including AIDS and organ transplants. Conversely, the incidence of HL has declined over the same time period, especially among older adults.

In general, lymphomas are the result of genetic mutations or viral infection. Globally, however, the incidence of lymphoma is increased in more developed countries (except for BL); therefore investigators are studying the following potential risk factors: diet, obesity, metabolic syndrome, sedentary lifestyle, stress, advances in medical care and access, increases in longevity, and exposure to compounds from industrialization. Malignant transformation produces a cell with uncontrolled and excessive growth that accumulates in the lymph nodes and other sites, producing tumor masses. Lymphomas usually start in the lymph nodes or lymphoid tissues of the stomach or intestines.

Hodgkin Lymphoma

Hodgkin lymphoma (HL) is a malignant lymphoma that progresses from one group of lymph nodes to another and includes the development of systemic symptoms and the presence of B cells called **Reed-Sternberg**

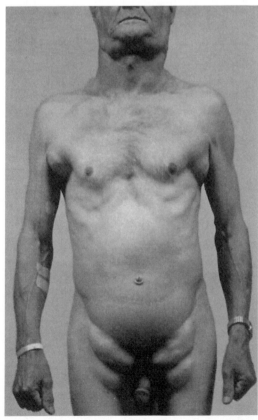

FIGURE 23.11 Lymphadenopathy. Individual with lymphocyte leukemia with extreme but symmetric lymphadenopathy. (Courtesy Dr. A.R. Kagan, Los Angeles. From del Regato JA et al: *Cancer: diagnosis, treatment, and prognosis*, ed 6, St Louis, 1985, Mosby.)

(RS) cells (see the Pathophysiology section). Estimates of new cases of HL include 8110 cases in 2019 and 1000 deaths.[12] The incidence of HL is higher in males, and the median age of diagnosis is 64 years. The incidence is greater in whites than blacks. Denmark, the Netherlands, and the United States have the highest incidence of HL, and Japan and Australia have the lowest incidence. HL peaks at two different ages: early in life in the second and third decades and later in life during the sixth and seventh decades. RS cells are infected with EBV in about 70% of cases. The incidence of HL is approximately 3.1/100,000 males and 2.4/100,000 females and peaks at two different times—during the second and third decades of life and later during the sixth and seventh decades.

PATHOPHYSIOLOGY   It is widely accepted that the RS cell represents the malignant transformed lymphocyte (Fig. 23.12). RS cells are often large and binucleate with occasional mononuclear variants. RS cells are necessary for the diagnosis of HL. In rare instances, cells resembling RS cells can be found in benign illnesses, as well as in other forms of cancer, including NHLs and solid tissue cancers and in IM.

The triggering mechanism for the malignant transformation of cells remains unknown. Classic HL appears to be derived from a B cell in the germinal center that has not undergone successful immunoglobulin gene rearrangement (see Chapter 7) and would normally be induced to undergo apoptosis. Survival of this cell may be linked to infection with EBV. Laboratory and epidemiologic studies have linked HL with EBV infections. The RS cells secrete and release cytokines (e.g., IL-10, transforming growth factor-beta [TGF-β]) that result in the accumulation of inflammatory cells, which produces the local and systemic effects. HL is subcategorized into two main types: classic Hodgkin and nodular lymphocyte–predominant Hodgkin. Classic HL is subclassified into four types: (1) nodular sclerosis Hodgkin lymphoma (grades 1 and 2), (2) lymphocyte rich classical Hodgkin lymphoma, (3) mixed cellularity Hodgkin lymphoma, and (4) lymphocyte depletion Hodgkin lymphoma. based on the structure of RS cells and the characteristics of the inflammatory cell infiltrate in the tumor. Lymphocyte-predominant disease presents with earlier stage disease, longer survival, and fewer treatment failures than classic HL. However, despite a more favorable prognosis, lymphocyte-predominant HL has a tendency to histologically transform into diffuse large B-cell lymphoma by 10 years in approximately 10% of people.

CLINICAL MANIFESTATIONS   Many clinical features of HL can be explained by the complex action of cytokines and other growth factors that are secreted and released by the malignant cells. These substances induce infiltration and proliferation of inflammatory cells, resulting in an enlarged, painless lymph node in the neck (often the first sign of HL) (Fig. 23.13). The discovery of an asymptomatic mediastinal mass on routine chest x-ray is not uncommon. The cervical, axillary, inguinal, and retroperitoneal lymph nodes are commonly affected in HL (Fig. 23.14). Local symptoms caused by pressure and obstruction of lymph nodes are the result of the lymphadenopathy.

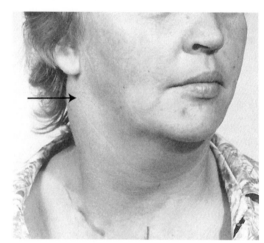

FIGURE 23.13 Hodgkin Lymphoma and Enlarged Cervical Lymph Node. Typical enlarged cervical lymph node in the neck *(arrow)* of a 35-year-old woman with Hodgkin lymphoma. (From del Regato JA et al: *Cancer: diagnosis, treatment, and prognosis,* ed 6, St Louis, 1985, Mosby.)

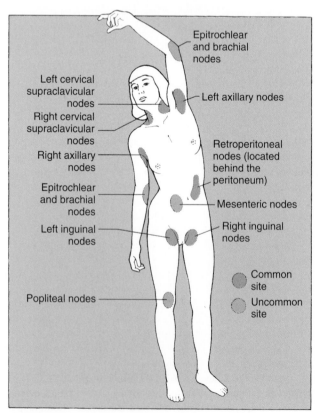

FIGURE 23.14 Common and Uncommon Involved Lymph Node Sites for Hodgkin Lymphoma.

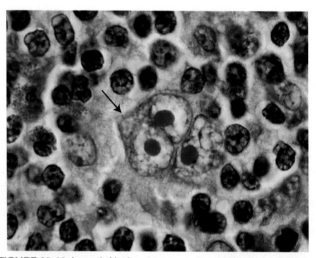

FIGURE 23.12 Lymph Nodes. Diagnostic Reed-Sternberg cell *(arrow).* A large multinucleated or multilobed cell with inclusion body–like nucleoli surrounded by a halo of clear nucleoplasm. (From Damjanov I, Linder J, editors, *Anderson's pathology,* ed 10, St Louis, 1996, Mosby.)

About one-third of individuals will have some common systemic symptoms, such as intermittent fever, without other symptoms of infection, drenching night sweats, itchy skin (pruritus), and fatigue. These constitutional symptoms accompanied by weight loss are associated with a poor prognosis.

Although HL rarely arises in the lung, mediastinal and hilar node adenopathy can cause secondary involvement of the trachea, bronchi, pleura, or lungs. Retroperitoneal nodes can involve vertebral bodies and nerves and also can cause displacement of ureters. Spinal cord involvement is more common in the thoracic and lumbar regions than in the cervical region. Skin lesions, although uncommon, include psoriasis and eczematoid lesions, causing itching and scratching.

As a result of direct invasion from mediastinal lymph nodes, pericardial involvement can cause pericardial friction rub, pericardial effusion, and engorgement of neck veins. The GI tract and urinary tract are rarely involved. Anemia is often found in individuals with HL accompanied by a low serum iron level and reduced iron-binding capacity. Other laboratory findings include elevated sedimentation rate, leukocytosis, and eosinophilia. Leukopenia occurs in advanced stages of HL.

Splenic involvement in HL depends on histologic type. In mixed cellularity and lymphocytic deletion types of HL, the spleen is involved in 60% of cases. With lymphocyte and nodular sclerosis types, 34% of cases involve the spleen.

EVALUATION AND TREATMENT   Because of the variability in symptoms, early definitive detection may be challenging. Asymptomatic lymphadenopathy can progress undetected for several years. Diagnosis is made from physical examination and history; complete blood count (CBC); and blood chemistry studies, including sedimentation rate, lymph node biopsy, pathology review for RS cells, and immunophenotyping for disease markers. Highly indicative of HL is a lymph node biopsy with scattered RS cells and cellular infiltrate. The current staging system for HL is the Ann Arbor staging system with Cotswolds modifications.[20] Clinical staging includes personal history; physical examination; laboratory studies, including sedimentation rate; and thoracic and abdominal/pelvic computed tomography (CT) scans[21] (Table 23.9). Bone marrow biopsy is not recommended in the staging of disease in most individuals with HL.[20] Positron emission tomography (PET) scans, usually combined with CT scans, have replaced gallium scans and lymphangiography for clinical staging.[22] Staging laparotomy is no longer recommended; it should be considered only when the results will allow substantial reduction in treatment. It should not be done in individuals who require chemotherapy. If the laparotomy is required for treatment decisions, the risks of potential morbidity should be considered.[22] For those at high risk of relapse, conventional CT scans are employed for screening to avoid the increased false-positive test results and increased radiation exposure of serial PET-CT scans.[23] Prognostic indicators include clinical stage, histologic type, tumor cell concentration and tumor burden, constitutional symptoms, and age of the individual.

The effectiveness of treatment is related to the age, sex, and general health of the individual; signs and symptoms; stage of the disease; blood test results; type of HL; and classification of the disease as recurrent or progressive. HL in adults usually can be cured with early diagnosis and treatment.[21] Three types of treatment are used: chemotherapy, radiation therapy, and surgery. Treatment for pregnant women includes watchful waiting and steroid therapy. Newer treatments undergoing testing include chemotherapy and radiation therapy with stem cell transplant and monoclonal antibody therapy.[21] Treatment with chemotherapy or radiation therapy, or both, may increase the risk of second cancers, cardiovascular disease, and other health problems for many months or years after treatment.

TABLE 23.9   Definitions of Stages of Hodgkin Disease

Stage	Criteria
I	Involvement of a single lymph node region (I) or localized involvement of a single extralymphatic organ or site (I_E)*
II	Involvement of two or more lymph node regions on same side of diaphragm (II) or localized involvement of a single associated extralymphatic organ or site and its regional lymph node(s), with or without involvement of other lymph node regions on same side of diaphragm (II_E)
III	Involvement of lymph node regions on both sides of diaphragm (III), which also may be accompanied by localized involvement of an associated extralymphatic organ or site (III_E), by involvement of the spleen (III_S) or by both (III_{E+S}).
IV	Disseminated (multifocal) involvement of one or more extralymphatic organs, with or without associated lymph node involvement, or isolated extralymphatic organ involvement with distant (nonregional) nodal involvement

A: No systemic symptoms present
B: Unexplained fevers >38° C (100.4° F), drenching night sweats, or weight loss >10% of body weight

*NOTE: The number of lymph node regions involved may be indicated by a subscript (e.g., II3).
From National Comprehensive Cancer Network: Hodgkin lymphoma. In *NCCN practice guidelines, Version 2.2014: Hodgkin lymphoma* (originally adapted from Carbono PP et al: *Cancer Res* 31[11]:1860-1861, 1971).

Non-Hodgkin Lymphomas

Non-Hodgkin lymphomas (NHLs) are a heterogeneous group of lymphoid tissue neoplasms with differing biologic and clinical patterns of activity and responses to treatment. For unknown reasons, NHL incidence rates increased worldwide from 1950 to 2000, tripling in adults older than 65 years of age. The previously used generic classification of NHL has been reclassified in the WHO/REAL scheme into (1) **B-cell neoplasms**, which include a variety of lymphomas and myelomas that originate from B cells at various stages of differentiation; and (2) **T-cell** and **NK-cell neoplasms**, which include lymphomas that originate from either T or NK cells. These cancers are differentiated from HL by lack of RS cells and other cellular changes not characteristic of HL.

More than 74,200 new cases of NHL and 19,970 deaths are predicted for 2019.[12] The median age of diagnosis is 67 years, with a higher occurrence in men than women. The highest incidences are in North America, Europe, Oceania, and several African countries. Part of the increased incidence has been attributed to diagnostic improvements as well as AIDS-related cancers after the HIV epidemic. Conversely, the mortality has risen at a slower rate. It is thought that newer treatment modalities are improving survival rates.

Risk factors for adult NHL include being older, male, or white and having one of the following: afflicted by certain inherited immune disorders, an autoimmune disease, or HIV/AIDS; exposure to a variety of mutagenic chemicals or certain pesticides; infection with certain cancer-related viruses (e.g., EBV, HIV, HTLV-1, hepatitis C, and human herpesvirus-8); and immune suppression related to organ transplantation. Gastric infection with *H. pylori* increases the risk for gastric lymphomas. NHL is a disease of middle age, usually found in persons more than 50 years old.

PATHOPHYSIOLOGY   NHL is a progressive clonal expansion of B cells, T cells, or NK cells. B cells account for 85% to 90% of NHLs, with most of the remainder being T cells and rarely NK cells. A very small percentage originates from macrophages. Oncogenes may be activated by chromosomal translocations or the tumor-suppressor loci may be inactivated by deletion or mutation of chromosomes. Certain subtypes may have altered genomes by oncogenic viruses. Various subtypes of NHL are identified by specific diagnostic markers related to various cytogenetic lesions. The most common type of chromosomal alteration in NHL is translocation, which disrupts the genes encoded at the breakpoints. Unlike HL, NHL spreads in a less predictable way and spreads widely early.

CLINICAL MANIFESTATIONS   Clinical manifestations of NHL usually begin as localized or generalized lymphadenopathy, similar to HL. Differences in clinical features are noted in Table 23.10. The cervical, axillary, inguinal, and femoral lymph node chains are the most commonly affected sites. Generally, the swelling is painless and the nodes have enlarged and transformed over a period of months or years. Other sites of involvement are the nasopharynx, GI tract, bone, thyroid, testes, and soft tissue. Some individuals have retroperitoneal and abdominal masses with symptoms of abdominal fullness, back pain, ascites (fluid in the peritoneal cavity), skin rash or itchy skin, fatigue, fever of unknown origin, drenching night sweats, and leg swelling.

Lymphomas are classified as low, intermediate, or high grade. A low-grade lymphoma, which also may be termed *indolent,* has a slow progression. Individuals with low-grade lymphoma commonly present with a painless, peripheral adenopathy. Spontaneous regression of these nodes may occur, mimicking the presence of an infection. Night sweats with an elevated temperature (more than 38° C [100.4° F]) and weight loss, as well as extranodular involvement, are not commonly present in the early stages but are common in advanced or end-stage disease. *Cytopenia,* or reduction in the number of blood cells, reflective of bone marrow involvement is often observed. Hepatomegaly is common; splenomegaly is present in approximately 40% of individuals. Fatigue and weakness are more prevalent with advanced stages.

Intermediate and high-grade lymphomas, which are more aggressive, have a more varied clinical presentation. A high-grade lymphoma also may be termed *aggressive.*

EVALUATION AND TREATMENT   The primary means for diagnosis of NHL is biopsy. A common finding in NHL is noncontiguous lymph node involvement, which is not common in HL. Staging is determined from radiologic studies, biopsy, and examination of bone marrow aspirate.

Treatment for NHL is quite diverse and depends on type (B cell or T cell), tumor stage, histologic status (low, intermediate, or high grade), symptoms, age, and presence of comorbidities. Depending on the type (B cell or T cell) of the tumor, stage of disease, and aggressiveness of the tumor, treatment is usually initiated at the time of diagnosis. However, because treatment is not curative for some low-grade indolent lymphomas that are widely disseminated, observation without treatment may be the most appropriate choice. These indolent tumors are often not symptomatic for the individual, and this approach improves quality of life. In some cases the disease may be so slow growing that treatment is not needed for an extended period of time.

Treatment with chemotherapy alone may be adequate for many individuals, although radiation therapy is often included. Low-dose chemotherapy has been followed by autologous stem cell transplantation in some NHLs or for recurrent disease. Treatment using monoclonal antibody alone or in combination with radiation therapy (radioimmunotherapy) also is being used.

Individuals with NHL can survive for extended periods. A partial remission may be achieved in some cases in which evidence of the disease remains but the disease does not progress. Survival with nodular lymphoma ranges up to 15 years, but those with diffuse disease generally do not survive as long. Overall, the survival rates of NHL are less than those for HL. Survival rates for NHL are 77% at 1 year, 59% at 5 years, and 42% at 10 years.

Burkitt lymphoma.   Burkitt lymphoma (BL) is a B-cell NHL with unique clinical and epidemiologic features. It is highly aggressive and is the fastest growing human tumor. There are three main types of BL: endemic, sporadic, and immunodeficiency-related. *Endemic* BL commonly occurs in Africa and is linked to the EBV, and *sporadic* BL occurs worldwide. *Immunodeficiency-related* BL is most often seen in individuals with AIDS. BL occurs most often in children and young adults. Endemic cases, usually from Africa, involve a rapidly growing tumor of the jaw and facial bones (Fig. 23.15). In the United States, BL is rare, usually

TABLE 23.10 Clinical Differences Between Non-Hodgkin Lymphoma and Hodgkin Lymphoma

Characteristics	Non-Hodgkin Lymphoma	Hodgkin Lymphoma
Nodal involvement	Multiple peripheral nodes	Localized to single axial group of nodes (i.e., cervical, mediastinal, paraaortic)
	Mesenteric nodes and Waldeyer ring commonly involved	Mesenteric nodes and Waldeyer ring rarely involved
Spread	Noncontiguous	Orderly spread by contiguity
B symptoms*	Uncommon	Common
Extranodal involvement	Common	Rare
Extent of disease	Rarely localized	Often localized

*Fever, weight loss, night sweats.

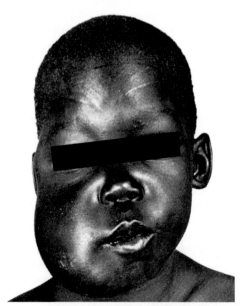

FIGURE 23.15 Burkitt Lymphoma. Burkitt lymphoma involving the jaw in a young African boy. (Courtesy I. Magrath, MD, Bethesda, MD. From Zitelli BJ et al: *Zitelli and Davis' atlas of pediatric physical diagnosis,* ed 6, Philadelphia, 2012, Saunders.)

involves the abdomen, and is characterized by extensive bone marrow invasion and replacement.

PATHOPHYSIOLOGY Almost all cases of BL are associated with EBV. Perhaps suppression of the immune system by other illnesses (e.g., HIV infection, chronic malaria) increases the individual's susceptibility to EBV. B cells are particularly sensitive because of specific surface receptors for EBV. As a result, the B cell undergoes chromosomal translocations that result in overexpression of the *c-MYC* proto-oncogene and loss of control of cell growth (Fig. 23.16). The most common translocation (75% of individuals) is between chromosomes 8 (containing the *c-MYC* gene) and 14 (containing the immunoglobulin heavy chain genes). Other translocations have been reported between chromosome 8 and chromosomes 2 or 22, which contain genes for immunoglobulin light chains.

CLINICAL MANIFESTATIONS In non-African BL the most common presentation is abdominal swelling. Manifestations of most tumors occur at extranodal sites. More advanced disease may involve the eye, ovaries, kidneys, or glandular tissue (breast, thyroid, tonsils) and presents with type B symptoms (night sweats, fever, weight loss). Common manifestations may include nausea and vomiting; loss of appetite or change in bowel habits, or both; GI bleeding; symptoms of an acute abdominal condition; intestinal perforation; and renal failure.

EVALUATION AND TREATMENT Usually indicative of BL is the presence of tumors in the jaw and facial bones, enlarged lymph nodes, and bone marrow containing malignant B cells. Laboratory studies include CBC, electrolytes, liver and renal function tests, lactate dehydrogenase, hepatitis B, HIV, and uric acid.[24] Treatment is aggressive multidrug regimens, such as combination chemotherapy. There is no role for radiation therapy in people with BL.[24]

Lymphoblastic lymphoma. Lymphoblastic lymphoma (LL) is a relatively rare variant of NHL overall (2% to 4%) but accounts for almost one-third of cases of NHL in children and adolescents, with a male predominance. The vast majority of LL (90%) is of T-cell origin; the remainder arises from B cells. LL is similar to acute lymphoblastic leukemia and may be considered a variant of that disease.

PATHOPHYSIOLOGY The disease arises from a clone of relatively immature T cells that becomes malignant in the thymus. As with most lymphoid tumors, LL is frequently associated with translocations, primarily of the chromosomes that encode for the T-cell receptor (chromosomes 7 and 14). These aberrations result in increased expression of a variety of transcription factors and loss of growth control.

CLINICAL MANIFESTATIONS The first sign of LL is usually a painless lymphadenopathy in the neck. Peripheral lymph nodes in the chest become involved in about 70% of individuals. Involved nodes are located mostly above the diaphragm. LL is a very aggressive tumor that presents as stage IV in most people. T-cell LL is associated with a unique mediastinal mass (up to 75%) because of the apparent origin of the tumor in the thymus. The mass results in dyspnea and chest pain and may cause compression of bronchi or the superior vena cava. The tumor may infiltrate the bone marrow in about half of those affected, and suppression of bone marrow hematopoiesis leads to increased susceptibility to infections. Other organs, including the liver, kidney, spleen, and brain, also may be affected. Many individuals express type B symptoms: fever, night sweats, and significant weight loss.

EVALUATION AND TREATMENT The most common therapeutic approach is combined chemotherapy (intensive therapy). In early stages of the disease, the response rate is high, with increased survival; the 5-year survival in children is 80% to 90% and 45% to 55% in adults. Although LL is easily treated, there is a high relapse rate: 40% to 60% of adults.

Plasma Cell Malignancy
Multiple Myeloma

Multiple myeloma (MM) is a clonal plasma cell cancer characterized by the slow proliferation of tumor cell masses in the bone marrow (Fig. 23.17). These masses are associated with *lytic bone lesions* (round, punched out regions of bone) (Fig. 23.18). Uncommon variants include *solitary myeloma (plasmacytoma)* with a single mass in bone or soft tissue and *smoldering myeloma*, which is defined by a lack of symptoms and a high plasma abnormal antibody called the M protein.

Myeloma cells reside in the bone marrow and are usually not found in the peripheral blood. As the number of myeloma cells increases, fewer red blood cells, white blood cells, and platelets are produced. It may occasionally spread to other tissues, especially in very advanced stages of the disease. For unknown reasons, the reported incidence of MM has doubled in the past 2 decades. About 32,110 new cases and

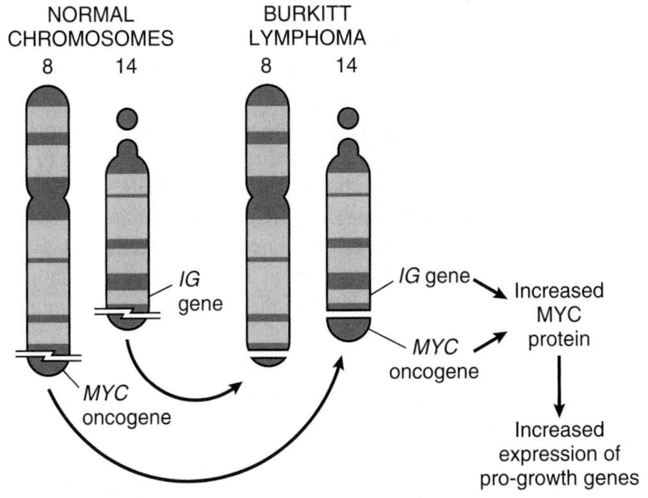

FIGURE 23.16 Burkitt Lymphoma Cells. The 8,14 chromosomal translocation and associated oncogenes in Burkitt lymphoma.

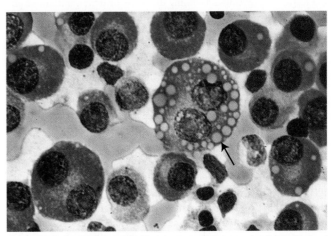

FIGURE 23.17 Multiple Myeloma, Bone Marrow Aspirate. Normal marrow cells are largely replaced by plasma cells, including atypical forms with multiple nuclei *(arrow)*, and cytoplasmic droplets *containing immunoglobulin.* (From Kumar V et al: *Robbins and Cotran pathologic basis of disease,* ed 9, Philadelphia, 2015, Saunders.)

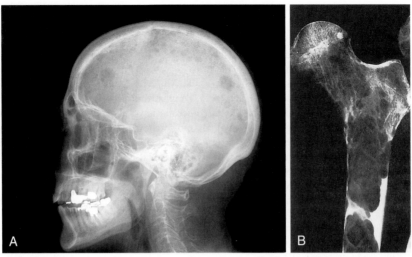

FIGURE 23.18 Osteolytic Lesions in Individuals With Multiple Myeloma. **A,** Radiograph showing skull lesions in a client with myeloma. **B,** Radiograph of femur showing extensive bone destruction caused by tumor. Note absence of reactive bone formation. (**A** from Abeloff M et al: *Abeloff's clinical oncology,* ed 4, Philadelphia, 2008, Churchill Livingstone. **B** from Kissane JM, editor: *Anderson's pathology,* ed 9, St Louis, 1990, Mosby.)

12,960 deaths are estimated for 2019.[12] MM occurs in all races, but the incidence in blacks is about twice that of whites. It rarely occurs before the age of 40 years—the peak age of incidence is between 65 and 70 years. It is slightly more common in men (7.7 estimated new cases per 100,000 persons) than in women (4.9 new cases per 100,000 persons). Other risk factors include exposure to radiation or certain chemicals, including pesticides, and a history of monoclonal gammopathy of undetermined significance (MGUS; see Clinical Manifestations) or plasmacytoma.

PATHOPHYSIOLOGY   MM is a plasma cell neoplasia that causes lytic bone lesions (bony disease; radiologically appears as punched-out defects), hypercalcemia, renal failure, anemia, and immune abnormalities. It is a biologically complex disease with significant heterogeneity (wide range of genetic abnormalities, differences in clinical response, and survival in those with the same treatment). Multiple mutations in different pathways alter the intrinsic biology of the plasma cell, generating the features of myeloma. Defining the main, or driver, mutations and heterogeneity is essential for treatment decisions. Many myelomas are aneuploid and, in most individuals with myeloma, chromosomal translocations are the most common. Development of further secondary genetic alterations increases progression to an aggressive MM. Investigators are studying various epigenetic alterations and interactions with extracellular matrix proteins. For example, myeloma cells interact and secrete peptides that adhere to stromal cells, inducing cytokines that possibly promote inflammation. Myeloma cells are prone to the accumulation of misfolded protein, such as unpaired immunoglobulin chains. Misfolded proteins activate apoptosis.

Malignant plasma cells arise from one clone of B cells that produce abnormally large amounts of one class of immunoglobulin (usually IgG, occasionally IgA, and rarely IgM, IgD, or IgE). The malignant transformation may begin early in B-cell development, possibly before encountering antigen in the secondary lymphoid organs. The myeloma cells return either to the bone marrow or to other soft tissue sites. Cytokines, particularly IL-6, have been identified as essential factors that promote the growth and survival of MM cells. (Lymphocytes and cytokines are described in Chapter 6.) IL-6 in particular acts as an osteoclast-activating factor and stimulates osteoclasts to reabsorb bone.

This process results in bone lesions and hypercalcemia (high calcium levels in the blood) attributable to the release of calcium from the breakdown of bone.

The antibody produced by the transformed plasma cell is frequently defective, containing truncations, deletions, and other abnormalities, and is often referred to as a *paraprotein* (abnormal protein in the blood). Because of the large number of malignant plasma cells, the abnormal antibody, or M protein, becomes the most prominent protein in the blood (see Fig. 23.19). Suppression of normal plasma cells by the myeloma results in diminished or absent normal antibodies. The excessive amount of M protein also may contribute to many of the clinical manifestations of the disease. Frequently, the myeloma produces free immunoglobulin light chain (Bence Jones protein) that is present in the blood and urine and contributes to damage of renal tubular cells.

CLINICAL MANIFESTATIONS   MM is characterized by elevated levels of calcium in the blood (hypercalcemia), renal failure, anemia, and bone lesions. The hypercalcemia and bone lesions result from infiltration of the bone by malignant plasma cells and stimulation of osteoclasts to reabsorb bone. This process results in the release of calcium (hypercalcemia) and the development of lytic lesions of bone (see Fig. 23.18). Destruction of bone tissue causes pain, the most common presenting symptom, and pathologic fractures. The bones most commonly involved, in decreasing order of frequency, are the vertebrae, ribs, skull, pelvis, femur, clavicle, and scapula. Spinal cord compression, because of the weakened vertebrae, occurs in about 10% of individuals.

A condition called amyloidosis may occur, in which antibody proteins increase and stick together in peripheral nerves and organs, such as the kidney and heart. Signs and symptoms of amyloidosis include fatigue, purple spots on the skin, enlarged tongue, diarrhea, edema, and numbness or tingling in the legs and feet.

Proteinuria is observed in 90% of individuals. Renal failure may be either acute or chronic and is usually secondary to the hypercalcemia. Bence Jones protein may lead to damage of the proximal tubules. Anemia is usually normocytic and normochromic and results from inhibited erythropoiesis caused by tumor cell infiltration of the bone marrow.

The high concentration of paraprotein in the blood may lead to hyperviscosity syndrome. The increased viscosity interferes with blood

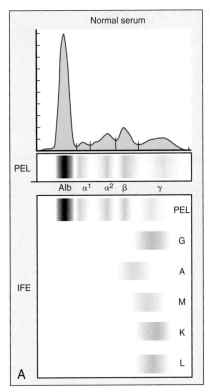
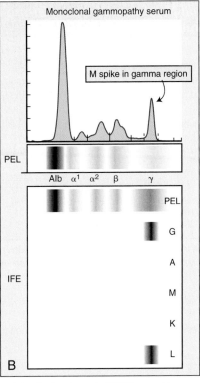
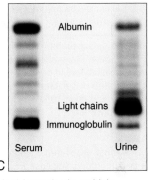

FIGURE 23.19 M Protein. Serum protein electrophoresis *(PEL)* is used to screen for M proteins in multiple myeloma (MM). **A,** In normal serum the proteins separate into several regions between albumin *(Alb)* and a broad band in the gamma *(γ)* region, where most antibodies (gamma globulins) are found. Immunofixation *(IFE)* can identify the location of IgG *(G)*, IgA *(A)*, IgM *(M)*, and kappa *(κ)*, and lambda *(λ)* light chains. **B,** Serum from an individual with MM contains a sharp M protein *(M spike)*. The M protein is monoclonal and contains only one heavy chain and one light chain. In this instance the IFE identifies the M protein as an IgG containing a lambda light chain. **C,** Serum and urine protein electrophoretic patterns in an individual with MM. Serum demonstrates an M protein *(Immunoglobulin)* in the gamma region, and the urine has a large amount of the smaller sized light chains with only a small amount of the intact immunoglobulin. (**A** and **B** from Abeloff M et al: *Abeloff's clinical oncology,* ed 4, Philadelphia, 2008, Churchill Livingstone. **C** from McPherson R, Pincus M: *Henry's clinical diagnosis and management by laboratory methods,* ed 22, Edinburgh, 2012, Saunders.)

circulation to various sites (brain, kidneys, extremities). Hyperviscosity syndrome is observed in up to 20% of persons. Additional neurologic symptoms (e.g., confusion, headaches, blurred vision) may occur secondary to hypercalcemia or hyperviscosity.

Suppression of the humoral (antibody-mediated) immune response results in repeated infections, primarily pneumonias, and pyelonephritis. The most commonly involved microorganisms are encapsulated bacteria that are particularly sensitive to the effects of antibody; pneumonia caused by *Streptococcus pneumoniae, Staphylococcus aureus,* or *Klebsiella pneumoniae;* or pyelonephritis caused by *Escherichia coli* or other gram-negative organisms. Cell-mediated (T-cell) function is relatively normal. Overwhelming infection is the leading cause of death from MM.

MM is a progressive disorder and is often preceded by a condition known as monoclonal gammopathy of undetermined significance (MGUS). MGUS is diagnosed by the presence of an M protein in the blood or urine without additional evidence of MM.[25] MGUS is present in approximately 1% of the general population and in 3% of individuals older than 70 years. Although MGUS is considered nonpathologic and requires no treatment, about 2% of individuals with MGUS progress to malignant plasma cell disorders. Progression of MM after MGUS advances to asymptomatic MM and finally symptomatic MM. Asymptomatic MM also may be referred to as smoldering myeloma and indolent myeloma.[25] Smoldering myeloma is usually characterized by the presence of an M protein and clonal bone marrow plasma cells, but with no indication of end-organ damage.

EVALUATION AND TREATMENT Diagnosis of MM is made by symptoms and radiographic and laboratory studies; a definitive diagnosis requires a bone marrow biopsy. The International Myeloma Working Group's new criteria[25] for the diagnosis of MM and smoldering MM is presented in Box 23.2. Several types of radiologic studies document the presence of bone lesions and areas of destruction. Quantitative measurements of immunoglobulins (IgG, IgM, IgA) are usually done, and serum electrophoretic analysis reveals increased levels of M protein. Bence Jones protein may be observed in the urine or serum by immunoelectrophoresis, or in the serum using available enzyme-linked immunosorbent assays (ELISAs). However, variants of MM include individuals in which only free light chain is produced and a rare variant that produces only free heavy chain; about 1% of cases are nonsecretory so that neither M protein nor Bence Jones protein is produced. Measurement of another protein, free β2-microglobulin, is used as an indicator of prognosis or effectiveness of therapy.

Treatment options include combinations of chemotherapy; other drug therapy; targeted therapy; high-dose chemotherapy with stem cell transplant; biologic therapy; radiation therapy (bone lesions of the spine); and, sometimes, surgery. New therapies, called *proteasome*

BOX 23.2 Revised International Myeloma Working Group Diagnostic Criteria for Multiple Myeloma and Smoldering Multiple Myeloma

Definition of Multiple Myeloma

Clonal bone marrow plasma cells ≥10% or biopsy-proven bony or extramedullary plasmacytoma* and any one or more of the following myeloma defining events:

Evidence of end organ damage that can be attributed to the underlying plasma cell proliferative disorder, specifically:

Hypercalcemia: serum calcium >0.25 mmol/L (>1 mg/dL) higher than the upper limit of normal or >2.75 mmol/L (>11 mg/dL)

Renal insufficiency: creatinine clearance >40 mL per min[†] or serum creatinine >177 μml/L (>2 mg/dL)

Anemia: hemoglobin value of >20 g/L below the lower limit of normal, or a hemoglobin value <100 g/L

Bone lesions: one or more osteolytic lesions on skeletal radiography, CT, or PET-CT[‡]

Any one or more of the following biomarkers of malignancy:

Clonal bone marrow plasma cell percentage* ≥60%

Involved/uninvolved serum free light chain ratio[§] ≥100

>1 focal lesion on MRI studies[¶]

Definition of Smoldering Multiple Myeloma

Both criteria must be met:

Serum monoclonal protein (IgG or IgA) ≥30 g/L or urinary monoclonal protein ≥500/24 hr and/or clonal bone marrow plasma cells 10% to 60%

Absence of myeloma-defining events or amyloidosis

*Clonality should be established by showing κ/λ-light-chain restriction on flow cytometry, immunohistochemistry, or immunofluorescence. Bone marrow plasma cell percentage should preferably be estimated from a core biopsy specimen; in case of disparity between the aspirate and core biopsy, the highest value should be used.

[†]Measured or estimated by validated equations.

[‡]If bone marrow has less than 10% clonal plasma cells, more than one bone lesion is required to distinguish from solitary plasmacytoma with minimal marrow involvement.

[§]These values are based on the serum Freelite assay (The Binding Site Group, Birmingham, UK). The involved free light chain must be ≥100 mg/L.

[¶]Each focal lesion must be ≥5 mm or more in size.

PET-CT, ^{18}F-Labeled fluorodeoxyglucose PET with CT.

From Rajkumar SV et al: *Lancet Oncol* 15(12):e538-e548, 2014.

---

inhibitors, are emerging. Dose intensification improves outcomes in younger persons; however, long-term remissions occur in a minority of people. Gene expression profiling (GEP) helps improve the treatment of MM because it identifies prognostic subgroups and defines the molecular pathways associated with these subgroups. Newer agents (e.g., bortezomib, lenalidomide) have expanded therapeutic regimens for end-stage myeloma. The median survival for all stages of MM is 3 years. Approval of new drugs has changed the management of MM, and research for survival improvement is ongoing.

✔**QUICK CHECK 23.4**

1. What are the risk factors for adult NHL?
2. Discuss why multiple myeloma (MM) causes bone lesions and increases the risk of fractures.
3. What are the main pathologic features of MM?

ALTERATIONS OF SPLENIC FUNCTION

The complexities of splenic function are not totally understood, and its mysteries are still being studied. The normal functions of the spleen that may affect disease states include (1) phagocytosis of blood cells and particulate matter (e.g., bacteria), (2) antibody production, (3) hematopoiesis, and (4) sequestration of formed blood elements. The spleen is part of the mononuclear phagocyte system and is involved in all systemic inflammations, hematopoietic disorders, and many metabolic disorders.

In the past, splenomegaly (enlargement of the spleen) has been associated with various disease states. It is now recognized that splenomegaly is not necessarily pathologic; an enlarged spleen may be present in certain individuals without any evidence of disease. Splenomegaly may be, however, one of the first physical signs of underlying conditions,

and its presence should not be ignored. In conditions in which splenomegaly is present, the normal functions of the spleen may become overactive, producing a syndrome known as hypersplenism.

Current criteria indicating the presence of hypersplenism include (1) cytopenias (anemia, leukopenia, thrombocytopenia, or combinations of these), (2) cellular bone marrow, (3) splenomegaly, and (4) improvement after splenectomy. Some individuals may seek treatment for problems even though they have not met all of these clinical criteria; therefore the relevance and significance of hypersplenism are still uncertain. Primary hypersplenism is recognized when no etiologic factor has been identified; secondary hypersplenism occurs in the presence of another condition.

PATHOPHYSIOLOGY Specific conditions causing splenomegaly and resulting hypersplenism are many (Box 23.3). Different pathologic processes that produce splenomegaly are described briefly.

Acute inflammatory or infectious processes cause splenomegaly because of an increased demand for defensive activities. An acutely enlarged spleen secondary to infection may become so filled with erythrocytes that their natural rubbery resilience is lost and they become fragile and vulnerable to blunt trauma. Splenic rupture is a complication associated with IM; rupture occurs mostly in males between days 4 and 21 of acute illness.

Congestive splenomegaly is accompanied by ascites, portal hypertension, and esophageal varices and is most commonly seen in those with hepatic cirrhosis. Splenic hyperplasia develops in disorders that increase splenic workload and is associated most commonly with various types of anemia (hemolytic) and CMPDs (i.e., PV).

Infiltrative splenomegaly is caused by engorgement by the macrophages with indigestible materials associated with various "storage diseases." Tumors and cysts cause actual growth of the spleen. Metastatic tumors in the spleen are rare and may result from primary tumors of the skin, lung, breast, and cervix.

CLINICAL MANIFESTATIONS Overactivity of the spleen results in hematologic alterations that affect all blood components. Sequestering of red blood cells, granulocytes, and platelets results in a reduction of all circulating blood cells. The spleen may sequester up to 50% of the red blood cell population, thereby upsetting the normal physiologic concentration of red blood cells in the circulation. The rate of splenic pooling is directly related to spleen size and the degree of increased blood flow through it. Sequestering exposes the red blood cells to splenic conditions that accelerate destruction, further contributing to the decreased red blood cell concentration. Anemia is the result of these combined activities. Anemia may be further potentiated by an increase in blood volume, which produces a *dilutional effect* on the already reduced concentration of red blood cells. The dilutional effect, as well as the removal and destruction of red blood cells, depends primarily on the degree of splenomegaly.

White blood cells and platelets also are affected by sequestering, although not to the same degree as the red blood cell. Again, the size of the spleen is the determining factor in the number of cells sequestered.

EVALUATION AND TREATMENT Treatment for hypersplenism is splenectomy; however, it may not be always indicated. A splenectomy is considered necessary to alleviate the destructive effects on red blood cells. Clinical indicators should determine the need for splenectomy, not necessarily specific conditions. Splenectomy for splenic rupture is no longer considered mandatory because of the possibility of overwhelming sepsis after removal. Repair and preservation are now considered before the decision to remove the spleen. Splenectomy also may be performed as treatment for hairy cell leukemia, Felty syndrome, agnogenic myeloid metaplasia, thalassemia major, Gaucher disease, hemodialysis, splenomegaly, splenic venous thrombosis, and thrombotic thrombocytopenia purpura (TTP).

Individuals are able to lead normal lives after splenectomy but blood cell abnormalities often exist after removal of the spleen (i.e., red blood cells become thinner, broader, and wrinkled; white blood cell counts initially increase and then plateau; platelet counts rise after surgery and then stabilize). A major postoperative complication after splenectomy is OPSI. Unless treated in time, OPSI may rapidly progress to septic shock and possibly disseminated intravascular coagulation (DIC).

> ✓ **QUICK CHECK 23.5**
> 1. Contrast the principal features of Hodgkin lymphoma with those of non-Hodgkin lymphoma.
> 2. What is Burkitt lymphoma?
> 3. Identify the major causes of splenomegaly. How does it differ from hypersplenism?

HEMORRHAGIC DISORDERS AND ALTERATIONS OF PLATELETS AND COAGULATION

The arrest of bleeding, or hemostasis, depends on adequate numbers of platelets, normal levels of coagulation factors, and absence of defects in vessels walls. The spectrum of abnormal bleeding varies widely from massive bleeds, such as rupture of large vessels such as the aorta, to small bleeds in skin or mucosal membranes. Diminished or excessive levels of coagulation factors can lead to defective hemostasis or spontaneous and unnecessary clotting. (Hemostasis is discussed in Chapter 22.) Diminished hemostasis results in either internal or external hemorrhage, defined as copious or heavy discharge of blood from blood vessels. A classification of hemorrhagic disorders is included in Table 23.11.

Purpuric disorders, red or purple discolored spots on skin, occur when there is a deficiency of normal platelets necessary to plug damaged vessels or prevent leakage from the tiny tears that occur daily in capillaries. More serious internal bleeding occurs from events that simply overwhelm hemostatic mechanisms, such as rupture of large blood vessels, trauma, and diseases associated with massive hemorrhage including abdominal aneurysm (also see the Anemias of Blood Loss section). Between these smaller bleeds and massive bleeds are deficiencies of coagulation factors found with the hemophilias (see Chapter 22). Disorders that result in spontaneous clotting can develop from genetic disorders of the clotting system components or from acquired diseases that activate clotting. These disorders are known collectively as thromboembolic disease.

BOX 23.3 Diseases Related to Classification of Splenomegaly

Inflammation or Infection
Acute: viral (hepatitis, infectious mononucleosis, cytomegalovirus), bacterial (*Salmonella*, gram negative), parasitic (typhoid)
Subacute or chronic: bacterial (subacute bacterial endocarditis, tuberculosis), parasitic (malaria), fungal (histoplasmosis), Felty syndrome, systemic lupus erythematosus, rheumatoid arthritis, thrombocytopenia

Congestive
Cirrhosis, heart failure, portal vein obstruction (portal hypertension), splenic vein obstruction

Infiltrative
Gaucher disease, amyloidosis, diabetic lipemia

Tumors or Cysts
Malignant: polycythemia rubra vera, chronic or acute leukemias, Hodgkin lymphoma, metastatic solid tumors

Nonmalignant: Hamartoma
Cysts: true cysts (lymphangiomas, hemangiomas, epithelial, endothelial); false cysts (hemorrhagic, serous, inflammatory)

TABLE 23.11 Classification of Hemorrhagic Disorders

Type of Defect	Example	Manifestation
Defects of primary hemostasis	Platelet defects or von Willebrand disease	Usually present with small bleeds in skin or mucosal membrane; bleeds are usually petechiae (<3-mm minute hemorrhages) or purpuras (>3-mm red-purple discolorations); common in capillaries; also includes epistaxis (nose bleeds), GI bleeds, or excessive menstruation
Defects of secondary hemostasis	Coagulation factor defects	Bleeds into soft tissue, muscle, or joints; intracranial bleeds may occur
Generalized defects of small vessels	Palpable purpura and ecchymoses	Extravasated blood creates a palpable mass (or palpable purpura), ecchymoses (simply called a *bruise*), or a larger palpable lesion (or hematoma); systemic disorders disrupt small blood vessels, called vasculitis

Additionally, any disorder of the blood that predisposes to clotting of blood or thrombosis is called hypercoagulability (thrombophilia).

Disorders of Platelets

Quantitative or qualitative abnormalities of platelets can interrupt normal blood coagulation and prevent hemostasis. The quantitative abnormalities are *thrombocytopenia,* a decrease in the number of circulating platelets, and *thrombocythemia,* an increase in the number of platelets. Qualitative disorders affect the structure or function of individual platelets and can coexist with the quantitative disorders. Qualitative disorders usually prevent platelet adherence and aggregation, preventing formation of a platelet plug.

Thrombocytopenia

Thrombocytopenia is defined as a platelet count less than 150,000 platelets/µl of blood, although most health care providers do not consider the decrease significant unless it falls below 100,000 platelets/µl of blood.[26] Hemorrhage associated with minor trauma does not appreciably increase until the count falls below 50,000 platelets/µl. Spontaneous bleeding without trauma can occur with counts ranging from 10,000 platelets/µl to 15,000 platelets/µl, resulting in skin manifestations (i.e., petechiae, ecchymoses, and larger purpuric spots) or frank bleeding from mucous membranes. Severe spontaneous bleeding may result if the count is less than 10,000 platelets/µl and can be fatal if it occurs in the GI tract, respiratory tract, or CNS.

Before the diagnosis of thrombocytopenia is made, pseudothrombocytopenia must be ruled out. This phenomenon occurs in approximately 1 in 1000 to 1 in 10,000 laboratory samples and results from an error in platelet counting when a blood sample is analyzed by an automated cell counter. Platelets in the blood sample may become nonspecifically agglutinated by immunoglobulins in the presence of ethylenediaminetetraacetic acid (EDTA), a preservative in banked blood. The agglutinated platelets are not counted, thus giving an apparent, but false, thrombocytopenia. Thrombocytopenia also may be falsely diagnosed because of a dilutional effect observed after massive transfusion of platelet-poor packed cells to treat a hemorrhage. This occurs when more than 10 units of blood have been transfused within a 24-hour period. The hemorrhage that necessitated the transfusion also accelerates the loss of platelets, contributing to the pseudothrombocytopenic state. Splenic sequestering of platelets in hypersplenism (congestive) also induces an apparent thrombocytopenia, as does hypothermia (less than 25° C [77° F]), which is reversed when temperatures return to normal, suggesting an increased platelet sequestration in response to chilling.

PATHOPHYSIOLOGY Thrombocytopenia results from decreased platelet production, increased consumption, or both. The condition may be either congenital or acquired and may be either primary or secondary to other acquired or congenital conditions. Thrombocytopenia secondary to congenital conditions occurs in a large number of different diseases, although each is relatively rare.

Acquired thrombocytopenia is more common and may occur as a result of decreased platelet production secondary to viral infections (e.g., EBV, rubella, CMV, HIV), drugs (e.g., thiazides, estrogens, quinine-containing drugs, chemotherapeutic agents, ethanol), nutritional deficiencies (vitamin B_{12} or folic acid in particular), chronic renal failure, bone marrow hypoplasia (e.g., AA), radiation therapy, or bone marrow infiltration by cancer. Most common forms of thrombocytopenia are the result of increased platelet consumption. Examples include heparin-induced thrombocytopenia, idiopathic (immune) TTP, TTP, and DIC (discussed in the Disorders of Coagulation section).

Heparin-induced thrombocytopenia. Heparin is a common cause of drug-induced thrombocytopenia. Approximately 4% of individuals

treated with unfractionated heparin develop heparin-induced thrombocytopenia (HIT). The incidence is lower (about 0.1%) with the use of low-molecular-weight heparin. HIT is an immune-mediated, adverse drug reaction caused by IgG antibodies against the heparin–platelet factor 4 complex leading to platelet activation through platelet Fc γIIa receptors. The release of additional platelet factor 4 from activated platelets and activation of thrombin lead to increased platelet consumption and a decrease in platelet counts beginning 5 to 10 days after administration of heparin.

CLINICAL MANIFESTATIONS The hallmark of HIT is thrombocytopenia. A decrease of approximately 50% in the platelet count is observed in more than 95% of individuals. However, 30% or more of those with thrombocytopenia are also at risk for venous or arterial thrombosis because a *prothrombotic state* is caused by antibody binding to platelets, inducing activation, aggregation, and consumption (thus the term *thrombocytopenia* in the syndrome name) of platelets. Venous thrombosis is more common and results in deep venous thrombosis (DVT) and pulmonary emboli. Arterial thrombosis affects the lower extremities, causing limb ischemia. Arterial thrombosis may lead to cerebrovascular accidents and myocardial infarctions. Other major arteries also may be affected (e.g., renal, mesenteric, upper limb). Although platelet counts are low, bleeding is uncommon.

EVALUATION AND TREATMENT Diagnosis is primarily based on clinical observations. The individual presents with dropping platelet counts after 5 days or longer of heparin treatment. On average, platelet counts may fall to 60,000/µl. Because most individuals have undergone surgery and the onset of symptoms, including thrombosis, may be delayed until after release from the hospital, other possible causes of thrombocytopenia (e.g., infection, other drug reactions) must be considered. Tests are available to measure anti-heparin–platelet factor 4 antibodies. The sensitivity of this test is extremely high (>90%), but the specificity is less because of false-positive reactions (e.g., those receiving dialysis). Treatment is the withdrawal of heparin and use of alternative anticoagulants.

Immune thrombocytopenia purpura. The most common cause of thrombocytopenia secondary to increased platelet destruction is immune thrombocytopenic purpura (ITP). The incidence of ITP is estimated to range from 5.8 to 6.6 per 100,000 in the general population and tends to increase with age. ITP may be acute or chronic. The acute form is frequently observed in children and typically lasts 1 to 2 months with a complete remission. In some instances it may last for up to 6 months, and some children (7% to 28%) may progress to the chronic condition (see Chapter 24). Acute ITP is usually secondary to infections (particularly viral) or other conditions that lead to large amounts of antigen in the blood, such as drug allergies or SLE. Under these conditions, the antigen usually forms immune complexes with circulating antibody; it is thought that the immune complexes bind to Fc receptors on platelets, leading to their destruction in the spleen. The acute form of ITP usually resolves as the source of antigen is resolved (infection) or removed (drugs).

Chronic ITP is caused by autoantibodies against platelet-specific antigens. This form is more commonly observed in adults, being most prevalent in women between 20 and 40 years of age, although it can be found in all ages. The chronic form tends to get progressively worse. It can occur from a variety of predisposing conditions or exposures (secondary) or have no known risk factors (primary). The autoantibodies are generally of the IgG class and are against one or more of several platelet glycoproteins (e.g., GPIIb/IIIa, GPIIb/IX, GPIa/IIa). The antibodies bind directly to the platelet antigens, after which the antibody-coated platelets are recognized and removed from the circulation by macrophages in the spleen.

CLINICAL MANIFESTATIONS Initial manifestations range from minor bleeding problems (development of petechiae and purpura) over the course of several days to major hemorrhage from mucosal sites (epistaxis, hematuria, menorrhagia, bleeding gums). Rarely will an individual present with intracranial bleeding or other sites of internal bleeding.

During pregnancy, a woman with ITP may have a newborn that is also thrombocytopenic. If the fetal platelets express the same antigen as the mother, the maternal antibody will coat the platelets, potentially resulting in thrombocytopenia in utero. A variant of neonatal thrombocytopenia *(neonatal alloimmune thrombocytopenia)* occurs when the mother does not have ITP but makes IgG antibodies against an antigen inherited from the father found on fetal platelets but not on maternal platelets.

EVALUATION AND TREATMENT Diagnosis of ITP is based on a history of bleeding and associated symptoms (weight loss, fever, headache). Physical examination includes notations on the type, location, and severity of bleeding. In addition, evidence of infections (bacterial, HIV and other viral), medication history, family history, and evidence of thrombosis are assessed. Other diagnostic tests include CBC and peripheral blood smear. Unlike some other forms of thrombocytopenia, there is usually no evidence of splenectomy. Testing for antiplatelet antibodies is usually not helpful. Although most cases of ITP are associated with elevated levels of IgG on platelets, other forms of thrombocytopenia also have a high incidence of platelet-associated antibodies; thus the specificity is low (50% to 65%).[27] In addition, some cases of ITP will not present with elevated platelet-associated antibodies. The sensitivity is 75% to 94%; therefore a negative test does not rule out ITP.

The acute form of ITP usually resolves without major clinical consequences, but the chronic form, like many autoimmune diseases, is variable with multiple remissions and exacerbations. Treatment is palliative, not curative, and focuses on prevention of platelet destruction. Initial therapy for ITP is glucocorticoids (e.g., prednisone), which suppress the immune response and prevent sequestering and further destruction of platelets. If steroid therapy is ineffective, other reagents have been used. Treatment with intravenous immunoglobulin (IVIG) is used to prevent major bleeding. The response rate is 80%, but the effects are transient, lasting only days to a few weeks. Anti-Rh$_o$(D) immune globulin (anti-D) has been used with limited success to treat individuals who are Rh-positive. Newer drug therapies are now available.

If other therapies are ineffective, splenectomy is considered to remove the site of platelet destruction. However, splenectomy is not without risks and approximately 10% to 20% of individuals who undergo a splenectomy suffer a relapse and require further treatment. In that situation, it is thought that the liver has become the site for platelet destruction. If splenectomy is unsuccessful and life-threatening thrombocytopenia persists, more aggressive immunosuppressive medications (e.g., azathioprine, cyclophosphamide) are usually recommended. Because of potential complications, these medications are reserved for individuals who are severely thrombocytopenic and refractory to other therapies.

Thrombotic thrombocytopenia purpura. Thrombotic thrombocytopenia purpura (TTP; also known as Moschcowitz disease) is a multisystem disorder characterized by thrombotic microangiopathy (TMA) (small or microvessel disease) in which platelets aggregate and cause occlusion of arterioles and capillaries within the microcirculation. Aggregation may lead to increased platelet consumption and organ ischemia. TTP is relatively uncommon, occurring in about 5 per 1 million individuals per year. The incidence is increasing and does appear to be an actual increase and not just the result of improved recognition. One suspected etiologic factor for TMA, thrombotic thrombocytopenic

purpura, and hemolytic-uremic syndrome is drug-induced, and a recent report found definite evidence from three drugs: quinine, cyclosporine, and tacrolimus.[28]

There are two types of TTP: familial and acquired idiopathic. The familial type is the more rare type and is usually chronic, relapsing, and typically seen in children. When the disease is recognized and treated early, the child experiences predictable recurring episodes at approximately 3-week intervals that are responsive to treatment. Acquired TTP is more common and more acute and severe. It occurs mostly in females in their thirties and is rarely observed in infants or older adults.

Platelet aggregation and microthrombi formation is found throughout the entire vascular system, causing damage to multiple organs. The most susceptible organs for damage include the kidney, brain, and heart. Also affected are the pancreas, spleen, and adrenal glands. The thrombi are composed of platelets with minimal fibrin and red cells, differentiating them from thrombi secondary to intravascular coagulation. Most cases of TTP are related to a dysfunction of the plasma metalloprotease ADAMTS13 (Fig. 23.20). This enzyme is responsible for digesting large precursor molecules of von Willebrand factor (vWF) produced by endothelial cells into smaller molecules. Defects in ADAMTS13 result in expression of large-molecular-weight vWF on the endothelial cell surface and the formation of large aggregates of platelets, which can break off and form occlusions in smaller vessels. People with TTP (about 80%) have less than 5% of normal plasma ADAMTS13 levels. Most individuals with familial TTP are homozygous for mutations in ADAMTS13. Acquired TTP of unexplained origin is associated in most people with an IgG autoantibody against ADAMTS13 that is able to neutralize the enzyme's activity and accelerate its clearance from the plasma.

CLINICAL MANIFESTATIONS Chronic relapsing TTP is a rare familial form of TTP observed in children and usually recognized and successfully treated. The acquired acute idiopathic TTP is much more common and more severe. Early diagnosis and treatment is essential because TTP may prove fatal within 90 days of onset. TTP is clinically related to and must be distinguished from other thrombotic microangiopathic conditions, including hemolytic uremic syndrome (HUS), malignant hypertension, preeclampsia, and pregnancy-induced HELLP (*h*emolysis, *e*levated *l*iver enzymes, *l*ow *p*latelet count) syndrome.

Acute idiopathic TTP is characterized by a *pathognomonic pentad* (characteristic for a particular disease; group of five). However, only 20% to 30% of those with acute idiopathic TTP present with the classic pentad. These include (1) extreme thrombocytopenia (less than 20,000 platelets/µl), (2) intravascular hemolytic anemia, (3) ischemic signs and symptoms most often involving the CNS (about 65% present with memory disturbances, behavioral irregularities, headaches, or coma), (4) kidney failure (affecting about 65% of individuals), and (5) fever (present in about 33% of individuals with TTP). It is not mandatory that all five be present to begin treatment.

EVALUATION AND TREATMENT A routine blood smear usually shows fragmented red cells (*schizocytes*) produced by shear forces when red cells are in contact with the fibrin mesh in clots that form in the vessels. As a result of tissue injury, serum levels of lactate dehydrogenase (LDH) may be very high, and low-density lipoprotein (LDL) levels may be elevated. Tests for antibody on red cells are negative, excluding immune hemolytic anemia.

Importantly, prompt treatment can significantly reduce the death rate. Plasma exchange with fresh frozen plasma, which replenishes functional ADAMTS13, is the treatment of choice, achieving a 70% to 85% response rate. Additionally, steroids (glucocorticoids) are administered. In the absence of major organ damage, this approach may lead

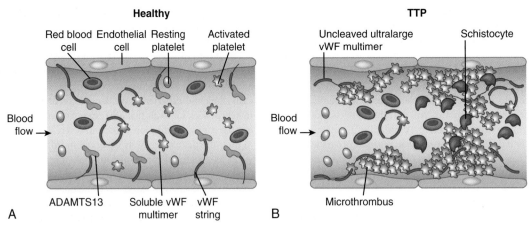

FIGURE 23.20 Thrombotic Thrombocytopenic Purpura. A, A microvessel (arteriole or capillary) in a healthy individual. Normal proteolysis by ADAMTS13 of ultra-large von Willebrand factor *(vWF)* strings anchored to or secreted from stimulated microvascular endothelial cells. **B,** A microvessel in thrombotic thrombocytopenic purpura *(TTP)*. Cleavage of secreted or anchored ultralarge vWF is severely reduced when ADAMTS13 activity is less than 10% of normal level. The results include excessive microthrombi formation, shear stress injury to red blood cells (schistocytes) flowing through microvessels that are partially occluded by platelet clumps (producing hemolysis), and perhaps damage from activation of the alternative complement pathway on the uncleaved ultralarge vWF strings. (From Kremer Hovinga JA et al: *Nat Rev Dis Primers* 3:17020, 2017.)

to complete recovery with no long-term complications. The anti-CD20 monoclonal antibody rituximab has shown some success in people who are refractory to plasma exchange.[29] Relapses do occur at a rate of 13% to 36%, and recurrences have been reported, sometimes delayed until 9 years after treatment. Individuals who do not respond to conventional treatment may be candidates for splenectomy; however, postoperative hemorrhage remains a dangerous complication. Immunosuppression therapy has been successful in some individuals.

Thrombocythemia

Thrombocythemia (also called thrombocytosis) is defined as a platelet count greater than 450,000/μl of blood.[30] Thrombocythemia may be primary or secondary (reactive) and is usually asymptomatic until the count exceeds 1 million/μl. Then intravascular clot formation (thrombosis), hemorrhage, or other abnormalities can occur.

PATHOPHYSIOLOGY Essential (primary) thrombocythemia (ET) is a chronic, myeloproliferative neoplasm (MPN) characterized by excessive platelet production resulting from a defect in the bone marrow megakaryocyte progenitor cells. Abnormal blood clotting commonly occurs in individuals with essential thrombocythemia causing many clinical manifestations. Other disease features include leukocytosis, splenomegaly, thrombosis, bleeding, microcirculatory symptoms, itching (or pruritus), and risk of leukemic or bone marrow fibrotic transformation. The most common mutated genes in ET are the Janus kinase 2 *(JAK2)* and calreticulin *(CALR)* genes. Other mutated genes also can occur and contribute to ET. The *JAK2* mutation induces overactivity in cell signaling from JAK2 protein. JAK2, a tyrosine kinase, is an essential player downstream of cytokine receptors, such as the thrombopoietin (TPO, affects platelet proliferation) and erythropoietin (EPO, affects erythrocyte proliferation) receptors. More simply, both EPO and TPO convey their signals and consequent proliferation through JAK2. Along with increased platelets, there may be a concomitant increase in the number of red cells, indicating a myeloproliferative disorder; however, the increase in red cells is not to the extent seen in PV. Red blood cells in ET tend to aggregate and adhere to the endothelium and contribute to the blockage of flow in the microvasculature and altered interactions between platelets

and the vascular endothelium. The *JAK2* (V617F) mutation is present in 50% to 60% of persons with ET. It is more common in middle-age individuals, with the majority of cases occurring between ages 50 and 60 years. There is no known sex preference. There also is a rare hereditary type of ET called *familial essential thrombocythemia (FET)* that is inherited in an autosomal dominant pattern.

Secondary thrombocythemia may occur after splenectomy because platelets that normally would be stored in the spleen remain in circulating blood. The increase in platelets may be gradual, with thrombocythemia not occurring for up to 3 weeks after splenectomy. Reactive thrombocythemia may occur during some inflammatory conditions, such as rheumatoid arthritis and cancers. In these conditions, excessive production of some cytokines (e.g., IL-6, IL-11) may induce increased production of thrombopoietin in the liver, resulting in increased megakaryocyte proliferation. Reactive thrombocythemia also may occur during a variety of physiologic conditions, such as after exercise.

CLINICAL MANIFESTATIONS Clinical manifestations vary among individuals. Those with ET are at risk for large-vessel arterial or venous thrombosis, although the most common complication is microvasculature thrombosis leading to ischemia in the fingers, toes, or cerebrovascular regions. The primary presenting symptoms of microvasculature thrombosis are erythromelalgia, headache, and paresthesias. Erythromelalgia is unilateral or bilateral warm, congested, red hands and feet with painful burning sensations, particularly in the forefoot sole and one or more toes. The lower extremities are affected more often, and only one side may be involved. The pain is initiated by standing, exercise, or warmth and relieved by elevation and cooling. In extreme situations, acrocyanosis (bluish or purple coloring of hands or feet) and gangrene may result.

Arterial thrombosis is more common than venous thrombosis and may involve the coronary and renal arteries. DVT of the lower extremities and pulmonary embolism are the major sites for venous involvement. Other common venous sites include intra-abdominal venous thrombosis (portal and hepatic). People older than 60 years of age or those with prior history of thrombotic events have as much as a 25% chance of developing a cerebral, cardiac, or peripheral arterial thrombus and, less often, developing a pulmonary embolism or DVT.[31,32] Conversion to acute leukemia is found in less than 10%.[33] Symptoms related to microvascular thrombosis in the CNS include headache, dizziness with paresthesias, transient ischemic attacks (TIAs), strokes, visual disturbances, and seizures. Major thrombotic events, not directly related to the platelet count, occur in about 20% to 30% of individuals with ET. Prior history of thrombotic events, advanced age, and duration of thrombocytosis are predictors of future thrombotic complications. Individuals older than age 60 are at greatest risk.

Although thrombosis is the more common symptom, hemorrhage can also occur. Sites for bleeding include the GI tract, skin, mucous membranes, urinary tract, gums, teeth sockets after extraction, joints, eyes, and brain. GI bleeding may be mistaken for a duodenal ulcer. Hemorrhage is not severe and generally occurs in the presence of very high platelet counts; transfusions are required only occasionally. Bleeding and clotting may occur simultaneously, and individuals will not necessarily be "bleeders" or "clotters."

EVALUATION AND TREATMENT Initial diagnosis is not difficult, and as many as two-thirds of cases are diagnosed from a routine CBC. Secondary thrombocytosis also may occur as a moderate rise in the platelet count that resolves with treatment or resolution of the underlying condition. The WHO criteria for the diagnosis of ET require the following four criteria be met: (1) sustained platelet count of at least 450×10^9/L; (2) bone marrow biopsy showing proliferation of enlarged mature megakaryocytes and no increase of granulocyte or erythrocyte precursors; (3) failure to meet the criteria of PV, myelofibrosis, CML, or other myelodysplastic syndrome; and (4) presence of JAK2 617F or another clonal marker or evidence of reactive thrombocytosis.[34] Because ET can be mistaken for CML, careful differentiation is necessary because treatment varies significantly.

Treatment of ET is directed toward preventing thrombosis or hemorrhage. Reducing the platelet count remains a significant treatment issue. Hydroxyurea, a nonalkylating myelosuppressive agent, has been the drug of choice to suppress platelet production; however, long-term use may cause progression to other myelodysplastic disorders, particularly AML or myelofibrosis.[35] Another drug used to treat ET is IFN. IFN has a response rate of 80% but may not be effective for everyone because of side effects. Anagrelide interferes with platelet maturation rather than production, thus not interfering with red and white cell growth and development. Low-dose aspirin may be effective to alleviate erthromyalgia and transient neurologic manifestations. ET is not necessarily considered life-threatening but, in those older than age 60 and who have had previous incidences of thrombosis, complications are more common and have a higher risk of mortality.

Alterations of Platelet Function

Qualitative alterations in platelet function are characterized by an increased bleeding time in the presence of a normal platelet count. Associated clinical manifestations include spontaneous petechiae and purpura, and bleeding from the GI tract, genitourinary tract, pulmonary mucosa, and gums. Congenital alterations in platelet function (thrombocytopathies) are quite rare and may be categorized into several types of disorders (also see Chapter 24).

Acquired disorders of platelet function are more common than the congenital disorders and may be categorized into three principal causes: (1) drugs, (2) systemic inflammatory conditions, and (3) hematologic alterations.

Multiple drugs are known to interfere with platelet function in several ways: inhibition of platelet membrane receptors, inhibition of prostaglandin pathways, and inhibition of phosphodiesterase activity. Aspirin is the most commonly used drug that affects platelets. It irreversibly inhibits cyclooxygenase function for several days after administration. Nonsteroidal antiinflammatory drugs also affect cyclooxygenase, although in a reversible fashion.

Systemic disorders that affect platelet function are chronic renal disease, liver disease, cardiopulmonary bypass surgery, and severe deficiencies of iron or folate and antiplatelet antibodies associated with autoimmune disorders. Hematologic disorders associated with platelet dysfunction include CMPDs, MM, leukemias, myelodysplastic syndromes, and dysproteinemias.

Disorders of Coagulation

Disorders of coagulation are usually caused by defects or deficiencies of one or more of the clotting factors. (Normal function of the clotting factors is described in Chapter 22.) Qualitative or quantitative abnormalities interfere with or prevent the enzymatic reactions that transform clotting factors, circulating as plasma proteins, into a stable fibrin clot (see Fig. 22.17). Some clotting factor defects are inherited and involve a single factor, such as the hemophilias and von Willebrand disease, caused by deficiencies of specific clotting factors. Other coagulation defects are acquired and tend to result from deficient synthesis of clotting factors by the liver. Causes include liver disease and dietary deficiency of vitamin K.

Other coagulation disorders are attributed to pathologic conditions that trigger coagulation inappropriately, engaging the clotting factors and causing detrimental clotting within blood vessels. For example, any cardiovascular abnormality that alters normal blood flow by acceleration or deceleration or obstruction can create conditions in which coagulation proceeds within the vessels. An example of this is thromboembolic disease, in which blood clots obstruct blood vessels. Coagulation is also stimulated by the presence of *tissue factor* that is released by damaged or dead tissues. Vasculitis, or inflammation of the blood vessels, along with vessel damage activates platelets, which in turn activates the coagulation cascade. In extensive or prolonged vasculitis, blood clot formation can suppress mechanisms that normally control clot formation and dissolution, leading to clogging of the vessels. In each of these acquired conditions, normal hemostatic function proves detrimental to the body by consuming coagulation factors excessively or by overwhelming normal control of clot formation and breakdown (fibrinolysis) (see Fig. 22.19).

Impaired Hemostasis

Impaired hemostasis, or the inability to promote coagulation and the development of a stable fibrin clot, is commonly associated with liver dysfunction, which may be caused by either specific liver disorders or lack of vitamin K.

Vitamin K deficiency. Vitamin K, a fat-soluble vitamin, is required for the synthesis and regulation of prothrombin, the procoagulant factors (VII, IX, X), and the anticoagulant factors within the liver (proteins C and S).[36] Unknown is the contribution of vitamin K to the overall supply by the intestinal flora. The primary source of vitamin K is found in green leafy vegetables. The most common cause of vitamin deficiency is parenteral nutrition in combination with antibiotics that destroy normal gut flora. Rarely is the deficiency caused by a lack of dietary intake; however, bulimia can suppress vitamin K–dependent activity. Parenteral administration of vitamin K is the treatment of choice and usually results in correction of the deficiency within 8 to 12 hours. Fresh frozen plasma also may be administered but is usually reserved for individuals with life-threatening hemorrhages or those who require emergency surgery.

Liver disease. Liver disease (e.g., acute or chronic hepatocellular diseases, cirrhosis), vitamin K deficiency, or liver surgery includes hemostatic derangements with defects in the clotting or fibrinolytic systems and platelet function. The hepatic (parenchyma) cells produce most of the factors involved in hemostasis; therefore damage to the liver frequently results in diminished production of factors involved in clotting. Factor VII level is the first to decline after liver damage because of its rapid turnover. Factor IX levels are less affected and do not decline until the liver destruction is well advanced. The liver also is a major site for production of plasminogen and α_2-antiplasmin of the fibrinolytic system, as well as thrombopoietin and the metalloprotease ADAMTS13. Diminished thrombopoietin may lead to thrombocytopenia from decreased platelet production. Decreased production of ADAMTS13 results in increased levels of large precursor molecules of vWF, which leads to the formation of large aggregates of platelets.

With severe liver disease, such as cirrhosis, most clotting factors are significantly depressed. Levels of clotting system regulators, such as antithrombin, protein C, protein S, and fibrinogen, also are diminished. The fibrolytic system is commonly active because of plasmin inhibitor and other activators that are unaffected. Thrombocytopenia occurs in affected individuals because of diminished thrombopoietin and ADAMTS13, as well as increased sequestration (pooling) of platelets in the spleen, which is frequently enlarged in cirrhosis and is associated with portal hypertension. Thus these individuals may appear to have a condition similar to DIC (see the Consumptive Thrombohemorrhagic Disorders section).

Treatment of hemostasis alterations in liver disease must be comprehensive to cover all aspects of dysfunctions. Fresh frozen plasma administration is the treatment of choice; however, not all individuals tolerate the volume needed to adequately replace all deficient factors. Alternative modalities include the addition of exchange transfusions and platelet concentrate to plasma administration.

Consumptive Thrombohemorrhagic Disorders

Consumptive thrombohemorrhagic disorders are a heterogeneous group of conditions that demonstrate the entire spectrum of hemorrhagic and thrombotic pathologic findings. Symptoms range from the subtle to the devastating and generally are considered to be intermediary disease processes that complicate a vast number of primary disease states. These disorders are also characterized by confusion and controversy related to their diagnosis, treatment, and management. No one definition can cover all possible varieties of these disorders; however, DIC is most commonly used in the clinical setting to describe a pathologic condition associated with hemorrhage and thrombosis.

Disseminated intravascular coagulation. Disseminated intravascular coagulation (DIC) is an acquired clinical syndrome characterized by widespread activation of coagulation resulting in formation of fibrin clots in medium and small vessels or microvasculature throughout the body. Widespread clotting may lead to blockage of blood flow to organs, resulting in multiple organ failure. The excess clotting may result in consumption of platelets and clotting factors, leading to tendency to bleed despite widespread clots.

The clinical course of DIC is largely determined by the stimulus intensity, host response, and comorbidities and ranges from an acute, severe, life-threatening process that is characterized by massive hemorrhage and thrombosis to a chronic, low-grade condition. The chronic condition includes subacute hemorrhage and diffuse microcirculatory thrombosis. DIC may be localized to one specific organ or generalized, involving multiple organs.

The diagnosis of DIC has been challenging because of the complexity and wide variations in clinical manifestations. Diagnostic criteria have been established and include a systemic thrombohemorrhagic disorder with laboratory evidence of (1) clotting activation, (2) fibrinolytic activation, (3) coagulation inhibitor consumption, and (4) biochemical evidence of end-organ damage or failure.

DIC is secondary to a wide variety of well-defined clinical conditions, specifically those capable of activating the clotting cascade (see Pathophysiology).

Sepsis is the most common condition associated with DIC. Gram-negative microorganisms, as well as some gram-positive microorganisms, fungi, protozoa (malaria), and viruses (influenza, herpes), are capable of precipitating DIC by causing damage to the vascular endothelium. Gram-negative endotoxins are the primary cause of endothelial damage; DIC may occur in up to 50% of individuals with gram-negative sepsis. DIC occurs in approximately 10% to 20% of individuals with metastatic cancer or acute leukemia. The adenocarcinomas most frequently associated with DIC include the lung, pancreas, colon, and stomach. Direct tissue damage (e.g., massive trauma, extensive surgery, severe burns) also results in release of tissue factor (TF), an initiator of DIC, by the endothelium. Severe trauma, especially to the brain, can induce DIC. DIC occurs in about two-thirds of individuals with a systemic inflammatory response to trauma. Some complications of pregnancy also are associated with DIC; incidences range from 50% for women with placental abruptions to less than 10% for severe preeclampsia. Other causes of DIC have been identified, most notably blood transfusion. Transfused blood dilutes the clotting factors, as well as circulating naturally occurring antithrombins. In hemolytic transfusion reactions, the endothelium is damaged by complement-mediated reactions.

PATHOPHYSIOLOGY DIC results from abnormally widespread and ongoing activation of clotting—*coagulopathy*—in small and midsize vessels that alters the microcirculation, leading to ischemic necrosis in various organs, particularly the kidney and lung. Concomitantly, DIC can be caused by the imbalance between the coagulant system and the fibrinolytic system (which generates plasmin) to maintain normal circulation. DIC can cause widespread deposition of fibrin in the microcirculation that leads to ischemia, microvascular thrombotic obstruction, and organ failure (Fig. 23.21).

Seemingly paradoxical, DIC involves both widespread clotting and bleeding because of simultaneous procoagulant activation, fibrinolytic activation, and consumption of platelets and coagulation factors, which results directly in serious bleeding (see Fig. 23.21).

DIC is not a disease but is secondary to a variety of conditions (Box 23.4) because of activation of the clotting cascade. The common pathway for DIC appears to be excessive and widespread exposure to TF. This may occur by several mechanisms:

1. Damage to the vascular endothelium results in exposure to TF.
2. When stimulated by inflammatory cytokines, endothelial cells and monocytes express surface TF.
3. Endotoxin triggers the release of many cytokines that can both promote and cause progression of DIC.
4. Sepsis is associated with many cytokines, interleukins, and platelet activating factor (PAF) that promote DIC as well as activate endothelial cells that stimulate thrombi development.
5. TF may be released directly into the bloodstream from circulating white blood cells.

TF binds clotting factor VII, which leads to conversion of prothrombin to thrombin and formation of fibrin clots (see Fig. 22.19). This pathway appears to be the primary route by which DIC is initiated.

Not only is the clotting system extensively activated in DIC, but also the activities of the predominant natural anticoagulants (tissue factor pathway inhibitor, antithrombin III, protein C) are greatly diminished. During DIC, the activation of clotting is prolonged and is a result of certain conditions (e.g., bacteremia or endotoxemia); thrombin generation is increased and is insufficiently balanced by impaired anticoagulant systems, such as antithrombin and protein C.

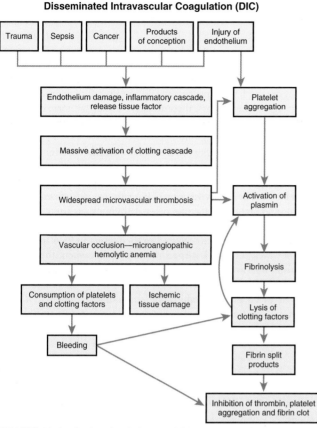

Disseminated Intravascular Coagulation (DIC)

FIGURE 23.21 Pathophysiology of Disseminated Intravascular Coagulation. See text.

The overall result is fibrin generation and deposition in the vascular system. In early DIC, plasmin (naturally occurring clot busting or fibrinolytic agent) produced from endothelial cells causes fibrinolysis to maintain circulation. Bleeding can occur with excess fibrinolytic activity. However, fibrinolysis becomes blunted by high levels of plasminogen activator inhibitor-1 (PAI-1), a fibrinolytic inhibitor. Over time the activity of plasmin is diminished by PAI-1. Although some fibrinolytic activity remains, the level is inadequate to control the systemic deposition of fibrin. The slow breakdown of fibrin by plasmin produces **fibrin split products (FSPs)** (also known as **fibrin degradation products [FDPs]**). These products are powerful anticoagulants that are normally removed from blood by fibronectin and macrophages. FSPs, along with thrombin, induce further cytokine release from monocytes, contributing to endothelial damage and TF release. During DIC, the presence of FSPs is prolonged. Low levels of fibronectin suggest a poor prognosis.

Although thrombosis is generalized and widespread, individuals with DIC are paradoxically at risk for hemorrhage. Hemorrhage is secondary to the abnormally high consumption of clotting factors and platelets, as well as the anticoagulant properties of FSPs, which interfere with fibrin mesh formation or polymerization. Both thrombin and FSPs have a high affinity for platelets and cause platelet activation and aggregation—an event that occurs early in the development of DIC—which facilitates microcirculatory coagulation and obstruction in the initial phase. However, platelet consumption exceeds production, resulting in a thrombocytopenia that increases bleeding.

Activation of clotting also leads to activation of other inflammatory pathways, including the kallikrein-kinin and complement systems (see Chapter 6). Activation of these systems contributes to increased vascular permeability, hypotension, and shock. Activated complement components also induce platelet destruction, which initially contributes to the thrombosis and later to the thrombocytopenia.

The deposition of fibrin clots in the circulation interferes with blood flow, causing widespread organ hypoperfusion. This condition may lead to ischemia, infarction, and necrosis, further potentiating and

---

BOX 23.4   Clinical Conditions Associated With Disseminated Intravascular Coagulation

Sepsis or Severe Infection
Potentially from any microorganism, including malaria

Trauma
Serious head injury
Head injury
Fat metabolism
Burns

Liver Diseases
Fulminant hepatitis
Severe liver cirrhosis

Heat Stroke
Organ Destruction
Severe pancreatitis

Malignancy
Solid tumors
Hematologic cancers

Obstetrical Calamities
Preeclampsia or eclampsia
Placental abruption
Amniotic fluid embolism
HELLP (hemolysis, elevated liver enzymes, and low platelet count) syndrome
Acute fatty liver
Sepsis during pregnancy

Vascular Abnormalities
Hemangioma
Leaking or ruptured aneurysm (such as in the aorta)
Aortic aneurysm
Kasabach-Merritt syndrome
Other vascular malformations

Severe Toxic or Immunologic Reactions
Snake bite
Recreational drug use
Severe transfusion reaction
Transplant rejection

Data from Gando S et al: *Nat Rev Dis Primers* 2:16037, 2016.

complicating the existing DIC process by causing further release of TF and eventually organ failure. Manifestations of multisystem organ dysfunction and failure ultimately result.

In addition to initiation of clotting by TF, DIC may be precipitated by direct proteolytic activation of factor X. This has been described as "thrombin mimicry" and is the result of proteases directly converting fibrinogen to fibrin. These proteases may come from snake venom, some tumor cells, or the pancreas and liver, where they are respectively released during episodes of pancreatitis and various stages of liver disease. Direct proteolytic activity appears to be independent of any type of damage to the endothelium or tissue.

Whatever initiates the process of DIC, the cycle of thrombosis and hemorrhage persists until the underlying cause of the DIC is removed or appropriate therapeutic interventions are used.

CLINICAL MANIFESTATIONS Clinical signs and symptoms of DIC present a wide spectrum of possibilities, depending on the underlying disease process that initiates DIC and whether the DIC is acute or chronic (see Box 23.4). Most symptoms are the result of either bleeding or thrombosis. Acute DIC presents with rapid development of hemorrhaging (oozing) from venipuncture sites, arterial lines, or surgical wounds or development of ecchymotic lesions (purpura, petechiae) and hematomas. Other sites of bleeding include the eyes (sclera, conjunctiva), the nose, and the gums. Most individuals with DIC demonstrate bleeding at three or more unrelated sites, and any combination may be observed. Shock of variable intensity, out of proportion to the amount of blood loss, also may be observed. Hemorrhaging into closed compartments of the body can occur and may precede the development of shock.

Manifestations of thrombosis are not always as evident, even though it is often the first pathologic alteration to occur. The initial observations may be bleeding and sometimes very extensive hemorrhage. Several organ systems are susceptible to microvascular thrombosis associated with dysfunction: cardiovascular, pulmonary, central nervous, renal, and hepatic systems. Acute and accurate clinical interpretations are critical to preventing progression of DIC that may lead to multisystem organ dysfunction and failure. (Multiple organ dysfunction and failure are discussed further in Chapter 26.) Indicators of multisystem dysfunction include changes in level of consciousness or behavior, confusion, seizure activity, oliguria, hematuria, hypoxia, hypotension, hemoptysis, chest pain, and tachycardia. Symmetric cyanosis of fingers and toes (blue finger/toe syndrome), nose, and breast may be observed and indicates macrovascular thrombosis. This may lead to infarction and gangrene that may require amputation. Jaundice also is observed and most likely results from red cell destruction rather than liver dysfunction.

Individuals with chronic or low-grade DIC do not present with the overt manifestations of hemorrhaging and thrombosis but instead have subacute bleeding and diffuse thrombosis; these individuals are described as having *compensated DIC*, or *non-overt DIC*. The major characteristic of this state is an increased turnover and decreased survival time of the components of hemostasis: platelets and clotting factors. Occasionally, diffuse or localized thrombosis develops, but this is infrequent.

EVALUATION AND TREATMENT No single laboratory test can be used to effectively diagnose DIC. Diagnosis is based primarily on clinical symptoms and confirmed by a combination of laboratory tests. The person must present with a clinical condition that is known to be associated with DIC. The most commonly used combination of laboratory tests usually confirms thrombocytopenia or a rapidly decreasing platelet count on repeated testing, prolongation of clotting times, the presence of fibrin split products, and decreased levels of

coagulation inhibitors. Platelet counts below 100,000/μl or a progressive decrease in platelet counts is very sensitive for DIC, although not greatly specific. These changes usually indicate consumption of platelets.

The standard coagulation tests (e.g., prothrombin time [PT], activated partial thromboplastin time [aPTT]) also have a high degree of sensitivity, but they are not highly specific for DIC. As a result of consumption of circulating clotting factors, these tests are usually abnormal, ranging from shortened to prolonged times. However, conditions other than DIC may prolong clotting times.

Detection of fibrin split products is more specific for DIC. Detection of D-dimers is a widely used test for DIC. A **D-dimer** is a molecule produced by plasmin degradation of cross-linked fibrin in clots. D-Dimers in the blood can be quantified using ELISA tests that include commercially available and highly specific monoclonal antibody against the D-dimer. Agglutination tests for other fibrin split products are available. Levels of fibrin split products are elevated in the plasma in 95% to 100% of cases; however, they are less specific and only document the presence of plasmin and its action on fibrin. ELISAs for markers of thrombin activity are sometimes used.

Levels of coagulation inhibitors (e.g., antithrombin III [AT-III], protein C) can be measured by assays that rely on function or by ELISAs that quantify the amount of the specific inhibitor. AT-III levels can provide key information for diagnosing and monitoring therapy of DIC. Initial levels of functional AT-III are low in DIC because thrombin is irreversibly complexed with activated clotting factors and AT-III.

Treatment of DIC is directed toward (1) eliminating the underlying pathologic condition, (2) controlling ongoing thrombosis, and (3) maintaining organ function. Elimination of the underlying pathologic condition is the initial intervention in the treatment phase in order to remove the trigger for activation of clotting. Once the stimulus is gone, production of coagulation factors in the liver leads to restoration of normal plasma levels within 24 to 48 hours.

Control of thrombosis is more difficult to attain. Heparin has been used for this; however, its use is controversial because its mechanism of action is binding to and activating AT-III, which is deficient in many types of DIC. Currently, heparin is indicated only in certain types of situations related to DIC. For instance, heparin seems to be effective in DIC caused by a retained dead fetus or associated with acute promyelocytic leukemia. Organ function is compromised by microthrombi, and there is a risk of losing an extremity because of vascular occlusion; thus heparin is also indicated in these conditions. Heparin's usefulness, however, for DIC that is precipitated by septic shock has not been established and so is contraindicated in that instance; heparin is also contraindicated when there is evidence of postoperative bleeding, peptic ulcer, or CNS bleeding.

Replacement of deficient coagulation factors, platelets, and other coagulation elements is gaining recognition as an effective treatment modality. Their use is not without controversy, however, because a major concern with replacement therapy is the possible risk of adding components that will increase the rate of thrombosis. Clinical judgment is the key factor in determining whether replacement is to be used as a treatment modality. Several clinical trials are evaluating replacement of anticoagulants (i.e., AT-III, protein C). Antifibrinolytic drugs also are used in treatment but are limited to instances of life-threatening bleeding that have not been controlled by blood component replacement therapy.

Maintenance of organ function is achieved by fluid replacement to sustain adequate circulating blood volume and maintain optimal tissue and organ perfusion. Fluids may be required to restore blood pressure, cardiac output, and urine output to normal parameters.

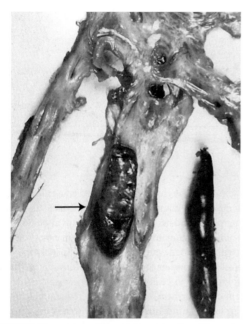

FIGURE 23.22 Thrombus. Thrombus arising in valve pocket at upper end of superficial femoral vein *(arrow)*. Postmortem clot on the right is shown for comparison. (From McLachlin J, Paterson JC: *Surg Gynecol Obstet* 93[1]:1-8, 1951.)

Thromboembolic Disorders

Certain conditions within the blood vessels predispose an individual to develop clots spontaneously. A stationary clot attached to the vessel wall is called a **thrombus** (Fig. 23.22). A thrombus is composed of fibrin and blood cells and can develop in either the arterial or the venous system. **Arterial thrombi** form under conditions of high blood flow and are composed mostly of platelet aggregates held together by fibrin strands. **Venous thrombi** form under conditions of low flow and are composed mostly of red cells with larger amounts of fibrin and few platelets.

A thrombus eventually reduces or obstructs blood flow to tissues or organs, such as the heart, brain, or lungs, depriving them of essential nutrients critical to survival. A thrombus also has the potential to detach from the vessel wall and circulate within the bloodstream (referred to as an **embolus**). The embolus may become lodged in smaller blood vessels, blocking blood flow into the local tissue or organ and leading to ischemia. Whether episodes of thromboembolism are life-threatening depends on the site of vessel occlusion.

Therapy consists of removal or dissolution of the clot and supportive measures. Anticoagulant therapy is effective in treating or preventing venous thrombosis; it is not as useful in treating or preventing arterial thrombosis. Parenteral heparin is the major anticoagulant used to treat thromboembolism. Oral coumarin drugs also are widely used, including a newer direct factor Xa inhibitor (rivaroxaban). More aggressive therapy may be indicated for such conditions as pulmonary embolism, coronary thrombosis, or thrombophlebitis. Streptokinase, tissue plasminogen activator (t-PA), and urokinase activate the fibrinolytic system and are administered to accelerate the lysis of known thrombi. These drugs are known as fibrinolytic or thrombolytic therapy and are prescribed with a high degree of caution because they can cause hemorrhagic complications.

The risk for developing spontaneous thrombi is related to several factors, referred to as the **Virchow triad**: (1) injury to the blood vessel endothelium, (2) abnormalities of blood flow, and (3) hypercoagulability of the blood.

Endothelial injury to blood vessels can result from atherosclerosis (plaque deposits on arterial walls) (see Chapter 26). Atherosclerosis initiates platelet adhesion and aggregation, promoting the development of atherosclerotic plaques that enlarge, causing further damage and occlusion. Other causes of vessel endothelial injury may be related to hemodynamic alterations associated with hypertension and turbulent blood flow. Injury is also caused by radiation injury, exogenous chemical agents (e.g., toxins from cigarette smoke), endogenous agents (e.g., cholesterol), bacterial toxins or endotoxins, or immunologic mechanisms.

Sites of turbulent blood flow in the arteries and stasis of blood flow in the veins increase the risk for thrombus formation. In areas of turbulence, platelets and endothelial cells may be activated, leading to thrombosis. In sites of stasis, platelets may remain in contact with the endothelium for prolonged lengths of time, and clotting factors that would normally be diluted with fresh flowing blood are not diluted and may become activated. The most common clinical conditions that predispose to venous stasis and subsequent thromboembolic phenomena are major surgery (e.g., orthopedic surgery), acute myocardial infarction, CHF, limb paralysis, spinal injury, malignancy, advanced age, the postpartum period, and bed rest longer than 1 week. Turbulence and stasis occur with ulcerated atherosclerotic plaques hyperviscosity (polycythemia) and conditions with deformed red cells (sickle cell anemia).

Hypercoagulability, or thrombophilia, increases the risk for venous thrombosis. Hypercoagulability is differentiated according to whether it results from primary (hereditary) or secondary (acquired) causes.

Hereditary thrombophilias. Thrombophilias can result from both inherited conditions and, more commonly, acquired conditions. Several inherited conditions increase the risk of developing thrombosis, and most are autosomal dominant. Thus individuals who are homozygous for the mutation are at greatest risk for thrombosis. These include mutations in platelet receptors, coagulation proteins, fibrinolytic proteins, and other factors. The particular mutations that have been most strongly linked as risk factors for venous thrombosis or for arterial thrombosis involving coronary artery disease or stroke include those that affect fibrinogen, prothrombin (G20210A variant), and factor V (factor V Leiden) of the coagulation system. Other inherited thrombophilias are risk factors mostly for venous thrombosis and include deficiencies in protein C, protein S, and AT-III.[37,38] Other hereditary thrombophilias are less common.

Tests to diagnose inherited thrombophilias include prothrombin time; partial thromboplastin time; and levels of protein C, protein S, and AT-III. More elaborate tests to detect precise mutations in factor V, prothrombin, or MTHFR may be indicated.

Acquired hypercoagulability. Deficiencies in proteins S and C and AT-III may be acquired and contribute to a hypercoagulable state. Conditions associated with an acquired protein deficiency include DIC, liver disease, infection, DVT, acute respiratory distress syndrome, L-asparaginase therapy, HUS, and TTP. The postoperative state also predisposes an individual to protein C or S deficiency; however, its role in contributing to DVT remains unclear.

Acquired hypercoagulable states include antiphospholipid syndrome (APS). APS is an autoimmune syndrome characterized by autoantibodies against plasma membrane phospholipids and phospholipid-binding proteins. As with most autoimmune diseases, the predominantly affected individual is female and of reproductive age. Those with APS are at risk for both arterial and venous thrombosis and a variety of obstetric complications, including pregnancy loss and preeclampsia/eclampsia. In severe cases the individual may die from recurrent major thrombus formation. The pathophysiology is related to autoantibodies directly reacting with platelets or endothelial cells (increasing the risk for thrombosis) or the placental surface (resulting in damage to the placenta). The predominant diagnostic tests measure prolongation of laboratory blood coagulation tests related to an antibody inhibitor (lupus anticoagulant) and specific ELISAs for antibodies against phospholipids (e.g., anticardiolipin antibody) or proteins that bind to phospholipids (e.g., β_2-glycoprotein I). Highly effective therapy (i.e., unfractionated or low-molecular-weight heparin with low-dose aspirin) is available to prevent the obstetric complications.

✔ **QUICK CHECK 23.6**
1. Identify three pathologic causes of DIC, and describe the manifestations associated with DIC.
2. Compare and contrast thrombocytopenia with thrombocytosis.
3. Why does vitamin K deficiency predispose an individual to a coagulation disorder?
4. Compare and contrast a thrombus with an embolus.

SUMMARY REVIEW

Anemia

1. Anemia is defined as a reduction in the number or volume of circulating red cells or a decrease in the quality or quantity of hemoglobin.
2. The most common classification of anemias is based on changes in the cell size—represented by the cell suffix *-cytic*—and changes in the cell's hemoglobin content—represented by the suffix *-chromic.*
3. Clinical manifestations of anemia can be found in all organs and tissues throughout the body. Decreased oxygen delivery to tissues causes fatigue, dyspnea, dizziness, compensatory tachycardia, and organ dysfunction.
4. Posthemorrhagic anemia is caused by acute blood loss, often caused by trauma. Complete recovery is possible if acute blood loss is not severe.
5. Macrocytic (megaloblastic) anemias are characterized by unusually large stem cells (megaloblasts) in the marrow that mature into very large erythrocytes (macrocytic). Macrocytic anemias are caused most commonly by deficiency of vitamin B_{12} or folate. Pernicious anemia can be fatal, usually because of heart failure, unless vitamin B_{12} replacement is given (lifelong replacement is required). Folate deficiency anemia is treated with folate supplements, but long-term therapy is not necessary if dietary adjustments are made to increase folate intake.
6. Microcytic-hypochromic anemias are characterized by abnormally small red cells with unusually reduced hemoglobin content. The most common cause is iron deficiency.
7. Iron deficiency anemia (IDA) is the most common nutritional disorder worldwide. The causes of IDA include (1) dietary deficiency, (2) impaired absorption, (3) increased requirement, (4) chronic blood loss, (5) impaired absorption, and (6) chronic diarrhea.
8. IDA usually develops slowly, with a gradual, insidious onset of nonspecific symptoms, including fatigue, weakness, shortness of breath, and pale earlobes, palms, and conjunctivae. Once the source of blood loss is identified and corrected, iron replacement therapy can be initiated.
9. Anemia of chronic disease results from decreased production of red blood cells and impaired iron utilization in people with chronic systemic diseases or inflammation. It is a common anemia found in hospitalized individuals and is usually in the mild to moderate range of anemias.
10. Normocytic-normochromic anemias are characterized by insufficient numbers of normal erythrocytes. Aplastic anemia is caused by a reduction in the effective production of mature cells by the bone marrow, causing a reduction or absence of all three blood cell types (pancytopenia). Hemolytic anemia is the premature accelerated destruction of erythrocytes.

Myeloproliferative Red Cell Disorders

1. Myeloproliferative disorders involve an overproduction of cells resulting from abnormal regulation of hematopoietic stem cells. Polycythemia is an excessive red cell production.
2. Polycythemia vera is a slow-growing blood cancer in which the bone marrow makes too many red blood cells. It is a stem cell disorder with hyperplastic and neoplastic bone marrow alterations characterized by abnormal uncontrolled proliferation of erythrocytes, frequently with increased white blood cells and platelets. Polycythemia is responsible for most of the clinical symptoms, including increased blood volume and viscosity.
3. Treatment of polycythemia vera includes frequent phlebotomies and aspirin in low-risk individuals. Hydroxyurea is the drug of choice for myelosuppression. Use of radioactive phosphorus has been helpful in suppressing erythropoiesis. Polycythemia vera may spontaneously convert to acute myelogenous leukemia.
4. Hereditary hemochromatosis is a common inherited disorder of iron metabolism characterized by increased gastrointestinal iron absorption with subsequent iron deposition in the liver, pancreas, heart, joints, and endocrine glands. Periodic phlebotomy is effective at removing excess iron.

Alterations of Leukocyte Function

1. Quantitative alterations of leukocytes (too many or too few) can be caused by bone marrow dysfunction or premature destruction of cells in the circulation. Many quantitative changes in leukocytes occur in response to invasion by microorganisms.
2. Leukocytosis is a condition in which the leukocyte count is higher than normal and is usually a response to physiologic stressors and pathologic conditions, such as malignancies and hematologic disorders.
3. Leukopenia is present when the leukocyte count is lower than normal and is caused by radiation, anaphylactic shock, autoimmune disease, immune deficiencies, and certain drugs. A decrease in neutrophils increases the risk for infection.
4. Granulocytosis (or neutrophilia) is an increase in circulating granulocytes—neutrophils, eosinophils, or basophils—that occurs in response to infection and inflammation. Granulocytopenia (or neutrophilia), a significant decrease in the number of neutrophils, is often caused by chemotherapeutic agents, severe infection, and radiation. Agranulocytosis is a complete absence of granulocytes in the blood.
5. Eosinophilia (increase in circulating eosinophils) results most commonly from allergic disorders and parasitic invasion. Eosinopenia (decrease in circulating eosinophils) is generally caused by the migration of eosinophils into inflammatory sites.
6. Basophilia (increase in circulating basophils) is rare and generally is a response to inflammation and immediate hypersensitivity reactions. Basopenia (decrease in circulating basophils) is seen in hyperthyroidism, acute infection, ovulation and pregnancy, and long-term steroid therapy.
7. Monocytosis (increase in circulating monocytes) is often transient and occurs during the late or recuperative phase of infection. Monocytopenia (decrease in circulating monocytes) is rare but may occur with hairy cell leukemia and prednisone therapy.

8. Lymphocytosis is an increase in the number or proportion of lymphocytes in the blood and is most commonly caused by viral infections. Lymphocytopenia is a decrease in the number of circulating lymphocytes and is associated with neoplasias, immune deficiencies, and destruction by drugs, viruses, or radiation.

9. Infectious mononucleosis (IM) is an acute, self-limiting infection of B lymphocytes most commonly associated with the Epstein-Barr virus (EBV), which is transmitted through saliva from close personal contact. The classic symptoms of IM are pharyngitis, lymphadenopathy, and fever. The proliferation of infected B cells may be uncontrolled and lead to B-cell lymphomas. Treatment of IM consists of rest and symptomatic treatment.

10. The common pathologic feature of all forms of leukemia is an uncontrolled proliferation of malignant leukocytes, overcrowding the bone marrow and resulting in decreased production and function of the other blood cell lines.

11. The classification of leukemias is complex, because the once discrete categories of lymphoma and leukemia have been blurred.

12. The World Health Organization (WHO) groups lymphoid neoplasms into five categories defined by cell of origin: (1) precursor B-cell neoplasms (immature B cells), (2) peripheral B-cell neoplasms (mature B cells), (3) precursor T-cell neoplasms (immature T cells), (4) peripheral T-cell and NK (natural killer)-cell neoplasms (mature T cells and NK cells), and (5) Hodgkin lymphoma (Reed-Sternberg cell and variants).

13. Acute leukemia is characterized by undifferentiated or immature cells. The onset of disease is abrupt and rapid, and, without treatment, disease progression results in a short survival time. In chronic leukemia, the predominant cell is more differentiated but does not function normally, with a relatively slow progression.

14. All leukemias have certain pathophysiologic features in common. Abnormal immature white blood cells, called leukemic blasts, fill the bone marrow and spill into the blood. The blasts overcrowd the marrow and cause cellular proliferation of the other cell lines to cease.

15. Acute leukemias include acute lymphocytic leukemia (ALL) and acute myelogenous leukemia (AML).

16. Increased risk for ALL has been linked to prenatal exposure to x-rays, postnatal exposure to ionizing radiation, past treatment with chemotherapy, and certain genetic conditions. AML is the most frequently reported secondary cancer after high doses of chemotherapy.

17. The major clinical manifestations of acute leukemia include fatigue caused by anemia, bleeding caused by thrombocytopenia, fever secondary to infection, anorexia, and weight loss.

18. Treatment varies depending on the type of leukemia and includes chemotherapy, radiation therapy, stem cell transplant, and other drug therapy.

19. Chronic leukemias include chronic lymphocytic leukemia (CLL) and chronic myelogenous leukemia (CML).

20. The only known cause of CML is exposure to ionizing radiation, and the cause of CLL is unknown.

21. Most individuals with chronic leukemia are asymptomatic at the time of diagnosis, but the most common finding is lymphadenopathy.

22. Treatment of CLL ranges from periodic observation with treatment of infection, hemorrhage, or immunologic complications. Treatments for CML do not cure the disease, but include chemotherapy, biologic response modifiers, and stem cell transplant.

Alterations of Lymphoid Function

1. Lymphadenopathy is enlarged lymph nodes. Lymphadenopathy results from four types of conditions: (1) neoplastic disease, (2) immunologic or inflammatory conditions, (3) endocrine disorders, or (4) lipid storage diseases.

2. Lymphomas consist of a diverse group of neoplasms that develop from the proliferation of malignant lymphocytes in the lymphoid system. The WHO classification of lymphomas based on the cell type it originated from include Hodgkin lymphoma (HL) and non-Hodgkin lymphoma (NHL). Classification based on morphology and cell lineage include B-cell neoplasms, T-cell neoplasms, and natural killer (NK) cell neoplasms. Two *basic* categories of lymphomas are HL and NHL.

3. In general, lymphomas are the result of genetic mutations or viral infection. Malignant transformation produces a cell with uncontrolled and excessive growth that accumulates in the lymph nodes and other sites, producing tumor masses.

4. HL is a malignant lymphoma that progresses from one group of lymph nodes to another and is characterized by abnormal cells called Reed-Sternberg cells, which are infected with EBV in most cases.

5. An enlarged, painless lymph node, most commonly in the neck, is an initial sign of HL; however, asymptomatic lymphadenopathy can progress undetected for years.

6. Treatment of HL includes chemotherapy, radiation therapy, and surgery. Treatment with chemotherapy or radiation therapy, or both, may increase the risk of second cancers, cardiovascular disease, and other health problems months or years after treatment.

7. The NHLs are a heterogeneous group of lymphoid tissue neoplasms. NHL is a progressive clonal expansion of B cells, T cells, or NK cells, with B cells accounting for the majority of NHLs. Oncogenes may be activated by chromosomal translocation or by deletion of tumor-suppressor genes. Certain subtypes may have altered genomes by oncogenic viruses.

8. Generally, with NHL, the swelling of lymph nodes is painless and the nodes enlarge and transform over a period of months or years. The cervical, axillary, inguinal, and femoral lymph node chains are the most commonly affected sites.

9. Treatment for NHL may include chemotherapy, radiation therapy, monoclonal antibody therapy, and watchful waiting.

10. Burkitt lymphoma (BL) is a B-cell NHL. It is highly aggressive and is the fastest growing human tumor. There are three main types of BL: endemic (common in Africa and linked to EBV), sporadic (occurs worldwide), and immunodeficiency-related (found in individuals with AIDS). The rapidly growing tumor involves the jaw and facial bones and sometimes the abdomen.

11. Treatment for BL is aggressive multidrug regimens, such as combination chemotherapy.

12. Lymphoblastic lymphoma is a rare variant of NHL, with the vast majority originating from the T cell. Painless lymphadenopathy in the neck is the first sign; peripheral lymph nodes in the chest become involved in most people. The most common treatment is combined chemotherapy.

13. Multiple myeloma (MM) is a clonal plasma cell cancer in the bone marrow. It is characterized by multiple malignant tumor masses of plasma cells scattered throughout the skeletal system (lytic bone lesions) and sometimes found in soft tissue. The common presentation of MM is characterized by elevated levels of calcium in the blood, renal failure, anemia, and lytic bone lesions.

14. Multiple mutations in different pathways alter the intrinsic biology of the plasma cell, generating the features of myeloma. The exact cause of MM is unknown, but risk factors include radiation, certain chemicals, and a history of monoclonal gammopathy of undetermined significance (MGUS).

15. Treatment options for MM include combinations of chemotherapy; other drug therapy; targeted therapy; high-dose chemotherapy with

stem cell transplant; biologic therapy; radiation therapy; and, sometimes, surgery.

Alterations of Splenic Function

1. Splenomegaly (enlargement of the spleen) may be considered normal in certain individuals, but its presence is associated with various diseases.
2. Splenomegaly results from (1) acute inflammatory or infectious processes, (2) congestive disorders, (3) infiltrative processes, and (4) tumors or cysts.
3. Hypersplenism (overactivity of the spleen) results from splenomegaly. Hypersplenism results in sequestering of the blood cells, causing increased destruction of red blood cells, leukopenia, and thrombocytopenia.

Hemorrhagic Disorders and Alterations of Platelets and Coagulation

1. The arrest of bleeding is called hemostasis. Copious or heavy discharge of blood from blood vessels is called hemorrhage.
2. Quantitative or qualitative abnormalities of platelets can interrupt normal blood coagulation and prevent hemostasis.
3. Thrombocytopenia is characterized by a platelet count below 150,000/μl of blood; this is considered significant when the count is less than 100,000 platelets/μl, and a count less than 50,000/μl increases the potential for hemorrhage associated with minor trauma. A count less than 15,000 platelets/μl can cause spontaneous bleeding without trauma.
4. Thrombocytopenia exists in primary or secondary forms and can be congenital or acquired. Acquired thrombocytopenia is associated with viral infections, drugs, nutritional deficiencies, chronic renal failure, cancer, radiation therapy, and bone marrow hypoplasia.
5. Common forms of thrombocytopenia include heparin-induced thrombocytopenia, idiopathic (immune) thrombocytopenia purpura, thrombotic thrombocytopenia purpura, and disseminated intravascular coagulation.
6. Thrombocythemia is characterized by a platelet count more than 450,000 platelets/μl of blood and is symptomatic when the count exceeds 1 million/μl, at which time the risk for intravascular clotting (thrombosis) is high.
7. Thrombocythemia is a myeloproliferative neoplasm characterized by excessive platelet production resulting from a defect in the bone marrow megakaryocyte progenitor cells. It also can include an increase in red blood cell production.
8. Qualitative alterations in normal platelet function prevent platelet plug formation and may result in prolonged bleeding times. Acquired disorders of platelet function are more common than congenital disorders.
9. Disorders of coagulation are usually caused by defects or deficiencies of one or more clotting factors. Coagulation is stimulated by the presence of tissue factor that is released by damaged or dead tissues.
10. Coagulation is impaired when there is a deficiency of vitamin K because of insufficient production of prothrombin and synthesis of clotting factors VII, IX, and X, often associated with liver diseases.
11. Disseminated intravascular coagulation (DIC) is an acquired clinical syndrome characterized by widespread activation of coagulation, resulting in formation of fibrin clots in medium and small vessels or microvasculature throughout the body. Widespread clotting may lead to blockage of blood flow to organs, resulting in multiple organ failure. The excessive clotting may result in consumption of platelets and clotting factors, leading to a tendency to bleed despite widespread clots.
12. DIC is secondary to a wide variety of clinical conditions, with sepsis being the most common.
13. For a diagnosis of DIC, the person must present with a clinical condition that is known to be associated with DIC. The most commonly used combination of laboratory tests usually confirms thrombocytopenia, or a rapidly decreasing platelet count on repeated testing, prolongation of clotting times, the presence of fibrin split products, and decreased levels of coagulation inhibitors.
14. Treatment of DIC is directed toward (1) eliminating the underlying pathologic condition, (2) controlling ongoing thrombosis, and (3) maintaining organ function.
15. Thromboembolic disease results from a fixed (thrombus) or moving (embolus) clot that blocks flow within a vessel, denying nutrients to tissues distal to the occlusion; death can result when clots obstruct blood flow to the heart, brain, or lungs.
16. The Virchow triad refers to three factors that influence the risk of developing spontaneous thrombi: (1) injury to the blood vessel endothelium, (2) abnormalities of blood flow, and (3) hypercoagulability of the blood.

■ KEY TERMS

Absolute polycythemia, 514
Acute idiopathic TTP, 537
Acute leukemia, 521
Acute lymphocytic leukemia (ALL), 523
Acute myelogenous leukemia (AML), 523
Agranulocytosis, 518
Amyloidosis, 532
Anemia, 505
Anemia of chronic disease (ACD; anemia of inflammation [AI]), 512
Anisocytosis, 505
Aplastic anemia (AA), 514
Apoferritin, 513
Arterial thrombus (pl., thrombi), 543

β₂-Microglobulin, 533
Basopenia, 518
Basophilia, 518
B-cell neoplasm, 529
Bence Jones protein, 532
Blast cell, 521
Burkitt lymphoma, 530
Chronic leukemia, 521
Chronic lymphocytic leukemia (CLL), 525
Chronic myelogenous leukemia (CML), 525
Chronic relapsing TTP, 537
Congestive splenomegaly, 534
Consumptive thrombohemorrhagic disorder, 540
D-Dimer, 542

Disseminated intravascular coagulation (DIC), 540
Embolus, 543
Eosinopenia, 518
Eosinophilia, 518
Eryptosis, 507
Erythromelalgia, 538
Essential (primary) thrombocythemia (ET), 538
Fibrin degradation product (FDP), 541
Fibrin split product (FSP), 541
Folate (folic acid), 511
Granulocytopenia, 518
Granulocytosis, 518
Hemochromatosis, 516
Hemolysis, 507
Hemolytic anemia, 514

Hemorrhage, 535
Hemostasis, 535
Heparin-induced thrombocytopenia (HIT), 536
Hepcidin, 517
Hereditary hemochromatosis (HH), 516
Hodgkin lymphoma (HL), 527
Hypercoagulability (thrombophilia), 536
Hypersplenism, 534
Hypoxemia, 507
Immune thrombocytopenic purpura (ITP), 536
Impaired hemostasis, 539
Infectious mononucleosis (IM), 520

REFERENCES

1. Rossaint R, et al: The European guideline on management of major bleeding and coagulopathy following trauma: fourth edition, *Crit Care* 20:100, 2016.
2. World Health Organization (WHO): Injuries and violence: the facts, 2010. Available from: http://whqlibdoc.who.int/publications/2010/97892415 99375_eng.pdf. (Accessed 22 April 2017).
3. Lang E, et al: Killing me softly—suicidal erythrocyte death, *Int J Biochem Cell Biol* 44(8):1236-1243, 2012.
4. Ainger E, Feldman A, Datz C: Obesity as an emerging risk factor for iron deficiency, *Nutrients* 6(9):3587-3600, 2014.
5. Drüeke TB: Anemia treatment in patients with chronic kidney disease, *N Engl J Med* 368(4):387-389, 2013.
6. Jing Z, et al: Hemoglobin targets for chronic kidney disease patients with anemia: a systematic review and meta-analysis, *PLoS ONE* 7(8):1-9, 2012.
7. Asare K: Anemia of critical illness, *Pharmacotherapy* 28(10):1267-1282, 2008.
8. U.S. Department of Health & Human Services (USDHHS), National Institutes of Health: *Genetics home reference hereditary hemochromatosis*, Bethesda, MD, 2018, Author.
9. U.S. Department of Health & Human Services (USDHHS), National Institutes of Health: *Genetics home reference HFE gene*, Bethesda, MD, 2018, Author.
10. Genetic Testing Registry: Hereditary hemochromatosis, Bethesda MD, National Center for Biotechnology Information, U.S. National Library of Medicine. Accessed 10/21/2018.
11. Thorley-Lawson DA, Gross A: Persistence of the Epstein-Barr virus and the origins of associated lymphomas, *N Engl J Med* 350(13):1328-1337, 2004.
12. American Cancer Society (ACS): *Cancer facts & figures 2019*, Atlanta, Ga, 2019, Author.
13. SEER cancer statistics review 1975-2008, Bethesda MD. National Institutes of Health, U.S. Department of Health and Human Services. 2011.
14. Talpaz M, et al: Dasatinib in imatinib-resistant Philadelphia chromosome-positive leukemias, *N Engl J Med* 354(24):2531-2541, 2006.
15. Wakeford R, Little MP, Kendall GM: Risk of childhood leukemia after low-level exposure to ionizing radiation, *Expert Rev Hematol* 3(3):251-254, 2010.

16. PDQ® Adult Treatment Editorial Board: PDQ adult acute lymphoblastic leukemia treatment, Bethesda, MD, National Cancer Institute. Updated 03/16/2017. Available from: https://www.cancer.gov/types/leukemia/hp/adult-all-treatment-pdq. (Accessed 6 February 2017).
17. Friese CR, et al: Timeliness and quality of diagnostic care for Medicare recipients with chronic lymphocytic leukemia, *Cancer* 117(7):1470-1477, 2011.
18. National Cancer Institute (NCI): Chronic lymphocytic leukemia treatment (PDQ®), Bethesda MD, National Cancer Institute, National Institutes of Health. Date last modified December 30, 2004. 2014. Available from: http://cancer.gov/cancertopics/pdq/treatment/CLL/Patient. (Accessed 12 January 2015).
19. Helgason GV, Young GAR, Holyoake TL: Targeting chronic myeloid leukemic stem cells, *Curr Hematol Malig Rep* 5(2):81-87, 2010.
20. Canellos GP, Freedman AS, Rosmarin AG: *Staging and prognosis of Hodgkin lymphoma*, UpToDate, 2018, Wolters Kluwer.
21. PDQ® Adult Treatment Editorial Board: Adult Hodgkin lymphoma treatment (PDQ®), Bethesda MD, National Cancer Institute. Date last modified February 25, 2015. Available from: http://cancer.gov/cancertopics/pdq/treatment/adulthodgkins/HealthProfessional. (Accessed 2 March 2015).
22. PDQ® Adult Treatment Editorial Board: Adult Hodgkin lymphoma treatment (PDQ®), Bethesda MD, National Cancer Institute. Date last modified January 9, 2015. Available from: http://cancer.gov/cancertopics/pdq/treatment/adulthodgkins/Patient. (Accessed 23 February 2015).
23. PDQ® Adult Treatment Editorial Board: PDQ adult Hodgkin lymphoma treatment, Bethesda, MD, National Cancer Institute. Updated 08/15/2018. Available from: https://www.cancer.gov/types/lymphoma/hp/adult-hodgkin-treatment-pdq. (Accessed 29 October 2018).
24. Freedman AS, Friedberg JW: *Treatment of Burkitt leukemia/lymphoma*, UpToDate, 2018, Wolters Kluwer. Accessed 11/01/2018.
25. Rajkumar SV, et al: Haematological cancer: redefining myeloma, *Nat Rev Clin Oncol* 9(9):494-496, 2012.
26. Thrombocytopenia, Bethesda MD, National Institutes of Health, U.S. Department of Health and Human Services. 2008. Available from: http://

www.nhlbi.nih.gov/health/dci/Diseases/thcp/thcp_all.html. (Accessed 1 September 2012).
27. Bennett CM, et al: Targeted ITP strategies: do they elucidate the biology of ITP and related disorders?, *Pediatr Blood Cancer* 47(Suppl 5):706-709, 2006.
28. Al-Nouri ZL, et al: Drug-induced thrombotic microangiopathy: a systematic review of published reports, *Blood* 125(4):616-618, 2015.
29. Scully M, et al: A phase 2 study of the safety and efficacy of rituximab with plasma exchange in acute acquired thrombotic thrombocytopenic purpura, *Blood* 118(7):1746-1753, 2011.
30. National Institutes of Health (NIH): Thrombocytopenia & thrombocytosis, Bethesda MD, National Institutes of Health, U.S. Department of Health and Human Services. 2008. Available from: http://www.nhlbi.nih.gov/health/dci/Diseases/thrm/thrm_all.html. (Accessed 1 September 2012).
31. Harrison C, et al: JAK inhibition with ruxolitinib versus best available therapy for myelofibrosis, *N Engl J Med* 366(9):787-798, 2012.
32. Passamonti F, et al: A prognostic model to predict survival in 867 World Health Organization-defined essential thrombocythemia at diagnosis: as study by the International Working Group on Myelofibrosis Research and Treatment, *Blood* 120(6):1197-1201, 2012.
33. Wolanskyj AP, et al: Essential thrombocythemia beyond the first decade: life expectancy, long-term complication rates, and prognostic factors, *Mayo Clin Proc* 81(2):159-166, 2006.
34. Tefferi A, et al: The 2008 World Health Organization classification system for myeloproliferative neoplasms: order out of chaos, *Cancer* 115(17):3842-3847, 2009.
35. Barbui T, et al: Front-line therapy in polycythemia vera and essential thrombocythemia, *Blood Rev* 26(5):205-211, 2012.
36. Lisman T, et al: Hemostasis and thrombosis in patients with liver disease: the ups and downs, *J Hepatol* 53(2):362-371, 2010.
37. Nakashima MO, Rogers HJ: Hypercoagulable states: an algorithmic approach to laboratory testing and update on monitoring of direct oral anticoagulants, *Blood Res* 49(2):85-94, 2014.
38. Bruce A, Massicotte MP: Thrombophilia screening: whom to test, *Blood* 120(7):1353-1355, 2012.

24

Alterations of Hematologic Function in Children

Lauri A. Linder, Kathryn L. McCance

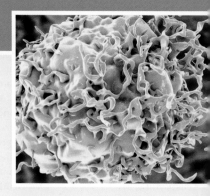

CHAPTER OUTLINE

This chapter will include conditions in children that affect red blood cells, the coagulation process and platelets, as well as disorders involving white blood cells. Discussions of both acquired conditions and inherited conditions also are presented.

DISORDERS OF ERYTHROCYTES

Anemia is the most common blood disorder in children. As do adult anemias, anemias occurring in children result from inadequate erythropoiesis or early destruction of erythrocytes. Iron deficiency is the most common cause of inadequate erythropoiesis. Iron deficiency can result from insufficient dietary intake or chronic loss of iron caused by bleeding. The hemolytic anemias of childhood are either inherited or acquired. They may be divided into disorders that result from destruction caused by (1) intrinsic abnormalities of the erythrocytes and (2) damaging factors external to the erythrocytes.

The most dramatic form of acquired congenital hemolytic anemia is hemolytic disease of the fetus and newborn (HDFN), also termed *erythroblastosis fetalis*. HDFN results when maternal blood and fetal blood are incompatible, causing the mother's immune system to produce antibodies against fetal erythrocytes. Intracellular defects in red blood cells include enzyme deficiencies, the most common of which is glucose-6-phosphate dehydrogenase (G6PD) deficiency, and defects of hemoglobin synthesis, which manifest as sickle cell disease or thalassemia, depending on which component of hemoglobin is defective. These and other causes of childhood anemia are listed in Table 24.1.

Acquired Disorders

Iron Deficiency Anemia

Iron deficiency anemia (IDA) is the most common nutritional disorder worldwide, with the highest incidence occurring between 6 months and 2 years of age. Its prevalence in the United States is greatest among toddlers, adolescent girls, and women of childbearing age. Iron is *critical* to the developing child, especially for normal brain development. Without it the damage from the periods of IDA is irreversible. The clinical manifestations of IDA are mostly related to inadequate hemoglobin synthesis.

IDA can result from (1) dietary lack of iron, (2) problems with iron absorption, (3) blood loss, and (4) increased requirement for iron. During the first few years of life, IDA most often results from inadequate iron intake. During childhood and adolescence, blood loss is the most common cause of IDA.

Dietary lack of iron is not common in developed countries, where iron is readily absorbed from heme found in meat. In developing countries, food may be less available. Although iron is found in plants, it is a more poorly absorbed form.[1] Infants are at increased risk for IDA because milk has only very small amounts of iron. The bioavailability of iron from breast milk is higher than that from cow's milk. Impaired absorption is found in chronic diarrhea, fat malabsorption, and sprue (see *Did You Know?* A Significant Number of Children Develop and Suffer from Severe Iron Deficiency Anemia).

Blood loss may not always be obvious; for example, blood loss caused by a gastrointestinal lesion, parasitic infestation, or hemorrhagic disease can be occult (hidden) and result in chronic IDA. Chronic parasitic infections are an important risk factor for IDA among children in developing countries. Treating these parasitic infections results in improved appetite and growth, as well as reduction of anemia.

Infants and young children who consume excessive amounts of cow's milk also may develop IDA as a result of chronic intestinal blood loss. A heat-labile protein in cow's milk may induce inflammation that damages the intestinal mucosa causing diffuse, chronic microhemorrhage. Cellular components of both innate and adaptive immunity may play significant roles in the development of cow's milk allergy.

TABLE 24.1 Anemias of Childhood

Cause	Examples of Anemic Condition
Blood Loss	
Trauma	Iron deficiency anemia
Gastrointestinal lesion	
Parasitic infestation	
Hemorrhagic disease	
Decreased Red Cell Production or Hemoglobin Synthesis	
Decreased stem cell population in marrow (congenital or acquired pure red cell aplasia)	Normocytic-normochromic anemia
Decreased erythropoiesis despite normal stem cell population in marrow (infection, inflammation, cancer, chronic renal disease, congenital dyserythropoiesis)	Normocytic-normochromic anemia
Deficiency of a Factor or Nutrient Needed for Erythropoiesis	
Cobalamin (vitamin B_{12}), folate	Megaloblastic anemia
Iron	Microcytic-hypochromic anemia
Increased or Premature Hemolysis	
Alloimmune disease (maternal-fetal Rh, ABO, or minor blood group incompatibility)	Autoimmune hemolytic anemia
Autoimmune disease (idiopathic autoimmune hemolytic anemia, symptomatic systemic lupus erythematosus, lymphoma, drug-induced autoimmune processes)	Autoimmune hemolytic anemia
Inherited defects of plasma membrane structure (spherocytosis, elliptocytosis, stomatocytosis) or cellular size or both (pyknocytosis)	Hemolytic anemia
Infection (bacterial sepsis, congenital syphilis, malaria, cytomegalovirus infection, rubella, toxoplasmosis, disseminated herpes)	Hemolytic anemia
Intrinsic and inherited enzymatic defects (deficiencies) of G6PD, pyruvate kinase, 5'-nucleotidase, glucose phosphate isomerase	Hemolytic anemia
Inherited Defects of Hemoglobin Synthesis	
Structurally abnormal globins	Sickle cell anemia
Deficient globin synthesis	Thalassemia
Other Anemias	
Disseminated intravascular coagulation (see Chapter 23)	Hemolytic anemia
Galactosemia	Hemolytic anemia
Prolonged or recurrent respiratory or metabolic acidosis	Hemolytic anemia
Blood vessel disorders (cavernous hemangiomas, large vessel thrombus, renal artery stenosis, severe coarctation of aorta)	Hemolytic anemia

ABO; type A, type B, type O blood; *G6PD*; glucose-6-phosphate dehydrogenase

DID YOU KNOW?

A Significant Number of Children Develop and Suffer From Severe Iron Deficiency Anemia

A recent study in the United States found that children aged 36 months to 15 years are particularly vulnerable to iron deficiency anemia (IDA), especially those consuming excessive quantities of whole cow's milk. The prevalence of IDA in infancy has not changed in the past four decades and remains about 7%. Several children who were not anemic at 12 months of age went on to develop IDA as their iron stores became depleted. These children had typical signs of anemia, although their parents were not aware of the abnormalities. Chronic severe IDA in the first years of life increases the risk of irreversible cognition problems, as well as affective and motor development. The American Academy of Pediatrics (AAP) recommends screening for IDA with hemoglobin concentration and clinical assessment at about 1 year of age, and the Centers for Disease Control and Prevention (CDC) recommends that all children aged 2 through 5 years be assessed annually for risk factors for IDA and screened appropriately. IDA is a preventable disease.

Data from Paoletti G et al: *Pediatrics* 53(4):1352-1358, 2014.

The association between IDA and lead poisoning is controversial. Newer areas of investigation include iron deficiency in overweight children and the association of *Helicobacter pylori* infection with IDA.

PATHOPHYSIOLOGY No matter the cause, a deficiency of iron produces a hypochromic-microcytic anemia. In the early stages, however, the body may respond by increasing red blood cell activity in the bone marrow, which may temporarily prevent the development of anemia. As the body's iron stores are depleted, anemia develops. Low serum levels of ferritin and transferrin saturation lead to lowered hemoglobin and hematocrit levels.

CLINICAL MANIFESTATIONS The symptoms of mild anemia—listlessness and fatigue—may go unnoticed in infants and young children, who are unable to describe these symptoms. Clinical indicators of anemia also are nonspecific, such as general irritability, decreased activity tolerance, weakness, and lack of interest in play, and may be attributed to other causes. As a result, parents may not note persistent changes in the child's behavior until moderate anemia has developed. Other clinical manifestations, such as pallor, anorexia, tachycardia, and systolic murmurs, are often not present until hemoglobin levels fall below 5 g/dl.

Other symptoms and signs of chronic IDA include splenomegaly, widened skull sutures, decreased physical growth, developmental delays, *pica* (a behavior in which nonfood substances, such as clay, are eaten), and altered neurologic and intellectual functions, especially those involving attention span, alertness, and learning ability.

EVALUATION AND TREATMENT The diagnosis of IDA is confirmed by laboratory tests. These tests include hemoglobin, hematocrit, serum iron, and ferritin levels and determination of the total iron binding capacity. Obtaining a thorough history of the child's present illness and dietary history and performing a complete physical examination also are essential to the evaluation and subsequent clinical management of IDA. Treatment of IDA is similar in children and adults (see Chapter 23). Oral administration of a simple ferrous salt is usually sufficient. Taking iron supplements with a vitamin C source helps promote absorption.[2] If liquid iron supplements are used, they should be given with a straw or a dropper placed back on the tongue to prevent staining the teeth. Dietary modification, including increasing intake of iron-rich food sources, is required to prevent recurrences of iron deficiency anemia. The intake of cow's milk should be restricted to the recommended daily allowance for age.

Hemolytic Disease of the Fetus and Newborn

The most common cause of hemolytic anemia in newborns is alloimmune disease. Hemolytic disease of the fetus and newborn (HDFN) (erythroblastosis fetalis) can occur only if antigens on fetal erythrocytes differ from antigens on maternal erythrocytes. Most cases are caused by ABO incompatibility, which occurs if the mother and fetus have different ABO blood types. About 1 in 3 cases of HDFN is caused by Rh incompatibility, which occurs when the fetus is Rh-positive and the mother is Rh-negative. Some minor blood antigens also may be involved (see Chapter 8).

ABO incompatibility occurs in about 20% to 25% of all pregnancies. Only 1 in 10 of these cases results in HDFN. Rh incompatibility occurs in less than 10% of pregnancies. It rarely causes HDFN in the first incompatible fetus. During this first pregnancy, erythrocytes from the fetus cause the mother's immune system to produce antibodies. These antibodies can affect fetuses in subsequent incompatible pregnancies. Even after five or more pregnancies, however, only 5% of women have babies with hemolytic disease.

PATHOPHYSIOLOGY Three conditions need to be met for HDFN to occur:
1. the mother's blood contains preformed antibodies against fetal erythrocytes or produces them when exposed to fetal erythrocytes,
2. sufficient amounts of antibody (usually immunoglobulin G [IgG] class) cross the placenta and enter fetal blood, and
3. IgG binds with sufficient numbers of fetal erythrocytes to cause widespread antibody-mediated hemolysis or splenic removal (antibody-mediated cellular destruction is described in Chapter 8).

In most cases of HDFN, the mother has blood type O and the fetus has blood type A or B. Maternal antibodies also may be formed against type B erythrocytes if the mother is type A or against type A erythrocytes if the mother is type B.

ABO incompatibility can cause HDFN even if fetal erythrocytes do not escape into the maternal circulation during pregnancy. This occurs because the blood of most adults already contains anti-A or anti-B antibodies. These antibodies are produced on exposure to certain foods or infection by gram-negative bacteria. As a result, IgG

against type A or B erythrocytes is usually already present in maternal blood and can enter the fetal circulation during the first incompatible pregnancy. Anti-O antibodies do not exist because type O erythrocytes are not antigenic.

Anti-Rh antibodies, on the other hand, form only in response to the presence of Rh-positive erythrocytes from the fetus in the blood of an Rh-negative mother. This exposure typically occurs when fetal blood is mixed with the mother's blood at the time of delivery. Exposure may also occur through transfused blood, and, rarely, previous sensitization of the mother by her own mother's incompatible blood (Fig. 24.1).

The first Rh-incompatible pregnancy generally presents no difficulties for the fetus. This is because few fetal erythrocytes cross the placental barrier during the pregnancy. When the placenta detaches at birth, a large number of fetal erythrocytes often enter the mother's bloodstream. If the mother is Rh-negative and the fetus is Rh-positive, the mother produces anti-Rh antibodies. These anti-Rh antibodies persist in the mother's bloodstream for a long time. If the next offspring is Rh-positive, the mother's anti-Rh antibodies can enter the bloodstream of the fetus and destroy the erythrocytes.

Antibody-coated fetal erythrocytes are usually destroyed in the spleen. As hemolysis proceeds, the fetus becomes anemic. Erythropoiesis accelerates, particularly in the liver and spleen. Immature nucleated cells (erythroblasts) are released into the bloodstream (hence the name *erythroblastosis fetalis*). The degree of anemia depends on several factors: (1) the length of time the antibody has been in the fetal circulation, (2) the concentration of the antibody, and (3) the ability of the fetus to compensate for increased hemolysis. During the pregnancy, unconjugated (indirect) bilirubin, which forms during the breakdown of hemoglobin, is transported across the placental barrier into the maternal circulation and is excreted by the mother. Hyperbilirubinemia occurs in the neonate after birth because bilirubin is no longer excreted through the placenta.

HDFN is typically more severe in Rh incompatibility than in ABO incompatibility. Rh incompatibility is more likely to result in severe or even life-threatening anemia, death in utero, or damage to the central nervous system. Severe anemia alone can cause death as a result of cardiovascular complications. Extensive hemolysis can result in increased levels of unconjugated bilirubin in the neonate's circulation. If bilirubin levels exceed the liver's ability to conjugate and excrete bilirubin, it can be deposited in the brain, a condition known as kernicterus, causing cellular damage and, eventually, death if the neonate does not receive exchange transfusions.

Fetuses that do not survive anemia in utero are usually stillborn, with gross edema in the entire body, a condition called hydrops fetalis. Death can occur as early as 17 weeks' gestation and results in spontaneous abortion.

CLINICAL MANIFESTATIONS Neonates with mild HDFN may appear healthy or slightly pale, with slight enlargement of the liver or spleen. Pronounced pallor, splenomegaly, and hepatomegaly indicate severe anemia, which predisposes the neonate to cardiovascular failure and shock. Life-threatening symptoms as a consequence of Rh incompatibility, however, are rare, largely because of the routine use of Rh immunoglobulin.

Because the maternal antibodies remain in the neonate's circulatory system after birth, erythrocyte destruction can continue. Without exchange transfusions, in which the neonate receives Rh-negative red blood cells, severe hyperbilirubinemia and icterus neonatorum (neonatal jaundice) can develop shortly after birth. If kernicterus develops, it can cause cerebral damage, including intellectual disabilities, cerebral palsy, or high-frequency deafness. It may even cause death (icterus gravis neonatorum).

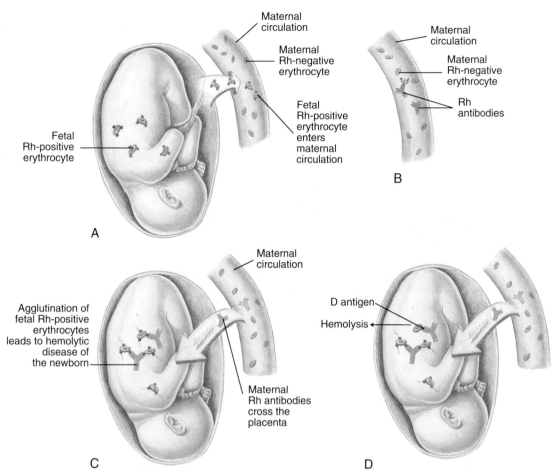

FIGURE 24.1 Hemolytic Disease of the Fetus and Newborn (HDFN). A, Before or during delivery, Rh-positive erythrocytes from the fetus enter the blood of an Rh-negative woman through a tear in the placenta. **B,** The mother is sensitized to the Rh antigen and produces Rh antibodies. Because this usually happens after delivery, there is no effect on the fetus in the first pregnancy. **C,** During a subsequent pregnancy with an Rh-positive fetus, Rh-positive erythrocytes cross the placenta, enter the maternal circulation, and **(D)** stimulate the mother to produce antibodies against the Rh antigen. (Modified from Seeley RR et al: *Anatomy and physiology,* ed 3, St Louis, 1995, Mosby.)

EVALUATION AND TREATMENT Fetuses and neonates with ABO incompatibility typically do not require additional monitoring or treatment. Fetuses and infants at risk for HDFN as a consequence of Rh incompatibility may require additional monitoring and treatment. Routine evaluation of fetuses at risk for HDFN includes the Coombs test. The indirect Coombs test measures antibody in the mother's circulation and indicates whether the fetus is at risk for HDFN. The direct Coombs test measures antibody already bound to the surfaces of fetal erythrocytes. It is used primarily to confirm the diagnosis of antibody-mediated HDFN. If a prior history of fetal hemolytic disease is present, additional diagnostic tests are done to determine risk with the current pregnancy. These include maternal antibody titers, fetal blood sampling, amniotic fluid spectrophotometry, and ultrasound fetal assessment.

Prevention is the key to managing HDFN that results from Rh incompatibility. Immunoprophylaxis through the use of Rh immune globulin (RhoGAM), a preparation of antibody against Rh antigen D (anti-D Ig), prevents an Rh-negative woman from producing antibodies.

If an Rh-negative woman is given Rh immune globulin within 72 hours of exposure to Rh-positive erythrocytes, she will not produce antibody against the D antigen. As a result, the next Rh-positive baby she conceives will be protected. Updated United States and United Kingdom guidelines also state that if anti-D Ig is not given within 72 hours, every effort should be made to administer it within 10 days.[3,4]

Inherited Disorders
Sickle Cell Disease
Sickle cell disease is a group of autosomal recessive disorders characterized by the production of hemoglobin S (Hb S; sickle hemoglobin) within the erythrocytes. Hb S is formed as a result of a genetic mutation in which one amino acid (valine) replaces another (glutamic acid) (Fig. 24.2). Under conditions of decreased oxygen tension and dehydration, Hb S stretches and elongates, causing the erythrocyte to assume a characteristic sickle shape. These sickled cells also die prematurely, resulting in hemolytic anemia (Fig. 24.3).

The most prevalent types of sickle cell disease are sickle cell anemia, sickle cell–thalassemia disease, and sickle cell–Hb C disease (Table 24.2). (See Chapter 2 for a discussion of genetic inheritance of disease.) Sickle cell anemia, a homozygous form, is the most severe. It results when the individual inherits two copies of Hb S. Sickle cell–thalassemia and sickle cell–Hb C disease are compound heterozygous forms in which the child inherits Hb S from one parent and another type of abnormal hemoglobin from the other parent. Sickle cell trait occurs when the

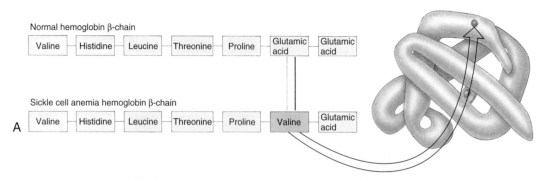

Normal hemoglobin β-chain

| Valine | Histidine | Leucine | Threonine | Proline | Glutamic acid | Glutamic acid |

Sickle cell anemia hemoglobin β-chain

A

| Valine | Histidine | Leucine | Threonine | Proline | Valine | Glutamic acid |

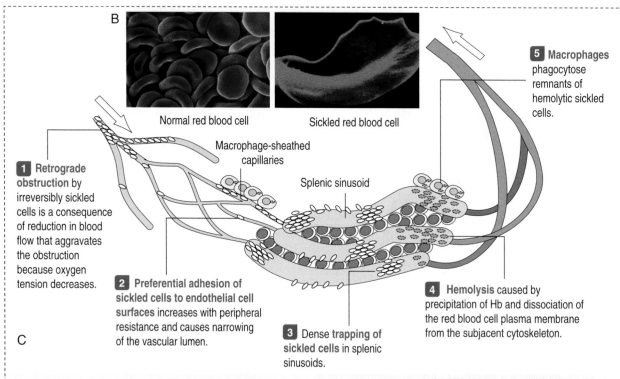

B

Normal red blood cell   Sickled red blood cell

1 **Retrograde obstruction** by irreversibly sickled cells is a consequence of reduction in blood flow that aggravates the obstruction because oxygen tension decreases.

Macrophage-sheathed capillaries

Splenic sinusoid

5 **Macrophages** phagocytose remnants of hemolytic sickled cells.

2 **Preferential adhesion of sickled cells to endothelial cell surfaces** increases with peripheral resistance and causes narrowing of the vascular lumen.

3 Dense **trapping of sickled cells** in splenic sinusoids.

4 **Hemolysis** caused by precipitation of Hb and dissociation of the red blood cell plasma membrane from the subjacent cytoskeleton.

C

Sickle cell anemia is determined by the substitution of normal hemoglobin (Hb A) by hemoglobin S (Hb S) caused by a point mutation (replacement of the nucleotide triplet CTC coding glutamic acid at the mRNA level [GAG] by the CAC triplet [GUG] coding for valine) that modifies the physicochemical properties of the β-globin chain of hemoglobin. All hemoglobin is abnormal in homozygous individuals for the mutant gene, and red blood cells show a sickling deformity and hemolytic anemia in the presence or absence of normal oxygen tension. Heterozygous individuals contain a mixture of Hb A and Hb S, and sickling and anemia are observed when the tension of oxygen decreases.

Irreversibly sickled red blood cells are trapped within the splenic sinusoids and are destroyed by adjacent macrophages. Hemolysis may also occur in the macrophage-sheathed capillaries of the red pulp.

FIGURE 24.2 Sickle Cell Hemoglobin. A, Sickle cell hemoglobin is produced by a recessive allele of the gene encoding the β-chain of the protein hemoglobin. It represents a single amino acid change—from glutamic acid to valine at the sixth position of the chain. In this model of a hemoglobin molecule, the position of the mutation can be seen near the end of the upper arm. **B,** Color-enhanced electron micrograph shows normal erythrocytes and sickled blood cell. **C,** Brief summary of the process of cell sickling. (**A** from Raven PH, Johnson GB: *Biology,* ed 3, St Louis, 1992, Mosby; **B** copyright Dennis Kunkel Microscopy, Inc; **C** from Kierszenbaum A, Tres L: *Histology and cell biology: an introduction to pathology,* ed 3, St Louis, 2012, Mosby.)

child inherits Hb S from one parent and normal hemoglobin (Hb A) from the other. This heterozygous carrier state rarely has clinical manifestations. All forms of sickle cell disease are lifelong conditions.

Sickle cell disease is most common among persons with ancestry from sub-Saharan Africa. Although less common, it also is present among individuals with ancestry from Mediterranean countries, the Arabian Peninsula, parts of India, and Spanish-speaking areas of South America.

In the United States, sickle cell anemia is most common in black people, with a reported incidence of around 1:365 live births.[5] In the general population, the risk of two black parents having a child with sickle cell anemia is 0.7%. Sickle cell–Hb C disease occurs in 1 in 800 births, and sickle cell–thalassemia is even less common (1 in 1700 births).

Sickle cell trait occurs in 7% to 13% of African Americans. Its prevalence in African countries, such as Nigeria and the Democratic

Republic of Congo, may be as high as 30%.[6] The sickle cell trait may provide protection against lethal forms of malaria. This results in a genetic advantage for carriers who reside in regions of the world that are endemic for malaria, such as sub-Saharan Africa and some Mediterranean countries.

PATHOPHYSIOLOGY Hb S is soluble and usually causes no problem when it is properly oxygenated. When oxygen tension decreases, the abnormal β-globin chain of Hb S polymerizes, forming abnormal fluid polymers. As these polymers realign, they cause the red cell to form into the sickle shape. Decreased oxygenation (hypoxemia) and pH, as well as dehydration, trigger the sickling process. Acute illness, stress, temperature changes, and living at altitude can cause decreased oxygen tension, leading to sickling.

Sickled erythrocytes tend to plug the blood vessels. This increases the viscosity of the blood, which slows circulation, and causes vascular occlusion, pain, and organ infarction. The increased blood viscosity also increases the time that erythrocytes are exposed to less oxygenation, which promotes further sickling. Sickled cells undergo hemolysis in the spleen or become sequestered there, causing blood pooling and infarction of splenic vessels. The anemia that follows these sickling episodes triggers erythropoiesis in the marrow and, in extreme cases, in the liver (Fig. 24.4).

Sickling usually is not permanent. Most sickled erythrocytes regain a normal shape after reoxygenation and rehydration. Irreversible sickling is caused by irreversible plasma membrane damage caused by sickling.

In persons with sickle cell anemia, in which the erythrocytes contain a high percentage of Hb S (75% to 95%), up to 30% of the erythrocytes can become irreversibly sickled.

CLINICAL MANIFESTATIONS The clinical manifestations of sickle cell disease can vary. Some individuals have mild symptoms; others suffer from repeated vasoocclusive crises. The general manifestations of hemolytic anemia from the sickling process include pallor, fatigue, jaundice, and irritability. Extensive sickling can precipitate four types of acute crises:

1. **Vasoocclusive crisis (thrombotic crisis).** This crisis type begins with sickling in the microcirculation. As blood flow is obstructed by sickled cells, vasospasm occurs and a logjam effect blocks all blood flow through the vessel. Unless the process is reversed, thrombosis and infarction of local tissue occur. Vasoocclusive crisis is extremely painful and may last for days or even weeks, with an average duration of 4 to 6 days. The frequency of this type of crisis is variable and unpredictable. Vasoocclusion in vessels to the brain can result in stroke. Chronic vasoocclusion in vessels to the kidneys results in end-stage renal disease.

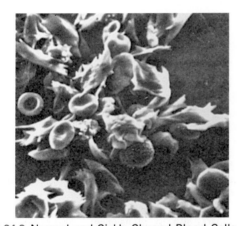

FIGURE 24.3 Normal and Sickle-Shaped Blood Cells. Scanning electron micrograph of normal and sickle-shaped red blood cells. The irregularly shaped cells are the sickle cells; the circular cells are the normal blood cells. (From Raven PH, Johnson GB: *Biology*, ed 3, St Louis, 1992, Mosby.)

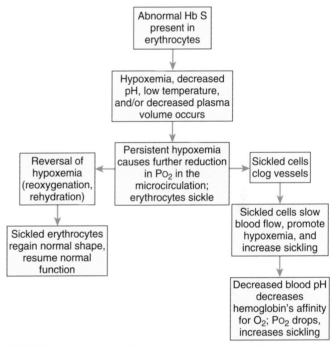

FIGURE 24.4 Sickling of Erythrocytes. O_2, Oxygen; Po_2, partial pressure of oxygen

TABLE 24.2 Inheritance of Sickle Cell Disease

Hemoglobin Inherited From First Parent	Hemoglobin Inherited From Second Parent	Form of Sickle Cell Disease in Child
Hb S (an abnormal hemoglobin)	Hb S	Sickle cell anemia: homozygous inheritance in which child's hemoglobin is mostly Hb S, with remainder Hb F (fetal hemoglobin)
Hb S	Defective or insufficient α- or β-chains of Hb A (alpha- or beta-thalassemia)	Sickle cell–thalassemia disease (heterozygous inheritance of Hb S and alpha- or beta-thalassemia)
Hb S	Hb C or D (both abnormal hemoglobins)	Sickle cell–hemoglobin C (or D) disease (heterozygous inheritance of hemoglobin S and either C or D)
Hb S	Normal hemoglobins (mostly Hb A)	Sickle cell trait, carrier state (heterozygous inheritance of Hb S and normal hemoglobin)

2. **Sequestration crisis.** This type of crisis is typically seen only in children less than 5 years of age. Large amounts of blood become acutely pooled in the liver and spleen. Because the spleen can hold as much as one-fifth of the body's blood supply at one time, the risk of mortality is high if the condition is not recognized and managed appropriately. Approximately half of children who experience sequestration crises will have recurrent episodes.

3. **Aplastic crisis.** Profound anemia is caused by lowered erythropoiesis despite an increased need for new erythrocytes. In sickle cell anemia, erythrocyte survival is only 10 to 20 days. Normally the bone marrow is able to compensate to replace the cells lost through premature hemolysis. When this compensatory response is compromised, often after a viral infection, aplastic crisis develops. This type of crisis typically lasts 7 to 10 days.

4. **Hyperhemolytic crisis.** Although unusual, this type of crisis may occur in association with certain drugs or infections. It has also been reported as an acute or chronic reaction following a blood transfusion.

The clinical manifestations of sickle cell disease usually do not appear until the infant is at least 6 months old. At this time, postnatal concentrations of Hb F decrease, causing concentrations of Hb S to rise (Fig. 24.5). Infection is the most common cause of death related to sickle cell disease. Sepsis and meningitis develop in as many as 10% of children with sickle cell anemia during the first 5 years of life. Advances in identification of sickle cell disease and supportive care have improved survival of children with sickle cell disease.

Sickle cell–Hb C disease is usually milder than sickle cell anemia. The main clinical problems are related to vasoocclusive crises, which are thought to result from higher hematocrit values and viscosity. In older children, sickle cell retinopathy, renal necrosis, and aseptic necrosis of the femoral heads can occur along with obstructive crises.

Sickle cell–thalassemia has the mildest clinical manifestations of all the sickle cell diseases. The normal hemoglobins, particularly Hb F, inhibit sickling. The erythrocytes tend to be small (microcytic) and to contain relatively little hemoglobin (hypochromic), making them less likely to occlude the microcirculation, even when in a sickled state.

EVALUATION AND TREATMENT   The parents' hematologic history and clinical manifestations may suggest that a child has sickle cell disease, but hematologic tests are necessary for diagnosis. If the sickle solubility test confirms the presence of Hb S in peripheral blood, hemoglobin electrophoresis provides information about the amount of Hb S in erythrocytes. Prenatal diagnosis can be made after chorionic villus sampling as early as 8 to 10 weeks' gestation or by amniotic fluid analysis at 15 weeks' gestation (Fig. 24.6). Hemoglobinopathies, including sickle cell disease, are now included as part of routine newborn screening in all 50 states and the District of Columbia.

Sickle cell trait typically does not affect life expectancy or interfere with daily activities. On rare occasions, however, severe hypoxia caused by shock, vigorous exercising at high altitudes, flying at high altitudes in unpressurized aircraft, or undergoing anesthesia is associated with

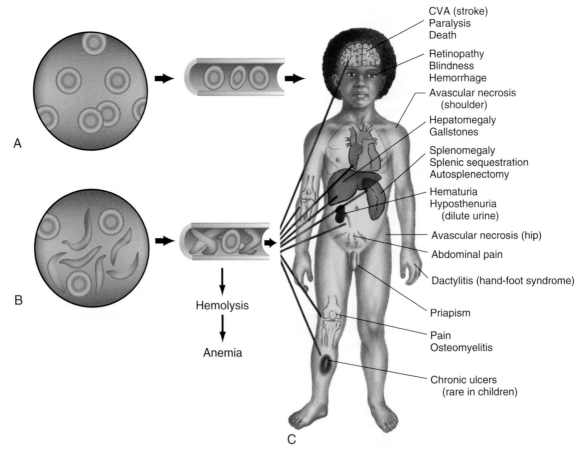

FIGURE 24.5 Differences between effects of normal (**A**) and sickled (**B**) red blood cells on blood circulation and selected consequences in a child. **C,** Tissue effects of sickle cell anemia. *CVA,* Cerebrovascular accident. (**A** and **B** adapted from Hockenberry MJ et al, editors: *Wong's nursing care of infants and children,* ed 10, St Louis, 2015, Mosby.)

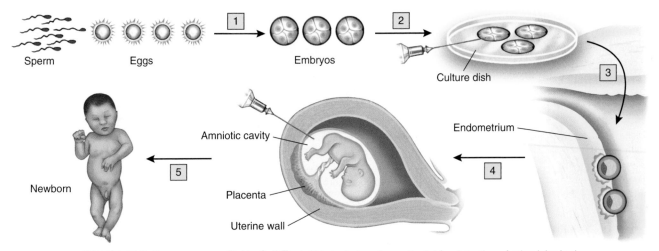

FIGURE 24.6 Prepregnancy Sickle Cell Test. This technique has potential for detection of other inherited diseases. **1,** Fertilization produces several embryos. **2,** The embryos are tested for the presence of the gene. **3,** The embryos without the gene are implanted. **4,** Amniocentesis confirms whether the fetus (or fetuses) has the sickle cell gene. **5,** Woman has a normal child.

vasoocclusive episodes in persons with sickle cell trait. These cells form an ivy shape instead of a sickle shape.

Advances in supportive care have led to decreased morbidity and mortality among children with sickle cell disease. Supportive care emphasizes preventing consequences of anemia and avoiding crises, including adequate hydration, infection prevention, and pain management. Genetic counseling and psychologic support are important for the child and family.

A common treatment for sickle cell disease is hydroxyurea. Hydroxyurea inhibits deoxyribonucleic acid (DNA) synthesis, which causes an increase in Hb F concentration. It also provides an antiinflammatory effect by decreasing leukocyte production. These outcomes are thought to decrease crises.

Transfusion therapy can decrease morbidity and mortality associated with sickle cell disease, particularly in those at increased risk for stroke.[7] Despite these benefits, it can result in iron overload, which can cause liver damage and fibrosis, delayed physical and sexual development, and heart disease. Chelation therapy to remove excess iron is often required.

Hematopoietic stem cell transplantation offers the only cure for sickle cell disease; however, it is not without important risks. Current research is seeking to reduce the toxicities associated with transplantation while optimizing long-term outcomes.

Thalassemias

The alpha- and beta-thalassemias are autosomal recessive disorders that result in impaired synthesis of one of the two chains—α or β—of adult hemoglobin (Hb A). Beta-thalassemia is most prevalent among Greek, Italian, some Arab, and Sephardic Jewish people. Alpha-thalassemia is most common among Chinese, Vietnamese, Cambodian, and Laotian people. Both alpha- and beta-thalassemias are common among Black people.

Beta-thalassemias are more common than alpha-thalassemias. Both types are further classified as major or minor. The classification is based on the number of genes that control α- or β-chain synthesis. It also is based on the combination of mutations and whether they are homozygous (thalassemia major) or heterozygous (thalassemia minor). The anemic manifestation of both alpha- and beta-thalassemia is microcytic-hypochromic hemolytic anemia.

PATHOPHYSIOLOGY The beta-thalassemias are caused by mutations that decrease the synthesis of β-globin chains, leading to anemia, tissue hypoxia, and red cell hemolysis. β-Globin chain production is depressed moderately in the heterozygous form, beta-thalassemia minor, and severely in the homozygous form, beta-thalassemia major (also called Cooley anemia). As a result, erythrocytes have a reduced amount of hemoglobin and free α-chains accumulate (Fig. 24.7). Free α-chains are unstable and easily precipitate in the cell. Most erythroblasts that contain precipitates are destroyed by mononuclear phagocytes in the marrow. Destruction results in ineffective erythropoiesis and anemia. Some of the precipitate-carrying cells mature and enter the bloodstream. These cells are destroyed prematurely in the spleen, resulting in mild hemolytic anemia.

There are four forms of alpha-thalassemia: (1) alpha trait (the heterozygous carrier state), in which a single α-chain–forming gene is defective; (2) alpha-thalassemia minor, in which two genes are defective; (3) hemoglobin H disease, in which three genes are defective; and (4) alpha-thalassemia major, in which all four α-forming genes are defective. Alpha-thalassemia major is fatal, often in utero, because α-chains are not produced and oxygen cannot be released to the tissues.

CLINICAL MANIFESTATIONS Beta-thalassemia minor causes mild to moderate microcytic-hypochromic anemia. The degree of reticulocytosis depends on the severity of the anemia and results in skeletal changes. Hemolysis of immature (and therefore fragile) erythrocytes may cause a slight elevation in serum iron and indirect bilirubin levels. Persons with beta-thalassemia minor may experience mild splenomegaly, bronze coloring of the skin, and hyperplasia of the bone marrow, but they are less likely to experience life-threatening complications.

Persons with beta-thalassemia major may become quite ill and show impaired physical growth and development. The severe anemia resulting from this condition can cause a significant cardiovascular burden with high-output congestive heart failure. In the past, death resulted from cardiac failure, often by age 20. Today, blood transfusions can increase the life span by one to two decades. Death is usually caused by consequences of hemochromatosis resulting from chronic transfusions. Liver enlargement occurs as a result of progressive hemosiderosis, and enlargement of the spleen is caused by extramedullary hemopoiesis and increased destruction of red blood cells. Skeletal changes begin in

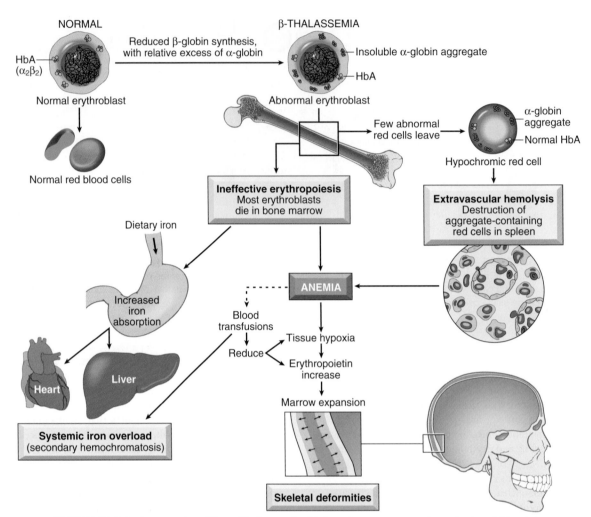

FIGURE 24.7 Pathogenesis of Beta-Thalassemia Major. The aggregates of unpaired α-globin chains are a hallmark of the disease. Blood transfusions can diminish the anemia, but they add to the systemic iron overload. (From Kumar V et al: *Robbins & Cotran pathologic basis of disease,* ed 9, Philadelphia, 2015, Saunders.)

infancy and include spinal impairment that retards linear growth and subsequent upper and lower limb-length discrepancy. Deformity of the facial bones in response to hyperplastic marrow results in a characteristic chipmunk-like facial appearance.

Persons who inherit the mildest form of alpha-thalassemia (the alpha trait) usually are symptom free or have mild microcytosis. Alpha-thalassemia minor has clinical manifestations that are virtually identical to those of beta-thalassemia minor: mild microcytic-hypochromic reticulocytosis, bone marrow hyperplasia, increased serum iron concentrations, and moderate splenomegaly.

Signs and symptoms of alpha-thalassemia minor are similar to those of beta-thalassemia minor but milder. Moderate microcytic-hypochromic anemia, enlargement of the liver and spleen, and bone marrow hyperplasia are evident.

Alpha-thalassemia major causes **hydrops fetalis,** whereby the developing fetus suffers from severe tissue anoxia and may develop fulminant intrauterine congestive heart failure. Signs of fetal distress became evident by the third trimester of pregnancy. In the past, severe tissue anoxia led to death in utero; now many such infants are saved by intrauterine transfusions.

EVALUATION AND TREATMENT Evaluation of thalassemia is based on the familial disease history, clinical manifestations, and blood tests.

Diagnostic tests include peripheral blood smears that show microcytosis and hemoglobin electrophoresis that demonstrates diminished amounts of α- or β-chains. Prenatal diagnosis is sometimes done, and families are referred for genetic counseling. Identification of thalassemia is now included as part of routine newborn screening for hemoglobinopathies in all 50 states and the District of Columbia. Molecular genetic testing of at-risk siblings should be offered to allow for early diagnosis and appropriate treatment.

Treatment is largely supportive and involves a regular transfusion program and chelation therapy to reduce transfusion iron overload. Milder forms of thalassemia rarely require transfusion. The only available definitive cure for thalassemia major is allogeneic hematopoietic stem cell transplantation (HSCT) from a matched family or unrelated donor or cord blood transplantation from a related donor.[8] Optimal clinical management may decrease the need for splenectomy.

✔ QUICK CHECK 24.1
1. Why is Rh incompatibility rare today?
2. Why do clinical manifestations of sickle cell disease not appear until the infant is at least 6 months old?
3. Why do children with thalassemia major develop cardiovascular complications?

DISORDERS OF COAGULATION AND PLATELETS

Inherited Hemorrhagic Disease

Hemophilias

The hemophilias are a group of inherited bleeding disorders resulting from mutations in coagulation factors. The focus of this section will be hemophilia A and hemophilia B, both of which are X-linked recessive conditions. A third type of hemophilia, hemophilia C, is an autosomal recessive condition that results from a deficiency of factor XI. Table 24.3 lists the coagulation factors and deficiencies associated with clinical bleeding.

Hemophilia A results from a mutation in the *F8* gene, which codes for factor VIII, an essential cofactor for factor IX in the coagulation cascade. It is the most common hereditary disease associated with life-threatening bleeding. Hemophilia B results from a mutation in the *F9* gene, which codes for factor IX. Because both factors VIII and IX function together to activate factor X, hemophilia A and B are clinically indistinguishable.

The incidence of hemophilia A is approximately 1 in 5000 male births. Hemophilia B is five times less common, with an incidence of approximately 1 in 30,000 male births. The worldwide prevalence of hemophilia it is estimated to be at more than 400,000 people.[9] All racial groups are equally affected.

PATHOPHYSIOLOGY   As X-linked recessive conditions, hemophilia A and B are most frequently inherited from a mother who is heterozygous for a mutation in either the *F8* or *F9* gene. Approximately 30% of cases, however, result from a new mutation. This new mutation can occur in either a carrier female or in an affected male. More than 1300 mutations have been associated with factor VIII and IX deficiency. Affected individuals within the same family will have the same mutation; however, the mutation causing hemophilia may be different across families.[10]

The *F8* and *F9* genes are located on the long arm of the X chromosome. A mutation in either of these genes typically results in either deficient or abnormal function of the corresponding clotting factor. Because males have only one copy of the X chromosome, the mutation results in the clinical manifestations of hemophilia. In females, the second copy of the X chromosome usually produces a sufficient quantity of normal functioning clotting factor. Females who are heterozygous carriers typically do not experience excessive bleeding. Because X-inactivation, or lyonization (see Chapter 2), is a random process, phenotypes of women who are heterozygous carriers can vary. Fifty percent of female carriers have lower than normal clotting factor levels. Although very uncommon, it is plausible for a female to be homozygous for mutations in the *F8* or *F9* gene and therefore have hemophilia.[10]

CLINICAL MANIFESTATIONS   The clinical manifestations and severity of hemophilia depend largely on the level of factor VIII and IX activity. Joint bleeding is the most characteristic type of bleeding in hemophilia. The joints most often affected are the knees, ankles, and elbows. Bleeding into muscles, usually from trauma, also can occur. Oral bleeding is common in the setting of dental surgery. Spontaneous painless hematuria is relatively common in hemophilia; it does not result in significant blood loss but requires evaluation. Hematuria accompanied by pain requires prompt evaluation and treatment.

Intracranial bleeds, bleeding of internal organs, and bleeding into the tissues of the neck, chest, or abdomen are all life-threatening. Delayed or suboptimal treatment of these bleeds may lead to permanent brain injury, loss of organ function, or death.

EVALUATION AND TREATMENT   A positive family history may expedite a diagnosis of hemophilia. When a mother who is a known or suspected carrier is pregnant, prenatal genetic testing through chorionic villus sampling (CVS) or amniocentesis may reveal a diagnosis of hemophilia. In the absence of a positive family history, a personal bleed history, laboratory testing, family history, and physical assessment contribute to a thorough evaluation and accurate diagnosis. In general, those with hemophilia A or B will have a prolonged partial thromboplastin time (PTT) and the prothrombin time (PT) will be normal. Measuring factor VIII and factor IX levels also is necessary for diagnosis.

The majority of children with hemophilia A can be treated with recombinant factor VIII. The majority of children with hemophilia B can be treated with recombinant factor IX. Recombinant factor is reconstituted in a small volume of diluent, administered by slow intravenous push, and raises the factor level almost immediately. Emerging therapies for hemophilia include the use of PEGylated factor. Adding a polyethylene glycol (PEG) molecule results in an extended half-life of the involved factor.[11]

Antibody-Mediated Hemorrhagic Disease

Antibody-mediated hemorrhagic diseases are caused by the immune response. Antibody-mediated destruction of platelets or antibody-mediated inflammatory reactions to allergens damage blood vessels and cause seepage into tissues. The thrombocytopenic purpuras may be intrinsic or idiopathic. They also may be transient phenomena transmitted from mother to fetus. The inflammatory, or "allergic," purpuras, although rare, occur in response to allergens in the blood. All of these disorders first appear during infancy or childhood.

Primary Immune Thrombocytopenia

Primary immune thrombocytopenia (ITP) (previously referred to as idiopathic thrombocytopenic purpura) is the most common disorder of platelet consumption. Autoantibodies bind to the plasma membranes of platelets, causing platelet sequestration and destruction by mononuclear phagocytes in the spleen and other lymphoid tissues at a rate

Clotting Factors	Synonym	Disorder
I	Fibrinogen	Congenital deficiency (afibrinogenemia) and dysfunction (dysfibrinogenemia)
II	Prothrombin	Congenital deficiency or dysfunction
V	Labile factor or proaccelerin	Congenital deficiency (parahemophilia)
VII	Stable factor or proconvertin	Congenital deficiency
VIII	AHF	Congenital deficiency is hemophilia A (classic hemophilia)
IX	Christmas factor	Congenital deficiency is hemophilia B
X	Stuart-Prower factor	Congenital deficiency
XI	Plasma thromboplastin antecedent	Congenital deficiency, sometimes referred to as hemophilia C
XII	Hageman factor	Congenital deficiency is *not* associated with clinical symptoms
XIII	Fibrin-stabilizing factor	Congenital deficiency

TABLE 24.3 The Coagulation Factors and Associated Disorders

AHF; antihemophilic factor.

that exceeds the ability of the bone marrow to produce them. The destruction of platelets is triggered by drugs, infections, lymphomas, or an unknown cause.

PATHOPHYSIOLOGY   The autoantibodies that produce the destruction are often of the IgG class and are usually against the platelet membrane glycoproteins (IIb-IIIa or Ib-IX). Approximately 70% of cases of ITP are preceded by a viral illness (e.g., cytomegalovirus [CMV], Epstein-Barr virus [EBV], parvovirus, or respiratory tract infection) prior to the eruption of petechiae or purpura by 1 to 3 weeks.

CLINICAL MANIFESTATIONS   Bruising and a generalized petechial rash often occur about 1 to 3 weeks after a viral illness. Petechiae can develop into ecchymoses. Asymmetric bruising is typical and is found most often on the legs and trunk. Hemorrhagic bullae of the gums, lips, and other mucous membranes may be prominent. Epistaxis (nose bleeding) may be severe and difficult to control. Except for signs of bleeding, the child appears well. The principal changes are found in the spleen, bone marrow, and blood. The acute phase lasts 1 to 2 weeks, but thrombocytopenia often persists. Intracranial hemorrhage is the most serious complication of ITP, however, the incidence is less than 1%. In some cases, the onset is more gradual, and clinical manifestations consist of moderate bruising and a few petechiae.

EVALUATION AND TREATMENT   Laboratory examination reveals an isolated low platelet count. The few platelets observed on a smear are large, reflecting increased bone marrow production. The Ivy bleeding time is prolonged. Bone marrow aspiration is not recommended for children with typical features of ITP. The primary treatment for children with ITP is observation regardless of the platelet count. When bleeding is present, primary treatment is with an infusion of intravenous immune globulin (IVIG) or a short course of corticosteroids.

Even without treatment, the prognosis for children with ITP is excellent: 75% recover completely within 3 months. After the initial acute phase, spontaneous clinical manifestations subside. By 6 months after onset, 80% to 90% of affected children have regained normal platelet counts. ITP that persists longer than 12 months in children is considered chronic, and immunosuppressive therapies are used.

✔ **QUICK CHECK 24.2**
1. List the major disorders of coagulation and platelets found in children.
2. What is the mechanism of inheritance associated with hemophilia and how does it contribute to the clinical manifestations associated with factor VIII or IX deficiency in males and females?
3. What are the most common sites of bleeding in individuals with hemophilia?
4. What is the primary abnormality in primary immune thrombocytopenia (ITP)?

NEOPLASTIC DISORDERS

Leukemia

Leukemia is cancer of the blood-forming tissues, such as the bone marrow, that most often produces abnormal white blood cells called leukemic cells. Once in the blood, leukemic cells can spread to other organs, such as the lymph nodes, spleen, and brain. Leukemia is the most common malignancy in children and teens. The four most common types of leukemia are (1) acute lymphoblastic leukemia (ALL), (2) acute myeloid leukemia (AML), (3) chronic lymphocytic leukemia (CLL), and (4) chronic myeloid leukemia (CML)[12] (see Chapter 23).

About 75% of leukemias among children and teens are ALL; the remaining cases are classified as AML and related neoplasms. Chronic leukemias are rare in children and account for fewer than 5% of cases.

ALL is most common in early childhood, peaking between 2 and 4 years of age. AML is slightly more common during the first 2 years of life and during the teenage years and occurs about equally among boys and girls of all races. ALL is more common in boys than girls and among Hispanic and white children than among black and Asian American children.

The cause of most childhood cancer, including leukemia, is unknown. About 5% of all childhood cancers are caused by inherited mutations. Genetic mutations that predispose the child to cancer development can occur during fetal development. Genetic conditions associated with leukemia include Down syndrome, neurofibromatosis, Shwachman-Diamond syndrome, Bloom syndrome, and ataxia-telangiectasia. Epigenetic modifications, including DNA methylation, have been proposed as mediating events between environmental exposures and subsequent disease development.[13]

Many studies have shown that exposure to ionizing radiation (prenatal exposure to x-rays and postnatal exposure to high doses) can lead to the development of childhood leukemia and possibly other cancers.[14] There is recent concern for performing computed tomography (CT) scans in children. The increased use of these scans combined with wide variability in radiation doses has resulted in many children receiving a high dose of radiation.[15] Studies of other possible environmental risk factors, including parental exposure to cancer-causing chemicals, prenatal exposure to pesticides, childhood exposure to common infectious agents, and living near a nuclear power plant, have so far produced inconsistent results. Higher risks of cancer have not been seen in children of individuals treated for sporadic cancer (cancer not caused by an inherited mutation).[16,17]

PATHOPHYSIOLOGY   ALL is composed of immature B (pre-B) or T (pre-T) cells called lymphoblasts. As leukemia develops, the bone marrow becomes dense with lymphoblasts that replace the normal marrow and disrupt normal function. Many of the chromosomal abnormalities documented in ALL cause dysregulation of the expression and function of transcription factors required for normal B-cell and T-cell development.[18] The mutations can include both gain of function and loss of function that are required for normal development.

AML is caused by acquired oncogenic mutations that impair differentiation, resulting in the accumulation of immature myeloid blasts in the marrow and other organs. Epigenetic alterations are frequent in AML and have a central role. The bone marrow crowding by blast cells produces marrow failure and complications, including anemia, thrombocytopenia, and neutropenia. AML is very heterogeneous because myeloid cell differentiation is very complex. Leukemia, ALL or AML, is typically distinguished from lymphoma by the presence of greater than 20% leukemic blasts in the bone marrow.

CLINICAL MANIFESTATIONS   The onset of leukemia may be abrupt or insidious. Children with leukemia may present with symptoms only 1 week before diagnosis. Regardless of how leukemia develops, the most common symptoms reflect consequences of bone marrow failure. These include decreased levels of red blood cells and platelets, as well as changes in white blood cells. Pallor, fatigue, petechiae, purpura, bleeding, and fever generally are present. Approximately 45% of children present with a hemoglobin level below 7 g/dl. Epistaxis often occurs in children with severe thrombocytopenia.

Fever can be present as a result of (1) infection associated with the decrease in functional neutrophils and (2) hypermetabolism associated with the ongoing rapid growth and destruction of leukemic cells. White blood cell counts greater than 200,000/mm^3 can cause leukostasis, an intravascular clumping of cells resulting in infarction and hemorrhage, usually in the brain and lung.

Renal failure as a result of hyperuricemia (high uric acid levels) can be associated with ALL, particularly at diagnosis or during the initial phase of treatment. Extramedullary invasion with leukemic cells can occur in nearly all body tissue. The central nervous system (CNS) is a common site of infiltration of extramedullary leukemia. Less than 10% of children with ALL, however, will have CNS involvement at diagnosis. The most common symptoms of CNS involvement relate to increased intracranial pressure, causing early morning headaches, nausea, vomiting, irritability, and lethargy. Gonadal involvement, with testicular infiltration, also may occur.

Leukemic infiltration into bones and joints is common. Reports of bone or joint pain actually lead to the diagnosis of leukemia in some children. In most children, bone pain is characterized as migratory, vague, and without areas of swelling or inflammation. In some cases, however, joint pain is the primary symptom and some swelling is associated with the pain. Occasionally, these children are initially misdiagnosed as having rheumatoid arthritis. Other organs reported to be sites of leukemic invasion include the kidneys, heart, lungs, thymus, eyes, skin, and gastrointestinal tract.

EVALUATION AND TREATMENT Leukemia is diagnosed through blood tests and examination of peripheral blood smears. A bone marrow aspiration is usually performed to further characterize the leukemia. The blast cell is the hallmark of acute leukemia (Fig. 24.8). Healthy children have less than 5% blast cells in the bone marrow and none in the peripheral blood. In ALL, the bone marrow often is replaced by 80% to 100% blast cells. Counts of normally developing red blood cells, granulocytes, and platelets are typically reduced. Occasionally, the marrow appears hypocellular, making the diagnosis difficult to differentiate from aplastic anemia. When this occurs, bone marrow biopsy or biopsy of extramedullary sites is necessary to confirm the diagnosis.

Approximately 85% of children with ALL will become 5-year survivors of their illness. Chemotherapy, using a combination of medications, is the treatment of choice for acute leukemia. Radiation of the CNS is used only in selected cases. Identification of various risk groups among children with ALL has led to the development of different intensities of drug protocols. As a result, treatment can be targeted specifically for a particular risk group. For children who experience relapses of ALL,

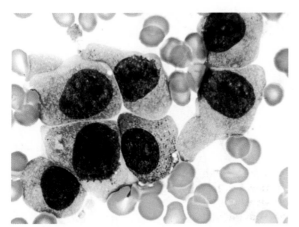

FIGURE 24.8 Monoblasts From Acute Monoblastic Leukemia. Monoblasts in a marrow smear from an individual with acute monoblastic leukemia. The monoblasts are larger than myeloblasts and usually have abundant cytoplasm, often with delicate scattered azurophilic granules (an element that stains well with blue aniline dyes). (From Damjanov I, Linder J, editors: *Anderson's pathology,* ed 10, St Louis, 1996, Mosby.)

treatment with chimeric antigen receptor T cells (CAR-T cells) is showing promise.[19,19a]

AML is more difficult to treat than ALL. Combination chemotherapy is the most common approach to treatment. Those children with unfavorable cytogenetic markers and those who experience a relapse of their disease will often undergo hematopoietic stem cell transplantation.[20]

CML accounts for less than 5% of childhood leukemias. Biologically targeted therapies, specifically tyrosine kinase inhibitors (TKIs), are becoming the mainstay of treatment, specifically for individuals whose disease has the *BCR/ABL* translocation[21] (see Chapter 23). TKIs are administered orally, and several are now approved for use in children. Treatment requires continued adherence to the medication regimen, and the health impact of long-term TKI therapy is not yet known.[21]

Lymphomas

Lymphoma (Hodgkin lymphoma [HL] and non-Hodgkin lymphoma [NHL]) develops from the proliferation of malignant lymphocytes in the lymphoid system (see Chapters 12 and 23). Lymphomas arise from discrete tissue masses. Lymphoid neoplasms involve some recognizable stage of lymphocyte B- or T-cell differentiation.

Some lymphomas occasionally have leukemic presentations, and evolution to "leukemia" is not unusual during the progression of incurable "lymphomas." The terms therefore merely reflect the usual tissue distribution. The World Health Organization (WHO) provides a classification scheme for lymphoma that was updated in 2016[22] (also see Chapter 23).

NHL and HL constitute about 11% of all cases of childhood cancer. Approximately 1800 children younger than 20 years of age are diagnosed with lymphoma in the United States each year.[23] NHL (including Burkitt lymphoma) occurs more often than Hodgkin lymphoma. Either group of diseases is rare before the age of 5 years, and the relative incidence increases throughout childhood. Boys are more likely to be diagnosed with lymphoma than are girls. Children with inherited or acquired immunodeficiency syndromes, such as Wiskott-Aldrich syndrome, ataxia-telangiectasia, and Bloom syndrome, are at particular risk for developing NHL.

Non-Hodgkin Lymphoma

Non-Hodgkin lymphomas (NHLs) are cancers of immune cells. NHLs are a large and diverse group of tumors. Some tumors develop more slowly, whereas others develop more quickly and aggressively. Childhood NHL typically becomes evident as a diffuse disease and can be further subdivided into four major types: (1) B-cell non-Hodgkin lymphoma (Burkitt and Burkitt-like lymphoma and Burkitt leukemia); (2) diffuse large B-cell lymphoma; (3) lymphoblastic lymphoma; and (4) anaplastic large cell lymphoma.[24] The common types of NHL in children are different from those in adults. The most common types of NHL in children are Burkitt lymphoma (40%), lymphoblastic lymphoma (25% to 30%), and large cell lymphoma (10%).

PATHOPHYSIOLOGY Burkitt lymphoma will be discussed as an example of the pathogenesis of NHL in children. All forms of Burkitt lymphoma are associated with translocations of the *MYC* gene on chromosome 8 that lead to increased MYC protein levels.[25] MYC is a transcriptional regulator that increases the expression of genes required for aerobic glycolysis, called the *Warburg effect* (see Chapter 11). Most Burkitt lymphomas are latently infected with the EBV.[26] EBV also is present in about 25% of tumors associated with human immunodeficiency virus (HIV) infection and in 15% to 20% of sporadic cases.[27]

CLINICAL MANIFESTATIONS NHL can arise from any lymphoid tissue. Signs and symptoms therefore are specific for the involved site. Associated signs of NHL include swelling of the lymph nodes in the neck, underarm, stomach, or groin; trouble swallowing; a painless lump or swelling in a testicle; weight loss for unknown reason; night sweats; and possibly trouble breathing. Involvement of facial bones, particularly the jaw, is common in African Burkitt lymphoma.

EVALUATION AND TREATMENT Diagnosis is made by physical exam and health history, followed by a needle biopsy of disease sites, usually the involved lymph nodes, tonsils, spleen, liver, bowel, or skin. Burkitt lymphoma is very aggressive and responds well to treatment. With intensive chemotherapy, most children and young adults can be cured.

Hodgkin Lymphoma

Hodgkin lymphoma (HL) is a group of lymphoid cancers. In contrast to NHL, HL arises in a single chain of lymph nodes and spreads first in a contiguous way to lymphoid tissue. HL is characterized by the presence of *Reed-Sternberg* cells, which are large cells derived from the germinal center of B cells (Fig. 24.9; also see Chapter 23). WHO has identified five types of HL: (1) nodular sclerosis, (2) mixed cellularity, (3) lymphocyte rich, (4) lymphocyte depletion, and (5) lymphocyte predominance. The first four types are considered the *classic* types of HL with similar expression of Reed-Sternberg cells. In the lymphocyte-predominance type, the Reed-Sternberg cell is distinctive but different from the others. HL is more common among adolescents, relative to younger childhood, and young adults.

PATHOPHYSIOLOGY The Reed-Sternberg cells fail to express most of the normal B-cell markers, as well as those of T-cells. The causes of the genetic rearrangements or reprogramming are not fully known but are thought to be the result of widespread epigenetic changes.

The abnormal pattern of gene expression in Reed-Sternberg cells suggests that the activity of many transcription factors is also altered.[28] Abnormalities in the activation of the transcription factor nuclear factor-kappa B (NF-κB) may be influenced by EBV infection. NF-κB is involved in many biologic processes, including inflammation, immunity, cell growth, differentiation, and apoptosis. EBV-infected B cells, resembling Reed-Sternberg cells, are found in lymph nodes in individuals with infectious mononucleosis, suggesting that the EBV proteins may have a role in changes of the B cells into Reed-Sternberg cells.[29]

Loss-of-function mutations in major histocompatibility class I antigens may allow Reed-Sternberg cells to avoid the normal host immune response.[30]

CLINICAL MANIFESTATIONS Painless lymphadenopathy in the lower cervical chain, with or without fever, is the most common symptom in children. Other lymph nodes and organs also may be involved (Fig. 24.10). Mediastinal involvement can cause pressure on the trachea or bronchi, leading to airway obstruction. Extranodal primary sites in Hodgkin lymphoma are rare. Initial symptoms consist of anorexia, malaise, and fatigue. Intermittent fever is present in 30% of children, and weight loss also may be present. Hodgkin lymphoma has a well-defined staging system that considers the extent and location of disease and the presence of fever, weight loss, or night sweats at diagnosis.

EVALUATION AND TREATMENT Treatment for Hodgkin lymphoma includes chemotherapy and radiation therapy. Historically, survivors had a much greater risk of developing a secondary cancer, such as lung cancer, melanoma, and breast cancer. Treatment protocols have been modified to minimize the use of radiotherapy and use less toxic chemotherapy. Targeted therapies, including monoclonal antibodies such as brentuximab vedotin and immune checkpoint inhibitors, may have a greater role in treating Hodgkin lymphoma.

✔ QUICK CHECK 24.3
1. List the childhood leukemias in order of incidence.
2. Why do children with leukemia experience bone or joint pain?
3. What are the common types of non-Hodgkin lymphoma (NHL) in children?

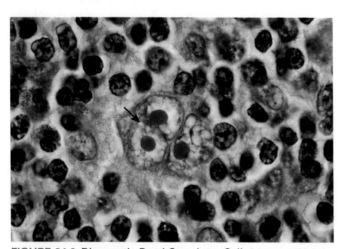

FIGURE 24.9 Diagnostic Reed-Sternberg Cell. A large multinucleated or multilobated cell with inclusion body–like nucleoli *(arrow)* surrounded by a halo of clear nucleoplasm. (From Damjanov I, Linder J: *Pathology: a color atlas,* St Louis, 2000, Mosby.)

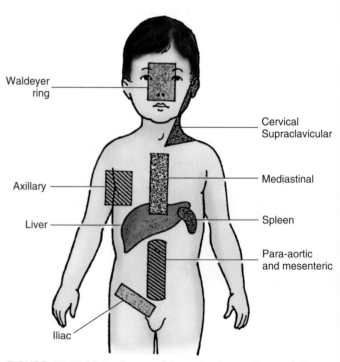

FIGURE 24.10 Main Areas of Lymphadenopathy and Organ Involvement in Hodgkin Lymphoma. (From Hockenberry MJ et al, editors: *Wong's nursing care of infants and children,* ed 10, St Louis, 2015, Mosby.)

SUMMARY REVIEW

Disorders of Erythrocytes

1. Anemia is the most common blood disorder in children. Like the anemias of adulthood, the anemias of childhood are caused by ineffective erythropoiesis or premature destruction of erythrocytes.

2. Iron deficiency anemia (IDA) is the most common nutritional disorder worldwide. Its incidence is greatest among children between 6 months and 2 years of age. Iron is critical for the developing child and without it damage from the periods of IDA is irreversible.

3. Regardless of its cause, IDA produces a hypochromic-microcytic anemia. Symptoms of mild anemia are often nonspecific, so parents may not notice changes until moderate anemia has developed.

4. Hemolytic disease of the fetus and newborn (HDFN) results from incompatibility between the maternal and the fetal Rh factors or blood type (ABO)Maternal antibodies (anti-Rh antibodies) form in response to the presence of fetal incompatible (Rh-positive) erythrocytes in the blood of an Rh-negative mother. The maternal antibodies then enter the fetal circulation and cause hemolysis of fetal erythrocytes. ABO incompatibility can cause HDFN even if fetal erythrocytes do not escape into the maternal circulation during pregnancy.

5. The key to treatment of HDFN resulting from Rh incompatibilities lies in prevention or immunoprophylaxis.

6. Sickle cell disease is a group of disorders characterized by the production of abnormal hemoglobin S (Hb S) within the erythrocytes. It is most common among people with ancestry from sub-Saharan Africa.

7. Sickle cell disease is an inherited, autosomal recessive disorder expressed as sickle cell anemia, sickle cell–thalassemia disease, or sickle cell–Hb C disease, depending on mode of inheritance. Sickle cell anemia, in which the individual is homozygous for Hb S, is the most severe. Sickle cell–thalassemia and sickle cell–Hb C disease are compound heterozygous forms in which the child inherits Hb S from one parent or another type of abnormal hemoglobin from the other parent. All forms of sickle cell disease are lifelong conditions.

8. Sickle cell trait, in which the child inherits Hb S from one parent and normal hemoglobin (Hb A) from the other, is a heterozygous carrier state that rarely has clinical manifestations.

9. Sickle cell disease causes a change in the shape of red blood cells into the sickle shape. Sickling is triggered by decreased oxygen or dehydration. Most sickled erythrocytes regain a normal shape after reoxygenation and rehydration.

10. The alpha- and beta-thalassemias are inherited autosomal recessive disorders. These conditions result in an impaired rate of synthesis of one of the two chains—α or β—of adult hemoglobin (Hb A).

Disorders of Coagulation and Platelets

1. Hemorrhagic diseases can be either inherited (hemophilias) or antibody-mediated (primary immune thrombocytopenia [ITP]).

2. The hemophilias are a group of inherited bleeding disorders resulting from mutations in coagulation factors.

3. Hemophilia A (factor VIII deficiency) and hemophilia B (factor IX deficiency) are caused by mutations in the genes coding for factors VIII and IX, factors essential in the coagulation cascade. Because factors VIII and IX function together, hemophilia A and B are clinically indistinguishable. Hemophilia A is the most common hereditary disease associated with life-threatening bleeding.

4. Hemophilias A and B are inherited as X-linked recessive conditions. Approximately one-third of cases, however, are the result of a spontaneous mutation in the involved gene.

5. The antibody-mediated hemorrhagic diseases are a group of disorders caused by the immune response. Antibody-mediated destruction of platelets or antibody-mediated inflammatory reactions to allergens damage blood vessels and cause seepage into tissues.

6. ITP is the most common disorder of platelet consumption in which antiplatelet antibodies bind to the plasma membranes of platelets. ITP results in platelet sequestration and destruction by mononuclear phagocytes at a rate that exceeds the ability of the bone marrow to produce them.

Neoplastic Disorders

1. Leukemia is cancer of the blood-forming tissues, such as the bone marrow, that most often produces abnormal white blood cells called leukemic cells.

2. About 75% of childhood leukemias are acute lymphoblastic leukemia (ALL). The remaining cases are classified as acute myeloid leukemia (AML) and related neoplasms. Chronic leukemias are rare in children.

3. The cause of most childhood cancer, including leukemia, is unknown. About 5% of all childhood cancers are caused by inherited mutations. Genetic mutations that predispose the child to cancer development can occur during fetal development.

4. Exposure to ionizing radiation can lead to the development of childhood leukemia and possible other cancers.

5. ALL causes dysregulation of the expression and function of transcription factors required for normal B-cell and T-cell development.

6. Epigenetic alterations are frequent in AML and have a central role in its development.

7. The onset of leukemia may be abrupt or insidious. The most common symptoms reflect consequences of bone marrow failure and can include decreased levels of red blood cells and platelets, as well as changes in white blood cells.

8. Lymphomas are proliferations of malignant lymphocytes that arise from discrete tissue masses. Lymphoid neoplasms involve some recognizable stage of lymphocyte B- or T-cell differentiation.

9. Some lymphomas occasionally have leukemic presentations, and evolution to leukemia is not unusual during the progression of incurable lymphoma.

10. The lymphomas of childhood are Hodgkin lymphoma (HL) and non-Hodgkin lymphoma (NHL).

11. NHLs are cancers of immune cells. Children with inherited or acquired immunodeficiency syndromes have an increased risk of developing NHL.

12. The most common types of NHL in children are Burkitt lymphoma, lymphoblastic lymphoma, and large cell lymphoma. Most Burkitt lymphomas are latently infected with the Epstein-Barr virus (EBV).

13. HL is a group of lymphoid cancers. HL arises in a single chain of lymph nodes and spreads first in a contiguous way to lymphoid tissue.

14. HL is characterized by the presence of Reed-Sternberg cells, which are large cells derived from the germinal center of B cells.

KEY TERMS

REFERENCES

1. Cerami C: Iron nutriture of the fetus, neonate, infant, and child, *Ann Nutr Metab* 71(Suppl 3):8-14, 2017.
2. Shah M, et al: Effect of orange and apple juice on iron absorption in children, *Arch Pediatr Adolesc Med* 157:1232-1236, 2003.
3. American College of Obstetricians and Gynecologists (ACOG) Committee on Practice Bulletins: Obstetrics, practice bulletin no 181: prevention of RhD alloimmunization, *Obstet Gynecol* 130:e57-e70, 2017.
4. McBain RD, et al: Anti-D Anti-D administration in pregnancy for preventing Rhesus alloimmunization, *Cochrane Database Syst Rev* (9):CD000020, 2015.
5. National Heart, Lung, & Blood Institute (NHLBI): Sickle cell disease. Available at: https://www.nhlbi.nih.gov/health-topics/sickle-cell-disease. (Accessed 9 October 2018).
6. DeBaun MR, Galadanci NA: Sickle cell disease in sub-Saharan Africa. UpToDate. Available at: https://www.uptodate.com/contents/sickle-cell-disease-in-sub-saharan-africa. Topic last updated April 23, 2018.
7. Fortin PM, et al: Red blood cell transfusion to treat or prevent complications in sickle cell disease: an overview of Cochrane reviews, *Cochrane Database Syst Rev* (8):CD012082, 2018.
8. Caocci G, et al: Long term survival of beta-thalassemia major patients treated with hematopoietic stem cell transplantation compared with survival with conventional treatment, *Am J Hematol* 92:1303-1310, 2017.
9. National Hemophilia Foundation (NHF): *Fast facts: about bleeding disordes,* New York, NY, 2018, Author. Available at: https://www.hemophilia.org/About-Us/Fast-Facts. (Accessed 18 October 2018).
10. Johnsen JM, et al: Novel approach to genetic analysis and results in 3000 hemophilia patients enrolled in the My Life, Our Future initiative, *Blood Adv* 1:824-834, 2017.
11. Wynn TT, Gumuscu B: Potential role of a new PEGylated recombinant factor VIII for hemophilia A, *J Blood Med* 7:121-128, 2016.
12. American Cancer Society (ACS): *What is childhood leukemia,* Atlanta, GA, 2018, Author. Available at: https://www.cancer.org/cancer/leukemia-in-children/about/what-is-childhood-leukemia.html. (Accessed 19 October 2018).
13. Timms JA, et al: DNA methylation as a potential mediator of environmental risks in the development of childhood acute lymphoblastic leukemia, *Epigenomics* 8:519-536, 2016.
14. Berrington de Gonzalez A, et al: Relationship between paediatric CT scans and subsequent risk of leukaemia and brain tumours: assessment of the impact of underlying conditions, *Br J Cancer* 114:388-394, 2016.
15. Baysson H, et al: Exposure to CT scans in childhood and long-term cancer risk: a review of epidemiological studies, *Bull Cancer* 103:190-198, 2016.
16. Kenney LB, et al: Improving male reproductive health after childhood, adolescent, and young adult cancer: progress and future directions for survivorship research, *J Clin Oncol* 36:2160-2168, 2018.
17. van Dorp W, et al: Reproductive function and outcomes in female survivors of childhood, adolescent, and young adult cancer: a review, *J Clin Oncol* 36:2169-2180, 2018.
18. Weimels JL, et al: GWAS in childhood acute lymphoblastic leukemia reveals novel genetic associations at chromosomes 17q12 and 8q24.21, *Nat Commun* 9(1):286, 2018.
19. Santiago R, et al: Novel therapy for childhood acute lymphoblastic leukemia, *Expert Opin Pharmacother* 18:1081-1099, 2017.
19a. PDQ® Pediatric Treatment Editorial Board: PDQ Childhood Acute Lymphoblastic Leukemia Treatment. Bethesda, MD: National Cancer Institute. Updated 23 July 2019. Available at: https://www.cancer.gov/types/leukemia/patient/child-all-treatment-pdq. (Accessed 9 August 2019). [PMID: 26389385].
20. National Cancer Institute (NCI): *PDQ® childhood acute lymphoblastic leukemia treatment,* Bethesda, Md, 2018, Author. Available at: http://cancer.gov/cancertopics/pdq/treatment/childALL/HealthProfessional. (Accessed 19 October 2018). Date last modified September 28, 2018.
21. National Cancer Institute (NCI): *PDQ® childhood acute myeloid leukemia/other myeloid malignancies treatment,* Bethesda, MD, 2018, Author. Available at: http://cancer.gov/cancertopics/pdq/treatment/childAML/HealthProfessional. (Accessed 17 October 2018). Date last modified August 28, 2018.
22. Swerdlow SH, et al: The 2016 revision of the World Health Organization classification of lymphoid neoplasms, *Blood* 127:2375-2390, 2016.
23. American Cancer Society (ACS): *What are the key statistics for non-Hodgkin lymphoma in children?* Atlanta, GA, 2017, Author. Available at: https://www.cancer.org/cancer/childhood-non-hodgkin-lymphoma/about/key-statistics.html. (Accessed 17 October 2018). Date last modified August 1, 2017.
24. National Cancer Institute (NCI): *PDQ® childhood non-Hodgkin lymphoma treatment,* Bethesda, MD, 2018, Author. Available at: https://www.cancer.gov/types/lymphoma/patient/child-nhl-treatment-pdq. (Accessed 19 October 2018). Last modified September 28, 2018.
25. Haberl S, et al: MYC rearranged B-cell neoplasms: impact of genetics on classification, *Cancer Genet* 209:431-439, 2016.
26. Naeini YB, et al: Aggressive B-cell lymphomas: frequency, immunophenotype, and genetics in a reference laboratory population, *Ann Diagn Pathol* 25:7-14, 2016.
27. Mbulaiteye SM, et al: Epstein-Barr virus patterns in U.S. Burkitt lymphoma tumors from the SEER Residual Tissue Repository during 1979-2009, *APMIS* 122:5-15, 2014.
28. Mata E, et al: Analysis of the mutational landscape of classic Hodgkin lymphoma identifies disease heterogeneity and potential therapeutic targets, *Oncotarget* 8:111386-111395, 2017.
29. Carbone A, et al: The impact of EBV and HIV infection on the microenvironmental niche underlying Hodgkin lymphoma pathogenesis, *Int J Cancer* 140:1233-1245, 2017.
30. Reichel J, et al: Flow sorting and exome sequencing reveal the oncogenome of primary Hodgkin and Reed-Sternberg cells, *Blood* 125:1061-1072, 2015.

25

Structure and Function of the Cardiovascular and Lymphatic Systems

Kathryn L. McCance

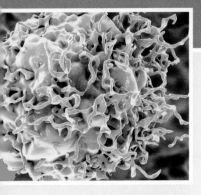

CHAPTER OUTLINE

The functions of the circulatory system include delivery of oxygen, nutrients, hormones, immune system components, and other substances to body tissues and removal of the waste products of metabolism. Delivery and removal are achieved by an extensive array of tubes—the blood and lymphatic vessels—connected to a pump—the heart. The heart continuously pumps blood through the blood vessels in collaboration with other systems, particularly the nervous and endocrine systems, which regulate the heart and blood vessels. Immune system components, nutrients, and oxygen are supplied by the immune, digestive, and respiratory systems; gaseous wastes of metabolism are expired through the lungs; and other wastes are removed by the kidneys and digestive tract.

The vascular endothelium also is a key component of the circulatory system and is sometimes considered a separate endocrine organ. This endothelium is a multifunctional tissue whose health is essential to normal vascular, immune, and hemostatic system function. Endothelial dysfunction is a critical factor in the development of vascular and other diseases.[1]

CIRCULATORY SYSTEM

The heart is composed of two conjoined pumps moving blood through two separate circulatory systems in sequence: one pump supplies blood to the lungs, whereas the second pump delivers blood to the rest of the body. Structures on the right side, or **right heart**, pump blood through the lungs. This system is termed the **pulmonary circulation** and is described in Chapter 28. The left side, or **left heart**, sends blood throughout the **systemic circulation**, which supplies all of the body

except the lungs (Fig. 25.1). These two systems are serially connected; thus the output of one becomes the input of the other.

Arteries carry blood from the heart to all parts of the body, where they branch into arterioles and even smaller vessels, ultimately becoming a fine meshwork of capillaries. Capillaries allow the closest contact and exchange between the blood and the interstitial space, or interstitium—the environment in which cells live. Venules and then veins next carry blood from the capillaries back to the heart. Some of the plasma or liquid part of the blood passes through the walls of the capillaries into the interstitial space. This fluid, lymph, is returned to the cardiovascular system by vessels of the lymphatic system. The lymphatic system is a critical component of the immune system as described in Chapters 6 and 7.

HEART

The adult heart is about the size of a fist and weighs between 200 and 350 grams. The heart lies obliquely (diagonally) in the mediastinum, the area above the diaphragm and between the lungs. Heart structures can be categorized by function:

1. *Structural support of heart tissues and circulation of pulmonary and systemic blood through the heart.* This category includes the heart wall and fibrous skeleton enclosing and supporting the heart and dividing it into four chambers; the valves directing flow through the chambers; and the great vessels conducting blood to and from the heart.
2. *Maintenance of cardiac metabolism.* This category includes all the vessels of the coronary circulation—the arteries and veins that serve

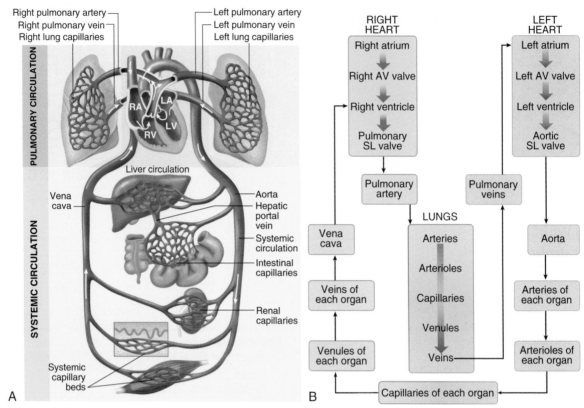

FIGURE 25.1 Diagram of the Pulmonary and Systemic Circulatory Systems and Flow Chart of the Direction of Blood Flow. A, The right heart pumps unoxygenated blood *(blue)* through the pulmonary circulation, where oxygen enters the blood and carbon dioxide is exhaled, and the left heart pumps oxygenated *(red)* blood to and from all the other organ systems in the body. **B,** Blood flow begins at the left ventricle of the heart; the blood flows to the arteries, arterioles, capillaries of each body organ, venules, veins, right atrium, right ventricle, pulmonary artery, lung capillaries, pulmonary veins, and left atrium and then returns to the left ventricle (**A** from Patton KT, Thibodeau GA, Douglas MM: *Essentials of anatomy & physiology,* St Louis, 2012, Elsevier. **B** adapted from Patton KT, Thibodeau GA: *The human body in health & disease,* ed 7, St Louis, 2018, Mosby).

the metabolic needs of all the heart cells—and the heart's lymphatic vessels.

3. *Stimulation and control of heart action.* Among these structures are the nerves and specialized muscle cells that direct the rhythmic contraction and relaxation of the heart muscles, propelling blood throughout the pulmonary and systemic circulatory systems.

Structures That Direct Circulation Through the Heart
Heart Wall

The three layers of the heart wall—the epicardium, myocardium, and endocardium—are enclosed in a double-walled membranous sac, the pericardium (Fig. 25.2, *B*). The pericardial sac has three main functions: it prevents displacement of the heart during gravitational acceleration or deceleration, it serves as a physical barrier to protect the heart against infection and inflammation coming from the lungs and pleural space, and it contains pain receptors and mechanoreceptors that can cause reflex changes in blood pressure and heart rate. The two layers of the pericardium, the parietal and the visceral pericardia (see Fig. 25.2), are separated by a fluid-containing space called the pericardial cavity. The pericardial fluid (about 20 ml) is secreted by cells of the mesothelial layer of the pericardium and lubricates the membranes that line the pericardial cavity, enabling them to slide smoothly over one another with minimal friction as the heart beats. The amount and character of

the pericardial fluid are altered if the pericardium is inflamed (see Chapter 26).

The smoothness of the outer layer of the heart, the epicardium, also minimizes the friction between the heart wall and the pericardial sac. The thickest layer of the heart wall, the myocardium, is composed of cardiac muscle and is anchored to the heart's fibrous skeleton. The heart muscle cells, cardiomyocytes, provide the contractile force needed for blood to flow through the heart and into the pulmonary and systemic circulations. About 0.5% to 1% of the cardiomyocytes are replaced annually; thus over a lifetime only about half of these muscle cells are replaced.[2] There is great interest in finding therapies that will increase the rate of cardiomyocyte replacement for persons who have suffered a myocardial infarction or have heart failure from another cause because the limited myocyte turnover is insufficient to restore contractile function.

The internal lining of the myocardium, the endocardium, is composed of connective tissue and squamous cells (see Fig. 25.2, *B*). This lining is continuous with the endothelium that lines all the arteries, veins, and capillaries of the body, creating a continuous, closed circulatory system.

Great Vessels

Blood moves into and out of the heart through several large veins and arteries (see Fig. 25.2). The right heart receives venous blood from the

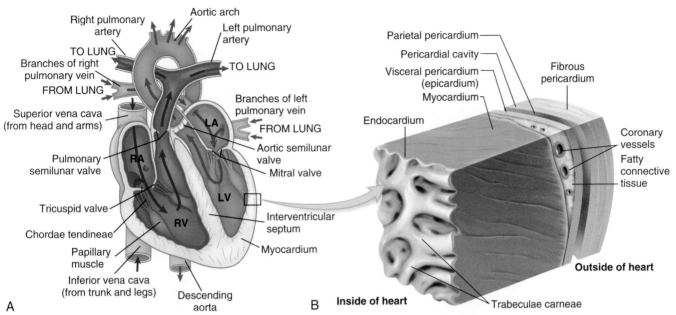

FIGURE 25.2 Structures That Direct Blood Flow Through the Heart and Wall of the Heart. A, The arrows indicate the path of blood through the chambers, valves, and major vessels. **B,** This section of the heart wall shows the fibrous pericardium, the parietal and visceral layers of the serous pericardium (with the pericardial space between them), the myocardium, and the endocardium. Note the fatty connective tissue between the visceral layer of the serous pericardium (epicardium) and the myocardium. Note also that the endocardium covers tubular projections of myocardial muscle tissue called *trabeculae.* (Revised from Applegate E: *The anatomy and physiology learning system,* ed 4, St Louis, 2011, Saunders.)

systemic circulation through the superior and inferior venae cavae, which join and then enter the right atrium. Blood leaving the right ventricle enters the pulmonary circulation through the pulmonary artery, which divides into right and left branches to transport deoxygenated blood from the right heart to the lungs. The pulmonary arteries branch further into the pulmonary capillary beds, where oxygen and carbon dioxide exchange occurs.

Four pulmonary veins, two from the right lung and two from the left lung, carry oxygenated blood from the lungs to the left side of the heart. The oxygenated blood moves through the left atrium and ventricle, out into the aorta that subsequently branches into the systemic arteries that supply the body.

Chambers of the Heart

The heart has four chambers: the left atrium, the right atrium, the right ventricle, and the left ventricle. These chambers form two pumps in series: the right heart is a low-pressure system pumping blood through the lungs, and the left heart is a high-pressure system pumping blood to the rest of the body (see Fig. 25.2, *A*). The atria are smaller than the ventricles and have thinner walls. The ventricles have a thicker myocardial layer and constitute much of the bulk of the heart. The ventricles are formed by a continuum of muscle fibers originating from the fibrous skeleton at the base of the heart.

The wall thickness of each cardiac chamber depends on the amount of pressure or resistance it must overcome to eject blood. The two atria have the thinnest walls because they are low-pressure chambers that serve as storage units and channels for blood that is emptied into the ventricles. Normally, there is little resistance to flow from the atria to the ventricles. The ventricles, on the other hand, must propel the blood all the way through the pulmonary or systemic vessels. The mean pulmonary artery pressure, the force the right ventricle must overcome, is only 15 mm Hg, whereas the mean arterial pressure the left ventricle

must pump against is about 92 mm Hg. Because the pressure is markedly higher in the systemic circulation, the wall of the left ventricle is about three times thicker than that of the right ventricle.

The right ventricle is shaped like a crescent or triangle, enabling a bellows-like action that efficiently ejects large volumes of blood through the pulmonary semilunar valve into the low-pressure pulmonary system. The larger left ventricle is bullet shaped, which allows it to generate enough pressure to eject blood through a relatively larger aortic semilunar valve into the high-pressure systemic circulation.

Blood normally does not flow between the chambers of the right and left sides of the heart. The atria are separated by the interatrial septum, and the ventricles by the interventricular septum. However, because the fetus does not depend on the lungs for oxygenation, there is an opening before birth between the right and left atria, called the *foramen ovale,* that facilitates circulation. This opening closes functionally at the time of birth as the higher pressure in the left atrium pushes a flap, the septum primum, over the hole. In 75% to 80% of infants these septa are permanently fused within the first year of life[3,4] (see Chapter 27).

Valves of the Heart

Four valves in the heart direct blood flow in one direction through the heart chambers (Fig. 25.3). The atrioventricular (AV) valves are termed such because they fall between the atria and ventricles. The AV valve openings are composed of tissue flaps called *leaflets* or *cusps,* which are attached at the upper margin to a ring in the heart's fibrous skeleton and by the chordae tendineae at the lower end to the papillary muscles (see Fig. 25.2, *A*). The papillary muscles, extensions of the myocardium, help hold the cusps together and downward at the onset of ventricular contraction, thus preventing their backward expulsion or prolapse into the atria. The AV valve in the right heart is called the tricuspid valve because it has three cusps. The left atrioventricular valve is a bicuspid

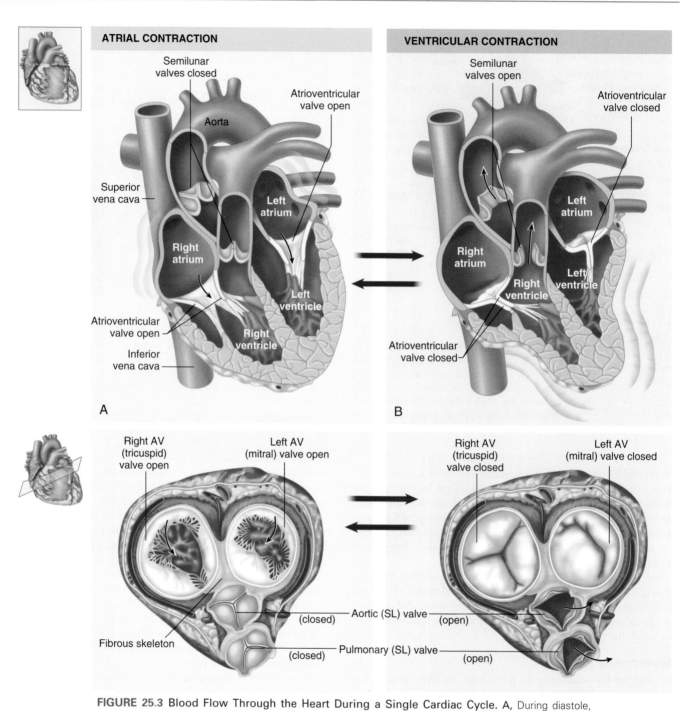

FIGURE 25.3 Blood Flow Through the Heart During a Single Cardiac Cycle. A, During diastole, blood flows into atria, the atrioventricular valves are pushed open, and blood begins to fill the ventricles. Atrial systole squeezes the blood remaining in the atria into the ventricles. **B,** During ventricular systole, the ventricles contract, pushing the blood out through the semilunar valves into the pulmonary artery (right ventricle) and the aorta (left ventricle). (From Patton KT, Thibodeau GA: *Structure & function of the body,* ed 15, St Louis, 2016, Elsevier.)

(two-cusp) valve called the mitral valve. The tricuspid and mitral valves function as a unit because the atria, fibrous rings, valvular tissue, chordae tendineae, papillary muscles, and ventricular walls are connected. Collectively, these six structures are known as the mitral and tricuspid complex. Damage to any one of the six components of this complex can alter function significantly and contribute to heart failure.

The other two valves in the heart are called the semilunar valves. These valves have three cup-shaped cusps that arise from the fibrous skeleton. Blood leaves the right ventricle through the pulmonary semilunar valve, and it leaves the left ventricle through the aortic semilunar valve (see Figs. 25.2 and 25.3).

Fibrous Skeleton of the Heart

Four rings of dense fibrous connective tissue provide a firm anchorage for the attachments of the atrial and ventricular musculature, as well as the valvular tissue (see Fig. 25.3). The fibrous rings are adjacent and form a central, fibrous supporting structure collectively termed the *annuli fibrosi cordis.*

Intracardiac Pressures

Four heart valves, four chambers, and the pressure gradients they maintain ensure that blood only flows one way through the heart. When the ventricles are relaxed, the two AV valves open and blood flows from the relatively higher pressure in the atria to the lower pressure in the ventricles. As the ventricles contract, ventricular pressure increases and causes these valves to close and prevent backflow into the atria. The semilunar valves of the heart open when intraventricular pressure exceeds aortic and pulmonary pressures, and blood flows out of the ventricles and into the pulmonary and systemic circulations. After ventricular contraction and ejection, intraventricular pressure decreases and the pulmonary and aortic semilunar valves close when the pressure in the vessels is greater than the pressure in the ventricles, thus preventing backflow into the right and left ventricles, respectively. The actions of the heart valves are shown in Figs. 25.2 and 25.3. Normal intracardiac pressures are shown in Table 25.1.

Blood Flow during the Cardiac Cycle

The pumping action of the heart consists of contraction and relaxation of the heart muscle, or myocardium. Each ventricular contraction and the relaxation that follows it constitute one cardiac cycle. (Blood flow through the heart during a single cardiac cycle is illustrated in Fig. 25.3.) During the period of relaxation, termed diastole, blood fills the ventricles. The ventricular contraction that follows, termed systole, propels the blood out of the ventricles and into the pulmonary and systemic circulations. Contraction of the left ventricle occurs slightly earlier than contraction of the right ventricle.

The five phases of the cardiac cycle are said to begin with the opening of the mitral and tricuspid valves and atrial contraction (Figs. 25.4 and 25.5). Closing of the mitral and tricuspid valves as passive ventricular filling begins marks the end of one cardiac cycle.

✔ **QUICK CHECK 25.1**
1. Why are the two separate circulatory systems said to be "serially connected"?
2. What are the functions of the pericardial sac?
3. Why is the thickness of the myocardium different in the right and left ventricles?
4. Trace the flow of blood through the heart during one cardiac cycle.

Structures That Support Cardiac Metabolism: Coronary Circulation

The myocardium and other heart structures are supplied with oxygen and nutrients by the coronary circulation, which is the part of the systemic circulation that occurs within the blood vessels of the heart

muscles. The coronary arteries originate at the upper edge of the aortic semilunar valve cusps (Fig. 25.6, *A* and *B*) and receive blood through openings in the aorta called the coronary ostia. The cardiac veins empty into the right atrium through another ostium, the opening of a large vein called the coronary sinus (see Fig. 25.6, *C*). (The Regulation of the Coronary Circulation section describes the regulation of this mechanism, which is similar to regulation of flow through systemic and pulmonary vessels.)

Coronary Arteries

The major coronary arteries, the right coronary artery (RCA) and the left coronary artery (LCA) (see Fig. 25.6, *A*), traverse the epicardium, myocardium, and endocardium and branch to become arterioles and then capillaries. The LCA arises from a single ostium behind the left cusp of the aortic semilunar valve. It generally divides into the left anterior descending (LAD) artery, or anterior interventricular artery

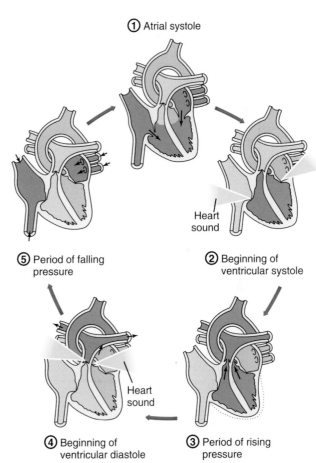

① Atrial systole

⑤ Period of falling pressure

Heart sound

② Beginning of ventricular systole

Heart sound

④ Beginning of ventricular diastole

③ Period of rising pressure

FIGURE 25.4 The Five Phases of the Cardiac Cycle. 1, Atrial systole. The atria contract, pushing blood through the open tricuspid and mitral valves into the ventricles. The semilunar valves are closed. **2,** Beginning of ventricular systole. The ventricles contract, increasing pressure within the ventricles. The tricuspid and mitral valves close, causing the first heart sound. **3,** Period of rising pressure. The semilunar valves open when pressure in the ventricle exceeds that in the arteries. Blood spurts into the aorta and pulmonary arteries. **4,** Beginning of ventricular diastole. Pressure in the relaxing ventricles drops below that in the arteries. The semilunar valves snap shut, causing the second heart sound. **5,** Period of falling pressure. Blood flows from the veins into the relaxed atria. The tricuspid and mitral valves open when pressure in the ventricles falls below that in the atria. (Adapted from Solomon E: *Introduction to human anatomy and physiology*, ed 4, St Louis, 2016, Saunders.)

TABLE 25.1	**Normal Intracardiac Pressures**	
	Mean (mm Hg)	**Range (mm Hg)**
Right atrium	4	0-8
Right Ventricle		
Systolic	24	15-28
End-diastolic	4	0-8
Left atrium	7	4-12
Left Ventricle		
Systolic	130	90-140
End-diastolic	7	4-12

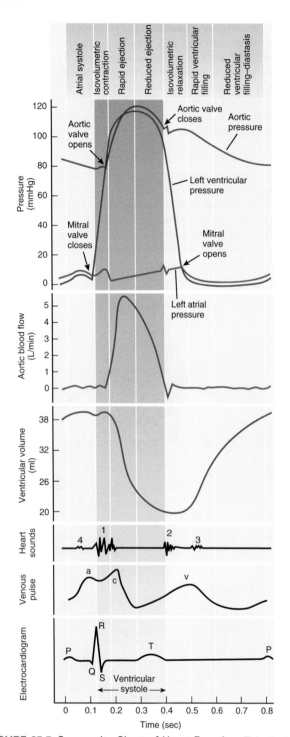

FIGURE 25.5 Composite Chart of Heart Function. This chart is a composite of several diagrams of heart function (cardiac pumping cycle, blood pressure, blood flow, volume, heart sounds, venous pulse, and an electrocardiogram [ECG]), all on the same time scale.

(supplies blood to portions of the left and right ventricles and much of the interventricular septum), and the circumflex artery (supplies blood to the left atrium and the lateral wall of the left ventricle). The RCA originates from an ostium behind the right aortic cusp. It branches into the conus (supplies blood to the upper right ventricle), right marginal branch (supplies the right ventricle to the apex), and posterior descending branch (supplies smaller branches to both ventricles). Because women's

hearts weigh proportionally less than men's hearts, the coronary arteries are smaller in women.

Collateral Arteries

Collateral arteries are connections, or *anastomoses*, between branches of the same coronary artery or connections of branches of the right coronary artery with branches of the left. The epicardium contains more collateral vessels than the endocardium. New collateral vessels are formed through two processes: arteriogenesis (new artery growth branching from preexisting arteries) and angiogenesis (growth of new capillaries within a tissue). This collateral growth is stimulated by shear stress, an increased blood flow speed within and just beyond areas of stenosis, or narrowing, as well as the production of growth factors and cytokines. The collateral circulation assists in supplying blood and oxygen to myocardium that has become ischemic following gradual stenosis of one or more major coronary arteries (coronary artery disease). Unfortunately, diabetes, which predisposes to coronary artery disease, also impedes collateral formation because of increased production of antiangiogenic factors, such as endostatin and angiostatin.

Coronary Capillaries

The heart requires an extensive capillary network to function. Blood travels from the arteries to the arterioles and then into the capillaries, where oxygen and other nutrients enter the myocardium while waste products enter the blood. At rest, the heart extracts 70% to 80% of the oxygen delivered to it, and coronary blood flow is directly correlated with myocardial oxygen consumption. Any alteration of the cardiac muscles dramatically affects blood flow in the capillaries.

Coronary Veins and Lymphatic Vessels

After passing through the capillary network, blood from the coronary arteries drains into the cardiac veins located alongside the arteries. Most of the venous drainage of the heart occurs through veins in the visceral pericardium. The veins then feed into the great cardiac vein and coronary sinus on the posterior surface of the heart, between the atria and ventricles, in the coronary sulcus (see Fig. 25.6, *C*).

There is an extensive system of lymphatic capillaries and collecting vessels within the layers of the myocardium and the valves. With cardiac contraction, the lymphatic vessels drain fluid to lymph nodes in the anterior mediastinum that empty into the superior vena cava. The lymphatics are important for protecting the myocardium against infection and injury.

Structures That Control Heart Action

Life depends on continuous repetition of the cardiac cycle (systole and diastole), which requires the transmission of electrical impulses, termed cardiac action potentials, through the myocardium.[5] (Action potentials are described in Chapters 1 and 5.) The muscle fibers of the myocardium are electrically coupled so that action potentials pass from cell to cell rapidly and efficiently.

The myocardium contains its own conduction system—a collection of specialized cells that enable the myocardium to generate and transmit action potentials without input from the nervous system (Fig. 25.7). Cells that initiate signals are called pacemakers. The pacemaker cells are concentrated at two sites in the myocardium, called *nodes*: the sinoatrial node and the atrioventricular node. The cardiac cycle is stimulated by these nodes of specialized cells. Although the heart is innervated by the autonomic nervous system (both sympathetic and parasympathetic fibers), neural impulses are not needed to maintain the cardiac cycle. Thus the heart will beat in the absence of any innervation, one of the many factors that allow heart transplantation to be successful.

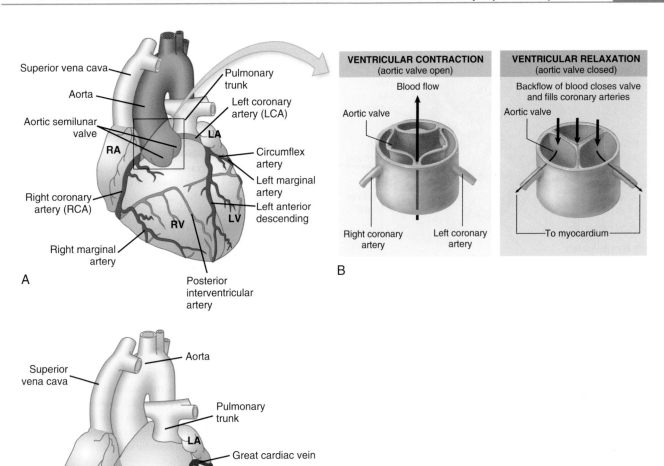

FIGURE 25.6 Coronary Circulation. A, Arteries. **B,** Coronary artery openings from the aorta. **C,** Veins. Both **A** and **C** are anterior views of the heart. Vessels near the anterior surface are more darkly colored than vessels of the posterior surface seen through the heart. (**A** and **C** from Patton KT, Thibodeau GA: *Anatomy & physiology,* ed 7, St Louis, 2010, Mosby. **B,** Patton KT, Thibodeau GA: *The human body in health & disease,* ed 6, St Louis, 2014, Mosby.)

Heart action is also influenced by substances delivered to the myocardium in coronary blood. Nutrients and oxygen are needed for cellular survival and normal function. Hormones and biochemical substances, including medications, can affect the strength and duration of myocardial contraction and the degree and duration of myocardial relaxation. Normal or appropriate function depends on the supply of these substances, which is why coronary artery disease can seriously disrupt heart function.

Conduction System

Normally, electrical impulses arise in the sinoatrial (SA) node (sinus node), the usual pacemaker of the heart. The SA node is located at the junction of the right atrium and superior vena cava, just superior to the tricuspid valve. The SA node is heavily innervated by both sympathetic and parasympathetic nerve fibers.[6] In the resting adult the SA node generates about 60 to 100 action potentials per minute, depending on the age and physical condition of the person. Each action potential travels rapidly from cell to cell and through the atrial myocardium, carrying the action potential onward to the

atrioventricular (AV) node, as well as causing both atria to contract, beginning systole.[6]

The AV node, located in the right atrial wall superior to the tricuspid valve and anterior to the ostium of the coronary sinus, conducts the action potentials onward to the ventricles. It is innervated by nerves from the autonomic parasympathetic ganglia that serve as receptors for the vagus nerve and cause slowing of impulse conduction through the AV node.

Conducting fibers from the AV node converge to form the bundle of His (atrioventricular bundle), within the posterior border of the interventricular septum. The bundle of His then gives rise to the right and left bundle branches. The right bundle branch (RBB) is thin and travels without much branching to the right ventricular apex. Because of its thinness and relative lack of branches, the RBB is susceptible to interruption of impulse conduction by damage to the endocardium. The left bundle branch (LBB) divides into two branches, or fascicles. The left anterior bundle branch (LABB) passes the left anterior papillary muscle and the base of the left ventricle and crosses the aortic outflow tract. Damage to the aortic valve or the left ventricle can interrupt this

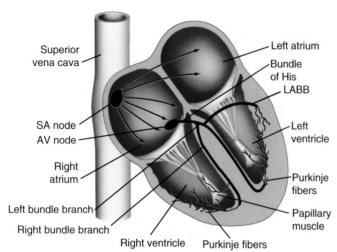

FIGURE 25.7 The Cardiac Conduction System. Specialized cardiac muscle cells in the heart wall rapidly conduct an electrical impulse throughout the myocardium. The signal is initiated by the sinoatrial (SA) node (pacemaker) and spreads through the atrial myocardium to the atrioventricular (AV) node. The AV node then initiates a signal that is conducted through the ventricular myocardium by way of the atrioventricular bundle (of His) and Purkinje fibers. (From Koeppen BM, editor: *Berne & Levy physiology,* ed 6, St Louis, 2010, Mosby.)

branch. The left posterior bundle branch (LPBB) travels posteriorly, crossing the left ventricular inflow tract to the base of the left posterior papillary muscle. This branch spreads diffusely through the posterior inferior left ventricular wall. Blood flow through this portion of the left ventricle is relatively nonturbulent, so the LBB is somewhat protected from injury caused by wear and tear.

The Purkinje fibers are the terminal branches of the RBB and LBB. They extend from the ventricular apexes to the fibrous rings and penetrate the heart wall to the outer myocardium. The first areas of the ventricles to be excited are portions of the interventricular septum. The septum is activated from both the RBB and the LBB. The extensive network of Purkinje fibers promotes the rapid spread of the impulse to the ventricular apexes. The basal and posterior portions of the ventricles are the last to be activated.

Propagation of cardiac action potentials. Electrical activation of the muscle cells, termed depolarization, is caused by the movement of ions, including sodium, potassium, calcium, and chloride, across cardiac cell membranes. Deactivation, called repolarization, occurs the same way. (Movement of ions across cell membranes is described in Chapter 1; electrical activation of muscle cells is described in Chapter 40.)

Movement of ions into and out of the cell creates an electrical (voltage) difference across the cell membrane, called the *membrane potential.* During depolarization, the inside of the cell becomes less negatively charged as positive ions move inside. In cardiac cells, as in other excitable cells, when the resting membrane potential (in millivolts) becomes less negative with depolarization and reaches the threshold potential for cardiac cells, a cardiac action potential is fired. The various phases of the cardiac action potential are related to changes in the permeability of the cell membrane to sodium, potassium, chloride, and calcium. *Threshold* is the point at which the cell membrane's selective permeability to these ions is temporarily disrupted, leading to an "all or nothing" depolarization. Drugs that alter the movement of these ions (e.g., calcium) have profound effects on the action potential and can alter heart rate. If the resting membrane potential becomes more

negative because of a decrease in the extracellular potassium concentration (hypokalemia), it is termed *hyperpolarization.*

Refractory periods, during which no new cardiac action potential can be initiated by a normal stimulus, follow depolarization. Abnormal refractory periods as a result of disease can cause abnormal heart rhythms or dysrhythmias, including ventricular fibrillation and cardiac arrest (see Chapter 26).

The electrocardiogram. An electrocardiogram originates from myocardial cell electrical activity as recorded by skin electrodes and is the summation of all the cardiac action potentials (Fig. 25.8). The P wave represents atrial depolarization. The PR interval is a measure of time from the onset of atrial activation to the onset of ventricular activation. The PR interval represents the time necessary for electrical activity to travel from the sinus node through the atrium, AV node, and His-Purkinje system to activate ventricular myocardial cells. The QRS complex represents the sum of all ventricular muscle cell depolarization. The configuration and amplitude of the QRS complex may vary considerably among individuals. During the ST interval, the entire ventricular myocardium is depolarized. The QT interval is sometimes called the "electrical systole" of the ventricles but the time it takes varies inversely with the heart rate. The T wave represents ventricular repolarization.

Automaticity. Automaticity, or the property of generating spontaneous depolarization to threshold, enables the SA and AV nodes to generate cardiac action potentials without any external stimulus. Cells capable of spontaneous depolarization are called automatic cells. The automatic cells of the cardiac conduction system can stimulate the heart to beat even when it is transplanted and thus has no innervation. Spontaneous depolarization is possible in automatic cells because the membrane potential of these special cells does not actually "rest" during return to the resting membrane potential. Instead, it slowly depolarizes toward threshold during the diastolic phase of the cardiac cycle. Because threshold is approached during diastole, return to the resting membrane potential in automatic cells is called diastolic depolarization. The electrical impulse normally begins in the SA node because its cells depolarize more rapidly than other automatic cells.

Rhythmicity. Rhythmicity is the regular generation of an action potential by the heart's conduction system. The SA node sets the pace because normally it has the fastest rate. The SA node depolarizes spontaneously 60 to 100 times per minute. If the SA node is damaged, the AV node can become the heart's pacemaker at a rate of about 40 to 60 spontaneous depolarizations per minute. Eventually, however, conduction cells in the atria usually take over from the AV node. Purkinje fibers are capable of spontaneous depolarization but at an even slower rate than the AV node.

✔ **QUICK CHECK 25.2**
1. Describe the structures and importance of coronary circulation.
2. What are the pathways of conduction through the heart?
3. What do the P wave, QRS complex, and T wave on the electrocardiogram represent?
4. Define automaticity and rhythmicity.

Cardiac Innervation: Sympathetic and Parasympathetic Nerves

Although the heart's nodes and conduction system are able to generate action potentials independently, the autonomic nervous system influences both the *rate* of impulse generation (firing), depolarization, and repolarization of the myocardium; and the *strength* of atrial and

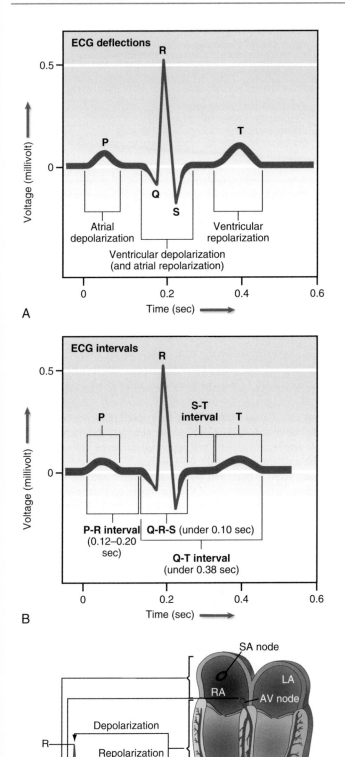

FIGURE 25.8 Electrocardiogram (ECG) and Cardiac Electrical Activity. A, Normal ECG. Depolarization and repolarization. **B,** ECG intervals among P, QRS, and T waves. **C,** Schematic representation of ECG and its relationship to cardiac electrical activity. *AV,* Atrioventricular; *LA,* left atrium; *LBB,* left bundle branch; *LV,* left ventricle; *RA,* right atrium; *RBB,* right bundle branch; *RV,* right ventricle.

ventricular contraction. Autonomic neural transmission produces changes in the heart and circulatory system faster than metabolic or humoral agents. Speed is important, for example, in stimulating the heart to increase its pumping action with increased physical activity or during times of stress and fear—the so-called fight or flight response. Although increased delivery of oxygen, glucose, hormones, and other blood-borne factors sustains increased cardiac activity, the rapid initiation of increased activity depends on the sympathetic and parasympathetic fibers of the autonomic nervous system.

Sympathetic and parasympathetic nerve fibers innervate all parts of the atria and ventricles and the SA and AV nodes. In general, sympathetic stimulation increases electrical conductivity and the strength of myocardial contraction, and vagal parasympathetic nerve activity does the opposite, slowing the conduction of action potentials through the heart and reducing the strength of contraction. Thus the sympathetic and parasympathetic nerves affect the speed of the cardiac cycle (**heart rate**, or beats per minute) (Fig. 25.9). Sympathetic nervous activity enhances myocardial performance. Stimulation of the SA node by the sympathetic nervous system rapidly increases heart rate. The sympathetic nervous system may also induce an increased influx of calcium (Ca^{2+}), which increases the contractile strength of the heart and the speed of electrical impulses through the heart muscle and the nodes. Finally, sympathetic nerves influence the diameter of the coronary vessels. Increased sympathetic discharge dilates the coronary vessels by causing the release of vasodilating metabolites resulting from increased myocardial contraction.

The parasympathetic nervous system affects the heart through the vagus nerve, which releases acetylcholine. Acetylcholine causes a decreased heart rate and slows conduction through the AV node.

Myocardial Cells

Cardiomyocytes are composed of long, narrow fibers that contain bundles of longitudinally arranged myofibrils; a nucleus; mitochondria; an internal membrane system (the sarcoplasmic reticulum); cytoplasm (sarcoplasm); and a plasma membrane (the sarcolemma), which encloses the cell (Fig. 25.10). Cardiac and skeletal muscle cells also have an "external" membrane system made up of transverse tubules (T tubules) formed by inward pouching of the sarcolemma. The sarcoplasmic reticulum forms a network of channels that surrounds the muscle fiber.

Because the myofibrils in both cardiac and skeletal fibers consist of alternating light and dark bands of protein, the fibers appear striped, or striated. The dark and light bands of the myofibrils create repeating longitudinal units, called *sarcomeres*, which are between 1.6 and 2.2 μm long (Fig. 25.11). The length of these sarcomeres determines the limits of myocardial stretch at the end of diastole and subsequently the force of contraction during systole. Alterations in sarcomere size are seen in both physiologic and pathologic myocardial hypertrophy.

There are a number of differences between cardiac and muscle cells. Cardiac cells are arranged in branching networks throughout the myocardium, whereas skeletal muscle cells tend to be arranged in parallel units throughout the length of the muscle. Cardiac fibers have only one nucleus, whereas skeletal muscle cells have many nuclei. Differences between cardiac and skeletal muscle often relate to heart function. Some of these functions include:

1. *Transmit action potentials quickly from cell to cell.* Electrical impulses are transmitted rapidly from cardiac fiber to cardiac fiber because the network of fibers connects at **intercalated disks**, which are thickened portions of the sarcolemma. The intercalated disks contain three junctions: desmosomes, or macula adherens; fascia adherens, which mechanically attach one cell to another; and gap junctions,

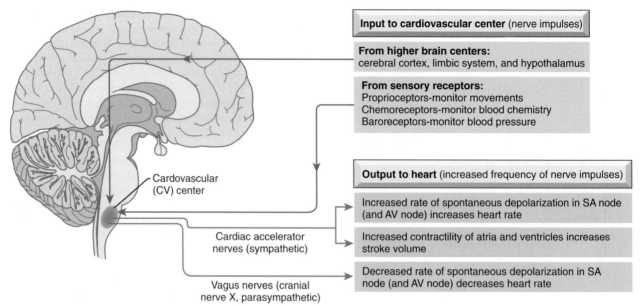

FIGURE 25.9 Autonomic Innervation of the Cardiovascular System. Input to the cardiovascular center and output to the heart.

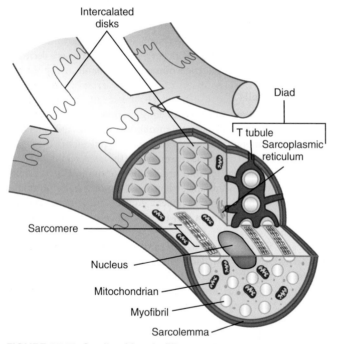

FIGURE 25.10 Cardiac Muscle Fiber. Unlike other types of muscle fibers, cardiac muscle fibers are typically branched with junctions, called *intercalated disks*, between adjacent myocytes. Like skeletal muscle cells, cardiac muscle cells contain sarcoplasmic reticula and T tubules, although these structures are not as highly organized as in skeletal muscle fibers.

which allow the electrical impulse to spread from cell to cell through a low-resistance pathway (see Chapter 1). Changes in the function of these junctional elements may cause an increased risk of arrhythmias.[6]

2. *Maintain high levels of energy synthesis.* Unlike skeletal muscle, the heart cannot rest and is in constant need of energy, which is supplied by molecules such as adenosine triphosphate (ATP). Therefore, the cytoplasm surrounding the bundles of myofibrils in each

cardiomyocyte contains a large number of mitochondria (25% to 35% of cell volume, versus 3% to 8% of cell volume in skeletal muscle). Cardiac muscle cells have more mitochondria than do skeletal muscle cells to provide the necessary respiratory enzymes for aerobic metabolism and supply quantities of ATP sufficient for the constant action of the myocardium.[7]

3. *Gain access to more ions, particularly sodium and potassium, in the extracellular environment.* Cardiac fibers contain more T tubules than do skeletal muscle fibers (see Fig. 25.10). This increased closeness to the T tubules gives each myofibril in the myocardium faster access to molecules needed for the transmission of action potentials, a process that involves transport of sodium and potassium through the walls of the T tubules. Because the T tubule system is continuous with the extracellular space and the interstitial fluid, it facilitates the rapid transmission of the electrical impulses from the surface of the sarcolemma to the myofibrils inside the fiber. This rapid transmission activates all the myofibrils of one fiber simultaneously. The sarcoplasmic reticulum is located around the myofibrils. As an action potential is transmitted through the T tubules, it induces the sarcoplasmic reticulum to release its stored calcium, thus activating the contractile proteins actin and myosin.

The sarcomere. Within each myocardial sarcomere are myosin and actin molecules that are grouped together to form filaments. Myosin molecules resemble golf clubs with two large, ovoid heads at one end of the shaft (see Fig. 25.11, *B*). About 200 myosin molecules are bundled together with their heads facing outward, forming a single thick filament. Actin molecules resemble beads, and they are strung into two chains that wind around each other, forming a thin filament. A tropomyosin molecule (a relaxing protein) lies alongside actin molecules. Troponin, another relaxing protein, associates with the tropomyosin molecule. The sarcomere also contains a giant elastic protein, titin, which attaches myosin to the Z line, acts as a spring, and influences myocardial stiffness.[7] The titin structure affects myocardial diastolic filling and has been found to play a role in heart failure.[8]

Where thick filaments overlap with thin filaments, a central dark band is formed, called the A band (see Fig. 25.11, *A*). The light bands of the sarcomere, called I bands, contain only actin molecules and no myosin. The center of the sarcomere is a less dense region called the

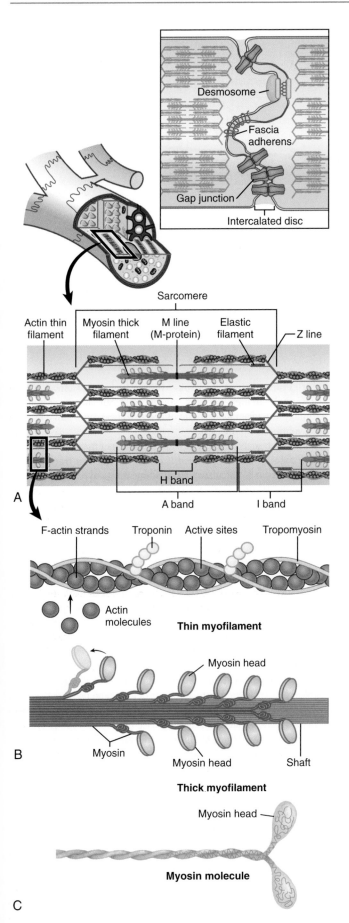

FIGURE 25.11 Structure of a Sarcomere, Myofilaments, and Myosin. A, The sarcomere is the basic contractile unit of a muscle cell. The Z disk is the anchor for the contractile elements actin and myosin. Actin attaches directly to the Z disk, whereas myosin is attached to it by elastic titin filaments. The myosin filaments are connected to each other by M-protein at the M line. The A, H, and I bands refer to parts of the sarcomere as they were originally seen by light microscopy. **B,** Thin myofilaments and thick myofilament. **C,** Mysosin molecule.

H band, which contains only myosin molecules and no actin. Thick filaments are held together by M-protein molecules that form a central thin, dark **M line.**[7] Thin filaments of actin extend from each side of the **Z line,** a dense fibrous structure at the center of each I band. The area from one Z line to the next Z line defines one **sarcomere.**

Myocardial metabolism. Cardiomyocytes depend on the constant production of ATP, which is synthesized within the mitochondria mainly from glucose, fatty acids, and lactate. If the myocardium is underperfused because of coronary artery disease, anaerobic metabolism must be used for energy (see Chapter 1). Energy produced by metabolic processes fuels muscle contraction and relaxation, electrical excitation, membrane transport, and synthesis of large molecules. Normally, the amount of ATP produced supplies sufficient energy to pump blood throughout the system.

Cardiac work is expressed as **myocardial oxygen consumption** ($M\dot{V}O_2$), which is closely correlated with total cardiac energy requirements. The $M\dot{V}O_2$ is determined by three major factors: (1) the amount of wall stress during systole, estimated by measuring the systolic blood pressure; (2) the duration of systolic wall tension, measured indirectly by the heart rate; and (3) the contractile state of the myocardium, which is not measured clinically.

The coronary arteries deliver oxygen (O_2) to the myocardium. Approximately 70% to 75% of this O_2 is used immediately by cardiac muscle, leaving little O_2 in reserve. Because the O_2 content of the blood and the amount of O_2 extracted from the blood cannot be increased under normal circumstances, any increased energy needs can be met only by increasing coronary blood flow. The $M\dot{V}O_2$ increases with exercise and decreases with hypotension and hypothermia. As myocardial metabolism and consumption of O_2 increase, the local concentration of local vasoactive metabolic factors increases. Some of these, such as adenosine, nitric oxide, and prostaglandins, dilate coronary arterioles, thus increasing coronary blood flow.[9]

Myocardial Contraction and Relaxation

Myocardial contractility is a change in developed tension at a given resting fiber length, which basically is the ability of the heart muscle to shorten. Each sarcomere serves as the basic contractile unit of a muscle cell. The outward-facing heads of myosin molecules are called *cross-bridges* because they can form force-generating bridges by binding with exposed actin molecules. Once bound, the myosin molecules effectively pull the thin filaments toward the center of the sarcomere, shortening the sarcomere and resulting in contraction. This process is known as the **cross-bridge theory of muscle contraction** (Fig. 25.12). The degree of shortening depends on the amount of overlap between the thick and thin filaments.

Calcium and excitation-contraction coupling. Excitation-contraction coupling is the process by which an action potential arriving at the muscle fiber plasma membrane triggers the cycle, leading to cross-bridge formation and contraction. Cycle activation depends on

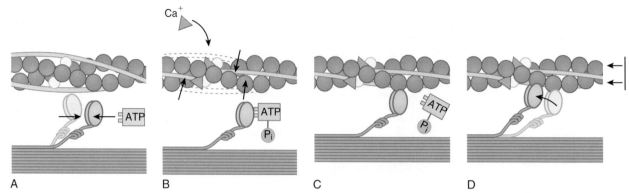

FIGURE 25.12 Cross-Bridge Theory of Muscle Contraction. A, Each myosin cross-bridge in the thick filament moves into a resting position after an adenosine triphosphate (ATP) molecule binds and transfers its energy. **B,** Calcium ions released from the sarcoplasmic reticulum bind to troponin in the thin filament, allowing tropomyosin to shift from its position blocking the active sites of actin molecules. **C,** Each myosin cross-bridge then binds to an active site on a thin filament, displacing the remnants of ATP hydrolysis—adenosine diphosphate (ADP) and inorganic phosphate (Pi). **D,** The release of stored energy from step A provides the force needed for each cross-bridge to move back to its original position, pulling actin along with it. Each cross-bridge will remain bound to actin until another ATP molecule binds to it and pulls it back into its resting position (**A**). (Adapted from Thibodeau GA, Patton KT: *Anatomy & physiology,* ed 4, St Louis, 1999, Mosby.)

calcium availability, and the amount of force developed is regulated by how much the concentration of calcium ions increases within the cardiomyocytes. Calcium enters the myocardial cell from the interstitial fluid after electrical excitation that increases membrane calcium permeability. Calcium entering the cell triggers the release of additional calcium from the two storage sites within the sarcomere. Calcium ions then diffuse toward the myofibrils, where they bind with troponin.

The calcium-troponin complex interaction facilitates the contraction process. In the resting state, troponin is bound to actin and the tropomyosin molecule covers the sites where the myosin heads bind to actin, thereby preventing interaction between actin and myosin. Calcium binds to troponin, which ultimately results in tropomyosin moving troponin, thus uncovering the binding sites. Myosin and actin can now form cross-bridges, and ATP can be dephosphorylated to adenosine diphosphate (ADP). Under these circumstances, sliding of the thick and thin filaments can occur, and the muscle contracts.[7]

Myocardial relaxation. Relaxation is as vital to optimal cardiac function as contraction; and calcium, troponin, and tropomyosin also facilitate relaxation. After contraction, free calcium ions are actively pumped out of the cell back into the interstitial fluid or taken back into storage by the sarcoplasmic reticulum and tubule system. As the concentration of calcium within the sarcomere decreases, troponin releases its bound calcium. The tropomyosin complex moves and blocks the active sites on the actin molecule, preventing cross-bridge formation with the myosin heads. If the ability of the myocardium to relax is impaired, it can lead to increased diastolic filling pressures and eventually heart failure.[10]

> ✔ **QUICK CHECK 25.3**
> 1. What features distinguish myocardial cells from skeletal cells?
> 2. Describe the interactions of actin and myosin in controlling heart function.
> 3. Define excitation-contraction coupling.

Factors Affecting Cardiac Output

Cardiac performance can be evaluated by measuring the cardiac output. Cardiac output is calculated by multiplying the heart rate in beats per

minute (beats/min) by the stroke volume (volume of blood ejected during systole) in liters per beat. Normal adult cardiac output is about 5 L/min at rest, given a heart rate of about 70 beats/min and a normal stroke volume of about 70 ml.

With each heartbeat, the ventricles eject much of their blood volume, and the amount ejected per beat is called the ejection fraction. The ejection fraction is calculated by dividing the stroke volume by the end-diastolic volume. The end-diastolic volume of the normal ventricle is about 70 to 80 ml/m^2, and the normal ejection fraction of the resting heart, measured with gated myocardial perfusion imaging, was 66% ± 8% for women and 58% ± 8% for men.[11]

The ejection fraction is increased by factors that increase contractility, such as increased sympathetic nervous system activity. A decrease in the ejection fraction may indicate ventricular failure. The effects of aging on cardiovascular function are summarized in Table 25.2.

The factors that determine cardiac output are (1) preload, (2) afterload, (3) myocardial contractility, and (4) heart rate. Preload, afterload, and contractility all affect stroke volume (Fig. 25.13).

Preload

Preload is the volume and pressure inside the ventricle at the end of diastole (ventricular end-diastolic volume [VEDV] and pressure [VEDP]). Preload is determined by two primary factors: (1) the amount of blood left in the ventricle after systole (end-systolic volume) and (2) the amount of venous blood returning to the ventricle during diastole. *End-systolic volume* is dependent on the strength of ventricular contraction and the resistance to ventricular emptying. *Venous return* is dependent on blood volume and flow through the venous system and the atrioventricular valves. Clinically, preload is estimated by measuring the central venous pressure (CVP) for the right side of the heart and the pulmonary artery wedge pressure (cross-sectional pressure) for the left side. Normal values for these two estimates are 1 to 5 mm Hg and 4 to 12 mm Hg, respectively.[12]

The Laplace law states that wall tension generated in the wall of the ventricle (or any chamber or vessel) to produce a given intraventricular pressure depends directly on ventricular size (internal radius) and inversely on ventricular wall thickness. The VEDV, which determines the size of the ventricle and the stretch of the cardiac muscle fibers, therefore affects the tension (or force) for contraction. The Frank-Starling law of the heart indicates that the volume of blood in the heart at the end of diastole, as the volume determines the length of its muscle fibers, is directly related to the force of contraction during the next systole. Muscle fibers have an optimal resting length from which to generate the maximum amount of contractile strength. Within a physiologic range of muscle stretching, increased preload increases stroke volume (and therefore cardiac output and stroke work) (Fig. 25.14, curve *B*). Excessive ventricular filling and preload (increased VEDV) stretches the heart muscle beyond optimal length, and stroke volume begins to fall. Factors that increase contractility cause the heart to operate on a higher length-tension curve (see Fig. 25.14, curve *A*). Factors that decrease contractility cause the heart to operate at a lower length-tension curve (see Fig. 25.14, curve *C*).

Increases in preload (VEDV) may not only cause a decline in stroke volume, but also result in increases in the VEDP. These changes can lead to heart failure (see Chapter 26). An increased VEDP causes pressures to increase, or "back up," into the pulmonary or systemic venous circulation, thus increasing the movement of plasma out through vessel walls, causing fluid to accumulate in lung tissues (pulmonary edema; see Chapter 29) or in peripheral tissues (peripheral edema).

Afterload

Ventricular afterload is the resistance to ejection of blood from the ventricle. It is the load the muscle must move during contraction. The aortic systolic pressure is an index of afterload. Pressure in the ventricle must exceed the aortic pressure before blood can be pumped out during

Determinant	Resting Cardiac Performance	Exercise Cardiac Performance*
Cardiac output	Unchanged	Decreases because of a decrease in maximum heart rate
Heart rate	Slight decrease	Increases less than in younger people
Stroke volume	Slight increase	No change
Ejection fraction	Unchanged	Decreased
Afterload	Increased	Increased
End-diastolic volume	Unchanged	Increased
End-systolic volume	Unchanged	Increased
Contraction	Decreased velocity	Decreased
Myocardial wall stiffness	Increased	Increased
Maximum oxygen consumption	Not applicable	Decreased
Plasma catecholamines	—	Increased

TABLE 25.2   Cardiovascular Function in Elderly Adults

*Changes in healthy men and women up to age 80 years as compared to those 20 years of age.
Data from Lakatta EG et al: Aging and cardiovascular disease in the elderly. In Fuster V et al, editors: *Hurst's the heart*, ed 13, Philadelphia, 2011, McGraw-Hill.

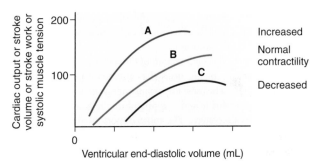

FIGURE 25.14 Frank-Starling Law of the Heart. The relationship between length and tension in the heart. The end-diastolic volume determines the end-diastolic length of ventricular muscle fibers and is proportional to tension generated during systole, as well as to cardiac output, stroke volume, and stroke work. A change in myocardial contractility causes the heart to perform on a different length-tension curve. *A,* Increased contractility; *B,* normal contractility; *C,* heart failure or decreased contractility. (See text for further explanation.)

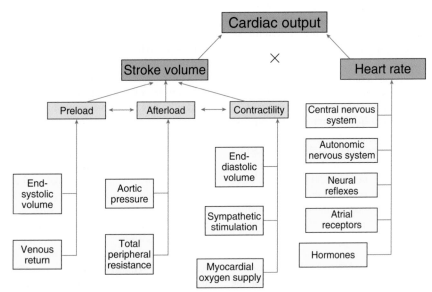

FIGURE 25.13 Factors Affecting Cardiac Performance. Cardiac output, the amount of blood (in liters) ejected by the heart per minute, depends on the heart rate (beats per minute) and stroke volume (milliliters of blood ejected during ventricular systole).

systole. Low aortic pressures (decreased afterload) enable the heart to contract more rapidly and efficiently, whereas high aortic pressures (increased afterload) slow contraction and cause higher workloads against which the heart must function to eject blood. Increased aortic pressure is usually the result of increased systemic vascular resistance (SVR), sometimes referred to as total peripheral resistance (TPR). In individuals with hypertension, increased SVR means that afterload is chronically elevated, resulting in increased ventricular workload and hypertrophy of the myocardium. SVR is calculated by dividing the mean arterial pressure by the cardiac output; the normal range is 700 dyne/sec/cm^{-5}.[5,12] The most sensitive measure of afterload is SVR.

Myocardial Contractility

Stroke volume, or the volume of blood ejected per beat during systole, also depends on the *force* of contraction, myocardial contractility, or the degree of myocardial fiber shortening. Three major factors determine the force of contraction (see Fig. 25.13):

1. *Changes in the stretching of the ventricular myocardium caused by changes in VEDV (preload)*. As discussed previously, increased venous return to the heart distends the ventricle, thus increasing preload, which increases the stroke volume and, subsequently, cardiac output, up to a certain point. However, an excessive increase in preload leads to decreased stroke volume.

2. *Alterations in the inotropic stimuli of the ventricles.* Hormones, neurotransmitters, or medications that affect contractility are called inotropic agents. The most important endogenous positive inotropic agents are epinephrine and norepinephrine released from the sympathetic nervous system. The most important negative inotropic agent is acetylcholine released from the vagus nerve. Many medications have positive or negative inotropic properties that can have significant effects on cardiac function. In sepsis, a variety of cytokines, including tumor necrosis factor-alpha (TNF-α), and interleukin-1β, have been shown to impair myocardial contractility.[13]

3. *Adequacy of myocardial oxygen supply.* O_2 and carbon dioxide levels (tensions) in the coronary blood also influence contractility. With severe hypoxemia (arterial O_2 saturation less than 50%), contractility is decreased. Moderate degrees of hypoxemia may increase contractility by enhancing the myocardial response to circulating catecholamines.[14]

Preload, afterload, and contractility all interact with one another to determine stroke volume and cardiac output. Changes in any one of these factors can result in deleterious effects on the others, resulting in heart failure (see Chapter 26).

Heart Rate

As described previously, SA node activity is the primary determinant of the heart rate. The average heart rate in healthy adults is about 70 beats/min. This rate diminishes by 10 to 20 beats/min during sleep and can accelerate to more than 100 beats/min during muscular activity or emotional excitement. In well-conditioned athletes, the resting heart rate is normally about 50 to 60 beats/min. In highly trained or elite athletes, the resting heart rate can be below 50 beats/min; these athletes also have a greater stroke volume and lower peripheral resistance in active muscles than they had before training. The control of heart rate includes activity of the central nervous system, autonomic nervous system, neural reflexes, atrial receptors, and hormones (see Fig. 25.13).

Cardiovascular control centers in the brain. The cardiovascular vasomotor control center is in the medulla and pons areas of the brainstem, with additional areas in the hypothalamus, cerebral cortex, and thalamus.[15] The hypothalamic centers regulate cardiovascular responses to changes in temperature, the cerebral cortex centers adjust cardiac reaction to a variety of emotional states, and the brainstem control center regulates heart rate and blood pressure.

The nerve fibers from the cardiovascular control center synapse with autonomic neurons that influence the rate of firing of the SA node. As previously discussed, an increased heart rate occurs with sympathetic (adrenergic) stimulation. When the parasympathetic nerves to the heart are stimulated (primarily via the vagus nerve), the heart rate slows and the sympathetic nerves to the heart, arterioles, and veins are inhibited.[6] At rest, the heart rate in healthy individuals is primarily under the control of parasympathetic stimulation. Administration of drugs that block parasympathetic function (anticholinergic) or physical interruption of the vagus nerve causes significant tachycardia (abnormally fast heart rate) because this inhibitory parasympathetic influence is lost.

Neural reflexes. Output from the baroreceptor reflexes influences short-term regulation of the vascular smooth muscle of resistance arteries, myocardial contractility, and heart rate, all components of blood pressure control. The baroreceptors or pressoreceptors are located in the aortic arch and carotid arteries. If blood pressure decreases, the baroreceptor reflex accelerates the heart rate, increases myocardial contractility, and increases vascular smooth muscle contraction in the arterioles, thus raising blood pressure. This reflex is critical to maintaining adequate tissue perfusion. When the blood pressure increases, the baroreceptors increase their rate of discharge, sending neural impulses over a branch of the glossopharyngeal nerve (cranial nerve IX) and through the vagus nerve to the cardiovascular control centers in the medulla. These reflexes increase parasympathetic activity and decrease sympathetic activity, causing the resistance arteries to dilate, decreasing myocardial contractility and the heart rate. The role of baroreceptors in influencing blood pressure is discussed in more detail later in this chapter.

Atrial receptors. Mechanoreceptors that influence the heart rate exist in both atria. They are located where the veins, venae cavae, and pulmonary veins enter their respective atria. The Bainbridge reflex is the name for the changes in the heart rate that may occur after intravenous infusions of blood or other fluid. The change in heart rate is thought to be caused by a reflex mediated by these atrial volume receptors that are innervated by the vagus nerve (volume receptors are thought to respond to increased plasma volume). Although this reflex can be elicited in humans, its relevance is uncertain at this time.[16] Stimulation of these atrial receptors also increases urine volume, presumably because of a neurally mediated reduction in antidiuretic hormone. In addition, peptides of the atrial natriuretic family are released from atrial tissue in response to the increases in blood volume. These peptides have diuretic and natriuretic (salt excretion) properties, resulting in decreased blood volume and pressure. The atrial natriuretic peptides also have been shown to relax vascular smooth muscle and oppose myocardial hypertrophy, leading to measurement of blood levels to evaluate clinical status and raising interest in their use as therapeutic agents.[17]

Hormones and biochemicals. Hormones and other biochemically active substances affect the arteries, arterioles, venules, capillaries, and contractility of the myocardium. Norepinephrine, mainly released as a neurotransmitter from the adrenal medulla, dilates vessels of the liver and skeletal muscle and also causes an increase in myocardial contractility. Some adrenocortical hormones, such as hydrocortisone, increase the effects of the catecholamines—norepinephrine and epinephrine.

Thyroid hormones enhance sympathetic activity and increase cardiac output. Growth hormone, working together with insulin-like growth factor-1 (IGF-1), also has been shown to increase myocardial contractility.[18] Decreases in levels of growth hormone or thyroid hormone may result in bradycardia (heart rate below 60 beats/min), reduced cardiac output, and low blood pressure. (Other hormones are discussed in the Regulation of Blood Pressure section.)

SYSTEMIC CIRCULATION

The arteries and veins of the systemic circulation are illustrated in Fig. 25.15. Oxygenated blood leaves the left side of the heart through the aorta and flows into the systemic arteries. These arteries branch into small arterioles, which branch into the smallest vessels, the capillaries, where nutrient and waste product exchange between the blood and tissues occurs. Blood from the capillaries then enters tiny venules that join to form the larger veins, which return venous blood to the right heart (see Fig. 25.1, *B*). Peripheral vascular system is the term used to describe the part of the systemic circulation that supplies the skin and the extremities, particularly the legs and feet.

Structure of Blood Vessels

Blood vessel walls are composed of three layers: (1) the tunica intima (innermost, or intimal, layer), (2) the tunica media (middle, or medial, layer), and (3) the tunica externa or adventitia (outermost, or external, layer), which also contains nerves and lymphatic vessels. These layers are illustrated in Fig. 25.16. Blood vessel walls vary in thickness, depending on the thickness or absence of one or more of these three layers. Cells of the larger vessel walls are nourished by the vasa vasorum, small vessels located in the tunica externa.

Arterial Vessels

An artery is a thick-walled, pulsating blood vessel transporting blood away from the heart. In the systemic circulation, arteries carry oxygenated blood. When the iron in hemoglobin is oxygenated, it turns bright red, which is why arterial vessels are often color-coded red in illustrations. Arterial walls are composed of elastic connective tissue, fibrous connective tissue, and smooth muscle. There are two types of arteries: elastic and muscular. Elastic arteries have a thick tunica media with more elastic fibers than smooth muscle fibers. Elastic arteries are located close to the heart and include the aorta and its major branches and the pulmonary trunk. Elasticity allows the vessel to absorb energy and stretch as blood is ejected from the heart during systole. During diastole, elasticity promotes recoil of the arteries, maintaining blood pressure within the vessels.

Muscular arteries, medium and small size arteries, are farther from the heart than the elastic arteries. They contain more muscle fibers and fewer elastic fibers than the elastic arteries and they function to distribute blood to arterioles throughout the body (see Fig. 25.16, *A*). Because their smooth muscle can contract or relax, they play a role in blood flow control and in directing flow to body parts with the highest need at any point in time. Contraction narrows the vessel lumen (the internal cavity of the vessel), which diminishes flow through the vessel (vasoconstriction). When the smooth muscle layer relaxes, more blood flows through the vessel lumen (vasodilation).

An artery becomes an arteriole where the diameter of its lumen narrows to less than 0.5 mm. Arterioles are mainly composed of smooth muscle and regulate the flow of blood into the capillaries by constricting or dilating to either slow or increase the flow of blood into the capillaries (Fig. 25.17). The thick smooth muscle layer of the arterioles is a major determinant of the resistance blood encounters as it flows through the systemic circulation.

The capillary network is composed of connective channels called metarterioles and "true" capillaries (see Fig. 25.17). Metarterioles have discontinuous smooth muscle cells in their tunica media, whereas capillaries have no smooth muscle cells. There is a ring of smooth muscle called the precapillary sphincter at the point where capillaries branch from metarterioles. As the sphincters contract and relax, they regulate blood flow through the capillary beds. The precapillary sphincters help to maintain arterial pressure and regulate selective flow to vascular beds.

Capillaries are composed solely of a layer of endothelial cells surrounded by a basement membrane. Their thin walls and unique structure make possible the rapid exchange of water; small soluble molecules; some larger molecules, such as albumin; and cells of the innate and adaptive components of the immune system between the blood and the interstitial fluid. In some capillaries, the endothelial cells contain oval windows or pores termed fenestrations covered by a thin diaphragm.

Substances pass between the capillary lumen and the interstitial fluid (1) through junctions between endothelial cells, (2) through fenestrations in endothelial cells, (3) in vesicles moved by active transport across the endothelial cell membrane, or (4) by diffusion through the endothelial cell membrane. A single capillary may be only 0.5 to 1 mm in length and 0.01 mm in diameter, but the capillaries are so numerous their total surface area may be more than 600 m^2 (about 100 football fields).

Endothelium

The vascular endothelium, or blood vessel lining, is important to several body functions and is sometimes considered a separate endocrine organ. All tissues depend on a blood supply, and the blood supply depends on endothelial cells, which form the lining, or endothelium, of the blood vessel (Fig. 25.18). In addition to substance transport, the vascular endothelium has important roles in coagulation, antithrombogenesis, and fibrinolysis; immune system function; tissue and vessel growth and wound healing; and vasomotion, the contraction and relaxation of vessels. Table 25.3 summarizes some of the more important endothelial functions. Endothelial injury and dysfunction are central processes in many of the most common and serious cardiovascular disorders, including hypertension and atherosclerosis (see Chapter 26).

Veins

Compared with arteries, veins are thin walled with more fibrous connective tissue and have a larger diameter (see Fig. 25.16, *B*). Veins also are more numerous than arteries. The smallest venules downstream from the capillaries have an endothelial lining and are surrounded by connective tissue. The largest venules have some smooth muscle fibers in their thin tunica media. The venous tunica externa has less elastic tissue than that in arteries, so veins do not recoil as much or as rapidly after distention. Like arteries, veins receive nourishment from tiny vasa vasorum.

Veins contain valves to facilitate the one-way flow of blood toward the heart (Fig. 25.19). These valves are folds of the tunica intima and resemble the semilunar valves of the heart. When a person stands up, contraction of the skeletal muscles of the legs compresses the deep veins of the legs and assists the flow of blood toward the heart. This important mechanism of venous return is called the muscle pump (see Fig. 25.19, *B*).

Factors Affecting Blood Flow

Blood flow, the amount of fluid moved per unit of time, is usually expressed as liters or milliliters per minute (L/min or ml/min). Factors

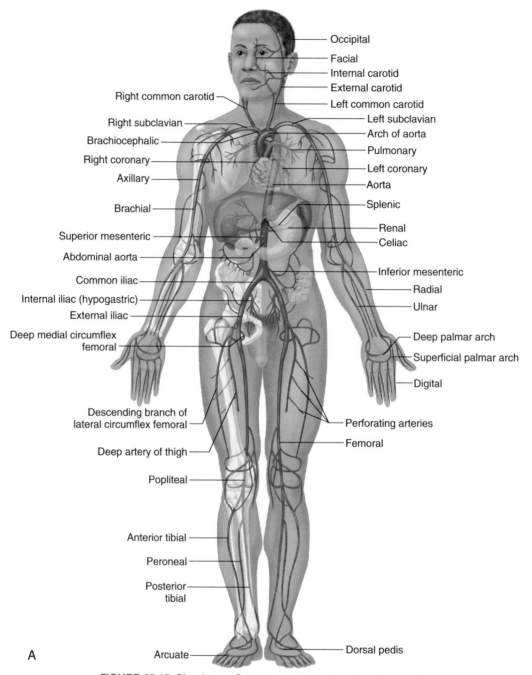

Occipital
Facial
Internal carotid
External carotid
Left common carotid
Right common carotid
Left subclavian
Right subclavian
Arch of aorta
Brachiocephalic
Pulmonary
Right coronary
Left coronary
Axillary
Aorta
Splenic
Brachial
Renal
Superior mesenteric
Celiac
Abdominal aorta
Inferior mesenteric
Common iliac
Radial
Internal iliac (hypogastric)
Ulnar
External iliac
Deep medial circumflex femoral
Deep palmar arch
Superficial palmar arch
Digital
Descending branch of lateral circumflex femoral
Perforating arteries
Femoral
Deep artery of thigh
Popliteal
Anterior tibial
Peroneal
Posterior tibial

A   Arcuate   Dorsal pedis

FIGURE 25.15 Circulatory System. A, Principal arteries of the body.

that influence blood flow include pressure, resistance, velocity, laminar versus turbulent flow, and compliance, with the most important of these being pressure and resistance.

Pressure and Resistance

Pressure in a liquid system is the force exerted on the liquid per unit area and is expressed clinically as millimeters of mercury (mm Hg), or torr (1 torr = 1 mm Hg). Blood flow to an organ depends partly on the pressure difference between the arterial and venous vessels supplying that organ. Fluid moves from the arterial "side" of the capillaries where the pressure is higher to the venous side where the pressure is lower.

Resistance is the opposition to blood flow. Most opposition to blood flow results from the diameter and length of the vessels. Changes in blood flow through an organ result from changes in the vascular resistance within the organ because of increases or decreases in vessel diameter and the opening or closing of vascular channels. Resistance in a vessel is inversely related to blood flow—that is, increased resistance leads to decreased blood flow. The Poiseuille law indicates that resistance is directly related to tube length and blood viscosity and inversely related to the radius of the tube to the fourth power (r^4). Because blood flow is inversely related to resistance, the greater the resistance the lower the blood flow will be. Resistance to flow cannot be measured directly, but it can be calculated if the pressure difference and flow volumes are known. Resistance to blood flow in a single vessel is determined by the radius and length of the blood vessel and by the blood viscosity.

Clinically, the most important factor determining resistance *in a single vessel* is the radius or diameter of the vessel's lumen. Small changes in the lumen's radius or diameter lead to large changes in vascular

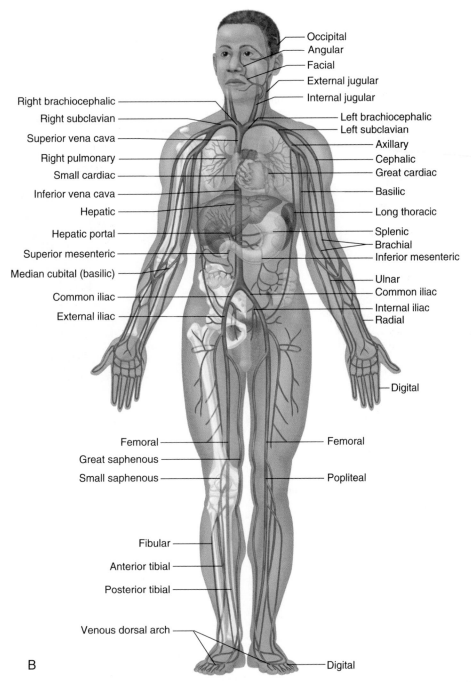

Occipital
Angular
Facial
External jugular
Internal jugular

Right brachiocephalic
Right subclavian
Superior vena cava
Right pulmonary
Small cardiac
Inferior vena cava
Hepatic
Hepatic portal
Superior mesenteric
Median cubital (basilic)
Common iliac
External iliac

Left brachiocephalic
Left subclavian
Axillary
Cephalic
Great cardiac
Basilic
Long thoracic
Splenic
Brachial
Inferior mesenteric
Ulnar
Common iliac
Internal iliac
Radial

Digital

Femoral
Great saphenous
Small saphenous

Femoral

Popliteal

Fibular
Anterior tibial
Posterior tibial

Venous dorsal arch

Digital

B

FIGURE 25.15, cont'd B, Principal veins of the body. (From Patton KT, Thibodeau GA, Douglas MM: *Essentials of anatomy & physiology,* St Louis, 2012, Elsevier.)

resistance. Clinically, vasoconstriction will contribute to an increase in resistance, whereas vasodilation will cause a decrease in resistance that may be reflected by a fall in blood pressure. Because vessel length is relatively constant but lumen size is quite variable, length is not as important as lumen size in determining flow through a single vessel.

Blood vessel radius is usually the key factor in determining the TPR because viscosity, the consistency of the fluid, is relatively constant. Thick fluids move more slowly and cause greater resistance to flow than thin fluids—just think of honey as compared to water. The viscosity of blood depends on the red cell content. The greater the percentage of red cells in the blood, the more viscous the blood. This relationship is expressed as the hematocrit. A high hematocrit value reduces flow through the blood vessels, particularly the microcirculation (arterioles,

capillaries, venules). An elevated hematocrit level is relatively rare. Conditions with elevated hematocrits include a lack of body water, cyanotic congenital heart disease (see Chapter 27), or polycythemia (see Chapter 23), and can lead to increased cardiac work as a result of increased vascular resistance.

Resistance to flow through a *system of vessels,* or total resistance, depends not only on characteristics of individual vessels, but also on whether the vessels are arranged in *series* (end to end) or in *parallel* (side to side) and on the total cross-sectional area of the system. Vessels arranged in parallel provide less resistance than vessels arranged in series. Blood flowing through the distributing arteries, beginning with branches off the aorta and ending at arterioles in the capillary bed, encounters more resistance than blood flowing through the capillary

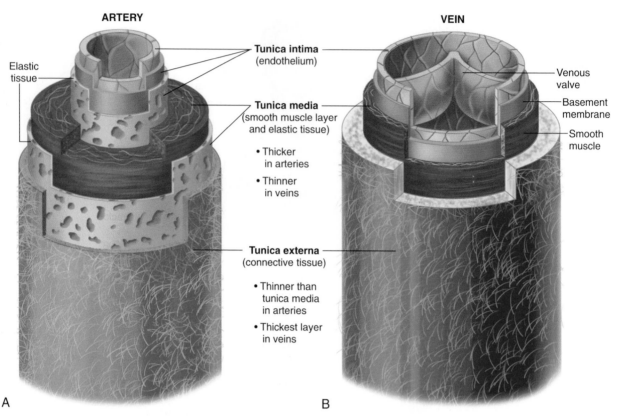

FIGURE 25.16 Structure of the Blood Vessels. The tunica externa of the veins *(blue)* and the arteries *(red).* (From Patton KT, Thibodeau GA: *Structure & function of the body,* ed 15, St Louis, 2016, Elsevier.)

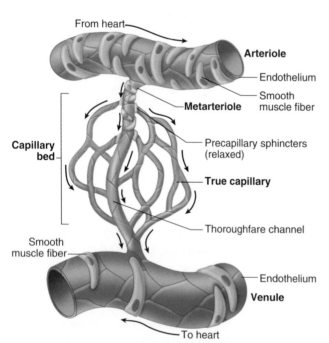

FIGURE 25.17 Microcirculation. Control of local blood flow through a capillary network is regulated by altering the tone of precapillary sphincters surrounding arterioles and metarterioles. In the diagram, the sphincters are relaxed, permitting blood flow to enter the capillary bed. (From Patton KT, Thibodeau GA, Douglas MM: *Essentials of anatomy & physiology,* St Louis, 2012, Elsevier.)

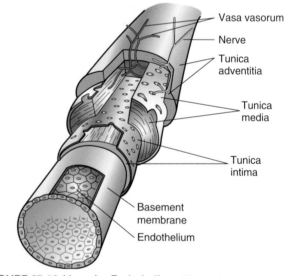

FIGURE 25.18 Vascular Endothelium. The endothelial cells arrange themselves as a single-layer lining that has numerous critical functions (see Table 25.3).

bed itself, where flow is distributed among many short, tiny branches arranged in parallel (Fig. 25.20). The total cross-sectional area of the arteriolar system is greater than that of the arterial system, yet the greater number of arterioles arranged in series leads to great resistance to flow in the arteriolar system. In contrast, the capillary system has a larger number of vessels arranged in parallel than the arteriolar system, and the total cross-sectional area is much greater; thus there is lower resistance overall through the capillary system. The resulting slow velocity of flow in each capillary is optimal for capillary-tissue exchange.

TABLE 25.3 Functions of the Endothelium

Function	Actions Involved
Filtration and permeability	Facilitates transport of large molecules via vesicular transport movement through intercellular junctions Facilitates transport of small molecules via movement of vesicles, through opening of tight junctions, and across cytoplasm
Vasomotion	Stimulates vascular relaxation through production of nitric oxide, prostacyclin, and other vasodilators Stimulates vascular constriction through production of endothelin-1 and of angiotensin II by the action of endothelial angiotensin-converting enzyme on angiotensin I
Hemostatic balance	Endothelial surface is normally antithrombotic and maintains a balance between procoagulant and anticoagulant factors, as well as profibrinolytic and antifibrinolytic factors Anticoagulant factors include prostacyclin, nitric oxide, antithrombin, thrombomodulin, tissue factor pathway inhibitor, and heparins Procoagulant factors include tissue factor (factor VII), factor VIII, factor V, and plasminogen activator inhibitor-1 (PAI-1) Profibrinolytic factors are tissue- and urokinase-type plasminogen activating factor and PAI-1 Antifibrinolytic factor is tissue plasminogen activator
Inflammation/immunity	Expresses chemotactic agents and adhesion molecules that support white blood cells (including monocytes, neutrophils, and lymphocytes) moving into tissues Expresses receptors for oxidized lipoproteins, allowing them to enter vascular intima
Angiogenesis/vessel growth	Releases growth factors, such as endothelin-1, and heparins for vascular smooth muscle cells
Lipid metabolism	Expresses receptors for lipoprotein lipase and low-density lipoproteins (LDLs)

From Griendling KK et al: Biology of the vessel wall. In Fuster et al, editors: *Hurst's the heart*, ed 13, Philadelphia, 2011, McGraw-Hill; Rajendran P et al: *Int J Biol Sci* 9(10):1057-1069, 2013.

Velocity

Blood velocity, or speed, is the *distance* blood travels in a unit of time, usually centimeters per second (cm/sec). It is directly related to blood flow (the *amount* of blood moved per unit of time) and inversely related to the cross-sectional area of the vessel in which the blood is flowing (see Fig. 25.20). As blood moves from the aorta to the capillaries, the total cross-sectional area of the vessels increases and the velocity decreases.

Laminar Versus Turbulent Flow

Flow through a tubular system can be either laminar or turbulent. Blood flow through the vessels, except where vessels split or branch, is usually laminar. In laminar flow, concentric layers of molecules move "straight ahead," with each layer flowing at a slightly different velocity (Fig. 25.21, *A*). The cohesive attraction between the fluid and the vessel wall prevents the molecules of blood that are in contact with the wall from moving at all. The next thin layer of blood is able to slide slowly past the stationary layer and so on until, at the center, the blood velocity is greatest. Large vessels have room for a large center layer; therefore they have less resistance to flow and greater flow and velocity than smaller vessels.

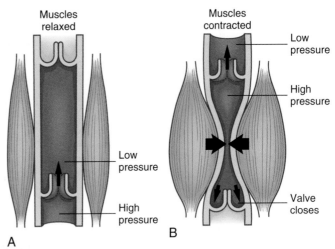

FIGURE 25.19 Venous Valves and the Muscle Pump. In veins, one-way valves aid circulation by preventing backflow of venous blood when pressure in a local area is low. **A,** Blood is moved toward the heart as valves in the veins are forced open by pressure from volume of blood downstream and the neighboring muscles are relaxed. **B,** When pressure below the valve drops, blood begins to flow backward but fills the "pockets" formed by the valve flaps, pushing the flaps together and thus blocking further backward flow. Contraction in the adjacent muscles and the valves of the systemic veins assist in the return of unoxygenated blood to the right heart.

Where flow is obstructed, the vessel turns or branches, or blood flows over rough surfaces, the flow becomes turbulent with whorls or eddy currents that produce noise, causing a murmur to be heard on auscultation (see Fig. 25.21, *B*). Resistance increases with turbulence, which frequently occurs in areas with atherosclerotic plaque (see Chapter 26).

Vascular Compliance

Vascular compliance is the increase in volume a vessel can accommodate with a given increase in pressure. Compliance depends on factors related to the nature of a vessel wall, such as the ratio of elastic fibers to muscle fibers in the wall. Elastic arteries are more compliant than muscular arteries. The veins are more compliant than either type of artery, and they can serve as storage areas for the circulatory system.

Compliance determines a vessel's response to pressure changes. For example, a large volume of blood can be accommodated by the venous system with only a small increase in pressure. In the less compliant arterial system, where smaller volumes and higher pressures are normal, even small changes in blood volume can cause significant changes in arterial pressure.

Stiffness is the opposite of compliance. Several conditions and disorders can cause stiffness, with the most common being aging and atherosclerosis (see Chapter 26).

> **QUICK CHECK 25.5**
> 1. What is the function of the arterioles?
> 2. Identify the functions of the endothelium.
> 3. Why does the total cross-sectional area in the capillary system lower the resistance to flow?

Regulation of Blood Pressure
Arterial Pressure

The arterial blood pressure is determined by the cardiac output multiplied by the peripheral resistance (Fig. 25.22). The systolic blood pressure is the highest arterial blood pressure after ventricular contraction or

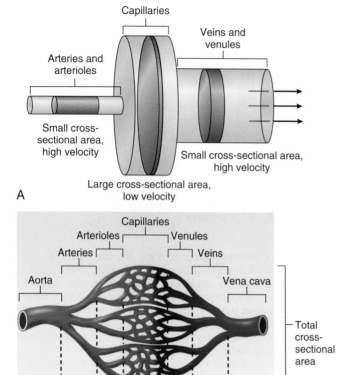

FIGURE 25.20 Relationship between Cross-Sectional Area and Velocity of Blood Flow. **A,** Small and large cross-sectional areas and their relationship to velocity changes. **B,** Total cross-sectional area of different kinds of blood vessels with velocity of blood flow (ml/sec). Blood flows with great speed in the large arteries. However, branching of arterial vessels increases the total cross-sectional area of the arterioles and capillaries, reducing the flow rate. When capillaries merge into venules and venules merge into veins, the total cross-sectional area decreases, causing the flow rate to increase. (From Patton KT, Thibodeau GA: *Anatomy & physiology,* ed 9, St Louis, 2016, Elsevier.)

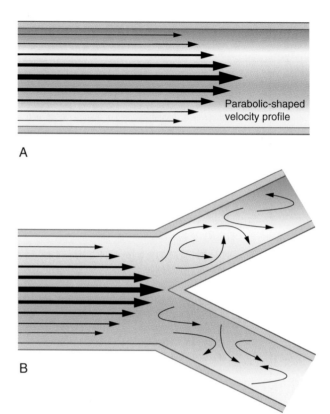

FIGURE 25.21 Laminar and Turbulent Blood Flow. **A,** Laminar flow. Fluid flows in long, smooth-walled tubes as if it is composed of a large number of concentric layers. **B,** Turbulent flow. Turbulent flow is caused by numerous small currents flowing crosswise or oblique to the long axis of the vessel, resulting in flowing whorls and eddy currents.

systole. The diastolic blood pressure is the lowest arterial blood pressure that occurs during ventricular filling or diastole. The mean arterial pressure (MAP), which is the average pressure in the arteries throughout the cardiac cycle, depends on the elastic properties of the arterial walls and the mean volume of blood in the arterial system. MAP can be approximated from the measured values of the systolic (P_s) and diastolic (P_d) pressures as follows:

$$MAP = P_d + \frac{1}{3}(P_s - P_d)$$

The normal range for MAP is 70 to 110 mm Hg. The difference between the systolic pressure and the diastolic pressure ($P_s - P_d$) is called the pulse pressure and typically is between 40 and 50 mm Hg. The pulse pressure is directly related to arterial wall stiffness and stroke volume.

During a wide range of physiologic conditions, including changes in body position, muscular activity, and circulating blood volume, arterial pressure is regulated within a fairly narrow range to maintain tissue perfusion, or blood supply to the capillary beds. The major factors

and relationships that regulate arterial blood pressure are summarized in Fig. 25.22.

Effects of Cardiac Output

The cardiac output (minute volume) of the heart can be changed by alterations in the heart rate, stroke volume (volume of blood ejected during each ventricular contraction), or both. An increase in cardiac output without a decrease in peripheral resistance will cause the MAP and flow rate to increase. The higher arterial pressure increases blood flow through the arterioles. On the other hand, a decrease in the cardiac output causes a drop in the MAP and arteriolar flow if peripheral resistance stays constant.

Effects of Total Peripheral Resistance

Total resistance in the systemic circulation, known as either SVR or TPR, is primarily a function of arteriolar diameter. If cardiac output remains constant, arteriolar constriction raises the MAP by reducing the flow of blood into the capillaries, whereas arteriolar dilation has the opposite effect. Reflex control of total cardiac output and peripheral resistance includes (1) sympathetic stimulation of the heart, arterioles, and veins; and (2) parasympathetic stimulation of the heart (Fig. 25.23). The cardiovascular center in the medulla receives input from arterial baroreceptors and chemoreceptors throughout the vascular system and then modifies vagal and sympathetic output to control heart rate and contractility, plus vascular diameter. Vasoconstriction is regulated by an area of the brainstem that maintains a constant (tonic) output of norepinephrine from sympathetic fibers in the peripheral arterioles. This tonic activity is essential for maintenance of blood pressure.

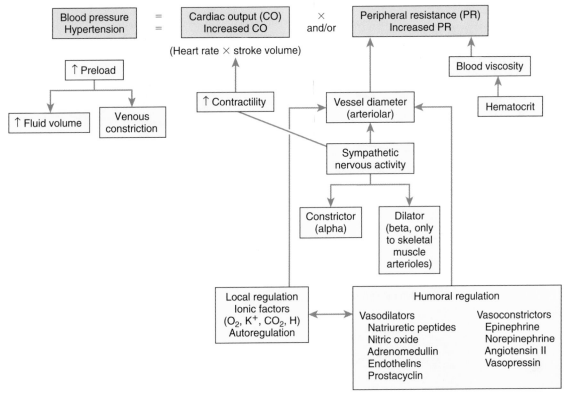

FIGURE 25.22 Factors Regulating Blood Pressure. O_2, Oxygen; K^+, potassium; CO_2, carbon dioxide; H, hydrogen.

Baroreceptors. As discussed previously, baroreceptors are stretch receptors located predominantly in the aorta and in the carotid sinus (see Fig. 25.23, *A*). They respond to changes in smooth muscle fiber length by altering their rate of discharge and supply sensory information to the cardiovascular center in the brainstem. When activated (stretched), the baroreceptors decrease cardiac output by lowering the heart rate, stroke volume, and peripheral resistance, and thus lower blood pressure.

Arterial chemoreceptors. Specialized areas within the aortic arch and carotid arteries are sensitive to concentrations of O_2, carbon dioxide (CO_2), and hydrogen ions (pH) in the blood (see Fig. 25.23, *B*). Although these chemoreceptors are most important for respiratory control, they also transmit impulses to the medullary cardiovascular centers that regulate blood pressure. A decrease in arterial oxygen concentration (hypoxemia), an increase in arterial $PaCO_2$ concentration, or to a lesser extent a decrease in arterial blood pH causes a reflexive increase in heart rate, stroke volume, and blood pressure.

Effects of Hormones

Hormones influence blood pressure regulation through their effects on vascular smooth muscle and blood volume. By constricting or dilating the arterioles in organs, hormones can (1) increase or decrease the flow in response to the body's needs, (2) redistribute blood volume during hemorrhage or shock, and (3) regulate heat loss. The key vasoconstrictor hormones include angiotensin II, vasopressin (or antidiuretic hormone), epinephrine, and norepinephrine. The main vasodilator hormones are the atrial natriuretic hormones. By causing fluid retention or loss, aldosterone, vasopressin, and the natriuretic hormones can influence stroke volume and thus blood pressure.

Vasoconstrictor hormones. The vasoconstrictor hormones include epinephrine; norepinephrine; angiotensin II, which is part of the renin-angiotensin-aldosterone system; and vasopressin (also known as antidiuretic hormone). Epinephrine, the catecholamine

hormone released from the adrenal medulla, causes vasoconstriction in most vascular beds except the coronary, liver, and skeletal muscle circulations. Norepinephrine mainly acts as a neurotransmitter; however, some also is released from the adrenal medulla. When released into the circulation, it is a more potent vasoconstrictor than epinephrine. Although angiotensin II and vasopressin are vasoconstrictors, they are not thought to have a major role in blood pressure control in normal circumstances.

Vasopressin and aldosterone, however, affect blood pressure by increasing blood volume through their influence on fluid reabsorption in the kidney and by stimulating thirst. Vasopressin causes the reabsorption of water from tubular fluid in the distal tubule and collecting duct of the nephron. Aldosterone, the end product of the renin-angiotensin-aldosterone system, stimulates the reabsorption of sodium, chloride, and water from the same locations in the kidney (Fig. 25.24; also see Chapters 5 and 20).

Vasodilator hormones. The natriuretic peptides (NPs) or hormones (see Fig. 25.24), including atrial natriuretic peptide (ANP), B-type natriuretic peptide (BNP), C-type natriuretic peptide (CNP), and urodilatin, function as both vasodilators and regulators of sodium and water excretion (natriuresis and diuresis). Increased pressure or diastolic volume in the heart stimulates the release of these peptide hormones. Increased levels of BNP predict increased risk of a poor outcome in heart failure, pulmonary embolism, valvular heart disease, and chronic coronary artery disease.[19]

Effects of Other Mediators

A variety of other mediators have been demonstrated to cause arteriolar vasodilation or vasoconstriction. Some of the vasodilating mediators include nitric oxide (NO), adrenomedullin (ADM), the endothelins, and prostacyclin. These mediators are being investigated to determine if they or their inhibitors might be useful drugs for the treatment of

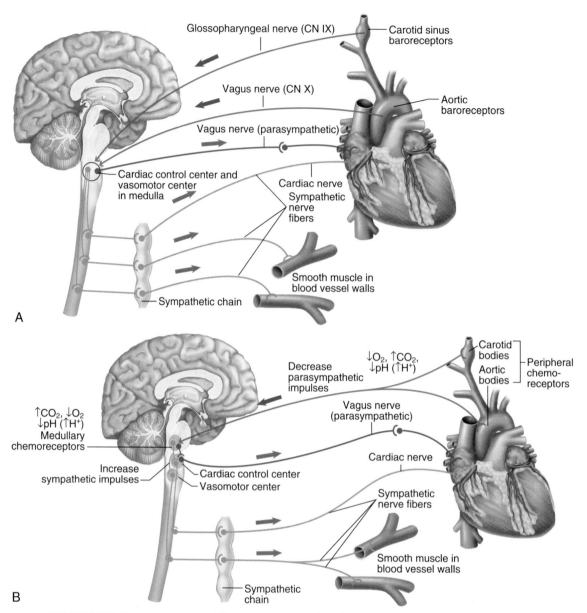

FIGURE 25.23 Baroreceptors and Chemoreceptor Reflex Control of Blood Pressure. A, Baroreceptor reflexes. **B,** Vasomotor chemoreflexes. *CN,* Cranial nerve; O_2, oxygen; CO_2, carbon dioxide; H^+, hydrogen. (Modified from Patton KT, Thibodeau GA: *Anatomy & physiology,* ed 9, St Louis, 2016, Elsevier.)

cardiovascular diseases or if their levels might be useful in determining the prognosis of persons with known disease.

Nitric oxide (NO), an intercellular and intracellular signaling molecule produced in endothelial cells, has a variety of roles in vascular function including acting as a vasodilator and inhibitor of smooth muscle proliferation. NO also has been called endothelium-derived relaxing factor (EDRF). One way that diabetes may contribute to hypertension is through inhibition of NO production by impeding a family of enzymes—the NO synthases. Understanding the role of NO in producing vasodilation explains why sublingual nitroglycerin has been a useful treatment for coronary artery spasm.

Adrenomedullin (ADM), a peptide with powerful vasodilatory activity, is present in numerous tissues. Although it has been found to have numerous cardiovascular effects, including a role in fetal cardiovascular system development and vasodilation, its exact role in adult human cardiovascular function and disease is unclear. Some research indicates that elevated ADM levels may be useful disease indicators.

The endothelins are a family of three structurally similar peptides (ET-1, ET-2, and ET-3) and four receptors produced in cells in the vascular smooth muscle, the endothelium, the kidneys, and other organs. Understanding the physiologic and pathologic roles of these peptides has been complicated by the fact that endothelin binding to some receptors causes vasodilation and natriuresis, whereas binding to other receptors causes the opposite response—vasoconstriction plus sodium and water retention. Inhibitors to ET-1 have been approved for the treatment of pulmonary hypertension.

Prostacyclin is a vasodilator that is produced by the actions of cyclooxygenases (COX-1 and COX-2) on arachidonic acid. It has the additional properties of opposing clot formation (antithrombotic), decreasing platelet activity, and inhibiting the release of growth factors from macrophages and the endothelial cells. Nonsteroidal antiinflammatory drugs (NSAIDs) that inhibit these cyclooxygenases have been associated with cardiovascular disease risk in healthy people and in those with a known cardiovascular disease.[20,21]

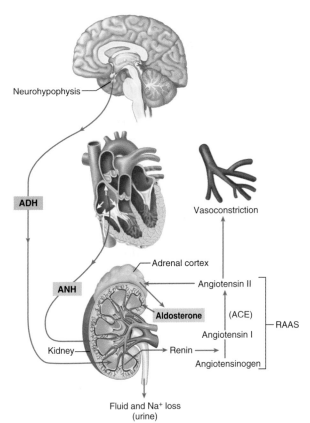

Neurohypophysis

ADH

Vasoconstriction

ANH

Adrenal cortex

Angiotensin II

Aldosterone (ACE)

RAAS

Angiotensin I

Kidney

Renin

Angiotensinogen

Fluid and Na⁺ loss
(urine)

FIGURE 25.24 Three Mechanisms That Influence Total Plasma Volume. Antidiuretic hormone *(ADH)* mechanism and renin-angiotensin-aldosterone system *(RAAS)* tend to increase water, sodium, and chloride retention and thus increase total plasma volume. The atrial natriuretic hormone *(ANH)* mechanism antagonizes these mechanisms by promoting water, sodium, and chloride loss, thus promoting a decrease in total plasma volume. *ACE,* Angiotensin-converting enzyme; *Na⁺,* sodium. (Modified from Patton KT, Thibodeau GA: *Anatomy & physiology,* ed 9, St Louis, 2016, Elsevier.)

Venous Pressure

The main determinants of venous blood pressure are (1) the volume of fluid within the veins and (2) the compliance (distensibility) of the vessel walls. The venous system typically accommodates about 66% of the total blood volume at any time, with venous pressure averaging less than 10 mm Hg. The systemic arteries accommodate about 11% of the total blood volume, with an average arterial pressure (blood pressure) of about 100 mm Hg; the remainder of the blood volume is within the heart, capillaries, and pulmonary circulation.

The sympathetic nervous system controls venous compliance. The walls of the veins are highly innervated by sympathetic fibers that control venous smooth muscle. Rather than constriction that would occur in the arteries, smooth muscle contraction in the veins results in stiffening of the vessel walls. This stiffening reduces venous distensibility and increases venous blood pressure, thus forcing more blood through the veins and into the right heart.

Two other mechanisms that increase venous pressure and venous return to the heart are (1) the skeletal muscle pump and (2) the respiratory pump. During skeletal muscle contraction, the veins within the muscles are partially compressed, causing decreased venous capacity and increased return to the heart (see Fig. 25.19, *B*). The respiratory pump acts during inspiration, when the veins of the abdomen are partially compressed by the downward movement of the diaphragm. Increased abdominal pressure moves blood toward the heart.

Regulation of the Coronary Circulation

Coronary blood flow is directly proportional to the perfusion pressure and inversely proportional to the vascular resistance of the coronary bed. Coronary perfusion pressure is the difference between pressure in the aorta and pressure in the coronary vessels. Thus, aortic pressure is the driving pressure for the arteries and arterioles that perfuse the myocardium. Vasodilation and vasoconstriction maintain coronary blood flow despite stresses imposed by the constant contraction and relaxation of the heart muscle and despite shifts (within a physiologic range) of coronary perfusion pressure.

Several unique anatomic factors influence coronary blood flow. Because of their anatomic location, the aortic valve cusps can obstruct coronary blood flow by occluding the openings of the coronary arteries during systole. Also during systole, the coronary arteries are compressed by ventricular contraction. The resulting systolic compressive effect is particularly evident in the subendocardial layers of the left ventricular wall and can greatly increase resistance to coronary blood flow, with the result that most left ventricular coronary blood flow occurs during diastole. During the period of systolic compression, when flow is slowed or stopped, myoglobin, a protein in heart muscle that binds O_2, provides the supply of O_2 to the myocardium. Myoglobin's O_2 levels are replenished during diastole.

Autoregulation

Autoregulation (automatic self-regulation) enables organs to regulate blood flow by altering the resistance (diameter) in their arterioles. Autoregulation in the coronary circulation maintains the blood flow at a nearly constant rate at perfusion pressures (MAP) between 60 and 140 mm Hg when other influencing factors are held constant. Thus autoregulation helps to ensure constant coronary blood flow despite shifts in the perfusion pressure within the stated range.

Given that blood flow is directly related to pressure and inversely related to resistance, for flow to stay constant as pressure decreases, resistance also has to decrease; therefore the mechanisms underlying autoregulation must be related to control of smooth muscle contraction in the arteriolar walls.

Autonomic Regulation

Although the coronary vessels themselves contain sympathetic (α- and β-adrenergic) and parasympathetic neural receptors, coronary blood flow during regular activity is regulated locally by the factors that cause autoregulation. During exercise, however, the vasodilating effects of β₂-receptors on the smaller coronary resistance arteries are responsible for about 25% of any increase in blood flow. At the same time, α-adrenergic receptors in larger arteries cause vasoconstriction to direct the blood flow to the inner layers of the myocardium.

> ✔ **QUICK CHECK 25.6**
> 1. Identify the factors regulating blood pressure.
> 2. Why is capillary flow increased with increased mean arterial pressure?
> 3. Define natriuretic peptides and adrenomedullin.

THE LYMPHATIC SYSTEM

The lymphatic system is a one-way network of lymphatic vessels and the lymph nodes (Figs. 25.25 and 25.26) that is important for immune function, fluid balance, and transport of lipids, hormones, and cytokines and is considered to be part of the circulatory system. Every day about 3 liters of fluid filters out of venous capillaries in body tissues and is not reabsorbed. This fluid becomes the lymph that is carried by the

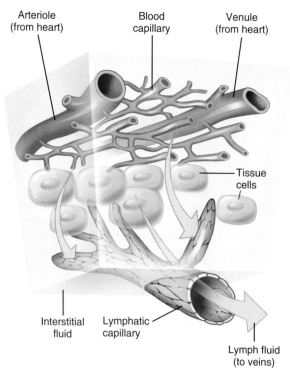

FIGURE 25.25 Role of the Lymphatic System in Fluid Balance.
Fluid from plasma flowing through the capillaries moves into interstitial spaces. Although most of this interstitial fluid is either absorbed by tissue cells or reabsorbed by blood capillaries, some of the fluid tends to accumulate in the interstitial spaces. This lymph then diffuses into the lymphatic vessels that carry it to the lymph nodes and then into the systemic venous blood. Green is used to diagram the lymphatic vessels although the lymphatic vessels, particularly the smaller ones, are almost transparent. (Modified from Thibodeau GA, Patton KT: *Structure & function of the body*, ed 13, St Louis, 2008, Elsevier.)

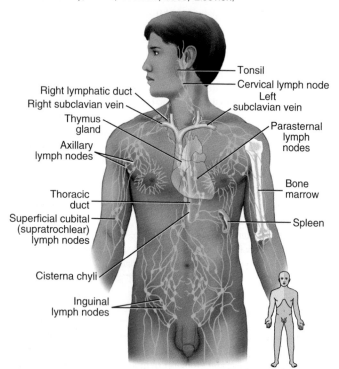

FIGURE 25.26 Principal Organs of the Lymphatic System. (From VanMeter KC, Hubert RJ: *Microbiology for the healthcare professional*, St Louis, 2010, Mosby.)

lymphatic vessels to the chest, where it enters the venous circulation. The lymphatic vessels run in the same sheaths with the arteries and veins. (Lymph nodes and lymphoid tissues are described in Chapter 7.) The lymphatic capillaries are closed at the distal ends, as shown in Fig. 25.27.

In this pumpless system, a series of valves ensures one-way flow of the excess interstitial fluid (now called *lymph*) toward the heart. Lymph consists primarily of water and small amounts of dissolved proteins, mostly albumin, that are too large to be reabsorbed into the less permeable blood capillaries. Lymph also carries two types of immune system cells: lymphocytes and antigen-presenting cells. The antigen-presenting cells are carried to the next lymph node in the system, whereas lymphocytes traffic between lymph nodes. Once within the lymphatic system, lymph travels through lymphatic venules and veins that drain into one of two large ducts in the thorax: the right lymphatic duct and the thoracic duct. The right lymphatic duct drains lymph from the right arm and the right side of the head and thorax, whereas the larger thoracic duct receives lymph from the rest of the body (see Fig. 25.23). The right lymphatic duct and the thoracic duct drain lymph into the right and left subclavian veins, respectively.

Lymphatic veins are thin walled like the veins of the cardiovascular system. In larger lymphatic veins, endothelial flaps form valves similar

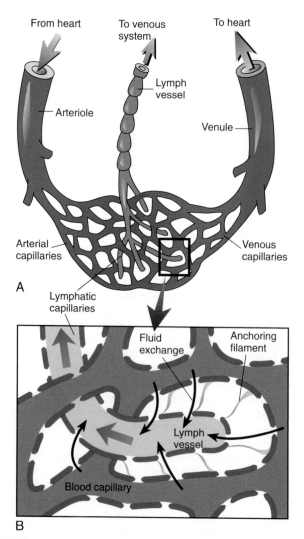

FIGURE 25.27 Lymphatic Capillaries. A, Schematic representation of lymphatic capillaries. **B,** Anatomic components of microcirculation.

to those in blood-carrying veins (see Fig. 25.27). The valves allow lymph to flow in only one direction, because lymphatic vessels are compressed intermittently by skeletal muscle contraction, pulsating expansion of the artery in the same sheath, and contraction of the smooth muscles in the walls of the lymphatic vessels.

As lymph is transported toward the heart, it is filtered through thousands of bean-shaped lymph nodes clustered along the lymphatic vessels (see Fig. 25.26). Lymph enters the nodes through afferent lymphatic vessels, filters through the sinuses in the node, and leaves by way of efferent lymphatic vessels. Lymph flows slowly through a node, allowing phagocytosis of foreign substances within the node and delivery of lymphocytes. (Phagocytosis is described in Chapter 6.)

> ✔ QUICK CHECK 25.7
> 1. Why is the lymphatic system considered a circulatory system?
> 2. What happens to lymph in lymph nodes?

▋ SUMMARY REVIEW

Circulatory System

1. The circulatory system is part of the body's transport and communication systems. It delivers O_2, nutrients, metabolites, hormones, neurochemicals, proteins, and blood cells, including lymphocytes and leukocytes, throughout the body and carries metabolic wastes to the kidneys, lungs, and liver for excretion.
2. The circulatory system consists of the heart and the blood and lymphatic vessels and is made up of two separate but conjoined, serially connected pump systems: the pulmonary circulation and the systemic circulation. The lymphatic system is a one-way network consisting of lymphatic vessels and lymph nodes.
3. The low-pressure pulmonary circulation is driven by the right side of the heart; its function is to deliver blood to the lungs for oxygenation.
4. The higher pressure systemic circulation is driven by the left side of the heart and functions to provide oxygenated blood, nutrients, and other key substances to body tissues and transport waste products to the lungs, kidneys, and liver for excretion.
5. The lymphatic vessels collect fluids from the interstitium and return the fluids to the circulatory system; lymphatic vessels also deliver antigens, microorganisms, and cells to the lymph nodes.

Heart

1. The heart consists of four chambers (two atria and two ventricles), four valves (two atrioventricular valves and two semilunar valves), a muscular wall, a fibrous skeleton, a conduction system, nerve fibers, systemic vessels (the coronary circulation), and openings where the great vessels enter the atria and ventricles.
2. The heart wall, which encloses the heart and divides it into chambers, is made up of three layers: the epicardium (outer layer), the myocardium (muscular layer), and the endocardium (inner lining). The heart lies within the pericardium, a double-walled sac.
3. The myocardial layer of the two atria, which receive blood entering the heart, is thinner than the myocardial layer of the ventricles, which have to be stronger to squeeze blood out of the heart.
4. The right and left sides of the heart are separated by portions of the heart wall called the *interatrial septum* and the *interventricular septum*.
5. Deoxygenated (venous) blood from the systemic circulation enters the right atrium through the superior and inferior venae cavae. From the right atrium, the blood passes through the right atrioventricular (tricuspid) valve into the right ventricle. In the ventricle, the blood flows from the inflow tract to the outflow tract and then through the pulmonary semilunar valve (pulmonary valve) into the pulmonary artery, which delivers it to the lungs for oxygenation.
6. Oxygenated blood from the lungs enters the left atrium through the four pulmonary veins (two from the left lung and two from the right lung). From the left atrium, the blood passes through the left atrioventricular valve (mitral valve) into the left ventricle. In the ventricle, the blood flows from the inflow tract to the outflow tract and then through the aortic semilunar valve (aortic valve) into the aorta, which delivers it to systemic arteries of the entire body.
7. There are four heart valves. The atrioventricular valves ensure one-way flow of blood from the atria to the ventricles. The semilunar valves ensure one-way blood flow from the right ventricle to the pulmonary artery and from the left ventricle to the aorta. The valves are supported by a fibrous skeleton.
8. The pumping action of the heart consists of two phases: diastole, during which the myocardium relaxes and the ventricles fill with blood; and systole, during which the myocardium contracts, forcing blood out of the ventricles. A cardiac cycle consists of one systolic contraction and the diastolic relaxation that follows it. Each cardiac cycle represents one heartbeat.
9. Coronary circulation provides O_2 and nutrients to the myocardium and other heart structures. Oxygenated blood enters the coronary arteries through openings from the aorta, and deoxygenated blood from the coronary veins enters the right atrium through the coronary sinus.
10. The conduction system of the heart generates and transmits electrical impulses (cardiac action potentials) that stimulate systolic contractions. The autonomic nerves (sympathetic and parasympathetic fibers) can adjust heart rate and force of contraction, but they do not originate the heartbeat.
11. The normal electrocardiogram is the sum of all cardiac action potentials. The P wave represents atrial depolarization; the QRS complex is the sum of all ventricular cell depolarizations. The ST interval occurs when the entire ventricular myocardium is depolarized.
12. Cardiac action potentials are generated by the sinoatrial node at a rate of 60 to 100 impulses per minute. The impulses can travel through the conduction system of the heart, stimulating myocardial contraction as they go.
13. Each cardiac action potential travels from the SA node to the AV node to the bundle of His (atrioventricular bundle), through the bundle branches, and finally to the Purkinje fibers and ventricular myocardium, where the impulse stops. It is prevented from reversing its path by the refractory period of cells that have just been polarized. The refractory period ensures that diastole (relaxation) will occur, thereby completing the cardiac cycle.
14. Cells of the cardiac conduction system have the properties of automaticity and rhythmicity. Automatic cells return to threshold and depolarize rhythmically without an outside stimulus. The cells of the sinoatrial node depolarize faster than other automatic cells, making it the natural pacemaker of the heart. If the SA node is disabled, the next fastest pacemaker, the AV node, takes over.
15. Adrenergic receptor number, type, and function govern autonomic (sympathetic) regulation of heart rate, contractile force, and the

dilation or constriction of coronary arteries. The presence of specific receptors on the myocardium and coronary vessels determines the effects of the neurotransmitters norepinephrine and epinephrine.

16. Unique features that distinguish myocardial cells from skeletal cells enable myocardial cells to transmit action potentials faster (through intercalated disks), synthesize more ATP (because of a large number of mitochondria), and have readier access to ions in the interstitium (because of an abundance of transverse tubules). These combined differences enable the myocardium to work constantly, which is not required by skeletal muscle.

17. Cross-bridges between actin and myosin enable contraction. Calcium ions interacting with the troponin complex help initiate the contraction process. Subsequently, myocardial relaxation begins as troponin releases calcium ions.

18. Cardiac performance is affected by preload, afterload, myocardial contractility, and heart rate.

19. Preload, or pressure generated in the ventricles at the end of diastole, depends on the amount of blood in the ventricle. Afterload is the resistance to ejection of the blood from the ventricle. Afterload depends on pressure in the aorta.

20. Myocardial stretch determines the force of myocardial contraction; thus the greater the stretch, the stronger the contraction up to a certain point. This relationship is known as the Frank-Starling law of the heart.

21. Contractility is the potential for myocardial fiber shortening during systole. It is determined by the amount of stretch during diastole (i.e., preload) and by sympathetic stimulation of the ventricles.

22. The heart rate is determined by the sinoatrial node and by components of the autonomic nervous system, including cardiovascular control centers in the brain, receptors in the aorta and carotid arteries, and hormones, including catecholamines (epinephrine, norepinephrine).

Systemic Circulation

1. Blood flows from the left ventricle into the aorta and from the aorta into arteries that eventually branch into arterioles and capillaries, the smallest of the arterial vessels. O_2, nutrients, and other substances needed for cellular metabolism pass from the capillaries into the tissues, where they are taken up by the cells. Capillaries also absorb metabolic waste products from the tissues.

2. Venules, the smallest veins, receive capillary blood. From the venules, the venous blood flows into larger and larger veins until it reaches the venae cavae, through which it enters the right atrium.

3. Vessel walls have three layers: the tunica intima (inner layer), the tunica media (middle layer), and the tunica externa (the outer layer).

4. Layers of the vessel wall differ in thickness and composition from vessel to vessel, depending on the vessel's size and location within the circulatory system. In general, the tunica media of arteries close to the heart has more elastic fibers (elastic arteries) because these arteries must be able to distend during systole and recoil during diastole. Arteries farther from the heart contain more smooth muscle fibers (muscular arteries) because they constrict and dilate to control blood pressure and volume within specific capillary beds.

5. Blood flow into the capillary beds is controlled by the contraction and relaxation of smooth muscle bands (precapillary sphincters) at junctions between metarterioles and capillaries.

6. Endothelial cells line the blood vessels. The endothelium is a life-support tissue; it functions as a filter (altering permeability), changes in vasomotion (constriction and dilation), and is involved in clotting and inflammation.

7. Blood flow through the veins is assisted by the contraction of skeletal muscles (the muscle pump), and backward flow is prevented by one-way valves, which are particularly important in the deep veins of the legs.

8. Blood flow is affected by blood pressure, resistance to flow within the vessels, velocity of the blood, anatomic features that may cause turbulent or laminar flow, and compliance (distensibility) of the vessels.

9. The Poiseuille law states that resistance is directly related to tube length and blood viscosity, and inversely related to the radius of the tube.

10. Total resistance, or the resistance to flow within the entire systemic circulatory system, depends on the combined lengths and radii of all the vessels within the system and on whether the vessels are arranged in series (greater resistance) or in parallel (lesser resistance).

11. Blood flow is also influenced by neural stimulation (vasoconstriction or vasodilation) and by autonomic features that cause turbulence within the vascular lumen (e.g., protrusions from the vessel wall, twists and turns, vessel branching).

12. Arterial blood pressure is influenced and regulated by factors that affect cardiac output (heart rate, stroke volume), total resistance within the system, and blood volume.

13. ADH, the RAAS system, and NPs can all alter blood volume and thus blood pressure.

14. Venous blood pressure is influenced by blood volume within the venous system and compliance of the venous walls.

15. Blood flow through the coronary circulation is governed by the same principles as flow through other vascular beds plus two adaptations dictated by cardiac dynamics. First, blood flows into the coronary arteries during diastole rather than systole, because during systole the cusps of the aortic semilunar valve block the openings of the coronary arteries. Second, systolic contraction inhibits coronary artery flow by compressing the coronary arteries.

16. Autoregulation enables the coronary vessels to maintain optimal perfusion pressure despite systolic compression.

17. Myoglobin in heart muscle stores O_2 for use during the systolic phase of the cardiac cycle.

The Lymphatic System

1. The vessels of the lymphatic system run in the same sheaths as the arteries and veins.

2. Lymph (interstitial fluid) is absorbed by lymphatic venules in the capillary beds and travels through ever larger lymphatic veins until it empties through the right lymphatic duct or thoracic duct into the right or left subclavian veins, respectively.

3. As lymph travels toward the thoracic ducts, it passes through thousands of lymph nodes clustered around the lymphatic veins. The lymph nodes are sites of immune function and are ideally placed to sample antigens and cells carried by the lymph from the periphery of the body into the central circulation.

KEY TERMS

A band, 572
Actin, 572
Adrenomedullin (ADM), 584
Afferent lymphatic vessel, 587
Afterload, 575
Angiogenesis, 568
Aorta, 565
Aortic semilunar valve, 566
Arteriogenesis, 568
Arteriole, 577
Artery, 577
Atrioventricular node (AV) node, 569
Atrioventricular (AV) valve, 565
Automatic cell, 570
Automaticity, 570
Autoregulation, 585
Bainbridge reflex, 576
Baroreceptor reflex, 576
Blood flow, 577
Blood velocity, 581
Bundle of His (atrioventricular bundle), 569
Capillary, 577
Cardiac action potential, 568
Cardiac cycle, 567
Cardiac output, 574
Cardiac vein, 567
Cardiomyocyte, 564
Cardiovascular vasomotor control center, 576
Chordae tendineae, 565
Circumflex artery, 568
Collateral artery, 568
Conduction system, 568
Coronary artery, 567
Coronary circulation, 567
Coronary ostium (pl., ostia), 567
Coronary perfusion pressure, 585
Coronary sinus, 567
Cross-bridge theory of muscle contraction, 573

Depolarization, 570
Diastole, 567
Diastolic blood pressure, 582
Diastolic depolarization, 570
Efferent lymphatic vessel, 587
Ejection fraction, 574
Elastic artery, 577
Endocardium, 564
Endothelial cell, 577
Endothelium, 577
Epinephrine, 583
Excitation-contraction coupling, 573
Fenestration, 577
Frank-Starling law of the heart, 575
Great cardiac vein, 568
H band, 573
Heart rate, 571
Hematocrit, 579
I band, 572
Inferior vena cava (pl., cavae), 565
Inotropic agent, 576
Intercalated disk, 571
Laminar flow, 581
Laplace law, 574
Left anterior descending (LAD) artery, 567
Left atrium, 565
Left bundle branch (LBB), 569
Left coronary artery (LCA), 567
Left heart, 563
Left ventricle, 565
Lumen, 577
Lymph, 586
Lymph node, 587
Lymphatic vein, 586
Lymphatic venule, 586
M line, 573
Mean arterial pressure (MAP), 582
Mediastinum, 563

Metarteriole, 577
Mitral and tricuspid complex, 566
Mitral valve, 566
Muscle pump, 577
Muscular artery, 577
Myocardial contractility, 573
Myocardial oxygen consumption ($M\dot{V}O_2$), 573, 573
Myocardium, 564
Myoglobin, 585
Myosin, 572
Natriuretic peptide (NP), 583
Nitric oxide (NO), 584
P wave, 570
Pacemaker, 568
Papillary muscle, 565
Perfusion, 582
Pericardial cavity, 564
Pericardial fluid, 564
Pericardial sac, 564
Pericardium, 564
Peripheral vascular system, 577
Poiseuille law, 578
PR interval, 570
Precapillary sphincter, 577
Preload, 574
Pressure, 578
Prolapse, 565
Pulmonary artery, 565
Pulmonary circulation, 563
Pulmonary semilunar valve, 566
Pulmonary vein, 565
Pulse pressure, 582
Purkinje fiber, 570
QRS complex, 570
QT interval, 570
Radius (diameter), 578
Refractory period, 570
Repolarization, 570
Resistance, 578
Rhythmicity, 570
Right atrium, 565

Right bundle branch (RBB), 569
Right coronary artery (RCA), 567
Right heart, 563
Right lymphatic duct, 586
Right ventricle, 565
Sarcomere, 573
Semilunar valve, 566
Shear stress, 568
Sinoatrial node (SA node, sinus node), 569
Stenosis, 568
ST interval, 570
Stroke volume, 574
Superior vena cava (pl., cavae), 565
Systemic circulation, 563
Systemic vascular resistance (SVR), 576
Systole, 567
Systolic blood pressure, 581
Systolic compressive effect, 585
T wave, 570
Thoracic duct, 586
Titin, 572
Total peripheral resistance (TPR), 576
Total resistance, 579
Tricuspid valve, 565
Tropomyosin molecule, 572
Troponin, 572
Tunica externa (adventitia), 577
Tunica intima, 577
Tunica media, 577
Turbulent (flow), 581
Vasa vasorum, 577
Vascular compliance, 581
Vasoconstriction, 577
Vasodilation, 577
Vein, 577
Venule, 577
Viscosity, 579
Z line, 573

REFERENCES

1. Rajendran P, et al: The vascular endothelium and human diseases, *Int J Biol Sci* 9(10):1057-1069, 2013.
2. Lin Z, Pu WT: Strategies for cardiac regeneration and repair, *Sci Transl Med* 6(239):239rv1, 2014.
3. Kutty S, et al: Patent foramen ovale: the known and the to be known, *J Am Coll Cardiol* 59(19):1665-1671, 2012.
4. Tobis J, Shenoda M: Percutaneous treatment of patent foramen ovale and atrial septal defects, *J Am Coll Cardiol* 60(19):1722-1732, 2012.
5. Klabunde RE: *Cardiovascular physiology concepts*, ed 2, Baltimore, 2012, Lippincott, Williams & Wilkins.
6. Rubart M, Zipes DP: Genesis of cardiac arrhythmias. In Mann DL, et al, editors: *Braunwald's heart disease: a textbook of cardiovascular medicine*, ed 10, Philadelphia, 2015, Saunders, pp 629-661. pp 33.

7. Opie LH, Bers DM: Mechanisms of cardiac contraction and relaxation. In Mann DL, et al, editors: *Braunwald's heart disease: a textbook of cardiovascular medicine*, ed 10, Philadelphia, 2015, Saunders, pp 429-453.
8. Linke WA, Hamdani N: Gigantic business: titin properties and function through thick and thin, *Circ Res* 114:1052-1068, 2014.
9. Deussen A, et al: Mechanisms of metabolic coronary flow regulation, *J Mol Cell Cardiol* 52(4):794-801, 2012.
10. Sakata Y, et al: Left ventricular stiffening as therapeutic target for heart failure with preserved ejection fraction, *Circ J* 77(4):886-892, 2013.
11. Ababneh AA, et al: Normal limits for left ventricular ejection fraction and volumes estimated with gated myocardial perfusion imaging in patients with normal exercise test results: influence of tracer,

gender, and acquisition camera, *J Nucl Cardiol* 7(6):661-668, 2000.
12. Davidson CJ, Bonow RO: Cardiac catheterization. In Mann DL, et al, editors: *Braunwald's heart disease: a textbook of cardiovascular medicine*, ed 10, Philadelphia, 2015, Saunders, pp 364-391.
13. Flynn A, et al: Sepsis-induced cardiomyopathy: a review of pathophysiologic mechanisms, *Heart Fail Rev* 15(6):605-611, 2010.
14. Goegel B, et al: Impact of acute normobaric hypoxia on regional and global myocardial function: a speckle tracking echocardiography study, *Int J Cardiovasc Imaging* 29(3):561-567, 2013.
15. Hoit BD, Walsh RA: Normal physiology of the cardiovascular system. In Fuster V, et al, editors: *Hurst's the heart*, ed 13, Philadelphia, 2011, McGraw-Hill.
16. Crystal GJ, Salem MR: The Bainbridge and the "reverse" Bainbridge reflexes: history, physiology, and

clinical relevance, *Anesth Analg* 114(3):520-532, 2012.

17. Volpe M, et al: Natriuretic peptides in cardiovascular diseases: current use and perspectives, *Eur Heart J* 35(7):419-425, 2014.

18. Perkel D, et al: The potential effects of IGF-1 and GH on patients with chronic heart failure, *J Cardiovasc Pharmacol Ther* 17(1):72-78, 2012.

19. Bergler-Klein J, et al: The role of biomarkers in valvular heart disease: focus on natriuretic peptides, *Can J Cardiol* 30(9):1027-1034, 2014.

20. Schjerning Olsen AM, et al: The impact of NSAID treatment on cardiovascular risk—insight from Danish observational data, *Basic Clin Pharmacol Toxicol* 115(2):179-184, 2014.

21. Singh BK, et al: Assessment of nonsteroidal anti-inflammatory drug-induced cardiotoxicity, *Expert Opin Drug Metab Toxicol* 10(2):143-156, 2014.

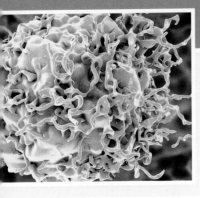

26

Alterations of Cardiovascular Function

Valentina L. Brashers

EVOLVE WEBSITE

http://evolve.elsevier.com/Huether/
Student Review Questions
Audio Key Points

Case Studies
Animations
Quick Check Answers

Our understanding of the pathophysiology of cardiovascular diseases is evolving rapidly. Neurohumoral, genetic, inflammatory, and metabolic factors are now the focus. This new information is leading to improvements in prevention and treatment.

DISEASES OF THE VEINS

Varicose Veins and Chronic Venous Insufficiency

A varicose vein is a vein in which blood has pooled, producing distended, tortuous, and palpable vessels (Fig. 26.1). Risk factors include age, female sex, family history of varicose veins, obesity, pregnancy, deep venous thrombosis (DVT), and previous leg injury. Varicose veins typically involve the saphenous veins of the leg and are caused by (1) injury or disease involving the saphenous veins that damages one or more valves or (2) gradual venous distention caused by the action of gravity on blood in the legs.

If a valve is damaged, volume and pressure increase within the vessel. The vein swells as it becomes engorged and surrounding tissue becomes edematous because increased hydrostatic pressure pushes plasma through the stretched vessel wall. Venous distention develops over time, especially in individuals who habitually stand for long periods, wear constricting garments, or cross the legs at the knees, which diminishes the action

of the muscle pump (see Fig. 25.19). Eventually the pressure in the vein damages venous valves, rendering them incompetent and unable to maintain normal venous pressure.

Varicose veins and valvular incompetence can progress to chronic venous insufficiency, especially in obese individuals. Chronic venous insufficiency (CVI) is inadequate venous return over a long period. Venous hypertension, circulatory stasis, and tissue hypoxia cause an inflammatory reaction in vessels and tissue leading to fibrosclerotic remodeling of the skin and then to ulceration. Symptoms include edema of the lower extremities and hyperpigmentation of the skin of the feet and ankles. Poor circulation makes tissues vulnerable to trauma and infection resulting in the formation of venous stasis ulcers (Fig. 26.2) and cellulitis.

Treatment of varicose veins and CVI begins conservatively with elevating the legs, wearing compression stockings, and performing physical exercise. Invasive management includes endovenous ablation, sclerotherapy or surgical ligation, and conservative vein resection.

Thrombus Formation in Veins

A thrombus is a blood clot that remains attached to a vessel wall (see Fig. 23.22). A detached thrombus is a thromboembolus. Venous thrombi are more common than arterial thrombi because flow and pressure are

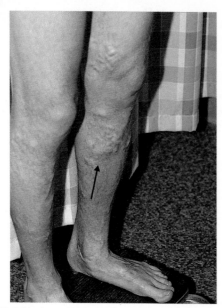

FIGURE 26.1 Varicose Veins of the Leg *(Arrow).* (From Kumar V et al: *Robbins and Cotran pathologic basis of disease,* ed 8, Philadelphia, 2010, Saunders. Courtesy Dr. Magruder C. Donaldson, Brigham and Women's Hospital, Boston, Mass.)

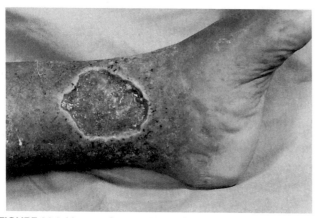

FIGURE 26.2 Venous Stasis Ulcer. (From Rosai J: *Ackerman's surgical pathology,* ed 7, vol 2, St Louis, 1989, Mosby.)

lower in the veins than in the arteries. **Deep venous thrombosis (DVT)** occurs primarily in the lower extremity. Three factors (triad of Virchow) promote venous thrombosis: (1) venous stasis (e.g., immobility, age, heart failure), (2) venous endothelial damage (e.g., trauma, surgery, intravenous medications), and (3) hypercoagulable states (e.g., inherited disorders, malignancy, pregnancy, use of oral contraceptives or hormone replacement therapy). Orthopedic trauma or surgery, spinal cord injury, and obstetric/gynecologic conditions are associated with a high likelihood of DVT. Inherited hypercoagulability states increase the risk for DVT, especially in association with other risk factors, such as immobility or pregnancy. The most common inherited abnormality is factor V Leiden mutation, which affects 3% to 8% of the population. Other inherited hypercoagulability states are caused by prothrombin mutations and deficiencies of protein C, protein S, and antithrombin.

Accumulation of clotting factors and platelets leads to thrombus formation in the vein, often near a venous valve. Inflammation around the thrombus promotes further platelet aggregation, and the thrombus propagates (grows) proximally. This inflammation may cause pain and redness, but is usually not accompanied by clinical symptoms or signs. If the thrombus creates significant obstruction to venous blood flow, increased pressure in the vein behind the clot may lead to edema of the extremity. Most thrombi will eventually dissolve without treatment; however, untreated DVT is associated with a high risk of thromboembolization to the lung (pulmonary embolism) (see Chapter 29). Persistent venous obstruction may lead to CVI and postthrombotic syndrome with associated pain, edema, and ulceration of the affected limb.

Because DVT is usually asymptomatic and difficult to detect clinically, prevention is important in at-risk individuals and includes early ambulation, pneumatic devices, and prophylactic anticoagulation. If thrombosis does occur, diagnosis is confirmed by a combination of serum D-dimer measurement and Doppler ultrasonography. Management most often consists of anticoagulation therapy using heparin (low-molecular-weight heparin) and warfarin. New oral anticoagulant therapies, such as factor Xa inhibitors and direct thrombin inhibitors, have been shown to have a more favorable benefit-to-risk ratio and are rapidly becoming the treatments of choice.[1] Thrombolytic therapy or placement of an inferior vena cava filter may be indicated in selected individuals.

Superior Vena Cava Syndrome

Superior vena cava syndrome (SVCS) is a progressive occlusion of the superior vena cava (SVC) that leads to venous distention in the upper extremities and head. The most common cause is bronchogenic cancer followed by lymphomas and metastasis of other cancers. Other less common causes include tuberculosis, mediastinal fibrosis, and cystic fibrosis. Invasive therapies (pacemaker wires, central venous catheters, and pulmonary artery catheters) with associated thrombosis now account for nearly half of cases. The SVC is a relatively low-pressure vessel that lies in the closed thoracic compartment; therefore space-occupying lesions can easily compress the SVC. The SVC is surrounded by lymph nodes and abuts the right mainstem bronchus, which commonly becomes involved in thoracic cancers and compresses the SVC during tumor growth.

Clinical manifestations of SVCS are edema and venous distention in the upper extremities and face, including the ocular beds. Affected persons complain of a feeling of fullness in the head or tightness of shirt collars, necklaces, and rings. Cerebral edema may cause headache, visual disturbance, and impaired consciousness. The skin of the face and arms may become purple and taut, and capillary refill time is prolonged. Respiratory distress may be present because of bronchial compression. In infants, SVCS can lead to hydrocephalus.

Diagnosis is made by chest X-ray, Doppler studies, computed tomography (CT), magnetic resonance imaging (MRI), and ultrasound. SVCS is an oncologic emergency. Treatment for malignant disorders can include radiation therapy, surgery, chemotherapy, and the administration of diuretics, steroids, and anticoagulants, as necessary. Treatment for nonmalignant causes may include bypass surgery using various grafts, thrombolysis (both locally and systemically), balloon angioplasty, and placement of intravascular stents.

✔ **QUICK CHECK 26.1**

1. What is chronic venous insufficiency, and how does it present clinically?
2. What are the major risk factors for deep venous thrombosis?
3. Name three causes of superior vena cava syndrome.

DISEASES OF THE ARTERIES

Hypertension

Hypertension is consistent elevation of systemic arterial blood pressure. It has recently been redefined as a sustained systolic blood pressure (SBP) of 130 mm Hg or a diastolic blood pressure (DBP) of 80 mm

TABLE 26.1 Classification of Blood Pressure for Adults Age 18 Years and Older

Category	Systolic (mm Hg)		Diastolic (mm Hg)
Normal	<120	AND	<80
Elevated	120-129	AND	<80
Stage 1 hypertension	130-139	OR	80-89
Stage 2 hypertension	≥140	OR	≥90
Hypertensive crisis	≥180	AND/OR	>120

Data from Whelton PK et al: *Hypertension* 71(6):e13-e115, 2018.

Hg or greater[2] (Table 26.1). One in three Americans has hypertension, and more than two thirds of those older than age 60 are affected.[3] The chance of developing primary hypertension increases with age, although children are being diagnosed with increasing frequency (see Chapter 27). The prevalence of hypertension is higher in African Americans and in those with diabetes. Those who fall into the new category called elevated blood pressure are at risk for developing hypertension unless lifestyle modification and treatment are instituted. All stages of hypertension are associated with increased risk for target organ disease events, such as myocardial infarction (MI), kidney disease, and stroke.

Most cases (92%-95%) of hypertension are diagnosed as primary hypertension (also called essential or idiopathic hypertension). Secondary hypertension is caused by an underlying disorder such as renal disease. This form of hypertension accounts for only 5% to 8% of cases.

Factors Associated With Primary Hypertension

A specific cause for primary hypertension has not been identified, and a combination of genetic and environmental factors is thought to be responsible for its development. Genetic predisposition to hypertension is thought to be polygenic and associated with epigenetic changes influenced by diet and lifestyle. These changes include defects in renal sodium excretion, insulin sensitivity, activity of the sympathetic nervous system (SNS) and the renin-angiotensin-aldosterone system (RAAS), and cell membrane sodium or calcium transport. Risk factors for primary hypertension relate to age, sex, race, and dietary factors (see *Risk Factors: Primary Hypertension*). Many of these factors are also risk factors for other cardiovascular disorders. In fact, obesity, hypertension, dyslipidemia, and glucose intolerance often are found together in a condition called the metabolic syndrome (see Chapter 20).

RISK FACTORS

Primary Hypertension

Family history
Advancing age
Cigarette smoking
Obesity
Heavy alcohol consumption
Sex (men > women before age 55, women > men after 55)
Black race
High dietary sodium intake
Low dietary intake of potassium, calcium, magnesium
Glucose intolerance

PATHOPHYSIOLOGY Hypertension results from a sustained increase in peripheral vascular resistance (PVR), an increase in circulating blood volume, or both.

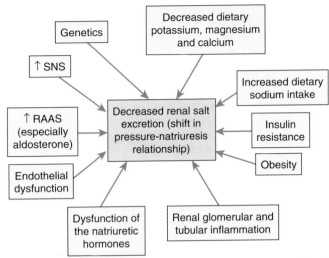

FIGURE 26.3 Factors That Cause a Shift in the Pressure-Natriuresis Relationship. Numerous factors have been implicated in the pathogenesis of sodium retention in individuals with hypertension. These factors cause less renal excretion of salt than would normally occur with increased blood pressure. This is called a shift in the pressure-natriuresis relationship and is thought to be a central process in the pathogenesis of primary hypertension. *RAAS,* Renin-angiotensin-aldosterone system; *SNS,* sympathetic nervous system.

Primary Hypertension

Primary hypertension is the result of an extremely complicated interaction of genetics and the environment mediated by a host of neurohumoral effects that influence intravascular volume and PVR. Multiple pathophysiologic mechanisms mediate these effects, including the SNS, the RAAS, and natriuretic peptides. Inflammation, endothelial dysfunction, obesity-related hormones, and insulin resistance also contribute. Increased vascular volume is related to a decrease in renal excretion of salt, often referred to as a shift in the pressure-natriuresis relationship (Fig. 26.3). This means that for a given blood pressure, individuals with hypertension tend to secrete less salt in their urine.

Increased SNS activity causes increased heart rate and systemic vasoconstriction. This increases both cardiac output and peripheral vascular resistance, thus raising the blood pressure. Additional mechanisms of SNS-induced hypertension include structural changes in blood vessels (vascular remodeling), renal sodium retention (shift in pressure-natriuresis curve), insulin resistance, increased renin and angiotensin levels, and procoagulant effects.

In hypertensive individuals, overactivity of the RAAS directly causes salt and water retention and increased vascular resistance (see Fig. 25.24). High levels of renin, angiotensin II (Ang II), and aldosterone also contribute to endothelial dysfunction, insulin resistance, platelet aggregation, and arteriolar remodeling. Remodeling is structural change in vessel walls that results in permanent increases in PVR and contributes to atherogenesis. The RAAS is associated with end-organ effects of hypertension, including coronary artery disease (CAD), renal disease, cardiac hypertrophy, and heart failure. Medications, such as angiotensin-converting enzyme (ACE) inhibitors, angiotensin receptor blockers (ARBs), and aldosterone blockers oppose the activity of the RAAS and are effective in reducing blood pressure and protecting against target organ damage. A second RAAS also has been described that has cardiovascular, cerebrovascular, and metabolic protective effects. Its discovery may lead to new and more effective medications (see *Did You Know? The Renin-Angiotensin-Aldosterone System [RAAS] and Cardiovascular Disease*).

The Renin-Angiotensin-Aldosterone System (RAAS) and Cardiovascular Disease

The RAAS has multiple effects on the cardiovascular system. There are two primary RAA systems. The best known includes the release of renin, the synthesis of Ang II through ACE, stimulation of the AT1 receptor (AT1R), and secretion of aldosterone. This system contributes to systemic vasoconstriction, renal salt and water retention, and remodeling of blood vessels, kidney, and the heart. Drugs that block this RAAS include ACE inhibitors, direct renin inhibitors, Ang II receptor blockers (ARBs), and aldosterone inhibitors. In contrast, the second RAAS serves a counterregulatory system. Activation of a second ACE pathway (ACE2) leads to the synthesis of angiotensin 1-7 from Ang II. Angiotensin 1-7 stimulates Mas receptors and has vasodilatory, antiproliferative, antifibrotic, and antithrombotic effects. These protective effects lead to lower blood pressure, less vascular inflammation and clotting, and decreased tissue remodeling and damage to target organ tissues. Research is underway to develop pharmacologic interventions, such as synthetic Mas agonists, Ang(1-7) formulations, and ACE2 activators that will stimulate these protective RAAS pathways.

Data from Bahramali E et al: *Clin Exp Hypertens* 39(4):371-376, 2017; Carey RM: *Am J Hypertens* 30(4), 339-347, 2017; Mirabito Colafella KM, Danser AHJ: *Hypertension* 69(6):994-999, 2017; Schmull S et al: *Curr Hypertens Rev* 12(3):170-180, 2016; Williams B: *Ther Adv Cardiovasc Dis* 10(3):118-125, 2016.

The natriuretic hormones include atrial natriuretic peptide (ANP), B-type natriuretic peptide (BNP), C-type natriuretic peptide (CNP), and urodilatin. They modulate renal sodium (Na^+) excretion and require adequate potassium, calcium, and magnesium intake to function properly. Dysfunction of these hormones, along with alterations in the RAA system and the SNS, causes a shift in the pressure-natriuresis relationship leading to increased blood volume and blood pressure. With inadequate natriuretic function, a compensatory increase occurs in natriuretic peptide serum levels. High levels of these peptides therefore indicate dysfunction and are linked to an increased risk for ventricular hypertrophy, atherosclerosis, and heart failure in individuals with hypertension. Salt restriction combined with adequate intake of dietary potassium, magnesium, and calcium improves natriuretic peptide function.

Innate and adaptive immunity with associated inflammation play a role in the pathogenesis of hypertension. Activation of immunity results in chronic inflammation with damage to endothelial cells, decreased production of vasodilators (such as nitric oxide), vascular remodeling, and smooth muscle contraction. Inflammation also contributes to insulin resistance, decreased natriuresis, and autonomic dysfunction.

Obesity is recognized as an important risk factor for hypertension in both adults and children and contributes to many of the neurohumoral, metabolic, renal, and cardiovascular processes that cause hypertension. Obesity causes changes in the adipokines (i.e., leptin and adiponectin) and also is associated with increased activity of the SNS and RAAS. Obesity is linked to inflammation, endothelial dysfunction, insulin resistance, and an increased risk for cardiovascular complications from hypertension (see *Did You Know? Obesity and Hypertension*).

Insulin resistance is common in hypertension, even in individuals without clinical diabetes. Insulin resistance is associated with decreased endothelial release of nitric oxide and other vasodilators. It also affects renal function and causes renal salt and water retention. Insulin resistance promotes overactivity of the SNS and RAAS. The interactions among obesity, hypertension, insulin resistance, and lipid disorders in metabolic syndrome result in a high risk of cardiovascular disease.

Obesity and Hypertension

Obesity is a well-known risk factor for hypertension. Obesity and increased caloric intake contribute to adipocyte dysfunction and ectopic fat deposition throughout the cardiovascular system. Adipocytes secrete adipokines, including leptin and adiponectin. The primary function of leptin is to interact with the hypothalamus to control body weight through appetite inhibition and increased metabolic rate. Chronically high levels of leptin noted in obesity, however, result in resistance to these weight-reducing functions. Adiponectin is a protein produced by adipose tissue but is reduced in obesity. With obesity, increased leptin and decreased adiponectin have been found to increase sympathetic nervous system and renin-angiotensin-aldosterone system activity, contribute to insulin resistance, decrease renal sodium excretion, promote inflammation, and stimulate myocyte hypertrophy. Other adipokines that are altered in obesity-related cardiovascular diseases include resistin, omentin, visfatin, and perivascular adipose tissue–derived relaxing factor. Obesity also is linked with endothelial dysfunction and release of vascular growth factors, which contribute to arterial remodeling. Taken together, these obesity-related changes result in vasoconstriction, salt and water retention, and renal dysfunction that contribute to the development of hypertension. Weight loss is an essential treatment for obesity-related hypertension. In severe obesity, bariatric surgery has been shown to cause long-standing remission of hypertension in many individuals.

Data from Cabandugama PK et al: *Med Clin North Am* 101(1):129-137, 2017; Faulkner JL, Belin de Chantemele EJ: *Hypertension* 71(1):15-21, 2018; Jakobsen GS et al: *J Am Med Assoc* 319(3):291-301, 2018; Nizar JM, Bhalla V: *Curr Hypertens Rep* 19(8):60, 2017; Schutten MT et al: *Physiology* 32(3):197-209, 2017; Seravalle G, Grassi G: *Pharmacol Res* 122:1-7, 2017.

It is likely that primary hypertension is an interaction among many of these factors, leading to sustained increases in blood volume and PVR. The pathophysiology of primary hypertension is summarized in Fig. 26.4.

Secondary Hypertension

Secondary hypertension is caused by an underlying disease process or medication that raises PVR or cardiac output. Examples include renal vascular or parenchymal disease, adrenocortical tumors, adrenomedullary tumors (pheochromocytoma), and drugs (oral contraceptives, corticosteroids, antihistamines). If the cause is identified and removed before permanent structural changes occur, blood pressure returns to normal.

Complicated Hypertension

As hypertension becomes more severe and chronic, tissue damage can occur in the blood vessels and tissues leading to target organ damage in the heart, kidney, brain, and eyes. Cardiovascular complications of sustained hypertension include left ventricular hypertrophy, angina pectoris, heart failure, coronary artery disease, myocardial infarction, and sudden death. Myocardial hypertrophy is mediated by the SNS and RAAS. Hypertrophy is characterized by a myocardium that is thickened, scarred, and less able to relax during diastole, leading to heart failure with preserved ejection fraction. Over time, the increased size of the heart muscle increases demand for oxygen delivery, the contractility of the heart is impaired, and the individual is at risk for myocardial infarction and heart failure with reduced ejection fraction. Vascular complications include hyaline sclerosis and accelerated atherosclerosis that can affect perfusion to any vascular bed. Hypertension also can contribute to the formation, dissection, and rupture of aneurysms

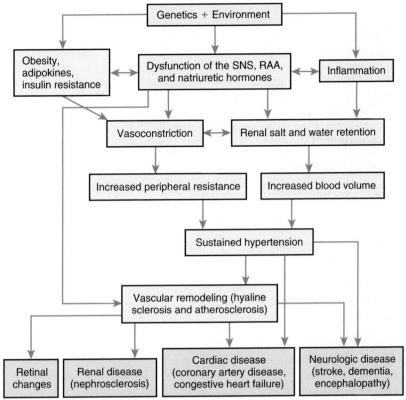

FIGURE 26.4 Pathophysiology of Hypertension. Numerous genetic vulnerabilities have been linked to hypertension and these, in combination with environmental risks, cause neurohumoral dysfunction (sympathetic nervous system *[SNS]*, renin-angiotensin-aldosterone *[RAA]* system, natriuretic hormones) and promote inflammation and insulin resistance. Insulin resistance and neurohumoral dysfunction contribute to sustained systemic vasoconstriction and increased peripheral vascular resistance. Inflammation contributes to renal dysfunction, which, in combination with the neurohumoral alterations, results in renal salt and water retention and increased blood volume. Increased peripheral vascular resistance and increased blood volume are two primary causes of sustained hypertension.

TABLE 26.2   Pathologic Effects of Sustained, Complicated Primary Hypertension

Site of Injury	Mechanism of Injury	Pathologic Effect
Heart		
Myocardium	Increased workload combined with diminished blood flow through coronary arteries	Left ventricular hypertrophy, myocardial ischemia, heart failure
Coronary arteries	Accelerated atherosclerosis (coronary artery disease)	Myocardial ischemia, myocardial infarction, sudden death
Kidneys	Reduced blood flow, increased arteriolar pressure, RAAS and SNS stimulation, and inflammation	Glomerulosclerosis and decreased glomerular filtration, end-stage renal disease
Brain	Reduced blood flow and oxygen supply; weakened vessel walls, accelerated atherosclerosis	Transient ischemic attacks, cerebral thrombosis, aneurysm, hemorrhage, acute brain infarction
Eyes (retinas)	Retinal vascular sclerosis, increased retinal artery pressures	Hypertensive retinopathy, retinal exudates and hemorrhages
Aorta	Weakened vessel wall	Dissecting aneurysm
Arteries of lower extremities	Reduced blood flow and high pressures in arterioles, accelerated atherosclerosis	Intermittent claudication, gangrene

RAAS, renin-angiotensin-aldosterone system; *SNS,* sympathetic nervous system.

(outpouchings in vessel walls). Renal manifestations of complicated hypertension include nephrosclerosis, renal arteriosclerosis, and renal insufficiency or failure. Microalbuminuria (small amounts of protein in the urine) occurs in many individuals with HTN and is now recognized as an early sign of impending renal dysfunction and increased risk for cardiovascular events. Complications specific to the retina include retinal vascular sclerosis, exudation, and hemorrhage. Cerebrovascular complications include transient ischemia, stroke, cerebral thrombosis, aneurysm, hemorrhage, and dementia. The pathologic effects of complicated hypertension are summarized in Table 26.2.

Hypertensive crisis is rapidly progressive hypertension in which systolic pressure is ≥180 mmHg and or diastolic pressure is ≥120 mmHg. It can occur in those with primary hypertension, but the reason why some people develop this complication and others do not is unknown. Other causes include complications of pregnancy, cocaine or amphetamine use, reaction to certain medications, adrenal tumors, and alcohol withdrawal. High arterial pressure renders the cerebral arterioles incapable of regulating blood flow to the cerebral capillary beds. High hydrostatic pressures in the capillaries cause vascular fluid to exude into the interstitial space. If blood pressure is not reduced, cerebral edema and cerebral dysfunction (encephalopathy) increase until death occurs. Besides encephalopathy, hypertensive crisis can cause papilledema, cardiac failure, uremia, retinopathy, and cerebrovascular accident and is considered a medical emergency.

CLINICAL MANIFESTATIONS The early stages of hypertension have no clinical manifestations other than elevated blood pressure; for this reason, hypertension is called a silent disease. Some hypertensive individuals never develop signs, symptoms, or complications, whereas others become very ill, and hypertension can be a cause of death. If elevated blood pressure is not detected and treated, it becomes established, setting the stage for the complications of hypertension that begin to appear during the fourth, fifth, and sixth decades of life.

Most clinical manifestations of hypertensive disease are caused by complications that damage organs and tissues outside the vascular system. Besides elevated blood pressure, the signs and symptoms therefore tend to be specific for the organs or tissues affected. Evidence of heart disease, renal insufficiency, central nervous system dysfunction, impaired vision, impaired mobility, vascular occlusion, or edema can all be caused by sustained hypertension.

EVALUATION AND TREATMENT Diagnosis of hypertension requires the measurement of blood pressure on at least two separate occasions, averaging two readings at least 2 minutes apart, with the following conditions: the person is seated, the arm is supported at heart level, the person must be at rest for at least 5 minutes, and the person should not have smoked or ingested any caffeine in the previous 30 minutes. Diagnostic tests for further evaluation of hypertension include 24-hour blood pressure monitoring in selected individuals; measurement of electrolytes, glucose, and lipids; and an electrocardiogram (ECG). Individuals who have elevated blood pressure are assumed to have primary hypertension unless their history, physical examination, or initial diagnostic screening indicates secondary hypertension. Once the diagnosis is made, a careful evaluation for other cardiovascular risk factors and for end-organ damage should be done.

Treatment of primary hypertension depends on its severity. Management begins with lifestyle modification including exercise, dietary modifications including reducing salt intake, smoking cessation, and weight loss. Pharmacologic treatment is recommended for individuals who have existing or are at high risk for atherosclerotic cardiovascular disease, or for those who have Stage 2 hypertension.[2] Commonly recommended medications include thiazide diuretics, ACE inhibitors or ARBs, and calcium channel blockers. Careful follow-up to support continued adherence, determine the response, and monitor for potential side effects of these medications is important.

Orthostatic (Postural) Hypotension

The term **orthostatic (postural) hypotension (OH)** refers to a decrease in SBP of at least 20 mm Hg or a decrease in DBP of at least 10 mm Hg within 3 minutes of moving to a standing position. OH is usually associated with disorders that affect autonomic nervous function, affects men more often than women, and usually occurs between the ages of

40 and 70 years. It is a significant risk factor for falls and associated injury and for increased mortality.

Normally when an individual stands, the gravitational changes on the circulation are compensated by a baroreceptor-mediated reflex that stimulates the SNS. This causes arteriolar and venous constriction and increased heart rate upon standing. Other compensatory mechanisms include mechanical factors, such as the closure of valves in the venous system, contraction of the leg muscles, and a decrease in intrathoracic pressure. These mechanisms are dysfunctional or inadequate in individuals with orthostatic hypotension; consequently, upon standing, blood pools in the lower extremities and normal arterial pressure cannot be maintained.

Orthostatic hypotension may be acute or chronic. **Acute orthostatic hypotension** is common in the elderly and occurs when the normal regulatory mechanisms are inadequate as a result of (1) altered body chemistry, (2) drug action (e.g., antihypertensives, antidepressants), (3) prolonged immobility, (4) starvation, (5) physical exhaustion, (6) volume depletion (e.g., dehydration, diuresis, potassium or sodium depletion), or (7) any condition that results in venous pooling (e.g., pregnancy, extensive varicosities of the lower extremities).

Chronic orthostatic hypotension may be (1) secondary to a specific disease or (2) primary (idiopathic). The conditions that cause secondary orthostatic hypotension are endocrine disorders (e.g., adrenal insufficiency, diabetes), metabolic disorders (e.g., porphyria), or diseases of the central or peripheral nervous systems (e.g., Parkinson disease, multiple system atrophy, intracranial tumors, cerebral infarcts, Wernicke encephalopathy, peripheral neuropathies). Cardiovascular autonomic neuropathy is a common cause of OH in persons with diabetes and is a serious and often overlooked complication.

OH is often accompanied by dizziness, blurring or loss of vision, and syncope or fainting. When possible, acute OH and secondary chronic OH are managed by correction of the underlying condition. Primary OH and irreversible secondary OH are managed with a combination of nondrug (fluid and salt intake, thigh-high stockings) and drug therapies (mineralocorticoids and vasoconstrictors).

> ✔ **QUICK CHECK 26.2**
> 1. What are the major risk factors for hypertension?
> 2. Summarize the pathophysiology of primary hypertension.
> 3. What are the causes of orthostatic hypotension?

Aneurysm

An **aneurysm** is a localized dilation or outpouching of a vessel wall or cardiac chamber (Fig. 26.5). The law of Laplace (discussed in detail in Chapter 25) can provide an understanding of the hemodynamics of an aneurysm. **True aneurysms** involve weakening in all three layers of the arterial wall (Fig. 26.6, *A*). Most are fusiform and circumferential, whereas *saccular aneurysms* are basically spherical in shape. **False aneurysms** are an extravascular hematoma that communicates with the intravascular space. A common cause of this type of lesion is a leak between a vascular graft and a natural artery.

Vascular aneurysms most commonly occur in the thoracic or abdominal aorta. The aorta is particularly susceptible to aneurysm formation because of constant stress on the vessel wall and the absence of penetrating vasa vasorum in the media layer. Atherosclerosis is the most common cause of arterial aneurysms because plaque formation erodes the vessel wall and contributes to inflammation and release of proteinases that can further weaken the vessel. Hypertension also contributes to aneurysm formation by increasing wall stress. Collagen-vascular disorders (e.g., Marfan syndrome), syphilis, and other infections that affect arterial walls also can cause aneurysms.

Cardiac aneurysms most commonly form after MI when intraventricular tension stretches the noncontracting infarcted muscle. The stretching produces infarct expansion, a weak and thin layer of necrotic muscle, and fibrous tissue that bulges with each systole.

Clinical manifestations depend on where the aneurysm is located. Aortic aneurysms often are asymptomatic until they rupture and then cause severe pain and hypotension. Thoracic aortic aneurysms can cause dysphagia (difficulty swallowing) and dyspnea (breathlessness). An aneurysm that impairs flow to an extremity causes symptoms of ischemia. Cerebral aneurysms, which often occur in the circle of Willis, are associated with signs and symptoms of increased intracranial pressure and stroke. (Cerebral aneurysms are described in Chapter 17.) Aneurysms in the heart present with dysrhythmias, heart failure, and embolism of clots to the brain or other vital organs.

The diagnosis of an aneurysm is usually confirmed by ultrasonography, CT, MRI, or angiography. Medical treatment is indicated for slow-growing aortic aneurysms, particularly in early stages, and includes cessation of smoking, reduction of blood pressure and blood volume, and implementation of β-adrenergic blockade. For aneurysms that are dilating rapidly or have become large, surgical treatment is indicated and usually includes replacement with a prosthetic graft.

Aortic aneurysms can be complicated by the acute aortic syndromes, which include aortic dissection, hemorrhage into the vessel wall, or vessel rupture. Dissection of the layers of the arterial wall occurs when there is a tear in the intima and blood enters the wall of the artery (see Fig. 26.6, B). Dissections can involve any part of the aorta (ascending, arch, or descending) and can disrupt flow through arterial branches. Symptoms include severe pain in the neck, jaw, chest, back, or abdomen. Emergent evaluation and surgical intervention is critical.

Thrombus Formation

As in venous thrombosis, arterial thrombi tend to develop when intravascular conditions promote activation of coagulation or when there is stasis of blood flow. These conditions include those in which there

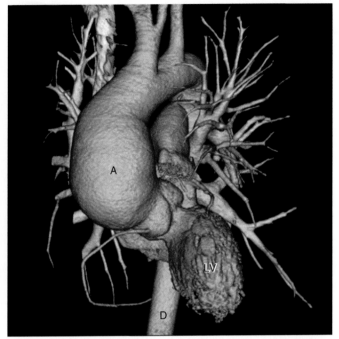

FIGURE 26.5 Aneurysm. A three-dimensional CT scan shows the aneurysm *(A)* involves the ascending thoracic aorta. *D,* Descending aorta; *LV,* left ventricle.

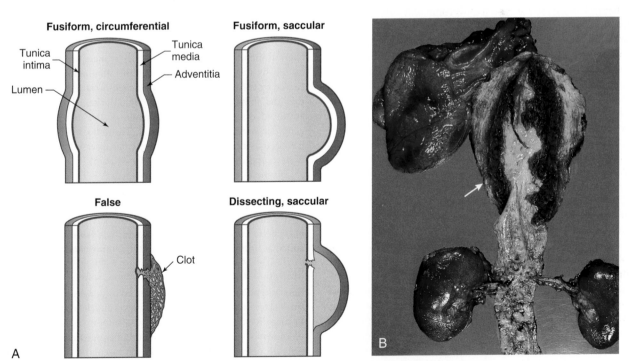

FIGURE 26.6 Longitudinal Sections Showing Types of Aneurysms. A, The fusiform circumferential and fusiform saccular aneurysms are true aneurysms, caused by weakening of the vessel wall. False and saccular aneurysms involve a break in the vessel wall, usually caused by trauma. **B,** Dissecting aneurysm of thoracic aorta *(arrow).* (B from Damjanov I, Linder J, editors: *Anderson's pathology,* ed 10, St Louis, 1996, Mosby.)

is intimal irritation or roughening (such as in surgical procedures and trauma), inflammation, infection, low intravascular volume and pressures, or obstructions that cause blood stasis and pooling within the vessels. (Mechanisms of coagulation are described in Chapter 22.) Inflammation of the endothelium leads to activation of the clotting cascade, causing platelets to adhere readily. An anatomic change in an artery (such as an aneurysm) can contribute to thrombus formation, particularly if the change results in a pooling of arterial blood. Valvular thrombi are most commonly associated with inflammation of the endocardium (endocarditis) and rheumatic heart disease. Widespread arterial thrombus formation can occur in shock when systemic inflammation activates the intrinsic and extrinsic pathways of coagulation, resulting in microvascular thrombosis throughout the systemic arterial circulation.

Arterial thrombi pose two potential threats to the circulation. First, the thrombus may grow large enough to occlude the artery, causing ischemia in tissue supplied by the artery. Second, the thrombus may dislodge, becoming a thromboembolus that travels through the vascular system until it occludes flow into a distal systemic vascular bed.

Diagnosis of arterial thrombi is usually accomplished through the use of Doppler ultrasonography and angiography. Pharmacologic treatment involves the administration of anticoagulants or thrombolytics. A balloon-tipped catheter can be used to remove or compress an arterial thrombus.

Embolism

Embolism is the obstruction of a vessel by an **embolus**—a bolus of matter circulating in the bloodstream. The embolus may consist of a dislodged thrombus; an air bubble; an aggregate of amniotic fluid; an aggregate of fat, bacteria, or cancer cells; or a foreign substance. The types of emboli are summarized in Table 26.3. Most emboli arise from venous or arterial thrombi and travel in the bloodstream until they reach a vessel through which they cannot pass. Pulmonary emboli originate on the venous system (mostly from the deep veins of the legs) or in the right heart; arterial emboli most commonly originate in the left heart and are associated with thrombus formation associated with MI, valvular disease, left heart failure, endocarditis, and dysrhythmias.

Embolism causes ischemia or **infarction** in tissues distal to the obstruction, producing organ dysfunction and pain. Infarction and subsequent necrosis of a central organ are life-threatening. For example, occlusion of a coronary artery will cause an MI whereas occlusion of a cerebral artery causes a stroke (see Chapter 17).

> ✔ **QUICK CHECK 26.3**
> 1. What are the major complications of aneurysms?
> 2. What is a thrombus?
> 3. Why are emboli dangerous?

Peripheral Vascular Disease
Thromboangiitis Obliterans (Buerger Disease)

Thromboangiitis obliterans (Buerger disease) is an autoimmune disease of the peripheral arteries. It is strongly associated with smoking. Thromboangiitis obliterans is characterized by the formation of thrombi filled with inflammatory and immune cells. Inflammatory cytokines and toxic oxygen free radicals contribute to accompanying vasospasm. Over time, these thrombi become organized and fibrotic and result in permanent occlusion of small- and medium-sized arteries in the feet and sometimes in the hands.

The chief symptom of thromboangiitis obliterans is pain and tenderness of the affected part, usually affecting more than one extremity.

TABLE 26.3	**Types of Emboli**
Type	**Characteristics**
Arteries	
Arterial thromboembolism	Dislodged thrombus; source is usually from heart; most common sites of obstruction are lower extremities (femoral and popliteal arteries), coronary arteries, and cerebral vasculature
Veins	
Venous thromboembolism	Dislodged thrombus; source is usually from lower extremities; obstructs branches of pulmonary artery
Air embolism	Bolus of air displaces blood in vasculature; source usually room air entering circulation through IV lines; trauma to chest also may allow air from lungs to enter vascular space
Amniotic fluid embolism	Bolus of amniotic fluid; extensive intra-abdominal pressure attending labor and delivery can force amniotic fluid into bloodstream of mother; introduces antigens, cells, and protein aggregates that trigger inflammation, coagulation, and immune responses
Bacterial embolism	Aggregates of bacteria in bloodstream; source is subacute bacterial endocarditis or abscess
Fat embolism	Globules of fat floating in bloodstream associated with trauma to long bones; lungs in particular are affected
Foreign matter	Small particles or fibers introduced during trauma or through an IV or intra-arterial line; coagulation cascade is initiated and thromboemboli form around particles

Clinical manifestations include rubor (redness of the skin), which is caused by dilated capillaries under the skin, and cyanosis, which is caused by tissue ischemia. Chronic ischemia causes the skin to become thin and shiny and the nails to become thickened and malformed. In advanced disease, profound ischemia of the extremities can cause gangrene necessitating amputation. Thromboangiitis obliterans also has been associated with cerebrovascular disease (stroke), mesenteric disease, and rheumatic symptoms (joint pain).

Diagnosis of thromboangiitis obliterans is made by identification of the following common features—age <45 years, smoking history, evidence of peripheral ischemia—and by exclusion of other causes of arterial insufficiency. The most important part of treatment is cessation of cigarette smoking. Other measures include vasodilators and exercises aimed at improving circulation to the foot or hand.

Raynaud Phenomenon

Raynaud phenomenon is characterized by attacks of vasospasm in the small arteries and arterioles of the fingers and, less commonly, the toes. Primary Raynaud phenomenon is a common vasospastic disorder of unknown origin. Secondary Raynaud phenomenon is associated with systemic diseases, particularly collagen vascular disease (scleroderma), vasculitis, malignancy, pulmonary hypertension, chemotherapy, cocaine use, hypothyroidism, thoracic outlet syndrome, trauma, serum sickness, or long-term exposure to environmental conditions such as cold temperatures or vibrating machinery in the workplace. Blood vessels in affected individuals demonstrate endothelial dysfunction with an imbalance in endothelium-derived vasodilators (e.g., nitric oxide) and vasoconstrictors (e.g., endothelin-1). Platelet activation also may play a role. It tends to affect young women and is characterized by vasospastic attacks triggered by brief exposure to cold, vibration, or emotional stress. Genetic predisposition may play a role in its development.

The clinical manifestations of the vasospastic attacks of either disorder are changes in skin color and sensation caused by ischemia. Attacks tend to be bilateral, and manifestations usually begin at the tips of the digits and progress to the proximal phalanges. Vasospasm causes pallor, numbness, and the sensation of coldness in the digits. Sluggish blood flow resulting from ischemia may cause the skin to appear cyanotic. Rubor, throbbing pain, and paresthesias follow as blood flow returns. Skin color returns to normal after the attack, but frequent, prolonged attacks interfere with cellular metabolism, causing the skin of the fingertips to thicken and the nails to become brittle. In severe, chronic Raynaud phenomenon, ischemia can eventually cause ulceration and gangrene.

The diagnosis of Raynaud phenomenon is based on clinical presentation and nailfold capillaroscopy. Treatment of Raynaud phenomenon begins with avoidance of stimuli that trigger attacks (e.g., cold temperatures, emotional stress) and cessation of cigarette smoking to eliminate the vasoconstricting effects of nicotine. If attacks of vasospasm become frequent or prolonged, vasodilators are administered. Sympathectomy may be indicated in severe cases. If ischemia leads to ulceration and gangrene, amputation may be necessary.

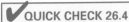

QUICK CHECK 26.4
1. What is thromboangiitis obliterans, and why does it occur?
2. What causes the physical manifestations of Raynaud phenomenon?

Atherosclerosis

Arteriosclerosis is a condition characterized by thickening and hardening of the vessel wall. Atherosclerosis is a form of arteriosclerosis that is caused by the accumulation of lipid-laden macrophages within the arterial wall, which leads to the formation of a lesion called a plaque. Atherosclerosis is a pathologic process that can affect vascular systems throughout the body and is the leading cause of peripheral artery disease, CAD, and cerebrovascular disease. (Atherosclerosis of the coronary arteries is described later in this chapter, and atherosclerosis of the cerebral arteries is described in Chapter 17.)

PATHOPHYSIOLOGY Atherosclerosis begins with injury to the endothelial cells that line artery walls. Pathologically, the lesions progress from endothelial injury and dysfunction to fatty streak to fibrotic plaque to complicated lesion (Fig. 26.7). Possible causes of endothelial injury include the common risk factors for atherosclerosis, such as smoking, hypertension, diabetes, increased levels of low-density lipoprotein (LDL), decreased levels of high-density lipoprotein (HDL), and autoimmunity. Other "nontraditional" risk factors include increased serum markers for inflammation and thrombosis (e.g., high-sensitivity C-reactive protein [hs-CRP]), troponin I, adipokines, infection, and air pollution. These risk factors are discussed in more detail in the following section on CAD (see the section on Coronary Artery Disease, Myocardial Ischemia, and Acute Coronary Syndromes).

Injured endothelial cells become inflamed. Inflamed endothelial cells cannot make normal amounts of antithrombic and vasodilating cytokines and express adhesion molecules that bind macrophages and other inflammatory and immune cells (Fig. 26.8). Macrophages release numerous inflammatory cytokines (e.g., tumor necrosis factor-alpha [TNF-α], interferons, interleukins, C-reactive protein) and enzymes that further injure the vessel wall. Toxic oxygen free radicals generated by the inflammatory process cause oxidation (i.e., addition of oxygen) of LDL that has accumulated in the vessel intima. Oxidized LDL causes additional adhesion molecule expression with the recruitment of monocytes that differentiate into macrophages. These macrophages penetrate into the intima, where they engulf oxidized LDL, and are then called foam cells. When they accumulate in significant amounts, they form a lesion called a fatty streak (see Figs. 26.8 and 26.9). Once formed, fatty streaks produce more toxic oxygen free radicals, recruit T cells leading to autoimmunity, and secrete additional inflammatory mediators resulting in progressive damage to the vessel wall.

Macrophages also release growth factors that stimulate smooth muscle cell proliferation. Smooth muscle cells in the region of endothelial injury proliferate, produce collagen, and migrate over the fatty streak, forming a fibrous plaque (see Fig. 26.9). The fibrous plaque may calcify, protrude into the vessel lumen, and obstruct blood flow to distal tissues (especially during exercise), which may cause symptoms (e.g., angina or intermittent claudication).

Many plaques, however, are "unstable," meaning they are prone to rupture. These plaques are clinically silent and do not affect luminal blood flow significantly until they rupture (see the section on Coronary Artery Disease, Myocardial Ischemia, and Acute Coronary Syndromes). Plaques that have ruptured are called complicated plaques. Once rupture occurs, exposure of underlying tissue results in platelet adhesion, initiation of the clotting cascade, and rapid thrombus formation. The thrombus may suddenly occlude the affected vessel, resulting in ischemia and infarction. Aspirin or other antithrombotic agents are used to prevent this complication of atherosclerotic disease.

CLINICAL MANIFESTATIONS Atherosclerosis presents with symptoms and signs that result from inadequate perfusion of tissues because of obstruction of the vessels that supply them. Partial vessel obstruction may lead to transient ischemic events, often associated with exercise or stress. As the lesion becomes complicated, increasing obstruction with superimposed thrombosis may result in tissue infarction. Obstruction of peripheral arteries can cause significant pain and disability. CAD caused by atherosclerosis is the major cause of myocardial ischemia. Atherosclerotic obstruction of the vessels supplying the brain is the major cause of stroke. Often, more than one vessel will become involved with this disease process such that an individual may present with symptoms from several ischemic tissues at the same time, and disease in one area may indicate that the individual is at risk for ischemic complications elsewhere.

EVALUATION AND TREATMENT In evaluating individuals for the presence of atherosclerosis, obtaining a complete health history (including risk factors and symptoms of ischemia) is essential. Physical examination may reveal arterial bruits and evidence of decreased blood flow to tissues. Laboratory data that include measurements of levels of lipids, blood glucose, and hs-CRP are also indicated. Judicious use of x-ray films, electrocardiography, ultrasonography, nuclear scanning, CT, MRI, and angiography may be necessary to identify affected vessels, particularly coronary vessels.

Current management of atherosclerosis is focused on detection and treatment of preclinical lesions with drugs aimed at stabilizing and reversing plaques before they rupture. Once a lesion obstructs blood flow, the primary goal in the management of atherosclerosis is to restore adequate blood flow to the affected tissues. If an individual has presented with acute ischemia (e.g., MI, stroke), interventions are specific to the diseased area (discussed further under those topics). In situations in which the disease process does not require immediate intervention, management focuses on reduction of risk factors and prevention of

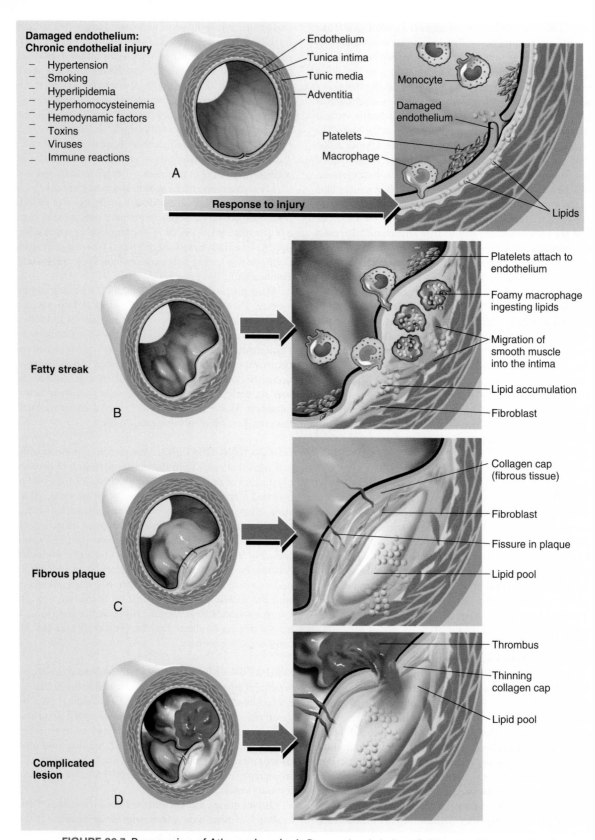

FIGURE 26.7 Progression of Atherosclerosis. A, Damaged endothelium. **B,** Diagram of fatty streak and lipid core formation (see Fig. 26.8 for a diagram of oxidized low-density lipoprotein [LDL]). **C,** Diagram of fibrous plaque. Raised plaques are visible: some are yellow; others are white. **D,** Diagram of complicated lesion; thrombus is red; collagen is blue. Plaque is complicated by red thrombus deposition.

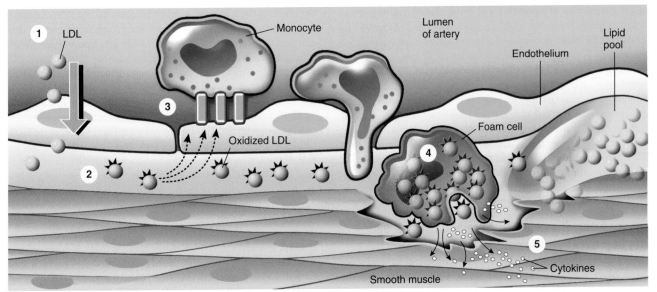

FIGURE 26.8 Low-Density Lipoprotein Oxidation. *(1)* Low-density lipoprotein (LDL) enters the arterial intima through an intact endothelium. *(2)* In hypercholesterolemia, the influx of LDL exceeds the eliminating capacity and an extracellular pool of LDL is formed. *(3)* Intimal LDL oxidized through the action of free oxygen radicals generates proinflammatory cytokines that induce endothelial expression of the adhesion molecules. Monocytes bind to the adhesion molecules and differentiate into macrophages, which then *(4)* internalize oxidized LDL and become foam cells. *(5)* Foam cells accumulate forming a fatty streak and release many inflammatory cytokines that damage the vessel wall. (Modified from Crawford MH et al: *Cardiology,* ed 3, London, 2010, Mosby.)

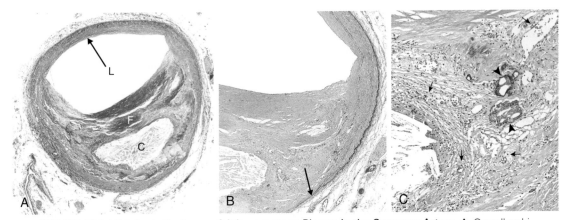

FIGURE 26.9 Histologic Features of Atheromatous Plaque in the Coronary Artery. A, Overall architecture demonstrating fibrous cap *(F)* and a central necrotic (largely lipid) core *(C)*. The lumen *(L)* has been moderately narrowed. Note that a segment of the wall is plaque free *(arrow)*, so that there is an eccentric lesion. In this section, collagen has been stained blue (Masson trichrome stain). **B,** Higher power photograph of a section of the plaque shown in **A,** stained for elastin *(black)*, demonstrating that the internal and external elastic membranes are destroyed and the media of the artery is thinned under the most advanced plaque *(arrow)*. **C,** Higher magnification photomicrograph at the junction of the fibrous cap and core, showing scattered inflammatory cells, calcification *(arrowhead)*, and neovascularization *(small arrows)*. (From Kumar V et al: *Robbins basic pathology,* ed 9, St Louis, 2007, Saunders.)

plaque progression. This includes implementation of an exercise program, cessation of smoking, and control of contributing factors such as hypertension, diabetes, and dyslipidemia. Management of atherosclerotic risk factors is discussed further in the Coronary Artery Disease, Myocardial Ischemia, and Acute Coronary Syndromes section.

Peripheral Artery Disease

Peripheral artery disease (PAD) refers to atherosclerotic disease of arteries that perfuse the limbs, especially the lower extremities. PAD affects an estimated 8.5 million Americans aged >40 years.[3] The risk factors for PAD are the same as those previously described for atherosclerosis. It is especially prevalent in smokers and elderly individuals with diabetes.

Lower extremity ischemia resulting from arterial obstruction in PAD can be gradual or acute. In most individuals, gradually increasing atherosclerotic obstruction to arterial blood flow in the iliofemoral vessels can result in leg pain with ambulation called intermittent claudication. If a thrombus forms over the atherosclerotic lesion, complete obstruction of blood flow can occur acutely, causing severe pain, loss of pulses, and skin color changes in the affected extremity.

Evaluation for PAD requires a careful history and physical examination that focuses on finding evidence of atherosclerotic disease (e.g., bruits), determining a difference in blood pressure measured at the ankle versus the arm (ankle-brachial index), and measuring blood flow using duplex ultrasound, CT angiography, or magnetic resonance angiography. Treatment includes risk factor reduction (smoking cessation, exercise, and treatment of diabetes, hypertension, and dyslipidemia) and anti-platelet therapy. Symptomatic PAD should be managed with vasodilators in combination with antiplatelet or antithrombotic medications and cholesterol-lowering medications.[4] If acute or refractory symptoms occur, emergent invasive catheterization followed by percutaneous or surgical revascularization may be indicated.

Coronary Artery Disease, Myocardial Ischemia, and Acute Coronary Syndromes

Coronary artery disease (CAD) caused by atherosclerosis is the primary cause of heart disease in the United States. CAD can diminish the myocardial blood supply until deprivation impairs myocardial metabolism enough to cause myocardial ischemia, a local state in which the cells are temporarily deprived of blood supply. The cells remain alive but cannot function normally. Persistent ischemia or the complete occlusion of a coronary artery causes the acute coronary syndromes, including MI *(heart attack)*.

Development of Coronary Artery Disease

CAD accounts for 1 in 7 deaths in the United States, with an estimated 366,800 deaths each year.[3] Risk factors for CAD are the same as those for atherosclerosis and can be categorized as conventional (major) versus nontraditional (novel) and as modifiable versus nonmodifiable. Conventional or major risk factors for CAD that are nonmodifiable include (1) advanced age, (2) male sex or women after menopause, and (3) family history. Aging and menopause are associated with increased exposure to risk factors and poor endothelial healing. Family history may contribute to CAD through genetics and shared environmental exposures. Many gene polymorphisms have been associated with CAD and its risk factors. Modifiable major risks include (1) dyslipidemia, (2) hypertension, (3) cigarette smoking, (4) diabetes and insulin resistance, (5) obesity, (6) sedentary lifestyle, and (7) atherogenic diet. Fortunately, modification of these factors can dramatically reduce the risk for CAD.

Dyslipidemia. The link between CAD and abnormal levels of lipoproteins is well documented. The term lipoprotein refers to lipids, phospholipids, cholesterol, and triglycerides bound to carrier proteins. The cycle of lipoprotein synthesis is complex. Dietary fat is packaged into particles known as chylomicrons in the small intestine. Chylomicrons primarily contain triglycerides. Some of the triglycerides may be removed and either stored by adipose tissue or used by muscle as an energy source. The chylomicron remnants, composed mainly of cholesterol,

are taken up by the liver. A series of chemical reactions in the liver results in the production of several lipoproteins that vary in density and function. These include very-low-density lipoproteins (VLDLs), primarily triglycerides and protein; low-density lipoproteins (LDLs), mostly cholesterol and protein; and high-density lipoproteins (HDLs), mainly phospholipids and protein. Although lipoproteins are necessary for many physiologic functions, they can accumulate in the serum.

Dyslipidemia (or dyslipoproteinemia) refers to abnormal concentrations of serum lipoproteins as defined by the Third Report of the National Cholesterol Education Program.[5] (Table 26.4). It is estimated that nearly half of the U.S. population has some form of dyslipidemia, especially among Caucasian and Asian populations.[3] These abnormalities are the result of a combination of genetic and dietary factors. Primary or familial dyslipoproteinemias result from genetic defects that cause abnormalities in lipid-metabolizing enzymes and abnormal cellular lipid receptors. Secondary causes of dyslipidemia include the existence of several common systemic disorders, such as diabetes, hypothyroidism, pancreatitis, and renal nephrosis, as well as the use of certain medications, such as some diuretics, glucocorticoids, interferons, and antiretrovirals.

LDL is responsible for the delivery of cholesterol to the tissues, and an increased serum concentration of LDL is a strong indicator of coronary risk. Serum levels of LDL are normally controlled by hepatic receptors that bind LDL and limit liver synthesis of this lipoprotein. Genetic predisposition to dysplidemias, in combination with a high dietary intake of saturated fats, result in high levels of LDL in the bloodstream. Excess LDL migration into the vessel wall, oxidation, and phagocytosis by macrophages are key steps in the pathogenesis of atherosclerosis (see Fig. 26.8). LDL also plays a role in endothelial injury, inflammation, and immune responses that have been identified as being important in atherogenesis. The term *LDL* actually describes several types of LDL molecules. Measurement of LDL subfractions allows for a better prediction of coronary risk. For example, LDL-C and apolipoprotein B (structural protein found in both LDL and VLDL) measurements allow for the detection of the small, dense LDL particles that are the most atherogenic. Guidelines from the American Heart Association and the American College of Cardiology focus on treating dyslipidemia in the context of other risk factors.[6] Diet and medication are the mainstays of treatment for elevated LDL. The most commonly used medications are the 3-hydroxy-3-methyl-glutaryl-CoA reductase medications (statins); however, side effects limit their use in some individuals. New medications, such as the proprotein convertase subtilisin/kexin 9 (PCKS9) inhibitors, also effectively lower LDL.

Low levels of HDL cholesterol also are a strong indicator of coronary risk. HDL is responsible for "reverse cholesterol transport," which returns excess cholesterol from the tissues to the liver for processing or elimination in the bile. HDL also participates in endothelial repair and decreases thrombosis. It can be fractionated into several particle densities (HDL-2 and HDL-3) that have different effects on vascular function. Exercise, weight loss, fish oil consumption, and moderate alcohol use result in modest increases in HDL level. Recent studies suggest that it is not only

TABLE 26.4	**Criteria for Dyslipidemia***						
	Optimal	Near-Optimal	Desirable	Low	Borderline	High	Very High
Total cholesterol			<200		200-239	≥240	
Low-density lipoprotein	<100	100-129			130-159	160-189	≥190
Triglycerides			<150		150-199	200-499	≥500
High-density lipoprotein				<40		≥60	

*All units are milligrams per deciliter.
Data from Expert Panel on Detection, Evaluation, and Treatment of High Blood Cholesterol in Adults, *JAMA* 285:2486-2497, 2001.

the serum levels of HDL that are key to determining CAD risk, but rather HDL functionality, which is harder to measure.

Other lipoproteins associated with increased cardiovascular risk include elevated levels of serum VLDLs (triglycerides) and increased lipoprotein(a) levels. Triglycerides are associated with an increased risk for CAD, especially in combination with other risk factors such as diabetes. Lipoprotein(a) (Lp[a]) is a genetically determined molecular complex between LDL and a serum glycoprotein called apolipoprotein A and has been shown to be an important risk factor for atherosclerosis, especially in women.

Hypertension. Hypertension is responsible for a twofold to threefold increased risk of atherosclerotic cardiovascular disease. It contributes to endothelial injury, a key step in atherogenesis. It also can cause myocardial hypertrophy, which increases myocardial demand for coronary flow. Overactivity of the RAAS commonly found in hypertension also contributes to the genesis of atherosclerosis, and treatment of hypertension with medications that block the RAAS reduces CAD risk.

Cigarette smoking. Both direct and passive (environmental) smoking increase the risk of CAD. Smoking has a direct effect on endothelial cells and the generation of oxygen free radicals that contribute to atherogenesis. Nicotine stimulates the release of catecholamines (epinephrine and norepinephrine), which increase heart rate and peripheral vascular constriction. As a result, blood pressure increases, as do cardiac workload and oxygen demand. Cigarette smoking is associated with an increase in LDL levels and a decrease in HDL levels. The risk of CAD increases with heavy smoking and decreases when smoking is stopped.

Diabetes mellitus. Insulin resistance and diabetes mellitus are extremely important risk factors for CAD. Insulin resistance and diabetes have multiple effects on the cardiovascular system, including damage to the endothelium, thickening of the vessel wall, increased inflammation, increased thrombosis, glycation of vascular proteins, and decreased production of endothelial-derived vasodilators, such as nitric oxide. Diabetes also is associated with dyslipidemia. Good diabetic control is linked to reduced risk for CAD.

Obesity/sedentary lifestyle. Abdominal obesity has a strong link with increased CAD risk and is related to inflammation, insulin resistance, decreased HDL level, increased blood pressure, and changes in hormones called adipokines (leptin and adiponectin). A sedentary lifestyle not only increases the risk of obesity but also has an independent effect on increasing CAD risk. Physical activity and weight loss offer substantial reductions in risk factors for CAD. Bariatric surgery procedures, such as gastric bypass, can provide sustained improvement in risk factors for cardiovascular disease, such as hypertension, dyslipidemia, and diabetes.

Atherogenic diet. Diet plays a complex role in atherogenic risk. Diets high in salt, fats, trans-fats, and carbohydrates all have been implicated. There are many recommendations regarding diet modification to reduce coronary risk; one of the most effective is called the Mediterranean Diet (see *Did You Know?* Mediterranean Diet).

Nontraditional risk factors. Nontraditional risk factors for CAD have been identified that can help with clinical decision-making about how best to manage individuals who also have established CAD or significant traditional risk factors.

Markers of inflammation and ischemia. Of the numerous markers of inflammation that have been linked to an increase in CAD risk, high-sensitivity C-reactive protein (hs-CRP) is the most important clinically. hs-CRP is a protein synthesized in the liver and is used as an indirect measure of atherosclerotic plaque–related inflammation. The primary use of hs-CRP is as an aid to decision-making about pharmacologic interventions for individuals with other risk factors for coronary disease.

Troponin I (TnI) is a serum protein whose measurement is used as a sensitive and specific diagnostic test to help identify myocardial

DID YOU KNOW?
Mediterranean Diet

A number of different kinds of studies—observational cohort, secondary prevention trial, and recent randomized intervention trials—show the Mediterranean diet patterns are associated with a reduced cardiovascular disease risk and cardiovascular events. The traditional Mediterranean diet is characterized by a high intake of olive oil, fruits, nuts, vegetables, and cereals; moderate intake of fish and poultry; low intake of dairy products, red meat, processed meats, and sweets; and moderate intake of wine consumed with meals.

A large prospective cohort study showed adherence to the Mediterranean diet was associated with a decrease in incidence of fatal and nonfatal coronary heart disease (CHD) in initially healthy middle-aged individuals. A recent large randomized trial (the Prevención con Dieta Mediterránea Study [PREDIMED]) among individuals at high cardiovascular risk showed that a Mediterranean diet supplemented with extra-virgin olive oil or nuts reduced the incidence of major cardiovascular events, especially stroke. The beneficial effects of the Mediterranean diet are hypothesized to include modulation of all of the following—inflammation and oxidative stress, glucose metabolism, lipid profile, and lipoprotein particle characteristics—and also favorable changes to the vascular endothelium. Additionally, effects may include a favorable interaction between diet and gene polymorphisms related to cardiovascular risk factors and events.

Data from Chiva-Blanch G et al: *Curr Atheroscler Rep* 16(10):446, 2014; Frolich S et al: *Nutr Metab Cardiovasc Dis* 27(11):999-1007, 2017; Liyanage T et al: *PLoS ONE* 11(8): e0159252, 2016; Tong TYN et al: *BMC Med* 14:135, 2016.

injury during acute coronary syndromes. Highly sensitive TnI assays are used in individuals without a history of CAD to assess risk for future CHD events, mortality, and heart failure.

Adipokines. Adipokines are a group of hormones released from adipose cells. Obesity causes increased levels of leptin and decreased levels of adiponectin that are associated with inflammation, endothelial injury, and thrombosis. Obesity-related changes in adipokines have been linked to hypertension, diabetes, and heart failure, as well as CAD. Weight loss, exercise, and healthy diet improve adipokine levels.

Chronic kidney disease. In individuals with chronic kidney disease (CKD), a decline in glomerular filtration rate is associated with an increasing risk for CAD. CKD is associated with dyslipidemia, endothelial injury, and vascular calcification, which contribute to atherogenesis.

Air pollution and ionizing radiation. Exposure to air pollution, especially roadway exposures, is strongly correlated with coronary risk. It is postulated that toxins in pollution contribute to macrophage activation, oxidation of LDL, thrombosis, and inflammation of vessel walls. Exposure to even low levels of ionizing radiation also has been linked to increased risk for CAD.

Medications. Medications may contribute to CAD through their effect on lipid metabolism (e.g., protease inhibitors, diuretics, antirejection medications), clotting (e.g., estrogens and progesterones), or other effects on vascular function and tone. Nonsteroidal antiinflammatory drugs (NSAIDs) are linked to an increase in CAD-related ischemic events that can occur within weeks of beginning their use. Likely mechanisms include increases in toxic oxygen radicals, vasoconstrictors, and thrombosis.

The microbiome. The microbiome is increasingly being recognized for its influence on cardiovascular disease risk. The impact of the microbiome on atherogenesis is likely related to its effects on underlying risk factors, as well as its role in modulating innate and adaptive immunity (see *Did You Know?* The Microbiome and Coronary Artery Disease).

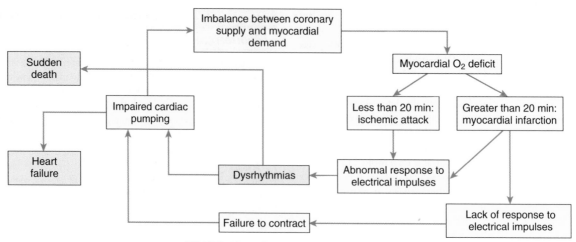

FIGURE 26.10 Cycle of Ischemic Events.

Transient Myocardial Ischemia

PATHOPHYSIOLOGY   Myocardial ischemia develops if the flow or oxygen content of coronary blood is insufficient to meet the metabolic demands of myocardial cells (Fig. 26.10). Imbalances between coronary blood supply and myocardial demand can result from a number of conditions. The most common cause of decreased coronary blood flow and resultant myocardial ischemia is the formation of atherosclerotic plaques in the coronary circulation (CAD). As the plaque increases in size, it may partially occlude the vessel lumina, thus limiting coronary flow and causing ischemia especially during exercise. As discussed earlier in this chapter, some plaques are "unstable," meaning they are prone to rupture. When this rupture occurs, underlying tissues of the vessel wall are exposed, resulting in platelet adhesion and thrombus formation (see Figs. 26.7 and 26.13). Thrombus formation can suddenly stop blood supply to the heart muscle, resulting in acute myocardial ischemia, and, if the vessel obstruction cannot be reversed rapidly, ischemia will

progress to infarction. Myocardial ischemia also can result from other causes of decreased blood and oxygen delivery to the myocardium, such as coronary spasm, hypotension, dysrhythmias, and decreased oxygen-carrying capacity of the blood (e.g., anemia, hypoxemia). Common causes of increased myocardial demand for blood include tachycardia, exercise, hypertension (hypertrophy), and valvular disease.

Myocardial cells become ischemic within 10 seconds of coronary occlusion, thus hampering pump function and depriving the myocardium of a glucose source necessary for aerobic metabolism. Anaerobic processes take over, and lactic acid accumulates. After several minutes, the heart cells lose the ability to contract and cardiac output decreases. Cardiac cells remain viable for approximately 20 minutes under ischemic conditions. If blood flow is restored, aerobic metabolism resumes, contractility is restored, and cellular repair begins. If perfusion is not restored, MI occurs (see Fig. 26.10).

CLINICAL MANIFESTATIONS   Individuals with transient myocardial ischemia present clinically in several ways. Chronic coronary obstruction results in recurrent predictable chest pain called *stable angina*. Abnormal vasospasm of coronary vessels results in unpredictable chest pain called *Prinzmetal angina*. Myocardial ischemia that does not cause detectable symptoms is called *silent ischemia*.

1. **Stable angina pectoris.** Angina is chest pain caused by myocardial ischemia. Atherosclerotic plaques partially obstruct coronary vessels, and affected vessels cannot dilate in response to increased myocardial demand associated with physical exertion or emotional stress. With rest, blood flow is restored and necrosis of myocardial cells does not occur. Angina pectoris is typically experienced as transient substernal chest discomfort, ranging from a sensation of heaviness or pressure to moderately severe pain. Individuals often describe the sensation by clenching a fist over the left sternal border. The discomfort may be mistaken for indigestion. The pain is caused by the buildup of lactic acid or abnormal stretching of the ischemic myocardium that irritates myocardial nerve fibers. These afferent sympathetic fibers enter the spinal cord from levels C3 to T4, accounting for a variety of locations and radiation patterns of anginal pain. Discomfort may radiate to the neck, lower jaw, left arm, and left shoulder, or occasionally to the back or down the right arm. Pallor, diaphoresis, and dyspnea may be associated with the pain. In stable angina, the pain is relieved by rest and nitrates. It is estimated that half of women with stable angina do not have obstructive CAD, but rather have "microvascular angina," which results from vasoconstriction

of small coronary arterioles deep in the myocardium (see *Did You Know?* Women and Microvascular Angina). This form of myocardial ischemia may present with atypical chest pain, palpitations, sense of unease, and severe fatigue rather than typical angina; thus many women with this disorder are misdiagnosed.

2. **Prinzmetal angina**. Prinzmetal angina (also called variant angina) is chest pain attributable to transient ischemia of the myocardium that occurs unpredictably and often at rest. Pain is caused by vasospasm of one or more major coronary arteries with or without associated atherosclerosis. The pain often occurs at night during rapid eye movement sleep and may have a cyclic pattern of occurrence. The angina may result from decreased vagal activity, hyperactivity of the SNS, or decreased nitric oxide activity. Other causes include altered calcium channel function in arterial smooth muscle or impaired production or release of inflammatory mediators, such as serotonin, histamine, endothelin, or thromboxane. Prinzmetal angina is usually a benign condition, but can occasionally cause serious dysrhythmias, especially if treatment is withdrawn; therefore vasodilator therapy should be continued even if clinical remission is achieved.

3. **Silent ischemia** and **mental stress–induced ischemia**. Myocardial ischemia may not cause detectable symptoms such as angina. Ischemia can be totally asymptomatic and referred to as silent ischemia, or individuals may complain of fatigue, dyspnea, or a feeling of unease. The primary cause of silent ischemia is abnormalities in autonomic innervation, most commonly associated with diabetes mellitus. Other causes include surgical denervation during coronary artery bypass graft (CABG) or cardiac transplantation. Also of interest is silent ischemia occurring in some individuals during mental stress. Chronic stress has been linked to an increase in the number of inflammatory cytokines and a hypercoagulable state that may contribute to acute ischemic events (see Chapter 10). Detection and management of silent ischemia is important because it may be an indicator of future serious cardiovascular events.

EVALUATION AND TREATMENT Many individuals with reversible myocardial ischemia will have a normal physical examination between events. Physical examination of those experiencing myocardial ischemia may disclose rapid pulse rate or extra heart sounds (gallops or murmurs), and pulmonary congestion indicating impaired left ventricular function. The presence of xanthelasmas (small fat deposits) around the eyelids or arcus senilis of the eyes (a yellow lipid ring around the cornea) suggests severe dyslipidemia and possible atherosclerosis. The presence of peripheral or carotid artery bruits suggests probable atherosclerotic disease and increases the likelihood that CAD is present.

Electrocardiography is a critical tool for the diagnosis of myocardial ischemia. Ischemic cells distort the electrical impulses that are measured across the myocardium during an ECG. Because many individuals have normal ECGs when there is no pain, diagnosis requires that an ECG be performed during an attack of angina or during exercise stress testing. The ST segment and the T wave segments of the ECG, respectively, correlate with ventricular contraction and relaxation (see Fig. 25.10). Transient ST segment depression and T wave inversion are characteristic signs of ischemia that involves only the inner wall of the myocardium (subendocardial ischemia). ST elevation is indicative of ischemia involving the full myocardial wall (transmural ischemia) (Fig. 26.11). The ECG tracings correlate with different parts of the myocardium and therefore can give some indication of which coronary artery is involved.

Normal ECG deflections

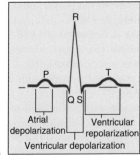

A

ECG alterations associated with ischemia

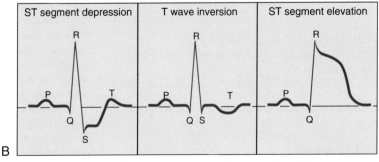

B

FIGURE 26.11 Electrocardiogram (ECG) and Ischemia. **A,** Normal ECG. **B,** Electrocardiographic alterations associated with ischemia.

Stress radionucleotide imaging is indicated to detect ischemic changes in asymptomatic individuals with multiple risk factors for coronary disease, such as diabetes and dyslipidemia, and for older individuals who plan to start vigorous exercise. Currently, the diagnostic modality of choice for the diagnosis of myocardial ischemia is single-photon emission computerized tomography (SPECT), which is effective at identifying ischemia and estimating coronary risk. Stress echocardiography is another technique used to diagnose CAD. Unfortunately these tests cannot detect the presence of vulnerable plaques that are the cause of the majority of acute coronary syndromes; therefore new diagnostic techniques are being evaluated. Other noninvasive tests for evaluating coronary atherosclerotic lesions include measurement of coronary artery calcium concentration by CT, noninvasive coronary angiography using electron beam CT, and protein-weighted MRI; however, the sensitivity and specificity of these tests vary widely. Coronary angiography helps determine the anatomic extent of CAD, but the procedure is expensive and carries some risk. It is used primarily to determine whether possible percutaneous coronary intervention (PCI) or CABG surgery is warranted for individuals whose noninvasive studies suggest severe disease.

The primary aims of therapy for myocardial ischemia and stable angina are to increase coronary blood flow and reduce myocardial oxygen consumption. Risk factor reduction is essential. Coronary blood flow is improved by reversing vasoconstriction, reducing plaque growth and rupture, and preventing clotting. Myocardial oxygen demand is reduced by manipulation of blood pressure, heart rate, contractility, and left ventricular volume. Several classes of drugs are useful for increasing coronary flow and decreasing myocardial demand, especially nitrates, β-blockers, and calcium channel blockers. Ranolazine represents a relatively new class of antianginal drugs known as sodium ion channel inhibitors and has been found to improve exercise tolerance, lessen anginal symptoms, and reduce the need for nitrates in many individuals with chronic stable angina. Antithrombotics are used to prevent thrombus formation. Recommendations for appropriate nonpharmacologic and pharmacologic management of stable ischemic heart disease have been published.[7]

Percutaneous coronary intervention (PCI) is a procedure in which stenotic (narrowed) coronary vessels are dilated with a catheter. The use of PCI for stable angina is associated with improvements in symptoms but does not reduce the risk for future MI or death. Indications for PCI include persistent symptoms despite optimal medical therapy or severe disease. Restenosis of the artery is the major complication of the procedure; however, placement of a coronary stent and the use of antithrombotics can reduce this risk. Severe CAD also can be surgically treated by a coronary artery bypass graft (CABG), usually using the saphenous vein from the lower leg. In selected individuals, a modified CABG procedure called minimally invasive direct coronary artery bypass (MIDCAB) can be used with much less surgical morbidity and more rapid recovery.

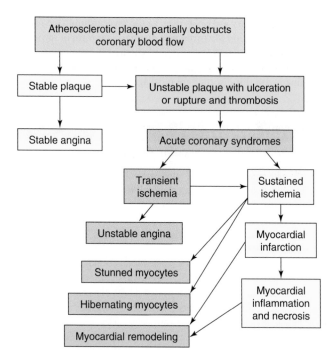

FIGURE 26.12 **Pathophysiology of Acute Coronary Syndromes.** The atherosclerotic process can lead to stable plaque formation and stable angina or can result in unstable plaques that are prone to rupture and thrombus. Thrombus formation on a ruptured plaque that disperses in less than 20 minutes leads to transient ischemia and unstable angina. If the vessel obstruction is sustained, myocardial infarction (MI) with inflammation and necrosis of the myocardium results. In addition, MI is associated with other structural and functional changes, including myocyte stunning and hibernation and myocardial remodeling (see Fig. 26.34).

---

formation over a ruptured atherosclerotic plaque, the acute coronary syndromes result (Fig. 26.12). Unstable angina is a reversible form of acute coronary syndrome that is a harbinger of impending infarction. Myocardial infarction (MI) results when there is prolonged ischemia causing irreversible damage to the heart muscle. MI can be further subdivided into non-ST elevation MI (non-STEMI) and ST elevation MI (STEMI). Sudden cardiac death can occur as a result of any of the acute coronary syndromes.

An unstable atherosclerotic plaque has a core that is especially rich in deposited oxidized LDL, has a thin fibrous cap, and is prone to rupture (Fig. 26.13). These unstable plaques may not extend into the lumen of the vessel and may be clinically silent until they rupture. Plaque rupture occurs because of the effects of shear forces, inflammation with release of multiple inflammatory mediators, secretion of macrophage-derived degradative enzymes, and apoptosis of cells at the edges of the lesions. Exposure of the plaque substrate activates the clotting cascade. The resulting thrombus can form very quickly (Fig. 26.14, *A*). Vessel obstruction is further exacerbated by the release of vasoconstrictors, such as thromboxane A_2 and endothelin. The thrombus may shatter before permanent myocyte damage has occurred (unstable angina), or it may cause prolonged ischemia with infarction of the heart muscle (MI) (Fig. 26.14, *B*).

Unstable angina. Unstable angina is a form of acute coronary syndrome that results from reversible myocardial ischemia. It is important to recognize this syndrome because it signals that the atherosclerotic plaque has begun to rupture and infarction may soon follow. Unstable angina occurs when a fairly small fissuring or superficial erosion of the plaque leads to transient episodes of thrombotic vessel occlusion and

✔ QUICK CHECK 26.5
1. Define atherosclerosis and briefly describe how it develops.
2. Why do hypertension and dyslipidemia increase the likelihood of developing coronary artery disease?
3. Discuss the relationships among myocardial ischemia, angina, and silent ischemia.

Acute Coronary Syndromes

The process of atherosclerotic plaque progression can be gradual. However, when there is sudden coronary obstruction caused by thrombus vasoconstriction at the site of plaque damage. This thrombus is labile and occludes the vessel for no more than 10 to 20 minutes, with return of perfusion before significant myocardial necrosis occurs. Unstable angina presents as new-onset angina, angina that is occurring at rest or angina that is increasing in severity or frequency (Box 26.1). Individuals may experience increased dyspnea, diaphoresis, and anxiety as the angina worsens. Physical examination may reveal evidence of ischemic myocardial dysfunction such as pulmonary congestion. The ECG most commonly shows ST segment depression and T wave inversion during pain that resolve as the pain is relieved. Unstable angina has traditionally been diagnosed by ECG changes without elevated serum cardiac isoenzyme evidence of myocyte necrosis. However, the advent of highly sensitive measurements of myocardial damage (hs-troponin I) that can identify tiny amounts of enzymes released from damaged myocytes has blurred the distinction between unstable angina and non-ST segment elevation MI. Therefore the current guidelines for the management of unstable angina and non-STEMI are identical. Management of unstable angina requires immediate hospitalization with administration of nitrates and antithrombotics. Anticoagulants, such as low-molecular-weight heparin or fondaparinux, also can be given. Beta-blockers and ACE inhibitors also may be used. Rapid intervention with PCI also may be indicated if the individual's condition is refractory to medical treatment.

Myocardial infarction. When coronary blood flow is interrupted for an extended period, infarction with myocyte necrosis occurs. This results in MI. Plaque progression, disruption, and subsequent clot formation are the same for MI as they are for unstable angina (see Figs. 26.12, 26.13, and 26.14). In this case, however, the thrombus is less labile and occludes the vessel for a prolonged period, such that myocardial ischemia progresses to myocyte necrosis and death. Pathologically, there are two major types of MI: subendocardial infarction and transmural infarction. Clinically, however, MI is categorized as non-ST segment elevation MI (non-STEMI) or ST segment elevation MI (STEMI).

If the thrombus disintegrates before complete distal tissue necrosis has occurred, the infarction will involve only the myocardium directly beneath the endocardium (subendocardial MI) (Fig. 26.15). This infarction will usually present with ST segment depression and T wave inversion

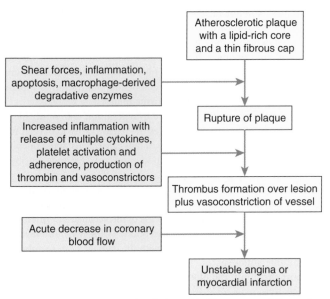

FIGURE 26.13 Pathogenesis of Unstable Plaques and Thrombus Formation.

BOX 26.1   **Three Principal Presentations of Unstable Angina**

1. Rest angina—Angina occurring at rest and prolonged, usually >20 minutes
2. New-onset angina—New-onset angina of at least CCS class III severity
3. Increasing angina—Previously diagnosed angina that has become distinctly more frequent, longer in duration, or lower in threshold (i.e., increased by ≥1 CCS class to at least CCS class III severity)

CCS, Canadian Cardiovascular Society.
From Anderson J et al: *J Am Coll Cardiol* 50:e1-e157, 2007; originally adapted from Braunwald E: *Circulation* 80:410-414, 1989.

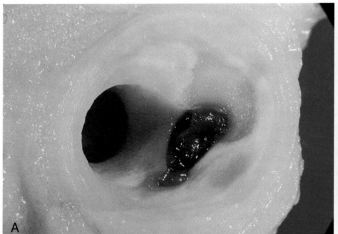

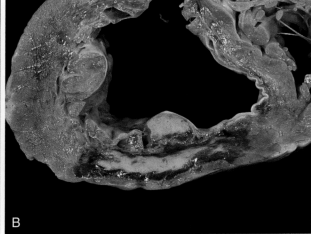

FIGURE 26.14 Plaque Disruption and Myocardial Infarction. A, Plaque disruption. The cap of the lipid-rich plaque has become torn, with the formation of a thrombus, mostly inside the plaque. B, Myocardial infarction. This infarct is 6 days old. The center is yellow and necrotic with a hemorrhagic red rim. The responsible arterial occlusion is probably in the right coronary artery. The infarct is on the posterior wall. (From Damjanov I, Linder J, editors: *Anderson's pathology,* ed 10, St Louis, 1996, Mosby.)

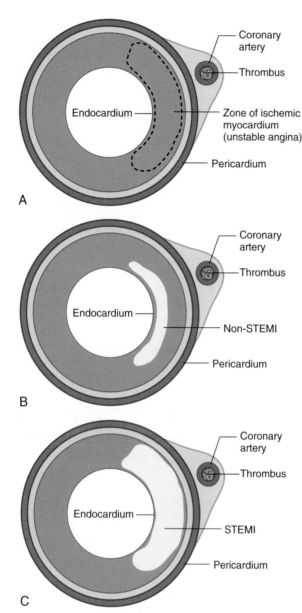

FIGURE 26.15 Unstable Angina, non-STEMI, and STEMI. A, Unstable angina. Coronary thrombosis leads to myocardial ischemia. B, Non-STEMI. Persistent coronary occlusion leads to infarction of the myocardium closest to the endocardium. C, STEMI. Continued coronary occlusion leads to transmural infarction extending from endocardium to pericardium.

without ST elevation; therefore it is termed non-STEMI. It is especially important to recognize this form of acute coronary syndrome because recurrent clot formation on the disrupted atherosclerotic plaque is likely. If the thrombus lodges permanently in the vessel, the infarction will extend through the myocardium all the way from endocardium to epicardium (transmural MI), resulting in severe cardiac dysfunction (see Fig. 26.15). Transmural myocardial infarction will usually result in ST segment elevation on ECG, so it is called STEMI. Clinically, it is important to identify individuals with STEMI because they are at highest risk for serious complications and should receive definitive intervention without delay.

PATHOPHYSIOLOGY After 8 to 10 seconds of decreased blood flow, myocardial oxygen reserves are used quickly. Glycogen stores decrease

as anaerobic metabolism begins. Unfortunately, glycolysis can supply only 65% to 70% of the total myocardial energy requirement and produces much less adenosine triphosphate (ATP) than aerobic processes. Hydrogen ions and lactic acid accumulate, making the myocardium more vulnerable to the damaging effects of lysosomal enzymes and may suppress impulse conduction and contractile function, thereby leading to heart failure.

Oxygen deprivation also is accompanied by electrolyte disturbances, specifically the loss of potassium, calcium, and magnesium from cells. Myocardial cells deprived of necessary oxygen and nutrients lose contractility, thereby diminishing the pumping ability of the heart. Ischemia causes the myocardial cells to release catecholamines, predisposing the individual to serious imbalances of sympathetic and parasympathetic function, irregular heartbeats (dysrhythmia), and heart failure. Catecholamines cause an increase in plasma concentrations of free fatty acids and glycerol, which can have a harmful detergent effect on cell membranes. Norepinephrine elevates blood glucose levels, which also contributes to myocardial dysfunction. Ang II is released during myocardial ischemia and causes peripheral vasoconstriction, coronary spasm, and fluid retention. It also is a growth factor for vascular smooth muscle cells, myocytes, and cardiac fibroblasts, resulting in structural changes in the myocardium called remodeling. Infiltration of inflammatory cells further contributes to tissue injury.

Ischemic injury can be exacerbated by reperfusion injury once blood flow is restored. This process involves the release of toxic oxygen free radicals, calcium flux, and pH changes that cause a sustained opening of mitochondrial permeability transition pores (mPTPs) and contribute to resultant cellular death.

Cardiac cells can withstand ischemic conditions for about 20 minutes before irreversible hypoxic injury causes cellular death (apoptosis) and tissue necrosis. This results in the release of intracellular enzymes, such as creatine phosphokinase-myocardial bound (CPK-MB), and myocyte proteins, such as the troponins, through the damaged cell membranes into the interstitial spaces. The lymphatics absorb the enzymes and transport them into the bloodstream, where they can be detected by serologic tests.

MI results in both structural and functional changes of cardiac tissues (Fig. 26.16). Gross tissue changes at the area of infarction may not become apparent for several hours, despite almost immediate onset (within 30 to 60 seconds) of electrocardiographic changes. Cardiac tissue surrounding the area of infarction also undergoes changes. Myocardial stunning is a temporary loss of contractile function that persists for hours to days after perfusion has been restored. This pathophysiologic state can occur both with MI and in individuals who suffer ischemia during cardiovascular procedures or during CNS trauma. Stunning is caused by the alterations in electrolyte pumps and calcium homeostasis and by the release of toxic oxygen free radicals and contributes to heart failure, shock, and dysrhythmias. Numerous interventions to limit the amount of stunning are being explored. Hibernating myocardium describes tissue that is persistently ischemic and undergoes metabolic adaptation to prolong myocyte survival until perfusion can be restored. PCI or surgery aimed at reperfusion of hibernating myocardium can restore significant cardiac function. Myocardial remodeling is a process mediated by Ang II, aldosterone, catecholamines, adenosine, and inflammatory cytokines that causes myocyte hypertrophy and loss of contractile function in the areas of the heart distant from the site of infarction. Remodeling can be limited through rapid restoration of coronary flow and the use of renin-angiotensin-aldosterone blockers and β-blockers after MI.

The severity of functional impairment depends on the size of the lesion and the site of infarction. Functional changes can include (1) decreased cardiac contractility with abnormal wall motion, (2) altered

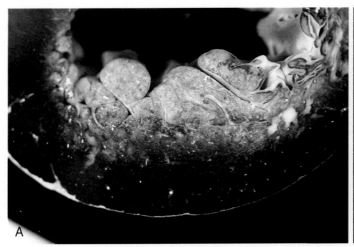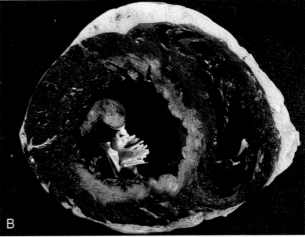

FIGURE 26.16 Myocardial Infarction. **A,** Local infarct confined to one region. **B,** Massive large infarct caused by occlusion of three coronary arteries. (From Damjanov I, Linder J, editors: *Anderson's pathology,* ed 10, St Louis, 1996, Mosby.)

left ventricular compliance, (3) decreased stroke volume and ejection fraction (EF), (4) increased left ventricular end-diastolic pressure (LVEDP), and (5) sinoatrial (SA) node malfunction. Life-threatening dysrhythmias and heart failure often follow MI.

With infarction, ventricular function is abnormal and the EF falls, resulting in increases in ventricular end-diastolic volume (VEDV). If the coronary obstruction involves the perfusion to the left ventricle, pulmonary venous congestion ensues; if the right ventricle is ischemic, increases in systemic venous pressures occur.

MI causes a severe inflammatory response that ends with wound repair (see Chapter 6). Damaged cells undergo degradation, fibroblasts proliferate, and scar tissue is synthesized. Within 24 hours, leukocytes infiltrate the necrotic area, and proteolytic enzymes released from scavenger neutrophils degrade the necrotic tissue. The collagen matrix that is deposited is initially weak, mushy, and vulnerable to reinjury. Unfortunately, it is at this time in the recovery period (10 to 14 days after infarction) that individuals feel more like increasing activities and may stress the newly formed scar tissue. After 6 weeks, the necrotic area is completely replaced by scar tissue, which is strong but cannot contract and relax like healthy myocardial tissue.

CLINICAL MANIFESTATIONS   The first symptom of acute MI is usually sudden, severe chest pain. The pain is similar to that of angina pectoris but more severe and prolonged. It may be described as heavy and crushing, such as a "truck sitting on my chest." Radiation to the neck, jaw, back, shoulder, or left arm is common. Some individuals, especially those who are elderly or have diabetes, experience no pain, thus having a "silent" infarction. Infarction often simulates a sensation of unrelenting indigestion. Nausea and vomiting may occur because of reflex stimulation of vomiting centers by pain fibers. Vasovagal reflexes from the area of the infarcted myocardium also may affect the gastrointestinal tract.

Various cardiovascular changes are found on physical examination:
1. The SNS is reflexively activated to compensate, resulting in a temporary increase in heart rate and blood pressure.
2. Abnormal extra heart sounds reflect left ventricular dysfunction.
3. Pulmonary findings of congestion, including dullness to percussion and inspiratory crackles at the lung bases, can occur if the individual develops heart failure.
4. Peripheral vasoconstriction may cause the skin to become cool and clammy.

The number and severity of postinfarction complications depend on the location and extent of necrosis, the individual's physiologic condition before the infarction, and the availability of swift therapeutic intervention. Table 26.5 lists the most common complications of MI. Sudden cardiac death can occur in individuals with myocardial ischemia even if infarction is absent or minimal. Risk factors for sudden death are related to an interaction among three factors: ischemia, left ventricular dysfunction, and electrical instability.

EVALUATION AND TREATMENT   The diagnosis of acute MI is made on the basis of history, physical examination, ECG results, and serial cardiac troponin elevations (Box 26.2).

MI can occur in various regions of the heart wall and may be described as anterior, inferior, posterior, lateral, subendocardial, or transmural, depending on the anatomic location and extent of tissue damage from infarction. Twelve-lead ECGs help localize the affected area through identification of changes in ST segments and T waves (Fig. 26.17). The infarcted myocardium is surrounded by a zone of hypoxic injury, which may progress to necrosis or return to normal, and adjacent to this zone of hypoxic injury is a zone of reversible ischemia (see Fig. 26.17). A characteristic Q wave often develops on ECG some hours later in STEMI.

Cardiac troponin I (cTnI) is the most specific indicator of MI, and measurement of its level should be performed on admission to the emergency department. cTnI level elevation is detectable 2 to 4 hours after onset of symptoms. Additional measurements within 6 to 9 hours and again at 12 to 24 hours are recommended if clinical suspicion is high and previous samples were negative. Troponin levels also can be used to estimate infarct size and therefore the likelihood of complications. Additional laboratory data may reveal leukocytosis and elevated C-reactive protein (CRP), both of which indicate inflammation. The individual's blood glucose level is usually elevated and the glucose tolerance level may remain abnormal for several weeks.

Acute MI requires admission to the hospital, often directly into a coronary care unit. The individual should be given an aspirin immediately (ticlopidine if allergic to aspirin) along with nitrates and morphine for pain. Continuous monitoring of cardiac rhythms and enzymatic changes is essential, because the first 24 hours after onset of symptoms is the time of highest risk for sudden death. Non-STEMI is treated in the same way as unstable angina including antithrombotics, anticoagulation or PCI, or both.[8] STEMI is best managed with emergent PCI or

TABLE 26.5 Complications With Myocardial Infarctions

Type	Characteristics
Dysrhythmias	Caused by alterations of impulse conduction because of ischemia and electrolyte disturbances; sudden onset of tachycardia or bradycardia, palpitations, syncope, shock, or sudden death
Left ventricular failure	Characterized by pulmonary congestion, reduced myocardial contractility, and abnormal heart wall motion; cardiogenic shock may develop
Pericarditis	Inflammation of the pericardium associated with anterior chest pain that worsens with respiratory effort and pericardial friction rub; occurs 2 to 3 days after infarction
Dressler postinfarction syndrome	Delayed form of pericarditis that occurs 1 week to several months after acute myocardial infarction and thought to be immunologic response to necrotic myocardium; marked by pain, fever, friction rub, pleural effusion, and arthralgias
Organic brain syndrome	Occurs if blood flow to brain is impaired
Rupture of chordae tendinae	Caused by necrosis of tissue in or around papillary muscles; acute onset of severe valvular regurgitation
Aneurysm and rupture of wall or septae of infarcted ventricle	Aneurysm formation resulting from high chamber pressures and volume pushing against weakened ventricular wall; rupture of ventricular wall or septae between chambers when pressure becomes too great; rapid onset of shock
Systemic arterial thromboembolism	May disseminate from debris and clots that collect inside dilated aneurysmal sacs or from infarcted endocardium; can affect any system but especially targets cerebrovascular system with transient ischemic attacks and stroke
Pulmonary thromboembolism	Usually from deep venous thrombi of legs; acute onset of dyspnea and hypoxemia
Sudden death	Dysrhythmias frequently causative, particularly ventricular fibrillation

BOX 26.2 The Fourth Universal Definition of Myocardial Infarction (2018)

The term *myocardial infarction* (MI) should be used when there is evidence of myocardial necrosis in a clinical setting with myocardial ischemia. Under these conditions any one of the following criteria meets the diagnosis for MI:

- Detection of an elevated high-sensitivity cardiac troponin (hs-cTn) value above the 99th percentile upper reference limit (URL) is defined as myocardial injury. The injury is considered acute if there is a rise and/or fall of cTn values.
- The criteria for type 1 MI include detection of a rise and/or fall of cTn with at least one value above the 99th percentile and with at least one of the following:
  - Symptoms of acute myocardial ischemia;
  - New ischemic electrocardiographic (ECG) changes;
  - Development of pathological Q waves;
  - Imaging evidence of new loss of viable myocardium or new regional wall motion abnormality in a pattern consistent with an ischemic etiology;
  - Identification of a coronary thrombus by angiography including intracoronary imaging or by autopsy.
- The criteria for type 2 MI include detection of a rise and/or fall of cTn with at least one value above the 99th percentile and evidence of an imbalance between myocardial oxygen supply and demand unrelated to coronary thrombosis, requiring at least one of the following:
  - Symptoms of acute myocardial ischemia;
  - New ischemic ECG changes;
  - Development of pathological Q waves;
  - Imaging evidence of new loss of viable myocardium, or new regional wall motion abnormality in a pattern consistent with an ischemic etiology.
- Cardiac procedural myocardial injury is arbitrarily defined by increases of cTn values (>99th percentile URL) in patients with normal baseline values (≤99th percentile URL) or a rise of cTn values >20% of the baseline value when it is above the 99th percentile, but it is stable or falling.
- Coronary intervention-related MI is arbitrarily defined by elevation of cTn values >5 times the 99th percentile URL in patients with normal baseline values. In patients with elevated pre-procedure cTn in whom the cTn levels are stable (≤20% variation) or falling, the post-procedure cTn must rise by

>20%. However, the absolute post-procedural value must still be at least five times the 99th percentile URL. In addition, one of the following elements is required:

- New ischemic ECG changes;
- Development of new pathological Q waves;
- Angiographic findings consistent with a procedural flow-limiting complication such as coronary dissection, occlusion of a major epicardial artery or a side branch occlusion/thrombus, disruption of collateral flow or distal embolization.
- Coronary artery bypass grafting (CABG)-related MI is arbitrarily defined as elevation of cTn values >10 times the 99th percentile URL in patients with normal baseline cTn values. In patients with elevated pre-procedure cTn in whom cTn levels are stable (≤20% variation) or falling, the post-procedure cTn must rise by >20%. However, the absolute post-procedural value still must be >10 times the 99th percentile URL. In addition, one of the following elements is required:
  - Development of new pathological Q waves;
  - Angiographic documented new graft occlusion or new native coronary artery occlusion;
  - Imaging evidence of new loss of viable myocardium or new regional wall motion abnormality in a pattern consistent with an ischemic etiology.
- It is increasingly recognized that there is a group of MI patients with no angiographic obstructive coronary artery disease (≥50% diameter stenosis in a major epicardial vessel), and the term "myocardial infarction with non-obstructive coronary arteries (MINOCA)" has been coined for this entity.
- Patients may have elevated cTn values and marked decreases in ejection fraction due to sepsis caused by endotoxin, with myocardial function recovering completely with normal ejection fraction once the sepsis is treated.

Arriving at a diagnosis of MI using the criteria set forth in this document requires integration of clinical findings, patterns on the ECG, laboratory data, observations from imaging procedures, and on occasion pathological findings, all viewed in the context of the time horizon over which the suspected event unfolds.

Data from Thygesen K et al: *J Am Coll Cardiol* 72(18):2231-2264, 2018.

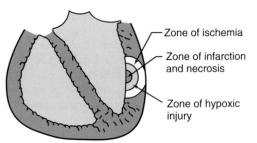
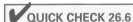

- Zone of ischemia
- Zone of infarction and necrosis
- Zone of hypoxic injury

Normal	Ischemia	Injury	Infarction/necrosis

FIGURE 26.17 Electrocardiographic Alterations Associated With the Three Zones of Myocardial Infarction.

thrombolytics and antithrombotics.[9] Hyperglycemia is treated with insulin. Once the person is stabilized, further management includes ACE inhibitors, beta-blockers, and statins. Individuals who are in shock require aggressive fluid resuscitation, ionotropic drugs, and possible emergent invasive procedures.

Bed rest, followed by gradual return to activities of daily living, reduces the myocardial oxygen demands of the compromised heart. Individuals not receiving thrombolytic or heparin infusion must receive DVT prophylaxis as long as their activity is significantly limited. Stool softeners are given to eliminate the need for straining. Education regarding appropriate diet and caffeine intake, smoking cessation, exercise, and other aspects of risk factor reduction is crucial for secondary prevention of recurrent myocardial ischemia.

✓ QUICK CHECK 26.6
1. Describe the coronary artery disease–myocardial ischemia continuum.
2. Describe the pathophysiology of myocardial infarction.
3. What complications are associated with the period after infarction?

DISORDERS OF THE HEART WALL

Disorders of the Pericardium

Pericardial disease is a localized manifestation of another disorder, such as infection (bacterial, viral, fungal, rickettsial, or parasitic); trauma or surgery; neoplasm; or a metabolic, immunologic, or vascular disorder (uremia, rheumatoid arthritis, systemic lupus erythematosus, periarteritis nodosa). The pericardial response to injury from these diverse causes may consist of acute pericarditis, pericardial effusion, or constrictive pericarditis.

Acute Pericarditis

Acute pericarditis is acute inflammation of the pericardium. The etiology of acute pericarditis is most often idiopathic or caused by viral infection by coxsackie, influenza, hepatitis, measles, mumps, varicella viruses, or human immunodeficiency virus (HIV). Other causes include MI, trauma, neoplasm, surgery, uremia, bacterial infection (especially tuberculosis), connective tissue disease (especially systemic lupus erythematosus and rheumatoid arthritis), or radiation therapy. The pericardial membranes become inflamed and roughened, and a pericardial effusion may develop that can be serous, purulent, or fibrinous (Fig. 26.18). Possible sequelae of pericarditis include recurrent pericarditis, pericardial constriction, and cardiac tamponade.

Symptoms may follow several days of fever and usually begin with the sudden onset of severe retrosternal chest pain that worsens with respiratory movements and when assuming a recumbent position. The

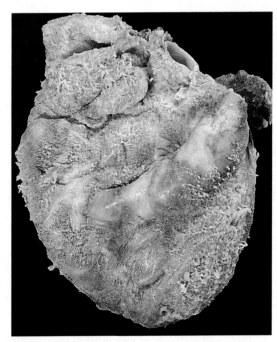

FIGURE 26.18 Acute Pericarditis. Note shaggy coat of fibers covering the surface of heart. (From Damjanov I, Linder J: *Pathology: a color atlas,* St Louis, 2000, Mosby.)

pain may radiate to the back as a result of irritation of the phrenic nerve (innervates the trapezius muscles) as it traverses the pericardium. Individuals with acute pericarditis also report dysphagia, restlessness, irritability, anxiety, weakness, and malaise.

Physical examination often discloses low-grade fever (<38° C [<100.4° F]) and sinus tachycardia. An intermittent friction rub—a scratchy, grating sound—may be heard at the cardiac apex and left sternal border and is highly suggestive of pericarditis. The rub is caused by the roughened pericardial membranes rubbing against each other. ECG findings may reflect inflammatory processes through PR segment depression and diffuse ST segment elevation without Q waves, and they may remain abnormal for days or even weeks. Ultrasound, CT scanning, and MRI may be used as diagnostic modalities. Acute pericarditis requires at least two of the following four criteria for diagnosis: (1) chest pain characteristics of pericarditis, (2) pericardial rub, (3) characteristic electrocardiographic changes, and (4) new or worsening pericardial effusion.

Treatment for uncomplicated acute pericarditis consists of administration of antiinflammatory agents, such as salicylates and NSAIDs, and colchicine. Exploration of the underlying cause is important. Approximately one third of cases will be complicated by the development of idiopathic recurrent pericarditis.

Pericardial Effusion

Pericardial effusion is the accumulation of fluid in the pericardial cavity and can occur in all forms of pericarditis. Most are idiopathic (20%), but other causes, such as neoplasm and infection, must be considered. Analysis of the fluid obtained through pericardiocentesis allows for identification of the likely source of the fluid. The fluid may be a transudate, such as the serous effusion that develops with left heart failure, overhydration, or hypoproteinemia. More often, however, the fluid is an exudate, which reflects pericardial inflammation like that seen with acute pericarditis, MI, heart surgery, some chemotherapeutic agents, infections, and autoimmune disorders such as systemic lupus erythematosus. (Types of exudate are described in Chapter 6.) If the fluid is serosanguineous, the underlying cause is likely to be tuberculosis, neoplasm, uremia, or radiation, although some remain idiopathic. Effusions of frank blood are generally related to aneurysms, trauma, or coagulation defects (Fig. 26.19). If chyle leaks from the thoracic duct, it may enter the pericardium and lead to cholesterol pericarditis.

If a pericardial effusion develops gradually, the pericardium can stretch to accommodate large quantities of fluid without compressing the heart. If the fluid accumulates rapidly, however, even a small amount (50-100 ml) may create sufficient pressure to cause cardiac compression, a serious condition known as tamponade. In tamponade, the pressure exerted by the pericardial fluid eventually equals or even exceeds diastolic pressure within the heart chambers, which interferes with right atrial filling. This causes increased venous pressure, systemic venous congestion, and signs and symptoms of right heart failure (distention of the jugular veins, edema, hepatomegaly). Decreased atrial filling also leads to decreased ventricular filling, decreased stroke volume, and reduced cardiac output. Life-threatening circulatory collapse may occur.

An important clinical finding is pulsus paradoxus, in which arterial blood pressure during expiration exceeds arterial pressure during inspiration by more than 10 mm Hg. Pulsus paradoxus in the setting of a pericardial effusion indicates tamponade and reflects impairment of diastolic filling of the left ventricle plus reduction of blood volume within all four cardiac chambers.

Other clinical manifestations of pericardial effusion are distant or muffled heart sounds, poorly palpable apical pulse, dyspnea on exertion, and dull chest pain. A chest x-ray film may disclose a "water-bottle configuration" of the cardiac silhouette. An echocardiogram can detect an effusion as small as 20 ml and is a reliable and accurate diagnostic test, although CT scans also may be done.

Treatment of pericardial effusion or tamponade generally consists of pericardiocentesis (aspiration of excessive pericardial fluid) and treatment of the underlying condition. Persistent pain may be treated with analgesics, antiinflammatory medications, or steroids. Surgery may be required if the underlying cause of tamponade is trauma or aneurysm. A pericardial "window" may be surgically created to prevent tamponade.

Constrictive Pericarditis

Constrictive pericarditis, or restrictive pericarditis (chronic pericarditis), is most commonly idiopathic or associated with viral infection, radiation exposure, collagen vascular disorders, sarcoidosis, neoplasm, uremia, or cardiac surgery. In constrictive pericarditis, fibrous scarring with occasional calcification of the pericardium causes the visceral and parietal pericardial layers to adhere, obliterating the pericardial cavity. The fibrotic lesions encase the heart in a rigid shell (Fig. 26.20). Like tamponade, constrictive pericarditis compresses the heart and eventually reduces cardiac output. Unlike tamponade, however, constrictive pericarditis always develops gradually.

Symptoms are exercise intolerance, dyspnea on exertion, fatigue, and anorexia. Clinical assessment shows edema, distention of the jugular vein, hepatic congestion, and systemic hypotension. Restricted ventricular filling may cause a pericardial knock (early diastolic sound).

ECG findings include nonspecific ST and T wave abnormalities and atrial fibrillation (AF). Chest x-ray films often disclose prominent pulmonary vessels and calcification of the pericardium. CT, MRI, and transesophageal echocardiography are used to detect pericardial thickening and constriction and to distinguish constrictive pericarditis from restrictive cardiomyopathy. Pericardial biopsy may be needed to determine the etiology.

Initial treatment for constrictive pericarditis consists of restriction of dietary sodium intake and administration of diuretics to improve

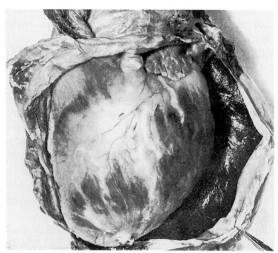

FIGURE 26.19 Exudate of Blood in the Pericardial Sac from Rupture of Aneurysm. (From Damjanov I, Linder J: *Pathology: a color atlas*, St Louis, 2000, Mosby.)

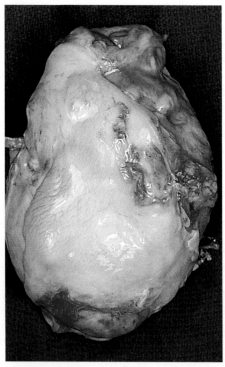

FIGURE 26.20 Constrictive Pericarditis. The fibrotic pericardium encases the heart in a rigid shell. (From Damjanov I, Linder J: *Pathology: a color atlas*, St Louis, 2000, Mosby.)

cardiac output. Management also may include use of antiinflammatory drugs and treatment of any underlying disorder. If these modalities are unsuccessful, surgical excision of the restrictive pericardium is indicated (pericardial decortication).

Disorders of the Myocardium: the Cardiomyopathies

The cardiomyopathies are a diverse group of diseases that affect the myocardium. Primary cardiomyopathies are disorders confined to the myocardium. Many primary cardiomyopathies are idiopathic; others are caused by ischemia, hypertension, inherited disorders, infections, toxins, myocarditis or autoimmunity. Secondary cardiomyopathies occur in the context of disorders that affect other organs as well as the heart, such as infectious disease, toxin exposure, systemic connective tissue disease, infiltrative and proliferative disorders, or nutritional deficiencies. The cardiomyopathies are further categorized as dilated, hypertrophic, or restrictive, depending on their physiologic effects on the heart (Fig. 26.21).

Dilated cardiomyopathy results from ischemic heart disease, valvular disease, diabetes, renal failure, alcohol or drug toxicity, peripartum complications, or infection. There is a strong genetic basis for dilated cardiomyopathy, and it can be associated with inherited disorders such as muscular dystrophy. It is characterized by impaired systolic function leading to increases in intracardiac volume, ventricular dilation, and heart failure with reduced EF (Fig. 26.22). Individuals complain of

dyspnea, fatigue, and pedal edema. Findings on examination include a displaced apical pulse, S_3 gallop, peripheral edema, jugular venous distention, and pulmonary congestion. Diagnosis is confirmed by chest x-ray and echocardiogram, and management is focused on reducing blood volume and increasing contractility. Further management is determined by the specific cause of the cardiomyopathy.[10] Heart transplant is required in severe cases.

Hypertrophic cardiomyopathy refers to two major categories of thickening of the myocardium: (1) hypertrophic obstructive cardiomyopathy (asymmetric septal hypertrophic cardiomyopathy or subaortic stenosis) and (2) hypertensive or valvular hypertrophic cardiomyopathy. Hypertrophic obstructive cardiomyopathy is the most commonly inherited cardiac disorder. It is characterized by thickening of the septal wall (Fig. 26.23), which may cause outflow obstruction to the left ventricle

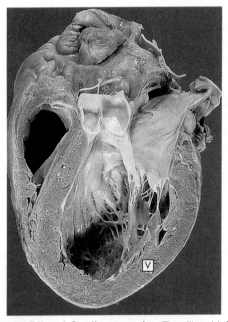

FIGURE 26.22 Dilated Cardiomyopathy. The dilated left ventricle has a thin wall *(V)*. (From Stevens A et al: *Core pathology,* ed 3, London, 2009, Mosby.)

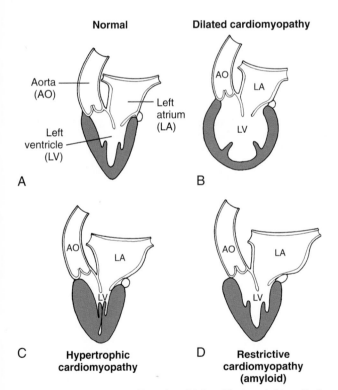

FIGURE 26.21 Diagram Showing Major Distinguishing Pathophysiologic Features of the Three Types of Cardiomyopathy. A, The normal heart. B, In the dilated type of cardiomyopathy, the heart has a globular shape and the largest circumference of the left ventricle is not at its base but midway between apex and base. C, In the hypertrophic type, the wall of the left ventricle is greatly thickened; the left ventricular cavity is small, but the left atrium may be dilated because of poor diastolic relaxation of the ventricle. D, In the restrictive (constrictive) type, the left ventricular cavity is normal size, but, again, the left atrium is dilated because of the reduced diastolic compliance of the ventricle. (From Kissane JM, editor: *Anderson's pathology,* ed 9, St Louis, 1990, Mosby.)

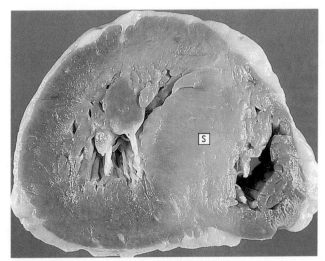

FIGURE 26.23 Hypertrophic Cardiomyopathy. There is marked left ventricular hypertrophy. This often affects the septum *(S)*. (From Stevens A et al: *Core pathology,* ed 3, London, 2009, Mosby.)

outflow tract. Obstruction of left ventricular outflow can occur when the heart rate is increased and the intravascular volume is decreased. This type of hypertrophic cardiomyopathy is a significant risk factor for serious ventricular dysrhythmias and sudden death. **Hypertensive hypertrophic cardiomyopathy** and **valvular hypertrophic cardiomyopathy** occur because of increased resistance to ventricular ejection, which is commonly seen in individuals with hypertension or valvular stenosis (usually aortic). In this case, hypertrophy of the myocytes is an attempt to compensate for increased myocardial workload. Long-term dysfunction of the myocytes develops over time, with diastolic dysfunction appearing first and leading eventually to systolic dysfunction of the ventricle (see the Heart Failure section). Individuals with hypertrophic cardiomyopathy may be asymptomatic or may complain of angina, syncope, dyspnea on exertion, and palpitations. Examination may reveal extra heart sounds and murmurs. Echocardiography and cardiac catheterization can confirm the diagnosis.

Restrictive cardiomyopathy is characterized by resistance to filling and increased diastolic pressure of either or both ventricles. Systolic function and wall thickness are normal. It may occur idiopathically or as a cardiac manifestation of systemic diseases, such as amyloidosis, scleroderma, sarcoidosis, lymphoma, and hemochromatosis, or a number of inherited storage diseases. The myocardium becomes rigid and noncompliant, impeding ventricular filling and raising filling pressures during diastole. The most common clinical manifestation of restrictive cardiomyopathy is right heart failure with systemic venous congestion. Cardiomegaly and dysrhythmias are common. A thorough evaluation for the underlying cause should be initiated (and may include myocardial biopsy). Treatment is aimed at the underlying cause. Death occurs as a result of heart failure or dysrhythmias.

> ✔ **QUICK CHECK 26.7**
> 1. Why does pericarditis develop?
> 2. What are the cardiomyopathies? List the major disorders.
> 3. Briefly describe the pathophysiologic effects of the cardiomyopathies.

Disorders of the Endocardium
Valvular Dysfunction

Disorders of the endocardium (the innermost lining of the heart wall) damage the heart valves, which are composed of endocardial tissue. Endocardial damage can be either congenital or acquired. The acquired forms are more common in adults and result from inflammatory, ischemic, traumatic, degenerative, or infectious alterations of valvular structure and function. One of the most common causes of acquired valvular dysfunction is degeneration or inflammation of the endocardium secondary to rheumatic heart disease (Table 26.6). Structural alterations of the heart valves are caused by remodeling changes in the valvular extracellular matrix and lead to stenosis, incompetence, or both.

In **valvular stenosis**, the valve orifice is constricted and narrowed, so blood cannot flow forward and the workload of the cardiac chamber proximal to the diseased valve increases (Fig. 26.24). Pressure (intraventricular or atrial) rises in the chamber to overcome resistance to flow through the valve, necessitating greater exertion by the myocardium and producing myocardial hypertrophy. Although all four heart valves may be affected, those of the left heart (mitral and aortic valves) in adults are far more commonly affected than those of the right heart (tricuspid and pulmonic valves).

TABLE 26.6 Clinical Manifestations of Valvular Stenosis and Regurgitation

Manifestation	Aortic Stenosis	Mitral Stenosis	Aortic Regurgitation	Mitral Regurgitation	Tricuspid Regurgitation
Most common cause	Congenital bicuspid valve, degenerative (calcific) changes with aging, rheumatic heart disease	Rheumatic heart disease	Infective endocarditis; aortic root disease (connective tissue diseases, Marfan syndrome); dilation of aortic root from hypertension and aging	Myxomatous degeneration (mitral valve prolapse)	Congenital; secondary to pulmonary hypertension with cor pulmonale
Cardiovascular outcome (untreated)	Left ventricular hypertrophy followed by left heart failure; decreased coronary blood flow with myocardial ischemia	Left atrial hypertrophy and dilation with fibrillation, followed by right ventricular failure	Left ventricular hypertrophy and dilation, followed by left heart failure	Left atrial hypertrophy and dilation, followed by left heart failure	Right heart failure
Pulmonary effects	Pulmonary edema with dyspnea on exertion	Pulmonary edema with dyspnea on exertion	Pulmonary edema with dyspnea on exertion	Pulmonary edema with dyspnea on exertion	Dyspnea (may be caused by underlying lung disease)
Central nervous system effects	Syncope, especially on exertion	Stroke resulting from emboli (e.g., hemiparesis)	Syncope	None	None
Pain	Angina pectoris	Atypical chest pain	Angina pectoris	Atypical chest pain	Palpitations
Heart sounds	Systolic murmur heard best at right parasternal second intercostal space and radiating to neck	Low, rumbling diastolic murmur heard best at apex and radiating to axilla; accentuated first heart sound, opening snap	Diastolic murmur heard best at right parasternal second intercostal space and radiating to neck	Murmur throughout systole heard best at apex and radiating to axilla	Murmur throughout systole heard best at left lower sternal border

With data from Mann DL et al, editors: *Braunwald's heart disease: a textbook of cardiovascular medicine*, ed 10, St Louis, 2014, Elsevier.

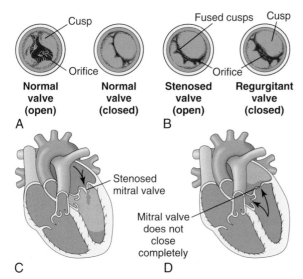

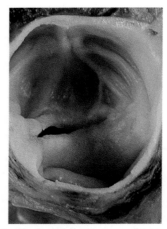

FIGURE 26.25 **Aortic Stenosis.** Mild stenosis in valve leaflets of a young adult. (From Damjanov I, Linder J: *Pathophysiology: a color atlas*, St Louis, 2000, Mosby.)

FIGURE 26.24 **Valvular Stenosis and Regurgitation. A,** Normal position of the valve leaflets, or cusps, when the valve is open and closed. **B,** Open position of a stenosed valve *(left)* and open position of a closed regurgitant valve *(right)*. **C,** Hemodynamic effect of mitral stenosis. The stenosed valve is unable to open sufficiently during left atrial systole, inhibiting left ventricular filling. **D,** Hemodynamic effect of mitral regurgitation. The mitral valve does not close completely during left ventricular systole, permitting blood to reenter the left atrium.

In valvular regurgitation (also called insufficiency or incompetence), the valve leaflets, or cusps, fail to shut completely, permitting blood flow to continue even when the valve is presumably closed (see Fig. 26.24). During systole or diastole, some blood leaks back into the chamber proximal to the diseased valve, which increases the volume of blood the heart must pump and increases the workload of both the atrium and the ventricle. Increased volume leads to chamber dilation, and increased workload leads to hypertrophy; both lead to cardiac dysfunction over time. Eventually, myocardial contractility diminishes, EF drops, diastolic pressure increases, and the ventricles fail from being overworked. Depending on the severity of the valvular dysfunction and the capacity of the heart to compensate, valvular alterations cause a range of symptoms and some degree of incapacitation (see Table 26.6).

In general, valvular disease is diagnosed by transthoracic echocardiography (TTE), which can be used to assess the severity of valvular obstruction or regurgitation before the onset of symptoms. CT or MRI may be indicated in certain settings. Valvular lesions are staged and appropriate management is determined by using four general categories: (1) at risk, (2) progressive, (3) asymptomatic severe, and (4) symptomatic severe.

Management almost always includes careful medical management, valvular repair, or valve replacement followed by long-term anticoagulation therapy and prophylaxis for endocarditis as needed.[11] The purpose of valvular intervention is to improve symptoms and prolong survival, as well as to minimize complications such as asymptomatic irreversible ventricular dysfunction, pulmonary hypertension, stroke, and AF.

Stenosis
Aortic stenosis. Aortic stenosis is the most common valvular abnormality, affecting nearly 2% of adults older than 65 years of age. It has three common causes: (1) congenital bicuspid valve, (2) degeneration with aging, and (3) inflammatory damage caused by rheumatic heart disease. Aortic stenosis is associated with many risk factors for CAD, including hypertension, smoking, and dyslipidemia. In aortic stenosis, the orifice of the valve narrows, causing resistance to blood

flow from the left ventricle into the aorta (Fig. 26.25). Outflow obstruction increases pressure within the left ventricle as it tries to eject blood through the narrowed opening. Left ventricular hypertrophy develops to compensate for the increased workload. Eventually, hypertrophy increases myocardial oxygen demand, which the coronary arteries may not be able to supply. Untreated aortic stenosis can lead to hypertrophic cardiomyopathy, dysrhythmias, myocardial ischemia or infarction, and heart failure.

Aortic stenosis usually develops gradually. Classic symptoms include angina, syncope, and dyspnea. Clinical manifestations include decreased stroke volume and narrowed pulse pressure (the difference between systolic and diastolic pressures). Heart rate is often slow, and pulses are delayed. Resistance to flow leads to a crescendo-decrescendo systolic heart murmur heard best at the right parasternal second intercostal space and may radiate to the neck. Echocardiography can be used to assess the severity of valvular obstruction before the onset of symptoms. Medical management includes vasodilator therapy to reduce resistance to ventricular ejection. Surgical valve replacement with either a mechanical or a bioprosthetic valve is indicated for both symptomatic and asymptomatic individuals with severe stenosis. Percutaneous placement of a prosthetic valve (transcatheter aortic valve implantation [TAVI]) avoids major heart surgery in selected individuals. Once individuals become symptomatic from aortic stenosis, the prognosis is poor.

Mitral stenosis. Mitral stenosis impairs the flow of blood from the left atrium to the left ventricle. Mitral stenosis is the most common form of rheumatic heart disease. Autoimmunity in response to group A β-hemolytic streptococcal M protein antigens leads to inflammation and scarring of the valvular leaflets. Scarring causes the leaflets to become fibrous and fused, and the chordae tendineae cordis become shortened (Fig. 26.26).

Impedance to blood flow results in incomplete emptying of the left atrium and elevated atrial pressure as the chamber tries to force blood through the stenotic valve. Continued increases in left atrial volume and pressure cause atrial dilation and hypertrophy. The risk of developing AF and dysrhythmia-induced thrombi is high. As mitral stenosis progresses, symptoms of decreased cardiac output occur, especially during exertion. Continued elevation of left atrial pressure and volume causes pressure to rise in the pulmonary circulation leading to pulmonary hypertension, pulmonary edema, and right ventricular failure.

Blood flow through the stenotic valve results in a rumbling decrescendo diastolic murmur heard best over the cardiac apex and radiating to the left axilla. If the mitral valve is forced open during diastole, it

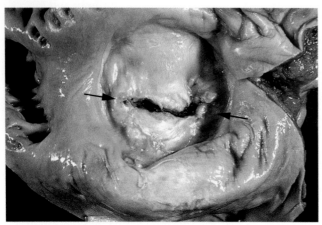

FIGURE 26.26 Mitral Stenosis With Classic "Fish Mouth" Orifice *(Arrows).* (From Kumar V et al: *Robins & Cotran pathologic basis of disease,* ed 9, St Louis, 2015, Elsevier.)

may make a sharp noise called an opening snap. The first heart sound (S_1) is often accentuated and somewhat delayed because of increased left atrial pressure. Other signs and symptoms are generally those of pulmonary congestion and right heart failure. Atrial enlargement and valvular obstruction are demonstrated by chest x-ray films, electrocardiography, and echocardiography. Management includes use of anticoagulation therapy and control of heart rate. Mitral stenosis often can be repaired with percutaneous balloon commissurotomy but may require valve replacement in advanced cases.

Regurgitation

Aortic regurgitation.   Aortic regurgitation results from an inability of the aortic valve leaflets to close properly during diastole because of abnormalities of the leaflets, the aortic root and annulus, or both. It can be primary, caused by congenital bicuspid valve or degeneration in the elderly; or secondary, resulting from chronic hypertension, rheumatic heart disease, bacterial endocarditis, syphilis, connective tissue disorders (e.g., Marfan syndrome and ankylosing spondylitis), appetite-suppressing medications, trauma, or atherosclerosis. During systole, blood is ejected from the left ventricle into the aorta. During diastole, some of the ejected blood flows back into the left ventricle through the leaking valve. Volume overload occurs in the ventricle because it receives blood from the left atrium and from the aorta during diastole. As the end-diastolic volume of the left ventricle increases, myocardial fibers stretch to accommodate the extra fluid. Compensatory dilation permits the left ventricle to increase its stroke volume and maintain cardiac output. Ventricular hypertrophy also occurs as an adaptation to the increased volume and because of increased afterload created by the high stroke volume and resultant systolic hypertension. Over time, ventricular dilation and hypertrophy eventually cannot compensate for aortic incompetence, and heart failure develops.

Clinical manifestations include widened pulse pressure resulting from increased stroke volume and diastolic backflow. Turbulence across the aortic valve during diastole produces a decrescendo murmur in the second, third, or fourth intercostal spaces parasternally and may radiate to the neck. Large stroke volume and rapid runoff of blood from the aorta cause prominent carotid pulsations and bounding peripheral pulses (Corrigan pulse). Other symptoms are usually associated with heart failure that occurs when the ventricle can no longer pump adequately. Dysrhythmias are a common complication of aortic regurgitation. The severity of regurgitation can be estimated by echocardiography, and valve replacement surgery may be delayed for many years through careful use of vasodilators and inotropic agents.

Mitral regurgitation.   Mitral regurgitation can be primary because of mitral valve prolapse (MVP), rheumatic heart disease, infective endocarditis, MI, connective tissue diseases (Marfan syndrome), and dilated cardiomyopathy. It also can be secondary because of ischemic or nonischemic myocardial disease, which damages the chordae tendineae or the mitral annulus. Mitral regurgitation permits backflow of blood from the left ventricle into the left atrium during ventricular systole. The left atrium and ventricle become dilated and hypertrophied to maintain adequate cardiac output. As the left atrium enlarges, stretching of the atrial myocardium often leads to AF. As mitral valve regurgitation progresses, left ventricular function may become impaired to the point of failure. Eventually, increased atrial pressure leads to pulmonary hypertension and failure of the right ventricle. Most clinical manifestations are caused by heart failure. A characteristic holosystolic (throughout systole) murmur, heard best at the apex and that radiates into the back and axilla, suggests the underlying valvular abnormality, which is then confirmed by echocardiography. Mitral incompetence is usually well tolerated—often for years—until heart failure occurs, at which time transcatheter or surgical repair or valve replacement become necessary. In acute mitral regurgitation caused by MI, surgical repair must be done emergently.

Tricuspid regurgitation.   Tricuspid regurgitation is more common than tricuspid stenosis. Primary tricuspid regurgitation can be caused by congenital defects, rheumatic heart disease, endocarditis, or trauma. However, 80% of the cases of tricuspid regurgitation in adults are the result of annular dilatation related to pulmonary hypertension and dilation of the right ventricle, which pulls the valve leaflets apart. Tricuspid valve incompetence leads to volume overload in the right atrium and ventricle, increased systemic venous blood pressure, and right heart failure. Pulmonic valve dysfunction can have the same consequences as tricuspid valve dysfunction.

Mitral Valve Prolapse Syndrome

In **mitral valve prolapse syndrome (MVPS)**, one or both of the cusps of the mitral valve billow upward (prolapse) into the left atrium during systole (Fig. 26.27). The most common cause of MVP is myxomatous degeneration of the leaflets in which the cusps are redundant, thickened, and scalloped because of changes in tissue proteoglycans, increased levels of proteinases, and infiltration by myofibroblasts. Mitral regurgitation occurs if the ballooning valve permits blood to leak into the atrium.

MVP is the most common valve disorder in the United States, with a prevalence of nearly 3% of adults. MVP can be associated with inherited connective tissue disorders (Marfan syndrome, Ehlers-Danlos syndrome, osteogenesis imperfecta), suggesting that it results from a genetic or environmental disruption of valvular development during the fifth or sixth week of gestation. There also may be a relationship between symptomatic MVP and hyperthyroidism.

Many cases of MVP are completely asymptomatic. Cardiac auscultation on routine physical examination may disclose a regurgitant murmur or midsystolic click, or echocardiography may demonstrate the condition in the absence of auscultatory findings. Symptomatic MVPS can cause palpitations, tachycardia, atypical chest pain, lightheadedness, syncope, fatigue, weakness, dyspnea, chest tightness, anxiety, depression, and panic attacks. Many symptoms are vague and puzzling and are unrelated to the degree of prolapse. Most individuals with MVP have an excellent prognosis, do not develop symptoms, and do not require any restriction in activity or medical management. Occasionally, β-blockers are needed to alleviate syncope, severe chest pain, or palpitations.

Acute Rheumatic Fever and Rheumatic Heart Disease

Rheumatic fever is a systemic inflammatory disease caused by a delayed exaggerated immune response to infection by the group A β-hemolytic

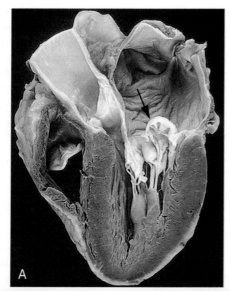

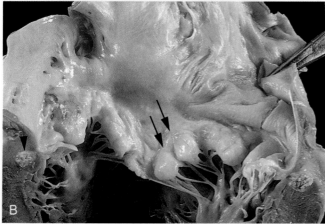

FIGURE 26.27 Mitral Valve Prolapse (MVP). A, Prolapsed mitral valve. Prolapse permits the valve leaflets to billow back *(arrow)* into the atrium during left ventricular systole. The billowing causes the leaflets to part slightly, permitting regurgitation into the atrium. **B,** Looking down into the mitral valve, the ballooning *(arrows)* of the leaflets is seen. (From Kumar V et al: *Robins & Cotran pathologic basis of disease,* ed 9, St Louis, 2015, Elsevier. **A** Courtesy William D. Edwards, MD, Mayo Clinic, Rochester, Minn.)

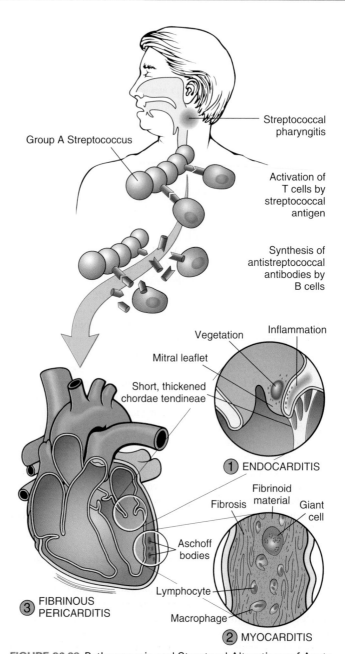

FIGURE 26.28 Pathogenesis and Structural Alterations of Acute Rheumatic Heart Disease. Beginning usually with a sore throat, rheumatic fever can develop only as a sequel to pharyngeal infection by group A β-hemolytic streptococcus. Suspected as a hypersensitivity reaction, it is proposed that antibodies directed against the M proteins of certain strains of streptococci cross-react with tissue glycoproteins in the heart, joints, and other tissues. The exact nature of cross-reacting antigens has been difficult to define, but it appears that the streptococcal infection causes an autoimmune response against self-antigens. Inflammatory lesions are found in various sites; the most distinctive within the heart are called Aschoff bodies. The chronic sequelae result from progressive fibrosis because of healing of the inflammatory lesions and the changes induced by valvular deformities. (From Damjanov I: *Pathology for the health professions,* ed 4, Philadelphia, 2012, Saunders.)

streptococcus. In its acute form, rheumatic fever is a febrile illness characterized by inflammation of the joints, skin, nervous system, and heart. If untreated, rheumatic fever can cause scarring and deformity of cardiac structures resulting in **rheumatic heart disease (RHD).** Acute rheumatic fever occurs most often in children between the ages of 5 and 15 years, whereas RHD is usually diagnosed in adults.

PATHOPHYSIOLOGY   Acute rheumatic fever can develop only as a sequel to pharyngeal infection by group A β-hemolytic streptococcus. Streptococcal skin infections do not progress to acute rheumatic fever because the strains of the microorganism that affect the skin do not have the same antigenic molecules in their cell membranes and do not elicit the same kind of immune response. Acute rheumatic fever is the result of an abnormal humoral and cell-mediated immune response to group A streptococcal cell membrane antigens called M proteins (Fig. 26.28). This immune response cross-reacts with molecularly similar self-antigens in the heart, muscle, brain, and joints, causing an autoimmune response that results in diffuse, proliferative, and exudative inflammatory lesions in these tissues. The inflammation may subside before treatment, leaving behind damage to the heart valves. Repeated attacks of acute rheumatic fever cause chronic proliferative changes with resultant tissue scarring, granuloma formation, and thrombosis.

Approximately 10% of individuals with rheumatic fever develop RHD, usually between the ages of 25 and 34. The primary lesion in RHD involves the endocardium. Endocardial inflammation causes swelling of the valve leaflets, with secondary erosion along the lines of leaflet contact. Small, beadlike clumps of vegetation containing platelets and fibrin are deposited on eroded valvular tissue and on the chordae tendineae cordis. These lesions can become progressively adherent, and the leaflets may adhere to each other. Scarring and shortening of the involved structures occur over time.

If inflammation penetrates the myocardium (myocarditis), localized fibrin deposits develop that are surrounded by areas of necrosis. These fibrinoid necrotic deposits are called Aschoff bodies. Pericarditis also can occur, characterized by serofibrinous effusion within the pericardial cavity. Cardiomegaly and left heart failure may occur during episodes of untreated acute or recurrent rheumatic fever. Conduction defects and AF often are associated with rheumatic heart disease.

CLINICAL MANIFESTATIONS The common symptoms of acute rheumatic fever are fever, lymphadenopathy, arthralgia, nausea, vomiting, epistaxis (nosebleed), abdominal pain, and tachycardia. The major clinical manifestations of acute rheumatic fever usually occur singly or in combination 1 to 5 weeks after streptococcal infection of the pharynx. They are (1) carditis: murmur, chest pain, pericardial friction rub, ECG changes, valvular dysfunction; (2) polyarthritis: heat, redness, swelling, and pain that migrate among the large joints of the extremities; (3) chorea: sudden, aimless, irregular, involuntary movements; (4) erythema marginatum: nonpruritic, erythematous macules on the trunk that may fade in the center; and (5) subcutaneous nodules: palpable nodules over bony prominences and extensor tendons.

EVALUATION AND TREATMENT Supportive evidence for the diagnosis of rheumatic fever include positive throat cultures and measurement of serum antibodies against the hemolytic factor streptolysin O. Several other antibody tests also are available. Elevated measurements of white blood cell count, erythrocyte sedimentation rate, and C-reactive protein indicate inflammation.

Appropriate antibiotic therapy given within the first 9 days of group A β-hemolytic streptococcus infection usually prevents rheumatic fever. Therapy for acute rheumatic fever is aimed at eradicating the streptococcal infection and involves a 10-day regimen of antibiotics. NSAIDs are used as antiinflammatory agents for both carditis and arthritis. Serious carditis may require corticosteroids and diuretics. Because recurrent rheumatic fever occurs in more than half of affected children, continuous prophylactic antibiotic therapy may be necessary for as long as 5 years. RHD may require surgical repair of damaged valves.

QUICK CHECK 26.8
1. Compare the effect of aortic stenosis with mitral stenosis on the left ventricle and atrium.
2. Describe aortic regurgitation, mitral regurgitation, and tricuspid regurgitation.
3. What are the common symptoms of mitral prolapse?
4. What is the cause of rheumatic heart disease?

Infective Endocarditis

Infective endocarditis is a general term used to describe infection and inflammation of the endocardium—especially the cardiac valves. Over 80% of cases are caused by bacteria, especially streptococci, staphylococci, and enterococci. Other causes include viruses, fungi, rickettsia, and parasites (see *Risk Factors:* Infective Endocarditis).

RISK FACTORS
Infective Endocarditis

- Acquired valvular heart disease
- Implantation of prosthetic heart valves
- Congenital lesions associated with highly turbulent flow (e.g., ventricular septal defect)
- Previous attack of infective endocarditis
- Intravenous drug use
- Long-term indwelling intravenous catheterization (e.g., for pressure monitoring, feeding, hemodialysis)
- Implantable cardiac pacemakers
- Heart transplant with defective valve

PATHOPHYSIOLOGY The pathogenesis of infective endocarditis requires at least three critical elements (Fig. 26.29):
1. *Endocardial damage.* Trauma, congenital heart disease, valvular heart disease, and the presence of prosthetic valves are the most common risk factors for endocardial damage that leads to infective endocarditis. Turbulent blood flow caused by these abnormalities usually affects the atrial surface of atrioventricular valves or the ventricular surface of semilunar valves. Endocardial damage exposes the endothelial basement membrane, which contains a type of collagen that attracts platelets and thereby stimulates sterile thrombus formation on the membrane. This causes an inflammatory reaction (nonbacterial thrombotic endocarditis).
2. *Adherence of blood-borne microorganisms to the damaged endocardial surface.* Bacteria may enter the bloodstream during injection drug use, trauma, dental procedures that involve manipulation of the gingiva, cardiac surgery, genitourinary procedures and indwelling catheters in the presence of infection, or gastrointestinal instrumentation, or they may spread from uncomplicated upper respiratory tract or skin infections. Bacteria adhere to the damaged endocardium using adhesins.
3. *Formation of infective endocardial vegetations* (Fig. 26.30). Bacteria infiltrate the sterile thrombi and accelerate fibrin formation by activating the clotting cascade. These vegetative lesions can form anywhere on the endocardium but usually occur on heart valves and surrounding structures. Although endocardial tissue is constantly bathed in antibody-containing blood and is surrounded by scavenging monocytes and polymorphonuclear leukocytes, bacterial colonies are inaccessible to host defenses because they are embedded in the protective fibrin clots. This also makes them difficult to treat with antibiotics. Embolization from these vegetations can lead to abscesses and characteristic skin changes, such as petechiae, splinter hemorrhages, Osler nodes, and Janeway lesions.

CLINICAL MANIFESTATIONS Infective endocarditis causes varying degrees of valvular dysfunction and may be associated with manifestations involving several organ systems, making diagnosis difficult. Signs and symptoms of infective endocarditis are caused by infection and inflammation, systemic spread of microemboli, and immune complex

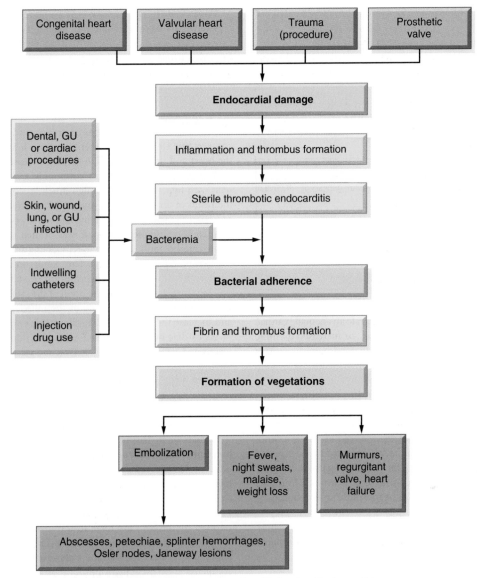

FIGURE 26.29 Pathogenesis of Infective Endocarditis.

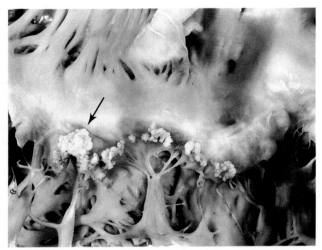

FIGURE 26.30 Bacterial Endocarditis of Mitral Valve. The valve is covered with large, irregular vegetations *(arrow)*. (From Damjanov I, Linder J: *Pathology: a color atlas,* St Louis, 2000, Mosby.)

deposition. Microemboli can spread to splenic, renal, pulmonary, peripheral arterial, coronary, bone, CNS, and ocular circulations. The classic findings are fever; new or changed cardiac murmur; and petechial lesions of the skin, conjunctiva, and oral mucosa. Characteristic physical findings include Osler nodes (painful erythematous nodules on the pads of the fingers and toes) and Janeway lesions (nonpainful hemorrhagic lesions on the palms and soles). CNS complications are the most severe extracardiac complications and include stroke, abscess, and meningitis. Other manifestations include weight loss, back pain, night sweats, and heart failure.

EVALUATION AND TREATMENT The Duke criteria for the diagnosis of infective endocarditis include blood cultures positive for bacteria, evidence for endocardial involvement (murmurs or documented regurgitation), recognized risk factors, fever, and vascular complications. Serum C-reactive protein is elevated. Echocardiography should be performed immediately. Antimicrobial therapy is generally given for several weeks, beginning with intravenous and ending with oral administration. Other drugs may be necessary to treat left heart failure secondary to valvular dysfunction. Surgery that involves excision of infected tissue with or without valve replacement may be needed for refractory infections.

Guidelines for the use of antibiotic prophylaxis before dental procedures to prevent infective endocarditis were updated in 2017. Indications include prosthetic valves (including transcatheter-implanted grafts), prosthetic material used for cardiac valve repair, a history of infective endocarditis, unrepaired cyanotic congenital heart disease, and heart transplant with valvular defect.[11]

> ✓ **QUICK CHECK 26.9**
> 1. What three critical elements are required for the pathogenesis of infective endocarditis?
> 2. Why does infective endocarditis involve several organ systems?

MANIFESTATIONS OF HEART DISEASE

Heart Failure

Heart failure is when the heart is unable to generate an adequate cardiac output, causing inadequate perfusion of tissues, or increased diastolic filling pressure of the left ventricle, or both, so that pulmonary capillary pressures are increased. It affects nearly 10% of individuals >65 years of age and is the most common reason for admission to the hospital in that age group.[3] Ischemic heart disease and hypertension are the most important predisposing risk factors. Other risk factors include age, obesity, diabetes, renal failure, valvular heart disease, cardiomyopathies, myocarditis, congenital heart disease, and excessive alcohol use. Numerous genetic polymorphisms have been linked to an increased risk for heart failure, including genes for cardiomyopathies, myocyte contractility, and neurohumoral receptors. Most heart failure results from dysfunction of the left ventricle (heart failure with reduced EF and heart failure with preserved EF). The right ventricle also may be dysfunctional, especially in pulmonary disease (right ventricular failure). Finally, some conditions cause inadequate perfusion despite normal or elevated cardiac output (high-output failure).

Left Heart Failure (Congestive Heart Failure)

Left heart failure is categorized as heart failure with reduced EF (systolic heart failure) or heart failure with preserved EF (diastolic heart failure). It is possible for these two types of heart failure to occur simultaneously in one individual.

Heart failure with reduced ejection fraction (HFrEF), or systolic heart failure, is defined as an EF of <40% and an inability of the heart to generate an adequate cardiac output to perfuse vital tissues. Cardiac output depends on the heart rate and stroke volume. Stroke volume is influenced by three major determinants: (1) contractility, (2) preload, and (3) afterload (see Chapter 25).

Contractility is reduced by diseases that disrupt myocyte activity. MI is the most common primary cause of decreased contractility. Other primary causes include myocarditis and cardiomyopathies, especially dilated cardiomyopathy and hypertensive hypertrophic cardiomyopathy. Myocardial ischemia and increased myocardial workload contribute to inflammatory, immune, and neurohumoral changes (activation of the SNS and RAAS) that mediate a process called ventricular remodeling. Ventricular remodeling results in disruption of the normal myocardial extracellular structure and causes progressive myocyte contractile dysfunction over time (Fig. 26.31). When contractility is decreased, stroke volume falls and left ventricular end-diastolic volume (LVEDV) increases. This causes dilation of the heart and an increase in preload.

Preload, or LVEDV, increases with decreased contractility or an excess of plasma volume (intravenous fluid administration, renal failure, mitral valvular disease). Increases in LVEDV stretch the heart and can actually improve cardiac output up to a certain point, but as preload continues to rise, dilation of the myocardium eventually leads to dysfunction of the sarcomeres and decreased contractility. This relationship is described by the Frank-Starling law of the heart (see Fig. 25.14). Dilation of the heart also stretches the coronary arteries causing them to narrow, diminishing blood flow to the myocardium and further compromising contractility. Decreased contractility means less blood is ejected from the heart and therefore leads to further increases in preload.

Increased afterload is most commonly a result of increased PVR seen with hypertension. Although much less common, it also can be the result of aortic valvular disease. With increased afterload, there is resistance to ventricular emptying and more workload for the ventricle (Fig. 26.32). Sustained afterload is associated with high levels of Ang II and catecholamines leading to remodeling and eventual hypertensive hypertrophic cardiomyopathy. This results in an increase in oxygen demand by the thickened myocardium. A state of relative ischemia develops that contributes to alteration of the cardiac extracellular matrix which can disrupt the integrity of the muscle, decrease contractility, and increase the likelihood that the ventricle will dilate and fail.

As cardiac output falls, renal perfusion diminishes and the RAAS is activated, which acts to increase PVR and plasma volume, thus further increasing afterload and preload. In addition, baroreceptors in the central circulation stimulate the SNS to cause yet more vasoconstriction and cause the hypothalamus to produce antidiuretic hormone. This vicious cycle of decreasing contractility, increasing preload, and increasing afterload causes progressive worsening of left heart failure (Fig. 26.33).

In addition to these hemodynamic interactions, HFrEF is characterized by a complex constellation of neurohumoral, inflammatory, and metabolic processes. Ang II and aldosterone have direct toxicity to the myocardium, contributing to remodeling, myocyte death, and fibrosis. Arginine vasopressin (antidiuretic hormone [ADH]) contributes to vasoconstriction, renal fluid retention, and hyponatremia. Catecholamines released by the SNS are toxic to the myocardium and contribute to remodeling. Natriuretic peptides, especially BNP, are released in an effort to improve renal salt and water excretion but are inadequate to compensate for these neurohumoral perturbations. Insulin resistance and diabetes not only contribute to heart failure but also are a complication of heart failure with changes in myocyte metabolism (see *Did You Know? Diabetes and Heart Failure*). Inflammatory cytokines, such as TNF-α, are released in heart failure, contributing to myocardial damage as well as systemic weight loss (cardiac cachexia). Finally, changes in the metabolic processes within the myocardium also are affected, with a decreased ability of the heart to produce energy and an increase in release of toxic metabolites. These neurohumoral, inflammatory, and metabolic aspects of left HFrEF have led to the routine use of combinations of medications that inhibit angiotensin, aldosterone, and catecholamines, and increase salt excretion in an effort to prevent long-term damage to the myocardium, as well as the exploration of new treatment modalities focused on reducing inflammation and improving myocardial metabolic function.

The clinical manifestations of left heart failure are the result of pulmonary vascular congestion and inadequate perfusion of the systemic circulation. Individuals experience dyspnea, orthopnea, cough of frothy sputum, fatigue, decreased urine output, and edema. Physical examination often reveals pulmonary edema (cyanosis, inspiratory crackles, pleural effusions), hypotension or hypertension, an S_3 gallop, and evidence of underlying CAD or hypertension. The diagnosis can be further confirmed with echocardiography showing decreased EF and cardiomegaly. The level of serum BNP is used to estimate the severity of heart failure.

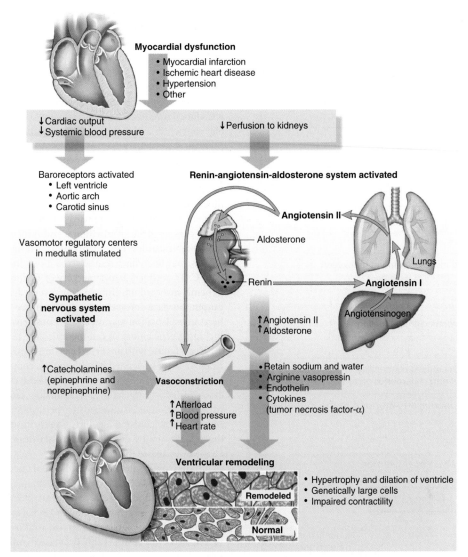

FIGURE 26.31 Pathophysiology of Ventricular Remodeling. Myocardial dysfunction activates the renin-angiotensin-aldosterone and sympathetic nervous systems, releasing neurohormones (angiotensin II, aldosterone, catecholamines, and cytokines). These neurohormones contribute to ventricular remodeling. (Redrawn from Carelock J, Clark AP: *Am J Nurs* 101[12]:27, 2001.)

DID YOU KNOW?

Diabetes and Heart Failure

The prevalence of diabetes in individuals with heart failure ranges from 25% to 40%, and two thirds of those with metabolic syndrome will eventually develop HFrEF. In addition to being a risk factor for coronary artery disease and hypertension, the deposition of damaging by-products of insulin resistance (advanced glycation end products [AGEs]) contributes to hypertrophic and fibrotic remodeling of the myocardium. In addition to structural changes, insulin resistance in type 2 diabetes leads to impairment of ATP production, which shifts myocyte metabolism toward fatty acid oxidation. In the failing heart, increased demand for oxygen and energy is coupled with a decreased ability to use fatty acids as an energy source and lipids are deposited into the myocardium causing lipotoxicity. Myocytes that cannot use glucose or fatty acids for energy cannot maintain contractility and cardiac output. Diabetes also contributes to autonomic dysfunction and inflammation in the heart, further compromising myocyte function. In addition to blocking renal reabsorption of glucose, the sodium-glucose cotransporter 2 (SLGT2) inhibitors increase renal sodium excretion and target many of the mechanisms implicated in diabetes and heart failure. They also increase the concentration of circulating ketone bodies, which might provide an alternative energy source for the diabetic heart in the presence of insulin resistance. Clinical studies demonstrate improved cardiovascular outcomes for individuals with diabetes who are treated with these medications.

Data from Lehrke M, Marx N: *Am J Cardiol* 120(Suppl):S37eS47, 2017; Leon BM, Maddox TM: *World J Diabetes* 6(13):1246-1258, 2015; Giuseppe MC et al: *Card Fail Rev* 3(1):52-55, 2017; Ritchie RH et al: *J Molec Endocrinol* 58(4):R225-R240, 2017; Trang A, Aguilar D: *Curr Heart Fail Rep* 14(6):445-453, 2017.

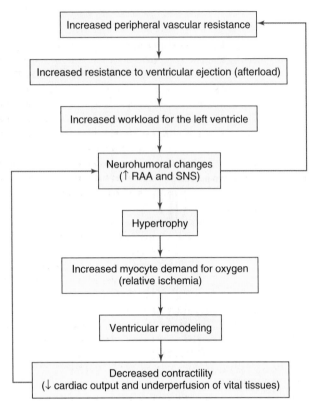

FIGURE 26.32 Role of Increased Afterload in the Pathogenesis of Heart Failure.

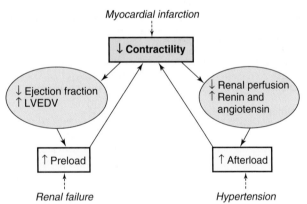

FIGURE 26.33 Vicious Cycle of Heart Failure With Reduced Ejection Fraction. Although the initial insult may be one of primary decreased contractility (e.g., myocardial infarction), increased preload (e.g., renal failure), or increased afterload (e.g., hypertension), all three factors play a role in the progression of left heart failure. *LVEDV,* Left ventricular end-diastolic volume.

Management of HFrEF is aimed at interrupting the worsening cycle of decreasing contractility, increasing preload, and increasing afterload. The acute onset of left heart failure is most often the result of acute myocardial ischemia and must be managed in conjunction with management of the underlying coronary disease. Oxygen, nitrate, and morphine administration improves myocardial oxygenation and helps relieve coronary spasm while lowering preload through systemic venodilation. Inotropic drugs, such as dopamine, dobutamine, and milrinone, increase contractility and can help raise the blood pressure in hypotensive individuals. Diuretics reduce preload. ACE inhibitors,

ARBs, and aldosterone blockers reduce both preload and afterload by decreasing aldosterone levels and reducing PVR. Finally, individuals with severe HFrEF failure may benefit from acute coronary bypass or PCI. These people often are supported with the intra-aortic balloon pump (IABP) or left ventricular assist devices (LVADs) until surgery can be performed.

Management of chronic left heart failure is based on current guidelines and clinical severity. The overall goals are to reduce preload and afterload. Salt restriction and diuretics (loop diuretics) are effective in reducing preload. A combination of ACE inhibitors (or ARBs) and aldosterone blockers are indicated, along with β-blockers.[12] Many patients are effectively managed with a new class of medications called angiotensin receptor–neprilysin inhibitors (ARNIs) that combine the effects of RAA blockade with a stimulus for increased BNP release from the myocardium.[13] Inotropic drugs are used for those with refractory symptoms or to control atrial dysrhythmias. Additional interventions, such as implantable cardioverter-defibrillators, cardiac resynchronization, and LVADs, may be indicated in selected individuals. For those individuals with CAD, coronary bypass surgery or PCI may improve perfusion to ischemic myocardium (hibernating myocardium) and improve cardiac output. Surgical interventions that improve ventricular geometry or heart transplantation may need to be considered. Experimental therapies, including gene and stem cell therapies, are being explored.

Heart failure with preserved ejection function (HFpEF), or **diastolic heart failure,** is defined as pulmonary congestion despite a normal stroke volume and cardiac output. It is the cause of nearly half of all cases of left heart failure. The major causes of HFpEF include hypertension-induced myocardial hypertrophy and myocardial ischemia–induced ventricular remodeling. Other causes include aortic valvular disease, mitral valve disease, pericardial diseases, and cardiomyopathies. Diabetes increases the risk for HFpEF.

HFpHF results from decreased compliance of the left ventricle and abnormal diastolic relaxation. These changes result from ventricular remodeling with alterations in the extracellular matrix and myocyte cytoskeletal changes. Hypertrophy and ischemia cause a decreased ability of the myocytes to actively pump calcium from the cytosol, resulting in impaired relaxation. With decreased compliance and inadequate relaxation, the ventricle lumen is smaller than normal during diastole and cannot accept filling with blood without causing an increase in wall tension. Thus a normal LVEDV results in an increased LVEDP. This pressure is reflected back into the pulmonary circulation and results in pulmonary edema, pulmonary hypertension, and right ventricular hypertrophy. The increase in pressure is made worse by rapid ventricular filling, so symptoms are worse with tachycardia (e.g., with exercise).

Individuals with HFpEF present with dyspnea on exertion and fatigue. Evidence of pulmonary edema (inspiratory crackles on auscultation, pleural effusions) is usually not present in resting individuals without tachycardia, but may develop over time. Late in diastole, atrial contraction with rapid ejection of blood into the noncompliant ventricle may give rise to an S_4 gallop. Electrocardiography often reveals evidence of left ventricular hypertrophy, and chest x-ray may show pulmonary congestion without cardiomegaly (Table 26.7). There also may be evidence of underlying coronary disease, hypertension, or valvular disease. Diagnosis is based on three factors: (1) signs and symptoms of heart failure, (2) normal left ventricular EF, and (3) evidence of diastolic dysfunction. The diagnosis is confirmed by clinical Doppler echocardiography, which demonstrates poor ventricular filling with normal EFs.

Management is aimed at improving ventricular relaxation and prolonging diastolic filling times to reduce diastolic pressure. Nitrates, β-blockers, ACE inhibitors, and ARBs have been used with only varying success, and current guidelines focus on treating hypertension, ischemia, or valvular disease.[12] Outcomes for individuals with HFpEF are as poor

TABLE 26.7   Comparison of Heart Failure With Reduced Ejection Fraction (HFrEF) and Heart Failure With Preserved Ejection Fraction (HFpEF)

Characteristic	HFrEF	HFpEF
Sex	Male > female	Female > male
Left ventricular ejection fraction	Decreased	Normal
Left ventricular chamber size	Increased	Decreased
Left ventricular hypertrophy on electrocardiogram	Possible	Probable
Chest radiography	Pulmonary congestion with cardiomegaly	Pulmonary congestion without cardiomegaly
Gallop	S_3	S_4

Modified from Jessup M, Brozena S: *N Engl J Med* 348(20):2007-2018, 2003.

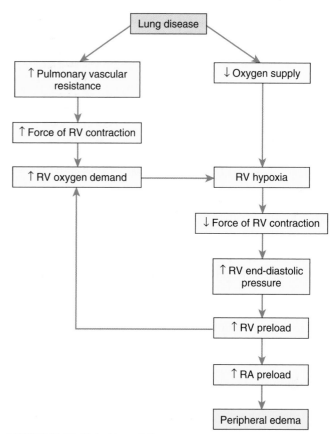

FIGURE 26.34 Right Heart Failure. *RA,* Right atrial; *RV,* right ventricular.

as those with HFrEF, and there has been little improvement in prognosis despite numerous new treatment trials.

Right Heart Failure

Right heart failure is defined as the inability of the right ventricle to provide adequate blood flow into the pulmonary circulation at a normal central venous pressure. It can result from left heart failure when an increase in left ventricular filling pressure is reflected back into the pulmonary circulation. As pressure in the pulmonary circulation rises, the resistance to right ventricular emptying increases (Fig. 26.34). The right ventricle is poorly prepared to compensate for this increased afterload and will dilate and fail. When this happens, pressure will rise in the systemic venous circulation, resulting in peripheral edema and hepatosplenomegaly. Treatment relies on management of the left ventricular dysfunction as just outlined.

When right heart failure occurs in the absence of left heart failure, it is typically attributable to diffuse hypoxic pulmonary disease such as chronic obstructive pulmonary disease (COPD), cystic fibrosis, and acute respiratory distress syndrome (ARDS). These disorders result in pulmonary vasoconstriction, pulmonary hypertension, and an increase in right ventricular afterload. The mechanisms for this type of right ventricular failure (cor pulmonale) are discussed in Chapter 29. Finally, MI, cardiomyopathies, and pulmonic valvular disease interfere with right ventricular contractility and can lead to right heart failure.

High-Output Failure

High-output failure is the inability of the heart to adequately supply the body with blood-borne nutrients, despite adequate blood volume and normal or elevated myocardial contractility. In high-output failure, the heart increases its output but the body's metabolic needs are still not met. Common causes of high-output failure are anemia, septicemia, hyperthyroidism, and beriberi (Fig. 26.35).

Anemia decreases the oxygen-carrying capacity of the blood. Metabolic acidosis occurs as the body's cells switch to anaerobic metabolism (see Chapter 5). In response to metabolic acidosis, heart rate and stroke volume increase in an attempt to improve tissue perfusion. If anemia is severe, however, even maximum cardiac output does not supply the cells with enough oxygen for metabolism.

In septicemia, disturbed metabolism, bacterial toxins, and the inflammatory process cause systemic vasodilation and fever. Faced with a lowered systemic vascular resistance (SVR) and an elevated metabolic rate, cardiac output increases to maintain blood pressure and prevent metabolic acidosis. In overwhelming septicemia, however, the heart may not be able to raise its output enough to compensate for vasodilation. Body tissues show signs of inadequate blood supply despite a high cardiac output.

Hyperthyroidism accelerates cellular metabolism through the actions of elevated levels of thyroxine from the thyroid gland. This may occur chronically (thyrotoxicosis) or acutely (thyroid storm). Because the body's increased demand for oxygen threatens to cause metabolic acidosis, cardiac output increases. If blood levels of thyroxine are high and the metabolic response to thyroxine is vigorous, even an abnormally elevated cardiac output may be inadequate.

In the United States, beriberi (thiamine deficiency) usually is caused by malnutrition secondary to chronic alcoholism. Beriberi actually causes a mixed type of heart failure. Thiamine deficiency impairs cellular metabolism in all tissues, including the myocardium. In the heart, impaired cardiac metabolism leads to insufficient contractile strength. In blood vessels, thiamine deficiency leads to peripheral vasodilation, which decreases SVR. Heart failure ensues as decreased SVR triggers increased cardiac output, which the impaired myocardium is unable to deliver. The strain of demands for increased output in the face of impaired metabolism may deplete cardiac reserves until low-output failure begins.

Dysrhythmias

A dysrhythmia, or arrhythmia, is a disturbance of heart rhythm. Normal heart rhythms are generated by the SA node and travel through the

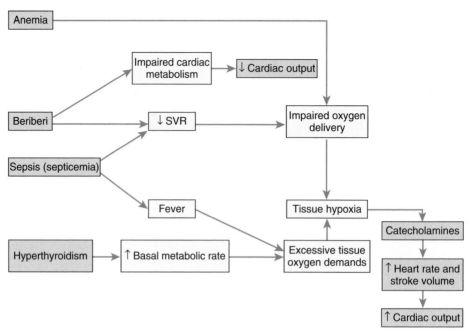

FIGURE 26.35 High-Output Failure. *SVR,* Systemic vascular resistance.

heart's conduction system, causing the atrial and ventricular myocardium to contract and relax at a regular rate that is appropriate to maintain circulation at various levels of physical activity (see Chapter 25). Dysrhythmias range in severity from occasional "missed" or rapid beats to serious disturbances that impair the pumping ability of the heart, contributing to heart failure and death. Dysrhythmias can be caused either by an abnormal rate of impulse generation (Table 26.8) from the SA node or other pacemaker or by the abnormal conduction of impulses (Table 26.9) through the heart's conduction system, including the myocardial cells themselves.

> ✔ **QUICK CHECK 26.10**
> 1. Why are changes in left ventricular end-diastolic volume important for left heart failure?
> 2. What is the vicious cycle of heart failure with reduced ejection fraction (EF)?
> 3. What are the mechanisms of heart failure with preserved EF?

SHOCK

In shock the cardiovascular system fails to perfuse the tissues adequately, resulting in widespread impairment of cellular metabolism. Because tissue perfusion can be disrupted by any factor that alters heart function, blood volume, or blood pressure, shock has many causes and various clinical manifestations. Ultimately, however, shock progresses to organ failure and death, unless compensatory mechanisms reverse the process or clinical intervention succeeds.

The term *multiple organ dysfunction syndrome* (MODS) describes the failure of two or more organ systems after severe illness and injury and is a frequent complication of severe shock. The disease process is initiated and perpetuated by uncontrolled inflammatory and stress responses. It is progressive and is associated with significant mortality.

Impairment of Cellular Metabolism

The final common pathway in shock of any type is impairment of cellular metabolism. Fig. 26.36 illustrates the pathophysiology of shock at the cellular level.

Impairment of Oxygen Use

In all types of shock, the cell either is not receiving an adequate amount of oxygen or is unable to use oxygen. An imbalance between tissue perfusion and cellular demand for oxygen results in impaired cellular metabolism. Without oxygen, the cell shifts from aerobic to anaerobic metabolism. Anaerobic metabolism is a less efficient method of extracting energy from carbon bonds, and the cell begins to use its stores of ATP faster than stores can be replaced. Without ATP, the cell cannot operate the sodium-potassium pump. Sodium, chloride, and water accumulate inside the cell causing cellular edema. Cellular edema disrupts cellular membranes and injures the cells internally. Cells of the nervous system and myocardium are profoundly and immediately affected. As water moves into cells, water is drawn from the vascular space. This decreases circulatory volume.

In addition to decreasing ATP stores, anaerobic metabolism produces lactate and metabolic acidosis develops. Enzymes necessary for cellular function dissociate under acid conditions, stopping cell function, repair, and division. As blood pH drops, there is reduced oxygen-carrying capacity of the blood (see Chapter 5). Further acidosis disrupts lysosomal membrane integrity causing cellular and tissue damage. Compensatory mechanisms, including inflammation and activation of the clotting cascade, further impair oxygen use and contribute to the complications of shock.

Impairment of Glucose Use

The reasons for inadequate glucose delivery are the same as those enumerated for inadequate oxygen delivery. Impaired glucose use can be caused by impaired glucose uptake by the cells (see Fig. 26.36). Stress hormones are released, including catecholamines, cortisol, and growth hormone. These cause hyperglycemia and insulin resistance. Cells shift

TABLE 26.8   Disorders of Impulse Formation

Type	Electrocardiogram	Effect	Pathophysiology	Treatment
Sinus bradycardia	P rate ≤60 PR interval normal QRS for each P	Increased preload Decreased mean arterial pressure	Hyperkalemia: slows depolarization Vagal hyperactivity: unknown Digoxin toxicity common Late hypoxia: lack of adenosine triphosphate (ATP)	If hypotensive, treat cause and support Follow with sympathomimetics, cardiotonics, and pacer Vagolytics
Simple sinus tachycardia	P rate 100-150 PR interval normal QRS for each P	Decreased filling times Decreased mean arterial pressure Increased myocardial demand	Catecholamines: rise in resting potential and calcium influx Fever: unknown Early failure and lung disease: hypoxic cell metabolism Hypercalcemia	Oxygen, bed rest Calcium channel blockers
Premature atrial contractions (PACs) or beats*	Early P waves that may have morphologic changes PR interval normal QRS for each P	Occasional decreased filling time and mean arterial pressure	Electrolyte disturbances: decrease in all phases Hypoxia and elevated preload: cell membrane disturbances Hypercalcemia	Treat underlying cause Digoxin
Sinus dysrhythmias	Rate varies P-P regularly irregular, short with inspiration, long with exhalation PR interval normal QRS for each P	Variable filling times Variable mean arterial pressure Variable oxygen demand	Unknown Common in young children and young adults	None
Atrial tachycardia (includes premature atrial tachycardia if onset is abrupt)	P rate 151-250; morphology may differ from sinus PPR interval normal P/QRS ratio variable	Decreased filling time Decreased mean arterial pressure Increased myocardial demand	Same as PACs: leads to increased atrial automaticity, atrial reentry Digoxin toxicity: common	Control ventricular rate Digoxin, calcium channel blockers, vagus stimulation Pace to override
Atrial flutter*	P rate 251-300; morphology may vary from sinus P PR interval usually not observable P/QRS ratio variable	Decreased filling time Decreased mean arterial pressure	Same as atrial tachycardia Aging	Same as atrial tachycardia Synchronous cardioversion
Atrial fibrillation*	P rate >300 and usually not observable No PR interval QRS rate variable and rhythm irregular	Same as atrial flutter	Same as atrial tachycardia Aging	Same as atrial tachycardia
Idiojunctional rhythm	P absent or independent QRS normal, rate 41-59, regular	Decreased cardiac output from loss of atrial contribution to ventricular preload Decreased mean atrial pressure as a result of bradycardia	Atrial and sinus bradycardia, standstill, or block	Same as sinus bradycardia
Junctional bradycardia	P absent or independent QRS normal, rate 40 or less	Same as idiojunctional rhythm	Same as idiojunctional rhythm Vagal hyperactivity	Same as sinus bradycardia
Premature junctional contractions (PJCs) or beats	Early beats without P waves QRS morphology normal	Decreased cardiac output from loss of atrial contribution to ventricular preload for that beat	Hyperkalemia (6-5.4 mEq/L) Hypercalcemia, hypoxia, and elevated preload (see PACs)	Same as PACs
Accelerated junctional rhythm	P absent or independent QRS morphology normal, rate 60-99	Decreased cardiac output from loss of atrial contribution to ventricular preload	Same as PJCs	Same as PACs
Junctional tachycardia	P absent or independent QRS morphology normal, rate 100 or more	Decreased cardiac output from loss of atrial contribution to ventricular preload Increased myocardial demand because of tachycardia	Same as PJCs	Same as PACs

Continued

TABLE 26.8 Disorders of Impulse Formation—cont'd

Type	Electrocardiogram	Effect	Pathophysiology	Treatment
Idioventricular rhythm[†]	P absent or independent QRS >0.11 and rate 20-39	Same as idiojunctional rhythm	Sinus, atrial, and junctional bradycardia, standstill, or block	Same as sinus bradycardia
Ventricular bradycardia[†]	P absent or independent QRS >0.11 and rate 60-21	Same as idiojunctional rhythm	Same as idiojunctional rhythm	Same as sinus bradycardia
Agonal rhythm/ electromechanical dissociation[†]	P absent or independent QRS >0.11 and rate ≤20	Absent or barely present cardiac output and pulse Not compatible with life	Depolarization and contraction not coupled: electrical activity present with little or no mechanical activity Usually caused by profound hypoxia	Vigorous pharmacologic treatment aimed at restoring rate and force Usually ineffective May attempt to pace
Ventricular standstill or asystole[†]	P absent or independent QRS absent	No cardiac output Not compatible with life	Profound ischemia, hyperkalemia, acidosis	Same as agonal rhythm, including electrical defibrillation
Premature ventricular contractions (PVCs) or depolarizations*	Early beats with P waves QRS occasionally opposite in deflection from usual QRS	Same as PJCs	Same as PJCs, including aging and induction of anesthesia Impulse originates in cell outside normal conduction system and spreads through intercalated disks	Pharmacology to change thresholds, refractory periods; reduce myocardial demand, increase supply Removal of cause
Accelerated ventricular rhythm	P absent or independent QRS >0.11 and rate of 41-99	Same as accelerated junctional rhythm	Same as PVCs	Same as PVCs
Ventricular tachycardia[†]	P absent or independent QRS >0.11 and rate 100 or more	Same as junctional tachycardia	Same as PVCs	Same as PVCs, including electrical cardioversion
Ventricular fibrillation[†]	P absent QRS >300 and usually not observable	Same as ventricular standstill	Same as PVCs Rapid infusion of potassium	Same as PVCs, including electrical defibrillation

*Most common in adults.
[†]Life-threatening in adults.

TABLE 26.9 Disorders of Impulse Conduction

Type	Electrocardiogram	Effect	Pathophysiology	Treatment
Sinus block	Occasionally absent P, with loss of QRS for that beat	Occasional decrease in cardiac output Increase in preload for following beat	Local hypoxia, scarring of intraatrial conduction pathways, electrolyte imbalances Increased atrial preload	Conservative Usually do not progress in severity Pharmacologic treatment includes vagolytics, sympathomimetics, pacing
First-degree block*	PRI interval >0.2	None	Same as sinus block Hyperkalemia (>7 mEq/L) Hypokalemia (<3.5 mEq/L) Formation of myocardial abscesses in endocarditis	Conservative Discovery and correction of cause
Second-degree block, Mobitz I, or Wenckebach*	Progressive prolongation of PRI interval until one QRS is dropped Pattern of prolongation resumes	Same as sinus block	Hypokalemia (<3.5 mEq/L) Faulty cell metabolism in atrioventricular (AV) node Severity increases as heart rate increases Supports theory that AV node is fatiguing Digoxin toxicity, beta-blockade Coronary artery disease (CAD), myocardial infarction (MI), hypoxia, increased preload, valvular surgery and disease, diabetes	Same as sinus block

TABLE 26.9 Disorders of Impulse Conduction—cont'd

Type	Electrocardiogram	Effect	Pathophysiology	Treatment
Second-degree block or Mobitz II	Same as sinus block	Same as sinus block	Hypokalemia (<3.5 mEq/L) Faulty cell metabolism below AV node Antidysrhythmics, cyclic antidepressants CAD, MI, hypoxia, increased preload, valvular surgery and disease, diabetes	More aggressively than Mobitz I because can progress to type III Pacemaker after pharmacologic treatment
Third-degree block†	P waves present and independent of QRS No observed relationship between P and QRS Always AV dissociation	Same as idiojunctional rhythm	Hypokalemia (<3.5 mEq/L) Faulty cell metabolism low in bundle of His MI MI, especially inferior wall, as nodal artery interrupted; results in ischemia of AV node	Pharmacologic until pacemaker inserted Temporary pacing if caused by inferior MI, because ischemia usually resolves
Atrioventricular dissociation	P waves present and independent of QRS, but not always because of block (e.g., ventricular tachycardia) AV dissociation not always third-degree block	Decreased cardiac output from loss of atrial contribution to ventricular preload Variable effect on myocardial demand, depending on ventricular rate	May result from third-degree block or accelerated junctional or ventricular rhythm or be caused by sinus, atrial, and junctional bradycardias	Treat according to cause Pacemaker or reducing rate of AV or ventricular discharge, or increasing rate of sinus or AV node discharge
Ventricular block	QRS >0.11 sec R-S-R′ in V₁, V₂, V₅, V₆	None	Faulty cell metabolism in right and left bundle branches RBBB more common than LBBB because of dual blood supply to left bundle branch Congestive heart failure, mitral regurgitation, especially anterior MI, because of infarct of fascicles Left anterior hemiblock more common than left posterior hemiblock, since posterior fascicles have dual blood supply	Isolated right bundle branch block (RBBB) or left bundle branch block (LBBB) or hemiblock not treated If acute and/or associated with acute anterior MI, treated with permanent pacer and vigorous pharmacologic
Aberrant conduction	QRS >0.11 sec	None unless ventricular rate abnormalities present	Conduction of impulse through intercalated disks because conduction system transiently blocked as a result of hypoxia, electrolyte imbalances, digoxin toxicity, excessively rapid rate of discharge	Correct underlying cause
Preexcitation syndromes (Wolff-Parkinson-White and Lown-Ganong-Levine)	P present with QRS for each P PR interval <0.12 and QRS <0.11 because of delta wave in PR interval	None	Congenital presence of accessory pathways (bundle of Kent and fiber of Mahaim) that conduct very rapidly and bypass AV node, causing early ventricular depolarization in relation to atrial depolarization Prone (reason unknown) to tachycardias and atrial fibrillation that can result in very rapid ventricular rates	Aimed at aligning refractory periods of accessory pathway and AV node to prevent reentry May slow rate with drug pharmacology May surgically cut pathways

*Most common in adults.
†Life-threatening in adults.

to glycogenolysis, gluconeogenesis, and lipolysis to generate fuel for survival (see Chapter 1). Total body stores can fuel the metabolism for only about 10 hours and, as energy stores are depleted, tissue damage and dysfunction begin. As proteins are consumed, serum albumin drops causing decreased capillary osmotic pressure leading to interstitial edema and decreased circulatory volume. Muscle wasting caused by protein breakdown weakens skeletal and cardiac muscle contributing to respiratory and cardiac dysfunction.

A final outcome of impaired cellular metabolism is the buildup of metabolic end products in the cell and interstitial spaces. As proteins are broken down anaerobically, ammonia and urea are produced at toxic levels, disrupting cellular function and membrane integrity. Once a sufficiently large number of cells from vital organs are damaged, shock can be irreversible.

Clinical Manifestations of Shock

The clinical manifestations of shock are variable depending on the type of shock. The individual may report feeling weak, cold, hot, nauseated, dizzy, confused, afraid, thirsty, and short of breath. Evidence of decreased tissue perfusion occurs well before systemic hypotension develops. Heart rate is usually elevated; however cardiac output and tissue perfusion decrease as the shock syndrome progresses. Respiratory rate is usually

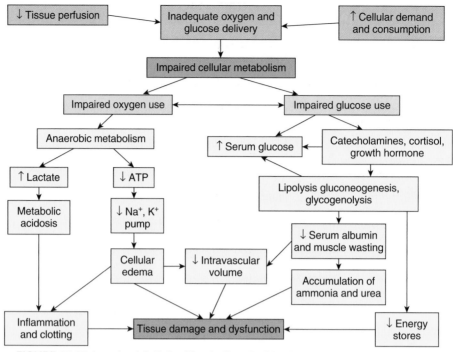

FIGURE 26.36 Impaired Cellular Metabolism in Shock. *ATP,* Adenosine triphosphate.

increased, and respiratory alkalosis may be an important early indicator of impending shock. Metabolic acidosis with associated electrolyte abnormalities develops as shock progresses. Other indicators of shock include hypothermia or hyperthermia, poor capillary refill, decreased urinary output, and altered sensorium. Decreased mixed venous oxygen saturation indicates poor tissue oxygenation and an alteration in cellular oxygen extraction and can be used to monitor response to therapy.

Treatment for Shock

The first treatment for shock is to discover and correct or remove the underlying cause. Simultaneously, management should begin directed at improvement in tissue perfusion. General supportive treatment includes administration of intravenous fluids to expand intravascular volume, use of vasopressors, supplemental oxygen, and control of glucose levels. Further treatment depends on the cause and severity of the shock syndrome, which is discussed with each type of shock. Prevention and very early treatment offer the best prognosis.

Types of Shock

Shock is classified by cause as cardiogenic (caused by heart failure), hypovolemic (caused by insufficient intravascular fluid volume), neurogenic (caused by neural alterations of vascular smooth muscle tone), anaphylactic (caused by immunologic processes), or septic (caused by infection). As described previously, each of these share similar effects on tissues and cells but can vary in their clinical manifestations and severity.

Cardiogenic Shock

Cardiogenic shock is defined as decreased cardiac output and evidence of tissue hypoxia in the presence of adequate intravascular volume. Most cases of cardiogenic shock follow MI, but shock also can follow left heart failure, dysrhythmias, acute valvular dysfunction, ventricular or septal rupture, myocardial or pericardial infections, massive pulmonary embolism, cardiac tamponade, and drug toxicity. Compensatory neurohumoral responses by the RAAS, SNS, and ADH systems contribute to the overall pathophysiology (Fig. 26.37).

The clinical manifestations of cardiogenic shock are caused by widespread impairment of cellular metabolism. They include impaired mentation, dyspnea and tachypnea, systemic venous and pulmonary edema, dusky skin color, marked hypotension, oliguria, and ileus. Management of cardiogenic shock includes careful fluid and vasopressor administration followed by early angiography, IABP counterpulsation, ventricular assist devices, extracorporeal membrane oxygenation, and early revascularization (PCI or bypass surgery). Cardiogenic shock is often unresponsive to treatment, with a high mortality.

Hypovolemic Shock

Hypovolemic shock is caused by loss of whole blood (hemorrhage), plasma (burns), or interstitial fluid (diaphoresis, diabetes mellitus, diabetes insipidus, emesis, diarrhea, or diuresis) in large amounts. Hypovolemic shock begins to develop when intravascular volume has decreased by about 15%.

Hypovolemia is offset initially by compensatory mechanisms (Fig. 26.38). Heart rate and SVR increase, boosting both cardiac output and tissue perfusion pressures. Interstitial fluid moves into the vascular compartment. The liver and spleen add to blood volume by disgorging stored red blood cells and plasma. In the kidneys, renin stimulates aldosterone release and the retention of sodium (and hence water), and antidiuretic hormone (ADH) from the posterior pituitary gland increases water retention. However, if the initial fluid or blood loss is great or if loss continues, compensation becomes inadequate, resulting in decreased tissue perfusion. As in cardiogenic shock, oxygen and nutrient delivery to the cells is impaired and cellular metabolism fails. Anaerobic metabolism and lactate production result in lactic acidosis and serum and cellular electrolyte abnormalities.

The clinical manifestations of hypovolemic shock include high SVR, poor skin turgor, thirst, oliguria, low systemic and pulmonary preloads, rapid heart rate, thready pulse, and mental status deterioration. The differences between the signs and symptoms of hypovolemic shock and those of cardiogenic shock are mainly caused by differences in fluid volume and cardiac muscle health. Management begins with rapid fluid

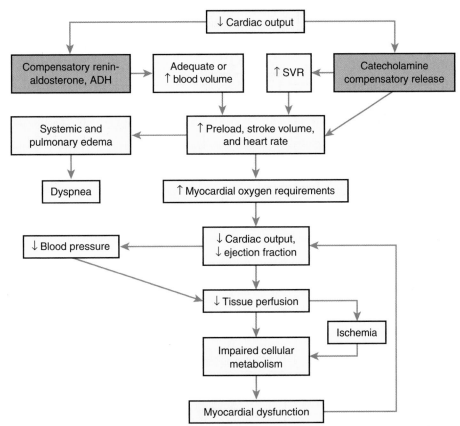

FIGURE 26.37 Cardiogenic Shock. Shock becomes life-threatening when compensatory mechanisms (in orange boxes) cause increased myocardial oxygen requirements. Renal and hypothalamic adaptive responses (i.e., renin-angiotensin-aldosterone and antidiuretic hormone [ADH]) maintain or increase blood volume. The adrenal gland releases catecholamines (e.g., mostly epinephrine, some norepinephrine), causing vasoconstriction and increases in contractility and heart rate. These adaptive mechanisms, however, increase myocardial demands for oxygen and nutrients. These demands further strain the heart, which can no longer pump an adequate volume, resulting in shock and impaired metabolism. *SVR,* Systemic vascular resistance.

replacement with crystalloids and blood products. Hypothermia and coagulopathies frequently complicate treatment. If adequate tissue perfusion cannot be restored promptly, systemic inflammation and multiple organ dysfunction are likely.

Neurogenic Shock

Neurogenic shock (sometimes called vasogenic shock) is the result of widespread and massive vasodilation that results from imbalances between parasympathetic and sympathetic stimulation of vascular smooth muscle (Fig. 26.39) (see Chapter 25). This type of shock can be caused by any factor that stimulates parasympathetic or inhibits sympathetic stimulation of vascular smooth muscle. Trauma to the spinal cord or medulla and conditions that interrupt the supply of oxygen or glucose to the medulla can cause neurogenic shock by interrupting sympathetic activity. Depressive drugs, anesthetic agents, and severe emotional stress and pain are other causes. The loss of vascular tone results in "relative hypovolemia," in which blood volume has not changed but SVR decreases drastically so that the amount of space containing the blood has increased. The pressure in the vessels falls below that needed to drive nutrients across capillary membranes to the cells. In addition, neurologic insult may cause bradycardia, which decreases cardiac output and further contributes to hypotension and underperfusion of tissues. As with other types of shock, this leads to impaired cellular metabolism. Management includes the careful use of fluids and vasopressors until blood pressure stabilizes.

Anaphylactic Shock

Anaphylactic shock results from a widespread hypersensitivity reaction known as anaphylaxis. The basic physiologic alteration is the same as that of neurogenic shock: vasodilation and relative hypovolemia, leading to decreased tissue perfusion and impaired cellular metabolism (Fig. 26.40). Anaphylactic shock is characterized by other effects that rapidly involve the entire body.

Anaphylactic shock begins with exposure of a sensitized individual to an allergen. Common allergens known to cause these reactions are insect venoms, shellfish, peanuts, latex, and medications such as penicillin. In genetically predisposed individuals, these allergens initiate a vigorous humoral immune response (type I hypersensitivity reaction) that results in the production of large quantities of immunoglobulin E (IgE) antibody (see Chapter 8). Allergen bound to IgE causes degranulation of mast cells. Mast cells release a large number of vasoactive and inflammatory cytokines. This provokes an extensive immune and inflammatory response, including vasodilation and increased vascular permeability, resulting in peripheral pooling and tissue edema. Extravascular effects include constriction of extravascular smooth muscle, often causing laryngospasm, bronchospasm, and cramping abdominal pain with diarrhea.

The onset of anaphylactic shock is usually sudden, and progression to death can occur within minutes unless emergency treatment is given. The primary clinical manifestations of anaphylaxis include anxiety, dizziness, difficulty breathing, stridor, wheezing, pruritus with hives

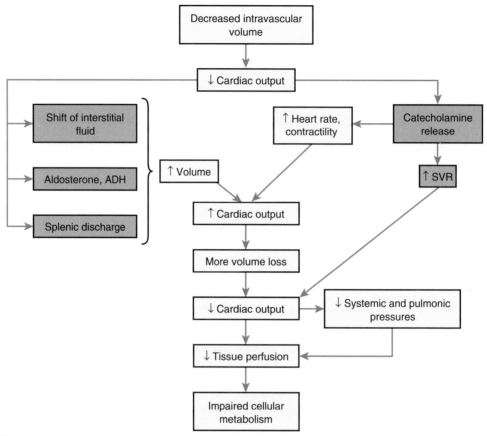

FIGURE 26.38 Hypovolemic Shock. This type of shock becomes life-threatening when compensatory mechanisms (in orange boxes) are overwhelmed by continued loss of intravascular volume. *ADH*, Antidiuretic hormone; *SVR*, systemic vascular resistance.

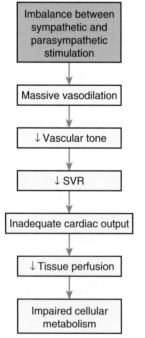

FIGURE 26.39 Neurogenic Shock. *SVR*, Systemic vascular resistance.

(urticaria), swollen lips and tongue, and abdominal cramping. A precipitous fall in blood pressure occurs, followed by impaired mentation. Other signs include decreased SVR, with high or normal cardiac output, and oliguria. The diagnosis can be confirmed by a number of serum markers, such as plasma histamine and tryptase. Treatment begins with removal of the antigen (if possible). Epinephrine is administered intramuscularly to cause vasoconstriction and reverse airway constriction. Fluids are given intravenously to reverse the relative hypovolemia, and antihistamines and corticosteroids are administered to stop the inflammatory reaction. Vasopressors and inhaled β-adrenergic agonist bronchodilators may also be necessary.

✔ QUICK CHECK 26.11

1. Describe the mechanisms operative in shock.
2. Why does myocardial infarction often cause cardiogenic shock?
3. How is hypovolemic shock manifested?
4. Why is anaphylactic shock considered a medical emergency?

Septic Shock

Septic shock begins with an infection that progresses from bacteremia to sepsis to septic shock, and finally to MODS. New definitions for sepsis, organ dysfunction, and septic shock were published in 2016[14] and are presented in Table 26.10.

Sepsis and septic shock are associated with high morbidity and mortality. Septic shock can be caused by community-acquired or health care–associated infections, especially pulmonary, intra-abdominal, and

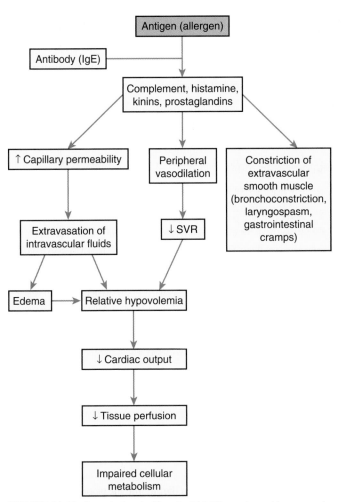

FIGURE 26.40 Anaphylactic Shock. *DIC,* Disseminated intravascular coagulation; *ECF-A,* eosinophil chemotactic factor anaphylaxis; *IgE,* immunoglobulin E; *SVR,* systemic vascular resistance.

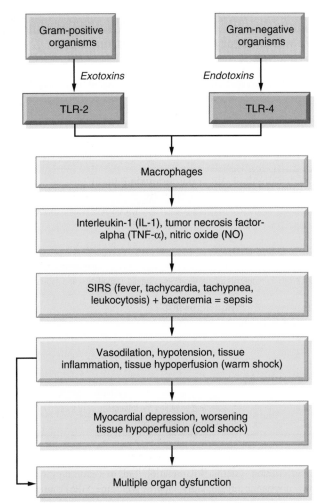

FIGURE 26.41 Septic Shock. *SIRS,* Systemic inflammatory response syndrome; *TLR,* toll-like receptor.

TABLE 26.10 Definitions of Sepsis, Organ Dysfunction, and Septic Shock

Cause	Definition
Bacteremia	Presence of viable bacteria in blood.
Sepsis	A life-threatening organ dysfunction caused by a dysregulated host response to infection.
Organ dysfunction	An acute change in the total SOFA score ≥2 points consequent to the infection.*
Septic shock	A subset of sepsis in which underlying circulatory and cellular/metabolic abnormalities are profound enough to substantially increase mortality. Clinically defined as sepsis with persisting hypotension requiring vasopressors to maintain MAP ≥65 mm Hg and having a serum lactate level >2 mmol/L (>18 mg/dL) despite adequate volume resuscitation.

*The SOFA score is based on respiratory function (partial pressure of arterial oxygen/fraction of inspired oxygen [PaO_2/FlO_2]), platelet count, liver function tests, blood pressure, Glasgow coma scale, and serum creatinine.
Data adapted from The Third International Consensus Definitions for Sepsis and Septic Shock (Sepsis-3): *J Am Med Assoc* 315(8):801-810, 2016.

urinary tract infections. Surgical wounds and indwelling arterial and central venous catheters also are an important source of infection. Sepsis can be caused by bacteria, fungi, and viruses. The source and virulence of the infectious microorganism, as well as the underlying health of the affected individual, significantly affect prognosis. Risk factors for septic shock include the individual's genetic composition, underlying chronic diseases, immune deficiency states, and timeliness of therapeutic interventions for infection.

Most septic shock begins when bacteria enter the bloodstream to produce bacteremia. Gram-negative microorganisms release endotoxins, and gram-positive microorganisms release exotoxins, lipoteichoic acids, and peptidoglycans. These bacteria and their associated toxins initiate an innate and adaptive immune response. Microorganismal pathogen-associated molecular patterns (PAMPs) trigger receptors on macrophages, such as toll-like receptor 2 (TLR-2) for gram-positive PAMPs and toll-like receptor 4 (TLR-4) for gram-negative PAMPs (Fig. 26.41). These macrophages release a large number of inflammatory mediators that trigger intense cellular responses and the subsequent release of secondary mediators, including cytokines, complement fragments, prostaglandins, platelet-activating factor, oxygen free radicals, nitric oxide, and proteolytic enzymes (see *Risk Factors:* Proinflammatory Mediators Contributing to Septic Shock). Polymorphonucleocytes also are activated in large numbers.

Proinflammatory Mediators Contributing to Septic Shock

More than 100 inflammatory mediators have been implicated in the pathogenesis of septic shock. The following are some of the most important contributors:

Tumor Necrosis Factor-Alpha (TNF-α)
Produced from macrophages, natural killer cells, and mast cells
Net effect: fever, vasodilation, cellular apoptosis, tissue damage

Interleukin-1β (IL-1β) and Interleukin-6 (IL-6)
Released by macrophages and lymphocytes
Net effect: produces fever, vasodilation and hypotension, edema, myocardial depression, and elevated white blood count

Nitric Oxide (NO)
Released by activated endothelial cells, macrophages, and neutrophils
Net effect: damages tissues and causes systemic vasodilation and hypotension

Platelet-Activating Factor (PAF)
Released from mononuclear phagocytes, platelets, and some endothelial cells
Net effect: contributes to widespread clotting and contributes to multiple organ failure

Complement
Serum protein activated by bacterial products and antigen/antibody complexes
Net effect: damages tissues and amplifies the inflammatory process by cellular chemotaxis and promotion of phagocytosis

Compensatory Antiinflammatory Syndrome and Sepsis

It has long been known that the profound inflammatory response to infection that accompanies sepsis contributes to the development of organ dysfunction with associated morbidity and mortality. Yet years of research failed to demonstrate consistent clinical benefit for the use of antiinflammatory agents, such as corticosteroids. It was also noted that many individuals survived the initial systemic inflammatory response only to succumb to secondary infections during their hospitalizations. More recent studies have identified numerous antiinflammatory cytokines that are released as a compensatory response in an effort to control overwhelming inflammation in individuals with sepsis. As the sepsis syndrome progresses, significant innate and adaptive immune cell dysfunction develops affecting polymorphonucleocytes (PMNs), macrophages, and T lymphocytes. Although PMNs increase in number in the bloodstream, both their ability to migrate into tissues and their phagocytic ability are impaired. Macrophages are less able to process and present antigens to T cells, and T cells undergo apoptosis and have diminished cytotoxicity needed to fight infection. This process of immunocompromise in sepsis has been called *immunoparalysis*. An understanding of the balance between proinflammatory and antiinflammatory/antiimmune processes during sepsis is leading to new therapies that have the potential to improve morbidity and mortality.

Data from Arts RJ et al: *J Leukoc Biol* 101(1):151-164, 2017; Girardot T et al: *Apoptosis* 22(2):295-305, 2017; Maestraggi Q et al: *BioMed Res Int* 2017:7897325, 2017; Prescott HC, Angus DC: *J Am Med Assoc* 319(1):62-75, 2018; Salluh JI, Povoa P: *Shock* 47(1S Suppl 1):47-51, 2017; van der Poll T et al: *Nat Rev Immunol* 17(7), 407-420, 2017; Zhuang Y et al: *Front Biosci (Landmark Ed)* 22:1344-1354, 2017.

The resultant systemic inflammation leads to a clinical presentation known as systemic inflammatory response syndrome (SIRS) characterized by fever, tachycardia, tachypnea, and elevated white blood count. Acute intense inflammation, especially through the action of nitric oxide, leads to widespread vasodilation with compensatory tachycardia and increased cardiac output in the early stages of septic shock (hyperdynamic phase). Later in the course of disease, complement and interleukins depress myocardial contractility such that cardiac output falls and tissue perfusion decreases. Tissue perfusion and cellular oxygen extraction also are affected by activation of the clotting cascade through the action of platelet-activating factor and depletion of the endogenous anticoagulant protein C. Furthermore, unresponsiveness to or depletion of vasoactive factors such as vasopressin contributes to hypotension and tissue hypoperfusion. The inflammatory response can become overwhelming, progressing to septic shock and MODS. The clinical outcomes of septic shock are not only a result of overwhelming inflammation. It has been determined that there is a parallel release of antiinflammatory mediators and impairment of immune cell function that causes a depression in the immune response to infection and contributes to the overall shock syndrome and mortality. This immune suppression is called the compensatory antiinflammatory syndrome (CARS) (see *Did You Know? Compensatory Antiinflammatory Syndrome and Sepsis*).

Clinical manifestations of septic shock are the result of inflammation, decreased perfusion of vital tissues, and an alteration in oxygen extraction by all cells. In early shock, tachycardia causes cardiac output to remain normal or become elevated, although myocardial contractility is reduced. Temperature instability is present, ranging from hyperthermia to hypothermia. Effects on other organ systems may result in decreased renal function, jaundice, clotting abnormalities with disseminated intravascular coagulation (DIC), deterioration of mental status, and ARDS. Gastrointestinal mucosa changes include stress ulceration and the translocation of bacteria from the gut into the bloodstream resulting in increased inflammation attributable to toxins carried by the intestinal lymphatics.

The diagnosis of septic shock rests on the recognition of the systemic manifestations of overwhelming inflammation (SIRS) in individuals with suspected or documented infection. Determining the cause and severity of septic shock can be aided by measurement of levels of serum lactate, troponin, CRP, and procalcitonin. The management of septic shock has improved outcomes by following the Surviving Sepsis Guidelines (see *Did You Know? The Surviving Sepsis Guidelines*). These guidelines include rapid resuscitation with fluids and vasopressors, antibiotic administration, and respiratory support. Control of hyperglycemia with insulin, treatment of complications associated with MODS, careful nutritional support, and prevention of stress ulcers and DVT are also essential. Despite improvements in septic shock–related mortality in recent years, mortality remains high and new treatments are being explored.

Multiple Organ Dysfunction Syndrome

Multiple organ dysfunction syndrome (MODS) is the progressive dysfunction of two or more organ systems resulting from an uncontrolled inflammatory response to a severe illness or injury. People at greatest risk for developing MODS are elderly individuals and persons with significant tissue injury or preexisting disease. The organ dysfunction can progress to organ failure and death (Fig. 26.42). Although sepsis and septic shock are the most common causes, any severe injury or disease process that activates a massive systemic inflammatory response can initiate MODS. These triggers include severe trauma, burns, acute renal failure, blood transfusion, liver failure, mesenteric ischemia, acute pancreatitis, obstetric complications, major surgery, circulatory shock, some drugs, and gangrenous or necrotic tissue.

The Surviving Sepsis Guidelines

Mortality rates for severe sepsis and septic shock have declined because of more rapid recognition of systemic infection and more effective management. Current Surviving Sepsis Guidelines for the management of sepsis were developed based on an in-depth analysis of the pathophysiology, clinical manifestations, and management outcomes reported over the past decade of sepsis care. The Guidelines provide a prioritized list of interventions that seek to quickly restore tissue perfusion, control infection, and support adequate oxygenation and ventilation. Intravenous infusion of fluids along with vasopressors, such as norepinephrine and vasopressin, is implemented quickly. Blood cultures, imaging modalities to determine the source of infection, and administration of appropriate antimicrobials are essential components of care. Respiratory support often includes mechanical ventilation, proper patient positioning, and careful monitoring of outcomes. Sedation is implemented as needed, and general supportive care includes glucose management with insulin, stress ulcer prevention, and nutrition. These Surviving Sepsis Guidelines have improved morbidity and mortality outcomes for individuals with septic shock.

Data from Rhodes A et al: *Crit Care Med* 45:486-552, 2017.

✔ QUICK CHECK 26.12

1. What are some of the important causes of sepsis and septic shock?
2. What is the role of inflammation in sepsis?
3. What are the basic steps in management of septic shock?

PATHOPHYSIOLOGY As a result of the initiating insult (sepsis, injury, or disease), the neuroendocrine system is activated with the release of the stress hormones cortisol, epinephrine, and norepinephrine into the bloodstream (see Chapter 10). Vascular endothelial damage occurs as a direct result of injury or from damage by bacterial toxins and inflammatory mediators such as nitric oxide, TNF, and IL-1, which are released into the circulation. The vascular endothelium becomes permeable, allowing fluid and protein to leak into the interstitial spaces, contributing to hypotension and hypoperfusion. Leakage of fluid into the lungs causes ARDS (see Chapter 29). When the endothelium is damaged, platelets and tissue thromboplastin are activated, resulting in systemic microvascular coagulation that may lead to DIC (see Chapter 23).

Because of the release of inflammatory mediators, four major plasma enzyme cascades are activated: complement, coagulation, fibrinolytic, and kallikrein/kinin. The overall effect of the activation of these cascades is a hyperinflammatory and hypercoagulant state that maintains the interstitial edema formation, cardiovascular instability, endothelial damage, and clotting abnormalities characteristic of MODS. A massive systemic immune/inflammatory response then develops involving neutrophils, macrophages, and mast cells that sets the stage for MODS.

The numerous inflammatory and clotting processes operating in MODS cause maldistribution of blood flow and hypermetabolism. Oxygen delivery to the tissues decreases for the following reasons:

1. Shunting of blood past selected regional capillary beds is caused when inflammatory mediators override the normal vascular tone.
2. Interstitial edema resulting from microvascular changes in permeability contributes to intravascular hypovolemia and poor tissue perfusion.
3. Capillary obstruction occurs because of formation of microvascular thrombi and the aggregation of white blood cells.
4. Myocardial depression with deceased cardiac output and tissue hypoperfusion results from inflammatory cytokines, bacterial products, and ischemia.

5. ARDS occurs because of systemic inflammation and capillary leakage with flooding of the alveoli resulting in decreased arterial oxygen levels.

Hypermetabolism in MODS with accompanying alterations in carbohydrate, fat, and lipid metabolism is initially a compensatory measure to meet the body's increased demands for energy. The alterations in metabolism affect all aspects of substrate utilization. The net result of hypermetabolism is depletion of oxygen and fuel supplies.

Decreased oxygen delivery and the hypermetabolic state combine to create an imbalance in oxygen supply and demand. This imbalance is critical in the pathogenesis of MODS because it results in a pathologic condition known as supply-dependent oxygen consumption, in which the tissues depend on oxygen delivery by the circulation, but this amount is inadequate in MODS. Therefore tissue hypoxia with cellular acidosis and impaired cellular function ensue and result in multiple organ failure.

CLINICAL MANIFESTATIONS There may be a lag time between the inciting event and the onset of symptoms that may last for as long as 24 hours. The individual develops a low-grade fever, tachycardia, dyspnea, altered mental status, and hyperdynamic and hypermetabolic states. ARDS is often an early manifestation of MODS and is characterized by tachypnea, pulmonary edema with crackles and diminished breath sounds, use of accessory muscles, and hypoxemia.

As the syndrome continues, hypermetabolic and hyperdynamic states intensify and signs of liver and kidney failure appear. Liver failure presents with jaundice, abdominal distention, liver tenderness, muscle wasting, and hepatic encephalopathy. All facets of metabolism, substance detoxification, and immune response are impaired; albumin and clotting factor synthesis decreases; protein wastes accumulate; and liver tissue macrophages (Kupffer cells) no longer function effectively. Progressive oliguria, azotemia, and edema mark the development of renal failure. Anuria, hyperkalemia, and metabolic acidosis may occur if renal shutdown is severe.

The gastrointestinal system is sensitive to ischemic and inflammatory injury. Clinical manifestations of bowel involvement are hemorrhage, ileus, malabsorption, diarrhea or constipation, vomiting, anorexia, and abdominal pain. Stress ulceration of the stomach lining can result in massive blood loss and death. Compounding the damage caused by injury to the bowel is the phenomenon of bacterial translocation. Bacteria translocate from the gut into the portal circulation where the overwhelmed liver is unable to clear these products and they move into the systemic circulation.

The signs and symptoms of cardiac failure in MODS are similar to those of septic shock: tachycardia, bounding pulse, increased cardiac output, decreased SVR, and hypotension. In the terminal stages, hypodynamic circulation with bradycardia, profound hypotension, and ventricular dysrhythmias may develop.

Ischemia and inflammation are responsible for the CNS manifestations, which include apprehension, confusion, disorientation, restlessness, agitation, headache, decreased cognitive ability and memory, and decreased level of consciousness. When ischemia is severe, seizures and coma can occur. Death may occur as early as 14 days or after a period of several weeks.

EVALUATION AND TREATMENT Early detection of organ failure is extremely important so that supportive measures can be initiated immediately. Frequent assessment of the clinical status of individuals at known risk is essential. Many different scoring systems are used to analyze the severity of disease and predict mortality. Once organ failure develops, monitoring of laboratory values and hemodynamic parameters also can be used to assess the degree of impairment.

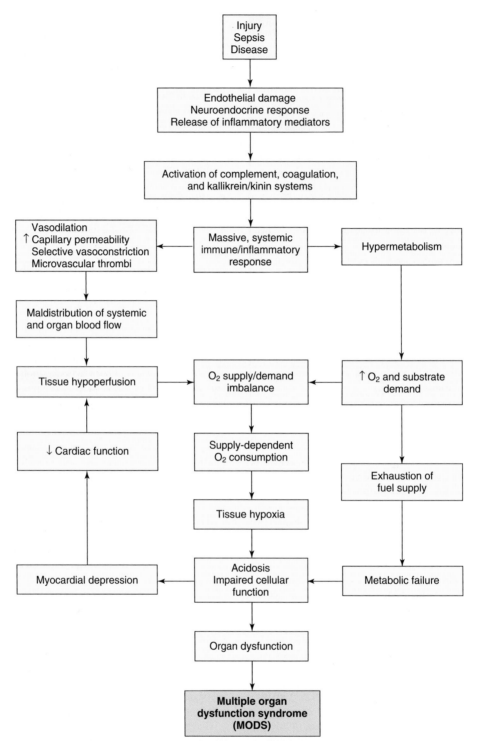

FIGURE 26.42 Pathogenesis of Multiple Organ Dysfunction Syndrome.

There is no specific treatment for MODS, and therapeutic management consists of prevention and support. Prevention consists of controlling the initial insult, treating infections quickly, and supporting healing. Management goals include controlling infection, restoring oxygenation and perfusion, and supporting organ function. Sources of infection are removed, and antimicrobials are administered. Ventilatory support is initiated to maintain adequate oxygen saturation, and fluids are administered to maintain vascular volume. Nutritional support must be provided to meet metabolic demand. Dialysis also may be required.

✔ **QUICK CHECK 26.13**
1. Why can MODS be initiated by either a septic or a nonseptic insult?
2. Why are inflammation and clotting triggered when the vascular endothelium is injured?
3. Describe the mechanisms that result in decreased oxygen delivery to the tissues in MODS.

SUMMARY REVIEW

Diseases of the Veins

1. Varicose veins are veins in which blood has pooled, usually in the saphenous veins of the leg. Varicose veins may be caused by damaged valves as a result of trauma to the valve or by chronic venous distention involving gravity and venous constriction.

2. Chronic venous insufficiency is inadequate venous return over a long period of time that causes pathologic ischemic changes in the vasculature, skin, and supporting tissues. Poor circulation makes tissues vulnerable to trauma and infection resulting in the formation of venous stasis ulcers.

3. A thrombus is a blood clot that remains attached to a vessel wall. Deep venous thrombosis results from stasis of blood flow, endothelial damage, or hypercoagulability. The most serious complication of deep venous thrombosis is pulmonary embolism.

4. Superior vena cava syndrome is a progressive occlusion of the superior vena cava that leads to venous distention in the upper extremities and head. Because this syndrome is usually caused by bronchogenic cancer, it is generally considered an oncologic emergency rather than a vascular emergency.

Diseases of Arteries

1. Hypertension is the elevation of systemic arterial blood pressure resulting from increases in cardiac output (blood volume), total peripheral vascular resistance, or both.

2. Hypertension can be primary, without a known cause, or secondary, caused by an underlying disease.

3. The risk factors for primary hypertension include a positive family history; male sex; advancing age; black race; obesity; high sodium intake; low magnesium, potassium, or calcium intake; diabetes mellitus; cigarette smoking; and heavy alcohol consumption.

4. Primary hypertension is the result of a complicated interaction of genetics and the environment mediated by neurohumoral effects that influence intravascular volume and peripheral vascular resistance. Pathophysiologic mechanisms include overactivity of the sympathetic nervous system; overactivity of the renin-angiotensin-aldosterone system; sodium and water retention by the kidneys; hormonal inhibition of sodium-potassium transport across cell walls; and complex interactions involving insulin resistance, inflammation, and endothelial function.

5. Secondary hypertension is caused by a disease process or medication that raises peripheral vascular resistance or cardiac output.

6. As hypertension becomes more severe and chronic, tissue damage can occur in the blood vessels and tissues leading to target organ damage in the heart, kidney, brain, and eyes. Hypertensive crisis is an extremely high blood pressure that can lead to cardiac failure, stroke, or death, and is considered a medical emergency.

7. Clinical manifestations of hypertension result from damage of organs and tissues outside the vascular system. These include heart disease, renal insufficiency, central nervous system dysfunction, impaired vision, impaired mobility, vascular occlusion, and edema.

8. Hypertension is managed with both pharmacologic and nonpharmacologic methods that lower the blood volume and the total peripheral vascular resistance.

9. Orthostatic hypotension is a drop in blood pressure that occurs upon standing. The compensatory vasoconstriction response to standing is replaced by a marked vasodilation and blood pooling in the muscle vasculature.

10. The clinical manifestations of orthostatic hypotension include dizziness, blurring or loss of vision, and syncope or fainting.

11. An aneurysm is a localized dilation of a vessel wall; the aorta is particularly susceptible.

12. Arterial thrombi develop similarly to venous thrombi. They may grow large enough to occlude the artery, or they can dislodge and become a thromboembolus that may occlude flow into a distal systemic vascular bed.

13. An embolus is a mobile aggregate of a variety of substances that occludes the vasculature. Sources of emboli include clots, air, amniotic fluid, bacteria, fat, and foreign matter. These emboli cause ischemia and necrosis when a vessel is totally blocked.

14. The most common source of arterial thrombotic emboli is the left heart and they are associated with thrombus formation associated with myocardial infarction, valvular disease, left heart failure, endocarditis, and dysrhythmias.

15. Peripheral vascular diseases include thromboangiitis obliterans and Raynaud phenomenon.

16. Thromboangiitis obliterans is an autoimmune disease of the peripheral arteries characterized by the formation of thrombi filled with inflammatory and immune cells. It is strongly associated with smoking.

17. Raynaud phenomenon is characterized by vasospastic attacks in the small arteries and arterioles of the fingers and the toes triggered by brief exposure to cold, vibration, or emotional stress.

18. Atherosclerosis is a form of arteriosclerosis that is characterized by thickening and hardening of the vessel wall. It is the leading cause of peripheral artery disease, coronary artery disease, and cerebrovascular disease.

19. Atherosclerosis is an inflammatory disease that begins with endothelial injury.

20. Following injury, important steps in atherogenesis include inflammation, adherence of macrophages, release of inflammatory mediators, oxidation of LDL, formation of foam cells and fatty streaks, and development of fibrous plaque.

21. Once a plaque has formed, it can rupture, resulting in clot formation and instability and vasoconstriction, which lead to obstruction of the lumen and inadequate oxygen delivery to tissues.

22. Peripheral artery disease is the result of atherosclerotic plaque formation in the arteries that supply the extremities, and it causes pain, loss of pulse, and skin color changes in the affected limb.

23. Coronary artery disease (CAD) caused by atherosclerosis can diminish the myocardial blood supply until deprivation impairs myocardial metabolism enough to cause myocardial ischemia, a local state in which the cells are temporarily deprived of blood supply.

24. Many risk factors contribute to the onset and escalation of CAD. Conventional (major) risk factors that are modifiable include dyslipidemia, smoking, hypertension, diabetes and insulin resistance, and obesity, sedentary lifestyle, and atherogenic diet. Conventional nonmodifiable risk factors include advanced age, male sex or women after menopause, and family history.

25. Nontraditional (novel) risk factors for CAD include markers of inflammation and ischemia, adipokines, chronic kidney disease, air pollution and ionizing radiation, medications, and the microbiome.

26. Myocardial ischemia develops if the flow or oxygen content of coronary blood is insufficient to meet the metabolic demands of myocardial cells. It is most commonly the result of coronary artery disease and the ensuing decrease in myocardial blood supply.

27. Atherosclerotic plaque progression can be gradual and cause stable angina pectoris, which is predictable chest pain caused by myocardial ischemia in response to increased demand (e.g., exercise) without infarction.

28. Prinzmetal angina, which results from coronary artery vasospasm, is chest pain attributable to transient ischemia of the myocardium that occurs unpredictably and often at rest.

29. Silent ischemia, myocardial ischemia that is asymptomatic, is an indicator of future serious cardiovascular events.

30. Sudden coronary obstruction because of thrombus formation on ruptured unstable atherosclerotic plaques causes the acute coronary syndromes. These include unstable angina and myocardial infarction.

31. Unstable angina results from rupture of an unstable plaque and subsequent thrombus formation with reversible myocardial ischemia.

32. Myocardial infarction is caused by rupture of an unstable plaque and thrombus formation leading to prolonged, unrelieved ischemia that interrupts blood supply to the myocardium. After about 20 minutes of myocardial ischemia, irreversible hypoxic injury causes cellular death and tissue necrosis.

33. Myocardial infarction is clinically classified as non-ST elevation myocardial infarction (non-STEMI) or ST elevation myocardial infarction (STEMI) based on electrocardiographic findings that suggest the extent of myocardial damage (subendocardial versus transmural).

34. An increase in plasma enzyme levels is used to diagnose the occurrence of myocardial infarction as well as indicate its severity. Elevations of the troponins are most predictive of a myocardial infarction.

35. Treatment of a myocardial infarction includes revascularization (thrombolytics or PCI) and administration of antithrombotics, ACE inhibitors, and beta-blockers. Pain relief and fluid management also are key components of care.

Disorders of the Heart Wall

1. Pericardial disease is a localized manifestation of another disorder, such as infection; trauma or surgery; neoplasm; or a metabolic, immunologic, or vascular disorder.

2. Acute pericarditis is acute inflammation of the pericardium. The pericardial membranes become inflamed and roughened, and a pericardial effusion may develop. Symptoms begin with sudden onset of severe chest pain that is worse with respirations or when lying down.

3. Pericardial effusion is the accumulation of fluid in the pericardial cavity. If the accumulation of fluid occurs rapidly, cardiac compression (tamponade) can occur.

4. In constrictive pericarditis, fibrous scarring with occasional calcification of the pericardium causes the pericardial layers to adhere. The fibrotic lesions encase the heart in a rigid shell which compresses the heart, reducing cardiac output.

5. Cardiomyopathies are a diverse group of diseases that affect the myocardium. The cardiomyopathies are categorized as dilated, hypertrophic, and restrictive. The size of the cardiac muscle walls and chambers may increase or decrease depending on the type of cardiomyopathy, thereby altering contractile activity.

6. Disorders of the endocardium damage the heart valves. Congenital or acquired disorders that result in stenosis (constricted or narrow valve), regurgitation (failure of valve to shut completely), or both can structurally alter the valves.

7. Characteristic heart sounds, cardiac murmurs, and systemic complaints assist in identification of an abnormal valve. If severely compromised function exists, a prosthetic heart valve may be surgically implanted to replace the faulty one.

8. Mitral valve prolapse (MVP) describes the condition in which the mitral valve leaflets do not position themselves properly during systole. MVP may be a completely asymptomatic condition or can result in unpredictable symptoms.

9. Rheumatic fever is an inflammatory disease that results from a delayed immune response to a streptococcal infection. Severe or untreated cases of rheumatic fever may progress to rheumatic heart disease, a potentially disabling cardiovascular disorder.

10. Infective endocarditis is a general term for infection and inflammation of the endocardium, especially the cardiac valves. Pathogenesis requires (1) endocardial damage, (2) adherence of blood-borne microorganisms to the damaged endocardial surface, and (3) formation of infective endocardial vegetations.

Manifestations of Heart Disease

1. Heart failure is when the heart is unable to generate an adequate cardiac output. Most causes of heart failure result from dysfunction of the left ventricle.

2. Left heart failure can be divided into heart failure with reduced ejection fraction (systolic) and heart failure with preserved ejection fraction (diastolic).

3. Left heart failure with reduced ejection fraction (systolic heart failure) is caused by increased preload, decreased contractility, or increased afterload. These processes result in increased left ventricular end-diastolic volume and pressure that cause increased pulmonary venous pressures and pulmonary edema.

4. In addition to the hemodynamic changes of left ventricular failure, there is a neuroendocrine response that tends to exacerbate and perpetuate the condition.

5. The neuroendocrine mediators of heart failure include the sympathetic nervous system and the renin-angiotensin-aldosterone system; thus diuretics, beta-blockers, and angiotensin-converting enzyme (ACE) inhibitors are important components of the pharmacologic therapy.

6. Left heart failure with preserved ejection fraction (diastolic heart failure) is a clinical syndrome characterized by the symptoms and signs of heart failure, a preserved ejection fraction, and abnormal diastolic function.

7. Diastolic dysfunction means that the left ventricular end-diastolic pressure is increased, even if volume and cardiac output are normal.

8. Right heart failure is the inability of the right ventricle to provide adequate blood flow into the pulmonary circulation and can result from left heart failure or pulmonary disease.

9. High-output failure is the inability of the heart to adequately supply the body with blood-borne nutrients, despite adequate blood volume and normal or elevated myocardial contractility

10. A dysrhythmia (arrhythmia) is a disturbance of heart rhythm. Dysrhythmias range in severity from occasional missed beats or rapid beats to disturbances that impair myocardial contractility and are life-threatening.

11. Dysrhythmias can occur because of an abnormal rate of impulse generation or an abnormal conduction of impulses.

Shock

1. Shock is a widespread impairment of cellular metabolism due to the cardiovascular system failing to perfuse tissues adequately. Shock progresses to organ failure and death unless compensatory mechanisms reverse the process or clinical intervention succeeds.

2. The final pathway common in all types of shock is impaired cellular metabolism—cells switch from aerobic to anaerobic metabolism through impairment in oxygen and glucose use. Energy stores drop, acidosis develops, cellular edema and decreased intravascular volume occurs, inflammation and clotting are initiated, and tissue dysfunction and damage ensue.

3. Anaerobic metabolism results in activation of the inflammatory response, decreased circulatory volume, and decreasing pH.

4. Impaired cellular metabolism results in cellular inability to use glucose because of impaired glucose uptake, resulting in a shift to glycogenolysis, gluconeogenesis, and lipolysis for fuel generation. As energy stores are depleted, tissue damage and dysfunction begin.

5. A final outcome of impaired cellular metabolism is the buildup of metabolic end products. As proteins are broken down anaerobically, ammonia and urea are produced at toxic levels, disrupting cellular function and membrane integrity. Once a sufficiently large number of cells from vital organs are damaged, shock can be irreversible.

6. Types of shock are cardiogenic, hypovolemic, neurogenic, anaphylactic, and septic. Multiple organ dysfunction syndrome can develop from all types of shock.

7. Cardiogenic shock is decreased cardiac output, tissue hypoxia, and the presence of adequate intravascular volume.

8. Hypovolemic shock is caused by loss of blood or fluid in large amounts. The use of compensatory mechanisms may be vigorous, but tissue perfusion ultimately decreases and results in impaired cellular metabolism.

9. Neurogenic shock results from massive vasodilation, causing a relative hypovolemia even though cardiac output may be high, and leads to impaired cellular metabolism.

10. Anaphylactic shock is caused by physiologic recognition of a foreign substance. The inflammatory response is triggered, and a massive vasodilation and relative hypovolemia occurs, leading to impaired cellular metabolism.

11. Septic shock begins with impaired cellular metabolism caused by uncontrolled septicemia. The infecting agent triggers the inflammatory and immune responses. This inflammatory response is accompanied by widespread changes in tissue and cellular function.

12. Multiple organ dysfunction syndrome (MODS) is the progressive failure of two or more organ systems after a severe illness or injury. It can be triggered by major surgery, necrotic tissue, severe trauma, burns, acute pancreatitis, and other severe injuries.

13. MODS involves the stress response; changes in the vascular endothelium resulting in microvascular coagulation; release of complement, coagulation, and kinin proteins; and numerous inflammatory processes. Consequences of all these mediators are a maldistribution of blood flow, hypermetabolism, hypoxic injury, and myocardial depression.

14. Clinical manifestations of MODS include inflammation, tissue hypoxia, and hypermetabolism. All organs can be affected including the kidney, lung, liver, gastrointestinal tract, and central nervous system.

KEY TERMS

Acute aortic syndrome, 597
Acute coronary syndrome, 602
Acute orthostatic hypotension, 596
Acute pericarditis, 611
Anaphylactic shock, 629
Anaphylaxis, 629
Aneurysm, 596
Aortic regurgitation, 616
Aortic stenosis, 615
Arteriolar remodeling, 593
Arteriosclerosis, 599
Atherosclerosis, 599
Cardiogenic shock, 628
Cardiomyopathy, 613
Chronic orthostatic hypotension, 596
Chronic venous insufficiency (CVI), 591
Chylomicron, 602
Complicated plaque, 599
Constrictive pericarditis (restrictive pericarditis [chronic pericarditis]), 612
Coronary artery bypass graft (CABG), 606
Coronary artery disease (CAD), 602
Deep venous thrombosis (DVT), 592
Dilated cardiomyopathy, 613
Dyslipidemia (dyslipoproteinemia), 602
Dysrhythmia (arrhythmia), 623
Embolism, 598

Embolus, 598
Endothelial injury, 599
False aneurysm, 596
Fatty streak, 599
Fibrous plaque, 599
Foam cell, 599
Heart failure, 620
Heart failure with preserved ejection fraction (HFpEF; diastolic heart failure), 622
Heart failure with reduced ejection fraction (HFrEF; systolic heart failure), 620
Hibernating myocardium, 608
High-output failure, 623
High-sensitivity C-reactive protein (hs-CRP), 603
Hypertension, 592
Hypertensive crisis, 596
Hypertensive hypertrophic cardiomyopathy, 614
Hypertrophic cardiomyopathy, 613
Hypertrophic obstructive cardiomyopathy, 613
Hypovolemic shock, 628
Infarction, 598
Infective endocarditis, 618
Intermittent claudication, 601
Left heart failure, 620
Lipoprotein, 602
Lipoprotein(a) (Lp[a]), 603
Mental stress–induced ischemia, 605

Microvascular angina (MVA), 605
Mitral regurgitation, 616
Mitral stenosis, 615
Mitral valve prolapse syndrome (MVPS), 616
Multiple organ dysfunction syndrome (MODS), 632
Myocardial infarction (MI), 606
Myocardial ischemia, 602
Myocardial remodeling, 608
Myocardial stunning, 608
Neurogenic shock (vasogenic shock), 629
Nonbacterial thrombotic endocarditis, 618
Non-ST elevation MI (non-STEMI), 606
Orthostatic (postural) hypotension (OH), 596
Percutaneous coronary intervention (PCI), 606
Pericardial effusion, 612
Peripheral artery disease (PAD), 601
Plaque, 599
Pressure-natriuresis relationship, 593
Primary hypertension, 593
Prinzmetal angina, 605
Raynaud phenomenon, 598
Restrictive cardiomyopathy, 614
Rheumatic fever, 616
Rheumatic heart disease (RHD), 617

Right heart failure, 623
Secondary hypertension, 593
Septic shock, 630
Shock, 624
Silent ischemia, 605
Stable angina pectoris, 604
ST elevation MI (STEMI), 606
Superior vena cava syndrome (SVCS), 592
Supply-dependent oxygen consumption, 633
Tamponade, 612
Thromboangiitis obliterans (Buerger disease), 598
Thromboembolus, 591
Thrombus, 591
Transmural myocardial infarction, 608
Tricuspid regurgitation, 616
Troponin I (TnI), 603
True aneurysm, 596
Unstable angina, 606
Valvular hypertrophic cardiomyopathy, 614
Valvular regurgitation (valvular insufficiency or valvular incompetence), 615
Valvular stenosis, 614
Varicose vein, 591
Venous stasis ulcer, 591
Ventricular remodeling, 620

REFERENCES

1. Kearon C, et al: Antithrombotic therapy for VTE disease: CHEST Guideline and Expert Panel Report, *Chest* 149(2):315-352, 2016.
2. Whelton PK, et al: 2017 ACC/AHA/AAPA/ABC/ ACPM/AGS/APhA/ASH/ASPC/NMA/PCNA guideline for the prevention, detection, evaluation and management of high blood pressure in adults: a report of the American College of Cardiology/ American Heart Association Task Force on Clinical Practice Guidelines, *Hypertension* 71(6):e13-e115, 2018.
3. Benjamin EJ, et al: Heart disease and stroke statistics—2018 update: a report from the American Heart Association, *Circulation* 137(12):e67-e492, 2018.
4. Gerhard-Herman MD, et al: 2016 AHA/ACC guideline on the management of patients with lower extremity peripheral artery disease: a report of the American College of Cardiology/American Heart Association Task Force on Clinical Practice Guidelines, *Circulation* 135:e726-e779, 2017.
5. Expert Panel on Detection: Evaluation and treatment of high blood cholesterol in adults: executive summary of the third report of the National Cholesterol Education Program (NCEP) Expert Panel on Detection, Evaluation, and Treatment of High Blood Cholesterol in Adults (Adult Treatment Panel III), *J Am Med Assoc* 285(19):2486-2497, 2001.
6. Stone NJ, et al: 2013 ACC/AHA guideline on the treatment of blood cholesterol to reduce atherosclerotic cardiovascular risk in adults: a report of the American College of Cardiology/American Heart Association Task Force on Practice Guidelines, *J Am Coll Cardiol* 63(25 Pt B): 3024-3025, 2014.
7. Fihn SD, et al: ACCF/AHA/ACP/AATS/PCNA/SCAI/ STS guideline for the diagnosis and management of patients with stable ischemic heart disease: a report of the American College of Cardiology Foundation/American Heart Association Task Force on Practice Guidelines, and the American College of Physicians, American Association for Thoracic Surgery, Preventive Cardiovascular Nurses Association, Society for Cardiovascular Angiography and Interventions, and Society of Thoracic Surgeons, *Circulation* 126:e354-e471, 2012.
8. Amsterdam EA, et al: AHA/ACC guideline for the management of patients with non-ST-elevation acute coronary syndromes: a report of the American College of Cardiology/American Heart Association Task Force on practice guidelines, *Circulation* 130(25):2354-2394, 2014.
9. O'Gara PT, et al: 2013 ACCF/AHA guideline for the management of ST-elevation myocardial infarction: a report of the American College of Cardiology Foundation/American Heart Association Task Force on practice guidelines, *Circulation* 127:e362-e425, 2013.
10. Bozkurt B, et al: Current diagnostic and treatment strategies for specific dilated cardiomyopathies: a scientific statement from the American Heart Association, *Circulation* 134:e579-e646, 2016.
11. Nishimura RA, et al: 2017 AHA/ACC focused update of the 2014 AHA/ACC guideline for the management of patients with valvular heart disease: a report of the American College of Cardiology/American Heart Association Task Force on Clinical Practice Guidelines, *Circulation* 135:e1159-e1195, 2017.
12. Yancy CW, et al: 2017 ACC/AHA/HFSA focused update of the 2013 ACCF/AHA guideline for the management of heart failure: a report of the American College of Cardiology/American Heart Association Task Force on Clinical Practice Guidelines and the Heart Failure Society of America, *Circulation* 136:e137-e161, 2017.
13. Yancy CW, et al: 2016 ACC/AHA/HFSA focused update on new pharmacological therapy for heart failure: an update of the 2013 ACCF/AHA guideline for the management of heart failure: a report of the American College of Cardiology/American Heart Association Task Force on Clinical Practice Guidelines and the Heart Failure Society of America, *Circulation* 134:e282-e293, 2016.
14. Singer M, et al: The Third International Consensus definitions for sepsis and septic shock (Sepsis-3), *J Am Med Assoc* 315(8):801-810, 2016.

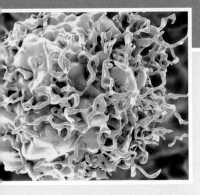

27

Alterations of Cardiovascular Function in Children

Nancy Pike, Jennifer Peterson

Cardiovascular disorders in children are classified as congenital or acquired. Congenital heart disease is the most common. The diagnosis and management of congenital heart disease continues to improve with the use of fetal echocardiography for early detection, early interventional catheterization, and refined surgical repair. Acquired heart disease in children continues to present challenges to the practitioner. Although guidelines for diagnosing acquired diseases are available, work is still needed in developing standards of treatment and long-term follow-up protocols.

CONGENITAL HEART DISEASE

The incidence of congenital heart disease (CHD), a heart disease present since birth, varies from 4 to 8 per 1000 live births and is the second leading cause of death in the first year of life, behind only prematurity. Several environmental and genetic risk factors are associated with the incidence of different types of CHD. The environmental factors are typically maternal and are listed with the associated congenital heart defect in Table 27.1.[1,2]

Genetic factors also have been implicated in the incidence of CHD, although the mechanism of causation is often unknown (Table 27.2). The incidence of CHD is three to four times higher in siblings of affected children, and chromosomal defects account for about 6% of all cases of CHD. Down syndrome, trisomies 13 and 18, Turner syndrome, and cri du chat syndrome (chromosome 5p deletion syndrome) have been associated with a relatively high incidence of heart defects. Only a small percentage of cases of CHD are clearly linked solely to genetic or environmental factors. There also are multiple hereditary and nonhereditary syndromes that are associated with cardiovascular abnormalities in children.[2] However, the cause of most defects is multifactorial.[1,2]

Congenital heart defects can be classified into four categories based on their blood flow patterns:
- Defects increasing pulmonary blood flow
- Defects causing obstruction of blood flow from the ventricles
- Defects decreasing pulmonary blood flow
- Defects causing mixed desaturated and saturated blood within the chambers or great arteries (Fig. 27.1).

The normal movement of blood through the right side of the heart and into the pulmonary system is separate from the blood flow through the left side of the heart into the systemic circulation (Fig. 27.2, *A*). Abnormal movement from one side of the heart to the other is termed a shunt. Shunting of blood flow from the left heart into the right heart is called a left-to-right shunt and occurs in conditions such as atrial septal defect and ventricular septal defect (see Fig. 27.2, *B*). This increases blood flow into the pulmonary circulation. Because blood continues to flow through the lungs before passing into the systemic circulation, there is no decrease in tissue oxygenation or cyanosis. Thus defects that cause left-to-right shunt are termed acyanotic heart defects. Other types of acyanotic heart defects obstruct blood flow from the ventricles but do not cause shunting. Cyanotic heart defects frequently cause shunting of blood from the right side of the heart directly into the left side of the heart (right-to-left shunt). A right-to-left shunt decreases blood flow through the pulmonary system, causing less-than-normal oxygen delivery to the tissues and resulting in a bluish discoloration of the skin called cyanosis (see Chapter 29). Tetralogy of Fallot is the most common cyanotic heart defect.[2] In this condition, narrowing of the pulmonary outflow tract increases right heart pressures, thus forcing blood through a defect in the ventricular septum into the left heart (see Fig. 27.2, *C*). Cyanosis also can be caused by other types of heart defects that result in the mixing of venous and arterial blood that enter the systemic circulation.

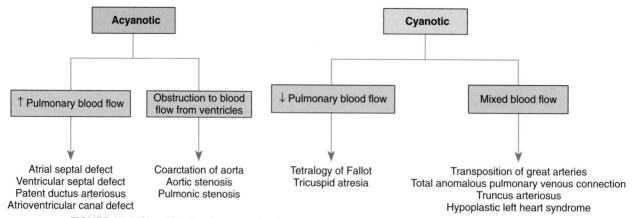

FIGURE 27.1 Classification Systems for Congenital Heart Disease. Individual diseases are discussed later in this chapter. (From Hockenberry MJ, Wilson D: *Wong's nursing care of infants and children*, ed 10, St Louis, 2016, Mosby.)

TABLE 27.1 Environmental Factors Associated With Congenital Heart Defects	
Cause	**Type of Congenital Heart Defect**
Infection	
Intrauterine	PDA, PS, COA
Systemic viral	PDA, PS, COA
Rubella	PDA, PS, COA
Coxsackie B5	Endocardial fibroelastosis
Herpesvirus, cytomegalovirus	Can infect endothelial cells and vascular endothelium
Radiation	Studies of cancer survivors reveal radiation can cause atherosclerosis; myocardial, endocardial, and pericardial disease; conduction disturbances; and endothelial vessel disease
Metabolic Disorders	
Diabetes	VSD, cardiomegaly, transposition of the great vessels
Phenylketonuria	COA, PDA
Hypercalcemia	Supravalvular AS, PS; aortic hyperplasia
Drugs	
Alcohol	TOF, ASD, VSD
Lithium	Exact effect not known
Phenytoin	Embryonic dysrhythmia and valvular heart disease
Warfarin	ASD, PDA
Peripheral Conditions	
Increased maternal age	VSD, TOF (relationship unclear)
Antepartal bleeding	Various defects (relationship unclear)
Prematurity	PDA, VSD
High altitude	PDA, ASD (increased incidence)

AS, Aortic stenosis; *ASD,* atrial septal defect; *COA,* coarctation of the aorta; *PDA,* patent ductus arteriosus; *PS,* pulmonary stenosis; *TOF,* tetralogy of Fallot; *VSD,* ventricular septal defect.

TABLE 27.2 Congenital Heart Disease in Selected Fetal Chromosomal Aberrations		
Conditions	**Incidence of CHD (%)**	**Common Defects (in Decreasing Order of Frequency)**
5p (cri du chat syndrome)	25	VSD, PDA, ASD
Trisomy 13 syndrome	90	VSD, PDA, dextrocardia
Trisomy 18 syndrome	99	VSD, PDA, PS
Trisomy 21 (Down syndrome)	50	AVSD, VSD
Turner syndrome (XO)	35	COA, AS, ASD
Klinefelter variant (XXXXY)	15	PDA, ASD

AS, Aortic stenosis; *ASD,* atrial septal defect; *AVSD,* atrioventricular septal defect; *COA,* coarctation of the aorta; *PDA,* patent ductus arteriosus; *PS,* pulmonary stenosis; *VSD,* ventricular septal defect. From Park MK: *Pediatric cardiology for practitioners,* ed 6, St Louis, 2014, Mosby.

Most congenital heart defects are named to describe the underlying defect (for example, valvular abnormalities are abnormal openings in the septa, and malformation or abnormal placement of the great vessels). Descriptions of the most common defects follow.

Defects With Increased Pulmonary Blood Flow
Patent Ductus Arteriosus

PATHOPHYSIOLOGY Patent ductus arteriosus (PDA) is failure of the fetal ductus arteriosus (artery connecting the aorta and pulmonary artery [PA]) to functionally close within hours after birth (Fig. 27.3). However, several weeks after birth may be needed for attainment of true anatomic closure, in which the ductus loses the ability to reopen. The continued patency of this vessel allows blood to flow from the higher pressure aorta to the lower pressure pulmonary artery, causing a left-to-right shunt.

CLINICAL MANIFESTATIONS Infants may be asymptomatic or show signs of pulmonary distress, such as dyspnea, fatigue, and poor feeding.

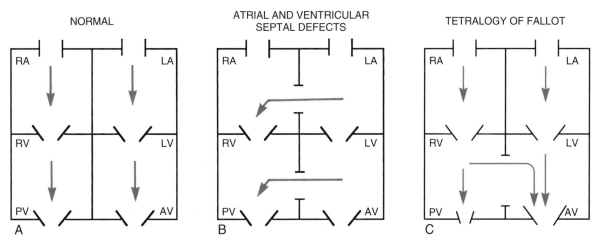

FIGURE 27.2 Shunting of Blood in Congenital Heart Disease. A, Normal. B, Acyanotic defect. C, Cyanotic defect. *AV,* Aortic valve; *LA,* left atrium; *LV,* left ventricle; *PV,* pulmonic valve; *RA,* right atrium; *RV,* right ventricle. (From Hockenberry MJ, Wilson D: *Wong's nursing care of infants and children,* ed 10, St Louis, 2016, Mosby.)

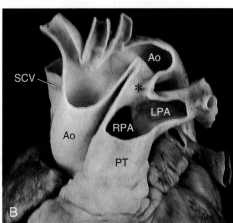

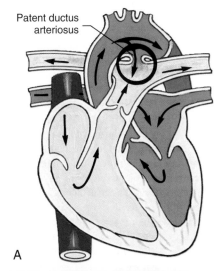

FIGURE 27.3 Patent Ductus Arteriosus (PDA). A, PDA with left-to-right shunt. B, PDA *(asterisk)* in an adult with pulmonary hypertension. *Ao,* Aorta; *LPA,* left pulmonary artery; *RPA,* right pulmonary artery; *SCV,* subclavian vein. (A from Hockenberry MJ, Wilson D: *Wong's essentials of pediatric nursing,* ed 10, St Louis, 2016, Mosby; B from Damjanov I, Linder J, editors: *Anderson's pathology,* ed 10, St Louis, 1996, Mosby.)

There is a characteristic continuous, machinery-like murmur in both systole and diastole, heard best at the left upper sternal border. Aortic flow (run-off) into the lower pressure pulmonary circulation produces low diastolic blood pressure, widened pulse pressure, and bounding pulses. Children are at risk for bacterial endocarditis and may develop pulmonary hypertension in later life from chronic excessive pulmonary blood flow.[2]

EVALUATION AND TREATMENT The diagnosis of PDA is confirmed by echocardiography and auscultation. Administration of intravenous indomethacin or ibuprofen (nonsteroidal antiinflammatory medications) has proved successful in closing a PDA in premature infants and some newborns. Surgical division of the PDA through a left thoracotomy or surgical incision to the chest wall also may be done; in some cases the procedure can be performed with video-assisted technology. Closure of the PDA with an occlusion device during cardiac catheterization is performed in select children older than 6 months of age. Both surgical and nonsurgical procedures are considered low risk.[2,3]

Atrial Septal Defect

PATHOPHYSIOLOGY An atrial septal defect (ASD) is an opening in the septal wall between the two atria. This opening allows blood to shunt from the left atrium (LA) to the right atrium (RA) (see the top half of Fig. 27.2, *B*). There are three types of ASDs:

- **Ostium primum atrial septal defect** is an opening low in the atrial septum and may be associated with abnormalities of the mitral valve.
- **Ostium secundum atrial septal defect** is an opening in the middle of the atrial septum and is the most common type.
- **Sinus venosus atrial septal defect** is an opening usually high in the atrial wall near the junction of the superior vena cava and may be associated with partial anomalous pulmonary venous connection.

Another opening in the atrial septal wall that is part of normal fetal communication and usually closes after birth is the foramen ovale. When the lungs become functional at birth, the pulmonary pressure decreases and the LA pressure exceeds that of the RA. The pressure change forces the septum to functionally close the foramen ovale. If it does not close, the condition is called a patent foramen ovale (PFO).

About 24% of adults have a PFO without CHD; however, in children with CHD the foramen ovale often remains open.[2]

CLINICAL MANIFESTATIONS Children with an ASD are usually asymptomatic. Infants with a large ASD may, in rare cases, develop pulmonary overcirculation and slow growth. Some older children and adults will experience shortness of breath with activity as the RV becomes less compliant with age. Pulmonary hypertension and stroke are associated rare complications. A systolic ejection murmur and a widely split second heart sound are the expected findings on physical examination.[2]

EVALUATION AND TREATMENT The diagnosis is confirmed by echocardiography. Surgical closure involves a pericardial patch or suture closure of the defect, depending on the size of the opening. Surgical repair involves open-heart surgery with cardiopulmonary bypass (mechanical bypass of the heart and lungs). Catheterization device closure offers a less invasive alternative for children with an ASD that meets anatomic and size criteria.[3] All options have low morbidity and mortality. Atrial dysrhythmias may persist in about 5% to 10% of individuals after closure.[3]

Ventricular Septal Defect

PATHOPHYSIOLOGY A ventricular septal defect (VSD) is an opening of the septal wall between the ventricles (see the bottom half of Fig. 27.2, *B*). VSDs are the most common type of congenital heart defect and account for 15% to 20% of all CHDs.[2] VSDs are classified by location. **Perimembranous ventricular septal defects** are located high in the ventricular septal wall underneath the atrioventricular (AV) valves, and VSDs located under the aortic valve are subarterial. **Muscular ventricular septal defects** are located low in the septal wall. VSDs also can be located in the inlet (AV canal type) or outlet (supracristal) portion of the ventricle. VSDs are similar to ASDs in that blood will shunt from left to right. Left-to-right shunting of blood can occur with a large VSD. Depending on the size and location, many VSDs close spontaneously, most often within the first 2 years of life.[2]

CLINICAL MANIFESTATIONS Depending on the size, location, and degree of shunting and pulmonary vascular resistance (PVR), children may have no symptoms or they may have clinical effects from excessive pulmonary blood flow. In the infant, excessive pulmonary blood flow from left-to-right shunting causes dyspnea and tachypnea symptoms, commonly referred to as heart failure (HF), even though the heart muscle functions well with a VSD. A loud, harsh, holosystolic (pansystolic) murmur and systolic thrill (a palpable tremor) is a classic finding on physical examination.

If the degree of shunting is significant and not corrected, the child is at risk for developing pulmonary hypertension. Irreversible pulmonary hypertension can result in **Eisenmenger syndrome**, in which shunting of blood is reversed because of high pulmonary pressure and resistance (right-to-left shunt with cyanosis).

EVALUATION AND TREATMENT The diagnosis is confirmed by echocardiogram and auscultatory findings. Cardiac catheterization may be needed to determine the hemodynamics and, in some instances, the location of other defects and additional VSDs. Smaller VSDs require minimal treatment and may close completely or become small enough that surgical closure is not required. If the infant has severe HF or failure to thrive (FTT) that is unmanageable with medical therapy, early surgical repair is performed. Surgical repair involves open-heart surgery with cardiopulmonary bypass. The opening is either sutured closed or covered with a patch of pericardium or artificial material. Nonsurgical

device closure in the catheterization laboratory is available, but only under restricted conditions, depending on the size and location of the defect.[3] Endocarditis prophylaxis is only recommended for 6 months after surgical or device closure and indefinitely with a residual VSD after patch closure.[2]

Atrioventricular Canal Defect

PATHOPHYSIOLOGY **Atrioventricular canal (AVC) defect**, or by the traditional term **endocardial cushion defect (ECD)**, is the result of incomplete fusion of endocardial cushions (Fig. 27.4). AVC defect consists of an ostium primum ASD and an inlet VSD with associated abnormalities of the AV valve tissue. These valve abnormalities range from a cleft in the mitral valve to a common mitral and tricuspid valve. The direction and pathways of flow are determined by pulmonary and systemic resistance, LV and RV pressures, and the compliance of each chamber. Flow is generally from left to right.[1,2] AVC is a common cardiac defect in children with trisomy 21, or Down syndrome. However, children with this defect can have a normal karyotype.

CLINICAL MANIFESTATIONS Infants with AVC often display moderate to severe HF attributable to left-to-right shunting and pulmonary overcirculation. Infants with pulmonary hypertension and high pulmonary resistance have less shunting and therefore minimal signs of HF. There may be mild cyanosis that increases with crying. Those with a large left-to-right shunt will have a holosystolic murmur, and those with minimal shunt may not have a murmur. Children with AVC are at risk for developing irreversible pulmonary hypertension if the condition is left surgically untreated.[2]

EVALUATION AND TREATMENT AVC is one of the most frequent diagnoses made with fetal echocardiography. Cardiac catheterization is rarely indicated but may be performed to evaluate the reversibility of pulmonary vascular disease. Initial treatment goals include aggressive medical management of HF and nutritional supplementation. Infants are followed closely for signs or symptoms of FTT. Pulmonary artery banding is occasionally performed in small infants with severe symptoms. However, complete surgical repair is most common and typically performed between 3 and 6 months of age to prevent irreversible

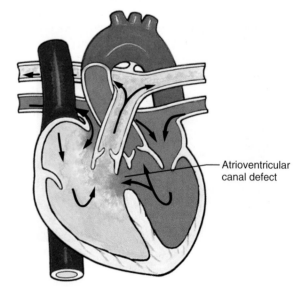

FIGURE 27.4 Atrioventricular Canal (AVC) Defect. (From Hockenberry MJ, Wilson D: *Wong's essentials of pediatric nursing*, ed 10, St Louis, 2016, Mosby.)

pulmonary hypertension. This procedure consists of patch closure of the septal defects and reconstruction of the AV valve tissue (either repair of the mitral valve cleft or fashioning of two AV valves). Postoperative complications include heart block, dysrhythmias, or mitral regurgitation requiring further surgical intervention or valve replacement.

Obstructive Defects

Coarctation of the Aorta

PATHOPHYSIOLOGY   Coarctation of the aorta (COA) is an abnormal localized narrowing of the aorta just proximal to the insertion of the ductus arteriosus. Before birth, the ductus arteriosus bypasses this obstruction and allows for blood to flow from the PA into the distal aorta. However, once the ductus functionally closes within hours after birth, blood flow to the lower extremities may be restricted by the coarctation. Clinically, there is increased blood pressure proximal to the defect (head and upper extremities, right greater than left) and decreased blood pressure distal to the obstruction (torso and lower extremities) (Fig. 27.5).

CLINICAL MANIFESTATIONS   The location and severity of the COA determine whether an infant will become symptomatic after the ductus arteriosus closes. If the COA is severe, infants will present with low cardiac output, poor tissue perfusion, acidosis, and hypotension. Physical examination of the infant will reveal weak or absent femoral pulses. Some infants with COA will remain asymptomatic after the closure of the ductus arteriosus. As they age, children with undiagnosed COA will present with unexplained upper extremity hypertension. Children may complain of leg pain or cramping with exercise. Although rare, they also may experience dizziness, headaches, fainting, or epistaxis from hypertension.

EVALUATION AND TREATMENT   Physical examination and measurement of upper and lower extremity blood pressures will often suggest the diagnosis. Echocardiography, magnetic resonance imaging (MRI), and cardiac catheterization may be needed to confirm the diagnosis. Initial treatment in the symptomatic newborn consists of continuous intravenous infusion of prostaglandin E_1 to maintain the patency of the ductus arteriosus. Once the symptomatic newborn is stabilized, surgical correction is indicated.

Surgical correction consists of either resection of the narrowed portion of the aorta with an end-to-end anastomosis (a surgical connection between vessels), arch augmentation, or enlargement of the constricted section using a portion of the left subclavian artery. Because this defect is outside the heart and pericardium, cardiopulmonary bypass usually is not required and a thoracotomy incision is used. However, COA repair may be part of a more complex operation, which might require a sternotomy incision and cardiopulmonary bypass. Postoperative hypertension is treated with intravenous medication, often a short-acting β-blocker, followed by oral medications, such as an angiotensin-converting enzyme (ACE) inhibitor. Residual hypertension after the repair of COA seems to be related to age and time of repair; therefore, surgical intervention is recommended at the time of diagnosis.

Percutaneous balloon angioplasty to dilate the vessel, with or without stent implantation, may be a less invasive option for treating native COA (infant >6 months of age) or for reducing residual postoperative COA in most children. However, aortic aneurysm formation and blood vessel injury from arterial access can be a complication of the procedure.

Aortic Stenosis

PATHOPHYSIOLOGY   Aortic stenosis (AS) is a narrowing or stricture of the outlet of the LV, causing resistance to blood flow from the LV

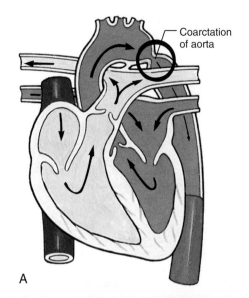

Coarctation of aorta

A

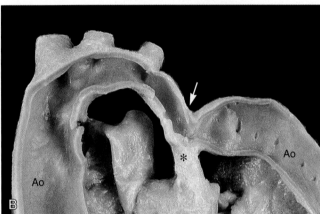

FIGURE 27.5   Postductal and Preductal Coarctation of the Aorta (COA). A, Postductal coarctation occurs distal to ("after") the insertion of the closed ductus arteriosus into the aortic arch. Preductal coarctation occurs proximal to ("before") the insertion of the patent ductus arteriosus. The coarctation consists of a flap of tissue that protrudes from the tunica media of the aortic wall. B, Coarctation of the aorta with typical indentation of the aortic wall (arrow) opposite the ductal arterial ligament (asterisk). Ao, Aorta. (A from Hockenberry MJ, Wilson D: Wong's essentials of pediatric nursing, ed 10, St Louis, 2016, Mosby; B from Damjanov I, Linder J, editors: Anderson's pathology, ed 10, St Louis, 1996, Mosby.)

into the aorta (Fig. 27.6). The physiologic consequence of severe AS is hypertrophy of the LV wall, which eventually leads to increased end-diastolic pressure, resulting in pulmonary venous and pulmonary arterial hypertension. If severe, there may be decreased cardiac output and pulmonary vascular congestion. Left ventricular hypertrophy impedes coronary artery perfusion and may result in subendocardial ischemia and associated papillary muscle dysfunction that cause mitral insufficiency.

There are three types of AS:
- Valvular aortic stenosis occurs because of malformed or fused cusps, resulting in a unicuspid or bicuspid valve. Valvular AS is a serious defect because the obstruction tends to be progressive. There may be sudden episodes of myocardial ischemia or low cardiac output that result in sudden death in late childhood or adolescence. This is one of the rare forms of CHD in which strenuous physical activity may be curtailed because of the cardiac condition until surgical intervention is accomplished.[1,2]

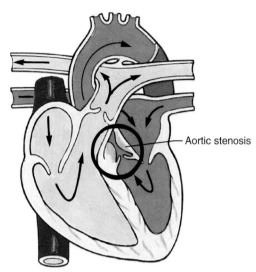

FIGURE 27.6 Aortic Stenosis (AS). Narrowing of the aortic valve causes resistance to blood flow in the left ventricle, decreased cardiac output, left ventricular hypertrophy, and pulmonary congestion. (From Hockenberry MJ et al: *Wong's essentials of pediatric nursing,* ed 10, St Louis, 2016, Mosby.)

- Subvalvular aortic stenosis is a stricture caused by a fibrous ring below a normal valve or by a narrowed LV outflow tract in combination with a small aortic valve annulus (diameter at the base of the aortic root).
- Supravalvular aortic stenosis, a narrowing of the aorta just above the valve, occurs infrequently. It can occur as a single defect or as a part of Williams syndrome, which also is characterized by an unusual elfin facial appearance and intellectual disability.[2]

CLINICAL MANIFESTATIONS Infants with significant AS demonstrate signs of decreased cardiac output, with faint pulses, hypotension, tachycardia, and poor feeding. A loud, harsh systolic ejection murmur is expected. Older children also may have complaints of exercise intolerance and, rarely, chest pain. Children are at risk for bacterial endocarditis, although prophylaxis with antibiotics is no longer routinely recommended (see *Did You Know?* Endocarditis Risk). Aortic stenosis, when severe, also can be complicated by coronary insufficiency, ventricular dysfunction, and, rarely, sudden death.

DID YOU KNOW?
Endocarditis Risk

Children with CHD are at risk for developing endocarditis. Although the risk is low, a transient bacteremia has been noted to follow dental and surgical procedures and dental instrumentation involving mucosal surfaces. A blood-borne pathogen can inhabit areas of the heart where there is high turbulence (e.g., an abnormal valve or vessel) or reside on artificial material (e.g., an artificial valve or a normal graft [called a *homograft*]). *Streptococcus viridans* is the most commonly found pathogen after dental or oral procedures. *Enterococcus faecalis* is the most common bacterium found after genitourinary and gastrointestinal tract surgery or instrumentation. The American Heart Association has provided updated guidelines for the prevention of bacterial endocarditis. Good dental hygiene, with daily brushing and flossing, is critical, along with regular dental checkups.

Data from the American Heart Association. Available at www. americanheart.org.

EVALUATION AND TREATMENT A diagnosis of valvular AS is confirmed by echocardiography. Mild to moderate valvular AS does not usually require intervention or restriction of activity. The treatment of severe valvular AS varies; the initial treatment of choice by many interventional cardiologists is nonsurgical methods to reduce symptoms. Dilation of the stenotic valve with balloon angioplasty, which is performed in the cardiac catheterization laboratory, still carries a high morbidity and mortality in the critically ill neonate. In older infants and children, it compares favorably with surgical cutting of a constricted cardiac valve, called *valvotomy.*[3] However, balloon angioplasty is associated with the risk of aortic regurgitation (insufficiency). Children undergoing this procedure almost always require surgical intervention at some time to relieve recurrent narrowing or worsening regurgitation.[3]

Surgical treatment for valvular AS depends on the severity of the stenosis, previous interventions, and the age of the child. Aortic valve commissurotomy (incision at the edges of the commissure, or joining point) or valvotomy may be used as an early intervention. Aortic valve replacement may be required if the valve is severely dysplastic. Mechanical valve replacement is usually deferred if possible to minimize the number of valve replacements related to growth. Aortic stenosis requires lifelong evaluation and treatment. Multiple surgical or catheterization interventions are expected. Mortality for sick infants and young children is higher than that for older children.[1,2]

Treatment for subvalvular AS and supravalvular AS involve surgical excision of the area causing the constriction. For subvalvular AS involving a small LV outflow tract and aortic annulus, a procedure may be required to enlarge this area with a patch and replace the aortic valve. Severe supravalvar AS may require balloon angioplasty and stent placement or surgical enlargement with coronary reimplantation.[1-3]

Pulmonic Stenosis
PATHOPHYSIOLOGY Pulmonic stenosis (PS) is a narrowing or stricture of the pulmonary valve that causes resistance to blood flow from the RV to the PA (Fig. 27.7). Generally moderate to severe stenosis causes RV hypertrophy. Pulmonary atresia is an extreme form of PS, with total fusion of the valve leaflets (blood cannot flow to the lungs); the RV may be hypoplastic. In some cases of RV outflow obstruction, the narrowing is below the valve (infundibular or subvalve PS).[1]

CLINICAL MANIFESTATIONS Most infants are asymptomatic if the PS is mild to moderate. Newborns with severe PS or pulmonary atresia will be cyanotic (from a right-to-left shunt through an ASD) and may have signs of decreased cardiac output. A harsh systolic murmur and ejection click with a potential thrill at the upper left sternal border is expected with PS.

EVALUATION AND TREATMENT Echocardiography confirms the diagnosis and determines the severity of the PS. The treatment of choice for infants with moderate to severe PS is balloon angioplasty (see Fig. 27.7, *B*). This procedure is considered highly effective in reducing the pressure gradient across the pulmonic valve.[3] In rare cases, surgical valvotomy may be required. Both valvotomy and balloon angioplasty may result in some pulmonary valve incompetence, and long-term follow-up may reveal the need for pulmonary valve replacement.

Treatment for pulmonary atresia depends on the size of the native/branch pulmonary arteries and associated cardiac defects. Initial treatment may consist of an aortopulmonary shunt to supply stable blood flow to the lungs and, later, a second procedure to connect the RV to the PA.[1,2]

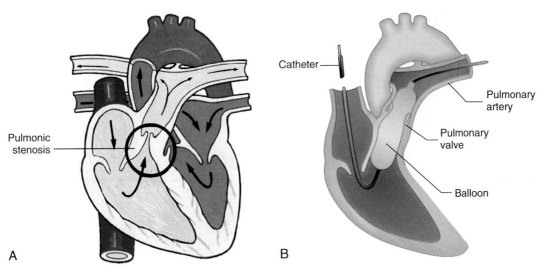

FIGURE 27.7 Pulmonic Stenosis (PS). A, The pulmonary valve narrows at the entrance of the pulmonary artery. **B,** Balloon angioplasty is used to dilate the valve. A catheter is inserted across the stenotic pulmonic valve into the pulmonary artery, and a balloon at the end of the catheter is inflated while it is positioned across the narrowed valve opening. **(A** from Hockenberry MJ et al: *Wong's essentials of pediatric nursing,* ed 10, St Louis, 2016, Mosby.)

Defects With Decreased Pulmonary Blood Flow
Tetralogy of Fallot

PATHOPHYSIOLOGY Tetralogy of Fallot (TOF) occurs in 5% to 10% of all CHD and is the most common cyanotic heart defect. The classic form of TOF consists of four defects: (1) a large VSD, (2) PS, (3) an overriding aorta that straddles the VSD, and (4) RV hypertrophy (Fig. 27.8). The pathophysiology associated with TOF varies widely, depending primarily on the degree of PS, the size of the VSD, and the pulmonary and systemic resistance to flow. If total resistance to pulmonary flow is greater than systemic resistance, the shunt is from right to left. If systemic resistance is more than pulmonary resistance, the shunt is from left to right (acyanotic; known as "pink tets"). PS decreases blood flow to the lungs and, consequently, the amount of oxygenated blood that returns to the left heart. Physiologic compensation for low oxygen saturation (hypoxemia) in the systemic circulation is the production of more red blood cells (polycythemia), the development of collateral bronchial vessels, and enlargement of the nail beds (clubbing).

CLINICAL MANIFESTATIONS Some infants may be acutely cyanotic at birth. In others, the progression of hypoxia and cyanosis may be more gradual over the first year of life as the pulmonary stenosis worsens. Acute episodes of cyanosis and hypoxia can occur, called *hypercyanotic spells* or *"tet" spells.* These spells (increased right-to-left shunt) may occur during crying or after feeding. Oxygen has little effect in improving hypoxemia. Placing the infant in a knee-chest position to increase peripheral resistance in the systemic circulation, thus causing an increase in pressures in the left heart, and administering morphine sulfate subcutaneously or intravenously is most commonly used to treat hypercyanotic spells. If prolonged or frequent, these spells are an indication for prompt evaluation and surgical treatment.

Chronic cyanosis may cause difficulty with feeding and poor growth in children. Squatting can temporarily help with cyanosis in these children because it increases peripheral resistance (e.g., so does the knee-chest position). The increased pressure reverses the shunting through the VSD and increases pulmonary blood flow. The pulmonary systolic ejection murmur can vary in intensity, depending on the degree of obstruction, or it may disappear during a hypercyanotic spell.[2]

EVALUATION AND TREATMENT The diagnosis is confirmed with echocardiography. Diagnostic cardiac catheterization is rarely indicated, except to define unusual coronary artery anatomy crossing the RV outflow tract that may complicate surgical palliation. Elective surgical repair is usually performed in the first year of life. Indications for earlier repair include increasing cyanosis or the development of hypercyanotic spells. Complete repair involves closure of the VSD, resection of the infundibular stenosis, and application of a pericardial patch to enlarge the RV outflow tract that can extend across the PV annulus (transannular patch). Some very small infants are unable to undergo primary repair as the initial procedure. In this case, a palliative shunt from the subclavian or innominate artery to the PA, known as the *modified Blalock-Taussig* (using a prosthetic graft) or *classic Blalock-Taussig* (using the native subclavian artery), is placed to increase pulmonary blood flow.[4]

Tricuspid Atresia

PATHOPHYSIOLOGY Tricuspid atresia is failure of the tricuspid valve to develop; consequently, there is no communication from the RA to the RV (Fig. 27.9). Blood flows through an ASD or a PFO to the LA and through a VSD to the hypoplastic RV and to the lungs. This condition is often associated with varying degrees of PS or less commonly with transposition of the great arteries. There is complete mixing of unoxygenated and oxygenated blood in the left side of the heart, resulting in systemic desaturation and mild cyanosis. Depending on the degree of PS and the size of the RV, a PDA is necessary to ensure blood flow into the pulmonary circulation.[1]

CLINICAL MANIFESTATIONS A murmur is noted, and cyanosis is usually seen in the newborn period. Tachycardia, dyspnea, fatigue, and poor feeding may be noted with excessive pulmonary blood flow. Older children may have signs of chronic hypoxemia with clubbing. Children are at risk for bacterial endocarditis, brain abscess, and stroke.[2]

EVALUATION AND TREATMENT After the diagnosis is confirmed by echocardiography, the neonate with decreased pulmonary blood flow is treated with a continuous infusion of prostaglandin E_1 to maintain the PDA until surgical intervention. If the ASD is restrictive, a balloon atrial

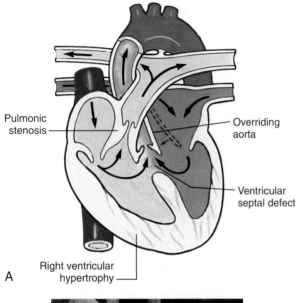

Pulmonic stenosis

Overriding aorta

Ventricular septal defect

Right ventricular hypertrophy

A

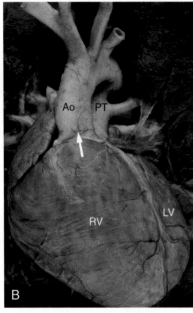

B

FIGURE 27.8 Tetralogy of Fallot (TOF). A, TOF hemodynamics. **B,** Right ventricular *(RV)* hypertrophy and overriding aorta *(arrow)*. (**A** from Hockenberry MJ, Wilson D: *Wong's essentials of pediatric nursing,* ed 10, St Louis, 2016, Mosby; **B** from Damjanov I, Linder J, editors: *Anderson's pathology,* ed 10, St Louis, 1996, Mosby.)

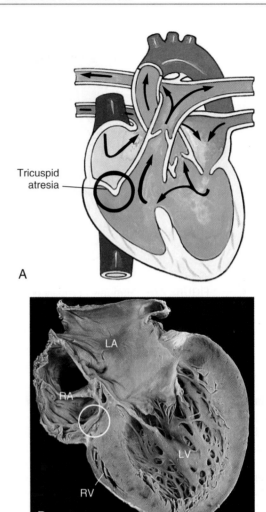

Tricuspid atresia

A

LA

RA

LV

RV

B

FIGURE 27.9 Tricuspid Atresia. A, Tricuspid atresia hemodynamics. **B,** Small right ventricle *(RV)* slit of ventricular septal defect; left ventricle *(LV)* is enlarged. (**A** from Hockenberry MJ, Wilson D: *Wong's essentials of pediatric nursing,* ed 10, St Louis, 2016, Mosby; **B** from Damjanov I, Linder J, editors: *Anderson's pathology,* ed 10, St Louis, 1996, Mosby.)

septostomy or creation of a hole between the chambers of the heart is performed during cardiac catheterization or under echocardiographic guidance at the bedside.[3] Treatment is accomplished in staged procedures. First, the newborn gets a shunt to increase blood flow to the lungs. Next, at 4 to 8 months of age, the superior vena cava is anastomosed to the PA, the PA is tied off, and the shunt from the first procedure is removed. Finally, at 2 to 4 years of age, the pulmonary circulation is fully separated from the systemic circulation by routing the inferior vena cava blood flow to the PA with a grafted or artificial tube.

Surgical outcomes are best in the child with normal ventricular function and a low PVR. For children with borderline PVR, a fenestration (opening) can be created in the tube to relieve high systemic pulmonary venous pressures if needed.[4] Postoperative complications that prolong a hospital stay include pleural and pericardial effusions, an elevated

PVR, and ventricular dysfunction. Exercise tolerance is limited in many children who had the final procedure, but general health is usually good.[2]

Mixing Defects
Transposition of the Great Arteries

PATHOPHYSIOLOGY In transposition of the great arteries (TGA), the PA leaves the LV and the aorta exits the RV (Fig. 27.10). Associated defects, such as ASD, VSD, or PDA, permit mixing of saturated and desaturated blood, which helps maintain adequate tissue oxygenation for a limited time.[1]

CLINICAL MANIFESTATIONS Clinical manifestations depend on the type and size of the associated defects. Children with limited communication between cardiac chambers are severely cyanotic, acidotic, and ill at birth. Those with large septal defects or a PDA may be less severely cyanotic but may have symptoms of pulmonary overcirculation. Classically, no murmur is heard unless there is an associated VSD.[2]

EVALUATION AND TREATMENT The diagnosis is suspected from the physical examination and confirmed with echocardiography. Administration of intravenous prostaglandin E_1 to maintain the patency of the

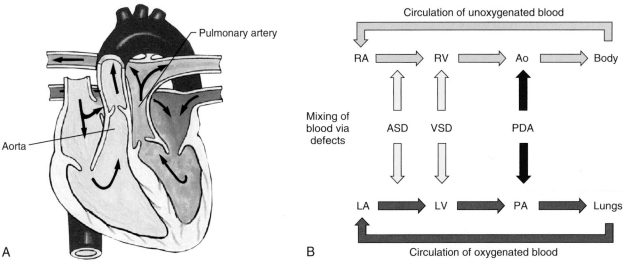

FIGURE 27.10 Hemodynamics in Transposition of the Great Arteries (TGA). **A,** Complete transposition of the great arteries with an intact interventricular septum. The aorta arises from the right ventricle and the pulmonary artery from the left ventricle. **B,** Oxygen saturation in the separate, parallel circuits with transposition of the great vessels (TGV). Mixing of blood occurs only with the defects associated with TGV. *Ao,* Aorta; *ASD,* atrial septal defect; *LA,* left atrium; *LV,* left ventricle; *PA,* pulmonary artery; *PDA,* patent ductus arteriosus; *RA,* right atrium; *RV,* right ventricle; *VSD,* ventricular septal defect. (**A** from Hockenberry MJ, Wilson D: *Wong's essentials of pediatric nursing,* ed 10, St Louis, 2016, Mosby.)

PDA may be initiated to increase oxygen delivery temporarily. Enlargement of the PFO by balloon atrial septostomy may be performed during cardiac catheterization or under echocardiographic guidance at the bedside to increase mixing and maintain cardiac output.[3]

The preferred type of surgical repair for TGA performed in the first weeks of life is the *arterial switch procedure,* which involves:

- transecting the great arteries and anastomosing the main PA to the native proximal aorta (just above the aortic valve) and anastomosing the ascending aorta to the native proximal PA, and,
- moving and reimplanting the coronary arteries with a *button* of tissue onto the new aortic outflow.

Reimplantation of the coronary arteries is critical to survival. The arteries must be reattached without torsion or kinking to provide oxygenated blood to the heart muscle. The advantage of the arterial switch procedure is the reestablishment of normal circulation, with the LV acting as the systemic pump. Potential complications of the arterial switch include narrowing at the great artery anastomoses, neoaortic valve regurgitation, or coronary artery insufficiency.[4] Long-term results for the arterial switch operation are usually good.

Total Anomalous Pulmonary Venous Connection

PATHOPHYSIOLOGY Total anomalous pulmonary venous connection (TAPVC), or *total anomalous pulmonary venous return (TAPVR),* is a rare defect characterized by failure of the pulmonary veins to join the left atrium during cardiac development (Fig. 27.11). The pulmonary venous return is connected to the right side of the circulation rather than to the LA. The type of TAPVC is classified according to the pulmonary venous point of attachment:

- *Supracardiac:* Attachment above the diaphragm, usually to the superior vena cava (most common form)
- *Cardiac:* Direct attachment to the heart, usually to the RA or coronary sinus
- *Infracardiac:* Attachment below the diaphragm, such as to the inferior vena cava (most severe and least common form)

The RA receives all the blood that normally would flow into the LA. As a result, the right side of the heart is enlarged and the left side,

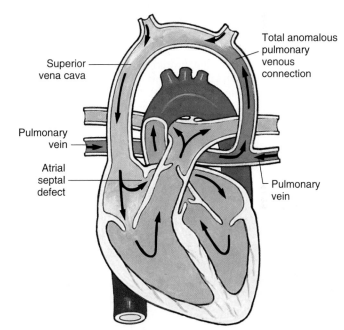

FIGURE 27.11 Total Anomalous Pulmonary Venous Connection (TAPVC).

especially the LA, is smaller than normal. An associated ASD or PFO allows systemic venous blood to shunt from the RA to the left side of the heart. As a result, the oxygen saturation of the blood in both sides of the heart (and, ultimately, in the systemic arterial circulation) is the same. If the pulmonary blood flow is increased, pulmonary venous return is also large, and the amount of saturated blood is relatively high. However, if there is obstruction to pulmonary venous drainage, the infant has severe cyanosis and low cardiac output. Infracardiac TAPVC often is associated with obstruction of pulmonary venous drainage and is a surgical emergency with higher mortality than the unobstructed types.[2]

CLINICAL MANIFESTATIONS   Most infants develop cyanosis early in life. The degree of cyanosis is inversely related to the amount of pulmonary blood flow. Children with unobstructed TAPVC may be asymptomatic until PVR decreases during infancy, increasing pulmonary blood flow, with resulting signs of pulmonary overcirculation. Cyanosis becomes worse with pulmonary vein obstruction; once obstruction occurs, the infant's condition deteriorates rapidly, necessitating immediate surgical intervention, or death will occur. Murmur is not a common feature of TAPVC.[2]

EVALUATION AND TREATMENT   The diagnosis is suspected with echocardiography but may require confirmative angiography. Corrective repair is usually required in early infancy. The surgical approach varies with the type of TAPVC or whether the defect is obstructed or unobstructed. In general, the common pulmonary vein (venous confluence) is sutured to the LA, the ASD is closed, and the anomalous pulmonary venous connection or vertical vein may be ligated. Potential complications include reobstruction at the anastomosis site; atrial dysrhythmias, including sick sinus syndrome; PA hypertension; and LV dysfunction.[4]

Truncus Arteriosus

PATHOPHYSIOLOGY   Truncus arteriosus (TA) is failure of normal septation and division of the embryonic outflow tract into a PA and an aorta, resulting in a single vessel that exits the heart (Fig. 27.12). There is always an associated VSD, with mixing of the systemic and arterial circulations causing some degree of cyanosis. Blood ejected from the heart flows preferentially to the lower pressure PAs, causing increased pulmonary blood flow. The three types are:

- *Type I:* A single pulmonary trunk arises near the base of the truncus and divides into the left and right PAs
- *Type II:* The left and right PAs arise separately from the posterior aspect of the truncus
- *Type III:* The PAs arise independently and from the lateral aspect of the truncus[1]

CLINICAL MANIFESTATIONS   Most infants are symptomatic with moderate HF and variable cyanosis, poor growth, and activity intolerance.

A harsh systolic regurgitant murmur is usually present as a result of the VSD, and a systolic click that indicates opening of the truncal valve. Children are at risk for brain abscess and bacterial endocarditis.[2]

EVALUATION AND TREATMENT   The diagnosis is made by echocardiography. Corrective repair is performed in the first few weeks or months of life. It involves closing the VSD so that the TA receives the outflow from the LV, and excising the PAs from the aorta and attaching them to the RV through a tissue homograft (cadaver conduit). These children require additional procedures to replace the homograft conduit since its size becomes inadequate in relation to growth or narrows because of calcification over time.[4]

Hypoplastic Left Heart Syndrome

PATHOPHYSIOLOGY   Hypoplastic left heart syndrome (HLHS) is underdevelopment of the left side of the heart. Features include a small LA and a small or absent mitral valve, LV, and AV (Fig. 27.13). Most blood from the LA flows across the PFO to the RA, to the RV, and out the PA. The descending aorta receives blood from the PDA supplying systemic blood flow and there is retrograde perfusion to the coronary arteries.[1]

CLINICAL MANIFESTATIONS   HLHS presents in the early newborn period as mild cyanosis, tachypnea, and low cardiac output, if it was not already detected by fetal echocardiogram. Support of the systemic circulation is accomplished with prostaglandin E_1 infusion. If HLHS is not suspected and the PDA closes, there is progressive deterioration with cyanosis and decreased cardiac output, leading to cardiovascular collapse. If left untreated, HLHS is usually fatal in the first months of life.[2]

EVALUATION AND TREATMENT   Echocardiography shows all the features of HLHS. Cardiac catheterization or echocardiographically guided balloon atrial septostomy may be necessary if the atrial septum is restrictive. Surgical intervention is a staged approach that includes:

- Anastomosis of the main PA to the aorta to create a new aorta, construction of shunt to provide pulmonary blood flow, and creation of a large ASD

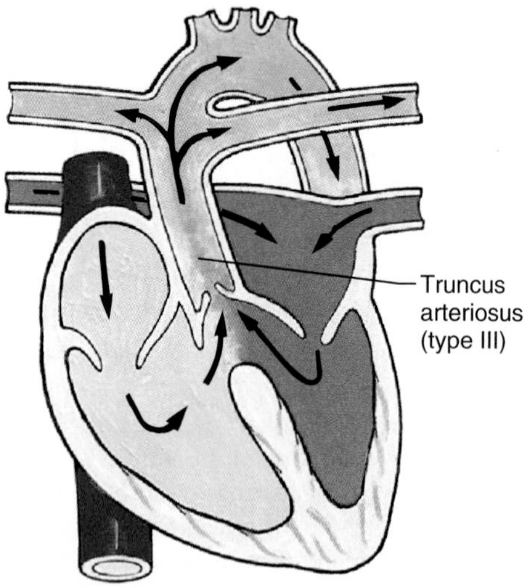

FIGURE 27.12 Truncus Arteriosus (TA). The TA fails to divide into the pulmonary artery and aorta, and the interventricular septum fails to close at the top. Blood from both ventricles mixes in the TA and then enters the pulmonary and systemic circuits. (From Hockenberry MJ, Wilson D: *Wong's essentials of pediatric nursing,* ed 10, St Louis, 2016, Mosby.)

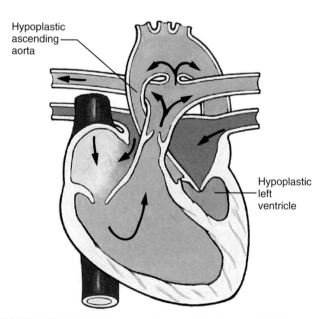

FIGURE 27.13 Hypoplastic Left Heart Syndrome (HLHS). (From Hockenberry MJ et al: *Wong's essentials of pediatric nursing,* ed 9, St Louis, 2016, Mosby.)

- Anastomosis of the superior vena cava to the PA
- Routing of the inferior vena cava blood flow to the PA with a grafted or artificial tube[4]

✓ QUICK CHECK 27.1

1. What are the four principal classifications of CHD?
2. Describe the different characteristics that determine whether the defects are cyanotic or acyanotic.
3. What is the most common type of congenital heart defect?

Heart Failure

Heart failure (HF) is a common complication of many congenital heart defects. HF occurs when the heart is unable to maintain sufficient cardiac output to meet the metabolic demands of the body. The most common congenital causes of HF in infancy and childhood are listed in Table 27.3. Classic HF in children also can be acquired, usually resulting from cardiomyopathies, dysrhythmias, or electrolyte disturbances. Pulmonary overcirculation from a large left-to-right shunt is often called congestive heart failure but is not usually associated with decreased ventricular function and failure to meet metabolic demands. However, the clinical manifestations are similar, such as FTT, tachypnea, tachycardia, and exercise intolerance.[2]

In general, the pathophysiologic mechanisms of HF in infants and children are similar to those in adults. It is most often a result of decreased LV systolic function and the associated LA and pulmonary venous hypertension and pulmonary venous congestion. The same compensatory mechanisms are activated in the face of inadequate cardiac output. RV failure is rare in childhood.[2,5]

Left heart failure in infants is manifested as poor feeding and sucking, often leading to FTT. In left heart failure, manifestations including dyspnea, tachypnea, and diaphoresis may be accompanied by retractions, grunting, and nasal flaring. Wheezing, coughing, and rales (a sound like crinkling paper from auscultation) are rare in childhood HF.[1,2] Common skin changes, such as pallor or mottling, are often present (Box 27.1). Signs of systemic venous congestion, such as enlarged liver, weight gain, ascites, and peripheral edema, can be present but could be suggestive of other medical conditions such as renal or nutritional deficiencies.[1,2]

A thorough physical examination with emphasis on cardiac and pulmonary findings will often reveal the degree of HF. Plotting a child's growth (height, weight, head circumference) is an important method of assessing a child's health. Infants with HF or pulmonary overcirculation usually have low weight with normal length and head circumference measurements. The FTT is usually the result of increased metabolic expenditure relative to caloric intake. An electrocardiogram (ECG) also should be performed to determine the presence of dysrhythmia or hypertrophy. A chest x-ray is useful in assessing the presence of an enlarged heart and signs of increased pulmonary circulation or pulmonary edema with echocardiogram to assess impaired function and possible etiology. B-type natriuretic peptide (BNP) has emerged as another diagnostic test of HF in children to confirm or exclude a cardiac cause for the symptoms.[5]

Treatment is aimed at decreasing cardiac workload and increasing the efficiency of heart function. Severe CHD is typically managed with surgical repair if applicable. Medical management initially consists of diuretics, such as furosemide. Depending on the degree of HF, other diuretics can be used in combination with furosemide to counteract potassium losses. Agents that reduce afterload, such as ACE inhibitors, angiotensin receptor blockers, and β-blockers, are used to further manage severe HF.[5] In severe cases of end-stage HF, anticoagulation and mechanical circulatory support may be indicated to support the failing myocardium while awaiting cardiac transplantation.[5]

TABLE 27.3 Congenital Heart Defects Causing Heart Failure

Age	Congenital Heart Defect
Time of birth	HLHS Volume overload caused by tricuspid regurgitation (rare) AV fistula
Birth to 1 week	HLHS Aortic atresia TGA with VSD COA TAPVC with obstruction PDA in small premature infants
First 4 weeks	COA TAPVC Large left-to-right shunt caused by VSD, PDA in premature infants Tricuspid atresia Persistent TA with large left-to-right shunt All previously mentioned defects
4 to 6 weeks	TGA with VSD Large left-to-right shunt caused by endocardial cushion defect
6 weeks to 6 months	VSD
6 months	Endocardial fibroelastosis

AV, Arteriovenous; *COA,* coarctation of the aorta; *HLHS,* hypoplastic left heart syndrome; *PDA,* patent ductus arteriosus; *TA,* truncus arteriosus; *TAPVC,* total anomalous pulmonary venous connection; *TGA,* transposition of the great arteries; *VSD,* ventricular septal defect. Modified from Park MK: *Pediatric cardiology for practitioners,* ed 6, St Louis, 2014, Mosby.

BOX 27.1 Clinical Manifestations of Heart Failure

Impaired Myocardial Function
Tachycardia
Sweating (inappropriate)
Decreased urinary output
Fatigue
Weakness
Restlessness
Anorexia
Pale, cool extremities
Weak peripheral pulses
Decreased blood pressure
Gallop rhythm
Cardiomegaly

Pulmonary Congestion
Tachypnea
Dyspnea

Retractions (infants)
Flaring nares
Exercise intolerance
Orthopnea
Cough, hoarseness
Cyanosis
Wheezing (rare)
Grunting

Systemic Venous Congestion
Weight gain
Hepatomegaly
Peripheral edema (rare)
Ascites
Neck vein distention (rare in children)

From Hockenberry MJ, Wilson D: *Wong's nursing care of infants and children,* ed 10, St Louis, 2015, Mosby.

ACQUIRED CARDIOVASCULAR DISORDERS

Acquired heart diseases refer to disease processes or abnormalities that occur after birth. They result from various causes, such as infection, genetic disorders, autoimmune processes in response to infection, environmental factors, or autoimmune diseases. Examples of acquired heart diseases include Kawasaki disease, myocarditis, rheumatic heart disease, cardiomyopathy, and systemic hypertension. This chapter discusses Kawasaki disease and systemic hypertension. Myocarditis, rheumatic heart disease, and cardiomyopathy are discussed in Chapter 26.

Kawasaki Disease

Kawasaki disease (KD), formerly known as mucocutaneous lymph node syndrome, is an acute, usually self-limiting systemic vasculitis that may result in cardiac sequelae without treatment. Although KD occurs throughout the world, the greatest incidence is seen in Japan.[6] This incidence reflects the genetic component of KD; the case rate is highest among Asians and lower among white and black children.

Kawasaki disease is primarily a condition of young children, with 80% of cases seen in children younger than 5 years of age, peaking in the toddler age group. Males are affected slightly more than females. The peak incidence is in the winter and spring.[6]

The etiology of KD remains unknown. Current etiologic theories center on an immunologic response to an infectious, toxic, or antigenic substance.[6]

PATHOPHYSIOLOGY Kawasaki disease progresses pathologically and clinically in these stages:

Stage I (days 1-12): Small capillaries, arterioles, and venules become inflamed, as does the heart itself.

Stage II (days 13-25): Inflammation spreads to larger vessels and aneurysms of the coronary arteries may develop.

Stage III (days 26-40): Medium-sized arteries begin the granulation process and may cause coronary artery thickening with increased risk for thrombosis.

Stage IV (day 41 and beyond): Inflammation wanes with potential scarring of the affected vessels, calcification, and stenosis.

CLINICAL MANIFESTATIONS KD progresses in three stages (acute, subacute, and convalescent):

- *Acute phase*: The child with classic or typical KD has fever, conjunctivitis, oral changes ("strawberry" tongue), rash, erythema of the palms and soles, and lymphadenopathy, and is often irritable. During this phase, myocarditis may develop.
- *Subacute phase*: Begins when the fever ends and continues until the clinical signs have resolved. It is at this time that the child is most at risk for coronary artery aneurysm development. Desquamation (skin peeling) of the palms and soles occurs at this time, as well as marked thrombocytosis.
- *Convalescent phase*: This phase is marked by the elevation of the erythrocyte sedimentation rate and C-reactive protein level, as well as by an increased platelet count. Arthritis or arthralgia of the joints may be present. This phase continues until all laboratory values return to normal—usually about 6 to 8 weeks after onset.[6]

EVALUATION AND TREATMENT The diagnosis of KD is based on clinical features, and the child must exhibit five of six criteria, including fever, presented in Box 27.2. These children usually have leukocytosis, increased erythrocyte sedimentation rates, thrombocytosis, and elevated liver enzymes. An echocardiogram is obtained at the time of diagnosis as a baseline measurement to assess for coronary aneurysms or

inflammation. Serial echocardiograms are obtained after treatment to assess for the development of coronary aneurysms or regression of those present early in the course of the disease. Treatment includes oral administration of aspirin and intravenous infusion of gamma globulin (most often only one dose). Aspirin is continued until the manifestations of inflammation are resolved, but it may be used indefinitely in children with residual coronary artery abnormalities.[6]

Atypical or "incomplete" KD can be seen in infants and children who lack the diagnostic criteria (have fewer than five signs) or "classic" physical findings. Recognition can be difficult and often results in delay of treatment, with possible cardiovascular sequelae.[6]

Treatment with aspirin and intravenous immunoglobulin during the acute phase has decreased the morbidity of KD and has reduced the incidence of coronary abnormalities from approximately 25% to less than 5% at 6 to 8 weeks after initiation of therapy. Most children recover completely from KD, including regression of aneurysms. The most common, although rare, cardiovascular sequela is coronary artery aneurysms and resulting thrombosis or myocardial infarction.[6]

Systemic Hypertension

Systemic hypertension (HTN) in children is defined as systolic and diastolic blood pressure levels greater than the 95th percentile for age, sex, and height on at least three occasions (Tables 27.4 and 27.5).[7]

Hypertension is classified into two categories:

- *primary (or essential) hypertension,* in which a specific cause cannot be identified
- *secondary hypertension,* in which a cause can be identified (Box 27.3)

BOX 27.2 Diagnostic Criteria for Kawasaki Disease

The child must exhibit five of these six criteria:
1. Fever for 5 or more days (often diagnosed with shorter duration of fever if other symptoms are present)
2. Bilateral conjunctival infection without exudation
3. Changes in the oral mucous membranes, such as erythema, dryness, and fissuring of the lips; oropharyngeal reddening; or "strawberry tongue"
4. Changes in the extremities, such as peripheral edema, peripheral erythema, and desquamation of the palms and soles, particularly periungual peeling
5. Polymorphous rash, often accentuated in the perineal area
6. Cervical lymphadenopathy (one lymph node >1.5 cm)

Modified from Hockenberry MJ et al: *Wong's nursing care of infants and children,* ed 10, St Louis, 2015, Mosby.

TABLE 27.4 Normative Blood Pressure Levels (Systolic/Diastolic Pressure [Mean]) by Dinamap Monitor in Children 5 Years Old or Younger

Age	Mean BP Levels (mm Hg)	90th Percentile	95th Percentile
1-3 days	64/41 (50)	75/49 (50)	78/52 (62)
1 mo to 2 yr	95/58 (72)	106/68 (83)	110/71 (86)
2-5 yr	101/57 (74)	112/66 (82)	115/68 (85)

BP, Blood pressure.
Data from Park MK: *Pediatric cardiology for practitioners,* ed 6, St Louis, 2014, Mosby; modified from Park MK, Menard SM: *Am J Dis Children* 143:860, 1989.

Hypertension (HTN) in children differs from adult HTN in etiology and presentation. Young children, when diagnosed with HTN, are often found to have secondary HTN caused by some underlying disease, such as renal disease or COA (see Box 27.3). An increased prevalence of primary HTN in older children has been noted. Researchers are now focusing on primary HTN in older children in relation to morbidity and the presence of early atherosclerotic disease. Certain factors influence blood pressure in children. Children who are overweight are often hypertensive[8] (see *Did You Know?* U.S. Childhood Obesity and Its Association With Cardiovascular Disease). Smoking and second-hand smoke are associated with an increased risk for HTN.[7]

TABLE 27.5 Suggested Normal Blood Pressure Values by Auscultatory Method (Systolic/Diastolic K5)

Age (Years)	Mean BP Levels (mm Hg)	90th Percentile	95th Percentile
6-7	104/55	114/73	117/78
8-9	106/58	117/76	120/82
10-11*	108/60	120/77	124/82
12-13*	112/62	124/78	128/83
14-15			
Boys	116/66	132/80	138/86
Girls	112/68	126/80	130/83
16-18			
Boys	121/70	136/82	140/86
Girls	110/68	125/81	127/84

*Values for ages 10 to 13 years have been extrapolated from these two studies using age-related increments from other studies.
BP, Blood pressure; *K5*, phase V of Korotkoff sound.
From Park MK: *Pediatric cardiology for practitioners*, ed 6, Philadelphia, 2014, Mosby; modified from Goldring D, et al: *J Pediatr* 91:884, 1977; Prineas RJ, et al: *Hypertension* 1(Suppl):18, 1980.

DID YOU KNOW?

U.S. Childhood Obesity and Its Association With Cardiovascular Disease

The prevalence of childhood obesity remains high in the United States. Approximately 18.5% (or 13.7 million) of children and adolescents ages 2 to 19 years are obese. This number increased by 1.5% compared to 17% in 2014. Obesity rates are higher in adolescents (12-19 years of age; 20.6%) and school-age children (6-11 years of age; 18.4%) compared to preschool-age children (2-5 years of age; 13.9%). Furthermore, there is no significant difference in obesity prevalence between boys and girls overall or by age group. However, non-Hispanic black and Hispanic youths had a higher prevalence of obesity compared with other racial groups. Obesity continues to be a major health concern in children and is linked to insulin resistance, diabetes, and increased cardiovascular risk, especially atherosclerosis, hypertension, and lipid abnormalities. The mechanisms by which insulin resistance and diabetes cause cardiovascular diseases include endothelial dysfunction, structural changes in arterial walls, abnormal vasoconstriction, and changes in renal function and salt transport. Research into genetics and insulin-regulated transcription factors suggests that obesity, insulin resistance, diabetes, and cardiovascular disease share important molecular etiologies and processes. These findings may lead investigators to important new treatments. For now, helping children develop good exercise and dietary habits has been shown to significantly improve arterial function and reduce cardiovascular risk.

Data from https://www.cdc.gov/obesity/data/childhood.html.

BOX 27.3 Conditions Associated With Secondary Hypertension in Children

Renal Disorders
Congenital defects
 Polycystic kidney, ectopic kidney, horseshoe kidney, etc.
 Obstructive anomalies
 Hydronephrosis
Renal tumor
 Wilms tumor
 Retrovascular tumor
Abnormalities of renal arteries
Renal vein thrombosis
Acquired disorders
 Glomerulonephritis, acute or chronic
 Pyelonephritis
 Nephritis associated with collagen disease

Cardiovascular Disease
Coarctation of the aorta
Arteriovenous fistulae
Patent ductus arteriosus
Aortic or mitral insufficiency

Metabolic and Endocrine Diseases
Adrenal tumors
 Adenoma
 Pheochromocytoma

Neuroblastoma
Cushing syndrome
Adrenogenital syndrome
Hyperthyroidism
Aldosteronism
Hypercalcemia
Diabetes mellitus

Neurologic Disorders
Space-occupying lesions of cranium (increased intracranial pressure)
 Tumors, cysts, hematoma
 Cerebral edema
 Encephalitis (including Guillain-Barré and Reye syndromes)

Miscellaneous Causes
Drugs (corticosteroids, oral contraceptives, pressor agents, amphetamines)
Burns
Genitourinary surgery
Trauma (e.g., stretching of femoral nerve with leg traction)
Insect bites (e.g., scorpion)
Intravascular overload (blood, fluid)
Hypernatremia
Toxemia of pregnancy
Heavy metal poisoning

From Hockenberry MJ, Wilson D: *Wong's essentials of pediatric nursing*, ed 10, St Louis, 2015, Mosby.

TABLE 27.6 Most Common Causes of Chronic Sustained Hypertension in Children

Age Group	Causes
Newborn	Renal artery thrombosis, renal artery stenosis, congenital renal malformation, coarctation of the aorta (COA), bronchopulmonary dysplasia
<6 years	Renal parenchymal disease, COA, renal artery stenosis
6-10 years	Renal artery stenosis, renal parenchymal disease, primary hypertension
>10 years	Primary hypertension, renal parenchymal disease

From Park MK: *Pediatric cardiology for practitioners*, ed 6, St Louis, 2014, Mosby.

PATHOPHYSIOLOGY In infants and children, a cause of HTN is almost always found. In general, the younger the child with significant HTN, the more likely a correctable cause can be determined. Therefore a thorough evaluation needs to be performed.[7]

The pathophysiology of primary HTN in children is not clearly understood but may result from a complex interaction of a strong predisposing genetic component with disturbances in sympathetic vascular smooth muscle tone, humoral agents (angiotensin, catecholamines), renal sodium excretion, and cardiac output. Studies have shown an increased level of leptin, a hormone produced by adipose tissue, to be associated with HTN in obese children.[2] Ultimately, these factors impair the ability of the peripheral vascular bed to relax.

CLINICAL MANIFESTATIONS Most children with systemic HTN are asymptomatic. It is necessary that a thorough history and physical examination be obtained. The examination should include an accurate blood pressure measurement obtained in the right arm with the arm supported at the level of the heart; three separate measurements using an appropriate-size cuff also are needed for an accurate blood pressure reading.[7]

EVALUATION AND TREATMENT In children, the history and physical examination should be directed at determining the etiology of HTN, such as COA or renal disease (Table 27.6). Table 27.7 includes routine and special laboratory tests for HTN. Blood pressure differential between upper and lower extremities and echocardiogram can be used to identify COA. If HTN is determined to be essential, or primary, in nature, nonpharmacologic therapy is used initially. Moderate weight loss and exercise can decrease systolic and diastolic pressures in many children. Appropriate diet, regular physical activity, and avoidance of smoking have been shown to be effective in reducing blood pressure.[1] Ambulatory blood pressure monitoring has the potential to become an important tool in the evaluation and management of childhood HTN.[7]

Medication therapy is controversial in children with primary HTN; however, when nonpharmacologic therapy fails, the approach is similar to the treatment of HTN in adults with the use of ACE inhibitors or angiotensin receptor blocker medications.[7] The current emphasis on preventive cardiology, especially for children, is significant because many investigators believe signs of atherosclerosis are present during childhood.[9]

TABLE 27.7 Routine and Special Laboratory Tests for Hypertension

Laboratory Tests	Significance of Abnormal Results
Urinalysis, urine culture, blood urea nitrogen, and creatinine levels	Renal parenchymal disease
Serum electrolyte levels (hypokalemia)	Hyperaldosteronism, primary or secondary Adrenogenital syndrome Renin-producing tumors
ECG, chest x-ray studies	Cardiac cause of hypertension, also baseline function
Intravenous pyelography (or ultrasonography, radionuclide studies, computed tomography of kidneys)	Renal parenchymal diseases Renovascular hypertension Tumors (neuroblastoma, Wilms tumor)
Plasma renin activity, peripheral	High-renin hypertension Renovascular hypertension Renin-producing tumors Some caused by Cushing syndrome Some caused by essential hypertension Low-renin hypertension Adrenogenital syndrome Primary hyperaldosteronism
24-hr urine collection for 17-ketosteroids and 17-hydroxycorticosteroids	Cushing syndrome Adrenogenital syndrome
24-hr urine collection for catecholamine levels and vanillylmandelic acid	Pheochromocytoma Neuroblastoma
Aldosterone	Hyperaldosteronism, primary or secondary Renovascular hypertension Renin-producing tumors
Renal vein plasma renin activity	Unilateral renal parenchymal disease Renovascular hypertension
Abdominal aortogram	Renovascular hypertension Abdominal COA Unilateral renal parenchymal diseases Pheochromocytoma
Intra-arterial digit subtraction angiography	Renovascular hypertension

COA, Coarctation of the aorta; *ECG*, electrocardiogram.
From Park MK: *Pediatric cardiology for practitioners*, ed 6, St Louis, 2014, Mosby.

✔ **QUICK CHECK 27.2**
1. Why are the infant's height and weight important in the assessment of HF?
2. Why is it critical to recognize and treat children during the acute phase of KD?
3. Discuss the cardiovascular effects of obesity in children.

SUMMARY REVIEW

Congenital Heart Disease

1. Congenital heart defects are heart defects present since birth, and some have associated causes, both environmental and genetic.

2. Environmental risk factors associated with the incidence of CHDs typically are maternal conditions and include infections, radiation, metabolic disorders, drug intake, and peripheral conditions.

3. Genetic factors associated with congenital heart defects include, but are not limited to, Down syndrome, trisomy 13, trisomy 18, cri du chat syndrome, and Turner syndrome.

4. Classification of congenital heart defects is based on whether they cause (1) increased pulmonary blood flow; (2) obstruction to flow; (3) decreased pulmonary blood flow; or (4) mixed desaturated and saturated blood within the chambers or great arteries of the heart.

5. Cyanosis, a bluish discoloration of the skin, indicates that the tissues are not receiving normal amounts of oxygenated blood. Cyanosis can be caused by defects that (1) restrict blood flow into the pulmonary circulation; (2) overload the pulmonary circulation, causing pulmonary overcirculation, pulmonary edema, and respiratory difficulty; or (3) cause large amounts of unoxygenated blood to shunt from the pulmonary to the systemic circulation.

6. Congenital defects that maintain or create direct communication between the pulmonary and systemic circulatory systems cause blood to shunt from one system to another, mixing oxygenated and unoxygenated blood and increasing blood volume and, occasionally, pressure on the receiving side of the shunt.

7. The direction of shunting through an abnormal communication depends on differences in pressure and resistance between the two systems. Flow is always from an area of high pressure to an area of low pressure.

8. If the abnormal communication between the left and right circuits is large, volume and pressure overload in the pulmonary circulation can lead to left-sided HF.

9. Acyanotic congenital defects that increase pulmonary blood flow consist of abnormal openings (ASD, VSD, PDA, or AVC) that permit blood to shunt from left (systemic circulation) to right (pulmonary circulation). Cyanosis does not occur because the left-to-right shunt

does not interfere with the flow of oxygenated blood through the systemic circulation.

10. An acyanotic defect caused by obstruction of ventricular outflow is commonly caused by PS or AS. In less severe obstruction, ventricular outflow remains normal because of compensatory ventricular hypertrophy stimulated by increased afterload and, in postductal COA, development of collateral circulation around the coarctation.

11. Cyanotic congenital defects in which saturated and desaturated blood mix within the heart or great arteries include TGA, TAPVC, TA, and HLHS.

12. In cyanotic heart defects that decrease pulmonary blood flow (TOF and tricuspid atresia), myocardial hypertrophy cannot compensate for restricted RV outflow. Flow to the lungs decreases, and cyanosis is caused by an insufficient volume of oxygenated blood and right-to-left shunt.

13. The initial treatment for CHD, depending on the defect, is aimed at controlling the level of HF symptoms or cyanosis. Interventional procedures in the cardiac catheterization laboratory and surgical palliation or repair are performed to establish a source of pulmonary blood flow or restore normal circulation.

14. Heart failure occurs when the heart is unable to maintain sufficient cardiac output to meet the metabolic demands of the body. HF is usually the result of congenital heart defects that increase blood volume in the pulmonary circulation. A clinical manifestation of HF unique to children is FTT.

Acquired Cardiovascular Disorders

1. Acquired heart diseases are those that develop after birth. They may result from infection, genetic disorders, autoimmune processes or diseases, or environmental factors.

2. Kawasaki disease (KD) is an acute systemic vasculitis, or inflammation of the blood vessels, that also may result in the development of coronary artery aneurysms and thrombosis if untreated.

3. Systemic hypertension in children differs from HTN in adults in etiology and presentation. When significant HTN is found in young children, they should be evaluated for the presence of secondary HTN, most commonly renal disease or COA.

KEY TERMS

Acquired heart disease, 650
Acyanotic heart defect, 639
Aortic stenosis (AS), 643
Atrial septal defect (ASD), 641
Atrioventricular canal (AVC) defect (endocardial cushion defect [ECD]), 642
Coarctation of the aorta (COA), 643
Congenital heart disease (CHD), 639
Cyanosis, 639
Cyanotic heart defect, 639
Eisenmenger syndrome, 642

Foramen ovale, 641
Heart failure (HF), 649
Hypoplastic left heart syndrome (HLHS), 648
Kawasaki disease (KD), 650
Left-to-right shunt, 639
Muscular ventricular septal defect, 642
Ostium primum atrial septal defect, 641
Ostium secundum atrial septal defect, 641
Patent ductus arteriosus (PDA), 640

Patent foramen ovale (PFO), 641
Perimembranous ventricular septal defect, 642
Pulmonary atresia, 644
Pulmonic stenosis (PS), 644
Right-to-left shunt, 639
Shunt, 639
Sinus venosus atrial septal defect, 641
Subvalvular aortic stenosis, 644
Supravalvular aortic stenosis, 644
Systemic hypertension (HTN), 650
Tetralogy of Fallot (TOF), 645

Total anomalous pulmonary venous connection (TAPVC), 647
Transposition of the great arteries (TGA), 646
Tricuspid atresia, 645
Truncus arteriosus (TA), 648
Valvular aortic stenosis, 643
Ventricular septal defect (VSD), 642

REFERENCES

1. Allen HD, editor: *Moss and Adams' heart disease in infants, children, and adolescents including the fetus and young adults*, ed 9, Philadelphia, 2016, Lippincott Williams & Wilkins.
2. Park MK: *Pediatric cardiology for practitioners*, ed 6, St Louis, 2014, Mosby. Available at: http://mdconsult/book.
3. Feltes TF, et al: Indications for cardiac catheterization and intervention in pediatric heart disease: a scientific statement from the American Heart Association, *Circulation* 123(22):2607-2625, 2011.
4. Jonas RA: *Comprehensive surgical management of congenital heart disease*, ed 2, Boca Raton FL, 2014, CRC Press, Taylor & Francis Group.
5. Stout KK, et al: Chronic heart failure in congenital heart disease: a scientific statement from the American Heart Association, *Circulation* 133(8):770-801, 2016.
6. McCrindle BW, et al: Diagnosis, treatment and long-term management of Kawasaki disease: a scientific statement for health professionals from the American Heart Association, *Circulation* 135(17):e927-e999, 2017.
7. Flynn JT, et al: Clinical practice guideline for screening and management of high blood pressure in children and adolescents, *Pediatrics* 140(3):2017.
8. Flynn JT: The changing face of pediatric hypertension in the era of the childhood obesity epidemic, *Pediatr Nephrol* 28(7):1059-1066, 2012.
9. Flynn JT, et al: Update: ambulatory blood pressure monitoring in children and adolescents: a scientific statement from the American Heart Association Atherosclerosis, Hypertension and Obesity in Youth Committee of the Council on Cardiovascular Disease in the Young, *Hypertension* 63(5):1116-1135, 2014.

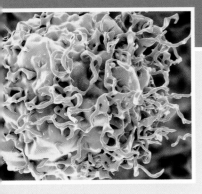

28

Structure and Function of the Pulmonary System

Valentina L. Brashers

CHAPTER OUTLINE

The primary function of the pulmonary system is the exchange of gases between the environmental air and the blood. The three steps in this process are (1) ventilation, the movement of air into and out of the lungs; (2) diffusion, the movement of gases between air spaces in the lungs and the bloodstream; and (3) perfusion, the movement of blood into and out of the capillary beds of the lungs to body organs and tissues. The first two functions are carried out by the pulmonary system and the third by the cardiovascular system (see Chapter 25). Normally the pulmonary system functions efficiently under a variety of conditions and with little energy expenditure.

STRUCTURES OF THE PULMONARY SYSTEM

The pulmonary system includes two lungs, the upper and lower airways, the blood vessels that serve these structures (Fig. 28.1), the diaphragm, and the chest wall (thoracic cage).[1] The lungs are divided into lobes: three in the right lung (upper, middle, lower) and two in the left lung (upper, lower). Each lobe is further divided into segments and lobules. The mediastinum is the space between the lungs and contains the heart, great vessels, and esophagus. A set of conducting airways, or bronchi, delivers air to each section of the lung. The lung tissue that surrounds the airways supports them, preventing distortion or collapse of the airways as gas moves in and out during ventilation. The diaphragm is a dome-shaped muscle that separates the thoracic and abdominal cavities and is involved in ventilation.

The lungs are protected from contaminants in inspired air by a series of mechanical barriers (Table 28.1). These defense mechanisms are so effective that, in the healthy individual, contamination of the lung tissue itself, particularly by infectious agents, is uncommon.

Conducting Airways

The conducting airways allow air into and out of the gas-exchange structures of the lung. The nasopharynx, oropharynx, and related structures are often called the *upper airway*[2] (Fig. 28.2). These structures are lined with a ciliated mucosa that warms and humidifies inspired air and removes foreign particles from it. The mouth and oropharynx are used for ventilation when the nose is obstructed or when increased flow is required (e.g., during exercise). Filtering and humidifying are not as efficient with mouth breathing.

The larynx connects the upper and lower airways and consists of the endolarynx and its surrounding triangular-shaped bony and cartilaginous structures. The endolarynx encompasses two pairs of folds: the false vocal cords (supraglottis) and the true vocal cords. The slit-shaped space between the true cords forms the glottis (see Fig. 28.2). The vestibule is the space above the false vocal cords. The laryngeal box is formed of three large cartilages (epiglottis, thyroid, cricoid) and three smaller cartilages (arytenoid, corniculate, cuneiform) connected by ligaments. The supporting cartilages prevent collapse of the larynx during inspiration and swallowing. The internal laryngeal muscles control vocal cord length and tension, and the external laryngeal muscles move the larynx as a whole. Both sets of muscles are important to swallowing, ventilation, and vocalization. The internal muscles contract during swallowing to prevent aspiration into the trachea. These muscles also contribute to voice pitch.

The trachea, which is supported by U-shaped cartilage, connects the larynx to the bronchi, the conducting airways of the lungs. The trachea branches into two bronchi (sing., bronchus) at the carina (see Fig. 28.1). The right and left main bronchi enter the lungs at the hila (sing., hilum), or "roots" of the lungs, along with the pulmonary blood

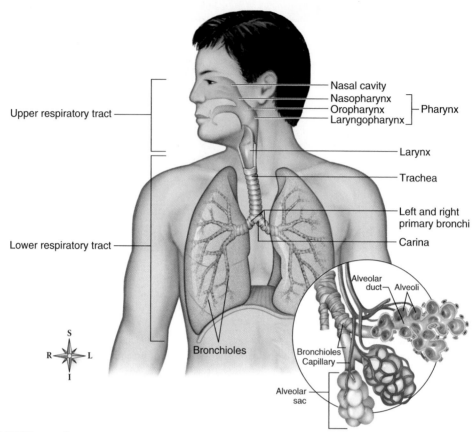

FIGURE 28.1 Structure of the Pulmonary System. The upper and lower respiratory tracts (airways) are illustrated. The enlargement in the circle depicts the acinus, where oxygen and carbon dioxide are exchanged. (From Patton KT, Thibodeau GA: *Structure & function of the body,* ed 15, St Louis, 2016, Mosby.)

TABLE 28.1 Pulmonary Defense Mechanisms

Structure or Substance	Mechanism of Defense
Upper respiratory tract mucosa	Maintains constant temperature and humidification of gas entering lungs; traps and removes foreign particles, some bacteria, and noxious gases from inspired air
Nasal hairs and turbinates	Trap and remove foreign particles, some bacteria, and noxious gases from inspired air
Mucous blanket	Protects trachea and bronchi from injury; traps most foreign particles and bacteria that reach lower airways
Cilia	Propel mucous blanket and entrapped particles toward oropharynx, where they can be swallowed or expectorated
Irritant receptors in nares (nostrils)	Stimulation by chemical or mechanical irritants triggers sneeze reflex, which results in rapid removal of irritants from nasal passages
Irritant receptors in trachea and large airways	Stimulation by chemical or mechanical irritants triggers cough reflex, which results in removal of irritants from lower airways
Alveolar macrophages	Ingest and remove bacteria and other foreign material from alveoli by phagocytosis, release inflammatory cytokines, and present antigens to the adaptive immune system (see Chapters 6 and 7)

and lymphatic vessels. From the hila the main bronchi branch farther, as shown in Fig. 28.3.

The bronchial walls have three layers: an epithelial lining, a smooth muscle layer, and a connective tissue layer. The epithelial lining of the bronchi contains single-celled mucous-secreting goblet cells and ciliated cells. The goblet cells produce a mucous blanket that protects the airway epithelium, and the ciliated epithelial cells rhythmically beat this mucous blanket toward the trachea and pharynx, where it can be swallowed or

expectorated by coughing. The layers of epithelium that line the bronchi become thinner with each successive branching (see Fig. 28.3).

Gas-Exchange Airways

The conducting airways terminate in the respiratory bronchioles, alveolar ducts, and alveoli (sing., alveolus). These thin-walled structures together are sometimes called the acinus (see Figs. 28.1 and 28.3), and all of them participate in gas exchange.[3]

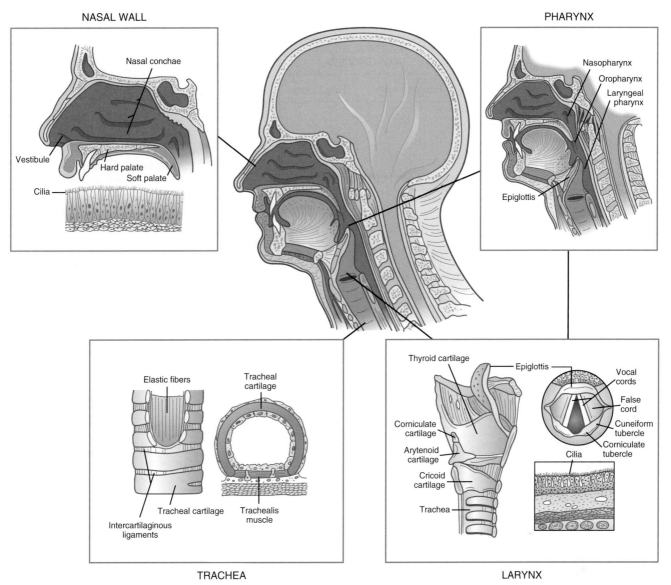

FIGURE 28.2 **Structures of the Upper Airway.** (Redrawn from Thompson JM et al: *Mosby's clinical nursing,* ed 5, St Louis, 2002, Mosby.)

The alveoli are the primary gas-exchange units of the lung, where oxygen (O_2) enters the blood and carbon dioxide (CO_2) is removed (Fig. 28.4). Tiny passages called *pores of Kohn* permit some air to pass through the septa from alveolus to alveolus, promoting collateral ventilation and even distribution of air among the alveoli. The lungs contain approximately 25 million alveoli at birth and 300 million by adulthood.

Alveolar cells provide a protective interface with the environment and are essential for adequate gas exchange, preventing entry of foreign agents, and maintaining mechanical stability of the alveoli. Two major types of epithelial cells appear in the alveolus. Type I alveolar cells provide structure, and type II alveolar cells secrete surfactant, a lipoprotein that coats the inner surface of the alveolus and lowers alveolar surface tension at end-expiration, thereby preventing lung collapse. Alveoli also contain cellular components of immunity and inflammation, particularly the mononuclear phagocytes (called *alveolar macrophages*). These cells ingest foreign material that reaches the alveolus and prepare it for removal through the lymphatics. (Phagocytosis and the mononuclear phagocyte system are described in Chapters 6 and 7.)

> **✔ QUICK CHECK 28.1**
> 1. List the major components of the pulmonary system.
> 2. What are conducting airways?
> 3. Describe an alveolus.
> 4. Which components of the pulmonary system contribute to the body's defense?

Pulmonary and Bronchial Circulation

The pulmonary circulation facilitates gas exchange, delivers nutrients to lung tissues, acts as a reservoir for the left ventricle, and serves as a filtering system that removes clots, air, and other debris from the circulation.[4]

Although the entire cardiac output from the right ventricle goes into the lungs, the pulmonary circulation has a lower pressure and resistance than the systemic circulation. Pulmonary artery pressure is about 18 mm Hg, compared to 90 mm Hg in the aorta. Usually about

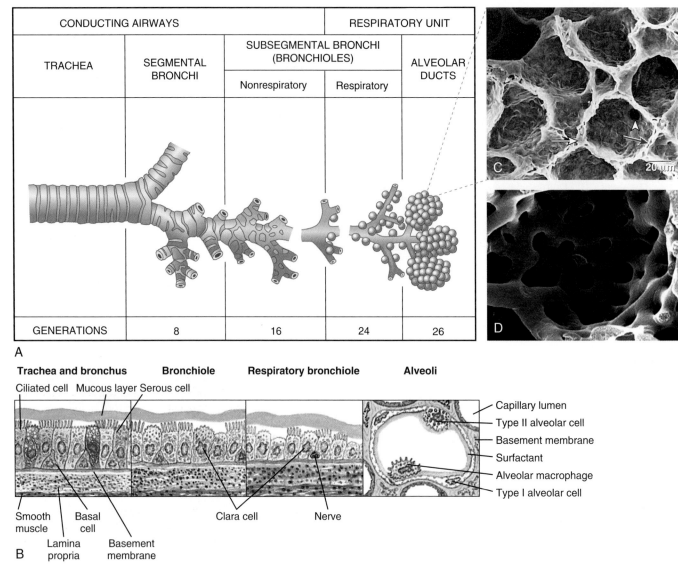

FIGURE 28.3 Structures of the Lower Airway. A, Structures of the lower respiratory airway. **B,** Changes in the bronchial wall with progressive branching. Clara (club) cells secrete protective surfactant type proteins. **C,** Electron micrograph of alveoli: long white arrow identifies type II pneumocyte (secretes surfactant); white arrowhead identifies pores of Kohn; red arrow identifies alveolar capillary. **D,** Plastic cast of pulmonary capillaries at high magnification. (**A** redrawn from Thompson JM et al: *Mosby's clinical nursing,* ed 5, St Louis, 2002, Mosby; **B** from Wilson SF, Thompson JM: *Respiratory disorders,* St Louis, 1990, Mosby; **C** from Mason RJ et al: *Murray and Nadel's textbook of respiratory medicine,* ed 5, Philadelphia, 2010, Saunders; **D** courtesy A. Churg, MD, and J. Wright, MD, Vancouver, Canada. From Leslie KO, Wick MR: *Practical pulmonary pathology: a diagnostic approach,* ed 2, Philadelphia, 2011, Saunders.)

one third of the pulmonary vessels are filled with blood (perfused) at any given time. More vessels become perfused when right ventricular cardiac output increases. Therefore increased delivery of blood to the lungs does not normally increase the mean pulmonary artery pressure significantly.

The pulmonary artery divides and enters the lung at the hila, branching with each main bronchus and with all bronchi at every division. Thus, every bronchus and bronchiole has an accompanying artery or arteriole. The arterioles divide at the terminal bronchioles to form a network of pulmonary capillaries around the acinus. Capillary walls consist of an endothelial layer and a thin basement membrane. Consequently, there is very little separation between blood in the capillary and gas in the alveolus. The shared alveolar and capillary walls compose the alveolocapillary membrane (Fig. 28.5). Gas exchange occurs across this membrane. Any disorder that thickens the membrane impairs gas exchange.

Each pulmonary vein drains several pulmonary capillaries. Unlike the pulmonary arteries, pulmonary veins are dispersed randomly throughout the lung and then leave the lung at the hila and enter the left atrium.

The bronchial circulation is part of the systemic circulation, and it both moistens inspired air and supplies nutrients to the conducting airways, large pulmonary vessels, lymph nodes, and membranes (pleurae) that surround the lungs. The bronchial circulation does not participate in gas exchange.

The lung vasculature also includes deep and superficial pulmonary lymphatic capillaries through which fluid and alveolar macrophages

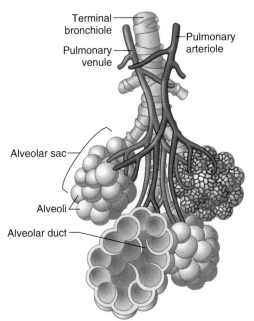

FIGURE 28.4 Alveoli. Bronchioles subdivide to form tiny tubes called *alveolar ducts,* which end in clusters of alveoli called *alveolar sacs.* (From Patton KT, Thibodeau GA: *The human body in health & disease,* ed 6, St Louis, 2014, Mosby.)

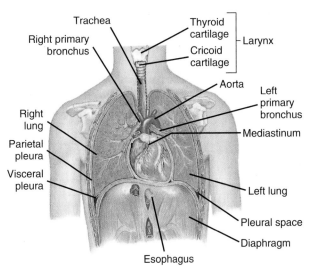

FIGURE 28.6 Thoracic (Chest) Cavity and Related Structures. The thoracic (chest) cavity is divided into three subdivisions (left and right pleural divisions and mediastinum) by a partition formed by a serous membrane called the *pleura.* (From Thibodeau GA, Patton KT: *Anatomy & physiology,* ed 3, St Louis, 1996, Mosby.)

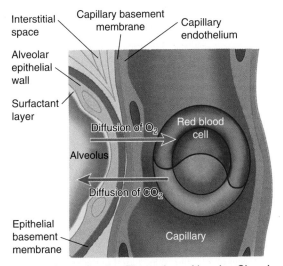

FIGURE 28.5 Cross-Section Through an Alveolus Showing Histology of the Alveolar-Capillary Membrane (Respiratory Membrane). The dense network of capillaries forms an almost continuous sheet of blood in the alveolar walls, providing a very efficient arrangement for gas exchange. *CO_2,* Carbon dioxide; *O_2,* oxygen. (Adapted from Montague SE, Watson R, Herbert R: *Physiology for nursing practice,* ed 3, London, 2005, Elsevier.)

can leave the alveoli and enter the lymphatic system. Both deep and superficial lymphatic vessels leave the lung at the hilum through a series of mediastinal lymph nodes. The lymphatic system plays an important role in both providing immune defense and keeping the lung free of fluid. (The lymphatic system is described in Chapter 25.)

Control of the Pulmonary Circulation
The caliber of pulmonary artery lumina decreases as smooth muscle in the arterial walls contracts. Contraction increases pulmonary artery

pressure. Caliber increases as these muscles relax, decreasing blood pressure. Contraction (vasoconstriction) and relaxation (vasodilation) occurs in response to both local humoral conditions and by the autonomic nervous system (ANS), as is the systemic circulation.

The most important cause of pulmonary artery constriction is a low alveolar partial pressure of oxygen ($P_{A_{O2}}$), often termed **hypoxic pulmonary vasoconstriction**. This results from an increase in intracellular calcium levels in vascular smooth muscle cells in response to a low O_2 concentration and the presence of charged O_2 molecules, called *oxygen radicals.* It can affect only one portion of the lung or the entire lung. If only one segment of the lung is involved, the arterioles to that segment constrict, shunting blood to other, well-ventilated portions of the lung. This reflex improves the lung's efficiency by better matching ventilation and perfusion. If all segments of the lung are affected, however, vasoconstriction occurs throughout the pulmonary vasculature and pulmonary hypertension (elevated pulmonary artery pressure) can result. The pulmonary vasoconstriction caused by a low $P_{A_{O2}}$ is reversible if the $P_{A_{O2}}$ is corrected. Chronic alveolar hypoxia can result in structural changes in pulmonary arterioles, causing permanent pulmonary artery hypertension, which eventually leads to right heart failure (cor pulmonale).

Acidemia also causes pulmonary artery constriction. If the acidemia is corrected, the vasoconstriction is reversed. (Respiratory acidosis and metabolic acidosis are described in Chapter 5.) Other biochemical factors that affect the caliber of vessels in the pulmonary circulation are histamine, prostaglandins, serotonin, nitric oxide, and bradykinin (see *Geriatric Considerations:* Aging & the Pulmonary System).

Chest Wall and Pleura
The chest wall (skin, ribs, intercostal muscles) protects the lungs from injury. The intercostal muscles of the chest wall, along with the diaphragm, accessory muscles, and abdominal muscles, perform the muscular work of breathing. The **thoracic cavity** is contained by the chest wall and encases the lungs (Fig. 28.6). A serous membrane called the **pleura** adheres firmly to the lungs and then folds over itself and attaches firmly to the chest wall. The membrane covering the lungs is the *visceral pleura;* that lining the thoracic cavity is the *parietal pleura.* The area between the two

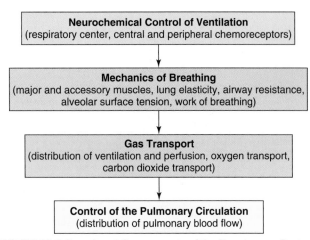

FIGURE 28.7 Functional Components of the Respiratory System. The central nervous system responds to neurochemical stimulation of ventilation and sends signals to the chest wall musculature. The response of the respiratory system to these impulses is influenced by several factors that affect the mechanisms of breathing and, therefore, the adequacy of ventilation. Gas transport between the alveoli and pulmonary capillary blood depends on a variety of physical and chemical activities. Finally, the control of the pulmonary circulation plays a role in the appropriate distribution of blood flow.

pleurae is called the pleural space, or pleural cavity. Normally, only a thin layer of fluid secreted by the pleura (pleural fluid) fills the pleural space, lubricating the pleural surfaces and allowing the two layers to slide over each other without separating. Pressure in the pleural space is usually negative or subatmospheric (-4 to -10 mm Hg).

✔ QUICK CHECK 28.2

1. What are the functions of the pulmonary circulation and of the bronchial circulation?
2. What is the most important factor causing pulmonary artery constriction? What other factors are involved?
3. What are the visceral and parietal pleurae?
4. What are the characteristics of the pleural space?

FUNCTION OF THE PULMONARY SYSTEM

The pulmonary system (1) ventilates the alveoli, (2) diffuses gases into and out of the blood, and (3) perfuses the lungs so that the organs and tissues of the body receive blood that is rich in O_2 and deficient in CO_2. Each component of the pulmonary system contributes to one or more of these functions.[5] (Fig. 28.7).

Ventilation

Ventilation is the mechanical movement of gas or air into and out of the lungs. It is often misnamed *respiration,* which is actually the exchange of O_2 and CO_2 during cellular metabolism. The "respiratory rate" is actually the ventilatory rate, or the number of times gas is inspired and expired per minute. The volume of ventilation is calculated by multiplying the ventilatory rate (breaths per minute) by the volume or amount of air per breath (liters per breath, or tidal volume). This is called the minute volume (or minute ventilation [$\dot{V}$]) and is expressed in liters per minute. The effective ventilation is calculated by multiplying ventilatory rate by the tidal volume minus the dead-space. Dead-space

ventilation (VD) is the volume of air per breath that does not participate in gas exchange. It is ventilation without perfusion.[6] *Anatomic dead-space* is the volume of air in the conducting airways. *Alveolar dead-space* is the volume of air in unperfused alveoli. The dead space is approximately equivalent to ideal body weight in pounds.

Carbon dioxide (CO_2), the gaseous form of carbonic acid (H_2CO_3), is produced by cellular metabolism. The lung eliminates about 10,000 milliequivalents (mEq) of H_2CO_3 per day in the form of CO_2, which is produced at the rate of approximately 200 ml/min. CO_2 is eliminated to maintain a normal arterial CO_2 pressure (Pa_{CO_2}) of 40 mm Hg and normal acid-base balance (see Chapter 5 for a discussion of acid-base regulation). Adequate ventilation is necessary to maintain normal Pa_{CO_2} levels. Diseases that limit the ventilatory rate or tidal volume, or both, decrease ventilation and result in CO_2 retention. The adequacy of alveolar ventilation *cannot* be accurately determined by observation of the ventilatory rate, pattern, or effort. If a healthcare professional needs to determine the adequacy of ventilation, an arterial blood gas analysis or capnography must be performed to determine if there is CO_2 retention.

Neurochemical Control of Ventilation

Breathing is usually involuntary, because homeostatic changes in the ventilatory rate and volume are adjusted automatically by the nervous system to maintain normal gas exchange. Voluntary breathing is necessary for talking, singing, laughing, and deliberately holding one's breath. The mechanisms that control respiration are complex (Fig. 28.8).

The respiratory center in the brainstem controls respiration by transmitting impulses to the respiratory muscles, causing them to contract and relax. The respiratory center is composed of several groups of neurons: the dorsal respiratory group (DRG), the ventral respiratory group (VRG), the pneumotaxic center, and the apneustic center.

The basic automatic rhythm of respiration is set by the DRG, which receives afferent input from peripheral chemoreceptors in the carotid and aortic bodies; from mechanical, neural, and chemical stimuli; and from receptors in the lungs. The VRG contains both inspiratory and expiratory neurons and is almost inactive during normal, quiet respiration, becoming active when increased ventilatory effort is required. The pneumotaxic center and apneustic center, situated in the pons, do not generate primary rhythm but, rather, act as modifiers of the rhythm established by the medullary centers. The pattern of breathing can be influenced by emotion, pain, and disease.

Lung Receptors

Three types of lung receptors send impulses from the lungs to the DRG:
1. Irritant receptors (C fibers) are found in the epithelium of all conducting airways. They are sensitive to noxious aerosols (vapors), gases, and particulate matter (e.g., inhaled dusts), which cause them to initiate the cough reflex. When stimulated, irritant receptors also cause bronchoconstriction and increased ventilatory rate.
2. Stretch receptors are located in the smooth muscles of airways and are sensitive to increases in the size or volume of the lungs. They decrease the ventilatory rate and volume when stimulated, an occurrence sometimes referred to as the *Hering-Breuer expiratory reflex.* This reflex is active in newborns and assists with ventilation. In adults, this reflex is active only at high tidal volumes (e.g., with exercise) and may protect against excess lung inflation. Bronchopulmonary C fibers and a subset of stretch-sensitive, pH-sensitive myelinated sensory nerves mediate the cough reflex.
3. J-receptors (juxtapulmonary capillary receptors) are located near the capillaries in the alveolar septa. They are sensitive to increased pulmonary capillary pressure, which stimulates them to initiate rapid, shallow breathing; hypotension; and bradycardia.

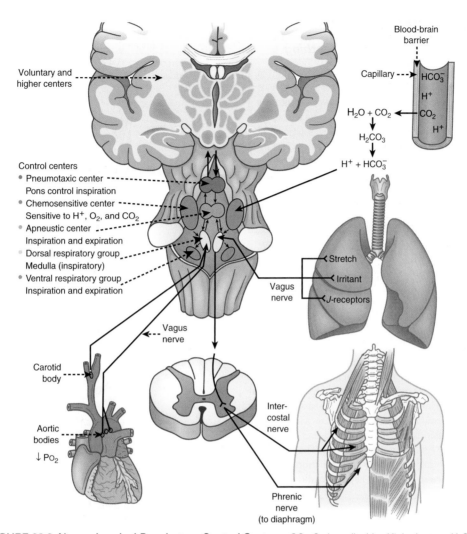

FIGURE 28.8 Neurochemical Respiratory Control System. *CO₂*, Carbon dioxide; *H⁺*, hydrogen; *H₂CO₃*, carbonic acid; *HCO₃⁻*, bicarbonate; *PO₂*, partial pressure of oxygen.

The lung is innervated by the ANS. Fibers of the sympathetic division in the lung branch from the upper thoracic and cervical ganglia of the spinal cord. Fibers of the parasympathetic division of the ANS travel in the vagus nerve to the lung. (The structures and function of the ANS are discussed in detail in Chapter 14.) The parasympathetic and sympathetic divisions control airway caliber (interior diameter of the airway lumen) by stimulating bronchial smooth muscle to contract or relax. The parasympathetic receptors cause smooth muscle to contract, whereas sympathetic receptors cause it to relax. Constriction occurs if the irritant receptors in the airway epithelium are stimulated by irritants in inspired air, by inflammatory mediators (e.g., histamine, serotonin, prostaglandins, leukotrienes), by many drugs, and by humoral substances. Dilation occurs in response to catecholamine release during physiologic stress and in response to medications (e.g., β-agonists) that stimulate sympathetic receptors.

Chemoreceptors

Chemoreceptors monitor the pH, Pa_{CO_2}, and Pa_{O_2} of arterial blood. **Central chemoreceptors** are located near the respiratory center and monitor arterial blood indirectly by sensing changes in the pH of cerebrospinal fluid (CSF) (see Fig. 28.8). As CO_2 accumulates in blood because of decreased ventilation, it diffuses across the blood-brain barrier (the capillary wall separating blood from cells of the central nervous system) into the CSF. CO_2 that has entered the CSF combines with water (H_2O) to form H_2CO_3, which subsequently dissociates into hydrogen ions (H^+) and lowers the pH. As the central chemoreceptors sense the decrease in pH, they stimulate the respiratory center to increase the depth and rate of ventilation. Increased ventilation causes the partial pressure of carbon dioxide (Pa_{CO_2}) in the arterial blood to decrease below that of the CSF, and CO_2 diffuses out of the CSF, returning its pH to normal.

The central chemoreceptors are sensitive to very small changes in the pH of the CSF (equivalent to a 1-2 mm Hg change in P_{CO_2}) and can maintain a normal Pa_{CO_2} under many different conditions, including strenuous exercise. If inadequate ventilation, or hypoventilation, is long term (e.g., in chronic obstructive pulmonary disease), these receptors become insensitive to small changes in Pa_{CO_2} ("reset") and regulate ventilation poorly. In addition, prolonged increases in Pa_{CO_2} result in renal compensation through bicarbonate (HCO_3^-) retention. This HCO_3^- gradually diffuses into the CSF, where it normalizes the pH and limits the effect on ventilatory drive (see *Did You Know?* Changes in the Chemical Control of Breathing).

DID YOU KNOW?

Changes in the Chemical Control of Breathing

There are multiple sites of central carbon dioxide and pH chemosensitivity in the brainstem. It has long been known that chemical control of ventilation is blunted in individuals who have chronic hypercapnia. Newer evidence has demonstrated that decreased sensitivity of the respiratory center also occurs during sleep, congestive heart failure, hypertension, obesity, sudden infant death syndrome, depression, anxiety, and sleep apnea. Proposed mechanisms for these changes in respiratory sensitivity include dysfunction of orexins (neurohormones that control feeding, vigilance, and sleep), altered neurohumoral control of the locus coeruleus, and abnormal gliotransmitters. Changes in the chemical control of breathing may contribute to morbidity and mortality seen in individuals with these disorders.

Data from Eugenin Leòn J, Olivares MJ, Beltrán-Castillo S: *Adv Exp Med Biol* 949:109-145, 2016; Fung ML: *Respir Physiol Neurobiol* 209:6-12, 2015; Hernandez AB, Patil SP: *Sleep Breath* 20(2):467-82, 2016; Lancien M et al: *Sleep Med* 33:57-60, 2017; Pan S et al: *Curr Heart Fail Rep* 14(2):100-105, 2017; Quintero MC, Putnam RW, Cordovez JM: *PLoS Comput Biol* 13(12):e1005853, 2017.

The peripheral chemoreceptors are only somewhat sensitive to changes in pH and instead are sensitive primarily to Pa_{O_2} levels. As the Pa_{O_2} and pH decrease, peripheral chemoreceptors, particularly in the carotid bodies, send signals to the respiratory center to increase ventilation. However, the Pa_{O_2} must drop well below normal (to approximately 60 mm Hg) before the peripheral chemoreceptors have much influence on ventilation. If the pH is decreased as well, ventilation increases much more than it would in response to either abnormality alone. The peripheral chemoreceptors become the major stimulus to ventilation when the central chemoreceptors are reset by chronic hypoventilation.

✔ **QUICK CHECK 28.3**

1. What are the functions of the pulmonary system?
2. How do ventilation and respiration differ?
3. Describe three functions of the respiratory center in the brainstem.
4. What are the three types of lung receptors?
5. How do the functions of central and peripheral chemoreceptors differ?

Mechanics of Breathing

The mechanical aspects of inspiration and expiration are known collectively as the *mechanics of breathing* and involve (1) major and accessory muscles of inspiration and expiration, (2) elastic properties of the lungs and chest wall, and (3) resistance to airflow through the conducting airways. Alterations in any of these properties increase the work of breathing or the metabolic energy needed to achieve adequate ventilation and oxygenation of the blood.

Major and Accessory Muscles

The major muscles of inspiration are the diaphragm and the external intercostal muscles (muscles between the ribs) (Fig. 28.9). The diaphragm is a dome-shaped muscle that separates the abdominal and thoracic cavities. When it contracts and flattens downward, it increases the volume of the thoracic cavity, creating a negative pressure that draws gas into the lungs through the upper airways and trachea. Contraction of the external intercostal muscles elevates the anterior portion of the ribs and increases the volume of the thoracic cavity by increasing its front-to-back (anterior-posterior [AP]) diameter. Although the external intercostals may contract during quiet breathing, inspiration at rest is usually assisted by the diaphragm only.

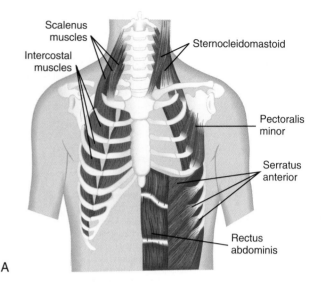

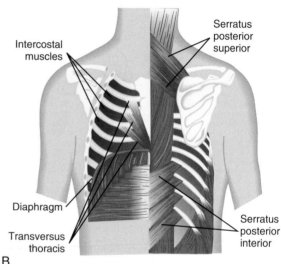

FIGURE 28.9 Muscles of Ventilation. A, Anterior view. **B,** Posterior view. (Modified from Thompson JM et al: *Mosby's clinical nursing,* ed 5, St Louis, 2002, Mosby.)

The accessory muscles of inspiration are the sternocleidomastoid and scalene muscles. Like the external intercostals, these muscles enlarge the thorax by increasing its AP diameter. The accessory muscles assist inspiration when the minute volume (volume of air inspired and expired per minute) is high, as during strenuous exercise, or when the work of breathing is increased because of disease. The accessory muscles do not increase the volume of the thorax as efficiently as the diaphragm does.

There are no major muscles of expiration because normal, relaxed expiration is passive and requires no muscular effort. The accessory muscles of expiration, the abdominal and internal intercostal muscles, assist expiration when minute ventilation is high, during coughing, or when airway obstruction is present. When the abdominal muscles contract, intra-abdominal pressure increases, pushing up the diaphragm and decreasing the volume of the thorax. The internal intercostal muscles pull down the anterior ribs, decreasing the AP diameter of the thorax.

Alveolar Surface Tension

Surface tension occurs at any gas-liquid interface and refers to the tendency for liquid molecules that are exposed to air to adhere to one another. This phenomenon can be seen in the way liquids "bead" when splashed on a waterproof surface.

Within a sphere, such as an alveolus, surface tension tends to make expansion difficult. According to the law of Laplace, the pressure (P) required to inflate a sphere is equal to two times the surface tension (2T) divided by the radius (r) of the sphere, or $P = 2T/r$. As the radius of the sphere (or alveolus) decreases, more and more pressure is required to inflate it. If the alveoli were lined only with a water-like fluid, taking breaths would be extremely difficult.

Alveolar ventilation, or distention, is made possible by surfactant, which lowers surface tension by coating the air-liquid interface in the alveoli. Surfactant, a lipoprotein (90% lipids and 10% protein) produced by type II alveolar cells, includes two groups of *surfactant* proteins. One group consists of small hydrophobic molecules that have a detergent-like effect that separates the liquid molecules, thereby decreasing alveolar surface tension. The decrease in surface tension caused by surfactant also is responsible for keeping the alveoli free of fluid. If surfactant is not produced in adequate quantities, alveolar surface tension increases, causing alveolar collapse, decreased lung expansion, increased work of breathing, and severe gas-exchange abnormalities. The second group of surfactant proteins consists of large hydrophilic molecules called collectins that are capable of inhibiting foreign pathogens (see Chapter 6).

Elastic Properties of the Lung and Chest Wall

The lung and chest wall have elastic properties that permit expansion during inspiration and return to resting volume during expiration. The elasticity of the lung is caused both by elastin fibers in the alveolar walls and surrounding the small airways and pulmonary capillaries, and by surface tension at the alveolar air-liquid interface. The elasticity of the chest wall is the result of the configuration of its bones and musculature.

Elastic recoil is the tendency of the lungs to return to the resting state after inspiration. Normal elastic recoil permits passive expiration, eliminating the need for major muscles of expiration. Passive elastic recoil may be insufficient during labored breathing (high minute ventilation), when the accessory muscles of expiration may be needed. The accessory muscles are used also if disease compromises elastic recoil (e.g., in emphysema) or blocks the conducting airways.

Normal elastic recoil depends on an equilibrium between opposing forces of recoil in the lungs and chest wall. Under normal conditions, the chest wall tends to recoil by expanding outward. The tendency of the chest wall to recoil by expanding is balanced by the tendency of the lungs to recoil or inward collapse around the hila. The opposing forces of the chest wall and lungs create the small negative intrapleural pressure. During inspiration, the diaphragm and intercostal muscles contract, air flows into the lungs, and the chest wall expands. During expiration, the muscles relax and the elastic recoil of the lungs causes the thorax to decrease in volume until a balance between the chest wall and lung recoil forces is reached (Fig. 28.10).

Compliance is the measure of lung and chest wall distensibility and is defined as volume change per unit of pressure change. It represents

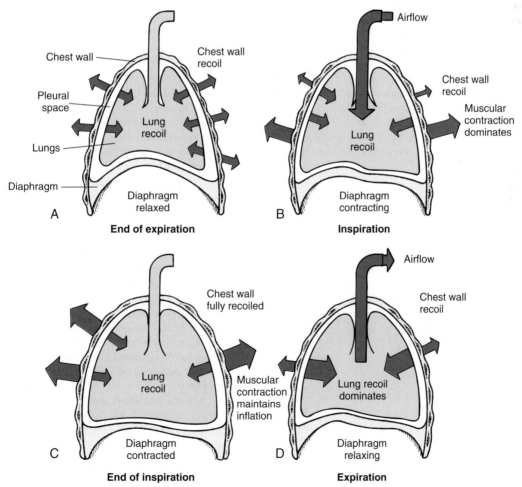

FIGURE 28.10 Interaction of Forces During Inspiration and Expiration. A, Outward recoil of the chest wall equals inward recoil of the lungs at the end of expiration. **B,** During inspiration, contraction of respiratory muscles, assisted by chest wall recoil, overcomes the tendency of lungs to recoil. **C,** At the end of inspiration, respiratory muscle contraction maintains lung expansion. **D,** During expiration, respiratory muscles relax, allowing elastic recoil of the lungs to deflate the lungs.

the relative ease with which these structures can be stretched and is, therefore, the opposite of elasticity. Compliance is determined by the alveolar surface tension and the elastic recoil of the lung and chest wall.

Increased compliance indicates that the lungs or chest wall is abnormally easy to inflate and has lost some elastic recoil. A decrease in compliance indicates that the lungs or chest wall is abnormally stiff or difficult to inflate. Compliance increases with normal aging and with disorders such as emphysema; it decreases in individuals with acute respiratory distress syndrome, pneumonia, pulmonary edema, and fibrosis. (These disorders are described in Chapter 29.)

Airway Resistance

Airway resistance, which is similar to resistance to blood flow (described in Chapter 25), is determined by the length, radius, and cross-sectional area of the airways and by the density, viscosity, and velocity of the gas. One half to two thirds of total airway resistance occurs in the nose. The next highest resistance is in the oropharynx and larynx. There is very little resistance in the conducting airways of the lungs because of their large cross-sectional area. Bronchodilation, which decreases resistance to airflow, is caused by β_2-adrenergic receptor stimulation. Bronchoconstriction, which increases airway resistance, can be caused by the stimulation of parasympathetic receptors in the bronchial smooth muscle and by numerous irritants and inflammatory mediators. Airway resistance can also be increased by edema of the bronchial mucosa and by airway obstructions, such as mucus, tumors, or foreign bodies. Pulmonary function tests (PFTs) measure lung volumes and flow rates and can be used to measure airway resistance and help diagnose certain lung diseases (Fig. 28.11).

Work of Breathing

The work of breathing is determined by the muscular effort (and therefore oxygen and energy) required for ventilation. Normally very low, the work of breathing may increase considerably in diseases that disrupt the equilibrium between forces exerted by the lung and chest wall. More muscular effort is required when lung compliance decreases (e.g., in

pulmonary edema), chest wall compliance decreases (e.g., in spinal deformity or obesity), or airways are obstructed (e.g., in asthma or chronic obstructive pulmonary disease). An increase in the work of breathing can result in a marked increase in O_2 consumption and an inability to maintain adequate tidal volume and minute ventilation.

> ### ✓ QUICK CHECK 28.4
> 1. Describe the work of the diaphragm in ventilation.
> 2. What is surfactant? What is its function?
> 3. How is elastic recoil related to compliance?
> 4. What causes changes in airway resistance?

Gas Transport

Gas transport is the delivery of O_2 to the cells of the body and the removal of CO_2. It has four steps: (1) ventilation of the lungs, (2) diffusion of O_2 from the alveoli into the capillary blood, (3) perfusion of systemic capillaries with oxygenated blood, and (4) diffusion of O_2 from systemic capillaries into the cells. Steps in the transport of CO_2 occur in reverse order: (1) diffusion of CO_2 from the cells into the systemic capillaries, (2) perfusion of the pulmonary capillary bed by venous blood, (3) diffusion of CO_2 into the alveoli, and (4) removal of CO_2 from the lung by ventilation. If any step in gas transport is impaired by a respiratory or cardiovascular disorder, gas exchange at the cellular level is compromised.

Measurement of Gas Pressure

The amount of O_2 that is available for diffusion from the alveoli into the blood is called the $P_{A}O_2$ and is determined by (1) the barometric pressure, (2) water vapor, (3) the fraction of inspired oxygen (FIO_2), and (4) the adequacy of ventilation. At sea level, the barometric pressure (P_B) is 760 mm Hg and is the sum of the pressures exerted by each gas in the air. At sea level the air consists of O_2 (20.9%), nitrogen (78.1%), and a few other trace gases. The **partial pressure** of oxygen (PO_2) is equal to the percentage of O_2 in the air (20.9%) times the total barometric pressure (760 mm Hg at sea level), or 159 mm Hg. At higher elevations, the barometric pressure falls and the amount of gases in the air decreases.

The amount of water vapor contained in a gas mixture is determined by the temperature of the gas and is unrelated to the barometric pressure. Gas that enters the lungs becomes saturated with water vapor (humidified) as it passes through the upper airway. At body temperature (37° C [98.6° F]), water vapor exerts a pressure of 47 mm Hg regardless of the total barometric pressure.

The percentage of O_2 in the inspired air is equal to the PO_2 (20.9%) and is called the **fraction of inspired oxygen (FIO_2)** in room air. The adequacy of ventilation to deliver O_2 to the alveoli cannot be measured directly but can be estimated by measuring the removal of CO_2 from the blood, as calculated by dividing the $PaCO_2$ by the respiratory quotient (0.8).

Thus, in order to calculate the PO_2 available for diffusion into the blood, one must determine the barometric pressure, subtract the water vapor pressure, multiply the result by the FIO_2, and subtract the $PaCO_2$ divided by the respiratory quotient. For example, in saturated air at sea level in an individual with normal ventilation, the PO_2 entering the alveoli and available for gas diffusion into the blood is $(760 - 47) \times (0.209) - (40 \div 0.8) = 99$ mm Hg (Fig. 28.12). All pressure and volume measurements made in pulmonary function laboratories specify the temperature and humidity of a gas at the time of measurement. Symbols used in the measurement of gas pressures and pulmonary ventilation are defined in Table 28.2.

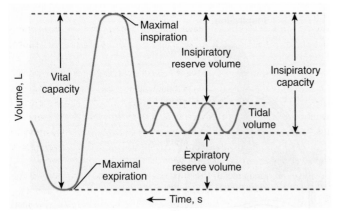

FIGURE 28.11 Pulmonary Ventilation and Lung Volumes. The chart shows a tracing like that produced with a spirometer. During normal, quiet breathing, about 500 ml of air is moved into and out of the respiratory tract (tidal volume). During forceful breathing (such as during and after heavy exercise), an extra 3300 ml can be inspired (inspiratory reserve volume), and an extra 1000 ml or so can be expired (expiratory reserve volume). The largest volume of air that can be moved in and out during ventilation is called the vital capacity (VC). (Modified from Patton KT, Thibodeau GA: *The human body in health & disease,* ed 4, St Louis, 2010, Mosby.)

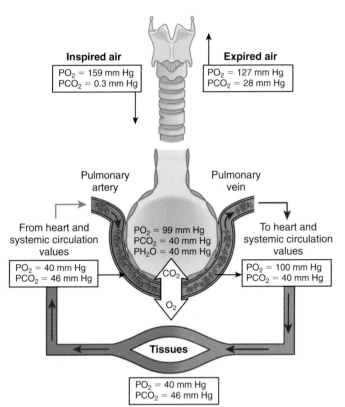

FIGURE 28.12 Partial Pressure of Respiratory Gases in Normal Respiration. The numbers shown are average values near sea level. (Modified from Thompson JM et al: *Mosby's clinical nursing*, ed 5, St Louis, 2002, Mosby.)

TABLE 28.2   Common Pulmonary Abbreviations

Symbol	Definition
V	Volume or amount of gas
Q	Perfusion or blood flow
P	Pressure (usually partial pressure) of a gas
Pao_2	Partial pressure of oxygen in arterial blood
$P_{A}o_2$	Partial pressure of oxygen in alveolar gas
$Paco_2$	Partial pressure of carbon dioxide in arterial blood
Pvo_2	Partial pressure of oxygen in mixed venous or pulmonary artery blood
$P(A-a)o_2$	Difference between alveolar and arterial partial pressure of oxygen (A–a gradient)
P_B	Barometric or atmospheric pressure
Sao_2	Saturation of hemoglobin (in arterial blood) with oxygen
Svo_2	Saturation of hemoglobin (in mixed venous blood) with oxygen
V_A	Alveolar ventilation
V_D	Dead-space ventilation
$\dot{V}$	Minute volume
V_T	Tidal volume or average breath
$\dot{V}/\dot{Q}$*	Ratio of ventilation to perfusion
Fio_2	Fraction of inspired oxygen
FRC	Functional residual capacity
FVC	Forced vital capacity
FEV_1	Forced expiratory volume in 1 second

*An overhead dot means measurement over time, usually 1 minute.

Distribution of Ventilation and Perfusion

Effective gas exchange depends on an approximately even distribution of gas (ventilation) and blood (perfusion) in all portions of the lungs. The lungs are suspended from the hila in the thoracic cavity. When an individual is in an upright position (sitting or standing), gravity pulls the lungs down toward the diaphragm and compresses their lower portions, or bases. The alveoli in the upper portions, or apices, of the lungs contain a greater residual volume of gas and are larger and less numerous than those in the lower portions. Because surface tension increases as the alveoli become larger, the larger alveoli in the upper portions of the lung are more difficult to inflate (less compliant) than the smaller alveoli in the lower portions of the lung. Therefore, during ventilation most of the tidal volume is distributed to the bases of the lungs, where compliance is greater.

The heart pumps against gravity to perfuse the pulmonary circulation. As blood is pumped into the lung apices of a sitting or standing individual, some blood pressure is dissipated in overcoming gravity. As a result, blood pressure at the apices is lower than that at the bases. Because greater pressure causes greater perfusion, the bases of the lungs are better perfused than the apices (Fig. 28.13). Thus, ventilation and perfusion are greatest in the same lung portions—the lower lobes—and depend on body position. If a standing individual assumes a supine or side-lying position, the areas of the lungs that are then most dependent become the best ventilated and perfused.

The distribution of perfusion in the pulmonary circulation also is affected by the alveolar pressure (gas pressure in the alveoli). The pulmonary capillary bed differs from the systemic capillary bed in that it is surrounded by gas-containing alveoli. If the gas pressure in the alveoli exceeds the blood pressure in the capillary, the capillary collapses and flow ceases. This is most likely to occur in portions of the lung where blood pressure is lowest and alveolar gas pressure is greatest—that is, at the apex of the lung.

The lungs are divided into three zones on the basis of relationships among all the factors affecting pulmonary blood flow. Alveolar pressure and the forces of gravity, arterial blood pressure, and venous blood pressure affect the distribution of perfusion, as shown in Fig. 28.14.

In zone I, the alveolar pressure exceeds the pulmonary arterial and venous pressures. The capillary bed collapses, and normal blood flow ceases. Normally zone I is a very small part of the lung at the apex. In zone II, the alveolar pressure is greater than the venous pressure but not the arterial pressure. Blood flows through zone II, but it is impeded to a certain extent by the alveolar pressure. Zone II is normally above the level of the left atrium. In zone III, both the arterial and venous pressures are greater than the alveolar pressure, and blood flow is not affected by the alveolar pressure. Zone III is in the base of the lung. Blood flow through the pulmonary capillary bed increases in regular increments from the apex to the base.

Although both blood flow and ventilation are greater at the base of the lungs than at the apices, they are not perfectly matched in any zone. Perfusion exceeds ventilation in the bases, and ventilation exceeds perfusion in the apices of the lung. The relationship between ventilation and perfusion is expressed as a ratio called the **ventilation-perfusion ratio** ($\dot{V}/\dot{Q}$). The normal $\dot{V}/\dot{Q}$ is called the respiratory quotient and is 0.8. This is the amount by which perfusion exceeds ventilation under normal conditions.

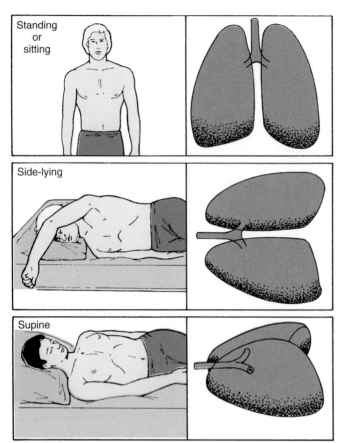

FIGURE 28.13 Pulmonary Blood Flow and Gravity. The greatest volume of pulmonary blood flow normally will occur in the gravity-dependent areas of the lung. Body position has a significant effect on the distribution of pulmonary blood flow. The shaded areas represent gravity-dependent pulmonary blood flow.

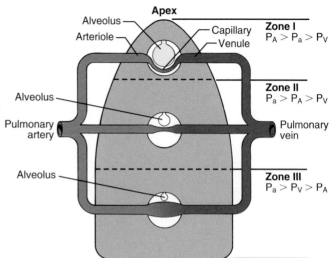

FIGURE 28.14 Gravity and Alveolar Pressure. Effects of gravity and alveolar pressure on pulmonary blood flow in the three lung zones. In zone I, the alveolar pressure (P_A) is greater than the arterial pressure (P_a) and the venous pressure (P_V), and no blood flow occurs. In zone II, the P_a exceeds the P_A, but the P_A exceeds the P_V. Blood flow occurs in this zone, but the P_A compresses the venules (venous ends of the capillaries). In zone III, both the P_a and P_V are greater than the P_A, and blood flow fluctuates, depending on the difference between the P_A arterial pressure and the P_V.

Oxygen Transport

Approximately 1000 ml (1 L) of O_2 is transported to the cells of the body each minute. O_2 is transported in the blood in two forms: a small amount dissolves in plasma, and the remainder binds to hemoglobin molecules. Without hemoglobin, O_2 would not reach the cells in amounts sufficient to maintain normal metabolic function. (Hemoglobin is discussed in detail in Chapter 22, and cellular metabolism is explored in Chapter 1.)

Diffusion across the alveolocapillary membrane. The alveolocapillary membrane is ideal for O_2 diffusion because it has a large total surface area (70-100 m²) and is very thin (0.5 micrometer [μm]). In addition, the P_{AO_2} (approximately 99 mm Hg at sea level) is much greater than that in capillary blood (approximately 40 mm Hg), a condition that promotes rapid diffusion down the concentration gradient from the alveolus into the capillary. Therefore, a pressure gradient of nearly 60 mm Hg facilitates the diffusion of O_2 from the alveolus into the capillary (see Fig. 28.12).

Blood remains in the pulmonary capillary for about 0.75 second, but only 0.25 second is required for the O_2 concentration to equilibrate (equalize) across the alveolocapillary membrane. Therefore, O_2 has ample time to diffuse into the blood, even during increased cardiac output, which speeds blood flow and shortens the time the blood remains in the capillary.

Determinants of arterial oxygenation. As O_2 diffuses across the alveolocapillary membrane, it dissolves in the plasma, where it exerts pressure (Pao_2). As the Pao_2 increases, O_2 moves from the plasma into the red blood cells (erythrocytes) and binds with hemoglobin molecules. O_2 continues to bind with hemoglobin until the hemoglobin-binding sites are filled, or *saturated*. O_2 then continues to diffuse across the alveolocapillary membrane until the Pao_2 (oxygen dissolved in plasma) and P_{AO_2} (oxygen in the alveolus) equilibrate, eliminating the pressure gradient across the alveolocapillary membrane. At this point, diffusion ceases (see Fig. 28.12).

The majority (97%) of the O_2 that enters the blood is bound to hemoglobin. The remaining 3% stays in the plasma and creates the Pao_2. The Pao_2 can be measured in the blood by obtaining an arterial blood gas measurement. The oxygen saturation (Sao_2) is the percentage of the available hemoglobin that is bound to O_2 and can be measured using a device called an *oximeter*.

Because hemoglobin transports all but a small fraction of the O_2 carried in arterial blood, changes in the hemoglobin concentration affect the O_2 content of the blood. Decreases in the hemoglobin concentration below the normal value of 15 g/dl of blood reduce the O_2 content, and increases in the hemoglobin concentration may increase O_2 content. An increased hemoglobin concentration is a major compensatory mechanism in pulmonary diseases that impair gas exchange. For this reason, measurement of the hemoglobin concentration is important in assessing individuals with pulmonary disease. If cardiovascular function is normal, the body's initial response to low O_2 content is to accelerate cardiac output. In individuals who also have cardiovascular disease, this compensatory mechanism is ineffective, making an increased hemoglobin concentration an even more important compensatory mechanism. (Hemoglobin structure and function are described in Chapter 22.)

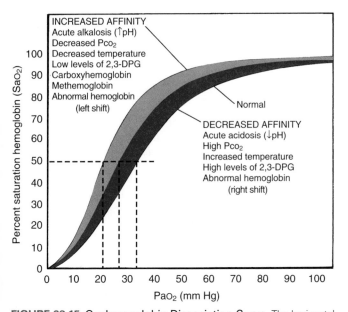

FIGURE 28.15 Oxyhemoglobin Dissociation Curve. The horizontal or flat segment of the curve at the top of the graph is the arterial or association portion, or that part of the curve where oxygen (O_2) is bound to hemoglobin and occurs in the lungs. This portion of the curve is flat because partial pressure changes of O_2 between 60 and 100 mm Hg do not significantly alter the percentage saturation of hemoglobin with O_2 and allow adequate hemoglobin saturation at a variety of altitudes. If the relationship between the oxygen saturation of hemoglobin in arterial blood (SaO_2) and the partial pressure of oxygen in the arterial blood (PaO_2) were linear (in a downward sloping straight line) instead of flat between 60 and 100 mm Hg, there would be inadequate saturation of hemoglobin with O_2. The steep part of the oxyhemoglobin dissociation curve represents the rapid dissociation of O_2 from hemoglobin that occurs in the tissues. During this phase there is rapid diffusion of O_2 from the blood into tissue cells. The P_{50} is the PaO_2 at which hemoglobin is 50% saturated, normally 26.6 mm Hg. A lower than normal P_{50} represents increased affinity of hemoglobin for O_2; a high P_{50} is seen with decreased affinity. Note that variation from the normal is associated with decreased (low P_{50}) or increased (high P_{50}) availability of O_2 to tissues (dashed lines). The shaded area shows the entire oxyhemoglobin dissociation curve under the same circumstances. 2,3-DPG, 2,3-Diphosphoglycerate; PaO_2, arterial pressure of oxygen; PCO_2, partial pressure of carbon dioxide. (From Lane EE, Walker JF: Clinical arterial blood gas analysis, St Louis, 1987, Mosby.)

Oxyhemoglobin association and dissociation. When hemoglobin molecules bind with O_2, oxyhemoglobin (HbO_2) forms. Binding occurs in the lungs and is called *oxyhemoglobin association* or *hemoglobin saturation with oxygen* (SaO_2). The reverse process, in which O_2 is released from hemoglobin, occurs in the body tissues at the cellular level and is called *hemoglobin desaturation*. When hemoglobin saturation and desaturation are plotted on a graph, the result is a distinctive S-shaped curve known as the oxyhemoglobin dissociation curve (Fig. 28.15).

Several factors can change the relationship between the PaO_2 and the SaO_2, causing the oxyhemoglobin dissociation curve to shift to the right or left (see Fig. 28.15). A shift to the right depicts hemoglobin's decreased affinity for O_2 or an increase in the ease with which oxyhemoglobin dissociates and O_2 moves into the cells.

A shift to the left depicts hemoglobin's increased affinity for O_2, which promotes association in the lungs and inhibits dissociation in the tissues.

The oxyhemoglobin dissociation curve is shifted to the right by acidosis (low pH) and hypercapnia (increased $PaCO_2$). In the tissues, the increased levels of CO_2 and H^+ produced by metabolic activity decrease the affinity of hemoglobin for O_2, and O_2 is released into the tissues. The curve is shifted to the left by alkalosis (high pH) and hypocapnia (decreased $PaCO_2$). In the lungs, as CO_2 diffuses from the blood into the alveoli, the blood CO_2 level is reduced and the affinity of hemoglobin for O_2 is increased so that more O_2 can be transported from the lungs into the tissues. The shift in the oxyhemoglobin dissociation curve caused by changes in the CO_2 and hydrogen ion concentrations in the blood is called the Bohr effect.

The oxyhemoglobin curve is also shifted by changes in body temperature and increased or decreased levels of 2,3-diphosphoglycerate (2,3-DPG), a substance normally present in erythrocytes. Hyperthermia and increased 2,3-DPG levels shift the curve to the right so that more O_2 is released into the tissues. Hypothermia and decreased 2,3-DPG levels shift the curve to the left.

Carbon Dioxide Transport

CO_2 is 20 times more soluble than O_2 and diffuses quickly from the tissue cells into the blood. As CO_2 diffuses out of the cells into the blood, it dissolves in the plasma. CO_2 is carried in the venous blood ($P_{V}CO_2$) and the arterial blood ($PaCO_2$) in three ways: (1) dissolved in plasma (PCO_2), (2) as bicarbonate (HCO_3^-), and (3) as carbamino compounds. The amount of CO_2 able to enter the blood is enhanced by the diffusion of O_2 out of the blood and into the cells. Reduced hemoglobin (hemoglobin that is dissociated from O_2) can carry more CO_2 than can hemoglobin saturated with O_2. Therefore, the drop in O_2 saturation at the tissue level increases the ability of hemoglobin to carry CO_2 back to the lung.

The diffusion gradient for CO_2 in the lung is only approximately 6 mm Hg ($P_{V}CO_2$ = 46 mm Hg; $P_{A}CO_2$ = 40 mm Hg) (see Fig. 28.12). Yet CO_2 is so soluble in the alveolocapillary membrane that the CO_2 in the blood quickly diffuses into the alveoli, where it is removed from the lung with each expiration. Diffusion of CO_2 in the lung is so efficient that diffusion defects that cause hypoxemia (low O_2 content of the blood) do not as readily cause hypercapnia (excessive CO_2 in the blood).

The diffusion of CO_2 out of the blood and into the lungs also is enhanced by O_2 binding with hemoglobin. As hemoglobin binds with O_2, the amount of CO_2 carried by the blood decreases and it is released into the alveoli. Thus, in the tissue capillaries, O_2 dissociation from hemoglobin facilitates the pickup of CO_2, and the binding of O_2 to hemoglobin in the lungs facilitates the release of CO_2 from the blood. This effect of O_2 on CO_2 transport is called the Haldane effect.

✔ QUICK CHECK 28.5

1. What are the eight steps of gas transport?
2. Describe the relationship between ventilation and pulmonary blood flow.
3. What is the alveolocapillary membrane? How does it function in ventilation and perfusion?
4. Describe the process of oxyhemoglobin association and dissociation.
5. What is barometric pressure? How is it related to physiologic pressure measurements?

GERIATRIC CONSIDERATIONS

Aging and the Pulmonary System

Elasticity/Chest Wall

Chest wall compliance decreases because ribs become ossified and joints are stiffer, which results in increased work of breathing.

Kyphoscoliosis may curve the vertebral column, decreasing lung volumes.

Intercostal muscle strength decreases.

Elastic recoil diminishes, possibly the result of loss of elastic fibers.

Result: Lung compliance increases and ventilatory capacity (VC) declines, residual volume (RV) increases, total lung capacity (TLC) is unchanged, ventilatory reserves decline, and ventilation-perfusion ratios fall.

Gas Exchange

Pulmonary capillary network decreases.

Alveoli dilate, and peripheral airways lose supporting tissues.

Surface area for gas exchange decreases.

pH and the partial pressure of carbon dioxide (Pco_2) do not change much, but the partial pressure of oxygen (Po_2) declines.

Sensitivity of respiratory centers to hypoxia or hypercapnia decreases.

Ability to initiate an immune response against infection decreases.

Note: The maximum partial pressure of oxygen in arterial blood (Pao_2) at sea level can be estimated by multiplying the person's age by 0.3 and subtracting the product from 100.

Exercise

Decreased Pao_2 and diminished ventilatory reserve lead to decreased exercise tolerance.

Early airway closure inhibits expiratory flow.

Changes depend on activity and fitness levels earlier in life.

An active, physically fit individual has fewer changes in function at any age than does a sedentary individual.

Respiratory muscle strength and endurance decrease but can be enhanced by exercise.

Lung Immunity

Alterations in alveolar complement and surfactant and an increase in proinflammatory cytokines increase the risk for pulmonary disease and infection.

NORMAL LUNG **AGING LUNG**

Inspiratory reserve volume

Tidal volume

Expiratory reserve volume

Residual volume

Total lung capacity

Vital capacity

Changes in Lung Volumes With Aging. With aging, note particularly the decreased vital capacity and the increase in residual volume.

Data from Carpagnano GE et al: *Aging Clin Exp Res* 25(3):239-245, 2013; Kim J et al: *PLoS ONE* 12(8): e0183654, 2017; Lalley PM: *Respir Physiol Neurobiol* 187(3):199-210, 2013; Lowery EM et al: *Clin Interv Aging* 8:1489-1496, 2013; Moliva JI et al: *Age (Dordr)* 36(3):9633, 2014; Ramly E et al: *Surg Clin North Am* 95(1):53-69, 2015; Skloot GS: *Clin Geriatr Med* 33(4):447-457, 2017.

SUMMARY REVIEW

Structures of the Pulmonary System

1. The pulmonary system consists of the lungs, upper and lower airways, chest wall, and pulmonary and bronchial circulation.

2. Air is inspired and expired through the conducting airways: nasopharynx, oropharynx, trachea, bronchi, and bronchioles.

3. Gas exchange occurs in structures beyond the respiratory bronchioles: in the alveolar ducts and the alveoli. Together these structures compose the acinus.

4. The chief gas-exchange units of the lungs are the alveoli. The membrane that surrounds each alveolus and contains the pulmonary capillaries is called the alveolocapillary membrane.

5. The gas-exchange airways are perfused by the pulmonary circulation, a separate division of the circulatory system. The bronchi and other lung structures are perfused by a branch of the systemic circulation called the bronchial circulation.

6. The pulmonary circulation is innervated by the autonomic nervous system (ANS), but vasodilation and vasoconstriction are controlled mainly by local and humoral factors, particularly arterial oxygenation and acid-base status.

7. The chest wall, which contains and protects the contents of the thoracic cavity, consists of the skin, ribs, and intercostal muscles, which lie between the ribs.

8. The chest wall is lined by a serous membrane called the parietal pleura; the lungs are encased in a separate membrane called the visceral pleura. The pleural space is the area where these two pleurae contact and slide over one another.

Function of the Pulmonary System

1. The pulmonary system (1) ventilates the alveoli, (2) diffuses gases into and out of the blood, and (3) perfuses the lungs so that the organs and tissues of the body receive blood that is rich in oxygen and deficient in carbon dioxide.

2. Ventilation is the process by which air flows into and out of the gas-exchange airways.

3. Most of the time, ventilation is involuntary. It is controlled by the sympathetic and parasympathetic divisions of the autonomic nervous system, which adjust airway caliber (by causing bronchial smooth muscle to contract or relax) and control the rate and depth of ventilation.

4. Neuroreceptors in the lungs (lung receptors) monitor the mechanical aspects of ventilation. Irritant receptors sense the need to expel unwanted substances, stretch receptors sense lung volume (lung expansion), and J-receptors sense pulmonary capillary pressure.

5. Chemoreceptors in the circulatory system and brainstem sense the effectiveness of ventilation by monitoring the pH status of cerebrospinal fluid and the oxygen content (PO_2) of arterial blood.

6. Successful ventilation involves the mechanics of breathing: the interaction of forces and counterforces involving the muscles of inspiration and expiration, alveolar surface tension, elastic properties of the lungs and chest wall, and resistance to airflow.

7. The major muscle of inspiration is the diaphragm. When the diaphragm contracts, it moves downward in the thoracic cavity, creating a vacuum that causes air to flow into the lungs.

8. The type II alveolar cells produce surfactant, a lipoprotein that lines the alveoli. Surfactant reduces alveolar surface tension and permits the alveoli to expand as air enters.

9. Elastic recoil is the tendency of the lungs and chest wall to return to their resting state after inspiration. The elastic recoil forces of the lungs and chest wall are in opposition and pull on each other, creating the normally negative pressure of the pleural space.

10. Compliance is the ease with which the lungs and chest wall expand during inspiration. Lung compliance is ensured by an adequate production of surfactant, whereas chest wall expansion depends on elasticity.

11. The work of breathing is determined by the muscular effort required for ventilation and is normally very low. Work increases when lung or chest wall compliance decreases or airways are obstructed.

12. Gas transport depends on ventilation of the lungs, diffusion of oxygen across the alveolocapillary membrane, perfusion of systemic capillaries with oxygenated blood, and diffusion between systemic capillaries and tissue cells.

13. Efficient gas exchange depends on an even distribution of ventilation (gas) and perfusion (blood) within the lungs. Both ventilation and perfusion are greatest in the bases of the lungs because the alveoli in the bases are more compliant (their resting volume is low) and perfusion is greater in the bases as a result of gravity.

14. Almost all the oxygen that diffuses into pulmonary capillary blood is transported by hemoglobin, a protein contained within red blood cells. The remainder of the oxygen is transported dissolved in plasma.

15. Oxygen enters the body by diffusing down the concentration gradient, from high concentrations in the alveoli to lower concentrations in the capillaries. Diffusion ceases when alveolar and capillary oxygen pressures equilibrate.

16. Oxygen is loaded onto hemoglobin by the driving pressure exerted by Pao_2 in the plasma. As pressure decreases at the tissue level, oxygen dissociates from hemoglobin and enters tissue cells by diffusion, again down the concentration gradient.

17. Compared with oxygen, carbon dioxide is more soluble in plasma. Therefore carbon dioxide diffuses readily from tissue cells into plasma and from plasma into the alveoli. Carbon dioxide returns to the lungs dissolved in plasma, as bicarbonate, or in carbamino compounds (e.g., bound to hemoglobin).

Geriatric Considerations: Aging and the Pulmonary System

1. Aging affects the mechanical aspects of ventilation by decreasing chest wall compliance and elastic recoil of the lungs. Changes in these elastic properties reduce the ventilatory reserve.

2. With aging, the surface area for gas exchange and capillary perfusion may decrease, reducing exercise capacity.

3. Level of fitness and associated systemic disease affect individual lung function.

KEY TERMS

Acinus, 656
Alveolar duct, 656
Alveolar ventilation, 660
Alveolocapillary membrane, 658
Alveolus (pl., alveoli), 656, 656
Bohr effect, 667
Bronchus (pl., bronchi), 655, 655
Carina, 655
Central chemoreceptor, 664
Collectin, 663
Compliance, 663
Dead-space ventilation (V_D), 660

Effective ventilation, 660
Elastic recoil, 663
Fraction of inspired oxygen (FIO_2), 664
Goblet cell, 656
Haldane effect, 667
Hilum (pl., hila), 655, 655
Hypoxic pulmonary vasoconstriction, 659
Irritant receptor, 660
J-receptor, 660
Larynx, 655
Mediastinum, 655

Minute volume (minute ventilation), 660, 660
Nasopharynx, 655
Oropharynx, 655
Oxygen saturation (Sao_2), 666
Oxyhemoglobin (HbO_2), 667
Oxyhemoglobin dissociation curve, 667
Partial pressure, 664
Peripheral chemoreceptor, 662
Pleura (pl., pleurae), 659
Pleural space (pleural cavity), 660, 660

Respiratory bronchiole, 656
Respiratory center, 660
Stretch receptor, 660
Surface tension, 662
Surfactant, 663
Thoracic cavity, 659
Trachea, 655
Ventilation, 660
Ventilation-perfusion ratio ($\dot{V}/\dot{Q}$), 665

REFERENCES

1. Chaudhry R, et al: *Lungs, StatPearls [Internet]*, Treasure Island (FL), 2018, StatPearls Publishing. Available from: http://www.ncbi.nlm.nih.gov/books/NBK470197/.
2. Ball M, Bhimji SS: *Anatomy, airway, StatPearls [Internet]*, Treasure Island (FL), 2018, StatPearls Publishing. Available from: http://www.ncbi.nlm.nih.gov/books/NBK459258/.
3. Hsia CC, Hyde DM, Weibel ER: Lung structure and the intrinsic challenges of gas exchange, *Compr Physiol* 6(2):827-895, 2016.
4. Suresh K, Shimoda LA: Lung circulation, *Compr Physiol* 6(2):897-943, 2016.
5. Brinkman JE, Sharma S: *Physiology, pulmonary, StatPearls [Internet]*, Treasure Island (FL), 2018, StatPearls Publishing. Available from: http://www.ncbi.nlm.nih.gov/books/NBK482426/.
6. Intagliata S, Rizzo A: *Physiology, lung, dead space, StatPearls [Internet]*, Treasure Island (FL), 2018, StatPearls Publishing. Available from: http://www.ncbi.nlm.nih.gov/books/NBK482501/.

29

Alterations of Pulmonary Function

Valentina L. Brashers, Sue E. Huether

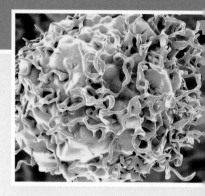

EVOLVE WEBSITE

http://evolve.elsevier.com/Huether/
Student Review Questions
Audio Key Points

Case Studies
Animations
Quick Check Answers

CHAPTER OUTLINE

Pulmonary disease is often classified as acute or chronic, obstructive or restrictive, infectious or noninfectious, and malignant or benign. Symptoms of lung disease are common and associated not only with primary lung disorders, but also with diseases of other organ systems, particularly the heart.

CLINICAL MANIFESTATIONS OF PULMONARY ALTERATIONS

Signs and Symptoms of Pulmonary Disease

Pulmonary disease is associated with many signs and symptoms, the most common of which are dyspnea and cough. Others include abnormal sputum, hemoptysis, altered breathing patterns, hypoventilation and hyperventilation, cyanosis, clubbing, and chest pain.

Dyspnea

Dyspnea is a subjective experience of breathing discomfort. It is often described as breathlessness, air hunger, shortness of breath, labored breathing, and preoccupation with breathing. Dyspnea may be the result of pulmonary disease or many other conditions, such as pain, heart disease, trauma, and anxiety.[1]

Dyspnea derives from interactions among multiple physiologic, psychological, social, and environmental factors. The severity of the experience of dyspnea may not directly correlate with the severity of underlying disease. Either diffuse or focal damage to lung tissue (lung parenchyma) or disturbances of ventilation can cause dyspnea. Stimulation of many receptors can contribute to the sensation of dyspnea, including afferent receptors in the brain and brainstem, mechanoreceptors in the chest wall and upper airway, and central and peripheral chemoreceptors that sense the effectiveness of gas exchange. Dyspnea also may be caused by a real or perceived increased work (effort) needed to breathe, which can be caused by stiffness of the lungs or pleura, weakness or stiffness of the thoracic musculoskeletal system, or anxiety.

The more severe signs of dyspnea include flaring of the nostrils and use of accessory muscles of respiration. Retraction (pulling back) of the supracostal or intercostal muscles may occur in children but is uncommon in adults. Dyspnea can be quantified by asking the individual to rate the level of dyspnea using an ordinal or visual analog scale.

Dyspnea may occur transiently or can become chronic. Dyspnea often first presents during exercise and is called *dyspnea on exertion*. Orthopnea is dyspnea that occurs when an individual lies flat, which causes the abdominal contents to exert pressure on the diaphragm. Paroxysmal nocturnal dyspnea (PND) occurs when individuals with pulmonary or cardiac disease awake at night, gasping for air, and have to sit or stand to relieve the dyspnea. Dyspnea may be unrecognized in mechanically ventilated individuals and is often accompanied by pain and anxiety.

Cough

Cough is a protective reflex that helps clear the airways by an explosive expiration. Inhaled particles, accumulated mucus, inflammation, or the presence of a foreign body initiates the cough reflex by stimulating the irritant receptors in the airway. There are few such receptors in the most distal bronchi and the alveoli; thus it is possible for significant amounts of secretions to accumulate in the distal respiratory tree without cough being initiated. The cough reflex consists of inspiration, closure of the glottis and vocal cords, contraction of the expiratory muscles, and reopening of the glottis, causing a sudden, forceful expiration that removes the offending matter. The effectiveness of the cough depends on the strength of the respiratory muscles, which affects the depth of the inspiration. Those with an inability to cough effectively are at greater risk for pneumonia.

Acute cough is cough that resolves within 2 to 3 weeks of the onset of illness or resolves with treatment of the underlying condition. It can be caused by any upper or lower respiratory disease. It is most commonly the result of upper respiratory tract infections, allergic rhinitis, acute bronchitis, pneumonia, congestive heart failure, pulmonary embolus, or aspiration. *Chronic cough* is defined as cough that is persistent. In individuals who do not smoke, chronic cough is commonly caused or triggered by postnasal drainage, asthma, bronchitis or bronchiectasis, the use of angiotensin-converting enzyme inhibitors, and gastroesophageal reflux disease (or there may be no identifiable underlying cause).[2] In persons who smoke, chronic bronchitis is the most common cause of chronic cough, although lung cancer must always be considered.

Abnormal Sputum

Changes in the amount, color, and consistency of sputum provide information about the cause and progression of disease and the effectiveness of therapy. Expectorated sputum may look clear, foamy, purulent (puslike), or bloody. The gross and microscopic appearances of sputum enable the clinician to identify cellular debris or microorganisms, which aids in diagnosis and choice of therapy.

Hemoptysis

Hemoptysis is the coughing up of blood or bloody secretions. This is sometimes confused with hematemesis, which is the vomiting of blood. Blood produced with coughing is usually bright red, has an alkaline pH, and is mixed with frothy sputum. Blood that is vomited is dark, has an acidic pH, and is mixed with food particles.

Hemoptysis usually indicates infection or inflammation that damages the bronchi (bronchitis, bronchiectasis) or the lung parenchyma (pneumonia, tuberculosis, lung abscess). Other causes include cancer or pulmonary embolism. The amount and duration of bleeding provide important clues about its source. Chest imaging, often combined with bronchoscopy, is used to confirm the site of bleeding.

Abnormal Breathing Patterns

Normal breathing (eupnea) is rhythmic and effortless. In the adult, the resting ventilatory rate is 8 to 16 breaths per minute, and tidal volume ranges from 400 to 800 ml with occasional deeper breaths or sighs. Sigh breaths, which help to maintain normal lung function, are usually 1.5 to 2 times the normal tidal volume and occur approximately 10 to 12 times per hour.

The rate, depth, regularity, and effort of breathing undergo characteristic alterations in response to physiologic and pathophysiologic conditions. Patterns of breathing automatically adjust to minimize the work of respiratory muscles. Strenuous exercise or metabolic acidosis induces Kussmaul respiration (hyperpnea), which is characterized by a slightly increased ventilatory rate and very large tidal volumes.

Labored breathing occurs whenever there is an increased work of breathing, especially if the airways are obstructed. In large airway obstruction, a slow ventilatory rate, large tidal volume, increased effort, prolonged inspiration and expiration, and stridor or audible wheezing (depending on the site of obstruction) are typical. In small airway obstruction, such as that seen in asthma and chronic obstructive pulmonary disease, a rapid ventilatory rate, small tidal volume, increased effort, prolonged expiration, and wheezing are often present. *Restricted breathing* is commonly caused by disorders, such as pulmonary fibrosis, that stiffen the lungs or chest wall and decrease compliance, resulting in small tidal volumes and a rapid ventilatory rate (tachypnea).

Shock and severe cerebral hypoxia (insufficient oxygen in the brain) contribute to gasping respirations that consist of irregular, quick inspirations with an expiratory pause. Cheyne-Stokes respirations are characterized by alternating periods of deep and shallow breathing. Apnea lasting from 15 to 60 seconds is followed by ventilations that increase in volume until a peak is reached; then ventilation (tidal volume) decreases again to apnea. Cheyne-Stokes respirations result from any condition that reduces blood flow to the brainstem, which in turn slows impulses sending information to the respiratory centers of the brainstem. Neurologic impairment above the brainstem is also a contributing factor. Anxiety can cause sighing respirations, which consist of irregular breathing characterized by frequent, deep sighing inspirations.

Hypoventilation and Hyperventilation

Hypoventilation is inadequate alveolar ventilation in relation to metabolic demands. Hypoventilation occurs when minute ventilation (respiratory rate × tidal volume) is reduced. It is caused by alterations in the drive to breathe (neurologic control) or the ability to respond to that drive (pulmonary mechanics). When alveolar ventilation is normal, carbon dioxide (CO_2) is removed from the lungs at the same rate as it is produced by cellular metabolism; the arterial CO_2 pressure (Pa_{CO_2}) and alveolar CO_2 pressure ($P_{A_{CO_2}}$) values remain at normal levels. With hypoventilation, CO_2 removal does not keep up with CO_2 production, and the Pa_{CO_2} increases, causing hypercapnia (Pa_{CO_2} >44 mm Hg) (see Table 28.2 for a definition of gas partial pressures and other pulmonary abbreviations). This results in a fall in the pH of the blood (respiratory acidosis) that can affect the function of many tissues throughout the body. Hypoventilation is often overlooked until it is severe because the breathing pattern and ventilatory rate may appear to be normal, and changes in the tidal volume can be difficult to detect clinically. Measurement of the Pa_{CO_2} (i.e., blood gas analysis) or in the inspired and expired air (capnography) reveals the hypoventilation. Severe hypoventilation can cause secondary hypoxemia, somnolence, and disorientation.

Hyperventilation is alveolar ventilation exceeding metabolic demands. The lungs remove CO_2 faster than it is produced by cellular metabolism, resulting in a decreased Pa_{CO_2}, or hypocapnia (Pa_{CO_2} <36 mm Hg). Hypocapnia results in an increase in the pH of the blood (respiratory alkalosis) that can interfere with tissue function. Hyperventilation commonly occurs with severe anxiety, acute head injury, pain, and in response to conditions that affect the lung and chest wall, especially those that cause hypoxemia. Like hypoventilation, hyperventilation can be determined by arterial blood gas analysis.

Cyanosis

Cyanosis is a bluish discoloration of the skin and mucous membranes caused by increasing amounts of desaturated or reduced hemoglobin (which is bluish) in the blood. *Peripheral cyanosis* (slow blood circulation in the fingers and toes) is most often caused by poor circulation resulting from heart disease, intense peripheral vasoconstriction (such as that observed in persons who have Raynaud disease), or cold environments. Peripheral cyanosis is best seen in the nail beds. *Central cyanosis* is caused by decreased arterial oxygenation (low Pa_{O_2}) from decreased inspired oxygen (e.g., at high altitudes), central nervous system disorders that affect respiration, pulmonary diseases, or cardiac diseases. Central cyanosis is best detected in the buccal mucous membranes and lips.

Lack of cyanosis does not necessarily indicate that oxygenation is normal. In adults, cyanosis is not evident until severe hypoxemia is present and, therefore, is an insensitive indicator of respiratory failure. Severe anemia (inadequate hemoglobin concentration) and carbon monoxide poisoning (in which hemoglobin binds to carbon monoxide instead of to oxygen) can cause inadequate oxygenation of tissues without causing cyanosis. Individuals with polycythemia (an abnormal increase in the number of red blood cells), however, may have cyanosis when oxygenation is adequate. Therefore, cyanosis must be interpreted in relation to the underlying pathophysiologic condition. If cyanosis is suggested, the Pao_2 should be measured.

Clubbing

Clubbing is the selective bulbous enlargement of the end (distal segment) of a digit (finger or toe) (Fig. 29.1); its severity can be graded from 1 to 5 based on the extent of nail bed hypertrophy and the number of changes in the nails themselves. It is usually painless. Clubbing is commonly associated with diseases that cause chronic hypoxemia, such as bronchiectasis, cystic fibrosis, pulmonary fibrosis, lung abscess, and congenital heart disease, and is rarely reversible. Although the exact cause of clubbing is unknown, it is proposed that platelet clumps escape filtration by the pulmonary bed and enter the systemic circulation. These platelets then release platelet-derived growth factor (PDGF), which causes periosteal changes near the nail bed. Clubbing can sometimes be seen in individuals with lung cancer even without hypoxemia because of the effects of inflammatory cytokines and growth factors (*hypertrophic osteoarthropathy*).

Pain

Pain caused by pulmonary disorders originates in the pleurae, airways, or chest wall. Infection and inflammation of the pleura (pleurisy or pleuritis) cause sharp or stabbing pain (pleurodynia) when the pleura stretches during inspiration. The pain is usually localized to a portion of the chest wall, where a unique breath sound called a *pleural friction rub* may be heard over the painful area. Laughing or coughing makes pleural pain worse.

Infection and inflammation of the trachea or bronchi (tracheitis or tracheobronchitis, respectively) can cause central chest pain that is pronounced after coughing. High blood pressure in the pulmonary circulation (pulmonary hypertension) can cause pain during exercise that is often mistaken for cardiac pain (angina pectoris).

Pain in the chest wall is muscle pain or rib pain. Excessive coughing (which makes the muscles sore) and rib fractures or thoracic surgery produce such pain. Inflammation of the costochondral junction (costochondritis) also can cause chest wall pain. Chest wall pain can often be reproduced by pressing on the sternum or ribs.

Conditions Caused by Pulmonary Disease or Injury
Hypercapnia

Hypercapnia, or an increased CO_2 concentration in the arterial blood (increased $Paco_2$), is caused by hypoventilation of the alveoli (Fig. 29.2). As discussed in Chapter 28, CO_2 is easily diffused from the blood into the alveolar space, but it must be removed from the alveoli by ventilation in order to maintain a normal $Paco_2$. Thus, minute ventilation (respiratory rate × tidal volume) determines not only the alveolar ventilation, but also the $Paco_2$. Hypoventilation is often overlooked because the breathing pattern and ventilatory rate may appear to be normal; therefore it is important to obtain blood gas analysis or capnography to determine the severity of the hypercapnia and resultant respiratory acidosis (acid-base balance is described in Chapter 5).

There are many causes of hypercapnia. Most are a result of a decreased drive to breathe or an inadequate ability to respond to ventilatory stimulation. Some of these causes include (1) depression of the respiratory center by drugs; (2) diseases of the medulla, including infections of the central nervous system or trauma; (3) abnormalities of the spinal conducting pathways, as in spinal cord disruption or poliomyelitis; (4) diseases of the neuromuscular junction or of the respiratory muscles themselves, as in myasthenia gravis or muscular dystrophy; (5) thoracic cage abnormalities, as in chest injury or congenital deformity; (6) large airway obstruction, as in tumors or sleep apnea; and (7) increased work of breathing or physiologic dead space, as in emphysema.

Hypercapnia and the associated respiratory acidosis result in electrolyte abnormalities that may cause dysrhythmias. High levels of arterial CO_2 cause cerebral vasodilation, resulting in somnolence and even coma. Alveolar hypoventilation with an increased alveolar CO_2 concentration limits the amount of oxygen available for diffusion into the blood, thereby leading to secondary hypoxemia.

Hypoxemia

Hypoxemia, or reduced oxygenation of arterial blood (reduced Pao_2), is caused by respiratory alterations, whereas hypoxia (or ischemia) is reduced oxygenation of cells in tissues. Although hypoxemia can lead to tissue hypoxia, tissue hypoxia can result from other abnormalities unrelated to alterations of pulmonary function, such as cardiac disease with poor tissue perfusion or anemia.

Hypoxemia results from problems with one or more of the major mechanisms of oxygenation (see Fig. 29.2):
1. Oxygen delivery to the alveoli
   a. Minute ventilation (respiratory rate × tidal volume)
   b. Oxygen content of the inspired air (Fio_2)
2. Diffusion of oxygen from the alveoli into the blood
   a. Balance between alveolar ventilation and perfusion ($\dot{V}/\dot{Q}$ match)
   b. Diffusion of oxygen across the alveolar capillary barrier
3. Perfusion of the pulmonary system

The amount of oxygen in the alveoli is the P_Ao_2 and is dependent on two factors. The first factor is the amount of alveolar minute ventilation (tidal volume × respiratory rate), as discussed previously in the Hypoventilation section. Hypoventilation results in an increase in the P_Aco_2 and a decrease in the amount of oxygen available in the alveoli for diffusion into the blood. This type of secondary hypoxemia is associated with hypercapnia and respiratory acidosis and can be corrected if alveolar ventilation is improved by increases in the rate and depth of breathing. The second factor is the presence of adequate oxygen

Clubbing — early

Clubbing — moderate

Clubbing — severe

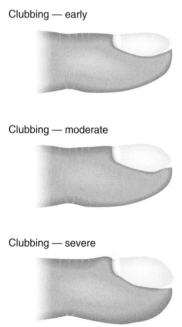

FIGURE 29.1 Clubbing of Fingers Caused by Chronic Hypoxemia. (Modified from Seidel HM et al: *Mosby's guide to physical examination,* ed 7, St Louis, 2011, Mosby.)

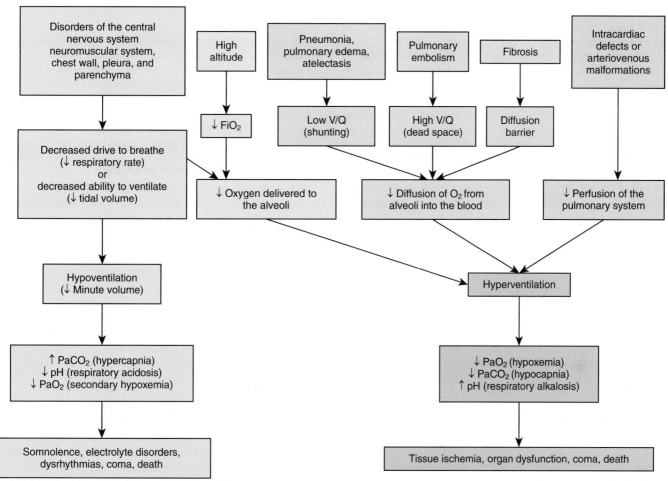

FIGURE 29.2 Hypercapnia and Hypoxemia. Disorders that diminish the respiratory rate or tidal volume lead to hypoventilation, hypercapnia, and respiratory acidosis. Disorders that decrease the amount of oxygen delivered to the alveoli, the diffusion of oxygen from the alveoli into the blood, or perfusion of the pulmonary system are associated with hyperventilation, hypoxemia, and a respiratory alkalosis.

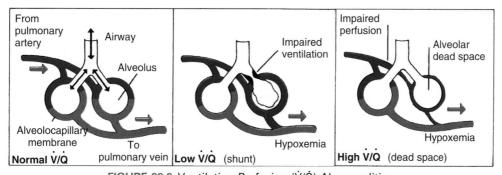

FIGURE 29.3 Ventilation-Perfusion ($\dot{V}/\dot{Q}$) Abnormalities.

content of the inspired air. The amount of oxygen in inspired air is expressed as the percentage or fraction of air that is composed of oxygen, the Fio_2. The Fio_2 of air at sea level is 20.9%. Anything that decreases the Fio_2 (e.g., high altitude) decreases the P_{AO_2}.

Diffusion of oxygen from the alveoli into the blood is also dependent on two factors. The first is the balance between the amount of air that enters alveoli ($\dot{V}$) and the amount of blood perfusing the capillaries around the alveoli ($\dot{Q}$). An abnormal ventilation-perfusion ratio ($\dot{V}/\dot{Q}$) is the most common cause of hypoxemia (Fig. 29.3). The normal $\dot{V}/\dot{Q}$ is

0.8 (also called the respiratory quotient) because some blood is normally shunted to the bronchial circulation. $\dot{V}/\dot{Q}$ mismatch refers to an abnormal distribution of ventilation and perfusion. Hypoxemia can be caused by inadequate ventilation of well-perfused areas of the lung (low $\dot{V}/\dot{Q}$), resulting in wasted perfusion. Mismatching of this type, called shunting, occurs in atelectasis, in asthma as a result of bronchoconstriction, and in pulmonary edema and pneumonia when alveoli are filled with fluid. Hypoxemia also can be caused by poor perfusion of well-ventilated portions of the lung (high $\dot{V}/\dot{Q}$), resulting in wasted ventilation. The most common cause of high $\dot{V}/\dot{Q}$ is a pulmonary embolus that impairs blood flow to a segment of the lung. An area where alveoli are ventilated but not perfused is termed alveolar dead space.

The second factor affecting diffusion of oxygen from the alveoli into the blood is the alveolocapillary membrane. Diffusion of oxygen through the alveolocapillary membrane is impaired if the membrane is thickened or the surface area available for diffusion is decreased. Thickened alveolocapillary membranes, as occur with edema (tissue swelling) and fibrosis (formation of fibrous lesions), increase the time required for oxygen to diffuse from the alveoli into the capillaries. If diffusion is slowed enough, the oxygenation levels (P_{O_2}) of alveolar gas and capillary blood do not have time to equilibrate during the fraction of a second that blood remains in the capillary. Hypercapnia is seldom produced by impaired diffusion because CO_2 diffuses so easily from capillary to alveolus.

Finally, hypoxemia can result when there is poor perfusion of the pulmonary system. Blood flow may bypass the lungs when there are intracardiac defects that cause right-to-left shunting or because of intrapulmonary arteriovenous malformations.

Hypoxemia is most often associated with a compensatory hyperventilation and the resultant respiratory alkalosis (i.e., decreased Pa_{CO_2} and increased pH). However, in individuals with associated ventilatory difficulties, hypoxemia may be complicated by hypercapnia and respiratory acidosis. Hypoxemia results in widespread tissue dysfunction and, when severe, can lead to organ infarction. In addition, hypoxic pulmonary vasoconstriction can contribute to increased pressures in the pulmonary artery (pulmonary artery hypertension) and lead to right heart failure, or *cor pulmonale* (see the Pulmonary Artery Hypertension section). Clinical manifestations of acute hypoxemia may include cyanosis, confusion, tachycardia, edema, and decreased renal output.

> ✔**QUICK CHECK 29.1**
> 1. List the primary signs and symptoms of pulmonary disease.
> 2. What abnormal breathing patterns are seen with pulmonary disease?
> 3. What mechanisms produce hypercapnia?
> 4. What mechanisms produce hypoxemia?

Acute Respiratory Failure

Respiratory failure is defined as inadequate gas exchange, which is characterized as $Pa_{O_2} \leq 60$ mm Hg (hypoxemic respiratory failure) and/or $Pa_{CO_2} \geq 50$ mm Hg, pH ≤ 7.25 (hypercapnic respiratory failure). Respiratory failure can result from direct injury to the lungs, airways, or chest wall or indirectly because of disease or injury involving another body system, such as the brain, spinal cord, or heart. If the respiratory failure is primarily hypercapnic, it is the result of inadequate alveolar ventilation and the individual requires ventilatory support, such as with a bag-valve mask, noninvasive positive pressure ventilation, or intubation and the use of mechanical ventilation. If the respiratory failure is primarily hypoxemic, it is the result of inadequate exchange of oxygen between the alveoli and the capillaries and the individual must receive supplemental oxygen therapy. Many people will have combined hypercapnic and hypoxemic respiratory failure and will require both kinds of support.

Of the many possible causes of respiratory failure, it is especially important to recognize that it is a potential complication of any major surgical procedure, especially those that involve the central nervous system, thorax, or upper abdomen. The most common postoperative pulmonary problems are atelectasis, pneumonia, pulmonary edema, and pulmonary emboli. People who smoke or are obese are at particular risk, especially if they have preexisting lung disease. Limited cardiac reserve, neurologic disease, chronic renal failure, chronic hepatic disease, and infection also increase the tendency to develop postoperative respiratory failure.

Prevention of respiratory failure includes the recognition of at-risk individuals and the initiation of deep-breathing exercises and early ambulation to prevent atelectasis and the accumulation of secretions. Incentive spirometry gives individuals immediate feedback about tidal volumes, which encourages them to breathe deeply. Humidification of inspired air can help loosen secretions. Antibiotics are given as appropriate to treat infection. If respiratory failure develops, the individual may require mechanical ventilation or extracorporeal membrane oxygenation.

Disorders of the Chest Wall and Pleura

There are many conditions that can affect the chest wall or pleura, or both, and influence the function of the respiratory system. Chest wall disorders primarily affect tidal volume resulting in hypoventilation and hypercapnia. Pleural diseases impact both ventilation and oxygenation.

Chest Wall Restriction

If the chest wall is deformed, traumatized, immobilized, or heavy from the accumulation of fat, the work of breathing increases and ventilation may be compromised because of a decrease in tidal volume. The degree of ventilatory impairment depends on the severity of the chest wall restriction. Grossly obese individuals are often dyspneic on exertion or when recumbent. Individuals with severe kyphoscoliosis (bending and rotation of the spinal column, with distortion of the thoracic cage) often present with dyspnea on exertion that can progress to respiratory failure. Other musculoskeletal abnormalities that can impair ventilation are ankylosing spondylitis (see Chapter 41) and pectus excavatum (a deformity characterized by depression of the sternum).

Impairment of respiratory muscle function caused by neuromuscular diseases, such as poliomyelitis, muscular dystrophy, myasthenia gravis, and Guillain-Barré syndrome (see Chapter 17), also can restrict the chest wall and impair pulmonary function. Muscle weakness can result in hypoventilation, inability to remove secretions, and hypoxemia.

Pain from chest wall injury, surgery, or disease can restrict the movement of the chest wall and cause significant hypoventilation, especially in those with underlying lung disease. Trauma to the thorax not only can restrict chest expansion because of pain, but also can cause structural and mechanical changes that impair the ability of the chest to expand normally. Flail chest results from the fracture of several consecutive ribs in more than one place or fracture of the sternum and several consecutive ribs. These multiple fractures result in instability of a portion of the chest wall, causing paradoxical movement of the chest with breathing. During inspiration the unstable portion of the chest wall moves inward and during expiration it moves outward, impairing movement of gas into and out of the lungs (Fig. 29.4).

An increase in the respiratory rate can compensate for small decreases in tidal volume, but many individuals will progress to hypercapnic respiratory failure. A diagnosis of chest wall restriction is made by pulmonary function testing (reduction in forced vital capacity [FVC]), arterial blood gas measurement and capnography (hypercapnia), and radiographs. Treatment is aimed at any reversible underlying cause but is otherwise supportive. In severe cases, mechanical ventilation may be indicated.

Pleural Abnormalities
Pneumothorax

Pneumothorax is the presence of air or gas in the pleural space caused by a rupture in the visceral pleura (which surrounds the lungs) or the parietal pleura and chest wall. As air separates the visceral and parietal pleurae, it destroys the negative pressure of the pleural space and disrupts the equilibrium between the elastic recoil forces of the

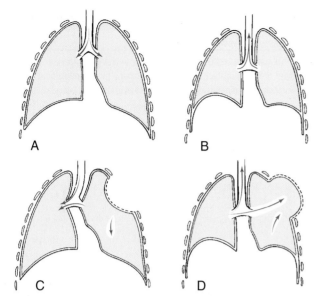

FIGURE 29.4 Flail Chest. Normal respiration: **A,** Inspiration; **B,** expiration. Paradoxical motion: **C,** inspiration, the area of the lung underlying the unstable chest wall flattens on inspiration; **D,** expiration, the unstable area inflates. Note the movement of the mediastinum toward the opposite lung during inspiration.

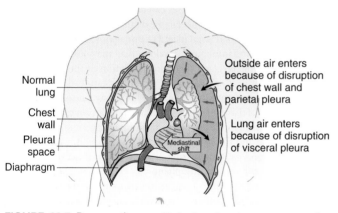

Normal lung
Chest wall
Pleural space
Diaphragm

Outside air enters because of disruption of chest wall and parietal pleura

Mediastinal shift

Lung air enters because of disruption of visceral pleura

FIGURE 29.5 Pneumothorax. Air in the pleural space causes the lung to collapse around the hilus and may push the mediastinal contents (heart and great vessels) toward the other lung.

lung and chest wall. The lung then tends to recoil by collapsing toward the hilum (Fig. 29.5).

Primary (spontaneous) pneumothorax occurs unexpectedly in healthy individuals (usually men) between 20 and 40 years of age and is caused by the spontaneous rupture of blebs (blister-like formations) on the visceral pleura. Bleb rupture can occur during sleep, rest, or exercise. The ruptured blebs are usually located in the apices of the lungs. The cause of bleb formation is not known, although there appears to be a genetic component, and more than 80% of these individuals have been found to have emphysema-like changes in their lungs even if they have no history of smoking. *Secondary pneumothorax* can be caused by chest trauma, such as a rib fracture or stab and bullet wounds that tear the pleura; rupture of a bleb or bulla (a larger vesicle), as occurs in emphysema; or mechanical ventilation (barotrauma). *Iatrogenic pneumothorax* is most commonly caused by transthoracic needle aspiration.

Primary pneumothorax and secondary pneumothorax can present as either the open or the tension type. In open (communicating) pneumothorax, air that is drawn into the pleural space during inspiration (through the damaged chest wall and parietal pleura or through the lungs and damaged visceral pleura) is forced back out during expiration and only partial lung collapse results. In tension pneumothorax, however, the site of pleural rupture acts as a one-way valve, permitting air to enter on inspiration but preventing its escape by closing during expiration. As more and more air enters the pleural space, air pressure in the pleural space increases. Air pressure in the pleural space pushes against the lung, causing compression atelectasis, and against the mediastinum, compressing and displacing the heart, great vessels, and trachea *(mediastinal shift)*. The pathophysiologic effects of tension pneumothorax are life-threatening (see Fig. 29.5).

Clinical manifestations of spontaneous or secondary pneumothorax begin with sudden pleural pain, tachypnea, and dyspnea. Depending on the size of the pneumothorax, the physical examination may reveal absent or decreased breath sounds and hyperresonance to percussion on the affected side. Tension pneumothorax may be complicated by severe hypoxemia, tracheal deviation away from the affected lung, and hypotension (low blood pressure). The diagnosis of pneumothorax is confirmed with chest radiographs, ultrasound, and computed tomography (CT). However, in the case of tension pneumothorax, deterioration occurs rapidly and immediate treatment is required. Pneumothorax is treated by aspiration, usually with insertion of a thoracostomy (chest) tube that is attached to a water-seal drainage system with suction. After the pneumothorax is evacuated and the pleural rupture has healed, the chest tube is removed. For individuals with persistent air leaks, other interventions may be needed, including thoracoscopic surgical techniques.[3]

Pleural Effusion

Pleural effusion is the presence of fluid in the pleural space. The source of the fluid is usually blood vessels or lymphatic vessels lying beneath the pleural space. Pleural effusions can be transudative (watery) or exudative (high concentrations of white blood cells and plasma proteins). Other types of pleural effusion are characterized by the presence of pus (empyema), blood (hemothorax), or chyle (chylothorax). Mechanisms of pleural effusion are summarized in Table 29.1.

Small collections of fluid may not affect lung function and may remain undetected. Most will be removed by the lymphatic system once the underlying condition is resolved. In larger effusions, dyspnea, compression of the lung with impaired ventilation, and pleural pain are common. Mediastinal shift and cardiovascular manifestations occur in a large, rapidly developing effusion. Physical examination shows decreased breath sounds and dullness to percussion on the affected side. A pleural friction rub may be heard over areas of inflamed pleura.

The diagnosis is confirmed by chest x-ray and thoracentesis (needle aspiration), which can determine the type of effusion and provide symptomatic relief. If the effusion is large, drainage usually requires the placement of a chest tube, and surgical interventions may be needed to prevent recurrence of the effusion.

Empyema

Empyema (infected pleural effusion) is the presence of pus in the pleural space and develops when the pulmonary lymphatics become blocked, leading to an outpouring of contaminated lymphatic fluid into the pleural space. Empyema occurs most commonly in older adults and children and usually develops as a complication of pneumonia, surgery, trauma, or bronchial obstruction from a tumor. Commonly documented infectious organisms include *Staphylococcus aureus, Escherichia coli,* anaerobic bacteria, and *Klebsiella pneumoniae.*

Individuals with empyema present clinically with cyanosis, fever, tachycardia (rapid heart rate), cough, and pleural pain. Breath sounds

TABLE 29.1 Mechanism of Pleural Effusion*

Type of Fluid/Effusion	Source of Accumulation	Primary or Associated Disorder
Transudate (hydrothorax)	Watery fluid that diffuses out of capillaries beneath pleura (i.e., capillaries in lung or chest wall)	Cardiovascular disease that causes high pulmonary capillary pressures; liver or kidney disease that disrupts plasma protein production, causing hypoproteinemia (decreased oncotic pressure in blood vessels)
Exudate	Fluid rich in cells and proteins (leukocytes, plasma proteins of all kinds; see Chapter 5) that migrates out of capillaries	Infection, inflammation, or malignancy of pleura that stimulates mast cells to release biochemical mediators that increase capillary permeability
Pus (empyema)	Microorganisms and debris of infection (leukocytes, cellular debris) accumulate in pleural space	Pulmonary infections, such as pneumonia; lung abscesses; infected wounds
Blood (hemothorax)	Hemorrhage into pleural space	Traumatic injury, surgery, rupture, or malignancy that damages blood vessels
Chyle (chylothorax)	Chyle (milky fluid containing lymph and fat droplets) that moves from lymphatic vessels into pleural space instead of passing from gastrointestinal tract to thoracic duct	Traumatic injury, surgical procedure, infection, or disorder that disrupts lymphatic transport

*The principles of diffusion are described in Chapter 1; mechanisms that increase capillary permeability and cause exudation of cells, proteins, and fluid are discussed in Chapter 5.

are decreased directly over the empyema. The diagnosis is made by chest radiographs, thoracentesis, and sputum culture. The treatment for empyema includes the administration of appropriate antimicrobials and drainage of the pleural space with a chest tube. Thoracoscopic or surgical intervention may be required.[4]

> **QUICK CHECK 29.2**
> 1. How does chest wall restriction affect ventilation?
> 2. How does pneumothorax differ from pleural effusion?
> 3. What causes empyema?

PULMONARY DISORDERS

Restrictive Lung Diseases

Restrictive lung diseases are characterized by decreased compliance (stiffness) of the lung tissue. This means that it takes more effort to expand the lungs during inspiration, which increases the work of breathing. Individuals with lung restriction have dyspnea, an increased respiratory rate, and a decreased tidal volume. Pulmonary function testing reveals a decrease in the FVC. Restrictive lung diseases can cause $\dot{V}/\dot{Q}$ mismatch and affect the alveolocapillary membrane, which reduces the diffusion of oxygen from the alveoli into the blood and results in hypoxemia. Some of the most common restrictive lung diseases in adults are aspiration, atelectasis, bronchiectasis, bronchiolitis, pulmonary fibrosis, inhalation disorders, pneumoconiosis, allergic alveolitis, pulmonary edema, and acute respiratory distress syndrome.

Aspiration

Aspiration is the passage of fluid and solid particles into the lung. It tends to occur in individuals whose normal swallowing mechanism and cough reflex are impaired by central or peripheral nervous system abnormalities. Predisposing factors include an altered level of consciousness caused by substance abuse, sedation, or anesthesia; seizure disorders; stroke; neuromuscular disorders that cause dysphagia; and feeding through a nasogastric tube. The right lung, particularly the right lower lobe, is more susceptible to aspiration than the left lung because the branching angle of the right mainstem bronchus is straighter than the branching angle of the left mainstem bronchus.

Aspiration of large food particles or acidic gastric fluid has serious consequences. Solid food particles can obstruct a bronchus, resulting in bronchial inflammation and collapse of airways distal to the obstruction. If the aspirated solid is not identified and removed by bronchoscopy, a chronic, local inflammation develops that may lead to recurrent infection and bronchiectasis (permanent dilation of the bronchus).

Aspiration of oral or pharyngeal secretions can lead to aspiration pneumonia. Aspiration of acidic gastric fluid may cause severe pneumonitis. Bronchial damage includes inflammation, loss of ciliary function, and bronchospasm. In the alveoli, acidic fluid damages the alveolocapillary membrane and diminishes surfactant production. Consequently, plasma and blood cells move from capillaries into the alveoli and the lung becomes stiff and noncompliant.

Clinical manifestations of aspiration include the sudden onset of choking and intractable cough with or without vomiting, fever, dyspnea, and wheezing. Some individuals have no symptoms acutely; instead they have recurrent lung infections, chronic cough, or persistent wheezing over months and even years.

Preventive measures for individuals at risk include use of a semirecumbent position, surveillance of enteral feeding, use of promotility agents, and avoidance of excessive sedation. Nasogastric tubes may be used to reduce stomach contents in order to prevent aspiration, but also can cause aspiration if fluid and particulate matter are regurgitated as the tube is being placed.

Treatment of aspiration pneumonitis includes use of supplemental oxygen with possible mechanical ventilation and administration of corticosteroids. Fluids are restricted to decrease blood volume and minimize pulmonary edema. Bacterial pneumonia may develop as a complication of aspiration pneumonitis and must be treated with antimicrobials.

Atelectasis

Atelectasis is the collapse of lung tissue. There are three types of atelectasis:
1. **Compression atelectasis** is caused by external pressure exerted by tumor, fluid, or air in the pleural space or by abdominal distention pressing on a portion of lung, causing alveoli to collapse.

2. **Obstructive (absorption) atelectasis** results from obstructed or hypoventilated alveoli as the air is gradually absorbed out of the alveoli and into the blood.

3. **Surfactant impairment (adhesive) atelectasis** results from decreased production or inactivation of surfactant, which is necessary to reduce surface tension in the alveoli and thus prevent lung collapse during expiration. Surfactant impairment can occur because of premature birth and from any serious lung injury, such as occurs with aspiration, acute respiratory distress syndrome, anesthesia induction, or mechanical ventilation.

Atelectasis is common after surgery or in individuals who are immobilized.[5] After surgery, individuals are often in pain, breathe shallowly, are reluctant to change position, and produce viscous secretions that tend to pool in dependent portions of the lung, causing obstruction of small airways. Atelectasis causes $\dot{V}/\dot{Q}$ mismatch (shunting), leading to perioperative hypoxemia.

Clinical manifestations of atelectasis include dyspnea, cough, fever, and leukocytosis and therefore may be mistaken for infection. Prevention and treatment of atelectasis usually include deep-breathing exercises (often with the aid of an incentive spirometer), frequent position changes, and early ambulation. Deep breathing promotes ciliary clearance of secretions, stabilizes the alveoli by redistributing surfactant, and promotes collateral ventilation through the *pores of Kohn,* promoting expansion of collapsed alveoli (Fig. 29.6).

Bronchiectasis

Bronchiectasis is persistent abnormal dilation of the bronchi. It usually occurs in conjunction with other respiratory conditions that are associated with chronic bronchial inflammation, such as obstruction of an airway with mucous plugs, atelectasis, aspiration of a foreign body, infection, cystic fibrosis (see Chapter 30), tuberculosis, or congenital weakness of the bronchial wall.[6] Bronchiectasis also is associated with a number of systemic disorders, such as rheumatologic disease, inflammatory bowel disease, and immunodeficiency syndromes (e.g., acquired immunodeficiency syndrome [AIDS]). There may be no known cause. Chronic inflammation of the bronchi leads to destruction of elastic and muscular components of their walls, obstruction of the bronchial lumen, fibrosis, and permanent dilation.

The primary symptom of bronchiectasis is a chronic productive cough. The disease is commonly associated with recurrent lower respiratory tract infections and expectoration of voluminous amounts of foul-smelling, purulent sputum (measured in cupfuls). Hemoptysis and clubbing of the fingers (from chronic hypoxemia) are common. Pulmonary function studies show decreases in the FVC and expiratory flow rates. The diagnosis is usually confirmed by the use of high-resolution CT. Bronchiectasis is treated with sputum culture, antibiotics, antiinflammatory drugs, bronchodilators, chest physiotherapy, and supplemental oxygen.

Bronchiolitis

Bronchiolitis is a diffuse, inflammatory obstruction of the small airways or bronchioles that occurs most commonly in children. In adults it usually occurs with chronic bronchitis but can occur in otherwise healthy individuals in association with an upper or lower respiratory tract viral infection or with inhalation of toxic gases. Bronchiolitis also is a serious complication of stem cell and lung transplantation and can progress to **bronchiolitis obliterans,** a fibrotic process that occludes airways and causes permanent scarring of the lungs. **Bronchiolitis obliterans organizing pneumonia (BOOP)** is a complication of bronchiolitis obliterans in which the alveoli and bronchioles become filled with plugs of connective tissue.

Clinical manifestations include a rapid ventilatory rate, use of accessory muscles, low-grade fever, and a nonproductive cough. A decrease in the $\dot{V}/\dot{Q}$ results in hypoxemia. The diagnosis of bronchiolitis obliterans is made by bronchoscopy with biopsy. Bronchiolitis is treated with antibiotics, corticosteroids, immunosuppressive agents, and chest physical therapy (humidified air administration, coughing and deep-breathing exercises, postural drainage).

Pulmonary Fibrosis

Pulmonary fibrosis is an excessive amount of fibrous or connective tissue in the lung. Pulmonary fibrosis can be idiopathic or caused by formation of scar tissue after active pulmonary disease (e.g., acute respiratory distress syndrome, inhalational injury), in association with a variety of autoimmune disorders (e.g., rheumatoid arthritis, progressive systemic sclerosis, sarcoidosis), by inhalation of harmful substances

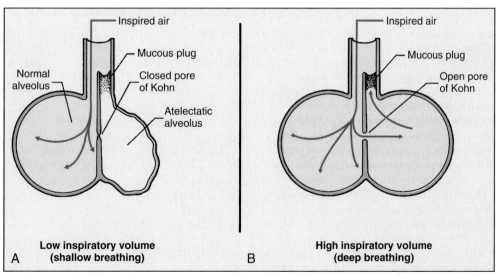

FIGURE 29.6 Pores of Kohn. A, Absorption atelectasis caused by a lack of collateral ventilation through the pores of Kohn. **B,** Restoration of collateral ventilation during deep breathing.

(e.g., coal dust, asbestos), or irradiation. Chronic inflammation leads to fibrosis and causes a marked loss of lung compliance. The lung becomes stiff and difficult to ventilate, and the diffusing capacity of the alveolocapillary membrane decreases, causing hypoxemia. Diffuse pulmonary fibrosis has a poor prognosis.

Idiopathic pulmonary fibrosis (IPF) is the most common idiopathic interstitial lung disorder.[7] There are associated genetic risks and presumed environmental insults, but a direct cause has not been identified. It is more common in men than in women, and most cases occur after age 60. IPF is characterized by chronic inflammation. Fibrosis of the interstitial lung tissue around the alveoli causes decreased oxygen diffusion across the alveolocapillary membrane and hypoxemia. As the disease progresses, decreased lung compliance leads to an increased work of breathing, a decreased tidal volume, and resultant hypoventilation with hypercapnia.

The primary symptom of pulmonary fibrosis is increasing dyspnea on exertion. The physical examination reveals diffuse inspiratory crackles. The diagnosis is confirmed by pulmonary function testing (a decreased FVC), x-rays, CT, and lung biopsy. Treatment includes oxygen, corticosteroids, antifibrotic and cytotoxic drugs, and lung transplantation.[8]

Inhalation Disorders

Exposure to toxic gases. Inhalation of gaseous irritants can cause significant respiratory dysfunction. Commonly encountered toxic gases include smoke, ammonia, hydrogen chloride, sulfur dioxide, chlorine, phosgene, and nitrogen dioxide. Inhalation injuries in burns can include toxic gases from household or industrial combustants, heat, and smoke particles. Inhaled toxins cause damage to the airway epithelium and promote mucus secretion, inflammation, mucosal edema, ciliary damage, pulmonary edema, and surfactant inactivation. The cellular effects of toxic gases and polluted air are described in Chapter 4. Acute toxic inhalation is frequently complicated by acute respiratory distress syndrome and pneumonia. Initial symptoms include burning of the eyes, nose, and throat; coughing; chest tightness; and dyspnea. Hypoxemia is common. Treatment includes administration of supplemental oxygen, mechanical ventilation, bronchodilators, corticosteroids, and support of the cardiovascular system. Most individuals respond quickly to therapy. Some, however, may improve initially and then deteriorate as a result of bronchiectasis or bronchiolitis.

Prolonged exposure to high concentrations of supplemental oxygen can result in a relatively rare condition known as oxygen toxicity. The basic underlying mechanism of injury is a severe inflammatory response mediated by oxygen free radicals. Damage to alveolocapillary membranes results in disruption of surfactant production, production of interstitial and alveolar edema, fibrosis, and a reduction in lung compliance. In infants this can lead to a condition known as *bronchopulmonary dysplasia,* in which there is severe scarring of the lung. Treatment involves a reduction of the inspired oxygen concentration as soon as tolerated.

Pneumoconiosis. Pneumoconiosis represents any change in the lung caused by inhalation of inorganic dust particles, usually occurring in the workplace. Pneumoconiosis often occurs after years of exposure to the offending dust, with progressive fibrosis of lung tissue.

The dusts of silica, asbestos, and coal are the most common causes of pneumoconiosis. Others include talc, fiberglass, clays, mica, slate, cement, and metals (cadmium, beryllium, tungsten, cobalt, aluminum, iron, indium, and titanium). Deposition of these materials in the lungs causes chronic inflammation with scarring of the alveolocapillary membrane, resulting in pulmonary fibrosis and progressive pulmonary deterioration. Clinical manifestations include cough, chronic sputum production, dyspnea, decreased lung volumes, and hypoxemia. In most cases, diagnosis is confirmed by performing chest radiography and

obtaining a complete occupational history. Treatment is usually palliative and focuses on preventing further exposure, management of associated hypoxemia and bronchospasm, and pulmonary rehabilitation.

Hypersensitivity pneumonitis. Hypersensitivity pneumonitis (extrinsic allergic alveolitis) is an allergic, inflammatory disease of the lungs caused by inhalation of organic particles. Many allergens can cause this disorder, including grains, silage, bird droppings or feathers, wood and cork dust, animal pelts, coffee beans, fish meal, mushroom compost, and molds that grow on sugarcane, barley, and straw. Lymphocytes and inflammatory cells infiltrate the interstitial lung tissue, releasing autoimmune and inflammatory cytokines and antibodies with damage to lung tissue.

Hypersensitivity pneumonitis can be acute, subacute, or chronic. The acute form causes fever, cough, and chills a few hours after exposure. Tachypnea and inspiratory crackles over the lower lung lobes are found on physical examination. With continued exposure, the disease becomes chronic and pulmonary fibrosis develops with dyspnea, fatigue, and weight loss. The diagnosis is made by obtaining a history of exposure and by performing serum antibody testing, chest radiography, bronchoscopy, and, in some cases, lung biopsy. Treatment consists of removal of the offending agent and administration of corticosteroids.

Pulmonary Edema

Pulmonary edema is excess water in the lung. The normal lung is kept dry by lymphatic drainage and a balance among capillary hydrostatic pressure, capillary oncotic pressure, and capillary permeability. In addition, surfactant lining the alveoli repels water, keeping fluid from entering the alveoli. Predisposing factors for pulmonary edema include heart disease, lung capillary injury, and processes that block the lymphatic vessels. The pathogenesis of pulmonary edema is shown in Fig. 29.7.

The most common cause of pulmonary edema is left-sided heart disease. When the left ventricle fails, caused by valvular or coronary disease, filling pressures on the left side of the heart increase and cause a concomitant increase in the pulmonary capillary hydrostatic pressure. When the hydrostatic pressure exceeds the oncotic pressure (which holds fluid in the capillary), fluid moves from the capillary into the interstitial space and alveoli. When the flow of fluid out of the capillaries exceeds the lymphatic system's ability to remove it, pulmonary edema develops.

Another cause of pulmonary edema is pulmonary capillary injury that increases capillary permeability, as in cases of adult respiratory distress syndrome or inhalation of toxic gases, such as ammonia. Capillary injury and inflammation causes water and plasma proteins to leak out of the capillary and move into the interstitial space, increasing the interstitial oncotic pressure (which is usually very low). As the interstitial oncotic pressure begins to exceed the capillary oncotic pressure, water moves out of the capillary and into the lung. (Mechanisms of edema are discussed in Chapter 5 and illustrated in Figs. 5.2 and 5.3.)

Pulmonary edema also can result from obstruction of the lymphatic system. This may occur during surgical procedures or because of the presence of tumors and fibrotic tissue.

Clinical manifestations of pulmonary edema include dyspnea, hypoxemia, and increased work of breathing. The physical examination may disclose inspiratory crackles (rales) and dullness to percussion over the lung bases. In severe edema, pink, frothy sputum is expectorated, hypoxemia worsens, and hypoventilation with hypercapnia may develop.

The treatment of pulmonary edema depends on its cause. If the edema is caused by increased hydrostatic pressure resulting from heart failure, therapy is directed toward improving cardiac output with diuretics, vasodilators, and drugs that improve the contraction of the heart muscle. If the edema is the result of increased capillary permeability resulting from injury, the treatment is focused on removing the offending

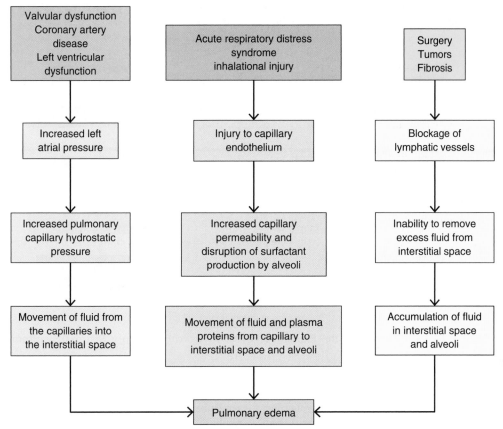

FIGURE 29.7 Pathogenesis of Pulmonary Edema.

agent and implementing supportive therapy to maintain adequate ventilation and circulation. Individuals with either type of pulmonary edema require supplemental oxygen. Lymphatic blockage is managed by treating the underlying condition but may not be reversible. Mechanical ventilation may be needed if edema significantly impairs ventilation and oxygenation.

Acute Respiratory Distress Syndrome

Acute respiratory distress syndrome (ARDS) is a form of acute lung inflammation and diffuse alveolocapillary injury that results from direct pulmonary injury or from severe systemic inflammation. ARDS is defined as (1) the acute onset of bilateral infiltrates on a chest radiograph (i.e., pulmonary edema) and (2) a low ratio of Pao_2 to Fio_2 (i.e., persistent hypoxemia despite supplemental oxygen). It is a common complication of intensive care unit ICU) admissions, and mortality remains high. The most common predisposing factors are sepsis and multiple trauma. There are many other causes, including pneumonia, burns, aspiration, cardiopulmonary bypass surgery, pancreatitis, blood transfusions, drug overdose, inhalation of smoke or noxious gases, fat emboli, radiation therapy, and disseminated intravascular coagulation.

PATHOPHYSIOLOGY   All disorders causing ARDS result in inflammation and acute injury to the alveolocapillary membrane. The alveolocapillary membrane consists of the epithelial cells that line the alveoli and the endothelial cells that line the capillaries, separated by the interstitial space. Damage to the alveolocapillary membrane causes pulmonary edema, often referred to as *noncardiogenic pulmonary edema*. ARDS progresses through three overlapping phases, characterized by microscopic changes in the lung: exudative (inflammatory), proliferative, and fibrotic.

Exudative phase (within 72 hours): Lung injury damages both endothelial cells of the pulmonary capillaries and alveolar epithelial cells (type II pneumocytes) (Fig. 29.8). Endothelial damage activates neutrophils, macrophages, and platelets with the release of inflammatory cytokines, resulting in greatly increased capillary membrane permeability. Fluids, proteins, and blood cells leak from the capillary bed into the pulmonary interstitium and flood the alveoli (hemorrhagic exudate). Alveolar ventilation is severely reduced, resulting in $\dot{V}/\dot{Q}$ mismatch (shunt) and hypoxemia. Epithelial cell damage to type II pneumocytes causes a reduction in surfactant production, resulting in atelectasis. Lung compliance declines, with associated decreases in tidal volume and hypercapnia. The result of this overwhelming inflammatory response by the lungs is acute respiratory failure.

Proliferative phase (within 4 to 21 days): After the initial lung injury, there is resolution of the pulmonary edema and proliferation of type II pneumocytes, fibroblasts, and myofibroblasts. The intraalveolar hemorrhagic exudate becomes a cellular granulation tissue, appearing as hyaline membranes that form a diffusion barrier for oxygen exchange and resulting in progressive hypoxemia.

Fibrotic phase (within 14 to 21 days): The final stage consists of remodeling and fibrosis of the lung tissue. In severe cases, the fibrosis progressively obliterates the alveoli, respiratory bronchioles, and interstitium, leading to long-term respiratory compromise.

CLINICAL MANIFESTATIONS   The clinical manifestations of ARDS are progressive:

1. Dyspnea and hypoxemia with poor response to oxygen supplementation
2. Hyperventilation and respiratory alkalosis

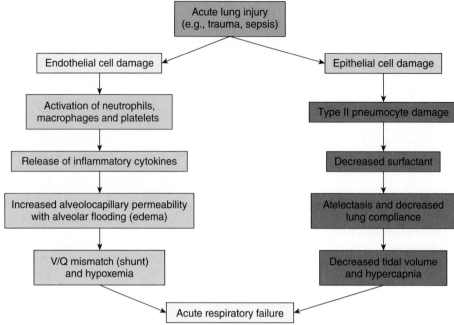

FIGURE 29.8 Pathogenesis of the Exudative Phase of Acute Respiratory Distress Syndrome (ARDS).

3. Decreased tissue perfusion, metabolic acidosis, and organ dysfunction
4. Increased work of breathing, decreased tidal volume, and hypoventilation
5. Hypercapnia, respiratory acidosis, and worsening hypoxemia
6. Respiratory failure, decreased cardiac output, hypotension, and death

EVALUATION AND TREATMENT   The diagnosis is based on a history of the lung injury, physical examination, blood gas analysis, and radiologic examination. Measurement of serum biomarkers (i.e., surfactant proteins, B-type natriuretic peptide [BNP], C-reactive protein [CRP], and interleukins) may aid in the diagnosis and prognosis of ARDS. Treatment is based on early detection, supportive therapy, and prevention of complications. Supportive therapy is focused on maintaining adequate oxygenation and ventilation while preventing infection. This often requires various modes of mechanical ventilation.[9,10] Pharmacologic therapy continues to be explored.

✔QUICK CHECK 29.3
1. Contrast aspiration and atelectasis.
2. What are some of the causes of pulmonary fibrosis?
3. What symptoms are produced by inhalation of toxic gases?
4. Describe pneumoconiosis, and give two examples.
5. Briefly describe the role of neutrophils in acute respiratory distress syndrome (ARDS).

Obstructive Lung Diseases

Obstructive lung disease is characterized by narrowing of the airways, resulting in airway obstruction that is worse with expiration. More force is required to expire a given volume of air, thus individuals must use their accessory muscles of expiration and have an increased work of breathing. Emptying of the lungs is slowed, as measured by a decreased forced expiratory volume in 1 second (FEV_1). Changes in alveolar

ventilation result in $\dot{V}/\dot{Q}$ mismatching and hypoxemia. Air trapping results in hypoventilation and hypercapnia. The unifying symptom of obstructive lung diseases is dyspnea, and the unifying sign is wheezing. The most common obstructive diseases are asthma, chronic bronchitis, and emphysema. Because many individuals have chronic bronchitis with emphysema, these diseases together are often called *chronic obstructive pulmonary disease (COPD)*.

Asthma

Asthma, as defined by the Global Initiative for Asthma (GINA) 2018 report, is a "…heterogenous disease, usually characterized by chronic airway inflammation. It is defined by the history or respiratory symptoms, such as wheeze, shortness of breath, chest tightness, and cough that vary over time and in intensity, together with variable expiratory limitation."[11] The chronic inflammation causes bronchial hyperresponsiveness, constriction of the airways, and variable airflow obstruction that is reversible. Asthma occurs at all ages, affecting 8.3% of children (see Chapter 30) and 20.4 million adults in the U.S.[12]

Asthma is a familial disorder, and more than 100 genes have been identified that may play a role in the susceptibility, pathogenesis, and treatment response of asthma. Specific gene expressions may impart associated *phenotypes* (e.g., eosinophilic [allergic], neutrophilic [nonallergic], late-onset, fixed airflow limitation, obesity-related asthma, and asthma-COPD overlap syndrome) or *endotypes*, such as clinical characteristics, biomarkers, lung physiology, genetics, histopathology, epidemiology, and treatment response.[11] Other risk factors include levels of allergen exposure, urban residence, exposure to indoor and outdoor air pollution, tobacco smoke, recurrent respiratory tract viral infections, obesity, use of acetaminophen containing medications, and gastroesophageal reflux disease.

Exposure to high levels of certain allergens during childhood increases the risk for asthma. Furthermore, decreased exposure to certain infectious microorganisms appears to create an immunologic imbalance that favors the development of allergy and asthma. This complex relationship has been called the *hygiene hypothesis*. Recently, the relationship between the microbiome and asthma risk is shedding light on these complex interactions (see *Did You Know? The Microbiome and Asthma*). Exposure to inhaled irritants, such as occurs in urban settings or during occupational exposures, can cause inflammation and damage to airways independent of allergen sensitivity. This leads to neutrophilic (nonallergic) asthma and also increases the hyperresponsiveness of the airways to allergens in those with eosinophilic (allergic) asthma.

Recurrent respiratory tract viral infections and obesity result in chronic inflammatory states that sensitize the bronchial mucosa to allergen and irritant exposure. Acetaminophen depletes glutathione levels in the respiratory tract, leading to oxidative stress, airway inflammation, and bronchoconstriction. Gastroesophageal reflux disease causes stimulation of the vagus nerve with the release of acetylcholine, which causes bronchoconstriction.

PATHOPHYSIOLOGY Airway epithelial exposure to antigen initiates both an innate and an adaptive immune response in sensitized individuals (see Chapter 8). Many cells and cellular elements contribute to the persistent inflammation of the bronchial mucosa and hyperresponsiveness of the airways, including dendritic cells (antigen-presenting macrophages), T-helper 2 (Th2) lymphocytes, B lymphocytes, mast cells, neutrophils, eosinophils, and basophils (see Chapter 8). There is both an immediate (early asthmatic response) and a late (delayed) response.

During the *early asthmatic response,* antigen exposure to the bronchial mucosa activates dendritic cells, which present antigen to T-helper cells. T-helper cells differentiate into Th2 cells, which release interleukins that activate B lymphocytes (plasma cells), and eosinophils. Plasma cells produce antigen-specific immunoglobulin E (IgE), which binds to the surface of mast cells. Subsequent cross-linking of IgE molecules with the antigen causes mast cell degranulation with the release of inflammatory mediators, including histamine, bradykinins, leukotrienes and prostaglandins, platelet-activating factor, and interleukins (see Figs. 8.1 and 8.2 for additional details). These inflammatory mediators cause vasodilation, increased capillary permeability, mucosal edema, bronchial smooth muscle contraction (bronchospasm), and mucus secretion from mucosal goblet cells with narrowing of the airways and obstruction to airflow. Eosinophils release toxic neuropeptides that contribute to increased bronchial hyperresponsiveness (Figs. 29.9, 29.10, and 29.11).

The *late asthmatic response* begins 4 to 8 hours after the early response. Chemotactic recruitment of eosinophils, neutrophils, and lymphocytes during the acute response causes a release of inflammatory mediators, again inciting bronchospasm, edema, and mucus secretion with obstruction to airflow. Synthesis of leukotrienes contributes to prolonged smooth muscle contraction. Eosinophils cause direct tissue injury with fibroblast proliferation and airway scarring. Damage to ciliated epithelial cells contributes to the accumulation of mucus and cellular debris forming plugs in the airways. Untreated inflammation can lead to long-term airway damage that is irreversible and is known as *airway remodeling* (subepithelial fibrosis, smooth muscle hypertrophy) (see Fig. 29.11).

Airway obstruction increases resistance to airflow and expiratory flow rates. Impaired expiration causes air trapping, hyperinflation distal to obstructions, and an increased work of breathing. Changes in resistance to airflow are not uniform throughout the lungs, and the distribution of inspired air is uneven, resulting in $\dot{V}/\dot{Q}$ mismatch and hypoxemia. Hyperventilation is triggered by lung receptors responding to increased lung volume and obstruction. The result is early hypoxemia with decreased Pa_{CO_2} and increased pH (respiratory alkalosis). With progressive obstruction of expiratory airflow, air trapping becomes more severe and the lungs and thorax become hyperexpanded, positioning the respiratory muscles at a mechanical disadvantage. This leads to a decrease in tidal volume, hypoventilation with increased Pa_{CO_2}, and respiratory acidosis. Respiratory acidosis signals respiratory failure.

CLINICAL MANIFESTATIONS Individuals are usually asymptomatic between attacks, and pulmonary function tests are normal. At the beginning of an attack, the individual experiences chest constriction, expiratory wheezing, dyspnea, nonproductive coughing, prolonged expiration, use of accessory muscles of respiration, tachycardia, and tachypnea. A **pulsus paradoxus** (decrease in systolic blood pressure during inspiration of more than 10 mm Hg) may be noted. Peak flow measurements should be obtained. Because the severity of blood gas alterations is difficult to evaluate by clinical signs alone, arterial blood gas tensions should be measured if oxygen saturation falls below 90%.

If bronchospasm is not reversed by usual treatment measures, the individual is considered to have acute severe bronchospasm or **status asthmaticus**. If status asthmaticus continues, hypoxemia worsens, expiratory flows and volumes decrease further, and effective ventilation decreases. Acidosis develops as the Pa_{CO_2} level begins to rise. Asthma becomes life-threatening at this point if treatment does not reverse this process quickly. A silent chest (no audible air movement) and a Pa_{CO_2} >70 mm Hg are ominous signs of impending death.

EVALUATION AND TREATMENT The diagnosis of asthma is supported by a history of allergies and recurrent episodes of wheezing, dyspnea, and cough or exercise intolerance. Further evaluation includes spirometry, which may document reversible decreases in FEV_1 during an induced attack. Many other conditions may be mistaken for asthma, including heart disease, cystic fibrosis, vocal cord dysfunction, and medication-related cough.

The evaluation of an acute asthma attack requires the rapid assessment of arterial blood gases and expiratory flow rates (using a peak flow meter) and a search for underlying triggers, such as infection. Hypoxemia and respiratory alkalosis are expected early in the course of an acute attack. The development of hypercapnia with respiratory acidosis signals the need for mechanical ventilation. Management of the acute asthma attack requires immediate administration of oxygen, inhaled β-agonist

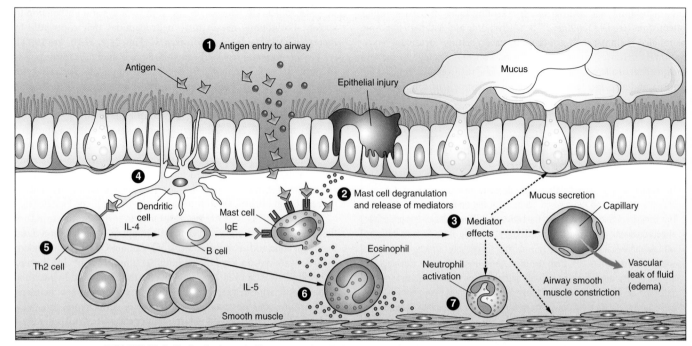

FIGURE 29.9 Early Asthmatic Response. Inhaled antigen (1) binds to mast cells covered with preformed IgE. Mast cells degranulate (2) and release inflammatory mediators such as histamine, bradykinins, leukotrienes, prostaglandins, platelet-activating factor, and interleukins. Secreted mediators (3) induce active bronchospasm (airway smooth muscle constriction), edema from increased capillary permeability, and airway mucus secretion from goblet cells. At the same time, antigen is detected by (4) dendritic cells that process and present it to Th2 cells (5), which produce interleukin-4 (IL-4) and many other interleukins (see text). IL-4 promotes switching of B cells to favor immunoglobulin E (IgE) production. Th2 cells also produce IL-5 (6), which activates eosinophils. Eosinophil products, such as major basic protein and eosinophilic cationic protein, damage the respiratory epithelium. Many inflammatory cells, including neutrophils (7), also contribute to the inflammatory process and airway obstruction. IgE, Immunoglobulin E.

bronchodilators, and oral corticosteroids. Careful monitoring of gas exchange and airway obstruction in response to therapy provides information necessary to determine whether hospitalization is necessary. Antibiotics are not indicated for acute asthma unless there is a documented bacterial infection.

Management of chronic asthma begins with avoidance of allergens and irritants. Individuals with asthma tend to underestimate the severity of their asthma, and extensive education is important, including the use of a peak flow meter and adherence to an action plan. Current guidelines for asthma management recommend the use of low-dose corticosteroids and short-acting beta-agonist inhalers for even the mildest forms of asthma (GINA 2019 https://ginasthma.org/reports/). For all categories of more severe asthma, anti-inflammatory medications are essential, and inhaled corticosteroids are the mainstay of therapy. In individuals who are not adequately controlled with inhaled corticosteroids, long-acting beta-agonist inhalers or leukotriene antagonists can be considered. Immunotherapy (allergy shots) has been shown to be an important tool in reducing asthma exacerbations and can now be given sublingually. Monoclonal antibodies to IgE (omalizumab) have been found to be helpful as adjunctive therapy to inhaled steroids. Exhaled nitric oxide (FENO) levels increasingly are used to follow response to therapy.

Chronic Obstructive Pulmonary Disease

Chronic obstructive pulmonary disease (COPD) is defined by the Global Initiative for Chronic Obstructive Lung Disease (GOLD) 2019 report as "…a common preventable and treatable disease characterized by persistent airflow limitation that is usually progressive and associated with an enhanced chronic inflammatory response in the airways and the lung to noxious particles or gases."[13] COPD is the most common chronic lung disease in the world, and the fourth leading cause of death in the United States, affecting as many as 9% of individuals in states where cigarette smoking is prevalent.[14] Risk factors for COPD include tobacco smoke (cigarette, pipe, cigar, and environmental tobacco smoke), occupational dusts and chemicals (vapors, irritants, and fumes), indoor air pollution from biomass fuel used for cooking and heating (in poorly vented dwellings), outdoor air pollution, and any factor that affects lung growth during gestation and childhood (low birth weight, respiratory tract infections). Genetic and epigenetic susceptibilities have been identified. An inherited mutation in the α_1-antitrypsin gene results in the development of COPD at an early age, even in individuals who do not smoke. The clinical phenotypes of COPD discussed here are chronic bronchitis and emphysema.

Chronic Bronchitis

Chronic bronchitis is defined as hypersecretion of mucus and a chronic productive cough for at least 3 months of the year (usually the winter months) for at least 2 consecutive years.

PATHOPHYSIOLOGY   Inspired irritants result in airway inflammation with infiltration of neutrophils, macrophages, and lymphocytes into the bronchial wall. Continual bronchial inflammation causes bronchial edema, an increase in the size and number of mucous glands and goblet cells in the airway epithelium, smooth muscle hypertrophy with fibrosis,

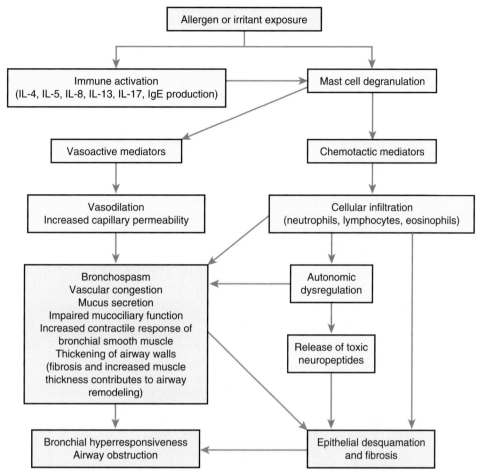

FIGURE 29.10 Pathophysiology of Asthma. Allergen or irritant exposure results in a cascade of inflammatory events, leading to acute and chronic airway dysfunction. *IgE,* Immunoglobulin E; *IL,* interleukin.

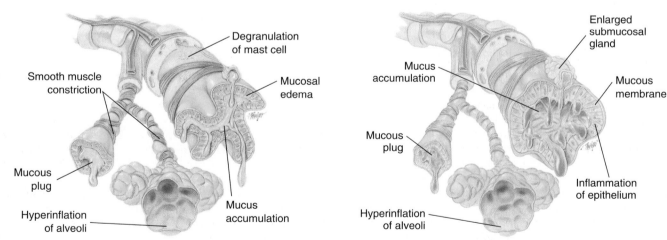

FIGURE 29.11 Bronchial Asthma. Thick mucus, mucosal edema, and smooth muscle spasm cause obstruction of small airways; breathing becomes labored and expiration is difficult. (Modified from Des Jardins T, Burton GG: *Clinical manifestations and assessment of respiratory disease,* ed 3, St Louis, 1995, Mosby.)

FIGURE 29.12 Chronic Bronchitis. Inflammation and thickening of the mucous membrane, with accumulation of mucus and pus, leading to obstruction characterized by a productive cough. (Modified from Des Jardins T, Burton GG: *Clinical manifestations and assessment of respiratory disease,* ed 3, St Louis, 1995, Mosby.)

and narrowing of airways. Thick, tenacious mucus is produced and cannot be cleared because of impaired ciliary function (Fig. 29.12). The lung's defense mechanisms are, therefore, compromised, increasing susceptibility to pulmonary infection and injury and ineffective repair. Frequent infectious exacerbations from bacterial colonization of damaged

airways are complicated by bronchospasm with dyspnea and productive cough. Exacerbations contribute to the overall severity and progression of disease. The pathogenesis of chronic bronchitis is shown in Fig. 29.13.

This process initially affects only the larger bronchi, but eventually all airways are involved. The thick mucus and hypertrophied bronchial

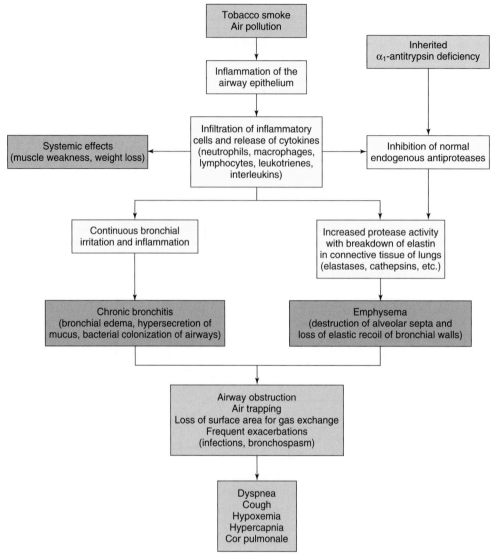

FIGURE 29.13 Pathogenesis of Chronic Bronchitis and Emphysema (Chronic Obstructive Pulmonary Disease).

smooth muscle constrict the airways and lead to obstruction, particularly during expiration when the airways are narrowed (Fig. 29.14). This expiratory obstruction traps air in the distal portions of the lung (hyperinflation), which expands the thorax and positions the respiratory muscles at a mechanical disadvantage. This leads to decreased tidal volume, hypoventilation, and hypercapnia. Obstruction also leads to $\dot{V}/\dot{Q}$ mismatch with hypoxemia.

CLINICAL MANIFESTATIONS Table 29.2 lists the common clinical manifestations of chronic obstructive lung disease, chronic bronchitis, and emphysema.

EVALUATION AND TREATMENT The diagnosis is based on a history of symptoms, physical examination, chest imaging, pulmonary function tests (i.e., a decreased FEV_1), and blood gas analyses. These tests reflect the progressive nature of the disease. Prevention of chronic bronchitis is essential because pathologic changes are not reversible. By the time an individual seeks medical care for symptoms, considerable airway damage is present. If the individual stops smoking, disease progression

TABLE 29.2 Clinical Manifestations of Chronic Obstructive Lung Disease

Clinical Manifestations	Bronchitis	Emphysema
Productive cough	Classic sign	With infection
Dyspnea	Late in course	Common
Wheezing	Intermittent	Common
History of smoking	Common	Common
Barrel chest	Occasionally	Classic
Prolonged expiration	Always present	Always present
Cyanosis	Common	Uncommon
Chronic hypoventilation	Common	Late in course
Polycythemia	Common	Late in course
Cor pulmonale	Common	Late in course

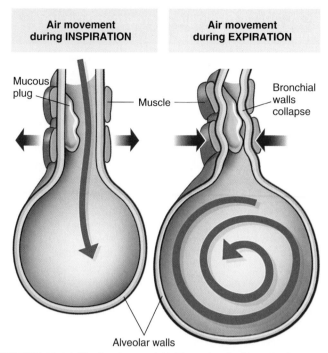

Air movement during INSPIRATION

Air movement during EXPIRATION

Mucous plug

Muscle

Bronchial walls collapse

Alveolar walls

FIGURE 29.14 Mechanisms of Air Trapping in Chronic Obstructive Pulmonary Disease. Mucous plugs and narrowed airways cause air trapping and hyperinflation of alveoli on expiration. During inspiration, the airways are pulled open, allowing gas to flow past the obstruction. During expiration, decreased elastic recoil of the bronchial walls results in collapse of the airways and prevents normal expiratory airflow.

can be halted. Influenza and pneumococcal vaccinations should be up-to-date.

The recommendations for management of chronic bronchitis include bronchodilators, mucolytics, antioxidants, and antiinflammatory drugs are prescribed as needed to control cough and reduce dyspnea.[13] Chest physical therapy may be helpful and includes deep breathing and postural drainage. During acute exacerbations (infection and bronchospasm), individuals require treatment with antibiotics and corticosteroids and may need mechanical ventilation. Antibiotics may need to be continued indefinitely in individuals who suffer frequent exacerbations. Chronic use of oral corticosteroids may be needed late in the course of the disease but should be considered a last resort. Individuals with severe hypoxemia will require home oxygen therapy. Teaching includes nutritional counseling, respiratory hygiene, recognition of the early signs of infection, and techniques that relieve dyspnea, such as pursed-lip breathing. In addition, many comorbidities accompany COPD and require monitoring and therapy, including cardiovascular disorders, metabolic diseases, bone disease, stroke, lung cancer, cachexia, skeletal muscle weakness, anemia, depression, and cognitive decline.

Emphysema

Emphysema is abnormal permanent enlargement of gas-exchange airways (acini) accompanied by destruction of alveolar walls without obvious fibrosis. Obstruction results from inflammatory and destructive changes in lung tissues, rather than mucus production as in chronic bronchitis. The major mechanism of airflow limitation is loss of elastic recoil with collapse of the airways during expiration.

Primary emphysema, which accounts for 1% to 3% of all cases of emphysema, is commonly linked to an inherited deficiency of the enzyme α_1-antitrypsin.[15] Normally α_1-antitrypsin inhibits the action of many proteolytic enzymes (i.e., elastases released by neutrophils) that serve

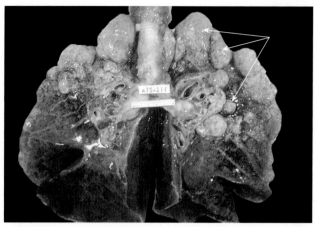

FIGURE 29.15 Bullous Emphysema With Large Apical and Subpleural Bullae *(arrows)*. (From Kumar V et al, editors: *Robbins basic pathology*, ed 8, Philadelphia, 2007, Saunders/Elsevier.)

to breakdown lung tissue; therefore α_1-antitrypsin deficiency (an autosomal recessive trait) increases the likelihood of developing emphysema because proteolysis in lung tissues is not inhibited. α_1-Antitrypsin deficiency is suggested in individuals who develop emphysema before 40 years of age and in individuals who do not smoke but still develop the disease. α_1-Antitrypsin augmentation therapy may be indicated for primary emphysema.

The major cause of secondary emphysema is the inhalation of cigarette smoke, although air pollution, occupational exposures, and childhood respiratory tract infections are known to be contributing factors. Many individuals are unaware that they have significant respiratory disease until irreversible lung disease has occurred.

PATHOPHYSIOLOGY Emphysema is characterized by inflammation and an imbalance between proteases and antiproteases, oxidative stress, and apoptosis (normal cell death) of lung structural cells. These processes lead to the destruction of alveoli through the breakdown of elastin within the septa (see Fig. 29.13). Alveolar destruction also produces large air spaces within the lung parenchyma (bullae) and air spaces adjacent to pleurae (blebs) (Fig. 29.15). Bullae and blebs are not effective in gas exchange and contribute to $\dot{V}/\dot{Q}$ mismatching and hypoxemia. Expiration becomes difficult because loss of elastic recoil reduces the rate at which air that can be expired and air is trapped in the lungs (see Fig. 29.14). Air trapping causes hyperexpansion of the chest, placing the muscles of respiration at a mechanical disadvantage. This results in an increased workload of breathing, so that many individuals will develop hypoventilation and hypercapnia late in the course of their disease. Persistent inflammation, along with acute infection or irritation of the airways, results in hyperreactivity of the bronchi and acute exacerbations with bronchoconstriction, which may be partially reversible with bronchodilators. Destruction of alveolar walls and pulmonary capillaries also causes pulmonary artery hypertension and cor pulmonale (see the Pulmonary Arterial Hypertension section). Chronic inflammation also can have significant systemic effects. including weight loss, muscle weakness, and increased susceptibility to comorbidities, such as infection.

CLINICAL MANIFESTATIONS The clinical manifestations of emphysema are listed in Table 29.2.

EVALUATION AND TREATMENT Emphysema is diagnosed and staged by pulmonary function measures. In COPD, pulmonary function tests indicate obstruction to gas flow during expiration with a marked decrease in the FEV_1. Chronic management of emphysema begins with smoking cessation. Prevention of acute exacerbations with pneumococcal and influenza vaccines, pulmonary rehabilitation, and improved nutrition is essential.[16] Pharmacologic management is based on clinical severity as described by the GOLD classification for COPD (mild, moderate, severe, or very severe).[13] Bronchodilators, including inhaled anticholinergic agents or β-agonists, should be prescribed for all symptomatic individuals and may be used in combination if needed. Roflumilast (phosphodiesterase E4 [PDE4] inhibitor) and mucolytics are added for those with moderate to severe COPD. Inhaled corticosteroids also may be used, although long-term therapy with oral steroids should be avoided if possible. Progressive pulmonary dysfunction with hypoxemia and hypercapnia require long-term oxygen therapy and noninvasive ventilation if indicated. Selected individuals with severe emphysema can benefit from lung volume reduction surgery.

> ✔ **QUICK CHECK 29.4**
> 1. What mechanisms cause airway obstruction in asthma?
> 2. How does emphysema affect oxygenation and ventilation?
> 3. Define chronic bronchitis.

Respiratory Tract Infections

Respiratory tract infections are the most common cause of short-term disability in the United States. Most of these infections—the common cold, pharyngitis (sore throat), and laryngitis—involve only the upper airways. Although the lungs have direct contact with the atmosphere, they usually remain sterile. Infections of the lower respiratory tract occur most often in the very young and very old or those with impaired immunity.

Acute Bronchitis

Acute bronchitis is acute infection or inflammation of the airways or bronchi and is usually self-limiting. The vast majority of cases of acute bronchitis are caused by viruses. Many of the clinical manifestations are similar to those of pneumonia (i.e., fever, cough, chills, malaise), but the physical examination does not reveal signs of pulmonary consolidation (i.e., dullness to percussion, crackles, egophony), and chest radiographs do not show infiltrates. Individuals with viral bronchitis usually have a nonproductive cough that occurs in paroxysms and is aggravated by cold, dry, or dusty air. Purulent sputum is produced in bacterial bronchitis. Chest pain often develops from the effort of coughing. Treatment consists of rest, aspirin, humidity, and a cough suppressant, such as codeine. Antibiotics are indicated for bacterial bronchitis.

Pneumonia

Pneumonia is infection of the lower respiratory tract caused by bacteria, viruses, fungi, protozoa, or parasites. It accounts for about 48,600 deaths per year in the United States.[17] Risk factors for pneumonia include advanced age, compromised immunity, underlying lung disease, alcoholism, altered consciousness, impaired swallowing, smoking, endotracheal intubation, malnutrition, immobilization, underlying cardiac or liver disease, and residence in a nursing home or other extended care facility. The causative microorganism influences the clinical presentation of the individual, the treatment plan, and the prognosis.

Pneumonia can be categorized as community-acquired (CAP), hospital-acquired (HAP), or ventilator-associated (VAP). CAP is one of the most common reasons for hospitalization in the United States. HAP denotes an episode of pneumonia not associated with mechanical ventilation; it is the second most common nosocomial infection (urinary tract infection [UTI] is the most common) and has the greatest mortality. VAP is a nosocomial infection that occurs in many individuals who require intubation and mechanical ventilation[18] (see *Did You Know? Ventilator-Associated Pneumonia*).The microorganisms that most

---

BOX 29.1 Etiologic Microorganisms for Pneumonia in Adults

CAP	HAP/VAP	Immunocompromised Individuals
Bacterial	Bacterial	Bacterial
Streptococcus pneumoniae	*Pseudomonas aeruginosa*	All CAP species
Moraxella catarrhalis	*Staphylococcus aureus*	*Mycobacterium tuberculosis*
Haemophilus influenzae	*Acinetobacter baumannii*	Atypical mycobacteria
Staphylococcus aureus	*Klebsiella pneumoniae*	Fungal
Legionella pneumophila	*Escherichia coli*	*Pneumocystis jirovecii*
Oral anaerobic bacteria		*Candida albicans*
Viral		*Cryptococcus neoformans*
Influenza virus		Viral
Respiratory syncytial virus		Cytomegalovirus
Atypical		Influenza
Chlamydia pneumoniae		Herpes simplex
Mycoplasma pneumoniae		Varicella zoster
		Parasitic
		Strongyloides
		Toxoplasmosis

CAP, Community-acquired pneumonia; *HAP,* hospital-acquired pneumonia; *VAP,* ventilator-associated pneumonia.

commonly cause CAP are different from those infections that cause HAP and VAP (Box 29.1). The mechanisms of viral and bacterial infection are reviewed in Chapter 9.

DID YOU KNOW?

Ventilator-Associated Pneumonia

Ventilator-associated pneumonia (VAP) is a common complication of mechanical ventilation and is the most serious infection in the intensive care unit. The principal determinant of VAP development is the presence of the endotracheal (ET) tube. Other risk factors include age greater than 65 years, presence of comorbidities, use of sedation, supine posture, poor oral hygiene, and immunocompromised status. Common etiologic microorganisms include *Staphylococcus aureus* and *Pseudomonas aeruginosa,* and multidrug-resistant strains are common. Bacterial colonization of the oropharynx occurs soon after placement of the ET tube, with pooling of bacteria near the ET tube cuff and subsequent aspiration. Many bacteria are capable of forming a protective coating, called a *biofilm,* on the surface of the ET tube that contributes to bacterial replication and makes microorganisms less vulnerable to antibiotics. Injury to the tracheal mucosa and decreased mucociliary clearance contribute to lower airway infection. Analgesic and sedation agents alter cellular function and reduce the immune response. Implementation of certain treatment protocols has shown improved outcomes regarding VAP prevention and mortality reduction, especially the use of a "bundle" of techniques, including raising the head of the bed, improving oral hygiene, providing continuous suction of subglottic secretions by antimicrobial-impregnated ET tubes, using checklists, and encouraging effective team communication. Recent studies have suggested that probiotics may reduce the risk of VAP, and the addition of aerosolized antibiotics may improve treatment outcomes.

Data from Álvarez-Lerma F et al: *Crit Care Med* 46(2):181-188, 2018; Guo R. Feng Y: *Crit Care Med* 46(1):199, 2018; Hellyer TP et al: *J Intensive Care Soc* 17(3):238-243, 2016; Kalil AC et al: *Clin Infect Dis* 63(5):e61-e111, 2016; Karakuzu Z et al: *Med Sci Monir* 24:1321-1328, 2018.

PATHOPHYSIOLOGY Aspiration of oropharyngeal secretions is the most common route of lower respiratory tract infection; thus, the nasopharynx and oropharynx constitute the first line of defense for most infectious agents. Another route of infection is through the inhalation of microorganisms that have been released into the air when an infected individual coughs, sneezes, or talks, or from aerosolized water, such as that from contaminated respiratory therapy equipment. In VAP, endotracheal tubes become colonized with bacteria that form biofilms (protected colonies of bacteria that are resistant to host defenses and treatment with antibiotics) and can seed the lung with microorganisms. Pneumonia also can occur when bacteria are spread to the lung from bacteremia that results from infection elsewhere in the body or from intravenous (IV) drug abuse.

In healthy individuals, pathogens that reach the lungs are expelled or controlled by mechanisms of self-defense (see Chapters 6 and 7). If a microorganism evades the upper airway defense mechanisms, such as the cough reflex and mucociliary clearance, the next line of defense is the airway epithelial cell, which can recognize some pathogens directly (e.g., *Pseudomonas aeruginosa* and *Staphylococcus aureus*) and prevent their growth. The most important guardian cell of the lower respiratory tract is the alveolar macrophage; it recognizes pathogens through its pattern-recognition receptors (e.g., Toll-like receptors; see Chapter 6). Macrophages phagocytose and present infectious antigens to the adaptive immune system, activating T cells and B cells with the induction of both cellular and humoral immunity (see Chapter 7). The release of tumor necrosis factor-alpha (TNF-α) and interleukin-1 (IL-1) from macrophages and of chemokines and chemotactic signals from mast cells and fibroblasts contributes to widespread inflammation in the lung and the recruitment of neutrophils from the capillaries of the lungs into the alveoli. The resulting inflammatory mediators and immune complexes can damage bronchial mucous membranes and alveolocapillary membranes, causing the alveoli and terminal bronchioles to fill with infectious debris and exudate. Some microorganisms release toxins from their cell walls that can cause further damage of lung tissue. The accumulation of exudate in the alveoli leads to dyspnea and to $\dot{V}/\dot{Q}$ mismatching and hypoxemia.

The most common cause of CAP is *Streptococcus pneumoniae* (also known as pneumococcus). Pneumococci most commonly infect the lungs through aspiration of colonized oropharyngeal secretions. These bacteria have capsules that make phagocytosis by alveolar macrophages more difficult. They also have the ability to release a variety of toxins, including pneumolysin, which damages airway and alveolar cells. An intense inflammatory response is initiated with release of TNF-α and IL-1. Neutrophils and inflammatory exudates cause alveolar edema, which leads to the other changes shown in Fig. 29.16.

The most common cause of viral CAP is influenza, which is a seasonal, usually mild, and self-limiting infection, however, it be fatal in elderly and debilitated individuals. It can set the stage for a secondary bacterial infection by damaging ciliated epithelial cells, which normally prevent pathogens from reaching the lower airways. Immunocompromised individuals are at risk for serious viral infections, such as pneumonia caused by cytomegalovirus. Viral pneumonia also can be a complication of another viral illness, such as chickenpox or measles (spread from the blood). New or atypical forms of viral infection, such as avian influenza A (H5N1) and severe acute respiratory syndrome (SARS), have affected previously healthy populations and pose a considerable threat for pandemics.

Viruses destroy the ciliated epithelial cells and invade the goblet cells and bronchial mucous glands. Sloughing of destroyed bronchial epithelium occurs throughout the respiratory tract, preventing mucociliary clearance. Bronchial walls become edematous and infiltrated with leukocytes. In severe cases, the alveoli are involved, with decreased compliance and increased work of breathing.

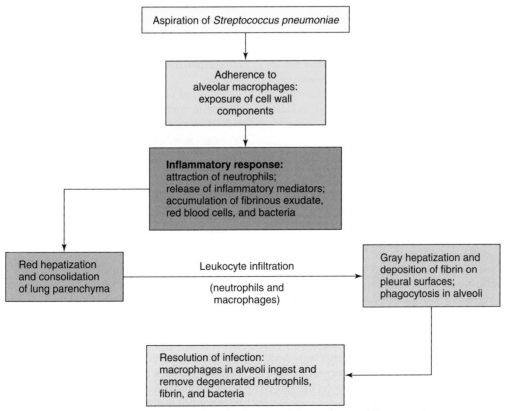

FIGURE 29.16 Pathophysiologic Course of Pneumococcal Pneumonia.

CLINICAL MANIFESTATIONS Most cases of pneumonia are preceded by a viral upper respiratory tract infection. Individuals then develop fever, chills, a productive or dry cough, malaise, pleural pain, and sometimes dyspnea and hemoptysis. The physical examination may show signs of pulmonary consolidation, such as dullness to percussion, inspiratory crackles, increased tactile fremitus (palpable chest vibrations when a person speaks), and egophony (a prolonged "a" heard on auscultation over consolidated lung tissue when the person says "e"). Individuals also may demonstrate symptoms and signs of underlying systemic disease or sepsis.

EVALUATION AND TREATMENT The diagnosis is made on the basis of the history and physical examination (tachypnea, tachycardia, crackles, bronchial breath sounds, findings of pleural effusion), white blood cell count, and chest x-rays. The white blood cell count is usually elevated, although it may be low if the individual is debilitated or immunocompromised. Serum procalcitonin, CRP, or soluble triggering receptor expressed on myeloid cells-1 (sTREM-1) obtained through bronchoscopy may help guide therapy. Chest radiographs show infiltrates that may involve a single lobe of the lung or may be more diffuse. Once the diagnosis of pneumonia has been made, the pathogen is identified by means of sputum characteristics (Gram stain, color, odor) and cultures. Because many pathogens exist in the normal oropharyngeal flora, the specimen may be contaminated with pathogens from oral secretions. If sputum studies fail to identify the pathogen, the individual is immunocompromised, or the individual's condition worsens, further diagnostic studies may include blood cultures, thoracentesis, bronchoscopy, or lung biopsy. Urine and serum antigen testing offers rapid pathogen identification for some microorganisms.

Prevention of pneumonia includes avoidance of aspiration (e.g., raising the head of the bed, endotracheal suctioning), respiratory isolation of infected individuals, and vaccination. The first step in the management of pneumonia is establishing adequate ventilation and oxygenation. Hydration and good pulmonary hygiene (e.g., deep breathing, coughing, chest physical therapy) also are important. Empiric antibiotics should be given promptly for bacterial pneumonia; however, resistant strains of microorganisms are becoming more prevalent and may require a change in antibiotics, especially in individuals with HAP or VAP.[18] Viral pneumonia is usually treated with supportive therapy alone, however, antivirals may be needed in severe cases. Opportunistic infections in immunocompromised individuals may be the result of several different microorganisms and require multiple drugs, including antifungals.

Tuberculosis

Tuberculosis (TB) is an infection caused by *Mycobacterium tuberculosis*, a bacillus that usually affects the lungs but may invade other body systems. TB is the leading cause of death in the world from a curable infectious disease. TB cases increased greatly during the mid-1990s as a result of AIDS, but both have decreased since 2000. Unfortunately, emerging multidrug-resistant strains are causing nearly 500,000 cases per year, especially in individuals from India, China, and Russia.[19] Emigration of infected individuals from high-prevalence countries, transmission in crowded institutional settings, homelessness, substance abuse, and lack of access to screening and medical care have contributed to the spread of TB.

PATHOPHYSIOLOGY TB is highly contagious and is transmitted from person to person in airborne droplets. In immunocompetent individuals, the microorganism is usually contained by the inflammatory and immune response systems. This results in latent TB infection (LTBI) and is associated with no clinical evidence of disease.

Once the bacilli are inspired, they lodge in the lung, usually in the upper lobe, and cause localized nonspecific pneumonitis (lung inflammation). Some bacilli migrate through the lymphatics and become lodged in the lymph nodes, where they encounter lymphocytes and initiate the immune response. Alveolar macrophages and neutrophils engulf and isolate the bacilli, preventing them from spreading. However, the bacterium is successful as a pathogen because it can survive and multiply within macrophages and resist lysosomal killing, forming a granulomatous lesion called a *tubercle* (see Chapter 6). Infected tissues within the tubercle die, forming cheeselike material called *caseation necrosis*. Collagenous scar tissue then grows around the tubercle, completing isolation of the bacilli. The immune response is complete after about 10 days, preventing further multiplication of the bacilli.

Once the bacilli are isolated in tubercles, tuberculosis may remain dormant for life. If the immune system is impaired, reactivation with progressive disease occurs and may spread through the blood and lymphatics to other organs. Infection with the human immunodeficiency virus (HIV), cancer, immunosuppressive medications (e.g., corticosteroids), poor nutritional status, and renal failure can reactivate the disease.

CLINICAL MANIFESTATIONS LTBI is asymptomatic. Symptoms of active disease often develop gradually and are not noticed until the disease is advanced. Common clinical manifestations include fatigue, weight loss, lethargy, anorexia (loss of appetite), and a low-grade fever that usually occurs in the afternoon. A cough that produces purulent sputum develops slowly and becomes more frequent over several weeks or months. Night sweats and general anxiety are often present. Dyspnea, chest pain, and hemoptysis may occur as the disease progresses. Extrapulmonary TB disease is common in HIV-infected individuals and may cause neurologic deficits, meningitis symptoms, bone pain, and urinary symptoms.

EVALUATION AND TREATMENT Screening for tuberculosis is usually conducted through the use of the tuberculin skin test (TST; purified protein derivative [PPD]), however, high-risk individuals instead should be screened with the interferon-gamma release assay (IGRA).[20] The diagnosis is confirmed through sputum stain and culture and chest radiographs. However, sputum culture can take up to 6 weeks to become positive.

Treatment consists of several months of combination antibiotic therapy to control active disease or prevent reactivation of LTBI.[21] Individuals must be kept in respiratory isolation until their sputum is no longer infectious. Multidrug-resistant TB requires a combination of second-line drugs for treatment success. Monitoring for adherence to and drug interactions and toxicities is essential.

Abscess Formation and Cavitation

An abscess is a circumscribed area of suppuration and destruction of lung parenchyma. Abscesses often occur because of aspiration associated with alcohol abuse, seizure disorders, general anesthesia, and swallowing disorders. Abscess formation follows consolidation of lung tissue, in which inflammation causes alveoli to fill with fluid, pus, and microorganisms. Necrosis (death and decay) of consolidated tissue may lead to cavitation in which the abscess empties into a bronchus and cavity formation. Abscess communication with a bronchus causes production of copious amounts of often foul-smelling sputum, and occasionally hemoptysis. Other clinical manifestations include fever, cough, chills, and pleural pain. The diagnosis is made by chest radiography and sputum analysis. Treatment includes appropriate antibiotics and chest physical therapy (chest percussion and postural drainage). Bronchoscopy may be performed to drain the abscess.

Pulmonary Vascular Disease

Blood flow through the lungs can be disrupted by disorders that occlude the vessels, increase pulmonary vascular resistance, or destroy the vascular bed. The consequences of altered pulmonary blood flow can result in severe and life-threatening changes in $\dot{V}/\dot{Q}$. Major disorders include pulmonary embolism, pulmonary hypertension, and cor pulmonale.

Pulmonary Embolism

Pulmonary embolism (PE) is occlusion of a portion of the pulmonary vascular bed by an embolus.[22] PE most commonly results from embolization of a clot from deep venous thrombosis involving the lower leg (see Chapter 26); this form of PE is often called *venous thromboembolism (VTE)*. Risk factors for PE caused by VTE include conditions and disorders that promote blood clotting as a result of venous stasis (immobilization, heart failure), injuries to the endothelial cells that line the vessels (trauma, infection, caustic IV infusions), and hypercoagulability (inherited coagulation disorders, malignancy, hormone replacement therapy, oral contraceptives). Inherited coagulation disorders include factor V Leiden, antithrombin II, protein S, protein C, and prothrombin gene mutations. Other, less common types of emboli include tissue fragments, lipids (fats), a foreign body, an air bubble, or amniotic fluid.

PATHOPHYSIOLOGY The effect of the embolus depends on the extent of pulmonary blood flow obstruction, the size of the affected vessels, the nature of the embolus, and the secondary effects. Pulmonary emboli that are relatively small cause $\dot{V}/\dot{Q}$ mismatch and associated hypoxemia without damaging the lung itself. However, larger emboli can cause pulmonary infarction or even massive occlusion of pulmonary vessels, resulting in shock. Some cases of PE involve multiple or recurrent emboli.

Significant obstruction of the pulmonary vasculature leads to pulmonary artery vasoconstriction, pulmonary hypertension, and an increased workload for the right ventricle. The pathogenesis of pulmonary embolism caused by VTE is summarized in Fig. 29.17.

If the embolus does not cause infarction, the clot is dissolved by the fibrinolytic system and pulmonary function returns to normal. If pulmonary infarction occurs, shrinking and scarring develop in the affected area of the lung.

CLINICAL MANIFESTATIONS In most cases, the clinical manifestations of PE are nonspecific and may be confused with many other pulmonary or cardiac conditions. Although most emboli originate from clots in the lower extremities, deep vein thrombosis is often asymptomatic, and clinical examination may not indicate the presence of clot, especially in the thigh and pelvis. Therefore, evaluation of risk factors and predisposing factors is an important aspect of diagnosis.

The classic clinical presentation of PE is the sudden onset of pleuritic chest pain, dyspnea, tachypnea, tachycardia, and unexplained anxiety. Occasionally syncope (fainting) or hemoptysis occurs. With large emboli, a pleural friction rub, pleural effusion, fever, and leukocytosis may be noted. Recurrent small emboli may not be detected until progressive incapacitation, precordial pain, anxiety, dyspnea, and right ventricular enlargement are exhibited. Massive occlusion causes severe pulmonary hypertension and shock.

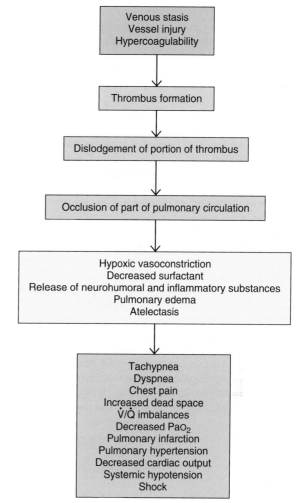

FIGURE 29.17 Pathogenesis of Pulmonary Embolism Caused by a Thrombus (Venous Thromboembolism). *PaO₂*, arterial oxygen pressure; $\dot{V}/\dot{Q}$, ventilation-perfusion.

EVALUATION AND TREATMENT Routine chest radiographs are not definitive for PE in the first 24 hours. Arterial blood gas analyses usually demonstrate hypoxemia and hyperventilation (respiratory alkalosis). The diagnosis of PE is made by measuring elevated levels of D-dimer in the blood (a product of thrombus degradation) in combination with CT arteriography or magnetic resonance arteriography (MRA). Measurement of the levels of BNP and troponin is useful in PE associated with right ventricular dysfunction.

Prevention of PE includes elimination of predisposing factors for individuals at risk. Venous stasis in hospitalized persons is minimized by leg elevation, bed exercises, position changes, early postoperative ambulation, and pneumatic calf compression. Clot formation is also prevented by prophylactic low-dose anticoagulant therapy.

Anticoagulant therapy is the primary treatment for PE. Initial anticoagulant therapy usually includes factor Xa inhibitors (e.g., fondaparinux, rivaroxaban) or low-molecular-weight heparins (e.g., enoxaparin).[23] If a massive life-threatening embolism occurs, a fibrinolytic agent, such as streptokinase, is sometimes used, and some individuals will require catheter-directed therapies or surgical thrombectomy. A filter in the inferior vena cava can prevent emboli from reaching the lungs. After stabilization, anticoagulation is continued for several months.

Pulmonary Arterial Hypertension

Pulmonary arterial hypertension (PAH) is defined as a mean pulmonary artery pressure greater than 25 mm Hg at rest (normal is 15 to 18 mm Hg).[24] PAH is classified into several groups based on its cause, including heritable defects, drugs, venoocclusive disease, lung or heart disease, systemic disorders, and chronic PE. COPD and interstitial fibrosis are the most common lung diseases associated with PAH, but any condition that causes chronic hypoxemia can result in pulmonary hypertension.

PATHOPHYSIOLOGY Many types of PAH are characterized by endothelial dysfunction with overproduction of vasoconstrictors, such as thromboxane and endothelin, and decreased production of vasodilators, such as prostacyclin and nitric oxide. Vascular growth factors are released, causing fibrosis and thickening of vessel walls (called *remodeling*) with arteriolar narrowing and abnormal vasoconstriction. Vasoconstriction causes resistance to pulmonary artery blood flow, thus increasing the pressure in the pulmonary arteries and right ventricle. As resistance and pressure increase, the workload of the right ventricle increases with subsequent right ventricular hypertrophy (cor pulmonale). Right heart failure may occur. The pathogenesis of PAH and cor pulmonale resulting from disease of the respiratory system is shown in Fig. 29.18.

CLINICAL MANIFESTATIONS Pulmonary arterial hypertension may not be detected until it is quite severe. The first indication of PAH may be an abnormality seen on a chest radiograph (enlarged right heart) or an electrocardiogram that shows right ventricular hypertrophy. Manifestations of fatigue, chest discomfort, tachypnea, and dyspnea (particularly with exercise) are common. The physical examination may reveal peripheral edema, jugular venous distention, a precordial heave, and accentuation of the pulmonary component of the second heart sound.

EVALUATION AND TREATMENT A definitive diagnosis of PAH is made by right heart catheterization. Common diagnostic modalities used to determine the cause include a chest x-ray, echocardiography, and CT.

General therapies for PAH include administration of oxygen, diuretics, and anticoagulants and avoidance of contributing factors, such as air travel, decongestant medications, nonsteroidal antiinflammatory medications, pregnancy, and tobacco use. The most effective treatments for pulmonary hypertension associated with lung respiratory disease are supplemental oxygen and treatment of the primary disorder. Medications used in the treatment of other forms of PAH include prostacyclin and its analogs, endothelin receptor antagonists, phosphodiesterase-5 inhibitors, prostanoids, and a soluble guanylate cyclase activator.[25] None of these drugs are curative, but they may improve morbidity and mortality. Individuals who do not achieve adequate clinical remission require lung transplantation.

Cor Pulmonale

Cor pulmonale occurs secondary to PAH and consists of right ventricular enlargement (hypertrophy, dilation, or both) (see Fig. 29.18).

PATHOPHYSIOLOGY Cor pulmonale develops as PAH exerts chronic pressure overload in the right ventricle. Pressure overload increases the work of the right ventricle, resulting in hypertrophy of the normally thin-walled heart muscle. This eventually progresses to dilation and failure of the ventricle.

CLINICAL MANIFESTATIONS The clinical manifestations of cor pulmonale may be obscured by underlying respiratory or cardiac disease and may appear only during exercise testing. The heart may appear normal at rest, but with exercise, cardiac output falls. The electrocardiogram may show right ventricular hypertrophy. The pulmonary component of the second heart sound (i.e., closure of the pulmonic valve) may be accentuated, and a pulmonic valve murmur also may be present. A tricuspid valve murmur may accompany the development of right ventricular failure. Increased pressures in the systemic venous circulation cause jugular venous distention, hepatosplenomegaly, and peripheral edema.

EVALUATION AND TREATMENT The diagnosis is based on the physical examination, thoracic imaging, and electrocardiography or echocardiography, or both. The goal of treatment for cor pulmonale is to decrease the workload of the right ventricle by lowering the pulmonary artery pressure. Treatment is the same as that for pulmonary hypertension, and its success depends on reversal of the underlying lung disease.

> **✔ QUICK CHECK 29.6**
> 1. What factors influence the impact of an embolus?
> 2. List three causes of pulmonary hypertension.
> 3. What is cor pulmonale?

Malignancies of the Respiratory Tract
Laryngeal Cancer

Cancer of the larynx (laryngeal cancer) represents less than 1% of all cancers in the United States, with an estimated 13,150 new cases and 3710 deaths in 2018.[26] Laryngeal cancer is much more common in men than women, and the primary risk factor is tobacco smoking. The risk

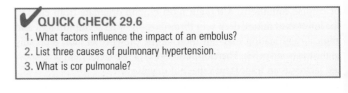

FIGURE 29.18 Pathogenesis of Pulmonary Hypertension and Cor Pulmonale. *COPD,* Chronic obstructive pulmonary disease;

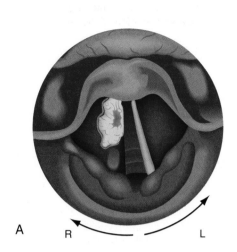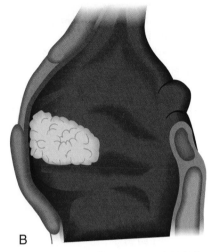

FIGURE 29.19 Laryngeal Cancer. A, Mirror view of carcinoma of the right false cord partially hiding the true cord. **B,** Lateral view. (Redrawn from del Regato JA et al: *Ackerman and del Regato's cancer,* ed 2, St Louis, 1985, Mosby.)

is heightened by the combination of smoking and alcohol consumption. The human papillomavirus (HPV 6 and HPV 11) also has been linked to both benign and malignant disease of the larynx.

PATHOPHYSIOLOGY Carcinoma of the true vocal cords (glottis) is more common than that of the supraglottic structures (epiglottis, aryepiglottic folds, arytenoids, false cords). Tumors of the subglottic area are rare. Squamous cell carcinoma is the most common cell type, although small cell carcinomas also occur (Fig. 29.19). Metastasis develops by spread to the draining lymph nodes, and distant metastasis is rare.

CLINICAL MANIFESTATIONS The presenting symptoms of laryngeal cancer include hoarseness, dyspnea, and cough. Progressive hoarseness can result in voice loss. Dyspnea is rare with supraglottic tumors but can be severe in subglottic tumors. Swallowing may initiate a cough reflex. Laryngeal pain is likely with supraglottic lesions.

EVALUATION AND TREATMENT Evaluation of the larynx includes external inspection and palpation of the larynx and the lymph nodes of the neck. Indirect or direct laryngoscopy with biopsy provides a definitive diagnosis. Imaging procedures facilitate the identification of tumor boundaries and the degree of extension to surrounding tissue.

Combined chemotherapy and irradiation or surgical resection can result in cure in selected cases, and larynx-preservation strategies are being used to preserve swallowing and speech whenever possible.[27] Swallowing and speech therapy after treatment can significantly improve recovery.

Lung Cancer

Lung cancer is the second most common cancer in the United States, comprising 13% of all new cancer cases in 2019, and is the leading cause of cancer deaths (24%).[26] Annual lung cancer mortality in the U.S. is roughly equal to breast, colon, pancreatic cancer, and lymphoma mortality combined. Despite emerging new therapies, the overall 5-year survival remains low, at about 20%.

Nearly 80% of lung cancers are caused by cigarette smoking. The reduction in smoking prevalence over the past 3 decades has led to a gradual decline in incidence, but many new cases of lung cancer occur in individuals who have already quit smoking. Smokers with COPD are at even greater risk. Other risk factors for lung cancer include

secondhand (environmental) smoke, radon gas exposure, occupational exposures to certain workplace toxins, radiation, and air pollution (see Chapter 12). Genetic risks include polymorphisms of the genes responsible for growth factor receptors, angiogenesis, apoptosis, deoxyribonucleic acid (DNA) repair, and detoxification of inhaled smoke.

Types of lung cancer. The vast majority of primary lung cancers arise from cells that line the bronchi within the lungs and are therefore called *bronchogenic carcinomas*. Lung cancers are classified by cell type and molecular profiling. Although there are many types of lung cancer, they can be divided into two major categories: non–small cell lung carcinoma (NSCLC) and neuroendocrine tumors of the lung. Characteristics of these tumors, including clinical manifestations, are listed in Table 29.3. The category of NSCLC accounts for about 85% of all lung cancers and can be subdivided into three types of lung cancer: squamous cell carcinoma, adenocarcinoma, and large cell undifferentiated carcinoma.

Neuroendocrine tumors of the lung also arise from the bronchial mucosa and include small cell carcinoma, large cell neuroendocrine carcinoma, and typical carcinoid and atypical carcinoid tumors. Small cell carcinoma is the most common of these neuroendocrine tumors, accounting for 15% to 20% of all lung cancers.

Other pulmonary tumors, such as mesotheliomas (associated with asbestos exposure), occur less commonly. Many cancers that arise in other organs of the body metastasize to the lungs; however, these are not considered lung cancers and are categorized by their primary site of origin.

Non–small cell lung cancer. Squamous cell carcinoma accounts for about 30% of bronchogenic carcinomas. These tumors are typically located near the hila and project into bronchi (Fig. 29.20, *A*). Because of this central location, symptoms of a nonproductive cough or hemoptysis are common. Pneumonia and atelectasis are often associated with squamous cell carcinoma (Fig. 29.20, *A*). Chest pain is a late symptom associated with large tumors. These tumors are often fairly well localized and tend not to metastasize until late in the course of the disease.

Adenocarcinoma (tumor arising from glands) of the lung constitutes 35% to 40% of all bronchogenic carcinomas (Fig. 29.20, *B*). Pulmonary adenocarcinoma develops in a stepwise fashion through atypical adenomatous hyperplasia, adenocarcinoma in situ, and minimally invasive adenocarcinoma to invasive carcinoma. These tumors, which are usually smaller than 4 cm, more commonly arise in the peripheral regions of

TABLE 29.3 Characteristics of Lung Cancers

Tumor Type	Growth Rate	Metastasis	Means of Diagnosis	Clinical Manifestations and Treatment
Non–Small Cell Carcinoma				
Squamous cell carcinoma	Slow	Late; mostly to hilar lymph nodes	Biopsy, sputum analysis, bronchoscopy, electron microscopy, immunohistochemistry	Cough, hemoptysis, sputum production, airway obstruction, hypercalcemia; treated surgically, chemotherapy, radiation and immunotherapy as adjunctive therapy
Adenocarcinoma	Moderate	Early; to lymph nodes, pleura, bone, adrenal glands, and brain	Radiography, fiberoptic bronchoscopy, electron microscopy	Pleural effusion; treated surgically, chemotherapy, and immunotherapy as adjunctive therapy
Large cell carcinoma	Rapid	Early and widespread	Sputum analysis, bronchoscopy, electron microscopy (by exclusion of other cell types)	Chest wall pain, pleural effusion, cough, sputum production, hemoptysis, airway obstruction resulting in pneumonia; treated surgically
Neuroendocrine Tumors of the Lung				
Small cell carcinoma	Very rapid	Very early; to mediastinum, lymph nodes, brain, bone marrow	Radiography, sputum analysis, bronchoscopy, electron microscopy, immunohistochemistry	Cough, chest pain, dyspnea, hemoptysis, localized wheezing, airway obstruction, signs and symptoms of excessive hormone secretion; treated by chemotherapy and ionizing radiation to thorax and central nervous system
Other Pulmonary Tumors				
Malignant pleural mesothelioma (MPM)	Rapid	Early; to lymph nodes, lungs, heart, bone	Radiography, thoracentesis	Chest pain, chronic cough, signs of pleural effusion; treated by surgery, chemotherapy, radiation, and immunotherapy

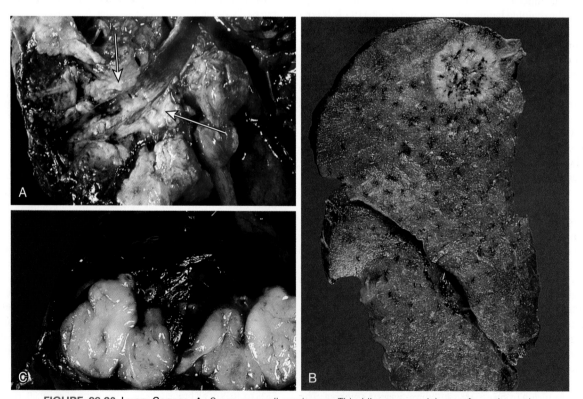

FIGURE 29.20 Lung Cancer. A, Squamous cell carcinoma. This hilar tumor originates from the main bronchus. **B,** Peripheral adenocarcinoma. The tumor shows prominent black pigmentation, suggestive of having evolved in an anthracotic scar. **C,** Small cell carcinoma. The tumor forms confluent nodules. On cross section, the nodules have an encephaloid appearance. (From Damjanov I, Linder J, editors: *Anderson's pathology,* ed 10, St Louis, 1996, Mosby.)

the pulmonary parenchyma. They may be asymptomatic and discovered by routine chest imaging in the early stages, or the individual may present with pleuritic chest pain and shortness of breath from pleural involvement by the tumor.

Included in the category of adenocarcinoma is bronchioloalveolar cell carcinoma. These tumors arise from terminal bronchioles and alveoli and are now being referred to as *adenocarcinoma in situ* or *minimally invasive adenocarcinoma*. They are slow-growing tumors with an unpredictable pattern of metastasis through the pulmonary arterial system and mediastinal lymph nodes.

Large cell carcinomas constitute approximately 10% of bronchogenic carcinomas. These transformed epithelial cells have lost clear evidence of maturation and are considered an undifferentiated non–small cell carcinoma. These tumors arise from squamous, glandular, or neuroendocrine precursor cells; commonly arise centrally; and can grow to distort the trachea and cause widening of the carina.

Neuroendocrine tumors. Small cell lung carcinoma (SCLC) is the most common type of neuroendocrine lung tumor and is the cause of nearly 25% of all lung cancer deaths. Small cell carcinoma arises from neuroendocrine cells that contain neurosecretory granules. Most of these tumors are central in origin (hilar and mediastinal) (see Fig. 29.20, C), have a rapid rate of growth, and tend to metastasize early and widely. Because these cells arise from neuroendocrine cells, they are often associated with ectopic hormone production. Ectopic hormone production is important to the clinician because resulting signs and symptoms, called *paraneoplastic syndromes,* may be the first manifestation of the underlying cancer. Examples include hyponatremia (antidiuretic hormone), Cushing syndrome (adrenocorticotropic hormone), hypocalcemia (calcitonin), gynecomastia (gonadotropins), carcinoid syndrome (serotonin), and Lambert-Eaton myasthenic syndrome (paneoplastic cerebellar degeneration).

Bronchial carcinoid tumors represent only about 1% of all lung tumors. They are unusual in that they are not related to smoking, may begin in childhood, and grow very slowly. They are usually discovered by chest imaging undertaken for an unrelated condition and can be cured by local surgical or bronchoscopic resection.

Other lung cancers. Mesotheliomas arise from the mesothelial cells that line the pleura. Nearly 80% have been linked to asbestos exposure, although it may take up to 40 years after exposure for the tumor to be diagnosed. Clinical manifestations include dyspnea and chest pain. Chest imaging may reveal a pleural effusion, with the diagnosis confirmed by CT scanning, thoracentesis, thoracoscopy, and cytology. Management includes surgery, chemotherapy, radiation, and immunotherapy.

PATHOPHYSIOLOGY Tobacco smoke contains more than 30 carcinogens, which, along with an inherited genetic predisposition to cancers, result in tumor development. Once lung cancer is initiated by these carcinogen-induced mutations, tumor development is promoted by growth factors that alter cell growth and differentiation and by the production of inflammatory mediators. The bronchial mucosa suffers multiple carcinogenic "hits" because of repetitive exposure to tobacco smoke and, eventually, epithelial cell changes begin progressing from metaplasia to carcinoma in situ and finally to invasive carcinoma. Further tumor progression includes invasion of surrounding tissues and finally metastasis to distant sites, including the brain, bone marrow, and liver (see Chapter 11 for the details of cancer biology).

CLINICAL MANIFESTATIONS Table 29.3 summarizes the characteristic clinical manifestations according to tumor type. Symptoms are nonspecific and often attributed to smoking; and when they are severe enough to motivate the individual to seek medical advice, the disease is often advanced.

EVALUATION AND TREATMENT Annual screening for lung cancer with low-dose CT scans is recommended for asymptomatic individuals age 55 to 77 who have 30 pack years or more of smoking history and either continue to smoke or have quit within the past 15 years.[28] Diagnostic tests for the evaluation of lung cancer include sputum cytologic studies, chest imaging, virtual bronchoscopy, radial probe endobronchial ultrasound, electromagnetic navigational bronchoscopy, and biopsy. Biopsy determines the cell type, and the evaluation of lymph nodes and other organ systems is used to determine the stage of the cancer. The current accepted system for the staging of non–small cell cancer is the TNM classification (*T* denotes the extent of the primary tumor, *N* indicates the nodal involvement, *M* describes the extent of metastasis) (see Chapter 11). In contrast, small cell lung cancers are only staged as either limited (confined to the area of origin in the lung) or extensive.

The histologic cell type, the genotype, and the stage of the disease are major factors that influence the choice of therapy. For all types of early-stage lung carcinoma, the preferred treatment is surgical resection. Once metastasis has occurred, total surgical resection is more difficult and survival rates dramatically decrease. For those for whom surgical removal is not an option, treatment modalities include chemotherapy, dose-intensified irradiation, radiofrequency ablation, microwave ablation, cryotherapy, and brachytherapy. Immunotherapies have been approved that can increase the survival time for selected individuals (see *Did You Know?* Molecular and Immune Therapies for Lung Cancer).

DID YOU KNOW?
Molecular and Immune Therapies for Lung Cancer

Better understanding of the genetic and immunologic features of lung cancer cells has led to new treatment options. Molecular gene therapies have improved treatment responses in non–small cell carcinoma. The most effective to date are epidermoid growth factor receptors (i.e., tyrosine kinase inhibitors), such as erlotinib, gefitinib, and afatinib. These drugs have increased overall response rates to treatment and have contributed to increased survival time. Other targets include drugs that block the effects of anaplastic lymphoma kinase (ALK) mutations (crizotinib, ceritinib) and angiogenesis (bevacizumab). New immune therapies have emerged that stop cancer growth by affecting "immune checkpoints." Cancer cells have the capacity to prevent effective adaptive immune responses by activating inhibitory molecules, such as PDL-1 and CTLA-4, on the surface of T cells, thus shutting these cells off. Monoclonal antibodies can be used to block these checkpoint inhibitors and thus restore the immune response to the cancer. Immunotherapies currently approved by the U.S. Food and Drug Administration (FDA) that block PDL-1 or CTLA-4 include nivolumab, pembrolizumab, atezolizumab, durvalumab, avelumab, and ipilimumab. These therapies can shrink tumors and prolong life but are rarely curative.

Data from Chee J et al: *Chest* 151(4), 891-897, 2017; Hirsch FR et al: *Lancet* 389(10066):299-311, 2017; Ke X, Shen L: *Front Lab Med* 1(2):69-75, 2017; Lievense LA et al: *Am J Respir Crit Care Med* 196(3):274-282, 2017; Remon J, Vilarino N, Reguart N: *Cancer Treat Rev* 64:21-29, 2018; Shroff GS et al: *Radiol Clin North Am* 56(3):485-495, 2018.

✓QUICK CHECK 29.7
1. Describe squamous cell carcinoma of the vocal cords.
2. Differentiate the two types of non–small cell lung cancer.
3. What are paraneoplastic syndromes?

SUMMARY REVIEW

Clinical Manifestations of Pulmonary Alterations

1. Dyspnea is the feeling of breathlessness and increased respiratory effort. Orthopnea is dyspnea that occurs when an individual lies flat, which causes the abdominal contents to exert pressure on the diaphragm.
2. Coughing is a protective reflex that expels secretions and irritants from the lower airways. It can be acute or chronic.
3. Changes in the sputum volume, consistency, or color may indicate underlying pulmonary disease.
4. Hemoptysis is expectoration of bloody mucus, usually due to infection or inflammation that damages the bronchi or lung parenchyma.
5. Abnormal breathing patterns are adjustments made by the body to minimize the work of respiratory muscles. They include Kussmaul, labored, restricted, gasping, and Cheyne-Stokes respirations as well as sighing.
6. Hypoventilation is decreased alveolar ventilation caused by altered pulmonary mechanics or neurologic control of breathing and results in increased $PaCO_2$ (hypercapnia).
7. Hyperventilation is increased alveolar ventilation produced by anxiety, head injury, pain, or severe hypoxemia and causes decreased $PaCO_2$ (hypocapnia).
8. Cyanosis is a bluish discoloration of the skin caused by desaturation of hemoglobin, polycythemia, or peripheral vasoconstriction.
9. Clubbing of the fingertips is associated with diseases that cause chronic hypoxemia, and it is rarely reversible.
10. Chest pain can result from infection and inflammation of the pleurae, trachea, bronchi, ribs, or respiratory muscles.
11. Hypercapnia is an increased $PaCO_2$ due to (1) depression of respiratory center by drugs, (2) diseases of the medulla, (3) abnormalities of the spinal conducting pathways, (4) diseases of the neuromuscular junction, (5) thoracic cage abnormalities, (6) large airway obstruction, and (7) increased work of breathing or physiologic dead space.
12. Hypoxemia is a reduced PaO_2 caused by (1) decreased oxygen content of inspired gas, (2) hypoventilation, (3) ventilation-perfusion mismatch, (4) diffusion abnormality, or (5) altered perfusion of the pulmonary system.
13. Respiratory failure is inadequate gas exchange that can result from direct injury to the lungs, airways, or chest wall or indirectly because of disease or injury involving another body system. It is classified as either hypoxemic or hypercapnic.
14. Chest wall compliance is diminished by obesity and kyphoscoliosis, which compress the lungs, and by neuromuscular diseases that impair chest wall muscle function.
15. Flail chest results from rib or sternal fractures that disrupt the mechanics of breathing.
16. Pneumothorax is the accumulation of air in the pleural space. It can be caused by spontaneous rupture of weakened areas of the pleura or can be secondary to pleural damage caused by disease, trauma, or mechanical ventilation.
17. Tension pneumothorax is a life-threatening condition caused by trapping of air in the pleural space, producing displacement of the great vessels and heart.
18. Pleural effusion is the accumulation of fluid in the pleural space resulting from disorders of the blood vessels or lymphatic vessels underlying the pleura. Pleural effusions can be transudative (watery) or exudative (high concentrations of white blood cells and plasma proteins).

19. Empyema is the presence of pus in the pleural space (infected pleural effusion); it usually occurs because of lymphatic drainage from sites of bacterial pneumonia.

Disorders of the Chest Wall and Pleura

1. Chest wall compliance is diminished by obesity and kyphoscoliosis, which compress the lungs, and by neuromuscular diseases that impair chest wall muscle function.
2. Flail chest results from rib or sternal fractures that disrupt the mechanics of breathing.
3. Pneumothorax is the accumulation of air in the pleural space. It can be caused by spontaneous rupture of weakened areas of the pleura or can be secondary to pleural damage caused by disease, trauma, or mechanical ventilation.
4. Tension pneumothorax is a life-threatening condition caused by trapping of air in the pleural space, producing displacement of the great vessels and heart.
5. Pleural effusion is the accumulation of fluid in the pleural space resulting from disorders that promote transudation or exudation from capillaries underlying the pleura or from blockage or injury to lymphatic vessels that drain into the pleural space.
6. Empyema is the presence of pus in the pleural space (infected pleural effusion); it usually occurs because of lymphatic drainage from sites of bacterial pneumonia.

Pulmonary Disorders

1. Pulmonary disorders can be restrictive (limiting lung volumes) or obstructive (limiting airflow) or both.
2. Restrictive lung diseases are characterized by decreased lung compliance meaning it takes more effort to expand the lungs during inspiration, which increases the work of breathing. Individuals with lung restriction have dyspnea, an increased respiratory rate, and a decreased tidal volume.
3. Aspiration of food particles or pharyngeal or gastric secretions can cause obstruction, inflammation, or pneumonia.
4. Atelectasis is the collapse of alveoli resulting from compression of lung tissue, absorption of gas from obstructed alveoli, or decreased production of surfactant.
5. Bronchiectasis is abnormal dilation of the bronchi secondary to another pulmonary disorder, usually infection or inflammation.
6. Bronchiolitis is the inflammatory obstruction of small airways. It is most common in children.
7. Pulmonary fibrosis is excessive connective tissue in the lung that diminishes lung compliance; it may be idiopathic or caused by disease and is associated with chronic inflammation.
8. Inhalation of noxious gases or prolonged exposure to high concentrations of oxygen can damage the bronchial mucosa or alveolocapillary membrane and cause inflammation or acute respiratory failure.
9. Pneumoconiosis, which is caused by inhalation of dust particles in the workplace, can cause pulmonary fibrosis and progressive pulmonary deterioration.
10. Hypersensitivity pneumonitis (extrinsic allergic alveolitis) is an allergic or hypersensitivity reaction to many allergens causing lung inflammation.
11. Pulmonary edema is excess water in the lung caused by increased capillary hydrostatic pressure, decreased capillary oncotic pressure, or increased capillary permeability. Causes include left heart failure that increases capillary hydrostatic pressure in the pulmonary circulation, inflammation of alveoli, or lymphatic obstruction.

12. Acute respiratory distress syndrome (ARDS) is a form of acute lung inflammation and diffuse alveolocapillary injury that results from direct pulmonary injury or from severe systemic inflammation. Endothelial damage results in increased capillary membrane permeability causing hypoxemia, and remodeling of the tissue causes fibrosis.

13. Obstructive lung disease is characterized by airway obstruction that causes difficult expiration. Accessory muscles of expiration must be used, which increases the work of breathing. The unifying symptom of obstructive lung diseases is dyspnea, and the unifying sign is wheezing.

14. Asthma is a chronic inflammation that causes bronchial hyperresponsiveness, constriction of the airways, and variable airflow obstruction that is reversible. Many cells contribute to the persistent inflammation including dendritic cells, T helper 2 lymphocytes, B lymphocytes, mast cells, neutrophils, eosinophils, and basophils.

15. In asthma, airway obstruction is caused by episodic attacks of bronchospasm, bronchial inflammation, mucosal edema, and increased mucus production.

16. Chronic obstructive pulmonary disease (COPD) is the coexistence of chronic bronchitis and emphysema and is an important cause of hypoxemic and hypercapnic respiratory failure.

17. Chronic bronchitis causes airway obstruction resulting from inflammation, bronchial smooth muscle hypertrophy, and production of thick, tenacious mucus.

18. In emphysema, destruction of the alveolar septa and loss of passive elastic recoil lead to alveolar enlargement, airway collapse, obstruction of gas flow, and air trapping during expiration.

19. Respiratory tract infections are the most common cause of short-term disability in the United States and most of these infections involve only the upper airways.

20. Acute bronchitis is usually a self-limiting viral infection.

21. Pneumonia is infection of the lower respiratory tract caused by bacteria, viruses, fungi, protozoa, or parasites.

22. Pneumococcal (*Streptococcus pneumoniae*) is the most common cause of community acquired pneumonia.

23. Viral pneumonia can be severe, but is more often an acute, self-limiting lung infection usually caused by the influenza virus.

24. Tuberculosis (TB) is a lung infection caused by *Mycobacterium tuberculosis* (tubercle bacillus). In tuberculosis, the inflammatory response proceeds to isolate colonies of bacilli by enclosing them in tubercles and surrounding the tubercles with scar tissue. TB bacilli escape immune defenses by surviving within macrophages.

25. An abscess is a circumscribed area of suppuration and destruction of lung parenchyma, often caused by aspiration. Necrosis of consolidated tissue may lead to cavitation in which the abscess empties into a bronchus and cavity formation.

26. Pulmonary vascular diseases are caused by embolism, hypertension, or cor pulmonale in the pulmonary circulation.

27. Pulmonary embolism is most often the result of embolism of part of a clot from deep venous thrombosis and causes vascular obstruction, $\dot{V}/\dot{Q}$ mismatch, hypoxemia, and pulmonary hypertension; it may or may not cause infarction.

28. Pulmonary artery hypertension (pulmonary artery pressure >25 mm Hg) can caused by heritable defects, drugs, venoocclusive disease, lung or heart disease, systemic disorders, and chronic pulmonary embolism.

29. Cor pulmonale is secondary to pulmonary artery hypertension and is right ventricular enlargement or failure.

30. Laryngeal cancer occurs primarily in men, represents less than 1% of all cancers, and presents with a clinical symptom of progressive hoarseness.

31. Lung cancer, the most common cause of cancer death in the United States, is usually caused by tobacco smoking.

32. Lung cancer (bronchogenic carcinomas) cell types include non–small cell carcinoma (squamous cell, adenocarcinoma, and large cell) and neuroendocrine tumors (small cell lung carcinoma and bronchial carcinoid tumors). Each type arises in a characteristic site or type of tissue, causes distinctive clinical manifestations, and differs in likelihood of metastasis and prognosis.

KEY TERMS

Abscess, 688
Acute bronchitis, 686
Acute respiratory distress syndrome (ARDS), 679
Adenocarcinoma, 691
Air trapping, 685
Alveolar dead space, 674
Aspiration, 676
Asthma, 680
Atelectasis, 676
Bronchial carcinoid tumor, 693
Bronchiectasis, 677
Bronchiolitis, 677
Bronchiolitis obliterans, 677
Bronchiolitis obliterans organizing pneumonia (BOOP), 677
Cancer of the larynx (laryngeal cancer), 690
Cavitation, 688
Cheyne-Stokes respiration, 671

Chronic bronchitis, 682
Chronic obstructive pulmonary disease (COPD), 682
Clubbing, 672
Compression atelectasis, 676
Cor pulmonale, 690
Cough, 670
Cyanosis, 671
Dyspnea, 670
Emphysema, 685
Empyema (infected pleural effusion), 675
Exudative effusion, 675
Flail chest, 674
Hemoptysis, 671
Hypercapnia, 672
Hypersensitivity pneumonitis (extrinsic allergic alveolitis), 678
Hyperventilation, 671
Hypocapnia, 671

Hypoventilation, 671
Hypoxemia, 672
Hypoxia (ischemia), 672
Idiopathic pulmonary fibrosis (IPF), 678
Kussmaul respiration (hyperpnea), 671
Large cell carcinoma, 693
Latent TB infection (LTBI), 688
Obstructive (absorption) atelectasis, 677
Open (communicating) pneumothorax, 675
Orthopnea, 670
Oxygen toxicity, 678
Paroxysmal nocturnal dyspnea (PND), 670
Pleural effusion, 675
Pneumoconiosis, 678
Pneumonia, 686
Pneumothorax, 674

Pulmonary artery hypertension (PAH), 690
Pulmonary consolidation, 688
Pulmonary edema, 678
Pulmonary embolism (PE), 689
Pulmonary fibrosis, 677
Pulsus paradoxus, 681
Respiratory failure, 674
Shunting, 673
Small cell lung carcinoma (SCLC), 693
Squamous cell carcinoma, 691
Status asthmaticus, 681
Surfactant impairment (adhesive) atelectasis, 677
Tension pneumothorax, 675
TNM classification, 693
Transudative effusion, 675
Tuberculosis (TB), 688

REFERENCES

1. Anzueto A, Miravitlles M: Pathophysiology of dyspnea in COPD, *Postgrad Med* 129(3):366-374, 2017.
2. Michaudet C, Malaty J: Chronic cough: evaluation and management, *Am Fam Physician* 96(9):575-580, 2017.
3. Tschopp JM, et al: ERS task force statement: diagnosis and treatment of primary spontaneous pneumothorax, *Eur Respir J* 46(2):321-335, 2015.
4. Shen KR, et al: The American Association for Thoracic Surgery consensus guidelines for the management of empyema, *J Thorac Cardiovasc Surg* 153(6):e129-e146, 2017.
5. Randtke MA, Andrews BP, Mach WJ: Pathophysiology and prevention of intraoperative atelectasis: a review of the literature, *J Perianesth Nurs* 30(6):516-527, 2015.
6. Boyton RJ, Altmann DM: Bronchiectasis: current concepts in pathogenesis, immunology, and microbiology, *Annu Rev Pathol* 11:523-554, 2016.
7. Sgalla G, Biffi A, Richeldi L: Idiopathic pulmonary fibrosis: diagnosis, epidemiology and natural history, *Respirology* 21(3):427-437, 2016.
8. Tolle LB, et al: Idiopathic pulmonary fibrosis: what primary care physicians need to know, *Cleve Clin J Med* 85(5):377-386, 2018.
9. Fan E, et al: An official American Thoracic Society/European Society of Intensive Care Medicine/Society of Critical Care Medicine clinical practice guideline: mechanical ventilation in adult patients with acute respiratory distress syndrome, *Am J Respir Crit Care Med* 195(9):1253-1263, 2017.
10. Howell MD, Davis AM: Management of ARDS in adults, *J Am Med Assoc* 319(7):711-712, 2018.
11. Global Initiative for Asthma: Global strategy for asthma management and prevention, (2018 update). Available at https://ginasthma.org/wp-content/uploads/2018/04/wms-GINA-2018-report-tracked_v1.3.pdf.
12. Center for Disease Control and Prevention (CDC): National center for health statistics. Fast stats asthma. Last reviewed January 19, 2017. Available at https://www.cdc.gov/nchs/fastats/asthma.htm.
13. Global Initiative for Chronic Obstructive Lung Disease: Global strategy for the diagnosis, management, and prevention of COPD 2019 report. Available at https://goldcopd.org/wp-content/uploads/2018/11/GOLD-2019-v1.7-FINAL-14Nov2018-WMS.pdf.
14. Centers for Disease Control and Prevention (CDC): Chronic obstructive pulmonary disease data and statistics. Available at https://www.cdc.gov/copd/data.html.
15. Greulich T, Vogelmeier CF: Alpha-1-antitrypsin deficiency: increasing awareness and improving diagnosis, *Ther Adv Respir Dis* 10(1):72-84, 2016.
16. Criner GJ, et al: Prevention of acute exacerbations of COPD: American College of Chest Physicians and Canadian Thoracic Society guideline, *Chest* 147(4):894-942, 2015.
17. Centers for Disease Control and Prevention (CDC): National center for health statistics. Last reviewed January 20, 2017. Available at https://www.cdc.gov/nchs/fastats/pneumonia.htm.
18. Kalil AC, et al: Management of adults with hospital-acquired and ventilator-associated pneumonia: 2016 clinical practice guidelines by the Infectious Diseases Society of America and the American Thoracic Society, *Clin Infect Dis* 63(5):e61-e111, 2016.
19. World Health Organizataion (WHO): WHO global tuberculosis report 2017. Available at http://www.who.int/tb/publications/global_report/en/.
20. Lewinsohn DM, et al: Official American Thoracic Society/Infectious Diseases Society of America/Centers for Disease Control and Prevention clinical practice guidelines: diagnosis of tuberculosis in adults and children, *Clin Infect Dis* 64:e1-e33, 2017.
21. Nahid P, et al: Executive Summary: official American Thoracic Society/Centers for Disease Control and Prevention/Infectious Diseases Society of America clinical practice guidelines: treatment of drug-susceptible tuberculosis, *Clin Infect Dis* 63(7):853-867, 2016.
22. Rali P, Gandhi V, Malik K: Pulmonary embolism, *Crit Care Nurs Q* 39(2):131-138, 2016.
23. Kearon C, et al: Antithrombotic therapy for VTE disease: CHEST guideline and expert panel report, *Chest* 149(2):315-352, 2016.
24. Ataya A, et al: Pulmonary arterial hypertension and associated conditions, *Dis Mon* 62(11):379-402, 2016.
25. Hahn SS, et al: A review of therapeutic agents for the management of pulmonary arterial hypertension, *Ther Adv Respir Dis* 11(1):46-63, 2017.
26. American Cancer Society (ACS): Cancer fact & figures 2019, Atlanta, 2019, Author. Available at https://www.cancer.org/research/cancer-facts-statistics/all-cancer-facts-figures/cancer-facts-figures-2019.html.
27. Forastiere AA, et al: Use of larynx preservation strategies in the treatment of laryngeal cancer: American Society of Clinical Oncology clinical practice guidelines, *J Clin Oncol* 36(11):1143-1169, 2018.
28. Mazzone PJ, et al: Screening for lung cancer: CHEST guideline and expert panel report, *Chest* 153(4):954-985, 2018.

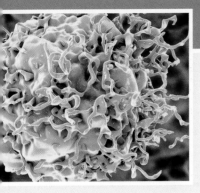

30

Alterations of Pulmonary Function in Children

Valentina L. Brashers

EVOLVE WEBSITE

http://evolve.elsevier.com/Huether/
Student Review Questions
Audio Key Points

Case Studies
Animations
Quick Check Answers

CHAPTER OUTLINE

Alterations of respiratory function in children are influenced by physiologic development, which is determined by age, genetics, and environmental conditions. Infants, especially premature infants, are particularly vulnerable to a variety of respiratory disorders because of incomplete development of the airways, circulation, chest wall, and immune system. A variety of upper and lower airway infections can cause respiratory compromise or play a role in the pathogenesis of more chronic pulmonary disease. Pulmonary dysfunction can be categorized into disorders of either the upper or the lower airways.

DISORDERS OF THE UPPER AIRWAYS

Disorders of the upper airways can cause significant obstruction to airflow. Common causes of upper airway obstruction (UAO) in children are infections, foreign body aspiration, obstructive sleep apnea, and trauma.

Infections of the Upper Airways

Table 30.1 compares some of the more common upper airway infections.

Croup

The two most common croup illnesses are viral croup and recurrent croup (spasmodic croup). Diphtheria can also be considered a croup illness but is now rare because of vaccinations. Croup illnesses are all characterized by obstruction of the upper airways.

Viral croup is an acute *laryngotracheobronchitis* and almost always occurs in children between 6 months and 5 years of age with a peak incidence at 2 years of age. It is most commonly caused by parainfluenza.

Other causes include respiratory syncytial virus, rhinovirus, adenovirus, rubella virus, or atypical bacteria. The incidence of croup is higher in males, and the disease is most common during the winter months. Recurrent (spasmodic) croup is two or more episodes of symptoms similar to viral croup except without symptoms of respiratory tract infection. It usually occurs in older children. The etiology is unknown but it is sometimes associated with underlying congenital obstruction or airway narrowing, gastroesophageal reflux, and allergies.[1]

PATHOPHYSIOLOGY The pathophysiology of viral croup is caused primarily by subglottic inflammation (the area containing the vocal cords) and edema from the infection. The mucous membranes of the larynx are tightly adherent to the underlying cartilage, whereas those of the subglottic space are looser and thus allow accumulation of mucosal and submucosal edema (Fig. 30.1). Furthermore, the cricoid cartilage is structurally the narrowest point of the airway, making edema in this area critical. Recurrent croup also causes obstruction but with less inflammation and edema. As illustrated in Fig. 30.2, increased resistance to airflow leads to increased work of breathing, which generates more negative intrathoracic pressure that, in turn, may exacerbate dynamic collapse of the upper airway.

CLINICAL MANIFESTATIONS Typically, a child with viral croup experiences rhinorrhea (runny nose), sore throat, and low-grade fever for a few days and then develops a harsh (seal-like), barking cough, a hoarse voice, and inspiratory stridor (a harsh, vibratory sound). The quality of the voice, cough, and stridor may suggest the location of the obstruction (Fig. 30.3). Most cases resolve spontaneously within 24 to 48 hours. A child with severe croup usually displays deep retractions

TABLE 30.1   Comparison of Upper Airway Infections

Condition	Age	Onset	Etiology	Pathophysiology	Symptoms
Acute laryngotracheobronchitis (croup)	6 months to 3 yr	Usually gradual	Viral (e.g., parainfluenza, respiratory syncytial virus)	Inflammation from larynx to bronchi	Harsh cough; stridor; low-grade fever; may have nasal discharge, conjunctivitis
Acute tracheitis	1 to 12 yr	Abrupt or after viral illness	*Staphylococcus aureus*/methicillin resistant *S. aureus* (MRSA) *Haemophilus influenzae* type B Group A streptococci	Inflammation of upper trachea	High fever; toxic appearance; harsh cough; purulent secretions; may prefer head elevation
Acute epiglottitis	2 to 6 yr	Abrupt	*Haemophilus influenzae*, group A streptococci	Inflammation of supraglottic structures	Severe sore throat; high fever; toxic appearance; muffled voice; may drool; sits erect or leans forward
Peritonsillar abscess	>9 yr	May be abrupt	*S. pyogenes* *S. aureus*/MRSA	Abscess within or around tonsil	Similar to epiglottis; may have trismus (locked jaw)

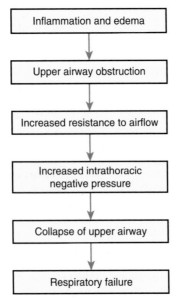

FIGURE 30.1 The Larynx and Subglottic Trachea. A, Normal epiglottis, laryngeal vocal cords, and trachea. B, Narrowing and obstruction of laryngeal tissue around false and true vocal cords from edema caused by croup. (From Hockenberry MJ, Wilson D: *Wong's nursing care of infants and children*, ed 10, St Louis, 2015, Mosby.)

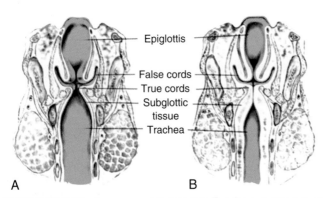

FIGURE 30.2 Upper Airway Obstruction With Croup.

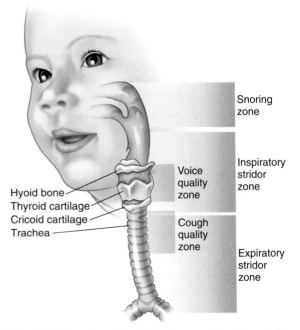

FIGURE 30.3 Listening Can Help Locate the Site of Airway Obstruction. A loud, gasping snore suggests enlarged tonsils or adenoids. In inspiratory stridor, the airway is compromised at the level of the supraglottic larynx, subglottic region and vocal cords which are behind the thyroid cartilage, or upper trachea. Expiratory stridor results from a narrowing or collapse in the trachea or bronchi. Airway noise during both inspiration and expiration often represents a fixed obstruction of the vocal cords or subglottic space. Hoarseness or a weak cry is a by-product of obstruction at the vocal cords. If a cough is croupy, suspect constriction below the vocal cords. (Redrawn from Eavey RD: *Contemp Ped* 3[6]:79, 1986; original illustration by Paul Singh-Roy.)

(Fig. 30.4), stridor, agitation, tachycardia, and sometimes pallor or cyanosis.

Recurrent croup is characterized by a similar hoarseness, barking cough, and stridor. It is of sudden onset and usually occurs at night and without prodromal symptoms. It usually resolves quickly.

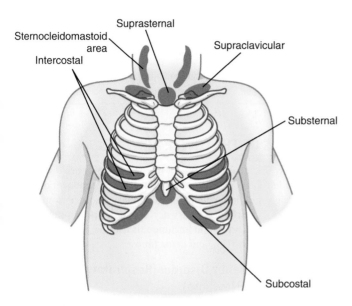

Sternocleidomastoid area
Intercostal
Suprasternal
Supraclavicular
Substernal
Subcostal

FIGURE 30.4 Areas of Chest Muscle Retraction.

EVALUATION AND TREATMENT   The degree of symptoms determines the level of treatment. The most common tool for estimating croup severity is the Westley Croup Score.[2] Few cases require hospitalization, and most children with croup receive outpatient evaluation and management. These children usually have only mild stridor or retractions and appear alert, playful, and able to eat. There has been much debate about the most effective outpatient treatments for croup. For example, humidified air does not improve symptoms in mild to moderate croup. Glucocorticoids—either injected, oral (dexamethasone), or nebulized (budesonide)—have been shown to improve symptoms because of their antiinflammatory action.

The presence of stridor at rest, moderate or severe retractions of the chest, or agitation suggests more severe disease and requires inpatient observation and treatment.[3] For acute respiratory distress, nebulized epinephrine stimulates α- and β-adrenergic receptors and decreases mucosal edema and airway secretions. Glucocorticoids and oxygen should be administered. Heliox (a helium-oxygen mixture) also can be used in severe cases. This works by improving gas flow and thus decreasing the flow resistance of the narrowed airway. In rare cases, croup and recurrent croup may require placement of an endotracheal tube.

Bacterial tracheitis. Bacterial tracheitis (pseudomembranous croup) is the most common potentially life-threatening upper airway infection in children. It is most often caused by *Staphylococcus aureus* (including methicillin-resistant *S. aureus* [MRSA] strains), *Haemophilus influenzae,* or group A beta-hemolytic *Streptococcus* (GABHS). The acute clinical presentation usually includes tachypnea, stridor, hoarse voice, fever, cough, and/or increased secretions from the nose or mouth. The presence of airway edema and copious purulent secretions leads to airway obstruction that can be worsened by the formation of a tracheal pseudomembrane and mucosal sloughing. Bacterial tracheitis is treated with immediate administration of antibiotics and endotracheal intubation to prevent total UAO.

Acute Epiglottitis

Historically, **acute epiglottitis** was caused by *H. influenzae* type B (HiB). Since the advent of the *H. influenzae* vaccine, the overall incidence of acute epiglottitis has decreased significantly; however, up to 25% of epiglottitis cases are still caused by HiB.[4] Current cases in children usually are related to vaccine failure or are caused by other pathogens.

PATHOPHYSIOLOGY   The epiglottis arises from the posterior tongue base and covers the laryngeal inlet during swallowing (see Fig. 30.1). Bacterial invasion of the mucosa with associated inflammation leads to the rapid development of edema, causing severe, life-threatening obstruction of the upper airway.

CLINICAL MANIFESTATIONS   In the classic form of the disease, a child between 2 and 6 years of age suddenly develops high fever, irritability, sore throat, inspiratory stridor, and severe respiratory distress. The child appears anxious and has a voice that sounds muffled ("hot potato voice"). Drooling, absence of cough, a preference to sit, and dysphagia (inability to swallow) are common. In addition to appearing ill, the child will generally adopt a position of leaning forward (tripoding) to try to improve breathing. Death can occur in a few hours. Pneumonia, cervical lymph node inflammation, otitis, and, rarely, meningitis or septic arthritis may occur during the course of epiglottitis.

EVALUATION AND TREATMENT   Acute epiglottitis is a life-threatening emergency. Efforts should be made to keep the child calm and undisturbed. Examination of the throat should not be attempted because it may trigger laryngospasm and cause respiratory collapse. With severe airway obstruction, the airway may be secured with intubation and prompt administration of broad-spectrum antibiotics. Corticosteroids also are generally indicated. Resolution with treatment is usually rapid. Postexposure prophylaxis with rifampin is recommended for all household unvaccinated contacts after a child is diagnosed.

Tonsillar Infections

Tonsillar infections (tonsillitis) are occasionally severe enough to cause upper airway obstruction. Viral infections, such as infectious mononucleosis, are the most common cause of tonsillitis, although the incidence of tonsillitis secondary to group A beta-hemolytic streptococcal (GABH) and MRSA infection has risen in the past 15 years. Significant swelling of the tonsils and pharynx occurs, and a tenacious membrane may cover the mucosa. The development of significant obstruction in tonsillar infections may require the use of corticosteroids, especially in the case of mononucleosis. The management of severe bacterial tonsillitis requires the use of antibiotics. Some children with recurrent tonsillitis benefit from adenotonsillectomy. Tonsillitis may be complicated by the formation of a **tonsillar abscess**, which can further contribute to airway obstruction.

Peritonsillar abscess is usually unilateral and is most often a complication of acute tonsillitis (see Table 30.1). Symptoms in children include fever, sore throat, dysphagia, trismus, pooling of saliva, and muffled voice. Peritonsillar bulging and cervical adenopathy on the same side are usually visible. The abscess must be drained, and the child given antibiotics. Death can occur from spontaneous abscess rupture with aspiration or airway obstruction.

Aspiration of Foreign Bodies

Aspiration of foreign bodies into the airways is most common in children 1 to 4 years of age. More than 100,000 cases and 100 deaths occur each year.[5] Most objects are expelled by the cough reflex, but some objects may lodge in the larynx, trachea, or bronchi. Large objects (e.g., hard candy, a bite of hot dog, nuts, seeds, popcorn, grapes, beans, toy pieces, fragments of popped balloons, or coins) may occlude the airway and become life-threatening. Items of particular concern are batteries (may result in acid erosion) and magnets (can cause loops of bowel to adhere to one another, causing perforation). The aspiration event often is not witnessed or is not recognized when it happens because the coughing, choking, or gagging symptoms may resolve quickly. Foreign bodies lodged in the larynx or upper trachea cause cough, stridor, hoarseness or inability to speak, respiratory distress, and agitation or panic; the presentation is often dramatic and frightening.

If the child is acutely hypoxic and unable to move air, immediate action, such as sweeping the oral airway or performing abdominal thrusts (formerly called the *Heimlich maneuver*), may be required to prevent death. Otherwise, bronchoscopic removal should be performed urgently. If an aspirated foreign body is small enough, it will be transferred to a bronchus before becoming lodged. If the foreign body is lodged in the airway for a longer period of time, local irritation, granulation, obstruction, and infection will ensue. Thus children may present with cough or wheezing, atelectasis, pneumonia, lung abscess, or blood-streaked sputum. These children are treated by prompt bronchoscopic removal of the object and administration of antibiotics as necessary.

Obstructive Sleep Apnea

Pediatric obstructive sleep apnea syndrome (OSAS) results from partial or complete UAO obstruction that occurs during sleep with associated snoring, labored or obstructed breathing, and disrupted sleep patterns.[6] OSAS has an estimated prevalence of 2% to 5% of children and can occur at any age. The prevalence is much higher in obese children, as well as in vulnerable populations (blacks, Hispanics, and preterm infants),[7] and there may be a family history of OSAS. Possible influences early in life may include passive smoke inhalation, socioeconomic status, and snoring, together with genetic modifiers that promote airway inflammation.

PATHOPHYSIOLOGY Airway narrowing, increased upper airway collapsibility, and airway inflammation are the common causes of OSAS. Adenotonsillar hypertrophy, gastroesophageal reflux, obesity, and craniofacial anomalies are associated with airway narrowing. Reduced motor tone of the upper airways may be seen in neurologic disorders, such as cerebral palsy and Down syndrome. Allergy, asthma, and obesity may contribute to inflammation. Obstruction of the upper airway during sleep results in cyclic episodes of increasing respiratory effort and changes in intrathoracic pressures with oxygen desaturation, hypercapnia, and arousal. The child goes back to sleep, and the cycle repeats. Infants are at risk because they have both anatomic and physiologic predispositions toward airway obstruction and gas exchange abnormalities.

CLINICAL MANIFESTATIONS Common manifestations of OSAS include snoring and labored breathing, sweating, and restlessness during sleep, which may be continuous or intermittent. There may be episodes of increased respiratory effort but no audible airflow, often terminated by snorting, gasping, repositioning, or arousal. Daytime sleepiness/napping is occasionally reported, as well as nocturnal enuresis. Cognitive and neurobehavioral impairment, excessive daytime sleepiness, impaired school performance, and poor quality of life are consequences of OSAS.

EVALUATION AND TREATMENT All parents should be asked if their child exhibits snoring, labored breathing, sweating, or restlessness during sleep. A variety of screening tools are available. The most definitive evaluation is the polysomnographic sleep study, during which the diagnosis of OSAS is confirmed by the presence of one or more obstructive events per hour of sleep, or obstructive hypoventilation resulting in hypercapnia for greater than 25% of sleep time.[6] Imaging of the upper airway may be used to rule out tonsillar enlargement or upper airway narrowing. If obstructive sleep apnea is caused by tonsillar enlargement, children are most often referred for tonsillectomy and adenoidectomy (T&A). For severely affected children who do not respond to T&A or who have different problems (e.g., obesity), the use of continuous positive airway pressure (CPAP), antiinflammatories, dental treatments, a high-flow nasal cannula, or weight loss can be considered. Treatment is important to minimize associated morbidities.[8]

DISORDERS OF THE LOWER AIRWAYS

Lower airway disease is one of the leading causes of morbidity in the first year of life and continues to be an important component of other illnesses progressing into childhood. Pulmonary disorders commonly observed include surfactant deficiency disorder, bronchopulmonary dysplasia, infections, aspiration pneumonitis, asthma, acute respiratory distress syndrome (ARDS), and cystic fibrosis.

Surfactant Deficiency Disorder (Respiratory Distress Syndrome of the Newborn)

Surfactant deficiency disorder (SDD), also known as respiratory distress syndrome (RDS) of the newborn, is a significant cause of neonatal morbidity and mortality. It occurs almost exclusively in premature infants because the immature lung has not yet developed adequate surfactant production, although rare mutations in one of the surfactant proteins can affect full-term babies. SDD (RDS) occurs in 50% to 60% of infants born at 29 weeks' gestation and decreases significantly by 36 weeks. Risk factors are summarized in *Risk Factors: Surfactant Deficiency Disorder (Respiratory Distress Syndrome of the Newborn)*. The incidence has increased in the United States over the past 2 decades,[9] however, death rates have declined significantly since the introduction of antenatal steroid therapy and postnatal surfactant therapy.

RISK FACTORS

Surfactant Deficiency Disorder (Respiratory Distress Syndrome of the Newborn)

- Premature birth/low birth weight
- Male sex
- Cesarean delivery without labor
- Diabetic mother
- Perinatal asphyxia

PATHOPHYSIOLOGY SDD (RDS) is caused by surfactant deficiency. Surfactant is a lipoprotein with a detergent-like effect that separates the liquid molecules inside the alveoli, thereby decreasing alveolar surface tension. Without surfactant, alveoli collapse at the end of each exhalation, decreasing the alveolar surface area available for gas exchange. Surfactant normally is not secreted by the alveolar cells until approximately 20 to 24 weeks' gestation (Fig. 30.5). Premature infants also are born with underdeveloped and small alveoli that are difficult to inflate and have thick walls and inadequate capillary blood supply such that gas exchange is significantly impaired. The net effect is *atelectasis* (collapsed alveoli), resulting in significant hypoxemia. Atelectasis is difficult for the neonate to overcome because it requires a significant amount of work to open the alveoli with each breath. The infant's chest wall is weak and highly compliant and, thus, the rib cage tends to collapse inward with increased respiratory effort. Increased work of breathing may result in hypercapnia. Hypoxia and hypercapnia

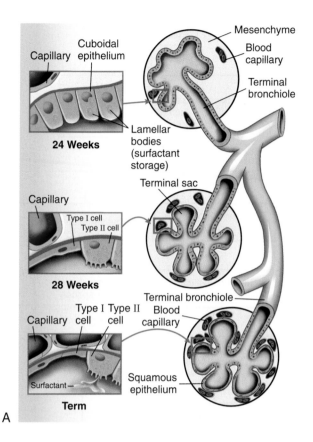

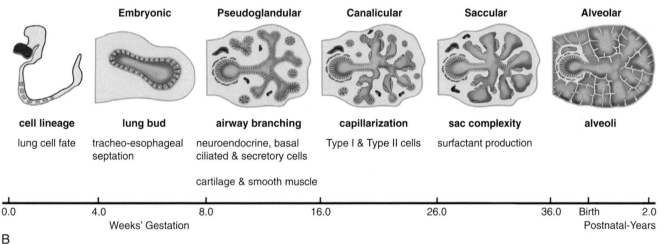

FIGURE 30.5 Prenatal Development of the Alveolar Unit. A, Epithelial cells differentiate into type II and type I cells. Mature type II cells (type II pneumocytes) store and secrete surfactant. Type I cells are derived from type II cells and consist of flattened epithelium overlying capillaries, thus forming part of the thin air-blood gas exchange membrane of the alveoli. **B,** Time line for gestational development of alveoli.

cause pulmonary vasoconstriction, which increases intrapulmonary resistance and pulmonary hypoperfusion. Increased pulmonary vascular resistance may cause a partial return to fetal circulation, with right-to-left shunting of blood through the ductus arteriosus and foramen ovale. Inadequate perfusion of tissues and hypoxemia contribute to metabolic acidosis.

Many premature infants with SDD (RDS) will require mechanical ventilation, which damages the alveolar epithelium, leading to leakage of plasma proteins into the alveoli. These proteins result

in fibrin deposits in the air spaces, which create the appearance of *hyaline membranes* (transparent or glassy appearance on microscopic examination) and contribute to the inactivation of any surfactant that may be present. The pathogenesis of SDD (RDS) is summarized in Fig. 30.6.

CLINICAL MANIFESTATIONS Signs of SDD (RDS) appear within minutes of birth and include tachypnea (respiratory rate greater than 60 breaths/min), expiratory grunting, intercostal and subcostal retractions

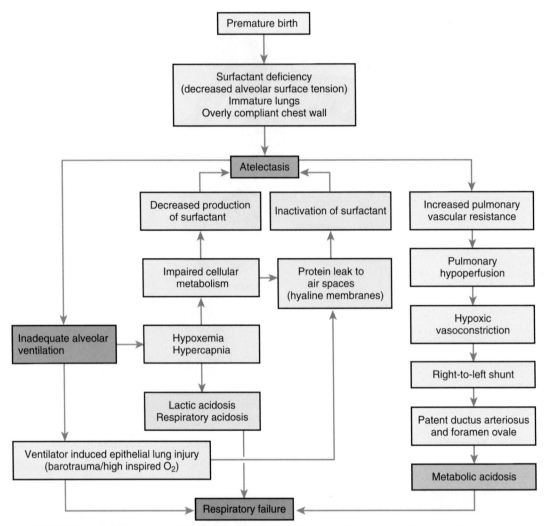

FIGURE 30.6 Pathogenesis of Surfactant Deficiency Disorder (Respiratory Distress Syndrome of the Newborn). O_2, Oxygen.

(see Fig. 30.4), nasal flaring, and cyanosis. The severity tends to increase over the first hours of life. Apnea and irregular respirations occur as the infant tires. The severity of hypoxemia and difficulty providing supplemental oxygenation have resulted in the Vermont Oxford Neonatal Network definition of RDS: an arterial pressure of oxygen (Pao_2) of less than 50 mm Hg in room air, central cyanosis in room air, or a need for supplemental oxygen to maintain a Pao_2 greater than 50 mm Hg, as well as a characteristic chest film appearance.[10] Clinical manifestations reach a peak within 3 days.

EVALUATION AND TREATMENT The diagnosis is made on the basis of premature birth or other risk factors, chest radiographs, pulse oximetry measurements, and, if needed, analysis of amniotic fluid or tracheal aspirates to estimate lung maturity. For women at risk of preterm birth, antenatal treatment with glucocorticoids induces a significant and rapid acceleration of lung maturation and stimulation of surfactant production in the fetus and significantly reduces the incidence of SDD (RDS) and death.[11] The ultimate prevention for SDD (RDS) would be the prevention of premature birth.

Administration of exogenous surfactant (either synthetic or natural) within 15 to 30 minutes of birth is recommended as a prophylactic or preventive treatment for infants weighing between 500 (1 lbs 1.65 oz) and 2000 g (4 lbs 6.5 oz). A thin catheter, nebulizer, or CPAP ventilation

is used for administration. Rescue surfactant therapy is given only to preterm infants with established SDD (RDS) and is most often administered within the first 12 hours after birth. There is usually a dramatic improvement in oxygenation, as well as a decreased incidence of death, pneumothorax, and pulmonary interstitial emphysema from SDD (RDS). Surfactant therapy also can be considered complementary to antenatal glucocorticoids. The two therapies together appear to have an additive effect on improving lung function.

Supportive care includes oxygen administration and often such measures as mechanical ventilation. Mechanical ventilation can result in a proinflammatory state that may contribute to the development of chronic lung disease, such as bronchopulmonary dysplasia. Strategies that are lung protective include greater reliance on nasal CPAP, permissive hypercapnia, lower oxygen saturation targets, modulation of tidal volume (V_t) settings, and use of high-frequency oscillation. Most infants survive SDD (RDS) and, in many cases, recovery may be complete within 10 to 14 days. However, the incidence of subsequent chronic lung disease (i.e., bronchopulmonary dysplasia) is significant among very low birth weight infants.

Bronchopulmonary Dysplasia

Bronchopulmonary dysplasia (BPD), also known as *chronic lung disease of prematurity*, is a chronic, inflammatory lung disease associated with arrested pulmonary development and a need for supplemental oxygen, It is the major cause of chronic pulmonary disease associated with premature birth (usually before 28 weeks' gestation and with birth weights less than 1500 g). It occurs most commonly in infants with severe SDD (RDS) who require prolonged perinatal supplemental oxygen (at least 28 days) and positive pressure ventilation. Each year in the United States, there are approximately 8000 infants affected, including about 40% of infants born weighing less than 1000 g.[12]

The widespread use of antenatal glucocorticoids and postnatal surfactant has lessened the incidence and severity of SDD (RDS) and BPD. BPD now is occurring primarily in the smallest premature infants (23 to 28 weeks' gestation) who have received mechanical ventilation or those with other complicating risks. Risk factors for BPD are summarized in *Risk Factors:* Bronchopulmonary Dysplasia (BPD).

RISK FACTORS

Bronchopulmonary Dysplasia (BPD)

- Premature birth (especially ≤28 weeks)
- Positive pressure ventilation
- Supplemental oxygen administration
- Antenatal chorioamnionitis
- Postnatal sepsis or pneumonia
- Patent ductus arteriosus
- Nutritional deficiencies
- Early adrenal insufficiency
- Genetic susceptibility

Data from Trembath A, Laughon MM: *Clin Perinatol* 39(3):585-601, 2012.

PATHOPHYSIOLOGY Lung immaturity and inflammation contribute to the development of BPD. Before the widespread use of surfactant therapy, BPD was a disease characterized by airway injury, inflammation, and parenchymal fibrosis *(classic BPD)*. With the initiation of surfactant therapy, what is called the *new BPD* is most common and is a form of arrested lung development. There is poor formation of the alveolar structure, with fewer and larger alveoli, and a decreased surface area for gas exchange. Persistent inflammation contributes to pulmonary capillary fibrosis, perfusion mismatch, pulmonary hypertension, and decreased exercise capacity. Table 30.2 compares the classic and new forms of BPD, and Fig. 30.7 illustrates the pathophysiology of the disease.

CLINICAL MANIFESTATIONS The clinical definition of BPD includes a need for supplemental oxygen at 36 weeks' gestational age (the time elapsed between the first day of the last normal menstrual period and the day of birth), and for at least 28 days after birth. The definition also includes a graded severity determination that is dependent on required respiratory support at term (mild, moderate, and severe, based on oxygen requirements and ventilatory needs). Clinically, the infant exhibits hypoxemia and hypercapnia caused by ventilation-perfusion mismatch and diffusion defects. The work of breathing increases, and the ability to feed may be impaired. Intermittent bronchospasm, mucus plugging, and pulmonary hypertension characterize the clinical course. Of the most severely affected infants, dusky spells may occur with agitation, feeding, or gastroesophageal reflux. Infants with mild BPD may demonstrate only mild tachypnea and difficulty handling respiratory tract infections.

EVALUATION AND TREATMENT Chest x-ray and echocardiography are used to rule out other causes of respiratory distress. Infants with

TABLE 30.2 Comparison of Classic and New Bronchopulmonary Dysplasia (BPD)

Classic BPD	New BPD
Metaplasia of respiratory epithelium	Less severe squamous metaplasia
Smooth muscle hypertrophy	Less smooth muscle hypertrophy
Significant fibrosis	Less fibrosis
Large vascular modifications	Abnormal pulmonary vascular structure
	Small number and increased diameter of alveoli
	Increase in elastic tissue

Adapted from Monte LF et al: *J Pediatr (Rio J)* 81(2):99-110, 2005 (Table 3). Available at www.scielo.br/scielo.php?pid=s0021-75572005000300004&script=sci_arttext&tlng=en.

severe BPD require prolonged assisted ventilation. Prevention of lung damage with noninvasive respiratory support, such as early nasal CPAP or nasal intermittent positive pressure ventilation (IPPV), should be used when possible. Compared with mechanical ventilation, CPAP use results in fewer days of oxygen and ventilator requirement by reducing the amount of lung injury. Diuretics are used to control pulmonary edema. Bronchodilators reduce airway resistance. Inhaled corticosteroids reduce the time that mechanical ventilation is required. Prophylactic caffeine citrate administration (to prevent apnea), vitamin A supplementation (necessary for normal lung development), and careful fluid and nutritional support are routinely used and have resulted in improved outcomes. Children with BPD will need to be monitored into adulthood for the development of chronic lung disease.[13]

QUICK CHECK 30.2
1. Why are premature infants susceptible to SDD (RDS)?
2. Describe the pathologic findings of "new BPD."

Respiratory Tract Infections

Respiratory tract infections are common in children and are a frequent cause for emergency department visits and hospitalizations. The clinical presentation, child's age, season of the year, and environmental exposures can often provide clues to the etiologic agent, even when the agent cannot be proved.

Bronchiolitis

Bronchiolitis is a common viral respiratory tract infection of the small airways that occurs almost exclusively in infants and young toddlers. It is the leading cause of hospitalization for infants during the winter season. The most common pathogen is respiratory syncytial virus (RSV), but bronchiolitis also may be caused by rhinovirus, adenovirus, influenza, parainfluenza virus, human metapneumovirus, and human bocavirus. Healthy infants usually make a full recovery from RSV bronchiolitis, but infants who were premature (birth weight <2500 g) or who have underlying BPD, heart disease, or immune deficiency have a higher risk for a more severe or even deadly course. Bronchiolitis has been linked to an increased risk for asthma later in childhood, particularly in those with a family history of asthma.

PATHOPHYSIOLOGY Viral infection causes necrosis of the bronchial epithelium and destruction of ciliated epithelial cells. There is infiltration

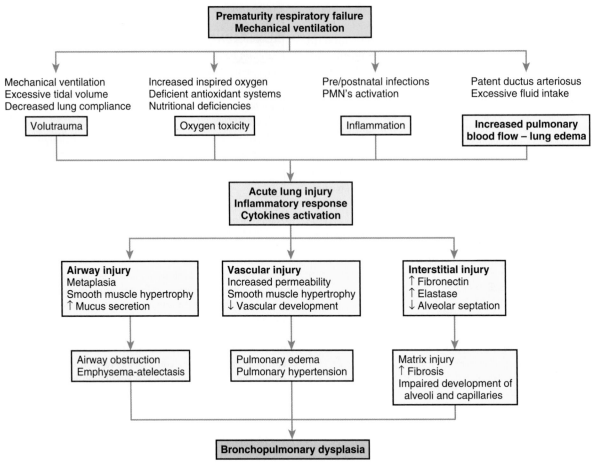

FIGURE 30.7 Pathophysiology of Bronchopulmonary Dysplasia. *PMN,* polymorphonuclear neutrophil.

with lymphocytes around the bronchioles and a cell-mediated hypersensitivity to viral antigens with the release of lymphokines causing inflammation, as well as activation of eosinophils, neutrophils, and monocytes. The submucosa becomes edematous, and cellular debris and fibrin form plugs within the bronchioles. Edema of the bronchiolar wall, accumulation of mucus and cellular debris, and bronchospasm narrow many peripheral airways. Other airways become partially or completely occluded. Atelectasis occurs in some areas of the lung and hyperinflation in others.

The mechanics of breathing are disrupted by bronchiolitis. Airway narrowing causes obstruction of airflow that is worse on expiration. This leads to air trapping, hyperinflation, and increased functional residual capacity. Airway resistance and hyperinflation result in increased work of breathing and the development of hypercapnia in severe cases.

CLINICAL MANIFESTATIONS Symptoms usually begin with significant rhinorrhea followed by a tight cough over the next several days, along with systemic signs of decreased appetite, lethargy, and fever. Infants typically have tachypnea, variable degrees of respiratory distress, and wheezing. inspiratory crackles, or rhonchi also may be present. Very young infants may present with severe apnea before lower respiratory tract symptoms appear, and these apneas frequently require mechanical ventilation. Many children also may present with conjunctivitis or otitis media.

EVALUATION AND TREATMENT Guidelines from the American Academy of Pediatrics are available for the evaluation, treatment, and prevention of bronchiolitis.[14] The diagnosis of bronchiolitis is made by reviewing the history, signs, and symptoms (e.g., rhinitis, cough, wheezing, chest retractions, tachypnea). Laboratory and radiologic examinations are not routinely performed.

Treatment for bronchiolitis is determined by the severity of the disease and the age of the child. Most cases are mild and require no specific treatment, and the child may be monitored as an outpatient. When treatment is indicated, it is primarily supportive in nature. Preventive treatment with RSV-specific monoclonal antibody (palivizumab) is recommended for high-risk infants younger than 2 years who meet specific criteria, although it is costly. Other preventive measures include the use of hand washing and alcohol-based decontamination, prevention of exposure to tobacco smoke, and promotion of infant breast feeding.

Pneumonia

Pneumonia is infection and inflammation in the terminal airways and alveoli. Community-acquired pneumonia (CAP) is a major cause of morbidity and mortality in children, particularly in developing countries. The most common agents are viruses, and then bacteria and atypical microorganisms (e.g., mycoplasma) (Table 30.3). Risk factors for developing CAP are age younger than 2 years, overcrowded living conditions, winter season, recent antibiotic treatment, daycare attendance, and passive smoke exposure. Nutritional status, age, and underlying disease process influence morbidity and mortality rates related to CAP. Hospital-acquired pneumonia (HAP) is a nosocomial infection that occurs most commonly in those who are immunocompromised or who experience prolonged hospitalization for treatment of malignancy, trauma, surgery, or underlying chronic illness (see Chapter 29).

TABLE 30.3 Common Types of Pneumonia in Children

Type	Causal Agent	Age	Onset	Signs/Symptoms
Viral pneumonia	Respiratory syncytial virus (RSV), influenza, adenovirus, others	Infants for RSV, all ages for others	Acute or gradual, winter and early spring	Mild to high fever, cough, rhinorrhea, malaise, rales, rhonchi, wheezing, or apnea; variable radiographic pattern
Pneumococcal pneumonia	Pneumococci (Streptococcus pneumoniae)	Usually 1 to 4 yr	Acute, occurs after an upper respiratory tract infection, winter and early spring	High fever, productive cough, pleuritic pain, increased respiration rate, decreased breath sounds in area of consolidation; lobar infiltrate or "round pneumonia" on radiograph
Staphylococcal pneumonia	Staphylococcus aureus (including methicillin-resistant strains)	1 wk to 2 yr	Acute, winter	High fever, cough, respiratory distress, toxic appearance, sepsis; empyema or pneumatoceles common
Streptococcal pneumonia	Group A beta-hemolytic streptococci	All ages	Acute, any season	High fever, chills, respiratory distress, sepsis, or shock; empyema, pneumatoceles
Mycoplasmal and chlamydial pneumonia	Mycoplasma pneumoniae, Chlamydophila pneumoniae	School-age and adolescents	Gradual	Low-grade fever, cough

PATHOPHYSIOLOGY AND CLINICAL MANIFESTATIONS Viral pneumonia is two to three times more likely to occur in children than in adults, and the incidence generally follows a seasonal pattern. RSV is the most common viral pneumonia in young children. A number of other viruses are important, including parainfluenza, influenza, human rhinovirus, human metapneumovirus, and adenoviruses. Acquisition of these viruses is by direct contact, droplet transmission, or aerosol exposure. There is initial destruction of the ciliated epithelium of the distal airway with sloughing of cellular material and initiation of an inflammatory response. Bacterial coinfections are common.

Viral pneumonia often presents with cough and no fever, the white blood cell count is often normal, and immunofluorescence tests may confirm the diagnosis. Development of safe agents to treat and prevent viral pneumonia continues to be a focus of much research.[15]

Bacterial pneumonia beyond the neonatal period is most commonly the result of infection with Streptococcus pneumoniae. Other causative bacteria include S. aureus and atypical bacteria (see Table 30.3). Childhood immunization with the pneumococcal and H. influenzae vaccines has decreased the incidence of these two types of bacterial pneumonia in children younger than 2 years of age.[16]

Bacterial pneumonia usually begins with aspiration of one's own nasopharyngeal bacteria. A preceding viral infection sometimes sets the stage for bacterial infection by causing epithelial damage, reduced mucociliary clearance in the trachea and major bronchi, and a reduced immune response. Once in the alveolar region, bacteria encounter local host defenses, such as antibodies, complement, and cytokines, which prepare bacteria for ingestion by alveolar macrophages. Alveolar macrophages recognize bacteria with their surface receptors and phagocytose them. If these mechanisms fail, the macrophages release numerous inflammatory cytokines, and neutrophils will be recruited into the lung. An intense, cytokine-mediated inflammation will ensue. Vascular engorgement, edema, and a fibrinopurulent exudate occur. Alveolar filling precludes gas exchange and, if extensive, can lead to respiratory failure. If sepsis occurs at the same time, shock and end-organ hypoperfusion will cause metabolic acidosis. Staphylococcal pneumonia and group A streptococcal pneumonia can be particularly fulminant (sudden, severe) and necrotizing (causing cell death), with a high incidence of accompanying empyema, pneumatocele (a lung lesion filled with air), and sepsis.

The clinical presentation of bacterial pneumonia, particularly pneumococcal, may include a preceding viral illness followed by fever with chills and rigors (shaking), shortness of breath, and an increasingly productive cough. Occasionally, there is blood streaking of the sputum. The respiratory rate and oxygen saturation also are important clinical indicators. Auscultation usually reveals crackles or decreased breath sounds. Other, less specific findings may include malaise, vomiting, abdominal pain, and chest pain. Absolute neutrophil counts and the percentage of bands (immature neutrophils) are usually elevated. Chest films may reveal dense pulmonary infiltrates.

Atypical pneumonia (*Mycoplasma pneumoniae, Chlamydophila pneumoniae*) is a common cause of CAP for school-age children and young adults. *Mycoplasma* can cause a wide spectrum of disease and is increasingly seen in infants and younger children. *Chlamydophila pneumoniae* pneumonia is clinically indistinguishable from and is typically grouped with *Mycoplasma pneumoniae* pneumonia as "atypical pneumonia." Transmission occurs person to person, and there is a 2- to 3-week incubation period.

Mycoplasma microorganisms lack cell walls but have a limiting membrane and a specialized receptor for attaching to ciliated respiratory epithelial cells. Local sloughing of cells occurs. Lymphocytic infiltration develops around the bronchi, along with neutrophil recruitment to the airway lumen. The pattern resembles bronchitis or bronchopneumonia. The onset is usually gradual, resembling a typical upper respiratory tract infection but with low-grade fever, cough, and chest pain. Most cases are not clinically severe, and full recovery should be expected. Complications, when they do occur, can include bronchopneumonia, parapneumonic pleural effusions, and necrotizing pneumonitis.

EVALUATION AND TREATMENT Guidelines have been developed to improve and aid assessment and management of pediatric pneumonia.[17] The diagnosis of pneumonia is based on clinical and laboratory findings. Identifying etiologic pathogens can be very difficult in children, especially because there is often overlap between bacterial and viral pathogens. The etiologic agent can sometimes be inferred from the age of the child and the clinical scenario. Chest x-rays can assist in determining the extent of pulmonary involvement. Biomarkers (i.e., procalcitonin) facilitate more rapid diagnosis and guide antibiotic therapy. Several more specific microbiologic tests, such as sputum and blood cultures, and antigen detection assays are available.

Many pneumonias may be treated on an outpatient basis; however, more severely ill children require oxygen supplementation and, occasionally, assisted ventilation. This is particularly true with infants who have a severe viral pneumonia that involves large portions of the lung, such as that seen with RSV. In addition, adequate hydration, proper nutrition, and supportive pulmonary therapy are required to reduce the duration and severity of illness. Many infected infants are markedly tachypneic and unable to coordinate their breathing with swallowing; they may require enteral feeding. Aspiration is always a risk with infants in respiratory distress.

Appropriate antibiotic administration for bacterial pneumonias is dependent on age and severity assessment. Local patterns of resistance must be considered when choosing appropriate antibiotics. Pneumococcal and mycoplasmal pneumonias present some unique treatment obstacles and may need a multifaceted approach to care, including immune adjuvant therapies in addition to antibiotics. Prevention with vaccines against influenza and pneumococcal pneumonias is important in infants and young children.

✔ **QUICK CHECK 30.3**

1. Describe the typical presentation of RSV bronchiolitis.
2. What are some of the most common causes of pneumonia and how do they differ?

Aspiration Pneumonitis

Aspiration pneumonitis is caused by a foreign substance, such as meconium, food, secretions (saliva or gastric), or environmental compounds, entering the lung and resulting in inflammation of the lung tissue. The aspiration of meconium from amniotic fluid can occur at birth. Children undergoing sedation or anesthesia also may aspirate oral secretions contaminated with anaerobic bacteria or acidic stomach contents. Neurologically compromised children or children with chronic lung disease may have chronic pulmonary aspiration (CPA), which can cause progressive lung disease, bronchiectasis (chronically enlarged and scarred bronchi), and respiratory failure. This is the leading cause of death in children who are neurologically compromised because of failure of protective reflexes and difficulty swallowing.

The severity of lung injury after an aspiration incident is determined by the volume and pH of the material aspirated and the presence of pathogenic bacteria. A very low or an extremely high pH will cause a significant inflammatory response. With hydrocarbon fluid ingestions, lung injury is determined by the volatility and viscosity of the aspirated substance. A low-viscosity substance, such as gasoline or lighter fluid, is the most toxic; high-viscosity hydrocarbons, such as petroleum jelly or mineral oil, are much less likely to cause a pneumonitis.

Treatment for aspiration pneumonitis depends on the material aspirated. In children who aspirate significant amounts of toxic chemicals or acidic gastric contents, hospitalization and management for respiratory failure may be needed. Secondary bacterial pneumonia requires the use of broad-spectrum antibiotics. Children with CPA benefit from feeding and swallowing therapy. Salivary gland injection with botulinum toxin A to suppress secretion may be indicated in selected children with neurologic disorders who have a large amount of upper respiratory tract secretions.

Asthma

Asthma is a chronic inflammatory disease characterized by bronchial hyperreactivity and reversible airflow obstruction, usually in response to an allergen (see Chapter 29). It is the most prevalent chronic disease in childhood, affecting about 8.3% of U.S. children between birth and 17 years of age, and the prevalence is increasing. Populations most affected include black and Puerto Rican children and those of low socioeconomic status.[18]

Childhood asthma results from a complex interaction between *genetic* susceptibility and *environmental* factors. Many genotypes are associated with multiple phenotypes of asthma, including early-onset mild allergic asthma, asthma with severe exacerbations, later-onset asthma associated with obesity, atopic (allergic) or nonatopic asthma, and corticosteroid-dependent asthma. Important risk factors include early exposure to environmental allergens (e.g., air pollution, dust mites, molds, cockroach antigen, cat exposure, and tobacco smoke), respiratory tract infections, gastroesophageal reflux, preterm birth, and childhood obesity. The *hygiene hypothesis* proposes that infants and children are more likely to develop allergic asthma if they are exposed to a highly hygienic environment and receive vaccinations to prevent certain infections. This lack of adequate exposure to common pathogens prevents the development of a balanced immune response as they mature.[19] The gut microbiome also plays a major role in influencing the development of immune function and asthma in children.[20]

Most acute wheezing episodes in children with asthma are associated with viral respiratory tract infection (i.e., RSV, human rhinoviruses, and parainfluenza viruses). In infants and toddlers younger than 2 years old, RSV is the most common. In older children and adults, rhinovirus (the "common cold" virus) is the major viral trigger. Bacterial respiratory tract infections also can trigger asthma.

PATHOPHYSIOLOGY The pathophysiology of asthma in children is similar to that for adults and is described in Chapter 29. Allergic asthma is initiated by a type I hypersensitivity reaction primarily mediated by T-helper 2 (Th2) lymphocytes, whose cytokines activate mast cells, eosinophilia, leukocytosis, and enhanced B-cell IgE production (see Chapter 8) (see Figs. 29.9, 29.10, and 29.11). As in adults, inflammation, bronchospasm, and mucus production in the airways both lead to ventilation and perfusion mismatch with hypoxemia and to expiratory airway obstruction with air trapping and increased work of breathing. In young children, airway obstruction can be more severe because of the smaller diameter of their airways.

CLINICAL MANIFESTATIONS Clinical manifestations of an acute asthma attack include coughing, expiratory wheezing, and shortness of breath. Breath sounds may become faint when air movement is poor. The child may speak in clipped sentences or not at all because of dyspnea. The respiratory rate and heart rate are elevated. Nasal flaring and the use of accessory muscles with retractions in the substernal, subcostal, intercostal, suprasternal, or sternocleidomastoid areas are evident (see Fig. 30.4). Infants may appear to be "head bobbing" because of sternocleidomastoid muscle use. Pulsus paradoxus (a decrease in the systolic blood pressure of more than 10 mm Hg during inspiration) may be present. The child may appear anxious or may be sweating heavily, important signs of respiratory compromise.

Findings in chronic asthma may include hyperinflation of the thorax (barrel chest) or pectus excavatum. Clubbing should not be seen with asthma and, if present, should trigger evaluation for other conditions, such as cystic fibrosis. Exercise intolerance may indicate underlying asthma (see *Did You Know?* Exercise-Induced Bronchoconstriction in Childhood Asthma).

EVALUATION AND TREATMENT Asthma is often underdiagnosed and undertreated, especially in preschool-age children because asthma symptoms overlap with other respiratory illnesses, such as bronchitis or upper respiratory tract infections. The diagnosis of asthma is based on episodes of wheezing as well as a variety of risk factors, including a parental history of asthma, atopic dermatitis, sensitization to aeroallergens or foods, blood eosinophilia, or wheezing not associated with upper respiratory tract illnesses. The modified Asthma Predictive Index (mAPI) can be used to help with asthma diagnosis and is recommended by the National Institutes of Health (NIH) guidelines.[21] Confirmation

Exercise-Induced Bronchoconstriction in Childhood Asthma

Exercise-induced bronchoconstriction (EIB) can occur in nonasthmatic individuals, but is far more common in those with asthma; it occurs in approximately half of children diagnosed with asthma. EIB is characterized by transient airway narrowing in association with strenuous exercise usually lasting 5 to 10 minutes, with a decline in pulmonary function by at least 10%. A proposed mechanism for EIB is epithelial injury and inflammation, which results from drying of the mucosa and changes in the osmolarity in the airway epithelium, leading to degranulation of mast cells. Another contributing factor is the inhalation of particles and toxins at high flow rates; this is of particular importance in urban areas and in swimmers in chlorinated pools. These changes result in increased type I hypersensitivity and airway hyperresponsiveness in those with asthma and are associated with an increase in leukotriene release. Eosinophil activation also plays a role in airway hyperreactivity and tissue damage. Symptoms are a poor indicator of the severity of bronchoconstriction, especially in obese children, and spirometry with exercise challenge testing is needed to make the diagnosis. Warm-up exercises and cooling down slowly after exercise, along with the use of facemasks in cold weather, can be helpful. Although bronchodilators remain the most commonly used medications for EIB, studies suggest that inhaled corticosteroids or leukotriene inhibitors are more effective and safer in children with EIB and asthma.

Data from Bonini M, Palange P: *Asthma Res Pract* 1:2, 2015; Lin LL et al: *J Microbiol Immunol Infect* 2017 Sep 6 [Epub ahead of print]; Randolph C: *Clin Rev Allergy Immunol* 34(2):205-216, 2008.

of the diagnosis of asthma relies on pulmonary function testing using spirometry, which can be accomplished only after the child is 5 to 6 years of age. For younger children, an empirical trial of asthma medications is commonly initiated.

The goal of asthma therapy is to achieve long-term control by reduction in impairment and risk. Child and family education and appropriate allergen avoidance techniques should begin immediately. Care providers need to periodically assess asthma control in children. Key features for assessment include nighttime awakenings, interference with normal activities, use of short-acting β₂-agonists, pulmonary function testing, and exacerbations requiring steroids. Peak flow meters are often used to help guide treatment. Before therapy is augmented, care providers need to assess medication administration techniques, environmental controls, and comorbidities. For a reduction in therapy, the asthma needs to be under good control for a minimum of 3 months.

The pharmacologic treatment of asthma in children is essentially the same as that for adults and is initiated in a stepwise sequence based on asthma severity and the response to treatment (see Chapter 29). The Global Initiative for Asthma (GINA) provides recommendations for the use of inhaled corticosteroids and leukotriene receptor antagonists in children.[22] Management of asthma medications in children is often difficult because fluctuation in the severity of the symptoms is common. Many children with less severe asthma outgrow the disease by adulthood.

QUICK CHECK 30.4

1. Why are neurologically compromised children at particular risk for aspiration pneumonitis?
2. Describe the key clinical features of childhood asthma.

Acute Respiratory Distress Syndrome

Acute respiratory distress syndrome (ARDS) is a clinical syndrome in which there is pulmonary edema that is not the result of cardiac disease (noncardiogenic pulmonary edema). It is often a life-threatening condition. ARDS results from a direct lung injury, such as pneumonia, aspiration, near-drowning, or smoke inhalation; or from a systemic insult, such as sepsis or multiple trauma. ARDS is characterized by an inflammatory response that causes alveolocapillary injury. ARDS accounts for approximately 10% of total admissions to pediatric intensive care units. Mortality in pediatric ARDS varies from 18% to 35%.[23]

PATHOPHYSIOLOGY The pathophysiology of ARDS in children is the same as that described for adults in Chapter 29 (see Fig. 29.8).[24]

CLINICAL MANIFESTATIONS Children with ARDS most commonly have suffered a known clinical insult, followed within 7 days by increasing dyspnea, hypoxemia, and pulmonary infiltrates on chest x-ray. Initially, hyperventilation occurs, but carbon dioxide (CO_2) retention may ultimately occur as well because of inadequate functional air space and respiratory muscle fatigue. The severity of the overall picture is modified by comorbid factors, such as the presence of sepsis or multiorgan failure, and by the presence or absence of complications, such as nosocomial pneumonia.

EVALUATION AND TREATMENT The evaluation of children with ARDS includes a physical examination, evaluation of blood gases, and imaging. The Pediatric Acute Lung Injury Consensus Conference[25] has developed diagnostic criteria for pediatric ARDS (pARDS). Perinatal causes of acute hypoxemia are excluded (i.e., lung disease related to prematurity, perinatal lung injury, congenital abnormalities, left ventricular failure, or fluid overload). A chest x-ray and arterial blood gas analysis are indicated. The degree of hypoxemia used to define the severity of pARDS uses the oxygenation index (OI), which is determined by the mean airway pressure and the ratio of supplemental oxygen to the Pao₂.

Treatment for ARDS remains supportive in nature, and the goals are to maintain adequate tissue oxygenation, minimize acute lung injury, and avoid iatrogenic pulmonary complications. Most children with ARDS require mechanical ventilation to promote alveolar ventilation and stabilization, and redistribution of alveolar edema fluid into the interstitium. Infants are at greater risk for ventilator-induced lung injury, and the use of lung-protective ventilation strategies may include measures to reduce barotrauma (low V_t and permissive hypercapnia) and oxygen toxicity (permissive hypoxemia). Extracorporeal membrane oxygenation (ECMO), in which a pump circulates blood through an artificial lung and then back into the body, can provide cardiac or respiratory support, or both, but does not heal the underlying condition. Use of corticosteroids in children with ARDS is controversial and remains at the discretion of the clinician. More research is needed regarding the long-term outcomes of ARDS.

Cystic Fibrosis

Cystic fibrosis (CF) is an autosomal recessive inherited disease that results from defective epithelial chloride ion transport. The CF gene is named the *cystic fibrosis transmembrane conductance regulator (CFTR)* and is located on chromosome 7. There are more than 2000 variants of this gene known to produce CF; they are divided into five classes with varying severity of disease expression.[26] Mortality correlates respectively with the severity of the class.

There are approximately 1000 new cases of CF diagnosed each year, and the median age at diagnosis is 6 months. CF primarily affects Caucasians (approximately 1 in 3000). The estimated carrier frequency for Caucasians is 1 in 29 in the United States. Carriers are not affected by the mutation. Among people with CF born between 2013 and 2017, half are predicted to live to 44 years old or more.[27]

PATHOPHYSIOLOGY CF is a multiorgan disease that affects the lungs, digestive tract (see Chapter 39), and reproductive organs. The *CFTR* gene mutation results in the abnormal expression of cystic fibrosis transmembrane conductance regulator (CFTCR) protein, which is an activated chloride channel present on the surface of many types of epithelial cells, including those lining airways, bile ducts, the pancreas, sweat ducts, paranasal sinuses, and vas deferens. Without adequate CFTCR function, chloride and water are not transported appropriately across epithelial membranes, resulting in thick, dehydrated mucus secretions. The most important effects are on the lungs, and respiratory failure is almost always the cause of death.

The typical features of CF lung disease are mucous plugging, chronic inflammation, and chronic infection of the small airways. The mucous plugging results from increased production of mucus from more numerous and larger goblet cells, altered physicochemical properties of the mucus, and impaired mucociliary clearance. The depleted fluid in the mucus and impaired mobility of the cilia allow mucus to adhere to the airway epithelium, along with bacteria and injurious by-products from neutrophils. Neutrophils are present in great excess in the airways and release oxidants and proteases (i.e., elastase) that cause direct damage to lung structural proteins. They also induce airway cells to produce inflammatory mediators that destroy immunoglobulin G (IgG) and complement components important for opsonization and phagocytosis of pathogens, thus contributing to chronic infection (see Fig. 30.8).

The CF airway microenvironment favors bacterial colonization, which leads to a bacterial biofilm that promotes chronic endobronchial infection. The biofilm resists beta-lactam antibiotics, and rapid mutation of the biofilm makes these children antibiotic resistant. Persistence of these microorganisms incites chronic local inflammation and airway damage, with microabscess formation, bronchiectasis, patchy consolidation and pneumonia, peribronchial fibrosis, and cyst formation (Fig. 30.9). Peripheral bullae may develop, and pneumothorax may occur. Hemoptysis (coughing up blood) is sometimes life-threatening and may occur because of the erosion of enlarged bronchial arteries. Over time, pulmonary vascular remodeling occurs because of localized hypoxia and arteriolar vasoconstriction. Pulmonary hypertension and cor pulmonale may develop in the late stages of the disease (see Chapter 29).

CLINICAL MANIFESTATIONS Clinical manifestations of CF can vary from mild to severe, depending on the degree of gene mutation. The most common presenting symptoms of CF involve the respiratory or gastrointestinal/digestive systems (see Chapter 39). Respiratory symptoms include persistent cough or wheeze, excessive sputum production, and recurrent or severe pneumonia. Physical signs that develop over time include barrel chest and digital clubbing. More subtle presentations include chronic sinusitis and nasal polyps.

EVALUATION AND TREATMENT According to the Cystic Fibrosis Foundation, guidelines for the diagnosis of CF include one or more clinical features, a history of CF in a sibling, or a positive newborn screen plus laboratory evidence of an abnormality in the *CFTR* gene or the CFTR protein.[28] The standard method of diagnosis (screening) uses the immunoreactive trypsinogen (IRT) blood test and the sweat test, which reveal a sweat chloride concentration in excess of 60 mEq/L. Alternative or supplemental methods include genotyping for *CFTR* mutations. Newborn screening for CF is universal throughout the United States and is essential to providing early, presymptomatic diagnosis and

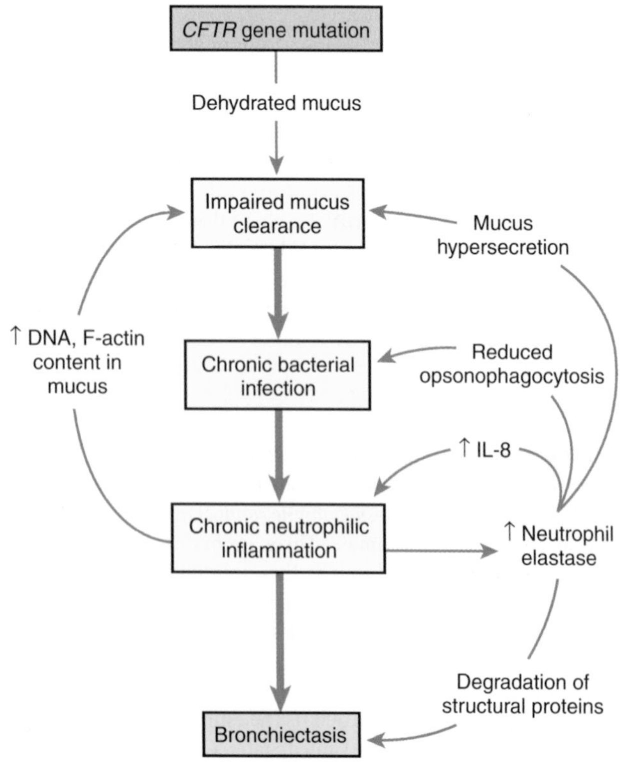

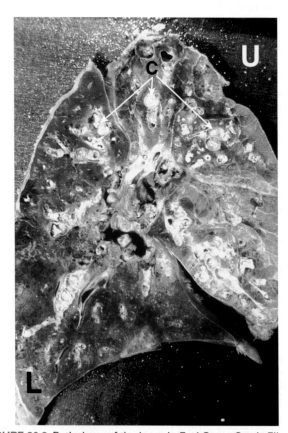

FIGURE 30.9 Pathology of the Lung in End-Stage Cystic Fibrosis. Key features are widespread mucus impaction of the airways and bronchiectasis, especially from the upper lobe *(U; white arrows)*, with hemorrhagic pneumonia in the lower lobe *(L)*. Small cysts are present at the apex of the lung *(C)*. (From Kleinerman J, Vauthy P: *Pathology of the lung in cystic fibrosis*, Atlanta, 1976, Cystic Fibrosis Foundation.)

FIGURE 30.8 Pathogenesis of Cystic Fibrosis Lung Disease. *CFTR,* Cystic fibrosis gene; *IL-8,* interleukin-8.

CFTR gene mutation
↓ Dehydrated mucus
Impaired mucus clearance ← Mucus hypersecretion
↑ DNA, F-actin content in mucus
Chronic bacterial infection ← Reduced opsonophagocytosis
↑ IL-8
Chronic neutrophilic inflammation → ↑ Neutrophil elastase
Degradation of structural proteins
Bronchiectasis

treatment (see *Did You Know?* Newborn Screening for Cystic Fibrosis). Carrier testing to detect adult heterozygotes is available and enables informed reproductive choices before the birth of the first child with CF (25% chance).[29]

Newborn screening for cystic fibrosis (CF) is now conducted in all 50 states in the United States and many other countries. The newborn screen for CF is a quantitative measure of immunoreactive trypsinogen (IRT) performed on a dried blood spot on a filter paper card. IRT is a pancreatic enzyme precursor that is persistently elevated in infants with CF. If a child is found to have an elevated IRT concentration, the next step is defined by state newborn screening protocols. Some states repeat the IRT level measurement, whereas others proceed to genetic testing for common mutations in the CF transmembrane conductance regulator (*CFTR*) gene. If the secondary testing is suggestive of a diagnosis of CF, the child is then referred to a Cystic Fibrosis Center for further evaluation and confirmatory sweat chloride testing. Research suggests that early diagnosis of CF has favorable effects on the outcome. Children who are diagnosed with CF in infancy have improved nutritional outcomes compared to children who are diagnosed later in life. Establishing good nutrition in infants with CF has been correlated with improved lung function later in life. It is these improved clinical outcomes that have led the Centers for Disease Control and Prevention to support universal screening for CF.

Data from Grosse SD et al: *MMWR Recomm Rep* 53:1-36, 2004; National Newborn Screening and Global Resource Center: http://genes-r-us.uthscsa.edu/sites/genes-r-us/files/nbsdisorders.pdf; Tridello G et al: *ERJ Open Res* 4(2), 2018; Wagener JS et al: *Curr Opin Pediatr* 24(3):329-335, 2014.

Treatment is primarily focused on pulmonary health and nutrition (see Chapter 39) and prevention of persistent cycles of lung infection and inflammation. Common pulmonary therapies include techniques to promote mucus clearance, such as chest physical therapy and related mechanical devices; use of bronchodilators; and the administration of solutions, which liquefy mucus (e.g., aerosolized dornase alfa [an enzyme] and hypertonic saline). Different classes of oral, inhaled, or intravenous antibiotics are used to treat different pathogens and to overcome antibiotic resistance. Individuals with end-stage lung disease may consider lung transplantation. Ivacaftor is a genetic therapy that can improve the function of the *CFTR* gene in individuals with certain types of mutations. Although this particular medication is indicated for only 4% to 5% of those with cystic fibrosis, new gene therapies are being developed.

SUDDEN INFANT DEATH SYNDROME

Sudden infant death syndrome (SIDS), also called sudden unexpected infant death, remains a disease of unknown cause, but it is the most common cause of unexplained infant death in Western countries. It is defined as "sudden death of an infant under 1 year of age which remains unexplained after a thorough case investigation, including performance of a complete autopsy, examination of the death scene, and review of the clinical history."[30]

The incidence of SIDS is low during the first month of life, with the peak incidence at 2 to 4 months of age. It is unusual after 6 months of age. In 2016, about 3600 infants died a sudden unexpected death, and 1500 of those were attributed to SIDS.[31] SIDS almost always occurs during nighttime sleep, when infants are least likely to be observed. A seasonal variation has been noted, with higher frequencies during the winter months. This has been related to a higher rate of respiratory tract infections during those months, and such infections are often reported to have preceded the death. The sleeping room also may be overheated or the infant overwrapped.

Clinical risk groups are summarized in *Risk Factors:* Sudden Infant Death Syndrome (SIDS). About 75% of all SIDS victims have no known predisposing clinical risk factor.[32] SIDS rates decreased where massive public campaigns warned against prone sleeping for infants (e.g., the Back-to-Sleep Campaign).[33]

RISK FACTORS
Sudden Infant Death Syndrome (SIDS)

- Prone and side-lying sleeping positions
- Sleeping on soft bedding
- Overheated sleeping environment
- Lower socioeconomic status
- Mothers younger than 20
- Blacks or African American, Native Americans, Alaska Natives
- Low birth weight or growth-restricted infants
- Male infants
- Preterm delivery
- Multiple gestations
- Sibling who died of SIDS
- Smoking during pregnancy
- Exposure to tobacco smoke
- Lack of prenatal care
- Illicit drug use or binge-drinking
- Larger family size

Data from Bergman NJ: *Pediatr Res* 77(1-1):10-19, 2015; Blackwell C et al: *Front Immunol* 6:44, 2015; Hakeem GF et al: *World J Pediatr* 11(1):41-47, 2015; Van Nguyen JM, Abenhaim HA: *Am J Perinatol* 30(9):703-714, 2013.

The etiology of SIDS remains unknown but probably involves a combination of predisposing factors, including a vulnerable infant and environmental stressors. There has been long-standing interest in hypotheses involving impaired autonomic regulation and failure of cardiovascular, ventilatory, and arousal responses. Other theories involve immune dysregulation, airway inflammation, and responses to bacterial pathogens from the nasopharynx or viral respiratory tract infections. Genetic factors may predispose certain individuals to SIDS. The most important risk factor genes include those involved in the regulation of the immune system and inflammation, cardiac abnormalities, and brainstem function.[34]

Currently, the best strategy for reducing SIDS and sudden unexpected infant death during sleep seems to be avoidance of risk factors. Other recommendations include breast feeding, recommended immunizations, and use of a pacifier at sleep time.[35] Parents of infants with clinical risk should be taught cardiopulmonary resuscitation (CPR) as a precaution. Some infants at risk for episodes of apnea and bradycardia may warrant cardiorespiratory monitoring after careful consideration of the individual situation.

✓ QUICK CHECK 30.5

1. How are the alveoli and capillaries affected by the inflammation of acute respiratory distress syndrome (ARDS)?
2. What aspects of lung disease in cystic fibrosis are the focus of current therapies?
3. What are the risk factors for sudden infant death syndrome (SIDS)?

SUMMARY REVIEW

Disorders of the Upper Airways

1. Viral croup is an acute laryngotracheobronchitis, usually caused by the parainfluenza virus. This infection causes swelling of the upper trachea. The typical sign is a seal-like barking cough, which appears after a few days of rhinorrhea, sore throat, and low-grade fever.
2. Recurrent (spasmodic) croup is characterized by a similar barking cough but occurs in older children and has a sudden onset at night, without fever. The etiology is unknown.
3. Acute epiglottitis is a potentially life-threatening airway infection; its incidence in children has decreased dramatically since the advent of the Hib vaccine. Now other pathogens, such as GABHS, *Candida* species, *S. aureus*, MRSA, and viral pathogens are usually the causative agents.
4. Tonsillar infections are usually caused by viral infections, such as infectious mononucleosis, and can be complicated by tonsillar and peritonsillar abscesses.
5. Aspiration of foreign bodies that lodge in the airways may cause cough, hoarseness, stridor or wheezing, and dyspnea. The severity depends on the location of the foreign body within the airway and the degree of obstruction. Blockage of the larynx or trachea can be fatal, whereas bronchial obstruction may not be diagnosed immediately.
6. OSAS results from partial or complete upper airway obstruction during sleep with associated snoring, labored or obstructed breathing, and disrupted sleep patterns.

Disorders of the Lower Airways

1. SDD (RDS of the newborn) usually occurs in premature infants who are born before surfactant production and alveolocapillary development are complete. Atelectasis and hypoventilation cause shunting, hypoxemia, and hypercapnia. Prenatal steroids and postnatal surfactant are beneficial preventive therapies.
2. BPD is the result of tissue injury and repair and disrupted alveolar development in the lungs of infants who required ventilatory support during a time when their lungs were underdeveloped because of their prematurity. Surfactant therapy has improved outcomes. Infants with BPD may require oxygen and additional therapies for many months.
3. Bronchiolitis is a viral lower respiratory tract infection that presents with a runny nose, wheezing, cough, and tachypnea in infants and is usually caused by infection with RSV. Infants with risk factors of prematurity or underlying lung or heart disease are at high risk and may receive RSV-specific monoclonal antibody to prevent RSV disease.
4. Pneumonia is infection and inflammation in the terminal airways and alveoli. Viral, bacterial, and atypical pneumonia cause varying degrees of illness in children. Bacterial CAP is one of the leading causes of hospitalization and is prevented with a polyvariant pneumococcal conjugate vaccine.
5. Aspiration pneumonitis is caused by inhalation of a foreign substance, such as food, milk, secretions, or environmental compounds, into the lung, resulting in inflammation.
6. Asthma is a chronic inflammatory disease characterized by bronchial hyperreactivity and reversible airflow obstruction, usually in response to an allergen. Its origins are multifactorial and include genetic, allergic, and viral-triggered mechanisms.
7. ARDS is a clinical syndrome in which there is pulmonary edema that is not the result of cardiac disease; it is often a life-threatening condition. ARDS results from direct lung injury. There is progressive respiratory distress with severe hypoxemia and respiratory failure.
8. Cystic fibrosis is an autosomal recessive genetic disease that affects the epithelial lining of many organ systems, especially the respiratory and gastrointestinal systems. Airway secretions are particularly thick and tenacious, and the airways develop a chronic bacterial infection. Chronic infection, plugged airways, and severe inflammation cause long-term lung damage and ultimately death.

Sudden Infant Death Syndrome (SIDS)

1. SIDS is the leading cause of postnatal death for infants outside of the hospital setting. It is associated with a low birth weight, a prone sleeping position, and other, environmental factors. There has been a significant reduction in SIDS cases since the widespread adoption of recommendations for supine positioning of infants during sleep.

KEY TERMS

Acute epiglottitis, 699
Acute respiratory distress syndrome (ARDS), 707
Aspiration of a foreign body, 699
Aspiration pneumonitis, 706
Asthma, 706
Atypical pneumonia (*Mycoplasma pneumoniae* pneumonia, *Chlamydophila pneumoniae* pneumonia), 705
Bacterial pneumonia, 705

Bacterial tracheitis (pseudomembranous croup), 699
Bronchiolitis, 703
Bronchopulmonary dysplasia (BPD), 702
Cystic fibrosis (CF), 707
Cystic fibrosis transmembrane conductance regulator (CFTR) protein, 708

Obstructive sleep apnea syndrome (OSAS), 700
Peritonsillar abscess, 699
Pneumonia, 704
Recurrent (spasmodic) croup, 697
Rhinorrhea, 697
Stridor, 697
Surfactant deficiency disorder (SDD) (respiratory distress syndrome (RDS) of the newborn), 700

Sudden infant death syndrome (SIDS)/sudden unexpected infant death, 709
Tonsillar abscess, 699
Tonsillar infection, 699
Upper airway obstruction (UAO), 697
Viral croup, 697
Viral pneumonia, 705

REFERENCES

1. Hiebert JC, Zhao YD, Willis EB: Bronchoscopy findings in recurrent croup: a systematic review and meta-analysis, *Int J Pediatr Otorhinolaryngol* 90:86-90, 2016.
2. Li SF: The Westley croup score, *Acad Emerg Med* 10(3):289, 2003. author reply 289.
3. Smith DK, McDermott AJ, Sullivan JF: Croup: diagnosis and management, *Am Fam Physician* 97(9):575-580, 2018.
4. Cirilli AR: Emergency evaluation and management of the sore throat, *Emerg Med Clin North Am* 31(2):501-515, 2013.
5. Kim IA, et al: The national cost burden of bronchial foreign body aspiration in children, *Laryngoscope* 125(5):1221-1224, 2015.
6. American Academy of Sleep Medicine: *International classification of sleep disorders*, 3rd edn, Darien, IL, 2014, Author.
7. Katz ES, D'Ambrosio CM: Pediatric obstructive sleep apnea syndrome, *Clin Chest Med* 31:221-234, 2010.
8. Brockbank JC: Update on pathophysiology and treatment of childhood obstructive sleep apnea syndrome, *Paediatr Respir Rev* 24:21-23, 2017.
9. Shapiro-Mendoza CK, Lackritz EM: Epidemiology of late and moderate preterm birth, *Semin Fetal Neonatal Med* 17(3):120-125, 2012.
10. Sweet D, et al: European consensus guidelines on the management of neonatal respiratory distress syndrome, *J Perinat Med* 35:175-186, 2007.
11. Booker WA, Gyamfi-Bannerman C: Antenatal corticosteroids: who should we be treating?, *Clin Perinatol* 45(2):181-198, 2018.
12. Islam JY, et al: Understanding the short- and long-term respiratory outcomes of prematurity and bronchopulmonary dysplasia, *Am J Respir Crit Care Med* 192(2):134-156, 2015.
13. Tracy MK, Berkelhamer SK: Bronchopulmonary dysplasia and pulmonary outcomes of prematurity, *Pediatr Ann* 48(4):e148-e153, 2019.
14. Ralston SL, et al: Clinical practice guideline: the diagnosis, management, and prevention of bronchiolitis, *Pediatrics* 134(5):e1474-e1502, 2014.

Available at: http://pediatrics.aappublications.org/content/134/5/e1474.full.pdf+html.
15. Pavia AT: What is the role of respiratory viruses in community-acquired pneumonia? What is the best therapy for influenza and other viral causes of community-acquired pneumonia? *Infect Dis Clin North Am* 27(1):157-175, 2013.
16. Durando P, et al: Improving the protection against *Streptococcus pneumoniae* with the new generation 13-valent pneumococcal conjugate vaccine, *J Prev Med Hyg* 53(2):68-77, 2012.
17. Bradley JS, et al: The management of community-acquired pneumonia in infants and children older than 3 months of age: clinical practice guidelines by the Pediatric Infectious Diseases Society and the Infectious Diseases Society of America, *Clin Infect Dis* 53:e25-e76, 2011.
18. Centers for Disease Control and Prevention (CDC): Most recent asthma data. Page last reviewed March 25, 2019. Available at: https://www.cdc.gov/asthma/most_recent_data.htm.
19. Prokopakis E, et al: The pathophysiology of the hygiene hypothesis, *Int J Pediatr Otorhinolaryngol* 77(7):1065-1071, 2013.
20. Pisi G, et al: The role of the microbiome in childhood asthma, *Immunotherapy* 9(15):1295-1304, 2017.
21. National Heart, Lung, and Blood Institute: National Asthma Education and Prevention Program Expert Panel Report 3: guidelines for the diagnosis and management of asthma, 2007. Available at: https://www.nhlbi.nih.gov/files/docs/guidelines/asthsumm.pdf. (Accessed 6 June 2019).
22. Global Initiative for Asthma: Global strategy for asthma management and prevention, 2018. Available from: www.ginasthma.org.
23. Yehya N, Thomas NJ: Relevant outcomes in pediatric acute respiratory distress syndrome studies, *Front Pediatr* 4:51, 2016.
24. Heidemann SM, et al: Pathophysiology and management of acute respiratory distress syndrome in children, *Pediatr Clin North Am* 64(5):1017-1037, 2017.
25. The Pediatric Acute Lung Injury Consensus Conference Group: Pediatric acute respiratory distress syndrome: consensus recommendations

from the Pediatric Acute Lung Injury Consensus Conference, *Pediatr Crit Care Med* 16(5):428-439, 2015.
26. Cystic Fibrosis Foundation: Types of CFTR mutations. Available at: https://www.cff.org/What-is-CF/Genetics/Types-of-CFTR-Mutations/.(Accessed 6 June 2019).
27. Cystic Fibrosis Foundation: 2017 Cystic fibrosis foundation patient registry highlights, Bethesda, MD, 2018. Available at: https://www.cff.org/Research/Researcher-Resources/Patient-Registry/Understanding-Changes-in-Life-Expectancy/.
28. Cystic Fibrosis Foundation: Testing for CF. Accessed June 6, 2019. Available at: https://www.cff.org/What-is-CF/Testing/.
29. Cystic Fibrosis Foundation: Carrier testing for cystic fibrosis. Available at: https://www.cff.org/What-is-CF/Testing/Carrier-Testing-for-Cystic-Fibrosis/.(Accessed 6 June 2019).
30. Centers for Disease Control and Prevention (CDC): Sudden unexpected infant death and sudden infant death syndrome. Page last reviewed January 3, 2019. Available at: www.cdc.gov/sids/index.htm.
31. Centers for Disease Control and Prevention (CDC): Sudden unexpected infant death and sudden infant death syndrome: data and statistics. Page last reviewed April 10, 2019. Available at: https://www.cdc.gov/sids/data.htm.
32. Bergman NJ: Proposal for mechanisms of protection of supine sleep against sudden infant death syndrome: an integrated mechanism review, *Pediatr Res* 77(1-1):10-19, 2015.
33. Trachtenberg FL, et al: Risk factor changes for sudden infant death syndrome after initiation of Back-to-Sleep campaign, *Pediatrics* 129(4):630-638, 2012.
34. Goldwater PN: Infection: the neglected paradigm in SIDS research, *Arch Dis Child* 102(8):767-772, 2017.
35. Moon RY, Task Force on Sudden Infant Death Syndrome: SIDS and other sleep-related infant deaths: evidence base for 2016 updated recommendations for a safe infant sleeping environment, *Pediatrics* 138(5):2016.

31

Structure and Function of the Renal and Urologic Systems

Sue E. Huether

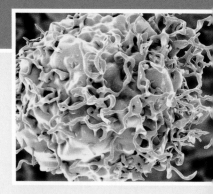

EVOLVE WEBSITE

CHAPTER OUTLINE

The renal system consists of the kidneys. The primary function of the kidney is to maintain a stable internal environment for optimal cell and tissue metabolism. The kidneys accomplish these life-sustaining tasks by balancing solute and water transport, excreting metabolic waste products, conserving nutrients, and regulating acids and bases. The kidney also has an endocrine function and secretes the hormones renin for regulation of blood pressure, erythropoietin for red blood cell production, and vitamin D_3 for calcium metabolism. The kidney also can release glucose into the circulation when needed. The formation of urine is achieved through the processes of glomerular filtration, tubular reabsorption, and secretion within the kidney. The bladder stores the urine received from the kidney by way of the ureters. Urine is then released from the bladder through the urethra.

STRUCTURES OF THE RENAL SYSTEM

Structures of the Kidney

The kidneys are paired organs located in the posterior region of the abdominal cavity behind the peritoneum. They lie on either side of the vertebral column with their upper and lower poles extending from the twelfth thoracic vertebra to the third lumbar vertebra (Fig. 31.1). The right kidney is slightly lower and is displaced downward by the overlying liver. Each kidney is approximately 11 cm long, 5 to 6 cm wide, and 3 to 4 cm thick. A tightly adhering renal capsule surrounds each kidney, which is embedded in a mass of perirenal fat. The capsule and fatty layer are covered with a double layer of renal fascia composed of fibrous tissue. A cushion of adipose tissue and the position of the kidney between the abdominal organs and muscles of the back protect it from trauma.

The internal structures of the kidney are summarized in Fig. 31.2. The hilum is a medial indentation in the kidney and is the location of the entry and exit for the renal blood vessels, nerves, lymphatic vessels, and ureter. The outer layer of the kidney is called the cortex. The medulla forms the inner part of the kidney and consists of regions called pyramids. Renal columns are an extension of the cortex and extend between the pyramids to the renal pelvis. The minor and major calyces are chambers receiving urine from the collecting ducts and form the entry into the renal pelvis. The renal pelvis is an extension of the upper ureter. The lobe is the structural unit of the kidney. Each lobe is composed of a pyramid and the overlying cortex. There are about 14 to 18 lobes in each kidney.

Nephron

The nephron is the functional unit of the kidney. Each kidney contains approximately 1.2 million nephrons. The nephron is a tubular structure with subunits that include the renal corpuscle, proximal tubule, loop of Henle, distal tubule, and collecting duct, all of which contribute to the formation of final urine (Fig. 31.3). The different structures of the epithelial cells lining various segments of the tubule facilitate the special functions of secretion and reabsorption (see Fig. 31.6). The cortex contains the renal corpuscle, most of the proximal tubules, and some segments of the distal tubule. The renal pyramids in the medulla contain the loops of Henle and collecting ducts. The kidney has three kinds of nephrons: (1) superficial cortical nephrons (85% of all nephrons), which extend partially into the medulla; (2) midcortical nephrons with short or long loops; and (3) juxtamedullary nephrons (about 12% of nephrons), which lie close to and extend deep into the medulla (about 40 mm) and are important for the concentration of urine (Fig. 31.4).

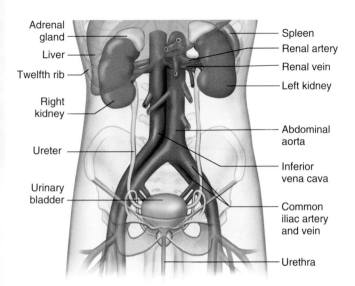

FIGURE 31.1 Organs of the Urinary System. (From Patton KT, Thibodeau GA: The human body in health & disease, ed 6, St Louis, 2014, Mosby.)

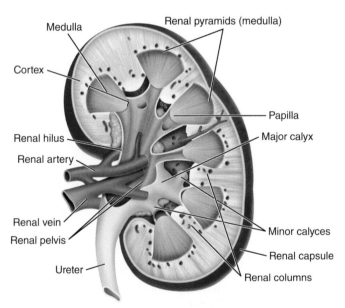

FIGURE 31.2 Internal Structure of the Kidney. (From Solomon E: Introduction to human anatomy and physiology, ed 4, St Louis, 2016, Saunders.)

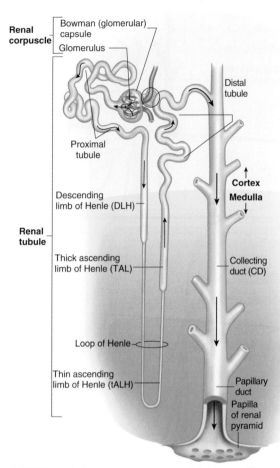

FIGURE 31.3 Components of the Nephron. (From Patton KT, Thibodeau GA, Douglas MM: Essentials of anatomy & physiology, St Louis, 2012, Mosby; Damjanov I: Pathology for the health professions, ed 4, St Louis, 2012, Mosby.)

The renal corpuscle is composed of the glomerulus, Bowman (glomerular) capsule, mesangial cells, and Bowman space. The glomerulus is a tuft of capillaries that loop into the Bowman space, like a fist pushed into bread dough. Mesangial cells (shaped like smooth muscle cells) secrete the mesangial matrix (a type of connective tissue) and lie between and support the glomerular capillaries (Fig. 31.5). Mesangial cells also have phagocytic abilities similar to monocytes, release inflammatory cytokines, and can contract to regulate glomerular capillary blood flow.

The glomerular filtration membrane has three layers: (1) an inner capillary endothelium, (2) a middle basement membrane, and (3) an outer layer of capillary or visceral epithelium (see Fig. 31.5, B). The capillary endothelium is composed of cells in continuous contact with the basement membrane and contains pores. The middle basement membrane is a selectively permeable membrane. The epithelium has

specialized cells called podocytes from which pedicles or projections radiate and adhere to the basement membrane. Pedicles from adjacent podocytes interlock, forming an elaborate network of intercellular clefts called filtration slits, or slit membranes. The endothelium, basement membrane, and podocytes are covered with protein molecules bearing negative (anionic) charges that retard the filtration of anionic proteins, preventing proteinuria. The glomerular filtration membrane separates the blood within the glomerular capillaries from the fluid (filtrate) in the Bowman space. The membrane allows all components of the blood to be filtered with the exception of blood cells and plasma proteins with a high molecular weight (most of the plasma proteins). The glomerular filtrate passes through the three layers of the glomerular membrane and forms the primary urine.

The glomerulus is supplied by the afferent arteriole and drained by the efferent arteriole. A group of specialized cells known as juxtaglomerular cells (renin-releasing cells) are located around the afferent arteriole where it enters the glomerulus (see Fig. 31.5). Between the afferent and efferent arterioles is the macula densa (sodium-sensing cells) of the distal tubule. Together the juxtaglomerular cells, macula densa cells, and mesangial cells form the juxtaglomerular apparatus. Control of renal blood flow, glomerular filtration, and renin secretion occurs at this site.

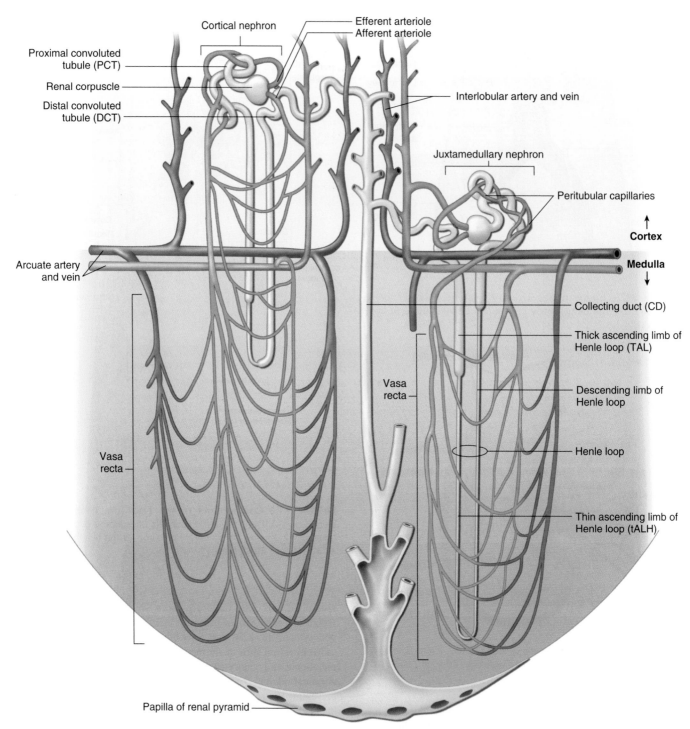

FIGURE 31.4 Nephron Unit with Its Blood Vessels. Blood flows through nephron vessels as follows: interlobular artery, afferent arteriole, glomerulus, efferent arteriole, peritubular capillaries (around the tubules), venules, interlobular vein. (From Patton KT, Thibodeau GA, Douglas MM: Essentials of anatomy & physiology, St Louis, 2012, Mosby.)

The proximal tubule continues from Bowman space and has an initial convoluted segment and then a straight segment that descends toward the medulla (see Fig. 31.3). The wall of the proximal tubule consists of one layer of cuboidal epithelial cells with a surface layer of microvilli (a brush border) that increases the reabsorptive surface area. This is the only surface inside the nephron where the cells are covered with a brush border of microvilli (Fig. 31.6). The proximal tubule joins the loop of Henle, which extends into the medulla. The cells of the thick segment are cuboidal and actively transport several solutes, but not water. The thin ascending segment of the loop of Henle narrows and is composed of thin squamous cells with no active transport function.

The distal tubule has straight and convoluted segments. It extends from the ascending loop of Henle to the collecting duct. The collecting

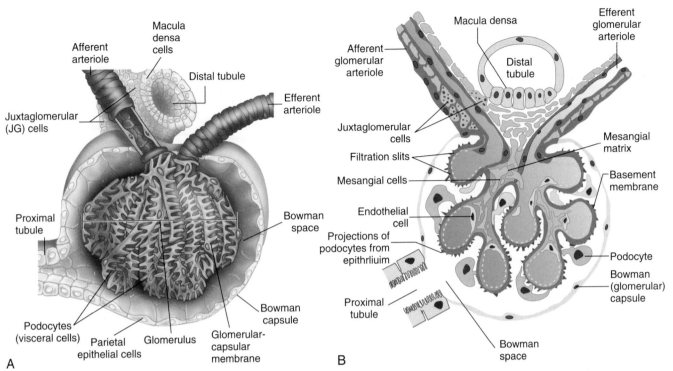

A

B

FIGURE 31.5 Anatomy of the Glomerulus and Juxtaglomerular Apparatus. A, Longitudinal cross section of glomerulus and juxtaglomerular apparatus (macula densa, juxtaglomerular cells and mesangial cells). **B,** Horizontal cross section of glomerulus.

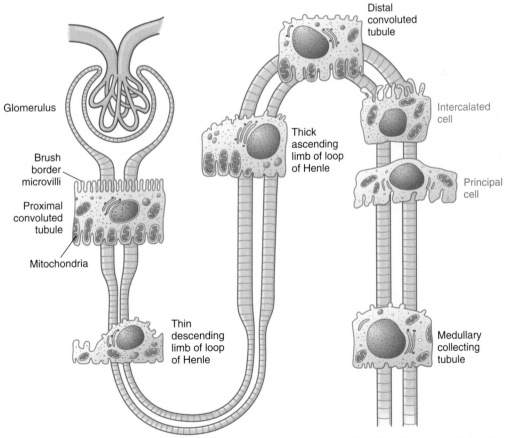

FIGURE 31.6 Epithelial Cells of the Various Segments of Nephron Tubules. The proximal tubule is the only segment of the nephron that has a brush border, and the increased surface area promotes reabsorption of 50% of the glomerular filtrate.

duct is a large tubule that descends down the cortex and through the renal pyramids of the inner and outer medullae, draining urine into the minor calyx. In the distal tubule, principal cells reabsorb sodium and secrete potassium, and intercalated cells secrete hydrogen and reabsorb potassium and bicarbonate (see Fig. 31.6). These cells are important for maintaining fluid and electrolyte and acid-base balance.

Blood Vessels of the Kidney

The blood vessels of the kidney closely parallel the nephron's structure (see Fig. 31.4). The major vessels are as follows:

1. Renal arteries (see Fig. 31.2) arise as the fifth branches of the abdominal aorta, divide into anterior and posterior branches at the renal hilum, and then subdivide into lobar arteries supplying blood to the lower, middle, and upper thirds of the kidney.
2. Interlobar arteries are lobar subdivisions that travel down renal columns and between pyramids to form afferent glomerular arteries.
3. Arcuate arteries consist of branches of interlobar arteries at the cortical-medullary junction; they arch over the base of the pyramids and run parallel to the surface.
4. Glomerular capillaries consist of four to eight vessels and are arranged in a fistlike structure; they arise from the afferent arteriole and empty into the efferent arteriole, which carries blood to the peritubular capillaries. They are the major resistance vessels for regulating intrarenal blood flow (see Autoregulation of Intrarenal Blood Flow in the Renal Blood Flow section).
5. Peritubular capillaries surround convoluted portions of the proximal and distal tubules and the loop of Henle; they are adapted for cortical and juxtamedullary nephrons.
6. Vasa recta is a network of capillaries that forms loops and closely follows the loops of Henle; it is the only blood supply to the medulla (important for formation of concentrated urine).
7. Renal veins follow the arterial path in reverse direction and have the same names as the corresponding arteries; they eventually empty into the inferior vena cava. The lymphatic vessels also tend to follow the distribution of the blood vessels.

✔ **QUICK CHECK 29.1**
1. What is the major structural difference between the cortex and the medulla of the kidney?
2. What is the function of the nephron?
3. Why are proteins not filtered at the glomerulus?

Urinary Structures

Ureters

The urine formed by the nephrons flows from the distal tubules and collecting ducts through the papillary ducts to the renal papillae (projections of the ducts) into the calyces, where it is collected in the renal pelvis (see Figs. 31.2 and 31.4). The urine is then funneled into the ureters (Fig. 31.7). Each adult ureter is approximately 30 cm long and is composed of long, intertwining smooth muscle bundles. The lower ends pass through the posterior aspect of the bladder wall. The close approximation of smooth muscle cells in the ureter permits the direct transmission of electrical stimulation from one cell to another, resulting in downward peristaltic contraction, which propels urine into the bladder. Contraction of the bladder during micturition (urination) compresses the lower end of the ureter, preventing reflux. Peristalsis is maintained even when the ureter is denervated, so ureters can be transplanted.

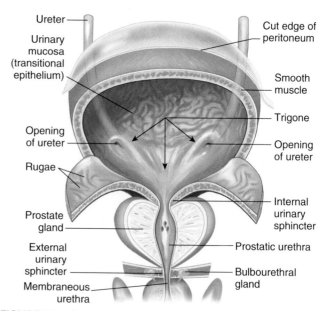

FIGURE 31.7 Structure of the Urinary Bladder. Frontal view of a dissected urinary bladder (male) in a fully distended position. No prostate is present in females. (From Patton KT, Thibodeau GA: The human body in health & disease, ed 6, St Louis, 2014, Mosby.)

Sensory innervation of the ureter arises from neural inputs from the tenth thoracic nerve to the second lumbar nerve. Ureteral pain (e.g., pain from a kidney stone in the ureter) can be referred pain to the flank, umbilicus, vulva, or penis. The ureters have a rich blood supply. The primary arteries for the ureters come from the kidney, with contributions from the lumbar and superior vesical (bladder) arteries.

Bladder and Urethra

The bladder is a bag made of smooth muscle fibers that forms the detrusor muscle with its smooth lining of uroepithelium. As the bladder fills with urine, it distends and the layers of uroepithelium within the lining slide past each other and become thinner as bladder volume increases. The uroepithelium forms the interface between the urinary space and the underlying vasculature and connective, nervous, and muscle tissue. Uroepithelium also lines the urinary tract from the renal pelvis to the urethra. The uroepithelium maintains an important barrier function to prevent movement of water and solutes between the urine and the blood. It communicates information about urine pressure and composition to surrounding nerve and muscle cells. The trigone is a triangular area of smooth muscle between the openings of the two ureters and the urethra (see Fig. 31.7). The position of the bladder varies with sex and age. In females, the bladder is anterior to the vagina and inferior to the uterus. In males, the bladder lies between the pubic symphysis and rectum. The bladder is positioned higher in infants and young children. The bladder has a profuse blood supply, accounting for the bleeding that readily occurs with trauma, surgery, or inflammation.

The urethra extends from the inferior side of the bladder to the outside of the body. A ring of smooth muscle forms the internal urethral sphincter at the junction of the urethra and bladder and is under involuntary muscle control. The external urethral sphincter is composed of striated skeletal muscle and is under voluntary motor control. The entire urethra is lined with mucus-secreting glands. The female urethra is short (3 to 4 cm). The male urethra is long (18 to 20 cm) and has three main segments: prostatic, membranous, and penile. The prostatic urethra is closest to the bladder. It passes through the prostate gland and contains the openings of the ejaculatory ducts. Prostatic enlargement can obstruct the flow of urine in this segment. The membranous urethra passes through the floor of the pelvis. The penile segment forms the remainder of the tube. It is surrounded by the corpus spongiosum erectile tissue (see Fig. 34.12).

The innervation of the bladder and internal urethral sphincter is supplied by the autonomic nervous system. The detrusor muscle is innervated by sympathetic nervous system fibers from the lumbar spinal cord and parasympathetic fibers from the sacral spinal cord. The reflex arc required for micturition is stimulated by mechanoreceptors that respond to stretching of tissue, sensing bladder fullness and sending impulses to the sacral level of the cord. When the bladder accumulates 250 to 300 ml of urine, the bladder contracts and the internal urethral sphincter relaxes through activation of the spinal reflex arc (known as the *micturition reflex*). At this time, a person feels the urge to void. The reflex can be inhibited or facilitated by impulses coming from the brain, resulting in voluntary control of micturition by the relaxation or contraction of the external sphincter.

RENAL BLOOD FLOW AND GLOMERULAR FILTRATION

The kidneys are highly vascular organs and usually receive 1000 to 1200 ml of blood per minute, or about 20% to 25% of the cardiac output. With a normal hematocrit of 45%, about 600 to 700 ml of blood flowing through the kidney per minute is plasma. Of the renal plasma flow (RPF), 20% (approximately 120 to 140 ml/min) is filtered at the glomerulus and passes into the Bowman capsule. (The remaining 80% of plasma flows through the efferent arterioles to the peritubular capillaries.) The filtration of the plasma per unit of time is known as the glomerular filtration rate (GFR) (e.g., 120 to 140 ml/min), which is directly related to the perfusion pressure of the glomerular capillaries. The ratio of glomerular filtrate to renal plasma flow per minute (e.g., 120/600 = 0.20) is called the *filtration fraction*. Normally all but 1 to 2 ml/min of the glomerular filtrate is reabsorbed from nephron tubules and returned to the circulation by the peritubular capillaries.

The GFR is directly related to the renal blood flow (RBF), which is regulated by intrinsic autoregulatory mechanisms, by neural regulation, and by hormonal regulation. In general, blood flow to any organ is determined by the arteriovenous pressure differences across the vascular bed. If the mean arterial pressure decreases or the vascular resistance increases, the RBF declines and urinary output decreases.

Autoregulation of Intrarenal Blood Flow

In the kidney, the autoregulation of the glomerular blood flow helps keep the GFR fairly constant over a range of systemic arterial pressures between 80 and 180 mm Hg[1] (Fig. 31.8). This is necessary to maintain the clearance of metabolic wastes and the reabsorption of filtered electrolytes and nutrients by the renal tubules with the normal variations in systemic blood pressure. For example, blood pressure increases during exercise and decreases during rest. This mechanism is known as the autoregulation of intrarenal blood flow. It is maintained by two mechanisms controlling the afferent arteriole:

1. When the blood pressure in the afferent arteriole increases, an *intrinsic autoregulatory myogenic mechanism* of arteriole contraction increases resistance, thus maintaining a constant flow and GFR. The opposite occurs with a decrease in the systemic blood pressure.
2. The tubuloglomerular feedback mechanism involves the macula densa cells at the juxtaglomerular apparatus in the distal tubule. As the blood pressure increases or decreases, the macula densa cells sense the resulting increase or decrease in the amounts of filtered sodium. When the GFR and sodium concentration increase, the macula densa cells stimulate afferent arteriolar vasoconstriction and

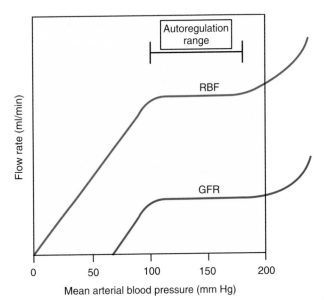

FIGURE 31.8 Renal Autoregulation. Renal blood flow (RBF) and glomerular filtration rate (GFR) are stabilized in the face of changes in perfusion pressure.

decrease GFR. The opposite occurs with decreases in the GFR and sodium concentration at the macula densa. This mechanism, combined with the intrinsic myogenic mechanism, prevents large fluctuations in body water and salt with variations in blood pressure.

Neural Regulation of Renal Blood Flow

The blood vessels of the kidney are innervated by sympathetic nerve fibers located primarily on afferent arterioles. When the systemic arterial pressure decreases, the renal sympathetic nerves release catecholamines. This stimulates afferent renal arteriolar vasoconstriction and decreases the RBF and GFR, increases renal tubular sodium and water reabsorption, and increases the systemic blood pressure. Decreased afferent renal sympathetic nerve activity produces the opposite effects. Renalase is a hormone released by the kidney, heart, and other organs that promotes the metabolism of catecholamines and in this way participates in lowering the blood pressure and GFR.[2] The sympathetic nervous system also participates in hormonal regulation of the RBF (i.e., stimulates the renin-angiotensin-aldosterone system). There is no significant parasympathetic innervation. The innervation of the kidney arises primarily from the celiac ganglion and greater splanchnic nerve.

Hormones and Other Factors Regulating Renal Blood Flow

Hormones and other mediators can alter the resistance of the renal vasculature by stimulating vasodilation or vasoconstriction. A major hormonal regulator of RBF is the renin-angiotensin-aldosterone system (RAAS), which can increase the systemic arterial pressure and change the RBF. Renin is an enzyme formed and stored in the cells of the arterioles of the juxtaglomerular apparatus (see Fig. 31.5). Renin release is triggered by a decreased blood pressure in the afferent arterioles, a decreased sodium chloride concentration in the distal convoluted tubule, sympathetic nerve stimulation of β-adrenergic receptors on the juxtaglomerular cells, and the release of prostaglandins.[3] Numerous physiologic effects of the RAAS stabilize the systemic blood pressure and preserve the extracellular fluid volume during hypotension or hypovolemia. Actions include sodium reabsorption, systemic vasoconstriction, sympathetic nerve stimulation, and thirst stimulation, with an increased fluid intake. The effects of aldosterone combine with those of antidiuretic hormone in regulating blood volume and are summarized in Fig. 31.9 (also see Fig. 5.5).

Natriuretic peptides are synthesized and released from the heart and are natural antagonists to the RAAS (see Fig. 5.6). Natriuretic peptides cause vasodilation and also increase sodium and water excretion and decrease the blood pressure. They assist in protecting the heart from volume overload. Urodilatin is a renal natriuretic peptide produced by cells in the distal tubule and collecting duct. It increases RBF, causing diuresis.

✓ **QUICK CHECK 29.2**
1. Where is pain from the ureters referred?
2. How do the bladder and urethra function in urine regulation?
3. What is the purpose of autoregulation of renal blood flow?
4. What triggers the activation of the renin-angiotensin-aldosterone system?

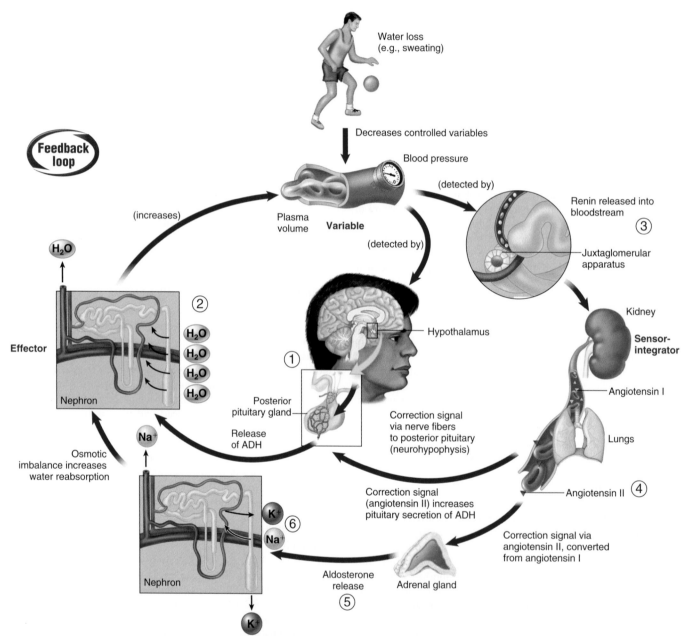

FIGURE 31.9 Cooperative Roles of Antidiuretic Hormone (ADH) and Aldosterone in Regulating Urine and Plasma Volume. The drop in blood pressure that accompanies loss of fluid from the internal environment triggers the hypothalamus to rapidly release ADH from the posterior pituitary gland **(1)**. ADH increases water reabsorption by the kidney by increasing water permeability of the distal tubules and collecting ducts **(2)**. The drop in blood pressure also is detected by each nephron's juxtaglomerular apparatus, which responds by secreting renin **(3)**. Renin triggers the formation of angiotensin II **(4)**, which stimulates release of aldosterone from the adrenal cortex **(5)**. Aldosterone then slowly boosts water reabsorption by the kidneys by increasing reabsorption of Na+ **(6)**. Because angiotensin II also stimulates secretion of ADH, it serves as an additional link between the ADH and aldosterone mechanisms. (From Patton KT: Anatomy & physiology, ed 10, St Louis, 2019, Mosby.)

KIDNEY FUNCTION

Nephron Function

The major function of the nephron is urine formation, which it does by performing many functions simultaneously (Fig. 31.10):

1. Filtering plasma at the glomerulus
2. Reabsorbing and secreting different substances along the tubular structures
3. Forming a filtrate of protein-free fluid (ultrafiltration)
4. Regulating the filtrate to maintain the body fluid volume, electrolyte composition, and pH within narrow limits

Glomerular filtration is the movement of fluid and solutes across the glomerular capillary membrane into the Bowman space. Tubular reabsorption is the movement of fluids and solutes from the tubular lumen into the peritubular capillary plasma. Tubular secretion is the transfer of substances from the plasma of the peritubular capillary to the tubular lumen (Fig. 31.11). The transport mechanisms are both active and passive (processes defined in Chapter 1). Excretion is the elimination of a substance in the final urine.

Glomerular Filtration

The fluid filtered across the glomerular capillary filtration membrane is protein free but contains electrolytes (e.g., sodium, chloride, and potassium) and organic molecules (e.g., creatinine, urea, and glucose) in the same concentrations as are found in plasma. As are other capillary membranes, the glomerulus is freely permeable to water and relatively impermeable to large colloids, such as plasma proteins. The molecule's size and electrical charge and the small size of the filtration slits in the glomerular epithelium affect the permeability of substances crossing the glomerulus and entering the proximal tubule.

In addition to permeability, capillary pressures also affect glomerular filtration. The hydrostatic pressure within the capillary is the major force for pushing water and solutes across the filtration membrane and into the Bowman capsule. Two forces oppose the filtration effects of the glomerular capillary hydrostatic pressure: (1) the hydrostatic pressure in the Bowman space and (2) the effective oncotic pressure of the glomerular capillary blood. Remember, hydrostatic pressure is a pushing pressure, and oncotic pressure is a pulling pressure in relation to water. Because the fluid in the Bowman space normally contains only very small amounts of protein, it does not usually have an oncotic influence on the plasma of the glomerular capillary (Fig. 31.12).

The combined effect of forces favoring and forces opposing filtration determines the filtration pressure. The net filtration pressure (NFP) is the sum of forces favoring and opposing filtration. The estimated values contributing to the forces of net filtration are presented in Fig. 31.12.

As the protein-free fluid is filtered into the Bowman capsule, the plasma oncotic pressure increases and the hydrostatic pressure decreases in the glomerular capillary. The increase in the glomerular capillary oncotic pressure is great enough to reduce the net filtration pressure to zero at the efferent end of the capillary and to stop the filtration process effectively. The low hydrostatic pressure and the increased oncotic pressure in the efferent arteriole then are transferred to the peritubular capillaries. This facilitates the reabsorption of fluid from the proximal tubules back into the circulating blood.

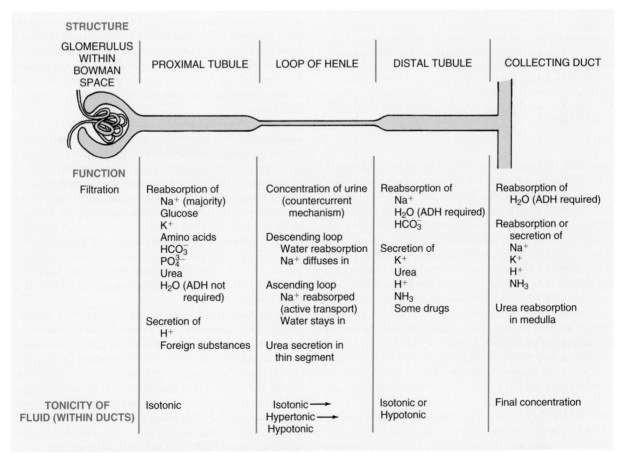

STRUCTURE				
GLOMERULUS WITHIN BOWMAN SPACE	PROXIMAL TUBULE	LOOP OF HENLE	DISTAL TUBULE	COLLECTING DUCT
FUNCTION				
Filtration	Reabsorption of Na$^+$ (majority) Glucose K$^+$ Amino acids HCO$_3^-$ PO$_4^{3-}$ Urea H$_2$O (ADH not required) Secretion of H$^+$ Foreign substances	Concentration of urine (countercurrent mechanism) Descending loop Water reabsorption Na$^+$ diffuses in Ascending loop Na$^+$ reabsorped (active transport) Water stays in Urea secretion in thin segment	Reabsorption of Na$^+$ H$_2$O (ADH required) HCO$_3^-$ Secretion of K$^+$ Urea H$^+$ NH$_3$ Some drugs	Reabsorption of H$_2$O (ADH required) Reabsorption or secretion of Na$^+$ K$^+$ H$^+$ NH$_3$ Urea reabsorption in medulla
TONICITY OF FLUID (WITHIN DUCTS)	Isotonic	Isotonic ⟶ Hypertonic ⟶ Hypotonic	Isotonic or Hypotonic	Final concentration

FIGURE 31.10 Major Functions of Nephron Segments. *ADH,* Antidiuretic hormone. (Modified from Hockenberry MJ et al: Wong's nursing care of infants and children, ed 8, St Louis, 2007, Mosby.)

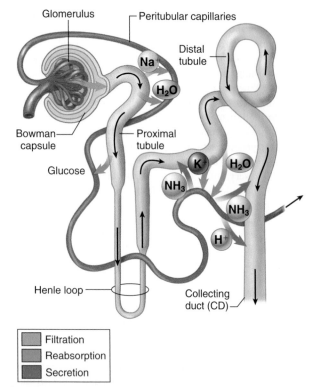

FIGURE 31.11 Urine Formation: Glomerular Filtration, Tubular Reabsorption, and Tubular Secretion. These are the three processes by which the kidneys excrete urine. Water, electrolytes, glucose, and organic molecules are filtered at the glomerulus. Sodium and glucose are reabsorbed into peritubular capillaries by active transport from the proximal convoluted tubules, and water reabsorption follows by osmosis. Sodium is reabsorbed by active transport from distal convoluted tubules; more sodium is conserved when aldosterone is secreted. Osmotic reabsorption of water from the distal tubules occurs when antidiuretic hormone is present. Secretion of ammonia (NH_3), hydrogen, and potassium occurs from peritubular capillaries into distal tubules by active transport. (From Patton KT, Thibodeau GA: The human body in health & disease, ed 7, St Louis, 2018, Mosby.)

Filtration rate. The total volume of fluid filtered by the glomeruli averages 180 L/day, or approximately 120 ml/min, a phenomenal amount considering the size of the kidneys. Because only 1 to 2 L of urine is excreted per day, 99% of the filtrate is reabsorbed into the peritubular capillaries and returned to the blood. The factors determining the GFR are directly related to the pressures that favor or oppose filtration (see Fig. 31.12). Obstruction of the outflow of urine (e.g., caused by strictures, stones, or tumors along the urinary tract) can cause a retrograde increase in hydrostatic pressure at the Bowman space and a decrease in the GFR. Low levels of plasma protein in the blood can also result in a decrease in the glomerular capillary oncotic pressure, which increases the GFR. Excessive loss of *protein-free fluid* as a result of vomiting, diarrhea, use of diuretics, or excessive sweating can increase the glomerular capillary oncotic pressure and decrease the GFR. Renal disease also can cause changes in pressure relationships by altering capillary permeability and the surface area available for filtration (see Chapter 32).

Proximal tubule. By the end of the proximal tubule, approximately 60% to 70% of filtered sodium and water and about 50% of urea have been actively reabsorbed, along with 90% or more of potassium, glucose, bicarbonate, calcium, phosphate, amino acids, and uric acid. Chloride, water, and urea are reabsorbed passively but linked to the active

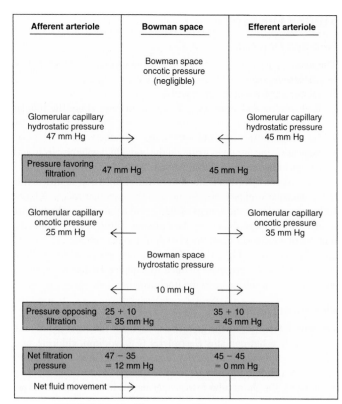

FIGURE 31.12 Glomerular Filtration Pressures.

transport of sodium (a cotransport mechanism). For some molecules, active transport in the renal tubules is limited as the carrier molecules become saturated, a phenomenon known as transport maximum (T_m). For example, when the carrier molecules for glucose reabsorption in the proximal tubule become saturated (i.e., with the development of hyperglycemia), the excess will be excreted in the urine, causing glucosuria.

Active reabsorption of sodium is the primary function of the convoluted segment of the proximal tubule. Water, most other electrolytes, and organic substances are cotransported with sodium. The osmotic force generated by active sodium transport promotes the passive diffusion of water out of the tubular lumen and into the peritubular capillaries. Passive transport of water is further enhanced by the elevated oncotic pressure of the blood in the peritubular capillaries, which is created by the previous filtration of water at the glomerulus. The reabsorption of water leaves an increased concentration of urea within the tubular lumen, creating a gradient for its passive diffusion to the peritubular plasma. As the positively charged sodium ions leave the tubular lumen, negatively charged chloride ions passively follow to maintain electroneutrality.

Bicarbonate is completely filtered at the glomerulus, and approximately 90% is reabsorbed in the proximal tubule. In the tubular lumen, hydrogen ions are actively exchanged for sodium. The hydrogen ions combine with bicarbonate ions and form carbonic acid (H_2CO_3), which rapidly breaks down, or dissociates, to carbon dioxide (CO_2) and water (H_2O). The CO_2 and H_2O then diffuse into the tubular cell, where the enzyme carbonic anhydrase again catalyzes the CO_2 and H_2O to form HCO_3^- and H^+. The H^+ is secreted into the tubular lumen again, and HCO_3^- combines with sodium and is transported to the peritubular capillary blood as $NaHCO_3$ (a sodium bicarbonate buffer). Bicarbonate is thus conserved. The hydrogen combines with hydroxide ion (OH^-) and is reabsorbed as water. Therefore, in the proximal tubule these ions normally do not contribute to the urinary excretion of acid or the addition of acid to the blood.

In the proximal tubule, secretory transport mechanisms exist for creatinine, other organic bases, and endogenous and exogenous organic acids, including *para*-aminohippurate (PAH) and penicillin (Box 31.1). These secretory mechanisms eliminate drugs and other exogenous chemical products from the body, often after first conjugating (combining) them with sulfate and glucuronic acid in the liver. Many drugs and their metabolites are eliminated from the body in this way. When the renal tubules are damaged, metabolic by-products and drugs may accumulate, causing toxic levels in the body.

Normally, 99% of the glomerular filtrate is reabsorbed. When the GFR spontaneously decreases or increases, the renal tubules, primarily the proximal tubules, automatically adjust their rate of reabsorption of sodium and water to balance the change in the GFR. This prevents wide fluctuations in the excretion of sodium and water into the urine, known as glomerulotubular balance.

Loop of Henle and distal tubule. Urine can be hypotonic, isotonic, or hypertonic, depending on the concentration or dilution of the urine. Urine concentration or dilution occurs principally in the loop of Henle, distal tubules, and collecting ducts. The structural features of the

medullary hairpin loops allow the kidney to concentrate urine and conserve water for the body. The transition of the filtrate into the final urine reflects the concentrating ability of the loops. Final adjustments in urine composition are made by the distal tubule and collecting duct according to the body's needs.

Production of concentrated urine involves a countercurrent exchange system, in which fluid flows in opposite directions through the parallel tubes of the loop of Henle. A concentration gradient causes fluid to be exchanged across the parallel pathways. The longer the loop, the greater the concentration gradient. The concentration gradient increases from the cortex to the tip of the medulla. The *loops of Henle multiply the concentration gradient,* and the vasa recta blood vessels (located around the loops of Henle) act as a *countercurrent exchanger* for maintaining the gradient. The process is initiated in the thick ascending limb of the loop of Henle with the active transport of chloride and sodium out of the tubular lumen and into the medullary interstitium (Fig. 31.13). Because the lumen of the ascending limb is impermeable to water, water cannot follow the sodium-chloride transport. This causes the ascending tubular fluid to become hypoosmotic and the medullary interstitium to become hyperosmotic.

The descending limb of the loop, which receives fluid from the proximal tubule, is highly permeable to water, but it is the only place in the nephron that does not actively transport either sodium or chloride. The hyperosmotic medullary interstitium causes water to move out of the descending limb, and the remaining fluid in the descending tubule becomes increasingly concentrated as it flows toward the tip of the medulla. When the tubular fluid rounds the loop and enters the ascending limb, sodium and chloride are removed and water is retained as described previously. The fluid then becomes more and more dilute as it encounters the distal tubule.

The slow rate of blood flow and the hairpin structure of the vasa recta blood vessels allow blood to flow through the medullary tissue without disturbing the osmotic gradient. When blood flows into the descending limb of the vasa recta, it encounters the increasing osmotic concentration gradient of the medullary interstitium. Water moves out, and sodium and chloride diffuse into the descending vasa recta. The plasma becomes increasingly concentrated as it flows toward the tip of the medulla.

BOX 31.1	**Substances Transported by Renal Tubules**
Reabsorption	**Secretion**
Albumin	Choline
Ascorbate	Creatinine
Fructose	Histamine
Galactose	Methylguanidine
Glutamate	*para*-Aminohippurate
Glucose	Penicillin and many other drugs
Phosphate	Steroid glucuronides
Sulfate	Thiamine
Xylose	

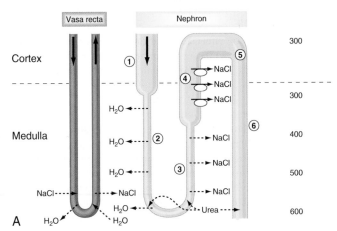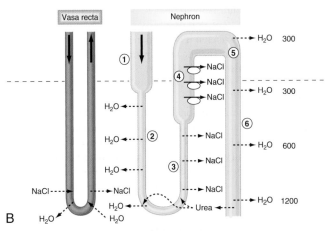

FIGURE 31.13 Countercurrent Mechanism for Concentrating and Diluting Urine. A, Urine dilution; **B,** urine concentration. **1,** Filtrate isotonic to plasma. **2,** Descending thin limb permeable to water. **3,** Ascending thin limb impermeable to water; permeable to ions. **4,** Ascending thick limb actively transports NaCl; impermeable to water and urea. **5,** Distal tubule actively resorbs NaCl; resorbs water in presence of antidiuretic hormone. **6,** Medullary collecting duct actively resorbs NaCl, and slightly permeable to water and urea. (**Note:** Numbers on illustration represent milliosmoles [mOsm]). *H₂O,* water; *NaCl,* sodium chloride. See text for details. (From Koeppen BM, Stanton BA: Berne and Levy physiology [updated], ed 6, St Louis, 2010, Mosby.)

As blood flows away from the tip of the medulla and toward the cortex, the surrounding interstitial fluid becomes comparatively more dilute. Water then moves back into the vasa recta, and sodium and chloride diffuse out and the plasma again becomes more dilute. The net result is a preservation of the medullary osmotic gradient. If blood were to flow rapidly through the vasa recta, as occurs in some renal diseases, the medullary concentration gradient would be washed away and the ability to concentrate urine and conserve water would be lost. The efficiency of water conservation is related to the length of the loops of Henle: the longer the loops, the greater the ability to concentrate the urine.

Urea is the major constituent of urine, along with water. The glomerulus freely filters urea, and tubular reabsorption depends on the urine flow rate, with less reabsorption at higher flow rates. Approximately 50% of urea is excreted in the urine, and 50% is recycled within the kidney. This recycling contributes to the osmotic gradient within the medulla and is necessary for the concentration and dilution of urine (see Fig. 31.13). Because urea is an end product of protein metabolism, individuals with protein deprivation cannot maximally concentrate their urine.

Another function of the ascending loop of Henle is the production of uromodulin (also known as Tamm-Horsfall protein [THP]), the most abundant protein in human urine. This protein binds to uropathogens to prevent urinary tract infection, protects the uroepithelium from injury, protects against kidney stone formation and is involved in sodium transport.[4]

The convoluted portion of the distal tubule is poorly permeable to water but readily reabsorbs ions and contributes to the dilution of the tubular fluid. The later, straight segment of the distal tubule and the collecting duct are permeable to water as controlled by antidiuretic hormone released from the posterior pituitary gland. Sodium is readily reabsorbed by the later segment of the distal tubule and collecting duct under the regulation of the hormone aldosterone (see Chapter 19). Potassium is actively secreted in these segments and is also controlled by aldosterone and other factors related to the concentration of potassium in body fluids (see Chapter 5).

Hydrogen is secreted by the distal tubule and combines with non-bicarbonate buffers (i.e., ammonium and phosphate) for the elimination of acids in the urine (see Fig. 5.12). The distal tubule thus contributes to the regulation of acid-base balance by excreting hydrogen ions into the urine and by adding new bicarbonate to the plasma. The mechanism is similar to the conservation of bicarbonate by the proximal tubule, except that the hydrogen ion is excreted in the urine and influences the acid-base balance. The specific mechanisms of acid-base balance and acid excretion are described in Chapter 5.

Urine Composition

Urine is normally clear yellow or amber in color. Cloudiness may indicate the presence of bacteria, cells, or a high solute concentration. The pH ranges from 4.6 to 8, but it is normally acidic, providing protection against bacterial survival. The specific gravity ranges from 1.001 to 1.035. Normal urine does not contain glucose or blood cells and only occasionally contains traces of protein, usually in association with rigorous exercise.

Hormones and Nephron Function
Antidiuretic Hormone
The distal tubule in the cortex receives the hypoosmotic urine from the ascending limb of the loop of Henle. The specific gravity, or concentration, of the final urine is controlled by antidiuretic hormone (ADH), which is secreted from the posterior pituitary or neurohypophysis. ADH increases water permeability and reabsorption in the last segment

of the distal tubule and along the entire length of the collecting ducts, which pass through the inner and outer zones of the medulla. The water diffuses into the ascending limb of the vasa recta and returns to the systemic circulation to maintain fluid balance. The excreted urine can have a high osmotic concentration, up to 1400 mOsm. The volume is normally reduced to about 1% of the amount filtered at the glomerulus. (The mechanism for the regulation of ADH and plasma osmolality is described in Chapters 5 and 19.)

Aldosterone
Aldosterone is synthesized and secreted by the adrenal cortex under the regulation of the RAAS (see Chapter 19 and the previous discussion of the RAAS in this chapter). Aldosterone stimulates the epithelial cells of the distal tubule and collecting duct to reabsorb sodium (promoting water reabsorption) and increases the excretion of potassium and hydrogen ion.

Natriuretic Peptides
Natriuretic peptides are a group of peptide hormones that promote sodium and water excretion, including atrial natriuretic peptide (ANP or A-type natriuretic peptide), secreted from myocardial cells in the atria, and brain natriuretic peptide (BNP or B-type natriuretic peptide), secreted from myocardial cells in the cardiac ventricles.[5] When the heart dilates during volume expansion or heart failure, ANP and BNP inhibit sodium and water absorption by the kidney tubules, inhibit secretion of renin and aldosterone, vasodilate the afferent arterioles, and constrict the efferent arterioles. The result is increased urine formation, leading to a decrease in blood volume and blood pressure. *C-type natriuretic peptide* is secreted from the vascular endothelium; it causes vasodilation in the nephron and complements the action of ANP and BNP. *Urodilatin* is a natriuretic peptide secreted by the distal convoluted tubules and collecting ducts that causes vasodilation and natriuretic and diuretic effects.

Diuretics as a Factor in Urine Flow
A diuretic is any agent enhancing the flow of urine. Clinically, diuretics interfere with renal sodium reabsorption and reduce the extracellular fluid volume. Diuretics are commonly used to treat hypertension and edema caused by heart failure, cirrhosis, and nephrotic syndrome. However, side effects may include dehydration, hypokalemia, systemic acidosis, metabolic alkalosis, nausea, and headache.

Renal Hormones
Certain hormones are either activated or synthesized by the kidney. These hormones have significant systemic effects and include urodilatin (see earlier text), the active form of vitamin D, and erythropoietin.

Vitamin D
Vitamin D is a hormone that is necessary for the absorption of calcium and phosphate by the small intestine.[6] The normal serum concentration is 50 nmol/L (i.e., 20 ng/mL). It can be obtained in the diet or synthesized by the action of ultraviolet radiation (sun exposure) on cholesterol in the skin. These forms of vitamin D_3 (cholecalciferol) are inactive and require two hydroxylations (which adds an OH^- group to a compound) to establish a metabolically active form. The first hydroxylation occurs in the liver and the second in the kidneys. The renal hydroxylation step is stimulated by parathyroid hormone (see Chapter 19). A decreased plasma calcium level (less than 10 mg/dl) stimulates the secretion of parathyroid hormone. Parathyroid hormone then stimulates a sequence of events to help return the plasma calcium concentration toward normal levels (9 to 10.5 mg/dl):
1. Calcium mobilization from bone
2. Synthesis of 1,25-dihydroxy-vitamin D_3

3. Absorption of calcium from the intestine
4. Increased renal calcium reabsorption
5. Decreased renal phosphate reabsorption

Fluctuations in the serum phosphate concentration also influence the renal hydroxylation of vitamin D. Decreased levels stimulate active 1,25-dihydroxy-vitamin D_3 formation, and increased levels inhibit formation. This results in compensatory changes in phosphate absorption from the bones and intestine. Individuals with renal disease have a deficiency of 1,25-dihydroxy-vitamin D_3 (1,25-OH_2D_3) and manifest symptoms of disturbed calcium and phosphate balance (see Chapters 5, 19, and 32).

Erythropoietin

Erythropoietin (Epo) stimulates the bone marrow to produce red blood cells in response to tissue hypoxia and may have tissue protective effects (see *Did You Know?* The Many Effects of Erythropoietin). Erythrocyte production is discussed in Chapter 22. The stimulus for Epo release is decreased oxygen delivery in the kidneys. Oxygen-sensing erythropoietin-producing cells are peritubular fibroblast-like cells located in the juxtamedullary cortex. The anemia of chronic renal failure, in which kidney cells have become nonfunctional, can be related to the lack of this hormone (see Chapter 32).

DID YOU KNOW?

The Many Effects of Erythropoietin

Receptors for Erythropoietin (Epo) are found in many body cells other than hematopoietic cells (i.e., neurons, immune cells, cancer cells, endothelial cells, bone marrow, myocardium, skeletal muscle, skin cells, kidney cells, pancreatic cells, and cells of the reproductive system and gastrointestinal tract). Epo has protective effects that limit injury and promote tissue repair. Mechanisms include antiapoptotic (prevents programmed cell death), antiinflammatory, and angiogenic (new blood vessel growth) actions. In acute kidney injury, Epo reduces ischemia, oxidative stress, and inflammation, protecting cells from injury. These same effects, including angiogenesis, limit myocardial infarction size and left ventricular remodeling. Epo inhibits inflammation in chronic inflammatory diseases. Epo is neuroprotective in conditions associated with hypoxia, neurodegeneration, and inflammation. Epo is used for the treatment of anemia in chronic kidney disease and anemia related to cancer chemotherapy.

Data from Kimáková P et al: Int J Mol Sci 18(7):pii: E1519, 2017; Korzeniewski SJ, Pappas A: Vitam Horm 105:39-56, 2017; Nekoui A, Blaise G: Am J Med Sci 353(1):76-81, 2017; Ostrowski D, Heinrich R: J Clin Med 7(2):pii: E24, 2018; Shih HM, Wu CJ, Lin SL: J Formos Med Assoc 117(11):955-963, 2018.

Kidney function changes throughout the life span; major changes are summarized in the boxes *Pediatric Considerations:* Pediatrics & Renal Function and *Geriatric Considerations:* Aging & Renal Function.

✔ QUICK CHECK 29.3

1. Outline the process of glomerular filtration.
2. What types of absorption/reabsorption take place in the proximal tubule, the loops of Henle, and the distal tubule?
3. What is the countercurrent exchange system? What substances are involved?
4. What hormones are activated or synthesized by the kidney?

TESTS OF RENAL FUNCTION

Renal Clearance

A number of specific renal functions can be measured by renal clearance. Renal clearance techniques or formulas determine how much of a substance can be cleared from the blood by the kidneys per given unit of time. The application of this principle permits an indirect measure of the GFR, tubular secretion, tubular reabsorption, and the RBF.

Clearance and Glomerular Filtration Rate

The GFR provides the best estimate of functioning renal tissue and is important for assessing or monitoring kidney damage and drug dosing. Damage to the glomerular membrane or loss of nephrons leads to a corresponding decrease in the GFR. Measurement of the GFR requires the use of a substance that has a stable plasma concentration; is freely filtered at the glomerulus; is not secreted, reabsorbed, or metabolized by the tubules; is constantly infused to maintain a stable plasma level; and is easy to measure. Therefore the clearance of **creatinine**, a natural substance produced by muscle and released into the blood at a relatively constant rate, is commonly used as an estimate clinically. It is freely filtered at the glomerulus, but a small amount is secreted by the renal tubules, meaning creatinine clearance overestimates the GFR, but within tolerable limits. Creatinine clearance provides a good clinical measure of the GFR because only one blood sample is required, in addition to an accurately collected 24-hour volume of urine. **Cystatin C** is a stable protein in serum filtered at the glomerulus and metabolized in the tubules. Serum levels of cystatin C also are a marker for estimating the GFR, particularly for mild to moderate impaired renal function. Formulas are used to estimate the GFR. Calculators for estimates of the GFR use a variety of formulas and are readily available on the internet (see an example at http://touchcalc.com/ip_epi_gfr/ip_ckd_epi). Normal GFR values are 90 to 120 ml/min.

Plasma Creatinine Concentration

A chronic decline in the GFR over weeks or months is reflected in the **plasma creatinine (P_{cr}) concentration** (normal value = 0.7 to 1.2 mg/dl). The P_{cr} concentration has a stable value when the GFR is stable because creatinine has a constant rate of production as a product of muscle metabolism. The amount filtered is approximately equal to the amount excreted. When the GFR declines, the P_{cr} increases proportionately. Thus the GFR and P_{cr} are inversely related. If the GFR were to decrease by 50%, the filtration and excretion of creatinine would be reduced by 50% and creatinine would accumulate in the plasma to twice the normal value. Therefore, elevated P_{cr} values represent a decreasing GFR. In the new steady state, however, the total amount of creatinine excreted in the urine would remain the same because of the proportionate decrease in the GFR and increase in the P_{cr}.

The application of this principle is simple and useful for monitoring progressive changes in renal function. The test is most valuable for monitoring the progress of chronic rather than acute renal disease because it takes 7 to 10 days for the plasma creatinine level to stabilize when the GFR declines. Serial measures can be obtained over a long time and plotted as a curve of glomerular function. The P_{cr} also becomes elevated during trauma or the breakdown of muscle tissue. In such instances, the value is then not useful for estimating the GFR.

Blood Urea Nitrogen

The concentration of urea nitrogen in the blood reflects glomerular filtration and urine-concentrating capacity. Because urea is filtered at the glomerulus, blood urea nitrogen (BUN) levels increase as glomerular filtration drops. Urea is reabsorbed by the blood through the permeable tubules, so the BUN value rises in states of dehydration and with acute and chronic renal failure when the passage of fluid through the tubules slows. BUN values also change as a result of altered protein intake and protein catabolism. The normal range for the BUN level in adults is 10 to 20 mg/dl of blood.

Clearance and Renal Blood Flow

A clearance formula also can be devised to estimate the RPF and RBF using the PAH molecule. When PAH is administered intravenously, some of it is filtered at the glomerulus, and most of the remainder is secreted into the tubules in one circulation through the kidney. A blood sample and urine sample are obtained simultaneously to measure the amount of PAH in each sample. If all the PAH is removed from the plasma during a single pass through the kidney, the total RPF can be determined. Because the supporting and nonsecreting structures of the kidney receive 10% to 15% of the effective renal blood flow (ERBF), the clearance of PAH measures only what is known as the effective renal plasma flow (ERPF), which is 85% to 90% of the true renal plasma flow.

Urinalysis

Urinalysis is a noninvasive and relatively inexpensive diagnostic procedure. The best results are obtained from a fresh, cleanly voided specimen because decay permits changes in the composition of the urine. Urinalysis includes evaluation of the color, turbidity, protein, pH, specific gravity, sediment, and supernatant. Urine tests are listed in Table 31.1.

✔ QUICK CHECK 29.4

1. Why is creatinine clearance a good estimate of the glomerular filtration rate?
2. What is the relationship between the plasma creatinine concentration and the glomerular filtration rate?

TABLE 31.1   Renal Function Test Results

Test	Normal Value	Interpretation of Abnormal Result
Urine		
Color	Amber-yellow	Drugs and foods may change color
Turbidity	Clear	Purulent matter causes cloudiness
pH	4.6-8	Bacteria create an alkaline urine
Specific gravity	*Adults:* 1.010-1.025 *Infants:* 1.010-1.018	Represents concentrating ability or density of urine in relation to density of water (1.000) (i.e., higher when contains glucose or protein; lower with dilute urine)
Blood	Negative	Bleeding along urinary tract
Microscopic Urine		
Bacteria	None	Infection
Red blood cells	Negative	Bleeding along urinary tract
White blood cells	Negative	Urinary tract infection
Crystals	Negative	May have potential for stones
Fat	Negative	Can be associated with nephrosis
Casts	Occasional	A few are normal; may represent renal disease
Urinary Chemistry		
Bilirubin	Negative	Increases may cause dark orange color
Urobilinogen	Less than 4 mg/24 hr	Increases may indicate red blood cell hemolysis
Ketones	Negative	Indicate an increase in fat metabolism
Glucose	Negative	Usually signifies hyperglycemia
Sodium	100-260 mEq/24 hr	Can increase or decrease with renal disease
Potassium	25-100 mEq/24 hr	Can increase or decrease with renal disease, potassium intake, aldosteronism, or diuretic use
Protein	Negative-trace	Dysfunction of glomerulus
Normal Serum Values		
Blood urea nitrogen (BUN)	7-18 mg/dl	Elevated with diseased kidneys
Creatinine	*Male:* 0.6-1.5 mg/dl *Female:* 0.6-1.1 mg/dl	Elevated with decreased glomerular filtration rate (GFR)
Cystatin C	0.8-2.1 mg/L	Early detection of decreased GFR
Potassium		Elevated in renal failure

PEDIATRIC CONSIDERATIONS

Pediatrics & Renal Function

All the nephrons are present at birth, and their numbers do not increase as the kidney grows and matures. The glomerular filtration rate (GFR) in infants does not reach adult levels until 1 to 2 years of age, and newborns have a decreased ability to efficiently remove excess water and solutes. Their shorter loops of Henle also decrease concentrating ability and produce a more dilute urine than that produced by adults. Risks for metabolic acidosis are increased during the first few months of life, while the mechanisms for excreting acid and retaining bicarbonate are maturing. These normal developmental processes result in a narrow safety margin for fluid and electrolyte balance when there is any disturbance, such as diarrhea, infection, fever, fasting for diagnostic tests, improper feeding, fluid replacement, or drug administration. Newborns diurese 2 to 3 days after birth, which is reflected by a decrease in total body water and body weight. An increased risk of toxicity accompanies drug administration. Low birth weight infants have a delay in achieving full renal function and may not have a full GFR until 8 years of age. They also are at greater risk for low nephron numbers and chronic kidney disease as adults. Maturation of nephrons is complete by adolescence.

Data from.Filler G et al: *Pediatr Nephrol* 29(2):183-192, 2014; Hoseini R et al: *Iran J Kidney Dis* 6(3):166-172, 2012; Lankadeva YR et al: *Am J Physiol Renal Physiol* 306(8):F791-F800, 2014; Starr MC, Hingorani SR: Curr Opin Pediatr 30(2):228-235, 2018; Sulemanji M, Vakili K: *Semin Pediatr Surg* 22(4):195-198, 2013.

GERIATRIC CONSIDERATIONS

Aging & Renal Function

- Structural changes commonly occur in the kidney with aging, including loss of renal mass, arterial sclerosis, an increased number of sclerotic glomeruli, loss of tubules, and interstitial fibrosis. These changes contribute to a slow decline in the glomerular filtration rate (GFR) and a reduction in creatinine clearance in most individuals, but it generally is not significant enough to lead to severe loss of renal function in healthy individuals. As the number of nephrons decreases and degenerative changes occur, nephrons are less able to concentrate urine and less able to tolerate dehydration, excessive water loads, or electrolyte imbalances, particularly with physiologic stress. Up to 45% of people older than 70 years of age have chronic kidney disease.
- The presence of comordid conditions, such as hypertension and diabetes mellitus, accelerates the decline of renal function.
- Response to acid-base changes and reabsorption of glucose may be delayed.
- Drugs eliminated by the kidney can accumulate in the plasma, causing toxic reactions; the GFR and drug dosages should be carefully evaluated.
- A decreased thirst sensation and diminished water intake may alter water balance.
- Impairment of renal blood flow, hormonal regulatory systems, and metabolism of medications may alter the sodium and water balance.
- Older donor kidneys show decreased regenerative capacity and response to renal injury.

Data from Gekle M: *Exp Gerontol* 87(Pt B):153-155, 2017; Hommos MS, Glassock RJ, Rule AD: *J Am Soc Nephrol* 28(10):2838-2844, 2017; O'Sullivan ED, Hughes J, Ferenbach DA: *J Am Soc Nephrol* 28(2):407-420, 2017; Rowland J et al: Kidney Blood Press Res 43(1):55-67, 2018; Sobamowo H, Prabhakar SS: *Prog Mol Biol Transl Sci* 146:303-340, 2017; Sturmlechner I et al: *Nat Rev Nephrol* 13(2):77-89, 2017.

SUMMARY REVIEW

Structures of the Renal System

1. The kidneys are paired structures lying bilaterally between the twelfth thoracic and third lumbar vertebrae and behind the peritoneum of the abdominal cavity.
2. The kidney is surrounded by the renal capsule and is composed of an outer cortex and an inner medulla. The cortex contains the glomerulus, proximal tubule, and parts of the distal tubule. The medulla contains the loops of Henle and collecting ducts.
3. The calyces are chambers that receive urine from the distal tubules and join to form the renal pelvis, which is continuous with the upper end of the ureter.
4. The nephron is the urine-forming unit of the kidney and is composed of the renal corpuscle (glomerulus, Bowman capsule, mesangial cells), proximal tubule, loops of Henle, distal tubule, and collecting duct.
5. The glomerulus contains loops of capillaries (afferent and efferent arterioles) supported by mesangial cells. The capillary walls serve as a filtration membrane for the formation of the primary urine.
6. The juxtaglomerular apparatus is located in the glomerulus and is composed of renin-secreting juxtaglomerular cells (around the afferent arteriole) and sodium-sensing macula densa cells (distal tubule) and mesangial cells (between the glomerular capillaries).
7. The proximal tubule is lined with microvilli to increase the surface area and enhance reabsorption of water, solutes, and electrolytes.
8. The loops of Henle transport solutes and water, contributing to the hypertonic state of the medulla, and are important for the concentration and dilution of urine.
9. The distal tubule adjusts acid-base balance by excreting acid into the urine and forming new bicarbonate ions.
10. The ureters extend from the renal pelvis to the posterior wall of the bladder. Urine flows through the ureters and into the bladder by means of peristaltic contraction of the ureteral muscles.
11. The bladder is a bag composed of the detrusor and trigone muscles and innervated by the autonomic nervous system. When the accumulation of urine reaches 250 to 300 ml, mechanoreceptors, which respond to stretching of tissue, stimulate the micturition reflex and elimination of urine through the urethra.

Renal Blood Flow and Glomerular Filtration

1. Renal blood flows at about 1000 to 1200 ml/min, or 20% to 25% of the cardiac output.

2. The GFR is the filtration of plasma per unit of time and is directly related to the perfusion pressure of RBF.
3. Blood flow through the glomerular capillaries is maintained at a constant rate in spite of a wide range of arterial pressures by auto-regulation of the glomerular capillaries.
4. Renin is an enzyme secreted from the juxtaglomerular apparatus in response to decreased blood pressure and causes the generation of angiotensin II, a potent vasoconstrictor. The RAAS is thus a regulator of renal blood flow.

Kidney Function

1. The major function of the nephron is urine formation, which involves the processes of glomerular filtration, tubular reabsorption, and tubular secretion and excretion.
2. Glomerular filtration is favored by capillary hydrostatic pressure and opposed by oncotic pressure in the capillary and hydrostatic pressure in the Bowman capsule. The NFP is the balance of favoring and opposing filtration forces.
3. The GFR is approximately 120 ml/min to 140 ml/min, and 99% of the filtrate is reabsorbed.
4. The proximal tubule reabsorbs about 60% to 70% of the filtered sodium and water and 90% of other electrolytes.
5. Because most molecules are reabsorbed by active transport, the carrier mechanism can become saturated at a point known as the *transport maximum*. Molecules not reabsorbed are excreted with the urine.
6. The concentration or specific gravity of the final urine is a function of the level of ADH. This hormone stimulates the distal tubules and collecting ducts to reabsorb water. The countercurrent exchange system of the long loops of Henle and their accompanying capillaries establishes a concentration gradient within the renal medulla to facilitate the reabsorption of water from the collecting duct.

7. The kidney secretes or activates a number of hormones having systemic effects, including vitamin D, erythropoietin, and the natriuretic hormone urodilatin.

Tests of Renal Function

1. Creatinine, a substance produced by muscle, is measured in both plasma and urine to calculate a commonly used clinical measurement of the GFR.
2. The plasma creatinine concentration, cystatin C level, and BUN level are estimates of glomerular function. The BUN value also is an indicator of hydration status.
3. Urinalysis involves evaluation of the color, turbidity, protein, pH, specific gravity, sediment, and supernatant. The presence of bacteria, red blood cells, white blood cells, casts, or crystals in the urine sediment may indicate a renal or bladder disorder.

Pediatric Considerations: Pediatrics & Renal Function

1. Compared with adults, infants and children have a more dilute urine because of higher blood flow and shorter loops of Henle.
2. Children are more affected than adults by fluid imbalances resulting from diarrhea, infection, or improper feeding because of their limited ability to quickly regulate changes in pH or osmotic pressure.

Geriatric Considerations: Aging & Renal Function

1. Older adults have a decreased ability to concentrate urine and are less able to tolerate dehydration or water loads because they have fewer nephrons.
2. Responses to acid-base changes and reabsorption of glucose are delayed in older adults.
3. In older adults, drugs eliminated by the kidney can accumulate in the plasma, causing toxic reactions.

KEY TERMS

Afferent arteriole, 716
Aldosterone, 722
Antidiuretic hormone (ADH), 722
Arcuate artery, 716
Atrial natriuretic peptide (ANP, A-type natriuretic peptide), 722
Autoregulation of intrarenal blood flow, 717
Bladder, 716
Bowman space, 713
Brain natriuretic peptide (BNP, B-type natriuretic peptide), 722
Collecting duct, 714
Cortex, 712
Cortical nephron, 712
Countercurrent exchange system, 721
Creatinine, 723
Cystatin C, 723
Detrusor muscle, 716
Distal tubule, 714
Diuretic, 722

Effective renal blood flow (ERBF), 724
Effective renal plasma flow (ERPF), 724
Efferent arteriole, 716
Erythropoietin (Epo), 723
Excretion, 719
External urethral sphincter, 716
Filtration slit, 713
Glomerular capillary, 716
Glomerular filtration, 719
Glomerular filtration membrane, 713
Glomerular filtration rate (GFR), 717
Glomerulotubular balance, 721
Glomerulus, 713
Hilum, 712
Intercalated cell, 716
Interlobar artery, 716
Internal urethral sphincter, 716
Juxtaglomerular apparatus, 713
Juxtaglomerular cell, 713
Juxtamedullary nephron, 712
Kidney, 712

Lobe, 712
Loop of Henle, 714
Macula densa, 713
Medulla, 712
Major calyx (pl., calyces), 712
Mesangial cell, 713
Mesangial matrix, 713
Micturition, 716
Midcortical nephron, 712
Minor and major calyces, 712
Natriuretic peptide, 718, 722
Nephron, 712
Net filtration pressure (NFP), 719
Peritubular capillary, 716
Plasma creatinine (P_{cr}) concentration, 723
Podocyte, 713
Principal cell, 716
Proximal tubule, 714
Pyramid, 712
Renal artery, 716
Renalase, 717
Renal capsule, 712
Renal column, 712

Renal corpuscle, 713
Renal fascia, 712
Renal papilla (pl., papillae), 716
Renal vein, 716
Renin-angiotensin-aldosterone system (RAAS), 717
Tamm-Horsfall protein (THP), 722
Transport maximum (T_m), 720
Trigone, 716
Tubular reabsorption, 719
Tubular secretion, 719
Tubuloglomerular feedback mechanism, 717
Urea, 722
Ureter, 716
Urethra, 716
Urinalysis, 724
Urine concentration, 721
Urine dilution, 721
Urodilatin, 718
Uroepithelium, 716
Uromodulin, 722
Vasa recta, 716
Vitamin D, 722

REFERENCES

1. Wang Y, et al: Extracellular renalase protects cells and organs by outside-in signaling, *J Cell Mol Med* 21(7):1260-1265, 2017.
2. Castrop H, et al: Physiology of kidney renin, *Physiol Rev* 90(2):607-673, 2010.
3. Wu TH, et al: Tamm-Horsfall protein is a potent immunomodulatory molecule and a disease biomarker in the urinary system, *Molecules* 23(1):pii: E200, 2018.
4. Maisel AS, Duran JM, Wettersten N: Natriuretic peptides in heart failure: atrial and B-type natriuretic peptides, *Heart Fail Clin* 14(1):13-25, 2018.
5. Wasung ME, Chawla LS, Madero M: Biomarkers of renal function, which and when?, *Clin Chim Acta* 438:350-735, 2015.
6. Levey AS, et al: GFR estimation: from physiology to public health, *Am J Kidney Dis* 63(5):820-834, 2014.

32

Alterations of Renal and Urinary Tract Function

Sue E. Huether

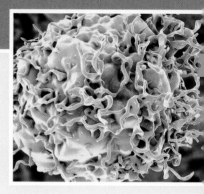

EVOLVE WEBSITE

http://evolve.elsevier.com/Huether/

CHAPTER OUTLINE

Kidney and urinary tract function can be affected by a variety of disorders. Infection of the bladder is the most common disorder, and stones, tumors, or inflammation can obstruct the urinary tract. Disease may be limited to only the kidney and urinary tract or include systemic diseases that cause acute or chronic kidney disease or difficulty eliminating urine (e.g., infection neurologic injury or diabetes mellitus). Because the kidney filters the blood, it is directly linked to every other organ system. Therefore kidney failure, whether acute or chronic, can affect other organs and become life-threatening.

URINARY TRACT OBSTRUCTION

Urinary tract obstruction is an interference with the flow of urine at any site along the urinary tract (Fig. 32.1). An obstruction may be anatomic (structural) or functional. The obstruction impedes flow and dilates structures proximal to the blockage, increases the risk for infection, and compromises renal function. Anatomic changes in the urinary system caused by obstruction are referred to as obstructive uropathy. The severity of an obstructive uropathy is determined by:
1. the location of the obstructive lesion,
2. the involvement of ureters and kidneys,
3. the severity (completeness) of the blockage,
4. the duration of the blockage, and
5. the nature of the obstructive lesion.

Obstructions may be relieved or partially alleviated by correction of the obstruction, although permanent impairments occur if a complete or partial obstruction persists over a period of weeks to months or longer.

Upper Urinary Tract Obstruction

Common causes of upper urinary tract obstruction include kidney stones (calculi) or tumor within the kidney or a stricture or compression from a tumor, stone, or fibrosis (stricture) along the ureter or at the ureterovesical (ureter-bladder) junction.

Obstruction of the upper urinary tract causes a "backing up" of urine and dilation of the ureter, renal pelvis, calyces, and renal parenchyma proximal to the site of urinary blockage. Dilation of the ureter is referred to as hydroureter (accumulation of urine in the ureter). Dilation of the renal pelvis and calyces proximal to a blockage is referred to as hydronephrosis or ureterohydronephrosis (dilation of both the ureter and the pelvicaliceal system) (see Fig. 32.1, *B*). The increased pressure from the backup of urine is transmitted to the glomerulus, which decreases the glomerular filtration rate (GFR). This occurs because the increase in hydrostatic pressure from the backup of urine into the Bowman space opposes the hydrostatic pressure of glomerular filtration (see Chapter 5 for forces that affect net filtration pressure). Unless the obstruction is relieved, the dilation leads to tubulointerstitial fibrosis with deposition of excessive amounts of collagen and other proteins.

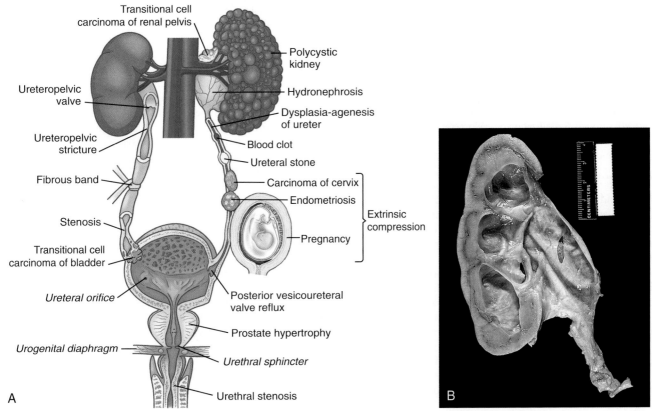

FIGURE 32.1 Urinary Tract Obstruction and Hydronephrosis. A, Major sites of urinary tract obstruction. **B,** Hydronephrosis of the kidney. There is marked dilation of the renal pelvis and calyces with thinning of the overlying cortex and medulla due to compression atrophy. (B From Kumar V et al: *Robbins and Cotran pathologic basis of disease*, ed 9, Philadelphia, 2015, Saunders.)

These changes occur in the nephrons and affect renal function within approximately 7 to 28 days. Tubular damage decreases the kidney's ability to concentrate urine, causing an increase in urine volume despite a decrease in GFR. The affected kidney has diminished ability to conserve sodium, reabsorb bicarbonate, excrete ammonia, and excrete hydrogen or potassium. Regulation of metabolic acid-base and fluid and electrolyte balance is thus diminished.

When there is unilateral obstruction, the body is able to partially counteract the negative consequences by a process called compensatory hypertrophy and hyperfunction. The compensatory response is guided by growth factors that cause the unobstructed kidney to increase the size and function of individual glomeruli and tubules but not the total number of functioning nephrons. The ability of the body to engage in compensatory hypertrophy and hyperfunction diminishes with age, and the process is reversible when relief of obstruction results in recovery of function by the obstructed kidney. Consequently the obstructed kidney can remain silent for a long time.

Relief of upper urinary tract obstruction is usually followed by a brief period of diuresis, commonly called postobstructive diuresis. Postobstructive diuresis is a physiologic response and is typically mild, representing a restoration of fluid and electrolyte imbalance caused by retention of fluid related to the obstructive uropathy. Occasionally, relief of obstruction will cause rapid excretion of large volumes of water, sodium, or other electrolytes, resulting in a urine output of 10 L/day or more. Rapid postobstructive diuresis causes dehydration and fluid and electrolyte imbalances that must be promptly corrected. Risk factors for severe postobstructive diuresis include chronic, bilateral obstruction; impairment of one or both kidneys' ability to concentrate urine or reabsorb sodium; hypertension; edema and weight gain; congestive heart failure; and uremic encephalopathy.

Kidney Stones

Kidney stones (nephrolithiasis, calculi, or urinary stones) are masses of crystals, protein, or other substances that are a common cause of urinary tract obstruction in adults. Stones can be located in the kidneys, ureters, and urinary bladder. The prevalence of stones in the United States is approximately 1 in 11 individuals over a lifetime, and the incidence has increased in the past 15 years.[1] The recurrence rate is approximately 30% to 50% within 5 years.[2] Most stones are unilateral. The risk of stone formation is influenced by a number of factors, including age, sex, race, geographic location, seasonal factors, fluid intake, diet, occupation, and genetic predisposition. Most persons develop their first stone before age 50 years. Geographic location influences the risk of stone formation because of indirect factors, including average temperature, humidity, and rainfall and their influence on fluid intake and dietary patterns. Persons who regularly consume an adequate volume of water and those who are physically active are at reduced risk when compared with persons who are inactive or consume lower volumes of water.

Stones can be classified according to the primary minerals (salts) that make up the stones. The most common stone types include calcium oxalate or phosphate (70% to 80%), struvite (magnesium-ammonium-phosphate) (15%), and uric acid (7%). Cystine stones are rare (<1%).[3]

Stones also can be classified according to location and size. *Staghorn calculi* are large and fill the minor and major calyces. *Nonstaghorn calculi* are of variable size and are located in the calyces, in the renal pelvis, or at various sites along the ureter.

PATHOPHYSIOLOGY Stone formation is complex and related to:
1. supersaturation of one or more salts in the urine,
2. precipitation of the salts from a liquid to a solid state,
3. growth through crystallization or agglomeration (sometimes called *aggregation*), and
4. the presence or absence of stone inhibitors (e.g., uromodulin [Tamm-Horsfall protein]).

Supersaturation is the presence of a higher concentration of a salt within a fluid (in this case, the urine) than the volume of fluid is able to dissolve to maintain equilibrium. Human urine contains many ions capable of *precipitating* from solution and forming a variety of salts. The salts form crystals that are retained and grow into stones. *Crystallization* is the process by which crystals grow from a small nucleus, or nidus, to larger stones in the presence of supersaturated urine. Although supersaturation is essential for free stone formation, the urine need not remain continuously supersaturated for a stone to grow once its nucleus has precipitated from solution. Intermittent periods of supersaturation after the ingestion of a meal or during times of dehydration from limited oral intake or secondary to continued use of diuretics are sufficient for stone growth in many individuals. In addition, the renal tubules and papillae have many surfaces that may attract a crystalline nidus (known as a Randall plaque) and add biologic material (matrix) forming a stone. *Matrix* is an organic material (i.e., mucoprotein) in which the components of a kidney stone are embedded.

The pH of the urine also influences the risk of stone formation. An alkaline urinary pH (pH >7.0) significantly increases the risk of calcium phosphate stone and struvite stone formation. An acidic urine (pH <5.0) increases the risk of uric acid stone formation. Cystine and xanthine also precipitate more readily in acidic urine.

Stone or *crystal growth inhibiting substances,* such as potassium citrate, Tamm-Horsfall protein, pyrophosphate, and magnesium, are capable of crystal growth inhibition. These substances reduce the risk of calcium phosphate or calcium oxalate precipitation in the urine and prevent subsequent stone formation.

The size of a stone determines the likelihood that it will pass through the urinary tract and be excreted through micturition. Stones smaller than 5 mm have about a 50% chance of spontaneous (painful) passage, whereas stones that are 1 cm have almost no chance of spontaneous passage.

Retention of *crystal particles* occurs primarily at the papillary collecting ducts. Most crystals are flushed from the tract through the normal flow of urine. Urinary stasis (i.e., from benign prostatic hyperplasia, neurogenic bladder), anatomic abnormalities (strictures), or inflamed epithelium within the urinary tract may prevent prompt flushing of crystals from the system, thus increasing the risk of stone formation.

CLINICAL MANIFESTATIONS Renal colic is pain related to dilation and spasms of smooth muscle related to ureteral obstruction. Moderate to severe pain often originates in the flank and radiates to the groin, and usually indicates obstruction of the renal pelvis or proximal ureter. Colic that radiates to the lateral flank or lower abdomen typically indicates obstruction in the midureter. Bothersome lower urinary tract symptoms (urgency, frequent voiding, urge incontinence) indicate obstruction of the lower ureter or ureterovesical junction. The pain can be agonizing and incapacitating and may be accompanied by nausea and vomiting. Gross or microscopic hematuria may be present.

EVALUATION AND TREATMENT The evaluation and diagnosis of kidney stones is based on presenting symptoms and history combined with a focused physical assessment. Imaging studies determine the location of the stone, the severity of obstruction, and associated obstructive uropathy. The history queries dietary habits, the age of the first stone episode, stone analysis, and presence of complicating factors, including hyperparathyroidism or recent gastrointestinal or genitourinary surgery. Urinalysis (including pH) is obtained and a 24-hour urine is completed to identify calcium oxalate, calcium citrate, and other significant constituents. In addition, every effort is made to retrieve and analyze stones that are passed spontaneously or retrieved through aggressive intervention. To diagnose and manage underlying metabolic disorders, additional tests are completed for those with suspected hyperparathyroidism (elevated serum calcium levels) or cystine or uric acid (high purine diet) stones.

The goals of treatment are to manage acute pain, promote stone passage, reduce the size of stones already formed, and prevent new stone formation. The components of treatment include:
1. managing pain (can require narcotic medication),
2. reducing the concentration of stone-forming substances by increasing urine flow rate with high fluid intake,
3. adjusting the pH of the urine (e.g., make it more alkaline with potassium citrate administration or more acid with potassium acid phosphate),
4. decreasing the amount of stone-forming substances in the urine by decreasing dietary intake or endogenous production or by altering urine pH, and
5. removing stones using percutaneous nephrolithotomy, ureteroscopy, or ultrasonic or laser lithotripsy to fragment stones for excretion in the urine.

Prevention of recurrent stones includes increasing fluid intake to generate 2.5 L of urine per day, avoiding intake of colas and other soft drinks acidified with phosphoric acid, avoiding dietary oxalate (e.g., chocolate, beets, nuts, rhubarb, spinach, strawberries, tea, wheat bran), eating less animal protein, and limiting sodium intake. Maintaining a dietary calcium intake of 1000 to 1200 mg/day is helpful for calcium stone prevention. Potassium citrate may be used to prevent calcium stone aggregation and to raise urinary pH.

✓ **QUICK CHECK 32.1**
1. How does obstruction of urine flow out of the kidney effect glomerular filtration?
2. What is the effect of tubulointerstitial fibrosis on renal tubular function?
3. What are three mechanisms that promote kidney stone formation?

Lower Urinary Tract Obstruction

Obstructions of the lower urinary tract (LUT) include both structural or anatomic disorders and alterations in neurologic function (neurogenic bladder), or both. These disorders are related to alterations of urine storage in the bladder or emptying of urine through the bladder outlet.[4,5] Incontinence is a common symptom associated with LUT obstructions. The types of incontinence are summarized in Table 32.1.

TABLE 32.1 Types of Incontinence

Type	Description
Urge incontinence (most common in older adults)	Involuntary loss of urine associated with abrupt and strong desire to void (urgency); often associated with involuntary contractions of detrusor; when associated with neurologic disorder, this is called *detrusor hyperreflexia;* when no neurologic disorder exists, this is called *detrusor instability;* may be associated with decreased bladder wall compliance
Stress incontinence (most common in women <60 years and men who have had prostate surgery)	Involuntary loss of urine during coughing, sneezing, laughing, or other physical activity associated with increased abdominal pressure
Overflow incontinence	Involuntary loss of urine with overdistention of bladder; associated with neurologic lesions below S1, polyneuropathies, and urethral obstruction (e.g., enlarged prostate)
Mixed incontinence (most common in older women)	Combination of both stress and urge incontinence
Functional incontinence	Involuntary loss of urine attributable to dementia or immobility

Data from Agency for Health Care Policy and Research, National Guideline Clearing House: *Assessment and diagnosis.* In *Guidelines on urinary incontinence.* Updated March 4, 2014. Available from <http://www.guideline.gov/content.aspx?id=47640&search=urinary+incontinence>; Khandelwal C, Kistler C: Diagnosis of urinary incontinence, *Am Fam Physician* 87(8):543-550, 2013.

Anatomic Obstructions to Urine Flow

Anatomic causes of resistance to urine flow include urethral stricture, prostatic enlargement in men, pelvic prolapse (bladder and uterus) in women, and tumor compression. A urethral stricture is a narrowing of its lumen and occurs when infection, injury, or surgical manipulation produces a scar that reduces the caliber of the urethra. The severity of obstruction is influenced by its location within the urethra, its length, and the severity of the stricture. Strictures that are longer than 1 centimeter and in the proximal urethra cause more severe obstruction. They are more common in men because of their longer urethra. Urethral stricture is treated with urethral dilation accomplished by using a steel instrument shaped like a catheter (urethral sound) or a series of incrementally increasing catheter-like tubes (filiforms and followers). Long, dense strictures typically require surgical repair to prevent recurrence. Prostate enlargement is caused by acute inflammation, benign prostatic hyperplasia, or prostate cancer (see Chapter 36). Severe pelvic organ prolapse (see Chapter 35) in a woman causes bladder outlet obstruction when a cystocele (the downward protrusion/herniation of the bladder into the vagina) or the uterus descends into the vagina below the level of the urethral outlet. In men, the bladder may rarely herniate into the scrotum, causing a similar type of obstruction. Each of these disorders can cause compression of the urethra with obstruction to urine flow.

Partial obstruction of the bladder outlet or urethra initially causes an increase in the force of detrusor contraction. If the obstruction persists, afferent nerves within the bladder wall are adversely affected, leading to urinary urgency and, in some cases, overactive detrusor contractions (a myogenic cause of overactive bladder). When obstruction persists, there is an increased deposition of collagen within the smooth muscle bundles of the detrusor muscle *(trabeculation).* Ultimately, the bladder wall loses its ability to stretch and accommodate urine, a condition called low bladder wall compliance (loss of elasticity), and the detrusor loses its ability to contract efficiently, resulting in urine retention. This is an underactive bladder syndrome and also can occur as a consequence of bladder radiation treatment. Low bladder wall compliance chronically elevates intravesicular pressure, greatly increasing the likelihood of hydroureter, hydronephrosis, impaired renal function, incontinence, and urinary tract infection (UTI).

Symptoms of obstruction include:

1. frequent daytime voiding (urination more than every 2 hours while awake);
2. nocturia (awakening more than once each night to urinate for adults younger than 65 years of age or more than twice for older adults);
3. poor force of stream;
4. intermittency of urinary stream;
5. bothersome urinary urgency, often combined with hesitancy; and
6. feelings of incomplete bladder emptying despite micturition.

Overactive Bladder Syndrome

Overactive bladder syndrome (OAB), non-neurogenic or idiopathic OAB, is a symptom complex characterized by urinary urgency, frequency, and nocturia with or without incontinence in the absence of UTI or other known pathology (i.e., neurologic disorders). The specific cause is unknown (idiopathic). The symptoms are usually associated with involuntary contractions of the detrusor muscle resulting in urge incontinence. The symptoms are more common in females and individuals 65 years of age and older. Risk factors in women include vaginal birth with episiotomy or use of forceps, surgery for pelvic organ prolapse, and decreased estrogen associated with menopause or hysterectomy. Loss of estrogen results in thinning and loss of urethral muscle strength. Risk factors in men include enlarged prostate with urinary obstruction and surgical treatment for prostate cancer. Risk factors also include use of medications, such as diuretics, antidepressants, alpha-agonists, beta-antagonists, sedatives, anticholinergics, and analgesics.

Diagnosis of LUT obstructions requires a detailed history; physical examination, including neurologic and pelvic examinations; urinalysis; and determining if pathologic causes of urgency and frequency, such as prostatic enlargement, pelvic organ prolapse, urethral strictures, and neurologic disorders or systemic disease, are present. Diaries and questionnaires are helpful to determine the pattern and severity of incontinence. However, no symptom or cluster of symptoms has been identified that accurately differentiates the various causes of these disorders. For example, symptoms such as urgency, urge incontinence, frequent urination, and nocturia may develop because of overactive bladder or either increased or decreased bladder outlet resistance. Reduced resistance is associated with the symptom of stress incontinence (incontinence with coughing or sneezing), and symptoms of increased resistance are similar to bladder outlet obstruction, including poor force of urinary stream, hesitancy, and feelings of incomplete bladder emptying. Various urodynamic tests (Box 32.1) assist with evaluation of how efficient the bladder, sphincters, and urethra are in storing and releasing urine. An evaluation of renal function, including functional imaging studies and measurement of serum creatinine level, is completed particularly when obstruction is severe and associated with elevated residual urine or UTI.

Treatment of LUT obstruction includes treating pathologic conditions when present. Both behavioral and pharmacologic therapy are first- and second-line treatments for idiopathic OAB. Behavioral therapy includes pelvic floor (Kegel) exercises (detrusor contraction can be inhibited by pelvic floor muscle contraction providing time to get to the toilet), bladder training with timed voiding, management of fluid intake and use of caffeine and alcohol, managing constipation, and biofeedback techniques. Drug therapy to manage incontinence includes topical vaginal estrogen in women, and drugs that increase urethral sphincter contraction or relax the bladder wall. Because the bladder sphincter muscle has cholinergic (muscarinic) and the detrusor muscle has α-adrenergic innervation, OAB may be managed by anticholinergic therapy (antimuscarinic) and adrenergic medications (i.e., anticholinergics increase urethral pressure and β$_3$-adrenergic agonists relax the bladder wall), although side effects must be monitored. When these therapies are not successful, neuromodulation therapy is considered, including intradetrusor onabotulinumtoxin A (inhibits release of acetylcholine), peripheral tibial nerve stimulation, and sacral neuromodulation.[6] Low bladder wall compliance (loss of elasticity) may be managed by antimuscarinic drugs, intradetrusor onabotulinumtoxin A injections, and intermittent catheterization.

Many individuals are reluctant to discuss OAB syndrome with their health care provider, and it should be a topic of evaluation during health assessments. Untreated OAB is an economic burden, impairs health and quality of life, and causes symptoms such as skin breakdown because of leakage, sleep disturbance, fall-related injuries, depression, prolonged hospital stays, and admission to a nursing home.

Neurogenic Bladder

Neurogenic bladder is a general term for bladder dysfunction caused by neurologic disorders (Table 32.2).[7] The types of dysfunction are related to the sites in the nervous system that control sensory and motor bladder function (Fig. 32.2). Lesions in the upper motor neurons of the brain and spinal cord result in detrusor hyperreflexia (overactive bladder) and bladder dyssynergia (loss of coordinated neuromuscular contraction). Lesions in the sacral area of the spinal cord or peripheral nerves result in underactive, hypotonic, or atonic (flaccid) bladder function, often with loss of bladder sensation. Chapter 14 discusses upper and lower motor neuron function.

Neurologic disorders that develop above the pontine micturition center (located near the posterior pons) result in detrusor (bladder muscle) hyperreflexia (overactivity), also known as an uninhibited or reflex bladder or neurogenic overactive bladder. This is an upper motor neuron disorder in which the bladder empties automatically (without voluntary control) when it becomes full and the urethral sphincter functions normally. Because the pontine micturition center remains intact, there is coordination between detrusor muscle contraction and relaxation of the urethral sphincter. Stroke, traumatic brain injury, dementia, and brain tumors are examples of disorders that result in detrusor hyperreflexia. Symptoms include urine leakage and incontinence.

Neurologic lesions that occur below the pontine micturition center but above the sacral micturition center (between C2 and S1) are also upper motor neuron lesions and result in detrusor hyperreflexia with vesicosphincter dyssynergia (loss of coordinated function between the bladder and sphincter). There is loss of pontine coordination of detrusor muscle contraction and external sphincter relaxation, so both the bladder and the sphincter are contracting at the same time (dyssynergia), causing a functional obstruction of the bladder outlet. Spinal cord injury, multiple sclerosis, Guillain-Barré syndrome, and vertebral disk problems are causes of this disorder. There is diminished bladder relaxation during storage with small urine volumes and high intravesicular (inside the bladder) pressures. The result is an overactive bladder syndrome with symptoms of frequency, urgency, urge incontinence, and increased risk for UTI. Diagnosis includes a medical history, physical examination, urinalysis, and urodynamic testing (see Box 32.1). Detrusor sphincter dyssynergia may be managed by intermittent catheterization in combination with higher dose antimuscarinic drugs to prevent overactive detrusor contractions and associated dyssynergia while ensuring regular, complete bladder evacuation by catheterization. Transurethral botulinum toxin

---

BOX 32.1 Urodynamic Tests

1. *Postvoid residual urine* measures the amount of urine remaining in the bladder after urination.
2. *Uroflowmetry* provides a graphic representation of urine flow rate and voiding time (the force of the urinary stream expressed as milliliters voided per second) and evaluates the presence of obstruction.
3. *Cystometric test* uses a catheter and manometer to evaluate bladder urine volume and pressure in relation to the occurrence of involuntary bladder contraction (the leak point pressure) and the urge to void.
4. Electromyography uses sensors to measure detrusor and sphincter muscle contraction strength during urination.
5. *Multichannel urodynamic testing* measure pressure in both the bladder and rectum during urination.
6. *Video-urodynamic recording* takes pictures and videos of the bladder using ultrasound or x-rays during bladder filling and emptying and can demonstrate overactive bladder and detrusor sphincter dyssynergia (lack of coordination between the bladder and sphincter).

TABLE 32.2 Causes of Neurogenic Bladder

Site of Lesion	Cause (Symptoms)	Diseases
Lesions above C2 involve pontine micturition center (UMN disorder)	Detrusor hyperreflexia (urgency and urine leakage)	Stroke, traumatic brain injury, multiple sclerosis (MS), hydrocephalus, cerebral palsy, Alzheimer disease, brain tumors
Lesions between C2 and S1 (UMN disorder)	Detrusor hyperreflexia with vesicosphincter dyssynergia (functional bladder outlet obstruction)	Spinal cord injury C2-T12, MS, transverse myelitis, Guillain-Barré syndrome, disk problems
Lesions below S1 (cauda equina syndrome) (LMN disorder)	Acontractile detrusor, with or without urethral sphincter incompetence (stress urinary incontinence)	Myelodysplasia, peripheral polyneuropathies, MS, tabes dorsalis, spinal injury T12-S1, cauda equina syndrome, herpes simplex/zoster

LMN, Lower motor neuron; *UMN,* upper motor neuron.

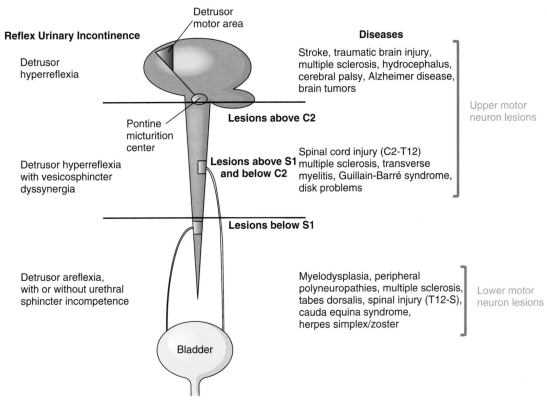

FIGURE 32.2 Sites of Neurologic Injury Associated with Neurogenic Bladder. (Adapted from Doughty DB, editor: *Urinary and fecal incontinence management concepts*, ed 3, Philadelphia, 2006, Mosby.)

A injection has shown temporary efficacy in reducing bladder outlet obstruction. Urinary sphincterotomy can be beneficial.[8]

Neurologic lesions involving the sacral micturition center (below S1, also termed *cauda equina syndrome*) or peripheral nerve lesions result in detrusor areflexia (acontractile detrusor, atonic bladder, or underactive bladder), a lower motor neuron disorder. The atonic bladder causes retention of urine and distention with stress and overflow incontinence. There is prolonged urination time with or without a sensation of incomplete bladder emptying, usually with hesitancy; reduced sensation on filling; and a slow stream. If the *sensory innervation* of the bladder is intact, the full bladder will be sensed but the detrusor may not contract. Myelodysplasia, multiple sclerosis, tabes dorsalis (deterioration of the posterior columns of the spinal cord associated with untreated syphilis), spinal cord injury, and peripheral polyneuropathies (i.e., diabetic neuropathy) are associated with this disorder.

Diagnosis includes disease history, clinical examination, urinalysis, and urodynamic studies (see Box 32.1). Bethanechol chloride (Urecholine) is a cholinergic agent (muscarinic agonist) that stimulates the bladder to empty and can be helpful in some cases. Intermittent catheterization or indwelling catheters are commonly required.[9]

Tumors
Kidney (Renal) Tumors
Kidney (Renal) Tumors Were Estimated at 73,820 (4.2%) of New Cancer Cases and 14,770 Deaths for 2019.[10] **Renal Cell Carcinoma (RCC)** (Also Known as **Renal Cell Adenocarcinoma**) Usually Occurs in Men (About Three Times More Often Than in Women) Between 50 and 60 Years of Age. Risk Factors Include Cigarette Smoking, Obesity, and Uncontrolled Hypertension. With Surgical Resection, 5-Year Survival Is About 93% for Stage I (Encapsulated) Cancer.

PATHOPHYSIOLOGY   There are a number of different types of RCCs. They are classified according to subtypes and extent of metastasis. *Clear cell RCC* is the most common renal neoplasm (85% of all renal neoplasms) and represents about 2% of cancer deaths.[10] It occurs primarily in the renal cortex. Other types include papillary and chromophobe RCC and both occur in the tubules of the kidneys.[11] Confinement within the renal capsule, together with treatment, is associated with a better survival rate. The tumors usually occur unilaterally (Fig. 32.3). Renal transitional cell carcinoma (RTCC) is rare and primarily arises in the renal parenchyma and renal pelvis near the ureteral orifice. Renal adenomas (benign tumors) are uncommon but are increasing in number. The tumors are encapsulated and are usually located near the cortex of the kidney. Because the tumors can become malignant, they are usually surgically removed.

CLINICAL MANIFESTATIONS   The classic clinical manifestations of renal tumors are hematuria, dull and aching flank pain, palpable flank mass, and weight loss, but all of these symptoms occur in fewer than 10% of cases. Further, they represent an advanced stage of disease, whereas earlier stages are often silent (painless hematuria). About 25% of individuals with RCC present with metastasis.[12] The most common sites of distant metastasis are the lung, lymph nodes, liver, bone, thyroid gland, and central nervous system.

EVALUATION AND TREATMENT   Diagnosis is based on the clinical symptoms and imaging procedures. The tumor, node, metastasis (TNM) classification is used to stage RCC. Staging systems using molecular

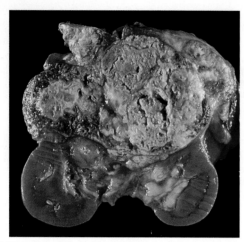

FIGURE 32.3 Renal Cell Carcinoma. Renal cell carcinomas usually are spheroidal masses composed of yellow tissue mottled with hemorrhage, necrosis, and fibrosis. (From Damjanov I, Linder J, editors: *Anderson's pathology*, ed 10, St Louis, 1996, Mosby.)

tumor markers are rapidly improving.[13] Treatment for localized disease is surgical removal of the affected kidney (radical nephrectomy) or partial nephrectomy for smaller tumors, with combined use of chemotherapeutic agents. Radiofrequency ablation also may be used for early stage tumors when surgery is not an option. Metastatic disease is treated with immunotherapy and targeted molecular therapies.[14] Survival is related to tumor grade, tumor cell type, and extent of metastasis.

Bladder Tumors

Bladder tumors represent about 4.5% of all malignant tumors with 80,470 new cases each year and 17,670 deaths.[10] The development of bladder cancer is most common in men older than 60 years. Smoking and exposure to occupational chemicals are the most common risk factors. *Transitional cell (urothelial) carcinoma* is the most common bladder malignancy, and tumors are usually superficial. More advanced tumors are muscle invasive. Less common forms are squamous cell and adenocarcinoma (cells that produce mucus).

PATHOPHYSIOLOGY The risk of primary bladder cancer is greater among people who smoke or are exposed to metabolites of aniline dyes, high levels of arsenic in drinking water, or heavy consumption of phenacetin or have uroepithelial schistosomiasis infection or a genetic predisposition. Metastasis is usually to lymph nodes, liver, bones, or lungs. The TNM classification is used for staging bladder carcinoma. Secondary bladder cancer develops by invasion of cancer from bordering organs, such as cervical carcinoma in women or prostatic carcinoma in men.

CLINICAL MANIFESTATIONS Gross painless hematuria is the archetypal clinical manifestation of bladder cancer. Episodes of hematuria tend to recur, and they are often accompanied by bothersome LUT symptoms including daytime voiding frequency, nocturia, urgency, and urge urinary incontinence, particularly for carcinoma in situ. Flank pain may occur if tumor growth obstructs one or both ureterovesical junctions.

EVALUATION AND TREATMENT Urine cytologic study (pathologic analysis of sloughed cells within the urine) is used for screening. Cystoscopy with tissue resection and biopsy is the first stage of treatment and confirms the diagnosis of bladder cancer. Use of biologic markers for bladder cancer diagnosis and treatment prognosis are available.[15] Transurethral resection or laser ablation, combined with intravesical

chemotherapy or immunotherapy, is effective for superficial tumors. Radical cystectomy (removal of the prostate and seminal vesicles in men and removal of the uterus, ovaries, and part of the vagina in women) with urinary diversion and adjuvant chemotherapy is required for locally invasive tumors.

> ✔**QUICK CHECK 32.2**
> 1. What are the symptoms of idiopathic overactive bladder syndrome?
> 2. What type of bladder dysfunction is associated with upper motor neuron lesions?
> 3. What are the common manifestations of renal tumors?
> 4. What are three risk factors for bladder cancer?

URINARY TRACT INFECTION

Causes of Urinary Tract Infection

A **urinary tract infection (UTI)** is an inflammation of the urinary epithelium (mucosa) usually caused by bacteria from gut flora. A UTI can occur anywhere along the urinary tract, including the urethra, prostate, bladder, ureter, or kidney (pyelonephritis). At risk are premature newborns; prepubertal children; sexually active and pregnant women; women treated with antibiotics that disrupt vaginal flora; spermicide users; estrogen-deficient postmenopausal women; individuals with indwelling catheters; and persons with diabetes mellitus, neurogenic bladder, or urinary tract obstruction. Cystitis is more common in women because of the shorter urethra and the closeness of the urethra to the anus (increasing the possibility of bacterial contamination). Up to 50% of women may have a lower UTI at some time in their life.[16]

Several factors normally combine to protect against UTIs. Most bacteria are washed out of the urethra during micturition. The low pH and high osmolality of urea, the presence of Tamm-Horsfall protein or uromodulin (secreted by renal tubular cells in the distal loop of Henle), and secretions from the uroepithelium provide a bactericidal effect. The ureterovesical junction closes during bladder contraction, preventing reflux of urine to the ureters and kidneys. Both the longer urethra and the presence of prostatic secretions decrease the risk of infection in men. A UTI occurs when a pathogen circumvents or overwhelms the host's defense mechanisms and rapidly reproduces.

Uncomplicated UTIs are mild and without complications and occur in individuals with a normal urinary tract. A *complicated UTI* develops when there is an abnormality in the urinary system or a health problem that compromises host defenses, such as human immunodeficiency virus (HIV), renal transplant, diabetes, or spinal cord injury. UTI may occur alone or in association with pyelonephritis, prostatitis, or kidney stones. Up to 30% of cases of septic shock are caused by urosepsis (a systemic response to an infection in the urogenital tract that can include symptoms of shock).[17] Factors associated with UTI include bacterial and human factors and are summarized in Fig. 32.4.

Types of Urinary Tract Infection
Cystitis

Cystitis is an inflammation of the bladder and is the most common site of UTI. The appearance of the bladder through a cystoscope describes the different types of cystitis:
1. *Mild cystitis* shows a hyperemic (red) mucosa.
2. *Hemorrhagic cystitis* shows diffuse mucosal hemorrhages and occurs with more advanced inflammation.
3. *Suppurative cystitis* shows mucosal pus formation or suppurative exudates.

Bacterial factors

Capsular antigens resist phagocytosis

Hemolysin damages epithelium

Urease positive bacteria promote infection i.e. *Proteus* and *Kebsiella*

Adhesins: *E. coli* type I and P fimbria bind to uroepithelium

Host factors

Kidney stones

Diabetes mellitus

Immunosuppression

Ureteral reflux

Pregnancy
Neurogenic bladder

P blood group antigens

Prostatic hypertrophy

Short urethra in women
Indwelling catheters

Escherchia coli... contamination from colon

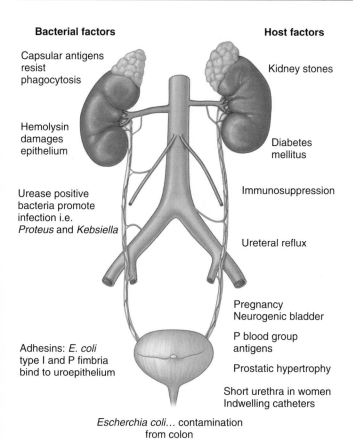

FIGURE 32.4 Mechanisms of Urinary Tract Infection.

4. *Ulcerative cystitis* results from prolonged infection with ulcers that may lead to sloughing of the mucosa.
5. *Gangrenous cystitis* is necrosis of the bladder wall and occurs with the most severe infections.

PATHOPHYSIOLOGY The most common infecting microorganisms are uropathic strains of *Escherichia coli,* and the second most common is *Staphylococcus saprophyticus.* Less common microorganisms include *Klebsiella, Proteus, Pseudomonas,* fungi, viruses, parasites, or tubercular bacilli. Schistosomiasis is the most common parasitic invasion of the urinary tract on a global basis and has a strong association with bladder cancer.[18] Bacterial contamination of the normally sterile urine usually occurs by retrograde (backward) movement of gastrointestinal gram-negative bacilli into the urethra and bladder from the opening of the urethra. The microorganisms can then move into the ureter and kidney. Uropathic strains of *E. coli* have *type-1 fimbriae* (also termed pili or finger-like projections) that bind to receptors on the uroepithelium. Consequently, they resist flushing during normal micturition. They also can bind to latex catheters used for urinary drainage. Some women may be genetically susceptible to certain strains of *E. coli* attachment. In these cases, women have P blood group antigen that binds to *P fimbriae* (pyelonephritis-associated fimbriae) of *E. coli* on the uroepithelium and they readily ascend the urinary tract (Fig. 32.5). Hematogenous (blood) infections are uncommon and often preceded by septicemia (bacterial infection of the blood). Infection initiates an inflammatory response and the symptoms of cystitis. The inflammatory edema in the bladder wall stimulates activation of stretch receptors. The activated stretch receptors initiate symptoms of bladder fullness with small volumes of urine, producing the urgency and frequency of urination associated with cystitis.

CLINICAL MANIFESTATIONS Clinical manifestations of cystitis are related to the inflammatory response and usually include frequency, urgency, dysuria (painful urination), and suprapubic and low back pain. Hematuria, cloudy urine, and flank pain are more serious symptoms. Many individuals with bacteriuria are asymptomatic, and the elderly have the highest risk and may have only confusion or vague abdominal discomfort. Individuals with asymptomatic bacteriuria require treatment if urine cultures are positive.[19]

EVALUATION AND TREATMENT Cystitis in symptomatic individuals is diagnosed by urine culture of specific microorganisms with counts of 10,000/ml or more from freshly voided urine. Urine dipstick testing that is positive for leukocyte esterase or nitrite reductase can be used for the diagnosis of uncomplicated UTI. Risk factors, such as urinary tract obstruction, should be identified and treated. Evidence of bacteria from urine culture and antibiotic sensitivity warrants treatment with a microorganism-specific antibiotic. Acute uncomplicated cystitis in nonpregnant women can be diagnosed without an office visit or urine culture. If a urine culture and sensitivity are ordered, the urine specimen must be obtained before the initiation of any antibiotic therapy; 3 to 7 days of treatment is most common.[20] Complicated UTI requires 7 to 14 days of treatment. Relapsing infection within 7 to 10 days requires prolonged antibiotic treatment. Follow-up urine cultures should be obtained 1 week after initiation of treatment and at monthly intervals for 3 months. Clinical symptoms are frequently relieved, but bacteriuria may still be present. Repeat cultures should be obtained every 3 to 4 months until 1 year after treatment for evaluation and treatment of recurrent infection. Guidelines are available for the treatment of complicated cystitis and for the prevention of catheter-associated cystitis (see *Did You Know?* Urinary Tract Infection and Antibiotic Resistance).

Painful Bladder Syndrome/Interstitial Cystitis

Interstitial cystitis/painful bladder syndrome (IC/PBS) is defined as an unpleasant sensation (pain, pressure, discomfort) perceived to be related to the urinary bladder associated with LUT symptoms of more than 6 weeks' duration in the absence of infection (sterile urine) or other identifiable causes.[21] It occurs most commonly in women ages 20 to 40 years of age.

The cause of IC/PBS is unknown. An autoimmune reaction may be responsible for the inflammatory response, which includes mast cell activation, altered uroepithelial permeability, and increased sensory nerve sensitivity. Inflammation and fibrosis of the bladder wall (uroepithelium) are accompanied by pain and the presence of hemorrhagic ulcers (Hunner ulcers). Bladder volume may decrease as a result of fibrosis. Alteration of the bladder uroepithelial proteoglycan layer (the layer that maintains impermeability of the bladder) makes it more susceptible to penetration by bacteria.

Characteristic symptoms of IC/PBS include bladder fullness, urinary frequency (including nocturia), small urine volume, and chronic pelvic pain with symptoms lasting longer than 6 weeks. Diagnosis of IC/PBS requires the exclusion of other diagnoses, and extensive evaluations are completed. No single treatment is effective. Oral and intravesical therapies, sacral nerve stimulation, and onabotulinumtoxinA (Botox) are used for symptom relief. Surgery is used in refractory cases.[22]

Acute Pyelonephritis

Pyelonephritis is an infection of one or both upper urinary tracts (ureter, renal pelvis, and kidney interstitium). Common causes are summarized in Table 32.3. Urinary obstruction and reflux of urine from the bladder (vesicoureteral reflux) are the most common underlying risk factors. One or both kidneys may be involved. Most cases occur in women.

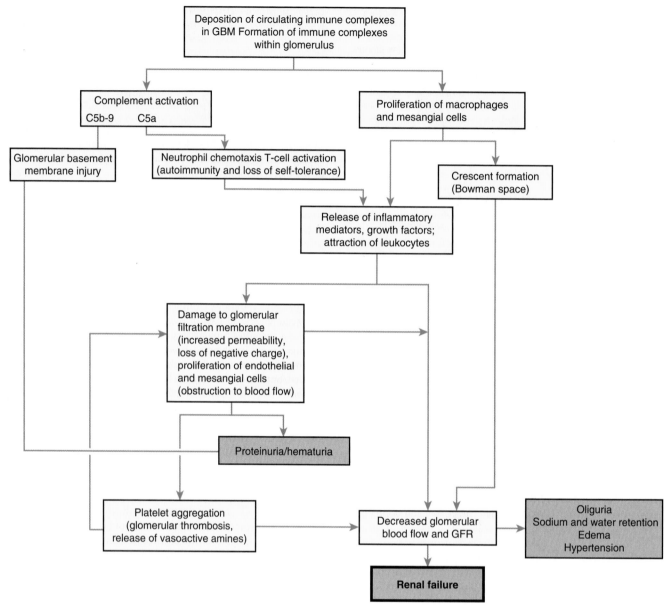

FIGURE 32.5 Mechanisms of Glomerular Injury. *Ab,* Antibody; *GBM,* glomerular basement membrane; *GFR,* glomerular filtration rate; *NO,* nitric oxide.

PATHOPHYSIOLOGY Microorganisms usually associated with acute pyelonephritis include *E. coli, Proteus,* or *Pseudomonas.* The latter two microorganisms are more commonly associated with infections after urethral instrumentation or urinary tract surgery. These microorganisms also split urea into ammonia, making an alkaline urine that increases the risk of stone formation. The infection is probably spread by ascending uropathic microorganisms along the ureters. Dissemination also may occur by way of the bloodstream. The inflammatory process primarily affects the pelvis, calyces, and medulla of the kidney. The infection causes infiltration of white blood cells with renal inflammation, renal edema, and purulent urine. In severe infections, localized abscesses may form in the medulla and extend to the cortex. Primarily affected are the tubules. The glomeruli usually are spared. Necrosis of renal papillae can develop. After the acute phase, healing occurs with fibrosis and atrophy of affected tubules. The number of bacteria decreases until the urine again becomes sterile. Acute pyelonephritis rarely causes renal failure.

CLINICAL MANIFESTATIONS The onset of symptoms is usually acute, with fever, chills, and flank or groin pain. Symptoms characteristic of a UTI, including frequency, dysuria, and costovertebral tenderness, may precede systemic signs and symptoms. Older adults may have nonspecific symptoms, such as low-grade fever and malaise.

EVALUATION AND TREATMENT Differentiating symptoms of cystitis from those of pyelonephritis by clinical assessment alone is difficult. The specific diagnosis is established by urine culture, urinalysis, and clinical signs and symptoms. White blood cell casts formed in the renal tubules and flushed into the urine indicate pyelonephritis. However, they are not always present in the urine. Complicated pyelonephritis requires blood cultures and urinary tract imaging.[23] Uncomplicated acute pyelonephritis responds well to 2 to 3 weeks of microorganism-specific antibiotic therapy. Follow-up urine cultures are obtained at 1 and 4 weeks after treatment if symptoms recur. Antibiotic-resistant

Urinary Tract Infection and Antibiotic Resistance

Uncomplicated urinary tract infection (UTI) is one of the most common bacterial infections. Worldwide, emergence of bacterial strains resistant to specific antibiotics in both hospital- and community-acquired UTIs is causing increased cost, hospitalization, morbidity, and mortality. The resistance is caused in part by overuse of antibiotics. Risks for resistance are highest in regions with the highest rates of prescription and in those who have received trimethoprim-sulfamethoxazole (TMP-SMX) treatment within the last 3 months, have a diagnosis of diabetes mellitus, have been recently hospitalized, and have community-specific antibiotic resistance rates of greater than 20%. The leading cause of UTI is uropathogenic *Escherichia coli (E. coli),* followed by *Klebsiella* and *Proteus,* and antibiotics are the mainstay of treatment. These bacteria and other gram-negative species produce β-lactamases and carbapenemases, causing resistance to penicillins, cephalosporins, and carbapenems (used for complicated UTI). TMP-SMX and fluoroquinolone have a high rate of resistance. Multidrug-resistant extended-spectrum β-lactamase (ESBL)–producing *E. coli* are occurring with no known risk factors. First-time uncomplicated lower UTI can be treated empirically with a 1- to 5-day regimen of nitrofurantoin, TMP-SMX, pivmecillinam, or a single dose of fosfomycin. Recurrent and complicated infection requires individualized assessment of risk factors for drug resistance and drug tolerability and includes history, physical examination, urine culture and sensitivity, and possible imaging evaluation. Asymptomatic bacteriuria requires treatment only in exceptional cases. The Agency for Healthcare Research and Quality has a tool-kit for reducing catheter-associated UTI in hospitals. Awareness of drug resistance and knowledgeable prescribing are essential to prevent inappropriate use of antibiotics. New drugs are being discovered that overcome bacterial resistance, and old drugs in new combinations are being tested.

Data from Agency for Healthcare Research and Quality (AHRQ): *Toolkit for reducing CAUTI in hospitals,* 2015, Agency for Healthcare Research and Quality, Rockville, MD, available at https://www.ahrq.gov/sites/default/files/publications/files/implementation-guide_0.pdf; Millner R, Becknell B: *Pediatr Clin North Am* 66(1):1-13, 2019; Grabe MJ, Resman F: *Eur Urol Focus* 5(1):46-49, 2019; Waller TA et al: *Prim Care.* 45(3):455-466, 2018.

TABLE 32.3 Common Causes of Pyelonephritis

Predisposing Factor	Pathologic Mechanisms
Kidney stones	Obstruction and stasis of urine contributing to bacteriuria and hydronephrosis; irritation of epithelial lining with entrapment of bacteria
Vesicoureteral reflux	Chronic reflux of urine up the ureter and into kidney during micturition, contributing to bacterial infection
Pregnancy	Dilation and relaxation of ureter with hydroureter and hydronephrosis; partly caused by obstruction from enlarged uterus and partly from ureteral relaxation caused by higher progesterone levels
Neurogenic bladder	Neurologic impairment interfering with normal bladder contraction with residual urine and ascending infection
Instrumentation	Introduction of organisms into urethra and bladder by catheters and endoscopes introduced into urinary tract for diagnostic purposes
Female sexual trauma	Movement of organisms from urethra into bladder with infection and retrograde spread to kidney

CLINICAL MANIFESTATIONS The early symptoms of chronic pyelonephritis are often minimal and may include hypertension, frequency, dysuria, and flank pain. Progression can lead to kidney failure, particularly in the presence of obstructive uropathy or diabetes mellitus.

EVALUATION AND TREATMENT Urinalysis, intravenous pyelography, and ultrasound are used diagnostically. Treatment is related to the underlying cause. Obstruction must be relieved. Antibiotics may be given, with prolonged antibiotic therapy for recurrent infection.

✔ QUICK CHECK 32.3
1. Why is cystitis more common in women?
2. What causes the urgency associated with cystitis?
3. What is interstitial cystitis/painful bladder syndrome?
4. How does pyelonephritis differ from cystitis?

microorganisms or reinfection may occur in cases of urinary tract obstruction or reflux. Intravenous pyelography and voiding cystourethrography identify surgically correctable lesions.

Chronic Pyelonephritis

Chronic pyelonephritis is a persistent or recurrent infection of the kidney leading to scarring of the kidney. One or both kidneys may be involved. The specific cause of chronic pyelonephritis may be unknown (idiopathic) or associated with chronic UTIs, vesicoureteral reflux, or kidney stone obstructive uropathy. Other causes include drug toxicity from analgesics, such as nonsteroidal antiinflammatory drugs, ischemia, irradiation, and immune-complex diseases

PATHOPHYSIOLOGY Chronic urinary tract obstruction prevents elimination of bacteria and starts a process of progressive inflammation. There is destruction of the tubules and diffuse scarring, with impaired urine-concentrating ability. The lesions of chronic pyelonephritis are sometimes termed *chronic interstitial nephritis* because the inflammation and fibrosis are located in the interstitial spaces between the tubules.

GLOMERULAR DISORDERS

Glomerulonephritis

Acute glomerulonephritis is an inflammation of the glomerulus caused by *primary glomerular injury* and is isolated to the kidney. *Secondary glomerular injury* is a glomerular injury that occurs as a consequence of systemic diseases, including diabetes mellitus, hypertension, bacterial toxins, systemic lupus erythematosus, congestive heart failure, and HIV-related kidney disease.

PATHOPHYSIOLOGY Immune mechanisms are a major component of both primary and secondary glomerular injury and will be the focus here (see Fig. 32.5). The injury damages the glomerular capillary filtration membrane. The most common type of immune injury is related to the presence of antigen-antibody complexes within the glomerulus.

Immune injury is caused by activation of the inflammatory response (i.e., complement activation, leukocyte recruitment, and release of cytokines from leukocytes). Injury begins after the antigen-antibody complexes have deposited or formed in the glomerulus. Complement is deposited with the antibodies, and complement activation can cause cell injury or serve as a chemotactic stimulus for attraction of leukocytes (neutrophils, monocytes, and T lymphocytes). These phagocytes, along with activated platelets, further the inflammatory reaction by releasing cytokines that injure the glomerular filtration membrane. The injury increases glomerular filtration membrane permeability and reduces glomerular membrane surface area.

There also may be swelling and proliferation of mesangial cells and expansion of the extracellular matrix in the Bowman space. The deposition of these substances and cell proliferation form a crescent shape within the Bowman space that can be seen under a microscope and assist with diagnosis if a biopsy is performed. The result of these processes is compression of glomerular capillaries, decreased glomerular blood flow, hypoxic injury, decreased driving glomerular hydrostatic pressure, alteration in the filtration membrane, and decreased GFR.

Loss of the normal negative electrical charge across the glomerular filtration membrane and increase in filtration pore size enhance movement of proteins into the urine. Proteins are normally repelled because they also have a negative charge and thus are not filtered into the urine. Red blood cells also escape if pore size is large enough. Consequently proteinuria or hematuria, or both, develops. The severity of glomerular damage and decline in glomerular function is related to the duration of exposure of antigen-antibody complexes formed and the size, number, and location (i.e., focal [affecting some glomeruli] or diffuse [affecting glomeruli throughout the kidney]) of cells injured and lesion characteristics (Table 32.4).

CLINICAL MANIFESTATIONS The onset of glomerulonephritis may be sudden or gradual, and significant loss of nephron function can occur before symptoms develop. Acute glomerulonephritis may be silent, mild, moderate, or severe in symptom presentation. Severe or progressive glomerular disease causes oliguria (urine output of 30 ml/hr or less), hypertension, and renal failure. Focal lesions tend to produce less severe clinical symptoms. Salt and water are reabsorbed, contributing to fluid volume expansion, edema, and hypertension.

Two major symptoms distinctive of more severe glomerulonephritis (i.e., associated with rapidly progressive glomerulonephritis) are (1) hematuria with red blood cell casts (the red blood cells accumulate in the kidney tubules and are washed into the urine in the form of a cast of the tubule) and (2) proteinuria exceeding 3 to 5 g/day with albumin (macroalbuminuria) as the major protein. Different types of acute glomerulonephritis may be associated with different patterns of urinary sediment (i.e., presence of various cells, casts, crystals, and microbes) and nephrotic or nephritic syndrome (see the Nephrotic and Nephritic Syndromes section).

EVALUATION AND TREATMENT The diagnosis of glomerular disease is confirmed by the progressive development of clinical manifestations and laboratory findings. There is an abnormal urinalysis with proteinuria, red blood cells, white blood cells, and casts in the urine. Microscopic evaluation from renal biopsy can provide a specific determination of renal injury and the type of pathologic lesion (i.e., the formation of glomerular crescents as previously described and location and character of glomerular lesions.) Patterns of antigen-antibody complex deposition within the glomerular capillary filtration membrane have been established using light, electron, and immunofluorescent microscopy for different disease processes. The findings with microscopy provide information about the distribution and extent of immune response

TABLE 32.4 Types of Glomerular Lesions

Lesion	Characteristics
Glomerular Lesions	
Diffuse	Relatively uniform involvement of most or all glomeruli; most common form of glomerulonephritis
Focal	Changes in only some glomeruli, whereas others are normal
Segmental-local	Changes in one part of glomerulus with other parts unaffected
Lesion Characteristics	
Mesangial	Deposits of immunoglobulins in mesangial matrix, mesangial cell proliferation
Membranous	Thickening of glomerular capillary wall with immune deposits
Proliferative	Increase in number of glomerular cells
Sclerotic	Glomerular scarring from previous glomerular injury
Crescentic	Accumulation of proliferating cells within Bowman space, making crescent appearance
Interstitial fibrosis	Scarring between glomerulus and tubules

injury and guide therapy. Some examples of mechanisms of immune injury are summarized in Table 32.5.

Reduced GFR during glomerulonephritis is evidenced by elevated plasma urea, cystatin C, and creatinine concentrations, or by reduced creatinine clearance (see Tests of Renal Function in Chapter 31). Edema, caused by excessive sodium and water retention and or loss of plasma proteins (see Chapter 5 for the pathophysiology of edema), may require the use of diuretics or dialysis.

Management principles for treating glomerulonephritis are related to treating the primary disease, preventing or minimizing immune responses, and correcting accompanying problems. Accompanying problems include edema, hypertension, hypoalbuminemia, and hyperlipidemia. Specific treatment regimens are necessary for particular types of glomerulonephritis. Antibiotic therapy is essential for the management of underlying infections that may be contributing to ongoing antigen-antibody responses. Corticosteroids decrease antibody synthesis and suppress inflammatory responses. Cytotoxic agents (e.g., cyclophosphamide) may be used to suppress the immune response in corticosteroid-resistant cases. Anticoagulants may be useful for controlling fibrin crescent formation in rapidly progressive glomerulonephritis.

Types of Glomerulonephritis

The classification of glomerulonephritis can be described according to cause, pathologic lesions (see Table 32.4), disease progression (acute, rapidly progressive, chronic), or clinical presentation (nephrotic syndrome, nephritic syndrome, acute or chronic renal failure). In nearly all types of glomerulonephritis, the epithelial or podocyte layer of the glomerular capillary membrane is disturbed with loss of negative charges and changes in membrane permeability. Plasma proteins (albumin) and red blood cells can escape into the urine and can cause proteinuria and/ or hematuria. The mesangial matrix may be expanded or the basement membrane thickened decreasing blood flow through the glomerular capillaries and decreasing GFR. Features of the patterns of glomerular injury are summarized in Table 32.6. Many types of glomerular injury occur most often in children or young adults, including acute postinfectious glomerulonephritis and minimal change nephropathy (lipoid nephrosis). Details of these diseases are presented in Chapter 33.

TABLE 32.5   Immunologic Mechanisms of Glomerular Injury

Glomerular Injury	Mechanism
Soluble immune-complex glomerulonephritis (90%)	Formation of antibodies stimulated by presence of endogenous or exogenous antigens; results in circulating soluble antigen-antibody complexes deposited in glomerular capillaries or formation of complexes within the glomerular membrane; glomerular injury occurs with complement activation and release of immunologic substances that lyse cells and increase membrane permeability; severity of glomerular injury related to number of complexes formed; type III hypersensitivity reaction
Anti–glomerular basement membrane glomerulonephritis (5%)	Antibodies are formed and act directly against glomerular basement membrane; immune response causes accumulation of inflammatory cells in Bowman space (in shape of a crescent moon) surrounding and compressing glomerular capillaries; generally associated with rapidly progressive renal failure, such as Goodpasture syndrome (a rare disease in which antibodies attack basement membranes in glomeruli and lung alveoli); type II hypersensitivity reaction
Alternative complement pathway	Relatively rare mechanism associated with low levels of complement and membranoproliferative glomerulonephritis; type III hypersensitivity reaction
Cell-mediated immunity	Delayed hypersensitivity response with activation or suppression of T-cell subsets resulting in glomerular damage; type IV hypersensitivity reaction

TABLE 32.6   Features of the Common Types of Glomerulonephritis

Type and Cause	Pathophysiology
Associated With Nephritic Syndrome	
Acute postinfectious/infection-related glomerulonephritis (group A β-hemolytic streptococcus or staphylococcus) Occurs with untreated primary infection in throat or skin	Diffuse deposits of immune complexes (IgG and complement) in glomerular capillary wall; infiltration of leukocytes; endocapillary proliferation and mesangial proliferation Decreased capillary blood flow and GFR
Crescentic or rapidly progressive glomerulonephritis In situ formation of anti–glomerular basement membrane antibodies or immune complex deposition Nonspecific response to glomerular injury; can occur in any severe glomerular disease Can be associated with Goodpasture syndrome	Accumulation of immune deposits and inflammatory cells and debris that proliferate into Bowman space and form crescent-shaped lesions Decreased capillary blood flow and GFR Can result in renal failure within 3 months Formation of Ab against both pulmonary capillary and GBM
Mesangial proliferative glomerulonephritis IgA nephropathy	Deposits of immune complexes in mesangium with mesangial proliferation Decreased glomerular blood flow and GFR Abnormal glycosylated IgA-1 and complement bind to mesangial cells causing proliferation
Associated With Nephrotic Syndrome	
Minimal change disease (lipoid nephrosis) Glomerular basement membrane appears normal Usually idiopathic No immune deposits	Uniform diffuse thinning of epithelial (podocyte) foot processes; loss of negative charge in basement membrane and increased permeability Severe proteinuria and nephrotic syndrome
Focal segmented glomerulosclerosis Usually idiopathic	Similar to minimal change disease
Membranous nephropathy (autoimmune response to unknown renal antigen) Usually idiopathic Can be associated with systemic diseases (i.e., hepatitis B virus, systemic lupus erythematous, solid malignant tumors)	Thickening of glomerular capillary wall caused by antibody and complement deposition and release of inflammatory cytokines with focal segmental sclerosis and increased permeability, proteinuria, and nephrotic syndrome
Membranoproliferative glomerulonephritis Usually idiopathic; associated with low complement levels	Mesangial cell proliferation; thickening of basement membrane; subendothelial deposits of immune complex occlude glomerular capillary blood flow Decreased GFR
IgA nephropathy (Berger disease) Usually idiopathic; elevated IgA plasma levels	Mesangial deposits of IgA and proliferation of inflammatory cells into Bowman space, with sclerosis and fibrosis of glomerulus and crescent formation Decreased GFR and hematuria; usually focal, some diffuse lesions
Chronic glomerulonephritis Can be a consequence of any type of glomerulonephritis; more common with crescentic or rapidly progressive glomerulonephritis	Glomerular fibrosis and scarring, interstitial and tubular fibrosis and vascular sclerosis; original glomerular lesions may not be definable; progression to end-stage kidney disease with uremia

Ab, Antibody; *GBM*, glomerular basement membrane; *GFR*, glomerular filtration rate; *IgA*, immunoglobulin A; *IgG*, immunoglobulin G.

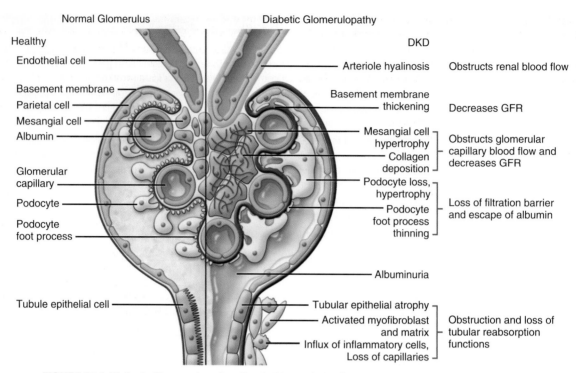

FIGURE 32.6 Diabetic Glomerulopathy. (Used with permission from Reidy K et al: *J Clin Invest* 124[6]:2333-2340, 2014.)

Complications of systemic diseases, such as diabetic nephropathy and systemic lupus erythematosus, can affect the entire nephron with significant glomerular injury. Different patterns of injury develop over the course of these diseases. Diabetic nephropathy develops from metabolic and vascular complications related to chronic hyperglycemia (see Chapter 20). Changes in the glomerulus are characterized by progressive thickening and fibrosis of the glomerular basement membrane, and expansion of the mesangial matrix with albuminuria, injury and loss of podocytes and tubular epithelial cells, and progression to chronic renal failure (CRF) (Fig. 32.6). Diabetic nephropathy is the most common cause of chronic kidney disease (CKD) and end-stage renal failure. Glomerular structure and function can return to normal after pancreatic transplantation and years of normoglycemia.[24] Lupus nephritis is caused by glomerular deposition of immune complexes and alteration in B cell and T cell lymphocytes. There is complement activation and a cascade of inflammatory events resulting in damage to the glomerular membrane with mesangial expansion, which can ultimately decrease glomerular filtration and blood flow and lead to renal failure.[25]

Chronic Glomerulonephritis

Chronic glomerulonephritis encompasses several glomerular diseases with a progressive course leading to chronic kidney failure. There may be no history of kidney disease before the diagnosis. Hypercholesterolemia and proteinuria have been associated with progressive glomerular and tubular injury. The proposed mechanism is related to those observed in glomerulosclerosis and interstitial injury, such as inflammatory processes and glomerular hyperfiltration. The primary cause may be difficult to establish because advanced pathologic changes may obscure specific disease characteristics. Diabetes mellitus and lupus erythematosus are examples of secondary causes of chronic glomerular injury. Renal insufficiency usually begins to develop after 10 to 20 years of disease, followed by nephrotic syndrome (see next section) and an accelerated

progression to end-stage renal failure. Symptom patterns vary depending on the underlying cause and the areas of the kidney that are damaged. The specific pathologic changes are identified by renal biopsy, which is best performed in early stages of CKD to identify specific treatment options. Management of the underlying disease and use of steroids and immunosuppressive agents can prolong remissions and preserve renal function. Dialysis or kidney transplantation ultimately may be needed.

Nephrotic and Nephritic Syndromes

Nephrotic and nephritic syndromes are consequences of glomerular injury and present with a pattern of clinical manifestations. Nephrotic syndrome is the excretion of 3.5 g or more of protein in the urine per day. It occurs when glomerular filtration of plasma proteins, particularly albumin, exceeds tubular reabsorption. Nephrotic syndrome is more common in children than adults[26] (see Chapter 33). *Primary causes of nephrotic syndrome* include particular types of glomerular injury including minimal change nephropathy (lipoid nephrosis) (see Chapter 33), membranous glomerulonephritis, and focal segmental glomerulosclerosis (see Table 32.6). *Secondary forms of nephrotic syndrome* occur in systemic diseases, including diabetes mellitus (see Chapter 20), amyloidosis, systemic lupus erythematosus (see Chapter 8), and Henoch-Schönlein purpura (see Chapter 33). Nephrotic syndrome also is associated with certain drugs (e.g., nonsteroidal antiinflammatory drugs [NSAIDs]), infections, malignancies, and vascular disorders.

Nephritic syndrome is hematuria and red blood cell casts in the urine. Proteinuria also is present and is usually less severe than in nephrotic syndrome. It occurs primarily with infection-related glomerulonephritis and rapidly progressive crescentic glomerulonephritis.

PATHOPHYSIOLOGY In nephrotic syndrome, injury to the glomerular filtration membrane leads to increased permeability and loss of an electrical negative charge. Normally, plasma proteins, which carry a negative charge, are repelled by the negative charge at the glomerular filtration membrane and thus remain in the plasma. Movement of plasma proteins, particularly albumin and some immunoglobulins, occurs across the injured membrane. The plasma proteins are then lost into the urine, resulting in decreased plasma oncotic pressure and edema (Fig. 32.7). Hypoalbuminemia results from urinary loss of albumin combined with a diminished synthesis of replacement albumin by the liver. Albumin is lost in the greatest quantity because of its high plasma concentration and low molecular weight. Decreased dietary intake of protein from anorexia or malnutrition or accompanying liver disease may also contribute to lower levels of plasma albumin. Loss of albumin stimulates lipoprotein synthesis by the liver and hyperlipidemia and can promote progression of glomerular disease. Loss of immunoglobulins may increase susceptibility to infections. Sodium retention is common, further contributing to edema and hypertension.

In nephritic syndrome, hematuria (usually microscopic) is present and red blood cell casts are present in the urine in addition to proteinuria, which is not severe. It is caused by increased permeability of the glomerular filtration membrane with pore sizes large enough to allow the passage of red blood cells and protein. Nephritic syndrome is associated with postinfectious glomerulonephritis, rapidly progressive (crescentic) glomerulonephritis, immunoglobulin A (IgA) nephropathy, lupus nephritis, and diabetic nephropathy. The pathophysiology is related to immune injury of the glomerulus as previously described. Hypertension and uremia (accumulation of urea and other nitrogen-based metabolic products) occur in advanced stages of disease.

CLINICAL MANIFESTATIONS Many clinical manifestations of nephrotic and nephritic syndrome are related to loss of serum proteins and associated sodium retention (Table 32.7). The manifestations of both nephrotic and nephritic syndrome include edema, hypoproteinemia, proteinuria, hyperlipidemia, lipiduria, vitamin D deficiency, and hypothyroidism. In addition, hematuria is associated with nephritic syndrome. Vitamin D deficiency is related to loss of serum transport proteins and decreased vitamin D activation by the kidney. Hypothyroidism can result from urinary loss of thyroid-binding protein and thyroxine. Alterations in coagulation factors can cause hypercoagulability and may lead to thromboembolic events.

EVALUATION AND TREATMENT Nephrotic syndrome is diagnosed when the protein level in a 24-hour urine collection is greater than 3.5 g. Serum albumin level decreases (to <3 g/dl), and concentrations of serum cholesterol, phospholipids, and triglycerides increase. Fat bodies may be present in the urine.

Nephrotic syndrome is commonly treated by consuming a moderate protein restriction (i.e., 0.8 g/kg body weight/day), low-fat, salt-restricted diet, and by prescribing diuretics. Diuretics are used to control hypertension and eliminate fluid. Care must be taken to observe for hypovolemia and hypokalemia or potassium toxicity in the presence of renal insufficiency. Spironolactone may be combined with loop diuretics to suppress aldosterone activity to conserve potassium. Anticoagulants are used for prophylactic anticoagulation. Glucocorticoids are used to control immune-mediated disease or may be combined with immunosuppressive drugs. Angiotensin-converting enzyme (ACE) inhibitors or angiotensin receptor blockers (ARBs) lower urine protein excretion.

The evaluation and treatment of nephritic syndrome are similar to those described for nephrotic syndrome. Red blood cells and red blood cell casts will be found in the urine. The course of glomerulonephritis is usually more severe with nephritic syndrome. High-dose corticosteroids and cyclophosphamide represent the standard therapy for rapidly progressive crescentic glomerulonephritis. The addition of plasma exchange (plasmapheresis) also may be helpful. Dialysis may be required.

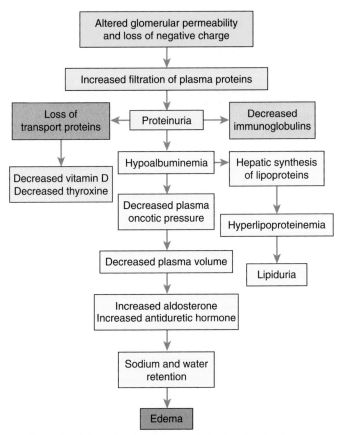

FIGURE 32.7 Pathophysiology of Nephrotic Syndrome.

TABLE 32.7 Clinical Manifestations of Nephrotic Syndrome

Manifestation	Contributing Factors	Result
Significant proteinuria	Increased glomerular permeability, decreased proximal tubule reabsorption	Edema, increased susceptibility to infection from loss of immunoglobulins
Hypoalbuminemia	Increased urinary losses of protein	Edema
Edema	Hypoalbuminemia (decreased plasma oncotic pressure, sodium and water retention, increased aldosterone and antidiuretic hormone [ADH] secretion), unresponsiveness to atrial natriuretic peptides	Soft, pitting, generalized edema
Hyperlipidemia	Decreased serum albumin level; increased hepatic synthesis of very-low-density lipoproteins; increased levels of cholesterol, phospholipids, triglycerides	Increased atherogenesis
Lipiduria	Sloughing of tubular cells containing fat (oval fat bodies); free fat from hyperlipidemia	Fat droplets that may float in urine

ACUTE KIDNEY INJURY

Classification of Kidney Dysfunction

Kidney injury may be acute and rapidly progressive (within hours). The process may be reversible. Kidney failure also can be chronic, progressing to end-stage kidney failure over a period of months or years. The terms *renal insufficiency, renal failure, uremia,* and *azotemia* are associated with decreasing kidney function but are not specific in relation to the cause of kidney disease. They are often used synonymously, although with some distinctions. Generally, renal insufficiency refers to a decline in renal function to about 25% of normal or a GFR of 25 to 30 ml/min. Levels of serum creatinine and urea are mildly elevated. The term *acute kidney injury* is preferred to the term *acute renal failure* because it captures the diverse nature of this syndrome, ranging from minimal or subtle changes in kidney function to complete kidney failure requiring renal replacement therapy. Kidney failure refers to significant loss of renal function. When less than 10% of kidney function remains, this is termed end-stage kidney disease (ESKD). Specific criteria for acute kidney dysfunction are discussed in the next section. Uremia (uremic syndrome) is a syndrome of renal failure and includes elevated blood urea and creatinine levels accompanied by fatigue, anorexia, nausea, vomiting, pruritus, and neurologic changes. Uremia represents numerous consequences related to kidney failure, including retention of toxic wastes, deficiency states, electrolyte disorders, and immune activation promoting a proinflammatory state. Azotemia is characterized by increased blood urea nitrogen (BUN) levels (normal is 8 to 20 mg/dl) and frequently increased serum creatinine levels (normal is 0.7 to 1.4 mg/dl). Renal insufficiency or kidney failure causes azotemia. Both azotemia and uremia indicate an accumulation of nitrogenous waste products in the blood, a common characteristic that explains the overlap in definitions of terms.

Acute Kidney Injury

Acute kidney injury (AKI) is a sudden decline in kidney function with a decrease in glomerular filtration and urine output with accumulation of nitrogenous waste products in the blood as demonstrated by an elevation in plasma creatinine and BUN levels. Classification criteria have been developed to guide the diagnosis of kidney injury and are described by the acronym RIFLE (*R* = risk, *I* = injury, *F* = failure, *L* = loss, and *E* = end-stage kidney disease [ESKD]), representing three levels of kidney dysfunction of increasing severity (Table 32.8). A similar set of criteria have been published by the Acute Kidney Injury Network and Kidney Disease Improving Global Outcomes.[27]

PATHOPHYSIOLOGY AKI results from ischemic injury related to extracellular volume depletion and decreased renal blood flow (perfusion), toxic injury from chemicals, or sepsis-induced injury. The injury initiates an inflammatory response, vascular responses, and cell death. Alterations in kidney function may be minimal or severe.[28] AKI can be classified as prerenal (renal hypoperfusion), intrarenal (disorders involving renal parenchymal or interstitial tissue), or postrenal (urinary tract obstructive disorders) (Table 32.9 and Fig. 32.8).

Prerenal acute kidney injury is the most common reason for AKI and is caused by inadequate kidney perfusion. Poor perfusion can result

TABLE 32.8 RIFLE Criteria for Acute Kidney Dysfunction/Failure

Category	GFR Criteria	Urine Output (UO) Criteria
Risk	Increased creatinine × 1.5 or GFR decrease >25%	UO <0.5 ml/kg/hr × 6 hr
Injury	Increased creatinine × 2 or GFR decrease >50%	UO <0.5 ml/kg/hr × 12 hr
Failure	Increased creatinine × 3 or GFR decrease >75%	UO <0.3 ml/kg/hr × 24 hr or anuria × 12 hr
Loss	Persistent ARF = complete loss of kidney function >4 weeks	
ESKD	End-stage kidney disease (>3 months)	

Adapted from Bellomo R et al: *Curr Opin Crit Care* 8(6):505-508, 2002; Bellomo R et al: *Crit Care* 8(4):R204-R212, 2004. *GFR,* glomerular filtration rate; *ARF,* acute renal failure; *ESKD,* end-stage kidney disease

TABLE 32.9 Classification of Acute Kidney Injury

Area of Dysfunction	Possible Causes

Prerenal	Hypovolemia
	  Hemorrhagic blood loss (trauma, gastrointestinal bleeding, complications of childbirth)
	  Loss of plasma volume (burns, peritonitis)
	  Water and electrolyte losses (severe vomiting or diarrhea, intestinal obstruction, uncontrolled diabetes mellitus, inappropriate use of diuretics)
	Hypotension or hypoperfusion
	  Septic shock
	  Cardiac failure or shock
	  Massive pulmonary embolism
	  Stenosis or clamping of renal artery

Intrarenal	Acute tubular necrosis (postischemic or nephrotoxic)
	  Glomerulopathies
	  Acute interstitial necrosis (tumors or toxins)
	  Vascular damage
	  Malignant hypertension, vasculitis
	  Coagulation defects
	  Renal artery/vein occlusion
	  Bilateral acute pyelonephritis

Postrenal	Obstructive uropathies (usually bilateral)
	  Ureteral destruction (edema, tumors, stones, clots)
	  Bladder neck obstruction (enlarged prostate)
	  Neurogenic bladder

from hypotension, hypovolemia associated with hemorrhage or fluid loss (e.g., burns), sepsis, inadequate cardiac output (e.g., myocardial infarct [heart attack]), or renal vasoconstriction (e.g., caused by NSAIDs or radiocontrast agents) or renal artery stenosis. The GFR declines because of the decrease in glomerular filtration pressure. Failure to restore blood volume or blood pressure and oxygen delivery can cause ischemic cell injury and acute tubular necrosis or acute interstitial necrosis, a more severe form of AKI. Reperfusion injury with cell death

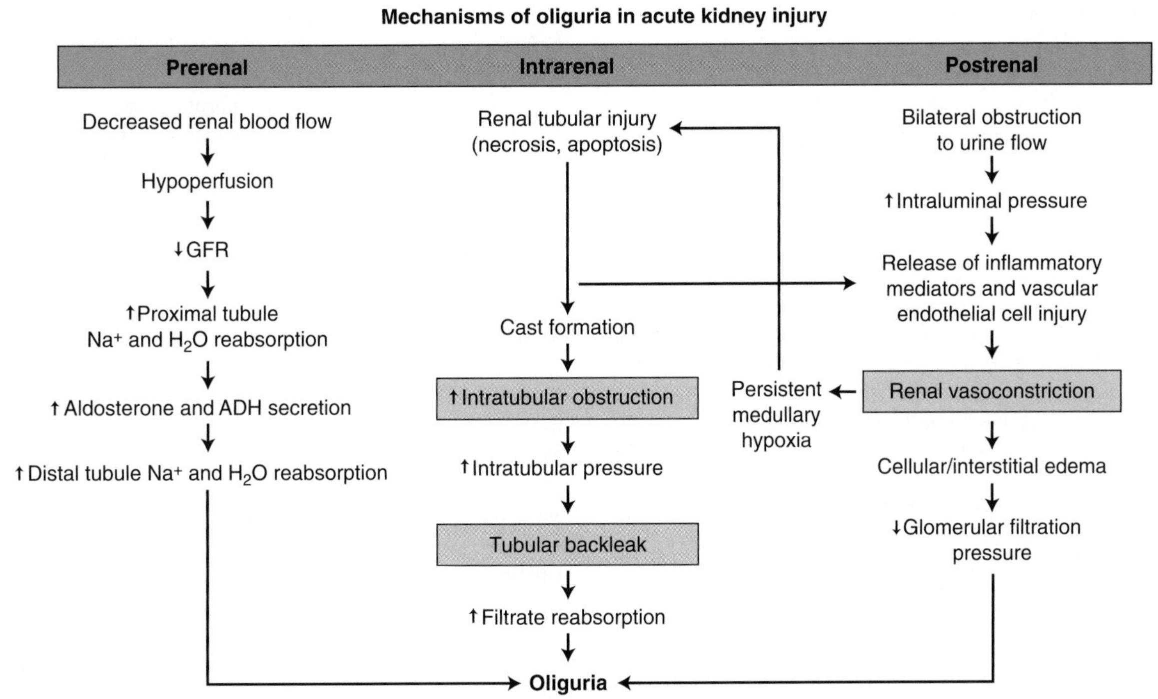

Mechanisms of oliguria in acute kidney injury

FIGURE 32.8 Acute Kidney Injury and Mechanisms of Oliguria. *ADH,* Antidiuretic hormone; *GFR,* glomerular filtration rate.

also can occur (see Fig. 4.10). AKI can occur during CRF if a sudden stress is imposed on already poorly functioning kidneys.

Intrarenal (intrinsic) acute kidney injury can result from ischemic **acute tubular necrosis (ATN)** related to prerenal AKI, nephrotoxic ATN, acute glomerulonephritis, vascular disease (malignant hypertension, disseminated intravascular coagulation, and renal vasculitis), allograft rejection, or interstitial disease (drug allergy, infection, tumor growth). ATN caused by ischemia occurs most often after surgery (40% to 50% of cases) but also is associated with sepsis, obstetric complications, and severe hemorrhagic trauma or severe burns. Hypotension associated with hypovolemia produces ischemia and the inflammatory response, generating toxic oxygen free radicals that cause cellular swelling, injury, and necrosis. Intrarenal microcirculatory vasoconstriction occurs in response to injury and inflammation and decreases blood flow. Ischemic necrosis results and tends to be patchy and may be distributed along any part of the nephron.

Nephrotoxic ATN can be produced by radiocontrast media and numerous antibiotics, particularly the aminoglycosides (neomycin, gentamicin, tobramycin) because these drugs accumulate in the renal cortex. Other substances, such as excessive myoglobin (oxygen-transporting substance from muscles released with crush injuries), carbon tetrachloride, heavy metals (mercury, arsenic), or methoxyflurane anesthetic, and bacterial toxins may promote kidney failure. Dehydration, advanced age, concurrent renal insufficiency, and diabetes mellitus tend to enhance nephrotoxicity. Necrosis caused by nephrotoxins is usually uniform and limited to the proximal tubules.

Postrenal acute kidney injury is rare and usually occurs with urinary tract obstruction that affects the kidneys bilaterally (e.g., bladder outlet obstruction, prostatic hypertrophy, bilateral ureteral obstruction), tumors, or neurogenic bladder. A pattern of several hours of anuria with flank pain followed by polyuria is a characteristic finding. The obstruction causes an increase in intraluminal hydrostatic pressure upstream from the site of obstruction with a gradual decrease in GFR. This type of kidney failure can occur after diagnostic catheterization of the ureters, a procedure that may cause edema of the tubular lumen.

Oliguria (<400 ml/24 hr) can occur in AKI. Three mechanisms have been proposed to account for the decrease in urine output. All three mechanisms probably contribute to oliguria in varying combinations and degrees throughout the course of the disease (see Fig. 32.8). These mechanisms are as follows:

1. *Alterations in renal blood flow.* Efferent arteriolar vasoconstriction may be produced by intrarenal release of angiotensin II or there may be redistribution of blood flow from the cortex to the medulla. Autoregulation of blood flow may be impaired, resulting in decreased GFR. Changes in glomerular permeability and decreased GFR also may result from ischemia.
2. *Tubular obstruction.* Necrosis of the tubules causes sloughing of cells, cast formation, and obstruction to urine flow. There can be ischemic edema that results in tubular obstruction. The obstruction causes a retrograde increase in hydrostatic pressure and opposes the hydrostatic pressure of glomerular filtration, thus reducing the GFR. Kidney failure can occur within 24 hours.
3. *Tubular backleak.* Tubular reabsorption of filtrate is accelerated as a result of increased permeability caused by ischemia and increased tubular pressure from obstruction. The increased reabsorption of filtrate results in oliguria.

CLINICAL MANIFESTATIONS   Oliguria begins within 1 day after a hypotensive event and lasts 1 to 3 weeks, but may regress in several hours or extend for several weeks, depending on the duration of ischemia or the severity of injury or obstruction. The clinical progression of AKI with recovery of renal function occurs in three overlapping phases: initiation phase, maintenance phase, and recovery phase. Each phase is described as follows:

1. The *initiation phase* is the phase of reduced perfusion or toxicity in which kidney injury is evolving. Prevention of injury is possible during this phase.
2. The *maintenance* or *oliguric phase* is the period of established kidney injury and dysfunction after the initiating event has been resolved. It may last from weeks to months with urine output

lowest during this phase. The serum creatinine and BUN levels both increase.

3. The *recovery* or *polyuric phase* is the interval when glomerular function returns but the regenerating tubules cannot yet concentrate the filtrate. Diuresis is common during this phase, with a decline in serum creatinine and urea concentrations and an increase in creatinine clearance.

Anuria (urine output <50 ml/day) is uncommon in ATN. It involves both kidneys and suggests bilateral renal artery occlusion, obstructive uropathy, or acute cortical necrosis. Kidney failure also can present with nonoliguric kidney failure and represents less severe injury, particularly with intrinsic kidney injury associated with nephrotoxins. The urine output may be normal or high in volume, but the BUN and plasma creatinine concentrations increase. Other manifestations of altered urine excretion include hyperkalemia, hyperphosphatemia, and metabolic acidosis. Edema and congestive heart failure can be associated with fluid retention.

As kidney function improves, the increase in urine volume (diuresis) is progressive. The tubules are still damaged early in the recovery phase and have not recovered secretion and reabsorption functions. Polyuria can result in excessive loss of sodium, potassium, and water during this phase. Fluid and electrolyte balance must be carefully monitored and excessive urinary losses replaced.

Serial measurements of plasma creatinine concentration provide an index of renal function during the *recovery phase*. Return to normal status may take 3 to 12 months, and some individuals do not have full recovery of a normal GFR or tubular function and their plasma creatinine concentration will remain higher than normal.

EVALUATION AND TREATMENT   The diagnosis of AKI is related to the cause of the disease. A history of surgery, trauma, or cardiovascular disorders is common, and exposure to nephrotoxins, obstructive uropathies (e.g., an enlarged prostate or kidney stones), or infection must be considered. The diagnostic challenge is to differentiate prerenal AKI from intrarenal AKI, and some evidence is available from urinalysis and measurement of plasma creatinine and BUN levels (Table 32.10). However, more than 50% of glomerular filtration must be lost before there is elevation of serum creatinine level. Cystatin C, a serum protein freely filtered at the glomerulus, can serve as a measure of GFR.

Biomarkers are being developed to assess the extent of kidney injury before elevation of the serum creatinine level.[29] Prevention of AKI is the most important therapeutic approach and involves avoidance of hypotension, hypovolemia, and nephrotoxicity.

The primary goal of therapy is to maintain the individual's life until kidney function has recovered. Management principles directly related to physiologic alterations generally include:

1. correcting fluid and electrolyte disturbances, particularly hyperkalemia;
2. managing blood pressure;
3. preventing and treating infections;
4. maintaining nutrition; and
5. remembering that certain drugs or their metabolites are not excreted and can be toxic.

Renal replacement therapy (hemodialysis or peritoneal dialysis) may be indicated for uncontrollable hyperkalemia, acidosis, or severe fluid overload.

CHRONIC KIDNEY DISEASE

Chronic kidney disease (CKD) is the progressive loss of renal function indicated by a decline in GFE to below 60 ml/min/1.73 m² for 3 months or more, irrespective of cause. AKI can progress to CKD. CKD is associated with systemic diseases, such as diabetes mellitus (most significant risk factor), hypertension, and systemic lupus erythematosus. CKD also is associated with intrinsic kidney diseases, such as AKI, chronic glomerulonephritis, chronic pyelonephritis, obstructive uropathies, or vascular disorders. The terms *renal insufficiency* and *chronic renal failure* are still often used to describe declining kidney function, but they do not have the specificity of the stages based on GFR recommended by the National Kidney Foundation (Table 32.11).

PATHOPHYSIOLOGY   The kidneys have a remarkable ability to adapt to loss of nephron mass. Symptomatic changes result from increased plasma levels of creatinine, urea, and potassium. Alterations in salt and water balance usually do not become apparent until renal function declines to less than 25% of normal when adaptive renal reserves have been exhausted.

Different theories have been proposed to account for the adaptation to loss of renal function. The *intact nephron hypothesis* proposes that

TABLE 32.10   Differentiation of Acute Oliguric Kidney Failure

	Urine Volume	Urine Specific Gravity	Urine Osmolality	Urine Sodium Concentration	BUN/Plasma Creatinine Ratio	FE_Na*
Normal values	800-2000 ml	1.010-1.030	500-800 mOsm	20 mEq/L	10:1-20:1	1%
Prerenal failure	<400 ml	1.016-1.020	>500 mOsm	<10 mEq/L	>20:1 BUN is elevated relative to plasma creatinine Dehydration or hypoperfusion is suspected	<1% (also seen in acute glomerulonephritis) Sodium is reabsorbed to increase plasma volume
Intrarenal failure (i.e., acute tubular necrosis)	<400 ml	1.010-1.012	<400 mOsm	>30 mEq/L	<10:1 Intrarenal damage causes reduced reabsorption of BUN	>1% (also seen in acute urinary tract obstruction and renal parenchymal disease) Sodium is lost due to tubular damage

$$* FE_{Na} = \frac{Urine\ Na/plasma\ Na}{Urine\ creatinine/plasma\ creatinine} = 100.$$

TABLE 32.11	Stages of Chronic Kidney Disease	
Stage	Description	Signs/Symptoms
I	Normal kidney function Normal or high GFR (>90 ml/min)	Usually none Hypertension common
II	Mild kidney damage, mild reduction in GFR (60-89 ml/min)	Subtle Hypertension Increasing creatinine and urea levels
III	Moderate kidney damage GFR 30-59 ml/min	Mild As above
IV	Severe kidney damage GFR 15-29 ml/min	Moderate As above Erythropoietin deficiency anemia Hyperphosphatemia Increased triglycerides Metabolic acidosis Hyperkalemia Salt/water retention
V	End-stage kidney disease Established kidney failure GFR <15 ml/min	Severe As above

GFR, glomerular filtration rate.

TABLE 32.12	Factors Representing Progression of Chronic Kidney Failure
Factor	Characteristics
Proteinuria	Glomerular hyperfiltration of protein contributes to tubular interstitial injury by accumulating in interstitial space and promoting inflammation and progressive fibrosis.
Creatinine and urea clearance	In chronic renal failure, the GFR falls and the plasma creatinine concentration increases by a reciprocal amount; because there is no regulatory adjustment for creatinine, plasma levels continue to rise and serve as an index of changing glomerular function. As GFR declines, urea clearance increases. (NOTE: Urea is both filtered and reabsorbed and varies with state of hydration.)
Sodium and water balance	In chronic renal failure, sodium load delivered to nephrons exceeds normal, so excretion must increase; thus less is reabsorbed. Obligatory loss occurs, leading to sodium deficits and volume depletion. As GFR is reduced, ability to concentrate and dilute urine diminishes.
Phosphate and calcium balance	Changes in acid-base balance affect phosphate and calcium balance. Major disorders associated with chronic renal failure are reduced renal phosphate excretion, decreased renal synthesis of 1,25-dihydroxy-vitamin D_3, and hypocalcemia. Hypocalcemia leads to secondary hyperparathyroidism, GFR falls, and progressive hyperphosphatemia, hypocalcemia, and dissolution of bone result.
Hematocrit	Because of anemia that accompanies chronic renal failure, lethargy, dizziness, and low hematocrit are common.
Potassium balance	In chronic renal failure, tubular secretion of potassium increases until oliguria develops. Use of potassium-sparing diuretics also may precipitate elevated serum potassium levels. As disease progresses, total body potassium levels can rise to life-threatening levels and dialysis is required.
Acid-base balance	In early renal insufficiency, acid excretion and bicarbonate reabsorption are increased to maintain normal pH. Metabolic acidosis begins when GFR reaches 30% to 40%. Metabolic acidosis and hyperkalemia may be severe enough to require dialysis when end-stage renal failure develops.
Dyslipidemia	Chronic hyperlipidemia may induce glomerular and tubulointerstitial injury, contributing to progression of chronic renal disease.

GFR, glomerular filtration rate.

loss of nephron mass with progressive kidney damage causes the surviving nephrons to sustain normal kidney function. These nephrons are capable of a compensatory hypertrophy and expansion or hyperfunction in their rates of filtration, reabsorption, and secretion and can maintain a constant rate of excretion in the presence of overall declining GFR. The intact nephron hypothesis explains adaptive changes in solute and water regulation that occur with advancing kidney failure. Although the urine of an individual with CKD may contain abnormal amounts of protein and red and white blood cells or casts, the major end products of excretion are similar to those of normally functioning kidneys until the advanced stages of renal failure, when there is a significant reduction of functioning nephrons.

The *particular location of kidney damage* also influences loss of kidney function. For example, tubular interstitial diseases damage primarily the tubular or medullary parts of the nephron, producing problems such as renal tubular acidosis, salt wasting, and difficulty diluting or concentrating the urine. When the damage is primarily vascular or glomerular, proteinuria, hematuria, and nephrotic syndrome are more prominent. With severe or repeated injury, interstitial capillary loss and fibroblast proliferation result in progressive glomerulosclerosis and tubulointerstitial fibrosis. These conditions contribute to CKD and ESKD. A summary of factors involved in the progression of CKD is outlined in Table 32.12 and Fig. 32.9.

Two factors that have consistently been recognized to advance renal disease are proteinuria and angiotensin II activity. Glomerular hyperfiltration, increased glomerular capillary permeability, and loss of negative charge lead to proteinuria. *Proteinuria* contributes to tubulointerstitial injury by accumulating in the interstitial space of the nephron tubules. There is activation of complement proteins and other mediators and cells, such as macrophages, that promote inflammation and progressive fibrosis. *Angiotensin II* (from activation of the renin-angiotensin-aldosterone system [RAAS]) causes efferent arteriolar vasoconstriction and promotes

glomerular hypertension and hyperfiltration. Hyperfiltration is also associated with hyperglycemia and diabetic nephropathy. The chronically high intraglomerular pressure increases glomerular capillary permeability, contributing to proteinuria. Angiotensin II also may promote systemic hypertension and the activity of inflammatory cells and growth factors that participate in tubulointerstitial fibrosis and scarring.

CLINICAL MANIFESTATIONS CKD decreases GFR and tubular functions with changes manifested throughout all organ systems. The

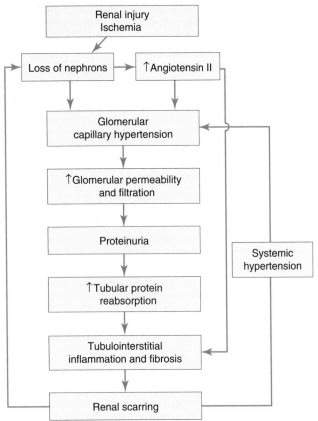

FIGURE 32.9 Mechanisms Related to the Progression of Chronic Kidney Disease.

manifestations are summarized in Table 32.13 and Fig. 32.9. Details of the systemic manifestations associated with CKD are discussed in the following sections.

Creatinine and Urea Clearance

Creatinine is constantly released from muscle and excreted primarily by glomerular filtration. In CKD, as GFR declines, the plasma creatinine level increases by a reciprocal amount to maintain a constant rate of excretion. With continuing decline in GFR, the plasma creatinine concentration increases. The clearance of *urea* follows a similar pattern, but urea is both filtered and reabsorbed, and its level varies with the state of hydration. Therefore urea concentration is not a good index of GFR. However, as the GFR decreases, plasma urea concentration also increases.

Fluid and Electrolyte Balance

Fluid and electrolyte and acid-base balance are significantly disturbed with CKD.[30] When the GFR decreases to 25%, there is an adaptive loss of 20 to 40 mEq of *sodium* per day with osmotic loss of water. Dietary intake must be maintained to prevent sodium deficits and volume depletion. As GFR continues to decline, there also is loss of tubular function to dilute and concentrate the urine and urine specific gravity becomes fixed at about 1.010. Ultimately the kidney loses its ability to regulate sodium and water balance and both sodium and water are retained, contributing to edema, proteinuria, and hypertension.

In early kidney failure, tubular secretion of *potassium* is maintained and larger amounts of potassium are lost through the bowel. With the onset of oliguria, total body potassium concentration can increase to life-threatening levels and must be controlled by dialysis.

Metabolic acidosis develops when the GFR decreases to less than 20% to 25% of normal. The causes of acidosis are primarily related to decreased hydrogen ion elimination and decreased bicarbonate reabsorption. With ESKD, metabolic acidosis may be severe enough to require alkali therapy and dialysis.

Calcium, Phosphate, and Bone

Bone and skeletal changes develop with alterations in calcium, phosphate, and vitamin D metabolism. These changes begin when the GFR decreases to 25% or less. *Hypocalcemia* is accelerated by impaired renal synthesis of 1,25-dihydroxy-vitamin D_3 (calcitriol) with decreased intestinal absorption of calcium. Renal phosphate excretion also decreases, and the increased serum phosphate binds calcium, further contributing to hypocalcemia. Acidosis also contributes to a negative calcium balance. Decreased serum calcium level stimulates parathyroid hormone secretion with mobilization of calcium from bone. The combined effect of *hyperparathyroidism* related to elevated phosphate levels and *vitamin D deficiency* can result in renal osteodystrophies (i.e., *osteoporosis, osteomalacia,* and *osteitis fibrosa*) with increased risk for fractures.

Protein, Carbohydrate, and Fat Metabolism

Protein, carbohydrate, and fat metabolism are altered in CKD. Proteinuria, metabolic acidosis, inflammation, and a catabolic state contribute to a negative nitrogen balance. Levels of serum proteins diminish, including albumin, complement, and transferrin, and there is loss of muscle mass. Insulin resistance and glucose intolerance are common and may be related to proinflammatory cytokines and alterations in adipokines (high leptin and low adiponectin levels) that interfere with insulin action.

Dyslipidemia is common among individuals with CKD. There is a high ratio of low-density lipoprotein (LDL) to high-density lipoprotein (HDL), a high level of triglycerides, and an accumulation of LDL particles. Uremia causes a deficiency in lipoprotein lipase and a decreased level of hepatic triglyceride lipase. Decreased lipolytic activity results in a reduction in HDL level. The concentration of apolipoprotein B is also elevated. The dyslipidemia accelerates atherogenesis and vascular calcification.

Cardiovascular System

Cardiovascular disease is a major cause of morbidity and mortality in CKD. Proinflammatory cytokines, oxidative stress, metabolic derangements, and uremic toxins are significant contributors.

Hypertension is the result of excess sodium and fluid volume and arteriosclerosis. Endothelial cell dysfunction and calcium deposits lead to a loss of vessel elasticity and vascular calcification. Elevated renin concentration also stimulates the secretion of aldosterone, increasing sodium reabsorption.

Dyslipidemia promotes atheromatous plaque formation. The resulting vascular disease increases the risk for *ischemic heart disease, left ventricular hypertrophy, congestive heart failure, stroke,* and *peripheral vascular disease* in individuals with uremia.

Pericarditis can develop from pericardial inflammation caused by the presence of uremic toxins. Accumulation of fluid in the pericardial space can compromise ventricular filling and cardiac output.[31] Fluid overload and hypertension can promote congestive heart failure (cardiorenal syndrome).

Anemia results from declining erythropoietin production, thereby increasing demands for cardiac output and adding to the cardiac workload.

Pulmonary System

Pulmonary complications are associated with fluid overload, congestive heart failure, and dyspnea. Pulmonary edema develops, and metabolic acidosis can cause Kussmaul respirations. Pulmonary hypertension can

TABLE 32.13   Systemic Effects of Chronic Kidney Failure

System	Manifestations	Mechanisms	Treatment
Skeletal	Spontaneous fractures and bone pain Deformities of long bones	Osteitis fibrosa: bone inflammation with fibrous degeneration related to hyperparathyroidism Osteomalacia: bone resorption associated with vitamin D and calcium deficiency	Control of hyperphosphatemia to reduce hyperparathyroidism; administration of calcium and aluminum hydroxide antacids, which bind phosphate in the gut, together with a phosphate-restricted diet; vitamin D replacement; avoidance of magnesium antacids because of impaired magnesium excretion
Cardiopulmonary	Pulmonary edema, Kussmaul respirations	Fluid overload associated with pulmonary edema and metabolic acidosis leading to Kussmaul respirations	ACE inhibitors; combination of propranolol, hydralazine, and minoxidil for those with high levels of renin; bilateral nephrectomy with dialysis or transplantation
Cardiovascular	Left ventricular hypertrophy, cardiomyopathy, and ischemic heart disease; hypertension, dysrhythmias, accelerated atherosclerosis; pericarditis with fever, chest pain, and pericardial friction rub	Extracellular volume expansion and hypersecretion of renin associated with hypertension; anemia increases cardiac workload; hyperlipidemia promotes atherosclerosis; toxins precipitate into pericardium	Volume reduction with diuretics that are not potassium sparing (to avoid hyperkalemia); dialysis
Neurologic	Encephalopathy (fatigue, reduced attention span, difficulty with problem solving); peripheral neuropathy (pain and burning in legs and feet, loss of vibration sense and deep tendon reflexes); loss of motor coordination, twitching, fasciculations, stupor, and coma with advanced uremia	Progressive accumulation of uremic toxins associated with end-stage renal disease Stroke or intracerebral hemorrhage associated with chronic dialysis	Dialysis or successful kidney transplantation
Hematologic	Anemia, usually normochromic-normocytic; platelet disorders with prolonged bleeding times	Reduced erythropoietin secretion and reduced red cell production; uremic toxins shorten red blood cell survival and alter platelet function	Dialysis; recombinant human erythropoietin and iron supplementation; conjugated estrogens; DDAVP (1-desamino-8-D-arginine vasopressin); transfusion
Gastrointestinal	Anorexia, nausea, vomiting; mouth ulcers, stomatitis, urine odor of breath (uremic fetor), hiccups, peptic ulcers, gastrointestinal bleeding, and pancreatitis associated with end-stage renal failure	Retention of metabolic acids and other metabolic waste products	Protein-restricted diet for relief of nausea and vomiting
Integumentary	Abnormal pigmentation and pruritus	Retention of urochromes, contributing to sallow yellow color; high plasma calcium levels and neuropathy associated with pruritus	Dialysis with control of serum calcium levels
Immunologic	Increased risk of infection that can cause death; increased risk of carcinoma	Suppression of cell-mediated immunity; reduction in number and function of lymphocytes, diminished phagocytosis	Routine dialysis
Reproductive	Sexual dysfunction: menorrhagia, amenorrhea, infertility, and decreased libido in women; decreased testosterone levels, infertility, and decreased libido in men	Dysfunction of ovaries and testes; presence of neuropathies	No specific treatment

ACE, angiotensin-converting enzyme.
With data from Almeras C, Argilés A: *Semin Dial* 22(4):329-333, 2009; Keane WF: *Kidney Int Suppl* 75:S27-S31, 2000; Thomas R et al: *Prim Care* 35(2):329-344, 2008.

develop because of left ventricular dysfunction or uremic-associated vascular changes.

Hematologic System

Hematologic alterations include *normochromic-normocytic anemia, impaired platelet function,* and *hypercoagulability.* Inadequate production of erythropoietin decreases red blood cell production, and uremia decreases red blood cell life span. Lethargy, dizziness, and low hematocrit values are common findings. Defective platelet aggregation, decreased platelet numbers, and altered vascular endothelium promote an increased bleeding tendency, increased risk for bruising, epistaxis, gastrointestinal bleeding, or cerebrovascular hemorrhage. Alterations in thrombin and other clotting factors contribute to hypercoagulability.

Immune System

Immune system dysregulation develops with the uremia of CRF. Chemotaxis, phagocytosis, antibody production, and cell-mediated immune responses are suppressed. Malnutrition, metabolic acidosis, and hyperglycemia may amplify immunosuppression. Release of inflammatory cytokines results in systemic inflammation. Failure of antioxidant systems also promotes inflammation. There are deficient responses to vaccination, increased risk for infection, and virus-associated cancers (e.g., human papillomavirus, hepatitis B and C viruses, Epstein-Barr virus).

Neurologic System

Neurologic symptoms are common and progressive with CKD. Symptoms may include headache, pain, drowsiness, sleep disorders, impaired concentration, memory loss, and impaired judgment (known as uremic encephalopathy). In advanced stages of kidney failure, symptoms may progress to seizures and coma. Neuromuscular irritation can cause hiccups, muscle cramps, and muscle twitching. Peripheral neuropathies associated with uremic toxins also can develop with impaired sensations, particularly in the lower limbs. Symptoms improve with hemodialysis.

Gastrointestinal System

Gastrointestinal complications are common in individuals with CKD. Uremic gastroenteritis can cause bleeding ulcer and significant blood loss. Nonspecific symptoms include anorexia, nausea, vomiting, constipation, or diarrhea. Uremic fetor is a form of bad breath caused by the breakdown of urea by salivary enzymes. Malnutrition is common.

Endocrine and Reproductive Systems

Endocrine and reproductive alterations develop with progression of CKD. Both males and females have a decrease in levels of circulating sex steroids. Males often experience a reduction in testosterone levels and may be impotent. Oligospermia and germinal cell dysplasia can result in infertility. Females have reduced estrogen levels, amenorrhea,

and difficulty maintaining a pregnancy to term.[32] A decrease in libido and fertility can occur in both sexes.

Insulin resistance is common in uremia, and as CKD progresses the ability of the kidney to degrade insulin is reduced and the half-life of insulin is prolonged. Individuals with diabetes mellitus and CRF need to carefully manage their insulin dosages.

CRF also causes alterations in thyroid hormone metabolism, particularly hypothyroidism, known as *nonthyroidal illness syndrome.* Uremia delays the response of thyroid-stimulating hormone receptors, and triiodothyronine (T_3) levels are often low.

Integumentary System

Skin changes are associated with other complications that develop with CKD. Anemia can cause pallor and bleeding into the skin and results in hematomas and ecchymosis. Retained urochromes manifest as a sallow skin color. Hyperparathyroidism and uremic skin residues (known as uremic frost) are associated with inflammation, irritation, and pruritus with scratching, excoriation, and increased risk for infection. Half-and-half nails (half white and half red or brown) are common.

EVALUATION AND TREATMENT   Early screening and evaluation of CKD is based on the risk factors, health history, presenting signs and symptoms, and diagnostic testing. Elevated serum creatinine and BUN concentrations are consistent with CKF. Markers of kidney damage include measurement of urine protein level, particularly albumin, and examination of urine sediment. Imaging will show small kidney size. Renal biopsy confirms the diagnosis.

Management involves dietary restriction of protein, sodium, potassium, and phosphate, supplementation with vitamin D or vitamin D receptor activators, maintenance of sodium and fluid balance, restriction of potassium, promotion of adequate caloric intake, management of dyslipidemias, and use of erythropoietin as needed. ACE inhibitors or ARBs are often used to control systemic hypertension, reduce proteinuria, provide renoprotection, and prevent progressive renal damage.

End-stage renal failure related to diabetic nephropathy can be significantly reduced with glycemic control. End-stage renal failure is treated with conservative care, continuous renal replacement therapy, supportive therapy, and renal transplantation. Portable and wearable dialysis devices are in development.[33]

> **✓ QUICK CHECK 32.5**
> 1. What mechanisms cause prerenal acute renal failure?
> 2. How does intrarenal acute renal failure differ from postrenal failure?
> 3. Briefly describe the causes of anemia, cardiovascular disease, and bone and neurologic changes associated with chronic renal failure.

SUMMARY REVIEW

Urinary Tract Obstruction

1. Obstruction can occur anywhere in the urinary tract. It may be anatomic (structural) or functional. Obstruction impedes flow and dilates structures proximal to the blockage, increases risk for infection, and compromises renal function.
2. Upper urinary tract obstructions are caused by kidney stones or tumors within the kidney; or compression from a tumor, stone, or fibrosis along the ureter or at the ureter-bladder junction,
3. Complications of upper urinary tract obstruction include hydronephrosis, hydroureter, ureterohydronephrosis, and tubulointerstitial fibrosis.

4. Hypertrophy of the unobstructed kidney compensates for loss of function of the kidney with obstructive disease.
5. Relief of obstruction is usually followed by postobstructive diuresis and may cause fluid and electrolyte imbalance.
6. Kidney stones are caused by supersaturation of the urine with precipitation of stone-forming substances and changes in urine pH.
7. Stones can be located in the kidneys, ureters, and urinary bladder. The most common kidney stone is formed from calcium oxalate.
8. Obstructions of the lower urinary tract include both structural or anatomic disorders and alterations in neurologic function (neurogenic bladder), or both. They are related to urine storage and emptying.

9. Anatomic causes of resistance to urine flow include urethral stricture, prostatic enlargement in men, pelvic prolapse in women, and tumor compression.
10. Partial obstruction of the bladder can result in an increase in the force of detrusor contraction. If obstruction persists, there is deposition of collagen in the bladder wall over time, resulting in decreased bladder wall compliance and ineffective detrusor muscle contraction.
11. Overactive bladder syndrome is an uncontrollable or premature contraction of the bladder that results in urgency with or without incontinence, frequency, and nocturia.
12. A neurogenic bladder is caused by a neural lesion that interrupts innervation of the bladder.
13. Upper motor neuron lesions result in overactive (hyperreflexive) bladder function and bladder dyssynergia (loss of coordinated neuromuscular contraction).
14. Lesions in the sacral area of the spinal cord or peripheral nerves result in underactive, hypotonic, or atonic bladder function.
15. Detrusor sphincter dyssynergia is failure of the urethrovesical junction smooth muscle to release urine during bladder contraction and causes a functional obstruction.
16. Kidney (renal) tumors classically present with hematuria, flank pain, flank mass, and weight loss. Renal tumors include renal cell carcinoma (the most common), renal adenomas, and renal transitional cell carcinomas. Renal cell carcinoma can metastasize to the lung, lymph nodes, liver, bone, thyroid gland, and central nervous system.
17. Bladder tumors are commonly composed of transitional cells and are usually superficial.

Urinary Tract Infection

1. Urinary tract infections (UTIs) are commonly caused by the retrograde movement of bacteria into the urethra and bladder and can ascend to the kidney. UTIs are uncomplicated when the urinary system is normal or complicated when there is an abnormality. Types of UTI include cystitis, interstitial cystitis, and acute or chronic pyelonephritis.
2. Cystitis is an inflammation of the bladder commonly caused by bacteria and may be mild, hemorrhagic, suppurative, ulcerative, or gangrenous.
3. Interstitial cystitis/painful bladder syndrome is an unpleasant sensation (pain, pressure, discomfort) perceived to be related to the bladder and associated with lower urinary tract symptoms of more than 6 weeks' duration in the absence of infection or other identifiable causes. It is likely related to autoimmune reaction.
4. Acute pyelonephritis is an inflammation of the upper urinary tracts (ureter, renal pelvis, and kidney interstitium). Infection due to urinary obstruction and reflux of urine from the bladder are the most common underlying risk factors. Severe infections may cause localized abscess formation.

5. Chronic pyelonephritis is a persistent or recurrent infection of the kidney leading to scarring of one or both kidneys and alteration in renal function. Untreated, chronic pyelonephritis can lead to kidney failure.

Glomerular Disorders

1. Acute glomerulonephritis is an inflammation of the glomerulus caused by primary or secondary glomerular injury, commonly immune injury, to the glomerular capillary filtration membrane.
2. Immune injury mechanisms in glomerulonephritis include (1) the deposition of circulating antigen-antibody complexes often with complement components that cause injury and/or (2) the attraction of leukocytes by complement that release cytokines that injure the glomerular filtration membrane.
3. Diabetic nephropathy is the most common cause of glomerular injury progressing to chronic kidney disease.
4. Chronic glomerulonephritis is related to a variety of diseases that cause deterioration of the glomerulus and a progressive course leading to chronic kidney failure.
5. Nephrotic syndrome is the excretion of at least 3.5 g of protein (primarily albumin) in the urine per day because of glomerular injury that causes glomerular filtration of plasma proteins to exceed tubular reabsorption.
6. Nephritic syndrome is characterized by hematuria and red blood cell casts with less severe proteinuria.
7. The manifestations of both nephrotic and nephritic syndrome include edema, hypoproteinemia, proteinuria, hyperlipidemia, lipiduria, vitamin D deficiency, and hypothyroidism.

Acute Kidney Injury

1. Acute kidney injury (AKI) is a sudden decline in kidney function with a decrease in glomerular filtration rate (GFR) and urine output and with an elevation in plasma creatinine and blood urea nitrogen levels.
2. Prerenal AKI is caused by decreased renal perfusion with ischemia, decreased GFR, and tubular necrosis.
3. Intrarenal AKI is associated with several systemic diseases but is commonly related to acute tubular necrosis.
4. Postrenal kidney injury is associated with diseases that obstruct the flow of urine from the kidneys.
5. Oliguria is urine output that is less than 400 ml/24 hr.

Chronic Kidney Disease

1. Chronic kidney disease (CKD) is the progressive loss of renal function for 3 months or more, irrespective of the causes. Plasma creatinine levels gradually become elevated as GFR declines; sodium is lost in the urine; potassium is retained; acidosis develops; calcium, phosphate, and vitamin D metabolism are altered; and erythropoietin production is diminished. All organs systems are affected by CKD.

KEY TERMS

REFERENCES

1. Scales CD, Jr, et al: Urinary stone disease: advancing knowledge, patient care, and population health, *Clin J Am Soc Nephrol* 11(7):1305-1312, 2016.
2. Lotan Y, et al: Primary prevention of nephrolithiasis is cost-effective for a national healthcare system, *BJU Int* 110(11 Pt C):E1060-E1067, 2012.
3. Sakhaee K, et al: Clinical review. Kidney stones 2012: pathogenesis, diagnosis, and management, *J Clin Endocrinol Metab* 97(6):1847-1860, 2012.
4. McDonough RC, 3rd, Ryan ST: Diagnosis and management of lower urinary tract dysfunction, *Surg Clin North Am* 96(3):441-452, 2016.
5. Nseyo U, Santiago-Lastra Y: Long-term complications of the neurogenic bladder, *Urol Clin North Am* 44(3):355-366, 2017.
6. Willis-Gray MG, Dieter AA, Geller EJ: Evaluation and management of overactive bladder: strategies for optimizing care, *Res Rep Urol* 8:113-122, 2016.
7. Amarenco G, et al: Diagnosis and clinical evaluation of neurogenic bladder, *Eur J Phys Rehabil Med* 53(6):975-980, 2017.
8. Stoffel JT: Detrusor sphincter dyssynergia: a review of physiology, diagnosis, and treatment strategies, *Transl Androl Urol* 5(1):127-135, 2016.
9. Chang YH, et al: Review of underactive bladder, *J Formos Med Assoc* 117(3):178-184, 2018.
10. American Cancer Society: *Cancer facts and figures 2019*, Atlanta, Georgia, 2019, Author.
11. Inamura K: Renal cell tumors: understanding their molecular pathological epidemiology and the 2016 WHO classification, *Int J Mol Sci* 18(10):2017. pii: E2195.

12. Bhatt JR, Finelli A: Landmarks in the diagnosis and treatment of renal cell carcinoma, *Nat Rev Urol* 11(9):517-525, 2014.
13. Ridge CA, et al: Epidemiology and staging of renal cell carcinoma, *Semin Intervent Radiol* 31(1):3-8, 2014.
14. Lalani AA, et al: Systemic treatment of metastatic clear cell renal cell carcinoma in 2018: current paradigms, use of immunotherapy, and future directions, *Eur Urol* 75(1):100-116, 2019.
15. Tan WS, et al: Novel urinary biomarkers for the detection of bladder cancer: a systematic review, *Cancer Treat Rev* 69:39-52, 2018.
16. McLellan LK, Hunstad DA: Urinary tract infection: pathogenesis and outlook, *Trends Mol Med* 22(11):946-957, 2016.
17. Wagenlehner FM, et al: Urosepsis: overview of the diagnostic and treatment challenges, *Microbiol Spectr* 3(5):2015.
18. Rinaldi G, et al: New research tools for urogenital schistosomiasis, *J Infect Dis* 211(6):861-869, 2015.
19. Cortes-Penfield NW, Trautner BW, Jump RLP: Urinary tract infection and asymptomatic bacteriuria in older adults, *Infect Dis Clin North Am* 31(4):673-688, 2017.
20. Gupta K, Grigoryan L, Trautner B: Urinary tract infection, *Ann Intern Med* 167(7):ITC49-ITC64, 2017.
21. Hanno PM, et al: Diagnosis and treatment of interstitial cystitis/bladder pain syndrome: AUA guideline amendment, *J Urol* 193(5):1545-1553, 2015.
22. Pazin C, et al: Treatment of bladder pain syndrome and interstitial cystitis: a systematic review, *Int Urogynecol J* 27(5):697-708, 2016.

23. Takhar SS, Moran GF: Diagnosis and management of urinary tract infection in the emergency department and outpatient settings, *Infect Dis Clin North Am* 28(1):33-48, 2014.
24. Fioretto P, et al: Is diabetic nephropathy reversible?, *Diabetes Res Clin Pract* 104(3):323-328, 2014.
25. Yap DY, Lai KN: Pathogenesis of renal disease in systemic lupus erythematosus—the role of autoantibodies and lymphocytes subset abnormalities, *Int J Mol Sci* 16(4):7917-7931, 2015.
26. Wang CS, Greenbaum LA: Nephrotic syndrome, *Pediatr Clin North Am* 66(1):73-85, 2019.
27. Thomas ME, et al: The definition of acute kidney injury and its use in practice, *Kidney Int* 87(1):62-73, 2014.
28. Maxwell RA, Bell CM: Acute kidney injury in the critically ill, *Surg Clin North Am* 97(6):1399-1418, 2017.
29. Malhotra R, Siew ED: Biomarkers for the early detection and prognosis of acute kidney injury, *Clin J Am Soc Nephrol* 12(1):149-173, 2017.
30. Dhondup T, Qian Q: Electrolyte and acid-base disorders in chronic kidney disease and end-stage kidney failure, *Blood Purif* 43(1-3):179-188, 2017.
31. Johnson RJ, et al: Cardiovascular disease in chronic kidney disease. In Johnson RJ, et al, editors: *Comprehensive clinical nephrology*, Philadelphia, 2015, Saunders, pp 949-966, (Chapter 82).
32. Vellanki K: Pregnancy in chronic kidney disease, *Adv Chronic Kidney Dis* 20(3):223-228, 2013.
33. van Gelder MK, et al: From portable dialysis to a bioengineered kidney, *Expert Rev Med Devices* 15(5):323-336, 2018.

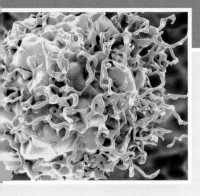

33

Alterations of Renal and Urinary Tract Function in Children

Patricia Ring, Sue E. Huether

EVOLVE WEBSITE

http://evolve.elsevier.com/Huether/
Student Review Questions
Audio Key Points

Case Studies
Animations
Quick Check Answers

The incidence and type of renal and urinary tract disorders experienced by children vary with age and maturation. Newborn disorders may involve congenital malformations. During childhood, the kidney and genitourinary structures continue to develop, so renal dysfunction may be associated with mechanisms and manifestations that differ from those found in adults.

STRUCTURAL ABNORMALITIES

Congenital abnormalities of the kidney and urinary tract (CAKUT) range from minor or easily correctable anomalies to those that are incompatible with life (Fig. 33.1). For example, the kidneys may fail to ascend from the pelvis to the abdomen, causing ectopic kidneys (abnormal location), which usually function normally. The kidneys may fuse as they ascend during fetal development, causing a single, U-shaped horseshoe kidney. Approximately one-third of individuals with horseshoe kidneys are asymptomatic, with the most common problems being infection, stone formation, hydronephrosis (from obstruction of urine flow), and, rarely, renal malignancies.[1] Collectively, structural anomalies of the renal system account for approximately 40% to 50% of cases of renal failure in children in developed countries.[2] Many are linked to gene defects and also may be associated with other structural malformations.

Hypoplastic/Dysplastic Kidneys

During embryologic development, the ureteric duct grows into the metanephric tissue, triggering the formation of the kidneys.[3] If this growth does not occur, the kidney is absent—a condition called renal aplasia. A hypoplastic kidney is small with a decreased number of nephrons. These conditions may be unilateral or bilateral. The occurrence may be incidental or familial. Bilateral hypoplastic kidneys are a common cause of chronic renal failure in children. Segmental hypoplasia (failure of parts of the renal cortex to develop)—the Ask-Upmark kidney—may be congenital or secondary to vesicoureteral reflux. Systemic hypertension is a common presentation.[4]

Renal dysplasia (abnormal development of renal tissue) usually results from abnormal differentiation of the renal tissues. For example, primitive glomeruli and tubules, cysts, and nonrenal tissue (such as cartilage) are found in the dysplastic kidney. Dysplasia may be secondary to antenatal obstruction of the urinary tract from ureteroceles (an outpouching of the ureter where it enters the bladder), posterior urethral valves (an obstructing membrane in the male urethra), or prune-belly syndrome (congenital absence of abdominal muscles).

Polycystic Kidney Disease

Polycystic kidney disease (PKD) is an inherited condition occurring in about 1 of 1000 live births.[5] PKD is associated with mutation of two genes: *PDK1* (autosomal dominant) or *PDK2* (autosomal recessive, more rare). Affected kidneys have multiple cysts that interfere with renal function. Autosomal dominant PKD (ADPKD) usually presents in late childhood or adulthood with the development of cysts. Defects in the formation of epithelial cells and their cilia result in cyst formation in all parts of the nephron. Cysts in other organs, including the liver, pancreas, and ovaries, may occur. Hypertension, aortic and intracranial aneurysms, and heart valve defects may develop. Autosomal recessive PKD (ARPKD) is often first suspected on a prenatal ultrasound. Epithelial

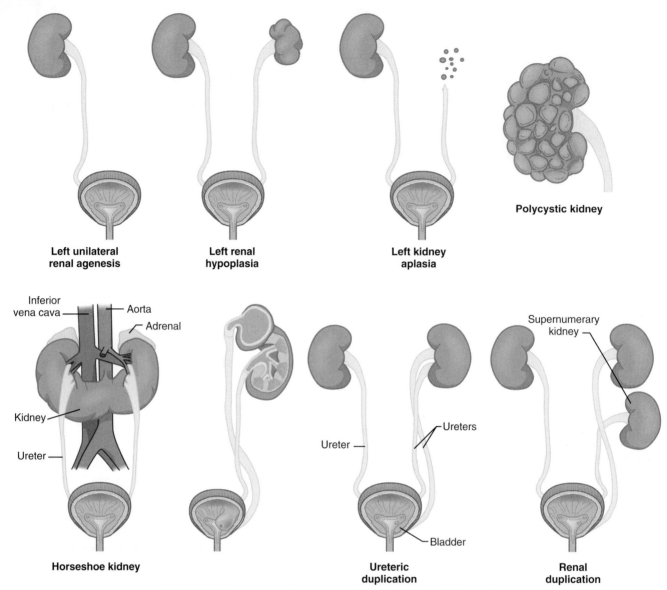

FIGURE 33.1 Congenital Anomalies of the Kidney and Urinary Tract.

hyperplasia and fluid secretion result in collecting duct cysts. Hepatic disease and hypertension typically accompany PKD. Renal dialysis is usually required during childhood or adolescence.

Renal Agenesis

Renal agenesis (the absence of one or both kidneys) may be unilateral or bilateral and may occur randomly or be hereditary. It may be an isolated entity or associated with anomalies in other organs.

Unilateral renal agenesis occurs in about 1 in 1000 live births in the United States. Males are more often affected, and it is usually the left kidney that is absent. The single remaining kidney is often completely normal so that the child can expect a normal, healthy life. By the time the child is several years old, the volume of this kidney may approach twice the normal size to compensate for the absence of a second kidney. In some instances, however, the single kidney is abnormally formed and associated with abnormalities of its collecting system. Because the child has a decreased number of nephrons, there is a risk of glomerular hyperfiltration injury, increasing the chance of developing proteinuria, hypertension, and chronic kidney disease (CKD).[6] Extrarenal congenital abnormalities of the urogenital, skeletal, cardiac, and other systems may coexist.

Bilateral renal agenesis is a rare disorder incompatible with extrauterine life. Approximately 75% of affected children are males. Oligohydramnios (low amount of amniotic fluid) resulting from inadequate fetal urine production leads to underdeveloped lungs. The term Potter syndrome refers to the association of a specific group of facial anomalies (wide-set eyes, parrot-beak nose, low-set ears, and receding chin). Approximately 40% of affected infants are stillborn. Infants with this condition rarely live more than 24 hours because of pulmonary insufficiency. Renal agenesis can be detected prenatally by ultrasound.

Ureteropelvic Junction Obstruction

Ureteropelvic junction (UPJ) obstruction is a blockage of the section where the renal pelvis transitions into the ureter. UPJ obstruction is the most common cause of hydronephrosis (distention of the renal pelvis and calyces with urine) in neonates. An intrinsic malformation of smooth muscle or urothelial development produces obstruction in the majority of cases. Extrinsic compression abnormalities are less common. Secondary ureteropelvic junction (UPJ) obstruction is caused by kinking or secondary scarring in the presence of high-grade vesicoureteral reflux. Children with UPJ obstruction have an increased risk of vesicoureteral reflux. Diagnosis of a UPJ obstruction can be made

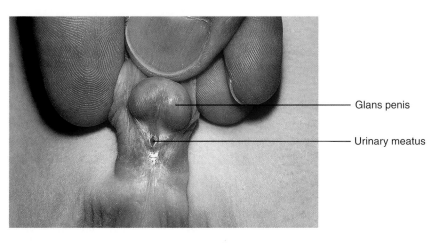

FIGURE 33.2 Hypospadias. (Courtesy H. Gil Rushton, MD, Children's National Medical Center, Washington, DC; from Hockenberry MJ, Wilson D: *Wong's nursing care of infants and children,* ed 10, St Louis, 2015, Mosby.)

by ultrasound. Obstruction of the distal ureter (**ureterovesical junction obstruction**) causes dilation of the entire ureter, renal pelvis, and calyceal system. A **ureterocele** is a ballooning dilation of the ureter where it enters into the bladder and impedes urine drainage. It often occurs when two ureters drain a kidney instead of one. Open or endoscopic surgery to relieve an obstruction is performed if there is decline of renal drainage or function.[7]

Hypospadias

Hypospadias is a congenital condition in which the urethral meatus is located on the ventral side or undersurface of the penis. The meatus can be located anywhere on the glans, on the penile shaft, at the base of the penis, at the penoscrotal junction, or in the perineum (Fig. 33.2). This is the most common anomaly of the penis; it occurs in about 1.86 to 5 per 10,000 infant boys.[8] The cause of this condition is multifactorial and includes genetic, endocrine, and environmental factors; advanced maternal age; and low birth weight. **Chordee**, or **penile torsion**, may accompany cases of hypospadias. In chordee, a shortage of skin on the ventral surface causes the penis to bend or "bow ventrally" (Fig. 33.3). Penile torsion is rotation, usually in a counterclockwise direction, of the penile shaft.

The goals for corrective surgery on the child with hypospadias are (1) a straight penis when erect to facilitate intercourse as an adult, (2) a uniform urethra of adequate caliber to prevent spraying during urination, (3) a cosmetic appearance satisfactory to the individual, and (4) repair completed in as few procedures as possible. Surgery is usually performed between 6 and 12 months of age.

Epispadias and Exstrophy of the Bladder

Epispadias and exstrophy of the bladder are the same congenital defect but expressed to a different degree. The dorsal urethra is not fused in epispadias and has failed to form a tube. In males, the urethral opening may be small and situated behind the glans (anterior epispadias), or a fissure may extend the entire length of the penis and into the bladder neck (posterior epispadias). In females, a cleft along the ventral urethra usually extends to the bladder neck. Continence is determined in part by the location of the defect, with urinary incontinence rates of up to 75% in children with distal epispadias.[9] Treatment is surgical reconstruction.

Exstrophy of the bladder is a rare, extensive congenital anomaly of herniation of the bladder through the abdominal wall. The bony part of the pelvis remains open (Fig. 33.4). The posterior portion of the bladder mucosa is exposed through the abdominal opening and appears bright red. The incidence of bladder exstrophy in the United States is about 1.7 per 100,000 live births.[10]

Exstrophy of the bladder is caused by intrauterine failure of the abdominal muscles and the anterior bladder to fuse during embryonic development. The pubic rami (bony projections of the pubic bone)

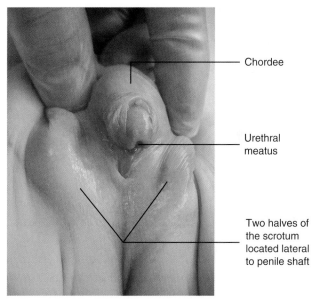

FIGURE 33.3 Hypospadias With Significant Chordee. (From Kliegman RM et al, editors: *Nelson textbook of pediatrics,* ed 19, Philadelphia, 2011, Saunders.)

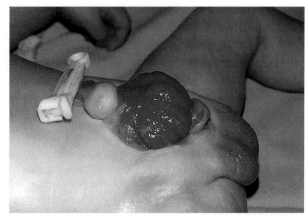

FIGURE 33.4 Exstrophy of Bladder. (Courtesy H. Gil Rushton, MD, Children's National Medical Center, Washington, DC; from Hockenberry MJ, Wilson D: *Wong's nursing care of infants and children,* ed 10, St Louis, 2015, Mosby.)

are not joined. This causes a waddling gait when the child first learns to walk, but most children quickly learn to compensate. The clitoris in girls is divided into two parts with the urethra between each half. The penis in boys is epispadiac. Urine seeps onto the abdominal wall from the ureters, causing a constant odor of urine and excoriation of the surrounding skin. Because the exposed bladder mucosa becomes hyperemic and edematous, it bleeds easily and is painful.

The unrepaired exstrophic bladder is prone to cancerous changes as soon as 1 year after birth. Ideally, the bladder and pubic defect should be closed before the infant is 72 hours old. Surgical reconstruction is usually performed within the first year either as a complete primary repair or as staged procedures. Staged procedures may include bladder augmentation, bladder neck reconstruction, and epispadias repair.[11] Objectives of management include preservation of renal function, attainment of urinary control, prevention of infection, and improvement of sexual function. Diagnosis is often made by prenatal ultrasound.

Cloacal exstrophy is the most rare and severe form of bladder exstrophy. The intestine and spine may be involved, and reconstruction with restored urine and fecal control is difficult.

Bladder Outlet Obstruction

Congenital causes of bladder outlet obstruction are rare and include urethral valves and polyps. A **urethral valve** is a thin membrane of tissue that occludes the urethral lumen and obstructs urinary outflow, usually in the posterior urethra in males. **Urethral polyps** are a benign fibroepithelial growth and are very rare in children. The timing and presentation of these conditions depend on the degree of obstruction they cause. Severe obstruction may impair renal embryogenesis and lead to renal failure. Urethral valves or polyps are resected as soon as they are diagnosed.

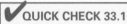

QUICK CHECK 33.1
1. Describe hypospadias.
2. What complications are associated with bladder exstrophy?
3. Contrast dysplastic kidney and hypoplastic kidney.

GLOMERULAR DISORDERS

The most common glomerular disorders in children are glomerulonephritis, nephrotic syndrome, and hemolytic uremic syndrome. Most glomerular diseases are acquired and immunologically mediated. The disease can be acute or chronic. The likelihood of developing renal failure depends on the specific condition.[12]

Glomerulonephritis

Acute glomerulonephritis includes a number of renal disorders in which inflammation of the glomeruli are secondary to an immune mechanism (the types of glomerulonephritis are described in Chapter 32 and Table 32.5). Chronic glomerulonephritis accounts for about 8% of the cases of CKD in children in the United States[13] and is the causative factor for 15% to 29% of end-stage renal disease in children worldwide.[14]

Acute Poststreptococcal Glomerulonephritis

Acute poststreptococcal glomerulonephritis (PSGN) is one of the most common immune complex–mediated renal diseases in children.[15] Glomerulonephritis develops with the deposition of antigen-antibody complexes or the formation of complexes in the glomerulus. The antigen-antibody complex activates complement and the release of inflammatory mediators that damage endothelial and epithelial cells lying on the glomerular basement membrane. Damage to the glomerular basement membrane alters membrane permeability and leads to hematuria and proteinuria.

Symptoms usually begin 1 to 2 weeks after an infection with a nephritogenic strain of group A β-hemolytic streptococci, such as an upper respiratory tract infection (pharyngitis, more common during cold weather), and up to 6 weeks after a skin infection (impetigo, more

common during warm weather). Occurrences have been observed after bacterial endocarditis, which may be associated with streptococcal or staphylococcal microorganisms, or after viral diseases, such as varicella-zoster virus and hepatitis B and C.

The onset of symptoms is abrupt, varying with disease severity. The child typically has gross or microscopic hematuria, proteinuria, edema, and renal insufficiency. Oliguria may be present. Hypertension occurs because of increased vascular volume. Acute hypertension may cause headache, vomiting, somnolence, and other central nervous system (CNS) manifestations. Cardiovascular symptoms, such as dyspnea, tachypnea, and an enlarged, tender liver, are related to circulatory overload and are compounded by hypertension. The most severely affected children develop acute renal failure with oliguria. As many as half of affected children are asymptomatic.

The disease usually runs its course in 1 month, but urine abnormalities may be found for up to 1 year or longer after the onset. Most children recover completely. Treatment is supportive and symptom specific.

Immunoglobulin A Nephropathy

Immunoglobulin A (IgA) nephropathy is the most common form of glomerulonephritis worldwide and occurs more often in males. It is an autoimmune disease characterized by deposition primarily of immunoglobulin A with activation of complement proteins initiating an inflammatory response in the mesangium of the glomerulus.[16] Children with the disease have recurrent gross hematuria concurrent with a respiratory tract infection. Most continue to have microscopic hematuria between the attacks of gross hematuria and have a mild proteinuria as well. Treatment is supportive. Some children recover completely, whereas 20% or more will eventually require dialysis and transplantation. IgA nephropathy may recur after transplantation.

Henoch-Schönlein purpura nephritis (immunoglobulin A vasculitis) is a particular form of IgA nephropathy that involves a systemic vasculitis. Symptoms include palpable purpura, and children may experience abdominal pain, arthralgia, hematuria, and/or proteinuria. Complete recovery usually occurs, but some children progress to end-stage kidney disease (ESKD).[17]

Nephrotic Syndrome

Nephrotic syndrome is a group of symptoms characterized by severe proteinuria, hypoalbuminemia, hyperlipidemia, and edema. The syndrome is more common in children than in adults. When no identifiable cause is found, the condition is called **primary (idiopathic) nephrotic syndrome**. If it results from a systemic disease or other causes (e.g., drugs, toxins), it is called **secondary nephrotic syndrome**. Primary nephrotic syndrome is found predominantly in the preschool-age child, with a peak incidence of onset between 2 and 3 years of age. It is rare after 8 years of age. Boys are affected more often than girls. No prevalent racial or geographic distributions are evident. The incidence is approximately 3 per 100,000 children per year.

PATHOPHYSIOLOGY The most common causes of primary nephrotic syndrome in children are minimal change nephropathy and focal segmental glomerulosclerosis. **Minimal change nephropathy (MCN, lipoid nephrosis)** is associated with an alteration in T cell function and is characterized by fusion of the glomerular podocyte foot processes, which are seen by electron microscopy. The glomeruli appear normal by light microscopy. Loss of the electrical negative charge and increased permeability within the glomerular capillary wall lead to albuminuria. Hypoalbuminemia (causing decreased plasma oncotic pressure) and sodium retention contribute to edema. Hyperlipidemia leads to lipiduria (fat bodies in the urine) and primarily results from increased hepatic lipid synthesis and decreased plasma lipid catabolism.[18]

In idiopathic focal segmental glomerulosclerosis (FSGS), there is segmental loss of glomerular capillaries with proliferation of the mesangial matrix and adhesion of the glomerular capillaries to Bowman capsule.[19]

CLINICAL MANIFESTATIONS Onset of nephrotic syndrome is often insidious, with periorbital edema as the first sign. The edema is most noticeable in the morning and subsides during the day as fluid shifts to the abdomen, genitalia, and lower extremities. Parents may notice diminished, frothy, or foamy urine output or, when edema becomes pronounced with ascites, respiratory difficulty from pleural effusion or labial or scrotal swelling (Fig. 33.5). Edema of the intestinal mucosa may cause diarrhea, anorexia, and poor absorption. Edema often masks the malnutrition caused by malabsorption and protein loss. Pallor, with shiny skin and prominent veins, also is common. Blood pressure is usually normal. The child has an increased susceptibility to infection, especially pneumonia, peritonitis, cellulitis, and septicemia. Irritability, fatigue, and lethargy are common. **Congenital nephrotic syndrome (Finnish type)** is caused by an autosomal recessive mutation of the *NPHS1* gene. *NPHS1* normally encodes an immunoglobulin-like protein, nephrin, at the podocyte filtration membrane. Lack of nephrin alters membrane permeability and causes heavy proteinuria, hypoproteinemia, and edema in the first 3 months of life. These babies do not respond to steroid treatment (termed steroid resistance) and require albumin infusion and diuretics to manage their fluid balance.

EVALUATION AND TREATMENT The diagnosis of nephrotic syndrome is evident from the findings of proteinuria, hyperlipidemia, and edema. Diagnostic testing, including kidney biopsy, may be required to determine whether the cause is an intrinsic renal disease or a consequence of systemic disease. Basic management of nephrotic syndrome includes administering glucocorticosteroids (prednisone); adhering to a low-sodium, well-balanced diet; performing good skin care; and, if edema becomes problematic, prescribing diuretics (furosemide, metolazone). Immunosuppressive agents (i.e., cyclophosphamide) may be used with children who have frequent relapses or who are resistant to steroid therapy (steroid-resistant nephrotic syndrome). Long-term outcomes depend on the underlying cause of the nephrotic syndrome. Children with minimal change disease tend to do very well, whereas those with other conditions may develop ESKD.

Hemolytic Uremic Syndrome

Hemolytic uremic syndrome (HUS) is an acute disorder characterized by hemolytic anemia, thrombocytopenia (a decrease in blood platelets), and acute renal failure. HUS is a thrombotic microangiopathy and the most common cause of acute renal failure in children. The disease occurs most often in infants and children younger than 4 years of age but has been known to occur in adolescents and adults.

PATHOPHYSIOLOGY HUS has been associated with bacterial and viral agents, as well as endotoxins, especially that from Shiga toxin-producing *Escherichia coli* (known as D^+ or diarrhea-positive HUS). Potential sources of exposure include animals, unpasteurized beverages, and contaminated meat and vegetables. Nondiarrhea, or atypical, HUS is known as D^- disease and is caused by other microorganisms or by an inherited abnormality in complement regulation.[20]

In HUS D^+, toxins are absorbed from the intestine into the blood and bind to white blood cells, which are transported to the kidney. In the kidney, the white blood cells cause damage to the glomerular filtration membrane, aggregation of platelets, and activation of the clotting cascade. Narrowed glomerular vessels damage passing erythrocytes. These damaged red blood cells are removed by the spleen, causing acute hemolytic anemia. Fibrinolysis, the process of dissolution of a clot, acts on precipitated fibrin, causing the fibrin split products to appear in serum and urine. Platelet thrombi develop within damaged vessels, and platelet removal produces thrombocytopenia. Varying degrees of renal vascular occlusion cause altered renal perfusion and renal insufficiency or failure.

CLINICAL MANIFESTATIONS A prodromal gastrointestinal illness (diarrhea with or without vomiting) or, less frequently, an upper respiratory tract infection often precedes the onset by 1 to 2 weeks. After a symptom-free 1- to 5-day period, there is sudden onset of pallor, bruising or purpura, irritability, and oliguria. Slight fever, anorexia, vomiting, diarrhea (with the stool characteristically watery and blood stained), abdominal pain, mild jaundice, and circulatory overload are accompanying symptoms. Seizures and lethargy indicate CNS involvement. In severe cases, renal failure is apparent within the first days of onset. The renal failure causes metabolic acidosis, azotemia (accumulated nitrogenous wastes in the blood), hyperkalemia, and often hypertension.

EVALUATION AND TREATMENT Clinical evaluation includes history of preexisting illness, presenting symptoms, and urine and blood analysis. Management is supportive. Blood transfusions with packed red cells are needed to maintain reasonable hemoglobin levels. Eculizumab, a complement inhibitor, has provided effective treatment for HUS.[21] Most children recover completely. Potential long-term sequelae include renal (hypertension, proteinuria, CKD, and ESKD) and nonrenal abnormalities (diabetes mellitus, neurologic manifestations). When renal failure occurs, dialysis is indicated.

NEPHROBLASTOMA

Nephroblastoma (Wilms tumor) is a rare embryonal tumor of the kidney arising from undifferentiated mesoderm. Approximately 500 children are diagnosed each year in the United States, most younger than 5 years of age.[22] The peak incidence occurs between 2 and 3 years of age. Nephroblastoma is slightly more common in African-American children than in white children.

PATHOGENESIS Nephroblastoma has both sporadic and inherited origins. The sporadic form occurs in children with no known genetic predisposition. Inherited cases, which are relatively rare, are transmitted in an autosomal dominant fashion. Syndromic and nonsyndromic causes of nephroblastoma have been linked to mutation of several

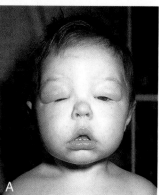
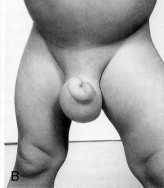

FIGURE 33.5 Nephrotic Syndrome. **A,** Facial edema. **B,** Gross edema of scrotum and legs with abdominal distention from ascites. (From Lissauer T, Clayden G: *Illustrated textbook of paediatrics,* ed 4, London, 2012, Mosby.)

tumor-suppressor genes (i.e., *WT1* and *WT2* mutations; these genes are important for development of the kidney).[23]

Some children who have nephroblastoma also have other congenital anomalies. The anomalies include aniridia (lack of an iris in the eye), hemihyperplasia (an asymmetry of the body), and genitourinary malformations (i.e., horseshoe kidneys, hypospadias, ureteral duplication, polycystic kidneys).

CLINICAL MANIFESTATIONS   Most children with nephroblastoma present with an enlarging asymptomatic abdominal mass before the age of 5 years. Many tumors are actually discovered by the child's parent, who feels or notices an abdominal swelling, usually while dressing or bathing the child. The child appears healthy and thriving. Other presenting complaints include vague abdominal pain, hematuria, anemia, and fever. Hypertension may be present, often as a result of excessive renin secretion by the tumor.[24]

Nephroblastoma may occur in any part of the kidney and varies greatly in size at the time of diagnosis. Bilateral tumors are very rare. The tumor generally appears as a solitary mass surrounded by a smooth, fibrous external capsule and also may contain cystic or hemorrhagic areas. A pseudocapsule generally separates the tumor from the renal parenchyma.

EVALUATION AND TREATMENT   On physical examination, the tumor feels firm, nontender, and smooth and is generally confined to one side of the abdomen. If the tumor is palpable past the midline of the abdomen, it may be large or may be arising from a horseshoe or ectopic kidney. Diagnostic imaging demonstrates a solid intrarenal mass.

Diagnosis is based on surgical biopsy. Imaging studies are used to evaluate the presence or absence of metastasis. The most common sites of metastasis are regional lymph nodes and the lungs, and less commonly the liver, brain, and bone.

Several staging systems for nephroblastoma have been developed and serve as guides to treatment. The most widely accepted system was developed by the National Wilms Tumor Study Group (Table 33.1). Primary treatment is usually surgical exploration and resection, including nephron sparing surgery or chemotherapy and then surgical resection. Radiation therapy may be used for children with higher stages of disease and metastases. Survival is greater than 90% for localized disease and more than 70% for higher stages. Heart failure, renal failure, and hypertension occur more frequently in long-term survivors than in the general population.[25]

> ✔ **QUICK CHECK 33.2**
> 1. What is the cause of proteinuria?
> 2. What is Wilms tumor?

TABLE 33.1   Staging of Nephroblastoma Tumor*

Stage	Tumor Characteristics
I	Tumor limited to kidney; can be completely resected
II	Tumor ascending beyond kidney but is totally resected
III	Residual nonhematogenous tumor confined to abdomen
IV	Hematogenous metastases to organs such as lungs, liver, bone, or brain
V	Bilateral disease either at diagnosis or later, then staged for each kidney

*Staging system of the National Wilms Tumor Study Group.

BLADDER DISORDERS

Urinary Tract Infections

Urinary tract infections (UTIs) are caused by colonization of a pathogen anywhere along the urinary tract (urethra, bladder, ureter, kidney) and occurs commonly in children. During the neonatal period, children with congenital renal abnormalities and noncircumcised males are at increased risk. UTIs in children are most common in 7- to 11-year-old girls and sexually active female adolescents as a result of perineal bacteria, especially *E. coli*, ascending the urethra. An abnormal urinary tract (presence of reflux, obstruction, stasis, or stones) is a risk factor for infection.

Cystitis, or infection of the bladder, results in mucosal inflammation and congestion. This causes detrusor muscle hyperactivity resulting in urgency and frequency and a decrease in bladder capacity. It may also cause distortion of the UVJ, leading to transient reflux of infected urine up the ureters, causing acute or chronic pyelonephritis.[26] Symptoms in children are nonspecific, and differentiating whether an infection is in the bladder or in the kidneys (pyelonephritis) is difficult based on symptoms alone. Infants may be asymptomatic or develop fever, lethargy, abdominal pain, vomiting, diarrhea, or asymptomatic jaundice. Children may present with fever of undetermined origin, frequency, urgency, dysuria, enuresis or incontinence in a previously dry child, flank or back pain, and sometimes hematuria. Acute pyelonephritis usually causes chills, high fever, and flank or abdominal pain, along with enlarged kidney(s) caused by inflammatory edema. Chronic pyelonephritis may be asymptomatic.

Diagnosis of UTIs is by urine culture before antibiotic therapy. Dipstick analyses for nitrite, leukocyte esterase, and blood may be used as a screening tool. Any positive or strong suspicion of a UTI, including unexplained jaundice in infants,[27] requires urine culture. Diagnostic imaging (e.g., ultrasound and cystogram) may be necessary to rule out obstructions, renal scarring, or functional abnormalities. With treatment, UTI symptoms are usually relieved in 1 to 2 days, and the urine becomes sterile. A 3- to 5-day course of oral antibiotics is effective for uncomplicated UTI.[28] Longer treatment may be required if the child has a history of recurrent UTIs, congenital abnormalities of the urinary tract, or upper UTI. If there is no improvement in 2 days, the child should be reevaluated (see *Did You Know?* Childhood Urinary Tract Infections).

> ### DID YOU KNOW?
> #### *Childhood Urinary Tract Infections*
>
> Childhood urinary tract infections (UTIs) are often seen in primary care settings and can cause significant longer term morbidity if not treated. Children younger than 2 years often have few nonspecific signs of infection, including fever, irritability, poor feeding, failure to thrive, and diarrhea. Obtaining a proper urine sample and culture is vital because true infections require further examination. Antibiotic prophylaxis may be considered for vesicoureteral reflux (VUR) or recurrent UTIs to prevent renal scarring and hypertension; however, this is a controversial issue because of the risk of antibiotic resistance. Current recommendations are to *consider* prophylaxis for children younger than 1 year of age with VUR and a history of febrile UTIs and in other children as individually evaluated. Circumcision status is controversial; however, recent studies have shown a decreased rate of UTIs in circumcised boys. Bowel and bladder abnormalities also must be managed because they can contribute to the development of UTIs.
>
> Data from Arlen AM, Cooper CS: *Curr Urol Rep* 16(9):64, 2015; Arshad M, Seed PC: *Clin Perinatol* 42(1):17-28, vii, 2015; Schlager TA: *Microbiol Spectr* 4(5), 2016; Schmidt B, Copp HL: *Urol Clin North Am* 42(4):519-526, 2015.

Vesicoureteral Reflux

Vesicoureteral reflux (VUR) is the retrograde flow of urine from the bladder into the kidney or ureters, or both. Reflux allows infected urine from the bladder to reach the kidneys. Vesicoureteral reflux occurs more often in girls and is uncommon in African-Americans. The actual incidence is unknown because VUR is often undiagnosed. An estimated 30% to 40% of children younger than 5 years who develop a UTI have VUR. Siblings of those affected have about a 27% to 51% chance of having reflux, and children with parents who had childhood reflux have almost a 70% chance of reflux.[29] Although reflux is considered abnormal at any age, the shortness of the submucosal tunnel of the ureter during infancy and childhood renders the antireflux mechanism relatively inefficient and delicate. Thus reflux is seen commonly in association with infections during early childhood but rarely in older children and adults.

PATHOPHYSIOLOGY The normal distal ureter enters the bladder through the detrusor muscle and passes through a submucosal tunnel before opening into the bladder lumen via the ureteral orifice. As the bladder fills with urine the ureter is compressed within the bladder wall, preventing reflux. *Primary reflux* results from a congenital abnormally short submucosal tunnel and ureter that permits reflux by the rising pressure of the filling bladder (Fig. 33.6). Urine sweeps up into the ureter and then flows back into the empty bladder. The reflux perpetuates infection by preventing complete emptying of the bladder and providing a reservoir for infection. With bladder filling, the intravesical pressure can be transmitted up the ureter to the renal pelvis and calyces. The combination of reflux lower UTI is an important cause of pyelonephritis. Renal parenchymal injury, scarring, hypertension, and chronic renal insufficiency can occur many years later, making early diagnosis and treatment important. *Secondary reflux* develops in association with acquired conditions (e.g., neurogenic bladder dysfunction, ureteral obstruction, voiding disorders, or surgery on the UVJ). Reflux may be unilateral or bilateral and is graded using the International Reflux Grading System[30] (Fig. 33.7):

Grade I: reflux into a nondilated distal ureter
Grade II: reflux into the upper collecting system without dilation
Grade III: reflux into a dilated ureter or blunting of calyceal fornices
Grade IV: reflux into a grossly dilated ureter and calyces
Grade V: massive reflux with urethral dilation and tortuosity and effacement of the calyceal details

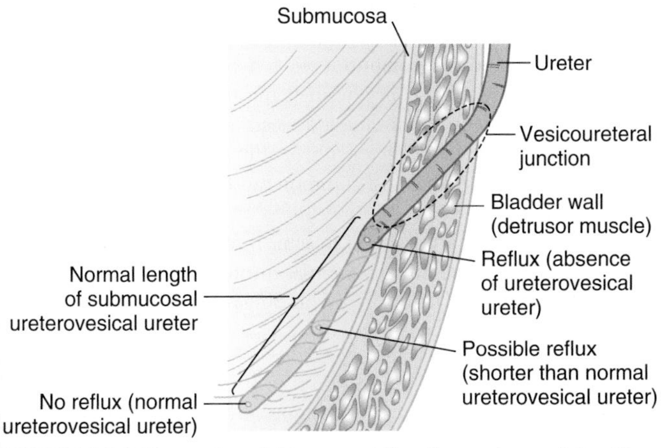

CLINICAL MANIFESTATIONS Children with reflux may be asymptomatic or have recurrent UTIs, unexplained fevers, poor growth and development, irritability, and feeding problems. The family history may reveal VUR or UTIs.

EVALUATION AND TREATMENT In addition to the history of recurrent UTI and other symptoms, a voiding cystourethrogram is the primary diagnostic procedure. Prompt treatment of UTIs in children with reflux is important to minimize the risk of pyelonephritis and renal scarring. Spontaneous remission of grades I, II, and III reflux may occur in 50% to 80% of children younger than 5 years. Approximately 20% of grades IV and V will resolve. Recurrent infection may require endoscopic, open, laparoscopic, and robotic procedures to stop the refluxing ureter.[31]

URINARY INCONTINENCE

Urinary incontinence refers to the involuntary passage of urine by a child who is beyond the age when voluntary bladder control should have been acquired. Bladder control is accomplished by most children before the age of 5 years, although this is largely influenced by cultural beliefs and parental toilet training practices. Wetness that occurs during the day is called **daytime incontinence**. Nighttime wetting is called **enuresis**. **Functional incontinence** is urinary incontinence in which no structural or neurologic abnormality can be identified.

The incidence of incontinence (enuresis) is difficult to determine because it is not a problem parents often discuss. Enuresis occurs in as many as 10% of 7-year-old males and resolves at a rate of 15% per year. Daytime incontinence occurs in up to 9% of early school-age children.[32]

PATHOPHYSIOLOGY A combination of factors is likely to be responsible for incontinence. A reasonable approach is to eliminate organic or physiologic causes before exploring psychological ones. Organic causes account for a minority of cases and include UTIs; neurologic disturbances; congenital defects of the meatus, urethra, or bladder neck; and allergies. Disorders that increase the normal output of urine, such as diabetes mellitus and diabetes insipidus, or disorders that impair the concentrating ability of the kidney, such as chronic renal failure or sickle cell disease, should be considered during evaluation. Other conditions that may be associated with incontinence include perinatal anoxia, CNS trauma, seizures, attention-deficit/hyperactivity disorder, developmental delay, imperforate anus, bladder trauma or surgery, obesity, and occult spinal

FIGURE 33.6 Normal and Abnormal Configurations of the Ureterovesical Ureter. A refluxing ureterovesical ureter has the same anatomic features as a nonrefluxing ureter, except for the shorter length of the intravesical ureter, which allows reflux of urine during filling of the bladder.

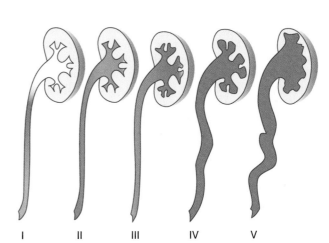

FIGURE 33.7 Grades of Vesicoureteral Reflux. (From Johnson JR, Feehally J, Floege J: *Comprehensive clinical nephrology,* ed 5, Philadelphia, Saunders.)

dysraphism. Altered sleep arousal or obstructive sleep apnea may be associated with enuresis. Stressful psychologic situations, such as a new sibling, may cause incontinence or enuresis to develop. Constipation is frequently present in children with urinary incontinence.

Genetic factors contribute to some types of incontinence. At least four gene loci associated with enuresis have been identified. Enuresis occurs with high frequency among parents, siblings, and other near relatives of symptomatic children. There is a high concordance rate in monozygotic twins with enuresis.[33]

CLINICAL MANIFESTATIONS   Primary incontinence (enuresis) means the child has never been continent. Secondary incontinence (enuresis) means the child has been continent for at least 6 months before wetting recurs. A child may have daytime incontinence, enuresis, or a combination of both. Types of incontinence and clinical manifestations are defined in Table 33.2.

EVALUATION AND TREATMENT   Evaluation of incontinence includes use of questionnaires, drinking and voiding charts, physical examination, and urinalysis. Underlying pathology, including kidney disease, VUR, UTI, or neurogenic bladder, is excluded. Radiologic and urodynamic evaluation may be required.[34]

Therapeutic management of incontinence begins with education. If the child and family understand the probable etiology of the child's condition, they are better able to choose and participate in therapies that are most likely to succeed. Treatment of daytime incontinence includes behavioral therapy, including timed voiding; fluid management; treatment of constipation, UTI, and other coexisting conditions if present; and medication (anticholinergic or alpha-blocker medications). Enuresis treatment also may include enuresis alarms.[35]

TABLE 33.2   Types of Incontinence

Type	Definition
Daytime voiding frequency	Decreased: 3 or fewer voids per day Increased: 8 or more voids per day
Dysfunctional voiding	Habitual contraction of urethral sphincter during voiding; observed by uroflow measurements
Enuresis	Incontinence of urine while sleeping
Incontinence, continuous	Continuous leakage, not in discrete portions
Incontinence, stress	Leakage with raised intra-abdominal pressure
Urgency	Sudden, unexpected, immediate need to void
Overactive bladder	Child with urgency; increased voiding frequency and/or incontinence may or may not be present
Underactive bladder	Decreased voiding frequency with use of raised intra-abdominal pressure to void
Urge incontinence	Incontinence in children with urgency

From Nevéus T et al: *J Urol* 176(1):312-324, 2006.

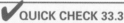

QUICK CHECK 33.3
1. How does the cause of urinary tract infections in newborns differ from that in older children?
2. How does vesicoureteral reflux occur?
3. What organic causes are operative in enuresis?

SUMMARY REVIEW

Structural Abnormalities

1. Congenital abnormalities of the kidney and urinary tract range in severity from minor conditions that need no treatment to those incompatible with life.
2. A hypoplastic kidney is small, with a decreased number of nephrons. A dysplastic kidney is the result of abnormal differentiation of renal tissues.
3. Polycystic kidney disease is a cystic genetic disorder resulting in multiple kidney cysts that interfere with renal function.
4. Renal agenesis is the absence of one or both kidneys and may occur as an isolated entity or in association with other disorders.
5. Ureteropelvic junction obstruction is blockage where the renal pelvis joins the ureter and is often caused by smooth muscle or urothelial malformation or by scarring that leads to hydronephrosis.
6. Hypospadias is a congenital condition in which the urethral meatus can be located anywhere on the ventral surface of the glans, the penile shaft, the midline of the scrotum, or the perineum.
7. Epispadias and exstrophy of the bladder are the congenital malformation expressed to a different degree. Epispadias involves the dorsal urethra failing to form a tube. In exstrophy, the pubic bones are separated and the posterior wall of the bladder is everted through the opening.
8. Urethral valves and polyps are congenital formations of tissue that block the urethra.

Glomerular Disorders

1. Glomerulonephritis is an inflammation of the glomeruli. The cause is unknown but is often immune mediated.

2. Acute poststreptococcal glomerulonephritis usually follows infection by strains of group A β-hemolytic streptococcus. Increases in glomerular capillary permeability lead to hematuria and proteinuria. Edema, hypertension, and renal insufficiency are also present.
3. Immunoglobulin A (IgA) nephropathy occurs with deposition of IgA in the glomerulus, causing glomerular injury with gross hematuria. Henoch-Schönlein purpura nephritis (immunoglobulin A vasculitis) is a particular form of IgA nephropathy that involves a systemic vasculitis.
4. Nephrotic syndrome is a group of symptoms characterized by severe proteinuria, hypoalbuminemia, hyperlipidemia, and edema. Metabolic, biochemical, or physiochemical disturbances in the glomerular basement membrane may lead to increased permeability to protein. Minimal change nephropathy and focal segmental glomerulosclerosis are the most common causes of nephrotic syndrome in children.
5. Hemolytic uremic syndrome is an acute thrombotic microangiopathy characterized by hemolytic anemia, thrombocytopenia, and acute renal failure and is associated with Shiga toxin of *Escherichia coli* infection.

Nephroblastoma

1. Nephroblastoma (Wilms tumor) is an embryonal tumor of the kidney that usually presents between birth and 5 years of age. Survival is high after treatment by surgery, a combination of drugs, and, for advanced disease, radiation therapy.

Bladder Disorders

1. Urinary tract infections (UTIs) result from bacteria ascending the urethra and occur anywhere along the urinary tract. The bladder alone is infected in cystitis. The infection ascends to one or both kidneys in pyelonephritis.
2. Vesicoureteral reflux is the retrograde flow of bladder urine into the kidney or ureter, or both, increasing the risk for pyelonephritis. It can be unilateral or bilateral; primary or secondary.

Urinary Incontinence

1. Urinary incontinence is the involuntary passage of urine by a child beyond the age when bladder control should have been acquired. It may occur during the day (daytime incontinence) or at night (enuresis), or both. Maturational delay, UTIs, constipation, and many other factors may contribute.

▮ KEY TERMS

Acute poststreptococcal glomerulonephritis (PSGN), 754
Acute pyelonephritis, 756
Ask-Upmark kidney, 751
Chordee (penile torsion), 753
Chronic pyelonephritis, 756
Congenital nephrotic syndrome (Finnish type), 755
Cystitis, 756
Daytime incontinence, 757
Enuresis, 757
Epispadias, 753
Exstrophy of the bladder, 753

Focal segmental glomerulosclerosis (FSGS), 755
Functional incontinence, 757
Hemolytic uremic syndrome (HUS), 755
Henoch-Schönlein purpura nephritis (immunoglobulin A vasculitis), 754
Horseshoe kidney, 751
Hypoplastic kidney, 751
Hypospadias, 753
Immunoglobulin A (IgA) nephropathy, 754
Minimal change nephropathy (MCN, lipoid nephrosis), 754

Nephroblastoma (Wilms tumor), 755
Nephrotic syndrome, 754
Oligohydramnios, 752
Polycystic kidney disease (PKD), 751
Potter syndrome, 752
Primary (idiopathic) nephrotic syndrome, 754
Primary incontinence, 758
Renal agenesis, 752
Renal aplasia, 751
Renal dysplasia, 751
Secondary incontinence, 758
Secondary nephrotic syndrome, 754

Secondary ureteropelvic junction (UPJ) obstruction, 752
Ureterocele, 753
Ureteropelvic junction (UPJ) obstruction, 752
Urethral polyp, 754
Urethral valve, 754
Urethrovesical junction obstruction, 753
Urinary incontinence, 757
Urinary tract infection (UTI), 756
Vesicoureteral reflux (VUR), 757

REFERENCES

1. Natsis K, et al: Horseshoe kidney: a review of anatomy and pathology, *Surg Radiol Anat* 36(6):517-526, 2013.
2. Capone VP, et al: Genetics of congenital anomalies of the kidney and urinary tract: the current state of play, *Int J Mol Sci* 18(4):2017.
3. Chen RY, Chang H: Renal dysplasia, *Arch Pathol Lab Med* 139(4):547-551, 2015.
4. Prasad S, et al: Ask-Upmark kidney: a report of 2 cases, *IJHSR* 3(1):61-64, 2013. Available at: www.ijhsr.org. Downloaded July 21, 2014.
5. Cordido A, Besada-Cerecedo L, García-González MA: The genetic and cellular basis of autosomal dominant polycystic kidney disease—a primer for clinicians, *Front Pediatr* 5:279, 2017.
6. Westland R, et al: Clinical implications of the solitary functioning kidney, *Clin J Am Soc Nephrol* 9(5):978-986, 2014.
7. Krajewski W, et al: Hydronephrosis in the course of ureteropelvic junction obstruction: an underestimated problem? Current opinions on the pathogenesis, diagnosis and treatment, *Adv Clin Exp Med* 26(5):857-864, 2017.
8. Springer A, van den Heijkant M, Baumann S: Worldwide prevalence of hypospadias, *J Pediatr Urol* 12(3):152.e1-152.e7, 2016.
9. Suzuki K, et al: Epispadias and the associated embryopathies: genetic and developmental basis, *Clin Genet* 91(2):247-253, 2017.
10. Lloyd JC, et al: Contemporary epidemiological trends in complex congenital genitourinary anomalies, *J Urol* 190(4 Suppl):1590-1595, 2013.
11. Roth E, et al: Postoperative immobilization and pain management after repair of bladder exstrophy, *Curr Urol Rep* 18(3):19, 2017.

12. Vogt B: Nephrology update: glomerular disease in children, *FP Essent* 444:30-40, 2016.
13. Vivante A, Hildebrandt F: Exploring the genetic basis of early-onset chronic kidney disease, *Nat Rev Nephrol* 12(3):133-146, 2016.
14. Ingelfinger FR, et al: World kidney day 2016, averting the legacy of kidney disease focus on childhood, *Clin Nephrol* 85(2):63-69, 2016.
15. VanDeVoorde RG, 3rd: Acute poststreptococcal glomerulonephritis: the most common acute glomerulonephritis, *Pediatr Rev* 36(1):3-12, 2015.
16. Mestecky J, et al: IgA nephropathy enigma, *Clin Immunol* 172:72-77, 2016.
17. Heineke MH, et al: New insights in the pathogenesis of immunoglobulin A vasculitis (Henoch-Schönlein purpura), *Autoimmun Rev* 16(12):1246-1253, 2017.
18. Vivarelli M, et al: Minimal change disease, *Clin J Am Soc Nephrol* 12(2):332-345, 2017.
19. Zand L, et al: What are we missing in the clinical trials of focal segmental glomerulosclerosis?, *Nephrol Dial Transplant* 32(suppl_1):i14-i21, 2017.
20. Talarico V, et al: Hemolytic uremic syndrome in children, *Minerva Pediatr* 68(6):441-455, 2016.
21. Vaisbich MH: Hemolytic-uremic syndrome in childhood, *J Bras Nefrol* 36(2):208-220, 2014.
22. Ward E, et al: Childhood and adolescent cancer statistics, 2014, *CA Cancer J Clin* 64(2):83-103, 2014.
23. National Cancer Institute (NCI): Wilms tumor and other childhood kidney tumors treatment for health professionals (PDQ®). Updated April 17, 2019. Available at: http://www.cancer.gov/types/kidney/hp/wilms-treatment-pdq#section/_1.
24. Romao RL, Lorenzo AJ: Renal function in patients with Wilms tumor, *Urol Oncol* 34(1):33-41, 2016.
25. Kieran K, Ehrlich PF: Current surgical standards of care in Wilms tumor, *Urol Oncol* 34(1):13-23, 2016.

26. Becknell B, et al: The diagnosis, evaluation and treatment of acute and recurrent pediatric urinary tract infections, *Expert Rev Anti Infect Ther* 13(1):81-90, 2015.
27. Mutlu M, et al: Urinary tract infections in neonates with jaundice in their first two weeks of life, *World J Pediatr* 10(2):164-167, 2014.
28. Okarska-Napierała M, Wasilewska A, Kuchar E: Urinary tract infection in children: diagnosis, treatment, imaging—comparison of current guidelines, *J Pediatr Urol* 13(6):567-573, 2017.
29. Hunziker M, Puri P: Familial vesicoureteral reflux and reflux related morbidity in relatives of index patients with high grade vesicoureteral reflux, *J Urol* 188(4 Suppl):1463-1466, 2012.
30. Lebowitz RL, et al: International system of radiographic grading of vesicoureteric reflux. International Reflux Study in Children, *Pediatr Radiol* 15(2):105-109, 1985.
31. Arlen AM, Cooper CS: Controversies in the management of vesicoureteral reflux, *Curr Urol Rep* 16(9):64, 2015.
32. Buckley BS, Lapitan MC: Prevalence of urinary incontinence in men, women, and children— current evidence: findings of the Fourth International Consultation on Incontinence, *Urology* 76(2):265-270, 2010.
33. von Gontard A, et al: Family history of nocturnal enuresis and urinary incontinence: results from a large epidemiological study, *J Urol* 185(6):2303-2306, 2011.
34. Maternik M, Krzeminska K, Zurowska A: The management of childhood urinary incontinence, *Pediatr Nephrol* 30(1):41-50, 2015.
35. Thurber S: Childhood enuresis: current diagnostic formulations, salient findings, and effective treatment modalities, *Arch Psychiatr Nurs* 31(3):319-323, 2017.

34

Structure and Function of the Reproductive Systems

George W. Rodway, Sue E. Huether

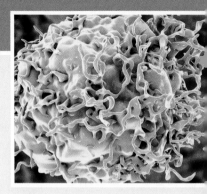

EVOLVE WEBSITE

http://evolve.elsevier.com/Huether/
Student Review Questions
Audio Key Points

Case Studies
Animations
Quick Check Answers

CHAPTER OUTLINE

The male and female reproductive systems have several anatomic and physiologic features in common. Most obvious is their major function—reproduction—through which a 23-chromosome female gamete, the ovum (pl., ova), and a 23-chromosome male gamete, the spermatozoon (sperm cell), unite to form a 46-chromosome zygote that is capable of developing into a new individual. The male reproductive system produces sperm that can be transferred to the female reproductive tract. The female reproductive system produces the ovum; if the ovum is fertilized, it is then called the embryo and developing fetus. These functions are determined not only by anatomic structures but also by complex hormonal and neurologic factors.

DEVELOPMENT OF THE REPRODUCTIVE SYSTEMS

The structure and function of both male and female reproductive systems depend on steroid hormones called sex hormones and their precursors. Cholesterol is the precursor for steroid hormones, including the sex hormones (e.g., estrogen and testosterone). Other hormones that are not steroid hormones (e.g., gonadotropins) also support reproduction. The actions of both sex and reproductive hormones are summarized in Table 34.1. Sex and reproductive hormones, like all hormones, act on target tissues by binding with cellular receptors (see Chapter 20). Hormonal effects on the reproductive systems begin during embryonic development and continue in varying degrees throughout life.

Sexual Differentiation in Utero

Initially, in embryonic development, the reproductive structures of male and female embryos are homologous (the same) or undifferentiated. They consist of one pair of primary sex organs, or gonads, and two pairs of ducts—the wolffian ducts and the müllerian ducts (Fig. 34.1). The müllerian ducts are the precursor of the internal female sex organs (oviducts, uterus, cervix, and upper vagina). The wolffian ducts are the precursor of male internal sex organs (secrete testosterone and promote development of the male sex organs).

The first sign of development of reproductive organs (male or female) occurs during the fifth week of gestation. Between 6 and 7 weeks' gestation, the male embryo differentiates under the influence of testes-determining factor (TDF), a protein expressed by a gene in the sex-determining region on the Y chromosome called *SRY*. When the *SRY* gene is expressed, male gonadal development prevails. TDF stimulates the male gonads to develop into the two testes, and by 8 weeks' gestation testosterone secretion begins. Müllerian inhibitory hormone (MIH), secreted by Sertoli cells in the testes, promotes degeneration of the müllerian ducts. The Leydig cells secrete testosterone and promote Wolffian duct development, which differentiates into the epididymis, vas deferens, seminal vesicles, and ejaculatory ducts. By 9 months' gestation, the male gonads (testes) have descended into the scrotum. The testes produce sperm after puberty.

Female gonadal development occurs in the absence of *SRY* expression and with the expression of other genes. The presence of *estrogen* and

TABLE 34.1   Summary of Female and Male Sex and Reproductive Hormones

Hormone (Source)	Action in Females	Action in Males
Dehydroepiandrosterone (DHEA) (adrenal gland, ovary, other tissues)	Converted to androstenedione and then to estrogens, testosterone, or both	Converted to androstenedione and then to estrogens, testosterone, or both
Estrogens (estrone, estradiol, estriol) (ovary and placenta, small amounts in other tissues)	Stimulates development of female sexual characteristics: maturation of breast, uterus, and vagina; promotes proliferative development of endometrium during menstrual cycle; during pregnancy promotes mammary gland development, fetal adrenal gland function, and uteroplacental blood flow (see Box 34.1)	Growth at puberty, growth plate fusion in bone, prevention of apoptosis of germ cells
Testosterone (adrenal glands from DHEA, testes)	Libido, learning, sleep, protein anabolism, growth of muscle and bone; growth of pubic and axillary hair; activation of sebaceous glands, accounting for some cases of acne during puberty	Stimulates spermatogenesis, stimulates development of primary and secondary sexual characteristics, promotes growth of muscle and bone (anabolic effect); growth of pubic and axillary hair; activates sebaceous glands, accounting for some cases of acne during puberty; maintains libido
Gonadotropin-releasing hormone (GnRH) (hypothalamus-neuroendocrine cells)	Stimulates secretion of gonadotropins (FSH and LH) from anterior pituitary	Stimulates secretion of gonadotropins (FSH and LH) from anterior pituitary
Follicle-stimulating hormone (FSH) (anterior pituitary, gonadotroph cells)	Gonadotropin; promotes development of ovarian follicle; stimulates estrogen secretion	Gonadotropin; promotes development and growth of testes and stimulates spermatogenesis by Sertoli cells
Luteinizing hormone (LH) (anterior pituitary, gonadotroph cells)	Gonadotropin; triggers ovulation; promotes development of corpus luteum	Gonadotropin; stimulates testosterone production by Leydig cells of testis
Inhibin (ovary and testes)	Inhibits FSH production in anterior pituitary (perhaps by limiting GnRH)	Inhibits FSH production in anterior pituitary
Human chorionic gonadotropin (hCG) (placenta)	Supports corpus luteum, which secretes estrogen and progesterone during first 7 weeks of pregnancy	
Activin (ovary)	Stimulates secretion of FSH and pituitary response to GnRH and FSH binding in dominant granulosa cells	
Progesterone (ovary and placenta)	Promotes secretory changes in endometrium during luteal phase of menstrual cycle; quiets uterine myometrium (muscle) activity and prevents lactogenesis during pregnancy	
Relaxin (corpus luteum, myometrium and placenta)	Inhibits uterine contractions during pregnancy and softens pelvic joints and cervix to facilitate childbirth	

the absence of *testosterone* and MIH cause degeneration in the wolffian ducts and maintenance of the müllerian ducts. At 6 to 8 weeks' gestation, the two female gonads develop into ovaries, which will produce ova. The upper ends of the müllerian ducts become the fallopian tubules, whereas the lower ends join to become the uterus, cervix, and upper two thirds of the vagina (see Fig. 34.1). The fallopian tubes will carry ova from the ovaries to the uterus during a female's reproductive years. Lack of testosterone and the presence of estrogen promote the development of external genitalia (lower end of vagina, labia, and clitoris).

Like the internal reproductive structures, the external structures develop from homologous embryonic tissues. During the first 7 to 8 weeks' gestation, both male and female embryos develop an elevated structure called the *genital tubercle* (Fig. 34.2). **Testosterone** is necessary for the genital tubercle to differentiate into external male genitalia; otherwise, female genitalia develop, which may occur even in the absence of ovaries, possibly because of the presence of placental estrogens.

Anterior pituitary development begins between the fourth and fifth weeks of fetal life, and the vascular connection between the hypothalamus and the pituitary is established by the twelfth week. **Gonadotropin-releasing hormone (GnRH)** is produced in the hypothalamus by 10 weeks' gestation and controls the production of two gonadotropins,

luteinizing hormone (LH) and follicle-stimulating hormone (FSH), by the anterior pituitary gland. In the female fetus, high levels of FSH and LH are excreted. FSH and LH stimulate the production of estrogen and progesterone by the ovary. The production of FSH and LH increases until about 28 weeks' gestation, when the production of estrogen and progesterone by the ovaries and placenta is high enough to result in the decline of gonadotropin production. Production of primitive female gametes (ova) occurs solely during fetal life. From puberty to menopause, one female gamete matures per menstrual cycle. Production of the male gametes (sperm) begins at puberty; after that, millions are produced daily, usually for life.

Puberty and Reproductive Maturation

Adolescence is the stage of human development between childhood and adulthood and includes social, psychologic, and biologic changes. **Puberty** is the onset of sexual maturation and differs from adolescence. Genetics, environment, ethnicity, general health, and nutrition can influence the timing of puberty. In females, puberty begins at about age 8 to 9 years with **thelarche** (breast development). In males, it begins later—at about age 11 years and occurs earlier with increased weight and body mass index.[1]

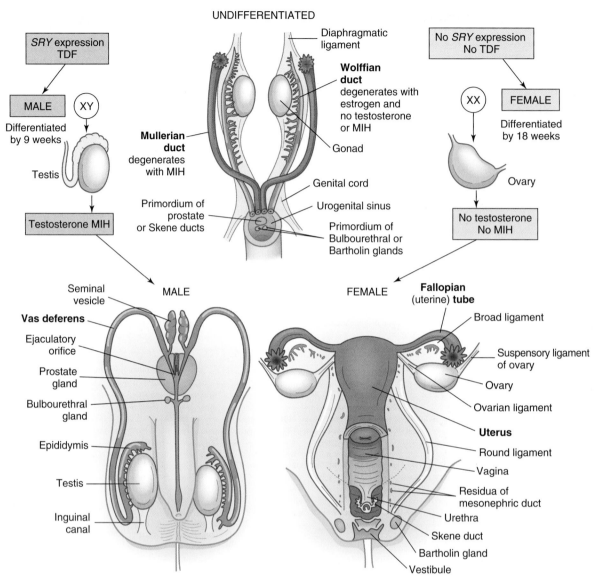

FIGURE 34.1 Embryonic Sexual Differentiation. Embryonic and fetal development of the internal genitalia. *MIH,* Müllerian inhibitory hormone; *SRY,* gene that produces TDF; *TDF,* testosterone development factor; see text for additional details.

Reproductive maturation involves the hypothalamic-pituitary-gonadal axis, the central nervous system, and the endocrine system (Fig. 34.3). There is a sequential series of hormonal events that promote sexual maturation as puberty approaches. Nocturnal gonadotropin secretion (i.e., LH and FSH) and an increased response in the pituitary to GnRH occur about 1 year before puberty. This, in turn, stimulates gonadal maturation (**gonadarche**) with estradiol secretion in females and testosterone secretion in males. Estradiol causes thelarche, maturation of the reproductive organs (vagina, uterus, ovaries), and deposition of fat in the female's hips. Estrogen and increased production of growth factors cause rapid skeletal growth in both males and females. Testosterone causes growth of the testes, scrotum, and penis. A positive feedback loop is created with gonadotropins stimulating the gonads to produce more sex hormones. The most important hormonal effects occur in the gonads. In males, the testes begin to produce mature sperm that are capable of fertilizing an ovum. Male puberty is complete with the first ejaculation that contains mature sperm. In females, the ovaries begin to release mature ova. Female puberty is complete at the time of

the first ovulatory menstrual period; however, this can take up to 1 to 2 years after menarche. Before puberty there also is an increase in adrenal androgen in both sexes, known as **adrenarche**. Adrenal androgens are converted to testosterone and estradiol and contribute to the growth of axillary and pubic hair and activation of sweat and sebaceous glands during puberty. In short, puberty is complete when an individual is capable of reproduction.

✔**QUICK CHECK 34.1**
1. What is the function of gonadotropin during puberty?
2. When do sex hormones first exhibit an effect on sexual development?

THE FEMALE REPRODUCTIVE SYSTEM

The function of the female reproductive system is to produce mature ova; then, if fertilization occurs, the female reproductive system provides protection and nourishment to the fetus until it is expelled at birth.

UNDIFFERENTIATED

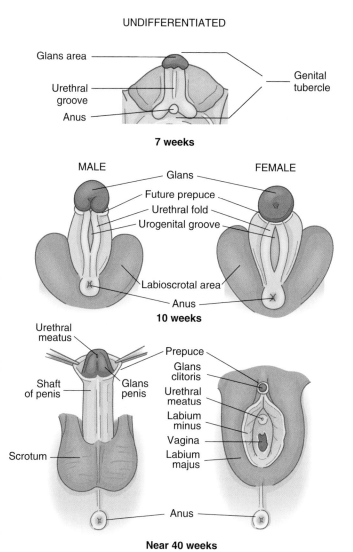

7 weeks

MALE   FEMALE

10 weeks

Near 40 weeks

FIGURE 34.2 External Genitalia Development. Embryonic and fetal development of the external genitalia.

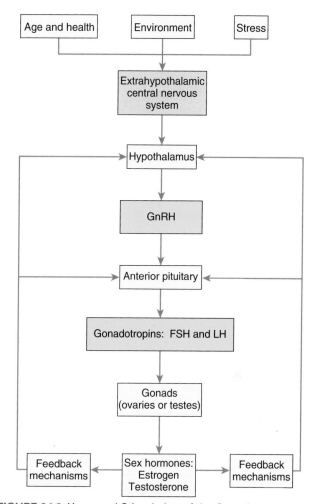

FIGURE 34.3 Hormonal Stimulation of the Gonads. The hypothalamic-pituitary-gonadal axis. *FSH,* follicle-stimulating hormone; *GnRH,* gonadotropin-releasing hormone; *LH,* luteinizing hormone.

External Genitalia

The external genitalia protect body openings and play an important role in sexual functioning. Fig. 34.4 shows the external female genitalia, known collectively as the **vulva**, or pudendum. The major structures are as follows:

- *Mons pubis:* A fatty layer of tissue with a moundlike shape over the pubic symphysis (joint formed by union of the pubic bones) that protects the joint during sexual intercourse. During puberty it becomes covered with pubic hair, and sebaceous and sweat glands become more active. Estrogen causes the fat to be deposited under the skin.
- *Labia majora (sing., labium majus):* Two folds of skin arising at the mons pubis and extending back to the fourchette, forming a cleft. During puberty the amount of fatty tissue increases, pubic hair grows on lateral surfaces, and sebaceous glands on hairless medial surfaces secrete lubricants. This structure is highly sensitive to temperature, touch, pressure, and pain and protects the inner structures of the vulva. It is homologous to the male scrotum.
- *Labia minora (sing., labium minus):* Two smaller, thinner, asymmetric folds of skin within the labia majora that form the clitoral hood (prepuce) and frenulum, then split to enclose the vestibule, and

converge near the anus to form the fourchette. The labia minora are hairless, pink, and moist; they are well supplied by nerves, blood vessels, and sebaceous glands that secrete bactericidal fluid with a distinctive odor that lubricates and waterproofs vulvar skin. The labia swell with blood during sexual arousal.

- *Clitoris:* A richly innervated erectile organ between the labia minora. It is a small, cylindric structure having a visible glans and a shaft that lies beneath the skin; the clitoris is homologous to the penis. It secretes smegma, which has a unique odor that may be sexually arousing to the male. Like the penis, the clitoris is a major site of sexual stimulation and orgasm. With sexual arousal, erectile tissue fills with blood, causing the clitoris to enlarge slightly.
- *Vestibule:* An area protected by the labia minora that contains the external opening of the vagina, called the *introitus* or vaginal orifice. A thin, perforated membrane, the *hymen,* may cover the introitus. The vestibule also contains the opening of the urethra, or *urinary meatus* (orifice). These structures are lubricated by two pairs of glands: Skene glands and Bartholin glands. The ducts of the *Skene glands* (also called the *lesser vestibular* or *paraurethral glands)* open on both sides of the urinary meatus. The ducts of the *Bartholin glands (greater vestibular* or *vulvovaginal glands)* open on either side of the introitus. In response to sexual stimulation, Bartholin glands secrete mucus that lubricates the inner labial surfaces, as well as enhances the viability and motility of sperm. Skene glands help

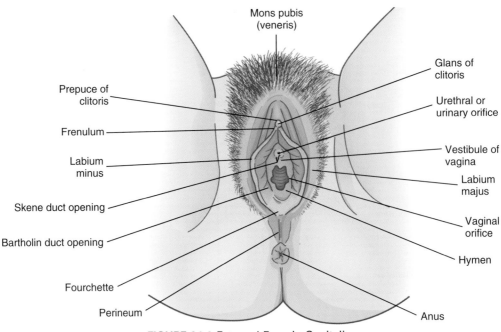

FIGURE 34.4 External Female Genitalia.

lubricate the urinary meatus and the vestibule. In response to sexual excitement, the highly vascular tissue just beneath the vestibule also fills with blood and becomes engorged.

- *Perineum:* An area with less hair, skin, and subcutaneous tissue lying between the vaginal orifice and anus. Unlike the rest of the vulva, this area has little subcutaneous fat so the skin is close to the underlying muscles. The perineum covers the muscular *perineal body,* a fibrous structure that consists of elastic fibers and connective tissue and serves as the common attachment for the bulbocavernosus, external anal sphincter, and levator ani muscles. The perineum varies in length from 2 to 5 cm or more and has elastic properties. The length of the perineum and the elasticity of the perineal body influence tissue resistance and injury during childbirth.

Internal Genitalia
Vagina
The **vagina** is an elastic, fibromuscular canal that is 9 to 10 cm long in a reproductive-age female. It extends up and back from the introitus to the lower portion of the uterus. As Fig. 34.5 shows, the vagina lies between the urethra (and part of the bladder) and the rectum. Mucosal secretions from the upper genital organs, menstrual fluids, and products of conception leave the body through the vagina. During coitus, the penis enters the vagina. During sexual arousal, the vagina lengthens and widens and the vaginal wall becomes engorged with blood, much like the labia minora and clitoris. Engorgement pushes some fluid to the surface of the mucosa, enhancing lubrication. The vaginal wall does not contain mucus-secreting glands; rather, secretions drain into the vagina from the endocervical glands or from the Bartholin and Skene glands of the vestibule. The vagina also functions as the birth canal during childbirth. Its elasticity and relatively sparse nerve supply enhance the vagina's function in this role. During childbirth, the pelvic floor muscles and rugae of the vagina stretch to facilitate the passage of the infant.

The vaginal wall is lined with a mucous membrane of squamous epithelial cells that thickens and thins in response to hormones, particularly estrogen. The squamous epithelial membrane is continuous with the membrane that covers the lower part of the uterus. In females of reproductive age, the mucosal layer is arranged in transverse wrinkles, or folds, called **rugae** (sing., **ruga**), that permit stretching during coitus and childbirth. Below the mucosal layer are three more layers: fibrous connective tissue containing numerous blood and lymphatic vessels, smooth muscle and connective tissue, and a rich network of blood vessels.

The upper part of the vagina surrounds the cervix, the lower end of the uterus (see Fig. 34.5). The recessed space around the cervix is called the **fornix** of the vagina. The posterior fornix is "deeper" than the anterior fornix because of the angle at which the cervix meets the vaginal canal. In most females this angle is about 90 degrees. A pouch called the **cul-de-sac** separates the posterior fornix and the rectum.

Two factors help maintain the self-cleansing action of the vagina and defend it from infection, particularly during the reproductive years. They are (1) an acid-base balance that discourages the proliferation of most pathogenic bacteria and (2) the thickness of the vaginal epithelium. Before puberty, vaginal pH is about 7.0 (neutral) and the vaginal epithelium is thin. At puberty, the pH becomes more acidic (4.0 to 5.0) and the squamous epithelial lining thickens. These changes are maintained until menopause (cessation of menstruation), when the pH rises again to more alkaline levels and the epithelium thins. Therefore protection from infection is greatest during the years when a female is most likely to be sexually active. Both defense factors are greatest when estrogen levels are high and the vagina contains a normal population of *Lactobacillus acidophilus,* a harmless resident bacterium that helps maintain pH at acidic levels. Any condition that causes vaginal pH to rise—such as douching or use of vaginal sprays or deodorants, the presence of low estrogen levels, or destruction of *L. acidophilus* by antibiotics—lowers vaginal defenses against infection.

Uterus
The **uterus** is a hollow, pear-shaped organ whose lower end opens into the vagina. It anchors and protects a fertilized ovum, provides an optimal environment while the ovum develops, and pushes the fetus out at birth. In addition, the uterus plays an important role in sexual response and conception. During sexual excitement, the opening of the lower uterus (the cervix) dilates slightly. At the same time, the uterus increases

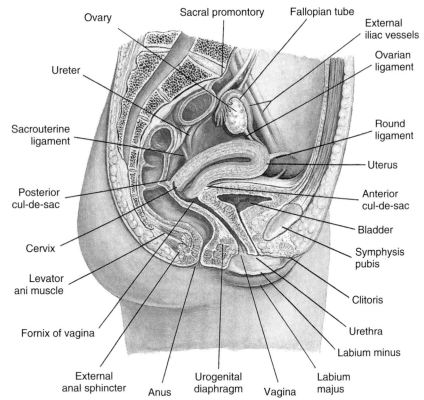

FIGURE 34.5 Internal Female Genitalia and Other Pelvic Organs. (From Ball JW et al: *Seidel's guide to physical examination,* ed 8, St Louis, 2015, Mosby.)

in size and moves upward and backward, creating a tenting effect in the midvagina that results in the cervix "sitting" in a pool of semen. During orgasm, rhythmic contractions facilitate movement of sperm through the cervical os while also enhancing physical pleasure.

At puberty, the uterus attains its adult size and proportions and descends from the abdomen to the lower pelvis, between the bladder and the rectum (see Fig. 34.5). The uterus of a mature, nonpregnant female is approximately 7 to 9 cm long and 6.5 cm wide, with muscular walls 3.5 cm thick, and enlarges about 1 cm in all dimensions after pregnancy.[2] It is loosely held in position by ligaments, peritoneal tissue folds, and the pressure of adjacent organs, especially the urinary bladder, sigmoid colon, and rectum. In most females, the uterus is tipped forward (anteverted) so that it rests on the urinary bladder. However, it may be tipped backward (retroverted) and various degrees of forward or backward flexion are normal (Fig. 34.6).

The uterus has two major parts: the corpus (body of the uterus) and the cervix (Fig. 34.7). The top of the corpus, above the insertion of the fallopian tubes, is called the fundus. The diameter of the uterine cavity is widest at the fundus and narrowest at the isthmus, just above the cervix (see Fig. 34.5). The cervix, or "neck of the uterus," extends from the isthmus to the vagina. The passageway between the upper opening (the internal os) and the lower opening (the external os) of the cervix is called the endocervical canal (see Fig. 34.7). The entire uterus, like the upper vagina, is innervated exclusively by motor and sensory fibers of the autonomic nervous system.

The uterine wall is composed of three layers (see Fig. 34.7). The perimetrium (parietal peritoneum) is the outer serous membrane that covers the uterus. The myometrium is the thick, muscular middle layer. It is thickest at the fundus, apparently to facilitate birth. The endometrium, or uterine lining, is composed of a functional layer

(superficial compact layer and spongy middle layer) and a basal layer. The functional layer of the endometrium responds to the sex hormones estrogen and progesterone. Between puberty and menopause, this layer proliferates and is shed monthly. The basal layer, which is attached to the myometrium, regenerates the functional layer after shedding (menstruation).

The endocervical canal does not have an endometrial layer but is lined with columnar epithelial cells. It is continuous with the lining of the outer cervix and vagina, which are lined with squamous epithelial cells. The point where the two types of cells meet is called the *transformation zone,* or squamous-columnar junction (see Fig. 35.16. The transformation zone is vulnerable to the human papillomavirus, which can lead to cervical dysplasia or carcinoma in situ. Cells of the transformation zone are removed for examination during a Papanicolaou (Pap test) smear.

The cervix acts as a mechanical barrier, protecting the uterus from infectious microorganisms from the vagina. The external cervical os is a very small opening that contains thick, sticky mucus (the mucous "plug") during the luteal phase of the menstrual cycle and throughout pregnancy. During ovulation, the mucus changes under the influence of estrogen and forms watery strands, or spinnbarkeit mucus, to facilitate the transport of sperm into the uterus. In addition, the downward flow of cervical secretions moves microorganisms away from the cervix and uterus. In females of reproductive age, the pH of these secretions is inhospitable to many bacteria. Further, mucosal secretions contain enzymes and antibodies (mostly immunoglobulin A [IgA]) of the secretory immune system. Uterine pathophysiologic disorders include infection, displacement of the uterus within the pelvis, benign growths (fibroids) of the uterine wall, hyperplasia of the endometrium, endometriosis, and cancer (see Chapter 35).

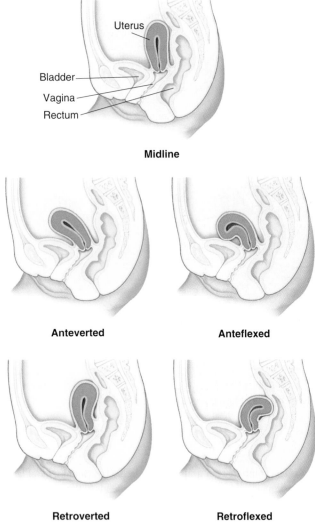

Midline

Anteverted

Anteflexed

Retroverted

Retroflexed

FIGURE 34.6 Variations in Uterine Positions.

Fallopian Tubes

The two **fallopian tubes (oviducts, uterine tubes)** enter the uterus bilaterally just beneath the fundus (see Fig. 34.7). They direct the ova from the spaces around the ovaries to the uterus. From the uterus, the fallopian tubes curve up and over the two ovaries. Each tube is 8 to 12 cm long and about 1 cm in diameter, except at its ovarian end, which resembles the bell of a trumpet and is fringed or fimbriated (**infundibulum**). The fimbriae (fringes) move, creating a current that draws the ovum into the infundibulum. Once the ovum enters the fallopian tube, cilia (hairlike structures) and peristalsis (muscle contractions) keep it moving toward the uterus.

The ampulla, or distal third, of the fallopian tube is the usual site of fertilization (see Fig. 34.7). Sperm released into the vagina travel upward through the endocervical canal and uterine cavity and enter the fallopian tubes. If an ovum is present in either tube, fertilization can occur. Whether or not the ovum encounters sperm, it continues to travel through the fallopian tube to the uterus. If fertilized, the ovum (then called a *blastocyst*) implants itself in the endometrial layer of the uterine wall. If not fertilized, the ovum fragments and leaves the uterus with menstrual fluids. Disorders that affect the fallopian tubes (e.g., congenital malformations, infection, and inflammation) block the path of both sperm and the ovum and may cause infertility or ectopic (tubal) pregnancy.

Ovaries

The **ovaries**, the female gonads, are the primary female reproductive organs (Fig. 34.8). Their two main functions are secretion of female sex hormones and development and release of female gametes, or ova.

The almond-shaped ovaries are located on both sides of the uterus and are suspended and supported by a portion of the broad ligament (the mesovarium component), ovarian ligaments, and suspensory ligaments (see Fig. 34.7). The ovaries are smaller than their male homologs, the testes. In females of reproductive age, each ovary is about 3 to 5 cm long, 2.5 cm wide, and 2 cm thick and weighs 4 to 8 g. Size and weight vary slightly during each phase of the menstrual cycle (see the Menstrual (Ovarian) Cycle section).

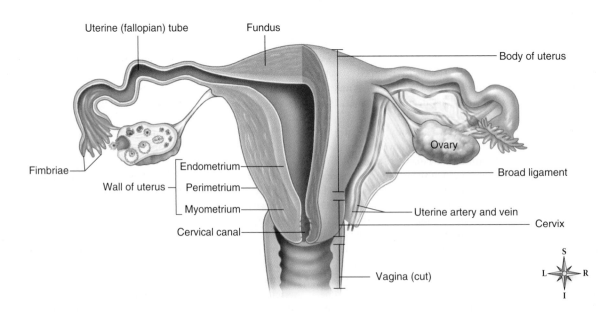

FIGURE 34.7 Cross Section of Uterus, Fallopian Tube, and Ovary. (From Ball JW et al: *Seidel's guide to physical examination*, ed 8, St Louis, 2015, Mosby.)

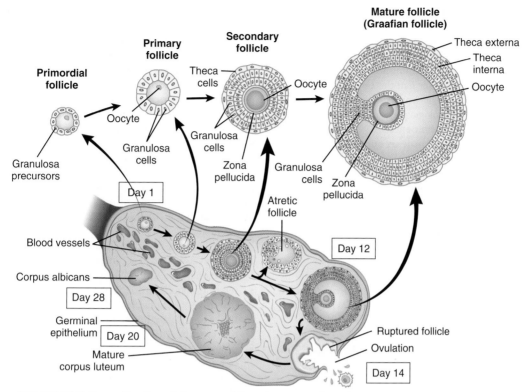

FIGURE 34.8 Cross Section of Ovary and Development of an Ovarian Follicle. Schematic representation (not to scale) of the structure of the ovary, showing the various stages in the development of the follicle and its successor structure, the corpus luteum. (Adapted from Berne RM, Levy MN, editors: *Physiology,* ed 5, St Louis, 2003, Mosby.)

At birth, the cortex of each ovary contains approximately 1 to 2 million ova within primordial (immature) **ovarian follicles**. By puberty, the number ranges between 300,000 and 500,000, and some of the follicles and the ova within them begin to mature. Between puberty and menopause, the ovarian cortex always contains follicles and ova in various stages of development (primary and secondary follicles). Once every menstrual cycle (about every 28 days), one of the follicles reaches maturation and discharges its ovum through the ovary's outer covering, the germinal epithelium. During the reproductive years, 400 to 500 ovarian follicles mature completely and release an ovum (ovulation). The remaining follicles either fail to develop at all or degenerate without maturing completely and are known as atretic follicles (see Fig. 34.8).

After release of the mature ovum (ovulation), the follicle develops into another structure, the **corpus luteum** (see Fig. 34.8). If fertilization occurs, the corpus luteum enlarges and begins to secrete hormones that maintain and support pregnancy. If fertilization does not occur, the corpus luteum secretes these hormones for approximately 14 days and then degenerates, which triggers the maturation of another follicle. The **ovarian cycle**—the process of follicular maturation, ovulation, corpus luteum development, and corpus luteum degeneration—is continuous from puberty to menopause, except during pregnancy or hormonal contraceptive use. At menopause, this process ceases and the ovaries atrophy to the point that they cannot be felt during a pelvic examination.

Sex hormones are secreted by cells present within the ovarian cortex, including two types of cells in the ovarian follicle—**theca cells** (produce androgens that migrate to granulosa cells) and **granulosa cells** (convert androgens to estradiol)—and cells of the corpus luteum (secrete primarily progesterone, estrogen, and inhibin) (see Fig. 34.8). These cells all contain receptors for the gonadotropins (LH, FSH) or for the sex hormones, which are discussed in the next section.

> **✓ QUICK CHECK 34.2**
> 1. Where are the Bartholin glands located? What is their function?
> 2. Name three functions of the uterus.
> 3. What is the name of the area in which cervical cancer is most likely to grow?
> 4. Why is the ovary the most essential female reproductive organ?

Female Sex Hormones

The sex hormones are all steroid hormones and are synthesized from cholesterol (see Chapter 20). Both male and female sex hormones are present in all adults. However, the female body contains low levels of testosterone and other androgens, and the male body contains low levels of estrogen. Individual effects of sex hormones depend on the amount and concentration in the blood.

Estrogens and Androgens

Estrogen is a generic term for any of three similar hormones derived from cholesterol: estradiol, estrone, and estriol. **Estradiol** (E_2) is the most potent and plentiful of the three and is principally produced (95%) by the ovaries (ovarian follicle and corpus luteum). Limited amounts are secreted by the cortices of the adrenal glands and the placenta during pregnancy. Androgens are converted to estrone in ovarian and adipose tissue; estriol is the peripheral metabolite of estrone and estradiol.

Estrogen has numerous biologic effects, many of which involve interactions with other hormones. It is needed for maturation of reproductive organs, development of secondary sex characteristics, growth, and maintenance of pregnancy. It also is needed for many nonreproductive effects, including closure of long bones after the pubertal growth spurt (in both males and females), maintenance of bone and skin, and systemic organ function (see Table 34.1 and Box 34.1). After menopause, the ovaries dramatically reduce production of estradiol and secretion of estrone is markedly diminished (see the Aging and the Female Reproductive System section). At this time, the majority of estradiol is derived from intracellular synthesis in peripheral tissues. Estradiol acts locally to meet physiologic needs according to cell type and is then inactivated without systemic effects.[3]

Although androgens are primarily male sex hormones produced in the testes, small amounts are produced in the adrenal cortex in both males and females and in the ovaries in females. Some androgens (dehydroepiandrosterone and its metabolite androstenedione) are precursors of estrogens (estrone, estradiol) (see Table 34.1). At puberty, androgens contribute to the skeletal growth spurt and cause growth of pubic and axillary hair. Androgens also activate sebaceous glands, accounting for some cases of acne during puberty, and play a role in libido.

Progesterone

LH from the anterior pituitary stimulates the corpus luteum to secrete progesterone, the second major female sex hormone. With estrogen, progesterone controls the ovarian menstrual cycle. LH surge occurs when there is a peak level of estrogen, about 24 to 36 hours before ovulation. LH promotes luteinization of the granulosa in the dominant follicle, resulting in progesterone production and the development of blood vessels and connective tissue. During the follicular phase, the ovary and adrenal glands each contribute approximately 50% of the progesterone production. Conversely, large amounts are cyclically secreted from the ovary while the corpus luteum is active for about 9 to 13 days after ovulation. (The complementary and opposing effects of progesterone and estrogen are listed in Table 34.2.) Progesterone secreted by the corpus luteum stimulates the thickened endometrium to become more complex in preparation for implantation of a blastocyte. If conception and implantation do occur, the corpus luteum persists and secretes progesterone (and estrogen) until the placenta is well established at approximately 8 to 10 weeks' gestation and undertakes progesterone production.

Progesterone is sometimes called the *hormone of pregnancy*. Progesterone's effects in pregnancy include:
- maintaining the thickened endometrium;
- relaxing smooth muscle in the myometrium, which prevents premature contractions and helps the uterus to expand;
- thickening (hypertrophy) the myometrium, which prepares it for the muscular work of labor;
- promoting growth of lobules and alveoli in the breast in preparation for lactation, but preventing lactation until the fetus is born and then promoting lactation in collaboration with prolactin after birth;
- preventing additional maturation of ova by suppressing FSH and LH, thereby stopping the menstrual cycle; and
- providing immune modulation, allowing tolerance against fetal antigens (the mother's immune system does not attack the fetus).

Menstrual (Ovarian) Cycle

In addition to pregnancy, the obvious manifestation of female reproductive functioning is menstrual bleeding (the menses), which starts with menarche (first menstruation) and ends with menopause (cessation of menstrual flow for 1 year). In the United States, the age of first menstruation is about 9 to 13 years.[4] Onset of menarche appears to be related to body weight, especially percentage of body fat (a high ratio of fat to lean tissue). The hormone leptin increases before the onset of menarche. Leptin (a regulatory hormone of appetite and energy metabolism) promotes the secretion of kisspeptin from the hypothalamus and leads to the release of GnRH, which in turn enhances release of FSH and LH and estradiol, triggering ovulation and the onset of puberty. A high percentage of body fat is associated with higher levels of leptin.

BOX 34.1   Summary of Nonreproductive Effects of Estrogen

- Estrogens (including estrone, estradiol, estriol) function through estrogen receptors alpha and beta, have different roles in different cells and tissues, and have paracrine or intracrine function.
- Maintains bone density by antagonizing effects of parathyroid hormone.
- Acts in liver to decrease cholesterol level, increase high-density lipoprotein (HDL) level, and decrease low-density lipoprotein (LDL) level (antiatherosclerotic); promotes fat deposition
- Maintains nervous system (neurotrophic and neuroprotective); facilitates memory and cognition.
- Increases collagen content, dermal thickness, elasticity, water content, and healing ability of skin.
- Protects against chronic kidney disease in individuals without diabetes.
- Prevents vascular injury and early atheroma formation through endothelial mechanisms.
- Inhibits platelet adhesiveness.
- Can promote inflammation and have variable effects on immunity.
- Promotes clotting; increased risk of thromboembolism (only estrogen associated with pregnancy or use in contraceptive pills or hormone replacement therapy).

TABLE 34.2   Complementary and Opposing Effects of Estrogen and Progesterone

Structure	Effect of Estrogen	Effect of Progesterone
Vaginal mucosa	Proliferation of squamous epithelium; increase in glycogen content of cells; layering (cornification) of cells	Thinning of squamous epithelium; decornification
Cervical mucosa	Production of abundant fluid secretions that favor survival and enhance motility of sperm	Production of thick, sticky secretions that tend to plug cervical os
Fallopian tube	Increase of motility and ciliary action	Decrease of motility and ciliary action
Uterine muscle	Increase of blood flow; increase of contractile proteins; increase of uterine muscle and myometrial excitability to action potential; increase of sensitization to oxytocin	Relaxation of myometrium; decrease of sensitization to oxytocin
Endometrium	Stimulation of growth; increase in number of progesterone receptors	Activation of glands and blood vessels; accumulation of glycogen and enzymes; decrease in number of estrogen receptors
Breasts	Growth of ducts; promotion of prolactin effects	Growth of lobules and alveoli; inhibition of prolactin effects

Childhood obesity is associated with an increase in leptin and with early menarche (age 11 years or younger).[5]

Cycles are not ovulatory at first and may vary in length from 10 to 60 days or more. As adolescence proceeds, regular patterns of menstruation and ovulation are established at intervals ranging between 21 and 45 days.[6] Menstruation continues to recur in a recognizable and characteristic pattern during adulthood, with the length of the menstrual cycle varying considerably among individuals. The commonly accepted cycle average is 28 (25 to 30) days, with rhythmic intervals of 21 to 35 days considered normal (Fig. 34.9). Approximately 2 to 8 years before menopause, cycles begin to lengthen again with variation related to changing hormone levels.[7]

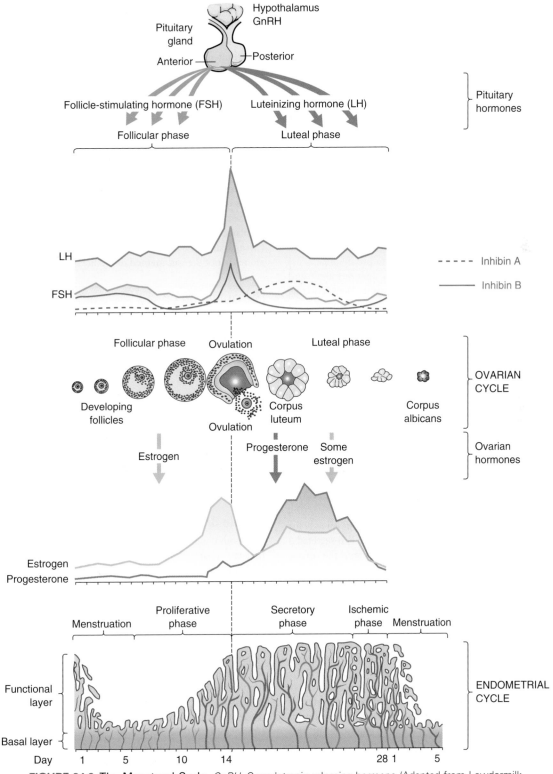

FIGURE 34.9 The Menstrual Cycle. *GnRH,* Gonadotropin-releasing hormone (Adapted from Lowdermilk DL, et al: *Maternity and women's health care,* ed 10, St Louis, 2012, Mosby.)

Phases of the Menstrual Cycle

The menstrual (ovarian) cycle (see Fig. 34.9) is the process of menstruation (menses) in the uterine endometrium and ovulation in the ovary. The cycle consists of the follicular/proliferative phase (postmenstrual) followed by the luteal/secretory phase (premenstrual) and then the ischemic/menstrual phase if conception does not occur. These are named for processes that occur in the ovary (follicular and luteal phases) and the uterine endometrium (proliferative, secretory, and ischemic phases) during the menstrual cycle.

During menstruation (menses), the functional layer of the endometrium disintegrates and is discharged through the vagina. Menstruation is followed by the follicular/proliferative phase. This phase is named for two simultaneous processes: maturation of an ovarian follicle and proliferation of the uterine endometrium (see Fig. 34.9). During this phase, GnRH and a balance between activin and inhibin levels from the granulosa cells contribute to the increase of FSH level, which stimulates a number of follicles. The result is a rescue of a dominant ovarian follicle from normal dissolution by days 5 to 7 of the cycle. Together, estrogen and FSH make the granulosa cells of the primary follicle more sensitive to FSH and promote LH stimulation, which causes a more rapid secretion of follicular estrogen. A surge in the levels of both LH and FSH then is required for final follicular growth and ovulation. Estrogen level increase and inhibin B inhibits the secretion of FSH level by the granulosa cells in the dominant follicle. This drop in FSH concentration decreases the growth of less developed follicles (see Fig. 34.8). Estrogen causes cells of the endometrium to proliferate.

Ovulation is the release of an ovum from a mature follicle and marks the beginning of the luteal/secretory phase of the menstrual cycle. The ovarian follicle begins its transformation into a corpus luteum (see Fig. 34.8), hence the name *luteal phase*. Pulsatile secretion of LH from the anterior pituitary stimulates the corpus luteum to secrete progesterone, estrogen, and inhibin A (suppresses FSH secretion), which in turn initiates the secretory phase of endometrial development. Estrogen maintains the thickness of the endometrium, and progesterone stimulates growth of glands and blood vessels in the endometrium. The glands begin to secrete a thin, glycogen-containing fluid, hence the name *secretory phase*. At this point, one of the following two paths occurs:

- If conception and implantation do not occur, the corpus luteum degenerates and ceases its production of progesterone and estrogen. Without progesterone or estrogen to maintain it, the endometrium enters the ischemic ("blood-starved") phase and disintegrates, hence the name ischemic/menstrual phase. Menstruation then occurs, marking the beginning of another cycle.
- If conception occurs, the nutrient-laden endometrium is ready for implantation. Human chorionic gonadotropin (hCG) is secreted 3 days after fertilization by the blastocytes and maintains the corpus luteum once implantation occurs at about day 6 or 7. hCG can be detected in maternal blood and urine 8 to 10 days after ovulation. The production of estrogen and progesterone will continue until the placenta can adequately maintain hormonal production.

Ovulatory cycles appear to have a minimum length of 24 to 26.5 days: the ovarian follicle requires 10 to 12.5 days to develop, and the luteal phase appears fixed at 14 days (±3 days). Menstrual blood flow usually lasts 3 to 7 days, but may be between 2 and 8 days and still be considered within normal limits. Bleeding is consistently scant to heavy and varies from 30 to 80 ml, with most blood loss occurring during the first 3 days of menses. Menstrual discharge consists of blood, mucus, and desquamated endometrial tissue and does not clot under normal circumstances. It is usually dark and produces a characteristic musty odor on oxidation. Environmental factors such as severe emotional stress, illness, malnutrition, obesity, and seasonal variation may affect the length of the menstrual cycle.[8-10]

Cervical mucus also undergoes cyclic changes during the menstrual cycle. During the proliferative phase, the cervical mucus is thin and watery. Peak estrogen levels occur just before ovulation and maximally stimulate the cervical glands to produce mucus. Cervical mucus becomes abundant and more elastic (spinnbarkeit) and provides access for sperm into the interior of the uterus. Changes in the consistency of cervical mucus can be used to identify fertile intervals.

The vaginal epithelium also responds to the cyclic hormonal changes of the menstrual cycle. Under the influence of estrogen, cells of the vaginal epithelium become thicker during the follicular/proliferative phase. After ovulation, layers of keratinized cells overgrow the basal epithelium (cells become larger and flatter), a process known as cornification. Near the end of the luteal phase, leukocytes invade vaginal epithelium, removing the outer layers in a process termed decornification with thinning of the epithelium.

Basal body temperature (BBT) undergoes characteristic biphasic changes during menstrual cycles in which ovulation occurs. During the follicular phase, the BBT fluctuates around 98° F (37° C). During the luteal phase, the average temperature increases by 0.4° to 1.0° F (0.2° to 0.5° C). At the end of the luteal phase, 1 to 3 days before the onset of menstruation, BBT declines to follicular-phase levels. The shift in temperature is related to ovulation, corpus luteum formation, and increased serum progesterone levels. Progesterone acts on the thermoregulatory center of the hypothalamus to increase body temperature. Changes in BBT are used to document ovulatory cycles but when used alone are not the best method to predict the exact timing of ovulation.[11]

✔ QUICK CHECK 34.3

1. What hormones does the ovary produce?
2. Why does menstruation occur?
3. What event is associated with the luteal/secretory phase of the menstrual cycle?

STRUCTURE AND FUNCTION OF THE BREAST

The breasts are modified sebaceous glands that lie on the ventral surface of the thorax, within the superficial fascia of the chest wall. They extend vertically from the second rib to the sixth or seventh intercostal space and laterally from the side of the sternum to the midaxillary line. Breast tissue also may extend into the axilla; this tissue is known as the *tail of Spence*.

Female Breast

The adult female breast is composed of 15 to 20 pyramid-shaped lobes that are separated and supported by Cooper ligaments (Fig. 34.10). Each lobe contains 20 to 40 lobules, which subdivide further into many functional units called acini (sing., acinus). Each acinus is lined with a layer of epithelial cells capable of secreting milk during lactation and a layer of subepithelial cells capable of contracting to squeeze milk from the acinus. The acini empty into a network of lobular collecting ducts, which empty into interlobular collecting and ejecting ducts. Ductal elongation and organized branching is achieved with collagen fiber alignment. The ducts reach the skin through openings (pores) in the nipple. The lobes and lobules are surrounded and separated by muscle strands and fatty connective tissue. The amount of fatty connective tissue varies among individuals, depending on weight and genetic and endocrine factors and contributes to the diversity of breast size and shape and the function of the mammary epithelium. Fat increases in the breast after menopause.[12]

An extensive capillary network surrounds the acini and is supplied by branches of the internal mammary, thoracoacromial, internal and

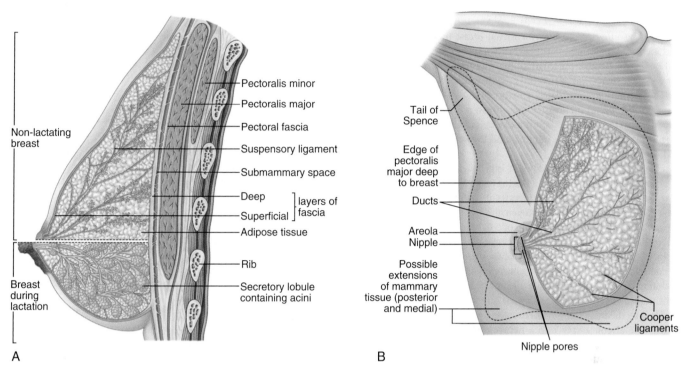

FIGURE 34.10 A, The structure of the breast. B, Changes in the breast during lactation. (From Standring S: *Gray's anatomy*, ed 41, London, 2016, Churchill Livingstone.)

lateral thoracic, and intercostal arteries. Venous return follows arterial supply, with relatively rapid emptying into the superior vena cava. The breasts receive sensory innervation from branches of the second through sixth intercostal nerves and the cervical plexus. This accounts for the fact that breast pain may be referred to the chest, back, scapula, medial arm, and neck. Lymphatic drainage of the breast occurs largely through axillary nodes, but there may be predominance of superficial mammary routes with resultant asymmetry between a person's breasts (Fig. 34.11).

The **nipple** is a pigmented cylindric structure usually located at the fourth or fifth intercostal space. It measures 0.5 to 1.3 cm in diameter and is approximately 10 to 12 mm in height when erect. On its surface lie multiple pores, one from each lobe. The **areola** is the pigmented circular area around the nipple. It may be 15 to 60 mm in diameter. A number of sebaceous glands, the **glands of Montgomery**, are located within the areola and aid in lubrication of the nipple during lactation. The nipple and areola contain smooth muscles, which receive motor innervation from the sympathetic nervous system. Breast-feeding, sexual stimulation, and exposure to cold cause the nipple to become erect.

The fetal and early postnatal development of breast tissue does not depend on hormones, although fetal breast tissue does become progressively responsive to hormonal stimulation. During childhood, breast growth is latent and growth of the nipple and areola keeps pace with body surface growth. At the onset of puberty in the female, growth hormone, insulin-like growth factor 1 (IGF1), and estrogen stimulate mammary growth. Thelarche is usually the first sign of puberty in the female. Full differentiation and development of breast tissue are mediated by the levels of several hormones, including estrogen, progesterone, prolactin, growth hormone, thyroid and parathyroid hormones, insulin, and cortisol.

During the reproductive years, the breast undergoes cyclic changes in response to changes in the levels of estrogen and progesterone associated with the menstrual cycle. Estrogen promotes development of the lobular ducts; progesterone stimulates development of cells lining

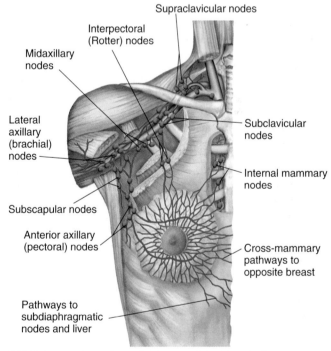

FIGURE 34.11 Lymphatic Drainage of the Female Breast. (From Ball JW, et al: *Seidel's guide to physical examination*, ed 8, St Louis, 2015, Mosby.)

the acini. During the follicular/proliferative phase of the menstrual cycle, high estradiol levels increase the vascularity of breast tissue and stimulate proliferation of ductal and acinar tissue. This effect is sustained into the luteal/secretory phase of the cycle. During this phase, progesterone levels increase and contribute to the breast changes induced by estradiol. Specific effects of progesterone include dilation of the ducts and conversion of the acinar cells into secretory cells. Most females experience some degree of premenstrual breast fullness, tenderness, and increased breast nodularity. Breast volume may increase as much as 10 to 30 ml. Because the length of the menstrual cycle does not allow for complete regression of new cell growth, breast growth continues at a slow rate until approximately 35 years of age. Because of the cyclic changes that occur in breast tissue, breast examination should be conducted at the conclusion of or a few days after the menstrual cycle, when hormonal effects are minimal and breasts are at their smallest and least tender.

The function of the female breast is primarily to provide a source of nourishment for the newborn. During pregnancy, the breast remodels into a milk-secreting organ and reaches its ultimate mature developmental stage. With increased levels of estrogen, the lobules further differentiate. Progesterone stimulates development of cells lining the alveoli to produce milk. Lactation (milk production) occurs after childbirth in response to increased levels of prolactin. Prolactin secretion, in turn, increases by continued breast-feeding. Oxytocin, another hormone released during and after delivery, controls milk ejection from alveolar cells. Milk is continuously secreted into the alveolar lumen and is stored there until suckling by the infant stimulates oxytocin, which triggers the let-down reflex. The alveoli empty into a network of lactiferous ducts. These ducts reach the skin through 9 or 10 pores in the nipple.

Physiologically, breast milk is the most appropriate nourishment for newborns. Colostrum, produced in low quantities in the first few days postpartum, is rich in immunologic components, including secretory IgA, lactoferrin, leukocytes, and developmental factors, such as epidermal growth factor. The nutrient composition changes over time to meet the changing digestive capabilities and nutritional requirements of the infant. Secretory IgA and nonspecific antimicrobial factors, such as lysosomes and lactoferrin, protect the infant against infection. During lactation, high prolactin levels interfere with hypothalamic-pituitary hormones that stimulate ovulation. This mechanism suppresses the menstrual cycle and can prevent ovulation.

Male Breast

Until puberty, development of the male breast is similar to that of the female breast. In the absence of sufficiently high levels of estrogen and progesterone, and with antagonistic effects of androgens, the male breast does not develop any further. The normal male breast consists mostly of fat with a small, underdeveloped nipple and a few ductlike structures in the subareolar area. The male breast may appear enlarged in obese males because of accumulation of fatty tissue. During puberty, some males experience benign gynecomastia (benign proliferation of male breast glandular tissue), a condition in which the breasts enlarge temporarily as a result of hormonal fluctuations, and which should be differentiated from any underlying systemic disorders.

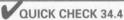
QUICK CHECK 34.4
1. What role does oxytocin play in the function of female breasts?
2. How does breast development differ between adult males and females?

THE MALE REPRODUCTIVE SYSTEM

The external genitalia in males perform the major functions of reproduction. Sperm are produced in the male gonads (testes) and delivered by the penis to the female vagina. The internal male genitalia consist of conducting tubes and fluid-producing glands, all of which aid in the transport of sperm from the testes to the urethral opening of the penis. The male reproductive and urinary structures are shown in Fig. 34.12.

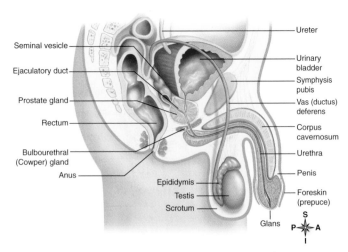

FIGURE 34.12 Structure of the Male Reproductive Organs. (From Patton KT, Thibodeau GA: *The human body in health and disease*, ed 6, St Louis, 2014, Mosby.)

External Genitalia
Testes

The testes (sing., testis) are the essential organs of male reproduction. Like the ovaries, the testes have two functions: (1) production of gametes (i.e., sperm) and (2) production of sex hormones (i.e., androgens and testosterone).

During embryonic and fetal life, the testes develop within the abdomen (see Fig. 34.1). About 3 months before birth, the testes start to descend toward the developing scrotum (Fig. 34.13). About 1 month before birth, they enter twin passageways called inguinal canals. Vaginal processes created by outpouchings of the peritoneum (lining of the abdominal cavity) also descend through the inguinal canals. When descent is complete, the abdominal end of each vaginal process closes and the scrotal end of each process becomes the outer covering of the testis, the tunica vaginalis. Failure of the testes to descend through the inguinal canal is known as cryptorchidism.

Fig. 34.14 shows a sagittal section of a mature testis. The adult testis is oval and varies considerably in length (3 to 6 cm), width (2 to 3.5 cm), depth (3 to 4 cm), and weight (10 to 40 g). The testis is almost entirely surrounded by the tunica vaginalis, which separates the testis from the scrotal wall, and the tunica albuginea. Inward extensions of the tunica albuginea form septa that separate the testis into about 250 compartments, or lobules, each of which contains several tortuously coiled ducts called seminiferous tubules. Sperm are produced in these tubules. (Sperm production is described in the Spermatogenesis section.) Tissue surrounding these ducts contains Leydig cells, which occur in clusters and produce androgens, chiefly testosterone.

The two ends of each seminiferous tubule join and leave the lobule through the tubulus rectus, which leads to the central portion of the testis, the rete testis. The sperm then move through the efferent tubules, or vasa efferentia, to the epididymis, where they mature.

The testes are innervated by adrenergic fibers whose sole function is to regulate blood flow to the Leydig cells. Arterial blood from the internal spermatic and differential arteries flows over the surface of the testes before entering the parenchyma (functional tissues). Surface flow cools the blood to temperatures that promote spermatogenesis, approximately 1° to 7° C (33.8° to 44.6° F) below body core temperature.[13] Additionally, the testes are suspended outside the pelvic cavity to facilitate cooling.

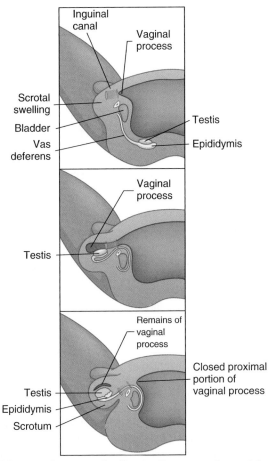

FIGURE 34.13 Descent of a Testis. The testes descend from the abdominal cavity to the scrotum during the last 3 months of fetal development.

Epididymis

The epididymis (pl., epididymides) is a comma-shaped structure that curves over the posterior portion of each testis (see Fig. 34.14). It consists of a single, densely packed and markedly coiled duct measuring 5 to 7 cm in length (but about 6 meters in length when uncoiled). The epididymis has structural and physiologic functions. Its structural function is to conduct sperm from the efferent tubules to the vas deferens, whereas physiologic functions include sperm maturation, mobility, and fertility. When sperm enter the head of the epididymis, they are not fully mature or motile, nor can they fertilize an ovum. During the 12 days (or more) sperm take to travel the length of the epididymis, they receive nutrients and testosterone and their capacity for fertilization is enhanced.[14] After traveling the length of the epididymis, sperm are stored in the epididymal tail and vas deferens. The vas deferens is a duct with muscular layers capable of powerful peristalsis that transports sperm toward the urethra (see Fig. 34.14). The vas deferens enters the pelvic cavity through the spermatic cord.

Scrotum

The testes, epididymides, and spermatic cord are enclosed and protected by the scrotum, a skin-covered, fibromuscular sac homologous to the female labia majora (see Fig. 34.2). The skin of the scrotum is thin and has rugae (wrinkles or folds), which enable it to enlarge or relax away from the body. At puberty the scrotal skin darkens, develops active sebaceous glands, and becomes sparsely covered with hair. Just under the skin lies a layer of connective tissue (fascia) and smooth muscle, the tunica dartos (see Fig. 34.14). The tunica dartos also forms a septum that separates the two testes. Exposure to cold temperatures causes the tunica dartos to contract, pulling the testes close to the warm body. In warm temperatures, the tunica dartos relaxes, suspending the testes away from body heat. These mechanisms promote optimal temperatures

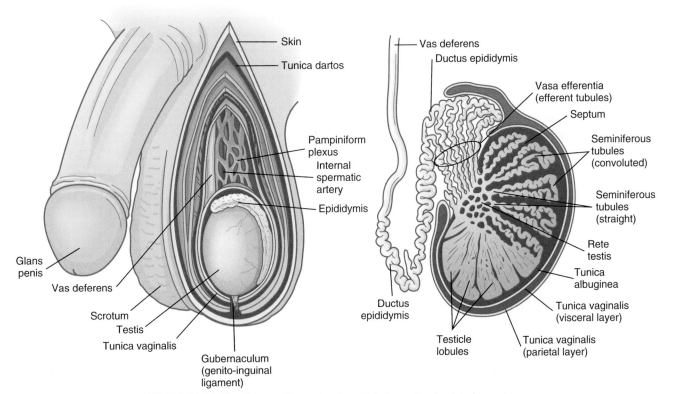

FIGURE 34.14 The Testes. External and sagittal views showing interior anatomy.

for spermatogenesis. In addition, scrotal sensitivity to touch, pressure, temperature, and pain protects the testes from potential harm. During sexual excitement, the scrotal skin and tunica thicken, the scrotum tightens and lifts, and the spermatic cords shorten, partially elevating the testes toward the body. As excitement plateaus, the engorged testes increase 50% in size, rotate anteriorly, and flatten against the body, signaling impending ejaculation.

Penis

The **penis** has two main functions: delivery of sperm to the female vagina and elimination of urine. Embryonically, the penis is homologous to the female clitoris (see Fig. 34.2).

Fig. 34.15 shows a sagittal section of the adult penis and its anatomic relation to other urogenital structures. Internally, the penis consists of the urethra and three compartments or sinusoids: two **corpora cavernosa** (sing., **corpus cavernosum**) and the **corpus spongiosum** separated by Buck fascia. Like the testes, these compartments are enclosed by the fibrous tunica albuginea. The **urethra** passes through the corpus spongiosum and ends at a sagittal slit in the glans.

Externally, the penis consists of a shaft with a tip (the **glans**) that contains the opening of the urethra (see Fig. 34.14). The skin of the glans folds over the tip of the penis, forming the **prepuce**, or **foreskin**. The skin of the penis is continuous with that of the groin, scrotum, and inner thighs. It is hairless, movable, and darker than surrounding skin.

Penetration of the female vagina is made possible by the **erectile reflex**, a process in which erectile tissues within the corpora cavernosa and corpus spongiosum become engorged with blood. The erectile tissues consist of vascular spaces, or chambers, supplied with blood by arterioles (small arteries). Usually, the arterioles are constricted, so that not much blood flows through the erectile tissues. Sexual stimulation, however, causes the arterioles to dilate and fill with blood, expanding the erectile tissues and causing an erection. The corpora cavernosa increases in length and width and becomes rigid. Erection apparently is maintained by compression or constriction of veins that drain the corpora cavernosa and corpus spongiosum. When sexual stimulation ceases or orgasm and ejaculation occur, these veins open, blood flows out of the arterioles, and the penis becomes flaccid (soft and pendulous). Erection is under the control of the autonomic nervous system but can be stimulated or inhibited by CNS input.

Stimulation of the glans, which is endowed with copious sensitive nerve endings, provides maximum erotic sensation. With sexual arousal, skin color deepens, the glans doubles in size, and the urethral meatus dilates. Ejaculation occurs with frequent, strong contractions of the vas

deferens, epididymis, seminal vesicles, prostate, urethra, and penis. Erection and ejaculation can occur independently of each other, but it is not common.[15,16]

Erections begin in utero and continue throughout life, but ejaculation does not occur until sperm production begins at puberty. Growth of the penis and scrotal contents continues well past puberty, however, and may not be complete until the late teens or early twenties. Penis size, when flaccid, varies considerably; with an erection, difference in penis size diminishes.

Internal Genitalia

Fig. 34.12 shows the anatomy of the internal genitalia and their relation to other pelvic organs. The internal genitalia consist of ducts and glands, as follows:

- *Ducts* consist of two vasa deferentia, the ejaculatory duct, and the urethra. They conduct sperm and glandular secretions from the testes to the urethral opening of the penis.
- *Glands* consist of the prostate gland, two seminal vesicles, and two Cowper (bulbourethral) glands. They secrete fluids that serve as a vehicle for sperm transport and create a nutritious alkaline medium that promotes sperm motility and survival. Together the sperm and the glandular fluids compose **semen**.

Sperm leaves the epididymides and travels rapidly through the internal ducts (**emission**). Emission occurs just seconds before ejaculation, at the moment when sexual arousal peaks. It always leads to ejaculation.

Emission occurs as smooth muscle in the walls of the epididymides and vasa deferentia begins to contract rhythmically, pushing sperm and epididymal secretions through the vasa deferentia. Each vas deferens is a firm, elastic, fibromuscular tube that begins at the tail of the epididymis, enters the pelvic cavity within the spermatic cord, loops up and over the bladder, and ends in the prostate gland (Fig. 34.16). Sperm are conducted by peristaltic contractions of smooth muscle in the walls of the vas deferens.

As sperm leave the ampulla (wide portion) of the vas deferens, the seminal vesicles secrete a nutritive, glucose-rich fluid into the ejaculate (semen). The **seminal vesicles** are glands about 4 to 6 cm long that lie behind the urinary bladder and in front of the rectum. The ducts of the seminal vesicles join the ampulla of the vas deferens to become the **ejaculatory duct**, which contracts rhythmically during emission and

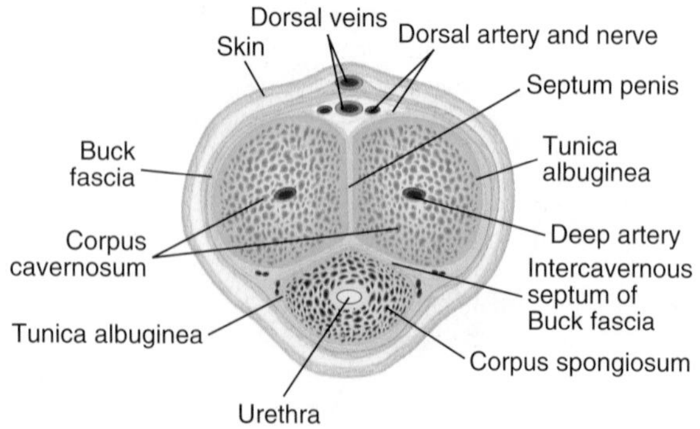

FIGURE 34.15 Cross Section of the Penis. The Buck fascia is the blue layer separating the corpora cavernosa from the corpus spongiosum. (From Thompson JM et al, editors: *Mosby's clinical nursing*, ed 5, St Louis, 2002, Mosby.)

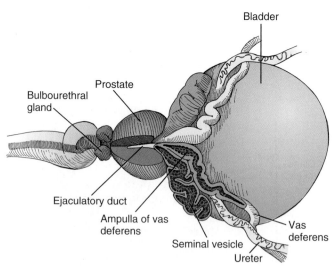

FIGURE 34.16 Prostate Gland, Seminal Vesicles, and Vas Deferens. (From Huguet J: *Hinman's atlas of urosurgical anatomy*, ed 2, pp 249-286, Philadelphia, 2012, Saunders.)

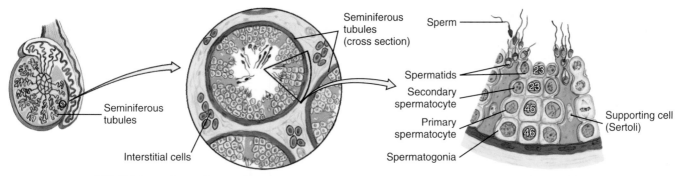

FIGURE 34.17 Seminiferous Tubule and Spermatogenesis. Cross section of a seminiferous tubule showing the different cell types. Interstitial cells that produce testosterone are between the seminiferous tubules. Spermatids in the lumen become sperm by a process called spermiogenesis. The numbers in white represent the number of chromosomes. (From Applegate E: *The anatomy and physiology learning system,* ed 4, St Louis, 2011, Saunders.)

ejaculation. As seen in Figs. 34.12 and 34.16, the ejaculatory duct joins the urethra, where both pass through the prostate gland. During emission and ejaculation, a sphincter (muscle surrounding a duct) closes, preventing urine from entering the prostatic urethra.

The **prostate gland** is about the size of a walnut, surrounds the urethra, and is composed of glandular alveoli and ducts embedded in fibromuscular tissue. Nerves required for penile erection travel along the posterolateral surface of the prostate. While semen moves through the prostatic portion of the urethra, the prostate gland contracts rhythmically and secretes prostatic fluid (a thin, milky substance with an alkaline pH that helps sperm survive in the acidic environment of the female reproductive tract) into the mixture. In addition, substances in seminal and prostatic fluids help to mobilize sperm after ejaculation.

Bulbourethral glands (Cowper glands) are the last pair of glands to add fluid to the ejaculate; their ducts secrete mucus into the urethra near the base of the penis. Ejaculation occurs as semen reaches the base of the penis, where muscles rhythmically contract and expel semen. Normally a male ejaculates between 2 and 6 ml of semen, containing 75 million to 400 million sperm. About 98% of the ejaculate consists of glandular fluids; 60% to 70% of the volume originates from the seminal vesicles; and 20% from the prostate.

Spermatogenesis

Spermatogenesis (the production of sperm) begins at puberty and continues for life. In this respect, spermatogenesis differs markedly from oogenesis (production of primordial ova), which occurs during fetal life only. Spermatogenesis takes place within the seminiferous tubules of the testes (Fig. 34.17). Each seminiferous tubule is lined with diploid (46-chromosome) germ cells called **spermatogonia** (sing., **spermatogonium**). Spermatogonia form primary and **secondary spermatocytes**, which undergo meiosis to become spermatids (see Fig. 34.17). **Spermatids** then differentiate into spermatozoa, or sperm, each of which contains 23 chromosomes (Fig. 34.18).

The development of spermatids into sperm depends on the presence of **Sertoli cells (nondividing support cells)** within the seminiferous tubules. Spermatids attach themselves to the Sertoli cells (see Fig. 34.17), where they receive nutrients and hormonal signals necessary to develop into sperm.

The process of spermatogenesis, from mitotic division of a spermatogonium to maturation of the spermatids, takes about 70 to 80 days. Mature sperm migrate from the seminiferous tubules to the epididymides, where their capacity for fertilization continues to develop. Although they are completely mature by the time they are ejaculated, the sperm do not become motile (capable of movement) until they are

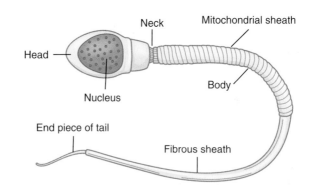

FIGURE 34.18 Anatomy of a Mature Sperm Cell (Spermatozoon).

activated by biochemicals in the epididymis and in the female reproductive tract (known as sperm capacitation).

Male Sex and Reproductive Hormones

The male sex hormones are androgens. Testosterone, the primary male sex hormone, and other androgens are produced mainly by Leydig cells of the testes, but they are also produced by the adrenal glands in both males and females and by the ovary in females (see Table 34.1 and discussion about adrenarche under Puberty and Reproductive Maturation). In males, sex hormone production is relatively constant and does not occur in a cyclic pattern, as it does in females.

The physiologic actions of androgen are related to the growth and development of male tissues and organs. Androgens are responsible for the fetal differentiation and development of the male urogenital system and have some effects on the fetal brain. After birth, the Leydig cells become dormant until activated by the gonadotropins during puberty. Then androgens cause the sex organs to grow and secondary sex characteristics to develop.

Testosterone affects nervous and skeletal tissues, bone marrow, skin and hair, and sex organs. It has an anabolic effect on skeletal muscle tissue, thereby contributing to the difference in body weight and composition between males and females. Testosterone also stimulates growth of the musculature and cartilage of the larynx, causing a permanent deepening of the voice. Testosterone directly stimulates the bone marrow and indirectly stimulates renal erythropoietin production to achieve increased hemoglobin and hematocrit levels. Because sebaceous gland activity is stimulated by testosterone, acne may develop. Hair becomes coarser in texture, and facial, axillary, and pubic hair grows in male patterns. Testosterone is required for spermatogenesis and for secretion of fluid by the prostate gland, seminal vesicles, and bulbourethral glands. Testosterone is also associated with libido (sex drive). Other, less-understood effects of testosterone include regulatory proteins involved in glycolysis, glycogen synthesis, insulin action, and lipid and cholesterol metabolism.

The regulation of androgen production and spermatogenesis is achieved by a complex feedback system involving the extrahypothalamic CNS, the hypothalamus, the anterior pituitary, the testes, and the androgen-sensitive end organs. These relationships are essentially the same in females (see Fig. 34.3).

✔ **QUICK CHECK 34.5**
1. Which cells produce testosterone?
2. Why do sperm take 12 days to travel the length of the epididymis?
3. What is the purpose of prostatic secretion?
4. What role do Sertoli cells play in spermatogenesis?

AGING AND REPRODUCTIVE FUNCTION

Aging and the Female Reproductive System

Menopause is a normal developmental and transitional event that is universally experienced by the average age of about 51 years with a range of 40 to 60 years. Changes are caused primarily by declining ovarian function and a resulting decrease in ovarian hormone secretion. The primary reproductive changes of menopause are as follows[17]:

- *Perimenopause:* This is the transitional period between reproductive and nonreproductive years and can last 1 to 8 years. About 5 to 10 years before menopause, approximately 90% of females note mild to extreme variability in frequency and quality of menstrual flow. Perimenopause usually begins with a shortening of the menstrual cycle, which correlates with a shorter follicular phase, followed by unpredictable or irregular ovulation and a lengthening of the menstrual cycle. The perimenopause varies between females and from cycle to cycle in the same person.
- *Menopause:* Menopause is defined by the point that marks 12 consecutive months of amenorrhea. This means that it is determined retrospectively, after a female has not had a menstrual period for 1 year. It is characterized by loss of ovarian function, low estrogen and progesterone levels, and high FSH and LH levels (Fig. 34.19). Early menopause is the 5 years after menopause onset. Late menopause follows and continues until death. The changes that take place are as follows:
  - *Ovarian changes:* Around 37 to 38 years of age, females experience accelerated follicular loss, which ends when the supply of follicles is depleted at menopause. This accelerated loss is correlated with increased FSH stimulation, declining inhibin production, and slightly elevated estradiol levels (see Fig. 34.19). The ovarian response to high FSH level recruits increasing numbers of follicles; these follicles only partially develop, with a net effect of irregular ovulation, lower progesterone levels, and depleted follicle reserve. The ovaries begin to decrease in size around age 30; this decrease accelerates after age 60.
  - *Uterine changes:* The increase in anovulatory cycles allows for proliferative growth of the endometrium. With this longer exposure to unopposed estrogen and greater thickness of the endometrium, 50% of perimenopausal females will experience dysfunctional uterine bleeding that is heavy and unpredictable. In the past, this has put them at high risk for hysterectomy or endometrial ablation. Medical or hormonal management is the first line of therapy if the uterus is normal.

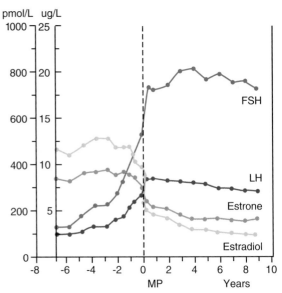

FIGURE 34.19 Perimenopausal Hormone Transition. Mean circulating hormone levels. *FSH*, Follicle-stimulating hormone; *LH*, luteinizing hormone; *MP*, menopause.

- *Breast tissue changes:* Breast tissue becomes involuted, fat deposits and connective tissue increase, and breasts are reduced in size and firmness.
- *Genitourinary tract changes:* The ovaries shrink; the uterus atrophies; and the vagina shortens, narrows, and loses some elasticity. Lubrication of the vagina diminishes and vaginal pH increases, creating higher incidence of vaginitis. The cervix atrophies; the cervical os shrinks; vaginal epithelium atrophies; labia major and minora become less prominent; some pubic hair is lost; urethral tone declines along with muscle tone throughout the pelvic area; urinary frequency or urgency, urinary tract infections, and incontinence may occur. Regular sexual activity and orgasm may diminish some of these changes. Sexually active females have less vaginal atrophy.
- *Hormonal changes:* Vasomotor flushes are characterized by a rise in skin temperature, dilation of peripheral blood vessels, increased blood flow in the hands, increased skin conductance, and transient increase in heart rate followed by a temperature drop and profuse perspiration over the area. This usually occurs in the face and neck and may radiate into the chest and other parts of the body. Dizziness, nausea, headaches, and palpitations may accompany the flush.[18] These flushes can vary in frequency, intensity, and duration and are experienced for 1 to 15 years by up to 85% of perimenopausal to postmenopausal females. Flushes are believed to be caused by rapid decreases in estrogen levels.

Rapid changes in estrogen levels also can increase emotional stress with unpredictable mood swings, depression and anxiety, weight gain, migraine headaches, and insomnia. Lower estrogen levels will decrease skin thickness and diminish skin elasticity, thereby causing increased skin dryness and wrinkling. There also is an increased risk for osteoporosis and cardiovascular disease after menopause. Hormone replacement therapy can relieve the symptoms of menopause, but risks and benefits must be evaluated for each person.

Menopause increases the risk of ovarian, breast, and uterine cancers. The risk is greater in females who began menstruating before age 12 or experience menopause after age 55. Females who menstruate longer than normal during a lifetime are exposed to more estrogen and have more ovulations. A longer exposure to estrogen increases the risk of uterine and breast cancers, and having more ovulations than normal increases the risk of ovarian cancer.

Aging and the Male Reproductive System

Males maintain reproductive capacity longer than females. No known discrete event, comparable to menopause, characterizes aging of the male reproductive system. Changes do occur, however, in testicular structure and function and sexual behavior. Emotional and physical changes associated with androgen deficiency in the aging male are known as andropause (also known as late-onset hypogonadism), but it occurs in only a small percentage of men and is a more gradual process than menopause. Contributing factors include decreased levels of testosterone, change in responsiveness of target tissues, decreased levels of sex hormone binding globulin, and changes in the hypothalamus and pituitary gland. Obesity also contributes to decreased testosterone production in aging males.

Male sexual behavior encompasses both sexual drive and erectile and ejaculatory capacity. Libido, or sexual drive, is a complex phenomenon that requires testosterone and is significantly influenced by health status and environmental, social, and psychologic factors. However, in males older than 40 years of age, chronic vascular, endocrine, and neurologic diseases are common causes of dysfunction of sexual capability. Primary changes are summarized as follows:

- *Erectile/ejaculatory capacity:* Longer stimulation needed to achieve full erection, slower and less forceful ejaculation, less pelvic muscle involvement; decreased vasocongestive response; longer refractory time, up to 24 hours.
- *Testicular changes:* Decreased weight, atrophy, softening of testes; seminiferous tubules thicken in basement membrane area, have germ cell arrest, decrease in spermatogenic activity, and collapse; then sclerosis and fibrosis cause complete obstruction; semen volume, sperm concentration, total sperm count, sperm motility, and number of motile sperm decrease; morphologic appearance of sperm changes. Fertility decreases.
- *Hormonal changes:* Hormone synthesis decreases and target tissues decline in responsiveness; testosterone levels decline as number of Leydig cells decreases; gonadotropin levels increase.
- *Associated change:* Functional deterioration of accessory sex organs occurs; loss of muscle mass, strength, and endurance and decrease in libido develop.

Hormone replacement therapy may be considered for men experiencing symptoms of low testosterone, but risks and benefits must be considered for each person.

> ✓ **QUICK CHECK 34.6**
> 1. What are the physical changes associated with menopausal decreases in estrogen level?
> 2. How does aging in males affect spermatogenesis?

SUMMARY REVIEW

Development of the Reproductive Systems

1. Differentiation of female and male genitalia begins around 7 to 8 weeks of embryonic development when the gonads of genetically male embryos begin to secrete male sex hormones, primarily testosterone, under the influence of *SRY* gene expression and testosterone-determining factor (TDF). Female gonadal development occurs in the absence of *SRY* gene expression. Until that time, the primitive reproductive organs of males and females are homologous (the same).

2. Production of primitive female gametes (ova) occurs solely during fetal life. From puberty to menopause, one female gamete matures per menstrual cycle. Production of male gametes (sperm) begins at puberty; after that, millions are produced daily, usually for life.

3. Puberty is the onset of sexual maturation. Adolescence is a stage of human development between childhood and adulthood and includes social, psychologic, and biologic changes.

4. The structure and function of both male and female reproductive systems depend on interactions among the central nervous system (hypothalamus), the endocrine system (anterior pituitary), the gonads (ovaries, testes), and the hypothalamic-pituitary-gonadal axis. A set of complex neurologic and hormonal interactions accelerate at puberty and lead to sexual maturation and reproductive capability.

5. One year before puberty, secretion of gonadotropin-releasing hormone (GnRH), follicle-stimulating hormone (FSH), and luteinizing hormone (LH) stimulate the gonads (ovaries and testes) to secrete female (estrogen and progesterone) or male sex hormones (testosterone). These stimulate maturation of the gonads, reproductive organs, and breasts (in females). Puberty is complete in females with the first ovulatory menstrual period and is complete in males with the first ejaculation that contains mature sperm.

The Female Reproductive System

1. The function of the female reproductive system is to produce mature ova and, when they are fertilized, to protect and nourish them through embryonic and fetal life and expel them at birth.

2. The external female genitalia are the mons pubis, labia majora, labia minora, clitoris, vestibule (urinary and vaginal openings), Bartholin and Skene glands, and perineum. They protect body openings and may play a role in sexual functioning.

3. The internal female genitalia are the vagina, uterus, fallopian tubes, and ovaries. Although all these organs are needed for reproduction, the ovaries are the most essential because they produce the female gametes and female sex hormones.

4. The vagina is a fibromuscular canal that receives the penis during sexual intercourse and is the exit route for menstrual fluids and products of conception. The vagina leads from the introitus (its external opening) to the cervical portion of the uterus.

5. The uterus is the hollow, muscular organ in which a fertilized ovum develops until birth. The uterine walls have three layers: the endometrium (lining), myometrium (muscular layer), and perimetrium (outer covering, which is continuous with the pelvic peritoneum). The endometrium proliferates (thickens) and is shed in response to cyclic changes in levels of female sex hormones. The cervix is the narrow, lower portion of the uterus that opens into the vagina.

6. The two fallopian tubes extend from the uterus to the ovaries. Their function is to direct ova from the spaces around the ovaries to the uterus. Fertilization normally occurs in the distal third of the fallopian tubes.

7. From puberty to menopause, the ovaries are the site of (1) ovum maturation and release and (2) production of female sex hormones (estrogen, progesterone) and androgens. The female sex hormones are involved in sexual differentiation and development, the menstrual cycle, pregnancy, and lactation. Although they are primarily male sex hormones, androgens in females are precursors of female sex hormones and contribute to the prepubertal growth spurt, pubic and axillary hair growth, and activation of sebaceous glands.

8. Estrogen (primarily estradiol) is produced by cells in the developing ovarian follicle (structure that encloses the ovum). Progesterone is produced by cells of the corpus luteum, the structure that develops from the ruptured ovarian follicle after ovulation (ovum release). Androgens are produced within the ovarian follicle, adrenal glands, and adipose tissue.

9. The average menstrual cycle lasts 25 to 30 days and consists of three phases, which are named for ovarian and endometrial changes: the follicular/proliferative phase, the luteal/secretory phase, and the ischemic menstrual phase.

10. The follicular/proliferative phase is the maturation of an ovarian follicle, the proliferation of the uterine endometrium, and the release of the ovum. FSH stimulates follicle and ovum maturation, then a surge of LH causes ovulation. Estrogen causes proliferation of the endometrium.

11. During the luteal/secretory phase, the ovum transforms into the corpus luteum. LH stimulates the corpus luteum to secrete progesterone and estrogen. Progesterone stimulates blood vessel and glandular growth, and estrogen maintains the thickened endometrium. Glands in the endometrium begin to secrete a thin, glycogen-containing fluid, hence the name *secretory phase*.

12. During the ischemic/menstrual phase, the corpus luteum degenerates, production of progesterone and estrogen drops sharply, and the "starved" endometrium degenerates and is shed, causing menstruation.

13. Cyclic changes in hormone levels also cause thinning and thickening of the vaginal epithelium, thinning and thickening of cervical secretions, and changes in basal body temperature.

Structure and Function of the Breast

1. The basic functional unit of the female breast is the lobe, a system of ducts that branches from the nipple to milk-producing units called *lobules*. Each breast contains 15 to 20 lobes, which are separated and supported by Cooper ligaments. The lobules contain *acini cells*, which are convoluted spaces lined with epithelial cells. Contraction of the subepithelial cells of each acinus moves milk into the system of ducts that leads to the nipple.

2. Until puberty, the female and male breasts are similar, consisting of a small, underdeveloped nipple and some fatty and fibrous tissue. At puberty, however, a variety of hormones (estrogen, progesterone, prolactin, growth hormone, insulin, cortisol) cause the female breast to develop into a system of glands and ducts that is capable of producing and ejecting milk.

3. During the reproductive years, breast tissue undergoes cyclic changes in response to hormonal changes of the menstrual cycle.

4. Milk production occurs in response to prolactin, a hormone that is secreted in larger amounts after childbirth. Milk ejection is under the control of oxytocin, another hormone of pregnancy and lactation.

5. The male breast does not develop because of the absence of sufficiently high levels of estrogen and progesterone and antagonistic effects of androgens.

The Male Reproductive System

1. The function of the male reproductive system is to produce male gametes (sperm) and deliver them to the female reproductive tract.

2. The external male genitalia are the testes, epididymides, scrotum, and penis. The internal genitalia are the vas deferens, ejaculatory duct, prostatic and membranous sections of the urethra, seminal vesicles, prostate gland, and bulbourethral glands.

3. The testes (male gonads) are paired glands suspended within the scrotum. The testes have two functions: spermatogenesis (sperm production) and production of male sex hormones (androgens, chiefly testosterone).

4. The epididymis is a long, coiled tube arranged in a comma-shaped compartment that curves over the top and rear of the testis. The epididymis receives sperm from the testis and stores them while they develop further. Sperm travel the length of the epididymis and then are ejaculated into the vas deferens, which transports sperm to the urethra.

5. The scrotum is a skin-covered, fibromuscular sac that encloses the testes and epididymides, which are suspended within the scrotum by the spermatic cord. The scrotum keeps these organs at optimal temperatures for sperm survival (about 1° to 2° C lower than body temperature) by contracting in cold environments and relaxing in warm environments.

6. The penis has two functions: delivery of sperm and elimination of urine.

7. The penis is a cylindric organ consisting of three longitudinal compartments (two corpora cavernosa and one corpus spongiosum) and the urethra. The urethra runs through the corpus spongiosum. The corpora cavernosa and corpus spongiosum consist of erectile tissue. Externally the penis consists of a shaft and a tip, which is called the *glans*.

8. Sexual intercourse is made possible by the erectile reflex, in which tactile or psychogenic stimulation of the parasympathetic nerves causes arterioles in the corpora cavernosa and corpus spongiosum to dilate and fill with blood, causing the penis to enlarge and become firm.

9. Emission, which occurs at the peak of sexual arousal, is the movement of semen from the epididymides to the penis. Ejaculation, which is a continuation of emission, is the pulsatile ejection of semen from the penis.

10. Spermatogenesis is a continuous process because spermatogonia, the primitive male gametes, undergo continuous mitosis within the seminiferous tubules of the testes. Some spermatogonia develop into primary spermatocytes, which divide meiotically into secondary spermatocytes and then spermatids. The spermatids develop into sperm with the help of nutrients and hormonal signals from Sertoli cells.

11. Production of the male sex hormones (androgens) is controlled by interactions among the hypothalamus, anterior pituitary, and gonads. The male hormones are produced steadily rather than cyclically, however.

Aging and Reproductive Function

1. Perimenopause is the transitional period between reproductive and nonreproductive years in females.

2. Menopause, the point that marks 12 consecutive months of amenorrhea, includes atrophic changes in the ovaries, vagina, and breast.

3. Andropause is androgen deficiency in the aging male. There is a decrease in testosterone production with testicular atrophy, decreased fertility, and some loss of muscle mass and strength.

KEY TERMS

Acinus (pl., acini) of breast, 770
Adrenarche, 762
Androgen, 768
Andropause, 777
Areola, 771
Breast, 770
Bulbourethral gland (Cowper gland), 775
Cervix, 765
Cornification, 770
Corpus (body of uterus), 765
Corpus cavernosum (pl., corpora cavernosa), 774
Corpus luteum, 767
Corpus spongiosum, 774
Cul-de-sac, 764
Decornification, 770
Efferent tubule, 772
Ejaculatory duct, 774
Emission, 774
Endocervical canal, 765
Endometrium, 765
Epididymis (pl., epididymides), 773
Erectile reflex, 774

Estradiol (E$_2$), 767
Estrogen, 767
Fallopian tube (oviduct, uterine tube), 766
Fimbriae, 766
Follicle-stimulating hormone (FSH), 761
Follicular/proliferative phase, 770
Fornix, 764
Fundus, 765
Glands of Montgomery, 771
Glans, 774
Gonad, 760
Gonadarche, 762
Gonadotropin-releasing hormone (GnRH), 761
Granulosa cell, 767
Infundibulum, 766
Inguinal canal, 772
Ischemic/menstrual phase, 770
Isthmus, 765
Lactation, 772
Leydig cell, 772
Libido, 776
Luteal/secretory phase, 770

Luteinizing hormone (LH), 761
Menarche, 768
Menopause, 768
Menstruation (menses), 770
Myometrium, 765
Nipple, 771
Ovarian cycle, 767
Ovarian follicle, 767
Ovary, 766
Oviduct, 766
Ovulation, 770
Ovum (pl., ova), 760
Oxytocin, 772
Penis, 774
Perimetrium (parietal peritoneum), 765
Prepuce (foreskin), 774
Primary spermatocyte, 778
Progesterone, 768
Prostate gland, 775
Puberty, 761
Rete testis, 772
Ruga (pl., rugae), 764
Scrotum, 773
Secondary spermatocyte, 775
Semen, 774

Seminal vesicle, 774
Seminiferous tubule, 772
Sertoli cell (nondividing support cell), 775
Sex hormone, 760
Spermatid, 775
Spermatogenesis, 775
Spermatogonium (pl., spermatogonia), 775
Spermatozoon (sperm cell), 760
Spinnbarkeit mucus, 765
Testis (pl., testes), 772
Testosterone, 761
Theca cell, 767
Thelarche, 761
Tubulus rectus, 772
Tunica albuginea, 772
Tunica dartos, 773
Tunica vaginalis, 772
Urethra, 774
Uterus, 764
Vagina, 764
Vas deferens, 773
Vasomotor flush, 776
Vulva, 763

REFERENCES

1. Tomova A, et al: Influence of the body weight on the onset and progression of puberty in boys, *J Pediatr Endocrinol Metab* 28(7-8):859-865, 2015.
2. Lenz GM, et al: *Comprehensive gynecology*, ed 6, St Louis, 2012, Mosby.
3. Labrie F: All sex steroids are made intracellularly in peripheral tissues by the mechanisms of intracrinology after menopause, *J Steroid Biochem Mol Biol* 145C:133-138, 2015.
4. Euling SY, et al: Examination of US puberty-timing data from 1940 to 1994 for secular trends: panel findings, *Pediatrics* 121(Suppl 3):S172-S191, 2008.
5. Karapanou O, Papadimitriou A: Determinants of menarche, *Reprod Biol Endocrinol* 8:115, 2010.
6. Rosenfield RL: Clinical review: adolescent anovulation: maturational mechanisms and implications, *J Clin Endocrinol Metab* 98(9):3572-3583, 2013.

7. Hall JE: Endocrinology of the menopause, *Endocrinol Metab Clin North Am* 44(3):485-496, 2015.
8. Pandey S, Bhattacharya S: Impact of obesity on gynecology, *Womens Health (Lond)* 6(1):107-117, 2010.
9. Scheid JL, De Souza MJ: Menstrual irregularities and energy deficiency in physically active women: the role of ghrelin, PYY and adipocytokines, *Med Sport Sci* 55:82-102, 2010.
10. Yamanoto K, et al: The relationship between premenstrual symptoms, menstrual pain, irregular menstrual cycles, and psychosocial stress among Japanese college students, *J Physiol Anthropol* 28(3):129-136, 2009.
11. Pallone SR, Bergus GR: Fertility awareness-based methods: another option for family planning, *J Am Board Fam Med* 22(2):147-157, 2009.
12. Jesinger RA: Breast anatomy for the interventionalist, *Tech Vasc Interv Radiol* 17(1):3-9, 2014.

13. Reyes JG, et al: The hypoxic testicle: physiology and pathophysiology, *Oxid Med Cell Longev* 2012:929285, 2012.
14. Dacheux JL, Dacheux F: New insights into epididymal function in relation to sperm maturation, *Reproduction* 147(2):R27-R42, 2013.
15. Giuliano F: Neurophysiology of erection and ejaculation, *J Sex Med* 8(Suppl 4):310-315, 2010.
16. Hsieh CH, et al: Advances in understanding of mammalian penile evolution, human penile anatomy and human erection physiology: clinical implications for physicians and surgeons, *Med Sci Monit* 18(7):RA 118-RA125, 2012.
17. Hale GE, et al: The perimenopausal woman: endocrinology and management, *J Steroid Biochem Mol Biol* 142:121-131, 2014.
18. Freedman RR: Menopausal hot flashes: mechanisms, endocrinology, treatment, *J Steroid Biochem Mol Biol* 142:115-120, 2014.

35

Alterations of the Female Reproductive System

Kathryn L. McCance

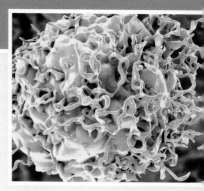

EVOLVE WEBSITE

CHAPTER OUTLINE

Alterations of the reproductive system span a wide range of concerns—from delayed sexual development and suboptimal sexual performance to structural and functional abnormalities. Many common reproductive disorders carry potentially serious physiologic or psychological consequences. For example, sexual or reproductive dysfunction, such as impotence or infertility, can dramatically affect self-concept, relationships, and overall quality of life. Conversely, organic and psychosocial problems, such as alcoholism, depression, situational stressors, chronic illness, and medications, can affect ovulation and menstruation, sexual performance, and fertility and may be risk factors for the development of some types of reproductive tract cancers. The diagnosis and treatment of reproductive system disorders, however, are often complicated by the stigma and symbolism associated with the reproductive organs and the emotion-laden beliefs and behaviors related to reproductive health. Treatment or diagnosis for any problem may be delayed because of embarrassment, guilt, fear, or denial.

ABNORMALITIES OF THE FEMALE REPRODUCTIVE TRACT

Normal development of the female reproductive tract requires the absence of testosterone during embryonic and fetal life (see Chapter 34). The resulting fusion of the two paramesonephric (müllerian) ducts produces the normal cervix and the uterus with an internal cavity. The distal portions of the paramesonephric ducts remain independent and form the two fallopian/uterine tubes. Alterations in the normal process include errors in cellular sensitivity to testosterone (androgen insensitivity) or failures of cell line migration, resulting in changes in the structure of the reproductive organs.

Androgen insensitivity occurs in its most extreme form in about 1 in 20,000 people[1] and is discussed briefly in this chapter because of the often-resulting female phenotype, despite a male genotype. Androgen insensitivity syndrome (AIS) is caused by an X-linked (recessive pattern) genetic mutation in cellular androgen receptors (ARs). ARs allow cells to respond to androgens, such as testosterone, and the mutation causes end-organ insensitivity to testosterone. Testosterone promotes embryonic male reproductive system development. The syndrome is characterized by a female phenotype or signs of both male and female sexual development in an individual with an XY karyotype or male genotype. The testes produce age-appropriate normal concentrations of androgens. Complete androgen insensitivity syndrome (CAIS) occurs when the body cannot use androgens at all.[2] Individuals with this condition have external sex characteristics of females but do not have a uterus, therefore they do not menstruate and are infertile. They are typically raised as females with a female sex identity. Affected children have male internal organs or testes (which may be palpable within the labia majora, inguinal ring, or abdominal cavity) that produce testosterone (and estrogen). Breast development may be normal, but pubic and axillary hair is often sparse. A short vagina that ends blindly also may be present.

Partial and milder forms of androgen insensitivity (also a common cause of male infertility) are much more common. Persons with partial androgen insensitivity (also called *Reifenstein syndrome*) can have genitalia that look typically female, genitalia that have both male and female characteristics, or genitalia that look typically male.[2] These individuals are raised as males or as females and may have a male or female sex identity. Those with mild androgen insensitivity are born with male sex characteristics but are often infertile and experience breast enlargement at puberty.[2]

Other abnormalities of the uterus, cervix, and fallopian/uterine tubes have multifactorial origins, often the result of an interaction between genetic predisposition and environmental factors. Such interactions result in müllerian duct abnormalities. Some medications, chemicals, and toxins have been implicated as a direct cause of uterine abnormalities.

About 5% of the general female population has some sort of uterine abnormality, but the rate is much higher in populations of women who have experienced infertility or miscarriage. Most uterine abnormalities stem from abnormal cell migration in the müllerian ducts during key moments in fetal development (Fig. 35.1). Uterine abnormalities are rarely diagnosed until the woman has trouble becoming pregnant or carrying a baby to term, because the uterus is capable of menstruation but may have difficulty supporting a growing fetus. Uterine malformations are usually diagnosed by ultrasound during pregnancy or with magnetic resonance imaging (MRI). The prognosis depends on the severity of the malformation and the location and size of the placenta and fetus. Some abnormalities can be surgically corrected to improve the outcome of subsequent pregnancies. Abnormalities of the lower genital tract also can result in women having two vaginas or a vaginal septum (a thin membrane dividing the vaginal vault). For most women this does not create functional problems, but it can be surgically corrected if needed.

ALTERATIONS OF SEXUAL MATURATION

The process of sexual maturation, or puberty, is marked by the development of secondary sex characteristics, rapid growth, and, ultimately, the ability to reproduce. A variety of congenital and endocrine disorders can disrupt the timing of puberty. These disorders may cause puberty to occur too late (delayed puberty) or too early (precocious puberty). Both types involve an inappropriate onset of sex hormone production by the gonads.

The age of puberty is multifactorial, involving genetic and environmental components. The onset of puberty is now 8 to 13 years of age and appears to be occurring earlier for girls. Girls of African descent and Hispanic/Latina girls begin puberty up to 1 year sooner than the average young female. The earlier onset appears primarily in breast development and not age of menarche. Obesity may accelerate the onset of puberty. Both precocious puberty and delayed puberty have implications for the child's social interactions and self-esteem.

Delayed or Absent Puberty

About 2% of children living in North America experience delayed development of secondary sex characteristics. One of the first signs of puberty in girls is thelarche, or breast development; which typically

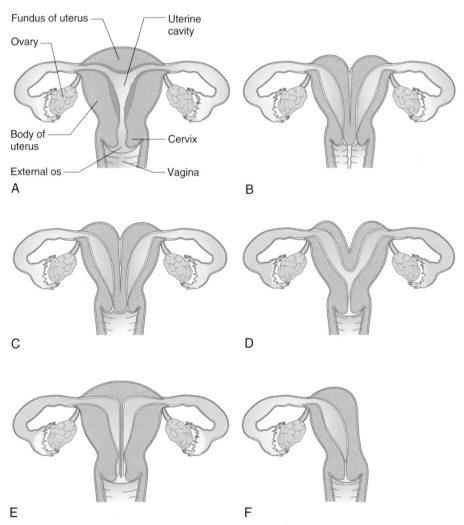

FIGURE 35.1 Uterine Malformations. Congenital uterine abnormalities. **A,** The normal configuration of the uterus and the ovaries. **B,** Double uterus with a double vagina. **C,** A single vagina. **D,** Bicornuate uterus. **E,** A uterus with a midline septum. **F,** Unicornuate uterus. (From de Bruyn R: *Pediatric ultrasound*, ed 2, London, 2010, Churchill Livingstone.)

TABLE 35.1   Frequency and Common Causes of Delayed Puberty Other Than Constitutional Delay of Growth and Puberty

Delayed Puberty	Hypergonadotropic Hypogonadism	Permanent Hypogonadotropic Hypogonadism	Functional Hypogonadotropic Hypogonadism
Boys	5%-10%	10%	20%
Girls	25%	20%	20%
Common causes	Turner syndrome, gonadal dysgenesis, chemotherapy, radiation therapy	Tumors or infiltrative diseases of the central nervous system, GnRH deficiency (isolated hypogonadotropic hypogonadism, Kallmann syndrome), combined pituitary-hormone deficiency, chemotherapy, or radiation therapy	Systemic illness (inflammatory bowel disease, celiac disease, anorexia nervosa, or bulimia), hypothyroidism, excessive exercise

GnRH, Gonadotropin-releasing hormone.
From Palmert MR, Dunkel L: *N Engl J Med* 366(5):443-453, 2012.

begins by 13 years of age. Normally, boys tend to mature later than girls, around 14 to 14.5 years of age. In boys, the first sign of maturity is enlargement of the testes and thinning of the scrotal skin. In delayed puberty, these secondary sex characteristics develop later.

In most cases, delayed puberty is a physiologic (constitutional) delay. Hormonal levels are normal, the hypothalamic-pituitary-gonadal (HPG) axis is intact, and maturation is slowly occurring. This physiologic delay tends to be familial, less common in girls than boys, and is diagnosed often retrospectively once pubertal progression is complete. Treatment is seldom needed unless the delayed puberty is causing psychosocial problems.

Less common, and a factor in a very small percentage of cases, is delayed puberty caused by a disruption of the HPG axis or by the outcomes of a systemic disease. Treatment depends on the cause (Table 35.1) and referral to a pediatric endocrinologist is recommended.

Precocious Puberty

Precocious puberty is a rare event, affecting about 29 in 100,000 girls (see Chapter 36 for boys). Precocious puberty is defined as the onset of clinical signs of puberty (breast or pubic hair development) before age 8. There are several postulated causes of precocious puberty (Box 35.1), including obesity, genetic factors, hypothyroidism, tumors, and the growing prevalence of the molecular compounds called *endocrine disruptors* in common household products (see *Did You Know?* Precocious Puberty). All cases of precocious puberty require thorough evaluation.

DID YOU KNOW?

Precocious Puberty

Studies implicate obesity, leptin, ghrelin, and environmental endocrine disruptor chemicals (EDCs) as possible contributors to precocious puberty in girls. Obesity may affect the production and secretion of leptin and ghrelin, powerful communicators of satiety, hunger, metabolic rate, and in the timing of puberty. EDCs may mimic, block, or alter the normal signaling systems involved in sex hormone secretion, uptake, and use. EDCs include agrochemicals, widespread industrial compounds, and persistent pollutants.

Data from Buluş AD et al: *Toxicol Mech Methods* 26(7):493-500, 2016; Rosenfield RL, Cooke DW, Radovick S: In Sperling Mark A, editor: *Pediatric endocrinology*, pp 569-663, Philadelphia, 2014, Elsevier Health Sciences; Sørensen K et al: *Horm Res Paediatr* 77(3):137-145, 2012; Trotman GEL *Curr Opin Obstet Gynecol* 28(5):366-372, 2016; Willemsen RH, Dunger DB: *Endocr Dev* 29:17-35, 2016.

BOX 35.1   Causes of Precocious Puberty

Central (Gonadotropin-Releasing Hormone [GnRH] Dependent)
Idiopathic
Central nervous system (CNS) disorders
   Congenital anomalies (hydrocephalus)
   Hypothalamic hamartoma
   Postinflammatory/infectious condition
   Trauma
   Tumors (hypothalamic, pineal, other)
   Imprinted gene (*MKRN3*)

Peripheral Puberty (GnRH Independent)
Adrenal hyperplasia or tumor
Environmental endocrine disruptions
Exogenous sex steroid exposure
Exogenous anabolic steroids
Familial Leydig cell hyperplasia
Gonadal tumors or cysts
Human chorionic gonadotropin (hCG)–secreting tumors (hepatoblastomas, intracranial lesions)
Hypothyroidism (severe)
McCune-Albright syndrome
Testotoxicosis

From Fuqua JS: *Clin Endocrinol Metab* 98(6):2198-2207, 2013; Rosenfeld RL et al: Puberty and its disorders in the female. In Sterling MA, editor: *Pediatric endocrinology*, Philadelphia, 2014, Elsevier Health Sciences; Schoelwer M, Eugster EA: *Endocr Dev* 29:230-239, 2016.

Precocious puberty may be the partial, complete, or mixed type (Box 35.2); it can be further classified as central (gonadotropin-releasing hormone [GnRH] dependent) and peripheral (GnRH independent; see Box 35.1). Complete precocious puberty is the onset and progression of all pubertal features (i.e., thelarche, pubarche, and menarche). Mixed precocious puberty (virilization of a girl or feminization of a boy) causes the child to develop secondary sex characteristics of the opposite sex. It is evident at birth and is rare in older children (see Box 35.2). Treatment for all forms of precocious puberty includes identifying and removing the underlying cause or administering appropriate hormones. If needed, precocious puberty can be reversed.

BOX 35.2 Causes of Mixed Precocious Puberty

Female (Virilization)
Congenital adrenal hyperplasia
Androgen-secreting tumors
    Adrenal
    Ovarian
    Teratoma
    Exogenous androgens

Male (Feminization)
Estrogen-producing tumors
    Adrenal
    Teratoma
    Hepatoma
    Testicular
Exogenous estrogens
Increased peripheral conversion of androgens to estrogens

Data from Rosenfield RL et al: Puberty and its disorders in the female. In Sperling MA, editor: *Pediatric endocrinology*, Philadelphia, 2014, Elsevier Health Sciences.

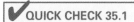

QUICK CHECK 35.1
1. Why does puberty occur too late or too early in some individuals?
2. What is the normal age range for the onset of puberty?

DISORDERS OF THE FEMALE REPRODUCTIVE SYSTEM

Hormonal and Menstrual Alterations

Primary Dysmenorrhea

Primary dysmenorrhea is painful menstruation associated with the release of prostaglandins in ovulatory cycles, but not with pelvic disease. Approximately 90% of all women experience dysmenorrhea, and 15% are incapacitated for 1 to 3 days because of pain severity. Primary dysmenorrhea begins with the onset of ovulatory cycles, and the prevalence is highest during adolescence. **Secondary dysmenorrhea** is related to pelvic pathologic conditions, manifests later in the reproductive years, and may occur any time in the menstrual cycle.

PATHOPHYSIOLOGY Primary dysmenorrhea results mostly from excessive prostaglandin $F_2\alpha$ ($PGF_2\alpha$), a potent myometrial stimulant and vasoconstrictor, found in secretory endometrium. Elevated levels of prostaglandins, especially $PGF_2\alpha$ and $PGE_2\alpha$, increase myometrial contractions, constrict endometrial blood vessels, and enhance nerve hypersensitivity, resulting in pain. These changes can lead to ischemia and endometrial shedding. Increased synthesis of prostaglandins may result from increased cyclooxygenase (COX) enzyme activity. Inflammatory mediators produced in leukocytes (leukotrienes) also contribute to increased levels of pain. The first 48 hours of menstruation correlate with higher prostaglandin levels. Women who are anovulatory because they use oral contraceptives rarely have primary dysmenorrhea. Secondary dysmenorrhea results from disorders such as endometriosis (most common cause), endometritis (infection), pelvic inflammatory disease, adhesions, obstructive uterine or vaginal anomalies, inflammation, uterine fibroids, polyps, tumors, cysts, or intrauterine devices (IUDs).

CLINICAL MANIFESTATIONS The chief symptom of dysmenorrhea is pelvic pain associated with the onset of menses. The severity is directly related to the length and amount of menstrual flow. The pain often radiates into the groin and may be accompanied by backache, anorexia, vomiting, diarrhea, syncope, insomnia, and headache. The latter symptoms are caused by the entry of prostaglandins and their metabolites into the systemic circulation. The discomfort commonly begins shortly before the onset of menstruation and rarely persists 1 to 3 days during menstrual flow.

EVALUATION AND TREATMENT A thorough medical history and pelvic examination can differentiate primary dysmenorrhea from secondary dysmenorrhea. Nonsteroidal antiinflammatory drugs (NSAIDs) (e.g., ibuprofen) are the treatment of choice because they reduce COX enzyme activity, and thus prostaglandin production. NSAIDs are effective in the majority of women with primary dysmenorrhea and are most effective if started at the first sign of bleeding or cramping. In women who desire contraception, dysmenorrhea may be relieved with hormonal contraceptives. Hormonal contraception stops ovulation and creates an atrophic endometrium, thereby decreasing prostaglandin synthesis and myometrial contractility. Regular exercise and stress reduction are thought to prevent or reduce symptoms. Other palliative approaches with some evidence of effectiveness in pain relief include local application of heat; acupuncture; high-frequency transcutaneous electrical nerve stimulation (TENS); supplements, such as thiamine and vitamin E; and Chinese herbal treatments.

Amenorrhea

Amenorrhea means lack of menstruation; the most common causes (aside from pregnancy) include hypothalamic dysfunction, polycystic ovarian syndrome, hyperprolactinemia, and ovarian failure. **Primary amenorrhea** is the failure of menarche and the absence of menstruation by age 13 years without the development of secondary sex characteristics or by age 15 years regardless of the presence of secondary sex characteristics (see the Alterations of Sexual Maturation section for a discussion of delayed puberty). **Secondary amenorrhea** is the absence of menstruation for a time equivalent to three or more cycles in women who have previously menstruated.

PATHOPHYSIOLOGY One approach to understanding the pathophysiology is to compartmentalize. *Compartment I disorders* are anatomic defects, including absence of the vagina and uterus. *Compartment II disorders* involve the ovary, primarily genetic disorders (e.g., Turner syndrome) and AIS. The target organs (e.g., ovaries) in AIS are completely resistant to the action of androgens, resulting in a lack of estrogen. *Compartment III disorders* are of the anterior pituitary gland, including tumors, and result in failure of signaling to the ovaries through follicle-stimulating hormone (FSH) and luteinizing hormone (LH) secretion. *Compartment IV disorders* include central nervous system (CNS) disorders and primarily involve hypothalamic defects that prevent secretion of GnRH; thus, there is no signaling to the pituitary to release FSH and LH.

CLINICAL MANIFESTATIONS The major clinical manifestation of primary amenorrhea is the absence of the first menstrual period. The cause of the amenorrhea determines whether secondary sex characteristics and height are affected.

EVALUATION AND TREATMENT Diagnosis of primary amenorrhea is based on the results of a history and physical examination and determination of the presence or absence of secondary sexual characteristics. Laboratory studies may be required to document abnormal

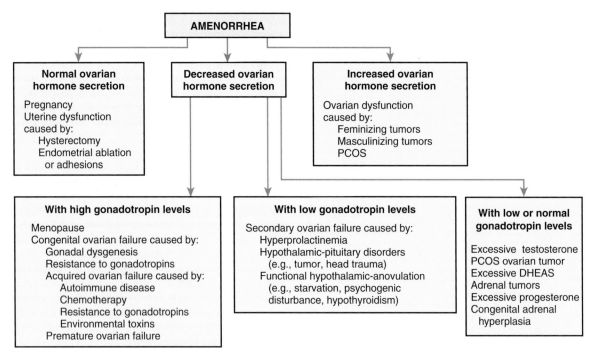

FIGURE 35.2 Causes of Secondary Amenorrhea. Of note, hypothyroidism is a relatively common condition and should be ruled out as the cause of hyperprolactinemia before more extensive evaluation (i.e., computed tomography or magnetic resonance imaging) occurs. *DHEAS,* Dehydroepiandrosterone sulfate; *PCOS,* polycystic ovary syndrome.

levels of gonadotropins or ovarian hormones, or the presence of genetic conditions. Diagnostic imaging, including ultrasonography and MRI, is used to document structural abnormalities.

Treatment involves correction of any underlying disorders and implementation of hormone replacement therapy to induce the development of secondary sex characteristics. Although surgical alteration of the genitalia may be undertaken to correct abnormalities, it should be postponed until the individual can make a truly informed decision.

Secondary Amenorrhea

Many disorders and physiologic conditions are associated with secondary amenorrhea. Secondary amenorrhea is common (normal) during early adolescence, pregnancy, lactation, and the perimenopausal period, primarily because of anovulation. The most common causes (after pregnancy) are thyroid disorders (e.g., hypothyroidism); hyperprolactinemia; hypothalamic-pituitary-ovarian (HPO) interruption secondary to excessive exercise, stress, or weight loss; and polycystic ovary syndrome (PCOS).

PATHOPHYSIOLOGY The pathophysiology is dependent on the causes of secondary amenorrhea. These causes are summarized in Fig. 35.2.

CLINICAL MANIFESTATIONS The major manifestation of secondary amenorrhea is the absence of menses after previous menstrual periods. Depending on the underlying cause of the amenorrhea, infertility, vasomotor flushes, vaginal atrophy, acne, osteopenia, and **hirsutism** (abnormal hairiness) may be present.

EVALUATION AND TREATMENT Pregnancy is the most common cause of secondary amenorrhea and must be ruled out before any further

evaluation. A thorough history and physical examination are important because the menstrual cycle may stop or become irregular in response to stress, extreme exercise, large dietary changes, eating disorders, or sleep abnormalities. Hypothyroidism also is a common cause and should be ruled out as well. Diagnosis of secondary amenorrhea involves identifying underlying hormonal or anatomic alterations. Evaluation of thyroid-stimulating hormone (TSH) or prolactin levels may be indicated. Depending on the cause of the amenorrhea, treatment may involve hormone replacement therapy or a corrective procedure, such as surgical removal of a pituitary tumor. The choice of treatment may be influenced by the woman's childbearing plans.

Abnormal Uterine Bleeding

Abnormal uterine bleeding (AUB) is bleeding that is abnormal in duration, volume, frequency, or regularity and has been present for the majority of 6 months. Menstrual irregularity or abnormal bleeding patterns (Table 35.2) account for approximately 33% of all gynecologic visits. Abnormal bleeding patterns have been inconsistently defined. A new system of definitions and classification has been adopted in the United States (see Table 35.2). AUB may be acute or chronic and is classified by the cause of bleeding using an internationally recognized PALM-COEIN system (Fig. 35.3).

Any bleeding is abnormal in premenstrual or menopausal women. For women of reproductive age, normal uterine bleeding occurs every 28 days, with variation up to 7 days. Abnormal is bleeding more frequently than every 21 days, less frequently than every 35 days, and menstrual bleeding longer than 7 days. In the United States, AUB (all etiologies) is the leading reason for hysterectomy.

PATHOPHYSIOLOGY The majority of AUB is associated with lack of ovulation. Although anovulatory AUB may occur at any time during

TABLE 35.2 Abnormal Uterine Bleeding

Current Terminology	Outdated Terminology	Definition
Chronic AUB	Menometrorrhagia, menorrhagia, menorrhea, polymenorrhea	Abnormal uterine bleeding for at least 4 out of 6 months, characterized by increased amount, irregularity, and/or timing
Acute AUB	—	Single episode of severe uterine bleeding that is sufficient to require immediate intervention to prevent further blood loss
Intermenstrual bleeding (AUB/IMB)	Metrorrhagia	Uterine bleeding that occurs between regular menstrual cycles; can be random or predictable
Heavy menstrual bleeding (AUB/HMB)	Hypermenorrhea	Increased menstrual volume that interferes with a woman's physical, emotional, and social quality of life

AUB, Abnormal uterine bleeding.
Data from Fraser IS et al: *Semin Reprod Med*, 29(5):383-390, 2011; Munro MG, et al: *Int J Gynecol Obstet* 113(1):3-13, 2011.

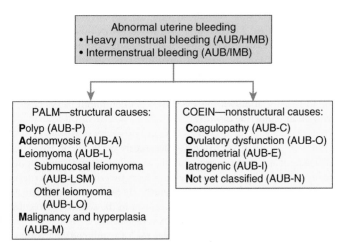

FIGURE 35.3 PALM-COEIN System for Classification of Abnormal Uterine Bleeding. *AUB*, Abnormal uterine bleeding. (Modified from Malcolm G, Munro et al: FIGO working group on menstrual disorders, *Int J Gynaecol Obstet* 113:3–13, 2011.)

the reproductive years and many conditions are associated with irregular ovulation, it tends to occur in adolescents and perimenopausal women more frequently. Women who fail to ovulate experience irregularities in their menstrual bleeding because of a lack of progesterone and, in some cases, an excess of estrogen. This results in excessive and irregular endometrial thickness and subsequent excessive and irregular bleeding. PCOS, obesity, and thyroid disease also are common contributors. Abnormal bleeding can result from defects of the corpus luteum that

result in progesterone deficiencies or from abnormalities of the uterus or cervix, such as endometrial polyps, uterine fibroids, or uterine or cervical cancers.

Abnormal menstrual bleeding in ovulatory cycles is less common, and mechanisms underlying the bleeding are unclear but can include defects of the corpus luteum and abnormalities of the uterus or cervix, such as polyps, fibroids, or cancer. Excessive fibrinolytic activity, use of anticoagulants, diseases of coagulation, infection, and changes in prostaglandin production may be implicated.

CLINICAL MANIFESTATIONS AUB is characterized by unpredictable and variable bleeding in terms of amount and duration. Especially during perimenopause, dysfunctional bleeding also may involve flooding and the passing of large clots, leading to excessive blood loss. Excessive bleeding can lead to iron deficiency anemia and associated symptoms, including fatigue or shortness of breath.

EVALUATION AND TREATMENT The first step in the evaluation of AUB is to establish the cause of bleeding. Evaluation includes a thorough history, physical examination, and transvaginal ultrasound. Laboratory evaluation includes a complete blood count, appropriate thyroid hormone tests, and coagulation studies, if indicated. If no cause is found, it is usually assumed that the bleeding is caused by lack of regular ovulation. NSAIDs are often first-line treatments for excessive menstrual bleeding because they reduce prostaglandin synthesis within the endometrial tissues, leading to vasoconstriction and decreased bleeding. For the best effect, they should be taken in the few days preceding the beginning of the menstrual period and be continued through the days of heaviest bleeding. NSAIDs are not as effective in controlling menstrual blood loss as hormonal therapies, but they are readily available without a prescription.

Goals of therapy are to control bleeding, prevent hyperplasia, prevent or treat anemia, and treat concurrent endocrine problems if present. Common treatments include administration of oral contraceptive pills that contain estrogen and progesterone, and prescription of long-term therapy with medroxyprogesterone (Depo-Provera). However, the black box warning required by the U.S. Food and Drug Administration (FDA) about potential bone loss with Depo-Provera has greatly curtailed the use of this therapy. Another treatment is placement of a levonorgestrel intrauterine device (LNG-IUD). The LNG-IUD has a dual indication from the FDA for both birth control and suppression of abnormal menstrual bleeding. The device releases a steady amount of progesterone directly into the uterus to stabilize and suppress the uterine lining. In addition, the progesterone works to suppress the HPG axis and prevent ovulation.

Women who do not wish to have future pregnancies also can opt for treatments that permanently suppress the uterine lining. These treatments include ablation, in which the lining is burned to prevent future proliferation of the endometrial cells, and complete removal of the uterus through hysterectomy. If a woman is menopausal and has not had a menstrual period for longer than 1 year, all vaginal bleeding should be investigated to rule out uterine and other cancers.

Polycystic Ovary Syndrome

Polycystic ovary syndrome (PCOS) remains one of the most common endocrine disturbances affecting women (Fig. 35.4). International criteria for the diagnosis of PCOS require at least two of these conditions: irregular ovulation, elevated levels of androgens (e.g., testosterone), and appearance of polycystic ovaries on ultrasound. Thus polycystic ovaries do not have to be present to diagnose PCOS, and their

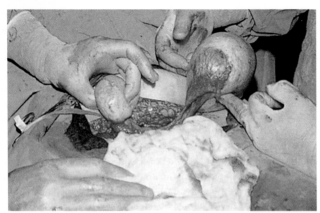

FIGURE 35.4 Polycystic Ovary. Surgical view of polycystic ovaries. (From Symonds EM, Macpherson MBA: *Diagnosis in color: obstetrics and gynecology,* London, 1997, Mosby-Wolfe.)

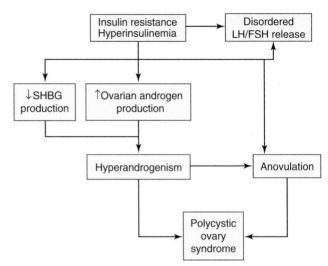

FIGURE 35.5 Insulin Resistance and Hyperinsulinemia in Polycystic Ovary Syndrome (PCOS). See text for explanation. *FSH,* Follicle-stimulating hormone; *LH,* luteinizing hormone; *SHBG,* sex hormone–binding globulin.

presence alone does not establish the diagnosis. The diagnosis is one of exclusion, and other disorders, such as thyroid dysfunction, hyperprolactinemia, and congenital adrenal hyperplasia, must be ruled out. PCOS is a leading cause of infertility in the United States. PCOS has a large incidence of inheritability. Signs and symptoms of PCOS can vary over time, with metabolic syndrome becoming more prominent with age.

PATHOPHYSIOLOGY No single factor accounts for the abnormalities of PCOS. PCOS is related to a genetic predisposition and an obesity-prone lifestyle related to insulin resistance and an excess of insulin and androgens. A hyperandrogenic state is a cardinal feature in the pathogenesis of PCOS. However, glucose intolerance/insulin resistance (IR) and hyperinsulinemia often occur concurrently and markedly aggravate the hyperandrogenic state, thus contributing to the severity of signs and symptoms of PCOS. PCOS predisposes to obesity, and preexisting obesity predisposes to more severe PCOS.

Insulin resistance and the resultant compensatory hyperinsulinemia overstimulate androgen secretion by the ovarian stroma and reduce hepatic secretion of serum sex hormone–binding globulin (SHBG). The net effect is an increase in free testosterone levels. Excessive androgens affect follicular growth, and insulin affects follicular decline by suppressing apoptosis and enabling the survival of follicles that would normally disintegrate (Fig. 35.5). Further, there seems to be a genetic ovarian defect in PCOS that makes the ovary either more susceptible to or more sensitive to insulin's stimulation of androgen production in the ovary.

Inappropriate gonadotropin secretion triggers the beginning of a vicious cycle that perpetuates anovulation. Typically, levels of FSH are low or below normal, and the LH level is elevated. Persistent LH level elevation causes an increase in the concentration of androgens (dehydroepiandrosterone sulfate [DHEAS] from the adrenal glands and testosterone, androstenedione, and dehydroepiandrosterone [DHEA] from the ovary). Androgens are converted to estrogen in peripheral tissues, and increased testosterone levels cause a significant reduction (approximately 50%) in the SHBG level, which in turn causes increased levels of free estradiol. Elevated estrogen levels trigger a positive feedback response in LH and a negative feedback response in FSH. Because FSH levels are not totally depressed, new follicular growth is continuously stimulated, but not to full maturation and ovulation (see Fig. 35.5).

Increased androgen secretion by the ovaries contributes to premature follicular failure (atresia) and persistent anovulation. Persistent

anovulation causes enlarged polycystic ovaries, characterized by a smooth, pearly white capsule. With advancing age, menstrual irregularities may improve, but the incidence of metabolic syndrome and type 2 diabetes mellitus increases. Women with PCOS have a three times greater incidence of uterine cancer later in life than normally cycling women because of an anovulatory lack of progesterone.

CLINICAL MANIFESTATIONS Clinical manifestations of PCOS usually appear within 2 years of puberty but may appear after a period of normal menstrual function and pregnancy. Symptoms are related to anovulation and hyperandrogenism and include dysfunctional uterine bleeding (DUB) or amenorrhea, hirsutism, acne, acanthosis nigricans, and infertility (Box 35.3). Approximately 60% of women with PCOS are obese. Hypertension, dyslipidemia, and sleep apnea also are frequently found in association with PCOS. PCOS is often found in association with other endocrine disorders.

EVALUATION AND TREATMENT Diagnosis of PCOS is based on evidence of androgen excess, chronic anovulation, and sonographic evidence of polycystic ovaries, with at least two of the three criteria present. Tests for impaired glucose tolerance are recommended. In female adolescents, evidence of hyperandrogenism in the setting of irregular menses must be present before PCOS is diagnosed.

Treatment of PCOS often includes use of combined oral contraceptives (COCs) for the management of symptoms (e.g., hirsutism, acne) and to establish regular menses. First-line treatments for obese or overweight women with PCOS include lifestyle modifications, such as regular exercise and weight loss. Reductions in weight can dramatically improve insulin sensitivity and the return of ovulatory cycles. Women with insulin resistance or those who do not respond to contraceptive therapy may benefit from the insulin sensitizer metformin. Progesterone therapy is recommended to oppose estrogen's effects on the endometrium and as a means to initiate monthly withdrawal bleeding if COCs are not used and pregnancy is not desired.

Premenstrual Disorders Syndrome

Premenstrual syndrome (PMS) and premenstrual dysphoric disorder (PMDD) are the cyclic recurrence (in the luteal phase of the menstrual cycle) of distressing physical, psychologic, or behavioral changes that impair interpersonal relationships or interfere with usual activities. The luteal phase of ovulatory cycles is linked with complex hormonal changes of the menstrual cycle. PMDD is often considered a severe, sometimes disabling extension of PMS. The prevalence of PMS and PMDD is difficult to determine, possibly because of the wide-ranging nature of accepted symptoms. Symptoms for PMS and PMDD begin after ovulation during the luteal phase and persist up to 4 days into the menstrual cycle. It has been estimated that 91% of women experience some form of distress around their menstrual period; 30% experience enough distress to interrupt their daily routine; but a much smaller number, as low as 3.1%, meet the criteria for PMDD.

PATHOPHYSIOLOGY   There are many theories to explain PMS/PMDD and the mechanisms, including an increased vulnerability to *fluctuations* in ovarian-derived hormones, and hypothalamic-pituitary-adrenal (HPA) axis changes. The neuroendocrine mechanisms of the

hormonal environment of the menopausal transition that might trigger depression are poorly understood. Erratic ovarian hormone fluctuation may be a mediator of risk for both vasomotor symptoms (hot flashes) and perimenopausal depression. Investigations are ongoing into the effects of changes in estradiol concentrations, the altered antiinflammatory and neuroprotective consequences, and modulation of limbic processing and memory. Neurotransmitters, such as serotonin, gamma-aminobutyric acid (GABA), and norepinephrine, have demonstrated interactions with estrogen and progesterone and have established mood and behavior effects, including negative mood, irritability, aggression, and impulse control. Additionally, neurotransmitters may have mediating or moderating roles on symptom manifestation. Sex steroids also interact with the renin-angiotensin-aldosterone system (RAAS), which could explain some PMS/PMDD signs and symptoms (e.g., water retention, bloating, weight gain). Levels of inflammatory mediators may be elevated with menstrual symptom severity and PMS.

A predisposition to PMS occurs in families, perhaps because of genetics or shared environment; however, no genes have been identified. A woman's menstrual experience is often similar to her mother's or her sister's experience. Evidence supports a relationship between the severity and frequency of PMS/PMDD and reports of low well-being, major affective disorder, and personal characteristics, such as increased stress, poor nutrition, lack of exercise, low self-esteem, perfectionism, history of sexual abuse, and family conflict. In turn, when PMS/PMDD is distressing, the quality of interpersonal relationships and self-image are negatively affected.

CLINICAL MANIFESTATIONS   The pattern of symptom frequency and severity is more important than specific complaints. Nearly 300 physical, emotional, and behavioral symptoms have been attributed to PMS/PMDD. Emotional symptoms, particularly depression, anger, irritability, and fatigue, have been reported as the most prominent and the most distressing, whereas physical symptoms seem to be the least prevalent and problematic. The presence of underlying physical or psychologic disease may be aggravated premenstrually and must be diagnosed and treated independently of PMS/PMDD.

EVALUATION AND TREATMENT   Diagnosis of PMS/PMDD is based on the health history and symptoms; a 2-month, prospective symptom questionnaire is used. Diagnostic criteria for PMDD are presented in Box 35.4. Current treatment is symptomatic because the cause is complex and cannot be reduced to a single biologic explanation; also, occurrence and severity are mediated by lifestyle, social, and psychologic factors. For many women, nonpharmacologic therapies, such as regular exercise, appropriate sleep, diet, stress reduction, acupuncture, and cognitive behavioral therapy with or without medication, may be effective in controlling symptoms. Two major forms of treatment are hormonal cycle regulation and selective serotonin reuptake inhibitor (SSRI) antidepressants. If a woman does not desire immediate fertility, the oral contraceptive pill containing estrogen and progesterone has shown benefits in decreasing PMS/PMDD.

BOX 35.3   Clinical Manifestations of Polycystic Ovary Syndrome

Presenting Signs and Symptoms (% of Women Affected)
Obesity (41%)
Menstrual disturbance (70% [e.g., dysfunctional uterine bleeding])
Oligomenorrhea (47%)
Amenorrhea (19%)
Regular menstruation (48%)
Hyperandrogenism (69%-74%)
Infertility (73% of anovulatory infertility)
Asymptomatic (20% of those with polycystic ovary syndrome [PCOS])

Hormonal Disturbances
Increased insulin (independent of obesity)
Decreased sex hormone–binding globulin (SHBG)
Increased androgens (testosterone, androstenedione)
increased dehydroepiandrosterone (DHEA) (occurs in 50% of women)
Increased luteinizing hormone (LH) (genetic variant LH-β subunit)
Increased prolactin
Increased leptin, especially in obesity (independent of insulin)
Suggested decreased insulin-like growth factor 1 (IGF-1) receptors on theca cells
Possible decreased estrogen receptors (intraovarian and along hypothalamic-pituitary axis)

Possible Late Sequelae
Dyslipidemia—increased low-density lipoproteins (LDLs), decreased high-density lipoproteins (HDLs), increased triglycerides
Diabetes mellitus (30% of women with or without obesity will develop type 2 diabetes mellitus by age 30)
Cardiovascular disease; hypertension
Endometrial hyperplasia and carcinoma (anovulatory women are hyperestrogenic)

Other
Women with PCOS are at increased risk of gestational diabetes mellitus, pregnancy-induced hypertension, preterm birth, and perinatal mortality

Adapted from Azziz R et al: *Fertil Steril* 91(2):456-488, 2009; Boomsma CM et al: *Semin Reprod Med* 26(1):72-84, 2008; Diamanti-Kandarakis E: *Expert Rev Mol Med* 10(2):e3, 2008; Spritzer PM et al: *Int J Clin Pract*, Aug. 19, 2015.

✓ QUICK CHECK 35.2
1. Why does amenorrhea occur?
2. Why do anovulatory cycles lead to abnormal uterine bleeding?
3. Discuss insulin resistance, hyperinsulinemia, anovulation, and androgen production in PCOS.
4. What are the current theories of pathophysiology for PMS/PMDD?

BOX 35.4 Diagnostic Criteria for Premenstrual Dysphoric Disorder

A. Five or more of the symptoms listed in this box—occur in most cycles during the week before menses onset, improve within a few days after menses onset, and diminish in the week postmenses

B. One (or more) of these symptoms must be present:
   a. Marked affective lability
   b. Marked irritability or anger or increased interpersonal conflicts
   c. Marked anxiety, tension

C. One (or more) of these symptoms must also be present:
   a. Decreased interest
   b. Difficulty concentrating
   c. Easy fatigability, low energy
   d. Increase or decrease in sleep
   e. Feelings of being overwhelmed
   f. Physical symptoms (e.g., breast tenderness, muscle or joint aches, "bloating" or weight gain)

NOTE: Criteria A through C must be present for most menstrual cycles in the preceding year.

D. Symptoms are associated with significant distress or interferences with work, school, and relationships.

E. The disturbance is not merely an exacerbation of another disorder, such as major depression, panic disorder, persistent depressive disorder, or a personality disorder.

F. Criterion A should be confirmed by prospective daily ratings in at least two symptomatic cycles.

G. The symptoms are not due to the physiological effects of a substance or another medical condition.

Data from the American Psychiatric Association: *Diagnostic and statistical manual of mental disorders—DSM V,* ed 5, Washington, 2013, Author.

Infection and Inflammation

Infections of the genital tract may result from exogenous or endogenous microorganisms. Exogenous pathogens are most often sexually transmitted. Endogenous causes of infection include microorganisms that are normally resident in the vagina, bowel, or vulva. Infection occurs if these microorganisms migrate to a new location or overproliferate when the immune system and other defense mechanisms are impaired.

Skin disorders that can affect the vulva include reactive dermatitis, contact dermatitis, psoriasis, and impetigo. (For a discussion of skin disorders, see Chapter 43.) Most infectious disorders that affect the vulva and vagina, however, are sexually transmitted. These currently recognized sexually transmitted infections are described in Table 36.1.

Pelvic Inflammatory Disease

Pelvic inflammatory disease (PID) is an acute inflammatory process caused by infection (Fig. 35.6). Data from the Centers for Disease Control and Prevention (CDC) showed a nationwide prevalence of self-reported PID diagnosis of 2.5 million cases among sexually experienced women ages 18 to 44.[3] The PID diagnosis varied by sexual behaviors and sexual health history and differed by race/ethnicity in women without a prior diagnosis of sexually transmitted infection (STI). PID may involve any organ, or combination of organs, of the upper genital tract—the uterus, fallopian tubes, or ovaries—and, in its most severe form, the entire peritoneal cavity. Inflammation of the fallopian tubes is termed salpingitis, and inflammation of the ovaries is called oophoritis. Most infectious disorders that affect the vulva and vagina are sexually transmitted, such as chlamydia and gonorrhea, which migrate from the vagina to the uterus, fallopian tubes, and ovaries. The risk factors for PID include infection by a *previous* STI that was not treated (delaying treatment increases complications from PID). Other risk factors for PID include multiple sex partners or a sex partner who has had multiple sex partners, previous PID, sexual activity before age 25, the use of douches, and the use of an IUD for birth control. Other causes of infection include spontaneous or induced abortions,

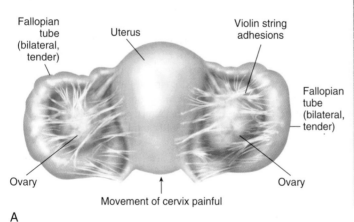
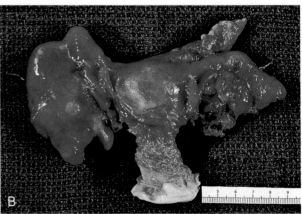

FIGURE 35.6 Pelvic Inflammatory Disease. A, The drawing depicts involvement of both ovaries and fallopian tubes. **B,** Total abdominal hysterectomy and bilateral salpingo-oophorectomy specimen showing unilateral pyosalpinx. (**A** from Ball JW et al: *Seidel's guide to physical examination,* ed 8, St Louis, 2015, Mosby; **B** from Morse SA et al: *Atlas of sexually transmitted diseases and AIDS,* ed 4, Edinburgh, 2010, Mosby.)

puerperal infections (infections occurring after normal or abnormal deliveries), and other surgical procedures; these infections are often polymicrobial.

PATHOPHYSIOLOGY   The development of upper genital tract infections is mediated by the failure of a number of defense mechanisms, including the virulence of the microorganism, the size of the inoculum, and the individual's immune defense status. The main infectious causes of PID are gonorrhea and chlamydia. The microorganisms that cause these infections can infect the vagina and cervix, and if the normal vaginal microbial flora is disrupted, the pathogens can more easily ascend through the cervix (Fig. 35.7). Many anaerobic bacteria have been implicated as increasing the risk of PID because they alter the pH of the vaginal environment and may decrease the integrity of the mucus blocking the cervical canal. Bacterial vaginosis (BV) is present in up to 66% of women with PID, and other anaerobes (e.g., *Bacteroides, Gardnerella vaginalis,* and *Haemophilus influenzae*) and genital tract mycoplasmas *(Mycoplasma hominis, Mycoplasma genitalis,* and *Ureaplasma urealyticum)* are frequently isolated from women with PID. *Escherichia coli* may contribute to pelvic infections in older women. Therefore, although *Neisseria gonorrhoeae* and *Chlamydia trachomatis* are the main pathogens in PID, the disease is actually polymicrobial in origin and is treated with a broad spectrum of antibiotics to ensure that all the causative agents are eliminated.

The infection may induce changes in the columnar epithelium lining of the upper reproductive tract, causing permanent damage. The subsequent inflammatory response causes localized edema and sometimes obstruction or necrosis of the area. Gonorrhea gonococci attach to the fallopian tubes and excrete a substance that is toxic to the tubal mucosa, increasing inflammation and damage. Chlamydiae enter the tubal cells and replicate, bursting the cell membrane as they reproduce and causing permanent scarring. Scarring increases the risk of a later ectopic pregnancy because the mobility of an egg through the fallopian tubes is slowed by damaged cilia. Gonococci and chlamydiae can spread to the abdominal cavity through the openings of the fallopian/uterine tubes. Other mechanisms that may contribute to PID include lymphatic drainage with parametrial spread of the infection, sexual intercourse, and retrograde menstruation. The acute complications of PID include peritonitis and bacteremia, which can increase the risk for endocarditis, meningitis, and infectious arthritis. The chronic consequences of PID include infertility and tubal obstruction, ectopic pregnancy, pelvic pain of varying degrees, and intestinal obstruction from adhesions between the bowel and pelvic organs.[4]

CLINICAL MANIFESTATIONS   The clinical manifestations of PID vary from sudden, severe abdominal pain with fever to no symptoms at all. An asymptomatic cervicitis may be present for some time before PID develops. The first sign of the ascending infection may be the onset of low bilateral abdominal pain, often characterized as dull and steady with a gradual onset. Symptoms are more likely to develop during or immediately after menstruation. The pain of PID may worsen with walking, jumping, or intercourse. Other manifestations of PID include dysuria (difficult or painful urination), dyspareunia (pain with sexual intercourse), and irregular bleeding.

EVALUATION AND TREATMENT   PID often has limited or vague clinical symptoms, leading to undertreatment and long-term health effects. Because PID is a substantial health risk to a woman, the CDC encourages clinicians to consider PID as a likely diagnosis when a sexually active woman has abdominal or pelvic tenderness and *one* of these conditions: cervical motion tenderness, uterine tenderness, or adnexal tenderness.[5] Box 35.5 lists the diagnostic criteria for PID. No laboratory tests or studies are needed to begin treatment; however, additional information can improve the specificity of the diagnosis. Abdominal pain in women can have many causes, and it is important to rule out other diagnoses; this can be done while the person is treated for PID.

The complications of PID can be significant, therefore, rapid treatment is recommended even before the causative pathogen can be identified. Because treatment is empiric, it needs to be effective against a broad range of pathogens, especially chlamydiae, gonococci and anaerobic bacteria. Treatment is usually done on an outpatient basis unless the woman has symptoms of advanced infection, cannot take oral medications, is pregnant, or exhibits other pathologies that cannot be excluded. The outpatient regimen recommended by the CDC is shown in Box 35.6.

To prevent recurrence, sexual partners of women with PID should also receive treatment, even if they are asymptomatic. Women receiving treatment should be reevaluated by their care provider in 3 days to ensure that the antibiotic treatment is effective. Because women with a history of PID are at increased risk for ectopic pregnancy, they should seek care as soon as they know they are pregnant, because ectopic

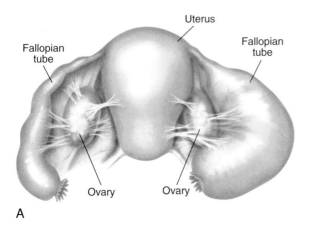

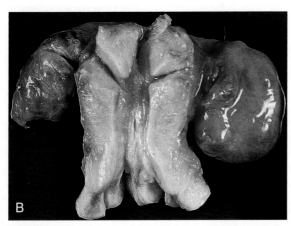

FIGURE 35.7 Salpingitis. A, Advanced pyosalpinx. Note the swollen fallopian tubes. **B,** Bilateral, retort-shaped, swollen, sealed tubes and adhesions of the ovaries are typical of salpingitis. (**A** from Ball JW et al: *Seidel's guide to physical examination,* ed 8, St Louis, 2015, Mosby; **B** from Damjanov I, Linder J, editors: *Anderson's pathology,* ed 10, St Louis, 1996, Mosby.)

BOX 35.5   Diagnostic Criteria for Pelvic Inflammatory Disease (PID)

Minimum Criteria (One or More Needed for Diagnosis)
Cervical motion tenderness, *or*
Uterine tenderness, *or*
Adnexal tenderness

Additional Criteria That Increase Specificity of Diagnosis
Fever >38.3° C (>101° F)
Mucopurulent cervical or vaginal discharge, or cervical friability
Numerous white blood cells on saline wet prep
Elevated C-reactive protein
Elevated erythrocyte sedimentation rate
Documented infection with *Chlamydia trachomatis* or *Neisseria gonorrhoeae*

Definitive Criteria (Not Needed for Treatment)
Transvaginal ultrasound, magnetic resonance imaging, *or*
Doppler studies showing thickened and fluid-filled tubes
Laparoscopic visualization of PID-related abnormalities
Endometrial biopsy with evidence of endometritis

From Centers for Disease Control and Prevention (CDC): *Pelvic inflammatory disease (PID) treatment and care*, Atlanta, 2015, U.S. Department of Health and Human Services.

BOX 35.6   CDC-Recommended Treatment for Pelvic Inflammatory Disease: Intramuscular/Oral Regimens

Ceftriaxone 250 mg IM in a single dose
Doxycycline 100 mg PO twice a day for 14 days
   WITH or WITHOUT
Metronidazole 500 mg PO twice a day for 14 days
Cefoxitin 2g IM in a single dose and **Probenecid,** 1 g orally administered concurrently
In a single dose
   PLUS
Doxycycline 100 mg orally twice a day for 14 days
   WITH or WITHOUT
Metronidazole 500 mg orally twice a day for 14 days
   OR
Other parenteral third-generation **cephalosporin** (e.g., ceftizoxime or cefotaxime)
   PLUS
Doxycycline 100 mg orally twice a day for 14 days
   WITH* or WITHOUT
Metronidazole 500 mg orally twice a day for 14 days

*The recommended third-generation cephalsporins are limited in the coverage of anaerobes. Therefore, until it is known that extended anaerobic coverage is not important for treatment of acute PID, the addition of metronidazole to treatment regimens with third-generation cephalosporins should be considered.
These regimens provide coverage against frequent etiologic agents of PID, but the optimal choice of a cephalosporin is unclear. Cefoxitin, a second-generation cephalosporin, has better anaerobic coverage than ceftriaxone, and in combination with probenecid and doxycycline has been effective in short-term clinical response in women with PID. Ceftriaxone has better coverage against *N. gonorrhoeae*. The addition of metronidazole also will effectively treat BV, which is frequently associated with PID.
CDC, Centers for Disease Control and Prevention; *IM,* intramuscularly; *PO,* orally.
Data from Centers for Disease Control and Prevention (CDC): *Pelvic inflammatory disease (PID) treatment and care*, Atlanta, 2015, U.S. Department of Health and Human Services; Walker CK, Wiesenfeld HC: Clin Infect Dis 28(Supp 1):S29–S36, 2007.

pregnancy is a major cause of maternal mortality. All sexually active women younger than age 25 should receive, at minimum, annual screening for chlamydia and gonorrhea, as should women older than age 25 who have a new sexual partner, more than one sexual partner, a partner who has been diagnosed with an STI, or a partner with more than one sexual partner.

Vaginitis

Vaginitis is irritation or inflammation of the vagina, typically caused by infection, irritants, pathologies, or disruption of the normal vaginal flora. Vaginitis is characterized by complaints of vaginal irritation, itching, burning, odor, or abnormal discharge. Clinically, it is characterized by an increase in white blood cells or abnormal cells, or both, observed on a saline wet prep examination. The major causes of vaginitis are overgrowth of normal flora, STIs, and vaginal irritation related to low estrogen levels during menopause (a condition known as *atropic vaginitis*). The primary forms of vaginitis are vulvovaginal candidiasis, or yeast vaginitis, and bacterial vaginosis, or trichomoniasis. **Bacterial vaginosis** is a noninflammatory condition resulting from an overgrowth of anaerobic bacteria. The overgrowth causes a shift in the composition of the vaginal flora and produces a malodorous vaginal discharge. Pain and itching are common manifestations.

The development of vaginitis is related to alterations in the vaginal environment. This includes changes with complications in local defense mechanisms, such as skin integrity, immune reaction and, particularly, vaginal pH. The pH of the vagina (normally 4 to 4.5) depends on cervical secretions and the presence of normal flora that help maintain an acidic environment. Changes in the vaginal pH may predispose a woman to infection. Variables that affect the vaginal pH, and therefore the bactericidal nature of secretions and the predisposition to infection, include semen and the use of douches, soaps, spermicides, feminine hygiene sprays, and deodorant menstrual pads or tampons. Another variable is having a condition associated with an increased glycogen content of vaginal secretions, such as pregnancy and diabetes. Antibiotics often destroy normal vaginal flora, facilitating the overgrowth of *Candida*

albicans and causing a yeast infection. Increased vaginal alkalinity also may enhance susceptibility to trichomoniasis and BV. Unusual changes in the amount, color, or texture of the vaginal discharge may signal an infection, especially if the discharge is malodorous, irritating, or copious.

The diagnosis is based on the history, physical examination, and examination of the discharge by wet mount. Infection is suggested by a marked change in color or by a discharge that becomes copious, malodorous, or irritating. Treatment involves developing and maintaining an acidic environment, relieving symptoms (usually pruritus and irritation), and administering antimicrobial or antifungal medications to eradicate the infectious organism. If the infection can be sexually transmitted, the woman's partner will also need to be treated. Research suggests that probiotics, especially *Lactobacillus rhamnosus,* can encourage the proliferation of normal vaginal flora and reduce the incidence of vaginitis in women at risk for this disease.

Cervicitis

Cervicitis is a nonspecific term used to describe inflammation of the cervix. The CDC defines cervicitis as having two major diagnostic signs:

a purulent or mucopurulent discharge from the cervical os, or endocervical bleeding (or both), induced by gently introducing a cotton swab into the cervix.[6] Cervicitis can have infectious or noninfectious causes; about half of all cases are caused by sexually transmitted pathogens. Chemicals and substances introduced into the vagina can cause cervicitis, as can disruptions in the normal vaginal flora. However, conflicting definitions of cervicitis are used clinically and in research. Age and risk factors are important in assessing a woman with cervicitis. Younger women are at risk for STIs and should be tested for chlamydia, gonorrhea, and trichomoniasis. Older women with cervicitis may have STIs but are at risk for irritation from abnormal vaginal flora related to low vaginal estrogen levels. Even if no infectious agent is identified, pharmacologic therapy may still be effective.

Mucopurulent cervicitis (MPC) is usually caused by one or more sexually transmitted pathogens, such as *Trichomonas, Neisseria, Chlamydia, Mycoplasma,* or *Ureaplasma spp.* Infection causes the cervix to become red and edematous. A mucopurulent (mucus and pus containing) exudate drains from the external cervical os, and the individual may report vague pelvic pain, bleeding, or dysuria. The cervix often becomes friable, and bleeding can occur during sexual intercourse or with pelvic examinations (or both) and Pap smears. Because mucopurulent cervicitis is a symptom of PID, women at risk for STIs, especially those younger than age 26, should receive treatment for PID while awaiting the results of microbial testing.[7] If the woman is not at risk for STIs, a thorough evaluation often reveals another cause for the inflammation.

Vulvodynia

Vulvodynia (VV) (also referred to as *vulvitis, vestibulitis,* or *vulvovestibulitis*) is chronic pain of at least 3 months duration and inflammation of the vulva or vaginal vestibule (entrance of vagina), or both. The classification of vulvodynia is based on the location of the pain, whether it is localized or generalized, and whether the pain is provoked, unprovoked, or mixed. *Localized* is characterized by pain from a cause that usually does not cause pain (allodynia) to the vulvar vestibule area. *Generalized* is a diffuse pain pattern involving all of the pudendal nerve distribution and beyond. *Provoked* means any touch or stimulation that elicits pain, *unprovoked* is pain that occurs in the absence of touch or stimulation, and *mixed* is pain that varies with or without touch or stimulation. Individuals describe the pain as burning, stinging, soreness, irritation, dyspareunia, throbbing, itching, or rawness. Vulvodynia is fairly common, with lifetime estimates of prevalence ranging from 10% to 28% among reproductive-age women, across races. It also can affect girls.

The cause of VV is unknown. Theories suggest it is multifactorial in origin, including embryonic factors, chronic inflammation, genetic immune factors, nerve pathways, increased sensitivity to environmental factors (infection, trauma, irritants), hormonal changes, human papillomavirus (HPV), and oxalates.[8] Although the inflammation of VV may be caused by contact dermatitis (i.e., exposure to soaps, detergents, lotions, sprays, shaving, menstrual pads/tampons, perfumed toilet paper, tight-fitting clothes), the condition may be more complex and represent abnormalities in three interdependent systems: the vestibular mucosa, pelvic floor musculature, and CNS pain regulatory pathways. The condition also may represent an autoimmune reaction or genetic and psychological links. Recent data suggest site-specific inflammatory responses and the production of proinflammatory mediators.[9] The mechanisms are poorly understood, making the condition difficult to evaluate and treat. An important trigger is chronic inflammation caused by contact irritants, recurrent infections, hormonal changes, and chronic skin conditions. Overall, with normal sensations there is a heightened sensitivity. VV can occur in the context of other pain conditions, such

as irritable bowel syndrome, interstitial cystitis, recurrent yeast infections, and fibromyalgia.

Cotton swab testing is used to identify painful areas. For vulvar pain, treatment is focused on identifying and treating any infectious cause or comorbid contributor. However, laboratory tests and imaging are rarely required for VV. Women are advised to avoid potential irritants; wear loose, cotton clothing; use mild soaps; and apply a vaginal emollient (e.g., coconut oil or vegetable oil) after bathing. Hot water may incite vulvar symptoms.

Studies on treatments are limited but suggest that women may benefit from topical lidocaine (Xylocaine), estrogen cream, topical or systemic antidepressants, or anxiolytics; Botox injections into the affected nerve; dietary modifications; physical therapy; behavioral or sexual counseling (or both); acupuncture; or vestibulectomy. Biofeedback may help to relax the muscles of the pelvic floor and reduce pain.

Bartholinitis

Bartholinitis, or Bartholin cyst, is an acute inflammation of one or both of the ducts that lead from the introitus (vaginal opening) to the Bartholin/greater vestibular glands (Fig. 35.8). Most lesions of the Bartholin gland are cysts or abscesses. The usual causes are microorganisms that infect the lower female reproductive tract, such as streptococci, staphylococci, and sexually transmitted pathogens. Acute bartholinitis may be preceded by an infection, such as cervicitis, vaginitis, or urethritis.

Infection or trauma causes inflammatory changes that narrow the distal portion of the duct, leading to obstruction and stasis of glandular secretions. The obstruction, or cyst, varies from 1 to 8 cm in diameter and is located in the posterolateral portion of the vulva. The affected area is usually red and painful, and pus may be visible at the opening of the duct. This exudate should be cultured. The individual may have fever and malaise. The diagnosis is based on the clinical manifestations and the identification of infectious microorganisms.

Chronic bartholinitis is characterized by the presence of a small cyst that is slightly tender but otherwise asymptomatic. Most Bartholin cysts require no treatment. However, if they are uncomfortable or show signs of infection, treatment is advised to prevent abscess formation.

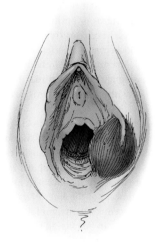

FIGURE 35.8 Inflammation of Bartholin Gland. (Modified from Gershenson DM et al: *Operative gynecology,* ed 2, Philadelphia, 2001, Saunders; Fuller JK: *Surgical technology,* ed 6, Philadelphia, 2013, Saunders.)

Treatment is controversial but involves broad-spectrum antibiotics. Some clinicians attempt to drain the cyst using hot soaks, needle aspiration, insertion of a catheter, or marsupialization (cutting a slit and suturing the edges) of the infected gland. No single treatment has proved superior for both relief and prevention of recurrence. Lesions in the form of carcinomas are a rare type of gynecologic tumor and are carefully monitored among postmenopausal women, who are more prone to Bartholin malignancy.

Pelvic Organ Prolapse

The bladder, urethra, and rectum are supported by the endopelvic fascia and perineal muscles. This muscular and fascial tissue loses tone and strength with aging and may fail to maintain the pelvic organs in the proper position. Progressive descent of the pelvic support structures may cause pelvic floor disorders, such as urinary and fecal incontinence, and pelvic organ prolapse. Pelvic organ prolapse (POP) is the descent of one or more of these structures: the vaginal wall, the uterus, or the apex of the vagina (after a hysterectomy). Although more than 50% of women have some version of POP on physical examination, most women have no symptoms. When prolapse becomes severe, the function of the surrounding organs can be altered. POP is thought be caused by direct trauma (e.g., childbirth); pelvic floor surgery; obesity; constipation; pelvic organ cancers; or damage to the pelvic innervation, particularly the pudendal nerve. Risk factors in nulliparous women, however, include occupational activities that require heavy lifting or chronic medical conditions, such as chronic lung disease or refractory constipation (chronically increased intra-abdominal pressure). The most frequently cited risk factors are aging, obesity, and hysterectomy. Other risk factors include a strong familial tendency (from family and twin studies) and possibly a multifactorial genetic component. Prolapse of the bladder, urethra, rectum, or uterus may occur many years after an initial injury to the supporting structure.

Uterine prolapse is descent of the cervix or entire uterus into the vaginal canal, and in severe cases the uterus falls completely through the vagina and protrudes from the introitus, creating ulceration and obvious discomfort. Fig. 35.9 illustrates the different degrees (grades) of uterine prolapse, showing descent of the cervix or the entire uterus into the vaginal canal. Grade 1 prolapse is not treated unless it causes discomfort. Grades 2 and 3 prolapse usually cause feelings of fullness, heaviness, and collapse through the vagina. Symptoms of other pelvic floor disorders also may be present.

A common first-line treatment is a pessary, a removable mechanical device that holds the uterus in position. The pelvic fascia may be strengthened through Kegel exercises (repetitive isometric tightening and relaxing of the pubococcygeal muscles) or by estrogen therapy in menopausal women. Maintaining a healthy body mass index, preventing constipation, and treating chronic cough may help prevent prolapse. Surgical repair, with or without hysterectomy, is the treatment of last resort.

Fig. 35.10 shows pelvic organ prolapse associated with cystocele and rectocele. Cystocele is descent of a portion of the posterior bladder wall and trigone into the vaginal canal and is usually caused by childbirth. In severe cases, the bladder and anterior vaginal wall bulge outside the introitus. Symptoms are usually insignificant in mild to moderate cases. Increased bulging and descent of the anterior vaginal wall and urethra can be aggravated by vigorous activity, prolonged standing, sneezing, coughing, or straining and can be relieved by rest or by assumption of a recumbent or prone position. If the prolapse is large, women may complain of vaginal pressure. Medical management can include a vaginal pessary, Kegel exercises, and estrogen therapy for postmenopausal women. Surgical treatment is used for severe injury that is unresponsive to medical treatment (see *Did You Know? Vaginal Mesh*).

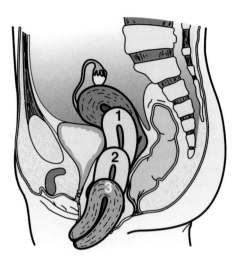

FIGURE 35.9 Degrees of Uterine Prolapse. Grade 1 prolapse is minimal and rarely requires correction. Grade 2 prolapse has moderate symptoms. Grade 3 prolapse is severe; the uterus is so low the cervix protrudes from the vagina. (From Phillips N: *Berry & Kohn's operating room technique,* ed 12, Philadelphia, 2013, Mosby.)

DID YOU KNOW?

Vaginal Mesh

Because pelvic organ prolapse is often a result of weakened pelvic fascia and musculature, a surgical mesh was developed to improve pelvic support. This mesh was designed to be placed surgically along the area needing support. The goal was to have the woman's tissues grow through the mesh and provide consistent, long-term support. However, women who received the surgical mesh had a high rate of complications, including infection and persistent postoperative pain. In many cases the mesh eroded through the tissue, protruding into the vagina and perforating other organs. In addition, the mesh may shrink over time, causing vaginal shortening, tightening, and pain.

Some large studies have shown a benefit from mesh use for some women. However, once implanted, the mesh is difficult to remove if it is ineffective, resulting in long-term pain and the need for intensive surgeries and repairs. The U.S. Food and Drug Administration has issued several warnings about the mesh to caution women and practitioners and encourage fully informed consent about the risks and benefits of mesh placement. On April 16, 2019, the FDA ordered the manufacturers of all remaining surgical mesh products for transvaginal repair of pelvic organ prolapse to stop selling and distributing their products in the U.S. immediately.

Data from Food and Drug Administration: *FDA takes action to protect women's health, orders manufacturers of surgical mesh intended for transvaginal repair of pelvic organ prolapse to stop selling all devices,* Silver Spring, MD, 2019, Author. Available at https://www.fda.gov/NewsEvents/Newsroom/PressAnnouncements/um636114.htm. Retrieved June 17, 2019; Maher C et al: *Cochrane Database Syst Rev* 4:CD004014, 2013; U.S. Food and Drug Administration: *FDA study communication: UPDATE on serious complications associated with transvaginal placement of surgical mesh for pelvic organ prolapse,* 2010. Available at www.fda.gov/MedicalDevices/Safety/AlertsandNotices/ucm2362435.htm.

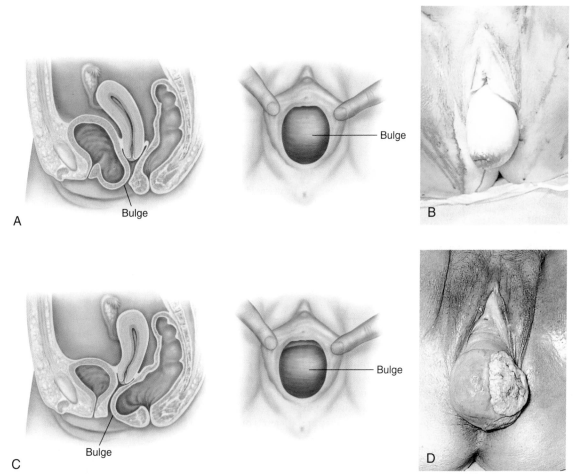

FIGURE 35.10 Cystocele and Rectocele. **A,** Grade 2 (moderate form): anterior vaginal wall prolapse (i.e., cystocele). **B,** Grade 4: prolapse. **C,** Grade 2: posterior wall prolapse (i.e., rectocele). **D,** Grade 4: associated with ulceration of the vaginal wall. Grades 1 and 3 are not shown. (**A** and **C** from Seidel HM et al: *Mosby's guide to physical examination,* ed 4, St Louis, 1999, Mosby; **B** and **D** from Symonds EM, Macpherson MBA: *Color atlas of obstetrics and gynecology,* London, 1994, Mosby-Wolfe.)

A rectocele is the bulging of the rectum and posterior vaginal wall into the vaginal canal. Childbirth may increase damage, ultimately leading to a rectocele, but symptoms may not appear until after menopause. Genetic and familial predisposition and bowel habits contribute to rectocele development. Lifelong chronic constipation and straining may produce or aggravate a rectocele. A large rectocele may cause vaginal pressure, rectal fullness, and incomplete bowel evacuation. Defecation may be difficult and can be facilitated by applying manual pressure to the posterior vaginal wall. Medical treatment focuses on the management and prevention of constipation and, if needed, the use of a pessary. Rectocele alone (without associated enterocele, uterine prolapse, and cystocele) seldom requires surgery.

An enterocele is a herniation of the rectouterine pouch into the rectovaginal septum (between the rectum and the posterior vaginal wall). It can be congenital or acquired. Congenital enterocele rarely causes symptoms or progresses in size, but an acquired enterocele can result from muscular weakness caused by previous surgery, especially those through the vagina, or from pelvic relaxation disorders, such as uterine prolapse, cystocele, and rectocele. Most large enteroceles are found in grossly obese and older adults. Treatment is surgical. Box 35.7 summarizes the symptoms and treatment of POP.

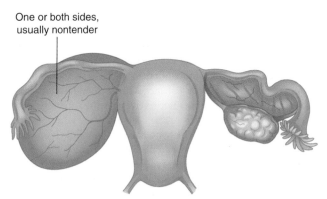

FIGURE 35.11 Depiction of an Ovarian Cyst.

Benign Growths and Proliferative Conditions
Benign Ovarian Cysts
Benign cysts of the ovary may occur at any time during the life span but are most common during the reproductive years and, in particular, at the extremes of those years (Fig. 35.11). An increase in benign ovarian cysts

---

BOX 35.7   Pelvic Organ Prolapse: Symptoms and Treatments

Symptoms	Treatment
Urinary	Depending on age of woman and cause and severity of condition:
Sensation of incomplete emptying of bladder	• Isometric exercises to strengthen pubococcygeal muscles (Kegel exercises)
Urinary incontinence	• Estrogen to improve tone and vascularity of fascial support (postmenopausal)
Urinary frequency/urgency	• Pessary (a removable device) to hold pelvic organs in place
Bladder "splinting" to accomplish voiding	**Surgical**
Bowel	Reconstructive: autologous grafts; synthetic mesh/sling
Constipation or feeling of rectal fullness or blockage	Obliterative (most extreme)
Difficult defecation	Weight loss
Stool or flatus incontinence	Avoidance of constipation
Urgency	Treatment of cough/lung conditions
Manual "splinting" of posterior vaginal wall to accomplish defecation	
Pain and Bulging	
Vaginal, bladder, rectum	
Pelvic pressure, bulging, pain	
Lower back pain	
Sexual	
Dyspareunia	
Decreased sensation, lubrication, arousal	

---

occurs when hormonal imbalances are more common, around puberty and menopause. Benign ovarian cysts are quite common, comprising one third of gynecologic hospital admissions. Two common causes of benign ovarian enlargement in ovulating women are follicular cysts and corpus luteum cysts. These cysts are called functional cysts because they are caused by variations of normal physiologic events. Follicular and corpus luteum cysts are unilateral. They are typically 5 to 6 cm in diameter but can grow as large as 8 to 10 cm. Most women are asymptomatic.

Benign cysts of the ovary are produced when a follicle or a number of follicles are stimulated but no dominant follicle develops and completes the maturation process. Every month about 120 follicles are stimulated, and generally, only 1 succeeds in ovulation of a mature ovum. Normally, in the early follicular phase of the menstrual cycle, follicles of the ovary respond to hormonal signals from the pituitary gland. The pituitary gland produces FSH to mature follicles in the ovary. If the dominant follicle develops properly before ovulation, the corpus luteum becomes vascularized and secretes progesterone. Progesterone arrests development of other follicles in both ovaries in that cycle. LH, proteolytic enzymes, and prostaglandins trigger follicular rupture and release of the ovum.

Follicular cysts (also called *ovarian* or *functional cysts*) are filled with fluid and can be caused by a transient condition in which the dominant follicle fails to rupture or one or more of the nondominant follicles fail to regress. This disturbance is not well understood. It may be that the hypothalamus does not receive or send a message strong enough to increase FSH levels to the degree necessary to develop or mature a dominant follicle. The hypothalamus monitors blood levels of estradiol and progesterone; when the FSH level is low, the estradiol concentration does not increase enough to stimulate LH. Research indicates that when progesterone is not being produced, the hypothalamus releases GnRH to increase the FSH level. FSH continues to stimulate follicles to mature; the granulosa cells grow and, presumably, the estradiol level increases. This abnormal cycle continues to stimulate follicular size and causes follicular cysts to develop. Although individuals may experience no symptoms, some have pelvic pain, a sensation of feeling bloated, tender breasts, and heavy or irregular menses. After several subsequent cycles in which hormone levels once again follow a regular cycle and progesterone levels are restored, cysts usually are absorbed or regress. Follicular cysts can be random or recurrent events.

A corpus luteum cyst may normally form by the granulosa cells left behind after ovulation. This cyst is highly vascularized but usually limited in size, and with the normal menstrual cycle it spontaneously regresses. With an imbalance in hormones, low LH and progesterone levels may cause an abnormal or hemorrhagic cyst. In some cases, large cysts can rupture and cause hemorrhage.

Corpus luteum cysts are less common than follicular cysts, but luteal cysts typically cause more symptoms, particularly if they rupture. Manifestations include dull pelvic pain and amenorrhea or delayed menstruation, followed by irregular or heavier than normal bleeding. Rupture occasionally occurs and can cause massive bleeding, with excruciating pain; immediate surgery may be required. Corpus luteum cysts usually regress spontaneously in nonpregnant women. Oral contraceptives may be used to prevent cysts from forming in the future.

Dermoid cysts are ovarian teratomas that contain elements of all three germ layers; they are common ovarian neoplasms. These growths may contain mature tissue including skin, hair, sebaceous and sweat glands, muscle fibers, cartilage, and bone. Dermoid cysts are usually asymptomatic and are found incidentally on pelvic examination. Dermoid cysts have malignant potential and need careful evaluation for removal.

Torsion of the ovary is a rare complication of ovarian cysts or tumors or enlargement of the ovary; it can occur in girls or women. If a cyst is sufficiently large, it can cause the ovary to twist on its ligaments, reducing the blood supply to the ovary and causing extreme pain. Ovarian torsion is rare, but it is a gynecologic emergency. It usually presents with acute, severe, unilateral abdominal or pelvic pain and is treated surgically.

> ✔ **QUICK CHECK 35.3**
> 1. Why is prompt treatment of pelvic inflammatory disease (PID) critical to reproductive health?
> 2. Why do benign ovarian cysts develop in women who ovulate?
> 3. What is the difference between a follicular cyst and a corpus luteum cyst?

Endometrial Polyps

An endometrial polyp is a benign mass of endometrial tissue that contains a variable amount of glands, stroma, and blood vessels.

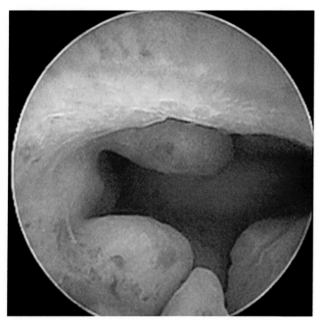

FIGURE 35.12 Uterine Polyps Visible Through Hysteroscopy. (From Cheng C et al: *J Minim Invasive Gynecol* 16[6]:739-342, 2009.)

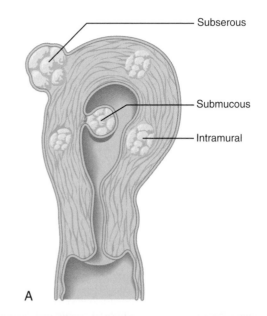

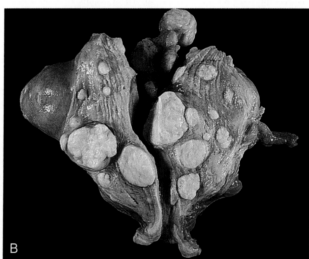

FIGURE 35.13 Leiomyomas. **A,** Uterine section showing the whorl-like appearance and locations of leiomyomas (also called *uterine fibroids*). **B,** Sagittal section showing multiple leiomyomas. Typical, well-circumscribed, solid, light gray nodules distort the uterus. (**B** from Damjanov I, Linder J: *Pathology: a color atlas*, St Louis, 2000, Mosby.)

Endometrial polyps are usually solitary and can occur anywhere within the uterus. Polyps are structurally diverse and are usually classified as hyperplastic, atrophic (or inactive), or functional. Hyperplastic polyps are often pedunculated (stalk or mushroom-like) and may be mistaken for endometrial hyperplasia or, if large, for adenosarcoma (Fig. 35.12). Although polyps most often develop in women between the ages of 40 and 50 years, they can occur at all ages. Risk factors include advancing age, obesity, nulliparity, early menarche or late menopause (or both), diabetes, estrogenic states (i.e., anovulatory cycles and unopposed estrogen), treatment with tamoxifen, and hypertension.

Endometrial polyps are a common cause of intermenstrual bleeding or even excessive menstrual bleeding. The diagnosis is made by transvaginal sonography or hysteroscopy. The lesions can be removed with small, curved forceps, but there is a high rate of spontaneous resolution. The coexistence of a separate endometrial atypical hyperplasia or adenocarcinoma is possible, but malignancy is extremely rare.

Leiomyomas

Leiomyomas, commonly called myomas or uterine fibroids, are benign tumors that develop from smooth muscle cells in the myometrium. Leiomyomas are the most common benign tumors of the uterus, affecting 70% to 80% of all women, and most remain small and asymptomatic. The prevalence increases in women ages 30 to 50 years but decreases with menopause. The incidence of leiomyomas in black and Asian women is two to five times higher than that in white women. On average, the age of onset for black women is 10 years earlier than it is for white women.

The cause of uterine leiomyomas is unknown, although their size appears to be related to estrogen and progesterone, growth factors, and reduced apoptosis. Because leiomyomas are estrogen and progesterone sensitive, uterine leiomyomas are not seen before menarche, are common during the reproductive years, and generally shrink after menopause. Tumors in pregnant women enlarge rapidly but often decrease in size after the end of the pregnancy. Risk factors include heredity, nulliparity, obesity, PCOS, black race, postmenopausal hormone use, and hypertension. Lifestyle factors are risk factors and include diet, caffeine and alcohol consumption, smoking, lack of physical activity, and stress.

PATHOPHYSIOLOGY Most leiomyomas occur in multiples in the fundus of the uterus, although they often can occur singly and throughout the uterus. Leiomyomas are classified as subserous, submucous, or intramural, according to their location within the various layers of the uterine wall (Fig. 35.13). Mutations in the Mediator Subcomplex 12 *(MED12)* gene have been identified in about 70% of uterine leiomyomas. Uterine leiomyomas are usually firm and surrounded by a connective tissue layer. Degeneration and necrosis may occur when the leiomyoma outgrows its blood supply, which is more common in larger tumors and is frequently accompanied by pain.

CLINICAL MANIFESTATIONS The major clinical manifestations of leiomyomas are abnormal vaginal bleeding, pain, and symptoms related to pressure on nearby structures. Fibroids also may contribute to infertility and subfertility, as well as obstruction during birth if the fibroids are large enough. The leiomyoma can make the uterine cavity larger, thereby increasing the endometrial surface area. This enlargement may account for the increased menstrual bleeding associated with leiomyomas. Although pain is not an early symptom, it occurs with the devascularization of larger leiomyomas and is associated with blood vessel compression that limits the blood supply to adjacent structures. Because the fibroid is relatively slow growing, enabling adjacent structures to adapt to pressure, symptoms of abdominal pressure develop slowly. Pressure on the bladder may contribute to urinary frequency, urgency, and dysuria. Pressure on the ureter may cause it to become distended "upstream" from the pressure point; rectosigmoid pressure may lead to constipation. Larger fibroids may cause a sensation of abdominal or genital heaviness.

EVALUATION AND TREATMENT   Uterine leiomyomas are suspected when bimanual examination discloses irregular, nontender nodularity of the uterus. Pelvic sonography or MRI confirms the diagnosis. Treatment depends on the symptoms and tumor size, and the woman's age, reproductive status, preference, and overall health. Most leiomyomas are asymptomatic and can be managed by observation only. Medical treatment is aimed at shrinking the myoma or reducing the symptoms. The use of hormonal contraceptives may shrink or enhance growth and should be closely monitored. Mifepristone (formerly RU-486), a progesterone receptor agonist, and ulipristal acetate may be useful in shrinking fibroids. Shrinking is sometimes done prior to surgical treatment. Nonpharmalogic therapies include green tea extract, curcumin (the active ingredient in turmeric), vitamin D, and herbal preparations used in Chinese medicines.

Surgical treatments are commonly used but may be decreasing in frequency. Hysterectomy is commonly performed for fibroid-related bleeding and pain. Myomectomy, or removal of the fibroid from the muscle of the uterus, may be less invasive than a full hysterectomy and remains the standard of cure for women wishing to preserve their fertility. Other treatments, such as uterine artery embolization (UAE), laser ablation, and the levonorgestrel-intrauterine system (LNG-IUS), all hold promise. A Cochrane review found that UAE appears to have an overall satisfaction rate similar to hysterectomy and myomectomy.[10] UAE is associated with a higher rate of minor complications and a much higher risk of requiring future surgical intervention within 2 to 5 years of the initial procedure.[10] Benefits and risks of all treatments should be carefully considered, as should a woman's desire for future pregnancy.

Adenomyosis

Adenomyosis is the presence of endometrial tissue within the uterine myometrium. Migration of endometrial cells into the myometrial layers occurs as a result of an unknown mechanism. The diagnosis of adenomyosis often is made during the late reproductive years, however, because it is commonly diagnosed after hysterectomy (30% to 60% of normal women), the time of diagnosis may not be associated with the onset. Incidence rates are higher for women taking tamoxifen. Parity also increases the risk for adenomyosis and for women who are pregnant; the outcomes can include preterm labor, preterm rupture of membranes, and low birth weight.

Adenomyosis may be asymptomatic or may be associated with abnormal menstrual bleeding, anemia, dysmenorrhea, uterine enlargement, uterine tenderness during menstruation, chronic pelvic pain, and infertility. Secondary dysmenorrhea becomes increasingly severe as the disease progresses. On examination, the uterus is enlarged, globular, and most tender just before or after menstruation. The diagnosis is confirmed by ultrasonography or MRI. Treatment is symptomatic and includes NSAIDs, hormonal contraceptives, and the LNG-IUD. Other promising treatments include estrogen receptor modulators, high-dose progestins, selective progesterone receptor modulators, aromatase inhibitors, and GnRH agonists. Surgical treatments include resection

or, if severe, hysterectomy. Further testing is needed for uterine artery embolization and uterine ablation. Treatment decisions are based on managing symptoms and preserving future fertility.

Endometriosis

Endometriosis is the presence of functioning endometrial tissue or implants outside the uterus. The ectopic (out of place) endometrium responds to the normal hormonal fluctuations of the menstrual cycle. Common sites of implantation of ectopic tissue include the pelvic peritoneum, ovaries, uterine ligaments, and rectovaginal septum. Many other sites of implantation have been identified (Fig. 35.14). Endometriosis primarily affects younger (premenopausal) women, with a peak incidence in the third decade. The incidence of endometriosis, however, is difficult to determine, especially in asymptomatic adolescent and fertile women. About 50% of women evaluated for pelvic pain, infertility, or a pelvic mass are diagnosed with endometriosis. It is the third most common reason for hysterectomy and is associated with a higher risk for cancers, especially ovarian cancer.

The cause of endometriosis is not known, and many theories exist. One commonly accepted theory, proposed in 1927, suggests that endometriosis results from the implantation of endometrial cells during retrograde menstruation, in which menstrual fluids move through the fallopian tubes and into the pelvic cavity. Women with obstructed menstrual flow do have a higher incidence of endometriosis. However, it is now known that retrograde menstruation occurs in almost all women, but not all women develop endometriosis. Other theories include alterations in cytokine and growth factor signaling, coelomic metaplasia (peritoneal mesothelium, the müllerian ducts, and the germinal epithelium of the ovary all are derived from coelomic wall epithelium), embryonic cell rest (primitive "at rest" embryonic cells become activated), possible spread of endometrial cells outside the uterus during fetal organogenesis, iatrogenic mechanical transplantation, and lymphatic and vascular dissemination.[11] A genetic predisposition to endometriosis has been documented, and genetic polymorphisms have been identified. Disruption of gene expression during embryogenesis may contribute to endometriosis.

PATHOPHYSIOLOGY   The growth of endometrial lesions depends on estrogen. Endometrial lesions are affected by ovarian hormones as endometrial tissue within the uterus, however, endometriosis cells have marked progesterone resistance. The cyclic changes are influenced by

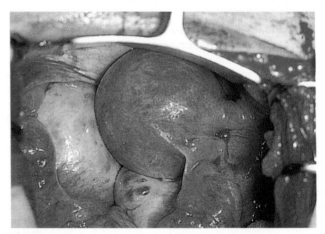

FIGURE 35.14 Endometriosis. The uterus is distended, and retrograde spillage of menstrual loss has led to the development of endometriosis *(dark purple patches).* (From Symonds EM, Macpherson MBA: *Color atlas of obstetrics and gynecology,* London, 1994, Mosby-Wolfe.)

blood supply and the presence of glandular and stromal cells. With an adequate blood supply. the ectopic endometrium proliferates, breaks down, and bleeds with the normal menstrual cycle. The response to the bleeding is inflammation triggering many inflammatory cascades, including cytokines, chemokines, growth factors, and protective factors (leukocyte protease inhibitor and superoxide dismutase). Eventually, the inflammation leads to fibrosis, scarring, adhesions, and pain.

CLINICAL MANIFESTATIONS The clinical manifestations of endometriosis vary in frequency and severity and can mimic other pelvic diseases (i.e., PID, ovarian cysts, and irritable bowel syndrome). Symptoms include infertility, pelvic pain, dyschezia (pain on defecation), dyspareunia, (pain on intercourse) and, less commonly, constipation and abnormal vaginal bleeding. If implants are located within the pelvis, an asymptomatic pelvic mass having irregular, movable nodules and a fixed, retroverted uterus are found on examination. Most symptoms can be explained by the proliferation, breakdown, and bleeding of the ectopic endometrial tissue, with subsequent formation of adhesions. In most instances, however, the degree of endometriosis is not related to the frequency or severity of symptoms. Dysmenorrhea, for example, does not appear to be related to the degree of endometriosis. With involvement of the rectovaginal septum or the uterosacral ligaments, dyspareunia develops. Dyschezia, a hallmark symptom of endometriosis, occurs with bleeding of ectopic endometrium in the rectosigmoid musculature and subsequent fibrosis.

About 25% to 40% of women with infertility have endometriosis. The relationship between endometriosis and infertility is strong; however, the *degree* of disease is not as closely associated. More simply, women with untreated minimal to mild disease may have high pregnancy rates or may experience infertility. The exact reason for infertility in women with endometriosis is unknown.

EVALUATION AND TREATMENT A presumptive diagnosis is based on the previously described symptoms, but pelvic laparoscopy is required for a definitive diagnosis. A uniform classification system that includes both extent and severity has been developed, including stage I, minimal; stage II, mild; and stage III, moderate. The classification, however, still does not correlate well with a woman's symptoms. Treatment is based on preventing progression of the disease, alleviating pain, and restoring fertility. Medical therapies include suppression of ovulation with various medications, such as the noncyclic estrogen-progestin–combined oral contraceptive pill, depot medroxyprogesterone acetate (DMPA), danazol, GnRH agonists/analogs, mifepristone or gestrinone, and promotion of atrophy of the endometrium with progestins or an LNG-IUD. Conservative surgical treatment includes laparoscopic removal of endometrial implants with conventional or laser techniques. All treatments have risks or side effects, and recurrent symptoms develop in most women within a few years, even with surgical treatments. Women should be fully informed of all options and understand the risk-to-benefit ratio of treatments, especially nonreversible treatments.

Cancer

Malignant tumors of the female reproductive system are common. Because the pelvis and abdomen are poorly innervated and designed to accommodate a growing fetus, cancers of the female reproductive tract can often grow large before causing pain. Reproductive cancers are likely to be diagnosed early if there are symptoms; for example, vaginal bleeding prompts women to seek treatment.

Cervical Cancer

Cancer of the cervix has the highest incidence in Africa, Latin America, and the Caribbean, and the lowest incidence in North America and Oceania.[12] In the United States in 2019, an estimated 13,170 new cases of invasive cervical cancer will be diagnosed with an estimated 4250 deaths.[13] Cervical cancer incidence rates declined by more than half between 1975 (14.8 per 100,000) and 2014 (6.9 per 100,000). The decline is attributed to the widespread use of screening, primarily with the Papanicolaou (Pap) test. In the United States, Hispanic women are most likely to get cervical cancer, followed by black women, Asians and Pacific Islanders, and whites. In the United States, American Indians and Alaskan Natives have the lowest risk of cervical cancer.[14]

Human papillomavirus (HPV) infection is almost exclusively the cause of cervical cancer. It is a necessary condition in the development of almost all precancerous and cancerous cervical lesions. Risk factors for cervical cancer include multiple sexual partners, a male partner with multiple previous or current sexual partners, young age at first sexual intercourse, high parity, persistent infection with HPV-16 or HPV-18, immunosuppression, a long history of the use of oral contraceptives, certain human leukocytic antigen (HLA) subtypes, and use of nicotine. Factors affecting the integrity of the immune system may affect a later risk of cervical cancer, including poor nutrition, chronic stress, and immunosuppressant medications. High-risk types of HPV (16 and 18) are found more frequently in women coinfected with chlamydia or gonorrhea. Women who use vaginal douches seemed to have a higher risk of HPV infections, possibly caused by the alteration in the cervicovaginal microbiome.[15] Healthy vaginal microbiomes, marked by adequate quantities of lactobacilli, seem to have a decreased prevalence and increased clearance of HPV.[16]

PATHOPHYSIOLOGY There are multiple subtypes of HPV, and the "high risk" (oncogenic) types of HPV (predominantly 16 and 18) have been most closely associated with high-grade dysplasia and cancer (also see Chapters 11 and 12). HPV-16 accounts for about 60% of cervical cancer cases and HPV-18 for about another 10%; other types contribute less than 5% of cases. The precancerous lesion, or dysplasia, also called *cervical intraepithelial neoplasia (CIN)* and *cervical carcinoma in situ (CIS)*, is a more advanced form of the cell changes and can progress to invasive cancer. Importantly, cervical dysplasia can be detected noninvasively through examination of the cervical cells. If dysplasia is detected early, treatment is available to prevent invasive cancer. Progress to invasive cancer can be very slow. About 30% to 70% of those untreated for CIS will develop invasive carcinoma over 10 to 12 years, however, in about 10% of women, progression from in situ to invasive cancer can occur in less than 1 year.[17]

The cervix is lined by two types of epithelial cells: squamous cells at the outer aspect and columnar glandular cells along the inner canal (Fig. 35.15). The site of the cellular **transformation zone**, called the *squamocolumnar junction*, is illustrated in Fig. 35.16. The transformation zone is very vulnerable to the oncogenic effects of HPV and is the site where CIS is most likely to develop. HPVs infect immature basal cells of the squamous epithelium in the areas of epithelial breaks or injury, or immature metaplastic squamous cells present at the squamocolumnar junction. Establishing HPV infection in the mature squamous cells that cover the ectocervix, vagina, or vulva requires damage to the surface epithelium. The cervix, with its large areas of immature epithelium, is very vulnerable to HPV infection.

Although HPV is a causative factor for cervical cancer, it is not the *only* factor. Other important cocarcinogens must play a role, because in spite of the high percentage of young women infected with one or more HPV types during their reproductive years, only a few develop cancer. The other factors that appear to be associated include immune responses, hormonal responses, and other environmental factors that determine regression or persistence of the HPV infection. Like other

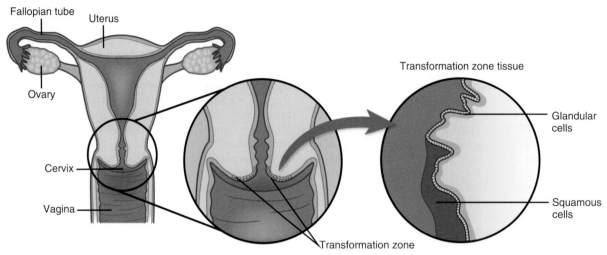

FIGURE 35.15 The Two Types of Epithelial Cells Lining the Cervix: Squamous Cells and Columnar Glandular Cells.

TABLE 35.3   International Federation of Gynecology and Obstetrics (FIGO) Clinical Staging of Cancer of the Cervix

Stage	Characteristics
0	Cancer in situ, intraepithelial carcinoma; earliest stage of cancer; cancer confined to its original site
I	Carcinoma confined to cervix (extension to corpus disregarded)
IA	Earliest form of stage I; very small amount of cancer, which is visible only under a microscope
IA1	Area of invasion is <3 mm (about ⅛ inch) deep and <7 mm (about ⅓ inch) wide
IA2	Area of invasion is between 3 and 5 mm (about 1/5 inch) deep, and <7 mm (about ⅓ inch) wide
IB	Includes cancers that can be seen without a microscope; also includes cancers seen only with a microscope that have spread deeper than 5 mm (about ⅕ inch) into the connective tissue of the cervix or are wider than 7 mm
IB1	IB cancer no larger than 4 cm (about 1⅓ inches)
IB2	IB cancer >4 cm
II	Cancer has spread beyond the cervix to the upper part of the vagina; cancer does not involve the lower third of the vagina
IIA	Involvement is limited to the upper two-thirds of the vagina, without the tissue next to the cervix or *parametrial* invasion
IIB	Cancer has spread to the parametrial tissue
III	Cancer has spread to the lower part of the vagina or the pelvic wall; cancer may be blocking the ureters (tubes that carry urine from the kidneys to the bladder)
IIIA	Cancer has spread to the lower third of the vagina but not to the pelvic wall
IIIB	Cancer extends to the pelvic wall, blocks urine flow to the bladder, or both
IV	Most advanced stage of cervical cancer; cancer has spread to other parts of the body
IVA	Cancer has spread to the bladder or rectum (i.e., organs close to the cervix)
IVB	Cancer has spread to distant organs beyond the pelvic area, such as the lungs

cancers, cervical cancer requires the accumulations of genetic alterations for carcinogenesis to occur.

Cervical cancer is a slowly progressive disease that moves from normal cervical epithelial cells to dysplasia to CIS and, eventually, to invasive cancer (see Fig. 35.16, *B*). Table 35.3 summarizes the staging of cervical cancer. Testing for high-risk HPV is often positive for many years (10 years or more) before dysplasia progresses to high-grade squamous intraepithelial lesions (HSILs) that can develop into invasive cervical cancer (CIN III, Table 35.4).

CLINICAL MANIFESTATIONS Because cervical neoplasms are predominantly asymptomatic, about 90% of cervical cancers can be detected early through the use of Pap and HPV testing. If symptoms exist, they may include a change in vaginal discharge or bleeding. Bleeding varies and may occur after intercourse or between menstrual periods. At times,

TABLE 35.4   Classification System for Squamous Cervical Precursor Lesions

Dysplasia/ Carcinoma in Situ	Cervical Intraepithelial Neoplasia	Squamous Intraepithelial Lesion, Current Classification
Mild dysplasia	CIN I	Low-grade SIL (LSIL)
Moderate dysplasia	CIN II	High-grade SIL (HSIL)
Severe dysplasia	CIN III	High-grade SIL (HSIL)
Carcinoma in situ	CIN III	High-grade SIL (HSIL)

CIN, Cervical intraepithelial neoplasia; *SIL,* squamous intraepithelial lesion.
From Kumar V et al: *Robbins & Cotran pathologic basis of disease,* ed 9, Philadelphia, 2015, Elsevier/Saunders.

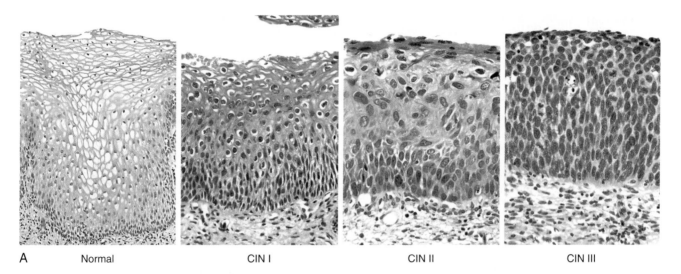

A   Normal   CIN I   CIN II   CIN III

Cervical Disease Progression[1-6]

Most HPV infections will clear, and most cervical lesions will not progress[1-3]

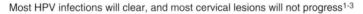

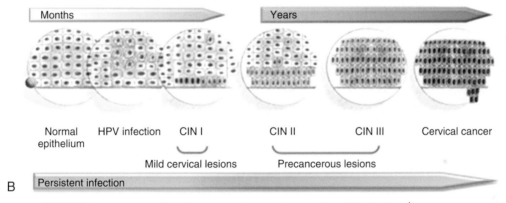

Normal   HPV infection   CIN I   CIN II   CIN III   Cervical cancer
epithelium

Mild cervical lesions   Precancerous lesions

B   Persistent infection

• CIN 2/3 lesions are more likely to progress to cervical cancer than CIN 1 lesions[1]

1. Oster A. *Int J of Gynecol Path*, 1993, 12:186-92. 2. Moscicki A et al, *Vaccine*, 2006, 2453:42-51. 3. Einstein M. *Cancer Immunol Immunother*, 2008, 57:443-51. 4. Winer R. et al. *J Int Dis*, 2005, 191:731-38. 5. Holowaty P. et al. *J Natl Cancer Inst*, 1999, 91:252-58. 6. Solomon D. et al. *JAMA*, 2002, 287:2114-19.

FIGURE 35.16 Cervical Intraepithelial Neoplasia (CIN). A, Normal multiparous cervix, including the transformation zone, where precancerous and cancerous changes occur. CIN stage I—note the white appearance of part of the anterior lip of the cervix; this is associated with neoplastic changes. CIN stage II—lesions also are reflected in distant capillaries. CIN stage III—lesions are predominantly around the external os. **B,** Normal epithelium, then human papillomavirus (HPV) infection progressing to CIN stage I. With more time, persistent HPV infections progress to precancerous lesions CIN II and CIN III and eventually to cervical cancer. Most cervical lesions do not progress to cervical cancer. (**A** from Kumar V et al: *Robbins & Cotran pathologic basis of disease,* ed 9, Philadelphia, 2015, Saunders; **B** from Symonds EM, Macpherson MBA: *Color atlas of obstetrics and gynecology,* London, 1994, Mosby.)

women will complain of abnormal menses or postmenopausal bleeding. A less common symptom may be a serosanguineous or yellowish vaginal discharge. A new or foul odor also may be present. Advanced disease may cause urinary or rectal symptoms and pelvic or back pain.

EVALUATION AND TREATMENT   Women should be screened for cervical cancer and their risk for future cervical cancer through Pap and HPV testing. The new U.S. Preventive Services Task Force (USPSTF) guidelines for screening are presented in Box 35.8. When dysplasia is detected, colposcopy is usually indicated to identify lesions and obtain needed biopsies. If invasive carcinoma is found, lymphangiography, a computed tomography (CT) scan, MRI, ultrasonography, or radioimmunodetection methods are used to further assess tissue involvement.

Treatment depends on the degree of neoplastic change, the size and location of the lesion, and the extent of metastatic spread. Treatment for invasive carcinoma depends on the stage of the tumor and includes surgery, radiation therapy, chemotherapy, and targeted treatment. The prognosis is excellent with early detection and treatment. The prevention of HPV infection through HPV vaccines is the key to substantially reducing the risk of cervical cancer (see *Did You Know?* Primary Prevention for Cervical Cancer). HPV also can cause anal cancer and mouth/throat (oropharyngeal) cancer, as well as cancer of the vulva, vagina, and penis. HPV vaccination is recommended for preteen girls and boys at age 11 or 12 years. Young women can get the HPV vaccine until they are 27 years old, and young men can get HPV vaccine until they are 22 years old.

BOX 35.8 Clinical Summary: Screening for Cervical Cancer

	Women 21-29 Years	Women 30-65 Years	Women <21 Years, Women >65 Years With Adequate Prior Screening, and Women Who Have Had a Hysterectomy
Recommendation	Screen for cervical cancer every 3 years with cytology alone. Grade: A	Screen for cervical cancer Every 3 years with cytology alone, every 5 years with high-risk human papillomavirus (hrHPV) testing alone, or every 5 years with cotesting. Grade: A	Do not screen for cervical cancer. Grade: D
Risk Assessment	All women age 21 to 65 years should be screened; they are at risk for cervical cancer because of potential exposure to hrHPV through sexual intercourse. Certain risk factors increase the risk for cervical cancer, including infection with the human immunodeficiency virus (HIV), a compromised immune system, in utero exposure to diethylstilbestrol, and previous treatment of a high-grade precancerous lesion or cervical cancer. Women with these risk factors should receive individualized follow-up.		
Screening Tests	Screening with cervical cytology alone, primary testing for hrHPV alone, or both at the same time (cotesting) can detect high-grade precancerous cervical lesions and cervical cancer. Clinicians should focus on ensuring that women receive adequate screening, appropriate evaluation of abnormal results, and indicated treatment, regardless of which screening strategy is used.		
Treatments and Interventions	High-grade cervical lesions may be treated with excisional and ablative therapies. Early-stage cervical cancer may be treated with surgery (hysterectomy) or chemotherapy.		

For a summary of the evidence systematically reviewed in making this recommendation, the full recommendation statement, and supporting documents, go to http://uspreventiveservicestaskforce.org.
From U.S. Preventive Services Task Force: *J Am Med Assoc* 320(7):674-686, 2018.

DID YOU KNOW?

Cervical Cancer Primary Prevention

Individuals who are not sexually active almost never develop genital human papillomavirus (HPV) infections. HPV vaccination before sexual activity can reduce the risk of infection by HPV types targeted by the vaccine.

The U.S. Food and Drug Administration (FDA) has approved three vaccines to prevent HPV infection: Gardasil, Gardasil 9, and Cervarix. Currently, Gardasil 9 is the only HPV vaccine available for use in the U.S. These vaccines provide strong protection against the HPV-targeted infections, but they are not effective for treating established infections or disease caused by HPV. All three vaccines prevent infections with HPV types 16 and 18, the two high-risk HPVs that cause about 70 percent of cervical cancers. Gardasil also prevents infection with HPV types 6 and 11, which causes about 90% of genital warts. Gardasil 9 prevents infection with the same four high-risk HPV types plus five additional high-risk types (31, 33, 45, 52, and 58)..

The current CDC recommendations for Gardasil 9 vaccination include:

- All children aged 11 or 12 years should get two HPV vaccine shots 6 to 12 months apart. If the two shots are given less than 5 months apart, a third shot will be needed. Changes in recommendations on dosing could change in the future.
- HPV vaccine is recommended for young women through age 26, and young men through age 21.
- Adolescents who get their first dose at age 15 or older need three doses of vaccine given over 6 months.
- Persons who have completed a valid series with any HPV vaccine do not need any additional doses.

Importantly, consistent and correct condom use is associated with reduced HPV transmission, and less frequent use is not. The virus can infect areas not covered by the condom.

Data from NIH National Cancer Institute: *Human papillomavirus (HPV) vaccines.* Reviewed May 16, 2018. Accessed 06/21/2019. Available at https://www.cancer.gov/about-cancer/causes-prevention/risk/infectious-agents/hpv-vaccine-fact-sheet.

Vaginal Cancer

Cancer of the vagina is the rarest of the female genital cancers (about 0.6 per 100,000 women yearly). In 2019, the number of new cases of vaginal cancer was estimated at 5350, with 1430 deaths.[13] Vaginal and cervical cancers are thought to have a similar epidemiology. They both start as intraepithelial lesions, occur in women who have been sexually active, and are associated with HPV infection. Prior carcinoma of the cervix or uterus increases a woman's risk for developing vaginal cancer. Another risk factor is in utero exposure to nonsteroidal estrogens such as diethylstilbestrol (DES), dienestrol, or hexestrol. For example, exposures from 1960 to 1971 were estimated to occur in 100,000 to 160,000 women.[18] Exposure to such hormones during the first 3 months of gestation can inhibit the normal replacement of columnar epithelium by squamous epithelium in the vagina of the fetus. Columnar epithelium, not normally found in the vagina, may then undergo malignant transformation. Other risk factors include smoking and previous radiation therapy in the vaginal area.

Vaginal cancer is usually diagnosed in women in their 60s and 70s, however, the cellular changes began many years before. More than 90% of women with vaginal cancer have squamous cell carcinoma. The remaining 10% are adenocarcinomas, sarcomas (rare), and melanomas (rare). Nonsquamous types of cancer are more common in younger women.

Vaginal cancer can be asymptomatic until late in the progression. The main clinical manifestations include vaginal bleeding or bloody discharge. Other manifestations include vaginal discharge, vulvar pruritus, rectal or bladder symptoms, pain, or leg edema.

Diagnosis of vaginal cancer includes Pap testing colposcopy, and biopsy. Once the diagnosis of cancer is known, the size and extent of the lesion are determined using MRI before surgery. Vaginal cancers are classified as intraepithelial neoplasia (dysplasia), CIS, or invasive carcinoma. Treatment depends on these findings and on the age of the individual. Treatments include laser therapy or removal, or both; chemotherapy; and radiation therapy. Recurrence and survival rates vary by the type and extent of the cancer. HPV vaccination is the primary form of prevention.

Vulvar Cancer

Cancer of the vulva most often affects the labia majora and less often the labia minora, clitoris, or vaginal glands. In 2019, the number of new cases was estimated as 6070, with 1280 deaths.[13] There has been a steady increase in the incidence of vulvar cancer over the past 30 years. The majority (90%) are squamous cell carcinomas. Risk factors for vulvar cancer include HPV type 16 (cause), infection with the human immunodeficiency virus (HIV), HPV-18 (probable cause), increasing age, previous cancer (untreated high-grade vulvar intraepithelial neoplasia [VIN]), cervical cancer survivor, previous CIN, women with certain autoimmune conditions (increased risk of HPV-associated tumors), organ transplant recipients (perhaps because of immunosuppression to clear HPV), and tobacco use (may relate to inability to clear HPV infection). Other possible risk factors include having many sexual partners, having the first sexual intercourse at a young age, and having a history of abnormal Pap test results. Risk factors for STIs are risk factors for vulvar cancer. The development of vulvar cancer is preceded by condyloma or squamous dysplasia. Early detection is critical. Treatment includes ablative or excisional surgery and, sometimes, radiation with or without chemotherapy.

Endometrial Cancer

Carcinoma of the endometrium is the most common type of uterine cancer (uterine corpus) and the most prevalent gynecologic malignancy (Fig. 35.17). Endometrial cancer begins in the cells lining the uterus or endometrium. Estimates in the United States include 61,880 new cases in 2019, with approximately 12,160 deaths.[13] Although the incidence rates for black women have historically been lower than those for white women, they may be equalizing because of risk factors. Death rates are still higher in black women, and these rates are the highest of any racial/ethnic group; black women are more frequently diagnosed at later stages with more aggressive subtypes of endometrial cancer. Most cases occur in postmenopausal women, with a peak incidence in the late 50s to early 60s. It is the sixth most common cancer worldwide, and the incidence is highest in North America and Europe and lowest in middle-income countries, such as India and South Africa. Incidence rates have

been increasing in 26 of 43 countries worldwide. The rise in incidence is thought to be caused by factors that affect hormones, such as rising rates of obesity and shifting reproductive trends (e.g., having fewer children). The primary risk factor for endometrial cancer is prolonged exposure to **unopposed estrogen** (without progesterone). Exposure to unopposed estrogen includes estrogen-only hormone replacement therapy, tamoxifen use, early menarche, late menopause, never having children, and failure to ovulate (i.e., PCOS and anovulatory cycles typical of the late reproductive years). Another risk factor is obesity, because it is a known source of endogenous estrogen. Although related to obesity, other risk factors include diabetes, chronic inflammation, and lack of physical activity (Fig. 35.18).

Controlling obesity, diabetes, and hypertension may reduce the risk of endometrial cancer. Another important factor for reducing the risk of endometrial cancer is exposure to progesterone for both immediate and long-term effect, however, it can increase the risk of breast cancer. So far, the lone dietary factor that may lower the risk of endometrial cancer is drinking coffee regularly.

PATHOPHYSIOLOGY Endometrial hyperplasia is associated with prolonged estrogenic stimulation of the endometrium. Endometrial

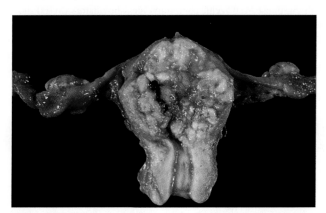

FIGURE 35.17 Endometrial Cancer. Tumor fills the endometrial cavity, and myometrial invasion is obvious. (From Damjanov I, Linder J, editors: *Anderson's pathology,* ed 10, St Louis, 1996, Mosby.)

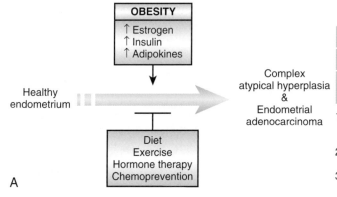

	ENDOMETRIAL CANCER	
	DECREASES RISK	INCREASES RISK
Convincing		Body fatness[1]
Probable	Physical activity[2] Coffee[3]	Glycemic load

1 The panel interpreted BMI (including BMI at age 18-25 years), measures of abdominal girth, and adult weight gain as interrelated aspects of body fatness as well as fat distribution
2 Physical activity of all types; occupational, household, transport and recreational
3 The effect is found in both caffeinated and decaffeinated coffee and cannot be attributed to caffeine

A

B

FIGURE 35.18 Food, Nutrition, Physical Activity, and Endometrial Cancer. A, Overview of obesity's contribution to the progression of endometrial cancer, and also preventive strategies. The T-shaped bar indicates factors that reduce the risk of endometrial cancer. (See the text for a full discussion.) **B,** Convincing and probable data on reducing and increasing the risk of endometrial cancer. (**A** from Schmandt RE et al: *Am J Obstet Gynecol* 205[6]:518-525, 2011; **B** from World Cancer Research Fund/American Institute for Cancer Research: *Continuous update project report: food, nutrition, physical activity, and the prevention of endometrial cancer,* 2013. Available at https://www.wcrf.org/dietandcancer.)

hyperplasia and carcinoma share acquired genetic alterations in genes linked to carcinogenesis (Table 35.5). Progesterone inhibits estrogen-driven growth in the uterus. The antagonistic effects of progesterone on the estrogen-induced proliferation and growth occur mostly during the luteal phase and are dependent on the presence of functional progesterone receptor (PR) expression. Investigators are studying the importance of stromal PR and its role in progesterone inhibition of epithelial proliferation (Fig. 35.19). The interactions between the epithelial and stromal cells of the endometrium may determine the eventual role in the actions of progesterone. The delicate balance of the PR isoforms can tip the scales to foster endometrial hyperplasia and atypia and enhance expression of uterine growth factors. Misregulation of isoform expression can lead to abnormal function and precancerous changes.

Two broad categories of endometrial carcinoma include type I and type II. Type I tumors are most common and result from estrogen exposure that leads to endometrial hyperplasia. Type II tumors are about 10% of endometrial tumors but are more likely to be invasive. Type I and type II endometrial carcinoma are summarized in Table 35.5.

CLINICAL MANIFESTATIONS AND EVALUATION AND TREATMENT
Abnormal vaginal bleeding is the most common clinical manifestation of endometrial cancer. Postmenopausal women, obese women, and women with unopposed estrogenic conditions (i.e., anovulatory cycles) should be evaluated in the event of unscheduled or persistent, irregular vaginal bleeding. Pain and weight loss are symptoms of more advanced disease. Transvaginal ultrasound (TVUS) may be used to measure endometrial thickness, and with the rising incidence of endometrial cancer, earlier

diagnosis is imperative. If the endometrium is abnormally thick (defined as >5 mm), then further testing, such as an endometrial biopsy, is done. Treatment is based on the extent of the disease and may include progestin therapy for simple hyperplasia (orally or through LNG-IUD), curettage for CIS, total abdominal hysterectomy, chemotherapy, and radiation. Metformin is being studied as a possible strategy for preventing and treating certain cancers, including endometrial cancer.

Ovarian Cancer

Ovarian cancer accounts for about 4% of the worldwide cancer incidence and mortality among women.[12] Ovarian cancer in the United States is a common gynecologic malignancy, with 50% of all cases occurring in women older than 65 years.[19] Globally, ovarian cancer is the seventh most common cancer and the eighth leading cause of death from cancer in women.[12] Incidence rates are highest in more developed regions and lowest in Sub-Saharan Africa.[12] In the United States, 22,530 new cases of ovarian cancer and 13,980 ovarian cancer deaths are estimated for 2019.[13] The understanding of incidence patterns both within and between populations is essential to revealing potential causes of and risk factors for ovarian cancer (Fig. 35.20). The highest age-adjusted incidence rates are observed in developed parts of the world, including North America and Central and Eastern Europe; the lowest such rates are seen in Asia and Africa. In the United States, racial differences in epidemiology mimic the observed international variation, with rates highest among whites, intermediate for Hispanics, and lowest among blacks and Asians.[20] Migration studies show that moving from countries with low rates to those with high rates results in greater risk, demonstrating the importance of nongenetic factors. Ovarian cancer has high morbidity and mortality. Based on global estimates, about 140,000 women die annually from the disease worldwide.[21] Risk factors for ovarian cancer are summarized in Table 35.6.

Despite study limitations, several factors related to ovulation have been consistently associated with an increased or a decreased risk of developing ovarian cancer. Risk is reduced by factors that suppress ovulation (pregnancy, breast-feeding, and combined hormonal contraceptive use). Ovarian cancer has been a very difficult disease to diagnose early and treat. The high mortality reflects a lack of early symptoms and a lack of effective screening tests.

PATHOPHYSIOLOGY   The biology of ovarian cancer is changing. and it is clear that ovarian cancer is diverse in character, or *heterogeneous.* Many genetic and epigenetic changes are evident in ovarian tumors. The majority of ovarian tumors are sporadic and are not caused by inherited genetic factors. These cancers are acquired as somatic mutations

TABLE 35.5	Type I and Type II Endometrial Carcinoma	
Characteristics	**Type I**	**Type II**
Age	55-65 yr	65-75 yr
Clinical setting	Unopposed estrogen	Atrophy
	Obesity	Thin physique
	Hypertension	
	Diabetes	
Morphology	Endometrioid	Serous
		Clear cell
		Mixed müllerian tumor
Precursor	Hyperplasia	Serous endometrial intraepithelial carcinoma
Mutated genes/genetic abnormalities	*PTEN*	*TP53*
	ARID1A (regulator of chromatin)	Aneuploidy
		PIK3CA (PI3K)
	PIK3CA (PI3K)	*FBXW7* (regulator of MYC, cyclin E)
	KRAS	
	FGF2 (growth factor)	*CHD4* (regulator of chromatin)
	MSI	
	CTNNB1 (Wnt signaling)	*PPP2R1A* (PP2A)
	TP53	
Behavior	Indolent	Aggressive
	Spreads via lymphatics	Intraperitoneal and lymphatic spread

CTNNB1, Beta-catenin gene; *MSI,* microsatellite instability.
From Kumar V et al: *Robbins & Cotran pathologic basis of disease,* ed 9, Philadelphia, 2015, Elsevier/Saunders.

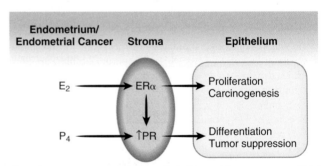

FIGURE 35.19 Actions of Estradiol (E₂) and Progesterone (P₄) in the Development of Endometrial Cancer. E₂ action through stromal estrogen receptor-α (ERα) is critical for the development of endometrial cancer. Progesterone (P₄) acts through stromal progesterone receptors (PRs) to oppose this carcinogenic effect of E₂. (From Kim JJ et al: *Endocr Rev* 34[1]:130-162, 2013.)

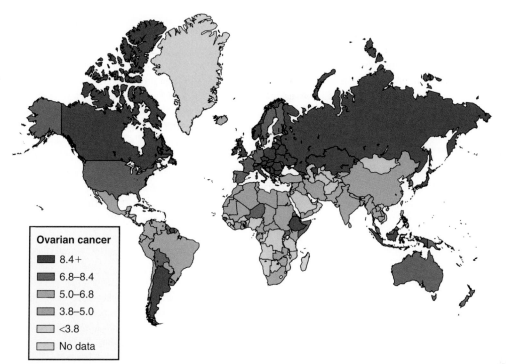

FIGURE 35.20 Map of Ovarian Cancer Worldwide. Rates are per 100,000 women and are age standardized to the 1960 world standard population. Data were not included for white areas on the map. (From Ferlay J et al: GLOBOCAN 2012 v1.0, *Cancer incidence and mortality worldwide: IARC CancerBase No. 11*, Lyon, France, 2013, International Agency for Research on Cancer. Available at http://globocan.iarc. fr/Default.aspx.)

that occur during a person's lifetime. In cases that cluster in families, the genetic basis for the disease and the pattern of inheritance is unclear.[22] Previously, the majority of ovarian cancers were thought to arise from just epithelial cells that cover the ovarian surface or line subserosal cysts. Newer evidence suggests that tumors arise from three ovarian components: (1) from the fimbriae of fallopian tubes and from deposits of endometriosis; (2) from germ cells, which are pluripotent and migrate to the ovary from the yolk sac; and (3) from stromal cells, including the sex cords, which precede endocrine changes of the postnatal ovary.[23] Some ovarian tumors remain too difficult to classify.

The normal ovary contains three major cell types: (1) germ cells, derived from the endoderm, which differentiate into oocytes; (2) hormone-producing cells (estrogen and progesterone) within the ovary; and (3) epithelial cells (derived from the müllerian duct) that cover the ovary and line inclusion cysts. Both benign and malignant tumors come from each of the three ovarian cell types[24] (Fig. 35.21). Epithelial ovarian cancers constitute about 90% of malignant ovarian tumors and generally develop after age 40. Sex cord–stromal tumors arise from connective tissue, often secrete hormones, can occur in women of all ages, and comprise about 7% of ovarian tumors.[24] Tumors that arise from germ cells occur in the second and third decades and account for about 3% to 5% of ovarian tumors.[24] Borderline tumors of low malignant potential can contain structural and molecular evidence of transformed epithelial cells that do not invade the underlying stromal tissue. Approximately 10% of borderline tumors can recur after surgical resection and prove lethal.[24]

There are three major histologic types of epithelial tumors: serous, mucinous, and endometrioid. These types all have a benign, borderline, and malignant category.[4] The most common histologic subtype is high-grade serous cancers, and they may originate from a precursor

lesion that arises from the fimbriae of the fallopian tubes. In women who underwent prophylactic salpingo-oophorectomies, fallopian tubal lesions were present in almost 100% of women with early serous cancers associated with familial *BRCA* gene mutations. Investigators recently proposed that the fallopian tube *is* the primary site of most serous carcinomas.[25] Although historically investigators proposed that the vast majority of serous carcinomas arose from cortical inclusion cysts, cysts may arise from implantation of detached fallopian tube epithelium at sites where ovulation has disrupted the surface of the ovary.[4] These findings have led to changes in the management of women at high risk for ovarian cancer (*BRCA* mutation carriers and women with a strong family history of breast/ovarian cancer); they are now recommended to have salpingo-oophorectomy and not just a simple oophorectomy.[4]

Additionally, histologically similar cancers diagnosed as primary peritoneal carcinomas share molecular findings (i.e., inactivation of p53 and BRCA1 and BRCA2 proteins). Therefore, tumors arising from fallopian tube and other locations from the peritoneal cavity, together with most ovarian epithelial cancers, are classified as "extrauterine adenocarcinomas of müllerian epithelial origin" and are included, staged, and treated similarly to ovarian cancer.[26]

Ovarian tumors are now classified as type I (low grade) and type II (high grade) (see Fig. 35.21, *B*). Endometrioid ovarian carcinomas may arise in the setting of endometriosis and are sometimes associated with borderline tumor.[4]

CLINICAL MANIFESTATIONS Generally, individuals with ovarian cancer have no *early* symptoms. Because there are no effective screening techniques to detect it, the disease is usually advanced by the time treatment is sought. Some women may experience *nonspecific* symptoms that include abdominal distention; loss of appetite; early

TABLE 35.6   Risk Factors for Ovarian Cancer

Risk Factor	Description
Advancing age	Incidence of ovarian cancer increases with advancing age. Most cases occur in postmenopausal women.
Genetic factors	About 5% to 15% of all ovarian cancers are inherited. Of these, the majority are related to mutations in *BRCA1* and *BRCA2* genes; other factors include mismatched repair genes (e.g., Lynch syndrome), TP53 in the germ line (e.g., Li-Fraumeni syndrome), and Peutz-Jeghers syndrome. Fallopian tube cancer and peritoneal carcinomas also are part of the *BRCA*-associated disease spectrum.
Family history	A family history of ovarian cancer in a first-degree relative (e.g., mother, daughter, or sister) is the most important risk factor. The highest risk appears in women who have two or more first-degree relatives with ovarian cancer. Risk may be higher if the affected relative was diagnosed at a younger age, previous breast cancer was diagnosed before the age of 40, and had previous breast cancer and a history of ovarian cancer. A cohort study showed ovarian cancer risk is higher in women whose sibling has/had liver, stomach, breast, prostate, connective tissue cancer, or melanoma; and in those whose parent has/had breast or liver cancer.
Overweight and obesity (body mass index [BMI])	Meta-analysis found higher risk of ovarian cancer in premenopausal women with a BMI >30 and no effect in postmenopausal women. Another meta-analysis found a link between a high BMI and ovarian cancer risk in women who had never used menopausal hormone therapy (MHT).
Height	Greater adult-attained height (reflects factors that promote childhood growth) is classified by the World Cancer Research Fund/American Institute for Cancer Research (WCRF/AICR) as a probable cause of ovarian cancer. A pooled analysis of Nordic data and meta-analyses showed ovarian cancer risk is 7% to 10% higher per 5-cm increment in height.
Reproductive/hormonal factors	Ovarian cancer risk is associated with factors affecting lifetime ovulations (and breaks between) or sex hormone levels (estrogens, progesterone, and androgens), or both. Early age at menarche and late age at menopause increases risk by increasing the number of ovulatory cycles. Structural changes to the ovary can occur with ovulation that may stimulate cancer development. These changes may be affected and enhanced by hormonal factors. Having more children, breast-feeding, or using oral contraceptives deceases the number of ovulations and therefore reduces the risk of ovarian cancer. Elevated risk with late age at first birth (>30 years of age).
Menopausal hormone therapy	Current use of postmenopausal hormone replacement therapy (HRT, also known as menopausal hormone therapy [MHT]) is classified by the International Agency for Research on Cancer (IARC) as a cause of ovarian cancer (see Table 12.1). A meta-analysis found women using MHT for just a few years were more likely to develop ovarian cancer than women who had never used MHT. For every 1000 women who take MHT for 5 years from about age 50, there will be one extra ovarian cancer. An estimated 1% of individuals with ovarian cancer in the United Kingdom are linked to MHT use. In long-term (5+ years) users of estrogen-only MHT, compared with never users, ovarian cancer risk is 53% higher. From a cohort study, ovarian cancer risk is 17% higher in long-term (5+ years) estrogen-progesterone MHT users when compared with never users.
Endometriosis	Recent studies have shown that women with endometriosis have an increase in ovarian cancer risk.
Diabetes	Meta-analyses have shown ovarian cancer risk is 20% to 55% higher in women with diabetes compared with those without diabetes.
Previous cancer	Ovarian cancer risk is 24% higher in breast cancer survivors compared with the general population (possibly reflects *BRCA* mutations and Lynch syndrome or shared hormonal factors). It is higher in those diagnosed with breast cancer at a younger age (40s and younger) versus those diagnosed older; the higher risk is limited to estrogen receptor (ER)–negative or ER-unknown breast cancer.
Smoking	An analysis showed an increased risk for mucinous ovarian tumors in current smokers. The risk decreased to normal after cessation of smoking. Recent results from the European Prospective Investigation into Cancer and Nutrition (EPIC) study showed smoking increases the risk of mucinous ovarian tumors.
Asbestos (occupational exposure)	Asbestos is classified by IARC as a cause of ovarian cancer (see Table 11.1).
Talc-based powder	Talc-based powder used peritoneally is classified by IARC as a probable cause of ovarian cancer (see Table 12.1). The risk of ovarian cancer with talc-based powders has been based on meta-analyses and pooled analyses of case control studies. Not all body powders contain talc.
Ionizing radiation	Use of x-radiation and gamma radiation is classified by IARC as a probable cause of ovarian cancer (see Table 12.1). A small number of cases of ovarian cancer may be associated with radiotherapy for previous cancer.
Factors that reduce the risk of ovarian cancer	Taking contraceptives is classified by IARC as protective against ovarian cancer. Breastfeeding is classified by WCRF/AICR as possibly protective against ovarian cancer. Ovarian cancer risk is lower in women with these factors (supported by meta-analyses and pooled analyses): higher parity, hysterectomy, tubal ligation, and use of statins. A meta-analysis estimated a 20% lower risk for the most physically active women compared to the least active. Certain drugs, for example, metformin and daily aspirin use has been associated with a lower risk. Avoidance of cumulative exposures, such as from cigarettes, may lower risk.

Data from Cancer Research UK: *Ovarian cancer risk factors*, London, Author; Cogliano VJ et al: *J Natl Cancer Inst* 103:1827-1839, 2011; Ferlay J et al: *GLOBOCAN 2008 v1.2, Cancer incidence and mortality worldwide: IARC CancerBase no. 10* [Internet], Lyon, France, 2010, International Agency for Research on Cancer; International Agency for Research on Cancer: *List of classifications by cancer sites with sufficient or limited evidence in humans*, vol 1-105; National Cancer Institute: *PDQ®ovarian epithelial, fallopian tube, and primary peritoneal cancer treatment*, Bethesda, Md, 2015, Author. Date last modified March 27, 2015. Available at http://cancer.gov/cancertopics/pdq/treatment/ovarianepithelial/HealthProfessional; Parkin DM et al: *Cancer* 105(S2):S77-S81, 2011; World Cancer Research Fund/American Institute for Cancer Research (WCR/AICR): *Food, nutrition, physical activity, and the prevention of cancer: a global perspective*, Washington, DC, 2007, Author; Reid BM et al: *Epidemiology of ovarian cancer: a review, Cancer Biol Med* 14(1):9-32, 2017.

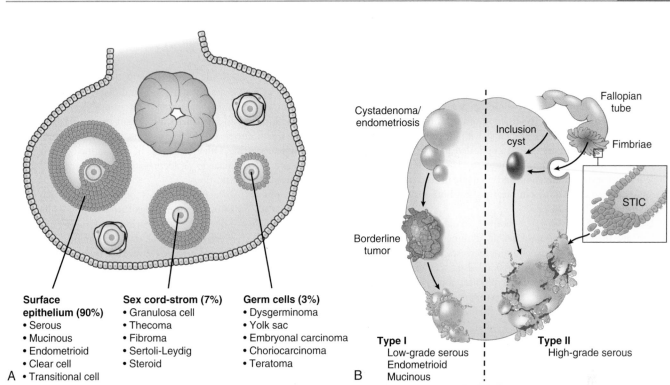

FIGURE 35.21 Heterogeneous Ovarian Tumors. A, Diverse ovarian tumors originate from different cell subtypes. B, Type I and type II ovarian tumors. Type I tumors progress from benign tumors through borderline tumors that give rise to low-grade carcinoma. Type II tumors arise from inclusion cysts/fallopian tube epithelium through intraepithelial precursors that often are unidentifiable. These tumors demonstrate high-grade features and are commonly of serous histology. *STIC*, Serous tubal intraepithelial carcinoma. (B from Kumar V et al: *Robbins & Cotran pathologic basis of disease*, ed 9, Philadelphia, 2015, Elsevier/Saunders.)

satiety; pelvic pain; vaginal bleeding, especially after menopause; vaginal discharge; and a lump in the pelvic area. To help decrease delays in diagnosis, efforts have been made to increase clinician and patient awareness of these symptoms. Symptoms of advanced disease include pain, abdominal swelling and distention, dyspepsia, vomiting, and alterations in bowel habits. There also can be a feeling of pressure in the pelvis and leg pain. Given the location of the ovaries, assessing abnormalities on routine gynecologic examination poses difficulty, especially in obese women. Ovarian cancer is generally considered a silent disease.

Tumor obstruction of vascular channels can cause venous and, occasionally, arterial thrombosis. Alterations in coagulation also occur, contributing to clot formation. Metastasis often causes pleural effusion (Fig. 35.22).

EVALUATION AND TREATMENT   There is no sensitive and specific test for ovarian cancer for screening low-risk women. Routine screening of women without risk factors has not been shown to be beneficial and may cause harm because more women have unnecessary surgical procedures.[27] Solid evidence indicates that screening with a CA-125 blood test and TVUS does not result in a decrease in ovarian cancer mortality after a research follow-up of 12.4 years.[26] Other tests include a pelvic exam, CT scan, positron emission tomography (PET), MRI, chest x-ray, and biopsy. The International Federation of Gynecologists and Obstetricians (FIGO) staging system is described in Table 35.7.

The initial approach to treatment is surgery to determine the stage of disease and to remove as much of the tumor as possible. Survival increases with the expertise of the surgeon. Understanding the biology of cancers and decreasing tumor implantation (seeding) have mandated highly

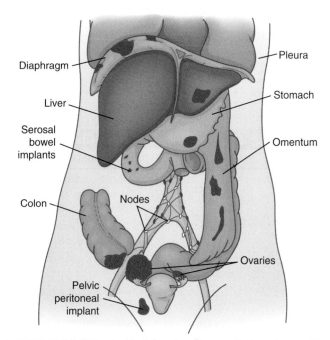

FIGURE 35.22 Metastasis of Ovarian Cancer. Pattern of spread for epithelial cancer of the ovary.

skilled surgical and biopsy techniques.[28,29] Treatment is then customized based on the stage of the cancer, the woman's desires, the cell type, and the sensitivity of the cancer cells. Radiation and chemotherapy are common treatments. New therapies under investigation include monoclonal antibodies, epidermal growth factor receptor, gene therapy, and small-molecular-weight inhibitors. Research into the prevention and treatment of ovarian cancer is ongoing and expanding.

Sexual Dysfunction

Sexual dysfunction is the lack of satisfaction with sexual function resulting from pain or a deficiency in sexual desire, arousal, or orgasm/climax. Sexual function and dysfunction result from a complex set of personal and biologic factors that interact with the culture. Both organic and psychosocial disorders can be implicated in sexual dysfunction. Additionally, studies have shown that up to 45% of adult women have some form of sexual dysfunction, and adequate research is still needed. Chronic medical conditions can greatly affect both sexual desire and sexual function (Table 35.8).

Disorders of desire (hypoactive sexual desire, decreased libido) are the most common sexual dysfunction in women. The prevalence of hypoactive sexual desire increases with age and may be a biologic manifestation of depression, dissatisfaction with partner relationships, a history of sexual or physical abuse, alcohol or other substance abuse, prolactin-secreting pituitary tumors, or testosterone deficiency. Medications, such as the β-adrenergic blockers used for

heart disease, may inhibit sexual desire. Treatment may include sexual and psychological therapy, flibanserin, exogenous testosterone, and antidepressants.

Anorgasmia (orgasmic dysfunction) is the inability of a woman to reach or achieve orgasm. It ranges from difficulty in arousal to lack of orgasm. Any chronic illness may affect arousal. Specific disorders that may block orgasm are diabetes, alcoholism, neurologic disturbances, hormonal deficiencies, and pelvic disorders, such as infections, trauma, and surgical scarring. Other inhibitors of orgasm include drugs, such as narcotics, tranquilizers, antidepressants (especially SSRIs), and antihypertensive medications.

Dyspareunia (painful intercourse) is common. Women may experience pain at any time from the beginning of arousal to after intercourse. The pain may have a burning, sharp, searing, or cramping quality and may be described as external, vaginal, deep abdominal, or pelvic. A variety of psychosocial and organic causes have been identified. Inadequate lubrication may make penetration or intercourse difficult or painful. Drugs with a drying effect (e.g., antihistamines, certain tranquilizers, and marijuana) and disorders (e.g., diabetes, vaginal infections, and estrogen deficiency) can decrease lubrication. Other causes include skin problems around the introitus or affecting the vulva; irritation or infection of the clitoris; disorders of the vaginal opening; disorders of the urethra or anus; disorders of the vagina, such as infections, thinning of the walls caused by aging or decreased estrogen level, or irritation caused by spermicides or douches; and pelvic disorders, such as infection, tumors, and cervical or uterine abnormalities.

Vaginismus is an involuntary muscle spasm in response to attempted penetration. Common psychological causes include prior sexual trauma and fear of sex. Organic causes are similar to those that cause dyspareunia, including VV. Even after the underlying organic problem is detected and successfully treated, vaginismus may persist.

Sexual dysfunction may develop as a coping mechanism. Women with a history of sexual trauma—rape, incest, or molestation—often have problems with desire, arousal, or orgasm or experience pain with sexual activity. In extreme cases, total sexual aversion may develop. At other times, sexual dysfunction may be a symptom of marital or relationship problems. Because sexual dysfunction has many causes, assessment and treatment should be holistic and culturally sensitive.

TABLE 35.7	FIGO* Staging of Carcinoma of the Ovary
Stage	**Characteristics**
I	Growth limited to ovaries
II	Growth involves one or both ovaries and also other organs (i.e., uterus, bladder, colon)
III	Cancer involves one or both ovaries, and one or both of these are present: (1) cancer has spread beyond pelvis to lining of abdomen, (2) cancer has spread to lymph nodes
IV	Growth involves one or both ovaries, with distant metastases to lungs, liver, or other organs outside peritoneal cavity
Recurrent	Cancer recurs after completion of treatment

*The International Federation of Gynecologists and Obstetricians.

TABLE 35.8	Possible Effects of Chronic Disease on Sexual Functioning in Women
Disease	**Sexual Function**
Cerebral palsy	Intact genital sensations, decreased lubrication; difficulty with sexual activity/positioning because of muscle spasticity, rigidity, or weakness; pain with positioning caused by contracture of knees and hips or because of increased spasms with arousal
Cerebrovascular accident (CVA)	Difficulties in sexual positioning and sensitivity because of impaired motor strength, coordination, or paralysis; decreased libido with stroke on dominant side of brain
Diabetes	Diminished intensity of orgasm and gradual decline in ability to achieve orgasm; decreased lubrication or recurrent vaginal infections with resultant dyspareunia
Chronic renal failure	Decreased arousal; increasingly rare and less intense orgasms; decreased lubrication
Rheumatoid arthritis (RA)	Painful sexual activity/positions because of swollen, painful joints, muscular atrophy, and joint contracture; decreased libido because of pain, fatigue, or medication; genital sensations remain intact
Systemic lupus erythematosus (SLE)	Similar to RA; decreased lubrication and vaginal lesions result in painful penetration
Myocardial infarction (MI)	Most literature male-oriented; problems related to medications
Multiple sclerosis (MS)	Diminished genital sensitivity; decreased lubrication; declining orgasmic ability; difficulty with sexual activity because of muscle weakness, pain, or incontinence
Spinal cord injury	Reflex sexual response with injury above sacral area; disrupted response with lesion at or below sacrum; loss of sensation, decreased lubrication; spasticity, incontinence, or pain with arousal; continued orgasmic sensations or sensations diffused in general or to specific body parts, such as breast or lips

Impaired Fertility

Infertility affects approximately 15% of all couples and is defined as the inability to conceive over 1 year of unprotected intercourse. Fertility can be impaired by factors in the man or in the woman, or in both partners. The rate of infertility may be increasing because of increased rates of STIs, environmental exposures, and delayed childbearing. Additionally, the rates of infertility may be increasing secondary to increased reporting from greater utilization of medical services for infertility.[30,31] Causes of infertility include ovulatory disorder, abnormal semen, blockage of the fallopian tubes, endometriosis, and unexplained infertility. Ovulatory disorders account for about 40% of female infertility. Ovulation can be disrupted by hormonal imbalances (e.g., TSH, estrogen, progesterone), chronic conditions, and stress. The regularity of ovulation and the quality of ova decrease with age. Approximately 20% of cases are because of abnormalities of the reproductive tract, such as tubal pathologies. The remaining cases are caused by rare disorders, or the etiology is unknown. Fallopian tube dysfunction may result from acute pelvic infections such as chlamydia or gonorrhea. Adhesions from a pelvic infection, abdominal surgery, or endometriosis may cause blockage of one or both fallopian tubes, preventing access of the sperm to the ovum. The fertilized ovum must implant on a receptive endometrium. Receptivity may be greatly diminished by fibroids or inadequate molecular or cellular preparation of the implantation site. Male infertility contributes to about 40% of cases of infertility (see Chapter 36).

Before the performance of basic fertility tests, a complete history is obtained that includes (1) coital timing and frequency; (2) an in-depth assessment and charting of the menstrual cycle; (3) a reproductive history, including previous pregnancies from both partners and their outcome; (4) a medical history of systemic disease; (5) current medications; (6) previous surgeries; (7) a sexual history, including any previous STIs; and (8) exposure to toxins. Testing starts with the least invasive test or procedure and advances in complexity and, possibly, invasiveness. The most common test for male infertility is the semen analysis. Hormonal assays may be helpful. Pelvic examination, ultrasound, and hysterosalpingogram help determine anatomy and fallopian/uterine tube patency. Chromosomal analyses of the couple may reveal mutations that result in early embryo loss.

To enable women and couples to conceive and bear children, assisted reproductive technologies (ARTs) have proliferated. Questions are being addressed about the health and long-term safety of infants conceived with assisted reproduction; for example, concerns about the high rate of twins and preterm births in pregnancies conceived with ARTs. Additionally, children born through ART have a higher rate of birth defects.[32] Several explanations of the causes of these outcomes suggest that the birth defects may be the result of epigenetic changes that occur when the expression of the embryo's DNA is affected by the very early environment of the blastocysts.[32] It is not clear, however, if damage done through the fertilization and implantation procedures themselves is caused by an underlying medical condition contributing to the infertility.[32] Importantly, research is ongoing in this area. It is essential to prevent STIs, which can result in scarring and adhesion formation in the reproductive tract of either the man or the woman.

> ✔ **QUICK CHECK 35.4**
> 1. Why is cervical cancer considered a sexually transmitted infection?
> 2. What are the risk factors and pathogenesis for endometrial cancer?
> 3. What factors reduce the risk of ovarian cancer?
> 4. Discuss the new hypothesis for the pathogenesis of ovarian cancer.

DISORDERS OF THE FEMALE BREAST

Galactorrhea

Galactorrhea (inappropriate lactation) is the persistent and sometimes excessive secretion of a milky fluid from the breasts of a woman who is not pregnant or nursing an infant. Galactorrhea, which also can occur in men, may involve one or both breasts and is not associated with breast cancer.

The incidence of galactorrhea is difficult to estimate because of differences among definitions of the condition, examination techniques, and populations of women who have been studied. The prevalence has been documented as 0.1% to 32% of all women.

PATHOPHYSIOLOGY Galactorrhea is a manifestation of pathophysiologic processes elsewhere in the body, rather than a primary breast disorder. These processes are chiefly hormone imbalances caused by hypothalamic-pituitary disturbances, pituitary tumors, or neurologic damage. Exogenous causes include drugs, estrogen, and manipulation of the nipples.

Galactorrhea caused by hyperprolactinemia is manifested by the spontaneous appearance of a milky secretion from multiple duct openings, usually from both breasts. Use of oral contraceptives (OCs), especially high-dose use, may cause galactorrhea that is characterized by a clear, serous, or milky discharge from multiple ducts. The discharge is noticeable during the drug-free interval between OC packets. In premenopausal women with unilateral or bilateral spontaneous multiple duct discharge that increases before menstruation, the condition is often caused by fibrocystic disease. Unilateral, spontaneous, serous, or serosanguineous discharge from a single duct usually is caused by an intraductal papilloma. Bloody discharge suggests cancer; bilateral, sticky, multicolored discharge from multiple ducts is often caused by ductal ectasia; and purulent discharge indicates a subareolar abscess.

The most common cause of galactorrhea is nonpuerperal prolactinemia, or excessive amounts of prolactin in the blood not related to pregnancy or childbirth. Nonpuerperal hyperprolactinemia can be caused by any factor that (1) stimulates or overstimulates the prolactin-secreting units of the pituitary gland; (2) interferes with production of prolactin-inhibiting factor (PIF), a neurotransmitter (probably dopamine) that inhibits prolactin secretion; or (3) interferes with pituitary receptors for PIF. Exogenous agents (e.g., certain drugs) can cause nonpuerperal hyperprolactinemia, as can certain disorders.

Hypothyroidism causes increased secretion of hypothalamic TSH, which stimulates prolactin release from the pituitary. Hypothyroidism also is associated with reduced metabolic clearance of prolactin, which prolongs its effects.

Many types of pituitary tumors cause hyperprolactinemia, particularly prolactinoma. Prolactinomas cause hyperprolactinemia by secreting prolactin, decreasing production of PIF, or applying pressure to the pituitary stalk, thus preventing delivery of PIF to the anterior pituitary. Growth hormone–secreting pituitary tumors may cause galactorrhea through the intrinsic lactogenic effect that growth hormone appears to have on mammary tissue. Prolactin-secreting lung and kidney tumors also cause hyperprolactinemia.

Chronic stress may cause hyperprolactinemia by inhibiting PIF release. Head trauma, cervical spinal injuries, encephalitis, meningitis, herpes zoster, or thoracotomy scars may stimulate the suckling reflex. The suckling reflex increases prolactin secretion.

CLINICAL MANIFESTATIONS Inappropriate lactation is manifested by the appearance of a milky breast secretion from one or both breasts of nonpregnant, nonlactating women. A small amount of breast milk expressed from the nipples of parous women is usually not a cancer.

Most women with galactorrhea experience menstrual abnormality. If a pituitary process is involved, the woman usually experiences hirsutism and infertility; if a hypothalamic lesion is present, she may report CNS symptoms, such as intractable headache, visual field disturbances, sleep disturbances, and abnormal temperature, thirst, or appetite.

EVALUATION AND TREATMENT　Galactorrhea in nulliparous women or in parous women who have not breast-fed for 12 months must be thoroughly evaluated. Evaluation includes a variety of diagnostic tests. Serum prolactin levels are measured, and at least two positive results are needed to diagnose hyperprolactinemia. Prolactin levels higher than 25 to 30 ng/ml (measured by radioimmunoassay) are considered elevated. Those in the range of 75 to 100 ng/ml are possibly caused by a pituitary tumor until proven otherwise. Serum thyroxine (T_4) and TSH levels are measured to rule out hypothyroidism, and LH and FSH levels are obtained if the individual is amenorrheic. MRI may assist in locating adenomas.

Treatment for galactorrhea consists of identifying and treating the cause. Medical therapy is typical, and surgical or radiation therapy is rarely required.

Benign Breast Disease and Conditions

Benign breast disease (BBD) is a range of noncancerous changes in the breast. Numerous benign alterations in ducts and lobules occur in the breast, including lumps, cysts, sensitive nipples, and itching. The most common symptoms reported by women are pain, a palpable mass, or nipple discharge; the majority of these prove to have a benign cause. Major determinants of the risk of breast cancer after a diagnosis of BBD include histologic or biologic features, or both; previous biopsy; and degree of family history.[33] Benign epithelial lesions can be broadly classified as (1) nonproliferative breast lesions, (2) proliferative breast disease without atypia, and (3) atypical (atypia) hyperplasia. The majority of nonproliferative benign lesions are not precursors of cancer and generally are not associated with an increased risk of breast cancer.[33]

Nonproliferative Breast Lesions

Nonproliferative epithelial breast lesions are usually not associated with an increased risk of breast cancer. The nonproliferative lesions include (1) simple breast cysts, (2) papillary apocrine change, and (3) mild hyperplasia of the usual type. Terms such as fibrocystic changes (FCCs); or physiologic nodularity and cysts), fibrocystic disease, chronic cystic mastitis, and mammary dysplasia refer to nonproliferative lesions but are not clinically useful because they are a heterogeneous group of diagnoses.[33] Simple cysts (fluid-filled sacs) are the most common nonproliferative breast lesion and are a specific type of lump that commonly occurs in women in their thirties, forties, and early fifties. Cysts feel "squishy" when they occur close to the surface of the breast, but when deeply embedded they can feel hard. An estimated 50% to 80% of women normally experience some of these changes. The prevalence of fibrocystic lesions is probably related to hormonal changes, which in turn are affected by genetic background, age, parity, history of lactation, and use of caffeine and exogenous hormones. Cystic changes can be induced in experimental animals by altering ratios of estrogens and progesterone. It is assumed, therefore, that breast cysts are the result of ovarian alterations, but the exact mechanism is unknown. Cysts also can be associated with unilateral nipple discharge. Cysts often rupture, with release of secretory material into the adjacent tissue. The resulting chronic inflammation and scarring fibrosis contribute to the palpable firmness of the breast. Fibrous tissue increases progressively until menopause and regresses thereafter.

Papillary apocrine change is an increase in ductal epithelial cells that has apocrine changes or an eosinophilic cytoplasm. Mild hyperplasia of the usual type is an increase in the number of epithelial cells within a duct that is more than two cells, but not more than four cells, in depth.[33]

Proliferative Breast Lesions Without Atypia

Proliferative breast lesions without atypia are characterized by the proliferation of ductal epithelium or stroma, or both, without cellular signs of abnormality (atypia, or deviation from normal). Five structurally diverse lesions are discussed next.

Usual ductal hyperplasia (UDH) is additional or proliferating epithelial cells that fill and distend the ducts and lobules. They are usually an incidental finding on mammography. The cells can vary in size and shape, but they retain features of benign cells.[33] No additional treatment is needed, and chemoprevention is not recommended.[33]

Intraductal papillomas can occur as solitary or multiple lesions. Solitary papillomas are a monotonous (sameness) array of papillary cells that grow from the wall of the cyst into the lumen of the duct. Growth occurs within a dilated duct often near or beside the nipple, causing benign nipple discharge. These papillomas *can* harbor areas of atypia or ductal carcinoma in situ (DCIS). Newer data suggest that not all papillomas diagnosed by core needle biopsy (CNB) require surgical excision, however, surgical excision is warranted when a CNB demonstrates papilloma with atypical cells.[33]

Diffuse papillomatosis (multiple papillomas) may present as breast masses, nodules on ultrasound, or the cause of nipple discharge. Diffuse papillomatosis is defined as a minimum of five papillomas within a localized segment of breast tissue.[33] Although the breast cancer risk is small, these lesions require surgical excision.

Sclerosing adenosis is a lobular lesion with increased fibrous tissue and scattered glandular cells.[33] No treatment is needed, and chemoprevention is not indicated.

Radial scar (RS) (also called *complex sclerosing lesions*) refers to an irregular, radial proliferation of ductlike small tubules entrapped in a dense central fibrosis. RSs are usually discovered when a breast lesion or radiologic abnormality is biopsied or removed. Rarely are radial scars discovered by mammography, which cannot reliably differentiate between these lesions and speculated carcinoma.[33] Although controversy exists about the need for surgical excision, there is some evidence that radial scars may be premalignant lesions and can slowly progress from scar to hyperplasia to carcinoma.[33]

Simple fibroadenomas are benign solid tumors that contain glandular and fibrous lesions.[33] In about 20% of cases, multiple fibroadenomas can occur in the same breast or bilaterally.[33] The etiology for fibroadenomas is unknown but appears to be hormonal because they persist during the reproductive years and can increase in size during pregnancy or with estrogen therapy. They usually regress after menopause.[33] They are more common among women between 15 and 35 years of age. Fibroadenomas are now considered proliferative lesions, and the histologic features influence the risk of breast cancer. There is no increased risk of breast cancer in the majority of women with a simple fibroadenoma. It is not necessary to excise all biopsy-proven fibroadenomas.[33] Disadvantages of excisional surgery include scarring at the incision site, dimpling of the breast from the removal of the tumor, damage to the breast's duct system, and mammographic changes (e.g., architectural distortion, skin thickening, increased focal density).[33] If a biopsy-proven fibroadenoma is asymptomatic, it can then be left in place, although some women wish to have the mass excised so that they will not worry further.[33]

Proliferative Breast Lesions With Atypia

Atypical hyperplasia (AH) is an increase in the number of cells (or proliferation) with the cells having some variation in structure—*atypia*.

AH is a high-risk benign lesion found in about 10% of biopsies with benign findings.[34] These proliferative breast lesions with some atypia include atypical ductal hyperplasia and atypical lobular hyperplasia. **Atypical ductal hyperplasia (ADH)** refers to abnormal proliferating cells in breast ducts. **Atypical lobular hyperplasia (ALH)** refers to proliferation of cells in the lumen of lobular units.

Much of the next discussion will refer just to "AH." Studies indicate that women with AH, especially multifocal lesions, have an increased risk (about fourfold) of breast cancer compared with women who have nonproliferative lesions. Ongoing studies will further determine risk estimates with such factors, for example, as family history, reproductive risk factors, alcohol, or breast density (Fig. 35.23). About 60% of the subsequent breast cancers in women with AH occur in the ipsilateral breast (same side) as the biopsy.[35-37] Long-term studies mentioned earlier have shown that atypical hyperplasia confers a relative risk of 4 for future breast cancer, and recently the *absolute risk* has been better defined with a cumulative incidence of breast cancer of about 30% at 25 years of follow-up.[38,39] Recent studies in women diagnosed with ADH by CNB and excisional biopsy had a slightly lower risk of invasive breast cancer than previously reported.[40]

It appears that menopausal status at the time of benign breast biopsy influences the magnitude of the subsequent breast cancer risk. For women who were premenopausal at the time of their breast biopsy, the risk of breast cancer was greater in those with ALH than among women

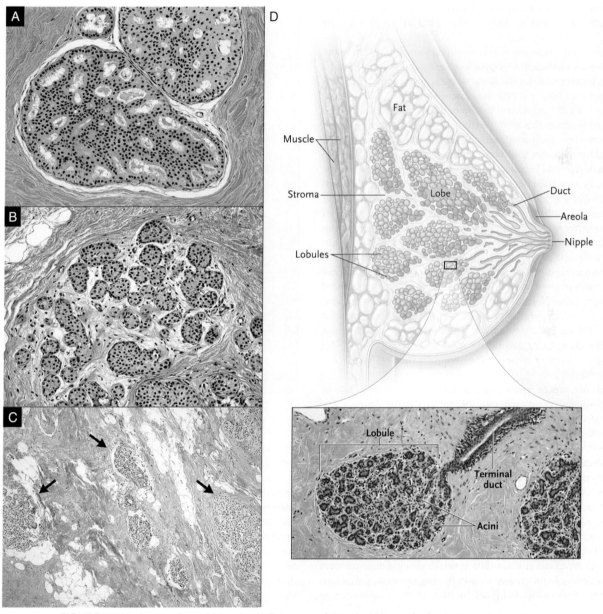

FIGURE 35.23 Anatomic and Histologic Features of Atypical Hyperplasia. A, Atypical ductal hyperplasia with proliferation of monotonous cells in architecturally complex patterns, including secondary lumens and micropapillary formations. **B,** Atypical lobular hyperplasia, with expanded acini filled with monotonous polygonal cells and a loss of acinar lumen. **C,** Multifocal atypical hyperplasia (in this case atypical lobular hyperplasia). Atypical lobular hyperplasia is present in more than one terminal duct lobular unit, and units are clearly separated from one another by interlobular mammary stroma *(arrows)*. **D,** Illustration of the microanatomy of the breast, including a photomicrograph of a terminal duct lobular unit. (From Hartmann LC, Degnim AC, Santen RJ et al: *N Engl J Med* 372[1]:1271-1272, 2015.)

with ADH.[37] Overall, the younger a woman is when she receives a diagnosis of atypical hyperplasia, the higher the risk that breast cancer will develop.[36,38,41] Among women who were postmenopausal at the time of benign breast biopsy, the risk was similar for ALH and ADH.[37] Overall, ADH and ALH are viewed best as "markers" of a generalized, bilateral increase in breast cancer risk.[33,37]

EVALUATION AND TREATMENT   Breast problems are diagnosed from a mutimodal approach that combines physical examination, mammography, ultrasonography, thermography, possibly MRI, and biopsy. The dense breast tissue often seen in young women can make mammographic interpretation extremely difficult (see *Did You Know? Breast Cancer Screening Mammography*). Surgical excision was historically recommended after a CNB identified ADH or ALH However, newer data suggest that routine excision of all atypical lesions may not be necessary.[33]

Treatment consists largely of relieving symptoms. Reduction in the consumption of caffeinated beverages (e.g., cola,) and chocolate, which can cause overstimulation for some women, may reduce pain and nodularity. Given time, the cysts may disappear without treatment.

Women with AH are advised to stop oral contraceptives and avoid hormone replacement therapy.[33] Certain selective estrogen modulators, such as tamoxifen and raloxifene, or an aromatase inhibitor may be considered for chemoprevention for women with AH after a thorough discussion of risks and benefits. Although still controversial, isoflavone exposure was associated with a decreased risk of proliferative benign fibrocystic changes, nonproliferative changes, and breast cancer.[42] Genistein, a soy isoflavone, has been reported to down-regulate an enzyme important in cancer progression (i.e., telomerase) and contributes to inhibition in both benign and cancer cells of the breast.[43] Toxicologists, in perhaps the first in vitro study quantifying the proliferative effects of isoflavone metabolites, conclude that soy supplementation will not induce proliferation of normal breast tissue and may even inhibit proliferation.[44] The North American Menopause Society found that soy foods generally appear to be breast protective and recommended moderate lifelong soy consumption.[45] Although quite controversial, another preventive factor may be iodine.[46]

Breast Cancer

Except for skin cancer, breast cancer is the most common cancer in American women, regardless of race and ethnicity. In the United States, it is estimated that 271,270 women were diagnosed with breast cancer, with 42,260 deaths in 2019.[13] It is the most common cause of death from cancer among Hispanic women, and the second most common cause of death from cancer among white, black, Asian/Pacific Islander, and American Indian/Alaska Native women.[47] The number of new cases worldwide of breast cancer in both sexes was estimated at 2,088,849 and the number of deaths as 626,679 for all ages and both sexes[48] (Fig. 35.24). Because DCIS is almost exclusively detected by mammography, the large increase in the incidence of DCIS over the past 20 years can be attributed to screening.

Although breast cancer is a multifactorial disease involving a complex web of interacting factors, risk is related to timing, duration, and pattern of exposures. Risk factors and possible causes of breast cancer can be classified broadly as reproductive, hormonal, environmental, and familial (Table 35.9). Another factor emerging as important is postpartum breast cancer with immune suppression and delayed involution (see the next section).

Reproductive Factors: Pregnancy

A clearer understanding of mammary gland structure (morphology) and function from fetal development to puberty, pregnancy, and aging

TABLE 35.9   Factors That Increase the Relative Risk for Breast Cancer in Women

Relative Risk	Factor
>4.0	Age (65+ versus <65 years, although risk increases across all ages until age 80)
	Biopsy-confirmed atypical hyperplasia
	Certain inherited genetic mutations for breast cancer (*BRCA1* and/or *BRCA2*)
	Ductal carcinoma in situ
	Lobular carcinoma in situ
	Mammographically dense breasts (compared to least dense)
	Personal history of early-onset (<40 years) breast cancer
	Two or more first-degree relatives with breast cancer diagnosed at an early age
2.1-4.0	Personal history of breast cancer (40+ years)
	High endogenous estrogen or testosterone levels (postmenopausal)
	High-dose radiation to chest
	One first-degree relative with breast cancer
1.1-2.0	Alcohol consumption
	Ashkenazi Jewish heritage
	Diethylstilbestrol (DES) exposure
	Early menarche (<12 years)
	Height (tall)
	High socioeconomic status
	Late age at first full-term pregnancy [>30 years])
	Late menopause (>55 years)
	Never breastfed a child
	No full-term pregnancies
	Obesity (postmenopausal/adult weight gain)
	Personal history of endometrial or ovarian cancer
	Proliferative breast disease without atypia (usual ductal hyperplasia and fibroadenoma)
	Recent and long-term use of menopausal hormone therapy containing estrogen and progestin
	Recent oral contraceptive use

Data from American Cancer Society (ACS): *Cancer facts & figures 2017-2018*, Atlanta, Ga, 2017, Author.

will help elucidate fundamental changes to breast development and disease. A key element in that process is "branching morphogenesis," in which the mammary gland fulfills its function by producing and delivering copious amounts of milk by forming a rootlike network of branched ducts from a rudimentary epithelial bud. Branching morphogenesis begins in fetal development, pauses after birth, starts again in response to estrogens at puberty, and is modified by cyclic ovarian hormonal action. This systemic hormonal action elicits local paracrine interactions between the developing epithelial ducts and their adjacent mesenchyme (embryonic) or postnatal stroma. The local cellular crosstalk then directs the tissue remodeling, ultimately producing a mature ductal tree.

A woman's age when her first child is born affects her risk for developing breast cancer—the younger she is, the lower the risk. Overall, the lifetime risk of breast cancer is reduced in parous women compared with nulliparous women, but pregnancy must occur at a young age. Delayed childbearing, observed in the United States and all developing countries, is expected to show a rise in diagnosed breast cancers. The influence of pregnancy on the risk of breast cancer also depends on

DID YOU KNOW?

Breast Cancer Screening Mammography

Joann G. Elmore, MD, MPH

The idea behind screening healthy individuals for disease is the hope that we can diagnose disease early, when more treatment options are available and when we can positively affect the life of the individual. Screening programs that cover the entire population of a country are a large undertaking and usually require extensive resources. Therefore we need to make certain the test has a high level of accuracy with reasonable costs and disadvantages, the disease is not too rare, and the treatment is effective for individuals who are diagnosed because of the screening.

Women have been encouraged to undergo breast cancer screening for many decades. Early screening programs encouraged women to perform self-breast exams and also to have their clinician perform a breast exam in the office—subsequent data have shown that these screening techniques lead to false-positive exams, and no studies have shown an association of these exams with a reduction in mortality. Most guideline groups no longer recommend breast self-exam or clinician breast exam for screening.

Breast cancer screening with mammography continues to be recommended by many groups, although the benefits are less than we had hoped and we are learning more about the harms. Mammography is an x-ray exam that takes views of each breast (see the following figure). The recommended age for the first mammogram and the frequency of screening vary among guidelines and countries. The U.S. Preventive Services Task Force periodically reviews the evidence and issues guidelines to help aid discussions with women about screening.

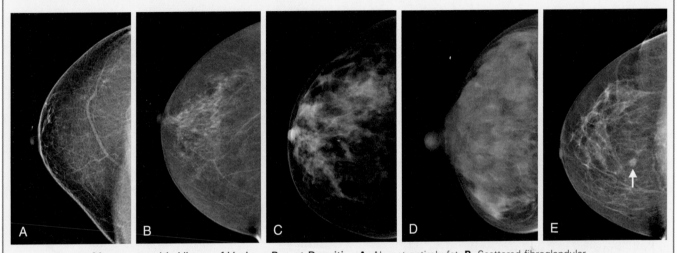

Mammographic Views of Various Breast Densities A, Almost entirely fat. **B,** Scattered fibroglandular densities. **C,** Heterogeneously dense. **D,** Extremely dense. **E,** Mammogram showing invasive cancer. (From Fuller MS et al: *Med Clin North Am* 99[3]:451-468, 2015; images provided by Christoph I. Lee, MD, MSHS.)

The benefits, risks, and accuracy of mammography screening depend on numerous factors, including a woman's age and breast density, and the time interval between screening exams. Possible risks of screening are important to consider, because screening at a population level involves testing healthy individuals; we are to "first, do no harm."

No medical test is perfect. About 10% of screening mammograms in the United States are interpreted as "abnormal," requiring additional testing. The great majority of women with these "abnormal" exams do not have breast cancer; this is called a *false-positive result*. The false-positive results lead to additional diagnostic testing, which can result in anxiety and morbidity for women. It is estimated that at least 50% of women in the United States, who are screened annually for a decade, will have experienced at least one false-positive examination.

Another harm of screening mammography is overdiagnosis—a *diagnosis* of cancer that would never have harmed the woman during her lifetime; such diagnoses can be either of a preinvasive lesion (e.g., DCIS) or of invasive breast cancer. With more women undergoing screening with mammography, we have seen a sharp increase in the number of women *diagnosed* with DCIS and early-stage breast cancer. By definition, DCIS is not an invasive carcinoma and not an immediate life-threatening cancer—it is confined to the duct—but DCIS is almost always treated as if it is an invasive early-stage breast cancer. Women with DCIS are at increased risk of a subsequent, invasive breast cancer *diagnosis;* however, most women with DCIS are never subsequently diagnosed with invasive

cancer and treatment of DCIS does not alter mortality. Women with DCIS have the same death rates as women without DCIS. Some discussion has centered on changing the name of DCIS lesions to better differentiate preinvasive DCIS from invasive cancer because the term *carcinoma* is similar to the term *cancer*. However, it is not likely that the name will be changed because of its current common usage.

Unfortunately, we are not able to identify which women with a new diagnosis of DCIS or invasive breast cancer have the type of lesion that is so low risk that it will never harm them during their lifetime. Thus, most women undergo treatment with either lumpectomy and radiation therapy or mastectomy. This is overtreatment if the DCIS or invasive cancer was overdiagnosed. Estimates of the prevalence of overdiagnosis vary in the literature from 10% to 50%, with many groups suggesting that about 1 in 5 women with a new diagnosis of breast cancer are overdiagnosed; more research is clearly needed.

Women with abnormalities noted on screening mammography are often offered the option of a breast biopsy versus watchful waiting with follow-up mammograms in 6 to 12 months. Some women think that a breast biopsy will provide an immediate and definitive diagnosis; however, this is not always the case. Pathologists have been noted to disagree on the diagnoses of atypia and DCIS.

Balancing the benefits and harms of breast cancer screening is not an easy task for women or their clinicians. Every woman should be encouraged to make an informed decision.

From Elmore JG: *N Engl J Med* 375(15):1483-1486, 2016; Elmore JG et al: *N Engl J Med* 338(16):1089-1096, 1998; Elmore JG et al: *J Am Med Assoc* 313(11):1122-1132, 2015; Fuller MS et al: *Med Clin North Am* 99(3):451-468, 2015; Katz DL et al: *Jekel's epidemiology, biostatistics, preventive medicine, and public health*, ed 4, Philadelphia, 2013, Elsevier Saunders; Pace LE, Keating NL: *J Am Med Assoc* 311(13):1327-1335, 2014; U.S. Preventive Services Task Force (USPSTF): *Ann Intern Med* 151(10):716-726, 2009; U.S. Preventive Services Task Force (USPSTF): *Final recommendation statement breast cancer: screening.* Available at https://www.uspreventiveservicestaskforce.org/Page/Document/RecommendationStatementFinal/breast-cancer-screening1.

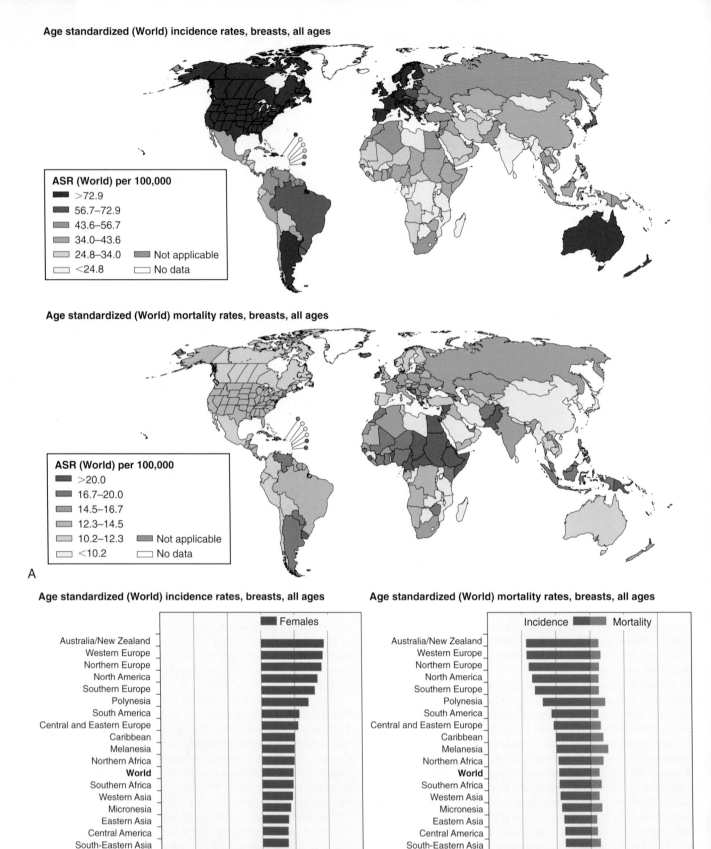

FIGURE 35.24 Breast Cancer Estimated Incidence and Mortality Worldwide in 2012. A, Estimated age-standardized rates (world) per 100,000 population. **B,** Incidence and mortality estimated age-standardized rates (world) per 100,000. These numbers represent a sharp rise in breast cancer incidence since the 2008 estimates by more than 20%. It is the most common cancer in women in both more and less developed regions, with slightly more cases in less developed regions (883,000 cases) than in more developed regions (794,000 cases). Incidence rates vary nearly fourfold across the world regions. (From Ferlay J et al: GLOBOCAN 2012 v1.0, *Cancer incidence and mortality worldwide: IARC CancerBase No. 11*, Lyon, France, 2018, International Agency for Research on Cancer. Available at http://globocan.iarc.fr/Default.aspx.)

the family history, lactation postpartum, and overall parity. Findings from a large prospective study found a *dual effect* from pregnancy—a transient postpartum increase in breast cancer risk, followed by a long-term reduction in risk (compared with nulliparous women).[49]

Pregnancy-associated breast cancer (PABC) is defined as breast cancer diagnosed up to 5 years after a completed pregnancy; however, risk may persist for a decade.[50,51] The transient increase in risk for breast cancer for all parous women includes events associated with pregnancy, such as pregnancy-related hormones (estrogen, progesterone, and growth hormone) that promote or initiate cancer cells; immune-suppressive effects of pregnancy; and breast tissue involution. A recent hypothesis for risk at any age is that gland *involution* after pregnancy and lactation uses some of the same tissue remodeling pathways that are activated during wound healing (i.e., proinflammatory pathways).[52] The proinflammatory environment, although physiologically normal, promotes tumor progression. The presence of macrophages in the involuting mammary gland may be contributing to carcinogenesis, and the normal involuting gland may be in an immunosuppressed state with T-cell suppression.[52,53] Involution is discussed in the next section.

Although many mechanisms have been proposed for the *protective effect* of pregnancy, newer data on the genomic profile of parous women have shown that pregnancy induces a long-lasting "genomic signature" that reveals chromatin remodeling derived from the early first pregnancy. The chromatin modifications are accompanied by higher expression of genes related to cell adhesion and differentiation, and genes activated only during the first 5 years after pregnancy may contribute to increased risk, however, the long-lasting genetic signature may explain pregnancy's preventive effect.[54]

Lobular Involution, Age, and Postlactational Involution

Part of the uniqueness of the mammary gland is its profound physiologic changes throughout the phases of a woman's life. These phases include puberty, pregnancy, lactation, postlactational involution, and aging. The human breast is organized into 15 to 20 major lobes, each with terminal lobules containing milk-forming acini (see Fig. 34.10). Terminal duct lobular units (TDLUs), the structures of the breast responsible for lactation, are the predominant source of breast cancers (Fig. 35.25).

With aging, breast lobules regress or involute, with a decrease in the number and size of acini per lobule and with replacement of the intralobular stroma with the denser collagen of connective tissue. With time, the glandular elements and collagen are replaced with fatty tissue. This process is called lobular involution, and over many years the parenchymal elements progressively atrophy and disappear. The first study of its kind found lobular involution was associated with a reduced risk of breast cancer.[55] Breast cancer risk decreased with an increasing *extent* of involution in both high- and low-risk subgroups defined by a family history of breast cancer, epithelial atypia, reproductive history, and age.[55] Based on pathologic and epidemiologic factors, these investigators propose that *delayed* involution (persistent glandular epithelium) is a major risk factor for breast cancer.[55] Tissue involution involves massive epithelial cell death, recruitment and activation of fibroblasts, stromal remodeling, and immune cell infiltration, including macrophages with similarities to microenvironments present during wound healing and tumor progression.[56]

Investigators suggest that the effect of lobular involution on breast cancer risk is a reduction in tissue from the involuting process, or the issue may be aging. Widely appreciated is that as women age, their risk of breast cancer increases. But, the *rate* of increase of breast cancer *slows* at about 50 years of age. This decline has been attributed to a reduction in ovarian hormone production; however, involution may contribute to this slowing rate. Importantly, investigators found an inverse association between lobular involution and parity.[55] Other investigators have reported that the more children a woman has, the more likely she is to have persistent lobular tissue,[57,58] which Milanese and colleagues[55] found was associated with an increased risk of breast cancer. However, multiparity also has been found to reduce the risk of breast cancer. This apparent contradiction may be explained by studies documenting that full-term pregnancies after 35 years of age are correlated with an increased risk of breast cancer. In the Milanese study, the age of the mother at each child's birth was unknown.

Late pregnancy, with its concomitant increase in the proliferation of the ductal-alveolar epithelium, is likely to interrupt the process of involution, which typically begins between 30 and 40 years of age. Failure to undergo TDLU involution among women with benign breast disease has been associated with progression to breast cancer, independent of other breast cancer risk factors.[59] The activated stromal environment (with the influx of immune cells similar to that which occurs during wound healing) in the process of involution is the "ideal niche" for carcinogenesis.

Major signaling pathways involved in mammary gland involution also are involved in breast cancer. Certain proteases activated during involution modify the extracellular matrix and are implicated in loss of cell anchoring, providing a microenvironment for tumor growth. Further, the normal involuting gland may be in an immunosuppressed state with the transient presence of immune-regulating cells that promote T-cell suppression.[60] Overall, for breast cancer, the long-term protective effects of pregnancy from hormones released (with consequent genetic and epigenetic changes) during pregnancy affect remodeling of the stromal microenvironment by causing apoptosis and involution. However, a transient increase in breast cancer risk after pregnancy may be caused by the *process* of mammary gland involution, which returns the tissue to its prepregnant state and is co-opted by the process of wound healing, resulting in a proinflammatory environment that, although physiologically normal, can promote carcinogenesis. In postlactational involution, the mammary gland regresses and remodels to its prepregnant state, whereby fibroblasts secrete proteases that degrade the extracellular matrix (ECM) proteins. Consequently, the increased release of bioactive matrix fragments can promote tumor growth, motility, and invasion.[61] The ECM is very different between nulliparous, lactating, and involuting glands as shown in Fig. 35.26. Understanding the factors from the microenvironment that control cell function, differentiation, and stem cell renewal is key—*the bottom line*—of developmental and cancer biology.

Hormonal Factors

The link between breast cancer and hormones is based on six factors that affect risk: (1) the protective effect of an early (i.e., in the twenties) first pregnancy; (2) the protective effect of removal of the ovaries and pituitary gland; (3) the increased risk associated with early menarche, late menopause, and nulliparity; (4) the relationship between types of fat, free estrogen levels, and oxidative changes in estrogen metabolism; (5) the hormone-dependent development and differentiation of mammary gland structures; and (6) the efficacy of antihormone therapies for treatment and prevention of breast cancer.

Throughout its existence, the mammary gland epithelium proceeds through critical "exposure periods" of rapid growth or cycles of proliferation, including neonatal growth, pubertal development, pregnancy, lactation, and involution after pregnancy and postmenopause (see the Lobular Involution, Age, and Postlactational Involution section).[53] Importantly, lack of TDLU involution has been associated with increased breast cancer risk, but the role of sex hormone levels and TDLU assessments has only begun to be studied (also see the Lobular Involution, Age, and Postlactational Involution section). Hormone levels may act, in part, to delay age-appropriate TDLU involution, resulting in a higher

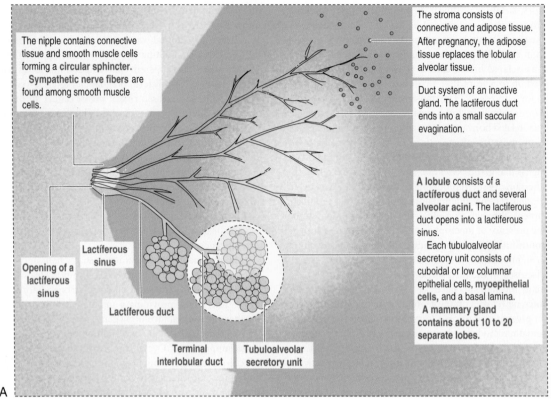

The nipple contains connective tissue and smooth muscle cells forming a **circular sphincter**.
Sympathetic nerve fibers are found among smooth muscle cells.

The stroma consists of connective and adipose tissue. After pregnancy, the adipose tissue replaces the lobular alveolar tissue.

Duct system of an inactive gland. The lactiferous duct ends into a small saccular evagination.

A lobule consists of a **lactiferous duct** and several **alveolar acini**. The lactiferous duct opens into a lactiferous sinus.
Each tubuloalveolar secretory unit consists of cuboidal or low columnar epithelial cells, **myoepithelial cells**, and a basal lamina.
A mammary gland contains about 10 to 20 separate lobes.

Lactíferous sinus

Opening of a lactíferous sinus

Lactíferous duct

Terminal interlobular duct

Tubuloalveolar secretory unit

A

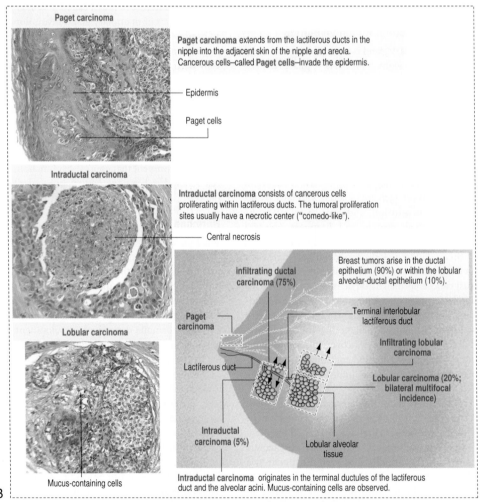

Paget carcinoma

Paget carcinoma extends from the lactiferous ducts in the nipple into the adjacent skin of the nipple and areola. Cancerous cells–called **Paget cells**–invade the epidermis.

Epidermis

Paget cells

Intraductal carcinoma

Intraductal carcinoma consists of cancerous cells proliferating within lactiferous ducts. The tumoral proliferation sites usually have a necrotic center ("comedo-like").

Central necrosis

Breast tumors arise in the ductal epithelium (90%) or within the lobular alveolar-ductal epithelium (10%).

infiltrating ductal carcinoma (75%)

Paget carcinoma

Terminal interlobular lactiferous duct

Infiltrating lobular carcinoma

Lactiferous duct

Lobular carcinoma (20%; bilateral multifocal incidence)

Lobular carcinoma

Intraductal carcinoma (5%)

Lobular alveolar tissue

Mucus-containing cells

Intraductal carcinoma originates in the terminal ductules of the lactiferous duct and the alveolar acini. Mucus-containing cells are observed.

B

FIGURE 35.25 Normal Breast and Breast Cancer. A, Normal breast. **B,** Breast cancer. (From Kierszenbaum AL: *Histology and cell biology: an introduction to pathology,* ed 2, Philadelphia, 2007, Mosby.)

quantity of at-risk epithelium.[59] Investigators found significant associations between higher TDLU counts, representing less involution, with higher levels of prolactin and lower levels of progesterone among premenopausal women, and higher levels of estradiol among postmenopausal women.[59] Higher testosterone levels were suggestively associated with higher TDLU counts among postmenopausal women.

The understanding of the role of systemic hormones as powerful regulators of mammary gland development is shifting. Evidence is pointing to the wide-ranging effects of systemic hormones, possibly not because of their *direct* hormone action, but rather because of their *induced* actions caused by multiple secondary paracrine effectors—thus the term *hierarchical*. Researchers are unraveling a complex model of hormone, paracrine, and adhesion molecule signaling pathways that affect the fate of both epithelial and stromal cells in both breast development and carcinogenesis. The key factor is the *tissue remodeling* that applies not only to pubertal growth but also immediately after pregnancy and during involution (see previous section).

The female reproductive hormones (estrogens, progesterone, and prolactin) have a major role and effect on mammary gland development and breast cancer (Fig. 35.27). The breast cancer risk increases with the number of menstrual cycles a woman has during her lifetime. Early menarche, late menopause, and short menstrual cycles all increase the risk; menopause slows the *rate* of increase of breast cancer; and ovariectomy reduces the risk. A vast majority of breast cancers are *initially* hormone dependent (estrogen positive [ER+] and/or progesterone positive [PR+]), with estrogens playing a crucial role in their development. Estrogens control processes critical for cellular functions by regulating activities and expression of key signaling molecules. These processes include regulation of receptor activity and receptor interaction with other intracellular proteins and deoxyribonucleic acid (DNA).

Endogenous estrogen. Much data has accrued on endogenous circulating estrogens and breast cancer risk in postmenopausal women. Increasing blood levels of estradiol increase the risk of breast cancer. Estrogen may promote the progression of ER-negative breast cancer by stimulating cancer-associated fibroblasts (CAFs) to secrete factors from the microenvironment, which can recruit bone marrow–derived cells to the tumor microenvironment. This recruitment of marrow-derived cells exerts tumor-promoting effects. Estrogens can modulate immune function in the mammary gland. For example, estradiol can promote a proinflammatory phenotype in macrophages, and estrogen can promote immunosuppression.

Endogenous progesterone. Several lines of evidence show that repeated exposure to the luteal phase of the menstrual cycle and, therefore endogenous increased serum progesterone (P) levels, increases the breast cancer risk. In the breast, cell proliferation occurs during the luteal phase and is accompanied by changes in the microenvironment. Proliferation happens in the TDLUs, where breast cancers originate. Progesterone is now recognized as a major proliferative hormone in both the mouse gland and the normal human breast epithelium.

Endogenous prolactin. Prolactin is the key regulator of lactation. Autocrine prolactin is required for terminal mammary epithelial differentiation during pregnancy, and the same signaling mechanisms for this function also may be important in breast carcinogenesis. Increased plasma levels of prolactin have been associated with the risk of cancer.

Endogenous testosterone. The association between circulating testosterone in postmenopausal women and the subsequent risk of breast cancer is now well established. Unclear is whether the association with testosterone is direct or indirect (i.e., enzyme conversion by aromatase of testosterone to estradiol) (Fig. 35.28).

Local in situ estrogens (paracrine). The formation of estrogens in breast tumors may be significant for the growth and survival of estrogen-dependent breast cancer in postmenopausal women. Stromal fibroblasts adjacent to the breast tumor express aromatase, actively induce local estrogen production, and signal crosstalk between estrogen and growth factors, all of which affect the progression of breast carcinoma.

Menopausal Hormone Therapy (MHT) and Breast Cancer Risk: Estrogen Plus Progesterone and Estrogen Only (ET)

The International Agency for Research on Cancer (IARC) lists estrogen-progestogen menopausal therapy and estrogen-progestogen contraceptives as carcinogenic agents with sufficient evidence in humans for breast cancer[62] (see Table 12.1). Evidence from the Agency for Healthcare Research and Quality (AHRQ, United States) published a systematic

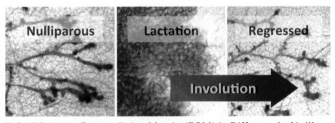

FIGURE 35.26 Extracellular Matrix (ECM) Is Different in Nulliparous, Lactating, and Involuting Glands. Several ECM differences between nulliparous, lactational, and involuting mammary glands are related to collagen fiber organization, cell motility and attachment, and cytokine regulation in a rodent model. Many protumorigenic ECM proteins are mediators of breast cancer progression specific to the involutional window; experimental treatment with systemic ibuprofen during involution reduced its tumor-promoting changes. (From O'Brien JH et al: *J Proteome Res* 11:4894-4905, 2012.)

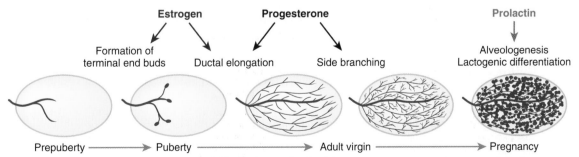

FIGURE 35.27 Mammary Gland Development in the Mouse. Schematic representation of distinct stages of postnatal mammary gland development. (From Brisken C, Hess, K, Jeitziner R: *Endocrinology* 156[10]:3442-3450, 2015.)

review from 283 trials comparing the effectiveness of treatments for menopausal symptoms.[63] From this report they stated, "Over the long term, estrogen combined with progestogen has both beneficial effects (fewer osteoporotic fractures) and harmful effects (increased risk of breast cancer, gallbladder disease, venous thromboembolic events, and stroke). Estrogens given alone do not appear to increase breast cancer risk, although endometrial cancer risk is increased." Only limited evidence is available from research on the route of administration of MHT, oral versus transdermal (gel or patch), and the risk of breast cancer.

Insulin and Insulin-Like Growth Factors

Insulin-like growth factors (IGFs) regulate cellular functions involving cell proliferation, migration, differentiation, and apoptosis. IGF-1 is a protein hormone with a structure similar to that of insulin. IGF-1 is a potent mitogen, and after binding to the IGF-1R (receptor), it triggers a signaling cascade that leads to proliferation and antiapoptosis. Many studies have shown IGF-1 is associated with breast cancer risk.

Diabetes is associated with a complex physiology of insulin resistance, increased insulin level, estrogen and growth hormone levels, inflammation, and signaling pathways leading to an increased risk of breast cancer. Insulin therapy and sulfonylurea were found to be mildly associated with an increased breast cancer risk.[64] A United Kingdom study showed that women treated with insulin glargine were not associated with breast cancer risk in the first 5 years; however, longer use may increase the risk.[65] Metformin appears to have a protective role. Much more investigation is needed to understand the role of insulin, insulin-like growth factors, and diabetes mellitus and the risk of breast cancer and recurrence of breast cancers.

Melatonin as a regulator of circadian rhythm is the main focus of shift work and light at night and breast cancer risk. However, tumor growth (in vivo) can be accelerated by light at night in part from continuous activation of IGF-1R signaling. A recent case-control study of 1679 women exposed to light at night during sleep was significantly associated with breast cancer risk.[66] Although inconclusive, shift work and its disruptive effects on circadian rhythms and sleep deprivation at night have been suggested as a risk factor for breast cancer.

Oral Contraceptives

The IARC Group confirmed that combined estrogen-progestogen OCs increase the risk for breast, cervix, and liver cancers.[62,67] However, the efficacy of OCs in protecting against ovarian cancer and endometrial cancer is well established. Hormones are discussed further in the Pathophysiology section.

Mammographic Breast Density

Mammographic density (MD) is the radiologic appearance of the breast, reflecting variations in breast composition (Fig. 35.29). Mammographic breast density (MBD) appears white or dense on a mammogram, is

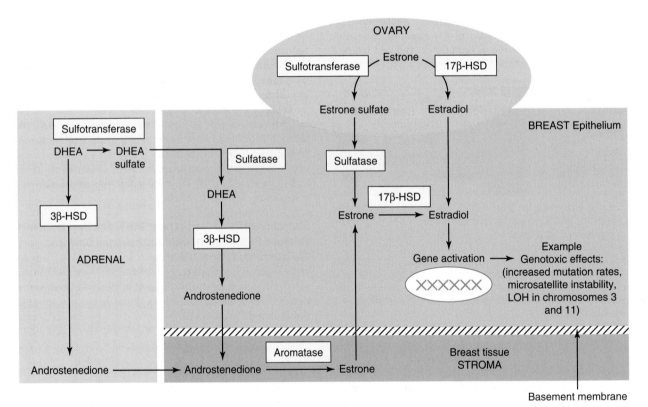

FIGURE 35.28 Local Biosynthesis of Estrogens. Three main enzyme complexes *(yellow)* are involved in estrogen formation in breast tissue: aromatase, sulfatase, and 17β-estradiol hydroxysteroid dehydrogenase *(17β-HSD).* Thus, despite low levels of circulating estrogens in postmenopausal women with breast cancer, the tissue levels are several-fold higher than those in plasma, suggesting tumor accumulation of these estrogens. Data suggest that the most abundant enzyme complex is sulfatase, in both premenopausal and postmenopausal women with breast cancer. Numerous agents can block the aromatase action. Exploration of progesterone and various progestins to inhibit sulfatase and 17β-HSD or stimulate sulfotransferase (breast cancer cells cannot inactivate estrogens because they lack sulfotransferase) may provide new possibilities for treatment. *LOH,* Loss of heterozygosity (see Chapter 11). (Adapted from Russo J, Russo I: *Molecular basis of breast cancer: prevention and treatment,* New York, 2004, Springer-Verlag.)

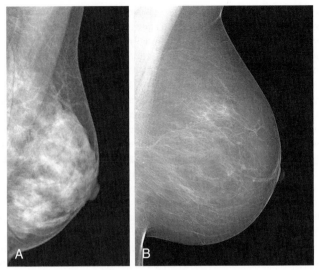

FIGURE 35.29 Breast Density Varies Among Women. The sensitivity of mammography for detecting malignancy is significantly reduced if the breast consists of a high proportion of fibroglandular (dense) breast tissue **(A)** compared with a breast that is fatty **(B)**. (From O'Malley FP et al, editors: *Breast pathology*, ed 2, Philadelphia, 2011, Saunders.)

expressed as a percentage of the mammogram, and is a strong and consistent risk factor for breast cancer. International and national studies have found that a significant increase in risk is associated with a higher percent of mammographic density (PMD). PMD is directly associated with height, parity, family history of breast cancer, and combined hormone therapy and inversely associated with age, weight, age of menopause, and use of tamoxifen. High breast density correlates with the collagen level. Investigators suggest COX-2 has a direct role in modulating tumor progression in tumors arising within collagen-dense microenvironments. An important implication of these findings is that inflammation contributes to the increased breast cancer in women with MBD. Finding tumors in women with MBD is a challenge because they both appear white; as Dr. Susan Love states, "…like trying to find a polar bear in a snow storm."

Environmental Factors and Lifestyle

The environmental causes of breast cancer possibly affect the breast the most during critical phases, or "windows," of development, including early differential stages—that is, undifferentiated cells to alveolar buds and then lobules, puberty, pregnancy and lactation, involution, and menopause. During these early phases, mitotic activity and cell division are more extensive than later in life.

Radiation. Ionizing radiation is a known mutagen and an established carcinogen for breast cancer. To date, only accidentally or medically induced radiation has been demonstrated to exert a carcinogenic effect on the breast. The Institute of Medicine (IOM) reports that the two most strongly associated environmental factors are exposure to ionizing radiation and combined postmenopausal hormone therapy (HT).[68] There are many sources of ionizing radiation, including x-rays, CT scans, fluoroscopy, and other medical radiologic procedures (see Chapter 12). Although only about 10% of diagnostic radiologic procedures in large U.S. hospitals are CTs, they contribute an estimated 65% of the effective radiation dose to the public from all medical x-ray examinations.[69] The IOM conclusion of a causal relationship between radiation exposure in the same range as CT and cancer is consistent with a large and varied literature.[70] The IOM makes it clear that avoidance of medical imaging is an important and concrete step that women (girls) can

take to reduce their risk of breast cancer.[71] Scientists and clinicians also have expressed concern about the increasing number of CT scans performed, including on children.[71,72] Radiologic exposure of the upper spine, heart, ribs, lungs, shoulders, and esophagus also exposes breast tissue to radiation. Breast tissue may be exposed from abdominal CT scans; x-rays and fluoroscopy of infants may constitute whole-body irradiation. The duration of increased risk from radiation is unknown, but increased risk appears to have lasted at least 35 years in women treated for mastitis, those treated with fluoroscopy, and those who survived the atomic bombs during World War II. Breast cancer rates in atomic bomb survivors in Japan were highest among women younger than 20 years of age at time of exposure; importantly, those who had early full-term pregnancies were at significantly lower risk than those who had not. Thus, interacting factors can modulate the risks from radiation. There is a linear relationship between radiation exposure and breast cancer risk in women treated for Hodgkin lymphoma, and women younger than age 20 years at the time of radiation exposure had the greatest risk of developing subsequent breast cancer.

An important topic currently is the effect of low-dose ionizing radiation. The debate is that low-energy x-rays may be more hazardous per unit dose than previously reported. Conventional x-ray mammography is one of the most valuable diagnostic tools for imaging of the breast. Currently, full-field digital mammography (FFDM) is frequently used. Continuous technical development has led to several new imaging techniques, including digital breast tomosynthesis (DBT), phase contrast x-ray imaging, and CT of the breast, as well as ultrasound and MRI. Despite technical innovations, except for ultrasound and MRI, these modalities require exposure of breast tissue to ionizing radiation, and the breast is considered a very radiosensitive organ.[73] Therefore, it is critical to compare delivered radiation doses to the breast and measure x-ray–induced DNA damage. A new technique for the detection and quantification of in vivo DNA damage has been developed. DNA double-strand breaks (DSBs) are the most relevant lesion induced by ionizing irradiation.[73] After induction of DSBs is the phosphorylation of the histone variant H2AX, named γ-H2AX. The γ-H2AX is a visible foci and a reliable and sensitive tool for the determination of DNA damage. Recently, investigators found mammography induces a slight but significant increase of γ-H2AX foci in systemic blood lymphocytes. A clear induction of DNA lesions was found both by FFDM and by DBT.[73] These data will be important for comparing different breast imaging techniques. Investigators are studying mammographic radiation–induced DNA damage in mammary epithelial cells from women with a low or high family risk of breast cancer, including comparisons with the number of views performed during screening.[74] Radiobiologic effects have been found in both low-risk and high-risk women, but the risks are greater in high-risk women.[74,75,76,77] Biologic understandings of low doses of radiation are presented in Chapter 12.

Women treated with chest radiation for a pediatric or young adult type of cancer have a substantially increased risk of breast cancer. Investigators from international studies have concluded that diagnostic chest irradiation or radiation therapy for benign or malignant diseases increases the risk of breast cancer for cumulative doses as low as 130 mGy. The breast cancer risk did not decrease when the number of radiologic treatment fractions was increased to deliver the same total dose, but the risk decreased greatly with increasing age of exposure to ionizing radiation.[76] The risk of secondary lung malignancy (SLM) is an important concern for women treated with whole-breast radiation therapy after breast-conserving surgery for early-stage breast cancer.[78] Investigators studied SLM risk associated with several common methods of delivering whole-breast radiation therapy (RT). Compared with supine whole-breast irradiation (WBI), prone breast irradiation is associated with a significantly lower predicted risk of secondary lung malignancy.[78]

A new, handheld breast-scanning device, called iBreastExam (iBE), can be used by community health workers to screen for breast abnormalities. With the increasing incidence of breast cancer worldwide, especially for low-resource countries, such a device is critical. iBE technology is free of radiation and uses Piezoelectric Sensor Array, which can measure tissue compression and stiffness by top-down touching of the skin surface. The device can enhance clinical breast examination (CBE) sensitivity by 19% while maintaining high specificity (94%) and a negative predictive value (NPV) of 98%. This is a promising tool for early detection of relevant lesions, and it is useful in younger women with dense breasts.[79-81] iBE received FDA approval as an aid in documenting palpable breast lesions from a CBE; it is to be used by qualified health care professionals and is not intended for home use. It currently is being used in low-resource countries.

The USPSTF has updated the recommendations for mammography because of overdiagnosis and overtreatment related to screening mammography (see *Did You Know? Breast Cancer Screening Mammography*).

Diet. Prospective epidemiologic studies on diet and breast cancer risk fail to show an association that is consistent, strong, and statistically significant except for alcohol intake, being overweight, and weight gain after menopause (see following discussion). Diet has been postulated as important for breast cancer risk because of the international correlations of consumption of specific dietary factors (e.g., fats) and breast cancer incidence and mortality. Additionally, migrant studies show a greater incidence of breast cancer among descendants who relocated to another country compared with those in the country of origin. International variations also can occur because of differences in reproductive history, physical activity, obesity, and other factors.

Dietary fat and breast cancer risk are the subject of much study, controversy, and debate. Potential biologic mechanisms between fat intake and breast cancer risk include (1) fat may stimulate endogenous steroid hormone production (also affects weight gain, age of menarche), (2) fat interferes with immune or inflammatory function, and (3) fat influences gene expression. Various studies on fat and breast cancer risk have been inconsistent; the concern has been that any association with fat intake may be because of total energy intake. Moreover, there is limited evidence that modest reductions in fat intake (less than 20% of caloric intake) reduce the breast cancer risk.

The association between individual foods and breast cancer is inconsistent, and new data on *dietary patterns* are emerging. The Mediterranean diet includes a high intake of vegetables, legumes, fruits, nuts, and minimally processed cereals; a moderately high intake of fish; and a high intake of monounsaturated lipids coupled with a low intake of saturated fat, low to moderate intake of dairy products, low intake of meat products, and moderate intake of alcohol. The Mediterranean diet may favorably influence the risk of breast cancer. The Western pattern includes a higher intake of red and processed meats, refined grains, sweets and desserts, and high-fat dairy products.

Dietary fiber can modify the estrogen concentration and stimulate intestinal microflora. A recent meta-analysis of prospective studies showed that every increment in dietary fiber of 10 g/day was associated with a significant reduction in breast cancer risk.[82] Lignans are found in fiber-rich foods and have been associated with a small risk reduction in postmenopausal breast cancer, but not premenopausal.

Alcohol consumption increases breast cancer risk. Beer, wine, and liquor all contributed to the positive association, and risks did not differ by menopausal status. In large prospective studies, high intake of folic acid appeared to decrease the enhanced risk for breast cancer caused by alcohol. The mechanisms by which alcohol intake increases the risk of breast cancer are unknown; however, physiologic studies have reported

an estrogen level increase in women taking HT, and IGF-1 level increases with alcohol intake. Alcohol may increase breast cancer risk by increasing mammographic breast density, especially in women at high risk. It is not known whether reducing or discontinuing alcohol consumption in midlife decreases the risk of breast cancer.

Soy products are a popular topic because of their consumption in Asian countries that have low rates of cancer. Soybeans are the main source of isoflavones. The isoflavone compounds, including daidzein and genistein, can bind estrogen receptors but are far less potent than estradiol. Soy may act like other antiestrogens (e.g., tamoxifen) by blocking the action of endogenous estrogens to reduce breast cancer risk. Thus, depending on the estradiol concentration, soy exhibits weak estrogenic or antiestrogenic activity. Many other mechanisms of action are proposed for isoflavones, including apoptosis and inhibition of angiogenesis. In 2011 the North American Menopause Society held a symposium to review the latest evidence-based science on the role of soy and found that soy foods generally appear to be breast protective and recommended moderate lifelong soy consumption.[45] A recent large study of both American and Chinese women suggested that a moderate intake of soy (≥10 mg of isoflavones/day) had a significant reduction in breast cancer recurrence, as well as a nonsignificant trend toward reduced all-cause mortality.[83] In addition, soy may optimize extrarenal 1,25-dihydroxycholecalciferol, or vitamin D_3 (a prodifferentiating vitamin D metabolite), which could result in growth control and, conceivably, inhibition of tumor progression.

Iodine deficiency is hypothesized to contribute to the development of breast pathology and cancer. Iodine plays a significant role in breast health. Evidence reveals that iodine is an antioxidant and antiproliferative agent contributing to the integrity of normal mammary tissue. Seaweed, which is iodine rich, is an important dietary item in Asian communities and has been associated with the *low* evidence of benign and breast cancer disease in Japanese women. Molecular iodine (I_2) supplementation exerts an inhibitory effect on the development and size of benign and cancerous tissue. Nutrition remains an important area of study.

Obesity. Excess body fatness is known to increase cancer risk from cellular pathways that involve hormonal regulation, cellular proliferation, and immunity. Obesity, measured as body mass index (BMI), has been associated with a reduced risk of premenopausal breast cancer. According to the Nurses' Health Studies, weight gain or weight loss since age 18 did not significantly decrease the risk of premenopausal breast cancer. Other data measuring adiposity, using the waist/hip ratio (WHR), have not found a reduced risk but rather no association (null) or an increased risk. Excess adiposity is positively associated with breast cancer recurrence and breast cancer–specific mortality among both premenopausal and postmenopausal women.

In 2002 IARC concluded that excess body weight (EBW) increased the risk of developing postmenopausal breast, colorectum, endometrium, kidney, and esophageal adenocarcinoma.[84] Evidence is increasing that a probable association exists between body fat and *postmenopausal* breast cancer, and *weight gain* may be more strongly related to postmenopausal breast cancer risk than attained weight.

Obesity is associated with poor survival among women with breast cancer. The increase in breast cancer risk with increasing BMI among postmenopausal women is most likely the result of increases in levels of estrogens by aromatase activity in adipose tissue. However, studies of hormones secreted by adipose tissue, *leptin* and *adiponectin,* may underlie the association between obesity and breast cancer risk. From molecular mechanism studies, leptin enhances breast cancer cell proliferation by inhibiting cell death (pro-apoptosis) signaling pathways and by increasing in vitro sensitivity to estrogens. Leptin secreted by adipocytes and fibroblasts in the microenvironment act on breast cancer cells in a paracrine fashion. Adiponectin has been shown to exert antiproliferative effects in vitro on human breast cancer cells. Additionally, factors that may be related to recurrence of breast cancer in women with excess adiposity at the time of diagnosis include cytokines, IGF or immune function, or both.

Environmental chemicals. Evidence linking synthetic chemicals to the cause of breast cancer is difficult to obtain. It is challenging because it is a life history of exposure that is important—not just a single chemical, but complex mixtures of chemicals and their interaction with endogenous hormones. With industrial development, breast cancer rates increase. An estimated 100,000 synthetic chemicals are registered for use in the United States, another 1000 or more are added each year, and toxicologic screening for these chemicals is minimal—only about 7%.[85] Current approaches to chemical screening are being reevaluated.

Chemicals persist in the environment, accumulate in adipose tissue, interact with local adipose tissue physiology in an endocrine/paracrine manner, and remain in breast tissue for decades. Estrogen receptors are some of the main targets of endocrine disruptor chemicals (EDCs), including the plasticizer bisphenol A and the flame retardant tetrachlorobisphenol A. Women who immigrate to the United States from Asian countries experience an enormous percent increase in risk within one generation. A generation later, the rate of their daughters' risk approaches that of women born in the United States. This change in risk suggests that in utero exposures affect subsequent disease risk. It is difficult to know whether these changes in risk come from nutritional content, pollutants, food additives, or other factors.

Xenoestrogens are synthetic chemicals that mimic the actions of estrogens and are found in many pesticides, fuels, plastics, detergents, and drugs. Because many factors correlated with breast cancer (e.g., early menarche, delayed pregnancy and breast-feeding, late menopause) are associated with lifetime exposure to estrogens, investigators reasoned that environmental chemicals affect estrogen metabolism and contribute to breast cancer. The most significant chemicals may be polychlorinated biphenyls (PCBs), such as dichlorodiphenyltrichloroethane (DDT), pesticides (dieldrin, aldrin, heptachlor, and others), bisphenol A (pervasive in polycarbonate plastics), tobacco smoke (active and passive), dioxins (vehicle exhaust, incineration, contaminated food supply), alkylphenols (detergents and cleaning products), metals, phthalates (makes plastics flexible, some cosmetics), parabens (antimicrobials), food additives (recombinant bovine somatotropin [rBST] and zeranol to enhance growth in cattle and sheep), MHT (i.e., hormone replacement therapy [HRT]), and others.

Physical activity. Physically active individuals have lower rates of many cancers and improved cancer outcomes. Physical activity has been associated with reduced breast cancer risk in both premenopausal and postmenopausal women. Activity also may reduce the invasiveness of breast cancer. A sedentary lifestyle may increase cancer risk through several mechanisms, including increased insulin resistance, increased inflammation, and decreased immune function. Epidemiologic studies demonstrate that physical activity lowered the risk of breast cancer mortality in breast cancer survivors and improved their physiologic and immune functions.

Inherited Cancer Syndromes, Genes, Epigenetic Considerations

The causes of breast cancer have been difficult to define because each woman has a different genetic profile, which is called genetic heterogeneity. Genetic heterogeneity is common among individuals but also at the level of the tumor itself, involving both genetic and epigenetic processes. Phenotypic heterogeneity is the result of tumor cell plasticity and, combined with genetic factors of the tumor, determines whether cells resist environmental stress, such as from the surrounding

microenvironment (e.g., hypoxia, entering dormancy) and metastasizing. These genetic factors interact with environmental factors. These facts are sobering and make the understanding of the genetic driving force behind tumor initiation, progression, and metastasis very complicated. Driver mutations are causally implicated in tumor development, and many new mutations have been identified.

A history of breast cancer in first-degree relatives (mother or sister) increases a woman's risk about two to three times. Risk increases even more if two first-degree relatives are involved, especially if the disease occurred before menopause and was bilateral. A small total proportion of breast cancers (5% to 10%, although the prevalence is significant) are the result of highly penetrant dominant genes (i.e., hereditary breast cancers). The most important of the dominant genes are the breast cancer susceptibility genes *(BRCA1, BRCA2)*. BRCA1 (breast cancer 1 gene), located on chromosome 17, is a tumor-suppressor gene; therefore any mutation in the gene may inhibit or retard its suppressor function, leading to uncontrolled cell proliferation. BRCA2 (breast cancer 2 gene) is located on chromosome 13. A family history of both breast cancer and ovarian cancer increases the risk that an individual with breast cancer carries a *BRCA1* mutation. Carriers of the *BRCA1* gene also are at higher risk for ovarian cancer. The risks for breast or ovarian cancer, or both, however, are not equal in all mutation carriers and have been found to vary by several factors, including type of cancer, age at onset, and mutation position. This observed variation in penetrance has led to the hypothesis that other genetic and/or environmental factors modify cancer risk in mutation carriers. Men who develop breast cancer are more likely to have a *BRCA2* mutation than a *BRCA1* mutation (see Chapter 36). Options for those who have a positive test for the *BRCA1* or *BRCA2* mutation include surveillance to find cancers early, prophylactic surgery (i.e., bilateral salpingo-oophorectomy), risk factor avoidance, promotion of breast-feeding, and chemoprevention. Several other genetic alterations can increase the risk of breast cancer.

PATHOPHYSIOLOGY Most breast cancers are adenocarcinomas and first arise from the ductal/lobular epithelium as CIS. Carcinoma in situ (CIS) is a proliferation of epithelial cells that is confined to the ducts and lobules by the basement membrane. DCIS and lobular LCIS are discussed in the following section. Tumors of the infiltrating (invasive) ductal type do not grow to a large size, but they metastasize early. This type accounts for 70% of breast cancers. Table 35.10 summarizes some types of breast cancer. Breast cancer is a heterogeneous—not a single—disease with diverse molecular, biologic, phenotypic, and pathologic changes. Tumor heterogeneity results from the genetic, epigenetic, and microenvironmental influences that occur as tumors progress. Cellular populations communicate through paracrine or contact-dependent signaling from ligands and mediated from components of the microenvironment, such as blood vessels, immune cells, and fibroblasts. Cancer cells behave as communities and the cooperative behavior of these groups of cells can influence cancer progression.

Gene expression profiling studies have identified major subtypes classified as luminal A, luminal B, HER2+, basal-like, Claudin-low, and normal breast. Tumors can be classified with gene expression profiles, such as Oncotype Dx, Prosigna, and MammaPrint, on the basis of genomic profiles. This information helps *personalize* breast cancer treatment and determine which women need aggressive systemic treatment for high-risk cancers and close surveillance for dormant tumors.

Many models of breast carcinogenesis have been suggested and include (1) gene addiction; (2) phenotype plasticity; and (3) cancer stem cells; and (4) hormonal outcomes affecting cell turnover of mammary epithelium, stem cells, ECM, and immune function (see previous sections Reproductive Factors: Pregnancy; Lobular Involution, Age, and Postlactational Involution; and Hormonal Factors). Cancer

TABLE 35.10 **Types of Breast Carcinomas and Major Distinguishing Features**

Histologic Type	Distinguishing Features
Carcinoma of the Mammary Ducts	
Papillary	Well-delineated cystic masses in multiple areas; hemorrhage often present; majority appear in 40- to 60-year age group; often involves skin
Intraductal (comedo)	Often accompanied by evidence of inflammation; well-circumscribed tumors within duct; well-differentiated tumor cells; rarely ulcerates skin
Infiltrating Carcinoma	
Ductal (no specific type [NST])	Fibrous, firm, glistening, gray-tan mass with chalky streaks, mixture of patterns; may cause discharge from nipple; represents about 70%-80% of all breast cancers
Mucinous	Usually large (>3 cm in diameter), circumscribed, and encapsulated, glistening appearance, varies in color; two types: pure and mixed; pure tumor is surrounded by mucin; infrequent; found in lateral half of breast; tends to occur in women after age 70
Medullary	Encapsulated and grows very large (7-8 cm in diameter); commonly surrounded by lymphocytic inflammatory infiltrate; occurs after age 50
Tubular	Well-differentiated with orderly tubules in center (stroma) of mass; can be associated with noninfiltrating ductal carcinoma; occurs in women about age 50; nodal metastasis infrequent; occurrence is rare
Adenoid cystic	Very rare; well-circumscribed, painless mass arising from nipple and areola
Metaplastic	Involves cartilage or bone, mixed tumors or osteogenic sarcomas
Squamous cell	Frequent in black people; originates in ductal epithelium
Carcinoma of the Mammary Lobules	
Lobular carcinoma in situ	Found in individuals with fibrocystic disease; localized to upper breast quadrants; 15%-35% risk of becoming invasive; occurs frequently in mid-40s; infiltrating variety occurs in early 50s
Infiltrating lobular	Infiltrates from duct; firm mass with chalky streaks
Paget disease	Eczema of nipple that extends to areola; cancer usually found underneath nipple; poorly circumscribed; large Paget cells arise from duct and directly invade nipple; history of scaly, red rash spreading from nipple; lesion palpable beneath nipple, often bilateral; occurs in middle age
Inflammatory carcinoma	Not a histologic type; fairly diffuse within breast tissue, diffuse edema of overlying skin; extremely undifferentiated, very rare; most metastasize to axilla
Sarcoma of the Breast	
Cystosarcoma phyllodes	Usually large (>17 cm in diameter); mostly localized but can rupture through skin; rarely metastasizes to lymph nodes; history of painless nodule present for years before it forms a large mass; ulceration and bleeding of skin often present; occurs in wide age range (13-77 years)
Fibrosarcoma	Well-circumscribed, firm, and usually does not involve skin or nipple; well-differentiated to extremely undifferentiated; arises from connective tissue; extremely rare (e.g., liposarcoma, angiosarcoma)

gene addiction includes oncogene addiction, whereby these driver genes (e.g., *HER2* and *MYC*) play key roles in breast cancer development and progression, and nononcogene addiction, whereby these genes may not initiate cancer but play roles in cancer development and progression.

Once a founding tumor clone is established, genomic instability may assist through the establishment of other subclones and contribute both to tumor progression and to therapy resistance. Phenotypic plasticity is exemplified by a distinctive phenotype called epithelial-to-mesenchymal transition (EMT) (see Chapter 11). EMT is involved in the generation of tissues and organs during embryogenesis, is essential for driving tissue plasticity during development, and is an unintentional process during cancer progression. The EMT-associated reprogramming is involved in many cancer cell characteristics, including suppression of cell death or apoptosis and senescence, is reactivated during wound healing, and is resistant to chemotherapy and radiation therapy. Remodeling or reprogramming of the breast during postpregnancy involution is important because it involves inflammatory and "wound healing–like" tissue reactions known as reactive stroma or inflammatory stroma. These tissue reactions increase the risk for tumor invasion and may facilitate the transition of CIS to invasive carcinoma. Activation of an

EMT program during cancer development often requires signaling between cancer cells and neighboring stromal cells. In advanced primary carcinomas, cancer cells recruit a variety of cell types into the surrounding stroma, including fibroblasts, myofibroblasts, granulocytes, macrophages, mesenchymal stem cells, and lymphocytes (Fig. 35.30). Overall, increasing evidence suggests that interactions of cancer cells with adjacent tumor-associated stromal cells induce malignant cell phenotypes (Fig. 35.31).

Research is ongoing to define cancer stem cells in breast carcinogenesis, including their origin and renewability properties. Studies have begun to identify the role of mammary stem cells (MaSCs) and to describe how they drive development of the gland and maintain homeostasis, the many cycles of proliferation and apoptosis needed to expand and maintain the breast during pregnancy, and return it to a quiet (quiescent) state after involution. EMT generates multiple epithelial cell subsets with different states of stemness relative to more differentiated cells. The ECM and the basement membrane (BM), in particular, are no longer just considered the "bricks and mortar" of a tissue but now a place where stem cells reside; and correct tissue architecture, together with the reservoir of growth factors, cytokines, and proteinases, is critical for mammary tissue to develop and function properly. Many of the

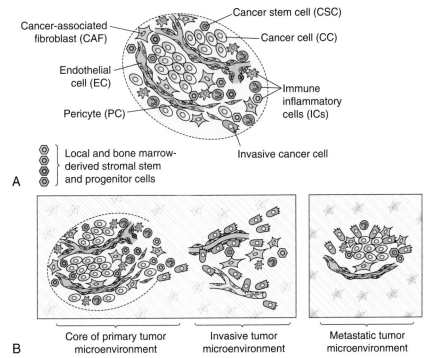

FIGURE 35.30 Cells of the Tumor Microenvironment. A, Distinct cell types constitute most solid tumors, including breast tumors. Both the main cellular tissue, called *parenchyma,* and the surrounding tissue, or stroma, of tumors contain cell types that enable tumor growth and progression. For example, the immune-inflammatory cells present in tumors can include both tumor-promoting and tumor-killing subclasses of cells. **B,** The microenvironment of tumors. Multiple stromal cell types create a succession of tumor microenvironments that change as tumors invade normal tissue, eventually seeding and colonizing distant tissues. The organization, numbers, and phenotypic characteristics of the stromal cell types and the extracellular matrix *(hatched background)* evolve during progression and enable primary, invasive, and metastatic growth. (The premalignant stages are not shown.) (Data from Hanahan D, Weinberg R: *Cell* 144:646-674, 2011.)

biologic traits of high-grade malignancy—motility, invasiveness, and self-renewal—have been traced to subpopulations of stem cells within carcinomas. Hormones may act as accelerators, as well as initiators, delay involution, and influence the susceptibility of the breast epithelium to environmental carcinogens because hormones control the differentiation of the mammary gland epithelium and, thereby, regulate the rate of stem cell division.

Invasion of cancer cells typically involves the collective migration of large unified groups of cells into adjacent tissue rather than the scattering of individual cancer cells (Fig. 35.32). Still unknown are the exact events that occur at the invasive edge of the tumor. It is critical to understand these events at the invasive edge as they relate to treatment. Displacement of tumor cells from a biopsy needle track is a concern and, although reported as low incidence, so is mechanical disruption from surgery that leads to displacement and seeding of tumor cells. Dormant cells appear to perpetuate carcinogenesis and form the precursors of eventual metastatic relapse and, sometimes, rapid recurrence. These dormant cells are called minimal residual disease (MRD). MRD may remain after initial chemotherapy, radiotherapy, and surgery. Current treatments preferentially kill proliferating cells, but dormant cells are not proliferating, which renders them more resistant to almost all current treatments.[86] The benefit of surgery is that it eliminates cancer bulk and the diversity of cancer cells, including therapy-resistant cells.[86]

Cancer metastases require that primary tumor cells evolve the ability to intravasate into the lymphatic system or vasculature, and extravasate into and colonize secondary sites. Investigators developed a mouse model of breast tumor heterogeneity and isolated a distinct clone of specialized cells that efficiently enter the vasculature and express two proteins, Serpine2 and Slpi, which were necessary and sufficient to program these cells for vascular mimicry. Vascular mimicry is a blood supply pathway in tumors that is formed by tumor cells and is independent of endothelial cell–lined blood vessels—thus it *mimics* real blood vessels (Fig. 35.33). This blood supply pathway facilitates perfusion of the primary tumors and correlates with a poor clinical outcome. The increase in these blood supply pathways was associated with an increase in circulating tumor cells (CTCs) and a subsequent increase in lung metastases. Additionally, treatment with the anticoagulant warfarin increased the number of CTCs and lung metastases, suggesting that the anticoagulant function of Serpine2 and Slpi both maintains blood flow through the extravascular network and promotes intravasation. These remarkable findings identify Serpine2- and Slpi-driven vascular mimicry as a critical mechanism or driver of metastatic progression in cancer.[87]

Carcinoma cells may promote the growth of lymphatic vessels through the process of *lymphoangiogenesis,* a process correlated with disease progression. Metastases may occur early in the process of neoplastic transformation. One explanation is the presence of preneoplastic cells living within inflammatory microenvironments and, from signaling, can activate EMT programs, causing the development of invasive phenotypes. In other cases, and traditionally understood, is metastases as a late event.

Ductal and Lobular Carcinoma in Situ

Ductal carcinoma in situ (DCIS) is a heterogeneous group of proliferative lesions limited to breast ducts and lobules without invasion of the

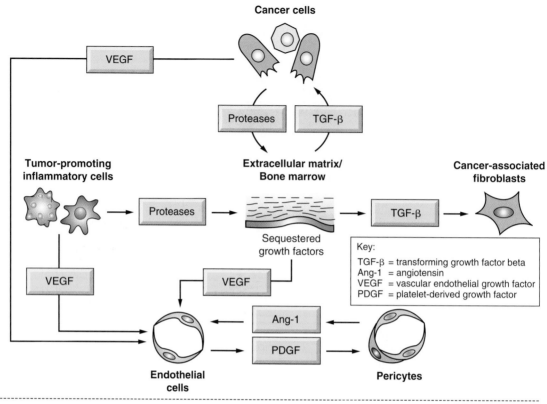

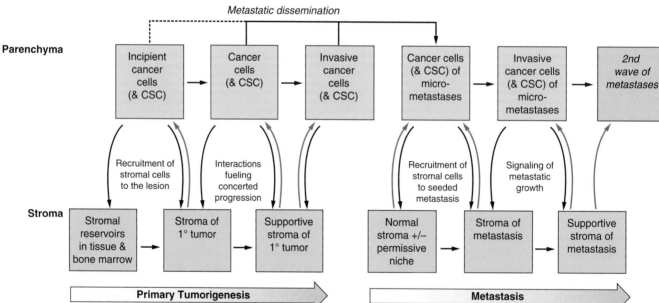

FIGURE 35.31 Signaling Interactions in the Tumor Microenvironment During Malignant Progression. *Upper panel,* Numerous cell types constitute the tumor microenvironment and are orchestrated and maintained by reciprocal interactions. *Lower panel,* The reciprocal interactions between the breast main tissue (parenchyma) and the surrounding stroma are important for cancer progression and growth. Certain organ sites of "fertile soil" or "metastasis niches" facilitate metastatic seeding and colonization. Cancer stem cells are involved in some or all stages of tumor development and progression. (Adapted from Hanahan D, Weinberg R: *Cell* 144:646-674, 2011.)

BM (Fig. 35.34). When DCIS breaches the BM and invades adjacent stroma, microinvasion (MI) is said to be present. About 84% of all in situ disease is DCIS; the remainder is mostly LCIS. DCIS occurs predominantly in females but can occur in males. Since 1980 the widespread adoption of screening mammography has led to an epidemic of

diagnoses of DCIS[88] (also see *Did You Know? Breast Cancer Screening Mammography*).

Perspectives on DCIS are changing. Because DCIS looks like invasive cancer, the presumption was that these lesions were the precursors of cancer and early removal and treatment would reduce cancer incidence

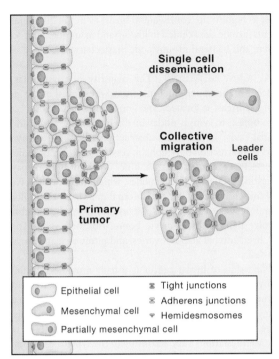

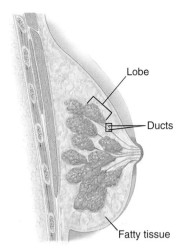

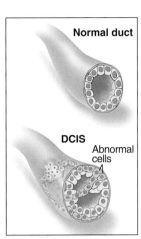

FIGURE 35.34 Ductal Carcinoma In Situ (DCIS). Illustration shows the location of DCIS. Given the low breast cancer mortality from DCIS, new approaches are needed for managing this disease. (From National Cancer Institute: *Risk of breast cancer death is low after a diagnosis of ductal carcinoma in situ,* Besthesda, Md, 2015, Author. With permission from Terese Winslow.)

FIGURE 35.32 Invasion. Invasion of carcinoma cells occurs through two mechanisms: by single cell dissemination through an epithelial-mesenchymal transition (EMT) *(gray arrow),* or by collective dissemination of a cluster of tumor cells. Emerging evidence suggests that the leader cells of tumor groups or clusters undergo EMT-associated phenotypic changes. Clusters of migrating cells are commonly noted at the borders of invasive carcinomas and are best documented in the breasts and lungs. (Adapted from Lambert AW, Pattabiraman DR, Weinberg RA: *Cell* 168[4]:670-691, 2017.)

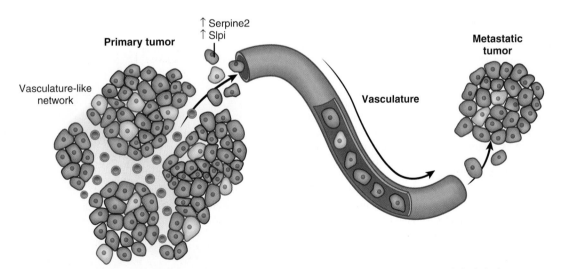

FIGURE 35.33 Vascular Mimicry Drives Metastasis. The steps to accomplish metastasis include *intravasation,* in which tumor cells escape from the primary tumor into the vasculature and move through the bloodstream; or *extravasation,* in which tumor cells escape from the vasculature to colonize in distant tissue. Metastasis is promoted by vascular mimicry, whereby tumor cells adopt characteristics similar to those of the endothelial cells that line blood vessels, and mimic vascular-like networks within tumors and between tumors and blood vessels. Wagenblast and colleagues found that two proteins, Serpine2 and Slpi, promoted metastasis by stimulating vascular mimicry. Tumor cells expressing these proteins *(green)* form the vascular-like network that allows other tumor cells *(purple, blue)* to move to secondary sites. (Adapted from Hendrix MJC: *Nature* 520:300-302, 2015; Wagenblast E et al: *Nature* 520:358-362, 2015.)

and mortality.[89] Long-term epidemiologic studies have demonstrated that the removal of 50,000 to 60,000 DCIS lesions annually has not been accompanied by a reduction in the incidence of invasive cancer.[90] The understanding is emerging that breast cancer has a range of behaviors, aggressive to indolent (idle), and screening mammography increases the likelihood of indolent lesions surfacing.[89]

A large study by Narod and colleagues has added to the growing concern to rethink the strategy for detecting and treating DCIS.[91] Their study of 100,000 women with a diagnosis of DCIS showed that the risk of dying from breast cancer was very low.[91] Less than 1% of women in this 20-year study died of breast cancer (compared to 5% of women who died of other causes). Surprisingly, the overall death rate for women with DCIS is lower than that for women in the population as a whole.[92,93] Aggressive treatment of almost all DCIS does not lead to a reduction in breast cancer mortality, confirming the conclusions from the NSABP trials.[94]

In summary, based on large numbers of subjects and long-term study follow-up, and given the low breast cancer mortality risk, DCIS is not an emergency. The detection and treatment of nonpalpable DCIS often represent overdiagnosis and overtreatment.[93] Data now suggest these measures:

1. In general, DCIS should be considered a "risk factor" for invasive cancer and should prompt targeting for preventive strategies.
2. Radiation therapy should not be routinely offered after lumpectomy for DCIS lesions that are not high-risk, because the absolute risk reduction in mortality was only 0.27% (relative risk reduction in mortality of 23%); Giannakease and colleagues state, "It is doubtful whether a benefit of this size is large enough to warrant radiotherapy."[95]
3. Low- to intermediate-grade DCIS does not need to be a target for screening or early detection.
4. Continuing study is needed, both for the biologic nature of the highest-risk DCIS (large, high-grade, hormone receptor negative) and protein HER2 positive, especially in very young and black women. Studies of target approaches to reduce death from breast cancer also are needed.[89]

DCIS represents an opportunity to alter the breast environment with increased exercise, decreased alcohol intake, and avoidance of postmenopausal hormone therapy with progesterone-containing regimens. Stratification of DCIS lesions may be accomplished through available tools, such as Oncotype DCIS; unfortunately genetic testing is performed only for about half of such women.

Lobular carcinoma in situ (LCIS) originates from the terminal duct lobular unit (see Fig. 35.25, *B*). Unlike DCIS, LCIS has a uniform appearance—the cells expand but do not distort involved spaces; thus the lobular structure is preserved. The cells grow in noncohesive (discohesive) clusters, usually because of a loss of the tumor-suppressive adhesion protein E-cadherin. LCIS is found as an incidental lesion from a biopsy and not from mammography because it is not associated with calcifications or stromal reactions that produce mammographic densities. LCIS has an incidence of about 1% to 6% of all carcinomas and does not increase with mammographic screening. With biopsies in both breasts, LCIS is bilateral in 20% to 40% of cases, compared with 10% to 20% of cases of DCIS. The cells of atypical hyperplasia, LCIS, and invasive lobular carcinoma are structurally identical. Loss of cellular adhesion because of dysfunction of E-cadherin results in a rounded shape without attachment to adjacent cells, increasing the risk of invasion. E-cadherin functions as a tumor-suppressor protein and may be lost in neoplastic proliferations from various mechanisms, including mutation.

LCIS is a risk factor for invasive carcinoma and develops in 25% to 35% of women over a period of 20 to 30 years. Unlike DCIS, the risk is almost as high in the contralateral breast as in the ipsilateral breast. Treatments include close clinical follow-up and mammographic screening, tamoxifen, and bilateral prophylactic mastectomy.

CLINICAL MANIFESTATIONS   The majority of carcinomas of the breast occur in the upper outer quadrant, where most of the glandular tissue of the breast is located. The lymphatic spread of cancer to the opposite breast, to lymph nodes in the base of the neck, and to the abdominal cavity is caused by obstruction of the normal lymphatic pathways or destruction of lymphatic vessels by surgery or radiotherapy (see Fig. 34.11). The less common, inner quadrant tumors may spread to mediastinal nodes or Rotter nodes, which are located between the pectoral muscles (see Fig. 34.11). Internal mammary chain nodes also are common sites of metastasis. Metastases from the vertebral veins can involve the vertebrae, pelvic bones, ribs, and skull. The lungs, kidneys, liver, adrenal glands, ovaries, and pituitary gland are also sites of metastasis.

The first sign of breast cancer is usually a painless lump. Lumps caused by breast tumors do not have any classic characteristics. Other presenting signs include palpable nodes in the axilla, retraction of tissue (dimpling) (Fig. 35.35), or bone pain caused by metastasis to the vertebrae. Table 35.11 summarizes the clinical manifestations of breast cancers. Manifestations vary according to the type of tumor and stage of disease.

EVALUATION AND TREATMENT   Clinical breast examination, mammography, ultrasound, thermography, MRI, biopsy, hormone receptor assays, and gene expression profiling are used in evaluating breast alterations and cancer. Most states in the U.S. enacted laws mandating that mammography facilities report breast density, but inconsistent guidelines have caused confusion and anxiety among individuals and health care providers.[96] Case-control and cohort studies provide indirect evidence for the effectiveness of screening, yet they can be limited by selection bias and healthy volunteer bias. Individuals who undergo screening have been shown to have lower mortality from causes unrelated

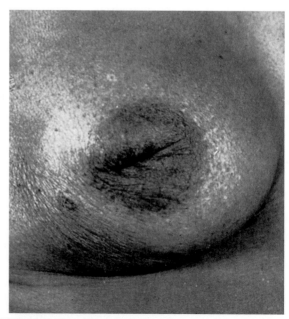

FIGURE 35.35 Retraction of Nipple Caused by Carcinoma. (From del Regato JA et al: *Ackerman and del Regato's cancer: diagnosis, treatment, and prognosis,* ed 6, St Louis, 1985, Mosby.)

TABLE 35.11   Clinical Manifestations of Breast Cancer

Clinical Manifestation	Pathophysiology
Local pain	Local obstruction caused by tumor
Dimpling of skin	Can occur with invasion of dermal lymphatics because of retraction of Cooper ligament or involvement of pectoralis fascia
Nipple retraction	Shortening of mammary ducts
Skin retraction	Involvement of suspensory ligament
Edema	Local inflammation or lymphatic obstruction
Nipple/areolar eczema	Paget disease
Pitting of skin (similar to surface of an orange [peau d'orange])	Obstruction of subcutaneous lymphatics, resulting in accumulation of fluid
Reddened skin, local tenderness, and warmth	Inflammation
Dilated blood vessels	Obstruction of venous return by a fast-growing tumor; obstruction dilates superficial veins
Nipple discharge in a nonlactating woman	Spontaneous and intermittent discharge caused by tumor obstruction
Ulceration	Tumor necrosis
Hemorrhage	Erosion of blood vessels
Edema of arm	Obstruction of lymphatic drainage in axilla
Chest pain	Metastasis to lung

to that screening then do those who did not undergo screening, likely caused by better overall health behavior profiles; thus, observed differences in survival or mortality by screening history could be caused by these other factors and not the actual screening.[96,97]

Treatment is based on the extent or stage of the cancer. The extent of the tumor at the primary site, the presence and extent of lymph node metastases, and the presence of distant metastases are all evaluated to determine the stage of disease. Treatment can include surgery, radiation, chemotherapy, hormone, and targeted therapy.

QUICK CHECK 35.5
1. What types of fibrocystic breast changes increase the risk of breast cancer?
2. What is the role of hormones and growth factors in the pathophysiology of breast cancer?
3. Why are reproductive factors, such as early menarche and late menopause, important for the pathogenesis of breast cancer?
4. Why is complete breast involution important for reducing the risk of breast cancer?
5. Discuss the role of the microenvironment or stromal tissue on breast cancer development.

SUMMARY REVIEW

Abnormalities of the Female Reproductive Tract
1. Normal development of the female reproductive tract requires the absence of testosterone during embryonic and fetal life.
2. Alterations in the normal process include errors in cellular sensitivity to testosterone (androgen insensitivity) or failures of cell line migration that result in changes in the structure of the reproductive organs.
3. AIS is a disorder of hormone resistance characterized by a female phenotype in an individual with an XY karyotype or male genotype.
4. Other abnormalities of the uterus, cervix, and fallopian/uterine tubes have multifactorial origins, often the result of an interaction between genetic predisposition and environmental factors.

Alterations of Sexual Maturation
1. Sexual maturation, or puberty, is marked by the development of secondary sex characteristics, rapid growth and ultimately, the ability to reproduce. The normal range for the onset of puberty is now 8 to 13 years of age and can vary geographically.
2. Delayed puberty is the onset of sexual maturation after these ages; precocious puberty is the onset before these ages. Treatment depends on the cause.

Disorders of the Female Reproductive System
1. The female reproductive system can be altered by hormonal imbalances, infectious microorganisms, inflammation, structural abnormalities, and benign or malignant proliferative conditions.
2. Primary dysmenorrhea is painful menstruation not associated with pelvic disease. It results from excessive synthesis of $PGF_2\alpha$.

Secondary dysmenorrhea results from endometriosis, pelvic adhesions, inflammatory disease, uterine fibroids, or adenomyosis.
3. Primary amenorrhea is the continued absence of menarche and menstrual function by 13 years of age without the development of secondary sex characteristics or by 15 years of age if these changes have occurred.
4. Secondary amenorrhea is the absence of menstruation for a time equivalent to three or more cycles in women who have previously menstruated. Secondary amenorrhea is associated with many disorders and physiologic conditions.
5. DUB is heavy or irregular bleeding in the absence of organic disease.
6. PCOS is a condition in which excessive androgen production is triggered by inappropriate secretion of gonadotropins. This hormonal imbalance prevents ovulation and causes enlargement and cyst formation in the ovaries, excessive endometrial proliferation, and often hirsutism. Insulin resistance and hyperinsulinemia play a key role in androgen excess.
7. PMS is the cyclic recurrence of physical, psychological, or behavioral changes distressing enough to disrupt normal activities or interpersonal relationships. Emotional symptoms, particularly depression, anger, irritability, and fatigue, are reported as the most distressing symptoms; physical symptoms tend to be less problematic. Treatment is symptomatic and includes stress reduction, exercise, biofeedback, lifestyle changes, counseling, and medication.
8. Infection and inflammation of the female genitalia can result from microorganisms that are present in the environment and often are sexually transmitted or from overproliferation of microorganisms that normally populate the genital tract.

9. PID is an acute inflammatory process caused by infection. Many infections are sexually transmitted, and microorganisms that comprise the vaginal flora are implicated. PID is a substantial health risk to women and untreated PID can lead to infertility.

10. Vaginitis is irritation or inflammation of the vagina, typically caused by infection. It is usually caused by sexually transmitted pathogens or *Candida albicans,* which causes candidiasis.

11. Cervicitis, which is infection of the cervix, can be acute (mucopurulent cervicitis) or chronic. Its most common cause is a sexually transmitted pathogen.

12. VV is chronic vulvar pain lasting 3 months or longer. The cause of VV is unknown; theories include embryonic factors, chronic inflammation, genetic immune factors, nerve pathways, increased sensitivity to environmental factors, infection with HPV, and hormonal changes.

13. Bartholinitis, also called *Bartholin cyst,* is an infection of the ducts that lead from the Bartholin glands to the surface of the vulva. Infection blocks the glands, preventing the outflow of glandular secretions.

14. The pelvic relaxation disorders—uterine displacement, uterine prolapse, cystocele, rectocele, and urethrocele—are caused by the relaxation of muscles and fascial supports, usually as a result of advancing age or after childbirth or other trauma. They are more likely to occur in women with a familial or genetic predisposition.

15. Benign ovarian cysts develop from mature ovarian follicles that do not release their ova (follicular cysts) or from a corpus luteum that persists abnormally instead of degenerating (corpus luteum cyst). Cysts usually regress spontaneously.

16. Endometrial polyps consist of benign overgrowths of endometrial tissue and often cause abnormal bleeding in the premenopausal woman.

17. Leiomyomas, also called *myomas* or *uterine fibroids,* are benign tumors arising from the smooth muscle layer of the uterus, the myometrium.

18. Adenomyosis is the presence of endometrial glands and stroma within the uterine myometrium.

19. Endometriosis is the presence of functional endometrial tissue (i.e., tissue that responds to hormonal stimulation) at sites outside the uterus. Endometriosis causes an inflammatory reaction at the site of implantation and is a cause of infertility. Information is emerging on the relationship between endometriosis and ovarian cancer.

20. Cancers of the female genitalia involve the uterus (particularly the endometrium), the cervix, and the ovaries. Cancer of the vagina is rare.

21. Cervical cancer arises from the cervical epithelium and is triggered by HPV. The cellular transformational zone is called the *squamo-columnar junction.* The progressively serious neoplastic alterations are CIN (cervical intraepithelial neoplasia, also known as cervical dysplasia), cervical CIS (carcinoma in situ), and invasive cervical carcinoma. Cocarcinogens include immune responses, hormonal responses, and other environmental factors that determine regression or persistence of the HPV infection.

22. Primary cancer of the vagina is rare. Risk factors include age 60 or older, exposure to DES, infection with HPV type 16, infection with HIV, and genital warts. The relationship of developing precancerous cell changes (called vaginal intraepithelial neoplasia) is controversial.

23. Risk factors for vulvar cancer include infection with HPV type 16 (cause), HIV, HPV-18 (probable cause), advancing age, previous cancer (untreated high-grade VIN), cervical cancer survivor, previous CIN, certain autoimmune conditions, organ transplant recipients (perhaps because of immunosuppression to clear HPV), and tobacco use (may relate to inability to clear HPV infection).

24. Carcinoma of the endometrium is the most common type of uterine cancer and most prevalent gynecologic malignancy. Primary risk factors for endometrial cancer include exposure to unopposed estrogen (e.g. estrogen-only hormone replacement therapy, tamoxifen, early menarche, late menopause, nulliparity, failure to ovulate), chronic hyperinsulinemia, hyperglycemia, body fatness and adult weight gain, chronic inflammation, lack of physical exercise.

25. Risk factors for ovarian cancer include advancing age, genetic factors, family history, overweight and obesity, height, reproductive/hormonal factors, HRT, endometriosis, diabetes, previous cancer, smoking, asbestos, use of talc-based powder, and ionizing radiation. Ovarian cancer causes more deaths than any other genital cancer in women.

26. Ovarian cancer is heterogeneous, and the biology of this type of cancer is changing.

Sexual Dysfunction

1. Sexual dysfunction is the lack of satisfaction with sexual function as a result of pain or a deficiency in sexual desire, arousal, or orgasm/climax.

2. Sexual function and dysfunction result from a complex set of personal and biologic factors that interact with the culture. Both organic and psychosocial disorders can be implicated in sexual dysfunction.

Impaired Fertility

1. Infertility, or the inability to conceive after 1 year of unprotected intercourse, affects approximately 15% of all couples. Fertility can be impaired by factors in the male, female, or both partners.

2. Female infertility results from dysfunction of the normal reproductive process: menses and ovulation, fallopian tube function (transport of the egg to the uterus, and the tube as a site of fertilization), ovarian dysfunction, and implantation of the fertilized egg into a receptive endometrium.

Disorders of the Female Breast

1. Most disorders of the breast are disorders of the mammary gland—that is, the female breast.

2. Galactorrhea, or inappropriate lactation, is the persistent secretion of a milky substance by the breasts of a woman who is not in the postpartum state or nursing an infant. Its most common cause is nonpuerperal hyperprolactinemia—a rise in serum prolactin levels.

3. Benign breast conditions are numerous and involve both ducts and lobules. Benign epithelial lesions can be broadly classified according to their future risk of developing breast cancer as (1) nonproliferative breast lesions, (2) proliferative breast disease, and (3) atypical (atypia) hyperplasia.

4. Nonproliferative lesions include simple breast cysts, papillary apocrine change, and mild hyperplasia of the usual type.

5. Proliferative breast lesions without atypia are diverse and include usual ductal hyperplasia, intraductal papillomas, sclerosing adenosis, radial scar, and simple fibroadenoma.

6. Proliferative breast lesions with atypia include ADH and ALH.

7. DCIS refers to a heterogeneous group of proliferations limited to breast ducts and lobules without invasion of the basement membrane. LCIS originates from the duct lobular unit.

8. Breast cancer is the most common form of cancer in women and second to lung cancer as the most common cause of cancer death. However, the inclusion of DCIS with invasive breast cancer statistics

is controversial. Breast cancer is a heterogeneous disease with diverse molecular, phenotypic, and pathologic changes.

9. The major risk factors for breast cancer are reproductive factors, such as nulliparity; hormonal factors and growth factors (e.g., excessive estradiol and IGF-1), familial factors (e.g., a family history of breast cancer) and environmental factors (e.g.,ionizing radiation). Two factors that have emerged as important are delayed involution of the mammary gland and breast density. Physical activity and avoiding postmenopausal weight gain may be risk-reducing factors.

10. A dominating belief in the field of cancer research is that epithelial function depends on the *entire* tissue, including the stroma or microenvironment. Breast cancer is now known as a tissue-based disease with a possible abnormal, aberrant wound healing and inflammatory stromal (reactive stroma) component.

11. Models of breast carcinogenesis include three interrelated themes: gene addiction, phenotype plasticity, and cancer stem cells. The exact molecular events leading to breast cancer invasion are complex and not completely understood. These events involve genetic and epigenetic alterations and cancer cell and stromal interactions. New concepts for breast cancer metastases include tumor dormancy and vascular mimicry.

12. Most breast cancers arise from the ductal epithelium and then may metastasize to the lymphatics, opposite breast, abdominal cavity, lungs, bones, kidneys, liver, adrenal glands, ovaries, and pituitary glands.

13. The first clinical manifestation of breast cancer is usually a small, painless lump in the breast. Other manifestations include palpable lymph nodes in the axilla, dimpling of the skin, nipple and skin retraction, nipple discharge, ulcerations, reddened skin, and bone pain associated with bony metastases.

KEY TERMS

Abnormal uterine bleeding (AUB), 784
Adenomyosis, 796
Amenorrhea, 783
Androgen insensitivity syndrome (AIS), 780
Anorgasmia (orgasmic dysfunction), 806
Atypia, 808
Atypical ductal hyperplasia (ADH), 809
Atypical hyperplasia (AH), 808
Atypical lobular hyperplasia (ALH), 809
Bacterial vaginosis, 790
Bartholinitis (Bartholin cyst), 791
Benign breast disease (BBD), 808
BRCA1, 819
BRCA2, 819
Carcinoma in situ (CIS), 819
Cervicitis, 790
Complete androgen insensitivity syndrome (CAIS), 780
Complete precocious puberty, 782
Corpus luteum cyst, 794
Cyst, 793, 808
Cystocele, 792
Delayed puberty, 782
Dermoid cyst, 794
Diffuse papillomatosis, 808

Disorders of desire (hypoactive sexual desire, decreased libido), 806
Ductal carcinoma in situ (DCIS), 821
Dyspareunia (painful intercourse), 806
E-cadherin, 824
Endometrial polyp, 794
Endometriosis, 796
Enterocele, 793
Epithelial-to-mesenchymal transition (EMT), 820
Fibrocystic change (FCC), 808
Follicular cyst, 794
Functional cyst, 794
Galactorrhea (inappropriate lactation), 807
Genetic heterogeneity, 819
Human papillomavirus (HPV), 797
Hirsutism, 784
Infertility, 807
Inflammatory stroma, 820
Intraductal papilloma, 808
Leiomyoma (myoma, uterine fibroid), 795
Lobular carcinoma in situ (LCIS), 824
Lobular involution, 813

Mammographic density (MD), 816
Mild hyperplasia of the usual type, 808
Minimal residual disease (MRD), 821
Mixed precocious puberty, 782
Mucopurulent cervicitis (MPC), 791
Nonpuerperal hyperprolactinemia, 807
Nonpuerperal prolactinemia, 807
Oophoritis, 788
Ovarian torsion, 794
Papillary apocrine change, 808
Pelvic inflammatory disease (PID), 788
Pelvic organ prolapse (POP), 792
Pessary, 792
Phenotypic heterogeneity, 819
Polycystic ovary syndrome (PCOS), 785
Precocious puberty, 782
Pregnancy-associated breast cancer (PABC), 813
Premenstrual dysphoric disorder (PMDD), 786
Premenstrual syndrome (PMS), 786
Primary amenorrhea, 783
Primary dysmenorrhea, 783

Prolactin-inhibiting factor (PIF), 807
Proliferative breast lesion without atypia, 808
Puberty, 781
Radial scar (RS), 808
Reactive stroma, 820
Rectocele, 793
Retrograde menstruation, 796
Salpingitis, 788
Sclerosing adenosis, 808
Secondary amenorrhea, 783
Secondary dysmenorrhea, 783
Sexual dysfunction, 806
Simple fibroadenoma, 808
Terminal duct lobular unit (TDLU), 813
Thelarche, 781
Transformation zone, 797
Unopposed estrogen, 801
Usual ductal hyperplasia (UDH), 808
Uterine prolapse, 792
Vaginismus, 806
Vaginitis, 790
Vascular mimicry, 821
Vulvodynia (VV), 791
Xenoestrogen, 819

REFERENCES

1. Geffner ME: Androgen insensitivity syndrome (AIS). In Shahram Yazdano, et al, editors: *Chronic complex diseases of childhood: a practical guide for clinicians*, Boca Raton, Fla, 2011, Universal Publishers.
2. National Institutes of Health (NIH): *Genetics home reference: androgen insensitivity syndrome*, Bethesda MD, 2018, U.S. Department of Health & Human Services, National Institutes of Health, U.S. National Library of Medicine. (Accessed 24 July 2018).
3. Kreisel K, et al: Prevalence of pelvic inflammatory disease in sexually experienced women of reproductive age—United States, 2013-2014, *MMWR Morb Mortal Wkly Rep* 66:80-83, 2017.
4. Kumar V, et al: *Robbins & Cotran pathologic basis of disease*, ed 9, Philadelphia, 2015, Elsevier/Saunders.
5. Centers for Disease Control and Prevention (CDC): *Sexually transmitted diseases (STDs)*, Atlanta, 2015, Author.
6. Centers for Disease Control and Prevention (CDC): *Diseases characterized by urethritis and cervicitis, STD sexually transmitted disease treatment guidelines*, Atlanta, 2014, Author.
7. Centers for Disease Control and Prevention (CDC): *STD treatment guidelines*, Atlanta, 2014, Author.

8. Shah M, Hoffstetter S: Vulvodynia, *Obstet Gynecol Clin North Am* 41:453-464, 2014.

9. Falsetta ML, et al: A review of the available clinical therapies for vulvodynia management and new data implicating proinflammatory mediators in pain elicitation, *BJOG* 124(2):210-218, 2017.

10. Gupta JK, et al: Uterine artery embolization for symptomatic uterine fibroids, *Cochrane Database Syst Rev* (12):CD005073, 2014.

11. Forte A, et al: Genetic, epigenetic and stem cell alterations in endometriosis: new insights and potential therapeutic perspectives, *Clin Sci* 126:123-138, 2014.

12. Ferlay J, et al: *GLOBOCAN 2012 v1.1, cancer incidence and mortality worldwide: IARC CancerBase No. 11 [internet]*, Lyon, France, 2013, International Agency for Research on Cancer. Available from: http://globocan.iarc.fr. (Accessed 26 August 2018).

13. American Cancer Society (ACS): *Cancer facts & figures 2019*, Atlanta GA, 2019, Author.

14. American Cancer Society (ACS): *Key statistics for cervical cancer*, Atlanta GA, 2018, Author.

15. Bui TC, et al: Association between vaginal douching and genital human papillomavirus infection among women in the united states, *J Infect Dis* 214(9):1370-1375, 2016.

16. Mitra A, et al: The vaginal microbiota, human papillomavirus infection and cervical intraepithelial neoplasia: what do we know and where are we going next?, *Microbiome* 4(1):58, 2016.

17. National Cancer Institute (NCI): *PDQ® cervical cancer treatment*, Bethesda, Md, 2015, Author. Date last modified January 9, 2015. Available at: http://cancer.gov/cancertopics/pdq/treatment/cervical/HealthProfessional. (Accessed 19 February 2015).

18. Goodman A, Schorge J, Greene MF: The long-term effects of in utero exposures—the DES story, *N Engl J Med* 364(22):2083-2084, 2011.

19. National Cancer Institute (NCI), PDQ® Adult Treatment Editorial Board: *PDQ ovarian epithelial, fallopian tube, and primary peritoneal cancer treatment*, Bethesda MD, 2018, Author. Updated 07/19/2018. Available at: https://www.cancer.gov/types/ovarian/hp/ovarian-epithelial-treatment-pdq. (Accessed 3 September 2018).

20. Reid BM, Permuth JB, Sellers TA: Epidemiology of ovarian cancer: a review, *Cancer Biol Med* 14(1):9-32, 2017.

21. Ferlay J, et al: Estimates of worldwide burden of cancer in 2008: GLOBOCAN 2008, *Int J Cancer* 127:2893-2917, 2010.

22. U.S. Department of Health & Human Services, National Institutes of Health: *Genetics home reference ovarian cancer*, Bethesda MD, 2018, Author.

23. Desai A, et al: Epithelial ovarian cancer: an overview, *World J Transl Med* 3(1):1-8, 2014.

24. Romero I, Bast RC: Minireview: human ovarian cancer biology, current management, and paths to personalizing therapy, *Endocrinology* 153(4):1593-1602, 2012.

25. Nik NN, et al: Origin and pathogenesis of pelvic (ovarian, tubal, and primary peritoneal) serous carcinoma, *Annu Rev Pathol* 9:27-45, 2014.

26. National Cancer Institute: *PDQ® ovarian, fallopian tube, and primary peritoneal cancer screening*, Bethesda, Md, 2015, Author. Date last modified March 3, 2015. Available at: www.cancer.gov/types/ovarian/hp/ovarian-screening-pdq. (Accessed 12 June 2015).

27. U.S. Preventive Services Task Force (USPSTF): Screening for ovarian cancer: U.S. Preventive services task force reaffirmation recommendation statement, *Ann Intern Med* 157(12):900-904, 2012.

28. Giede KC, et al: Who should operate on patients with ovarian cancer? An evidence-based review, *Gynecol Oncol* 99(2):447-461, 2005.

29. Mercado C, et al: Quality of care in advanced ovarian cancer: the importance of provider specialty, *Gynecol Oncol* 117(1):18-22, 2010.

30. Barbieri RL: Female infertility. In Strauss JF, Barbieri RL, editors: *Yen and Jaffe's reproductive endocrinology*, ed 7, Philadelphia PA, 2014, Elsevier, pp 512-517.

31. Marshburn PB: Counseling and diagnostic evaluation for the infertile couple, *Obstet Gynecol Clin North Am* 42(1):1-14, 2015.

32. Boulet SL, et al: Assisted reproductive technology and birth defects among liveborn infants in Florida, Massachusetts, and Michigan, 2000-2010, *JAMA Pediatr* 170(6):e154934, 2016.

33. Sabel MS: Overview of benign breast disease, 2018. Available at UpToDate Individual Web: www.uptodate.com. (Accessed 11 September 2018).

34. Lester S: The breast. In Kumar V, et al, editors: *Robbins & Cotran pathologic basis of disease*, ed 9, Philadelphia, 2015, Elsevier Saunders.

35. Dupont WD, Page DL: Risk factors for breast cancer in women with proliferative breast disease, *N Engl J Med* 312:146-151, 1985.

36. Page DL, et al: Atypical hyperplastic lesions of the female breast. A long-term follow-up study, *Cancer* 55:2698-2708, 1985.

37. Sanders M, et al: Continued observation of the natural history of low-grade ductal carcinoma in situ reaffirms proclivity for local recurrence even after more than 30 years of follow-up, *Mod Pathol* 28(5):662-669, 2015.

38. Hartmann LC, et al: Benign breast disease and the risk of breast cancer, *N Engl J Med* 353:229-237, 2005.

39. Page DL, et al: Atypical lobular hyperplasia as a unilateral predictor of breast cancer risk: a retrospective cohort study, *Lancet* 361(9352):125-129, 2003. [Erratum: *Lancet* 361(9373), 1994.].

40. Menes TS, et al: Subsequent breast cancer risk following diagnosis of atypical ductal hyperplasia on needle biopsy, *JAMA Oncol* 3(1):36-41, 2017.

41. Hartmann LC, et al: Understanding the premalignant potential of atypical hyperplasia through its natural history: a longitudinal cohort study, *Cancer Prev Res (Phila)* 7:211-217, 2014.

42. Hollowell JG, et al: Iodine nutrition in the United States. Trends and public health implications: iodine excretion data from National Health and Nutrition Examination Surveys I and II (1971-1974 and 1988-1994), *J Clin Endocrinol Metab* 83(10):3401-3408, 1998.

43. Li Y, et al: Genistein depletes telomerase activity through cross-talk between genetic and epigenetic mechanism, *Int J Cancer* 125(2):286-296, 2009.

44. Islam MA, et al: Deconjugation of soy isoflavone glucuronides needed for estrogenic activity, *Toxicol In Vitro* 29(4):706-715, 2015.

45. North American Menopause Society (NAMS): The role of soy isoflavones in menopausal health: report of the North American Menopause Society/Wulf H. Utian Translational Science Symposium in Chicago, IL, *Menopause* 18(7):732-753, 2011.

46. Iodine monograph, *Altern Med Rev* 15(3):273-278, 2010.

47. Centers for Disease Control and Prevention (CDC): *Breast cancer statistics, updated June 12, 2018*, Atlanta GA, 2018, Division of Cancer Prevention and Control, Centers for Disease Control and Prevention. (Accessed 14 September 18).

48. International Agency for Research on Cancer (IARC): *Breast GLOBOCAN 2018*, Lyon, France, 2018, World Health Organization, International Agency for Research on Cancer, Global Cancer Observatory.

49. Albrektsen G, et al: The short-term and long-term effect of pregnancy on breast cancer risk: a prospective study of 802,457 parous Noregian women, *Br J Cancer* 72(2):480-484, 1995.

50. Callihan EB, et al: Postpartum diagnosis demonstrates a high risk for metastasis and merits an expanded definition of pregnancy-associated breast cancer, *Breast Cancer Res Treat* 138:549-559, 2013.

51. Johansson AL, et al: Increased mortality in women with breast cancer detected during pregnancy and different periods postpartum, *Cancer Epidemiol Biomarkers Prev* 20(9):1865-1872, 2011.

52. Schedin P, et al: Microenvironment of the involuting mammary gland mediates mammary cancer progression, *J Mammary Gland Biol Neoplasia* 12:71-82, 2007.

53. Martinson HA, et al: Wound healing-like immune program facilitates postpartum mammary gland involution and tumor progression, *Int J Cancer* 136(8):1803-1813, 2015.

54. Barton M, et al: Molecular pathways involved in pregnancy-induced prevention against breast cancer, *Front Endocrinol (Lausanne)* 5:213, 2014.

55. Milanese TR, et al: Age-related lobular involution and risk of breast cancer, *J Natl Cancer Inst* 98(2):1600-1607, 2006.

56. Jindal S, et al: Postpartum breast involution reveals regression of secretory lobules mediated by tissue-remodeling, *Breast Cancer Res* 16(2):R31, 2014.

57. Geschickter CD: *Diseases of the breast*, ed 2, Philadelphia, 1945, Lippincott.

58. Vorrherr H, editor: *The breast: morphology, physiology, and lactation*, New York, 1974, Academic Press.

59. Khodr ZG, et al: Circulating sex hormones and terminal duct lobular unit involution of the normal breast, *Cancer Epidemiol Biomarkers Prev* 23(12):2765-2773, 2014.

60. Martinson HA, et al: Wound healing-like immune program facilitates postpartum mammary gland involution and tumor progression, *Int J Cancer* 136(8):1803-1813, 2015.

61. Schedin P: Pregnancy-associated breast cancer and metastasis, *Nat Rev Cancer* 6:281-291, 2006.

62. World Health Organization (WHO): *A review of human carcinogens. B. Biological agents IARC monographs on the evaluation of carcinogenic risks to humans, IARC Monographs, vol 100(B)*, Geneva, Switzerland, 2015, Author.

63. Grant MD, et al: *Menopausal symptoms: comparative effectiveness of therapies, Blue Cross and Blue Shield Association Technology Evaluation Center, Evidence-Based Practice Center*, Rockville, Md, 2015, Agency for Healthcare Research and Quality.

64. Ahmadieh H, Azar ST: Type 2 diabetes oral diabetic medications, insulin therapy, and overall breast cancer risk, *ISRN Endocrinol* 2013:181240, 2013.

65. Suissa S, et al: Long-term effects of insulin glargine on the risk of breast cancer, *Diabetologia* 54(9):2254-2262, 2011.

66. Wu J, et al: Light at night activates IGF-1R/PDK1 signaling and accelerates tumor growth in human breast cancer xenografts, *Cancer Res* 71(7):2622-2631, 2011.

67. IARC Special Report: Policy: a review of human carcinogens—Part A: pharmaceuticals, *Lancet* 10:13-14, 2009.

68. Institute of Medicine (IOM) of the National Academies: *Breast cancer and the environment: a life course approach*, Washington, DC, 2011, The National Academies Press.

69. National Cancer Institute (NCI): *Radiation risks and pediatric computed tomography (CT): a guide for health care providers*, 2002. Available at: www.cancer.gov. (Accessed December 2012).

70. Ginsburg ON, et al: Mammographic density, lobular involution, and risk of breast cancer, *Br J Cancer* 4(99):1369-1374, 2008.

71. Smith-Bindman R: Environmental causes of breast cancer and radiation from medical imaging, *Arch Intern Med* 172(13):1023-1027, 2012.

72. Brenner DJ, Hall EJ: Computed tomography—an increasing source of radiation exposure, *N Engl J Med* 357(22):2277-2284, 2007.

73. Schwab SA, et al: X-ray induced formation of γ-H2AX foci after full-field digital mammography and digital breast tomosynthesis, *PLoS ONE* 8(7):e70660, 2013.

74. Colin C, et al: DNA double-strand breaks induced by mammographic screening procedures in human mammary epithelial cells, *Int J Radiat Biol* 87(11):1103-1112, 2011.

75. Colin C, Foray N: DNA damage induced by mammography in high family risk patients: only one single view in screening, *Breast* 21:409-410, 2012.

76. Colin C, et al: Update relevance of mammographic screening modalities in women previously treated with chest irradiation for Hodgkin disease, *Radiology* 265(3):669-676, 2012.

77. Frankenberg-Schwager M, et al: Chromosomal instability carriers, *Int J Radiat Biol* 88:846-857, 2012.

78. Ng J, et al: Predicting the risk of secondary lung malignancies associated with whole-breast radiation therapy, *Int J Radiat Oncol Biol Phys* 83(4):1101-1106, 2012.

79. Broach RB, et al: A cost-effective handheld breast scanner for use in low-resource environments: a validation study, *World J Surg Oncol* 14(1):277, 2016.

80. Somashekhar SP, et al: Noninvasive and low-cost technique for early detection of clinically relevant breast lesions using a handheld point-of–care medical device (iBreastExam): prospective three-arm triple-blinded comparative study, *Indian J Gynecologic Oncol* 14:26, 2016.

81. Xu X, et al: Breast tumor detection using piezoelectric fingers: first clinical report, *J Am Coll Surg* 216(6):1168-1173, 2013.

82. Aune D, et al: Dietary fiber and breast cancer risk: a systematic review and meta-analysis of prospective studies, *Ann Oncol* 23(6):1394-1402, 2012.

83. Nechuta SJ, et al: Soy food intake after diagnosis of breast cancer and survival: an in-depth analysis of combined evidence from cohort studies of U.S. and Chinese women, *Am J Clin Nutr* 96(1):123-132, 2012.

84. Vaino H, Bianchini F, editors: *IARC. International Agency for Research on Cancer. Weight control and physical activity*, Lyon, 2002, IARC Press.

85. Bennett LM, Davis BJ: Identification of mammary carcinogens in rodent bioassays, *Environ Mol Mutagen* 39(2-3):150-157, 2002.

86. Lambert AW, Pattabiraman DR, Weinberg RA: Emerging biological principles of metastasis, *Cell* 168(4):670-691, 2017.

87. Wagenblast E, et al: A model of breast cancer heterogeneity reveals vascular mimicry as a driver of metastasis, *Nature* 520:358-362, 2015.

88. Kerlikowske K: Epidemiology of ductal carcinoma in situ, *J Natl Cancer Inst Monogr* 41:139-141, 2010.

89. Esserman L, Yau C: Rethinking the standard for ductal carcinoma in situ treatment, *JAMA Oncol* 1(7):881-883, 2015.

90. Lin C, et al: The majority of locally advanced breast cancers are interval cancers, *J Clin Oncol* 27:2009, 1503.

91. Narod SA, et al: Breast cancer mortality after a diagnosis of ductal carcinoma in situ, *JAMA Oncol* 1(7):888-896, 2015.

92. Lester S: The breast. In Kumar V, Abbas AK, Fausto N, editors: *Robbins and Cotran pathologic basis of disease*, ed 9, Philadelphia, 2015, Elsevier Saunders.

93. National Cancer Institute (NCI): *PDQ® breast cancer screening*, Bethesda, Md, 2015, Author. Date last modified May 14, 2015. Available at: www.cancer.gov/ types/breast/hp/breast-screening-pdq. (Accessed 6 June 2015).

94. Wapnir IL, et al: Long-term outcomes of invasive ipsilateral breast tumor recurrences after lumpectomy in NSABP B-17 and B-24 randomized clinical trials for DCIS, *J Natl Cancer Inst* 103(6):478-488, 2011.

95. Giannakeas V, et al: Association of radiotherapy with survival in women treated for ductal carcinoma in situ with lumpectomy or mastectomy, *JAMA Netw Open* 1(4):e181100, 2018.

96. National Cancer Institute (NCI), PDQ® Screening and Prevention Editorial Board: *PDQ® cancer screening overview*, Bethesda, Md, 2019, Author. Updated 05/31/2019. Available at: https:// www.cancer.gov/about-cancer/screening/ hp-screening-overview-pdq. (Accessed 21 June 2019).

97. Pierre-Victor D, Pinsky PF: Association of nonadherence to cancer screening examinations with mortality from unrelated causes: a secondary analysis of the PLCO Cancer Screening Trial, *JAMA Intern Med* 179(2):196-203, 2019.

36

Alterations of the Male Reproductive System

George W. Rodway

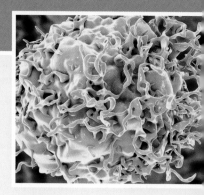

EVOLVE WEBSITE

http://evolve.elsevier.com/Huether/
Student Review Questions
Audio Key Points

Case Studies
Animations
Quick Check Answers

Alterations of the reproductive system span a wide range of concerns, from delayed sexual development and suboptimal sexual performance to structural and functional abnormalities. Many common male reproductive disorders carry potentially serious physiologic or psychological consequences. For example, sexual or reproductive dysfunction, such as impotence or infertility, can dramatically affect self-concept, relationships, and overall quality of life. Conversely, organic and psychosocial problems, such as alcoholism, depression, situational stressors, chronic illness, and medications, can affect sexual performance and may be risk factors for the development of some types of reproductive tract cancers. Aside from skin cancer, prostate cancer is the second leading cause of cancer deaths and is the most frequently diagnosed cancer in men. The incidence rates for prostate cancer changed substantially between the mid-1980s and the mid-1990s and have since fluctuated widely from year to year, in large part reflecting changes in prostate cancer screening with the prostate-specific antigen (PSA) blood test. As with disorders of the female reproductive system, the diagnosis and treatment of male reproductive system disorders are often complicated by the stigma and symbolism associated with the reproductive organs and emotion-laden beliefs and behaviors related to reproductive health. The diagnosis or treatment for any problem may be delayed because of embarrassment, guilt, fear, or denial.

ALTERATIONS OF SEXUAL MATURATION

The process of sexual maturation, or puberty, is marked by the development of secondary sex characteristics, rapid growth, and, ultimately, the ability to reproduce. A variety of congenital and endocrine disorders can disrupt the timing of puberty. Puberty that occurs too late (delayed puberty) or too early (precocious puberty) is caused by the inappropriate onset of sex hormone production. While the average age of pubertal onset appears to be decreasing for girls, the age of pubertal onset has remained essentially unchanged for boys.

Delayed or Absent Puberty

About 3% of children living in North America experience delayed development of secondary sex characteristics.[1] Normally, boys tend to mature later than girls, around 14 to 14.5 years of age. In boys, the first sign of maturity is enlargement of the testes and thinning of the scrotal skin. In delayed puberty, these secondary sex characteristics develop later.

In about 95% of cases, delayed puberty is a normal physiologic event. Hormonal levels are normal, the hypothalamic-pituitary-gonadal axis is intact, and maturation is slowly occurring. Treatment is seldom needed unless the delayed puberty is causing psychosocial problems.[2]

The other 5% of cases are caused by the disruption of the hypothalamic-pituitary-gonadal axis or by the outcomes of a systemic disease. Treatment depends on the cause (Box 36.1), and referral to a pediatric endocrinologist is necessary.

Precocious Puberty

Precocious puberty is a rare event, affecting fewer than 1 in 50,000 boys. Precocious puberty for boys of all ethnic and racial groups is defined as sexual maturation occurring before age 9.[3] The mean ages of beginning male genital and pubic hair growth and early testicular volumes are leaning toward younger ages than earlier studies have suggested, although this seems to be dependent on race and/or ethnicity. Precocious puberty may be caused by many conditions (Box 36.2), including lethal central nervous system tumors. All cases of precocious puberty require thorough evaluation.

BOX 36.1   Causes of Delayed Puberty

Hypergonadotropic Hypogonadism: Low Testosterone, Increased Follicle-Stimulating Hormone (FSH) and Luteinizing Hormone (LH)

1. Gonadal dysgenesis, most commonly Turner syndrome (45,X/46,XX; structural X or Y abnormalities, or mosaicism)
2. Klinefelter syndrome (47,XXY)
3. Bilateral gonadal failure
   a. Traumatic or infectious
   b. Postsurgical, postirradiation, or postchemotherapy
   c. Autoimmune
   d. Idiopathic empty scrotum or vanishing testes syndrome (congenital anorchia)

Hypogonadotropic Hypogonadism: Low Testosterone, Decreased LH, Depressed FSH

1. Reversible
   a. Physiologic delay
   b. Weight loss/anorexia
   c. Strenuous exercise
   d. Severe obesity
   e. Illegal drug use; also use of marijuana in particular
   f. Primary hypothyroidism
   g. Congenital adrenal hyperplasia
   h. Cushing syndrome
   i. Prolactinomas
2. Irreversible
   a. Gonadotropin-releasing hormone (GnRH) deficiency (Kallmann syndrome) or idiopathic hypogonadotropic hypogonadism (IHH)
   b. Hypopituitarism
   c. Congenital central nervous system defects
   d. Other pituitary adenomas
   e. Craniopharyngioma
   f. Malignant pituitary tumors

BOX 36.2   Primary Forms of Precocious Puberty

Complete Precocious Puberty
Premature development of appropriate characteristics for the child's sex
Hypothalamic-pituitary-ovarian axis functioning normally but prematurely
In about 10% of cases, lethal central nervous system tumor may be the cause

Partial Precocious Puberty
Partial development of appropriate secondary sex characteristics
Premature adrenarche (growth of axillary and pubic hair), which tends to occur between 5 and 8 years of age
Can progress to complete precocious puberty; may be caused by estrogen-secreting neoplasms or may be a variant of normal pubertal development

Mixed Precocious Puberty
Causes the child to develop some secondary sex characteristics of the opposite sex
Common causes: adrenal hyperplasia or androgen-secreting tumors

Data from Burchett MLR et al: Endocrine and metabolic diseases. In Burns CE et al, editors: *Pediatric primary care,* St Louis, 2009, Saunders; Jospe N: Disorders of pubertal development. In Osborn LM et al, editors: *Pediatrics,* Philadelphia, 2005, Mosby.

All forms of precocious puberty are treated by identifying and removing the underlying cause or administering appropriate hormones. In many cases, precocious puberty can be reversed. However, **complete precocious puberty** (development consistent with the sex of the individual) is difficult to treat and can cause long bones to stop growing before the child has reached normal height.

✔ **QUICK CHECK 36.1**
1. Why does puberty occur too late or too early in some individuals?
2. Why do all forms of precocious puberty require evaluation?

DISORDERS OF THE MALE REPRODUCTIVE SYSTEM

Disorders of the Urethra

Urethritis and urethral strictures are common disorders of the male urethra. Urethral carcinoma, an extremely rare form of cancer, can occur in men older than 60 years.

Urethritis

Urethritis is an inflammatory process that is usually, but not always, caused by a sexually transmitted microorganism. Infectious urethritis caused by *Neisseria gonorrhoeae* is often called *gonococcal urethritis (GU)*; urethritis caused by other microorganisms is called *nongonococcal urethritis (NGU)*. Nonsexual origins of urethritis include inflammation or infection as a result of urologic procedures, insertion of foreign bodies into the urethra, anatomic abnormalities, or trauma.

Noninfectious urethritis is rare and is associated with the ingestion of wood or ethyl alcohol or turpentine. It is also seen with reactive arthritis.

Symptoms of urethritis include urethral tingling or itching or a burning sensation, and frequency and urgency with urination. The individual may note a purulent or clear mucus-like discharge from the urethra. Nucleic acid detection amplification tests allow early detection of *N. gonorrhoeae* and *Chlamydia trachomatis* in urine studies. Treatment consists of appropriate antibiotic therapy for infectious urethritis and avoidance of future exposure or mechanical irritation.

Urethral Strictures

A **urethral stricture** is a narrowing of the urethra caused by scarring. The scars may be congenital but can be present at any age and have a wide range of etiologic factors, including untreated urethral infection, trauma, and urologic instrumentation. Infections also can occur from long-term use of indwelling catheters. Prostatitis and infection secondary to urinary stasis are common complications. Severe and prolonged obstruction can result in hydronephrosis and renal failure.

The clinical manifestations of urethral stricture are caused by bladder outlet obstruction. Urethral stricture often manifests itself as lower urinary tract symptoms or urinary tract infections with significant impairment in the quality of life. The primary symptom is diminished force and caliber of the urinary system; other symptoms include urinary frequency and hesitancy, mild dysuria, double urinary stream or spraying, and dribbling after voiding. Urethral stricture is diagnosed on the basis of the history, physical examination, flow rates, and cystoscopy. Treatment is usually surgical and may involve urethral dilation, urethrotomy, or a variety of open surgical techniques. The choice of surgical intervention depends on the age of the individual and the severity of the problem.

Disorders of the Penis
Phimosis and Paraphimosis

Phimosis and paraphimosis are both disorders in which the foreskin (prepuce) is "too tight" to move easily over the glans penis. **Phimosis** is a condition in which the foreskin cannot be retracted back over the

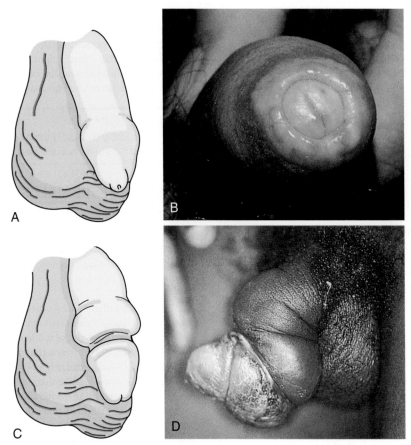

FIGURE 36.1 Phimosis and Paraphimosis. A, Phimosis: the foreskin has a narrow opening that is not large enough to permit retraction over the glans. **B,** Lesions on the prepuce secondary to infection cause swelling, and retraction of the foreskin may be impossible. Circumcision is usually required. **C,** Paraphimosis: the foreskin is retracted over the glans but cannot be reduced to its normal position. Here it has formed a constricting band around the penis. **D,** Ulcer on the retracted prepuce with edema. (**A** and **C** from Monahan FD et al: *Phipps' medical-surgical nursing: health and illness perspectives,* ed 8, St Louis, 2007, Mosby; **B** from Taylor PK: *Diagnostic picture tests in sexually transmitted diseases,* St Louis, 1995, Mosby; **D** from Morse SA et al: *Atlas of sexually transmitted diseases and AIDS,* ed 4, London, 2011, Saunders.)

glans, whereas paraphimosis is the opposite: the foreskin is retracted and cannot be moved forward (reduced) to cover the glans (Fig. 36.1). Both conditions can cause penile pathologic conditions.

The inability to retract the foreskin is normal in infancy and is caused by congenital adhesions. During the first 3 years of life, congenital adhesions (between the foreskin and glans) separate naturally with penile erections and are not an indication for circumcision. Phimosis can occur at any age and is most commonly caused by poor hygiene and chronic infection. It rarely occurs with normal foreskin.

Reasons for seeking treatment include edema, erythema, and tenderness of the prepuce and purulent discharge; inability to retract the foreskin is a less common complaint. Circumcision, if needed, is performed after infection has been eradicated. Complications of phimosis include inflammation of the glans (balanitis) or prepuce (posthitis) and paraphimosis. There is a higher incidence of penile carcinoma in uncircumcised males, but chronic infection and poor hygiene are usually the underlying factors in such cases. Approximately 60% of invasive penile carcinomas are attributable to human papillomavirus (HPV).[4]

Paraphimosis, in which the foreskin is retracted, can constrict the penis, causing edema of the glans. If the foreskin cannot be reduced manually, surgery must be performed to prevent necrosis of the glans caused by constricted blood vessels. Severe paraphimosis is a surgical emergency.

Peyronie Disease

Peyronie disease ("bent nail" syndrome) is a fibrotic condition that causes lateral curvature of the penis during erection (Fig. 36.2). Peyronie disease develops slowly and is characterized by tough fibrous thickening of the fascia in the erectile tissue of the corpora cavernosa. A dense, fibrous plaque is usually palpable on the dorsum of the penile shaft. The problem usually affects middle-aged men and is associated with painful erection, painful intercourse (for both partners), and poor erection distal to the involved area. In some cases, impotence or unsatisfactory penetration occurs. When the penis is flaccid, there is no pain.

A local vasculitis-like inflammatory reaction occurs, and decreased tissue oxygenation results in fibrosis and calcification. The exact cause is unknown. Peyronie disease is associated with Dupuytren contracture (a flexion deformity of the fingers or toes caused by shortening or fibrosis of the palmar or plantar fascia), diabetes, tendency to develop keloids, and, in rare cases, use of beta-blocker medications.

There is no definitive treatment for Peyronie disease; however, treatment can include pharmacologic agents and surgery. Spontaneous remissions occur in as many as 50% of individuals. However, men suffering with Peyronie disease who have a significant penile deformity that precludes successful coitus should be appraised for surgical correction.

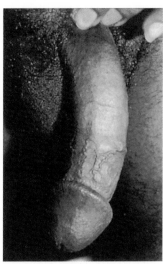

FIGURE 36.2 Peyronie Disease. This person complained of pain and deviation of his penis to one side on erection. (From Taylor PK: *Diagnostic picture tests in sexually transmitted diseases,* London, 1995, Mosby.)

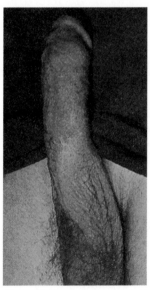

FIGURE 36.3 Priapism. (From Lloyd-Davies RW et al: *Color atlas of urology,* ed 2, London, 1994, Wolfe Medical.)

Priapism

Priapism is an uncommon condition of prolonged penile erection. It is usually painful and is not associated with sexual arousal (Fig. 36.3). Priapism is idiopathic in 60% of cases; the remaining 40% of cases can be associated with spinal cord trauma, sickle cell disease, leukemia, pelvic tumors, infections, or penile trauma.

Priapism must be considered a urologic emergency. Treatment within hours is effective and prevents impotence. Conservative approaches include iced saline enemas, ketamine administration, and spinal anesthesia. Needle aspiration of blood from the corpus through the dorsal glans is often effective and is followed by catheterization and pressure dressings to maintain decompression. More aggressive surgical treatments include the creation of vascular shunts to maintain blood flow. Erectile dysfunction results in up to 50% of prolonged cases.

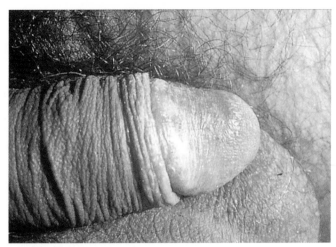

FIGURE 36.4 Balanitis. (From Taylor PK: *Diagnostic picture tests in sexually transmitted diseases,* London, 1995, Mosby.)

Balanitis

Balanitis is an inflammation of the glans penis (Fig. 36.4) that usually occurs in conjunction with posthitis, an inflammation of the prepuce. (Inflammation of the glans and the prepuce is called *balanoposthitis.*) Balanitis is associated with poor hygiene and phimosis. The accumulation under the foreskin of glandular secretions (smegma), sloughed epithelial cells, and *Mycobacterium smegmatis* can irritate the glans directly or lead to infection. Skin disorders (e.g., psoriasis, lichen planus, eczema) and candidiasis must be differentiated from inflammation resulting from poor hygienic practices. Balanitis is most commonly seen in men with poorly controlled diabetes and candidiasis. The infection is treated with antimicrobials. After the inflammation has subsided, circumcision can be considered to prevent recurrences.

Tumors of the Penis

Tumors of the penis are not common. The most frequent are the benign epithelial tumor condyloma acuminatum and penile carcinomas.

Condyloma acuminatum is a benign tumor caused by HPV, a microorganism that causes a sexually transmitted infection (STI). HPV type 6 and, less often, type 11, are the most frequent types and can cause a common wart and moist surface of the external genitalia. Giant condylomata (Buschke-Löwenstein) affect older men and may be 5 to 10 cm in size. Atypia may be evident in long-standing giant condylomata, and assessment of other HPV subtypes may be indicated to distinguish the lesion from a noninvasive warty carcinoma.

Penile Cancer

Carcinoma of the penis is rare in the United States, affecting about 1 in 100,000 men. However, it does account, for about 10% of cancers in African and South American men. It can affect men 40 to 70 years of age; two thirds of men are diagnosed at 65 years of age or older. In the United States about four out of five cases of the disease are diagnosed in men more than 55 years of age. Although the exact cause is unknown, risk factors may include HPV infection, AIDS (weakened immune system), smoking, and treatment (psoralens and ultraviolet A) for psoriasis. Circumcision at birth appears to decrease the risk of penile cancer, and penile cancer is more common in men with phimosis.[5]

Squamous cell carcinoma accounts for 95% of invasive penile cancers. Other premalignant lesions, or in situ forms of epidermal carcinoma, that occur on the penis include leukoplakia (white plaque), Paget disease (red, inflamed areas), erythroplasia of Queyrat (raised red areas), and Buschke-Löwenstein patches (large venous areas). HPV 6 and HPV 11 associated with genital warts (condylomata acuminata) have low cancer risks. At times, the penis might be the site of metastatic spread of solid tumors from the bladder, prostate, rectum, or kidney. Early squamous cell carcinoma and premalignant epidermal lesions are easily treated, but delays in seeking treatment are attributed to denial, embarrassment, failure to detect lesions under a phimotic foreskin, fear, guilt, and ignorance. When diagnosed early (stage 0, stage I, and stage II), penile cancer is highly curable.

Squamous cell carcinoma usually begins as a small, flat, ulcerative or papillary lesion on the glans or foreskin that grows to involve the entire penile shaft. Extensive lesions are associated with metastases and a poor prognosis. The regional femoral and iliac lymph nodes are common metastatic sites; the urethra and bladder are rarely involved. Weight loss, fatigue, and malaise accompany chronic suppurative lesions.

The specific diagnosis is made by biopsy after examination to document the location, size, and fixation of the lesion. After a positive biopsy, the extent of cancer spread is determined by imaging studies. Distant metastases are uncommon. Stages of carcinoma of the penis are presented in Box 36.3.

Penile carcinoma is managed primarily with surgery. Newer, innovative surgical techniques can preserve as much penile tissue as possible without compromising cancer control. A multimodal approach with chemotherapy is under study. Palliative treatment with radiation or chemotherapy may be used when the disease is inoperable and bulky inguinal metastases have occurred. Options for individuals with carcinoma in situ include local excision, radiation, laser surgery, cryosurgery, chemosurgery, or chemotherapy.

> ✔ **QUICK CHECK 36.2**
> 1. Why are priapism and severe paraphimosis considered urologic emergencies?
> 2. What are the risk factors for cancer of the penis?

Disorders of the Scrotum, Testis, and Epididymis
Disorders of the Scrotum

Men may seek treatment for painful or painless scrotal masses. Masses may be serious (cancer or torsion) or benign (hydrocele or cyst) and may require immediate surgical intervention or allow for careful observation. Varicocele, hydrocele, and spermatocele are common intrascrotal disorders. A varicocele is an abnormal dilation of the testicular vein and the pampiniform plexus within the scrotum; it is classically described as a "bag of worms" (Fig. 36.5). Varicoceles are one of the most commonly identified scrotal abnormalities and abnormal findings among infertile men. Advancements in diagnostic techniques indicate that the incidence of varicoceles is significantly greater than previously reported. Most (90%) occur on the left side because of discrepancies in venous drainage, and they may be painful or tender. Varicocele occurs in 10% to 15% of males and is seen most often after puberty.[6,7] Because most develop in adolescence, physiologic changes in testosterone level may contribute to increasing blood flow to the testicle, causing venous dilation. Unilateral right-sided varicoceles are rare and result from compression or obstruction of the inferior vena cava by a tumor or thrombus. Varicoceles may be less likely to be diagnosed among obese men.

The cause of varicocele is poorly understood. Blood pools in the veins rather than flowing into the venous system. Varicocele decreases blood flow through the testis, interfering with spermatogenesis and causing infertility. Varicoceles can alter testosterone and follicle-stimulating hormone levels, cause oxidative stress, decrease sperm count, and affect sperm quality. Varicocele surgical repair is generally done when the male has a grade II or III varicocele and

---

BOX 36.3 Staging for Penile Cancer

In this system, *T* stands for primary tumor size, *N* stands for regional lymph nodes, and *M* stands for distant metastasis.

Stage 0: Tis or Ta, N0, M0
The cancer has not grown into tissue below the top layers of skin and has not spread to lymph nodes or distant sites.

Stage I: T1a, N0, M0
The cancer has grown into tissue just below the superficial layer of skin but has not grown into blood or lymph vessels. It is a grade 1 or 2. It has not spread to lymph nodes or distant sites.

Stage II: Any of the Following:
T1b, N0, M0
The cancer has grown into tissue just below the superficial layer of skin and is high grade or has grown into blood or lymph vessels. It has not spread to lymph nodes or distant sites.
Or

T2, N0, M0
The cancer has grown into one of the internal chambers of the penis (the corpus spongiosum or corpora cavernosa). The cancer has not spread to lymph nodes or distant sites.
Or

T3, N0, M0
The cancer has grown into the urethra. It has not spread to lymph nodes or distant sites.

Stage IIIA: T1 to T3, N1, M0
The cancer has grown into tissue below the superficial layer of skin (T1). It also may have grown into the corpus spongiosum, the corpora cavernosa, or the urethra (T2 or T3). The cancer has spread to a single groin lymph node (N1). It has not spread to distant sites.

Stage IIIB: T1 to T3, N2, M0
The cancer has grown into the tissues of the penis and may have grown into the corpus spongiosum, the corpora cavernosa, or the urethra (T1 to T3). It has spread to two or more groin lymph nodes. It has not spread to distant sites.

Stage IV: Any of the Following:
T4, any N, M0
The cancer has grown into the prostate or other nearby structures. It may or may not have spread to groin lymph nodes. It has not spread to distant sites.
Or

Any T, N3, M0
The cancer has spread to lymph nodes in the pelvis or spread in the groin lymph nodes and grown through the lymph nodes' outer covering and into surrounding tissue. The cancer has not spread to distant sites.
Or

Any T, any N, M1
The cancer has spread to distant sites.

---

an abnormal semen analysis and the female has no known cause of infertility. If the varicocele is mild and fertility is not an issue, a scrotal support is usually sufficient to relieve symptoms of scrotal heaviness or "dragging." Color Doppler ultrasonography is used to confirm the diagnosis.

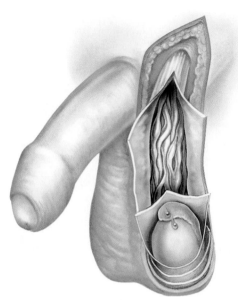

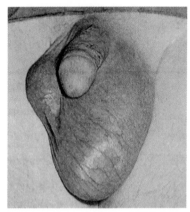

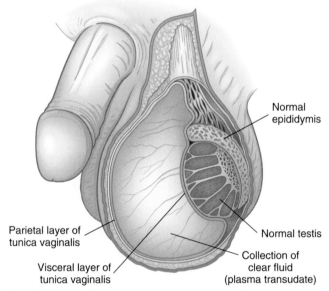

Normal epididymis

Normal testis

Collection of clear fluid (plasma transudate)

Parietal layer of tunica vaginalis

Visceral layer of tunica vaginalis

FIGURE 36.6 Hydrocele. Accumulation of clear fluid between the visceral (inner) and parietal (outer) layers of the tunica vaginalis.

A hydrocele is a collection of fluid between the layers of the tunica vaginalis (Fig. 36.6). It is the most common cause of scrotal swelling. Hydroceles occur in 6% of male newborns and are congenital malformations that often resolve spontaneously in the first year of life.[8] In North America, common infectious causes include epididymitis and viruses. Worldwide, however, filariasis is a major cause. especially with recent travel to tropical countries. Other causes include trauma, torsion of the testicle or testicular appendage, and recent scrotal surgery. A man presenting with a hydrocele in his third or fourth decade needs careful evaluation for testicular cancer.

Hydroceles vary in size, and most are asymptomatic. The most important feature on physical examination is a tense, smooth scrotal mass that easily transilluminates. Transillumination, or holding a light behind the scrotum, can help distinguish a hydrocele from a hernia or a solid mass. Treatment includes watchful waiting in infants and for those older than 1 year; 75% of hydroceles resolve within 6 months.[8] Symptomatic or communicating hydroceles need definitive treatment. Treatment includes surgical resection, aspiration, and sclerotherapy (injection of a sclerosing agent into the scrotal sac [cystic dilation]) to excise the tunica vaginalis.

Spermatoceles (epididymal cysts) are benign cystic collections of fluid of the epididymis located between the head of the epididymis and the testis. Spermatoceles are filled with a milky fluid containing sperm and are usually painless (Fig. 36.7). Spermatoceles that cause significant pain or discomfort are excised. Both spermatoceles and epididymal cysts present clinically as discrete, firm, freely mobile masses distinct from the testis that may be transilluminated. Usually, however, spermatoceles are asymptomatic or produce mild discomfort that is relieved by scrotal support. Neither hydroceles nor spermatoceles are associated with infertility.

Cryptorchidism and Ectopy

Cryptorchidism is a group of abnormalities in which the testis fails to descend completely; an ectopic testis has strayed from the normal pathway of descent. Ectopy may be caused by an abnormal connection at the distal end of the gubernaculum testis that leads the gonad to an abnormal position, usually at the superficial inguinal site. In cryptorchidism, the descent of one or both testes is arrested, with unilateral arrest occurring more often than bilateral arrest. The testes may remain in the abdomen, or testicular descent may be arrested in the inguinal canal or the puboscrotal junction. Cryptorchidism is a common congenital anomaly, with an incidence of approximately 3% in full-term infants. However, this rate increases significantly with low birth weight.[9,10] The incidence of cryptorchidism in adults is 0.7% to 0.8%.[11] Cryptorchidism is commonly associated with vasal or epididymal abnormalities. These congenital anomalies affect about 33% to 66% of newborns with cryptorchidism. Other structural anomalies include posterior urethral valves (less than 5%), upper genital tract abnormalities (less than 5%), and hypospadias. The presence of both hypospadias and cryptorchidism raises the suspicion of mixed gonadal dysgenesis (intersex infant). It has been hypothesized that cryptorchidism may result from an absence or abnormality of the gubernaculum—a cordlike structure that extends from the lower pole of the testis to the scrotum; a congenital gonadal or dysgenetic defect that makes the testis insensitive to gonadotropins (a likely explanation for unilateral cryptorchidism); or lack of maternal gonadotropins (a likely explanation for bilateral cryptorchidism of prematurity).[11]

Mechanical possibilities include a short spermatic cord, fibrous bands or adhesions in the normal path of the testes, or a narrowed inguinal canal. Chromosomal studies do not support a genetic component. Physiologic cryptorchidism, also called *retractile* or *migratory testis,* is an involuntary retraction of the testes out of the scrotum that occurs with excitement, physical activity, or exposure to cold and is caused by the small mass of prepubertal testis and the strength of the cremaster muscle. This is a common phenomenon that is self-limiting (descent occurs at puberty).

Physical examination discloses the absence of one or both testes in the scrotum and an atrophic scrotum on the affected side. If the undescended testis is in a vulnerable position, over the pubic bone for example, an individual may complain of severe pain secondary to trauma. The adult male with bilateral cryptorchidism may be infertile.

Testicular cancer also is a well-established complication of cryptorchidism. In men with a history of unilateral cryptorchidism, neoplasms also develop more commonly in the contralateral testis. This finding suggests cryptorchidism affects the testes and is a process more significant than simply the position of the testis in childhood. The risk of testicular cancer is 35 to 50 times greater for men with cryptorchidism or a history of cryptorchidism than for the general male population. Because definite histologic change occurs in the cryptorchid testis by 1 year of age, surgical correction is recommended around that age.[10] Treatment often begins with administration of gonadotropin-releasing hormone (GnRH) or human chorionic gonadotropin (hCG), hormones that may initiate descent and make surgery unnecessary. If hormonal therapy is not successful (success rates range from 6% to 75%), the testis is located and moved surgically (orchiopexy) in young children or removed (orchiectomy) in adults and children more than 10 years of age.[11] The testis that is properly placed in the scrotum provides adequate hormonal function and gives the scrotum a normal appearance. A successful operation does not ensure fertility if the testis is congenitally defective. Approximately 20% of males with unilateral undescended testis remain infertile even though orchiopexy is performed by age 1 year; most individuals with treated or untreated bilateral testicular maldescent have poor fertility.

Torsion of the Testis and Testicular Appendages

In **torsion of the testis**, the testis rotates on its vascular pedicle, interrupting its blood supply (Fig. 36.8). Torsion of the testis is one of several conditions that cause an acute scrotum, which is testicular pain and swelling. **Testicular appendages** include the appendix testis (a remnant of the müllerian duct) and the appendix epididymis (a remnant of the wolffian duct). Torsion of the appendages can also cause acute scrotum and be confused with testicular torsion, a urologic emergency.

Torsion of the testis can occur at any age but is most common among neonates and adolescents, particularly at puberty.[8] The onset may be spontaneous or may follow physical exertion or trauma. Torsion twists the arteries and veins in the spermatic cord, reducing or stopping circulation to the testis. Vascular engorgement and ischemia develop, causing scrotal swelling and pain not relieved by rest or scrotal support. Diagnostic testing includes urinalysis (to determine infection) and color Doppler ultrasonography.[11] Torsion of the testis is a surgical emergency. If it cannot be reduced manually (scrotal elevation), surgery must be performed within 6 hours after the onset of symptoms to preserve normal testicular function.

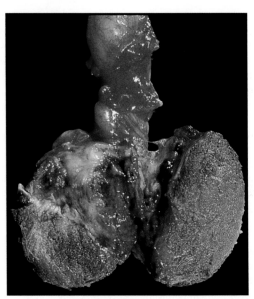

FIGURE 36.8 Torsion of the Testis. The testes appear dark red and partially necrotic as a result of hemorrhagic infarction. (From Damjanov I, Linder J, editors: *Anderson's pathology,* ed 10, St Louis, 1996, Mosby.)

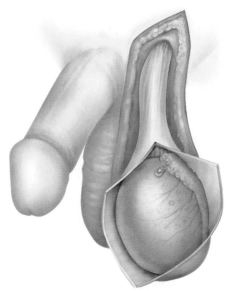

FIGURE 36.9 Orchitis. (From Ball JW et al: *Seidel's guide to physical examination,* ed 8, St Louis, 2015, Mosby.)

Orchitis

Orchitis is an acute inflammation of the testes (Fig. 36.9). It is uncommon except as a complication of systemic infection or as an extension of an associated epididymitis (see the section Epididymitis). Infectious organisms may reach the testes through the blood or the lymphatics or, most commonly, by ascent through the urethra, vas deferens, and epididymis. Most cases of orchitis are actually cases of epididymo-orchitis (inflammation of both the epididymis and testis). Occasionally in middle-aged men, a nonspecific, apparently noninfectious, inflammatory process (called *granulomatous orchitis*) can occur, presumably a granulomatous response to spermatozoa.

Mumps, the most common infectious cause of orchitis, usually affects postpubertal males. The onset is sudden, occurring 3 to 4 days after the onset of parotitis. Signs and symptoms include high fever, reaching 40° C (104° F), marked prostration, bilateral or unilateral erythema, edema and tenderness of the scrotum, and leukocytosis. An acute hydrocele may develop. Urinary signs and symptoms, which accompany epididymitis, are absent. Atrophy with irreversible damage to spermatogenesis may result in 30% of affected testes. Bilateral orchitis does not affect hormonal function but may cause permanent sterility.

Treatment is supportive and includes bed rest, scrotal support, elevation of the scrotum, hot or cold compresses, and analgesic agents for relief of pain. If an acute hydrocele develops, it is aspirated. Testicular abscess usually requires orchiectomy (removal of the testis). Appropriate antimicrobial drugs should be used for bacterial orchitis, and corticosteroids are indicated in proven cases of nonspecific granulomatous orchitis.

Cancer of the Testis

Testicular cancer is a highly treatable, usually curable cancer that most often develops in young and middle-aged men. For men with seminoma (all stages combined), the cure rate exceeds 90%. For men with low-stage seminoma or nonseminoma, the cure rate approaches 100%.[12] Overall, testicular cancers are uncommon, accounting for approximately 1% of all male cancers; yet they are the most common solid tumor of young adult men, and their incidence has risen over the past two decades in Western countries.[12,13] Cancer of the testis occurs most commonly in men between the ages of 15 and 35 years. In the United States, the lifetime probability of developing testicular cancer is 0.3% for white men, an incidence that is 4.5 times higher than that found in black men. Testicular tumors are slightly more common on the right side than on the left, a pattern that parallels the occurrence of cryptorchidism, and they are bilateral in 1% to 3% of cases (Fig. 36.10). Risk factors for testicular cancer include an undescended testicle, abnormal development of the testicles, a personal history of testicular cancer, a family history of testicular cancer (especially in father or brother), and being white.[14]

PATHOPHYSIOLOGY   Ninety percent of testicular cancers are germ cell tumors, arising from the male gametes. Germ cell tumors include

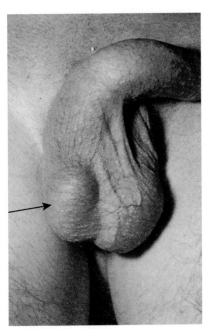

FIGURE 36.10 Testicular Tumor. (From Wolfe J: *400 self-assessment picture tests in clinical medicine*, London, 1984, Wolfe Medical.)

seminomas (most common), embryonal carcinomas, teratomas, yolk sac tumors, and choriocarcinomas. Testicular tumors also can arise from specialized cells of the gonadal stroma (Leydig, Sertoli, granulosa, theca cells).

The cause of testicular neoplasms is unknown. A genetic predisposition is suggested by the fact that the incidence is higher among brothers, identical twins, and other close male relatives. Genetic predisposition is supported statistically, showing that the disease is relatively rare among Africans, African Americans, Asians, and native New Zealanders.

CLINICAL MANIFESTATIONS   Painless testicular enlargement commonly is the first sign of testicular cancer. Occurring gradually, it may be accompanied by a sensation of testicular heaviness or a dull ache in the lower abdomen. Occasionally, acute pain occurs because of rapid growth resulting in hemorrhage and necrosis. Ten percent of affected men have epididymitis, 10% have hydroceles, and 5% have breast enlargement (gynecomastia). The testicular mass is usually discovered by the individual or by his sexual partner. At the time of initial diagnosis, approximately 10% of individuals already have symptoms related to metastases. Lumbar pain also may be present and usually is caused by retroperitoneal node metastasis. Signs of metastasis to the lungs include cough, dyspnea, and bloody sputum (hemoptysis). Supraclavicular node involvement may cause difficulty swallowing (dysphagia) and neck swelling. With metastasis to the central nervous system (CNS), alterations in vision or mental status, papilledema, and seizures may be experienced.

EVALUATION AND TREATMENT   An incorrect diagnosis at the initial examination occurs in as many as 25% of men with testicular cancer. Epididymitis and epididymo-orchitis are the most common misdiagnoses; others include hydrocele and spermatocele. Evaluation begins with careful physical examination, including palpation of the scrotal contents with the individual in the standing and supine positions. Signs of testicular cancer include abnormal consistency, induration, nodularity, or irregularity of the testis. The abdomen and lymph nodes are palpated to seek evidence of metastasis, and CT scanning is an important aspect of staging and treatment planning.[14] Although testicular self-examination has not been studied enough to be recommended by the American Cancer Society, many physicians recommend monthly examinations after puberty. Testicular biopsy is not recommended because it may cause dissemination of the tumor and increase the risk of local recurrence.

Primary testicular cancer can be assessed rapidly and accurately by scrotal ultrasonography. Tumor markers are higher than normal in the presence of a tumor and may help detect a tumor that is too small to be palpated during the physical examination or to be visualized on imaging. Serum tumor markers include alpha-fetoprotein (AFP), beta-human chorionic gonadotropin (beta-hCG), and lactate dehydrogenase (LDH) and are important for staging and monitoring germ cell tumors. Radiologic imaging and measurement of serum markers are used in clinical staging of the disease. Besides surgery, treatment involves radiation and chemotherapy singly or in combination. Radiation therapy, chemotherapy, and retroperitoneal lymph node dissection can all cause infertility problems so banking sperm may be recommended before undergoing any treatment. An increased risk of leukemia has been associated with platinum-based chemotherapy and radiation therapy.[14] Factors influencing the prognosis include histologic studies of the tumor stage of the disease and selection of appropriate treatment. Most individuals treated for cancer of the testis can expect a normal life span; some have persistent paresthesias, Raynaud phenomenon, or infertility. Approximately 10% of men treated for testicular cancer will experience a relapse; if the relapse is discovered early and treated, 99% can be cured. Orchiectomy does not affect sexual function.

Epididymitis

Epididymitis, or inflammation of the epididymis, generally occurs in sexually active young males (younger than 35 years) and is rare before puberty (Fig. 36.11). In young men, the usual cause is a sexually transmitted microorganism, such as *N. gonorrhoeae* or *C. trachomatis*. Coliform bacteria are the common pathogens in other age groups. Men who practice unprotected anal intercourse may acquire sexually transmitted epididymitis that results from infection with *Escherichia coli*, *Haemophilus influenzae*, tuberculosis, or *Cryptococcus* or *Brucella* species. In men older than 35 years, Enterobacteriaceae (intestinal bacteria) and *Pseudomonas aeruginosa* associated with urinary tract infections and prostatitis also may cause epididymitis. Epididymitis also may result from a chemical inflammation caused by the reflux of sterile urine into the ejaculatory ducts, which is then called chemical epididymitis. It is associated with urethral strictures, congenital posterior valves, and excessive physical straining in which increased abdominal pressure is transmitted to the bladder. Chemical epididymitis is usually self-limiting and does not require evaluation or intervention unless it persists.

PATHOPHYSIOLOGY The pathogenic microorganism usually reaches the epididymis by ascending the vasa deferentia from an already infected urethra or bladder. The resulting inflammatory response causes symptoms of bacterial epididymitis. Epididymitis caused by heavy lifting or straining results from the reflux of urine from the bladder into the vas deferens and epididymis. Urine is extremely irritating to the epididymis and initiates the inflammatory response called *chemical epididymitis*.

CLINICAL MANIFESTATIONS The main symptom of epididymitis is scrotal or inguinal pain caused by inflammation of the epididymis and surrounding tissues. The pain is usually acute and severe. Flank pain may occur if, as the urethra passes over the spermatic cord, edematous swelling of the cord obstructs the urethra. The individual may have pyuria, bacteriuria, and a history of urinary symptoms, including urethral discharge. The scrotum on the involved side is red and edematous. The tail of the epididymis near the lower pole of the testis usually swells first; swelling then ascends to the head of the epididymis. The spermatic cord also may be swollen and tender.

Complications include abscess formation, infarction of the testis, recurrent infection, and infertility. Infarction is probably caused by

thrombosis (obstruction by blood clots) of the prostatic vessels secondary to severe inflammation. Recurrent epididymitis may result from inadequate initial treatment or failure to identify or treat predisposing factors. Chronic epididymitis can cause scarring of the epididymal endothelium and infertility. Once scarring has occurred, treatment with antibiotics is ineffective because adequate antibiotic levels cannot be achieved within the epididymis.

EVALUATION AND TREATMENT A history of recent urinary tract infection or urethral discharge suggests the diagnosis of epididymitis. Common physical findings include a swollen, tender epididymis or testis located in the normal anatomic position with an intact same-side cremasteric reflex. The relief of pain when the inflamed testis and epididymis are elevated (Prehn sign) also is diagnostic. The definitive diagnosis is based on culture or Gram stain of a urethral swab. Epididymal aspiration may be necessary to obtain a specimen, especially if the individual has been taking antibiotics and has sterile urine.

Treatment includes antibiotic therapy for the infection itself. Analgesics, ice, and scrotal elevation can provide symptomatic relief. If the individual does not steadily improve, he should be reevaluated for possible complications, such as abscess formation, sepsis, or continued infection. Complete resolution of swelling and pain may take several weeks to months. The individual's sexual partner should be treated with antibiotics if the causative microorganism is a sexually transmitted pathogen.

> **✔ QUICK CHECK 36.3**
> 1. Why is a genetic predisposition suggested for testicular cancer?
> 2. Why is epididymitis rare in prepubescent males?
> 3. Why is testicular torsion considered a urologic emergency?

Disorders of the Prostate Gland
Benign Prostatic Hyperplasia

Benign prostatic hyperplasia (BPH), also called benign prostatic hypertrophy, is the enlargement of the prostate gland (Fig. 36.12). (Because the major prostatic changes are caused by hyperplasia, not hypertrophy, *benign prostatic hyperplasia* is the preferred term.) This condition becomes problematic when prostatic tissue compresses the urethra where it passes through the prostate, resulting in frequency of lower urinary tract symptoms. Similar to prostate cancer, BPH occurs more often in Westernized countries (e.g., United States, United Kingdom, and Canada). Overall, no clear patterns have emerged with risk of BPH and race.[15] In the United States studies of black men have observed an increased prostate transition zone and total volume compared with white men.[15] Being overweight or obese with central fat distribution (i.e., around the abdomen) increases the risk of developing BPH. Autopsy studies observe a histological prevalence of 8%, 50%, and 80% in the 4th, 6th, and 9th decades of life, respectively.[15] BPH is common and involves a complex pathophysiology with several endocrine and local factors and a remodeled microenvironment. Its relationship to aging is well documented. At birth the prostate is pea sized, and growth of the gland is gradual until puberty. At that time, there is a period of rapid development that continues until the third decade of life, when the prostate reaches adult size (see Chapter 34). Around age 40 to 45, benign hyperplasia begins and continues slowly until death. Although androgens, such as dihydrotestosterone (DHT), are necessary for normal prostatic development, their role in BPH remains unclear.

PATHOPHYSIOLOGY Current causative theories for BPH focus on aging and the levels and ratios of endocrine factors (e.g., androgens

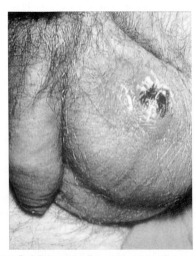

FIGURE 36.11 Epididymitis Secondary to Gonorrhea or Nongonococcal Urethritis. This infection has spread to the testes, and rupture through the scrotal wall is threatened. (From Taylor PK: *Diagnostic picture tests in sexually transmitted disease*, London, 1995, Mosby.)

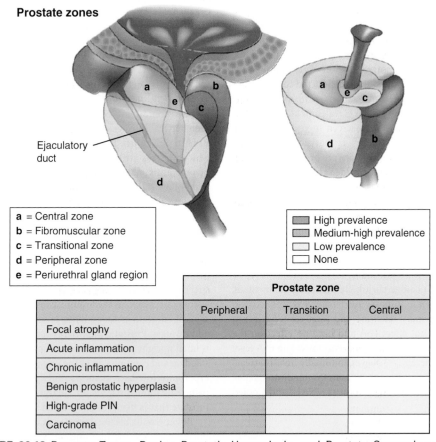

Prostate zones

a = Central zone
b = Fibromuscular zone
c = Transitional zone
d = Peripheral zone
e = Periurethral gland region

Ejaculatory duct

☐ High prevalence
☐ Medium-high prevalence
☐ Low prevalence
☐ None

	Prostate zone		
	Peripheral	Transition	Central
Focal atrophy			
Acute inflammation			
Chronic inflammation			
Benign prostatic hyperplasia			
High-grade PIN			
Carcinoma			

FIGURE 36.12 Prostate Zones, Benign Prostatic Hyperplasia, and Prostate Cancer Locations. Benign prostatic hyperplasia (BPH) occurs in the peripheral zone of the prostate gland that can enlarge (not shown). BPH nodules and atrophy are associated with inflammation in the transition zone. Most cancer lesions occur in the peripheral zone. Carcinoma can involve the central zone but rarely occurs in isolation, suggesting that prostatic intraepithelial neoplasia (PIN) lesions do not easily progress to carcinoma in this region. (Adapted from De Marzo AM et al: *Nat Rev Cancer* 7:256-269, 2007.)

and estrogens [androgen/estrogen ratio]), the role of chronic inflammation, and the effects of autocrine/paracrine growth-stimulating and growth-inhibiting factors. Recent data shows that human prostate stromal cells can actively contribute to the inflammatory process from the induction of inflammatory cytokines and chemokines (see the section Cancer of the Prostate).

With aging, circulating androgens are associated with BPH and enlargement. Other effects related to estrogens include apoptosis, aromatase expression, and paracrine regulation that may be important for stimulating inflammation. BPH is a multifactorial disease, and not all men respond well to currently available treatments, which suggests that factors are involved other than androgens. The prostate is an estrogen target tissue, and estrogens directly and indirectly affect growth and differentiation of the prostate. The precise role of endogenous and exogenous estrogens in directly affecting prostate growth and differentiation in the context of BPH is an understudied area. Estrogens and selective estrogen receptor modulators have been shown to promote or inhibit prostate proliferation, signifying potential roles in BPH. Taken together, these interactions lead to an increase in prostate volume. The remodeled stroma promotes local inflammation with altered cytokine, reactive oxygen/nitrogen species, and chemoattractants. The resultant increased oxygen demands of proliferating cells cause a local hypoxia that induces angiogenesis and changes to fibroblasts.

BPH begins in the periurethral glands, which are the inner glands or layers of the prostate. The prostate enlarges as nodules form and grow (nodular hyperplasia) and glandular cells enlarge (hypertrophy). The development of BPH occurs over a prolonged period, and changes within the urinary tract are slow and insidious.

CLINICAL MANIFESTATIONS As nodular hyperplasia and cellular hypertrophy progress, tissues that surround the prostatic urethra compress it, usually, but not always, causing bladder outflow obstruction. These symptoms are sometimes called the *spectrum of lower urinary tract symptoms* (LUTS). Symptoms include the urge to urinate often, some delay in starting urination, and decreased force of the urinary stream. As the obstruction progresses, often over several years, the bladder cannot empty all the urine, and the increasing volume leads to long-term urine retention. The volume of urine retained may be great enough to produce uncontrolled "overflow incontinence" with any increase in intra-abdominal pressure. At this stage, the force of the urinary stream is significantly reduced, and much more time is required to initiate and complete voiding. Hematuria, bladder or kidney infection, bladder calculi, acute urinary retention hydroureter, hydronephrosis, and renal insufficiency are common complications.

Progressive bladder distention causes diverticular outpouchings of the bladder wall. The ureters may be obstructed where they pass through the hypertrophied detrusor muscle, potentially causing hydroureter, hydronephrosis, and bladder or kidney infection.

EVALUATION AND TREATMENT The diagnosis is made from a medical history, physical examination, and laboratory tests, including urinalysis. Careful review of symptoms is necessary. A digital rectal examination (DRE) and measurement of the PSA level are conducted to determine hyperplasia. However, the PSA level alone cannot confirm symptoms attributable to BPH because the PSA level is elevated in both BPH and prostate cancer. Annual DREs are used to screen men older than 40 years for BPH, sooner in high-risk men.[16] If marked enlargement, moderate to severe symptoms, or complications are present, transrectal ultrasound (TRUS) is used to determine bladder and prostate volume and residual urine. Urinalysis, serum creatinine and blood urea nitrogen levels, uroflowmetry, postvoid residual (PVR) urine, a pressure-flow study, cystometry, and cystourethroscopy are used to determine kidney and bladder function. BPH has been treated successfully with drugs. α_1-Adrenergic blockers (prazosin and tamsulosin) are used to relax the smooth muscle of the bladder and prostate. Antiandrogen agents, such as finasteride (Proscar), selectively block androgens at the prostate cellular level and cause the prostate gland to shrink. By shrinking the prostate, these drugs have been shown to improve BPH-related symptoms and reduce the risk of future urinary retention and BPH-related surgery. α_1-Adrenergic blockers do not affect PSA and have no effect on the prostate cancer risk; however, antiandrogen agents lower the PSA level by 50% after 6 months of therapy.[17,18] Newer, minimally invasive treatments include interstitial laser treatment, transurethral radiofrequency procedures (e.g., transurethral needle ablation [TUNA]), and Cooled ThermoTherapy.

Prostatitis

Prostatitis is an inflammation of the prostate. The incidence and prevalence of prostatitis are not known. Inflammation is usually limited to a few of the gland's excretory ducts.

Prostatitis syndromes have been classified by the National Institutes of Health as (1) acute bacterial prostatitis (ABP), (2) chronic bacterial prostatitis (CBP), (3) chronic pelvic pain syndrome (CPPS), and (4) asymptomatic inflammatory prostatitis (Box 36.4). ABP and CBP are mostly caused by gram-negative Enterobacteriaceae and *Enterococci*

BOX 36.4 National Institutes of Health Classification of Prostatitis Syndrome

This system, developed for clinical research purposes, can be simplified for use in primary care practice (see text).

Category I, or acute bacterial prostatitis (ABP), is an acute infection of the prostate and is manifested by systemic signs of infection and a positive urine culture result.

Category II, or chronic bacterial prostatitis (CBP), is a chronic bacterial infection in which bacteria are received in significant numbers from a purulent prostatic fluid. These bacteria are thought to be the most common cause of recurrent urinary tract infection in men.

Category III, or chronic pelvic pain syndrome (CPPS), is diagnosed when no pathologic bacteria can be localized to the prostate (culture of expressed prostatic fluid or postprostatic massage urine specimen) and is further divided into IIIa and IIIb. Category IIIa is inflammatory CPPS, in which a significant number of white blood cells (WBCs) are localized to the prostate; category IIIb is noninflammatory.

Category IV is asymptomatic inflammatory prostatitis in which bacteria or WBCs are localized to the prostate, but individuals are asymptomatic.

---

species that originate in the gastrointestinal flora. The most common organism is *Escherichia coli,* which is identified in the majority of infections. *Klebsiella* species, *Pseudomonas aeruginosa,* and *Serratia* species are common gram-negative cultured microorganisms. Nonbacterial prostatitis (CP/CPPS) syndromes are caused by a cascade of inflammatory, immunologic, neuroendocrine, and neuropathic mechanisms, such that the initiating cause is unknown.

Bacterial prostatitis. Acute bacterial prostatitis (ABP, category I) is an ascending infection of the urinary tract that tends to occur in men between the ages of 30 and 50 years, but it is also associated with BPH in older men. Infection stimulates an inflammatory response in which the prostate becomes enlarged, tender, firm, or boggy. The onset of prostatitis may be acute and unrelated to previous illnesses, or it may follow catheterization or cystoscopy.

Clinical manifestations of acute bacterial prostatitis are those of urinary tract infection or pyelonephritis. A sudden onset of malaise, low back and perineal pain, high fever (up to 40° C [104° F]), and chills is common, as are dysuria, inability to empty the bladder, nocturia, and urinary retention. The individual also may have symptoms of lower urinary tract obstruction, such as a slow, small, "narrowed" urinary stream, which may be a medical emergency. Acute inflammatory prostatic edema can compress the urethra, causing urinary obstruction. Systemic signs of infection include sudden onset of a high fever, fatigue, arthralgia, and myalgia. Prostatic pain may occur, especially when the individual is in an upright position, because the pelvic floor muscles tighten with standing and compression of the prostate gland occurs. Some individuals experience low back pain, painful ejaculation, and rectal or perineal pain. Palpation discloses an enlarged, extremely tender and swollen prostate that is firm, indurated, and warm to the touch.

Because acute bacterial prostatitis is usually associated with a bladder infection caused by the same microorganism, urine cultures disclose its identity. Prostatic massage may express enough secretions from the urethra for direct bacterial examination, but massage may be painful and increases the risk that the infection will ascend to adjacent structures or enter the bloodstream and cause septicemia.

To resolve the infection and control its spread, individuals may require antibiotics. In severe cases, the individual is hospitalized and treated with intravenous antibiotics, followed by oral antibiotics. Analgesics, antipyretics, bed rest, and adequate hydration are also therapeutic. Complications include urinary retention that resolves with antibiotic therapy; prostatic abscess that may rupture into the urethra, rectum, or perineum; epididymitis; bacteremia; and septic shock. Urinary retention requiring drainage is best managed with a suprapubic catheter; Foley catheterization is contraindicated during acute infection.

Chronic bacterial prostatitis (CBP, category II) is characterized by recurrent urinary tract symptoms and persistence of pathogenic bacteria (usually gram negative) in urine or prostatic fluid. This form of prostatitis is the most common recurrent urinary tract infection in men. Symptoms may be similar to those of an acute bladder infection: frequency, urgency, dysuria, perineal discomfort, low back pain, myalgia, arthralgia, and sexual dysfunction. The prostate may be only slightly enlarged or boggy, but it may be fibrotic because repeated infections can cause it to be firm and irregular in shape.

When the initial urine sample is bacteria free, prostatic massage is used to express secretions. Subsequently, the first 10 ml of voided urine is collected and examined microscopically. Prostatic secretions showing more than 10 white blood cells (WBCs) per high-power field (hpf) and macrophages containing fat are indicative of bacterial infection; the diagnosis is confirmed by culture. A pelvic x-ray or transurethral ultrasound (TUUS may show prostatic calculi.

Treatment of CBP is difficult because it is often caused by prostatic calculi. Calculi are silent and are found in up to 50% of men with prostatitis. Infected calculi can serve as a source of bacterial persistence and relapsing urinary tract infection. Calculi harbor pathogens within the stone and, consequently, pathogens cannot be eradicated from the urinary tract. A permanent cure is achieved by surgical intervention.

Chronic prostatitis/chronic pelvic pain syndrome. Chronic prostatitis/chronic pelvic pain syndrome (CP/CPPS, category III) is diagnosed when no pathogenic bacteria can be localized to the prostate. It is further subdivided into categories IIIa and IIIb (see Box 36.4). Category IIIa refers to inflammatory CPPS in which the WBC count is elevated and localized to the prostate. Compared with category III, symptoms tend to be milder but are persistent and annoying. Presumably, noninfectious prostatitis or pain is caused by reflux of sterile urine into the ejaculatory ducts because of high-pressure voiding. Reflux may be triggered by spasms of the external or internal sphincters. Category IIIb is noninflammatory. Category IV exists when individuals are asymptomatic but have an increase in bacteria and WBCs localized to the prostate. Microorganisms suspected of causing CP/CPPS include *E. Enterobacter* organisms, *P. aeruginosa*, and *Helicobacter pylori*.

Men with nonbacterial prostatitis may complain of pain or a dull ache that is continuous or spasmodic in the suprapubic, infrapubic, scrotal, penile, or inguinal area. Other symptoms are pain on ejaculation and urinary symptoms, such as frequency of urination. The prostate gland generally feels normal on palpation.

Nonbacterial prostatitis is a diagnosis of exclusion. Digital examination of the prostate, bacterial cultures of the urogenital tract, microscopic examination of expressed prostatic fluid, urethroscopy, and urodynamic studies are used to verify the diagnosis of nonbacterial prostatitis.

There is no generally accepted treatment for nonbacterial prostatitis. Hot sitz baths, bed rest, and pharmacologic therapies, including anti-inflammatory drugs, can relieve symptoms.

Cancer of the Prostate

Prostate cancer is the most commonly diagnosed, non–skin cancer in men in the United States; the lifetime risk for this diagnosis currently is estimated at 15.9%.[19] The incidence varies greatly worldwide (Fig. 36.13), but prostate cancer is considered the third leading cause of cancer death globally, accounting for 7.1% of all cancer deaths. In the U.S., the lifetime risk of being diagnosed with prostate cancer is approximately 11%, with a 2.5% lifetime risk of dying from it.[19,20] An estimated 1.1 million cases of prostate cancer were diagnosed worldwide in 2012, accounting for 15% of the cancers diagnosed in men. Almost 70% of diagnosed cases of prostate cancer (759,000) were found to occur in more developed regions.[21] Importantly, incidence rates vary by more than 25-fold worldwide, with the highest rates recorded mostly in developed countries, such as Oceania, Europe, and North America, largely because of wide use or overuse of PSA testing. Screening with PSA can amplify the incidence of prostate cancer by allowing detection of prostate lesions that, although meeting the pathologic criteria for malignancy, may have low potential (e.g., latent, indolent, preclinical) for growth and metastasis. In countries with higher use of PSA testing, such as the United States, Canada, Australia, and the Nordic countries, trends in incidence rates follow similar patterns.

Unlike in Western countries, the incidence and death rates are rising in several Asian and Central and Eastern European countries, including Japan. Death rates have been decreasing in several countries, including Australia, Canada, the United Kingdom, the United States, Italy, and Norway, in part because of improved treatment. Males of African descent in the Caribbean region have the highest mortality from prostate cancer in the world. Most cases of prostate cancer have a good prognosis even without treatment, but some cases are aggressive. Prostate cancer is rare before age 50 years, and very few men die from this cancer before 60 years of age. Indeed, more than 75% of all prostate cancer is diagnosed in men older than 65.[19] With aging, most of the androgen-metabolizing enzymes undergo significant alteration and older age, race (black), and family history remain the well-established risk factors.

Dietary factors. Although evidence exists for a dietary role in prostate cancer, the epidemiologic evidence is inconsistent. The problem has been confounded by the lack of biomarkers for certain nutrients, difficulties in measuring and quantifying diet, and a limitation of clinical trials to study diet over time. An important factor is the effects of diet

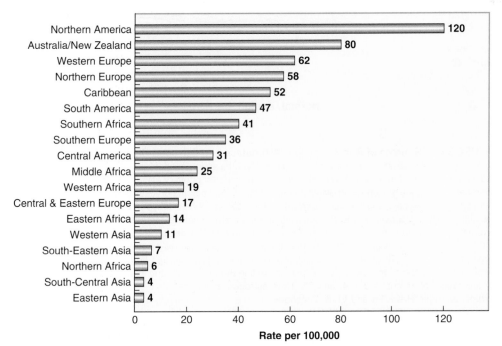

FIGURE 36.13 Selected World Population Age-Standardized (to the World Population) Incidence Rates of Prostate Cancer. (From Jemal A et al: *Biomark Prev* 19:1893, 2010.)

on signaling pathways, hormones, oxidative stress, and reactive oxygen species (ROS). The nutrients in the epidemiology of prostate cancer that have received the most attention include carotenoids, fat, vitamin E, vitamin D/calcium, and selenium. Less studied are isoflavones, curcumin, lycopene, green tea, omega-3 polyunsaturated fats, and sulforaphane (Box 36.5).

Associations between obesity and prostate cancer are not clear because there are some inconsistencies, but obesity seems to be negatively associated with more indolent prostate cancer and positively associated with more aggressive disease and a worse outcome. Because adipose tissue is increasingly being regarded as hormonally active tissue, high body fat and obesity need in-depth exploration to understand the associated risk of prostate problems. Adipose tissue is now known to affect circulating levels of several bioactive messengers and therefore could affect the risk of developing prostate problems in addition to several other well-recognized health problems. High-energy intake (consumption of excess calories) indicates that this may indeed increase insulin levels and levels of insulin-like growth factor 1 (IGF-1), a powerful carcinogenic agent.

Hormones. Prostate cancer develops in an androgen-dependent epithelium and is usually androgen sensitive. Androgens are synthesized not only in the testis, accounting for 50% to 60% of the total testosterone in the prostate, but also in the prostate gland itself. In a process called intraprostatic conversion, the hormone dehydroepiandrosterone (DHEA) produced by the adrenal glands is converted to testosterone and then into DHT in the prostate (Fig. 36.14). Additionally, prostate cancer cells have been reported to make androgens from cholesterol (i.e., de novo). However, these overall relative contributions from intratumoral sources remain to be determined. Population studies have not yet provided clear and convincing patterns involving associations between circulating hormone concentrations (i.e., not tissue concentrations) and the risk for prostate cancer. Thus, there is universal agreement that androgens are important for prostatic growth, development, and maintenance of tissue balance; but their role in cancer is controversial.

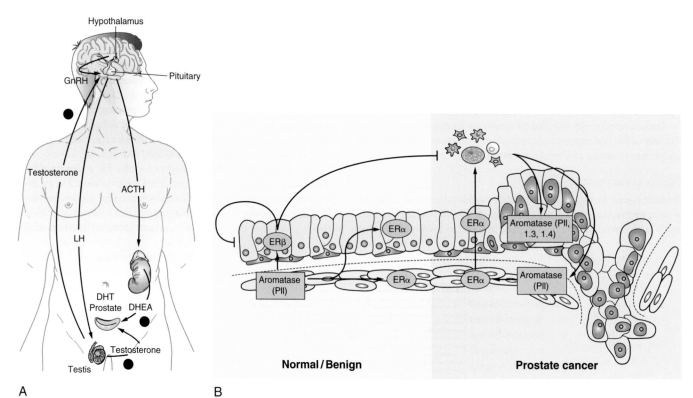

A   B

FIGURE 36.14 Sources of Androgens and Aromatase and Estrogen Signaling in the Prostate. A, Body sources of androgens in the prostate gland. Hypothalamic gonadotropin-releasing hormone (GnRH) causes the release of luteinizing hormone (LH) from the anterior pituitary gland. LH stimulates the testes to produce testosterone, which accumulates in the blood. Pituitary adrenocorticotropic hormone (ACTH) release stimulates the adrenal glands, which secrete the androgen precursor dehydroepiandrosterone (DHEA) into the blood. DHEA is converted into testosterone and then into dihydrotestosterone (DHT) in the prostate. **B,** Aromatase and estrogen signaling in the prostate. In normal and benign tissue, aromatase is expressed within the stroma and regulated by promoter PII. Estrogen then exerts its effects in an autocrine fashion through the stromal ER-α receptor and also in a paracrine fashion through both ER-α and ER-β receptors. With prostate cancer, aromatase is now expressed within the tumor cells and in stromal cells and is regulated by aromatase promoters 1.3, 1.4, and PII. Thus estrogen exerts its effects in an autocrine way through stromal and epithelial ER-α and ER-β. Consequently, the increased levels of estrogen and abnormal ER-α signaling promote inflammation, which increases aromatase expression and the development of a positive feedback cycle. Inflammation drives aromatase expression, thus increasing estrogen, which in turn promotes further inflammation. *ACTH,* Adrenocorticotropic hormone; *DHEA,* dehydroepiandrosterone; *DHT,* dihydrotestosterone; *GnRH,* gonadotropin-releasing hormone; *LH,* luteinizing hormone. (**A** adapted from Labrie F: *Nat Rev Urol* 8:73-80, 2011. **B** from Ellem SJ, Risbridger GP: *J Steroid Biochem Mol Biol* 118[4-5]:246-251, 2010.)

BOX 36.5 Summary of Diet for Prostate Cancer

- Lower rates of prostate cancer are found in countries whose residents consume a low-fat and high-vegetable diet. When men from a low-risk country move to the United States and eat a Western diet, their rates of prostate cancer increase significantly. Inconclusive are the exact culprits that increase this risk, including fat and sugar intake.
- Obesity is linked to advanced and aggressive prostate cancer.
- High body mass index (BMI) is associated with more aggressive disease and a worse outcome.
- A calorie-dense or an excessive carbohydrate intake and obesity, independent of dietary fat intake, may increase the risk of developing prostate cancer.
- Dietary fat may increase levels of androgens, increase oxidative stress, and increase reactive oxygen species (ROS).
- Monounsaturated fats may decrease the risk of prostate cancer.
- High levels of linoleic acid (found in corn oil) act as a proinflammatory eicosanoid, which is implicated in promotion of cell proliferation and angiogenesis, as well as inhibition of apoptosis.
- The Western diet has increased omega-6–to–omega-3 ratios and therefore is proinflammatory. Carcinogenic nitrosamines are formed after consumption of processed meat that contains nitrites and from heme iron present in large quantities of red meat.
- Even given this knowledge, it is important to realize that studies showing an association between meat intake and prostate cancers have been largely inconclusive. Some studies indicated that red meat is positively associated with an increased prostate cancer risk with an association with more aggressive disease states. Despite some studies showing a 43% elevation in prostate cancer risk with a diet excessively high in red meat, others show no association with prostate cancer risk.
- Although the role of red meat in prostate and breast cancer remains inconclusive, one explanation for the possible associations reported is the accumulation of carcinogens during the cooking process. Cooking meat at high temperatures produces heterocyclic amines and aromatic hydrocarbons that are carcinogenic.
- Vitamin E has long been considered a candidate for prostate cancer prevention from in vitro and in vivo animal studies. Vitamin E belongs to the family of tocopherols and tocotrienols that exist as α, β, γ, and δ isoforms. Among these, δ-tocopherol is the major dietary isoform, whereas supplements contain α-tocopherol. Vitamin E is a fat-soluble vitamin obtained from vegetable oils, nuts, and egg yolk. It is a potent intracellular antioxidant known to inhibit peroxidation and deoxyribonucleic acid (DNA) damage. The Alpha-Tocopherol, Beta-Carotene Cancer Prevention Study (ATBC) showed that supplementation with vitamin E could reduce the incidence of prostate cancer among men who smoked. In vitro studies demonstrate that α-tocopherol succinate induces cell cycle arrest in human prostate cancer cells (i.e., induces apoptosis) and inhibits the androgen receptor. Mouse studies show vitamin E can inhibit the growth-promoting effects of a high-fat diet; however, vitamin E in combination with selenium does not reduce the incidence of prostate cancer in Lady mice models. A prospective large clinical trial, the Selenium and Vitamin E Cancer Prevention Trial (SELECT), showed no reduction in prostate cancer period prevalence but an increased risk of prostate cancer with vitamin E alone.
- Selenium is a trace mineral and exists in food as selenomethionine and selenocysteine. It is essential for the functioning of many antioxidant enzymes and proteins in the body. Humans receive selenium in their diet through plant (dependent on soil concentrations) and animal products. The SELECT trial showed that neither selenium nor vitamin E, taken alone or together, helped to prevent prostate cancer.
- Vitamin D may play an important role in prostate cancer prevention.
- Soy's anticancer properties include inhibition of cell proliferation and angiogenesis and a reduction in prostate-specific antigen (PSA) and androgen receptor levels. Countries whose residents have a high intake of soy have much lower rates of prostate cancer.

- Tomatoes or tomato products ingested daily seem to reduce prostate cancer risk. In vitro studies show that the lycopene found in tomatoes inhibits DNA strand breaks. Unresolved is whether lycopene itself or a metabolic product is responsible for its biologic effect. In clinical studies tomato paste, which is high in lycopene, reduced plasma PSA levels in men with benign prostatic hyperplasia. Lycopene administration is associated with cell cycle arrest (apoptosis) and growth factor signaling. In 2007 the U.S. Food and Drug Administration (FDA) evaluated 13 available studies and found the relationship between lycopene and a reduced risk of prostate cancer inadequate.
- Vegetables such as broccoli, cabbage, cauliflower, brussels sprouts, Chinese cabbage, and turnips (all crucifers) may be protective (several epidemiologic studies) against prostate cancer. In particular, a diet high in broccoli reduced cancer risk. By contrast, four studies revealed no cancer preventive effects. Cruciforms have anticancer properties mediated by the phytochemicals phenethyl isothiocyanate, sulforaphane, and indole-3-carbinol. Sulforaphane is a naturally occurring isothiocyanate that was first isolated in broccoli. It protects against carcinogen-induced cancer in many rodents. Mice given 240 mg of broccoli sprouts per day showed a significant reduction in growth of prostate cancer cells. Sulforaphane treatment lowered androgen receptor protein and gene expression.
- Green tea contains polyphenols, including epigallocatechin gallate (EGCG). Green tea consumption has been associated with a reduced incidence of several cancers, including prostate cancer. Green tea consumed within a balanced, controlled diet in humans improved overall antioxidant potential. The anticancer effect potential of green tea from in vitro and experimental studies shows that these compounds bind directly to carcinogens and induce phase II enzymes that inhibit heterocyclic amines. EGCG administration decreased NF-κB activity. Green tea was shown to inhibit insulin-like growth factor 1 (IGF-1) and increase insulin-like growth factor binding protein 3 (IGFBP3), leading to inhibition of prostate cancer development and progression. Yet, in two small randomized studies in individuals with high-grade prostatic neoplasia, green tea showed no effects. However, treatment with a mixture of bioactive compounds that share molecular anticarcinogenic targets may enhance the effect on these targets at low concentrations of individual compounds.
- Epidemiologic studies have consistently shown that regular consumption of fruits and vegetables is strongly associated with a reduced risk of developing chronic diseases, such as cancer. It is now accepted that the actions of any specific phytonutrient alone do not explain the observed health benefits of diets rich in fruits and vegetables; also, clinical trials demonstrated that consumption of phytonutrients did not show consistent preventive effects. Synergistic inhibition of prostate cancer cell growth has been evident with the use of combinations of low concentrations of various carotenoids or carotenoids with retinoic acid and the active metabolite of vitamin D. Combinations of several carotenoids (e.g., lycopene, phytoene, and phytofluene) or carotenoids and polyphenols (e.g., carnosic acid and curcumin) and/or other compounds (e.g., vitamin E) synergistically inhibit the androgen receptor activity and activate the electrophile/antioxidant response element (EpRE/ARE) transcription system. The activation of EpRE/ARE is up to fourfold higher than the sum of activities of single ingredients.
- Examples of important potential processes that can be targeted in the regulation of tumorigenesis include cholesterol synthesis and metabolites, ROS and hypoxia, macrophage activation and conversion, indoleamine 2,3-dioxygenase regulation of dendritic cells, vascular endothelial growth factor regulation of angiogenesis, fibrosis inhibition, and endoglin and Janus kinase signaling.
- Curcumin has anticarcinogenic potential, with well-characterized antiinflammatory, antiangiogenic, and antioxidant properties. Recent studies report that curcumin modulates the Wingless signaling pathway (Wnt) that supports its antiproliferative potential. Curcumin is characteristic of regulating multiple targets, a desirable feature in current drug design and drug development. Together with its potential for treating castration-resistant prostate cancer

Continued

BOX 36.5   Summary of Diet for Prostate Cancer—cont'd

and its safety profile, this feature enables curcumin to serve as an ideal compound for the design and syntheses of agents with improved potential for enhancing clinical therapies used to treat prostate cancer.

- Overall, multiple signaling pathways are involved in prostate cancer development and progression, many of which are affected by dietary and lifestyle factors.

References

Alexander DD, et al: A review and meta-analysis of prospective studies of red and processed meat intake and prostate cancer, *Nutr J* 9:50, 2010.

Astorg P: Dietary N-6 and N-3 polyunsaturated fatty acids and prostate cancer risk: a review of epidemiological and experimental evidence, *Cancer Causes Control* 15:367-386, 2004.

Beier R, et al: Induction of cyclin E-cdk2 kinase activity, E2F-dependent transcription and cell growth by Myc are genetically separable events, *EMBO J* 19(21):5813-5823, 2000.

Casey SC, et al: Cancer prevention and therapy through the modulation of the tumor microenvironment, *Semin Cancer Biol* 35(Suppl):S199-S223, 2015.

Chen QH: Curcumin-based anti-prostate cancer agents, *Anticancer Agents Med Chem* 15(2):138-156, 2015.

Dagnelie PC, et al: Diet, anthropometric measures and prostate cancer risk: a review of prospective cohort and intervention studies, *BJ Int* 93(8):1139-1150, 2004.

Demark-Wahnefried W, Moyad MA: Dietary intervention in the management of prostate cancer, *Curr Opin Urol* 17:168-174, 737-743, 2001, 2007.

Freedland SJ, Aronson WJ: Obesity and prostate cancer, *Urology* 65:433-439, 2005.

Giovannucci E, et al: Risk factors for prostate cancer incidence and progression in the health professionals follow-up study, *Int J Cancer* 121:1571-1578, 2007.

Greenwald P: Clinical trials in cancer prevention: current results and perspectives for the future, *J Nutr* 134(12 Suppl):3507S-3512S, 2004.

Hill P, et al: Diet and urinary steroids in black and white North American men and black South African men, *Cancer Res* 39:5101-5105, 1979.

Kim DJ, et al: Premorbid diet in relation to survival from prostate cancer (Canada), *Cancer Causes Control* 11:65-77, 2000.

Kobayashi N, et al: Effect of altering dietary omega-6/omega-3 fatty acid ratios on prostate cancer membrane composition, cyclooxygenase-2, and prostaglandin E2, *Clin Cancer Res* 12(15):4660-4670, 2006.

Kolonel LN: Fat, meat, and prostate cancer, *Epidemiol Rev* 23:72-81, 2001.

Kristal AR, et al: Dietary patterns, supplement use, and the risk of symptomatic benign prostatic hyperplasia: results from the prostate cancer prevention trial, *Am J Epidemiol* 167:925-934, 2008.

Linnewiel-Hermoni K, et al: The anti-cancer effects of carotenoids and other phytonutrients resides in their combined activity, *Arch Biochem Biophys* 572:28-35, 2015.

Lloyd JC, et al: Effect of isocaloric low fat diet on prostate cancer xenograft progression in a hormone deprivation model, *J Urol* 183:1619-1624, 2010.

Matsumara K, et al: Involvement of the estrogen receptor beta in genistein-induced expression of p21 (waf1/cip1) in PC-3 prostate cancer cells, *Anticancer Res* 28:709-714, 2008.

Ngo TH, et al: Effect of diet and exercise on serum insulin, IGF-1, and IGFBP-1 levels and growth of LNCaP cells in vitro (United States), *Cancer Causes Control* 13:929-935, 2002.

Ngo TH, et al: Effect of isocaloric low-fat diet on human LAPC-4 prostate cancer xenografts in severe combined immunodeficient mice and the insulin-like growth factor axis, *Clin Cancer Res* 9:2734-2743, 2003.

Ni J, Yeh S: The roles of alpha-vitamin E and its analogues in prostate cancer, *Vitam Horm* 76:493-518, 2007.

Punnen S, et al: Impact of meat consumption, preparation, and mutagens on aggressive prostate cancer, *PLoS ONE* 6:e27711, 2011.

Rodriguez C, et al: Body mass index, weight change, and risk of prostate cancer in the Cancer Prevention Study II Nutrition Cohort, *Cancer Epidemiol Biomarkers Prev* 16:63-69, 2007.

Salem S, et al: Major dietary factors and prostate cancer risk: a prospective multicenter case-control study, *Nutr Cancer* 63:21-27, 2011, 2011.

Sinha R, et al: Meat and meat-related compounds and risk of prostate cancer in a large prospective cohort study in the United States, *Am J Epidemiol* 170:1165-1177, 2009.

Teiten M, et al: Anti-proliferative potential of curcumin in androgen dependent prostate cancer cells occurs through modulation of the Wingless signaling pathway, *Int J Oncol* 38:603-611, 2011.

Wang P, et al: Increased chemopreventive effect by combining arctigenin, green tea polyphenol and curcumin in prostate and breast cancer cells, *RSC Adv* 4(66):35242-35250, 2014.

Wright JL, et al: AMACR polymorphisms, dietary intake of red meat and dairy and prostate cancer risk, *Prostate* 71:498-506, 2011.

Zhou DY, et al: Curcumin analogues with high activity for inhibiting human prostate cancer cell growth and androgen receptor activation, *Mol Med Rep* 10(3):1315-1322, 2014.

In men younger than 50 years, circulating levels of androgens and estrogens appear to be higher in men of African descent than in European-American men.

Despite the well-documented importance of androgens, their pathophysiologic process in prostate diseases is incomplete. Androgens also are metabolized to estrogens (see Fig. 36.14, *B*) through the action of the enzyme aromatase, and a growing body of evidence implicates estrogens in the etiology of prostate disease (see the Pathogenesis section).

Vasectomy. Vasectomy has been identified as a possible risk factor for prostate cancer in both case-controlled studies and cohort studies. Three mechanisms by which vasectomy could increase the risk are (1) elevation of circulating androgens; (2) activation of immunologic mechanisms involving antisperm antibodies; and (3) reduction of seminal fluid levels of 5α-dihydrotestosterone, the active metabolite of testosterone in the prostate, in vasectomized men. These results suggest an elevation of circulating free testosterone level after vasectomy. However, with these combined mechanisms, it is unlikely that vasectomy plays a causal role.

Chronic inflammation. Certain metabolic comorbidities, including obesity, diabetes, sleep apnea, and erectile dysfunction, may be linked both to BPH and to inflammation. The causes of chronic inflammation are emerging (possible causes are shown in Fig. 36.15). Thus, chronic inflammation may be an important risk factor for prostatic adenocarcinoma. Chronic inflammation involves autocrine/paracrine growth-stimulating and growth-inhibiting factors. These factors include insulin-like growth factors (IGFs), epidermal growth factors, fibroblast factors, and transforming growth factor-beta (TGF-β), as well as several others. Recent data show that human prostate stromal cells can actively contribute to the inflammatory process from the induction of inflammatory cytokines and chemokines. Importantly, continuous input from TGF-β and IGF in the tumor microenvironment or stroma results in cancer progression. Understanding these events can help in the prevention, diagnosis, and therapy of prostate cancer (Fig. 36.16).

Genetic and epigenetic factors. Other possible causes are those of genetic predisposition (familial and hereditary forms). Genetic studies suggest that a strong familial predisposition may be responsible for 5% to 10% of prostate cancers.[5] Compared with men with no family history, those with one first-degree relative with prostate cancer have twice the risk and those with two first-degree relatives have five times the risk.[22] Germline mutations in the breast cancer predisposition gene 2 (*BRCA2*) are the genetic events known to date that confer the highest risk of prostate cancer (8.6-fold in men age 65 or older). Although the role of *BRCA2* and *BRCA1* in prostate tumorigenesis remains unrevealed, deleterious mutations in both genes have been associated with more aggressive disease and poor clinical outcomes. Men with *BRCA2* (tumor suppressor) germline mutations have a 20-fold increase in the risk of prostate cancer.[23] A common type of somatic mutation that develops into chromosomal rearrangements is the *ETS* gene. The most common epigenetic alteration in prostate cancer is hypermethylation of the glutathione *S*-transferase (*GSTP1*) gene located on chromosome 11. More than 30 independent, peer-reviewed studies have reported a consistently high sensitivity and specificity of *GSTP1* hypermethylation in prostatectomy or biopsy tissue. There is no clear evidence of a causal link between BPH and prostate cancer, even though

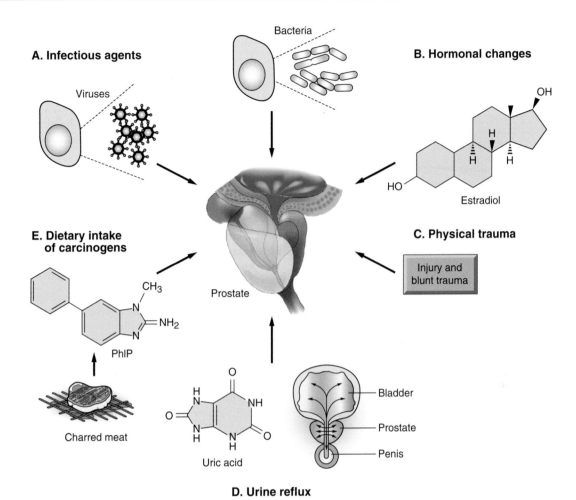

FIGURE 36.15 Possible Causes of Prostate Inflammation. A, Infection, including viruses, bacteria, fungi, and parasites. **B,** Hormones, for example, estrogen at key times during development. **C,** Physical trauma, any type of blunt physical injury. **D,** Urine reflex. **E,** Certain dietary factors (see text).

they may often occur together. Variations in several other genes related to inflammatory pathways might affect the probability of developing prostate cancer.

PATHOPHYSIOLOGY More than 95% of prostatic neoplasms are adenocarcinomas, and most occur in the periphery of the prostate (see Fig. 36.12 and Fig. 36.17). Prostatic adenocarcinoma is a heterogeneous group of tumors with a diverse spectrum of molecular and pathologic characteristics and, therefore, diverse clinical behaviors and challenges. The biologic aggressiveness of the neoplasm appears to be related to the degree of differentiation rather than the size of the tumor (Box 36.6). Several genetic alterations have been found for prostate carcinoma, including acquired genomic structural changes, somatic mutations, and epigenetic alterations.

Hormonal factors. Just as the testicles are the male equivalent of the female ovaries, the prostate is the male equivalent of the female uterus; in both situations they originate from the same embryonic cells. This may be important in understanding the role of the associated hormones testosterone (T), DHT, and estrogens in prostate cancer development. Testicular T synthesis and serum T levels fall as men age, but the levels of estradiol do not decline, remaining unchanged or increasing with age. The relationship between hormones and the pathophysiology of prostate carcinogenesis is incomplete and controversial. The main issues and controversies include (1) sources of

BOX 36.6 Determining the Grade of Prostate Cancer With the Gleason Score

Grade 1. The cancer cells closely resemble normal cells. They are small, uniform in shape, evenly spaced, and well differentiated (i.e., they remain separate from one another).

Grade 2. The cancer cells are still well differentiated, but they are arranged more loosely and are irregular in shape and size. Some of the cancer cells have invaded the neighboring prostate tissue.

Grade 3. This is the most common grade. The cells are less well differentiated (some have fused into clumps) and are more variable in shape.

Grade 4. The cells are poorly differentiated and highly irregular in shape. Invasion of the neighboring prostate tissue has progressed further.

Grade 5. The cells are undifferentiated. They have merged into large masses that no longer resemble normal prostate cells. Invasion of the surrounding tissue is extensive.

androgen production outside of the testes, or extratesticular sources (e.g., from adrenal DHEA and from prostate tissue cholesterol [de novo] itself); (2) the role of prostatic androgen receptor; (3) the role of estrogens, aromatase enzyme, and the estrogen receptors ERα and ERβ; and (4) the role of the surrounding microenvironment or stroma.

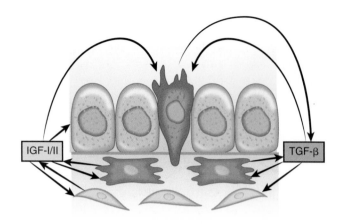

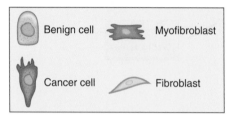

FIGURE 36.16 Working Model of Stromal-Epithelial Interaction in Prostate Cancer Development and Progression. Normally, signaling events between tumor growth factor β (TGF-β) and insulin-like growth factor (IGF) are tightly regulated, keeping the epithelial cells under homeostatic balance. TGF-β binds to co-receptors on the cell surface known as betaglycan *receptor type I (TbR-I)* and betaglycan *receptor type II* (TbR-II). A reduction in TbRs in the stromal cells results in an increase in IGF production. The increase in IGF has a proliferative effect on the prostate epithelial cells (which have already undergone a cancer initiation process as a result of the hormones testosterone and estradiol). TGF-β and IGF in the stromal cells adjacent to prostate epithelial cells perpetuate a vicious cycle to promote cancer progression. (Adapted from Lee C et al: *Biomed Res* 2014:502093, 2014.)

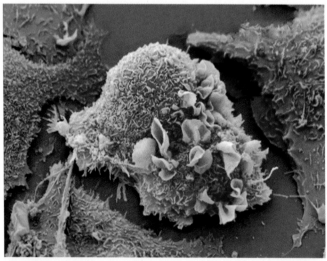

FIGURE 36.17 Photomicrograph of Prostate Cancer Cells. Pink ruffled cells are prostate cancer cells. (From Cancer Research UK, London Research Institute, Electron Microscopy Unit.)

Prostate cancer is considered a hormone-dependent disease; cell growth and survival of early stage prostate cancer can respond to androgens and this is the background evidence for androgen-deprivation therapy (ADT). However, evidence thus far is lacking to associate *plasma* androgens with prostate cancer progression. Prostatic tissue has the

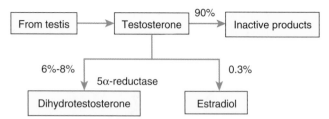

FIGURE 36.18 Testosterone and Conversion to Dihydrotestosterone.

ability to produce its own steroids, including androgens and estrogens. Therefore, the local tissue levels of sex steroids have become a major focus of intraprostatic hormonal profiles. Prostate tissue contains many metabolizing enzymes for the local production of active androgens and estrogens. Carcinogenesis can alter these intraprostatic enzymes and alter the normal balance.

The androgenic hormone responses in the normal prostate and prostate cancer are mediated by androgen receptor (AR) signaling. Exactly how AR drives the growth of prostate cancer cells is not fully known. Testicular T provides the main source of androgens in the prostate (see Fig. 36.14) and is the major *circulating* androgen, whereas DHT predominates in prostate tissue and binds to the AR with greater affinity than does T. The adrenal cortex contributes the far less potent DHEA, which promotes the synthesis of androgens in the prostate. In the target tissues and, to a lesser extent, in the testes themselves, T is converted to DHT by the enzyme 5α-reductase (Fig. 36.18). Thus, DHT is the most potent intraprostatic androgen.

Normally, a small amount of estrogen (i.e., estrone and estradiol) is produced daily by the aromatization of androstenedione and T, respectively. This reaction is catalyzed by the enzyme aromatase. A small quantity of estradiol is released by the testes (see Fig. 36.18); the rest of the estrogens in males are produced by adipose tissue, liver, skin, brain, and other nonendocrine tissue. Thus, T is a precursor of two hormones, DHT and estradiol.

Accumulating evidence shows that estrogens participate in the pathogenesis and development of BPH and prostate cancer by activating estrogen receptor α (ER-α). In contrast, estrogen receptor β (ER-β) is involved in the differentiation and maturation of prostatic epithelial cells and thus exerts antitumor effects in prostate cancer. The effect of estrogen is determined by the two receptors ER-α and ER-β. ER-α leads to abnormal proliferation, inflammation, and the development of premalignant lesions. In contrast, ER-β leads to antiproliferative, antiinflammatory, and potentially anticarcinogenic effects that act in concert or balance the actions of ER-α and androgens. Increased expression of ER-α has been found to be associated with prostate cancer progression, metastasis, and the so-called castration-resistant (i.e., medical treatment that suppresses androgens) phenotype. A specific oncogene is regulated by ERs, and hormones that stimulate the ER-α receptor–like (i.e., agonists) endogenous estrogens can stimulate oncogene expression.

Most of the androgen-metabolizing enzymes undergo a significant age-dependent alteration. In epithelium, both the blood levels of 5α-reductase activity and the DHT level decrease with age, whereas in stroma (prostate), not only the 5α-reductase activity but also the stromal DHT level is rather constant over the lifetime. In contrast to the relatively unaltered DHT level over time, the estrogen concentration follows an age-dependent increase. Thus the age-dependent decrease of the DHT accumulation in epithelium and the concomitant increase of the estrogen accumulation in stroma lead to a tremendous increase with age of the estrogen/androgen ratio in the human prostate. In animal studies, chronic exposure to T plus estradiol is strongly carcinogenic, whereas T alone is weakly carcinogenic. In mice studies, elevated T levels in the absence of estrogen leads to the development of hypertrophy and hyperplasia but not malignancy. High estrogen and low T levels have been shown to lead to inflammation with aging and the emergence of precancerous lesions. The mechanism is not clearly understood and may involve estrogen-generated oxidative stress and deoxyribonucleic acid (DNA) toxicity, and it requires androgen-mediated and estrogen receptor–mediated processes, such as changes in sex steroid metabolism and receptor status. In addition, there are changes in the balance between autocrine/paracrine growth-stimulatory and growth-inhibitory factors, such as the IGFs.

Investigators have summarized these key findings on hormones and prostate cancer: (1) androgens are clearly involved in the progression of prostate cancer; (2) it is only with the addition of estrogen to T in rats that cancer can be reliably induced; (3) in vivo and in vitro studies have identified multiple mechanisms involving hormonal involvement with genotoxicity, epigenetic toxicity, hyperprolactinemia, chronic inflammation, and estrogen receptor–mediated changes.

Prostate epithelial neoplasia. A precursor lesion, prostatic epithelial neoplasia (PIN), has been described. PIN may be more concentrated in prostates containing cancer and is noted in proximity to cancer. However, the final fate of PIN is unknown, including the possibilities of latency, invasion, and even regression. The current working model of prostate carcinogenesis suggests that repeated cycles of injury and cell death occur to the prostate epithelium as a result of damage (i.e., from oxidative stress) from inflammatory responses. The direct injury is hypothesized as a response to infections; autoimmune disease; circulating carcinogens or toxins, or both, from the diet; or urine that has refluxed into the prostate (see Fig. 36.15). The resultant manifestation of this injury is focal atrophy or prostate intraepithelial atrophy (PIA). Biologic responses cause an increase in proliferation and a massive increase in epithelial cells that have a phenotype intermediate between basal cells and mature luminal cells (Fig. 36.19). In a small subset of cells, some may contain "stem cell" or tumor-initiating properties and telomere shortening (see Chapter 11). A subset of PIN cells may activate telomerase enzyme, causing the cells to become immortal. Molecular genetic and epigenetic changes can increase genetic instability that might progress to high-grade PIN and early prostate cancer formation. This model of prostate carcinogenesis needs much more research.

Stromal environment. The prostate gland is composed of secretory luminal epithelium, basal epithelium, neuroendocrine cells, and various cell types comprising supportive tissue or stroma. Stroma, or tissue microenvironment, produces autocrine/paracrine factors as well as structural supporting molecules that help regulate normal cell behavior and organ homeostasis. Stromal components in the tumor microenvironment are important contributions to tumor progression and metastasis. Reciprocal interactions between tumor cells and stromal components influence the metastatic, dormancy-related, and stem cell–like potential of tumor cells. The stromal compartment of the tumor is complex and includes inflammatory/immune cells, vascular endothelial cells, pericytes, fibroblasts, adipocytes, and components of the extracellular matrix. Tumor-infiltrating inflammatory cells release a host of growth factors, chemokines, cytokines, and proinvasive matrix-degrading enzymes to promote tumor growth and progression. Angiogenesis occurs in response to factors secreted from tumor cells, resulting in continued growth and progression. Adipocytes in the tumor microenvironment produce adipokines, which are important for tumor growth. Fibroblasts in the tumor microenvironment provide the structural framework of the stroma; they remain quiet or dormant, but proliferate during wound healing, inflammation, and cancer. Tumor cells release paracrine factors that activate fibroblasts to become "cancer-associated fibroblasts" (CAFs). CAFs secrete factors that modulate tumor growth and modify the stroma to enhance metastasis and dampen responses to anticancer therapies. These findings suggest that alteration in the prostate microenvironment with therapeutic agents and approaches—in particular, natural products such as berberine, resveratrol, onionin A, EGCG, genistein, curcumin, naringenin, desoxyrhapontigenin, piperine, and zerumbone—warrants further investigation to target the tumor microenvironment for the treatment and prevention of cancer.

Epithelial-mesenchymal transition (EMT) was first described in embryonic development, and is observed in a number of solid tumors (see Chapter 11). Cells that undergo EMT become more migratory and invasive and gain access to vascular vessels. Numerous studies have shown that these transition states (EMT and mesenchymal-epithelial transition [MET]) are a consequence of tumor-stromal interactions.

Prostate cancer is known to be diverse and composed of multiple genetically distinct cancer cell clones. However, recent studies indicate that most metastatic cancers arise from a single precursor cancer cell.

From all these observations, a multifactorial general hypothesis of prostate carcinogenesis emerges: (1) androgens act as strong tumor promoters through androgen receptor–mediated mechanisms to enhance the carcinogenic activity of strong endogenous DNA toxic carcinogens,

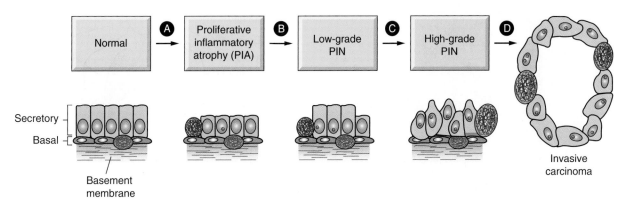

FIGURE 36.19 Cellular and Molecular Model of Early Prostate Neoplasia Progression. A, This stage includes infiltration of lymphocytes, macrophages, and neutrophils caused by repeated infections, dietary factors, urine reflux, injury, onset of autoimmunity (which triggers inflammation), and wound healing. **B,** Epigenetic alterations mediate telomere shortening. **C,** Genetic instability and accumulation of genetic alterations. **D,** Continued proliferation of genetically unstable cells, leading to cancer progression. *PIN,* Prostatic intraepithelial neoplasia.

including reactive estrogen metabolites and estrogen, and prostate-generated reactive oxygen species; (2) reciprocal interactions between tumor cells and the stromal microenvironment promote prostate cancer pathogenesis; and (3) possibly unknown environmental and lifestyle carcinogens may contribute to prostate cancer. All these factors are modulated by diet and genetic determinants, such as hereditary susceptibility genes and polymorphic genes, which encode receptors and enzymes involved in the metabolism and action of steroid hormones.

The most common sites of distant metastasis are the lymph nodes, bones, lungs, liver, and adrenals. The pelvis, lumbar spine, femur, thoracic spine, and ribs are the most common sites of bone metastasis. Local extension is usually posterior, although late in the disease the tumor may invade the rectum or encroach on the prostatic urethra and cause bladder outlet obstruction (Fig. 36.20). The spread of cancer through blood vessels is illustrated in Fig. 36.21.

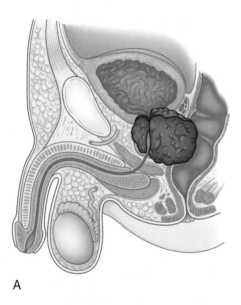

A

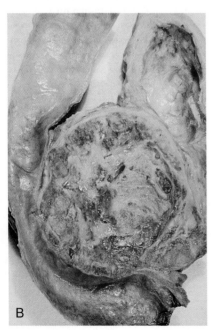

B

FIGURE 36.20 Carcinoma of the Prostate. A, Schematic of carcinoma of the prostate. **B,** Carcinoma of the prostate extending into the rectum and urinary bladder. (**B** from Damjanov I, Linder J, editors: *Pathology: a color atlas,* St Louis, 2000, Mosby.)

CLINICAL MANIFESTATIONS   Prostatic cancer often causes no symptoms until it is far advanced. The first manifestations of disease are those of bladder outlet obstruction: slow urinary stream, hesitancy, incomplete emptying, frequency, nocturia, and dysuria. Unlike the symptoms of obstruction caused by BPH, the symptoms of obstruction caused by prostatic cancer are progressive and do not remit. Local extension of prostatic cancer can obstruct the upper urinary tract ureters as well. Rectal obstruction also may occur, causing the individual to experience large bowel obstruction or difficulty in defecation. Symptoms of late disease include bone pain at sites of bone metastasis, edema of the lower extremities, enlargement of lymph nodes, liver enlargement, pathologic bone fractures, and mental confusion associated with brain metastases. Prostatic cancer and its treatment can affect sexual functioning.

EVALUATION AND TREATMENT   Screening for prostatic cancer includes DRE and also PSA blood tests. However, evidence is lacking on whether PSA screening or DRE reduces the mortality from prostate cancer.[24] It is unclear if the detection of prostate cancer at an early stage leads to any change in the natural history or outcome. Observational studies in some countries show a trend toward lower mortality, but the relationship between the intensity and trends of screening is not clear, and the associations with screening are inconsistent. Strong evidence shows implementation of PSA or DRE detects some prostate cancers that would never have caused significant clinical problems. These screening tests lead to some degree of overtreatment. The screening tests can harm patients, including radical prostatectomy and radiation therapy that lead to irreversible side effects in many men. The most common side effects are erectile dysfunction and urinary incontinence. The screening process can cause considerable anxiety, especially in men who have a prostate biopsy but no identified prostate cancer. Screening can lead to biopsies, which are associated with complications, including fever, pain, hematuria, hematospermia, positive urine cultures for bacteria, and, rarely, sepsis. About 20% to 70% of men who had no problems before radical prostatectomy or external beam radiation therapy will have reduced sexual function or urinary problems, or both.

Prostate cancer usually grows very slowly and is predominantly a tumor of older men; the median age at diagnosis is 72 years.[25] Until recently, many physicians and organizations encouraged yearly PSA screening for men beginning at age 50; however, as the benefits and detriments have become more clearly understood, a number of organizations now caution men against routine population screening (Fig. 36.22).

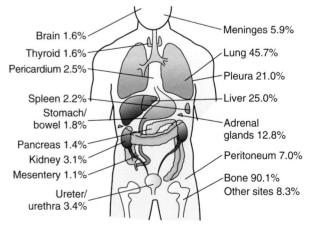

Brain 1.6%
Thyroid 1.6%
Pericardium 2.5%
Spleen 2.2%
Stomach/ bowel 1.8%
Pancreas 1.4%
Kidney 3.1%
Mesentery 1.1%
Ureter/ urethra 3.4%

Meninges 5.9%
Lung 45.7%
Pleura 21.0%
Liver 25.0%
Adrenal glands 12.8%
Peritoneum 7.0%
Bone 90.1%
Other sites 8.3%

FIGURE 36.21 Distribution of Hematogenous Metastases in Prostate Cancer. The results are from a study of 556 men with metastatic prostate cancer. (Adapted from Budendorf L et al: *Hum Pathol* 31:578, 2000.)

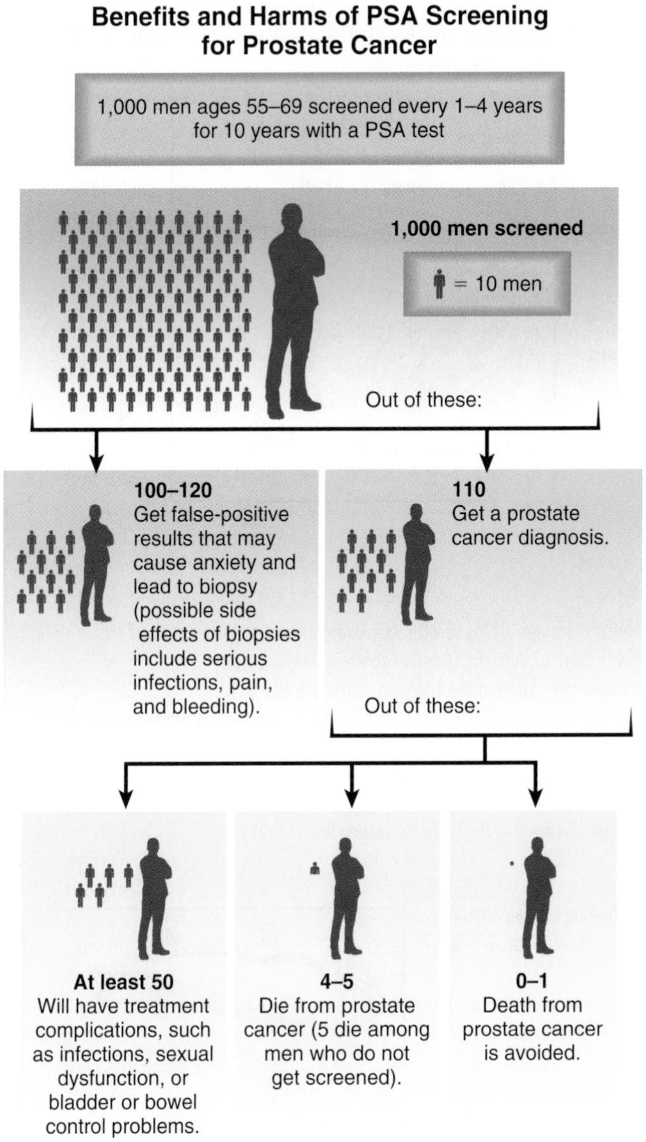

Benefits and Harms of PSA Screening for Prostate Cancer

1,000 men ages 55–69 screened every 1–4 years for 10 years with a PSA test

1,000 men screened

= 10 men

Out of these:

100–120
Get false-positive results that may cause anxiety and lead to biopsy (possible side effects of biopsies include serious infections, pain, and bleeding).

110
Get a prostate cancer diagnosis.

Out of these:

At least 50
Will have treatment complications, such as infections, sexual dysfunction, or bladder or bowel control problems.

4–5
Die from prostate cancer (5 die among men who do not get screened).

0–1
Death from prostate cancer is avoided.

FIGURE 36.22 Benefits and Harms of Prostate-Specific Antigen (PSA) Screening for Prostate Cancer. The U.S. Preventive Services Task Force (USPSTF) recommends against PSA-based screenings for prostate cancer (grade D recommendation). (Adapted from USPSTF Recommendation Statement, *Annals of Internal Medicine*, 2012.)

For men aged 55 to 69 years, the decision to undergo periodic PSA-based screening for prostate cancer should be an individual one and should include discussion of the potential benefits and harms of screening with their clinician. Screening offers a small potential benefit to reduce the chance of death from prostate cancer in some men.[19]

The sum of the current evidence suggests that PSA screening may reduce the prostate cancer mortality risk but is associated with false positive results, biopsy complications, and overdiagnosis. Compared with conservative approaches (e.g., watchful waiting), active treatments for screen-detected prostate cancer have unclear effects on long-term survival but are associated with sexual and urinary difficulties.[26] Supporting this evidence is the knowledge that some tumors found through PSA screening do not cause symptoms, grow slowly, and are unlikely to threaten a man's life.

Across age ranges, black men and men with a family history of prostate cancer have an increased risk of developing and dying of prostate

cancer. Black men are approximately twice as likely to die of prostate cancer compared with men of other races in the United States, and the reason for this disparity is unknown. Black men represent a very small minority of participants in randomized clinical trials of screening, and thus no firm conclusions can be made about the balance of benefits and harms of PSA-based screening in this population. As such, it is questionable practice to selectively recommend PSA-based screening for black men in the absence of data that support a more favorable balance of risks and benefits. Because of this "overtreatment" phenomenon, active surveillance with delayed intervention is gaining traction as a viable management approach in contemporary practice. Individuals and clinicians are increasingly considering the balance of benefits and harms of prostate cancer screening on the basis of family history, race/ethnicity, comorbid medical conditions, and other health needs. The current US Preventive Services Task Force (USPSTF) recommendation statement[19] has added an opinion that clinicians should not screen men who do not express a preference for screening, and it also recommends against PSA-based screening for prostate cancer in any man 70 years or older.

Treatment of prostatic cancer depends on the stage of the neoplasm, the anticipated effects of treatment, and the age, general health, and life expectancy of the individual. Options include no treatment; surgical treatments, such as total prostatectomy, transurethral resection of the prostate (TURP), or cryotherapy; nonsurgical treatments, such as radiation therapy, hormone therapy, or chemotherapy; watchful waiting; and any combination of these treatment modalities. In addition, new approaches are using immunotherapy. Palliative treatment is aimed at relieving urinary, bladder outlet, or colon obstruction; spinal cord compression; and pain. Box 36.7 shows the staging for prostate cancer. Prognosis and survival rates have improved steadily over the past 50 years. Over the past 25 years, the 5-year relative survival rate for all stages combined has increased from 68% to almost 100%. According to the most recent data, the 10-year relative survival rate is 98% for all stages combined (local, regional, and distant).[5]

Stress incontinence can occur after surgery and mild urge incontinence can occur after radiation therapy. Prostate cancer and its treatment can affect sexual functioning. The sensation of orgasm is not usually affected, but smaller amounts of ejaculate will be produced or men may experience a "dry" ejaculate because of retrograde ejaculation.

Sexual Dysfunction

In males, the normal sexual response involves erection, emission, and ejaculation. Sexual dysfunction is the impairment of any or all of these processes and can be caused by various physiologic, psychological, and emotional factors.

Until the late 1970s, most cases of male sexual dysfunction were considered psychogenic. Now there is evidence that 89% to 90% of cases involve organic factors and include (1) vascular, endocrine, and neurologic disorders; (2) chronic disease, including renal failure and diabetes; (3) penile diseases and penile trauma; and (4) iatrogenic factors, such as surgery and pharmacologic therapies. Most of these disorders cause erectile dysfunction (ED).

PATHOPHYSIOLOGY Sexual dysfunction can have a specific physiologic cause, can be associated with many chronic diseases and their treatment, or may be related to low energy levels, stress, or depression. For example, vascular disease may cause impotence, and endocrine disorders or conditions that cause decreased T levels or testicular atrophy can diminish sexual functioning or libido. In addition, neurologic disorders and spinal cord injuries can interfere with sympathetic, parasympathetic, and CNS mechanisms required for erection, emission, and ejaculation.

BOX 36.7 Staging for Prostate Cancer

Stage I

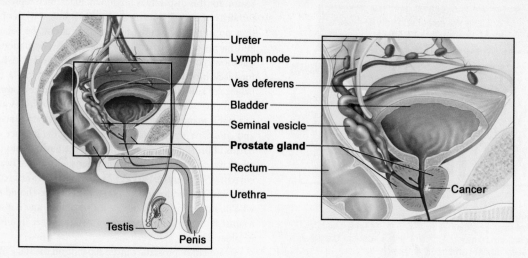

In stage I, cancer is found in the prostate only. In addition:

- The cancer is found by performing a needle biopsy (done for a high prostate-specific antigen [PSA] level) or by examining a small amount of tissue during surgery for other reasons (e.g., benign prostatic hyperplasia). The PSA level is lower than 10, and the Gleason score is 6 or lower; *or*
- The cancer is found on half or less of one lobe of the prostate. The PSA level is lower than 10, and the Gleason score is 6 or lower; *or*
- The cancer cannot be felt during a digital rectal exam and cannot be seen in imaging tests. Cancer is found in half or less of one lobe of the prostate. The PSA level and the Gleason score are not known.

Stage II

In stage II, cancer is more advanced than in stage I but has not spread outside the prostate. Stage II is divided into stages IIA and IIB.

Stage IIA

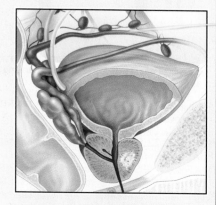

- The cancer is found by performing a needle biopsy (done for a high PSA level) or by examining a small amount of tissue during surgery for other reasons (e.g., benign prostatic hyperplasia). The PSA level is lower than 20, and the Gleason score is 7; *or*
- The cancer is found by performing a needle biopsy (done for a high PSA level) or by examining a small amount of tissue during surgery for other reasons (e.g., benign prostatic hyperplasia). The PSA level is at least 10 but lower than 20, and the Gleason score is 6 or lower; *or*
- The cancer is found in half or less of one lobe of the prostate. The PSA level is at least 10 but lower than 20, and the Gleason score is 6 or lower; *or*
- The cancer is found in half or less of one lobe of the prostate. The PSA level is lower than 20, and the Gleason score is 7; *or*
- The cancer is found in more than half of one lobe of the prostate.

Stage IIB

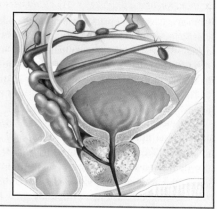

- The cancer is found on opposite sides of the prostate. The PSA can be any level, and the Gleason score can range from 2 to 10; *or*
- The cancer cannot be felt during a digital rectal examination and cannot be seen in imaging tests. The PSA level is 20 or higher, and the Gleason score can range from 2 to 10; *or*
- The cancer cannot be felt during a digital rectal examination and cannot be seen in imaging tests. The PSA can be any level, and the Gleason score is 8 or higher.

BOX 36.7 Staging for Prostate Cancer—cont'd

Stage III
- In stage III, the cancer has spread beyond the outer layer of the prostate and may have spread to the seminal vesicles. The PSA can be any level, and the Gleason score can range from 2 to 10.

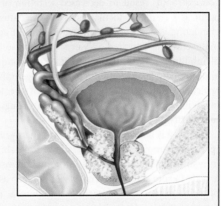

Stage IV
In stage IV, the PSA can be any level and the Gleason score can range from 2 to 10. Also:
- The cancer has spread beyond the seminal vesicles to nearby tissue or organs, such as the rectum, bladder, or pelvic wall; *or*
- The cancer may have spread to the seminal vesicles or to nearby tissue or organs, such as the rectum, bladder, or pelvic wall. The cancer has spread to nearby lymph nodes; *or*
- The cancer has spread to distant parts of the body, which may include lymph nodes or bones. Prostate cancer often spreads to the bones.

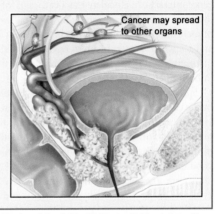

Cancer may spread to other organs

Data from National Cancer Institute: *PDQ prostate cancer treatment,* Bethesda, Md, 2015, Author. Updated April 16, 2015. Available at http://cancer.gov/cancertopics/pdq/treatment/prostate/Patient. Figures copyright Terese Winslow.

Drug-induced sexual dysfunction consists of decreased desire, decreased erectile ability, or decreased ejaculatory ability. Alcohol and other CNS depressants, antihypertensives, antidepressants, antihistamines, and hormonal preparations are commonly used drugs that affect sexual functioning. Other pharmacologic agents may diminish the quality or quantity of sperm or cause priapism.

CLINICAL MANIFESTATIONS, EVLAUATION, AND TREATMENT Evaluation of sexual dysfunction includes a thorough history and physical examination. Particular attention is given to the drug history and examination of the genitalia, prostate, and nervous system. Basic laboratory tests are used to identify the presence of endocrinopathies or other underlying disorders that can cause dysfunction. Psychological evaluation is indicated for younger men with a sudden onset of sexual dysfunction or for men of any age who can achieve but not maintain an erection. If no physiologic cause is found and the condition does not improve with psychotherapy, the man is referred for further investigation of organic causes.

Treatments for organic sexual dysfunction include both medical and surgical approaches. The advent of phosphodiesterase type 5 inhibitors (PDE5i) has revolutionized the ED treatment landscape and provided effective, minimally invasive therapies to restore male sexual function. The original PDE5i, Viagra (sildenafil), has created much enthusiasm over its ability to help a man maintain an erection. For a small percentage of men (1%), however, this improvement in sexual function is accompanied by heart attacks and death. Whether these effects are the result of sexual performance or Viagra has been controversial. Research has shown that Viagra increases blood concentrations of the enzyme cyclic guanosine monophosphate (cGMP)-dependent protein kinase G (PKG), which increases blood flow to the penis. PKG, however, plays a dual role: first, it increases platelet aggregation; and then, minutes later, it decreases clot size. The initial clot could cause some men with heart disease to experience cardiac arrest.

Currently available PDE5i medications in the United States include sildenafil, vardenafil, tadalafil, and avanafil, each of which has a unique side effects profile. For instance, sildenafil is associated with (in addition to the previously mentioned cardiac issues) an increased rate of visual changes, vardenafil with QT prolongation, and tadalafil with lower back pain. Nonsurgical approaches include correction of underlying disorders, particularly drug-induced dysfunction and endocrinopathy-related dysfunction (e.g., reduced T level associated with chronic renal failure). Use of vasodilators and cessation of smoking can benefit individuals with vasculogenic erectile dysfunction. Surgical approaches include penile implants, penile revascularization, and correction of other anatomic defects contributing to sexual dysfunction.

Impairment of Sperm Production and Quality

Spermatogenesis requires adequate secretion of follicle-stimulating hormone (FSH) and luteinizing hormone (LH) by the pituitary and sufficient secretion of T by the testes. Inadequate secretion of gonadotropins may be caused by numerous alterations (e.g., hypothyroidism, hyperadrenocortisolism, hyperprolactinemia, or hypogonadotropic hypogonadism). In the absence of adequate gonadotropin levels, the Leydig cells are not stimulated to secrete T, and sperm maturation is not promoted in the Sertoli cells. Spermatogenesis also depends on an appropriate response by the testes. Defects in testicular response to the gonadotropins result in decreased secretion of T and inhibin B and occur as a result of normal feedback mechanisms and high levels of circulating gonadotropins. In the absence of adequate T levels, spermatogenesis is impaired. Newer studies demonstrate the importance of inhibin B as a valuable marker of the competence of Sertoli cells and spermatogenesis. Impaired spermatogenesis also can be caused by testicular trauma, infection, atrophy of the testes, systemic illness involving high fever, ingestion of various drugs, exposure to environmental toxins, and cryptorchidism.

Fertility is adversely affected if spermatogenesis is normal but the sperm are chromosomally or morphologically abnormal or are produced in insufficient quantities. Chromosomal abnormalities are caused by genetic factors and by external variables, such as exposure to radiation or toxic substances. Because the Y chromosome plays a key role in testis determination and control of spermatogenesis, understanding how the genes interact can elucidate exact causes of infertility. Research related to mapping the critical genes and gene pathways is the current focus of male infertility. Common mechanisms may be involved in infertility and testicular cancer. In utero environmental exposure to endocrine disruptors modulates the genetic makeup of the gonad and may result in both infertility and testicular cancer.

Sperm motility also may affect fertility. Motility appears to be affected by the characteristics of the semen. Dysfunction of the prostate, excessive viscosity of the semen, presence of drugs or toxins in the semen, and presence of antisperm antibodies are associated with impaired sperm motility. However, new data show that motile density may not be a good indicator of infertility. Approximately 17% of infertile males have antisperm antibodies in their semen. These antibodies may be (1) cytotoxic antibodies, which attack sperm and reduce their number in the semen; or (2) sperm-immobilizing antibodies, which impair sperm motility and reduce their ability to traverse the endocervical canal.

Male infertility has a variety of causes, and many of the causes can be corrected. Hormonal disorders, such as thyroid disturbances or low T levels, can be diagnosed and corrected. During sperm creation and maturation, the testes must be kept cooler than body temperature. Temperature elevations caused by illness, abnormal testes placement, or exposure to high temperatures in hot tubs or saunas may kill or disable sperm. Male infertility is also linked to abnormalities of the seminal tract and sexual dysfunction that disrupts ejaculation.

The most common test for male infertility is semen analysis. A fresh semen sample is evaluated for volume and concentration, morphology, and motility of sperm. More advanced analysis may examine the function of the sperm, including ability to bind to and penetrate eggs. In addition, the sperm's DNA also may be analyzed for number and ability to merge with the egg's DNA.

Treatment for impaired spermatogenesis involves correcting any underlying disorders, avoiding radiation and possibly electromagnetic radiation (hypothesis from cell phones) and toxins, and using hormones to enhance spermatogenesis. In addition, semen can be modified to improve sperm motility; modifications are followed by artificial insemination.

✔ **QUICK CHECK 36.4**
1. What is the current understanding of hormones in the pathophysiology of prostate cancer?
2. Why is the worldwide variation of prostate cancer incidence important?
3. Describe what is meant by prostate cancer cell and stromal interactions for carcinogenesis.
4. What causes impaired spermatogenesis?

DISORDERS OF THE MALE BREAST

Gynecomastia

Gynecomastia is the overdevelopment of breast tissue in a male. Gynecomastia accounts for approximately 85% of all masses that develop in the male breast and affects 32% to 40% of the male population. If only one breast is involved, it is typically the left. The incidence is greatest among adolescents and men older than 50 years.

Gynecomastia results from hormonal alterations, which may be idiopathic or caused by systemic disorders, drugs, or neoplasms. Gynecomastia usually involves an imbalance of the estrogen/T ratio. The normal estrogen/T ratio can be altered in one of two ways. First, estrogen levels may be excessively high, although T levels are normal. This is the case in drug-induced and tumor-induced hyperestrogenism. Second, T levels may be extremely low, although estrogen levels are normal, as is the case in hypergonadism. Gynecomastia also can be caused by alterations in breast tissue responsiveness to hormonal stimulation. Breast tissue may have increased responsiveness to estrogen or decreased responsiveness to androgen. Alterations of responsiveness may cause many cases of idiopathic gynecomastia.

Besides puberty and aging, estrogen/T imbalances are associated with hypogonadism, Klinefelter syndrome, and testicular neoplasms. Hormone-induced gynecomastia is usually bilateral. Pubertal gynecomastia is a self-limiting phenomenon that usually disappears within 4 to 6 months. Senescent gynecomastia usually regresses spontaneously within 6 to 12 months.

Systemic disorders associated with gynecomastia include cirrhosis of the liver, infectious hepatitis, chronic renal failure, chronic obstructive lung disease, hyperthyroidism, tuberculosis, and chronic malnutrition. It may be that these disorders ultimately alter the estrogen/T ratio, initiating the gynecomastia.

Gynecomastia is often seen in males receiving estrogen therapy, either in preparation for a sex-change operation or in the treatment of prostatic carcinoma. Other drugs that can cause gynecomastia include digitalis, cimetidine, spironolactone, reserpine, thiazide, isoniazid, ergotamine, tricyclic antidepressants, amphetamines, vincristine, and busulfan. Gynecomastia is usually unilateral in these instances.

Malignancies of the testes, adrenals, or liver can cause gynecomastia if they alter the estrogen/testosterone ratio. Pituitary adenomas and lung cancer also are associated with gynecomastia.

PATHOPHYSIOLOGY   The enlargement of the breast consists of hyperplastic stroma and ductal tissue. Hyperplasia results in a firm, palpable mass that is at least 2 cm in diameter and located beneath the areola.

EVALUATION AND TREATMENT   The diagnosis of gynecomastia is based on physical examination. Identification and treatment of the cause are likely to be followed by resolution of the gynecomastia. The man should be taught to perform breast self-examination and is reexamined at 6- and 12-month intervals if the gynecomastia persists.

Carcinoma

Male breast cancer (MBC) accounts for 0.26% of all male cancers and 1.1% of all breast cancers. About 2550 new cases of breast cancer in men were estimated in 2018.[5] Global incidence rates were generally less than 1 per 100,000 man-years, in contrast to much higher rates in females.[27] It is seen most commonly after the age of 60 years, with the peak incidence between 60 and 69 years (men tend to be diagnosed at an older age than women). However, it has been reported in males as young as 6 years old and in adolescents. Klinefelter syndrome is the strongest risk factor for developing male breast carcinoma. Other risk factors include germline mutation in *BRCA1* or *BRCA2,* but familial cases usually have *BRCA2* rather than *BRCA1* mutations.[28] Obesity increases the risk of MBC. Testicular disorders, including cryptorchidism, mumps, orchitis, and orchiectomy, are related to risk. The relationship between these factors and the risk of disease is not clearly defined.

Recent data on the most frequent molecular subtypes of MBC appears to be different from those for female breast cancers. Luminal A and luminal B are most common; and basal-like, unclassifiable triple-negative, and *HER2*-driven male breast cancers are rare.[28] Male breast tumors often resemble carcinoma of the breast in women (see Breast Cancer in Chapter 35). The majority of MBCs express estrogen and progesterone receptors. The malignant male breast lesion is usually a unilateral solid mass located near the nipple. Because the nipple is commonly involved, crusting and nipple discharge are typical clinical manifestations. Other findings include skin retraction, ulceration of the skin over the tumor, and axillary node involvement. Patterns of metastasis are similar to those in females.

The diagnosis of cancer is confirmed by biopsy. Because of delays in seeking treatment, MBC tends to be advanced at the time of diagnosis and therefore is likely to have a poor prognosis. Treatment protocols are similar to those for female breast cancer, but endocrine therapy is used more often for males because a higher percentage of male tumors are hormone dependent. The mainstay of treatment is modified mastectomy with axillary node dissection to assess the stage and prognosis. Because 90% of tumors are hormonal receptor positive, tamoxifen is standard adjuvant therapy. Orchiectomy is performed to treat metastatic disease. For metastatic disease, hormonal therapy is the main treatment but chemotherapy also can provide palliation.

SEXUALLY TRANSMITTED INFECTIONS

Sexually transmitted infections (STIs) are a variety of clinical syndromes and infections caused by pathogens that can be acquired and transmitted through sexual activity. Sexually contracted infections affected approximately 2.5 million Americans in 2017.[29] Young women ages 15 to 24 account for about one half of the reported cases in the United States, and they face the most severe consequences of an undiagnosed infection[29] (Table 36.1). STIs can lead to severe reproductive health problems (e.g., infertility and ectopic pregnancy). Untreated or undertreated chlamydial infections are the primary cause of preventable infertility and ectopic pregnancy. In addition to ectopic pregnancy and infertility, other complications of STIs include pelvic inflammatory disease (PID), chronic pelvic pain, neonatal morbidity and mortality, genital cancer, and epidemiologic synergy with HIV transmission (Table 36.2). Long-term sequelae of untreated or undertreated STIs may be disastrous and can affect a person's physical, emotional, and financial well-being. Treatment guidelines for STIs can be found on the CDC website (http://www.cdc.gov/std/treatment/default.htm).

Anyone can become infected with an STI, but young people and gay and bisexual men are at greatest risk. Young people between the ages of 15 to 24 years continue to have the highest reported rates of chlamydia and gonorrhea compared with other groups. Both young men and women are heavily affected by STIs, but young women have the most serious long-term health consequences. Undiagnosed STIs cause 20,000 women to become infertile each year.[29] Men who have sex with men (MSM) account for about 75% of all primary and secondary

TABLE 36.1 Currently Recognized Sexually Transmitted Infections

Causal Microorganism	Infection
Bacteria	
Campylobacter	*Campylobacter enteritis*
Calymmatobacterium granulomatis	*Granuloma inguinale*
Chlamydia trachomatis	Urogenital infections; lymphogranuloma venereum
Polymicrobial	
Gardnerella vaginalis interaction with anaerobes (*Bacteroides* and *Mobiluncus spp.*) and genital mycoplasmas	Bacterial vaginosis
Haemophilus ducreyi	Chancroid
Mycoplasma	Mycoplasmosis
Neisseria gonorrhoeae	Gonorrhea
Shigella	Shigellosis
Treponema pallidum	Syphilis
Viruses	
Cytomegalovirus	Cytomegalic inclusion disease
Hepatitis B virus (HBV)	Hepatitis
Hepatitis C virus (HCV)	Hepatitis
Herpes simplex virus (HSV)	Genital herpes
Human immunodeficiency virus (HIV)	Acquired immunodeficiency syndrome (AIDS)
Human papillomavirus (HPV)	Condylomata acuminata, cervical dysplasia, and cervical cancer
Molluscum contagiosum virus	Molluscum contagiosum
Zika virus	Zika virus disease
Protozoa	
Entamoeba histolytica	Amebiasis; amebic dysentery
Giardia lamblia	Giardiasis
Trichomonas vaginalis	Trichomoniasis
Ectoparasites	
Phthirus pubis	Pediculosis pubis
Sarcoptes scabiei	Scabies
Fungus	
Candida albicans	Candidiasis

syphilis cases. Primary and secondary syphilis are the most infectious stages of the disease and, if not treated adequately, can lead to visual impairment and stroke. Syphilis infection raises the risk of acquiring and transmitting HIV infection. Half of MSM with syphilis also are infected with HIV.

Individual risk behaviors, such as higher numbers of lifetime sex partners and environmental, social, and cultural factors, contribute to health disparities of MSM (e.g., difficulty accessing health care). Homophobia and stigma also can make it difficult for gay and bisexual men to find culturally sensitive and appropriate care and treatment. STIs screening is critical. It is recommended that women who are sexually active and younger than 25 years of age or have multiple sex partners

TABLE 36.2   Photographs of STIs and Their Precursors

Bacterial Sources
Gonococcal Infections

Symptomatic gonococcal urethritis[a]

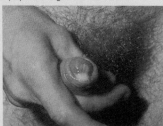

Endocervical gonorrhea[a]

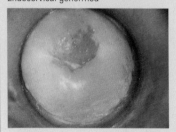

Skin lesions of disseminated gonococcal infection[a]

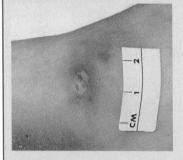

Bacterial Vaginosis
Vaginal examination showing mild bacterial vaginosis[a]

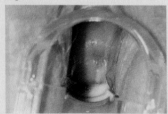

Syphilis
Erythematous penile plaques of secondary syphilis[b]

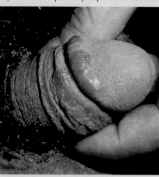

Multiple primary syphilitic chancres of the labia and perineum

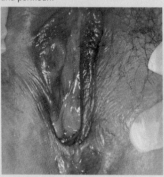

(Courtesy Barbara Romanowski, MD.)[a]
Papular secondary syphilis[a]

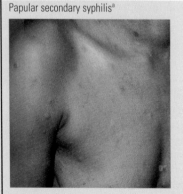

Lymphogranuloma
"Groove sign" in man with lymphogranuloma venereum (LV)[b]

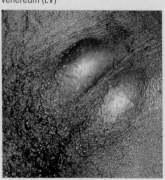

Chlamydial Infections
Beefy red mucosa in chlamydial infection[a]

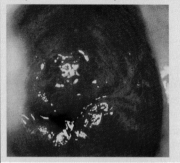

Chlamydial epididymitis

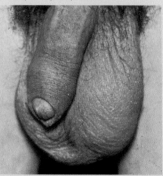

(Courtesy Richard E. Berger.)[a]
Chlamydial ophthalmia: erythematous conjunctiva in an infant[a]

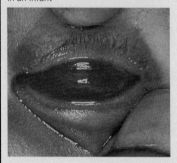

TABLE 36.2   Photographs of STIs and Their Precursors—cont'd

Viral Sources
Genital Herpes

Early lesions of primary genital herpes[a]

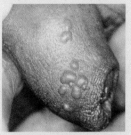

Primary vulvar herpes

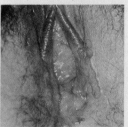

(Courtesy Barbara Romanowski, MD.)[a]

Generalized herpes simplex in patient with atopic dermatitis.

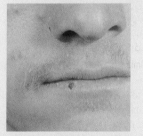

(Courtesy David Mandeville and Peter Lane, MD.)[a]

Human papillomavirus (HPV)

Human papillomavirus (HPV) infection of the cervix[b]

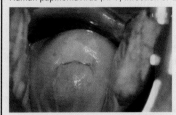

Exophytic (outward-growing) condyloma, subclinical human papillomavirus (HPV) infection, and high-grade cervical intraepithelial neoplasia (CIN)[b]

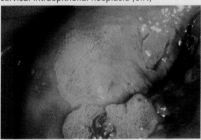

Subclinical HPV infection
Cervical os
Cervical intraepithelial neoplasia
Exophytic condyloma

Condylomata Acuminata

Condylomata acuminata: vulvar and perineal[a]

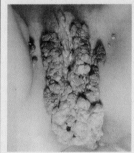

Condylomata acuminata: perianal[a]

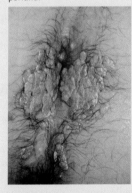

Condylomata acuminata: penile[a]

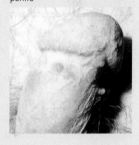

Parasite Sources
Trichomonisasis

"Strawberry cervix" seen with trichomoniasis[a]

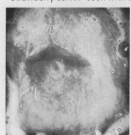

Scabies

Nodular lesions of scabies on male genitalia[b]

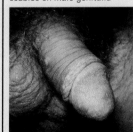

Scabies of the palm with secondary pyoderma in an infant[a]

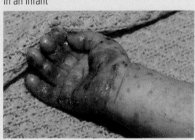

Pediculosis pubis (Phthirus pubis [crab louse])

Phthirus pubis feeding on its host[a]

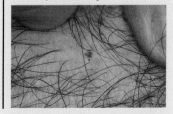

Pubic hair with multiple nits[a]

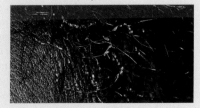

[a]From Morse SA, Ballard RC, Holmes KK, et al: *Atlas of sexually transmitted diseases and AIDS,* ed 4, London, 2010, Elsevier.
[b]From Morse SA, Moreland AA, Holmes KK: *Atlas of sexually transmitted diseases and AIDS,* ed 2, London, 1996, Elsevier.

be tested annually for chlamydia and gonorrhea. Pregnant women should request syphilis, HIV, chlamydia, and hepatitis B testing early in the pregnancy. These tests also should be requested if a woman has a new or multiple sex partners. Recommended tests include syphilis, chlamydia, gonorrhea, and HIV once a year for gay, bisexual, or other men who have sex with men. More frequent testing is recommended for men at high risk.

✔ **QUICK CHECK 36.5**

1. What is the cause of male gynecomastia?
2. What are the risk factors for male breast cancer?
3. What factors increase the incidence of STIs?
4. What are the serious long-term health consequences of STIs for young women?
5. What are the long-term health consequences for MSM who acquire syphilis?

SUMMARY REVIEW

Alterations of Sexual Maturation

1. Sexual maturation, or puberty, is marked by the development of secondary sex characteristics, rapid growth and ultimately, the ability to reproduce. Puberty begins later in boys than in girls, typically around 14 to 14.5 years.
2. Delayed puberty in boys is the onset of sexual maturation after 14 to 14.5 years and seldom requires treatment. Precocious puberty is the onset before these ages, and treatment depends on the cause.

Disorders of the Male Reproductive System

1. Disorders of the urethra include urethritis (infection of the urethra) and urethral strictures (narrowing or obstruction of the urethral lumen caused by scarring).
2. Most cases of urethritis result from sexually transmitted pathogens. Urologic instrumentation, foreign body insertion, trauma, or an anatomic abnormality can cause urethral inflammation with or without infection.
3. Urethritis causes urinary symptoms, including a burning sensation during urination (dysuria), frequency, urgency, urethral tingling or itching, and a clear or purulent discharge.
4. The scarring that causes urethral stricture can be attributed to trauma or severe untreated urethritis.
5. Manifestations of urethral stricture include those of bladder outlet obstruction: urinary frequency and hesitancy, mild dysuria, double urinary stream or spraying, and dribbling after voiding.
6. Phimosis and paraphimosis are penile disorders involving the foreskin (prepuce). In phimosis, the foreskin cannot be retracted over the glans. In paraphimosis, the foreskin is retracted and cannot be reduced (returned to its normal anatomic position over the glans). Phimosis is caused by poor hygiene and chronic infection and can lead to paraphimosis. Paraphimosis can constrict the penile blood vessels, preventing circulation to the glans.
7. Peyronie disease consists of fibrosis affecting the corpora cavernosa, which prevents engorgement on the affected side, causing a lateral curvature during erection. Peyronie disease can cause painful erection, painful intercourse for both partners, and poor erection distal to the involved area.
8. Priapism is a prolonged, painful erection that is not stimulated by sexual arousal. Priapism is idiopathic in the majority of cases but can be associated with spinal cord trauma, sickle cell disease, leukemia, pelvic tumors, infections, or penile trauma.
9. Balanitis is an inflammation of the glans penis, and it usually occurs in conjunction with posthitis, an inflammation of the prepuce. It is associated with phimosis, inadequate cleansing under the foreskin, skin disorders, and pathogens (e.g., *Candida albicans*).
10. Cancer of the penis is rare. Condyloma acuminatum is a benign tumor caused by HPV. Penile carcinoma in situ tends to involve the glans; invasive carcinoma of the penis involves the shaft as well.
11. Varicocele, hydrocele, and spermatocele are common disorders of the scrotum.

12. A varicocele is an abnormal dilation of the veins within the spermatic cord and is classically described as a "bag of worms." Varicoceles are one of the most commonly identified scrotal abnormalities and abnormal findings among infertile men.
13. A hydrocele is a collection of fluid between the testicular and scrotal layers of the tunica vaginalis. Hydroceles can be idiopathic or can be caused by trauma or infection of the testes.
14. A spermatocele is a cyst located between the testis and epididymis that is filled with fluid and sperm.
15. Cryptorchidism is a congenital condition in which one or both testes fail to descend into the scrotum completely, whereas an ectopic testis has strayed from the normal pathway of descent. Uncorrected cryptorchidism is associated with infertility and a significantly increased risk of testicular cancer.
16. Torsion of the testis is the rotation of a testis, which twists blood vessels in the spermatic cord. This interrupts the blood supply to the testis, resulting in edema and ischemia. Torsion of the testis is a surgical emergency and must be corrected within 6 hours to preserve normal testicular function.
17. Orchitis is an acute infection of the testes. Complications of orchitis include hydrocele and abscess formation.
18. Testicular cancer is uncommon but most often affects males 15 to 35 years of age. Although its cause is unknown, risk factors include genetic predisposition, history of cryptorchidism, abnormal testicular development, HIV and AIDS, Klinefelter syndrome, and a history of testicular cancer.
19. Epididymitis, an inflammation of the epididymis, is usually caused by a sexually transmitted pathogen that ascends through the vasa deferentia from an already infected urethra or bladder.
20. BPH, also called *benign prostatic hypertrophy*, is the enlargement of the prostate gland. This condition becomes symptomatic as the enlarging prostate compresses the urethra, causing symptoms of bladder outlet obstruction and urine retention.
21. Prostatitis is inflammation of the prostate. Prostatitis syndromes have been classified by the National Institutes of Health as (1) acute bacterial prostatitis (ABP), (2) chronic bacterial prostatitis (CBP), (3) chronic pelvic pain syndrome (CPPS), and (4) asymptomatic inflammatory prostatitis.
22. Prostate cancer is the most commonly diagnosed, non–skin cancer in American males, and the incidence varies greatly worldwide. Possible risk factors include genetic and epigenetic factors, environmental and dietary factors, inflammation, vasectomy, and alterations in levels of hormones (testosterone, dihydrotestosterone, and estradiol) and growth factors. Incidence is greatest in developed countries because of wide use or overuse of screening, which can amplify the incidence.
23. Most cancers of the prostate are adenocarcinomas that develop at the periphery of the gland.
24. Sexual dysfunction in males can be caused by any physical or psychological factor that impairs erection, emission, or ejaculation.

25. Spermatogenesis (sperm production by the testes) can be impaired by disruptions that reduce testosterone secretion and by testicular trauma, infection, atrophy from any cause, systemic illness involving high fever, ingestion of various drugs, exposure to environmental toxins, and cryptorchidism.

Disorders of the Male Breast

1. Gynecomastia is the overdevelopment (hyperplasia) of breast tissue in a male; it affects 32% to 40% of the male population. The incidence is greatest among adolescents and men older than 50 years of age. It is first seen as a firm, palpable mass at least 2 cm in diameter and is located in the subareolar area.

2. Gynecomastia is caused by hormonal or breast tissue alterations that cause estrogen to dominate. These alterations can result from systemic disorders, drugs, neoplasms, or idiopathic causes.

3. Breast cancer is relatively uncommon in males, but it has a poor prognosis because men tend to delay seeking treatment until the disease is advanced. The incidence is greatest in men in their sixties.

Sexually Transmitted Infections

1. STIs are contracted by intimate, as well as sexual, contact. STIs can lead to severe reproductive health problems, such as infertility, ectopic pregnancy, chronic pelvic pain, neonatal morbidity and mortality, and genital cancer. They include systemic infections, such as tuberculosis and hepatitis, which can spread to a sexual partner.

2. The etiology of an STI may be bacterial, viral, protozoan, parasitic, or fungal.

KEY TERMS

Acute bacterial prostatitis (ABP, category I), 840
Androgen receptor (AR) signaling, 846
Balanitis, 833
Benign prostatic hyperplasia (BPH, benign prostatic hypertrophy), 838, 838
Bladder outflow obstruction, 839
Chemical epididymitis, 838
Chronic bacterial prostatitis (CBP, category II), 840

Chronic prostatitis/chronic pelvic pain syndrome (CP/CPPS, category III), 841
Complete precocious puberty, 831
Condyloma acuminatum, 833
Cryptorchidism, 835
Delayed puberty, 830
Ectopic testis, 835
Epididymitis, 838
Fibroblast, 847
Gynecomastia, 852
Hydrocele, 835

Intraprostatic conversion, 842
Nonbacterial prostatitis, 841
Orchitis, 836
Paraphimosis, 832
Peyronie disease ("bent nail syndrome"), 832
Phimosis, 831
Precocious puberty, 830
Priapism, 833
Prostatic epithelial neoplasia (PIN), 847
Prostatitis, 840
Sexual dysfunction, 849

Sexually transmitted infection (STI), 853
Spermatocele (epididymal cyst), 835
Stroma, 847
Testicular appendage, 836
Torsion of the testis, 836
Urethral stricture, 831
Urethritis, 831
Varicocele, 834

REFERENCES

1. Jospe N: Disorders of pubertal development. In Osborn LM, et al, editors: *Pediatrics*, Philadelphia, 2005, Mosby.
2. Whittemore BJ, et al: Endocrine and metabolic disorders. In Burns CE, et al, editors: *Pediatric primary care*, St Louis, 2012, Saunders.
3. Euling SY, et al: Examination of US puberty-timing data from 1940 to 1994 for secular trends: panel findings, *Pediatrics* 12(Suppl 3):S172-S191, 2008.
4. Centers for Disease Control and Prevention (CDC): *How many cancers are linked with HPV each year?*, Atlanta, 2014, Author.
5. American Cancer Society (ACS): *Cancer facts & figures 2019*, Atlanta, 2019, Author.
6. Chen SS: Differences in the clinical characteristics between young and elderly men with varicocele, *Int J Androl* 35(5):695-699, 2012.
7. Hart RJ, et al: Testicular function in a birth cohort of young men, *Hum Reprod* 30(12):2713-2724, 2015.
8. Günther P, Rübben I: The acute scrotum in childhood and adolescence, *Dtsch Arztebl Int* 109(25):449-457, 2012.
9. Jensen MS, et al: Cryptorchidism and hypospadias in a cohort of 934,538 Danish boys: the role of birth weight, gestational age, body dimensions, and fetal growth, *Am J Epidemiol* 175(9):917-925, 2012.
10. John Radcliffe Hospital Cryptorchidism Study Group: Cryptorchidism: a prospective study of 7500 consecutive male births, 1984–8, *Arch Dis Child* 67:892-899, 1992.
11. Walsh TJ, Smith JF: Male infertility. In McAninch JW, Lue TF, editors: *Smith and Tanagho's general urology*, ed 18, Norwalk, Conn, 2012, McGraw Hill Lange.

12. National Cancer Institute (NCI): Testicular cancer incidence and mortality, 2014. Available at www.cancer.gov/cancertopics/pdq/treatment/testicular.
13. Cheng L, et al: Testicular cancer, *Nat Rev Dis Primers* 4(1):29, 2018.
14. PDQ Adult Treatment Editorial Board: *PDQ® testicular cancer treatment*, Bethesda, MD, 2019, National Cancer Institute. Available at: https://www.cancer.gov/types/testicular/patient/testicular-treatment-pdq. (Accessed 5 July 2019). PMID: 26389286. Updated <04/09/2019>.
15. Lim KB: Epidemiology of clinical benign prostatic hyperplasia, *Asian J Urol* 4(3):148-151, 2017.
16. Pearson R, Williams PM: Common questions about the diagnosis and management of benign prostatic hyperplasia, *Am Fam Physician* 90(11):769-774, 2014.
17. Jiwrajka M, et al: Review and update of benign prostatic hyperplasia in general practice, *Aust J Gen Pract* 47:471-475, 2018.
18. Kapoor A: Benign prostatic hyperplasia (BPH) management in the primary care setting, *Can J Urol* 19(5 Suppl 1):10-17, 2012.
19. U. S. Preventive Services Task Force (US PSTF): Screening for prostate cancer: U. S. Preventive Services Task Force recommendation statement, *J Am Med Assoc* 319:1901-1913, 2018.
20. Bray F, et al: Global cancer statistics 2018: GLOBOCAN estimates of incidence and mortality worldwide for 36 cancers in 185 countries, *CA Cancer J Clin* 68:394-424, 2018.
21. Ferlay J, et al: Cancer incidence and mortality worldwide: sources, methods and major patterns in GLOBOCAN 2012, *Int J Cancer* 136(5):E359-E386, 2015.

22. Albright F, et al: Significant evidence for a heritable contribution to cancer predisposition: a review of cancer familiality by site, *BMC Cancer* 12:138, 2012.
23. Leongamornlert D, et al: Germline BRCA1 mutations increase prostate cancer risk, *Br J Cancer* 106(10):1697-1701, 2012.
24. PDQ Screening and Prevention Editorial Board: *PDQ® prostate cancer screening*, Bethesda, Md, 2019, National Cancer Institute. Available at: https://www.cancer.gov/types/prostate/hp/prostate-screening-pdq. (Accessed 6 July 2019). Updated <03/22/2019>.
25. National Cancer Institute (NCI): *PDQ® prostate cancer treatment*, Bethesda, Md, 2015, Author. Available at: www.cancer.gov/types/prostate/hp/prostate-treatment-pdq. (Accessed 20 May 2015). Date last modified April 2, 2015.
26. Fenton JJ, et al: Prostate-specific antigen-based screening for prostate cancer: evidence report and systematic review for the US Preventive Services Task Force, *J Am Med Assoc* 319:1914-1931, 2018.
27. Ferzoco RM, Ruddy KJL: The epidemiology of male breast cancer, *Curr Oncol Rep* 18(1):1, 2016.
28. Deb S, et al: The cancer genetics and pathology of male breast cancer, *Histopathology* 68(1):110-118, 2016.
29. Centers for Disease Control and Prevention (CDC): *Fact sheet reported STDs in the United States 2017 national data for chlamydia, gonorrhea, and syphilis*, Atlanta, Ga, 2017, Author.

37

Structure and Function of the Digestive System

Sue E. Huether

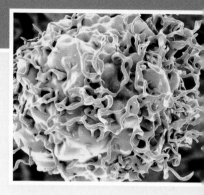

The digestive system includes the gastrointestinal (GI) tract and accessory organs of digestion: the liver, gallbladder, and exocrine pancreas (Fig. 37.1). The digestive system breaks down ingested food, prepares it for uptake by the body's cells, absorbs fluid, and eliminates wastes. The GI tract and gut microbiome also provide important immune and protective functions. Except for chewing, swallowing, and defecation of solid wastes, the movements of the digestive system (peristalsis) are all controlled by hormones and the autonomic nervous system.

Food breakdown begins in the mouth with chewing and continues in the stomach, where food is churned and mixed with acid, mucus, and enzymes. From the stomach, the fluid and partially digested food pass into the small intestine, where bile and enzymes secreted by the intestinal cells, liver, gallbladder, and exocrine pancreas break it down into absorbable components of proteins, carbohydrates, and fats. These nutrients pass through the walls of the small intestine into blood and lymphatic vessels, which carry them to the liver for storage or further processing. Ingested substances and secretions not absorbed in the small intestine pass into the large intestine, where fluid continues to be absorbed. Fluid wastes travel to the kidneys and are eliminated in the urine. Solid wastes pass into the rectum and are eliminated from the body through the anus. Aging can alter the structure and function of the gastrointestinal tract (see *Geriatric Considerations:* Aging & the Digestive System).

THE GASTROINTESTINAL TRACT

The gastrointestinal tract (alimentary canal) is a single, hollow tube that consists of the mouth, esophagus, stomach, small intestine, large intestine, rectum, and anus (see Fig. 37.1). It carries out these digestive processes:

1. Ingestion of food
2. Propulsion of food and wastes from the mouth to the anus
3. Secretion of mucus, water, and enzymes
4. Mechanical digestion of food particles
5. Chemical digestion of food particles
6. Absorption of digested food
7. Elimination of waste products by defecation
8. Immune and microbial protection against infection

Histologically, the GI tract consists of four layers. From the inside out they are the mucosa, submucosa, muscularis, and serosa or adventitia (Fig. 37.2). These concentric layers vary in thickness, and each layer has sublayers. A network of intrinsic nerves that controls mobility, secretion, sensation, and blood flow is located solely within the GI tract and controlled by local and autonomic nervous system stimuli through the enteric (intramural) plexus located in different layers of the gastrointestinal walls (see Fig. 37.2).

Mouth and Esophagus

The mouth is the site for mastication (chewing) and mixing of food with saliva. There are 32 permanent teeth in the adult mouth, and they are important for speech and mastication. As food particles become smaller and move around in the mouth, taste buds are continuously stimulated, adding to the satisfaction of eating. The tongue's surface and soft palate have thousands of taste buds that contain taste receptors. These can distinguish salty, sour, bitter, sweet, and savory (umami) tastes. Tastes and food odors, which stimulate the olfactory nerve, help to initiate salivation and the secretion of gastric juice in the stomach.

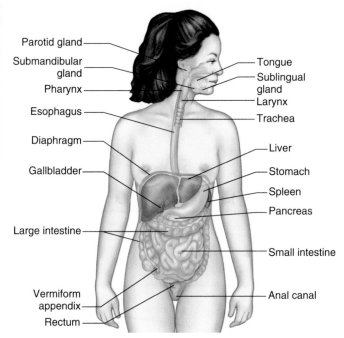

FIGURE 37.1 Structures of the Digestive System. (From Patton KT, Thibodeau GA: *The human body in health & disease,* ed 7, St Louis, 2018, Elsevier.)

Salivation

The three pairs of salivary glands—the submandibular, sublingual, and parotid glands (Fig. 37.3)—secrete about 1 L of saliva per day. Saliva consists mostly of water with mucus, sodium, bicarbonate, chloride, potassium, and salivary α-amylase (ptyalin), an enzyme that initiates carbohydrate digestion in the mouth and stomach.

The composition of saliva and other gastric juices depends on the rate of secretion (Fig. 37.4, *A*). Aldosterone can increase the epithelial exchange of sodium for potassium, increasing sodium conservation and potassium excretion. The bicarbonate concentration of saliva sustains a pH of about 7.4, which neutralizes bacterial acids and prevents tooth decay. Saliva also contains mucin, immunoglobulin A (IgA), and other antimicrobial substances, which help prevent infection. Mucin provides lubrication. Exogenous fluoride (e.g., fluoride in drinking water) is also secreted in the saliva, providing additional protection against tooth decay.

Both the sympathetic and parasympathetic divisions of the autonomic nervous system control salivation. Cholinergic parasympathetic fibers stimulate the salivary glands, and atropine (an anticholinergic agent) inhibits salivation and makes the mouth dry. β-Adrenergic stimulation from sympathetic fibers also increases salivary secretion. Salivary gland secretion is not regulated by hormones.

Swallowing

The esophagus is a hollow, muscular tube approximately 25 cm long that conducts substances from the oropharynx to the stomach (see Fig. 37.1). Swallowed food is moved to the stomach by peristalsis, the

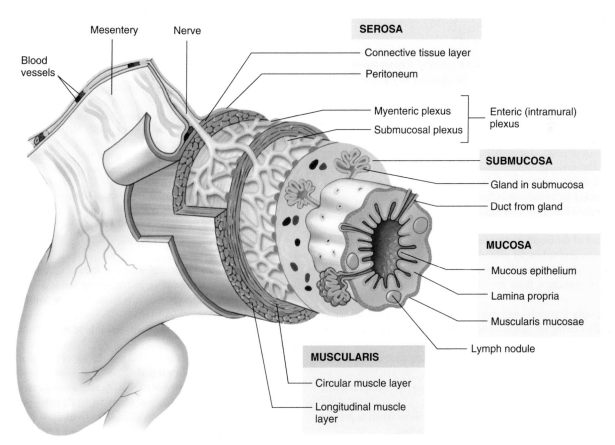

FIGURE 37.2 Wall of the Gastrointestinal Tract. The wall of the gastrointestinal tract is made up of four layers with a network of nerves between the layers. This generalized diagram shows a segment of the gastrointestinal tract. Note that the serosa is continuous with a fold of serous membrane called the *mesentery.* Note also that digestive glands may empty their products into the lumen of the gastrointestinal tract by way of ducts. (From Patton KT: *Anatomy & physiology,* ed 10, St Louis, 2019, Elsevier.)

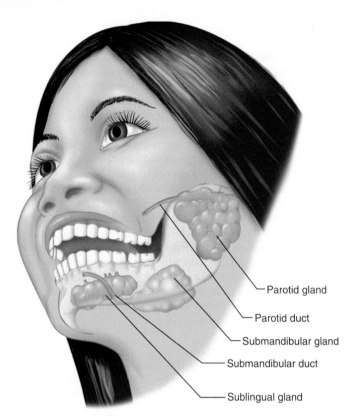

FIGURE 37.3 Salivary Glands. (From Patton KT, Thibodeau GA: *The human body in health & disease*, ed 7, St Louis, 2018, Elsevier.)

Parotid gland

Parotid duct

Submandibular gland

Submandibular duct

Sublingual gland

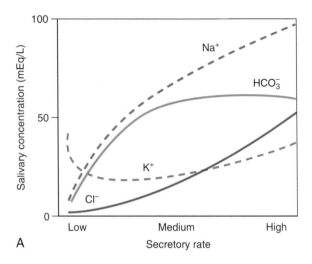

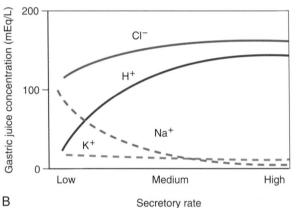

FIGURE 37.4 Electrolyte Concentrations and Flow Rate. A, Saliva. Changes in the concentrations of sodium (Na^+), potassium (K^+), chloride (Cl^-), and bicarbonate (HCO_3^-) increase the flow rate of saliva. At low rates of salivary flow (e.g., between meals), Na^+, Cl^-, and HCO_3^- are reabsorbed in the collecting ducts of the salivary glands and the saliva contains fewer of these electrolytes (i.e., is more hypotonic). At higher flow rates (e.g., when stimulated by food), reabsorption decreases and saliva is hypertonic. By this mechanism, Na^+, Cl^-, and HCO_3^- are recycled until they are released to help with digestion and absorption. **B,** Gastric juice. The Na^+ concentration is lower in the gastric juice than in the plasma, whereas the hydrogen (H^+), potassium (K^+), and Cl^- concentrations are higher.

coordinated, sequential contraction and relaxation of outer longitudinal and inner circular layers of muscles. The pharynx and upper third of the esophagus contain striated muscle (voluntary) that is directly innervated by skeletal motor neurons that control swallowing. The lower two thirds contain smooth muscle (involuntary) that is innervated by preganglionic cholinergic fibers from the vagus nerve. The fibers are activated in a downward sequence and coordinated by the swallowing center in the medulla. Peristalsis is stimulated when afferent fibers distributed along the length of the esophagus sense changes in wall tension caused by stretching as food passes. The greater the tension, the greater the intensity of esophageal contraction. Occasionally, intense contractions cause pain similar to "heartburn" or angina.

Each end of the esophagus is opened and closed by a sphincter. The **upper esophageal sphincter** prevents air from entering the esophagus during respiration. The **lower esophageal sphincter (cardiac sphincter)** prevents regurgitation from the stomach and caustic injury to the esophagus.

Swallowing is coordinated primarily by the swallowing center in the medulla. During the **oropharyngeal (voluntary) phase**, which takes place in less than 1 second, the following steps occur:

1. Food is segmented into a bolus by the tongue and forced posteriorly toward the pharynx.
2. The superior constrictor muscle of the pharynx contracts so the food cannot move into the nasopharynx.
3. Respiration is inhibited, and the epiglottis slides down to prevent the food from entering the larynx and trachea.

The **esophageal (involuntary) phase** takes 5 to 10 seconds and proceeds as follows:

1. The bolus of food enters the esophagus.
2. Waves of relaxation travel the esophagus, preparing for the movement of the bolus.

3. Peristalsis, the sequential waves of muscular contractions that travel down the esophagus, transports the food to the lower esophageal sphincter, which is relaxed at that point. The bolus moves at 2 to 6 cm/sec.
4. The bolus enters the stomach, and the sphincter muscles return to their resting tone.

Peristalsis that immediately follows the oropharyngeal phase of swallowing is called **primary peristalsis**. If a bolus of food becomes stuck in the esophageal lumen, **secondary peristalsis**—a wave of contraction and relaxation independent of voluntary swallowing—occurs. This is in response to stretch receptors stimulated by increased wall tension, which activate impulses from the swallowing center of the brain.

The muscle tone of the lower esophageal sphincter changes with neural and hormonal stimulation and relaxes with swallowing. Cholinergic vagal input and the digestive hormone gastrin increase sphincter tone. Nonadrenergic, noncholinergic vagal impulses relax the lower esophageal sphincter, as do the hormones progesterone, secretin, and glucagon.[1]

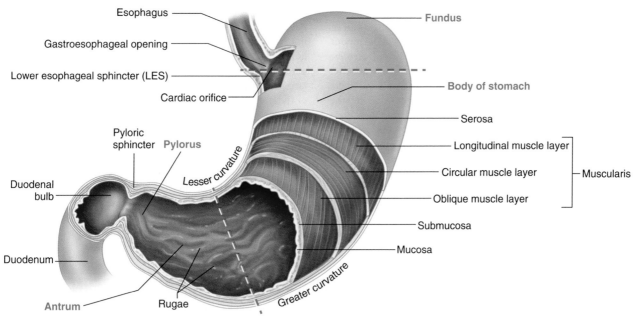

FIGURE 37.5 The Stomach. A portion of the anterior wall has been excised to reveal the muscle layers of the stomach wall. Note that the mucosa lining the stomach forms folds called *rugae*. The dashed lines distinguish the fundus, body, and antrum of the stomach. (Modified from Patton KT, Thibodeau GA: *The human body in health & disease,* ed 7, St Louis, 2018, Elsevier.)

✔ **QUICK CHECK 37.1**
1. What are the functions of saliva?
2. What are the phases of swallowing and how are they controlled?

Stomach

The **stomach** is a hollow, muscular organ just below the diaphragm (Fig. 37.5) that stores food during eating, secretes digestive juices, mixes food with these juices, and propels partially digested food, called **chyme**, into the duodenum of the small intestine. Functional areas are the **fundus** (upper portion), **body** (middle portion), and **antrum** (lower portion). Its major anatomic boundaries are:

- The lower esophageal sphincter, where food passes through the **cardiac orifice** at the gastroesophageal junction into the stomach.
- The **pyloric sphincter**, which relaxes as food is propelled through the **pylorus (gastroduodenal junction)** into the duodenum.

The stomach has three layers of smooth muscle: an outer, longitudinal layer; a middle, circular layer; and an inner, oblique layer (the most prominent) (see Fig. 37.5). These layers become progressively thicker in the body and antrum where food is mixed and pushed into the duodenum. The interior of the stomach is lined with mucosa. When the stomach is empty, this mucosal layer sits in folds called **rugae**. Few substances are absorbed in the stomach. The stomach mucosa is impermeable to water but can absorb alcohol and aspirin because they are lipid soluble.

The stomach's blood supply comes from a branch of the celiac artery (Fig. 37.6) and is so abundant that nearly all arterial vessels would need to be blocked before ischemic changes occur in the stomach wall. A series of small veins drain blood from the stomach toward the hepatic portal vein.

The sympathetic and parasympathetic divisions of the autonomic nervous system innervate the stomach. Some of the autonomic fibers are extrinsic—that is, they originate outside the stomach and are controlled by nerve centers in the brain. The vagus nerve provides

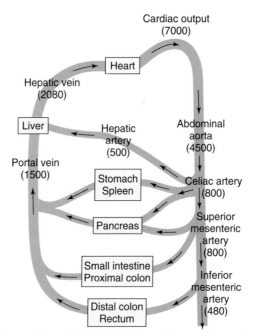

FIGURE 37.6 Major Blood Vessels and Organs Supplied With Blood in the Splanchnic Circulation. Numbers in parentheses reflect approximate blood flow values (ml/min) for each major vessel in an 80-kg (176 lb) normal, resting, adult human. Arrows indicate the direction of blood flow. (Modified from Johnson LR: *Gastrointestinal pathophysiology,* St Louis, 2001, Mosby.)

parasympathetic innervation and branches of the celiac plexus innervate the stomach sympathetically. The **myenteric (Auerbach) plexus** and **submucosal (Meissner) plexus** are intrinsic and part of the enteric (intramural) nervous system. They originate within the stomach and respond to local stimuli.

Gastric Motility

In its resting state, the stomach is small and contains about 50 ml of fluid. There is minimal wall tension, and the muscle layers in the fundus contract very little. Swallowing causes the fundus to relax (receptive relaxation) to receive a bolus of food from the esophagus. Relaxation is coordinated by efferent, nonadrenergic, noncholinergic vagal fibers and is facilitated by two polypeptide hormones secreted by the gastrointestinal mucosa—gastrin and cholecystokinin. (The actions of digestive hormones are summarized in Table 37.1.) Food is stored in vertical or oblique layers as it arrives in the fundus, whereas fluids flow relatively quickly down to the antrum.

Gastric (stomach) motility increases with the initiation of peristaltic waves, which sweep over the body of the stomach toward the antrum. The rate of peristaltic contractions is approximately three per minute and is influenced by neural and hormonal activity. Gastrin, motilin (an intestinal hormone), and the vagus nerve increase the rate of contraction by lowering the threshold potential of muscle fibers. (The neural and biochemical mechanisms of muscle contraction are described in Chapter 40.) Sympathetic activity and secretin (another intestinal hormone) are inhibitory and raise the threshold potential. The rate of peristalsis is mediated by pacemaker cells that initiate a wave of depolarization (basic electrical rhythm), which moves from the upper part of the stomach to the pylorus.

Gastric mixing and emptying of chyme from the stomach take several hours. Mixing occurs as food is propelled toward the antrum. As food approaches the pylorus, the velocity of the peristaltic wave increases. This forces the contents back toward the body of the stomach. This retropulsion effectively mixes food with digestive juices, and the oscillating motion breaks down large food particles. With each peristaltic wave, a small portion of the chyme passes through the pylorus and into the duodenum. The pyloric sphincter is about 1.5 cm long and is always open about 2 mm. It opens wider during contraction of the

TABLE 37.1	Selected Hormones* and Neurotransmitters of the Digestive System		
Source	**Hormone/Neuro Transmitter**	**Stimulus for Secretion**	**Action**
Mucosa of the stomach	Gastrin	Presence of partially digested proteins in the stomach	Stimulates gastric glands to secrete hydrochloric acid, pepsinogen, and histamine; growth of gastric mucosa
	Histamine	Gastrin	Stimulates acid secretion
	Somatostatin	Acid in stomach	Inhibits acid, pepsinogen, and histamine secretion and release of gastrin
	Acetylcholine	Vagus and local nerves in stomach	Stimulates release of pepsinogen and acid secretion
	Gastrin-releasing peptide (bombesin)	Vagus and local nerves in stomach	Stimulates gastrin and release of pepsinogen and acid secretion
	Ghrelin	High during fasting	Stimulates growth hormone secretion and hypothalamus to increase appetite
Mucosa of the small intestine	Motilin	Presence of acid and fat in the duodenum	Increases gastrointestinal motility
	Secretin	Presence of chyme (acid, partially digested proteins, fats) in duodenum	Stimulates pancreas to secrete alkaline pancreatic juice and liver to secrete bile; decreases gastrointestinal motility; inhibits gastrin and gastric acid secretion
	Serotonin (5-hydroxytryptamine)	Intestinal distention; vagal stimulation; presence of acids, amino acids, or hypertonic fluids; released from enterochromaffin cells throughout intestine	Stimulates intestinal secretion, motility and sensation (i.e., pain and nausea), vasodilation; activates gut immune responses
	Cholecystokinin	Presence of chyme (acid, partially digested proteins, fats) in duodenum	Stimulates gallbladder to eject bile and pancreas to secrete alkaline fluid; decreases gastric motility; constricts pyloric sphincter; inhibits gastrin
	Enteroglucagon	Intraluminal fats and carbohydrates	Weakly inhibits gastric and pancreatic secretion and enhances insulin release, lipolysis, ketogenesis, and glycogenolysis
	Gastric inhibitory peptide (GIP)	Fat and glucose in the small intestine	Inhibits gastric secretion and emptying; stimulates insulin release
	Peptide YY	Intraluminal fat and bile acids	Inhibits postprandial gastric acid and pancreatic secretion and delays gastric and small bowel emptying
	Pancreatic polypeptide	Protein, fat, and glucose in the small intestine	Decreases pancreatic bicarbonate and enzyme secretion
	Vasoactive intestinal peptide	Intestinal mucosa and muscle	Relaxes intestinal smooth muscle

*The digestive hormones are not secreted into the gastrointestinal lumen, but rather into the bloodstream, where they travel to target tissues. Multiple peptide hormone genes and more than 100 hormonally active peptides are expressed in the gastrointestinal tract.
Modified from Johnson LR: *Gastrointestinal physiology*, ed 8, St Louis, 2014, Mosby. Data from Feldman M et al: *Sleisenger and Fordtran's gastrointestinal and liver disease*, ed 10, Philadelphia, 2015, Saunders.

antrum. Normally there is no regurgitation from the duodenum into the antrum.

The rate of **gastric emptying** (movement of chyme into the duodenum) depends on the volume, osmotic pressure, and chemical composition of the gastric contents. Larger volumes of food increase gastric pressure, peristalsis, and rate of emptying. Solids, fats, and nonisotonic solutions (i.e., hypertonic or hypotonic gastric tube feedings) delay gastric emptying. (Osmotic pressure and tonicity are described in Chapters 1 and 5.) Products of fat digestion, which are formed in the duodenum by the action of bile from the liver and enzymes from the pancreas, stimulate the secretion of cholecystokinin. This hormone inhibits food intake, reduces gastric motility, and decreases gastric emptying so that fats are not emptied into the duodenum at a rate that exceeds the rate of bile and enzyme secretion. Osmoreceptors in the wall of the duodenum are sensitive to the osmotic pressure of duodenal contents. The arrival of hypertonic or hypotonic gastric contents activates the osmoreceptors, which delay gastric emptying to facilitate formation of an isosmotic duodenal environment. The rate at which acid enters the duodenum also influences gastric emptying. Secretions from the pancreas, liver, and duodenal mucosa neutralize gastric hydrochloric acid in the duodenum. The rate of emptying is adjusted to the duodenum's ability to neutralize the incoming acidity.[2]

Gastric Secretion

The stomach secretes large volumes of gastric juices or gastric secretions, including acid, pepsinogen, mucus, enzymes, hormones, intrinsic factor, and gastroferrin. **Intrinsic factor** is necessary for the intestinal absorption of vitamin B_{12}, and gastroferrin facilitates the absorption of iron in the small intestine. The hormones are secreted into the blood and travel to target tissues. The other gastric secretions are released directly into the stomach lumen.[3]

Gastric secretion is stimulated by the process of eating (gastric distention), by the actions of the hormone gastrin and paracrine pathways (e.g., histamine, ghrelin, somatostatin), and by the effects of the neurotransmitter acetylcholine and other chemicals (e.g., ethanol, coffee, protein). The secretion of gastric juice is influenced by numerous stimuli that together facilitate the process of digestion. There are three phases of gastric secretion, all of which promote the secretion of acid by the stomach:

- *Cephalic phase*—stimulated by the thought, smell, and taste of food
- *Gastric phase*—stimulated by distention of the stomach
- *Intestinal phase*—stimulated by histamine and digested protein

In the fundus and body of the stomach, the **gastric glands** of the mucosa are the primary secretory units (Fig. 37.7). The composition of gastric juice depends on volume and flow rate (see Fig. 37.4, *B*). The potassium level remains relatively constant, but its concentration is greater in gastric juice than in plasma. The rate of secretion varies with the time of day. Generally, the rate and volume of secretion are lowest in the morning and highest in the afternoon and evening. Loss of gastric juices through vomiting, drainage, or suction may decrease body stores of sodium and potassium and result in fluid, electrolyte (e.g., hyponatremia, hypokalemia, dehydration), and acid-base imbalances (e.g., metabolic alkalosis)[4] (see Chapter 5).

Gastric secretion is inhibited by somatostatin, by unpleasant odors and tastes, and by rage, fear, or pain. A discharge of sympathetic impulses inhibits parasympathetic impulses. Increased secretions are associated with aggression or hostility and may contribute to some forms of gastric pathology.

Acid. The major functions of gastric hydrochloric acid are to dissolve food fibers, act as a bactericide against swallowed microorganisms, and convert pepsinogen to pepsin. The production of acid by the **parietal**

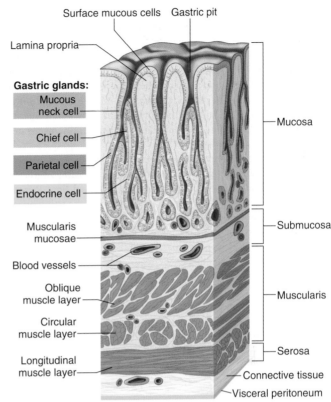

FIGURE 37.7 Gastric Pits and Gastric Glands. Gastric pits are depressions in the epithelial lining of the stomach. At the bottom of each pit are one or more tubular *gastric glands*. Chief cells produce pepsinogen, which is converted to pepsin (a proteolytic enzyme); parietal cells secrete hydrochloric acid and intrinsic factor; G cells produce gastrin; endocrine cells (enterochromaffin-like cells and D cells) secrete histamine and somatostatin. (From Patton KT, et al: *Essentials of anatomy & physiology,* St Louis, 2012, Mosby.)

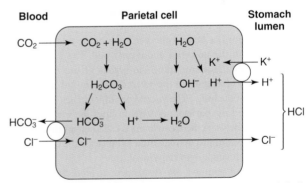

FIGURE 37.8 Hydrochloric Acid Secretion by Parietal Cell.

cells requires the transport of hydrogen and chloride from the parietal cells to the stomach lumen. Acid is formed in the parietal cells, primarily through the hydrolysis of water (Fig. 37.8). At a high rate of gastric secretion, bicarbonate moves into the plasma, producing an "alkaline tide" in the venous blood, which also may result in a more alkaline urine.[4]

Acid secretion is stimulated by the vagus nerve, which releases acetylcholine and stimulates the secretion of gastrin; gastrin then stimulates the release of histamine from enterochromaffin cells (mast cells; see Chapter 6) in the gastric mucosa. Histamine stimulates acid secretion by activating histamine receptors (H_2 receptors) on acid-secreting parietal cells. Caffeine, calcium, and ghrelin also stimulate acid secretion. Acid secretion is inhibited by somatostatin, secretin, and other intestinal hormones.[3]

Pepsin. Acetylcholine, gastrin, and secretin stimulate the chief cells to release pepsinogen during eating. Pepsinogen is quickly converted to pepsin in the acidic gastric environment (optimum pH for pepsin activation = 2). Pepsin is a proteolytic enzyme—that is, it breaks down protein and forms polypeptides in the stomach. Once chyme has entered the duodenum, the alkaline environment of the duodenum inactivates pepsin.

Mucus. The gastric mucosa is protected from the digestive actions of acid and pepsin by intercellular tight junctions, a coating of mucus called the mucosal barrier, and gastric mucosal blood flow. Prostaglandins protect the mucosal barrier by stimulating the secretion of mucus and bicarbonate and by inhibiting the secretion of acid. A break in the protective barrier may occur from ischemia or by exposure to *Helicobacter pylori*, aspirin, nonsteroidal antiinflammatory drugs (inhibit prostaglandin synthesis), ethanol, or regurgitated bile. Breaks cause inflammation and ulceration.

> ✔ **QUICK CHECK 37.2**
> 1. Why are there three layers of stomach muscle?
> 2. What hormones stimulate gastric motility?
> 3. What are the phases of gastric secretion?

Small Intestine

The small intestine is coiled within the peritoneal cavity and is about 5 to 6 meters long. Functionally, it is divided into three segments: the duodenum, jejunum, and ileum (Fig. 37.9, *A*). The duodenum begins at the pylorus and ends where it joins the jejunum at a suspensory ligament called the *Treitz ligament*. The end of the jejunum and the beginning of the ileum are not distinguished by an anatomic marker. These structures are not grossly different, but the jejunum has a slightly larger lumen than the ileum. The ileocecal valve, or sphincter, controls the flow of digested material from the ileum into the large intestine and prevents reflux into the small intestine.

The duodenum lies behind the peritoneum, or retroperitoneally, and is attached to the posterior abdominal wall. The peritoneum is the serous membrane surrounding the organs of the abdomen and pelvic cavity. It is analogous to the pericardium around the heart and the pleura around the lungs. The visceral peritoneum lies on the surface of the organs, and the parietal peritoneum lines the wall of the body cavity. The space between these two layers is called the peritoneal cavity and normally contains just enough fluid to lubricate the two layers and prevent friction during organ movement.

The ileum and jejunum are suspended in loose folds from the posterior abdominal wall by a peritoneal membrane called the mesentery. The mesentery facilitates intestinal motility and supports blood vessels, nerves, and lymphatics.

The arterial supply to the duodenum arises primarily from the gastroduodenal artery, a branch of the celiac artery. The jejunum and ileum are supplied by branches of the superior mesenteric artery (see Fig. 37.6). The superior mesenteric vein drains blood from the entire small intestine and empties into the hepatic portal circulation. The regional lymph nodes and lymphatics drain into the thoracic duct, which empties into the subclavian vein.

Enteric nerves from both divisions of the autonomic nervous system innervate the small intestine.[5] Secretion, motility, pain sensation, and intestinal reflexes (e.g., relaxation of the lower esophageal sphincter) are mediated parasympathetically by the vagus nerve. Sympathetic

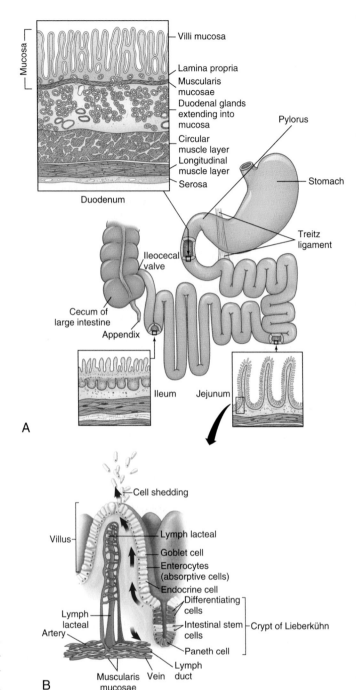

A

B

FIGURE 37.9 The Small Intestine. A, Segments of the small intestine. Inserts show longitudinal sections of the duodenum, jejunum, and ileum. **B,** Anatomy of a villus. Arrows show migration and then shedding of epithelial cells.

activity inhibits motility and produces vasoconstriction. Intrinsic reflexive activity is mediated by the myenteric (Auerbach) plexus and the submucosal (Meissner) plexus of the enteric nervous system.

The smooth muscles of the small intestine are arranged in two layers: a longitudinal outer layer and a thicker inner circular layer (see Figs. 37.2 and 37.9, *A*). Circular folds of the small intestine slow the passage of food, thereby providing more time for digestion and absorption. The folds are most numerous and prominent in the jejunum and proximal ileum (see Fig. 37.9, *A*).

Absorption occurs through villi (sing., villus), which cover the circular folds and are the functional units of the intestine. A villus is composed of absorptive columnar cells (enterocytes) and mucus-secreting goblet cells of the mucosal epithelium (see Fig. 37.9, B). Each villus secretes some of the enzymes necessary for digestion and absorbs nutrients. Near the surface, columnar cells closely adhere to each other at sites called *tight junctions*. Water and electrolytes are absorbed through these intercellular spaces. The surface of each columnar epithelial cell on the villus contains tiny projections called microvilli (sing., microvillus). Together the microvilli create a mucosal surface known as the brush border. The villi and microvilli greatly increase the surface area available for absorption. Coating the brush border is an "unstirred" layer of water that is important for the absorption of water-soluble substances including emulsified micelles of fat. The lamina propria (a connective tissue layer of the mucous membrane) lies beneath the epithelial cells of the villi and contains lymphocytes and plasma cells, which produce immunoglobulins (see The Gastrointestinal Tract and Immunity section).

Central arterioles ascend within each villus and branch into a capillary array that extends around the base of the columnar cells and cascades down to the venules that lead to the hepatic portal circulation. A central lacteal, or lymphatic capillary, also is contained within each villus and is important for the absorption and transport of fat molecules (see Fig. 37.9, B). The contents of the lacteals flow to regional nodes and channels that eventually drain into the thoracic duct.

Between the bases of the villi are the crypts of Lieberkühn, which extend to the submucosal layer. Undifferentiated cells arise from stem cells at the base of the crypt and move toward the tip of the villus, maturing to become columnar epithelial secretory cells (water, electrolytes, and enzymes) and goblet cells (mucus). After completing their migration to the tip of the villus, they function for a few days and then are shed into the intestinal lumen and digested. Discarded epithelial cells are an important source of endogenous protein. The entire epithelial population is replaced about every 4 to 7 days. Many factors can influence this process of cellular proliferation. Starvation, vitamin B_{12} deficiency, and cytotoxic drugs or irradiation suppress cell division and shorten the villi. Decreased absorption across the epithelial membrane can cause diarrhea and malnutrition. Nutrient intake and intestinal resection stimulate cell production.

Intestinal Digestion and Absorption

The process of digestion is initiated in the stomach by the actions of gastric hydrochloric acid and pepsin. The chyme that passes into the duodenum is a liquid with small particles of undigested food. Digestion of food components continues in the proximal portion of the small intestine by the action of pancreatic enzymes, intestinal enzymes, and bile salts. As seen in Fig. 37.10, in the proximal small intestine:

- carbohydrates are broken down to monosaccharides and disaccharides,
- proteins are degraded further to amino acids and peptides, and
- fats are emulsified and reduced to fatty acids (Box 37.1) and monoglycerides.

These nutrients, along with water, vitamins, and electrolytes, are absorbed across the intestinal mucosa by active transport, diffusion, or facilitated diffusion. Products of carbohydrate and protein breakdown move into villus capillaries and then to the liver through the hepatic portal vein. Digested fats move into the lacteals and reach the liver through the portal and systemic circulation. These components are metabolized within the liver (see the Metabolism of Nutrients section). Intestinal motility exposes nutrients to a large mucosal surface area by mixing chyme and moving it through the lumen. Different segments of the GI tract absorb different nutrients. Digestion and absorption of all major nutrients and many drugs occur in the small intestine. Sites of absorption are shown in Fig. 37.11. Box 37.2 outlines the major nutrients involved in this process.

Intestinal Motility

The movements of the small intestine facilitate digestion and absorption.[5] Chyme leaving the stomach and entering the duodenum stimulates intestinal movements that help blend secretions from the liver, gallbladder, pancreas, and intestinal glands. A churning motion brings the luminal contents into contact with the absorbing cells of the villi. Propulsive movements then advance the chyme toward the large intestine.

Intestinal motility is affected by the following two movements:

- Segmentation. Localized rhythmic contractions of circular smooth muscles divide and mix the chyme, enabling it to have contact with digestive enzymes and the absorbent mucosal surface, and then propel it toward the large intestine.
- Peristalsis. Waves of contraction along short segments of longitudinal smooth muscle allow time for digestion and absorption. The intestinal villi move with contractions of the muscularis mucosae, a thin layer of muscle separating the mucosa and submucosa, with absorption promoted by the swaying of the villi in the luminal contents.

Neural reflexes along the length of the small intestine facilitate motility, digestion, and absorption. The ileogastric reflex inhibits gastric motility when the ileum becomes distended. This prevents the continued movement of chyme into an already distended intestine. The intestinointestinal reflex inhibits intestinal motility when one part of the intestine is overdistended. Both of these reflexes require extrinsic

---

BOX 37.1   Dietary Fat

Saturated Fatty Acid (Palmitic Acid [$C_1 6H_{32}O_2$])
Each carbon atom in the chain is linked by single bonds to adjacent carbon and hydrogen atoms; atoms are solid at room temperature and found in animal fat and tropical oils (coconut and palm oils); they increase the blood levels of low-density lipoprotein (LDL) cholesterol ("bad" cholesterol) and also the risk of coronary artery disease.

Unsaturated Fatty Acid
Unsaturated fatty acids are soft or liquid at room temperature; omega-6 fatty acids are found in plants and vegetables (olive, canola, and peanut oils), and omega-3 fatty acids are found in fish and shellfish.
- Monounsaturated fatty acids (e.g., oleic acid [$C_{18}H_{34}O_2$]): Contain one double bond in the carbon chain and are found in plants and animals; may be beneficial

in reducing blood cholesterol, glucose levels, and systolic blood pressure; do not lower high-density lipoprotein (HDL) cholesterol ("good" cholesterol) level; low HDL levels have been associated with coronary heart disease.
- Polyunsaturated fatty acids (e.g., linoleic acid [$C_{18}H_{32}O_2$]): Contain two or more double bonds in the carbon chain and are found in plants and fish oils; omega-6 fatty acids lower total and LDL cholesterol blood levels; high levels of polyunsaturated fatty acids may lower the LDL level; omega-3 fatty acids lower blood triglyceride levels, reduce platelet aggregation and blood-clotting tendencies, are necessary for growth and development, and may prevent coronary artery disease, hypertension, cancer, and inflammatory and immune disorders.

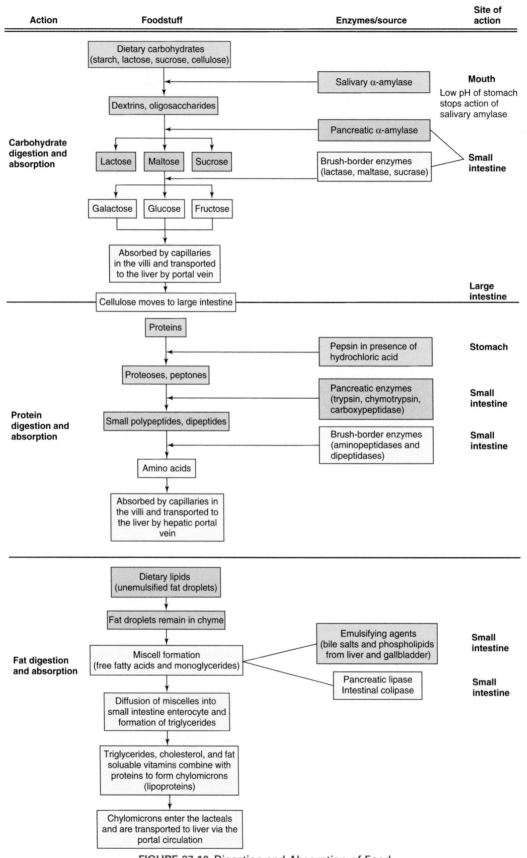

FIGURE 37.10 Digestion and Absorption of Food.

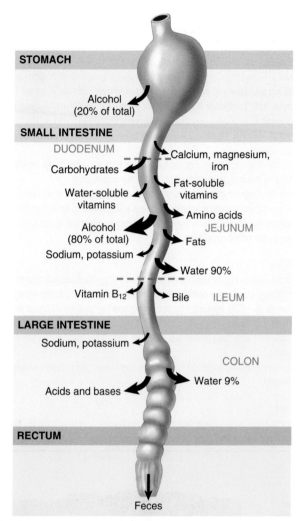

STOMACH

Alcohol
(20% of total)

SMALL INTESTINE

DUODENUM

Calcium, magnesium,
iron

Carbohydrates

Fat-soluble
vitamins

Water-soluble
vitamins

Amino acids

JEJUNUM

Alcohol
(80% of total)

Fats

Sodium, potassium

Water 90%

Vitamin B$_{12}$

Bile   ILEUM

LARGE INTESTINE

Sodium, potassium

COLON

Water 9%

Acids and bases

RECTUM

Feces

FIGURE 37.11 Sites of Absorption of Major Nutrients. (Modified from Patton KT: *Anatomy & physiology*, ed 10, St Louis, 2019, Elsevier.)

innervation. The gastroileal reflex, which is activated by an increase in gastric motility and secretion, stimulates an increase in ileal motility and relaxation of the ileocecal valve. This empties the ileum and prepares it to receive more chyme. The gastroileal reflex is probably regulated by the hormones gastrin and cholecystokinin.

During prolonged fasting or between meals, particularly overnight, slow waves sweep along the entire length of the intestinal tract from the stomach to the terminal ileum. This interdigestive myoelectric complex appears to propel residual gastric and intestinal contents into the colon.

The ileocecal valve (sphincter) marks the junction between the terminal ileum and the large intestine. This valve is intrinsically regulated and is normally closed. The arrival of peristaltic waves from the last few centimeters of the ileum causes the ileocecal valve to open, allowing a small amount of chyme to pass. Distention of the upper large intestine causes the sphincter to constrict, preventing further distention or retrograde flow of intestinal contents.

> ✔ **QUICK CHECK 37.3**
> 1. What cells arise from the crypts of Lieberkühn?
> 2. How are fats absorbed from the small intestine?
> 3. Which reflexes inhibit intestinal motility? Which promote it?

Large Intestine

The large intestine is approximately 1.5 meters long and consists of the cecum, appendix, colon, rectum, and anal canal (Fig. 37.12, *A*). The cecum is a pouch that receives chyme from the ileum. Attached to it is the vermiform appendix, an appendage having limited physiologic function. However, recent studies suggest it may have an important protective role in gut immunity.[6] From the cecum, chyme enters the colon, which loops upward, traverses the abdominal cavity, and descends to the anal canal. The four parts of the colon are the ascending colon, transverse colon, descending colon, and sigmoid colon. Two sphincters control the flow of intestinal contents through the cecum and colon: the ileocecal valve, which admits chyme from the ileum to the cecum; and the rectosigmoid canal, which controls the movement of wastes from the sigmoid colon into the rectum. A thick (2.5 to 3 cm) portion of smooth muscle surrounds the anal canal, forming the internal anal sphincter. Overlapping it distally is the striated skeletal muscle of the external anal sphincter (**anus**).

In the cecum and colon, the longitudinal muscle layer consists of three longitudinal bands called teniae coli (see Fig. 37.12, *B*). They are shorter than the colon and give it a gathered appearance. The circular muscles of the colon separate the gathers into outpouchings called haustra (sing., haustrum). The haustra become more or less prominent with the contractions and relaxations of the circular muscles. The mucosal surface of the colon has rugae (folds), particularly between the haustra, and crypts of Lieberkühn but no villi. Columnar epithelial cells and mucus-secreting goblet cells form the mucosa throughout the large intestine. The columnar epithelium absorbs fluid and electrolytes, and the mucus-secreting cells lubricate the mucosa.

In the large intestine, extrinsic parasympathetic innervation occurs through the vagus nerve. Vagal stimulation increases rhythmic contraction of the proximal colon from the cecum to the first part of the transverse colon. Vagal fibers reach the distal colon through the sacral parasympathetic splanchnic nerves. The internal anal sphincter is usually contracted, and its reflex response is to relax when the rectum is distended. The intrinsic myenteric plexus provides the major innervation of the internal anal sphincter, but responds to sympathetic stimulation to maintain contraction and parasympathetic stimulation that facilitates relaxation when the rectum is full. Sympathetic innervation of this sphincter arises from the celiac and superior mesenteric ganglia and the sphincter nerve. The external anal sphincter is innervated by the pudendal nerve arising from sacral levels of the spinal cord. Sympathetic activity in the entire large intestine modulates intestinal reflexes, conveys somatic sensations of fullness and pain, participates in the defecation reflex, and constricts blood vessels. The blood supply of the large intestine and rectum is derived primarily from branches of the superior and inferior mesenteric arteries[7] (see Figs. 37.6 and 37.12, *A*) and venous blood drains through the inferior mesenteric vein.

The primary type of colonic movement is segmental. The circular muscles contract and relax at different sites, shuttling the intestinal contents back and forth between the haustra, most commonly during fasting. The movements massage the intestinal contents, called the fecal mass at that point, and facilitate the absorption of water. Propulsive movement occurs with the proximal-to-distal contraction of several haustral units. Peristaltic movements also occur and promote the emptying of the colon. The gastrocolic reflex initiates propulsion in the entire colon, usually during or immediately after eating, when chyme enters from the ileum. The gastrocolic reflex causes the fecal mass to pass rapidly into the sigmoid colon and rectum, stimulating defecation. Gastrin may participate in stimulating this reflex. Epinephrine inhibits contractile activity, as do exogenous opioids.

BOX 37.2   Major Nutrients Absorbed in the Small Intestine

Water and Electrolytes
- Approximately 85% to 90% of the water that enters the gastrointestinal tract is absorbed in the small intestine.
- Sodium passes through tight junctions and is actively transported across cell membranes; it is exchanged for bicarbonate to maintain electroneutrality in the ileum; sodium absorption is enhanced by cotransport with glucose.
- Potassium moves passively across tight junctions with changes in the electrochemical gradient.

Carbohydrates
- Only monosaccharides are absorbed by the intestinal mucosa; therefore complex carbohydrates must be hydrolyzed to the simplest form.
- Salivary and pancreatic amylases break down starches to oligosaccharides (lactose, maltose, sucrose) in the stomach and duodenum; brush-border enzymes hydrolyze them in the small intestine so they can pass through the unstirred water layer by diffusion.
- Fructose diffuses into the bloodstream; glucose and galactose diffuse or are actively transported.
- Cellulose remains undigested and stimulates large intestine motility.

Proteins
- From 90% to 95% of protein is absorbed; major hydrolysis is accomplished in the small intestine by the pancreatic enzymes trypsin, chymotrypsin, and carboxypeptidase.
- Brush-border enzymes break down proteins into smaller peptides that can cross cell membranes. In the cytosol, they are metabolized into amino acids, specifically neutral amino acids, basic amino acids, and proline and hydroxyproline.

Fats
Digestion and absorption occur in four phases:
- Phase 1—Emulsification and lipolysis: Emulsifying agents (bile salts) cover small fat particles and prevent them from reforming into fat droplets; then lipolysis with pancreatic lipases divides them into monoglycerides and free fatty acids.
- Phase 2—Micelle formation: A spherical formation of lipid products that are water soluble.
- Phase 3—Fat absorption: Fat products move from micelles to the absorbing surface of the intestinal epithelium and enter enterocytes.
- Phase 4—Triglycerides are resynthesized and, along with cholesterol, fat-soluble vitamins and phospholipids, combine with proteins to form chylomicrons (lipoproteins). Chylomicrons leave the enterocyte, enter the lymphatics, and travel to the portal circulation.

Minerals
- Calcium—absorbed by passive diffusion and transported actively across cell membranes bound to a carrier protein; absorption primarily in the ileum.
- Magnesium—50% absorbed by active transport or passive diffusion in the jejunum and ileum.
- Phosphate—absorbed by passive diffusion and active transport in the small intestine.
- Iron—absorbed by epithelial cells of the duodenum and jejunum; vitamin C facilitates.

Vitamins
- Absorbed mainly by sodium-dependent active transport, with vitamin B_{12} bound to intrinsic factor and absorbed in the terminal ileum.

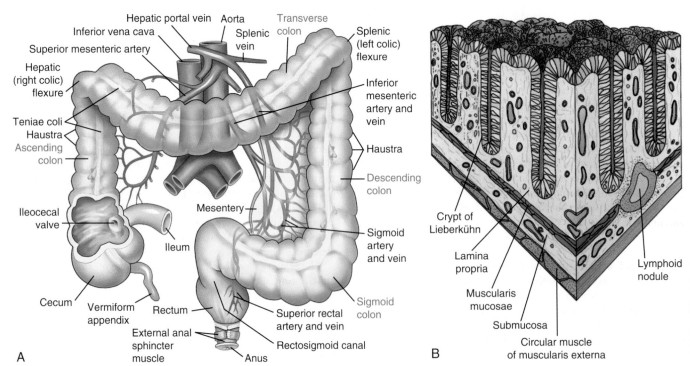

FIGURE 37.12 The Large Intestine. A, Structure of the large intestine. **B,** Microscopic cross section illustrating cellular structures of the large intestine. The wall of the large intestine is lined with columnar epithelium, in contrast to the villi characteristics of the small intestine. The longitudinal layer of muscularis is reduced to become the teniae coli. (**A** modified from Patton KT, Thibodeau GA: *The human body in health & disease,* ed 7, St Louis, 2018, Mosby; **B** from Gartner LP, Hiatt JL: *Color textbook of histology,* ed 3, Philadelphia, 2007, Saunders.)

Approximately 500 to 700 ml of chyme flows from the ileum to the cecum per day. Most of the water is absorbed in the colon by diffusion and active transport. Aldosterone increases membrane permeability to sodium, thereby increasing both the diffusion of sodium into the cell and the active transport of sodium to the interstitial fluid. (See Chapters 5 and 20 for a discussion of aldosterone secretion.) The colon does not absorb monosaccharides and amino acids, but some short-chain free fatty acids, which are produced by fermentation, are absorbed.

Absorption and epithelial transport occur in the cecum, ascending colon, transverse colon, and descending colon. By the time the fecal mass enters the sigmoid colon, the mass consists entirely of wastes, called the feces, and is composed of food residue, unabsorbed GI secretions, shed epithelial cells, and bacteria.

The movement of feces into the sigmoid colon and rectum stimulates the defecation reflex (rectosphincteric reflex). The rectal wall stretches, and the tonically constricted internal anal sphincter (smooth muscle with autonomic nervous system control) relaxes, creating the urge to defecate. The defecation reflex can be overridden voluntarily by contraction of the external anal sphincter and muscles of the pelvic floor. The rectal wall gradually relaxes, reducing tension, and the urge to defecate passes. Retrograde contraction of the rectum may displace the feces out of the rectal vault until a more convenient time for evacuation. Pain or fear of pain associated with defecation (e.g., rectal fissures or hemorrhoids) can inhibit the defecation reflex.

Squatting and sitting facilitate defecation because these positions straighten the angle between the rectum and anal canal and increase the efficiency of straining (increasing intra-abdominal pressure). Intra-abdominal pressure is increased by initiating the Valsalva maneuver—that is, inhaling and forcing the diaphragm and chest muscles against the closed glottis to increase both intrathoracic and intra-abdominal pressure, which is transmitted to the rectum.

The Gastrointestinal Tract and Immunity

The GI tract's gut-associated lymphoid tissue (GALT) plays a major role in immune defenses by killing many pathogenetic microorganisms and preventing reaction to foreign proteins (dietary antigens) ingested in the diet.[8] The mucosa of the intestine covers a large surface area, and mucosal secretions produce antibodies, particularly IgA, and enzymes that provide defenses against microorganisms. Small intestinal Paneth cells, located near the base of the crypts of Lieberkühn (see Fig. 37.9, B), produce defensins and other antimicrobial peptides and lysozymes important to mucosal immunity. Small intestinal Peyer patches (lymph nodules containing collections of lymphocytes, plasma cells, and macrophages) are most numerous in the ileum and produce antimicrobial peptides and IgA as a component of GALT in the small intestine (see Figs. 37.2 and 7.3). Peyer patches are important for antigen processing and immune defense (see Chapter 7).

Intestinal Microbiome

The type and number of bacterial flora vary greatly throughout the normal GI tract and among individuals. There are an increasing number of bacteria from the proximal to the distal GI tract, with the highest number in the colon. Genetics, diet, environmental pollution, personal hygiene, vaccination, infection, antibiotics and other drugs, and radiation affect the normal composition of bacterial flora. The intestinal bacteria do not have major digestive or absorptive functions, but they do play a role in the metabolism of bile salts, estrogens, androgens, lipids, carbohydrates, various nitrogenous substances, and drugs. They produce antimicrobial peptides, hormones, neurotransmitters, antiinflammatory metabolites, and vitamins; destroy toxins; prevent pathogen colonization; and alert the immune system to protect against infection. They are important to overall health and, when altered (dysbiosis) or translocated,

they cause disease.[9] The intestinal tract is sterile at birth but becomes colonized within a few hours. Within 3 to 4 weeks after birth, the normal flora are established. The number and diversity of bacteria decrease with aging, increasing the risk for infection. The normal flora do not have the virulence factors associated with pathogenic microorganisms, thus permitting immune tolerances.

Bacteria in the stomach are relatively sparse because of the secretion of acid that kills ingested pathogens or inhibits bacterial growth (with the exception of *H. pylori*). Bile acid secretion, intestinal motility, and antibody production suppress bacterial growth in the duodenum. In the duodenum and jejunum, there is a low concentration of aerobes, primarily streptococci, lactobacilli, staphylococci, and other enteric bacteria. Anaerobes are found distal to the ileocecal valve but not proximal to the ileum. They constitute about 95% of the fecal flora in the colon and contribute one third of the solid bulk of feces. *Bacteroides* (gram negative) and *Firmicutes* (gram positive) are the most common colon bacteria.

Splanchnic Blood Flow

The splanchnic (visceral) blood flow provides blood to the esophagus, stomach, small and large intestines, liver, gallbladder, pancreas, and spleen (see Fig. 37.6). Blood flow is regulated by cardiac output and blood volume, the autonomic nervous system, hormones, and local autoregulatory blood flow mechanisms. The GI circulation serves as an important reservoir of blood volume to maintain circulation to the heart and lungs when needed.

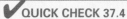

> ✓ **QUICK CHECK 37.4**
> 1. What is the major arterial blood supply to the large intestine?
> 2. What is the Valsalva maneuver?
> 3. What roles do bacterial flora play in the GI tract?

ACCESSORY ORGANS OF DIGESTION

The liver, gallbladder, and exocrine pancreas all secrete substances necessary for the digestion of chyme. These secretions are delivered to the duodenum through the sphincter of Oddi at the major duodenal papilla (of Vater) (Fig. 37.13). The liver produces bile, which contains salts necessary for fat digestion and absorption. Between meals, bile is stored in the gallbladder. The exocrine pancreas produces (1) enzymes needed for the complete digestion of carbohydrates, proteins, and fats; and (2) an alkaline fluid that neutralizes chyme, creating a duodenal pH that supports enzymatic action.

The liver also receives nutrients absorbed by the small intestine and metabolizes or synthesizes them into forms that can be absorbed by the body's cells. It then releases the nutrients into the bloodstream or stores them for later use.

Liver

The liver weighs 1200 to 1600 g. It is located under the right diaphragm and is divided into right and left lobes (Fig. 37.14). The larger, right lobe is divided further into the caudate and quadrate lobes. The *falciform ligament* separates the right and left lobes and attaches the liver to the anterior abdominal wall. The *round ligament (ligamentum teres)* extends along the free edge of the falciform ligament, extending from the umbilicus to the inferior surface of the liver. The *coronary ligament* branches from the falciform ligament and extends over the superior surface of the right and left lobes, binding the liver to the inferior surface of the diaphragm. The liver is covered by the Glisson capsule, which contains blood vessels, lymphatics, and nerves. When the liver is diseased or swollen, distention of the capsule causes pain because it is innervated by sensory neurons.

The metabolic functions of the liver require a large amount of blood. The liver receives blood from both arterial and venous sources. The **hepatic artery** is formed by the merging of superior mesenteric and splenic veins and receives blood from the inferior mesenteric, gastric, and cystic veins. It provides arterial oxygenated blood at the rate of about 400 to 500 ml/min or about 5% to 7% of the cardiac output (see Fig. 37.6). The **hepatic portal vein** receives deoxygenated blood from the inferior and superior mesenteric veins, the splenic vein, and the gastric and esophageal veins, and delivers about 1000 to 1500 ml/min to the liver. The hepatic portal vein, which carries 70% of the blood to the liver, is rich in nutrients that have been absorbed from the intestinal tract (Fig. 37.15).

Within the liver lobes are approximately 100,000 tiny anatomic units called **liver lobules** (Fig. 37.16). They are formed of cords or plates of **hepatocytes**, which are the functional cells of the liver. These cells can regenerate; therefore damaged or resected liver tissue can regrow. Small capillaries, or **sinusoids**, are located between the plates of hepatocytes. They receive a mixture of venous and arterial blood from branches of

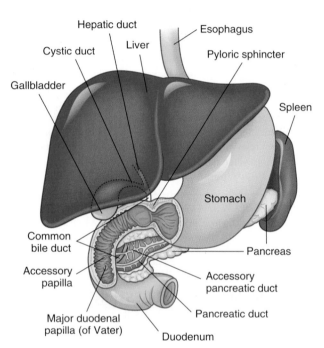

FIGURE 37.13 Accessory Organs of Digestion. Location of the liver, gallbladder, and exocrine pancreas.

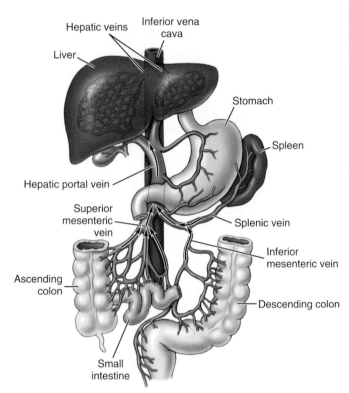

FIGURE 37.15 Hepatic Portal Circulation. In this unusual circulatory route, a vein is located between two capillary beds. The hepatic portal vein collects blood from capillaries in visceral structures located in the abdomen and empties into the liver. Hepatic veins return blood to the inferior vena cava. (From Herlihy B: *The human body in health and illness,* ed 5, St Louis, 2015, Saunders.)

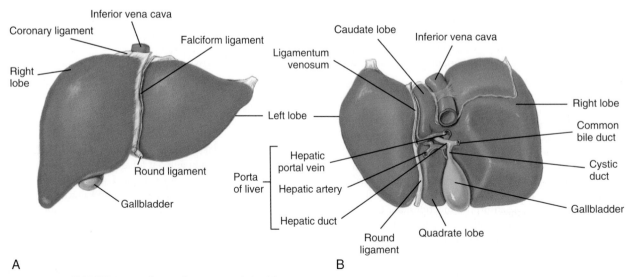

FIGURE 37.14 Gross Structure of the Liver. A, Anterior surface. **B,** Visceral surface. (From Applegate E: *The anatomy and physiology learning system,* ed 4, St Louis, 2011, Saunders.)

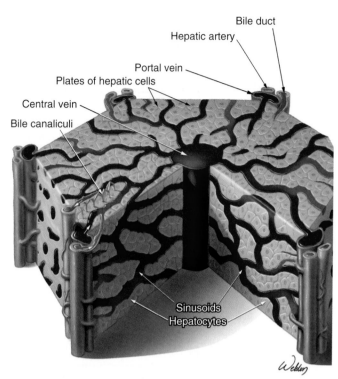

FIGURE 37.16 Schematic of the Liver Lobule. A cross section of a single liver lobule shows that, in whole, it is shaped like a hexagonal cylinder. The cut away area shows the central vein in the center of the lobule, separated by cords of hepatocytes forming sinusoids from six portal areas at the periphery. The portal areas contain a portal vein, hepatic artery, and bile duct. Blood flows toward the center of the lobule, whereas bile flows toward the portal triads at the margins. Note the hepatic artery providing oxygenated blood to the hepatic sinusoids. (From Polin RA, et al: *Fetal and neonatal physiology,* ed 4, St Louis, 2011, Saunders.)

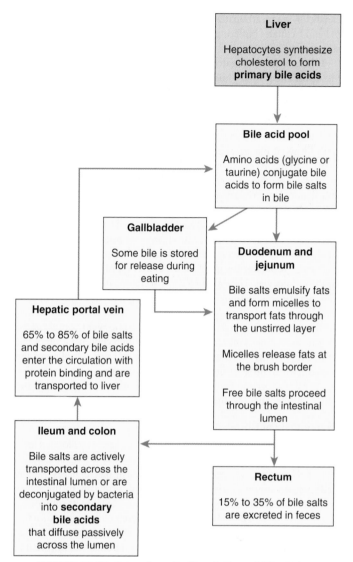

FIGURE 37.17 Enterohepatic Circulation of Bile Salts.

the hepatic artery and portal vein. Blood from the sinusoids drains to a central vein in the middle of each liver lobule. Venous blood from all the lobules then flows into the hepatic vein, which empties into the inferior vena cava. The sinusoids of the liver lobules are lined with highly permeable endothelium. This permeability enhances the transport of nutrients from the sinusoids into the hepatocytes, where they are metabolized.

The immune functions of the liver are carried out by various cells, including sinusoidal endothelial cells, Kupffer, stellate, and natural killer cells. Sinusoidal cells line the sinusoidal capillaries and, in addition to their barrier function, have immune functions including endocytosis, antigen presentation, and leukocyte recruitment. The sinusoids also are lined with phagocytic Kupffer cells (tissue macrophages) and are part of the mononuclear phagocyte system. Kupffer cells are important for healing injury to the liver, are bactericidal, and are important for bilirubin production and lipid metabolism. Stellate cells contain retinoids (vitamin A), are contractile in liver injury, regulate sinusoidal blood flow, may proliferate into myofibroblasts, participate in liver fibrosis, produce erythropoietin, can act as antigen-presenting cells, remove foreign substances from the blood, and trap bacteria. Natural killer cells (pit cells) also are found in the sinusoidal lumen; they produce interferon-γ and are important in tumor defense. Between the endothelial lining of the sinusoid and the hepatocyte is the Disse space, which drains interstitial fluid into the hepatic lymph system.

Secretion of Bile

The liver assists intestinal digestion by secreting 700 to 1200 ml of bile per day. Bile is an alkaline, bitter-tasting, yellowish green fluid that contains bile salts (conjugated bile acids), cholesterol, bilirubin (a pigment), electrolytes, and water. It is formed by hepatocytes and secreted into the bile canaliculi. Bile canaliculi are small channels that conduct bile outward to bile ducts and eventually drain into the common bile duct (see Figs. 37.13 and 37.16). This duct empties bile into the ampulla of Vater, and then into the duodenum through an opening called the major duodenal papilla (sphincter of Oddi). Bile salts are required for the intestinal emulsification and absorption of fats, including fat-soluble vitamins. Having facilitated fat emulsification and absorption, most bile salts are actively absorbed in the terminal ileum and returned to the liver through the portal circulation for resecretion. The pathway for recycling of bile salts is termed the enterohepatic circulation (Fig. 37.17).

Bile has two fractional components: the acid-dependent fraction and the acid-independent fraction. Hepatocytes secrete the bile acid–dependent fraction, which consists of bile acids, cholesterol, lecithin (a phospholipid), and bilirubin. The bile acid–independent fraction, which is secreted by the hepatocytes and epithelial cells of the bile canaliculi, is a bicarbonate-rich aqueous fluid that gives bile its alkaline pH and facilitates buffering of chyme entering the duodenum from the stomach.

Bile salts are conjugated in the liver from primary and secondary bile acids. The primary bile acids are cholic acid and chenodeoxycholic (chenic) acid. These acids are synthesized from cholesterol by the hepatocytes. The secondary bile acids are deoxycholic and lithocholic acid. These acids are formed in the small intestine by intestinal bacteria, after which they are absorbed and flow to the liver (see Fig. 37.17). Both forms of bile acids are conjugated with amino acids (glycine or taurine) in the liver to form bile salts. Conjugation makes the bile acids more water soluble, thus restricting their diffusion from the duodenum and ileum. The primary and secondary bile acids together form the bile acid pool.

Some bile salts are deconjugated by intestinal bacteria to secondary bile acids. These acids diffuse passively into the portal blood from both small and large intestines. An increase in the plasma concentration of bile acids accelerates the uptake and resecretion of bile acids and salts by the hepatocytes. The cycle of hepatic secretion, intestinal absorption, and hepatic resecretion of bile acids completes the enterohepatic circulation.

Bile secretion is called choleresis. A choleretic agent stimulates the liver to secrete bile. One strong stimulus is a high concentration of bile salts. Other choleretics include cholecystokinin, vagal stimulation, and secretin, which increase the rate of bile flow by promoting contraction of the gallbladder and the secretion of bicarbonate from canaliculi and other intrahepatic bile ducts.

Metabolism of Bilirubin

Bilirubin is a byproduct of the destruction of aged red blood cells. It gives bile a greenish black color and produces the yellow tinge of jaundice. Aged red blood cells are absorbed and destroyed by macrophages (Kupffer cells) of the mononuclear phagocyte system, primarily in the spleen and liver. Within these cells, hemoglobin is separated into its component parts: heme and globin (Fig. 37.18). The globin component is further degraded into its constituent amino acids, which go into the amino acid pool to form new protein. The heme component is converted to biliverdin by the enzymatic cleavage of iron. The iron attaches to transferrin in the plasma and can be stored in the liver or used by the bone marrow to make new red blood cells. The biliverdin is enzymatically converted to bilirubin in the Kupffer cell and then is released into the plasma where it binds to albumin and is known as unconjugated bilirubin, or free bilirubin, which is lipid soluble. Bilirubin also has a role as an antioxidant and provides cytoprotection.

In the liver, unconjugated bilirubin moves from plasma in the sinusoids into the hepatocyte. Within hepatocytes, unconjugated bilirubin joins with glucuronic acid to form conjugated bilirubin, which is water soluble and is secreted in the bile. When conjugated bilirubin reaches the distal ileum and colon, it is deconjugated by bacteria and converted to urobilinogen. Urobilinogen is then reabsorbed in the intestines and excreted in the urine as urobilin. A small amount is eliminated in feces, as stercobilin (an end-product of heme metabolism), which contributes to the stool's brown pigmentation. The elimination of bilirubin also is an important route for the elimination of cholesterol.

Vascular and Hematologic Functions

Because of its extensive vascular network, the liver can store a large volume of blood. The liver can release blood to maintain systemic circulatory volume in the event of hemorrhage. The liver also has hemostatic functions; it synthesizes most clotting factors (see Chapter 22). Vitamin K, a fat-soluble vitamin, is essential for the synthesis of the clotting factors. Because bile salts are needed for reabsorption of

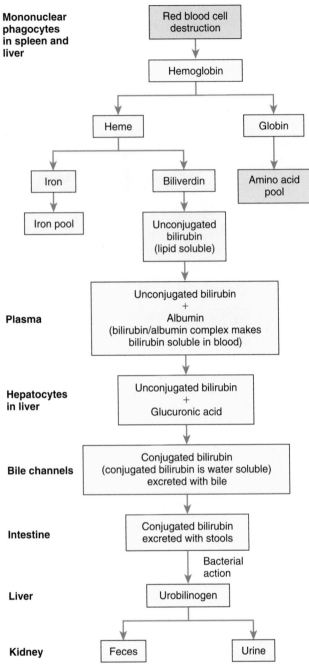

FIGURE 37.18 Bilirubin Metabolism. See text for further explanation.

fats, vitamin K absorption depends on adequate bile production in the liver.

Metabolism of Nutrients

Carbohydrates. The liver contributes to the stability of blood glucose levels by releasing glucose during hypoglycemia (low blood glucose level), absorbing glucose during hyperglycemia (high blood glucose level), and storing it as glycogen (glycogenesis) or converting it to fat. When all glycogen stores have been used, the liver can convert amino acids and glycerol to glucose (gluconeogenesis).

Proteins. Protein synthesis requires the presence of all the essential amino acids (obtained only from food), as well as nonessential amino acids. Proteins perform many important functions in the body; these are summarized in Table 37.2.

TABLE 37.2   Importance of Proteins in the Body

Function	Example
Contraction	Actin and myosin enable muscle contraction.
Energy	Proteins can be metabolized for energy.
Fluid balance	Albumin is a major source of plasma oncotic pressure.
Protection	Antibodies, complement, and C-reactive protein protect against infection and foreign substances.
Regulation	Enzymes control chemical reactions; hormones regulate many physiologic processes.
Structure	Collagen fibers provide structural support to many parts of the body; keratin strengthens skin, hair, and nails.
Transport	Hemoglobin transports oxygen and carbon dioxide in the blood; plasma proteins serve as transport molecules; proteins in cell membranes control movement of materials into and out of cells.
Coagulation	Hemostasis is regulated by clotting factors and proteins that balance coagulation and anticoagulation.

Within hepatocytes, amino acids are converted to carbohydrates (keto acids) by the removal of ammonia (NH_3), a process known as deamination. The ammonia is converted to urea by the liver and passes into the blood to be excreted by the kidneys. Depending on the nutritional status of the body, the keto acids either are converted to fatty acids for fat synthesis and storage or are oxidized by the Krebs tricarboxylic acid cycle (see Chapter 1) to provide energy for the liver cells.

The plasma proteins, including albumins and globulins (with the exception of gamma globulin, which is formed in lymph nodes and lymphoid tissue), are synthesized by the liver. They play an important role in preserving blood volume and pressure by maintaining plasma oncotic pressure. The liver also synthesizes several nonessential amino acids and serum enzymes, including aspartate aminotransferase (AST; previously SGOT), alanine aminotransferase (ALT; previously SGPT), lactate dehydrogenase (LDH), and alkaline phosphatase.

Fats. Ingested fat absorbed by lacteals in the intestinal villi enters the liver circulation through the lymphatics, primarily as triglycerides. In the liver, the triglycerides can be hydrolyzed to glycerol and free fatty acids and used to produce metabolic energy called adenosine triphosphate (ATP), or they can be released into the bloodstream bound to proteins (lipoproteins). The lipoproteins are carried by the blood to adipose cells for storage. The liver also synthesizes phospholipids and cholesterol, which are needed for the hepatic production of bile salts, steroid hormones, components of plasma membranes, and other special molecules.

Metabolic Detoxification

The liver alters exogenous and endogenous chemicals (e.g., drugs), foreign molecules, and hormones to make them less toxic or less biologically active. This process, called metabolic detoxification or biotransformation, diminishes intestinal or renal tubular reabsorption of potentially toxic substances and facilitates their intestinal and renal excretion. In this way alcohol, barbiturates, amphetamines, steroids, and hormones (including estrogens, aldosterone, antidiuretic hormone, and testosterone) are metabolized or detoxified, preventing excessive accumulation and adverse effects. Although metabolic detoxification is usually protective, the end products of metabolic detoxification sometimes become toxins (*Did You Know?* Paracetamol [Acetaminophen] and Acute Liver Failure) or active metabolites (see Chapter 4). Toxins of alcohol metabolism, for example, are acetaldehyde and hydrogen, which can damage the liver's ability to function.

Storage of Minerals and Vitamins

The liver stores certain vitamins and minerals, including iron and copper, in times of excessive intake and releases them in times of need. The liver can store vitamins B_{12} and D for several months and vitamin A for several years. The liver also stores vitamins E and K. Iron is stored in the liver as ferritin, an iron-protein complex, and is released as needed for red blood cell production. Common tests of liver function are listed in Table 37.3.

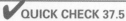

QUICK CHECK 37.5
1. Where does blood in the hepatic portal vein originate?
2. What is the function of hepatocytes?
3. Trace the route of bile salts and acids from formation to recycling.
4. What are the sources of the two types of bilirubin?

Gallbladder

The gallbladder is a saclike organ on the inferior surface of the liver (Fig. 37.19). Its primary function is to store and concentrate bile between meals.[10] During the interdigestive period, bile flows from the liver through the right or left hepatic duct into the common hepatic duct and meets resistance at the closed sphincter of Oddi (duodenal papilla), which controls flow into the duodenum and prevents backflow of duodenal contents into the pancreatobiliary system. Bile then flows through the cystic duct into the gallbladder, where it is concentrated and stored. The mucosa of the gallbladder wall readily absorbs water and electrolytes, leaving a high concentration of bile salts, bile pigments, and cholesterol. The gallbladder holds about 90 ml of bile.

Within 30 minutes after eating, the gallbladder begins to contract, forcing stored bile through the cystic duct and into the common bile duct. The sphincter of Oddi relaxes, and bile flows into the duodenum through the major duodenal papilla. During the cephalic and gastric phases of digestion, gallbladder contraction is mediated by cholinergic branches of the vagus nerve. Hormonal regulation of gallbladder contraction is derived primarily from the release of cholecystokinin secreted by the duodenal and jejunal mucosa in the presence of fat. Vasoactive intestinal peptide, pancreatic polypeptide, and sympathetic nerve stimulation relax the gallbladder.

TABLE 37.3   Common Tests of Liver Function

Test	Normal Value	Interpretation
Serum Enzymes		
Alkaline phosphatase	35-150 units/L	Increases with biliary obstruction and cholestatic hepatitis
Gamma-glutamyl transpeptidase	Male: 12-38 units/L Female: 9-31 units/L	Increases with biliary obstruction and cholestatic hepatitis
Aspartate aminotransferase (previously serum glutamate-oxaloacetate transaminase)	Male: 8-40 units/L Female: 6-34 units/L	Increases with hepatocellular injury and injury in other tissues (e.g., skeletal and cardiac muscle)
Alanine aminotransferase (previously serum glutamate-pyruvate transaminase)	Male: 10-40 units/L Female: 9-32 units/L	Increases with hepatocellular injury and necrosis
Lactate dehydrogenase	110-220 units/L	Isoenzyme LD5 is elevated with hypoxic and primary liver injury
5'-Nucleotidase	2-11 units/L	Increases with increase in alkaline phosphatase and cholestatic disorders
Bilirubin Metabolism		
Serum bilirubin		
Unconjugated (indirect)	0.1-1 mg/dL	Increases with hemolysis (lysis of red blood cells)
Conjugated (direct)	0.1-0.4 mg/dL	Increases with hepatocellular injury or obstruction
TOTAL	<1 mg/dL	Increases with biliary obstruction
Urine bilirubin	0	Increases with biliary obstruction
Urine urobilinogen	0-4 mg/24 hr	Increases with hemolysis or shunting of portal blood flow
Serum Proteins		
Albumin	3.5-5.5 g/dL	Reduced with hepatocellular injury
Globulin	2-4 g/dL	Increases with hepatitis
TOTAL	6-7 g/dL	
Albumin/globulin ratio	1.5:1 to 2.5:1	Ratio reverses with chronic hepatitis or other chronic liver disease
Transferrin	250-300 mcg/dL	Liver damage with decreased values, iron deficiency with increased values
Alpha fetoprotein	6-20 ng/mL	Elevated values in primary hepatocellular carcinoma
Blood-Clotting Functions		
Prothrombin time	10-13 sec or 90%-100% of control	Increases with chronic liver disease (cirrhosis) or vitamin K deficiency
Partial thromboplastin time	22-37 sec	Increases with severe liver disease or heparin therapy
Bromsulphthalein excretion	<6% retention in 45 min	Increased retention with hepatocellular injury

Exocrine Pancreas

The pancreas is approximately 20 cm long. Its head is tucked into the curve of the duodenum, and its tail touches the spleen. The body of the pancreas lies deep in the abdomen, behind the stomach (see Figs. 37.1 and 37.19). The pancreas is unique in that it has both endocrine and exocrine functions. The endocrine pancreas secretes hormones—insulin, glucagon, somatostatin, and pancreatic polypeptide—from cells in the pancreatic islets (see Chapter 20).

The exocrine pancreas is composed of acinar cells that secrete enzymes and networks of ducts that secrete alkaline fluids. Both have important digestive functions. The acinar cells are organized into spherical lobules, called acini, around small secretory ducts (see Fig. 37.19). Secretions drain into a system of ducts that leads to the pancreatic duct (Wirsung duct), which empties into the common bile duct at the ampulla of Vater, and then into the duodenum. In some individuals, an accessory duct (the duct of Santorini) branches off the pancreatic duct and drains directly into the duodenum at the minor duodenal papilla.

Arterial blood is supplied to the pancreas by branches of the celiac and superior mesenteric arteries (see Fig. 37.6). Venous blood leaves the head of the pancreas through tributaries to the portal vein, and the body and tail are drained through the splenic vein. All hormonal pancreatic secretions also pass through the hepatic portal vein into the liver.

Pancreatic innervation arises from parasympathetic neurons of the vagus nerve. These fibers activate postganglionic fibers, which stimulate enzymatic and hormonal secretion. Sympathetic postganglionic fibers from the celiac and superior mesenteric plexuses innervate the blood vessels, cause vasoconstriction, and inhibit pancreatic secretion.

The aqueous secretions of the exocrine pancreas are isotonic and contain potassium, sodium, bicarbonate, and chloride. The highly alkaline pancreatic juice neutralizes the acidic chyme that enters the duodenum from the stomach and provides the alkaline medium needed for the actions of digestive enzymes and intestinal absorption of fat.

In the pancreas, transport of water and electrolytes through the ductal epithelium involves both active and passive mechanisms. The ductal cells actively transport hydrogen into the blood and bicarbonate into the duct lumen. Potassium and chloride are secreted by diffusion according to changes in electrochemical potential gradients. As the secretion flows down the duct, water is osmotically transported into the juice until it becomes isosmotic. At low flow rates bicarbonate is exchanged passively for chloride, but at higher flow rates there is less time for this exchange and bicarbonate concentration increases. Because eating stimulates the flow of pancreatic juice, the juice is most alkaline when it needs to be: during digestion.

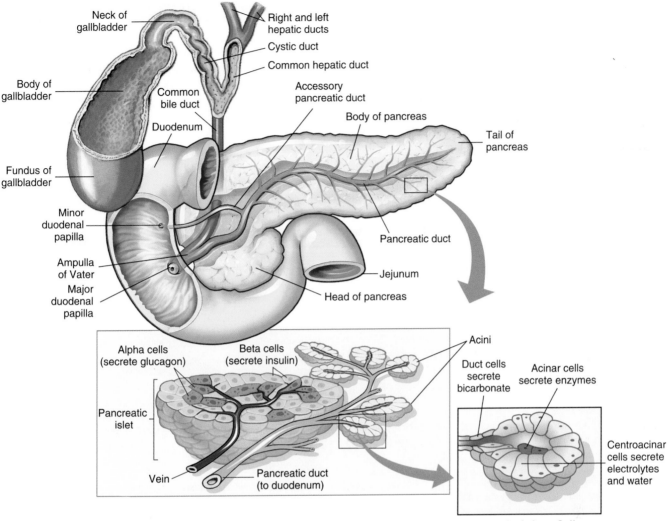

FIGURE 37.19 Associated Structures of the Gallbladder, Pancreas, and Pancreatic Acinar Cells and Duct. (Modified from Thibodeau GA, Patton KT: *Anatomy & physiology*, ed 6, St Louis, 2007, Mosby.)

The pancreatic enzymes can hydrolyze proteins (proteases), carbohydrates (amylases), and fats (lipases) (see Fig. 37.10). The proteolytic (protein-digesting) enzymes include trypsin, chymotrypsin, carboxypeptidase, and elastase. These enzymes are secreted in their inactive forms—that is, as trypsinogen, chymotrypsinogen, procarboxypeptidase, and proelastase, respectively—to protect the pancreas from the digestive effects of its own enzymes. For further protection, the pancreas produces **trypsin inhibitor**, which prevents the activation of proteolytic enzymes while they are in the pancreas. Once in the duodenum, the inactive forms (proenzymes) are activated by **enterokinase**, an enzyme secreted by the duodenal mucosa. Trypsinogen is the first proenzyme to be activated. Its conversion to trypsin stimulates the conversion of chymotrypsinogen to chymotrypsin and procarboxypeptidase to carboxypeptidase. Each of these enzymes cleaves specific peptide bonds to reduce polypeptides to smaller peptides.

Secretion of the aqueous and enzymatic components of pancreatic juice is controlled by hormonal and vagal stimuli. Secretin stimulates the acinar and duct cells to secrete the bicarbonate-rich fluid that neutralizes chyme and prepares it for enzymatic digestion. As chyme enters the duodenum, its acidity (pH of 4.5 or less) stimulates the S cells (secretin-producing cells) of the duodenum to release secretin, which is absorbed by the intestine and delivered

to the pancreas in the bloodstream. In the pancreas, secretin causes ductal and acinar cells to release alkaline fluid. Secretin also inhibits the actions of gastrin, thereby decreasing gastric hydrochloric acid secretion and motility. The overall effect is to neutralize the contents of the duodenum.

Enzymatic secretion follows, stimulated by cholecystokinin, which activates acetylcholine (ACh) from the vagus nerve and release of ACh from pancreatic stellate cells. Cholecystokinin is released in the duodenum in response to the essential amino acids and fatty acids already present in chyme. Once in the small intestine, activated pancreatic enzymes inhibit the release of more cholecystokinin and ACh. This feedback mechanism inhibits the secretion of more pancreatic enzymes. Pancreatic polypeptide is released after eating and inhibits postprandial pancreatic exocrine secretion. (See Table 37.1 for a summary of hormonal stimulation of pancreatic secretions.) Selected tests of pancreatic function are listed in Table 37.4.

✔ **QUICK CHECK 37.6**
1. What is the function of the gallbladder?
2. How does the endocrine pancreas differ from the exocrine pancreas?

TABLE 37.4   Selected Tests of Pancreatic Function

Test	Normal Value	Clinical Significance
Serum amylase	25-125 units/mL	Elevated levels with pancreatic inflammation
Serum lipase	20-240 units/mL	Elevated levels with pancreatic inflammation (may be elevated with other conditions; differentiates with amylase isoenzyme study)
Urine amylase	35-260 Somogyi units/hr	Elevated levels with pancreatic inflammation
Secretin test	Volume: 1.8 ml/kg/hr Bicarbonate concentration: >80 mEq/L Bicarbonate output: >10 mEq/L/30 sec	Decreased volume with pancreatic disease as secretin stimulates pancreatic secretion
Stool fat	2-5 g/24 hr	Measures fatty acids; decreased pancreatic lipase increases stool fat (malabsorption)
Fecal elastase	>200 μg/g of stool	Decreased in pancreatic insufficiency

GERIATRIC CONSIDERATIONS

Aging & the Digestive System

Age-related changes in digestive function vary among individuals and within organ systems. The following are some of the changes that can occur.

Oral Cavity and Esophagus
- Tooth enamel and dentin deteriorate, so cavities are more likely.
- Teeth are lost as a result of periodontal disease and brittle roots that break easily.
- Taste buds decline in number.
- Sense of smell diminishes.
- Salivary secretion decreases.

These changes may make eating less pleasurable, reduce the appetite, and result in food not being sufficiently chewed or lubricated; therefore swallowing is difficult (dysphagia).

Stomach
- Gastric motility, blood flow, and the volume and acid content of gastric juice may be reduced, particularly with gastric atrophy, and gastric emptying may be delayed.
- The protective mucosal barrier declines.

Intestines
- Changes in the composition of the intestinal microbiota result in increased susceptibility to disease.
- The size of Peyer patches and degree of mucosal immunity decline, resulting in an increased risk for infection and inflammation.

- The brain-gut axis (bidirectional neuroendocrine communication) may be disrupted, and enteric neurons may degenerate, with changes in GI motility, secretion, and absorption, as well as the elder person's appetite and overall nutritional status.
- Intestinal villi may become shorter and more convoluted, with diminished reparative capacity.
- Intestinal absorption, motility, and blood flow may decrease, prolonging transit time and altering nutrient and drug absorption.
- Rectal muscle mass decreases, and the anal sphincter weakens.
- Constipation, fecal impaction, and fecal incontinence may develop; these are related to immobility, a low-fiber diet, and changes in the enteric nervous system's structure and functions.

Liver
- Decreased hepatic regeneration leads to a decrease in the size and weight of the liver.
- The ability to detoxify drugs decreases.
- Blood flow decreases, influencing the efficiency of drug metabolism.

Pancreas and Gallbladder
- Fibrosis, fatty acid deposits, and pancreatic atrophy occur.
- Secretion of digestive enzymes, particularly proteolytic enzymes, decreases.
- No changes occur in the gallbladder and bile ducts, but the prevalence of gallstones and cholecystitis is increased.

Data from Soenen S et al: *Curr Opin Clin Nutr Metab Care*, 19(1):12-18, 2016; Tan JL et al: *Drugs Aging* 32(12):999-1008, 2015.

SUMMARY REVIEW

The Gastrointestinal Tract
1. The major functions of the GI tract are the mechanical and chemical breakdown of food and the absorption of digested nutrients.
2. Except for swallowing and defecation, which are controlled voluntarily, the functions of the GI tract are controlled by extrinsic and intrinsic autonomic nerves and intestinal hormones.
3. The GI tract is a hollow tube that extends from the mouth to the anus.
4. The walls of the GI tract have four layers. From the inside out they are the mucosa, submucosa, muscularis, and serosa.
5. Digestion begins in the mouth, with chewing and salivation. The digestive component of saliva is α-amylase, which initiates carbohydrate digestion.

6. The esophagus is a muscular tube that transports food from the mouth to the stomach. The tunica muscularis in the upper part of the esophagus is striated muscle, and that in the lower part is smooth muscle.
7. Food is propelled through the esophagus by peristalsis (waves of sequential relaxations and contractions of the layers of muscles).
8. Swallowing is controlled by the swallowing center in the medulla of the brain. The two phases of swallowing are the oropharyngeal phase (voluntary swallowing) and the esophageal phase (involuntary swallowing).
9. The lower esophageal sphincter opens to admit swallowed food into the stomach and then closes to prevent regurgitation of food back into the esophagus.

10. The stomach is a baglike structure that secretes digestive juices, mixes and stores food, and propels partially digested food (chyme) through the pylorus into the duodenum.

11. The vagus nerve stimulates gastric (stomach) secretion and motility.

12. The hormones gastrin and motilin stimulate gastric emptying; the hormones secretin and cholecystokinin delay gastric emptying.

13. The stomach secretes large volumes of gastric secretions, including acid, pepsinogen, mucus, enzymes, hormones, intrinsic factor (needed for vitamin B_{12} absorption), and gastroferrin (facilitates absorption of iron).

14. The three phases of gastric secretion by the stomach are the cephalic phase (anticipation and swallowing), the gastric phase (food in the stomach), and the intestinal phase (chyme in the intestine).

15. Parietal cells produce hydrochloric acid, which dissolves food fibers, kills microorganisms, and activates the enzyme pepsin. Acid secretion is stimulated by the vagus nerve, gastrin, and histamine and is inhibited by sympathetic stimulation and intestinal hormones.

16. Chief cells in the stomach secrete pepsinogen, which is converted to pepsin in the acidic environment created by hydrochloric acid. Pepsin breaks down proteins and forms polypeptides.

17. Mucus is secreted throughout the stomach and protects the stomach wall from acid and digestive enzymes.

18. The small intestine is 5 meters long and has three segments: the duodenum, jejunum, and ileum.

19. The peritoneum is a double layer of membranous tissue. The visceral layer covers the abdominal organs, and the parietal layer extends along the abdominal wall. The peritoneal cavity is the space between the two layers. The duodenum lies behind the peritoneum (retroperitoneal).

20. The ileocecal valve connects the small and large intestines and prevents reflux into the small intestine.

21. Villi are small fingerlike projections that extend from the small intestinal mucosa and increase its absorptive surface area.

22. Enzymes secreted by the small intestine (maltase, sucrase, lactase), pancreatic enzymes, and bile salts act in the small intestine to digest proteins, carbohydrates, and fats.

23. Digested substances are absorbed across the intestinal wall and then transported to the liver, where they are metabolized further. Carbohydrate and protein components move into villus capillaries and to the liver through the hepatic portal vein.

24. Bile salts emulsify and hydrolyze fats and incorporate them into water-soluble micelles. The fat content of the micelles diffuses through the epithelium into lacteals (lymphatic ducts) in the villi. From there, fats flow into lymphatics and into the systemic circulation, which delivers them to the liver.

25. Minerals and water-soluble vitamins are absorbed by both active and passive transport throughout the small intestine.

26. Contractions of the circular muscles (segmentation) mix the chyme, and peristaltic movements created by longitudinal muscles propel the chyme along the intestinal tract.

27. The ileogastric reflex inhibits gastric motility when the ileum is distended. The intestinointestinal reflex inhibits intestinal motility when one intestinal segment is overdistended. The gastroileal reflex increases intestinal motility when gastric motility increases.

28. The large intestine consists of the cecum, appendix, colon (ascending, transverse, descending, and sigmoid), rectum, and anal canal.

29. The teniae coli are three bands of longitudinal muscle that extend the length of the colon and give it a gathered appearance. Haustra are pouches of colon formed with alternating contraction and relaxation of the circular muscles.

30. The mucosa of the large intestine contains mucus-secreting cells and mucosal folds, but no villi.

31. The large intestine massages the fecal mass and absorbs water and electrolytes.

32. Distention of the ileum with chyme causes the gastrocolic reflex, or the mass propulsion of feces to the rectum.

33. Defecation is stimulated when the rectum is distended with feces. The tonically contracted internal anal sphincter relaxes, and if the voluntarily regulated external sphincter relaxes, defecation occurs.

34. The immune system of the GI tract consists of Paneth cells, which produce defensins and other antimicrobial peptides and lysozymes; and the lymph nodes of Peyer patches, which contain lymphocytes, plasma cells, and macrophages.

35. The largest number of intestinal bacteria (intestinal microbiome) is in the colon. The most numerous anaerobes are *Bacteroides* and *Firmicutes*. Intestinal bacteria are important for metabolism of bile salts, metabolism of selected drugs and hormones, destruction of pathogens, and prevention of pathogen colonization.

36. The intestinal tract is sterile at birth and becomes totally colonized within 3 to 4 weeks.

37. The splanchnic blood flow provides blood to the esophagus, stomach, small and large intestines, gallbladder, pancreas, and spleen.

Accessory Organs of Digestion

1. The liver, gallbladder, and exocrine pancreas secrete substances necessary for digestion. These secretions flow through an opening guarded by the sphincter of Oddi.

2. The liver sits under the diaphragm. It has digestive, metabolic, hematologic, vascular, and immunologic functions.

3. The liver is divided into the right and left lobes and is supported by the falciform, round, and coronary ligaments.

4. Plates of hepatocytes, which are the functional cells of the liver, together form anatomic units called liver lobules.

5. Hepatocytes synthesize bile and secrete it into the bile canaliculi, which are small channels between the hepatocytes. The bile canaliculi drain bile into the common bile duct and then into the duodenum through an opening called the major duodenal papilla (sphincter of Oddi).

6. Sinusoids are capillaries located between the plates of hepatocytes. Blood from the portal vein and hepatic artery flows through the sinusoids to a central vein in each lobule and then to the hepatic vein and inferior vena cava.

7. Kupffer cells, which are part of the mononuclear phagocyte system, line the sinusoids and destroy microorganisms in sinusoidal blood; they are important in bilirubin production and lipid metabolism.

8. The liver produces 700 to 1200 mL of bile per day. Bile is made up of bile salts, cholesterol, bilirubin, electrolytes, and water.

9. The primary bile acids are synthesized from cholesterol by the hepatocytes. The primary acids are then conjugated to form bile salts. The secondary bile acids are the product of bile salt deconjugation by bacteria in the intestinal lumen.

10. Most bile salts and acids are recycled. The absorption of bile salts and acids from the terminal ileum and their return to the liver are known as the enterohepatic circulation of bile.

11. Bilirubin is a pigment liberated by the lysis of aged red blood cells in the liver and spleen. Unconjugated bilirubin is fat soluble and can cross cell membranes. Unconjugated bilirubin is converted to water-soluble, conjugated bilirubin by hepatocytes and is secreted with bile.

12. The liver produces clotting factors and can store a large volume of blood.

13. The liver plays a major role in the metabolism of carbohydrates, proteins, and fats and stores minerals, vitamin B_{12}, and fat-soluble vitamins.

14. The liver metabolically transforms or detoxifies hormones, toxic substances, and drugs to less active substances. This process is known as metabolic detoxification.

15. The gallbladder is a saclike organ located on the inferior surface of the liver. The gallbladder stores bile between meals and ejects it when chyme enters the duodenum.

16. Stimulated by cholecystokinin, the gallbladder contracts and forces bile through the cystic duct and into the common bile duct. The sphincter of Oddi relaxes, enabling bile to flow through the major duodenal papilla into the duodenum.

17. The pancreas is a gland located behind the stomach. The endocrine pancreas produces hormones (glucagon, insulin) that facilitate the formation and cellular uptake of glucose. The exocrine pancreas secretes an alkaline solution and the enzymes (trypsin, chymotrypsin, carboxypeptidase, α-amylase, lipase) that digest proteins, carbohydrates, and fats.

18. Secretin stimulates pancreatic secretion of alkaline fluid, and cholecystokinin and acetylcholine stimulate secretion of enzymes. Pancreatic secretions originate in acini and ducts of the pancreas and empty into the duodenum through the common bile duct or an accessory duct that opens directly into the duodenum.

KEY TERMS

Acini, 874
Ampulla of Vater, 874
Antrum, 861
Ascending colon, 867
Bile, 871
Bile acid pool, 872
Bile acid–dependent fraction, 871
Bile acid–independent fraction, 871
Bile canaliculi, 871
Bile salt, 871
Bilirubin, 872
Body, 861
Brush border, 865
Cardiac orifice, 861
Cecum, 867
Chief cell, 864
Cholecystokinin, 862
Choleresis, 872
Choleretic agent, 872
Chyme, 861
Colon, 867
Common bile duct, 871
Conjugated bilirubin, 872
Crypts of Lieberkühn, 865
Cystic duct, 873
Deamination, 873
Defecation reflex (rectosphincteric reflex), 869
Descending colon, 867
Disse space, 871
Duodenum, 864
Enteric (intramural) plexus, 858

Enterocyte, 865
Enterohepatic circulation, 871
Enterokinase, 875
Esophageal (involuntary) phase, 860
Esophagus, 859
Exocrine pancreas, 874
External anal sphincter (anus), 867
Fecal mass, 867
Feces, 869
Fundus, 861
Gallbladder, 873
Gastric emptying, 863
Gastric gland, 863
Gastrin, 862
Gastrocolic reflex, 867
Gastroileal reflex, 867
Gastrointestinal tract (alimentary canal), 858
Glisson capsule, 869
Gut-associated lymphoid tissue (GALT), 869
Haustrum (pl., haustra), 867
Hepatic artery, 870
Hepatic portal vein, 870
Hepatic vein, 871
Hepatocyte, 870
Ileocecal valve (sphincter), 864
Ileogastric reflex, 865
Ileum, 864
Internal anal sphincter, 867
Intestinointestinal reflex, 865
Intrinsic factor, 863
Jejunum, 864

Kupffer cell (tissue macrophage), 871
Lacteal, 865
Lamina propria, 865
Large intestine, 867
Liver, 869
Liver lobule, 870
Lower esophageal sphincter (cardiac sphincter), 860
Major duodenal papilla (sphincter of Oddi), 871
Mastication (chewing), 858
Mesentery, 864
Metabolic detoxification (biotransformation), 873
Microvillus (pl., microvilli), 865
Motilin, 862
Mouth, 858
Mucosal barrier, 864
Myenteric (Auerbach) plexus, 861
Natural killer cell (pit cell), 871
Oropharyngeal (voluntary) phase, 860
Pancreas, 874
Pancreatic duct (Wirsung duct), 874
Paneth cell, 869
Pepsin, 864
Parietal cell, 863
Peristalsis, 865
Peritoneal cavity, 864
Peritoneum, 864
Peyer patch, 869
Primary bile acid, 872

Primary peristalsis, 860
Pyloric sphincter, 861
Pylorus (gastroduodenal junction), 861
Rectosigmoid canal, 867
Rectum, 869
Retropulsion, 862
Rugae, 861
S cell, 875
Saliva, 859
Salivary α-amylase (ptyalin), 859
Salivary gland, 859
Secondary bile acid, 872
Secondary peristalsis, 860
Secretin, 862
Segmentation, 865
Sigmoid colon, 867
Sinusoid, 870
Small intestine, 864
Splanchnic (visceral) blood flow, 869
Stellate cell, 871
Stomach, 861
Submucosal (Meissner) plexus, 861
Swallowing, 860
Teniae coli, 867
Transverse colon, 867
Trypsin inhibitor, 875
Unconjugated bilirubin, 872
Upper esophageal sphincter, 860
Urobilinogen, 872
Valsalva maneuver, 869
Vermiform appendix, 867
Villus (pl., villi), 865

REFERENCES

1. Woodland P, et al: The neurophysiology of the esophagus, *Ann N Y Acad Sci* 1300:53-70, 2013.
2. Hellström PM, et al: The physiology of gastric emptying, *Best Pract Res Clin Anaesthesiol* 20(3):397-407, 2006.
3. Chu S, Schuberft ML: Gastric secretion, *Curr Opin Gastroenterol* 28(6):587-593, 2012.

4. Niv Y, Fraser GM: The alkaline tide phenomenon, *J Clin Gastroenterol* 35(1):5-8, 2002.
5. Kumral D, Zfass AM: Gut movements: a review of the physiology of gastrointestinal transit, *Dig Dis Sci* 63(10):2500-2506, 2018.
6. Kooij IA, et al: The immunology of the vermiform appendix: a review of the literature, *Clin Exp Immunol* 186(1):1-9, 2016.
7. Bobadilla JL: Mesenteric ischemia, *Surg Clin North Am* 93(4):925-940, ix, 2013.

8. Ahluwalia B, Magnusson MK, Öhman L: Mucosal immune system of the gastrointestinal tract: maintaining balance between the good and the bad, *Scand J Gastroenterol* 52(11):1185-1193, 2017.
9. Cani PD: Human gut microbiome: hopes, threats and promises, *Gut* 67(9):1716-1725, 2018.
10. Housset C, et al: Functions of the gallbladder, *Compr Physiol* 6(3):1549-1577, 2016.

38

Alterations of Digestive Function

Sue E. Huether

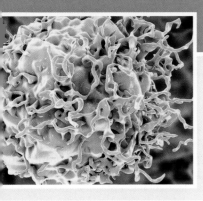

EVOLVE WEBSITE

CHAPTER OUTLINE

Disorders of the gastrointestinal (GI) tract disrupt one or more of its structures and functions. The GI tract is a continuous, hollow organ that extends from the mouth to the anus. It includes the esophagus, stomach, small intestine, large intestine, and rectum. The accessory organs of digestion include the salivary glands, liver, gallbladder, and pancreas. Structural and neural abnormalities can slow, obstruct, or accelerate the movement of intestinal contents at any level of the GI tract. Inflammatory and ulcerative conditions of the GI wall disrupt secretion, motility, and absorption. Inflammation or obstruction of the liver, pancreas, or gallbladder can alter metabolism and result in local and systemic symptoms. Many clinical manifestations of GI tract disorders are nonspecific and can be caused by a variety of impairments.

DISORDERS OF THE GASTROINTESTINAL TRACT

Clinical Manifestations of Gastrointestinal Dysfunction

Anorexia

Anorexia is the lack of a desire to eat despite physiologic stimuli that would normally produce hunger. This nonspecific symptom is often associated with nausea, abdominal pain, diarrhea, psychological stress, and weight loss. Side effects of drugs, cancer, heart disease, renal disease, and liver disease are often accompanied by anorexia.

Vomiting

Vomiting (emesis) is the forceful emptying of stomach and intestinal contents (chyme) through the mouth. The vomiting center lies in the medulla oblongata. Stimuli initiating the vomiting reflex include severe pain; distention of the stomach or duodenum; the presence of ipecac or copper salts in the duodenum; stimulation of the vestibular system through the eighth cranial nerve (motion sickness); side effects of many drugs; torsion or trauma affecting the ovaries, testes, uterus, bladder, or kidney; motion; and activation of the in the medulla (e.g., morphine). Nausea and retching (dry heaves) are distinct events that usually precede vomiting. Nausea is a subjective experience associated with various conditions, including abnormal pain and labyrinthine stimulation (i.e., spinning movement). Specific neural pathways have not been identified, but hypersalivation and tachycardia are common associated symptoms. Retching is the muscular event of vomiting without the expulsion of vomitus.

Vomiting begins with deep inspiration. The glottis closes, the intrathoracic pressure falls, and the esophagus becomes distended. Simultaneously, the abdominal muscles contract, creating a pressure gradient from abdomen to thorax. The lower esophageal sphincter (LES) and body of the stomach relax. The duodenum and antrum of the stomach produce reverse peristalsis, and the pressure gradient forces chyme from the stomach and duodenum up into the esophagus. Because the upper esophageal sphincter is closed, chyme does not enter the mouth. When the stomach is full of gastric contents, the diaphragm is forced high into the thoracic cavity by strong contractions of the abdominal muscles. The higher intrathoracic pressure forces the upper esophageal sphincter to open, and chyme is expelled from the mouth. Then the stomach relaxes, and the upper part of the esophagus contracts, forcing the remaining chyme back into the stomach. The lower esophageal sphincter then closes. The cycle is repeated if there is a volume of chyme remaining in the stomach. A diffuse sympathetic discharge causes the tachycardia, tachypnea, and diaphoresis that accompany retching and vomiting. The parasympathetic system mediates copious salivation, increased gastric motility, and relaxation of the upper and lower esophageal sphincters.

Spontaneous vomiting not preceded by nausea or retching is called **projectile vomiting**. It is caused by direct stimulation of the vomiting center by neurologic lesions (e.g., increased intracranial pressure, tumors, or aneurysms) involving the brainstem, or it can be a symptom of GI obstruction (pyloric stenosis). The metabolic consequences of vomiting are fluid, electrolyte, and acid-base disturbances including hyponatremia, hypokalemia, hypochloremia, and metabolic alkalosis (see Chapter 5).

Constipation

Constipation is difficult or infrequent defecation. It is a common problem, particularly among the elderly, and usually means a decrease in the number of bowel movements per week, hard stools, and difficult evacuation. The definition must be individually determined because normal bowel habits range from one to three evacuations per day to one per week. Constipation is not significant until it causes health risks or impairs the individual's quality of life.

PATHOPHYSIOLOGY Constipation can occur as a primary or secondary condition. Primary constipation is generally classified into three categories. *Normal transit (functional) constipation* involves a normal rate of stool passage but difficulty with stool evacuation. *Functional constipation* is associated with a sedentary lifestyle, low-residue diet (habitual consumption of highly refined foods), or a low fluid intake. *Slow-transit constipation* involves impaired colonic motor activity, with infrequent bowel movements, straining to defecate, mild abdominal distention, and palpable stool in the sigmoid colon.

Secondary constipation can be caused by diet, medications, or neurogenic disorders (e.g., stroke, Parkinson disease, spinal cord lesions, multiple sclerosis, Hirschsprung disease) in which neural pathways or neurotransmitters are altered and colon transit time is delayed. Rectal fissures, strictures, or hemorrhoids also may cause constipation. Antacids containing calcium carbonate or aluminum hydroxide, anticholinergics, iron, and bismuth tend to inhibit bowel motility. *Opioid-induced constipation* is caused by drugs that activate μ-opioid receptors in the gut and slow transit time. Endocrine or metabolic disorders associated with constipation include hypothyroidism, diabetes mellitus, hypokalemia, and hypercalcemia. Pelvic hiatal hernia (herniation of the bowel through the floor of the pelvis), diverticula, irritable bowel syndrome (constipation predominant), and pregnancy are associated with constipation. Aging may result in decreased mobility, changes in neuromuscular function, use of medications, and comorbid medical conditions causing constipation. Constipation as a notable change in bowel habits can be an indication of colorectal cancer.

CLINICAL MANIFESTATIONS Indicators of constipation include two of the following for at least 3 months: (1) straining with defecation at least 25% of the time; (2) lumpy or hard stools at least 25% of the time; (3) sensation of incomplete emptying at least 25% of the time; (4) manual maneuvers to facilitate stool evacuation for at least 25% of defecations; and (5) fewer than three bowel movements per week.[1] Changes in bowel evacuation patterns, such as less frequent defecation, smaller stool volume, hard stools, difficulty passing stools (straining), or a feeling of bowel fullness and discomfort, require investigation. Fecal impaction (hard, dry stool retained in the rectum) is associated with rectal bleeding, abdominal or cramping pain, nausea and vomiting,

weight loss, and episodes of diarrhea. Straining to evacuate stool may cause engorgement of the hemorrhoidal veins and hemorrhoidal disease or thrombosis with rectal pain, bleeding, and itching. Passage of hard stools can cause painful anal fissures.

EVALUATION AND TREATMENT The history, current use of medications, physical examination, and stool diaries provide precise clues regarding the nature of constipation. The individual's description of frequency, stool consistency, associated pain, and presence of blood or whether evacuation was stimulated by enemas or cathartics (laxatives) is important. Palpation may disclose colonic distention, masses, and tenderness. Digital examination of the rectum and anorectal manometry are performed to assess sphincter tone and detect anal lesions. Colonic transit time and imaging techniques can assist in identifying the cause of constipation. Colonoscopy is used to visualize the lumen directly.

The treatment for constipation is to manage the underlying cause or disease for each individual. Management of constipation usually consists of bowel retraining, in which the individual establishes a satisfactory bowel evacuation routine without becoming preoccupied with bowel movements. The individual also may need to engage in moderate exercise, drink more fluids, and increase fiber intake. Fiber supplements, stool softeners, and laxative agents are useful for some individuals. Enemas can be used to establish a bowel routine, but they should not be used habitually. Biofeedback may be beneficial in some instances for forming new bowel evacuation habits. When there is failure to respond to dietary or medical therapies, surgery (colectomy) is considered as a last resort.

Diarrhea

Diarrhea is the presence of loose, watery stools. Acute diarrhea is more than three loose stools developing within 24 hours and lasting less than 14 days. Persistent diarrhea lasts longer than 14 to 30 days, and chronic diarrhea lasts longer than 4 weeks. Diarrhea can have high rates of morbidity and mortality in children younger than 5 years of age, particularly in developing countries (see Chapter 39) and in the elderly. Many factors determine stool volume, including water content of the colon, diet, the presence of nonabsorbed food, nonabsorbable material, and intestinal secretions. Stool volume in the normal adult averages less than 200 g/day. Stool volume in children depends on age and size. An infant may pass up to 100 g/day. The adult intestine processes approximately 9 L of luminal contents per day: 2 L are ingested. and the remaining 7 L consist of intestinal secretions. Of this volume, most of the fluid is absorbed: (7 to 8 L) in the small intestine and a smaller amount (1 to 2 L) in the colon. Normally, approximately 150 ml of water is excreted daily in the stool.

PATHOPHYSIOLOGY Diarrhea in which the volume of feces is increased is called *large-volume diarrhea*. It generally is caused by excessive amounts of water or secretions or both in the intestines. *Small-volume diarrhea*, in which the volume of feces is not increased, usually results from excessive intestinal motility and may be caused by an inflammatory disorder of the intestine, such as ulcerative colitis, Crohn disease, or microscopic colitis, but also can result from colon cancer or fecal impaction.

The three major mechanisms of diarrhea are osmotic, secretory, and motile.

1. **Osmotic diarrhea.** A nonabsorbable substance in the intestine draws excess water into the intestine and increases stool weight and volume, producing large-volume diarrhea. Causes include lactase and pancreatic enzyme deficiency; excessive ingestion of synthetic, nonabsorbable sugars; full-strength tube-feeding formulas; or dumping syndrome associated with gastric resection (see the Postgastrectomy Syndromes section).

2. **Secretory diarrhea.** Excessive mucosal secretion of fluid and electrolytes produces large-volume diarrhea. Infectious causes include viruses (e.g., rotavirus), bacterial enterotoxins (e.g., *Escherichia coli* and *Vibrio cholerae*), exotoxins from overgrowth of *Clostridium difficile* after antibiotic therapy, or small bowel bacterial overgrowth.

3. **Motility diarrhea** is caused by resection of the small intestine (short bowel syndrome), surgical bypass of an area of the intestine, fistula formation between loops of intestine, irritable bowel syndrome–diarrhea predominant, diabetic neuropathy, hyperthyroidism, and laxative abuse. Excessive motility decreases transit time and the opportunity for fluid absorption, resulting in diarrhea.

CLINICAL MANIFESTATIONS Diarrhea can be acute or chronic, depending on its cause. Systemic effects of prolonged diarrhea are dehydration, electrolyte imbalance (hyponatremia, hypokalemia), and weight loss. Manifestations of acute bacterial or viral infection include fever, with or without vomiting or cramping pain. Most infectious diarrhea usually lasts less than 2 weeks. The exceptions are *Clostridium difficile*, *Aeromonas*, or *Yersinia enterocolitica*.[2] Fever, cramping pain, and bloody stools accompany chronic diarrhea caused by inflammatory bowel disease or dysentery. Anal and perineal skin irritation can occur.

EVALUATION AND TREATMENT A thorough history is taken to document the onset, frequency, volume of stools, duration of diarrhea, and presence of blood in the stools. Malabsorption syndromes usually manifest steatorrhea (fat in the stool), bloating, and diarrhea. Exposure to contaminated food or water is indicated if the individual has traveled in foreign countries or areas where drinking water might be contaminated. Iatrogenic diarrhea is suggested if the individual has undergone abdominal radiation therapy, intestinal resection, or treatment with selected drugs (e.g., antibiotics, diuretics, antihypertensives, laxatives, anticoagulants or chemotherapy). Physical examination helps identify underlying systemic disease. Stool studies, abdominal imaging, endoscopy, and intestinal biopsies provide more specific data, particularly for persistent diarrhea.

Treatment for diarrhea includes restoration of fluid and electrolyte balance, administration of antimotility (e.g., loperamide) and/or water-absorbent (e.g., attapulgite and polycarbophil) medications, and treatment of causal factors. Natural bran and commercial preparations of psyllium are inexpensive and effective treatments for mild diarrhea. Probiotics can be useful for preventing and treating *Clostridium difficile*–associated diarrhea as an approach to restoring normal microflora in addition to antibiotic therapy. Fecal transplantation can be used for cases that are resistant to conventional therapies, particularly *Clostridium difficile*–associated diarrhea. Nutritional deficiencies need to be corrected in cases of chronic diarrhea or malabsorption.[3]

Abdominal Pain

Abdominal pain is the presenting symptom of a number of GI diseases and can be acute or chronic. The causal mechanisms of abdominal pain are *mechanical, inflammatory,* or *ischemic.* Generally, the abdominal organs are not sensitive to mechanical stimuli, such as cutting, tearing, or crushing. However, these organs are sensitive to stretching and distention, which activate nerve endings in both hollow and solid structures. Pain accompanies rapid distention rather than gradual distention. Traction on the peritoneum caused by adhesions, distention of the common bile duct, or forceful peristalsis resulting from intestinal obstruction causes pain because of increased tension. Capsules that surround solid organs, such as the liver and gallbladder, contain pain fibers that are stimulated by stretching if these organs swell. Abdominal pain may be generalized to the abdomen or localized to a particular abdominal quadrant. The nature of the pain is often described as sharp, dull, or colicky.

Abdominal pain is usually associated with tissue injury and inflammation. Biochemical mediators of the inflammatory response, such as histamine, bradykinin, and serotonin, stimulate organic nerve endings and produce abdominal pain. The edema and vascular congestion that accompany chemical, bacterial, or viral inflammation also cause painful stretching. Hindrance of blood flow from the distention of bowel obstruction or mesenteric vessel thrombosis produces the pain of ischemia, and increased concentrations of tissue metabolites stimulate pain receptors.

Abdominal pain can be parietal (somatic), visceral, or referred. **Parietal pain,** from the parietal peritoneum, is more localized and intense than visceral pain, which arises from the organs themselves. Parietal pain lateralizes because, at any particular point, the parietal peritoneum is innervated from only one side of the nervous system.

Visceral pain arises from a stimulus (distention, inflammation, ischemia) acting on an abdominal organ. Inflammatory mediators associated with chronic low-grade inflammation can cause pain hypersensitivity. The pain is usually poorly localized, diffuse, or vague with a radiating pattern because nerve endings in abdominal organs are sparse and multisegmented. Pain arising from the stomach, for example, is experienced as a sensation of fullness, cramping, or gnawing in the midepigastric area. **Referred pain** is visceral pain felt at some distance from a diseased or affected organ. It is usually well localized and is felt in the skin dermatomes or deeper tissues that share a central afferent pathway with the affected organ. For example, acute cholecystitis may have pain referred to the right shoulder or scapula.

Gastrointestinal Bleeding

Upper gastrointestinal bleeding is bleeding in the esophagus, stomach, or duodenum and is characterized by frank, bright red bleeding or dark, grainy digested blood ("coffee grounds") that has been affected by stomach acids (Table 38.1). Upper GI bleeding is commonly caused by bleeding varices (varicose veins) in the esophagus, peptic ulcers, arteriovenous malformations, or a Mallory-Weiss tear at the esophageal-gastric junction caused by severe retching. **Lower gastrointestinal bleeding,** or bleeding from the jejunum, ileum, colon, or rectum, can be caused by polyps, diverticulitis, inflammatory disease, cancer, or hemorrhoids. **Occult bleeding** is usually caused by slow, chronic blood loss that is not obvious and results in iron deficiency anemia as iron

TABLE 38.1 Presentations of Gastrointestinal Bleeding

Presentations	Definition
Acute Bleeding	
Hematemesis	Bloody vomitus; either fresh, bright red blood or dark grainy digested blood with "coffee grounds" appearance
Melena	Black, sticky, tarry, foul-smelling stools caused by digestion of blood in gastrointestinal tract; should be distinguished from black stools caused by dietary iron supplements, blackberries, or bismuth (e.g., Pepto-Bismol)
Hematochezia	Fresh, bright red blood passed from rectum
Occult Bleeding	Trace amounts of blood in normal-appearing stools or gastric secretions; detectable only with positive fecal occult blood test (guaiac test)

stores in the bone marrow are slowly depleted. Acute, severe GI bleeding is life-threatening, depending on the volume and rate of blood loss, associated diseases and the age of the individual, and the effectiveness of treatment.

Physiologic response to GI bleeding depends on the amount and rate of the loss (Fig. 38.1). Changes in blood pressure and heart rate are the best indicators of massive blood loss in the GI tract. During the early stages of blood volume depletion, the peripheral arteries and arterioles constrict to shunt blood to vital organs, including the brain. Signs of large-volume blood loss are postural hypotension (a drop in blood pressure that occurs with a change from the recumbent position to a sitting or upright position), lightheadedness, and loss of vision.

Tachycardia develops as a compensatory response to maintain cardiac output and tissue perfusion. If blood loss continues, hypovolemic shock develops (see Chapter 26). Diminished blood flow to the kidneys causes decreased urine output and may lead to oliguria (low urine output), tubular necrosis, and renal failure. Ultimately, insufficient cerebral and coronary blood flow causes irreversible anoxia and death.

The presentations of GI bleeding are summarized in Table 38.1. The accumulation of blood in the GI tract is irritating and increases peristalsis, causing vomiting or diarrhea, or both. If bleeding is from the lower GI tract, the diarrhea is frankly bloody. Bleeding from the upper GI tract also can be rapid enough to produce hematochezia (bright red stools), but generally some digestion of the blood components will have occurred,

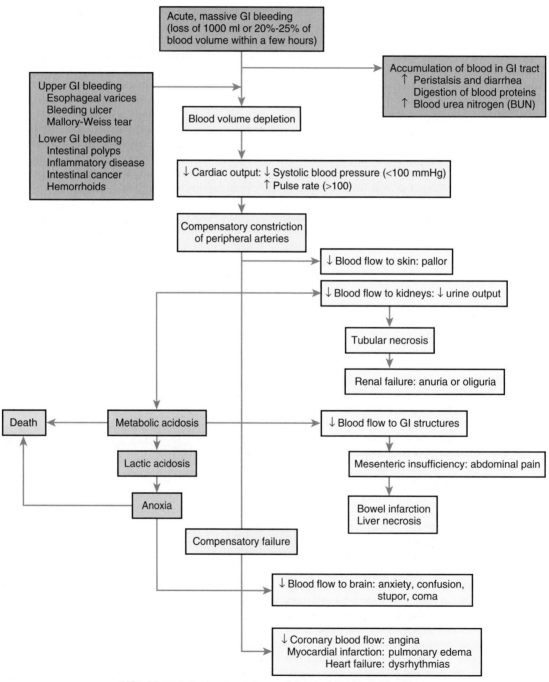

FIGURE 38.1 Pathophysiology of Gastrointestinal Bleeding.

producing melena—black or tarry stools that are sticky and have a characteristic foul odor. The digestion of blood proteins originating from massive upper GI bleeding is reflected by an increase in blood urea nitrogen (BUN) levels (see Fig. 38.1).

The hematocrit and hemoglobin values are not the best indicators of acute GI bleeding because plasma volume and red cell volume are lost proportionately. As the plasma volume is replaced, the hematocrit and hemoglobin values begin to reflect the extent of blood loss. The interpretation of these values is modified to account for exogenous replacement of fluids and the hydration status of the tissues.

✔ QUICK CHECK 38.1
1. How is visceral pain "referred"?
2. How does osmotic diarrhea differ from secretory diarrhea?
3. What are the best clinical indicators of acute GI bleeding blood loss?

Disorders of Motility
Dysphagia

PATHOPHYSIOLOGY   Dysphagia is difficulty swallowing. It can result from *mechanical obstruction* of the esophagus or from a functional disorder that impairs esophageal motility. Intrinsic obstructions originate in the wall of the esophageal lumen (esophageal dysphagia) and include tumors, strictures, and diverticular herniations (outpouchings). Extrinsic mechanical obstructions originate outside the esophageal lumen and narrow the esophagus by pressing inward on the esophageal wall. The most common cause of extrinsic mechanical obstruction is tumor.

Functional dysphagia is caused by neural or muscular disorders that interfere with voluntary swallowing or peristalsis. Disorders that affect the striated muscles of the hypopharyngeal area and upper esophagus interfere with the oropharyngeal (voluntary) phase of swallowing (oropharyngeal dysphagia). Typical causes are dermatomyositis (a muscle disease) and neurologic impairments caused by cerebrovascular accidents, Parkinson disease, multiple sclerosis, muscular dystrophy, or achalasia.

Achalasia is a rare form of dysphagia related to loss of inhibitory neurons in the myenteric plexus with smooth muscle atrophy in the middle and lower portions of the esophagus. The myenteric neurons are attacked by a cell-mediated and antibody-mediated immune response against an unknown antigen. This leads to altered esophageal peristalsis and failure of the lower esophageal sphincter (LES) to relax, causing functional obstruction of the lower esophagus with varying severity. Food accumulates above the obstruction, distends the esophagus, and causes dysphagia. Cough and aspiration can occur. As hydrostatic pressure increases, food is slowly forced past the obstruction into the stomach. Chronic esophageal distention requires dilation or surgical myotomy of the LES.

CLINICAL MANIFESTATIONS   Distention and spasm of the esophageal muscles during eating or drinking may cause a mild or severe stabbing pain at the level of obstruction. Discomfort occurring 2 to 4 seconds after swallowing is associated with upper esophageal obstruction. Discomfort occurring 10 to 15 seconds after swallowing is more common in obstructions of the lower esophagus. If obstruction results from a growing tumor, dysphagia begins with difficulty swallowing solids and advances to difficulty swallowing semisolids and liquids. If motor function is impaired, both solids and liquids are difficult to swallow. Regurgitation of undigested food, an unpleasant taste sensation, vomiting, aspiration, and weight loss are common manifestations of all types of dysphagia. Aspiration of esophageal contents can lead to cough and pneumonia.

EVALUATION AND TREATMENT   Knowledge of the person's history and clinical manifestations contributes significantly to a diagnosis of dysphagia. Imaging is used to visualize the contours of the esophagus and identify structural defects. Esophageal motility testing documents abnormal pressure changes associated with obstruction or loss of neural regulation. Esophageal endoscopy is performed to examine the esophageal mucosa and obtain biopsy specimens.

The individual is taught to manage symptoms by eating small meals slowly, taking fluid with meals, and sleeping with the head elevated to prevent regurgitation and aspiration. Food and medications may need to be formulated so they can be swallowed Anticholinergic drugs (e.g., botulinum toxin) may relieve symptoms of dysphagia. Mechanical dilation of the esophageal sphincter and surgical separation of the lower esophageal muscles with a longitudinal incision (myotomy) are the most effective treatments for achalasia.

Gastroesophageal Reflux Disease

Gastroesophageal reflux disease (GERD) is the reflux of acid and pepsin or bile salts from the stomach into the esophagus, causing esophagitis. The prevalence of GERD is estimated at 18% to 27% in North America.[4] Risk factors for GERD include older age, obesity, hiatal hernia, and drugs or chemicals that relax the LES (anticholinergics, nitrates, calcium channel blockers, nicotine). GERD may be a trigger for asthma or chronic cough. Gastroesophageal reflux that does not cause symptoms is known as *physiologic reflux*. In *nonerosive reflux disease (NERD)*, individuals have symptoms of reflux disease but no visible or minimal esophageal mucosal injury (functional heartburn).

PATHOPHYSIOLOGY   Abnormalities in LES function, esophageal motility, and gastric motility or emptying can cause GERD. The resting tone of the LES tends to be lower than normal from either transient relaxation or weakness of the sphincter. Vomiting, coughing, lifting, bending, obesity, or pregnancy increases abdominal pressure, contributing to the development of reflux esophagitis. A hiatal hernia can weaken the LES. Delayed gastric emptying can contribute to reflux esophagitis by (1) lengthening the period during which reflux is possible and (2) increasing gastric acid content. Disorders that delay emptying include gastroparesis; gastric or duodenal ulcers, which can cause pyloric edema; and strictures that narrow the pylorus.[5]

The severity of the esophagitis depends on the composition of the gastric contents and the esophageal mucosa exposure time. If the gastric content is highly acidic or contains bile salts and pancreatic or intestinal enzymes, reflux esophagitis can be severe. The refluxate causes mucosal injury and inflammation, with hyperemia, increased capillary permeability, edema, tissue fragility, and erosion. Fibrosis and thickening may develop. Precancerous lesions (Barrett esophagus; see the Esophageal Cancer section) can be a long-term consequence. Precancerous lesions can progress to adenocarcinoma.

CLINICAL MANIFESTATIONS   The clinical manifestations of erosive reflux esophagitis are heartburn (pyrosis), acid regurgitation, dysphagia, chronic cough, asthma attacks (see Chapter 29), laryngitis, hoarseness, and upper abdominal pain within 1 hour of eating. The symptoms worsen if the individual lies down or if intra-abdominal pressure increases (e.g., as a result of coughing, vomiting, or straining at stool). Edema, strictures, esophageal spasm, or decreased esophageal motility may result in dysphagia with weight loss. Alcohol or acid-containing foods, such as citrus fruits, can cause discomfort during swallowing.

EVALUATION AND TREATMENT   The diagnosis of GERD is based on the history and clinical manifestations. Esophageal endoscopy shows hyperemia, edema, erosion, and strictures. Dysplastic changes (Barrett esophagus) can be identified by tissue biopsy. Impedance/pH monitoring measures the movement of stomach contents upward into the esophagus and the acidity of the refluxate. Because heartburn also may be experienced as chest pain, cardiac ischemia must be ruled out.

Proton pump inhibitors are the agents of choice for controlling symptoms and healing esophagitis. Other therapies include histamine 2 (H_2)-receptor antagonists or prokinetics and antacids. Weight reduction, smoking cessation, elevation of the head of the bed 6 inches, and avoiding tight clothing also help to alleviate symptoms. Laparoscopic fundoplication is the most common surgical intervention when medical treatment fails.[6]

Eosinophilic esophagitis is an idiopathic chronic inflammatory disease of the esophagus characterized by infiltration of eosinophils associated with atopic disease, including asthma and food allergies. It occurs in adults and children. Dysphagia, food impaction, vomiting, and weight loss are common symptoms. Endoscopy with biopsy identifies the eosinophilic infiltration and differentiates this condition from GERD. Treatment is symptomatic and includes acid inhibitors, elimination diets, and swallowed steroids.

Hiatal Hernia

PATHOPHYSIOLOGY **Hiatal hernia** is a type of diaphragmatic hernia with protrusion (herniation) of the upper part of the stomach through the diaphragm and into the thorax[7] (Fig. 38.2). In **sliding hiatal hernia (type 1)** (the most common type), the proximal portion of the stomach moves into the thoracic cavity through the esophageal hiatus, an opening in the diaphragm for the esophagus and vagus nerves. A congenitally short esophagus, fibrosis or excessive vagal nerve stimulation, or weakening of the diaphragmatic muscles at the gastroesophageal junction

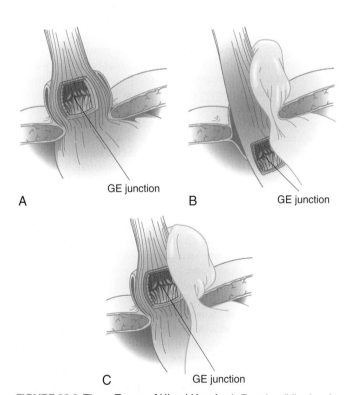

FIGURE 38.2 Three Types of Hiatal Hernia. A, Type I—*sliding hernia.* The visceral peritoneum remains intact and restrains the size of the hernia in sliding hiatal hernia. **B,** Type II—*paraesophageal* or *rolling hernia.* The membrane becomes thinner or defective in a paraesophageal hernia, allowing a true peritoneal sac to protrude into the posterior mediastinum, where negative intrathoracic pressure causes it to enlarge. **C,** Type III—*mixed hernia. GE,* Gastroesophageal. NOTE: Type IV—complex paraesophageal hernia is not shown. (From Townsend CM et al: *Sabiston textbook of surgery,* ed 19, Philadelphia, 2012, Saunders.)

contributes to the hernia. GERD is associated with this type of herniation. Coughing, bending, tight clothing, ascites, obesity, and pregnancy accentuate the hernia.

Paraesophageal hiatal hernia (type 2) is the herniation of the greater curvature of the stomach through a secondary opening in the diaphragm alongside the esophagus. The position of a portion of the stomach above the diaphragm causes congestion of mucosal blood flow, leading to gastritis and ulcer formation. Strangulation of the hernia is a major complication. It can present with vomiting and epigastric and retrosternal epigastric pain and is a surgical emergency.

Mixed hiatal hernia (type 3), less common, is a combination of sliding and paraesophageal hiatal hernias. It tends to occur in conjunction with several other diseases, including reflux esophagitis, peptic ulcer, cholecystitis (gallbladder inflammation), cholelithiasis (gallstones), chronic pancreatitis, and diverticulosis.

CLINICAL MANIFESTATIONS Hiatal hernias are often asymptomatic. Generally, a wide variety of symptoms develop later in life and are associated with other GI disorders, including GERD. Symptoms include heartburn, regurgitation, dysphagia, and epigastric pain. Ischemia from hernia strangulation causes acute, severe chest or epigastric pain, nausea, vomiting, and GI bleeding.

EVALUATION AND TREATMENT Diagnostic procedures include radiology with barium swallow, endoscopy, and high-resolution manometry. A chest x-ray film often will show the protrusion of the stomach into the thorax, indicating paraesophageal hiatal hernia.

Treatment for a sliding hiatal hernia is usually conservative. The individual can diminish reflux by eating small, frequent meals and avoiding the recumbent position after eating. Abdominal supports and tight clothing should be avoided, and weight control is recommended for obese individuals. Antacids alleviate reflux esophagitis. Individuals who are uncomfortable at night benefit from sleeping with the head of the bed elevated 6 inches. Surgery is performed if medical management fails to control symptoms.

Gastroparesis is delayed gastric emptying in the absence of a mechanical gastric outlet obstruction. It is most commonly associated with diabetes mellitus, surgical vagotomy, or fundoplication. It can be idiopathic. The pathophysiology is not well understood but involves abnormalities of the autonomic nervous system, smooth muscle cells, enteric neurons, and GI hormones. Diabetic gastroparesis represents a form of neuropathy involving the vagus nerve. Symptoms include nausea, vomiting, abdominal pain, and postprandial fullness or bloating. Treatment options include dietary management; prokinetic drugs; and, in some cases, gastric electrical stimulation; or surgical venting gastrostomy.[8]

Pyloric Obstruction

PATHOPHYSIOLOGY **Pyloric obstruction (gastric outlet obstruction)** is the narrowing or blocking of the opening between the stomach and the duodenum. This condition can be congenital (e.g., infantile hypertrophic pyloric stenosis; see Chapter 39) or acquired. Acquired obstruction is caused by peptic ulcer disease or carcinoma near the pylorus. Duodenal ulcers are more likely than gastric ulcers to obstruct the pylorus. Ulceration causes obstruction resulting from inflammation, edema, spasm, fibrosis, or scarring. Tumors cause obstruction by growing into the pylorus.

CLINICAL MANIFESTATIONS Early in the course of pyloric obstruction, the individual experiences vague epigastric fullness, which becomes more distressing after eating and at the end of the day. Nausea and epigastric pain may occur as the muscles of the stomach contract in attempts to

TABLE 38.2 **Common Causes of Intestinal Obstruction**

Cause	Pathophysiology
Hernia	Protrusion of intestine through weakness in abdominal muscles or through inguinal ring
Intussusception	Telescoping of one part of intestine into another; this usually causes strangulation of the blood supply; more common in infants 10-15 months of age than in adults (see Fig. 38.3, D)
Torsion (volvulus)	Twisting of the intestine on its mesenteric pedicle, with occlusion of the blood supply; often associated with fibrous adhesions; occurs most often in middle-aged and elderly men
Diverticulosis	Inflamed saccular herniations (diverticula) of mucosa and submucosa through tunica muscularis of the colon; diverticula are interspersed between thick, circular, fibrous bands; most common in obese individuals older than 60 years (see Fig. 38.8)
Tumor	Tumor growth into intestinal lumen; adenocarcinoma of the colon and the rectum is the most common tumoral obstruction; most common in individuals older than 60 years
Paralytic (adynamic) ileus	Loss of peristaltic motor activity in intestine; associated with abdominal surgery, peritonitis, hypokalemia, ischemic bowel, spinal trauma, or pneumonia
Fibrous adhesions	Peritoneal irritation from surgery, trauma, or Crohn disease leads to the formation of fibrin and adhesions that attach to intestine, omentum, or peritoneum and can cause obstruction; most common in small intestine

force chyme past the obstruction. These symptoms disappear when the chyme finally moves into the duodenum. As obstruction progresses, anorexia develops sometimes accompanied by weight loss. Severe obstruction causes gastric distention and atony (lack of muscle tone and gastric motility). Gastric distention stimulates gastric secretion, which increases the feeling of fullness. Rolling or jarring of the abdomen produces a sloshing sound called the *succussion splash*. At this stage, vomiting is a cardinal sign of obstruction. It is usually copious and occurs several hours after eating. The vomitus contains undigested food but no bile. Prolonged vomiting leads to dehydration, which is accompanied by a hypokalemic and hypochloremic metabolic alkalosis caused by loss of gastric potassium and acid, respectively. Because food does not enter the intestine, stools are infrequent and small. Prolonged pyloric obstruction causes severe malnutrition, dehydration, and extreme debilitation.

EVALUATION AND TREATMENT The diagnosis is based on clinical manifestations, a history of ulcer disease, and examination of residual gastric contents. Endoscopy is performed if gastric carcinoma is the suggested cause of pyloric obstruction.

Obstructions resulting from ulceration often resolve with conservative management. A large-bore nasogastric tube is used to aspirate stomach contents and relieve distention. Then nasogastric suction is maintained for 2 to 3 days to decompress the stomach and restore normal motility. Gastric secretions that contribute to inflammation and edema can be suppressed with proton pump inhibitors or H_2-receptor antagonists. Fluids and electrolytes (saline and potassium) are given intravenously to promote rehydration and correct hypokalemia and alkalosis (see Chapter 5). Severely malnourished individuals may require parenteral hyperalimentation (intravenous nutrition). Surgery or the placement of pyloric stents may be required to treat gastric carcinoma or persistent obstruction caused by fibrosis and scarring.[9]

Intestinal Obstruction and Paralytic Ileus

Intestinal obstruction can be caused by any condition that prevents the normal flow of chyme through the intestinal lumen (Table 38.2). Obstructions can occur in either the small or the large intestine (Table 38.3). The small intestine is more commonly obstructed because of its narrower lumen. Classifications of intestinal obstruction are summarized in Table 38.4. Intestinal obstruction is classified by cause as simple or functional. *Simple obstruction* is mechanical blockage of the lumen by a lesion and it is the most common type of intestinal obstruction. **Paralytic ileus**, or *functional obstruction*, is a failure of intestinal motility

TABLE 38.3 **Large and Small Bowel Obstruction**

Type of Obstruction	Cause
Small bowel obstruction	Adhesions: secondary to previous abdominal surgeries—75%
	Hernia: inguinal, ventral, or femoral—10%
	Tumors: may be associated with intussusception—10%
	Mesenteric ischemia—3%-5%
	Crohn disease—<1%
Large bowel obstruction	Colon/rectal cancer—90%
	Volvulus—4%-5%
	Diverticular disease—3-5%
	Other causes (inflammatory bowel disease, adhesions, hernia)

Data from Mizell JS, Turnage RH: Intestinal obstruction. In Feldman M et al, editors: *Sleisenger & Fordtran's gastrointestinal and liver disease*, ed 10, pp 2154-2170, Philadelphia, 2016, Saunders.

often occurring after intestinal or abdominal surgery, acute pancreatitis, or hypokalemia. Acute obstructions usually have mechanical causes, such as adhesions or hernias (Fig. 38.3). Chronic or partial obstructions are more often associated with tumors or inflammatory disorders, particularly of the large intestine.

PATHOPHYSIOLOGY The major pathophysiologic alterations are presented in Fig. 38.4. Postoperative paralytic ileus results from inhibitory neural reflexes associated with inflammatory mediators, and the influence of exogenous (i.e., meperidine or morphine) and endogenous opioids (endorphins) that affect the entire GI tract. **Small bowel obstruction (SBO)** is caused by postoperative adhesions, tumors, Crohn disease, and hernias. SBO leads to distention caused by impaired absorption and increased secretion with accumulation of fluid and gas inside the lumen proximal to the obstruction.[10] Distention decreases the intestine's ability to absorb water and electrolytes and increases the net secretion of these substances into the lumen. Copious vomiting or sequestration of fluids in the intestinal lumen prevents their reabsorption and produces severe fluid and electrolyte disturbances. Extracellular fluid volume and plasma volume decrease, causing dehydration, increased hematocrit

TABLE 38.4   Classifications of Intestinal Obstruction

Criteria for Classification	Definition
Onset	
Acute	Sudden onset; often caused by torsion, intussusception, or herniation
Chronic	Protracted onset; more commonly from tumor growth or progressive formation of strictures
Extent of Obstruction	
Partial	Incomplete obstruction of intestinal lumen
Complete	Complete obstruction of intestinal lumen
Location of Obstructing Lesion	
Intrinsic	Obstruction develops within intestinal lumen; examples: gut wall edema or hemorrhage, foreign bodies (gallstones), tumors, or gut wall fibrosis
Extrinsic	Obstruction originates outside intestine; examples: tumors, torsion, fibrosis, hernia, intussusception
Effects on Intestinal Wall	
Simple	Luminal obstruction without impairment of blood supply
Strangulated	Luminal obstruction with occlusion of blood supply
Closed loop	Obstruction at each end of a segment of intestine
Casual Factors	
Mechanical	Blockage of intestinal lumen by intrinsic or extrinsic lesions; usually treated surgically
Functional (paralytic ileus)	Paralysis of intestinal musculature caused by trauma, peritonitis, electrolyte imbalances, or spasmolytic agents; usually treated by decompression with suction or surgery if death of tissue

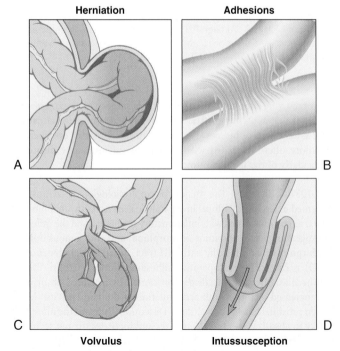

FIGURE 38.3 Intestinal Obstructions. A, Hernia. **B,** Constrictions from adhesions. **C,** Volvulus. **D,** Intussusception. (From Kumar V et al: Robbins basic pathology, ed 9, Philadelphia, 2013, Saunders.)

level, hypotension, and tachycardia. Severe dehydration leads to hypovolemic shock. Metabolic alkalosis initially develops as a result of excessive loss of hydrogen ions that would normally be reabsorbed from the gastric juice and vomiting. With prolonged obstruction or obstruction lower in the intestine, metabolic acidosis is more likely to occur because bicarbonate from pancreatic secretions and bile cannot be reabsorbed. Hypokalemia from vomiting and decreased potassium absorption can be extreme, promoting acidosis and atony of the intestinal wall. Metabolic acidosis also may be accentuated by ketosis, the result of declining carbohydrate stores caused by starvation. Lack of circulation permits the buildup of significant amounts of lactic acid, which worsen the metabolic acidosis. If pressure from the distention is severe enough, it occludes the arterial circulation and causes ischemia, necrosis, perforation, and peritonitis. Fever and leukocytosis are often associated with overgrowth of bacteria, ischemia, and bowel necrosis. Bacterial proliferation and translocation across the mucosa to the systemic circulation cause peritonitis or sepsis. The release of inflammatory mediators into the circulation causes remote organ failure.

Large bowel obstruction is less common and often related to cancer. Diverticulitis, inflammatory bowel disease, and other causes of obstruction are less common. **Acute colonic pseudo-obstruction (Ogilvie syndrome)** is a rare massive dilation of the large bowel that is related to excessive sympathetic motor input or decreased parasympathetic motor input with absence of mechanical obstruction. It occurs primarily in people who are critically ill and immobilized older adults.

CLINICAL MANIFESTATIONS   Signs and symptoms of *small intestine obstruction* include colicky pains caused by intestinal distention followed by nausea and vomiting. Pain intensifies for seconds or minutes as a peristaltic wave of muscle contraction meets the obstruction. Pain may be continuous with severe distention and then diminish in intensity. If ischemia occurs, the pain loses its colicky character and becomes more constant and severe. Sweating and tachycardia occur as a sympathetic nervous system response to hypotension. Fever, severe leukocytosis, abdominal distention, and rebound tenderness develop as ischemia progresses to necrosis, perforation, and peritonitis.

Obstruction at the pylorus causes early, profuse vomiting. Obstruction in the proximal small intestine causes mild distention and vomiting of bile-stained fluid. Lower obstruction in the small intestine causes more pronounced distention because a greater length of intestine is proximal to the obstruction. In this case, vomiting may not occur early but may occur later and contain fecal material. Partial obstruction can cause diarrhea or constipation, but complete obstruction usually causes constipation only. Complete obstruction increases the number of bowel sounds, which may be tinkly and accompanied by peristaltic rushes and crampy abdominal pain. Signs of hypovolemia and metabolic acidosis may be observed as early as 24 hours after the occurrence of complete obstruction. Distention may be severe enough to push against the diaphragm and decrease lung volume. This can lead to atelectasis and pneumonia, particularly in debilitated individuals.

Large bowel obstruction usually presents with hypogastric pain and abdominal distention. Pain can vary from vague to excruciating, depending on the degree of ischemia and the development of peritonitis. Vomiting occurs late in the obstructive process. Small and large intestinal perforation presents the same with acute, persistent abdominal pain, nausea, vomiting, and fever. *Acute colonic pseudo-obstruction* is characterized by abdominal distention, abdominal pain, and nausea and vomiting with the absence of mechanical obstruction. Bowel sounds are usually present.

EVALUATION AND TREATMENT   Evaluation is based on clinical manifestations and imaging studies. Successful management requires

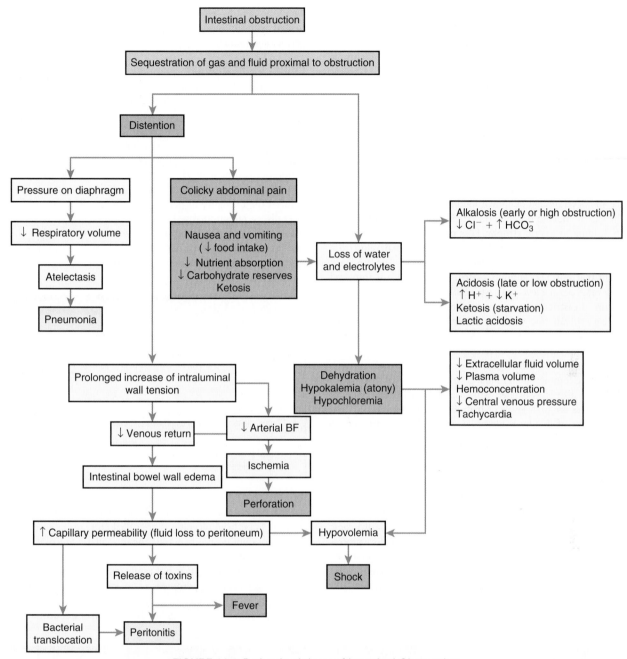

FIGURE 38.4 Pathophysiology of Intestinal Obstruction.

early identification of the site and type of obstruction. Replacement of fluid and electrolytes and decompression of the lumen with gastric or intestinal suction are essential forms of therapy. Laparoscopic procedures can release adhesions. Immediate surgical intervention is required for strangulation, complete obstruction, or perforation. Colonic stents may be placed for malignant obstruction. Neostigmine, a parasympathomimetic, is used for colonic pseudo-obstruction and colonoscopic decompression may be required.

> ✔ **QUICK CHECK 38.2**
> 1. Why is heartburn associated with gastroesophageal reflux?
> 2. How does peritonitis develop with bowel obstruction?
> 3. What causes postoperative paralytic ileus?

Gastritis

Gastritis is a nonspecific inflammatory disorder of the gastric mucosa. The most common causes are use of nonsteroidal antiinflammatory drugs (NSAIDs), *Helicobacter pylori* infection, and physiologic stress-related mucosal changes. Alcohol, digitalis, and metabolic disorders, such as uremia, also are contributing factors.

Acute gastritis is caused by injury of the protective mucosal barrier. NSAIDs (e.g., ibuprofen, naproxen, indomethacin, and aspirin) cause gastritis because they inhibit prostaglandin synthesis, which normally stimulates the secretion of mucus. Alcohol, histamine, digitalis, and metabolic disorders, such as uremia, are contributing factors. *H. pylori*–associated acute gastritis causes inflammation, increased gastric secretion in antral gastritis, decreased gastric secretion in fundal gastritis, pain, nausea, and vomiting. The clinical manifestations of acute gastritis can include vague abdominal discomfort, epigastric tenderness, and bleeding. Healing usually occurs spontaneously within a few days. Discontinuing injurious drugs, using antacids, or decreasing acid secretion with H$_2$-receptor antagonists facilitates healing.

Chronic gastritis tends to occur in older adults and causes chronic inflammation, mucosal atrophy, and epithelial metaplasia.[11,12] Chronic gastritis is classified as type A, immune (fundal), or type B, nonimmune (antral), depending on the pathogenesis and location of the lesions. When both types of chronic gastritis occur, it is known as type AB, or pangastritis, and the antrum is more severely involved. Type C gastritis is associated with reflux of bile and pancreatic secretions into the stomach, causing chemical injury.

Chronic immune (fundal) gastritis, the most rare form of gastritis, is a recessive, multigenetic disease. It is associated with loss of T-cell tolerance and development of autoantibodies to acid-secreting parietal cells. The gastric mucosa degenerates extensively in the fundus of the stomach, leading to gastric atrophy. Loss of parietal cells diminishes acid and intrinsic factor secretion. Pernicious anemia can develop from decreased vitamin B$_{12}$ absorption (see Chapter 23). The feedback mechanism that normally inhibits gastrin secretion also is impaired causing elevated plasma levels of gastrin (stimulates gastric secretion). Chronic fundal gastritis occurs in association with other autoimmune diseases (e.g., rheumatoid arthritis, autoimmune thyroid disease, or type 1 diabetes mellitus) and is a risk factor for gastric carcinoma, particularly in individuals who develop pernicious anemia.

Chronic nonimmune (antral) gastritis generally involves the antrum only and is more common than fundal gastritis. It is caused by *H. pylori* bacteria, and it also is associated with use of NSAIDs, alcohol, and smoking.[13] There are high levels of hydrochloric acid secretion, with an increased risk of duodenal ulcers. *H. pylori* also can progress to autoimmune atrophic gastritis and involve the fundus, thus becoming pangastritis. There is greater risk for the development of gastric cancer in these cases. The pathologic characteristics of *H. pylori* are summarized in Box 38.1.

Signs and symptoms of chronic gastritis often include vague symptoms: anorexia, fullness, nausea, vomiting, and epigastric pain. Gastric bleeding may be the only clinical manifestation of gastritis. Gastroscopic examination and biopsy may show a long-standing inflammatory process and gastric atrophy in an individual with no history of abdominal distress. Failure to stimulate acid secretion confirms achlorhydria (diminished secretion of hydrochloric acid). The gastric secretions also can be evaluated for the presence of intrinsic factor. Symptoms can usually be managed by eating smaller meals in conjunction with a soft,

bland diet and by avoiding alcohol and aspirin. *H. pylori* infection is treated with antibiotics, and vitamin B$_{12}$ is administered to correct pernicious anemia.

Peptic Ulcer Disease

A **peptic ulcer** is a break or ulceration in the protective mucosal lining usually located in the stomach or proximal duodenum, however, they can be found in the esophagus. Ulcers develop when mucosal protective factors are overcome by erosive factors commonly caused by NSAIDs and *H. pylori* infection. However, only a few people with *H. pylori* infection or those taking NSAIDs develop peptic ulcer disease. Successful antibiotic treatment of *H. pylori* infection and the use of mucosal protecting agents during NSAID and *H. pylori* treatment has significantly reduced the incidence of peptic ulcer disease. Risk factors for peptic ulcer disease are summarized in *Risk Factors:* Peptic Ulcer. Psychological stress may be a risk factor for peptic ulcer disease, but the exact mechanism of causation is not known.[14] The prevalence of peptic ulcer in 2011 in the United States was 15.5 million people.[15]

RISK FACTORS
Peptic Ulcer

- Infection of the gastric and duodenal mucosa with *Helicobacter pylori*
- Chronic use of nonsteroidal antiinflammatory drugs (NSAIDs)
- Alcohol
- Smoking
- Advanced age
- Chronic diseases, such as emphysema, rheumatoid arthritis, cirrhosis, obesity, and diabetes
- Type O blood (increases risk of binding to *H. pylori*)
- Psychological stress

Peptic ulcers can be single or multiple, acute or chronic, and superficial or deep. Superficial ulcerations are called *erosions* because they erode the mucosa but do not penetrate the muscularis mucosae (Fig. 38.5). True ulcers extend through the muscularis mucosae and damage blood vessels, causing hemorrhage but rarely perforate the GI wall.

Zollinger-Ellison syndrome is a rare syndrome that also is associated with peptic ulcers caused by a gastrin-secreting neuroendocrine tumor or multiple tumors (gastrinoma) of the pancreas or duodenum. Increased

---

BOX 38.1   Pathologic Characteristics of *Helicobacter Pylori*

Helicobacter pylori (H. pylori), a gram-negative spiral bacterium with a flagellum, is a major cause of acute and chronic gastritis, peptic ulcer disease in the duodenum and stomach, gastric adenocarcinoma, and gastric mucosa–associated lymphoid tissue (MALT) in about 20% of infected individuals. *H. pylori* is transmitted through the fecal-oral route and is usually acquired in childhood. Infection is asymptomatic in about 70% of cases. In other cases inflammation and immune responses promote mucosal ulcerations or prevent healing of injured tissue. Gene-environment interaction and different pathogenic strains of *H. pylori* increase the risk for disease. Patterns of gastritis and disease progression vary by site of infection and strain of *H. pylori*. Pathogenic and virulence factors include:

1. An ability to colonize and adhere to gastric epithelial cells.
2. The presence of flagella, which allow movement through the mucous layer to a site of higher pH.
3. A lipopolysaccharide membrane component, which evades immune protection and promotes inflammation.

4. Secretion of urease, which produces ammonia and carbon dioxide, resulting in a more alkaline environment and suppression of acid secretion. Both mechanisms improve survival.
5. Release of vacuolating cytotoxin (VacA), which promotes bacterial survival and causes epithelial injury.
6. The presence of cytotoxin-associated gene *(CagA)* strains that can escape normal immune responses and cause inflammation with the release of inflammatory cytokines that damage mucosal epithelial cells and loss of the protective mucosal barrier; they also promote tumor development by degrading *p53* tumor-suppression.
7. Recruitment and activation of inflammatory cells and cytokines that cause gastric epithelial cell death (apoptosis), which can result in atrophy, ulcers, dysplasia, or malignant growth.

Data from Mommersteeg MC et al: *Biochim Biophys Acta Rev Cancer* 1869(1):42-52, 2018; Nejati S et al: *Microb Pathog* 117:43-48, 2018.

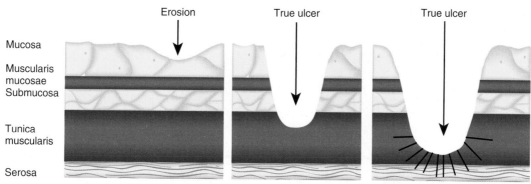

FIGURE 38.5 Lesions Caused by Peptic Ulcer Disease.

secretion of gastrin causes excess secretion of gastric acid, resulting in gastric and duodenal ulcers, gastroesophageal reflux with abdominal pain, and diarrhea.[16]

Duodenal Ulcers

Duodenal ulcers occur with greater frequency than other types of peptic ulcers and are caused by *H. pylori* infection (most commonly) and NSAID use. Idiopathic duodenal ulcers are rare and can be associated with altered mucosal defenses, rapid gastric emptying, elevated serum gastrin levels, or acid production stimulated by smoking.[17]

PATHOPHYSIOLOGY   Causative factors, singly or in combination, cause acid and pepsin concentrations in the duodenum to increase and penetrate the mucosal barrier, causing ulceration (Fig. 38.6). The host response to chronic stomach antral *H. pylori* infection is increased levels of gastrin resulting in increased stomach acid secretion and an increased acid load in the duodenum. The increased duodenal acid promotes gastric metaplasia in the duodenum and favors *H. pylori* colonization. Both the *H. pylori* and increased acid result in decreased duodenal bicarbonate production. Additionally the *H. pylori* infection activates immune cells (T and B lymphocytes with infiltration of neutrophils) and release of inflammatory cytokines which damage the mucosa. *H. pylori* also produces a toxin that causes loss of protective mucosal cells (see Box 38.1). The end result is ulceration. *H. pylori* mucosal infection can promote gastric cancer, but the incidence is lower for duodenal ulcer than for gastric ulcer, and the mechanism is unknown.[18]

CLINICAL MANIFESTATIONS   The characteristic manifestation of a duodenal ulcer is chronic intermittent pain in the epigastric area. The pain begins 2 or 3 hours after eating, when the stomach is empty. It is not unusual for pain to occur in the middle of the night and disappear by morning. Pain is relieved rapidly by ingestion of food or antacids, creating a typical pain-food-relief pattern. Some individuals with a duodenal ulcer may have no symptoms; the first manifestation may be hemorrhage or perforation, particularly with a history of NSAID or anticoagulant use.

Complications of a duodenal ulcer include bleeding, perforation, and obstruction of the duodenum or outlet of the stomach. Bleeding is the most common cause of mortality, particularly among the elderly. Bleeding from duodenal ulcers causes hematemesis or melena. Perforation occurs with destruction of all layers of the duodenal wall and causes sudden, severe epigastric pain. Obstruction may be the result of edema from inflammation or scarring from chronic injury. Duodenal ulcers often heal spontaneously but recur within months without treatment. Relief of pain accompanies healing.[19]

EVALUATION AND TREATMENT   Several diagnostic approaches are used to differentiate duodenal ulcers from gastric ulcers or gastric carcinoma. Endoscopic evaluation allows visualization of lesions and biopsy. Radioimmune assays of gastrin levels are evaluated to identify ulcers associated with gastric carcinomas. *H. pylori* is detected using the urea breath test, *H. pylori*–specific serum immunoglobulin G (IgG) and IgA antibodies, and measurement of *H. pylori* stool antigen levels.[20]

The management of duodenal ulcers is aimed at relieving the causes and effects of hyperacidity and pepsin and preventing complications. Antacids neutralize gastric contents and relieve pain. Acid secretion can be suppressed with drugs that block H_2 receptors and inhibit the secretion of acid. Proton pump inhibitors inhibit acid production. *H. pylori* is treated with a combination of antibiotics and proton pump inhibitors, but antibiotic resistance is an increasing problem. Surgical resection may be required for bleeding or perforating ulcers, obstruction, or peritonitis.

Gastric Ulcers

Gastric ulcers are ulcers of the stomach. They occur about equally in males and females, usually between the ages of 55 and 65 years. They are less common than duodenal ulcers (Table 38.5).

PATHOPHYSIOLOGY   Generally, gastric ulcers develop in the antral region, adjacent to the acid-secreting mucosa of the body. The primary defect is an abnormality that increases the mucosal barrier's permeability to hydrogen ions. Gastric secretion may be normal or less than normal, and there may be a decreased mass of parietal cells. Chronic gastritis is often associated with development of gastric ulcers and may precipitate ulcer formation by limiting the mucosa's ability to secrete a protective layer of mucus (Fig. 38.7). Other factors include:

- Decreased mucosal synthesis of prostaglandins
- Damage to the mucosal membrane from duodenal reflux of bile and pancreatic enzymes
- Use of NSAIDs (decreases prostaglandin synthesis)
- *H. pylori* infection

A break in the mucosal barrier permits hydrogen ions to diffuse into the mucosa, where they disrupt permeability and cellular structure. A vicious cycle can be established as the damaged mucosa liberates histamine, which stimulates the increase of acid and pepsinogen production, blood flow, and capillary permeability. The disrupted mucosa becomes edematous and loses plasma proteins. Destruction of small vessels causes bleeding.

CLINICAL MANIFESTATIONS   The clinical manifestations of gastric ulcers are similar to those of duodenal ulcers (see Table 38.5). The pattern of pain is common, but the pain of gastric ulcers also occurs

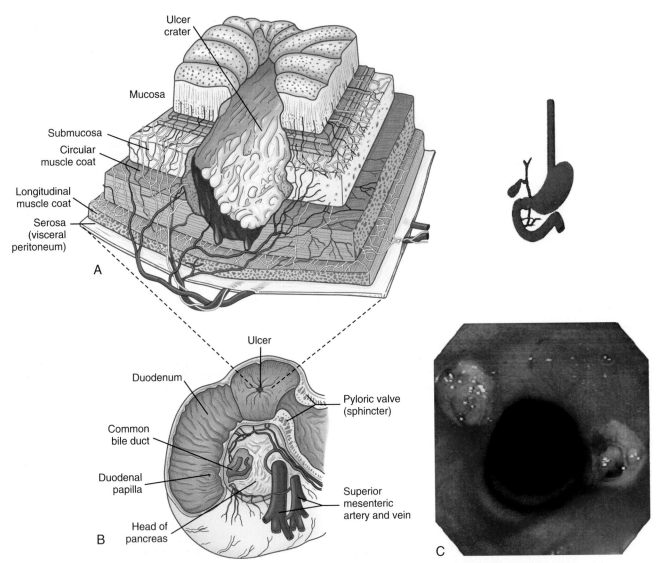

FIGURE 38.6 Duodenal Ulcer. A, A deep ulceration in the duodenal wall extending as a crater through the entire mucosa and into the muscle layers. **B,** Sequence of ulcerations from normal mucosa to duodenal ulcer. **C,** Bilateral (kissing) duodenal ulcers in a person using nonsteroidal antiinflammatory drugs (NSAIDs). (**C** courtesy David Bjorkman, MD, University of Utah School of Medicine, Department of Gastroenterology, Salt Lake City, Utah.)

immediately after eating. Gastric ulcers also tend to be chronic rather than alternating between periods of remission and exacerbation, and they cause more anorexia and vomiting than do duodenal ulcers. The pain associated with eating tends to suppress food intake, resulting in weight loss. The evaluation and treatment of gastric ulcers are similar to those for duodenal ulcers. However, long-term use of proton pump inhibitors is a reported risk factor for gastric cancer after H. pylori eradication and is related to hypergastrinemia and hyperplasia of enterochromaffin-like cells that promote the secretion of gastric acid.[21]

Stress-Related Mucosal Disease

A **stress-related mucosal disease (stress ulcer)** is an acute form of peptic ulcer that tends to accompany the physiologic stress of severe illness or major trauma. Usually multiple sites of ulceration are distributed within the stomach or duodenum. Stress ulcers may be classified as ischemic ulcers or Cushing ulcers.

Ischemic ulcers develop within hours of an event such as hemorrhage, multisystem trauma, severe burns, heart failure, or sepsis. Shock, anoxia,

inflammation, and sympathetic responses cause ischemia of the stomach and duodenal mucosa, disrupting the mucosal barrier. Stress ulcers that develop as a result of burn injury are often called **Curling ulcers. Cushing ulcer** is a stress ulcer associated with severe brain trauma or brain surgery. Decreased mucosal blood flow and hypersecretion of acid caused by overstimulation of the vagal nuclei damage the mucosal barrier, causing erosions and ulceration.

The primary clinical manifestation of stress-related mucosal disease is bleeding, which is uncommon, but occurs more readily with the presence of coagulopathy and more than 48 hours of mechanical ventilation. Prophylactic treatment regimens are used to prevent this disease. Stress ulcers seldom become chronic.[22]

Surgical Treatment of Ulcer

Advances in the medical treatment of peptic ulcer disease with acid suppression and eradication of *H. pylori* have reduced the number of cases requiring surgery. The most common indications for ulcer surgery are recurrent or uncontrolled bleeding and perforation of the stomach

TABLE 38.5 Characteristics of Gastric and Duodenal Ulcers

Characteristics	Gastric Ulcer	Duodenal Ulcer
Incidence		
Age at onset	50-70 years	20-50 years
Family history	Usually negative	Positive
Sex (prevalence)	Equal in women and men	Greater in men
Stress factors	Increased	Average
Ulcerogenic drugs	Normal use	Increased use
Cancer risk	Increased	Not increased
Pathophysiology		
Abnormal mucus	May be present	May be present
Parietal cell mass	Normal or decreased	Increased
Acid production	Normal or decreased	Increased
Serum gastrin	Increased	Normal
Serum pepsinogen	Normal	Increased
Associated gastritis	More common	Usually not present
Helicobacter pylori	May be present (60%-80%)	Often present (95%-100%)
	Stimulates reduced acid secretion, gastric atrophy, and risk of gastric cancer	Stimulates acid hypersecretion
Clinical Manifestations		
Pain	Located in upper abdomen	Located in upper abdomen
	Intermittent	Intermittent
	Pain-antacid-relief pattern	Pain-antacid/food-relief pattern
	Food-pain pattern (when food in stomach)	Pain when stomach empty
		Nocturnal pain common
Clinical course	Chronic ulcer without pattern of remission and exacerbation	Pattern of remissions and exacerbation for years
	Heals more slowly	Heals more quickly

or duodenum. The primary objectives of surgical treatment are to reduce stimuli for acid secretion, decrease the number of acid-secreting cells in the stomach, and correct complications of ulcer disease.

Acute complications of gastrectomy or anastomosis are relatively uncommon except in debilitated persons. Chronic complications, however, are likely to develop if a large portion of the stomach has been removed. These complications and their pathophysiologic mechanisms are described in the next section.

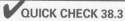

QUICK CHECK 38.3
1. What is the most common cause of chronic gastritis?
2. Compare duodenal, gastric, and stress ulcers.
3. What causes a stress ulcer?

Postgastrectomy Syndromes

Postgastrectomy syndromes are a group of signs and symptoms that occur after gastric resection for the treatment of peptic ulcer,

gastric carcinoma, or bariatric surgery for extreme obesity (metabolic surgery). They are caused by anatomic and functional changes in the stomach and upper small intestine[23] and include the following conditions.

Dumping syndrome is the rapid emptying of hypertonic chyme from the surgically residual stomach (the smaller stomach component remaining after surgical resection following gastric or bariatric surgery) into the small intestine 10 to 20 minutes after eating, is promoted by loss of gastric capacity, loss of emptying control when pylorus is removed, and loss of feedback control by duodenum when it is removed. Symptoms include cramping pain, nausea, vomiting, osmotic diarrhea, hypotension, weakness, and pallor. Dumping syndrome responds to dietary management. Late dumping syndrome occurs 1 to 3 hours after eating a high carbohydrate meal and is related to hyperinsulinemia with hypoglycemia.

Alkaline (bile) reflux gastritis occurs when stomach inflammation, caused by reflux of bile and alkaline pancreatic secretions containing proteolytic enzymes, disrupts the mucosal barrier in the remnant stomach. Symptoms include nausea, bilious vomiting, and sustained epigastric pain that worsens after eating and is not relieved by antacids. It responds somewhat to avoidance of aspirin and alcohol, but surgical correction may be required.

Afferent loop obstruction occurs with intermittent severe pain and epigastric fullness after eating as a result of volvulus, hernia, adhesion, or stenosis of the duodenal stump on the proximal side of the gastro-jejunostomy. Vomiting relieves symptoms. Management includes low-fat diet, but decompression or surgery revision is required for complete obstruction.

Diarrhea is frequent, persistent elimination of loose stools or intermittent, precipitous, and unpredictable elimination of a large volume of stool. It is related to rapid gastric emptying and osmotic attraction of water into the gut, especially after a large intake of high-carbohydrate liquids; small, dry meals and anticholinergic drugs are effective control measures.

Weight loss is commonly caused by inadequate caloric intake because the individual cannot tolerate carbohydrates or a normal-sized meal. The stomach also is less able to mix, churn, and break down food. In the case of bariatric surgery for extreme obesity, weight loss is the intended outcome, but nutrient deficiencies, including vitamins and minerals, must be supplemented.[24]

Anemia may occur if iron malabsorption results from decreased acid secretion or lack of duodenum after a Billroth II procedure (gastrojejunostomy). Deficiencies of iron and vitamin B_{12} or folate also may result.

Bone and mineral disorders are related to altered calcium absorption and metabolism with increased risk for fractures and deformity and malabsorption of vitamins and nutrients, such as vitamin D.

Malabsorption Syndromes

Malabsorption syndromes interfere with nutrient absorption in the small intestine. Historically they have been classified as maldigestion or malabsorption. **Maldigestion** is failure of the chemical processes of digestion that take place in the intestinal lumen or at the brush border of the intestinal mucosa. **Malabsorption** is failure of the intestinal mucosa to absorb (transport) the digested nutrients. Often these two syndromes are interrelated, or occur together, making classification difficult. Generally, however, maldigestion is caused by deficiencies of the enzymes needed for digestion or inadequate secretion of bile salts and inadequate reabsorption of bile in the ileum. Malabsorption is the result of mucosal disruption caused by gastric or intestinal resection, vascular disorders, or intestinal disease (also see Chapter 39).

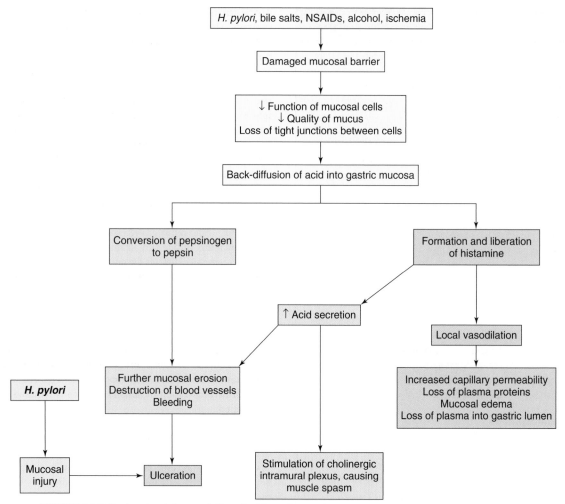

FIGURE 38.7 Pathophysiology of Gastric Ulcer Formation. *NSAIDs,* Nonsteroidal antiinflammatory drugs.

Pancreatic Exocrine Insufficiency

The pancreatic enzymes (lipase, amylase, trypsin, chymotrypsin) are required for the digestion of proteins, carbohydrates, and fats. **Pancreatic insufficiency** is the deficient production of these enzymes, particularly lipase, by the pancreas. Causes include chronic pancreatitis, pancreatic carcinoma, pancreatic resection, and cystic fibrosis. Significant damage to or loss of pancreatic tissue must occur before enzyme levels decrease sufficiently to cause maldigestion. Although pancreatic insufficiency causes poor digestion of all nutrients, fat maldigestion is the chief problem. Absence of pancreatic bicarbonate in the duodenum and jejunum causes an acidic pH that worsens maldigestion by precipitating bile salts and preventing activation of the pancreatic enzymes that are present. A large amount of fat in the stool (steatorrhea) is the most common sign of pancreatic insufficiency. There is also a deficit of fat-soluble vitamins (A, D, E, and K) and weight loss.

Lactase Deficiency (Lactose Intolerance)

A deficiency of disaccharidase at the brush border of the small intestine is caused by a genetic defect in which a single enzyme, usually lactase, is lacking. **Lactase deficiency** inhibits the breakdown of lactose (milk sugar) into monosaccharides and therefore prevents lactose digestion and absorption across the intestinal wall. Lactase deficiency is most common in blacks, Latinos, and Native Americans and usually does not develop until adulthood. Secondary (acquired) lactase deficiency can be caused by several diseases of the intestine, including gluten-sensitive enteropathy, enteritis, and bacterial overgrowth.

The undigested lactose remains in the intestine, where bacterial fermentation causes formation of gases. Undigested lactose also increases the osmotic gradient in the intestine, causing irritation and osmotic diarrhea. Clinical manifestations of lactose consumption with lactase deficiency are bloating, crampy pain, diarrhea, and flatulence. The disorder is diagnosed by a lactose-tolerance test. Avoiding milk products (more than 1 cup of milk) and adhering to a lactose-free diet relieve symptoms.[25]

Bile Salt Deficiency

Conjugated bile acids (bile salts) are necessary for the digestion and absorption of fats. Bile salts are conjugated in the bile that is secreted from the liver. When bile enters the duodenum, the bile salts aggregate with fatty acids and monoglycerides to form micelles. Micelle formation makes fat molecules more soluble and allows them to pass through the unstirred layer at the brush border of the small intestinal villi (see Chapter 37). A minimum concentration of bile salts, termed the *critical micelle concentration,* is required to allow formation of micelles. Therefore, conditions that decrease the production or secretion of bile result in decreased micelle formation and fat malabsorption. These conditions include advanced liver disease, which decreases the production of bile salts; obstruction of the common bile duct, which decreases flow of bile into the duodenum (cholestasis); intestinal stasis (lack of motility), which permits overgrowth of intestinal bacteria that deconjugate bile salts; and diseases of the ileum, which prevent the reabsorption and recycling of bile salts (enterohepatic circulation).[26]

Clinical manifestations of bile salt deficiency are related to poor intestinal absorption of fat and fat-soluble vitamins (A, D, E, and K). Increased fat in the stools (steatorrhea) leads to diarrhea and decreased levels of plasma proteins. The losses of fat-soluble vitamins and their effects include:

- Vitamin A deficiency results in night blindness.
- Vitamin D deficiency results in decreased calcium absorption with bone demineralization (osteoporosis), bone pain, and fractures.
- Vitamin K deficiency prolongs prothrombin time, leading to spontaneous development of purpura (bruising) and petechiae.
- Vitamin E deficiency has uncertain effects but may cause testicular atrophy and neurologic defects in children.

The most effective treatment for fat-soluble vitamin deficiency is to increase consumption of medium-chain triglycerides in the diet, for example, by using coconut oil for cooking. Vitamins A, D, and K are given parenterally. Oral bile salts are an effective therapy.

Inflammatory Bowel Disease

Ulcerative colitis and Crohn disease are major types of chronic relapsing inflammatory bowel diseases (IBDs). The prevalence of IBD is about 1.4 million people in the United States with about 30,000 new cases per year.[27] The disease is more prevalent among white populations and

Ashkenazi Jews.[28] Risk factors and theories of causation include susceptibility genes, environmental factors, alterations in epithelial-cell barrier functions, and an altered immune response to intestinal microflora[29] (Table 38.6). Environmental factors or infections are thought to alter the barrier function of the mucosal epithelium, leading to loss of immune tolerance to normal intestinal antigens. There is possible loss of discrimination of potentially harmful pathogens from commensal microorganisms in the intestinal mucosa. The loss of tolerance activates immune cells. Production of proinflammatory mediators damages the intestinal epithelium. The risk of colon cancer increases significantly after many years of inflammatory bowel disease, particularly in untreated disease.[30] Future research is directed at an integration of these factors to refine our understanding of disease cause and trajectory, particularly interactions between genetics, the microflora, mucosa, and immune responses.

Ulcerative Colitis

Ulcerative colitis (UC) is a chronic inflammatory disease that causes ulceration of the colonic mucosa, most commonly in the rectum and sigmoid colon. The lesions appear in susceptible individuals between 20 and 40 years of age. UC is less common in people who smoke.[31]

PATHOPHYSIOLOGY The primary lesion of UC begins with inflammation at the base of the crypt of Lieberkühn in the large intestine. The disease begins in the rectum (proctitis) and may extend proximally to the entire colon (pancolitis). The mucosa is inflamed and is involved in a continuous fashion. Small erosions form and coalesce into ulcers.

TABLE 38.6 Features of Ulcerative Colitis and Crohn Disease

Feature	Ulcerative Colitis	Crohn Disease
Incidence		
Age at onset	Any age; 10-40 years most common	Any age; 10-30 years most common
Family history	Less common	More common
Sex	Prevalence equal in women and men	Prevalence about equal in women and men
Cancer risk	Increased	Increased
Nicotine use	Later and less severe disease; nicotine withdrawal may cause exacerbation	Increases disease risk and greater disease severity
Pathophysiology		
Location of lesions	Large intestine, continuous lesions; Left side more common	Mouth to anus, "skip" lesions common; Right side more common
Inflammation	Mucosal layer involved	Entire intestinal wall involved
Granulomata	Rare	Transmural granulomata common; cobblestone appearance
Ulceration	Friable mucosa, superficial ulcers, crypt abscesses common	Deep fissuring ulcers and fistulae common
Anal and perianal fistulae	Rare	Common; abscesses
Narrowed lumen and possible obstruction	Rare	Common; obstruction
Clinical Manifestations		
Abdominal pain	Mild to severe	Moderate to severe
Diarrhea	Common; 4 times/day	May or may not be present
Bloody stools	Common	Less common
Weight loss	Less common	Common
Abdominal mass	Rare	Common
Small intestine malabsorption	None	Common
Clinical course	Remissions and exacerbations	Remissions and exacerbations
Comorbidities	Extraintestinal manifestations	Extraintestinal manifestations

Abscess formation, necrosis, and ragged ulceration of the mucosa ensue. Edema and thickening of the muscularis mucosae may narrow the lumen of the involved colon. Mucosal destruction and inflammation causes bleeding, cramping pain, and an urge to defecate. Frequent diarrhea, with passage of small amounts of blood and purulent mucus, is common. Loss of the absorptive mucosal surface and rapid colonic transit time cause large volumes of watery diarrhea.

CLINICAL MANIFESTATIONS The course of UC consists of intermittent periods of remission and exacerbation. Mild UC involves less mucosa, so the frequency of bowel movements, bleeding, and pain is minimal. Severe forms may involve the entire colon and are characterized by abdominal pain, fever, an elevated pulse rate, frequent diarrhea (10 to 20 stools/day), urgency, obviously bloody stools, and continuous, crampy pain. Dehydration, weight loss, anemia, and fever result from fluid loss, bleeding, and inflammation. Complications include anal fissures, hemorrhoids, and perirectal abscess. Severe hemorrhage is rare. Edema, strictures, or fibrosis can obstruct the colon. Perforation is an unusual but possible complication. Extraintestinal manifestations include cutaneous lesions (erythema nodosum), polyarthritis, episcleritis, uveitis, disorders of the liver, and alterations in coagulation.[32]

EVALUATION AND TREATMENT The diagnosis of UC is based on the medical history, clinical manifestations, and laboratory, serologic, imaging, endoscopic, and biopsy findings. Infectious causes are ruled out by stool culture. The symptoms of UC may be similar to those of Crohn disease, making differential diagnosis challenging. Treatment is individualized and depends on the severity of symptoms and the extent of mucosal involvement. A goal is to promote mucosal healing and avoid surgery. Mild to moderate disease is treated with 5-aminosalicylate therapy followed by steroids. Immunomodulatory agents are used for serious disease. Severe, unremitting disease can require hospital admission for administration of intravenous fluids and steroids. Extreme malnutrition may require total parenteral nutrition (TPN). Surgical resection of the colon may be performed if other forms of therapy are unsuccessful or if there are acute serious complications (sepsis, hemorrhage, perforation, or obstruction). Surgical approaches for severe UC include total proctocolectomy, with end ileostomy or ileorectal anastomosis, or ileal pouch–anal anastomosis (IPAA). *Pouchitis* is a complication of restorative proctocolectomy with ileal pouch–anal anastomosis performed as surgical treatment for both UC and Crohn disease. Antibiotic treatment is usually successful.[33]

Crohn Disease

Crohn disease (CD) (granulomatous colitis, ileocolitis, or regional enteritis) is an idiopathic inflammatory disorder that affects any part of the GI tract from the mouth to the anus. In a small percentage of cases, CD is difficult to differentiate from ulcerative colitis (see Table 38.6). Risk factor associated with CD include smoking, low fiber–high carbohydrate diet, medications, such as NSAIDs, and altered intestinal microbiome.[34]

PATHOPHYSIOLOGY Inflammation begins in the intestinal submucosa and spreads with discontinuous transmural involvement ("skip lesions") that can involve any part of the GI tract from the mouth to the perianal area. The distal small intestine and proximal large colon are most commonly involved. The ulcerations of CD can produce fissures that extend inflammation into lymphoid tissue. The typical lesion is a granuloma (a mass of inflammatory tissue) surrounded by ulceration. Fistulae may form in the perianal area between loops of intestine or extend into the bladder, rectum, or vagina. Strictures may develop, promoting obstruction. Smoking increases the risk of developing severe disease, and may cause a poorer response to treatment.

CLINICAL MANIFESTATIONS Individuals with CD may have no specific symptoms for several years. Symptoms vary according to the location of the disease but are similar to those for UC. Diarrhea is one of the most common symptoms and, occasionally, rectal bleeding if the colon is involved. Weight loss and abdominal pain accompany CD. If the ileum is involved, the individual may be anemic as a result of malabsorption of vitamin B_{12}. There also may be deficiencies in folic acid and vitamin D absorption. In addition, proteins may be lost, leading to hypoalbuminemia. Extraintestinal complications are similar to those occurring in ulcerative colitis.

EVALUATION AND TREATMENT The diagnosis and treatment of CD are similar to the diagnosis and treatment of ulcerative colitis; however, imaging of the small intestine is used in the diagnosis of CD, including either a small bowel series or a capsule endoscopy (camera pill). There are no specific biomarkers or definitive treatments. Smoking cessation is a component of therapy. Steroids and immunomodulators (i.e., anti-tumor necrosis factor [TNF]) are effective for initial therapy. Antiinflammatory drugs and immunomodulators are used for maintenance therapy. Surgery may be performed to manage complications such as fistula, abscess, or obstruction. Routine colonoscopy for cancer screening should be performed for long-standing colonic disease.[34]

Microscopic Colitis

Microscopic colitis is a relatively common cause of nonbloody diarrhea. Although the mucosa appears normal, there are two histologic forms: lymphocytic and collagenous. Lymphocytic colitis shows an increase in the number of intraepithelial lymphocytes in the wall of the colon. Collagenous colitis is characterized by a thickened subepithelial collagen layer, alteration of the vascular mucosal pattern, and mucosal nodularity. The cause is unknown. Risk factors include age 50 years or older, female sex, weight loss, smoking, use of proton pump inhibitors, nonsteroidal anti-inflammatory drugs, and selective serotonin reuptake inhibitors.[35]

The symptoms of frequent, chronic daily watery diarrhea are the same for both types and can be accompanied by abdominal pain and weight loss. Antidiarrheal agents and budesonide (an oral antiinflammatory steroid) are the best documented treatments. The disease is negatively associated with colorectal cancer.

Irritable Bowel Syndrome

Irritable bowel syndrome (IBS) currently is considered a disorder of brain-gut interaction characterized by recurrent abdominal pain with altered bowel habits. Worldwide prevalence is about 10% to 15%.[36] It is more common in women, with a higher prevalence during youth and middle age. Individuals with symptoms of IBS also are more likely to have anxiety, depression, and a reduced quality of life.

The pathophysiology of IBS is unknown, and there are no specific biomarkers for the disease. There is increasing evidence to explain a multisystem interaction with variables, including infection, gut microbiota, immune activation, serotonin dysregulation, psychological stress, and diet, as contributing factors to the varying symptom presentations. The presentations are summarized as follows:

- *Visceral hypersensitivity or hyperalgesia,* may originate in either the peripheral or the central nervous system. The mechanism may be related to a dysregulation of the bidirectional "brain-gut axis" (alterations in gut or central nervous system processing of gut-pain information). Factors include genetic-related changes in the function of serotonin-secreting cells of gut-brain pain modulation, alterations in gut microbiota metabolite production with activation of the gut immune system, increased visceral sensitivity and permeability, and altered motility and secretion.

- *Abnormal GI permeability, motility, secretion, and sensitivity* are associated with IBS. Individuals with diarrhea-type IBS have more rapid colonic transit times and increased intestinal permeability. Those with bloating and constipation have delayed transit times and decreased intestinal permeability. The mechanism may be related to dysregulation of the brain-gut axis, alterations in the function of gut neuroendocrine cells or dorsal root ganglion neurons, or changes in the activity of mast cells (produce histamine). Sex hormones may be a contributing factor.
- *Postinflammatory (infectious or noninfectious) IBS* is associated with intestinal infection (bacterial enteritis) and low-grade inflammation. Alterations in gut microbiota, immune activation in gut tissues, and changes in intestinal permeability have been proposed.
- *Alteration in gut microbiota (dysbiosis)* influences the sensory, motor, and immune systems of the gut and interacts with higher brain centers and may contribute to symptoms of IBS. Small intestine overgrowth of normal gut bacteria may be associated with IBS symptoms in some cases. Nonabsorbable antibiotics and prebiotics and probiotics may be helpful in some individuals.
- *Food allergy or food intolerance* is associated with IBS in some cases. Food antigens may activate the mucosal immune system, alter intestinal flora, or mediate hypersensitivity reactions and IBS symptoms. Food elimination approaches are helpful in some cases.
- *Psychosocial factors (epigenetic factors)*—including early life trauma or abuse or emotional stress interacting with neuroendocrine, neuroimmune, autonomic nervous system, and pain modulatory responses—contribute to the symptoms of IBS.

CLINICAL MANIFESTATIONS IBS is characterized by lower abdominal pain or discomfort and bloating. IBS can be grouped as diarrhea-predominant, constipation-predominant, or alternating diarrhea/constipation. Symptoms including gas, bloating, and nausea are usually relieved with defecation and do not interfere with sleep.

EVALUATION AND TREATMENT The diagnosis of IBS is based on signs, symptoms, and personal history and includes the exclusion of structural or biochemical causes of disease. Diagnostic procedures to rule out other causes of symptoms may include endoscopic evaluations, computed tomography (CT) scans or abdominal ultrasound, blood tests, and tests for lactose intolerance, celiac disease or other disorders. The person may be evaluated for food allergies, parasites, or bacterial growth. The Rome IV criteria for diagnosing IBS are presented in Box 38.2.

There is no cure for IBS, and treatment is individualized. Treatment of symptoms may include laxatives and fiber, antidiarrheals, antispasmodics, prosecretory drugs, low-dose antidepressants, visceral analgesics, and serotonin agonists or antagonists. Alternative therapies include prebiotics and probiotics to manipulate the microflora, hypnosis, acupuncture, yoga, cognitive behavioral therapy, and dietary interventions. Research continues to advance the management and understanding of the pathophysiology of this complex syndrome.[36]

Diverticular Disease of the Colon

Diverticula are herniations or saclike outpouchings of the mucosa and submucosa through the muscle layers, usually in the wall of the sigmoid colon (Fig. 38.8). They rarely occur in the small intestine. **Diverticulosis** is asymptomatic diverticular disease. **Diverticulitis** represents inflammation. The cause of diverticular disease is unknown. It is associated with increased intracolonic pressure, abnormal neuromuscular function,

---

BOX 38.2 Diagnostic Criteria* for Irritable Bowel Syndrome (IBS)

Rome IV Criteria

Recurrent abdominal pain, on average, at least 1 day per week in the past 3 months associated with two or more of the following criteria:
- Related to defecation
- Associated with a change in frequency of stool
- Associated with a change in form (appearance) of stool
- IBS subtypes include:
  - IBS with predominant constipation (IBS-C)
  - IBS with predominant diarrhea (IBS-D)
  - IBS with mixed bowel habits (IBS-M)
  - IBS unclassified (IBS-U)

*Criteria met for the past 3 months with symptom onset at least 6 months before diagnosis.
IBS, Irritable bowel syndrome.
Adapted from Drossman DA: *Gastroenterology* 150(6):1262-1297, 2016: Lacey BE et al: *Gastroenterology* 150(6):1393-1407, 2016.

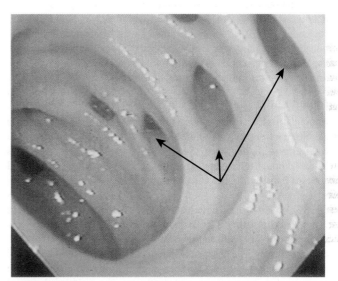

FIGURE 38.8 Diverticular Disease. In diverticular disease, the outpouches *(arrows)* of mucosa seen in the sigmoid colon appear as slitlike openings from the mucosal surface of the opened bowel. (From Townsend CM et al: *Sabiston textbook of surgery,* ed 19, Philadelphia 2012, Saunders)

and alterations in intestinal motility. Predisposing factors include older age, genetic predisposition, obesity, smoking, diet, lack of physical activity, and medication use, such as aspirin and nonsteroidal anti-inflammatory drugs. Lack of dietary fiber may or may not contribute to diverticular disease. Altered intestinal microbiota, visceral hypersensitivity, and abnormal colonic motility also may be contributing factors.[37]

PATHOPHYSIOLOGY Diverticula can occur anywhere in the GI tract, particularly at weak points in the colon wall, usually where arteries penetrate the tunica muscularis. The most common sites are the left sigmoid colon (prevalent in Western countries) and the right colon (prevalent in Asian countries). A common associated finding is thickening of the circular muscles and shortening of the longitudinal (teniae coli) muscles surrounding the diverticula. Increased collagen and elastin deposition, not muscle hypertrophy, is associated with muscle thickening, and this contributes to increased intraluminal pressure and herniation.

According to the law of Laplace (see Chapter 25), wall pressure increases as the diameter of a cylindrical structure decreases. Therefore, pressure within the narrow lumen can increase enough to rupture the diverticula, causing inflammation and diverticulitis. Bacteria and local ischemia also may be contributing factors. Complicated diverticulitis includes abscess, fistula, obstruction, bleeding, or perforation.

CLINICAL MANIFESTATIONS   Symptoms of uncomplicated diverticular disease may be vague or absent. Cramping pain of the lower abdomen can accompany constriction of the thickened colonic muscles. Diarrhea, constipation, distention, or flatulence may occur. If the diverticula become inflamed or abscesses form, the individual develops fever, leukocytosis (increased white blood cell count), and tenderness in the lower left quadrant.

EVALUATION AND TREATMENT   Diverticula are often discovered during diagnostic procedures performed for other problems. Ultrasound, sigmoidoscopy, or colonoscopy permits direct observation of the lesions. Abdominal CT is used for diagnosis of complicated cases.

An increase in dietary fiber intake often relieves symptoms by increasing bulk and lowering colonic pressure. Uncomplicated diverticulitis is usually treated with bowel rest and a clear, liquid diet and analgesia. Use of antibiotics is individually evaluated. Probiotics, nonabsorbable antibiotics, and 5-aminosalicylic acid are being evaluated. Laparoscopic resection and other minimally invasive approaches are implemented for more severe complications.[38]

Appendicitis

Appendicitis is an inflammation of the vermiform appendix, which is a projection from the apex of the cecum. It is the most common surgical emergency of the abdomen, usually occurring between 10 and 19 years of age (although it may develop at any age). The incidence in the United States is 7 to 10 cases per 10,000 persons.[39]

PATHOPHYSIOLOGY   The exact mechanism of the cause of appendicitis is not well understood. Obstruction of the lumen with stool, tumors, or foreign bodies, with consequent bacterial infection, is the most common theory. The obstructed lumen does not allow drainage of the appendix, and as mucosal secretion continues, intraluminal pressure increases. The increased pressure decreases mucosal blood flow, and the appendix becomes hypoxic. The mucosa ulcerates, promoting bacterial or other microbial invasion, with further inflammation and edema. Inflammation may involve the distal or entire appendix. Gangrene develops from thrombosis of the luminal blood vessels, followed by perforation in complex cases.[40]

CLINICAL MANIFESTATIONS   Epigastric or periumbilical pain is the typical symptom of an inflamed appendix. The pain may be vague at first and in the periumbilical area, increasing in intensity over 3 to 4 hours. It may subside and then migrate to the right lower quadrant, indicating extension of the inflammation to the surrounding tissues. Nausea, vomiting, and anorexia follow the onset of pain, and a low-grade fever is common. Diarrhea occurs in some individuals, particularly children; others have constipation. Perforation, peritonitis, and abscess formation are the most serious complications of appendicitis.

EVALUATION AND TREATMENT   In addition to clinical manifestations, there is pain with abdominal palpation and rebound tenderness, usually referred to the right lower quadrant. The white blood cell count is greater than 10,000 cells/mm^3, with increased neutrophils and C-reactive protein. Abdominal ultrasound, CT scans, and magnetic resonance imaging (MRI) (particularly for pregnant women and children) assist with diagnostic accuracy and help rule out nonappendiceal disease. Antibiotics or antibiotics and appendectomy are treatments for simple appendicitis. Complicated appendicitis (perforation, abscess formation, peritonitis) usually requires both antibiotics and surgery.[41]

Mesenteric Vascular Insufficiency

Mesenteric vascular insufficiency is rare, with an incidence of about 2 to 3 cases per 100,000 persons.[42] Three branches of the abdominal aorta supply the stomach and intestines: the celiac artery and the superior and inferior mesenteric arteries (see Fig. 37.6). The inferior mesenteric vein drains into the splenic vein, and the splenic vein and superior mesenteric vein join the portal vein. *Mesenteric venous thrombosis* is the least common of the causes of mesenteric vascular insufficiency. Malignancies, right-sided heart failure, and deep vein thrombosis are risk factors. Mesenteric venous thrombosis presents with abdominal pain and is treated with anticoagulants.

Acute mesenteric arterial insufficiency results in a significant reduction in mucosal blood flow to the large and small intestines.[43] Preexisting morbidities include dissecting aortic aneurysms, arterial thrombi, or emboli. Embolic obstruction is associated with atrial fibrillation, mitral valve disease, heart valve prostheses, and myocardial infarction. The superior mesenteric artery has a more direct line of flow from the aorta; therefore, emboli enter it more readily than the inferior branch, causing ischemia and necrosis of the small intestine. Ischemia and necrosis (intestinal infarction) alter membrane permeability. Initially, there is increased motility, nausea and vomiting, urgent bowel evacuation, and severe abdominal pain. Ischemia leads to decreased motility and distention. The damaged intestinal mucosa cannot produce enough mucus to protect itself from digestive enzymes. Mucosal alteration causes fluid to move from the blood vessels into the bowel wall and peritoneum. Fluid loss causes hypovolemia, and further decreases intestinal blood flow. As intestinal infarction progresses, shock, fever, bloody diarrhea, and leukocytosis develop. Bacteria invade the necrotic intestinal wall, causing gangrene and peritonitis

Chronic mesenteric ischemia is rare but can develop with atherosclerotic stenosis or occlusion, or secondary to congestive heart failure, acute myocardial infarction, hemorrhage, thrombus formation, or any condition that decreases arterial blood flow. Chronic occlusion is often accompanied by the formation of collateral circulation. The collateral vessels may be able to nourish the resting intestine, but after eating, when the intestine requires more blood, the arterial supply may be insufficient. Ischemia develops, causing cramping abdominal pain (abdominal angina), a cardinal symptom. Some individuals suffer significant weight loss because they stop eating to control the pain. Progressive vascular obstruction eventually causes continuous abdominal pain and necrosis of the intestinal tissue.

The diagnosis of acute and chronic mesenteric ischemia is based on clinical manifestations, laboratory findings, and imaging studies. A bruit can often be heard over a partially occluded artery. Treatment includes aggressive rehydration and the use of antibiotics, anticoagulants, vasodilators, and inhibitors of reperfusion injury. Surgery, including endovascular techniques, is required to remove necrotic tissue, repair sclerosed vessels, and revascularize affected tissue. Acute occlusion is a surgical emergency, and the mortality rate is high (50% to 90%). Early diagnosis and aggressive treatment result in the best survival rates.[44]

DISORDERS OF THE ACCESSORY ORGANS OF DIGESTION

The accessory organs of digestion (liver, gallbladder, pancreas) secrete substances necessary for digestion and, in the case of the liver, carry out metabolic functions needed to maintain life. Disorders of these organs include inflammatory disease, obstruction of ducts, and tumors. (Cancers of the digestive system are described at the end of this chapter.)

Common Complications of Liver Disorders

Of all the accessory organ disorders, acute or chronic liver disease leads to the most significant systemic, life-threatening complications. These complications are common to all liver disorders and include portal hypertension, ascites, hepatic encephalopathy, jaundice, and hepatorenal syndrome.

Portal Hypertension

Portal hypertension is abnormally high blood pressure in the portal venous system caused by resistance to blood flow. Pressure in this system is normally 3 mm Hg; portal hypertension is an increase to at least 10 mm Hg.

PATHOPHYSIOLOGY   Portal hypertension is caused by disorders that obstruct or impede blood flow through any component of the portal venous system or vena cava. *Intrahepatic causes* result from vascular remodeling with shunts, thrombosis, inflammation, or fibrosis of the sinusoids, as occurs in cirrhosis of the liver, biliary cirrhosis, viral hepatitis, or schistosomiasis (a parasitic infection). *Posthepatic causes* occur from hepatic vein thrombosis or cardiac disorders that impair the pumping ability of the right side of the heart. This causes blood to collect and increases pressure in the veins of the portal system. The most common cause of portal hypertension is fibrosis and obstruction caused by cirrhosis of the liver. Long-term portal hypertension causes several pathophysiologic problems that are difficult to treat and can be fatal. These problems include varices, splenomegaly, ascites, hepatic encephalopathy, and hepatopulmonary syndrome.

Varices are distended, tortuous collateral veins. Prolonged elevation of pressure in the portal vein cause collateral veins to open between the portal vein and systemic veins. The prolonged pressure results in transformation into varices, particularly in the lower esophagus and stomach, but also over the abdominal wall (known as the caput medusae [Medusa head]) and rectum (hemorrhoidal varices) (Fig. 38.9). Rupture of varices can cause life-threatening hemorrhage.[45]

Splenomegaly is enlargement of the spleen caused by increased pressure in the splenic vein, which branches from the portal vein. Thrombocytopenia is the most common symptom of congestive splenomegaly. The enlarged spleen can be palpated. Hepatopulmonary syndrome (vasodilation, intrapulmonary shunting, and hypoxia) and portopulmonary hypertension (pulmonary vasoconstriction and vascular remodeling) are complications of liver disease and portal hypertension. The pathophysiology is complex and involves different effects of vasoactive substances. There may be no clinical manifestations, although dyspnea, cyanosis, and clubbing may occur.

CLINICAL MANIFESTATIONS   Vomiting of blood (hematemesis) from bleeding esophageal varices is the most common clinical manifestation of portal hypertension. Bleeding is usually from varices that have developed slowly over a period of years. Slow, chronic bleeding from varices causes anemia or melena. Rupture of esophageal varices causes hemorrhage and voluminous vomiting of dark-colored blood. The ruptured varices are usually painless. Rupture is caused by a combination of erosion by gastric acid and elevated venous pressure. Mortality from ruptured esophageal varices ranges from 30% to 60%. Recurrent bleeding of esophageal varices indicates a poor prognosis. Hemorrhoidal varices present as hematochezia and copious rectal bleeding. Most individuals die within 1 year.

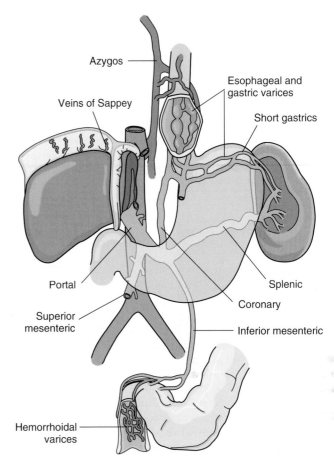

FIGURE 38.9 Varices Related to Portal Hypertension. The portal vein, its major tributaries, and the most important shunts (collateral veins) between the portal and caval systems. The shunted blood returns to the systemic venous system, bypassing the liver. (From Monahan FD et al: *Phipps' medical-surgical nursing: concepts and clinical practice,* ed 8, St Louis, 2007, Mosby.)

EVALUATION AND TREATMENT   Portal hypertension is often diagnosed at the time of variceal bleeding and confirmed by upper GI endoscopy and evaluation of portal venous pressure. The individual usually has a history of jaundice, hepatitis, alcoholism, or cirrhosis. Pressure in the portal venous system can be reduced with nonselective beta-blocking drugs to assist in preventing variceal bleeding.

Emergency management of bleeding varices includes use of vasopressors and compression of the varices with an inflatable tube or balloon, sclerotherapy, variceal ligation, or portacaval shunt. Surgical construction of transjugular intrahepatic portosystemic shunts (TIPS) and anastomosis of the portal vein to the inferior vena cava may decompress the varices. This treatment can precipitate encephalopathy. Liver transplantation is the most successful option for liver failure.

Ascites

Ascites is the accumulation of fluid in the peritoneal cavity. Ascites traps body fluid in the peritoneal space, from which it cannot escape. Ascites reduces the amount of body fluid available for normal physiologic functions. Cirrhosis is the most common cause of ascites, but other causes include heart failure, constrictive pericarditis, abdominal malignancies, nephrotic syndrome, and malnutrition. Of individuals who develop ascites caused by cirrhosis, 25% die within 1 year. Continued heavy drinking of alcohol is associated with this mortality and is related to cirrhosis.

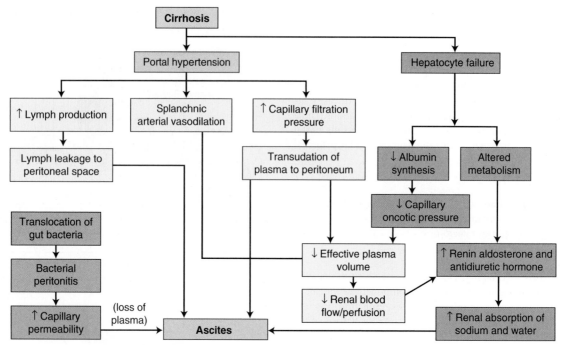

FIGURE 38.10 Mechanisms of Ascites Caused by Cirrhosis.

PATHOPHYSIOLOGY   Several factors contribute to the development of ascites, including portal hypertension, decreased synthesis of albumin by the liver, splanchnic arterial vasodilation, and renal sodium and water retention. Portal hypertension and reduced serum albumin levels cause capillary hydrostatic pressure to exceed capillary osmotic pressure (see Chapter 5), pushing water into the peritoneal cavity. Portal hypertension also increases the production of hepatic lymph, which "weeps" into the peritoneal cavity. Splanchnic arterial vasodilation, associated with increased nitric oxide produced by the diseased liver, can decrease effective circulating blood volume, activating aldosterone and antidiuretic hormone, which promote renal sodium and water retention. The sodium and water retention expands plasma volume, thereby accelerating portal hypertension and ascites formation. Translocation of bacteria and release of endotoxin cause peritonitis with an inflammatory response that increases mesenteric capillary permeability and fluid movement into the peritoneal cavity, promoting ascites. Fig. 38.10 summarizes the mechanisms by which cirrhosis of the liver cause ascites.

CLINICAL MANIFESTATIONS   The accumulation of ascitic fluid causes abdominal distention, increased abdominal girth, and weight gain (Fig. 38.11). Large volumes of fluid (10 to 20 L) displace the diaphragm and cause dyspnea by decreasing lung capacity. The respiratory rate increases, and the individual assumes a sitting position to relieve the dyspnea. Some peripheral edema is usually present. Approximately 10% of individuals with ascites develop bacterial peritonitis, which causes fever, chills, abdominal pain, decreased bowel sounds, and cloudy ascitic fluid.

EVALUATION AND TREATMENT   The diagnosis is usually based on clinical manifestations and identification of liver disease. Dietary salt restriction and diuretics can reduce ascites. Albumin may be given. Paracentesis is used to aspirate ascitic fluid for bacterial culture, biochemical analysis, and microscopic examination. The goal of treatment is to relieve discomfort. If the restoration of liver function is possible, the ascites diminishes spontaneously. Levels of serum electrolytes are monitored carefully because the individual is at risk for hyponatremia and hypokalemia.

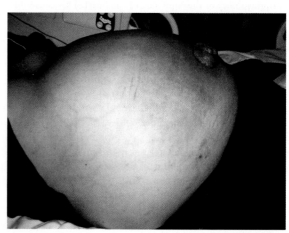

FIGURE 38.11 Massive Ascites in an Individual With Cirrhosis. Distended abdomen, dilated upper abdominal veins, and inverted umbilicus are classic manifestations. (From Goldman L, Schafer AI: *Goldman's Cecil medicine*, ed 24, Philadelphia, 2012, Saunders.)

Palliative measures include paracentesis to remove 1 or 2 L of ascitic fluid and relieve respiratory distress. However, the removal of too much fluid relieves pressure on blood vessels and carries the risk of hypotension, shock, or death. Despite repeated paracentesis, ascitic fluid reaccumulates because of the persistent portal hypertension and reduced plasma albumin levels associated with irreversible disease. Peritonitis is treated with antibiotics. Other procedures include peritoneovenous shunt (peritoneal fluid into veins) and transjugular intrahepatic portosystemic shunt (TIPS) (bypass of blood flow from the portal venous branch to the hepatic venous branch). Individuals with ascites and portal hypertension have a poor prognosis, and liver transplantation is the best treatment option.

Hepatic Encephalopathy

Hepatic encephalopathy (portal system encephalopathy) is a complex neurologic syndrome characterized by impaired behavioral, cognitive, and motor function. The syndrome may develop rapidly during acute fulminant hepatitis or slowly during the course of cirrhosis and the development of portal hypertension or after portosystemic bypass or shunting.

PATHOPHYSIOLOGY Hepatic encephalopathy results from a combination of biochemical alterations that affect neurotransmission and brain function.[46] Liver dysfunction and the development of collateral vessels that shunt blood around the liver to the systemic circulation permit toxins absorbed from the GI tract and normally removed by the liver, to accumulate and circulate freely to the brain. The accumulated toxins alter cerebral energy metabolism, interfere with neurotransmission, and cause edema. The most hazardous substances are end products of intestinal protein digestion, particularly ammonia, which cannot be converted to urea by the diseased liver. Other substances include inflammatory cytokines, short chain fatty acids, serotonin, tryptophan, and manganese. These substances cause astrocyte swelling and alter the blood-brain barrier, promoting cerebral edema. Infection, hemorrhage, and electrolyte imbalance (including zinc deficiency), constipation, and the use of sedatives and analgesics can precipitate hepatic encephalopathy in the presence of liver disease.

CLINICAL MANIFESTATIONS Subtle changes in personality, memory loss, irritability, disinhibition, lethargy, and sleep disturbances are common initial manifestations of hepatic encephalopathy. Symptoms then can progress to confusion, disorientation to time and space, flapping tremor of the hands (asterixis), slow speech, bradykinesia, stupor, convulsions, and coma. Coma is usually a sign of liver failure and ultimately results in death. Variceal bleeding and ascites may develop concurrently. Symptoms may be episodic, recurrent, or persistent. Hepatic encephalopathy is often associated with bleeding varices and ascites.

EVALUATION AND TREATMENT The diagnosis of hepatic encephalopathy is based on a history of liver disease, clinical manifestations, psychometric tests, and exclusion of other causes of brain dysfunction. Electroencephalography and blood chemistry tests provide supportive data. Tracking levels of serum ammonia assesses treatment effectiveness and liver function.

Correction of fluid and electrolyte imbalances and withdrawal of depressant drugs metabolized by the liver are the first steps in the treatment of hepatic encephalopathy. Dietary protein is maintained to prevent malnutrition but at levels that reduce blood ammonia levels. Lactulose prevents ammonia absorption in the colon. Neomycin eliminates ammonia-producing intestinal bacteria but can be nephrotoxic. Glutamase inhibitors reduce gut ammonia. Rifaximin decreases intestinal production of ammonia and is used for lactulose nonresponders. Extracorporeal liver support systems remove toxins from the blood and are an option for managing overt hepatic encephalopathy or as a bridge to liver transplantation.[47]

Jaundice

Jaundice, or icterus, is a yellow or greenish pigmentation of the skin caused by hyperbilirubinemia (plasma bilirubin concentrations greater than 2.5 to 3 mg/dl). Hyperbilirubinemia and jaundice can result from (1) extrahepatic (posthepatic) obstruction to bile flow, (2) intrahepatic obstruction, or (3) prehepatic excessive production of unconjugated bilirubin (i.e., excessive hemolysis of red blood cells) (Fig. 38.12). Jaundice

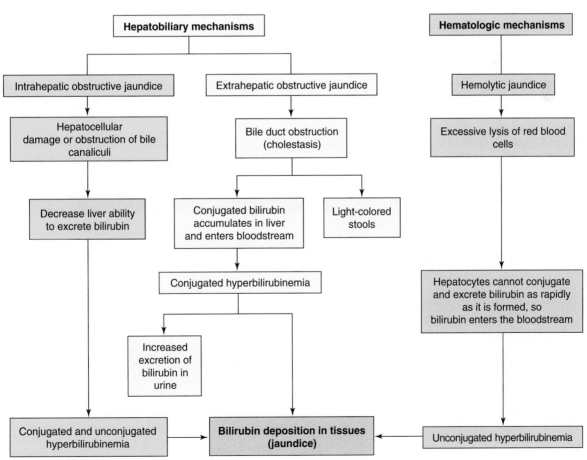

FIGURE 38.12 Mechanisms of Jaundice.

in newborns is caused by impaired bilirubin uptake and conjugation (see Chapter 39).

PATHOPHYSIOLOGY Obstructive jaundice can result from extrahepatic or intrahepatic obstruction.[48] *Extrahepatic obstructive jaundice* develops if the common bile duct is occluded (e.g., by a gallstone, tumor, or inflammation). Bilirubin conjugated by the hepatocytes cannot flow through the obstructed common bile duct into the duodenum. Therefore, it accumulates in the liver and enters the bloodstream, causing hyperbilirubinemia and jaundice. *Intrahepatic obstructive jaundice* involves disturbances in hepatocyte function and obstruction of bile canaliculi. The uptake, conjugation, or excretion of bilirubin can be affected with elevated levels of both conjugated and unconjugated bilirubin. Obstruction of bile canaliculi diminishes flow of conjugated bilirubin into the common bile duct. In mild cases, some of the bile canaliculi open. Consequently, the amount of bilirubin in the intestinal tract may be only slightly decreased.

Excessive hemolysis (destruction) of red blood cells can cause hemolytic jaundice *(prehepatic or nonobstructive jaundice)*. Increased unconjugated bilirubin is formed through metabolism of the heme component of destroyed red blood cells and exceeds the conjugation ability of the liver, causing blood levels of unconjugated bilirubin to rise. Decreased bilirubin uptake or conjugation also causes unconjugated hyperbilirubinemia, as occurs with reaction to some drugs (e.g., rifampin), and in genetic disorders, such as Gilbert syndrome (caused by lack of an enzyme that conjugates bilirubin). Because unconjugated bilirubin is not water soluble, it is not excreted in the urine. The causes of jaundice are summarized in Table 38.7.

CLINICAL MANIFESTATIONS Conjugated bilirubin is water soluble and appears in the urine. The urine may darken several days before the onset of jaundice. The complete obstruction of bile flow from the liver to the duodenum causes light-colored stools. With partial obstruction, the stools are normal in color and bilirubin is present in the urine.

Fever, chills, and pain often accompany jaundice resulting from viral or bacterial inflammation of the liver (e.g., viral hepatitis). Yellow discoloration may first occur in the sclera of the eye and then progress to the skin as bilirubin attaches to elastic fibers. Pruritus (itching) often accompanies jaundice because bilirubin accumulates in the skin, irritating itch receptors.

EVALUATION AND TREATMENT Laboratory evaluation of serum establishes whether elevated plasma bilirubin is conjugated or unconjugated, or both. The history and physical examination identify underlying disorders, such as cirrhosis, exposure to hepatitis virus, gallbladder, pancreatic disease, or hematologic disorders. The treatment for jaundice consists of correcting the cause.

Hepatorenal Syndrome

Hepatorenal syndrome is functional renal failure that develops as a complication of advanced liver disease. The renal failure is not caused by primary renal disease or other extrinsic factors, but rather by portal hypertension, cardiac impairment, and other circulatory alterations associated with advanced liver disease, such as cirrhosis or fulminant hepatitis with portal hypertension and decreased systemic vascular resistance. Manifestations include oliguria, sodium and water retention (usually with ascites and peripheral edema), hypotension, and peripheral vasodilation. The kidney usually has a normal structure.

PATHOPHYSIOLOGY *Type 1 hepatorenal syndrome* accompanies a sudden decrease in blood volume secondary to massive GI or variceal bleeding and hypotension caused by bleeding and peripheral vasodilation associated with failing liver function. Hypotension also can be caused by the excessive use of diuretics to treat ascites or decreased cardiac output. The decrease in blood volume and hypotension result in decreased renal perfusion, decreased glomerular filtration, and oliguria (see Chapter 32). *Type 2 hepatorenal syndrome* develops slowly and is related to ascites. Ineffective circulating blood volume causes decreased glomerular filtration and oliguria. Intrarenal vasoconstriction may result from the selective effects of vasoactive substances that accumulate in the blood because of liver failure or a compensatory response to portal hypertension and the pooling of blood in the splanchnic circulation.

CLINICAL MANIFESTATIONS The onset of hepatorenal manifestations may be acute or gradual. Oliguria and complications of advanced liver disease, including jaundice, ascites, peripheral edema, hypotension and GI bleeding, are usually present. Systolic blood pressure is usually below 100 mm Hg. Nonspecific symptoms of hepatorenal syndrome include anorexia, weakness, and fatigue.

EVALUATION AND TREATMENT Despite oliguria, serum potassium levels do not become dangerously elevated until the terminal stages of

TABLE 38.7	Common Types of Jaundice	
Type	**Mechanism**	**Causes**
Hemolytic (prehepatic) jaundice (predominantly unconjugated bilirubin)	Destruction of erythrocytes (increased bilirubin production)	Hemolytic anemias (e.g., sickle cell) Severe infection Toxic substances in circulation (e.g., snake venom) Transfusion of incompatible blood
Disorders of bilirubin metabolism (unconjugated bilirubin)	Decreased bilirubin uptake Decreased bilirubin conjugation	Drug induced (e.g., rifampin and cyclosporine) Hereditary disorder (e.g., Gilbert syndrome)
Obstructive (posthepatic) jaundice (predominantly conjugated bilirubin)	Obstruction of passage of conjugated bilirubin from liver to intestine	Obstruction of bile duct by gallstones or tumor (extrahepatic obstructive jaundice) Obstruction of bile flow through liver (intrahepatic obstructive jaundice) Drugs
Hepatocellular (intrahepatic) jaundice (both conjugated and unconjugated bilirubin)	Failure of liver cells (hepatocytes) to conjugate bilirubin and of bilirubin to pass from liver to intestine	Genetic defect of hepatocytes (decreased enzymes), such as occurs in premature infants (see Chapter 39) Severe infections (e.g., hepatitis) Alcoholic liver disease or biliary cirrhosis

the hepatorenal syndrome. Blood urea level increases, followed by an increase in creatinine concentration and metabolic acidosis. Urine osmolality increases, but urine sodium concentrations are below normal. Urine specific gravity is greater than 1.015.

The prognosis is usually poor and is related to a failing liver requiring liver transplantation. Bridge treatments include albumin administration and terlipressin (a vasopressin analogue).[49]

✔ QUICK CHECK 38.4

1. How does portal hypertension cause varices and promote the formation of ascites?
2. What are two factors that cause hepatic encephalopathy?
3. Why is the concentration of unconjugated bilirubin elevated in hemolytic jaundice?
4. Describe how failure of liver function causes renal failure (hepatorenal syndrome).

Disorders of the Liver
Acute Liver Failure

Acute liver failure (fulminant liver failure) is a rare clinical syndrome resulting in severe impairment or necrosis of liver cells without preexisting liver disease or cirrhosis. Acetaminophen overdose is a leading cause of acute liver failure in the United States[50] (see *Did You Know?* Paracetamol [Acetaminophen] and Acute Liver Failure in Chapter 37). N-acetyl cysteine is an available treatment for detoxification and should be given as soon as possible, preferably within 16 hours after the acetaminophen was taken. Acute liver failure also can occur with concurrent liver disease (acute on chronic liver failure), including complication of viral hepatitis, particularly hepatitis B virus (HBV) infection; compounded by infection with the delta virus; as well as metabolic liver disorders. Edematous hepatocytes and patchy areas of necrosis and inflammatory cell infiltrates disrupt liver tissue. The death of hepatocytes may be caused by viral or toxic injury or immunologic and inflammatory damage.

Acute liver failure usually develops 6 to 8 weeks after the initial symptoms of viral hepatitis or a metabolic liver disorder, or within 5 days to 8 weeks of acetaminophen overdose. Anorexia, vomiting, abdominal pain, and progressive jaundice are initial signs, followed by ascites and GI bleeding. Hepatic encephalopathy is manifested as lethargy, altered motor functions, seizures, and coma. Coma is related to cerebral edema, ischemia, and brainstem herniation. Liver function tests reflect liver injury and show elevations in the levels of both direct and indirect serum bilirubin, serum transaminases, and blood ammonia. The prothrombin time is prolonged. Renal failure and pulmonary distress can occur. Treatment of acute liver failure requires rapid evaluation and critical care. The hepatic necrosis is irreversible, and there can be significant mortality. Liver transplantation may be lifesaving. Artificial liver support devices can provide a bridge to transplantation.[47]

Cirrhosis

Cirrhosis is an irreversible inflammatory, fibrotic liver disease. It has a prevalence in the United States of about 633,323 with a death rate of about 26%.[51] Many disorders can cause cirrhosis, and they are summarized in Box 38.3. The process of cellular injury depends on the cause of cirrhosis, and the pathologic mechanisms are not all clearly understood. Structural changes result from injury (e.g., viruses or toxicity from alcohol) and fibrosis, which is a consequence of infiltration of leukocytes, release of inflammatory mediators, and activation of fibrotic processes. Chaotic fibrosis alters or obstructs biliary channels and blood flow, producing jaundice and portal hypertension. New vascular channels form shunts, and blood from the portal vein bypasses the liver,

---

BOX 38.3 Causes of Cirrhosis

Hepatitis viruses—B and C (common)
Excessive alcohol intake (common)
Idiopathic (common)
Nonalcoholic fatty liver disease (NAFLD), also known as nonalcoholic steato-
 hepatitis (NASH)
Autoimmune disorders
  Autoimmune hepatitis
  Primary biliary cirrhosis
  Primary sclerosing cholangitis
Hereditary metabolic disorder
  α-Antitrypsin deficiency
  Hemochromatosis
  Wilson disease
  Glycogen or lipid storage diseases
Prolonged exposure to drugs or toxins (e.g., carbon tetrachloride, cleaning and
 industrial solvents, copper salts)
Hepatic venous outflow obstruction
  Budd-Chiari syndrome
  Right-sided heart failure

---

contributing to portal hypertension, metabolic alterations, and toxin accumulation. The process of regeneration is disrupted by hypoxia, necrosis, atrophy, and (ultimately) liver failure. The formation of fibrous bands and regenerating nodules distorts the architecture of the liver parenchyma and gives the liver a cobbly appearance. The liver may be larger or smaller than normal and is usually firm or hard when palpated.[52]

Cirrhosis develops slowly over a period of years. Its severity and rate of progression depend on the cause. If toxins, such as alcohol metabolites, are involved, the rate of cell death and the severity of inflammation depend on the amount of toxin present. Removal of the toxin slows the progression of liver damage and enhances the process of regeneration.

Alcoholic liver disease. Alcoholic liver disease is related to the toxic effects of alcohol (see Chapter 4) and coexisting liver disease. Although alcoholic cirrhosis is the most prevalent of the various types of cirrhosis, the occurrence of cirrhosis among persons with alcoholism is relatively low (approximately 25%). The spectrum of alcoholic liver disease includes alcoholic fatty liver, alcoholic steatohepatitis, and alcoholic cirrhosis.[53]

PATHOPHYSIOLOGY Alcoholic fatty liver (steatosis) is the mildest form of alcoholic liver disease. It can be caused by relatively small amounts of alcohol, may be asymptomatic, and is reversible with the cessation of drinking. The fat deposition (deposition of triglycerides) within the liver is caused primarily by increased lipogenesis, cholesterol synthesis, and decreased fatty acid oxidation by hepatocytes. Lipids mobilized from adipose tissue or dietary fat intake may contribute to fat accumulation.

Alcoholic steatohepatitis (alcoholic hepatitis) is a precursor of cirrhosis characterized by increased hepatic fat storage, inflammation, and degeneration and necrosis of hepatocytes with infiltration of neutrophils and lymphocytes. The inflammation and necrosis caused by alcoholic steatohepatitis stimulate the irreversible fibrosis characteristic of the cirrhotic stage of disease.

Alcoholic cirrhosis is caused by the toxic effects of alcohol metabolism in the liver, immunologic alterations, inflammatory cytokines, oxidative stress from lipid peroxidation, and malnutrition. Alcohol is transformed to acetaldehyde, and excessive amounts significantly alter hepatocyte function and activate hepatic stellate cells, a primary cell involved in liver fibrosis. Enzyme and protein synthesis may be depressed or altered, and hormone and ammonia degradation is diminished. Acetaldehyde inhibits export of proteins from the liver, alters metabolism of vitamins and minerals, and induces malnutrition. Kupffer cell (macrophage) activation attracts neutrophils promoting inflammation, endotoxins accumulate from translocation of gut bacteria, and cell-mediated immunity is suppressed. Cellular damage initiates an inflammatory response that, along with necrosis, results in activation of hepatic stellate cells and excessive collagen formation. Fibrosis and scarring alter the structure of the liver and obstruct biliary and vascular channels.

CLINICAL MANIFESTATIONS Fatty infiltration causes no specific symptoms or abnormal liver function test results. The liver is usually enlarged, however, and the individual has a history of continuous alcohol intake during the previous weeks or months. Anorexia, nausea, jaundice, and edema develop with advanced fatty infiltration or the onset of alcoholic steatohepatitis (Fig. 38.13).

The clinical manifestations of alcoholic steatohepatitis can be mild or severe. Nonspecific symptoms include fatigue, weight loss, and anorexia. Manifestations of acute illness include nausea, anorexia, fever, abdominal pain, and jaundice. Cirrhosis is a multiple-system disease and causes hepatomegaly, splenomegaly, ascites, portal hypertension, GI hemorrhage, hepatic encephalopathy, and esophageal varices. Anemia results from blood loss, malnutrition, and hypersplenism. Renal failure is often a late complication of hepatorenal syndrome. Toxic effects of alcohol also can cause testicular atrophy, reduced libido, azoospermia, and decreased testosterone levels in men. The presence of numerous and severe manifestations increases the risk of death. Cirrhosis increases the risk of hepatocellular carcinoma.

EVALUATION AND TREATMENT The diagnosis of alcoholic steatohepatitis or cirrhosis is based on the individual's history and clinical manifestations. The results of liver function tests are abnormal, and serologic studies show elevated levels of serum enzymes and bilirubin, decreased levels of serum albumin, and a prolonged prothrombin time that is not easily corrected with vitamin K therapy. Liver biopsy can confirm the diagnosis of cirrhosis, but biopsy is not necessary if clinical manifestations of cirrhosis are evident.

There is no specific treatment for alcoholic steatohepatitis or cirrhosis. Rest, vitamin supplements, a nutritious diet, corticosteroids, antioxidants,

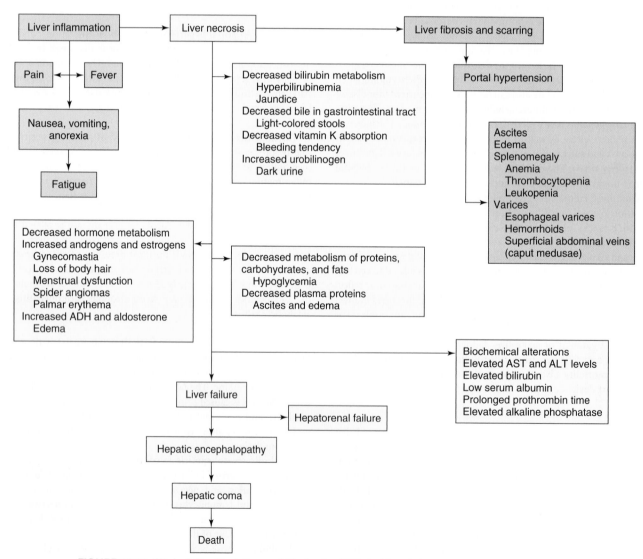

FIGURE 38.13 Clinical Manifestations of Cirrhosis. *ADH,* Antidiuretic hormone; *ALT,* alanine transaminase; *AST,* aspartate transaminase.

drugs that slow fibrosis, and management of complications (such as ascites, GI bleeding, and encephalopathy) slow disease progression. Cessation of alcohol consumption slows the progression of liver damage, improves clinical symptoms, and prolongs life. Although the liver damage is irreversible, measures that halt the inflammation and destruction of liver cells prolong life. Liver transplantation is the treatment of end-stage liver disease.

Nonalcoholic liver disease and nonalcoholic steatohepatitis. Nonalcoholic fatty liver disease (NAFLD) is the infiltration of hepatocytes with fat, primarily in the form of triglycerides, that occurs in the absence of alcohol intake. It is associated with obesity (including obese children), high levels of cholesterol and triglycerides, metabolic syndrome, and type 2 diabetes mellitus. NAFLD is the most common chronic liver disease in the United States. Some individuals with NAFLD will develop nonalcoholic steatohepatitis (NASH), with hepatocellular injury, inflammation, and fibrosis. NASH is difficult to distinguish from alcohol-induced liver fibrosis. NAFLD is usually asymptomatic and may remain undetected for years. The most severe forms of NASH progress to cirrhosis and end-stage liver disease. There can be progression to hepatocellular carcinoma. Treatment is individualized and includes the use of behavioral modification, dietary counseling, and regular exercise.[54]

Primary Biliary Cholangitis

Primary biliary cholangitis is a chronic, slowly progressive, autoimmune, cholestatic liver disease that begins in the bile canaliculi and bile ducts, rather than in the hepatocytes. It is caused by autoimmune T-lymphocyte and highly specific antimitochondrial antibody destruction of the small intrahepatic bile ducts and primarily affects middle-aged women. Primary biliary cholangitis often accompanies other autoimmune diseases. Pathogenesis includes inflammation, destruction, fibrosis, and obstruction of the intrahepatic bile ducts. Primary biliary cholangitis can be detected by biochemical evidence of cholestatic liver disease. Test findings include the presence of antinuclear antibodies, anticentromere antibodies, and the GP210 antinuclear antibody, as well as elevated alkaline phosphatase levels for at least 6 months. Ultrasound imaging of the liver, or liver biopsy, assists with diagnosis. Manifestations progress insidiously from pruritus, hyperbilirubinemia, jaundice, and light or clay-colored stools to cirrhosis, portal hypertension, and encephalopathy. Life expectancy is 5 to 10 years after the onset of symptoms if the condition is not treated. Treatment with ursodeoxycholic acid slows disease progression, and pruritus may be relieved by cholestyramine, which binds bile salts in the intestine. Liver transplantation is highly effective.[55]

> ✔ **QUICK CHECK 38.5**
> 1. How does alcohol damage the liver?
> 2. What kind of liver changes are common to alcoholic cirrhosis and nonalcoholic fatty liver disease?
> 3. What causes liver injury in primary biliary cholangitis?

Viral Hepatitis

Viral hepatitis is a relatively common systemic disease that affects primarily the liver. Different strains of viruses cause different types of hepatitis. In 2016 the infection types and estimated incidence in the United States were: 2007 cases of hepatitis A virus (HAV); 3218 cases of hepatitis B virus (HBV); unknown cases of hepatitis D virus (HDV) associated with HBV; 2967 cases of hepatitis C virus (HCV); and unknown cases of hepatitis E virus (HEV). Hepatitis A formerly was known as infectious hepatitis and hepatitis B as serum hepatitis.[56] Characteristics of the different types of viruses that cause hepatitis are presented in Table 38.8. Viral hepatitis in children is presented in Chapter 39.

PATHOPHYSIOLOGY   All five types of viral hepatitis (A, B, C, D, and E) can cause acute, icteric illness. HBV and HCV are the most common causes. In pregnant women HEV infection can be a serious disease.

TABLE 38.8 Characteristics of Viral Hepatitis

Characteristic	Hepatitis A	Hepatitis B	Hepatitis D	Hepatitis C	Hepatitis E
Size of virus	27 nm RNA virus	47 nm DNA virus	36 nm RNA virus, defective virus with HBsAg coat	30- to 60 nm RNA virus	32 nm RNA virus
Incubation phase	30 days	60-180 days	30-180 days; dependent on HBV for multiplication	35-72 days	15-60 days
Route of transmission	Fecal-oral, parenteral, sexual	Parenteral, sexual	Parenteral, fecal-oral, sexual	Parenteral	Fecal-oral
Onset	Acute with fever	Insidious	Insidious	Insidious	Acute
Carrier state	Negative	Positive	Positive	Positive	Negative
Severity	Mild	Severe; may be prolonged or chronic	Severe	Mild to severe	Severe in pregnant women
Chronic hepatitis	No	Yes	Yes	Yes	No
Age group affected	Children and young adults	Any	Any	Any	Children and young adults
Prophylaxis	Hygiene, immune serum globulin, HAV vaccine	Hygiene, HBV vaccine	Hygiene, HBV vaccine	Hygiene, screening of blood, interferon-alpha or combined with ribavirin; treatment also related to HCV genotype ± cirrhosis	Hygiene, safe water and meat

DNA, Deoxyribonucleic acid; *HAV,* hepatitis A virus; *HBsAg,* hepatitis B surface antigen; *HBV,* hepatitis B virus; *HCV,* hepatitis C virus; *RNA,* ribonucleic acid.

The pathologic lesions of hepatitis include hepatic cell necrosis, scarring (with chronic disease), and Kupffer cell hyperplasia; infiltration by mononuclear phagocytes occurs with varying severity. Cellular injury is promoted by cell-mediated immune mechanisms. Regeneration of hepatic cells begins within 48 hours of injury. The inflammatory process can damage and obstruct bile canaliculi, leading to cholestasis and obstructive jaundice. In milder cases, the liver parenchyma is not damaged. Damage tends to be most severe in cases of HBV and HCV disease. Acute fulminating hepatitis can cause acute liver failure and severe hepatic encephalopathy, which is manifested as confusion, stupor, coma, and coagulopathy.

Coinfection with HBV, HCV, HDV, and the human immunodeficiency virus (HIV) occurs because these viruses share the same route of transmission (contact between infected body fluids and broken skin or mucous membranes, or intravenously). Progression of liver disease is more rapid in these cases.

CLINICAL MANIFESTATIONS   The clinical manifestations of the various types of hepatitis are very similar. The spectrum of manifestations ranges from absence of symptoms to fulminating hepatitis, with rapid onset of liver failure and coma. Acute viral hepatitis causes abnormal liver function test results. The serum aminotransferase values, aspartate transaminase (AST) and alanine transaminase (ALT), are elevated but not consistent with the extent of cellular damage. The clinical course of hepatitis usually consists of three phases, preceded by an incubation phase. The incubation phase and manifestations vary depending on the virus (see Table 38.8). The other three phases are:

1. Prodromal (preicteric) phase begins about 2 weeks after exposure and ends with the appearance of jaundice; marked by fatigue, anorexia, malaise, nausea, vomiting, headache, hyperalgia, cough, and low-grade fever; the infection is highly transmissible during this phase.
2. Icteric phase begins 1 to 2 weeks after the prodromal phase and lasts 2 to 6 weeks; jaundice, dark urine, and clay-colored stools are common; the liver is enlarged, smooth, and tender, and percussion or palpation of the liver causes pain; GI and respiratory symptoms subside, but fatigue and abdominal pain may persist or become more severe. This is the actual phase of illness. Individuals who develop chronic HBV, HDV, or HCV infection do not become jaundiced and may not be diagnosed.
3. Recovery phase begins with resolution of jaundice, about 6 to 8 weeks after exposure; symptoms diminish, but the liver remains enlarged and tender; liver function returns to normal 2 to 12 weeks after the onset of jaundice.

Chronic active hepatitis is the persistence of clinical manifestations and liver inflammation after the acute stages of HBV, HBV/HDV coinfection, and HCV infection. Liver function tests remain abnormal for longer than 6 months, and the hepatitis B surface antigen (HBsAg) persists. Chronic, active HBV or HCV infection is a predisposition to cirrhosis and primary hepatocellular carcinoma. Chronic active hepatitis constitutes a carrier state, and HBV and HCV can be transmitted from mothers to infants.

EVALUATION AND TREATMENT   The diagnosis of HAV and HCV infections is based on the presence of anti-HAV and anti-HCV antibodies. The most specific diagnostic test for HBV is serologic analysis for specific hepatitis virus antigens (i.e., HBsAg, which is the marker for HBV). There are other markers for HBV, including hepatitis B surface antibody (anti-HBs), hepatitis B envelope antigen (HBeAg), hepatitis B envelope antibody, (anti-HBe), hepatitis B core antibody (anti-HBc), IgM and IgG, and HBV deoxyribonucleic acid (DNA). The assay for HDV is the measurement of total antibody to hepatitis D antigen (anti-HDV) and serum HDV ribonucleic acid (RNA). HCV RNA quantification is important for assessment of the viral load, to evaluate antiviral therapy for chronic HCV infection. HEV infection is diagnosed from the presence of serum anti-HEV IgG and HEV RNA. HEV infection is usually a self-limiting disease, except in undeveloped countries, where it causes chronic hepatitis with an increased risk in pregnant women. Liver enzyme levels and function tests also can indicate other viral liver diseases, drug toxicity, or alcoholic hepatitis.[57]

Prophylactic treatments for different types of viral hepatitis are summarized in Table 38.8. Physical activity may be restricted, and a low-fat, high-carbohydrate diet is beneficial if bile flow is obstructed. For chronic hepatitis, treatment is directed at suppressing viral replication before irreversible liver cell damage or hepatic carcinoma occurs. Cyclic and combination therapy may prevent drug resistance, and new agents are being developed.

After ingestion and GI uptake, HAV replicates in the liver and is secreted into the bile, feces, and sera. To prevent the transmission of HAV, proper hand hygiene and the use of gloves for disposing of bedpans and fecal matter are imperative. HAV may be shed in the feces for up to 3 months after the onset of symptoms. Molecular procedures are available for direct surveillance of HAV in food. Direct contact with blood or body fluids of individuals with HBV or HBV/HDV coinfection or HCV should be avoided. The administration of immune globulin before exposure or early in the incubation period can prevent HAV and HBV infection. A combined vaccine is available to protect against HAV and HBV infection. There is no vaccine for HCV or HEV in the United States. Preexposure vaccination is recommended for health care workers, liver transplant recipients, and others who are at risk for contact with infected body fluids, particularly children.

✔ **QUICK CHECK 38.6**
1. How does hepatitis A virus (HAV) differ from hepatitis B virus (HBV)?
2. What vaccines are available to prevent viral hepatitis?
3. What are the three phases of hepatitis viral infection?
4. What complications are associated with chronic active viral hepatitis?

Disorders of the Gallbladder

Obstruction and inflammation are the most common disorders of the gallbladder. Obstruction is caused by gallstones, which are aggregates of substances in the bile. The gallstones may remain in the gallbladder or may be ejected, with bile, into the cystic duct. Gallstones that become lodged in the cystic duct obstruct the flow of bile into and out of the gallbladder and cause inflammation. Gallstone formation is termed cholelithiasis. Inflammation of the gallbladder or cystic duct is known as cholecystitis.

Cholelithiasis

Cholelithiasis (gallstones) is a prevalent disorder in developed countries, where the incidence is 10% to 15% in white adults and 60% to 70% in Native Americans. Risk factors include obesity, middle age, female sex, use of oral contraceptives, rapid weight loss, Native American ancestry, genetic predisposition, and gallbladder, pancreatic, or ileal disease.[58]

PATHOPHYSIOLOGY   Gallstones are formed as a result of impaired metabolism of cholesterol, bilirubin, and bile acids.[59] All gallstones contain cholesterol, unconjugated bilirubin, bilirubin calcium salts, fatty acids, calcium carbonates and phosphates, and mucin glycoproteins. The three types of gallstones are determined by their chemical composition: cholesterol stones (70% cholesterol and the most common type [70% to 80%]); pigmented stones (black [hard] and brown [soft] with less than 30% cholesterol); and mixed stones. *Cholesterol gallstones* form in bile that is supersaturated with cholesterol produced by the liver. Supersaturation sets the stage for cholesterol crystal formation, or the formation of "microstones." More crystals then aggregate on the microstones, which grow to form "macrostones." This process usually occurs in the gallbladder, which may have decreased motility. The stones may lie dormant or may become lodged in the cystic or common duct, causing pain when the gallbladder contracts and cholecystitis. The stones can accumulate and fill the entire gallbladder (Fig. 38.14). *Pigmented brown gallstones* form from calcium bilirubinate and fatty acid soaps that bind with calcium. They are associated with biliary stasis, bacterial infections, and biliary parasites. *Black gallstones* are rare and are associated with chronic liver disease and hemolytic disease. They are composed of calcium bilirubinate with mucin glycoproteins.

CLINICAL MANIFESTATIONS   Cholelithiasis is often asymptomatic. Epigastric and right hypochondrium pain and intolerance to fatty foods are the cardinal manifestations of cholelithiasis. Vague symptoms include heartburn, flatulence, epigastric discomfort, and food intolerances, particularly to fats and cabbage. The pain (biliary colic) occurs 30 minutes to several hours after eating a fatty meal. It is caused by the lodging of one or more gallstones in the cystic or common duct during contraction of the gallbladder. It can be intermittent or steady and usually occurs in the right upper quadrant, radiating to the mid-upper area of the back. Jaundice indicates that the stone is located in the common bile duct.

EVALUATION AND TREATMENT   The diagnosis is based on the medical history, physical examination, and imaging evaluation. An oral cholecystogram usually outlines the stones. Intravenous cholangiography is used to differentiate cholelithiasis from other causes of extrahepatic biliary obstruction if the cholecystogram is negative. Endoscopic or percutaneous cholangiography and endoscopic or transabdominal ultrasonography are diagnostic options. Oral bile acids (ursodeoxycholic acid or chenodeoxycholic acid) may prevent or dissolve cholesterol stones, but the stones may recur when the drug is discontinued. Dietary factors may prevent the development of gallstones, including reducing the intake of polyunsaturated fat, monounsaturated fat, and caffeine and increasing the consumption of fiber. Endoscopic removal of gallstones is the preferred treatment for uncomplicated gallstones causing obstruction of the bile ducts. Large stones may be managed by extracorporeal shock wave lithotripsy.

Cholecystitis

Cholecystitis can be acute or chronic, but both forms are almost always caused by a gallstone lodged in the cystic duct. Obstruction causes the gallbladder to become distended and inflamed. The pain is similar to

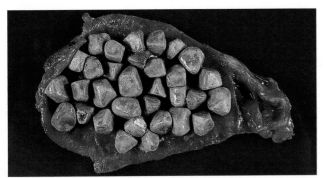

FIGURE 38.14 Resected Gallbladder Containing Mixed Gallstones. (From Kissane JM, editor: *Anderson's pathology*, ed 9, St Louis, 1990, Mosby.)

that caused by gallstones. Pressure against the distended wall of the gallbladder decreases blood flow and may result in ischemia, necrosis, and perforation. Fever, leukocytosis, rebound tenderness, and abdominal muscle guarding are common findings. Serum bilirubin and alkaline phosphatase levels may be elevated. Cholescintigraphy (a radiotracer scan of the gallbladder) is the most sensitive imaging for cholecystitis. The acute abdominal pain of cholecystitis must be differentiated from that caused by pancreatitis, myocardial infarction, and acute pyelonephritis of the right kidney. Narcotics may be required to control pain not responding to nonsteroidal anti-inflammatory drugs, and antibiotics are prescribed to manage bacterial infection in severe cases. Acute attacks usually require laparoscopic gallbladder resection (cholecystectomy). Obstruction also may lead to reflux of bile into the pancreatic duct, causing acute pancreatitis.[60]

Disorders of the Pancreas

Pancreatitis, or inflammation of the pancreas, is a relatively rare disease and potentially serious disorder. The incidence is about equal in men and women, is more common between 50 and 60 years of age, and is more likely to occur in blacks. Risk factors include obstructive biliary tract disease (particularly cholelithiasis), alcoholism, obesity, peptic ulcers, trauma, hyperlipidemia, hypercalcemia, smoking, certain drugs, and genetic factors (hereditary pancreatitis, cystic fibrosis). The cause is unknown in 15% to 25% of cases. Pancreatitis can be acute or chronic.

Acute Pancreatitis

Acute pancreatitis is usually a mild disease and resolves spontaneously, but about 20% of those with the disease develop a severe, acute pancreatitis requiring hospitalization. Pancreatitis develops because of obstruction to the outflow of pancreatic digestive enzymes caused by bile and pancreatic duct obstruction (e.g., gallstones). Acute pancreatitis also results from direct cellular injury from alcohol, drugs, or viral infection.[61]

PATHOPHYSIOLOGY   In obstructive disease, there is backup of pancreatic secretions and activation and release of enzymes (activated trypsin activates chymotrypsin, lipase, and elastase) within the pancreatic acinar cells. The activated enzymes cause autodigestion of pancreatic cells and tissues, resulting in inflammation. The autodigestion causes vascular damage, coagulation necrosis, fat necrosis (see Chapter 4), and the formation of pseudocysts (walled-off collections of pancreatic secretions). Edema within the pancreatic capsule leads to ischemia and can contribute to necrosis (Fig. 38.15). In cases of alcohol abuse, the pancreatic acinar cell metabolizes ethanol, with the generation of toxic metabolites that injure pancreatic acinar cells, causing release of activated enzymes. Chronic alcohol use may also cause formation of protein plugs in pancreatic ducts and spasm of the sphincter of Oddi, resulting in obstruction. The obstruction leads to intrapancreatic release of activated enzymes, autodigestion, inflammation, and pancreatitis.

Systemic effects of acute pancreatitis are related to the release of proinflammatory cytokines into the bloodstream. There is activation of leukocytes, injury to vessel walls, and coagulation abnormalities, with the development of vasodilation, hypotension, and shock. Complications can include acute respiratory distress syndrome (ARDS), heart failure, renal failure, coagulopathies, intra-abdominal hypertension, and systemic inflammatory response syndrome (SIRS). Paralytic ileus and GI bleeding can occur. Translocation of intestinal bacteria to the bloodstream may cause peritonitis or sepsis. Recurrent inflammation activates pancreatic stellate cells, causing pancreatic fibrosis, strictures, and duct obstruction that lead to chronic pancreatitis.

CLINICAL MANIFESTATIONS   The cardinal manifestation of acute pancreatitis is epigastric or midabdominal constant pain ranging from

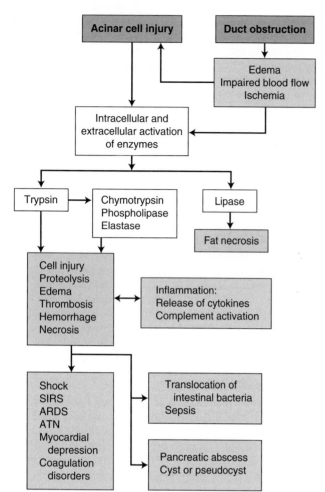

FIGURE 38.15 Pathophysiology of Acute Pancreatitis. *ARDS,* Acute respiratory distress syndrome; *ATN,* acute tubular necrosis; *SIRS,* systemic inflammatory response syndrome.

mild abdominal discomfort to severe, incapacitating pain. The pain may radiate to the back. Pain is caused by (1) edema, which distends the pancreatic ducts and capsule; (2) chemical irritation and inflammation of the peritoneum; (3) irritation or obstruction of the biliary tract; and (4) inflammation of nerves. Fever and leukocytosis accompany the inflammatory response. Nausea and vomiting are caused by paralytic ileus secondary to the pancreatitis or peritonitis. Jaundice can occur from obstruction of the bile duct (e.g., a gallstone) or from pancreatic edema pressing on the duct. Abdominal distention accompanies bowel hypomotility and the accumulation of fluids in the peritoneal cavity. Hypovolemia, hypotension, tachycardia, myocardial insufficiency, and shock occur because plasma volume is lost as inflammatory mediators released into the circulation increase vascular permeability and dilate vessels. Tachypnea and hypoxemia develop secondary to ascites, pulmonary edema, atelectasis, or pleural effusions. Hypovolemia can decrease renal blood flow sufficiently to impair renal function and can cause renal failure. Tetany may develop as a result of hypocalcemia when calcium is deposited in areas of fat necrosis or as a decreased response to parathormone. Transient hyperglycemia also can occur if glucagon is released from damaged alpha cells in the pancreatic islets. In severe acute pancreatitis, some individuals develop flank or periumbilical ecchymosis, a sign of a poor prognosis. Multiple organ failure or SIRS accounts for most deaths of those with severe acute pancreatitis.

EVALUATION AND TREATMENT The diagnosis is based on clinical findings, identification of associated disorders, laboratory studies, and imaging results. An elevated serum amylase concentration is characteristic but not diagnostic of the severity or specificity of disease. An elevated serum lipase level is the primary diagnostic marker for acute pancreatitis.

The goal of treatment for acute pancreatitis is to stop the process of autodigestion and prevent systemic complications. Narcotic medications may be needed to relieve pain. To decrease pancreatic secretions and "rest the gland," oral food and fluids may be withheld initially and continuous gastric suction instituted. Nasogastric suction may not be necessary with mild pancreatitis, but it helps to relieve pain and prevent paralytic ileus in individuals who are nauseated and vomiting. Feeding is usually initiated within 24 to 48 hours if ileus is not present. Parenteral fluids are essential to restore blood volume and prevent hypotension and shock. In severe pancreatitis enteral nutrition with use of jejunal tube feeding usually is well tolerated, may decrease pancreatic enzyme secretion, prevents gut bacterial overgrowth, and maintains gut barrier function. Drugs that decrease gastric acid production (e.g., H_2-receptor antagonists) can decrease stimulation of the pancreas by secretin. Antibiotics are used if there is infection. The risk of mortality increases significantly with the development of infection or pulmonary, cardiac, and renal complications.

Chronic Pancreatitis

Chronic pancreatitis is a process of progressive fibrotic destruction of the pancreas. Chronic alcohol abuse is the most common cause. Obstruction from gallstones, smoking, and genetic factors increase the risk of chronic pancreatitis.[62] Toxic metabolites and chronic release of inflammatory cytokines contribute to the destruction of acinar cells and islets of Langerhans. The pancreatic parenchyma is destroyed and replaced by fibrous tissues, strictures, calcification, ductal obstruction, and pancreatic cysts. The cysts are walled-off areas or pockets of pancreatic juice, necrotic debris, or blood within or adjacent to the pancreas.

Continuous or intermittent abdominal pain and weight loss are common. The pain is difficult to manage and is associated with increased intraductal pressure, ischemia, neuritis, intra-abdominal hypertension (compartment syndrome), ongoing injury, and both peripheral and central pain sensitization. Manifestations of pancreatic enzyme deficiency, such as steatorrhea or a malabsorption syndrome, are present in late stages of chronic pancreatitis. To correct enzyme deficiencies and prevent malabsorption, oral enzyme replacements are taken before and during meals. Loss of islet cells can cause insulin-dependent diabetes and requires treatment. Cessation of alcohol intake is essential for the management of both acute and chronic pancreatitis. Endoscopic or surgical drainage of cysts or partial resection of the pancreas may be required to relieve pain and to prevent cystic rupture. Chronic pancreatitis is a risk factor for pancreatic cancer.

CANCER OF THE DIGESTIVE SYSTEM

Cancer of the Gastrointestinal Tract

Table 38.9 presents information on the various GI cancers by organ, percentage of deaths compared with all cancer deaths, risk factors, type of cell, and common manifestations. The biology of cancer is presented in Chapter 11.

Cancer of the Esophagus

Carcinoma of the esophagus is a rare type of cancer with an estimated incidence of 17,650 new cases and 16,080 deaths in the United States in 2019.[63] Risk factors are summarized in *Risk Factors:* Esophageal Cancer.

TABLE 38.9   Cancer of the Gut, Liver, and Pancreas

Organ	Proportion of All Cancer Deaths*	Risks	Cell Type	Common Manifestations
Esophagus	2.6%	Malnutrition Alcohol Tobacco Chronic reflux	Squamous cell Adenocarcinoma	Chest pain Dysphagia
Stomach	1.8%	Salty food Fried red meat Nitrates-nitrosamines	Adenocarcinoma Squamous cell	Anorexia Malaise Weight loss Upper abdominal pain Vomiting Occult blood
Colon/rectum	8.4%	Polyps Long-term inflammatory bowel disease Diverticulitis Diets high in fat and refined carbohydrates; low in fiber	Adenocarcinoma (left colon grows as ring; right colon grows as mass)	Pain Mass Anemia Bloody stool Obstruction Distention
Liver	5.0%	HBV, HCV, HDV Cirrhosis Intestinal parasite Aflatoxin from moldy peanuts and corn	Hepatomas Cholangiomas	Pain Anorexia Bloating Weight loss Portal hypertension Ascites Jaundice
Pancreas	7.5%	Chronic pancreatitis Cigarette smoking Alcohol (?) Diabetic women	Adenocarcinoma (exocrine part of gland, ductal epithelium)	Weight loss Weakness Nausea Vomiting Abdominal pain Depression ± jaundice May have insulin-secreting tumors with symptoms of hypoglycemia

*The percentage of all cancer deaths combined.
HBV, Hepatitis B virus; *HCV,* hepatitis C virus; *HDV,* hepatitis D virus.
From the American Cancer Society: *Cancer facts & figures 2019,* Atlanta, 2019, Author. Available at https://www.cancer.org/content/dam/cancer-org/research/cancer-facts-and-statistics/annual-cancer-facts-and-figures/2019/cancer-facts-and-figures-2019.pdf.

RISK FACTORS

Esophageal Cancer

- Age greater than 65 years
- Tobacco use
- Alcoholism
- Dietary factors: deficiencies of trace elements and vitamins
- Malnutrition associated with poor economic conditions or special dietary habits (e.g., very hot drinks, fish preserved in lye; diet deficient in fruits and vegetables)
- Gastroesophageal reflux with dysplasia
- Sliding hiatal hernia
- Obesity

PATHOPHYSIOLOGY   Carcinoma of the esophagus includes squamous cell carcinoma and adenocarcinoma, which is more prevalent in the United States. Squamous cell carcinomas are more common in the thoracic and cervical areas of the esophagus and are associated with smoking tobacco and chronic alcohol consumption. Adenocarcinomas are associated with obesity, GERD, and smoking tobacco. The development of adenocarcinoma often occurs secondary to infiltration by a gastric carcinoma or to the presence of Barrett dysplasia (also known as **Barrett esophagus**; the mucosal lining becomes abnormal and more like the intestine) and it can progress to metaplasia, a precancerous lesion. The *CagA*-positive strain of *H. pylori* may be protective against esophageal carcinoma.[64]

CLINICAL MANIFESTATIONS   The two frequent symptoms of esophageal carcinoma are chest pain and dysphagia. The most common type of pain is heartburn. It is initiated by eating spicy or highly seasoned foods and by assuming the recumbent position. Odynophagia (pain on swallowing) may be initiated by the swallowing of cold liquids. Some individuals with esophageal cancer complain of a constant retrosternal pain that radiates to the back. Dysphagia (difficulty swallowing) is usually pressure-like and may radiate posteriorly between the scapulae. Dysphagia usually progresses rapidly. Esophageal carcinoma is asymptomatic during the early stages and presents at an advanced stage. Esophageal cancer metastasizes rapidly and, therefore, has a poor prognosis.

EVALUATION AND TREATMENT Individuals with dysphagia undergo endoscopy so that specimens can be obtained and examined for neoplastic change. Endoscopic ultrasound and CT studies of the thorax are used for diagnosis and staging. Prevention of gastroesophageal reflux and removal of high-grade dysplasia are essential to the management of Barrett esophagus. It is impossible to remove all lymph nodes with the tumor, but removal of the primary lesion and the local lymph nodes can benefit the individual with esophageal cancer. If the malignancy has not spread beyond these sites, cure is likely. If metastasis has occurred, however, an incomplete resection is of little survival benefit. Treatment is combined radiation and chemotherapy.

Cancer of the Stomach

The incidence of gastric adenocarcinoma is estimated at 27,510 new cases and 11,140 deaths in the United States in 2019.[63] Loss of tumor-suppressor genes and other genetic alterations may be important in gastric cancer.[65]

PATHOPHYSIOLOGY Gastric adenocarcinomas are associated with atrophic gastritis and *H. pylori*. *H. pylori* also causes gastric B-cell mucosa-associated lymphoid tissue lymphoma. Most adenocarcinomas are sporadic and associated with the consumption of heavily salted and preserved foods (e.g., nitrates in pickled or salted foods such as bacon), a low intake of fruits and vegetables, and the use of tobacco and alcohol. Dietary salt enhances the conversion of nitrates to carcinogenic nitrosamines in the stomach. Salt and nitrates converted to nitrites are caustic to the stomach, delay gastric emptying, and can cause chronic atrophic gastritis. Insufficient acid secretion by the atrophic mucosa creates a relatively alkaline environment that permits bacteria to multiply and act on nitrates. The resulting increase in nitrosamines damages the DNA of mucosal cells, further promoting metaplasia and neoplasia. Gastric adenocarcinoma usually begins in the glands of the distal stomach mucosa. Duodenal reflux also may contribute to an intestinal-like metaplasia. The reflux contains caustic bile salts that destroy the mucosal barrier that normally protects the stomach.[66]

CLINICAL MANIFESTATIONS The early stages of gastric cancer are generally asymptomatic or produce vague symptoms such as loss of appetite (especially for meat), malaise, and indigestion. Later manifestations of gastric cancer include unexplained weight loss, upper abdominal pain, vomiting, change in bowel habits, and anemia caused by persistent occult bleeding. The prognosis is poor because symptoms do not occur until the tumor has spread and caused distant metastases, particularly to the liver and peritoneal structures. Generally, the first manifestations of carcinoma are caused by distant metastases, and the disease is already in an advanced stage.

EVALUATION AND TREATMENT No specific biomarkers have been identified for gastric cancer. Most symptoms suggest a problem in the upper GI tract. Direct endoscopic visualization, lavage, and cellular examination or biopsy establish the diagnosis. Screening and treatment for *H. pylori* infection constitute the best preventive approach to gastric cancer. Surgery is the usual treatment for early stages of disease. Staging is determined by pathologic findings after resection. Early diagnosis and chemotherapy, combined with radiation, improve the postsurgical outcomes.

✔ QUICK CHECK 38.7
1. How do gallstones form?
2. Compare acute and chronic pancreatitis.
3. What factors are associated with cancer of the esophagus?
4. What dietary factors are associated with gastric cancer?

Cancer of the Colon and Rectum

Colorectal cancer (CRC) is the third most common cause of cancer and cancer death. An estimated 101,420 new cases of colon cancer and 44,180 new cases of rectal cancer, and 51,020 deaths, occurred in the United States in 2019.[63] The incidence has been declining over the past several years because of successful screening programs. CRC tends to occur in individuals older than 50 years and is rare in children. Risk factors for CRC can be reviewed in *Risk Factors:* Cancer of the Colon and Rectum. Regular use of aspirin and cyclooxygenase 2 (COX-2) selective inhibitors are associated with a decreased risk of CRC. Small intestinal carcinoma is more rare.[67]

RISK FACTORS

Cancer of the Colon and Rectum

- Advanced age
- Diet high in fat (especially egg consumption) and red and processed meats, low in fiber
- High consumption of alcohol
- Cigarette smoking
- Obesity
- Familial polyposis or family history of colorectal cancer
- Low levels of physical activity
- Inflammatory bowel disease
- Type 2 diabetes mellitus
- African-American race/ethnicity

PATHOPHYSIOLOGY Most CRCs are sporadic (acquired) or associated with a family history of colorectal cancer. They are caused by multiple gene alterations and environmental interactions (see Chapter 3 for epigenetics and Chapter 11 for mechanisms of oncogenesis). Familial adenomatous polyposis (FAP) is a mutation of the *APC* gene (adenomatous polyposis coli, a tumor-suppressor gene) and is the most common hereditary cause of colorectal cancer. Hereditary nonpolyposis colorectal cancer (HNPCC), or Lynch syndrome, is associated with several DNA mismatch repair (MMR) genes. Both FAP and HNPCC have a rare, family-linked autosomal dominant inheritance trait that accounts for about 3% to 5% of colorectal cancers.[68] Sporadic tumors are also thought to involve the loss of function or mutation of tumor-suppressor genes. CRC begins with the formation of an adenoma, termed "tumor initiation." The progression to carcinoma is termed "tumor progression" and is a multistep process of genetic mutations that may take 8 to 10 years.

Colorectal polyps are closely associated with the development of cancer. A polyp, or papilloma, is a projection arising from the mucosal epithelium. The most common types of polyps are benign. However, adenomatous polyps are neoplastic. Neoplastic polyps are premalignant lesions[69] (Fig. 38.16). The larger the polyp, the greater the risk of colorectal cancer. Although lesions larger than 1.5 cm occur less often, they are more likely to be malignant than those smaller than 1 cm. Thus, screening colonoscopy with polypectomy is performed when polyps are found.

Adenocarcinomas of the colon and rectum usually arise from adenomatous polyps and undergo a multistep cascade of genetic events that leads to carcinoma and metastasis (see Fig. 11.5 and 11.6). These tumors have a long preinvasive phase and when they invade, they tend to grow slowly. CRC begins from epithelial stem cells located in the colon mucosa. Because the lymphatic channels are located under the submucosae, the lesions must traverse this layer before the multistep process of metastasis can occur. Once the malignant cells of an adenoma traverse the submucosae, tumor cells enter the bloodstream and lymphatics and become invasive, spreading to other organs. Adenomas can be detected early, however, because the submucosa may not be penetrated for several years.

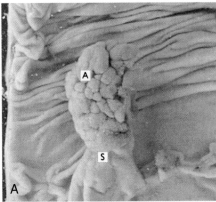

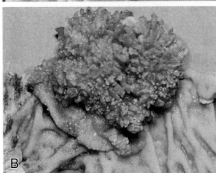

FIGURE 38.16 Neoplastic Polyps. A, Tubular adenomata *(A)* are rounded lesions 0.5 to 2 cm in size that are generally red and sit on a stalk *(S)* of normal mucosa that has been dragged up by traction of the polyp in the bowel lumen. B, Villous adenomata are velvety lesions about 0.6 cm thick that occupy a broad area of mucosa generally 1 to 5 cm in diameter. (From Stevens A et al: *Core pathology,* ed 3, London, 2009, Mosby.)

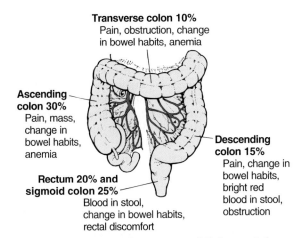

Transverse colon 10%
Pain, obstruction, change in bowel habits, anemia

Ascending colon 30%
Pain, mass, change in bowel habits, anemia

Descending colon 15%
Pain, change in bowel habits, bright red blood in stool, obstruction

Rectum 20% and sigmoid colon 25%
Blood in stool, change in bowel habits, rectal discomfort

FIGURE 38.17 Signs and Symptoms of Colorectal Cancer by Location of Primary Lesion. Clinical manifestations are listed under the order of frequency for each region.

CLINICAL MANIFESTATIONS Symptoms of CRC depend on the location, size, and shape of the lesion and are silent in the early stages (Fig. 38.17). Tumors of the right (ascending) colon and left (descending) colon evolve into two distinct tumor types.[70] On the right side (proximal colon), the lesions extend along one wall of the cecum and ascending colon. These tumors may be silent, evolving to pain, a palpable mass in the lower right quadrant, anemia, fatigue, and dark red or mahogany-colored blood mixed with the stool. These tumors can become

large and bulky with necrosis and ulceration, contributing to persistent blood loss and anemia. Obstruction is unusual because the growth does not readily encircle the colon. These tumors are more common in women.

Tumors of the left, or descending, colon (distal colon) start as small, elevated, buttonlike masses. This type grows circumferentially, encircling the entire bowel wall, and eventually ulcerating in the middle of the tumor as the tumor penetrates the blood supply. Obstruction is common but occurs slowly, and stools become narrow and pencil shaped. Manifestations include progressive abdominal distention, pain, vomiting, constipation, a need for laxatives, cramps, and bright red blood on the surface of the stool. These tumors are more common in men.

Systematic lymphatic distribution occurs along the aorta to the mesenteric and pancreatic lymph nodes. Liver metastasis is common and follows invasion of the mesenteric veins (left colon) or superior veins (right colon), which drain into the portal circulation.

Rectal carcinomas (about 20% of CRCs) are defined as tumors occurring up to 15 cm from the anal opening. Tumors of the rectum can spread through the rectal wall to nearby structures: the prostate in men and the vagina in women. Penetration occurs more readily in the lower third of the rectum because it has no serosal covering. Systemic and pulmonary metastases occur through the hemorrhoidal plexus, which drains into the vena cava.

EVALUATION AND TREATMENT Individuals with hereditary polyposis should begin screening at an early age (10 to 12 years); colonoscopy should be used, with the removal of polyps when they are found. Specific, sensitive, and affordable molecular markers are being evaluated to assist with early diagnosis and evaluation of therapy. Carcinoembryonic antigen (CEA) is evaluated during and after cancer treatment. Screening procedures for the detection of nonhereditary CRC are summarized in Box 38.4. Aspirin and celecoxib may reduce the incidence of CRC in the general population, but the risk of GI bleeding must be considered. Vitamin D, calcium, fiber, folate, dietary modification, weight control, exercise, and other nondietary lifestyle changes can reduce the risk of CRC.

The staging of CRC involves imaging and operative exploration. Physical examination of the abdomen detects liver enlargement and ascites; appropriate lymph nodes are palpated. Imaging is useful for pretreatment staging. Operative staging consists of careful exploration during surgery and biopsy of possible metastases. The National Cancer Institute's[71] tumor-node-metastasis (TNM) classification system is widely used for staging CRC (www.cancer.gov/cancertopics/pdq/treatment/colon/HealthProfessional; also see Chapter 11).

Treatment for all stages of cancer of the colon is surgical. Chemotherapy and radiation therapy may be given before surgery in the hope they will shrink the tumor or alter the malignant cells, or both, so that these cells will not survive after surgery. Resection and anastomosis can be performed for cancer of the ascending, transverse, descending, or sigmoid colon and upper rectum. These surgeries are performed through abdominal incisions and assisted with radiofrequency ablation. Natural defecation is preserved. Growths in the lower portion of the rectum require removal of the entire rectum with the formation of a permanent colostomy. Chemotherapy, including immunotherapy, is used to treat metastatic disease and cases with a high risk of recurrence. New therapeutic agents are improving personalized, first-line therapy. Immunotherapy, vaccines, and viral vectors for the treatment of colon cancer are under continuing investigation. Resection of liver metastases or hepatic intra-arterial chemotherapy may prolong survival.

Cancer of the Accessory Organs of Digestion
Cancer of the Liver

Cancer of the liver is a leading cause of cancer death worldwide. The estimated number of new cases is 42,030 with 31,780 deaths in the United States in 2019.[63] Primary liver cancer is rare before the age of 40 years and is most common after 60 years. Cancer in the liver is usually caused by metastatic spread from a primary site elsewhere in the body. Risk factors for primary liver cancer are summarized in *Risk Factors: Primary Liver Cancer*. Risks associated with HBV and HCV infection are decreasing with antiviral therapy.

RISK FACTORS
Primary Liver Cancer

- Exposure to mycotoxins (aflatoxins), including mold found on spoiled corn, peanuts, and grain
- Alcohol abuse
- Obesity
- Chronic liver disease, especially cirrhosis
- Infection with hepatitis B virus (HBV), hepatitis C virus (HCV), and hepatitis D virus (HDV), particularly in conjunction with cirrhosis; these infections act either as carcinogens or as co-carcinogens in chronically infected hepatocytes

---

PATHOPHYSIOLOGY Primary carcinomas of the liver are hepatocellular or cholangiocellular. **Hepatocellular carcinoma (HCC)** develops in the hepatocytes and can be nodular (consisting of multiple, discrete nodules), massive (consisting of a large tumor mass having satellite nodules), or diffuse (consisting of small nodules distributed throughout most of the liver). It is closely associated with chronic hepatitis and cirrhosis.[72] Because carcinoma of the liver invades the hepatic and portal veins, it often spreads to the heart and lungs. Other sites of metastases are the brain, kidney, and spleen.

Cholangiocellular carcinoma (cholangiocarcinoma) is rare (less than 1% of liver cancers) and develops in the bile ducts. It is associated with primary sclerosing cholangitis (a rare autoimmune disease often associated with ulcerative colitis) and is geographically associated with areas where liver fluke infestation is prevalent, such as Southeast Asia. Cholangiocellular carcinoma can occur anywhere along the bile duct and extend directly into the liver, usually as a solitary lesion. A combined form of HCC is known as combined (mixed) hepatocellular-cholangiocellular carcinoma. It is difficult to distinguish an invasion of cholangiocellular carcinoma from a metastatic adenocarcinoma except by neoplastic changes found in nearby ducts.

CLINICAL MANIFESTATIONS HCC is usually asymptomatic. Manifestations are often nonspecific, can develop slowly or abruptly, and include vague abdominal symptoms, such as nausea and vomiting, fullness, pressure, a dull ache in the right upper abdominal area, and weight loss. In individuals with cirrhosis, deepening jaundice or abrupt lack of appetite is a sign of HCC. Obstruction by the tumor can cause sudden worsening of portal hypertension and development of ascites. As the tumor enlarges, it causes pain. Cholangiocellular carcinoma more commonly presents insidiously as pain, loss of appetite, weight loss, and gradual onset of jaundice. Some carcinomas of the liver rupture spontaneously, causing hemorrhage. Others are discovered accidentally during laboratory evaluation, imaging, or surgery for other diseases or trauma.

EVALUATION AND TREATMENT There is no specific test for the diagnosis of liver cancer. For high-risk individuals, alpha fetoprotein associated with HBV infection and abdominal ultrasound are common screening tools. Diagnosis is based on clinical manifestations, laboratory findings, imaging, and exploratory laparotomy. In individuals without cirrhosis, liver scans can document filling defects. CT or ultrasonography is used to detect solid tumors, but neither can distinguish benign from malignant tumors. Biopsy is generally not performed because of risk for tumor seeding and bleeding. Primary prevention may be achieved by vaccinating against HBV, preventing and treating HBV and HCV infection, screening all donated blood for the presence of HBV, and reducing contamination of food with aflatoxins.

Surgical resection is possible only if the tumor is localized to a removable lobe of the liver. Surgery is hazardous and usually not undertaken if the individual has cirrhosis. Percutaneous or laparoscopic ablation and transplantation are effective for early stages of disease. Most individuals develop metastases after surgical resection, but long-term survival is possible. Chemoembolization, immunotherapy, and radiotherapy are treatment options. Targeted molecular therapy includes sorafenib and new drugs are under investigation. The prognosis for those with symptomatic liver cancer is poor.

Cancer of the Gallbladder

In 2019 in the United States, there were an estimated 12,360 new cases and 3960 deaths attributable to gallbladder cancer.[63] Risk factors include biliary reflux, gallstones, advancing age, female sex (2:1), anomalous pancreaticobiliary ductal junction, bacterial infection, exposure to heavy metals, and obesity. It occurs rarely before the age of 40 years and is most common between the ages of 50 and 60 years. Primary carcinoma of the gallbladder is rare and associated with larger gallstones. Most gallbladder cancer is caused by metastasis.

PATHOPHYSIOLOGY Most primary carcinomas of the gallbladder are adenocarcinomas, and more rarely squamous cell carcinomas. The pathogenesis is not clear. Chronic inflammation may trigger dysplasia and progression to metaplasia. The molecular mechanisms involve mutation of several genes, including tumor-suppressor genes and oncogenes, DNA repair genes, and alterations in the extracellular matrix.[73] Invasion of the liver and lymph nodes occurs early. Direct invasion of the stomach and the duodenum can cause pyloric obstruction. Infection often accompanies cancer of the gallbladder. Generalized peritonitis, gangrene, perforation, and liver abscesses are potential complications of infection.

CLINICAL MANIFESTATIONS Early stages of gallbladder carcinoma are asymptomatic, and the disease usually presents at an advanced stage. When symptoms develop, there is usually steady, upper right quadrant pain for about 2 months. Other manifestations include diarrhea, belching, weakness, loss of appetite, weight loss, and vomiting. Obstructive jaundice can occur if an enlarging tumor presses on the extrahepatic ducts and is a sign of an inoperable tumor.

EVALUATION AND TREATMENT Early diagnosis of cancer of the gallbladder is rare and is often found incidentally. Therefore, older adults with gallstones, particularly women, are evaluated for disease. Inflammatory disorders, such as cholangitis (bile duct inflammation) and peritonitis, often obscure an underlying malignancy. Diagnostic procedures include ultrasonography and further imaging with suspicious findings. Complete surgical resection of the gallbladder is the only effective treatment for early stages of disease, and recurrence is common. Complete removal of tumor tissue and lymph nodes with chemoradiation therapy is performed for more advanced stages. Because advanced malignancies cannot be resected, gallbladders containing stones are removed as a preventive measure. The prognosis of unresectable gallbladder cancer is extremely poor. Molecular therapies are under development.

Cancer of the Pancreas

Pancreatic cancer is the fourth leading cause of cancer deaths in the United States. An estimated 56,770 new cases and 45,750 deaths occurred in the United States in 2019.[63] The incidence of pancreatic cancer rises steadily with age. The cause of pancreatic cancer is not known, but there are modest risks associated with tobacco smoking, certain dietary factors (e.g., high-fat foods and processed meat), obesity, diabetes mellitus, chronic pancreatitis, family history of pancreatic cancer, HNPCC (Lynch syndrome), and several oncogenic and tumor-suppressor gene mutations.[74]

PATHOPHYSIOLOGY Pancreatic cancer can arise from exocrine or endocrine cells. Most pancreatic tumors arise from metaplastic exocrine cells in the ducts and are called *pancreatic ductal adenocarcinomas*. Chronic pancreatitis and inflammatory cytokines support tumor growth. There is significant expansion of the extracellular matrix (stroma) that contributes to therapeutic resistance. Tumors arising in small ducts invade nearby glandular tissue, penetrate the covering of the pancreas, and extend into surrounding tissues. Tumors of the head of the pancreas quickly spread to obstruct the common bile duct and portal vein. These tumors can then infiltrate the superior mesenteric artery, the vena cava, and the aorta and form emboli. Tumors of the body and tail of the pancreas infiltrate the posterior abdominal wall. Lymphatic invasion occurs early and rapidly. Venous invasion causes metastases to the liver. Tumor implants on the peritoneal surface can obstruct veins and promote development of ascites.

CLINICAL MANIFESTATIONS Early stages of pancreatic cancer are asymptomatic. When symptoms occur there usually has been obstruction and a malignant transformation. Typically, vague upper abdominal pain that radiates to the back or shoulder develops. Nonspecific symptoms include lethargy, nausea, vomiting, bloating, and changes in bowel habits. Jaundice arises in most cases, usually caused by obstruction of the bile duct. Because obstruction impairs enzyme secretion and flow to the duodenum, pancreatic cancer causes fat and protein malabsorption, resulting in weight loss. Distant metastases are found in the cervical lymph nodes, the lungs, and the brain. Most individuals die of hepatic failure, malnutrition, or systemic diseases.

EVALUATION AND TREATMENT The molecular pathogenic pathways associated with pancreatic cancer are very complex and there is no specific biomarker for pancreatic cancer. Several molecular markers are under investigation.[75] The diagnosis is usually made after the tumor has spread and is nonresectable. CT and endoscopic ultrasound are used initially for diagnosis. Laparotomy is often used to establish a definitive diagnosis, evaluate the extent of disease, and determine whether palliative bypass surgery (i.e., cholecystojejunostomy and gastrojejunostomy) is needed. Pancreaticoduodenectomy (Whipple procedure) is performed to decompress duct obstruction. Many surgeons recommend a total pancreatectomy because cancer of the pancreas seldom consists of a single lesion. Adjuvant chemotherapy, immunotherapy, radiochemotherapy, and combination therapy may produce favorable controls in locally advanced cancer. Supportive therapy involves pain management, nutritional support, and an interdisciplinary team. Five-year survival is about 15% to 20% with resectable disease (a small subset) and less than 6% for metastatic disease. There is a need for new approaches for earlier diagnosis and more effective treatment.

> ✔ **QUICK CHECK 38.8**
> 1. What are the primary risk factors for colorectal carcinoma?
> 2. Compare tumors of the right colon with those of the left colon.
> 3. What is the most common cause of liver cancer?

▌ SUMMARY REVIEW

Disorders of the Gastrointestinal Tract

1. Clinical manifestations of GI dysfunction include anorexia, vomiting, constipation, diarrhea, and abdominal pain and bleeding. They are nonspecific and can be caused by a variety of impairments.
2. Anorexia is the lack of a desire to eat despite physiologic stimuli that would normally produce hunger.
3. Vomiting is the forceful emptying of the stomach effected by GI contraction and reverse peristalsis of the esophagus. It is usually preceded by nausea and retching, with the exception of projectile vomiting, which is associated with direct stimulation of the vomiting center in the brain.
4. Constipation is difficult or infrequent defecation often caused by unhealthy dietary and bowel habits combined with lack of exercise. Constipation can result from a disorder that delays intestinal motility or obstructs the intestinal lumen.
5. Diarrhea is frequent loose, watery stools. It can be caused by excessive fluid drawn into the intestinal lumen by osmosis (osmotic diarrhea), excessive secretion of fluids by the intestinal mucosa (secretory diarrhea), or excessive GI motility (motility diarrhea).
6. Abdominal pain is caused by stretching, inflammation, or ischemia (insufficient blood supply) of abdominal organs. Abdominal pain originates in the organs themselves (visceral pain) or in the peritoneum (parietal pain) and can be acute or chronic. Visceral pain is often referred to the back.
7. Manifestations of GI bleeding are hematemesis (vomiting of blood), melena (dark, tarry stools), and hematochezia (frank bleeding from the rectum). Occult bleeding can be detected only by testing stools or vomitus for the presence of blood.
8. Disorders of GI motility include dysphagia, GERD, hiatal hernia, pyloric obstruction, and intestinal obstruction.

9. Dysphagia is difficulty swallowing. It can be caused by a mechanical or functional obstruction of the esophagus. Functional obstruction is an impairment of esophageal motility. Achalasia is a form of functional dysphagia caused by loss of esophageal innervation.

10. GERD is the regurgitation of chyme from the stomach into the esophagus, resulting in an inflammatory response (reflux esophagitis) when the esophageal mucosa is repeatedly exposed to acids and enzymes in the regurgitated chyme.

11. Hiatal hernia is the protrusion of the upper part of the stomach through the hiatus (esophageal opening in the diaphragm) at the gastroesophageal junction. Hiatal hernia can be sliding or paraesophageal, or both.

12. Gastroparesis is delayed gastric emptying in the absence of mechanical gastric outlet obstruction.

13. Pyloric obstruction is the narrowing or blockage of the pylorus, which is the opening between the stomach and the duodenum. It can be caused by a congenital defect, inflammation and scarring secondary to a gastric ulcer, or tumor growth.

14. Intestinal obstruction prevents the normal movement of chyme through the intestinal tract. It can be simple (caused by mechanical blockage) or functional (caused by paralytic ileus). The most severe consequences of intestinal obstruction are fluid and electrolyte losses, hypovolemia, shock, intestinal necrosis, and perforation of the intestinal wall.

15. Gastritis is an acute or chronic inflammation of the gastric mucosa. The most common causes are use of NSAIDs, *H. pylori* infection, and physiologic stress-related mucosal changes. Alcohol, digitalis, and metabolic disorders, such as uremia, also are contributing factors.

16. Acute gastritis is caused by injury to the protective mucosal barrier and leads to vague abdominal discomfort, epigastric tenderness, and bleeding. Healing usually occurs spontaneously within a few days.

17. Chronic gastritis of the fundus (immune) and antrum (nonimmune) is the most severe form of gastritis. In chronic immune gastritis, which is rare, the fundus of the stomach degenerates extensively, leading to gastric atrophy. Chronic nonimmune gastritis is more common and involves the antrum only.

18. A peptic ulcer is a circumscribed area of mucosal inflammation and ulceration in the stomach or proximal duodenum caused by excessive secretion of gastric acid, disruption of the protective mucosal barrier, or infection with *H. pylori*.

19. Zollinger-Ellison syndrome is a rare syndrome associated with peptic ulcers caused by a gastrin-secreting neuroendocrine tumor or multiple tumors (gastrinoma) of the pancreas or duodenum.

20. The three types of peptic ulcers are duodenal, gastric, and stress ulcers.

21. Duodenal ulcers, the most common peptic ulcer, are associated with *H. pylori* infection, chronic use of NSAIDs, altered mucosal defenses, rapid gastric emptying, elevated gastrin levels, and acid production stimulated by smoking. Pain occurs when the stomach is empty and is relieved with food or antacids. Duodenal ulcers tend to heal spontaneously and recur frequently.

22. Gastric ulcers develop near acid-secreting mucosa, generally in the antrum, and tend to become chronic. Gastric secretions may be normal or decreased, and pain may occur after eating.

23. Stress ulcers develop suddenly after severe illness, systemic trauma, or neural injury. Ulceration follows mucosal damage caused by ischemia (decreased blood flow to the gastric mucosa).

24. Curling ulcers are stress ulcers associated with burn trauma.

25. Cushing ulcer is a stress ulcer associated with head trauma. Ulceration follows hypersecretion of hydrochloric acid caused by overstimulation of the vagal nuclei.

26. Postgastrectomy syndromes are long-term complications that occur after gastrectomy (the resection of all or part of the stomach). The postgastrectomy syndromes include dumping syndrome, alkaline reflux gastritis, afferent loop obstruction, diarrhea, weight loss, and anemia.

27. Dumping syndrome is the rapid emptying of chyme into the small intestine.

28. Alkaline (bile) reflux gastritis is stomach inflammation caused by the reflux of bile and pancreatic secretions from the duodenum into the stomach.

29. Afferent loop obstruction is an obstruction of the duodenal stump on the proximal side of a gastrojejunostomy causing intermittent severe pain and epigastric fullness.

30. Malabsorption syndromes (pancreatic exocrine insufficiency, lactase deficiency, and bile salt deficiency) result in impaired digestion or absorption of nutrients.

31. Pancreatic exocrine insufficiency causes malabsorption associated with impaired digestion. The pancreas does not produce sufficient amounts of the enzymes that digest protein, carbohydrates, and fats. A large amount of fat in the stool (steatorrhea) is the most common sign of pancreatic insufficiency.

32. Deficient lactase production in the brush border of the small intestine inhibits the breakdown of lactose. This prevents lactose absorption and causes osmotic diarrhea.

33. Bile salt deficiency causes fat malabsorption and steatorrhea. Bile salt deficiency can result from inadequate secretion of bile, excessive bacterial deconjugation of bile, or impaired reabsorption of bile salts caused by ileal disease.

34. UC and CD are major types of chronic relapsing IBDs.

35. UC is a chronic IBD that causes ulceration, abscess formation, and necrosis of the colonic and rectal mucosa. Cramping pain, bleeding, frequent diarrhea, dehydration, and weight loss accompany severe forms of the disease. A course of frequent remissions and exacerbations is common.

36. CD is similar to UC, but it affects the GI tract from the mouth to the anus and tends to involve all the layers of the intestinal lumen. "Skip lesion" fissures and granulomata are characteristic of CD. Abdominal pain, diarrhea, and weight loss are the usual symptoms.

37. Microscopic colitis is an inflammation that involves either mucosal lymphocytic infiltration or a thickened subepithelial collagen layer of the colon with symptoms of watery diarrhea.

38. IBS is a disorder of brain-gut interaction with recurring abdominal pain and bloating. IBS can be diarrhea prevalent or constipation prevalent or may alternate between diarrhea and constipation. It is a multisystem interaction, and variables such as infection, gut microbiota, immune activation, serotonin dysregulation, psychological stress, and diet are contributing factors in the varying symptom presentations.

39. Diverticula are outpouchings of colonic mucosa through the muscle layers of the colon wall. Diverticulosis is asymptomatic diverticular disease; diverticulitis is inflammation of the diverticula.

40. Appendicitis is inflammation of the vermiform appendix and the most common surgical emergency of the abdomen. Obstruction of the lumen leads to increased pressure, ischemia, and inflammation of the appendix. Without surgical resection, inflammation may progress to gangrene, perforation, and peritonitis.

41. Mesenteric vascular insufficiency in the intestine is most often associated with occlusion or obstruction of the mesenteric vessels or insufficient intestinal arterial blood flow. The resulting ischemia

and necrosis produce abdominal pain, fever, bloody diarrhea, hypovolemia, and shock.

Disorders of the Accessory Organs of Digestion

1. Disorders of the accessory organs of digestion (liver, gallbladder, and pancreas) include inflammatory disease, obstruction of ducts, and tumors.

2. Portal hypertension, ascites, hepatic encephalopathy, jaundice, and hepatorenal syndrome are complications of many liver disorders.

3. Portal hypertension is an elevation of the portal venous pressure to at least 10 mm Hg (normal pressure is 3 mm Hg). It is caused by increased resistance to venous flow in the portal vein and its tributaries, including the sinusoids and hepatic vein. Portal hypertension is the most serious complication of liver disease because it can cause potentially fatal complications, such as bleeding varices, splenomegaly, ascites, hepatic encephalopathy, and hepatopulmonary syndrome.

4. Varices (esophageal, gastric, hemorrhoidal) are distended, tortuous, collateral veins resulting from prolonged elevation of pressure in the portal vein.

5. Splenomegaly is enlargement of the spleen caused by increased pressure in the splenic vein, which branches from the portal vein.

6. Hepatopulmonary syndrome and portopulmonary hypertension are complications of portal hypertension caused by release of nitric oxide and carbon monoxide in the presence of liver injury.

7. Ascites is the accumulation and sequestration of fluid in the peritoneal cavity, often as a result of portal hypertension and decreased concentrations of plasma proteins.

8. Hepatic encephalopathy (portal-systemic encephalopathy) is impaired cerebral function caused by blood-borne toxins (particularly ammonia) not metabolized by the liver because toxin-bearing blood bypasses the liver in collateral vessels opened as a result of portal hypertension. Manifestations of hepatic encephalopathy range from confusion and asterixis (flapping tremor of the hands) to loss of consciousness, coma, and death.

9. Jaundice (icterus) is a yellow or greenish pigmentation of the skin or sclera of the eyes caused by increases in plasma bilirubin concentration (hyperbilirubinemia).

10. Obstructive jaundice is caused by obstructed bile canaliculi (intrahepatic obstructive jaundice) or obstructed bile ducts outside the liver (extrahepatic obstructive jaundice). Bilirubin accumulates proximal to the sites of obstruction and enters the bloodstream, causing hyperbilirubinemia and jaundice.

11. Hemolytic jaundice is caused by destruction of red blood cells at a rate that exceeds the liver's ability to metabolize unconjugated bilirubin.

12. Hepatorenal syndrome is functional kidney failure caused by advanced liver disease, particularly cirrhosis with portal hypertension. Renal failure is caused by a sudden decrease in blood flow to the kidneys, usually caused by massive GI hemorrhage, liver failure, or inadequate circulating blood volume associated with ascites. The chief clinical manifestation is oliguria.

13. Acute liver failure is severe impairment or necrosis of liver cells with or without preexisting liver disease or cirrhosis. It is commonly associated with acetaminophen overdose or as a complication of viral hepatitis.

14. Cirrhosis is an inflammatory disease of the liver that causes disorganization of lobular structure, fibrosis, and nodular regeneration. The disease causes progressive irreversible liver damage, usually over a period of years.

15. Alcoholic liver disease includes fatty liver and alcoholic steatohepatitis from accumulations of fat in the liver and is a precursor to alcoholic cirrhosis.

16. Alcoholic cirrhosis impairs the hepatocytes' ability to synthesize enzymes and proteins and degrade hormones. The inflammatory response includes excessive collagen formation, fibrosis, and scarring, which obstruct bile canaliculi and sinusoids. Bile obstruction causes jaundice. Vascular obstruction causes portal hypertension, shunting, and varices.

17. NAFLD and NASH involve the accumulation of fat in the liver not associated with alcohol intake and are commonly associated with obesity.

18. Primary biliary cholangitis is an autoimmune inflammatory destruction of intrahepatic bile ducts.

19. Viral hepatitis is an infection of the liver caused by a strain of the hepatitis virus (i.e., hepatitis A virus [HAV], HBV, HCV, HEV, and HDV transmitted with HBV). Although they differ with respect to modes of transmission and severity of acute illness, all can cause hepatic cell necrosis and obstruct bile flow.

20. The clinical manifestations of viral hepatitis depend on the stage of infection. Fever, malaise, anorexia, and liver enlargement and tenderness characterize the prodromal phase. Jaundice marks the icteric phase. During the recovery phase symptoms resolve. Recovery takes several weeks.

21. Obstruction (by gallstones) and inflammation are the most common disorders of the gallbladder.

22. Cholelithiasis (the formation of gallstones) is a common disorder of the gallbladder. Gallstones form in the bile as a result of the aggregation of cholesterol crystals (cholesterol stones) or precipitates of unconjugated bilirubin (pigmented stones). Gallstones that fill the gallbladder or obstruct the cystic or common bile duct cause abdominal pain and jaundice.

23. Cholecystitis is an acute or chronic inflammation of the gallbladder usually associated with obstruction of the cystic duct by gallstones.

24. Pancreatitis (pancreatic inflammation) is a serious but relatively rare disorder. Acute pancreatitis results from pancreatic duct obstruction and injury that permits leakage of digestive enzymes into pancreatic tissue, where they become activated and begin the process of autodigestion, inflammation, and destruction of tissues. Release of pancreatic enzymes into the bloodstream or abdominal cavity causes damage to other organs.

25. Chronic pancreatitis results from structural or functional impairment of the pancreas. It causes recurrent abdominal pain and digestive disorders.

Cancer of the Digestive System

1. Cancer of the esophagus is rare and tends to occur in people older than 60 years of age. Alcohol and tobacco use, gastroesophageal reflux with dysplasia, and nutritional deficiencies are associated with esophageal carcinoma. Dysphagia and chest pain are the primary manifestations of esophageal cancer. Early treatment of tumors that have not spread into the mediastinum or lymph nodes results in a good prognosis.

2. Gastric adenocarcinoma is associated with *H. pylori*, a diet high in salt and food preservatives (nitrates, nitrites), and atrophic gastritis. Clinical manifestations of gastric cancer (weight loss, upper abdominal pain, vomiting, hematemesis, anemia) develop only after the tumor has penetrated the wall of the stomach.

3. CRC (colorectal cancer) is the third most common cause of cancer and cancer death in the United States. Colorectal polyps are highly associated with adenocarcinoma of the colon. Familial adenomatous polyposis accounts for about 3% to 5% of colorectal cancer cases.

4. Tumors of the right (ascending or proximal) colon are usually large and bulky; tumors of the left (descending, sigmoid or distal) colon develop as small, button-like masses. Manifestations of colon tumors include pain, bloody stools, and a change in bowel habits.

5. Rectal carcinoma is located up to 15 cm from the opening of the anus. The tumor spreads transmurally to the vagina in women or the prostate in men.

6. Metastatic invasion of the liver is more common than primary cancer of the liver.

7. Primary liver cancers are associated with chronic liver disease (cirrhosis, HBV infection). Hepatocellular carcinomas arise from the hepatocytes, whereas cholangiocellular carcinomas arise from the bile ducts. Primary liver cancer spreads to the heart, lungs, brain, kidney, and spleen through the circulation.

8. Cancer of the gallbladder is relatively rare and tends to occur in women older than 50 years. Adenocarcinoma is most common. Because clinical manifestations occur late in the disease, early diagnosis is rare. Advanced malignancies cannot be resected, resulting in a poor prognosis.

9. Cancer of the pancreas is the fourth leading cause of cancer deaths. Most tumors are adenocarcinomas that arise in the exocrine cells of ducts in the head, body, or tail of the pancreas. The 5-year survival rate is about 15% to 20% with resectable disease and less than 6% for metastatic disease.

KEY TERMS

Achalasia, 883
Acute colonic pseudo-obstruction (Ogilvie syndrome), 886
Acute gastritis, 887
Acute liver failure (fulminant liver failure), 901
Acute pancreatitis, 905
Afferent loop obstruction, 891
Alcoholic cirrhosis, 901
Alcoholic fatty liver (steatosis), 901
Alcoholic steatohepatitis (alcoholic hepatitis), 901
Alkaline (bile) reflux gastritis, 891
Anemia, 891
Anorexia, 879
Appendicitis, 896
Ascites, 897
Barrett esophagus, 907
Bone and mineral disorder, 891
Cholangiocellular carcinoma (cholangiocarcinoma), 910
Cholecystitis, 904
Cholelithiasis, 904
Chronic active hepatitis, 904
Chronic gastritis, 888
Chronic pancreatitis, 906
Cirrhosis, 901
Colorectal polyp, 908
Constipation, 880
Crohn disease (CD), 894

Curling ulcer, 890
Cushing ulcer, 890
Diarrhea, 880
Diverticula, 895
Diverticulitis, 895
Diverticulosis, 895
Dumping syndrome, 891
Duodenal ulcer, 889
Dysphagia, 883
Eosinophilic esophagitis, 884
Esophageal varices, 897
Familial adenomatous polyposis (FAP), 908
Gallstone, 904
Gastric ulcer, 889
Gastritis, 887
Gastroesophageal reflux disease (GERD), 883
Gastroparesis, 884
Hematochezia, 882
Hemolytic jaundice, 900
Hepatic encephalopathy, 898
Hepatocellular carcinoma (HCC), 910
Hepatopulmonary syndrome, 897
Hepatorenal syndrome, 900
Hereditary nonpolyposis colorectal cancer (HNPCC: Lynch syndrome), 908
Hiatal hernia, 884
Hyperbilirubinemia, 899
Icteric phase of hepatitis, 904

Incubation phase, 904
Intestinal obstruction, 885
Irritable bowel syndrome (IBS), 894
Ischemic ulcer, 890
Jaundice (icterus), 899
Lactase deficiency, 892
Large bowel obstruction, 886
Lower gastrointestinal bleeding, 881
Malabsorption, 891
Maldigestion, 891
Melena, 883
Microscopic colitis, 894
Mixed hiatal hernia (type 3), 884
Motility diarrhea, 881
Nausea, 879
Neoplastic polyp, 908
Nonalcoholic fatty liver disease (NAFLD), 903
Nonalcoholic steatohepatitis (NASH), 903
Obstructive jaundice, 900
Occult bleeding, 881
Osmotic diarrhea, 880
Pancreatic cancer, 911
Pancreatic insufficiency, 892
Pancreatitis, 905
Paraesophageal hiatal hernia (type 2), 884
Paralytic ileus, 885
Parietal pain, 881
Peptic ulcer, 888

Portal hypertension, 897
Portopulmonary hypertension, 897
Primary biliary cholangitis, 903
Prodromal (preicteric) phase of hepatitis, 904
Projectile vomiting, 880
Pyloric obstruction (gastric outlet obstruction), 884
Recovery phase of hepatitis, 904
Rectal carcinoma, 909
Referred pain, 881
Retching, 879
Secretory diarrhea, 881
Sliding hiatal hernia (type 1), 884
Small bowel obstruction (SBO), 885
Small intestinal carcinoma, 908
Splenomegaly, 897
Steatorrhea, 881
Stress-related mucosal disease (stress ulcer), 890
Ulcerative colitis (UC), 893
Upper gastrointestinal bleeding, 881
Varices, 897
Viral hepatitis, 903
Visceral pain, 881
Vomiting (emesis), 879
Weight loss, 891
Zollinger-Ellison syndrome, 888

REFERENCES

1. Forootan M, Bagheri N, Darvishi M: Chronic constipation: a review of literature, *Medicine (Baltimore)* 97(20):e10631, 2018.
2. Schiller LR: Definitions, pathophysiology, and evaluation of chronic diarrhea, *Best Pract Res Clin Gastroenterol* 26(5):551-562, 2012.
3. Schiller LR, Pardi DS, Sellin JH: Chronic diarrhea: diagnosis and management, *Clin Gastroenterol Hepatol* 15(2):182-193, 2017.
4. Boeckxstaens G, et al: Symptomatic reflux disease: the present, the past and the future, *Gut* 63(7):1185-1193, 2014.
5. Chatila AT, et al: Natural history, pathophysiology and evaluation of gastroesophageal reflux disease, *Dis Mon* 2019. Epub ahead of print.
6. Kellerman R, Kintanar T: Gastroesophageal reflux disease, *Prim Care* 44(4):561-573, 2017.
7. Roman S, Kahrilas PJ: The diagnosis and management of hiatus hernia, *BMJ* 349:g6154, 2014.
8. Camilleri M, et al: Clinical guideline: management of gastroparesis, *Am J Gastroenterol* 108(1):18-37, 2013.
9. No JH, et al: Long-term outcome of palliative therapy for gastric outlet obstruction caused by unresectable gastric cancer in patients with good performance status: endoscopic stenting versus surgery, *Gastrointest Endosc* 78(1):55-62, 2013.
10. Paulson EK, Thompson WM: Review of small-bowel obstruction: the diagnosis and when to worry, *Radiology* 275(2):332-342, 2015.
11. Sipponen P, Maaroos HI: Chronic gastritis, *Scand J Gastroenterol* 50(6):657-667, 2015.
12. Varbanova M, Frauenschläger K, Malfertheiner P: Chronic gastritis—an update, *Best Pract Res Clin Gastroenterol* 28(6):1031-1042, 2014.
13. Lahner E, Annibale B: Pernicious anemia: new insights from a gastroenterological point of view, *World J Gastroenterol* 15(41):5121-5128, 2009.
14. Levenstein S, et al: Psychological stress increases risk for peptic ulcer, regardless of *Helicobacter pylori* infection or use of nonsteroidal

anti-inflammatory drugs, *Clin Gastroenterol Hepatol* S1542-3565(14):1136-1137, 2014.

15. Schiller JS, et al: Summary health statistics for U.S. adults: National Health Interview Survey, 2011. Vital and Health Statistics, Series 10: Data from the National Health Interview Survey, Centers for Disease Control and Prevention. Available at www.niddk.nih.gov/health-information/health-statistics/Pages/digestive-diseases-statistics-for-the-united-states.aspx#18. (Accessed 17 June 2019).

16. De Angelis C, et al: Diagnosis and management of Zollinger-Ellison syndrome in 2018, *Minerva Endocrinol* 43(2):212-220, 2018.

17. Lanas A, Chan FKL: Peptic ulcer disease, *Lancet* 390(10094):613-624, 2017.

18. Graham DY: History of *Helicobacter pylori*, duodenal ulcer, gastric ulcer and gastric cancer, *World J Gastroenterol* 20(18):5191-5204, 2014.

19. Najm WI: Peptic ulcer disease, *Prim Care* 38(3):383-394, vii, 2011.

20. Patel SK, et al: Diagnosis of *Helicobacter pylori*: what should be the gold standard?, *World J Gastroenterol* 20(36):12847-12859, 2014.

21. Cheung KS, Leung WK: Long-term use of proton-pump inhibitors and risk of gastric cancer: a review of the current evidence, *Therap Adv Gastroenterol* 12:2019. 1756284819834511.

22. Toews I, et al: Interventions for preventing upper gastrointestinal bleeding in people admitted to intensive care units, *Cochrane Database Syst Rev* (6):CD008687, 2018.

23. Davis JL, Ripley RT: Postgastrectomy syndromes and nutritional considerations following gastric surgery, *Surg Clin North Am* 97(2):277-293, 2017.

24. Tack J, Deloose E: Complications of bariatric surgery: dumping syndrome, reflux and vitamin deficiencies, *Best Pract Res Clin Gastroenterol* 28(4):741-749, 2014.

25. Levitt M, et al: Clinical implications of lactose malabsorption versus lactose intolerance, *J Clin Gastroenterol* 47(6):471-480, 2013.

26. Johnston I, et al: New insights into bile acid malabsorption, *Curr Gastroenterol Rep* 13(5):418-425, 2011.

27. Crohn's and Colitis Foundation of America: *Fact sheet—about IBD*, New York, 2019, Author. Available at: http://www.crohnscolitisfoundation.org/news/for-the-media/media-kit/fact-sheet-about-ibd.html. (Accessed 17 June 2019).

28. Burisch J, Munkholm P: Inflammatory bowel disease epidemiology, *Curr Opin Gastroenterol* 29(4):357-362, 2013.

29. Zhang YZ, Li YY: Inflammatory bowel disease: pathogenesis, *World J Gastroenterol* 20(1):91-99, 2014.

30. Beaugerie L, Itzkowitz SH: Cancers complicating inflammatory bowel disease, *N Engl J Med* 372(15):1441-1452, 2015.

31. Ungaro R, et al: Ulcerative colitis, *Lancet* 389(10080):1756-1770, 2017.

32. Vavricka SR, et al: Extraintestinal manifestations of inflammatory bowel disease, *Inflamm Bowel Dis* 21(8):1982-1992, 2015.

33. Hata K, et al: Pouchitis after ileal pouch-anal anastomosis in ulcerative colitis: diagnosis, management, risk factors, and incidence, *Dig Endosc* 29(1):26-34, 2017.

34. Gajendran M, et al: A comprehensive review and update on Crohn's disease, *Dis Mon* 64(2):20-57, 2018.

35. Gentile N, Yen EF: Prevalence, pathogenesis, diagnosis, and management of microscopic colitis, *Gut Liver* 12(3):227-235, 2018.

36. Defrees DN, Bailey J: Irritable bowel syndrome: epidemiology, pathophysiology, diagnosis, and treatment, *Prim Care* 44(4):655-671, 2017.

37. Walker MM, Harris AK: Pathogenesis of diverticulosis and diverticular disease, *Minerva Gastroenterol Dietol* 63(2):99-109, 2017.

38. Elisei W, Brandimarte G, Tursi A: Management of diverticulosis: what's new?, *Minerva Med* 108(5):448-463, 2017.

39. Buckius MT, et al: Changing epidemiology of acute appendicitis in the United States: study period 1993-2008, *J Surg Res* 175(2):185-190, 2012.

40. Bhangu A, et al: Acute appendicitis: modern understanding of pathogenesis, diagnosis, and management, *Lancet* 386(10000):1278-1287, 2015.

41. Wagner M, Tubre DJ, Asensio JA: Evolution and current trends in the management of acute appendicitis, *Surg Clin North Am* 98(5):1005-1023, 2018.

42. Bobadilla JL: Mesenteric ischemia, *Surg Clin North Am* 93(4):925-940, ix, 2013.

43. Ehlert BA: Acute gut ischemia, *Surg Clin North Am* 98(5):995-1004, 2018.

44. Singh M, Long B, Koyfman A: Mesenteric ischemia: a deadly miss, *Emerg Med Clin North Am* 35(4):879-888, 2017.

45. Tayyem O, et al: EVALUATION and management of variceal bleeding, *Dis Mon* 64(7):312-320, 2018.

46. Butterworth RF: Hepatic encephalopathy in cirrhosis: pathology and pathophysiology, *Drugs* 79(Suppl 1):17-21, 2019.

47. Bunchorntavakul C, Reddy KR: Acute liver failure, *Clin Liver Dis* 21(4):769-792, 2017.

48. Fargo MV, Grogan SP, Saguil A: EVALUATION of jaundice in adults, *Am Fam Physician* 95(3):164-168, 2017.

49. de Mattos ÁZ, de Mattos AA, Méndez-Sánchez N: Hepatorenal syndrome: current concepts related to diagnosis and management, *Ann Hepatol* 15(4):474-481, 2016.

50. Chiew AL, et al: Interventions for paracetamol (acetaminophen) overdose, *Cochrane Database Syst Rev* (2):CD003328, 2018.

51. Scaglione S, et al: The epidemiology of cirrhosis in the United States: a population-based study, *J Clin Gastroenterol* 49(8):690-696, 2015.

52. Zhou WC, Zhang QB, Qiao L: Pathogenesis of liver cirrhosis, *World J Gastroenterol* 20(23):7312-7324, 2014.

53. Osna NA, Donohue TM, Jr, Kharbanda KK: Alcoholic liver disease: pathogenesis and current management, *Alcohol Res* 38(2):147-161, 2017.

54. Andronescu CI, Purcarea MR, Babes PA: Nonalcoholic fatty liver disease: epidemiology, pathogenesis and therapeutic implications, *J Med Life* 11(1):20-23, 2018.

55. Gonzalez RS, Washington K: Primary biliary cholangitis and autoimmune hepatitis, *Surg Pathol Clin* 11(2):329-349, 2018.

56. Centers for Disease Control and Prevention (CDC): Surveillance for viral hepatitis—United States, 2016. Available at https://www.cdc.gov/hepatitis/statistics/index.htm.

57. Easterbrook PJ, et al: Diagnosis of viral hepatitis, *Curr Opin HIV AIDS* 12(3):302-314, 2017.

58. Stinton LM, Shaffer EA: Epidemiology of gallbladder disease: cholelithiasis and cancer, *Gut Liver* 6(2):172-187, 2012.

59. Lammert F, et al: Gallstones, *Nat Rev Dis Primers* 2:16024, 2016.

60. Chung AY, Duke MC: Acute biliary disease, *Surg Clin North Am* 98(5):877-894, 2018.

61. Lankisch PG, Apte M, Banks PA: Acute pancreatitis, *Lancet* 386(9988):85-96, 2015.

62. Pham A, Forsmark C: Chronic pancreatitis: review and update of etiology, risk factors, and management, *F1000Res* 7:2018. F1000 Faculty Rev-607.

63. American Cancer Society (ACS): *Cancer facts and figures 2019*, Atlanta, 2019, Author.

64. Kuipers EJ, Spaander MC: Natural history of Barrett's esophagus, *Dig Dis Sci* 63(8):1997-2004, 2018.

65. Resende C, et al: Genetic and epigenetic alteration in gastric carcinogenesis, *Helicobacter* 15(Suppl 1):3434-3439, 2010.

66. Ajani JA, et al: Gastric adenocarcinoma, *Nat Rev Dis Primers* 3:17036, 2017.

67. Aparicio T, et al: Small bowel adenocarcinoma: epidemiology, risk factors, diagnosis and treatment, *Dig Liver Dis* 46(2):97-104, 2014.

68. Wells K, Wise PE: Hereditary colorectal cancer syndromes, *Surg Clin North Am* 97(3):605-625, 2017.

69. Meseeha M, Attia M: *Colon polyps, StatPearls [Internet]*, Treasure Island FL, 2017, StatPearls Publishing. Available at: http://www.ncbi.nlm.nih.gov/books/NBK430761/. Last updated November 18, 2018.

70. Lee GH, et al: Is right-sided colon cancer different to left-sided colorectal cancer? A systematic review, *Eur J Surg Oncol* 41(3):300-308, 2014.

71. National Cancer Institute (NCI): Stages of colon cancer, Updated December 11, 2014. Available at http://www.cancer.gov/types/colorectal/patient/colon-treatment-pdq#section/_112. Page updated May 15, 2019.

72. Dimitroulis D, et al: From diagnosis to treatment of hepatocellular carcinoma: an epidemic problem for both developed and developing world, *World J Gastroenterol* 23(29):5282-5294, 2017.

73. Sharma A, et al: Gallbladder cancer epidemiology, pathogenesis and molecular genetics: recent update, *World J Gastroenterol* 23(22):3978-3998, 2017.

74. Borazanci E, et al: Pancreatic cancer: "a riddle wrapped in a mystery inside an enigma, *Clin Cancer Res* 23(7):1629-1637, 2017.

75. Kunovsky L, et al: The use of biomarkers in early diagnostics of pancreatic cancer, *Can J Gastroenterol Hepatol* 2018:2018. 5389820.

39

Alterations of Digestive Function in Children

Sharon Sables-Baus, Sara J. Fidanza

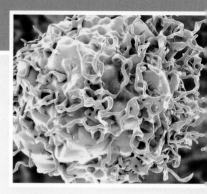

EVOLVE WEBSITE

CHAPTER OUTLINE

Disorders of the gastrointestinal (GI) tract and liver in children include congenital anomalies with structural and functional alterations, enzyme deficiencies, and infections. These disorders lead to impairment of normal digestive function and often affect growth and development.

CONGENITAL IMPAIRMENT OF MOTILITY IN THE GASTROINTESTINAL TRACT

Congenital impairments of motility can occur throughout the gastrointestinal tract. Here they are presented in order by location, starting with the mouth and esophagus, through the stomach and small intestine, and into the large intestine, rectum, and anus.

Mouth and Esophagus
Cleft Lip and Cleft Palate

There are numerous types of congenital orofacial anomalies, the most common of which is cleft lip (CL) or cleft palate (CP), or both (CLP). The incidence of CL, with or without CP, is about 1 in 940 live births. In the United States, the incidence varies significantly by racial group.[1,2] Asian and Native American populations have the highest prevalence, and African-derived populations have the lowest.[3] CL and CP can occur in isolation or as part of a broad range of chromosomal, mendelian, or teratogenic (substances that cause malformations) syndromes. When this occurs, the defect may be referred to as syndromic CLP. If CP occurs alone, the defect may be referred to as nonsyndromic (isolated)

CP and is more common in females. CL with or without CP is more common in males. Both anomalies can be unilateral or bilateral, or partial or complete.[4] Intake of B vitamins, folate, and folic acid and reduced tobacco and alcohol use before and during pregnancy may prevent orofacial clefts.[5]

PATHOPHYSIOLOGY CL and CP are embryonic developmental anomalies and vary in severity (Fig. 39.1). There may be genetic and environmental triggers for syndromic and nonsyndromic CLP. Epigenetic and genetic influences include maternal smoking and alcohol intake, steroid or statin use, B vitamin deficiency (B_6, folic acid, B_{12}), disordered metabolism, and gene mutations. (This phenomenon, called *multifactorial inheritance,* is discussed in Chapter 2.) CL and CP also may be associated with other malformations (i.e., cardiac, skeletal, or central nervous system). Together the genetic and epigenetic factors reduce the amount of neural crest mesenchyme that migrates into the area that will develop into the face of the embryo.[6]

Cleft lip is caused by the incomplete fusion of the nasomedial or intermaxillary process beginning the fourth week of embryonic development, a period of rapid development. The cleft causes structures of the face and mouth to develop without the normal restraints of encircling lip muscles. The facial cleft may affect not only the lip but also the external nose, nasal cartilages, nasal septum, and alveolar processes. The cleft is usually just beneath the center of one nostril. The defect may occur bilaterally and may be symmetrical or asymmetrical. The

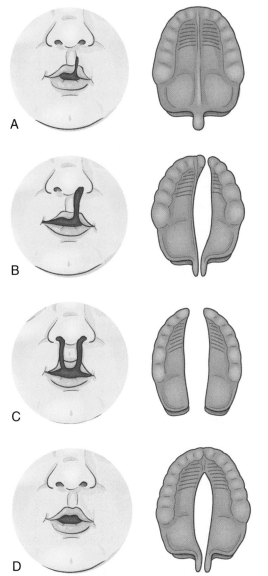

FIGURE 39.1 Variations in Clefts of the Lip and Palate. A, Notch in the vermilion border. **B,** Unilateral cleft lip and palate. **C,** Bilateral cleft lip and cleft palate. **D,** Cleft palate.

more complete the CL, the greater the chance that teeth in the line of the cleft will be missing or malformed.

Cleft palate is often associated with CL but may occur without it. The fissure may affect only the uvula and soft palate or may extend forward to the nostril and involve the hard palate and the maxillary alveolar ridge. It may be unilateral or bilateral, with the cleft occupying the midline posteriorly and as far forward as the alveolar process (the ridge of bone that holds the teeth), where it deviates to the involved side. Clefts involving the palate only are usually but not necessarily in the midline. In some cases, the vomer (the small, thin bone separating the left and right nasal cavities) and nasal septum are partly or completely undeveloped. When these facial bones are involved, the nasal cavity may freely communicate with the oral cavity.

CLINICAL MANIFESTATIONS Clefts of the lip or palate, or both, are immediately recognizable disruptions of normal facial structure. Feeding difficulty is the most significant clinical manifestation because of the oronasal communication and inability to generate negative pressure

needed for normal sucking. There also may be swallowing difficulty, and there is increased risk for middle ear infections.

EVALUATION AND TREATMENT Prenatal diagnosis is made by ultrasound, and postnatal imaging confirms the extent of bone deformity. Soft tissue alterations are evaluated by history and physical examination. The nature and extent of the cleft, the infant's condition, and the method of surgical correction proposed determine the course of treatment. Surgical correction is planned at about the third to sixth month and may be performed in stages.[7-9]

Feeding the infant with CL usually presents no difficulty if the CL is simple and the palate intact. An infant with a complete CP requires consultation with a feeding and swallowing specialist to ensure adequate and safe nutritional intake. Bottles with nipples specialized for feeding an infant with a cleft palate are required. Breast-feeding may be possible for some infants. An orthodontic prosthesis for the roof of the mouth may facilitate sucking for some infants. Parental education and support are required for the long-term care of children with CP. Longitudinal monitoring requires a cleft/orofacial multidisciplinary team, including a plastic surgeon, speech therapist, orthodontist, and nurse.

Esophageal Malformations

Congenital malformations of the esophagus are rare and often occur with other congenital malformations. **Esophageal atresia (EA)**, where the esophagus ends in a blind pouch, is the most common congenital malformation involving the esophagus. **Atresia** is an absence of embryonic development. EA is often accompanied by a fistula (an abnormal connection) between the esophagus and the trachea (**tracheoesophageal fistula [TEF]**). Either defect can occur alone (Fig. 39.2). Environmental risk factors include maternal exposure to methimazole (used to treat an overactive thyroid), exogenous sex hormones, infectious diseases, alcohol, or smoking; maternal diabetes; advanced maternal age; and maternal employment in agriculture. Many genes and chromosomal abnormalities have been implicated; 10% to 30% of infants with EA/TEF have associated *v*ertebral, *a*nal, *c*ardiovascular, *t*racheo*e*sophageal, *r*enal, and *l*imb anomalies (VACTERL).[10]

PATHOPHYSIOLOGY The pathogenesis of esophageal abnormalities is unknown, but post viral, infectious, environmental, and genetic factors have been suggested. Defective growth of endodermal cells and impaired embryonic foregut development of the trachea and esophagus lead to atresia.

CLINICAL MANIFESTATIONS The diagnosis of EA/TEF during pregnancy increases with the findings of polyhydramnios (excessive amniotic fluid) on ultrasound. Swallowed amniotic fluid is usually absorbed into the placental circulation; therefore if the fetus cannot swallow, amniotic fluid accumulates in the uterus. EA is diagnosed at birth on the basis of drooling, inability to swallow secretions or choking with feeding, and respiratory distress. Confirmation is established by inability to pass a gastric tube into the stomach. If a fistula connects the trachea with the distal esophagus, the abdomen fills with air and becomes distended, possibly interfering with breathing (Fig. 39.2, *C* to *E*). Intermittent cyanosis may result.

Pulmonary complications are compounded by reflux of air and gastric secretions into the tracheobronchial tree through the fistula, causing severe chemical irritation. Infants with EA but no fistulae have scaphoid (boat-shaped), gasless abdomens. In infants with fistulae but without atresia (see Fig. 39.2, *E*), the usual symptoms are recurrent aspiration, pneumonia, and atelectasis that remains unexpressed for days or even months.

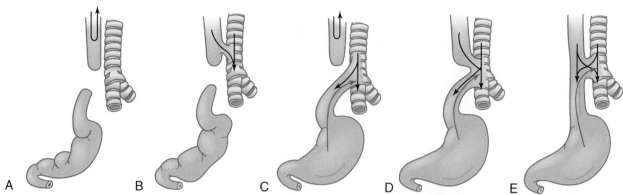

FIGURE 39.2 Five Types of Esophageal Atresia and Tracheoesophageal Fistulae. A, Simple esophageal atresia. The proximal esophagus and distal esophagus end in blind pouches, and there is no tracheal communication. Nothing enters the stomach; regurgitated food and fluid may enter the lungs. **B,** Proximal and distal esophageal segments end in blind pouches, and a fistula connects the proximal esophagus to the trachea. Nothing enters the stomach; food and fluid enter the lungs from the mouth. **C,** Proximal esophagus ends in a blind pouch, and a fistula connects the trachea to the distal esophagus. Air enters the stomach; regurgitated gastric secretions enter the lungs through the fistula. **D,** A fistula connects both proximal and distal esophageal segments to the trachea. Air, food, and fluid enter the stomach and the lungs from the mouth; regurgitated gastric secretions enter the lungs through the fistula. **E,** A simple tracheoesophageal fistula is present between an otherwise normal esophagus and trachea. Air, food, and fluid enter the stomach and the lungs from the mouth through the fistula; regurgitated gastric secretions enter the lungs through the fistula. Of esophageal anomalies, 85% to 90% are the type shown in **C;** 6% to 8% are the type shown in **A;** 3% to 5% are the type shown in **E;** and fewer than 1% are the types shown in **B** and **D.**

EVALUATION AND TREATMENT   Infants presenting with EA are evaluated with ultrasound, echocardiogram, and vertebral and limb radiographs. After diagnosis, a tube should be placed into the upper pouch and continuous suction applied to reduce the risk of aspiration. The head of the bed should be elevated slightly to assist drainage of the upper pouch. The infant should not be fed orally. Surgical repair is completed in the majority of cases. The overall survival rate for infants with esophageal defects is greater than 90%, and they need follow-up to assess growth and development and lung function.[11]

Stomach
Infantile Hypertrophic Pyloric Stenosis
Infantile hypertrophic pyloric stenosis (IHPS) is an acquired narrowing and distal obstruction of the pylorus and a common cause of postprandial (after a meal) vomiting. It is the most common cause of intestinal obstruction in infancy. The etiology of IHPS is unknown.

PATHOPHYSIOLOGY   Individual muscle fibers of the longitudinal and circular muscles thicken, so the entire pyloric sphincter becomes enlarged and inflexible. The mucosal lining of the pyloric opening is folded and narrowed by the encroaching muscle. Because of the extra peristaltic effort necessary to force the gastric contents through the narrow opening, the muscle layers of the stomach may become hypertrophied as well.

CLINICAL MANIFESTATIONS   Within 2 to 3 weeks after birth, an infant who has fed well and gained weight begins forceful, nonbilious vomiting immediately after feeding. The infant then demands to be refed. Constipation occurs because little food reaches the intestine.

In severe, untreated cases, increased gastric peristalsis and vomiting lead to dehydration and electrolyte imbalances, malnutrition, weight loss, and shock that can be life-threatening. Infants with pyloric stenosis are irritable because of hunger, and they may have esophageal discomfort caused by repeated vomiting and esophagitis. The vomitus may be blood streaked because of rupture of gastric and esophageal vessels.

EVALUATION AND TREATMENT   The diagnosis is based on the history, clinical manifestations, and findings on abdominal ultrasound. The force and timing of the vomiting can help distinguish IHPS from gastroesophageal reflux, for which episodes of vomiting are not forceful and occur 10 minutes or more after a feeding. The hypertrophied pylorus is palpable as a firm, small, movable mass, approximately the size of an olive, and is felt in the right upper quadrant in 70% to 90% of infants with pyloric stenosis. The hypertrophied pyloric muscles and narrowed pyloric channel are identified with ultrasound and radiographs.

The standard treatment for IHPS is a laparoscopic pyloromyotomy, in which the muscles of the pylorus are split and separated. Preoperative and postoperative medical management to correct fluid and electrolyte imbalance has been the key to the high success and low complication rates associated with this surgery.[12]

Small Intestine
Obstructions of the Duodenum, Jejunum, and Ileum
High intestinal obstruction should be considered whenever persistent vomiting occurs. With duodenal obstruction there will be upper abdominal distention, visible peristaltic waves, a decrease in the size and frequency of meconium stools, progressive weight loss, persistent vomiting, and dehydration. Congenital obstruction of the duodenum is rare and can be caused by intrinsic malformations, such as atresia (complete blockage), stenosis (partial obstruction or narrowing), or external pressure. Duodenal obstruction may be partial or complete and is usually located at or near the major duodenal papilla (the opening of the common bile duct and pancreatic duct into the duodenum). The classic "double bubble" sign is seen on imaging of the abdomen and represents dilation associated with duodenal obstruction. The larger, proximal "bubble" is air in a dilated stomach. The more distal, smaller "bubble" is air in a dilated proximal duodenum. There is usually little or no air in the bowel distal to the obstruction. Double bubble also may be seen on prenatal ultrasounds.

Congenital obstructions of the jejunum and ileum can be attributable to atresia, stenosis, meconium ileus, megacolon (Hirschsprung disease), intussusception, Meckel diverticulum, intestinal duplication, or strangulated hernia. In ileal or jejunal atresia, the intestine ends blindly, proximal and distal to an interruption in its continuity, with or without a gap in the mesentery. Stenosis (narrowing of the lumen) causes dilation proximal to the obstruction and luminal collapse distal to it.

Intestinal Malrotation

Intestinal malrotation is the most common congenital anomaly of the small intestine. It has an estimated incidence of about 0.5%. Associated abnormalities are common and include duodenal, jejunal, or biliary atresia; pancreatic malformations; and heart defects.[13]

PATHOPHYSIOLOGY   During normal embryonic development, the ileum and cecum rotate into the lower right abdominal quadrant and are fixed there by the mesentery. In malrotation, this rotation does not occur and the small intestine lacks a normal posterior attachment. The mobile loops of intestine can twist upon themselves (volvulus), leading to symptoms of bowel obstruction. The twisting can partly or completely occlude the superior mesenteric artery, causing infarction and necrosis of the entire midgut. Additionally, abnormal periduodenal (Ladd) bands may press against and obstruct the duodenum.

CLINICAL MANIFESTATIONS   Most cases of malrotation-associated volvulus and infarction develop during the neonatal period (90% are younger than 1 year). Some develop during childhood or adulthood. Classic symptoms in infants are intermittent or persistent bile-stained vomiting after feedings and epigastric distention. Dehydration and electrolyte imbalance may occur rapidly. Fever usually ensues, with pain and scanty stools. Diarrhea and bloody stools are associated with progressive volvulus, vascular compression, and infarction of the intestine. Intermittent or partial volvulus may be seen in older children and adults. It may be asymptomatic or cause minor abdominal discomfort and be discovered during unrelated abdominal surgery.

EVALUATION AND TREATMENT   The diagnosis of malrotation with volvulus and infarction is based on clinical manifestations. Radiographic films of the abdomen and barium studies show intestinal gas bubbles and distention proximal to the site of obstruction.

Treatment includes laparoscopic or open surgery to reduce the volvulus. Necrotic bowel may be resected and a primary anastomosis performed. An enterostomy, an opening from the outside of the abdominal wall directly into the intestine, may be created. Most children have a good outcome; however, there is risk for adhesion-related bowel obstruction in a small number of cases. Resection of large segments of the small intestine results in short bowel syndrome, a malabsorption syndrome with diarrhea, dehydration, and malnutrition.

Meckel Diverticulum

Diverticula are small outpouches, or sacs, that have formed and pushed outward through weak spots of the intestinal wall. Meckel diverticulum is a true diverticulum in that it contains all layers of the wall of the intestine, usually the ileum. It is a remnant of the embryonic yolk sac and is the most prevalent congenital abnormality of the small bowel. Ectopic (abnormal location) gastric mucosal cells are contained in the diverticula and may cause peptic ulcer and painless bleeding or mimic colonic diverticulitis. Often referred to as "the rule of 2s," a Meckel diverticulum occurs in approximately 2% of the general population, is typically located within 2 feet of the ileocecal valve (on the antimesenteric border of the ileum), is 2 inches in length on average, and its clinical symptomatology often occurs before 2 years of age. Although most

Meckel diverticula are asymptomatic, the most common symptom is painless rectal bleeding. Complications of Meckel diverticula include intestinal obstruction, intussusception, and volvulus.[14] The diagnosis is made by symptom presentation and imaging; imaging shows the gastric mucosal cells in the diverticula. Treatment is surgical resection.

> **QUICK CHECK 39.1**
> 1. What structures are affected in cleft palate and cleft lip?
> 2. How do EA and TEF affect the respiratory system?
> 3. What produces pyloric stenosis?

Meconium Syndromes

Meconium is a substance that fills the entire intestine before birth. It is a dark greenish mass of desquamated cells, mucus, and bile that accumulates in the bowel of a fetus and is typically discharged during the first 12 to 48 hours after birth.

Meconium ileus (MI) is an intestinal obstruction in the neonatal period caused by meconium formed in utero that is abnormally thick and sticky, which leads to a partial or complete obstruction at the level of the terminal ileum. There are two forms of MI: simple and complex. In simple MI, thickened meconium accumulates and obstructs the ileum causing proximal dilatation, bowel wall thickening, and congestion. Complex MI is associated with bowel atresia, volvulus, necrosis, or perforation and is a surgical emergency. MI occurs in up to 20% of infants with cystic fibrosis. It is thought to result from abnormal mucus production in the intestine or impaired pancreatic enzymes, or both.[15]

Meconium plug syndrome (MPS), also termed *functional immaturity of the colon*, is a transient disorder of the newborn colon characterized by delayed passage (>24 to 48 hours) of meconium and intestinal dilation. Plugs of meconium are found in the distal ileum and proximal colon, resulting in obstruction of passage of meconium from the rectum. Radiocontrast enema aids with both diagnosis and treatment.

Distal intestinal obstruction syndrome (DIOS), formerly called *meconium ileus equivalent*, is seen in a small number of children and adults with cystic fibrosis. It is characterized by partial or complete intestinal obstruction by abnormally viscous intestinal contents in the terminal ileum and proximal colon.

PATHOPHYSIOLOGY   The terminal ileum is plugged with thick, sticky meconium resulting from the formation of abnormal mucus. The segment of the ileum proximal to the obstruction is distended with liquid contents, and its walls may be hypertrophied. The segment distal to the obstruction is collapsed and filled with small pellets of pale-colored stool. Meconium in the obstructed segment has the consistency of thick syrup or glue. Peristalsis fails to propel this sticky material through the ileum, so it becomes impacted. Volvulus, atresia, or perforation of the bowel occurs in complicated MI.

CLINICAL MANIFESTATIONS   Abdominal distention usually develops during the first few days after birth. The distention increases as air is swallowed. The infant does not pass meconium and begins to vomit bile-stained material within hours or days of birth. Infants with cystic fibrosis may have signs of pulmonary involvement, such as tachypnea, intercostal retractions, and grunting respirations. The distended abdomen shows patterns of dilated intestinal loops that feel doughlike when palpated. Some of the loops contain scattered, firm, movable masses. Despite hyperactive peristalsis, the rectal ampulla is empty.

EVALUATION AND TREATMENT   Radiologic examination confirms the presence of meconium in the ileum or ileocecum. The sweat test, which measures the amount of chloride in the sweat, is performed to detect or rule out cystic fibrosis and is accurate in 90% of infants. In cases not complicated by volvulus or perforation, the obstruction is relieved by intestinal lavage and administration of oral laxatives. If this is not possible, the meconium is removed surgically. Survival of infants with simple meconium ileus is improving, with rates approaching 100%. Mortality of infants increases if the obstruction is complicated by peritonitis. DIOS is treated with hydration and stool softeners.

Large Intestine, Rectum, and Anus
Hirschsprung Disease

Hirschsprung disease, or congenital aganglionic megacolon, is a functional obstruction of the colon. It is rare but the most common cause of colon obstruction, and it accounts for about one third of all GI obstructions in infants. The incidence is higher in males, siblings of children with Hirschsprung disease, and children with Down syndrome or other congenital malformations.[16]

PATHOPHYSIOLOGY The cause of Hirschsprung disease is unknown, but it is associated with genetic mutations in some cases. Hirschsprung disease is characterized by the absence of parasympathetic nervous system intrinsic ganglion cells in the submucosal and myenteric plexuses along variable lengths of the colon (see Fig. 37.2 for normal colon structure). Lacking neural stimulation, muscle layers fail to propel feces through the colon, leading to functional obstruction. This causes the proximal colon to become distended, hence the term *megacolon* (Fig. 39.3). In most cases, the aganglionic segment is limited to the rectal end of the sigmoid colon. In rare cases, the entire colon lacks ganglion cells and the ileum may be involved.

CLINICAL MANIFESTATIONS The infant typically becomes symptomatic during the first 24 to 72 hours after birth with delayed passage of meconium. Mild to severe constipation is the usual manifestation of Hirschsprung disease, with poor feeding, poor weight gain, and progressive abdominal distention. However, diarrhea may be the first sign because only water can travel around the impacted feces.

The most serious complication in the neonatal period is enterocolitis related to fecal impaction. Bowel dilation stretches and partly occludes the encircling blood and lymphatic vessels, causing edema, ischemia, infarction of the mucosa, and significant outflow of fluid into the bowel lumen. Copious liquid stools result. Infarction and destruction of the mucosa enable enteric microorganisms to penetrate the bowel wall and gram-negative sepsis can occur accompanied by fever and vomiting. Severe and rapid fluid and electrolyte changes may take place, causing hypovolemic or septic shock or death.

EVALUATION AND TREATMENT Radiocontrast enema and anorectal manometry are screening tools for the diagnosis of Hirschsprung disease. The definitive diagnosis is made by rectal biopsy, showing an absence of ganglion cells in the submucosa of the colon. Surgery is the definitive treatment in all cases of Hirschsprung disease. In general, the prognosis of congenital megacolon is satisfactory for children who undergo surgical treatment. Bowel training may be prolonged; most children achieve bowel continence before puberty but some have long-term constipation or fecal incontinence.[17]

Anorectal Malformations

Anorectal malformations (ARMs) represent a spectrum of rare anomalies of the anus and rectum (Fig. 39.4). ARMs include anorectal stenosis, imperforate anus, anorectal atresia, and rectal atresia. Persistent cloaca (an embryonic component of the hind gut) is the most severe type of anorectal malformation and occurs exclusively in girls. The rectum, urethra, and vagina fail to develop separately; instead, they drain through a single, common channel onto the perineum. Infants with anorectal malformations may have other developmental anomalies (i.e., Down syndrome, Hirschsprung disease, duodenal atresia, neurogenic bladder, and spinal malformations).

Most ARMs are identified in routine physical examination during the neonatal period. Types of imperforate anus include an anal opening that is narrow or misplaced; a membrane (covering) may be present over the anal opening; the rectum may not connect to the anus; the rectum may connect to part of the urinary tract or to the reproductive system through a fistula; or the anal opening is not present. Treatment recommendations depend on the type of imperforate anus, the presence and type of associated abnormalities, and the child's overall health status. Anal stenosis can be treated by dilations. Infants with an imperforate anus and other anorectal malformations require surgical correction. Lower lesions have better functional outcomes than higher lesions. Continuing care is required to maintain bowel, bladder, and reproductive function.[18]

ACQUIRED IMPAIRMENT OF MOTILITY IN THE GASTROINTESTINAL TRACT

Gastroesophageal Reflux (GER) and Gastroesophageal Reflux Disease (GERD)

Gastroesophageal reflux (GER) is the passage of gastric contents into the esophagus independent of swallowing. GER is normal and nonpathologic in healthy infants and may be asymptomatic or exhibited by regurgitation and vomiting. The frequency of GER is highest in premature infants and declines during the first 6 to 12 months of life. Infants usually outgrow their reflux and do not require treatment.[19]

Gastroesophageal reflux disease (GERD) is different from GER. It occurs when it is the cause of troublesome symptoms or complications, or both, described as esophageal or extraesophageal in nature. Children at greatest risk for complicated GERD are those with prematurity, neurologic impairment, EA, obesity, hiatal hernia, achalasia, chronic lung diseases, and certain genetic disorders, including cystic fibrosis.

PATHOPHYSIOLOGY GERD is influenced by genetic, environmental, anatomic, hormonal, and neurogenic factors. Although transient lower

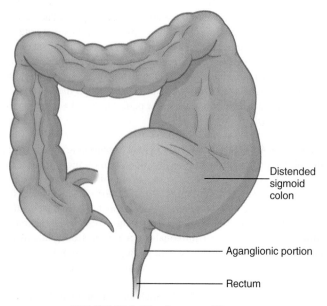

Distended sigmoid colon

Aganglionic portion

Rectum

FIGURE 39.3 Hirschsprung Disease.

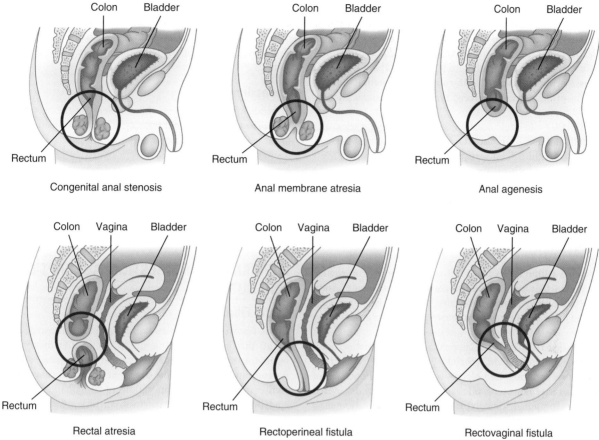

FIGURE 39.4 Anorectal Stenosis and Imperforate Anus. Except for the rectovaginal fistula, all of the malformations shown occur in both males and females.

esophageal sphincter relaxations (TLESRs) are the most common pathophysiologic cause of GERD, inadequate adaptation of sphincter tone to changes in abdominal pressure also may be implicated. Factors that maintain lower esophageal sphincter integrity in children include the location of the gastroesophageal junction in a high-pressure zone within the abdomen, mucosal gathering within the sphincter, and the angle at which the esophagus is inserted into the stomach. Reflux persists if any one of these pressure-maintaining factors is altered. Other mediators of GERD are esophageal peristalsis or clearance, mucosal resistance that mediates the noxiousness of the refluxate, and delayed gastric emptying. Reflux of acidic gastric contents results in inflammation of the esophageal epithelium (esophagitis) and stimulation of the vomiting reflex.

Esophageal inflammation resulting from GERD is differentiated from eosinophilic esophagitis (EoE), which can occur in children. EoE is thought to be an allergic esophageal disease involving both immediate and delayed hypersensitivity reactions to food ingestion. An eosinophilic infiltrate is associated with inflammation of the entire esophagus that is nonresponsive to acid-suppression therapy. The hallmark symptoms of EoE are dysphagia, food refusal or impaction, and throat and chest pain. Treatment involves elimination of problem foods from the diet and oral steroids.

CLINICAL MANIFESTATIONS   The clinical manifestations of GERD include excessive regurgitation or vomiting; food refusal/anorexia; unexplained crying, choking, or gagging; sleep disturbance; dysphagia; and abdominal or epigastric pain, or both. Esophageal complications of GERD can be significant, such as esophagitis, hemorrhage, stricture, Barrett esophagus (metaplasia) (see Chapter 38) and, rarely, adenocarcinoma.

Extraesophageal symptoms include cough and wheezing, laryngitis, pharyngitis, dental erosions, sinusitis, recurrent otitis media, and Sandifer syndrome (a neurologic disorder). This constellation of symptoms is often indistinguishable from those of cow's milk protein allergy, which may coexist with or overlap GERD.

EVALUATION AND TREATMENT   The clinical manifestations are often adequate to confirm a diagnosis of GERD. Esophageal pH monitoring with a probe for 24 hours and endoscopy with biopsy are routinely used for diagnosis.

In breast-fed babies, maternal elimination of cow's milk protein is recommended, whereas formula-fed infants may require feeding volume and frequency adjustments using extensively hydrolyzed protein or amino acid–based formulas. Using thickened feedings has been shown to improve symptoms of GERD. Prone positioning is recommended only for infants older than 1 year of age because of the risk of sudden infant death syndrome. Lifestyle changes for children and adolescents include weight loss, smoking cessation, sleeping position changes, and avoidance of caffeine, chocolate, alcohol, and spicy foods.

Medications are used to buffer or reduce gastric acid secretion, increase motility, or increase lower esophageal sphincter pressure to treat GERD. If no improvement is seen with medical management or the child has life-threatening events with reflux, an antireflux surgical procedure, including gastropexy and fundoplication, is performed.[20]

Intussusception

Intussusception is the telescoping of a proximal segment of intestine into a distal segment, causing an obstruction. It is rare but the most common cause of small bowel obstruction in children in the United States.[21] Most cases occur between 5 and 7 months of age. Intussusception is more common in males and can occur in children with polyps or tumors (lead points), cystic fibrosis, Meckel diverticulum, intestinal adhesions, or immediately after abdominal surgery. There is a small risk of intussusception associated with rotavirus vaccination, but the health benefits of the vaccine far exceed the risk of intussusception.[22]

PATHOPHYSIOLOGY In intussusception, the ileum commonly telescopes into the cecum and part of the ascending colon by collapsing through the ileocecal valve, although intussusception can occur anywhere from the duodenum to the rectum. The proximal portion of the intestine (the intussusceptum) telescopes into the distal portion (the intussuscipiens) in the direction of peristaltic flow (Fig. 39.5). The intussusceptum then drags its mesentery into the enveloping lumen, causing an intussusception. Initially, the mesentery is constricted, obstructing venous return. Compression of the mesenteric vessels between the two layers of intestinal wall and at the U-shaped angle at either end of the intussusceptum leads within hours to venous stasis, engorgement, edema, exudation, and further vascular compression. Edema and compression obstruct the flow of chyme through the intestine. Unless the intussusception is treated, bleeding, necrosis, and bowel perforation ensue.

CLINICAL MANIFESTATIONS The classic symptoms of intussusception include colicky abdominal pain, irritability, knees drawn to the chest, abdominal mass, vomiting, and bloody (currant jelly) stools. All of these symptoms may not occur. Intussusception has been discovered incidentally by computed tomography (CT) or magnetic resonance imaging (MRI) scan for other indications. Abdominal tenderness and distention develop as intestinal obstruction becomes more acute.

EVALUATION AND TREATMENT The diagnosis is based on clinical manifestations, the onset of symptoms, and ultrasonographic or radiologic imaging studies. An enema reduction is usually effective for

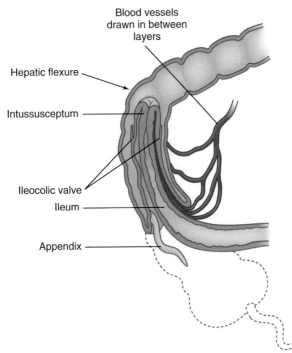

FIGURE 39.5 Ileocolic Intussusception. Dotted outline indicates normal anatomy.

large bowel intussusception and avoids the progression to ischemia and perforation. Laparotomy remains the treatment of choice for small bowel intussusception. Untreated intussusception in infants is nearly always fatal. Most infants recover if the intussusception is reduced within 24 hours.[23]

Appendicitis

Appendicitis is common in children between the ages of 10 and 11 years. The mechanisms of disease, symptoms, and treatment are similar to those for adults and can be reviewed in Chapter 38.

✔ QUICK CHECK 39.2
1. Describe the pathologic defect in meconium ileus.
2. Why is there poor bowel motility with Hirschsprung disease?
3. Describe the defect in intussusception.

IMPAIRMENT OF DIGESTION, ABSORPTION, AND NUTRITION

Cystic Fibrosis

Cystic fibrosis (CF) is an autosomal recessive disease of the exocrine glands that involves multiple organ systems but mostly the GI and respiratory systems. CF leads to death at a younger age; the prognosis is determined mainly by the degree of pulmonary involvement. This section focuses on GI complications of CF. (Chapter 30 discusses the epidemiology and pulmonary involvement.)

PATHOPHYSIOLOGY The GI presentation of CF is caused by a dysfunction of the CF transmembrane regulator (CFTR) protein, which is located on epithelial membranes and regulates chloride and sodium ion channels. It is found throughout the airways, sweat glands, digestive tract, pancreas, hepatobiliary system, and reproductive system. The hallmark pathophysiologic triad of CF is obstruction, infection, and inflammation that are evident throughout the GI tract and within the airways. The full spectrum of involvement is summarized in Table 39.1.

Dysfunction of the CFTR protein results in altered sodium, chloride, and potassium resorption, all of which remain external to the surface of the epithelial membrane, with reduced clearance from tubular structures lined by affected epithelia. Maldigestion of proteins, carbohydrates, fats, and fat-soluble vitamins occurs because mucus obstruction of the pancreatic ducts blocks the flow of pancreatic enzymes, causing intestinal malabsorption and degenerative and fibrotic changes in the pancreas and GI tract. Diabetes mellitus commonly develops from damage to insulin-producing beta cells and insulin resistance.

CLINICAL MANIFESTATIONS Clinical manifestations are summarized in Table 39.1. Gastrointestinal symptoms often precede pulmonary manifestations. Most of those with CF present early in life with pancreatic insufficiency (PI). PI is the cause of nutrient malabsorption and failure to thrive in children with CF. Steatorrhea (fatty stools) and abdominal distention are common symptoms with potential sequelae that include DIOS, fibrotic colonopathy, intussusception, or focal biliary cirrhosis. Children who are pancreatic sufficient (PS) are at greater risk of developing pancreatitis.

EVALUATION AND TREATMENT All states in the United States screen newborns for cystic fibrosis using a blood test to detect immunoreactive trypsinogen. Genetic screening and the sweat test are required for diagnosis. Evaluation of pancreatic sufficiency also is essential. The extent of pancreatic function is determined by 72-hour fecal fat

TABLE 39.1 Cystic Fibrosis—Pathophysiology, Clinical Manifestations, and Complications

Organ Involved	Secretory Dysfunction	Clinical Manifestations	Complications
Sweat Glands	Elevated concentrations of sodium and chloride in sweat	Hyponatremia; hypochloremia	Heat prostration; shock
Digestive System			
Esophagus	None	Gastroesophageal reflux	Risk for aspiration events
Intestine			
Newborn	Viscid meconium	Meconium ileus with intestinal obstruction	Meconium peritonitis
Older child and adult	Inspissated (dried out) mucofecal masses (intestinal sludging)	Partial intestinal obstruction with severe cramping pains	Gastroesophageal reflux Volvulus (obstruction), intussusception (prolapse) Distal intestinal obstruction syndrome
Pancreas (enzyme deficiency)	Inspissation and precipitation of pancreatic secretions, causing obstruction of pancreatic ducts Insulin deficiency	Absence of pancreatic enzymes, causing malabsorption of food; fatty, bulky stools Decreased vitamins A, D, E, and K absorption Growth failure Glucose intolerance	Hypoproteinemia; iron deficiency anemia; malnutrition Recurrent pancreatitis, pancreatic cysts Vitamins A, D, E, and K deficiency and rectal prolapse Decreased bone density and risk of fractures in adolescents and adults Diabetes mellitus
Liver	Inspissation and precipitation of bile in biliary system	Focal biliary cirrhosis; shrunken, "hobnail" liver	Portal hypertension with esophageal varices, hematemesis and hypersplenism Hepatic steatosis Focal biliary cirrhosis Steatorrhea from lack of bile salts
Salivary glands	Inspissation and precipitation of secretions in small ducts of submaxillary and sublingual salivary glands	Mild patchy fibrosis of salivary glands	None
Respiratory System			
Paranasal structures	Viscid mucus	Retention of mucus; clouding seen on sinus roentgenograms	Mucopyoceles (pus accumulations) with nasal deformity or orbital cavity extension
Nose	Nasal polyps	Obstruction of nasal airflow	None
Lungs	Viscid mucus in bronchioles and bronchi	Obstruction of bronchioles causing bronchiolectasis, bronchiectasis, and chronic lung infection	Hemoptysis; pneumothorax; cor pulmonale; atelectasis; chronic bacterial infection; respiratory failure
Reproductive System			
Male	Viscid genital tract secretions during embryologic development, causing failure of formation of normal vas deferens	Delayed puberty Sterility	None
Female	Distention of endocervical epithelial cells with cytoplasmic mucin	Delayed puberty Decreased fertility	Polypoid cervicitis (cervical inflammation) while taking oral contraceptives

Data from Assis DN, Freedman SD: *Clin Chest Med* 37(1):109–118, 2016; Lavelle LP et al: *Radiographics* 35(3):680–695, 2015; Leeuwen L, Fitzgerald DA, Gaskin KJ: *Paediatr Respir Rev* 15(1):69–74, 2014; Marcdante KJ, Kliegman RM, editors: *Nelson essentials of pediatrics,* ed 7, Philadephia, 2014, Saunders; Stalvey MS, Clines GA: *Curr Opin Endocrinol Diabetes Obes* 20(6):547–552, 2013.

measurements, which are not easily obtained. Therefore, the most common measurement of fat malabsorption is fecal elastase. A serum test for trypsinogen also can be used to detect pancreatic insufficiency in children older than 8 years of age.

The goal of treatment for PI is to reduce malabsorption of nutrients and improve growth. Most children with CF take pancreatic enzyme replacement therapy (PERT) for the rest of their lives. PERT is administered before or with every meal, snack, or enteral feeding supplementation. High doses of PERT are associated with DIOS;

therefore, minimal effective doses are indicated. High-caloric, high-protein diets with frequent snacks and vitamin supplements are used to treat malnutrition. Nutritional status and growth should be carefully monitored, and growth hormone may be included with nutritional supplements.[24]

Celiac Disease

Celiac disease (CD), also known as *celiac sprue* or *gluten-sensitive enteropathy*, is an autoimmune disease that damages small intestinal

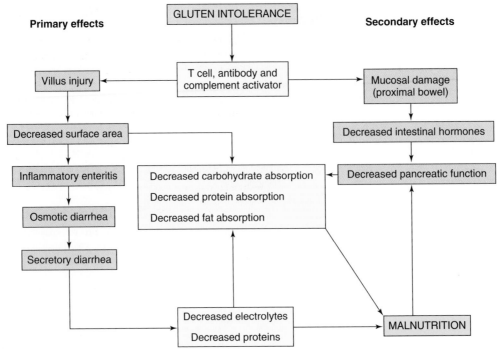

FIGURE 39.6 Pathophysiology of Celiac Disease.

villous epithelium when gluten (gliadin), the protein component of cereal grains, is ingested. CD is a common multiorgan disease with a strong genetic predisposition. It is associated with certain human leukocyte antigens (HLAs) and autoantibodies.[25] Nonceliac gluten sensitivity (GS) occurs in individuals who do not have celiac disease or wheat allergy, however, they do have intestinal symptoms or extraintestinal symptoms, or both, when they ingest foods that contain gluten. Symptoms improve on withdrawal of gluten.[26]

The pathogenesis of CD is complex and involves genetic and immunologic factors. Environmental factors include early infections, gut microbiota in infants, feeding patterns, and the timing and amount of gluten. CD presents with greater frequency in children with type 1 diabetes mellitus, autoimmune thyroid or liver disease, Down syndrome, Turner syndrome, Williams syndrome, selective immunoglobulin A (IgA) deficiency, and Addison disease, and in those with first-degree relatives with CD.

PATHOPHYSIOLOGY The major pathophysiologic characteristic of celiac disease is autoimmune injury to the small intestinal epithelial cells of genetically susceptible individuals. There are increased numbers of intraepithelial lymphocytes, atrophy and flattening of villi, crypt hyperplasia in the upper small intestine, and malabsorption of most nutrients in the presence of cereal gluten, particularly wheat, rye, and barley (Fig. 39.6).

Damage to the mucosa of the duodenum and jejunum exacerbates malabsorption. The secretion of intestinal hormones, such as secretin and cholecystokinin, may be diminished. Consequently, secretion of pancreatic enzymes and expulsion of bile from the gallbladder are reduced, contributing to malabsorption. Destruction of mucosal cells causes inflammation, and water and electrolytes are secreted, leading to watery diarrhea. Potassium loss leads to muscle weakness. Magnesium and calcium malabsorption can cause seizures or tetany. Unabsorbed fatty acids combine with calcium, and secondary hyperparathyroidism increases phosphorus excretion, resulting in bone reabsorption. Calcium is no longer able to bind oxalate in the intestine and is absorbed, which

causes hyperoxaluria. Gallbladder function may be abnormal, and bile salt conjugation may decrease.

Fat malabsorption in the jejunum is the major cause of steatorrhea. Deficiencies of fat-soluble vitamins are common in children with CD. Vitamin K malabsorption leads to hypoprothrombinemia. There can be iron and folic acid malabsorption manifested as cheilosis; anemia; and a smooth, red tongue. Vitamin B_{12} absorption is impaired in those with extensive ileal disease, and folate and iron deficiencies are common.

CLINICAL MANIFESTATIONS The onset of clinical manifestations of celiac disease depends on the age of the infant when gluten-containing substances are added to the diet. It is not uncommon for a person to be diagnosed later in life. The severity of the symptoms can vary tremendously; many untreated children older than 3 years of age present with nongastrointestinal symptoms related to malabsorption and malnutrition, and the effect of autoantibodies on nonintestinal tissues. GI and extraintestinal symptoms of CD are listed in Box 39.1.

An unusual complication of celiac disease in infancy is celiac crisis. Celiac crisis is characterized by severe diarrhea, dehydration, and hypoproteinemia as a result of malabsorption and protein deficiency.

EVALUATION AND TREATMENT The diagnosis includes confirmation with serologic autoantibody measurement against tissue transglutaminase IgA (most sensitive and specific), antiendomysium IgA, or deaminated gliadin peptides, which are more sensitive in children younger than 2 years of age. A negative genetic screening for HLA haplotypes rules out CD. If an autoantibody or genetic screen is positive, a small duodenal biopsy sample may be obtained to check for the classic mucosal changes caused by CD. A wide variety of screening tests for malabsorption also may be useful. Even though very useful screening tools are available to diagnose CD, many children remain undiagnosed.

Treatment consists of lifelong adherence to a gluten-free diet (GFD), which includes the elimination of wheat, rye, barley, and malt. Lactose (milk sugar) intolerance also may be present from

BOX 39.1   Symptoms of Celiac Disease

Gastrointestinal Symptoms

Diarrhea
Abdominal pain and distension
Vomiting
Anorexia
Constipation

Extraintestinal Symptoms

Fatigue
Iron deficiency anemia
Weight loss, growth failure
Delayed puberty
Infertility
Dermatitis herpetiformis
Dental enamel hypoplasia, aphthous stomatitis
Arthritis
Osteoporosis
Fractures
Neurologic manifestations: ataxia, neuropathy, seizures

Data from Jericho H, Guandalini S: *Nutrients* 10(6), 2018; Leonard MM et al: *JAMA* 318(7):647-656, 2017.

damage to villi; therefore, lactose also may be excluded from the diet but should be resumed after treatment. Infants are routinely given fat-soluble vitamins, iron, and folic acid supplements to treat deficiencies. Bone mineral density (BMD) screening is required. For most children the long-term prognosis is excellent. Refractory CD, which is resistant to a GFD treatment, is rare and may require steroids or immunosuppressants.

Malnutrition

Pediatric malnutrition is an imbalance between nutrient requirements (energy expenditure) and intake that results in energy, protein, and micronutrient deficits that impair growth and development. Malnutrition may involve impaired absorption, altered nutrient utilization, increased nutrient losses, or increased nutrient requirements (hypermetabolism). Severe or moderate acute or chronic illnesses can contribute to the development of malnutrition, including surgery, trauma, burns, and chronic diseases (e.g., cystic fibrosis, tuberculosis, chronic kidney disease, malignancies, congenital heart disease [CHD], GI diseases, and neuromuscular diseases). Malnutrition unrelated to illness develops from a lack of access to nutrients as a result of environmental factors (i.e., political/socioeconomic, inadequate food supplies, or food contaminated with parasites) or behavioral factors (e.g., anorexia nervosa). Malnutrition may be acute (less than 3 months' duration) or chronic (more than 3 months' duration).

Kwashiorkor (a deficiency of dietary protein) and marasmus (all forms of inadequate nutrient intake) are terms that have been used to describe types of malnutrition in children, particularly in developing countries. Collectively they are known as protein-energy malnutrition (PEM). PEM describes the effects of malnutrition but not the etiology or interactions that contribute to nutrient depletion. A definition of pediatric malnutrition that includes the etiology (illness or environmental), identification of pathogenesis and chronicity, associations with inflammation, and resulting impact on functional status is more directive for defining the risk of malnutrition, planning interventions, and assessing outcomes.[27]

States of long-term starvation are often the result of widespread nutritional deficiencies among children in developing countries and economically destitute populations, particularly when associated with human immunodeficiency virus (HIV) infection.[28] Malnutrition can occur in infants or children from 1 to 4 years of age who have been weaned from breast milk to a high-starch, protein-deficient diet or switched to overdiluted commercial formulas that lack adequate protein and carbohydrates.

Hospitalized children are at risk for malnutrition. Acute illness, trauma, surgery, or preexisting chronic diseases contribute to malnutrition and requires assessment and intervention. Acute and chronic inflammatory states also increase nutrient requirements. Treatments, including radiation therapy, chemotherapy, and longer times on mechanical ventilation, also can contribute to malnutrition with increased hospital length of stay, and increased morbidity and mortality rates.[29]

PATHOPHYSIOLOGY The pathogenesis of PEM (kwashiorkor) is uncertain but includes inadequate dietary protein, leaky gut syndrome (compromised gut barrier), and intestinal inflammation. The lack of sufficient plasma proteins results in hypoproteinemia and generalized edema with a substantial loss of potassium. The liver swells with stored fat because no hepatic proteins are synthesized to form and release lipoproteins. Pancreatic atrophy and fibrosis may be present. There is reduced bone density and impaired renal function. If the condition is not reversed, the prognosis is very poor and growth is severely retarded. Lack of all nutrients (proteins, carbohydrates, fats, and micronutrients [marasmus]) is more common in infants and leads to dehydration, weight loss, and growth restriction. There is wasting of muscle and fat but not the edema associated with PEM.

Alterations in gut microbiota also are involved in the pathophysiology of malnutrition.[30] Children with malnutrition show stunting of gut microbiota maturation, which may delay normal development of the gut, depress intestinal immune function, and promote inflammation and infection. Healthy gut bacteria also produces short-chain fatty acids, B vitamins, and vitamin K, and promotes the absorption of minerals important for maintaining the intestinal epithelium.[31]

CLINICAL MANIFESTATIONS Children with PEM have marked generalized edema, dermatoses, hypopigmented hair, a distended abdomen, hepatomegaly, and almost normal weight for age (because of edema). Children with malnutrition related to inadequate proteins, carbohydrates, fats, and micronutrients demonstrate greater wasting of protein and fat stores characterized by muscle wasting, diarrhea, dermatosis, low hemoglobin level, and infection. There is loss of subcutaneous fat and an absence of edema. Both conditions lead to delays in physical, behavioral, and cognitive development and academic performance. Lastly, micronutrient deficiencies, especially with zinc, selenium, iron, and antioxidant vitamins, can lead to immune deficiency and infections. Severe vitamin A deficiency commonly results in blindness.[32]

EVALUATION AND TREATMENT Evaluation of malnutrition is based on the nutritional history and clinical manifestations, including anthropometric measurements and use of appropriate growth charts. Laboratory monitoring is used to assess for macronutrient and micronutrient deficiencies, aminotransaminase alterations, the presence of inflammation, and response to refeeding. Treatment of underlying disease and provision of deficient nutrients will resolve clinical symptoms in 4 to 6 weeks.[33] Developmental sequelae of malnutrition may be irreversible; therefore early intervention is recommended. Nutritional rehabilitation with appropriate environmental stimulation for infants and young children has been shown to resolve or improve cerebral shrinkage, physical growth, and psychomotor development.

Faltering Growth (Failure to Thrive)

Faltering growth (previously known as failure to thrive [FTT]) is not a diagnosis but a physical sign demonstrating that a child has a slower rate of weight gain in childhood than expected for age and sex. It is manifested as a deceleration in weight gain, a low weight/height or body mass index (BMI) ratio, or a low weight/height/head circumference ratio. Faltering growth is a common problem and can present at any time in childhood but is usually present before 18 months of age.[34]

PATHOPHYSIOLOGY Faltering growth is considered a multifactorial condition that includes biologic, psychosocial, and environmental contributions that may or may not be related to illness (Box 39.2). In more than 80% of cases, an underlying medical condition is never found. Categories of faltering growth include inadequate caloric intake, inadequate caloric absorption, or excessive caloric expenditure. Infants and children are at risk if their parents or primary caregivers are unable to provide nurturance.

CLINICAL MANIFESTATIONS Clinical manifestations of faltering growth are delayed growth accompanied by manifestations of malnutrition or an underlying disease (e.g., diarrhea or infectious disease, or both). Infants who present with faltering growth frequently have feeding problems. Symptoms include pallid or dry, cracked skin; sparse hair; poorly developed musculature; decreased subcutaneous fat; swollen abdomen with malabsorption, diarrhea, or anorexia; and signs of vitamin deficiencies, such as rickets. Social or emotional manifestations include reduced energy level, reduced responsiveness and interaction with the environment, social isolation, spasticity and rigidity when held or touched, inability to make eye contact or smile, refusal to eat, and rejection of foods. There may be long-term adverse effects on cognitive, behavioral, and academic performance.

EVALUATION AND TREATMENT Faltering growth is suggested if a child falls below the 3rd percentile for weight, or shows stagnation in length or weight on appropriate growth charts. Underlying medical conditions are evaluated. If illness is ruled out, a thorough review of psychosocial, emotional, and environmental components of care is necessary. Screening tools are available to assist with evaluation of nutrition status and to guide therapy, particularly in hospitalized children.

BOX 39.2 Factors Associated With Faltering Growth

Poverty (food insecurity related to lack of money)

Premature birth; low birth weight

Inadequate caloric intake or caloric absorption (infant feeding problems, underlying chronic disease or malabsorption syndromes)

Incorrect preparation of formula (too diluted, too concentrated)

Mechanical feeding difficulties (oromotor dysfunction, congenital anomalies, central nervous system disorders)

Unsuitable feeding habits (food fads, excessive juice)

Behavior problems affecting eating

Disturbed parent-child relationship; parental stress, parental lack of knowledge; child neglect

Data from Krishna A et al: *Glob Health Action* 8:26523, 2015; National Guideline Alliance (UK): *Faltering growth–recognition and management*, London, 2017, National Institute for Health and Care Excellence (UK); available from https://www.ncbi.nlm.nih.gov/books/NBK458459/.

Treatment for faltering growth includes treating an underlying illness if found, increasing volume or caloric density of formula, increasing frequency of breast-feeding (if found to be insufficient), structuring meals and snacks, and adding high-calorie foods and additives. Eliminating fruit juice, soda, or excessive milk also will improve appetite and absorption of nutrients. Medications are used to stimulate appetite. Nutrient deficiencies are supplemented. If the child is unable to gain weight, an oral enteral supplement may be added to the diet or a nasogastric or gastrostomy tube can be used to supplement oral intake.

If the cause is not medical, management involves the immediate total care of the child and measures to address (1) the psychosocial and emotional problems of the caregivers and (2) parent-child interactions. Counseling, parental modeling, and long-term family support are sometimes required.

Hospital admission and evaluation are recommended if the diagnosis is unclear or the child is in nutritional or emotional jeopardy. Eating patterns, food preferences, caloric intake, and family interactions can be assessed and treatment plans implemented during the hospital stay.

Necrotizing Enterocolitis

Necrotizing enterocolitis (NEC) is an ischemic, inflammatory condition that causes bowel necrosis and perforation. NEC is not a specific diagnosis but a constellation of signs and symptoms with several proposed etiologies. It is the most common severe neonatal GI emergency that predominantly affects the smallest and most premature infants. Approximately 5% to 10% of infants born weighing less than 1500 g will develop NEC; of those, about 40% will not survive.[35]

PATHOPHYSIOLOGY The exact etiology of NEC is unclear.[36] Factors contributing to the development of NEC include infections, abnormal bacterial colonization, intestinal ischemia, immature immune responses, exaggerated inflammatory responses, immature intestinal motility, altered microcirculatory blood flow and barrier function, perinatal stress, effects of medications and feeding practices, and genetic predisposition. The immature mucosal barrier delays digestion and motility is slower, allowing for the accumulation of noxious substances that damage the intestine, increase permeability, and increase the risk for infection. Translocation of intestinal bacteria and other substances contributes to injury, with inflammation, vasoconstriction of mesenteric blood flow, development of systemic inflammatory disease, multiple organ failure and death. Immature intestinal innate immunity and an unfavorable balance between normal and pathogenic bacteria promote intestinal inflammation and release of proinflammatory cytokines. Accumulation of gas in the intestine can cause pressure that decreases blood flow, and an imbalance between vasodilator and vasoconstrictor inputs in the immature gut may lead to vasoconstriction promoting ischemia and oxidative stress, reperfusion injury, and necrosis.

CLINICAL MANIFESTATIONS Manifestations of NEC usually appear suddenly and within weeks of premature birth, and sooner for term neonates. Signs and symptoms of "classic" NEC include feeding intolerance, abdominal distention and bloody stools after 8 to 10 days of age, septicemia with an elevated white blood cell count, and falling platelet levels. An unstable temperature, bradycardia, and apnea are nonspecific signs. In late preterm or term infants, NEC is more likely to be associated with other predisposing factors, such as low Apgar scores, chorioamnionitis, exchange transfusions, prolonged rupture of membranes, congenital heart defects, or neural tube defects.

EVALUATION AND TREATMENT The diagnosis is based on the clinical manifestations, laboratory results, and plain films of the abdomen. Symptoms usually progress rapidly, often within hours, from subtle signs to abdominal discoloration, intestinal perforation, and peritonitis or even death. Abdominal radiographs show pneumoperitoneum, pneumatosis intestinalis (gas in the bowel wall), or unchanging "rigid" loops of small bowel. Systemic hypotension requires intensive medical support or bowel resection, or both. Efforts are in progress to identify predictive biologic markers for early diagnosis.

Preventive strategies include encouragement of breast milk feeding, preferential feeding of human milk, judicious fluid management to prevent vascular fluid overload, and confirmation of patent ductus arteriosus (see Chapter 27). Additional treatments include administration of amino acids (i.e., arginine and glutamine supplements) to support intestinal epithelial cell growth, and enteral probiotics to support normal gut bacteria. The rapid onset of symptoms makes primary prevention difficult.

Treatments include cessation of feeding, implementation of gastric suction to decompress the intestines, maintenance of fluid and electrolyte balance, and administration of antibiotics to control sepsis. Surgical resection is the treatment of choice for perforation, and peritoneal drainage may be used as an adjunct to laparotomy. Overall mortality is high, particularly for infants who have surgery.

> ✔ **QUICK CHECK 39.3**
> 1. Why do individuals with cystic fibrosis have pancreatic insufficiency?
> 2. Why does loss of villi occur with celiac disease?
> 3. Compare kwashiorkor and marasmus.

DIARRHEA

Diarrhea is an increase in the water content, volume, or frequency of stools and can be acute or chronic. Diarrhea is usually defined as three or more watery or loose stools in 24 hours. Children with acute gastroenteritis often remain mildly symptomatic for up to 4 weeks, therefore, diarrhea that persists longer than 4 weeks is considered chronic. Diarrhea is a common GI problem during infancy and early childhood and is the leading cause of death in young children, particularly among preterm infants and children in developing countries.[37] Severe, acute infectious diarrhea occurs one to three times during the first 3 years of life. Most episodes are self-limiting and resolve within 72 hours.

The pathophysiologic mechanisms of diarrhea in children are similar to those described for adults—osmotic, secretory, intestinal dysmotility, or inflammatory (see Chapter 38). Prolonged diarrhea is more dangerous in infants and children, however, because they have much smaller fluid reserves and more rapid peristalsis and metabolism than adults. Therefore dehydration in children can develop rapidly if any disturbance:

- increases fluid secretion into the GI lumen (secretory diarrhea).
- draws fluid into the lumen by osmosis (osmotic diarrhea).
- reduces intestinal transit time with luminal fluid retention (intestinal dysmotility).
- causes inflammation that results in malabsorption and an increased luminal osmotic load from nutrients, fluid, and blood, which may increase gut motility (inflammatory diarrhea).

Acute Infectious Diarrhea

Diarrhea in infants and young children has numerous causes, including bacterial and systemic infections, malabsorption syndromes, autoimmune disorders, congenital malformations, and genetic disorders. Acute infection is the most common cause of childhood diarrhea worldwide.[37]

Acute infectious diarrhea in infants and young children is usually associated with viral or bacterial gastroenteritis. Viruses include rotaviruses, noroviruses, and adenoviruses. Rotavirus is a common cause in young children and is associated with a higher death rate in low-income countries. Rotavirus vaccination is an effective preventive strategy. Numerous bacteria or parasites can contaminate food or water and cause diarrhea. Bacterial causes of diarrhea have geographic variation, and specific bacteria can be identified using molecular analysis or stool culture. *Clostridium difficile* is often associated with previous antibiotic therapy.

Infectious diarrhea has a rapid onset, with watery stools sometimes mixed with blood, abdominal cramping, fever, vomiting, and weight loss. Severe dehydration, acidosis, and shock can occur quickly from diarrhea and vomiting. Hemolytic uremic syndrome and renal failure can develop when diarrhea is associated with *Shigella* toxin and *Escherichia coli* infection (see Chapter 33). Other causes of acute diarrhea in the older child include antibiotic therapy, appendicitis, chemotherapy, inflammatory bowel disease, parasitic infestation, parenteral infections, and ingestion of toxic substances.

Treatment of diarrhea requires evaluation of the cause through the history, stool testing for common pathogens, and laboratory analysis. Treatment of underlying illness is warranted when identified. Other treatments include hydration, electrolyte replacement, nutrition maintenance, and antibiotics if a pathogen is found. Antispasmodics may relieve abdominal cramping, and selected probiotics can reduce the duration and improve morbidity and mortality.[38] Intravenous solutions are used only when oral solutions are not tolerated. Prevention includes clean water, environmental sanitation, and good hygiene.

Primary Lactose Intolerance

Lactose malabsorption and lactose intolerance, the inability to digest lactose, are caused by inadequate production or impaired activity of the enzyme lactase. It is a common cause of diarrhea, particularly in children under the age of 7 years. The malabsorption of lactose results in osmotic diarrhea accompanied by abdominal pain, bloating, and flatulence. Systemic manifestations include skin disease, rheumatologic complaints, chronic fatigue, and failure to thrive. Intolerance to other forms of carbohydrates and deficient enzymes can cause symptoms similar to lactose intolerance.[39]

The diagnosis can be made through elimination of dietary lactose or by performing a hydrogen lactose breath test or an oral lactose tolerance test. Treatment consists of reducing milk consumption or supplementing the diet with oral lactase. Some children can tolerate lactose in fermented forms, such as cheese and yogurt, or by adding soy food. A diet low in fermentable oligosaccharides, disaccharides, and monosaccharides and polyols (FODMAPs) or administration of probiotics to alter intestinal flora has been found to be effective in children with lactose intolerance and IBS who have persistent symptoms.

DISORDERS OF THE LIVER

Disorders of Biliary Metabolism and Transport

Neonatal Jaundice

Jaundice (icterus) is a yellow pigmentation of the skin caused by an increased level of bilirubin in the bloodstream (i.e., a total serum bilirubin [TSB] level that exceeds the 95th percentile for the infant's age in hours or greater than 20 mg/dl, except in the low birth weight population). Jaundice usually becomes clinically apparent when the serum bilirubin concentration is greater than 2 mg/dl (34 μmol/L). Physiologic jaundice (hyperbilirubinemia) of the newborn is a frequently encountered problem in otherwise healthy newborns caused by lack of maturity of bilirubin uptake and conjugation. Poor caloric intake or dehydration, or both, associated with inadequate breast-feeding also may contribute to the high levels of bilirubin. High bilirubin levels in the newborn period can be associated with hemolytic disease, metabolic and endocrine disorders, anatomic abnormalities of the liver, and infections. For older infants and children, the most common causes of unconjugated hyperbilirubinemia are hemolytic processes resulting in bilirubin overproduction.

Pathologic jaundice is a bilirubin concentration greater than 20 mg/dl in the newborn period associated with a severe illness, or a total serum bilirubin level that rises by more than 5 mg/dl during the newborn period. Risk factors for development of pathologic jaundice include fetal-maternal blood type incompatibility (ABO and Rh incompatibility, hemolytic disease in the newborn), premature birth, exclusive breast-feeding in some infants, maternal age greater than or equal to 25 years, male sex, delayed meconium passage, glucose-6-phosphate dehydrogenase deficiency, and excessive birth trauma, such as bruising or cephalohematomas.[40]

PATHOPHYSIOLOGY Pathologic jaundice results from the complex interaction of factors that cause (1) increased bilirubin production (e.g., hemolysis), (2) impaired hepatic uptake or excretion of unconjugated bilirubin, or (3) delayed maturation of liver bilirubin conjugating mechanisms. The most common cause is hemolytic disease of the newborn and all pregnant women should be tested for ABO and Rh incompatibility (see Chapters 8 and 24). Unconjugated bilirubin (indirect bilirubin) is lipid soluble and bound to albumin in the blood, and in the free form it readily crosses the blood-brain barrier in infants. Chronic bilirubin encephalopathy (kernicterus) is caused by the deposition of toxic, unconjugated bilirubin in brain cells and usually does not occur in healthy, full-term infants. The mechanism of injury is not clearly known. An elevated level of conjugated bilirubin is a sign of underlying disease.

CLINICAL MANIFESTATIONS Physiologic jaundice develops during the second or third day after birth and usually subsides in 1 to 2 weeks in full-term infants and in 2 to 4 weeks in premature infants. After this, increasing bilirubin values and persistent jaundice indicate pathologic hyperbilirubinemia. Manifestations include yellowing of the skin, dark urine, light-colored stools, and weight loss. Premature infants with respiratory distress, acidosis, or sepsis are at greater risk for kernicterus and the development of bilirubin-induced neurologic dysfunction (BIND) (e.g., neuromotor signs, hyperexcitable neonatal reflexes, and speech and hearing impairment).[41]

EVALUATION AND TREATMENT Jaundice is detected by clinical assessment. Both total and direct (conjugated) bilirubin levels are monitored. Other causes of jaundice must be eliminated to confirm physiologic jaundice. Treatment depends on the degree of hyperbilirubinemia. Physiologic jaundice is commonly treated by phototherapy and several techniques are available. Pathologic jaundice requires an exchange transfusion and treatment of the underlying disorder.

Biliary Atresia

Biliary atresia (BA) is a rare congenital malformation characterized by the absence or obstruction of extrahepatic bile ducts resulting in neonatal cholestasis. The etiology of duct injury is not clear but is thought to be related to an embryonic (or congenital) abnormality or an acquired anomaly (e.g., perinatal viral-induced progressive inflammation with innate autoimmune destruction). The disease expression is a continuum in which the principal process is one of bile duct destruction. The atresia of the bile ducts is associated with inflammation, fibrosis, loss of epithelial cells, and obstruction of the bile canaliculi. Progressive obstruction leads to secondary biliary cirrhosis (see Chapter 38), portal hypertension, or liver failure.

Jaundice is the primary clinical manifestation of BA, along with hepatomegaly and acholic (clay-colored) stools. Fat absorption is impaired because of the lack of bile salts. Abdominal distention caused by hepatomegaly and ascites may cause anorexia and faltering growth. Fat-soluble vitamin deficiencies (A, D, E, K) require supplementation. Manifestations

of cirrhosis and liver failure include ascites, hypoalbuminemia, hypercoagulation, pruritus, esophageal varices, and gastrointestinal bleeding that may lead to death.

Early diagnosis of BA is essential; the best outcome is achieved when the infant is diagnosed and treated in the first 30 to 45 days of life. BA that is diagnosed late does not respond well to current surgical treatment. The diagnosis of BA is based on the clinical manifestations, abnormal liver function test results, liver biopsy results, and an intraoperative cholangiogram. Serum aminotransaminase and alkaline phosphatase levels are elevated, and conjugated (direct) serum bilirubin levels rise progressively. BA can be relieved by hepatoportoenterostomy (HPE, or the Kasai procedure), in which a segment of the small intestine is used to create a bile duct. Even with initial restoration of bile flow, however, obliteration of intrahepatic bile ducts can continue and cirrhosis results. Liver transplantation is performed for 80% of children with BA and is the only long-term therapeutic option.[42]

Inflammatory Disorders
Hepatitis

Details related to viral hepatitis are presented in Chapter 38, including differentiation of the types of viruses (see Table 38.8).

Hepatitis A virus. HAV is transmitted through contact with the feces of people infected with HAV. Approximately 30% to 50% of the reported cases of hepatitis A virus (HAV) occur in children, particularly children of nursery school age. Outbreaks tend to occur in day-care centers with large numbers of children who are not toilet trained and with staff members who practice poor handwashing techniques.[43] Vertical transmission from mother to newborn or from a transfusion is rare. HAV in children is usually mild and asymptomatic, but it may involve nausea, vomiting, and diarrhea. Jaundice appears in more than 70% of older children. Almost all children recover from hepatitis A without residual liver damage, although relapse may occur. After HAV infection, the body produces antibodies that prevent reinfection. Vaccination programs have successfully reduced the incidence of HAV in the United States by 95%.[44]

Hepatitis B virus. Risk factors for hepatitis B virus (HBV) include infants of mothers who are chronic hepatitis B surface antigen (HBsAg) carriers, children from families that immigrated to the United States or are adopted from endemic areas, infection from HBsAg-positive household contacts, and children who abuse parenteral drugs or engage in unprotected sex. Maternal-fetal transmission (vertical transmission) is the most common route of HBV transmission in children. About 25% to 50% of children between the ages of 1 and 5 years of age who are acutely infected will develop chronic infection. Chronic hepatitis may develop more often in young children because their immune system is immature. The most serious consequence of HBV infection is fulminant hepatitis, which occurs in 1% of cases. Hepatitis D virus (HDV) infection depends on active infection with HBV. Exacerbation of HBV is more common in children with an HDV superinfection. There is evidence that the risk of fulminant hepatitis is higher in individuals with combined infection with HBV, HDV, HCV, or HIV than in those with HBV infection alone. There also is a higher risk of hepatocellular carcinoma and increased mortality in this group. Aggressive HBV vaccination programs have reduced the incidence of HBV; HDV reduction has mirrored this response. To prevent perinatal transmission of HBV, immunoprophylaxis and HBV vaccination within the first 12 hours of birth are recommended, with close follow-up visits. Treatment is conservative, and antivirals are used for chronic disease. Children ages 2 to 17 years who are HBsAg seropositive for more than 6 months with elevated serum alanine transaminase (ALT) and HBV deoxyribonucleic acid (DNA) levels for more than 3 months respond to treatment with antivirals. Maternal antiviral therapy during pregnancy and lactation reduces the HBV mother-to-child transmission rate.[45,46]

Hepatitis C virus. Hepatitis C virus (HCV) in children is most commonly transmitted vertically and is enhanced by maternal coinfection with HIV. Risk factors for vertical transmission include internal fetal monitoring, prolonged rupture of membranes, and fetal anoxia. HCV transmission also can occur through exposure to infected blood or contaminated materials (as in injection drug use or tattooing and body piercing) and, less commonly, after sexual encounters with partners infected with HCV. Transmission from blood transfusions has become a negligible risk with universal HCV screening of blood. With vertical transmission, spontaneous resolution of HCV is high; otherwise, the disease is usually mild in children and cirrhosis is rare. Because of adverse drug events, only children with persistently elevated serum aminotransferases or those with progressive liver disease are treated with antiviral drugs.[47]

Chronic hepatitis. HBV and HCV are the main causes of chronic hepatitis in children. Manifestations of chronic hepatitis include malaise, anorexia, fever, GI bleeding, hepatomegaly, edema, and transient joint pain. Often there are no symptoms. Serum alanine aminotransferase and bilirubin levels are elevated. There may be evidence of impairment of synthetic functions of the liver: prolonged prothrombin time, thrombocytopenia, and hypoalbuminemia. The diagnosis is based on the clinical manifestations and liver biopsy results. There is no curative therapy for chronic HBV or chronic HCV. Children are treated with antiviral drugs and should continue to be monitored. Liver transplant may ultimately be required for chronic hepatitis.

There is an autoimmune form of chronic hepatitis, known as *autoimmune hepatitis* (AIH) or *autoimmune primary sclerosing cholangitis* (PSC), which has an unknown etiology. The pathogenic mechanism is thought to be immunologic with loss of tolerance to hepatocyte-specific autoantigens, environmental, or genetic in nature. These diseases present with elevations in the levels of aminotransferases, autoantibodies, and immunoglobulin G (IgG). AIH is more common in female children. Both females and males are treated with immunosuppressive therapy; about 50% to 80% will achieve remission and long-term survival.[48]

Cirrhosis

Cirrhosis is fibrotic scarring of the liver, in response to inflammation and tissue damage, that results in obstruction to the flow of blood and bile. Most forms of chronic liver diseases in children can progress to cirrhosis, but they seldom do so. The complications of cirrhosis in children are the same as those in adults: portal hypertension, the opening of collateral vessels between the portal and systemic veins, and varices. In addition, children with cirrhosis experience growth failure caused by nutritional deficits, as well as developmental delay, particularly in gross motor function because of ascites and weakness. The cause of cirrhosis may influence its severity and course (i.e., biliary atresia and hepatitis). Some types of cirrhosis can be stabilized if the cause is identified and treated early.[49] The risk of cirrhosis is increasing in obese children with nonalcoholic fatty liver disease (see

Did You Know? Childhood Obesity and Nonalcoholic Fatty Liver Disease).

DID YOU KNOW?

Childhood Obesity and Nonalcoholic Fatty Liver Disease

Nonalcoholic fatty liver disease (NAFLD) is the most common cause of chronic liver disease in children. It is associated with obesity, insulin resistance, genetic predisposition, ethnicity, the gut microbiome, and environmental factors (diet and lack of exercise). NAFLD is associated with dyslipidemia, hypertension, and early cardiac dysfunction in children and can progress to cirrhosis and cardiometabolic syndrome within a few years if not treated. The rise in childhood obesity worldwide is contributing to the increasing prevalence of NAFLD. The disease usually presents in prepubertal children and is predominant in males and in children of Hispanic origin. The diagnosis is made by exclusion of other causes of the disease, usually by 12 to 13 years of age. Liver biopsy is required for definitive diagnosis of nonalcoholic steatohepatitis (NASH). Compared to adults, there are differences in the extent of fat, inflammation, and fibrosis in children, and there is no standard scoring system. There also is no consensus regarding treatment. Exercise and slow, consistent weight loss with a low glycemic index diet have been shown to be more effective than a low-fat diet in lowering body weight. Pharmacologic agents are being evaluated to control insulin resistance and prevent the progression of liver disease and cirrhosis. Omega-3 fatty acids, probiotics, and vitamin E may delay disease progression. Research is in progress to define the pathophysiology, noninvasive diagnostic procedures, and prevention measures.

Data from Fang YL et al: World J Gastroenterol 24(27):2974-2983, 2018; Goyal NP, Schwimmer JB: Clin Liver Dis 22(1):59-71, 2018; Selvakumar PKC et al: Pediatr Clin North Am 64(3):659-675, 2017.

Metabolic Disorders

More than 5000 genetically determined metabolic pathways have been identified in liver tissue. The earliest possible identification of metabolic disorders is essential because (1) early treatment may prevent permanent damage to vital organs, such as the liver or brain; (2) precise genetic counseling may be possible with prenatal diagnosis; and (3) complications can be minimized, even if cure is not possible. More common inborn errors of metabolism include galactosemia, fructosemia, and Wilson disease, which have treatable hepatic clinical manifestations. The mechanisms of disease, clinical manifestations, and evaluation and treatment of these disorders are reviewed in Table 39.2.

✓ QUICK CHECK 39.4

1. Why is diarrhea such a serious disorder in infants and children?
2. What is biliary atresia?
3. What are the three most common metabolic disorders that cause liver damage in children?

TABLE 39.2 Galactosemia, Fructosemia, and Wilson Disease

	Galactosemia	Fructosemia	Wilson Disease
Mechanism of disease	Deficiency of galactose-1-phosphate uridylyltransferase Autosomal recessive trait Cannot convert galactose to glucose Toxic accumulation of galactose in body tissues, liver, and brain	Deficiency of fructose-1-phosphate aldolase Autosomal recessive trait Cannot metabolize fructose, sucrose, or honey; occurs when breast milk is replaced with cow's milk Toxic accumulation of fructose in body tissues	Defect in copper excretion by liver Autosomal recessive: defect on chromosome 13 (ATP 7B) Impaired transport of copper into bile/blood caused by diminished transport protein (ceruloplasmin) Toxic accumulations of copper in liver, brain, kidney, corneas

Continued

TABLE 39.2   Galactosemia, Fructosemia, and Wilson Disease—cont'd

	Galactosemia	Fructosemia	Wilson Disease
Clinical manifestation	High levels of blood galactose Vomiting Hypoglycemia May have failure to thrive Symptoms of cirrhosis at 2-6 months—jaundice Intellectual disabilities if not treated Cataracts if not treated	High levels of blood fructose Vomiting Hypoglycemia May have failure to thrive Hepatomegaly Jaundice Seizures	Intention tremors Indistinct speech Dystonia Greenish yellow rings in cornea Hepatomegaly Jaundice Anorexia Renal tubular defects
Evaluation	Newborn screening Presence of reducing substances in urine when infant is receiving lactose	Detailed dietary history Liver or intestinal mucosa biopsy	Low plasma ceruloplasmin level
Treatment	Galactose-free diet	Fructose-, sucrose-, honey-free diet Vitamin C supplementation	Chelation therapy to remove copper from body Decreased dietary intake of copper Liver transplantation

SUMMARY REVIEW

Congenital Impairment of Motility in the Gastrointestinal Tract

1. Alterations of digestive function in children include congenital or acquired disorders of the intestinal tract; disorders of digestion, absorption, or nutrition; or liver disease.
2. CL and CP (failure of the bony palate to fuse in the midline) may occur separately or together. The fissure may affect the uvula, soft palate, hard palate, nostril, and maxillary alveolar ridge, with difficulty sucking and swallowing.
3. EA, a condition in which the esophagus ends in a blind pouch, may occur with or without a TEF. As the infant swallows oral secretions or ingests milk, the pouch fills, causing either drooling, regurgitation, or aspiration into the lungs.
4. IHPS is an obstruction of the pyloric outlet caused by hypertrophy of circular muscles in the pyloric sphincter.
5. In intestinal malrotation, the small intestine lacks a normal posterior attachment during fetal development, causing volvulus (twisting of the bowel on itself) that may partly or completely occlude the GI tract and its blood vessels.
6. Meckel diverticulum is a congenital malformation of the GI tract involving all layers of the small intestinal wall; it usually occurs in the ileum.
7. Meconium ileus is a newborn condition in which intestinal secretions and amniotic waste products produce a thick, sticky plug that obstructs the intestine; it occurs in up to 20% of newborns with cystic fibrosis.
8. Hirschsprung disease (congenital aganglionic megacolon) is caused by a malformation of the parasympathetic nervous system in a segment of the colon needed for peristalsis, resulting in colon obstruction.
9. Malformations of the anus and rectum range from mild congenital stenosis of the anus to complex deformities.

Acquired Impairment of Motility in the Gastrointestinal Tract

1. GERD is the presence of symptoms related to the return of stomach contents into the esophagus. This is caused by relaxation or incompetence of the lower esophageal sphincter that results from immaturity of the gastroesophageal sphincter.
2. Intussusception is the telescoping of a proximal segment of intestine into a distal segment, causing an obstruction.

3. Appendicitis is common in children 10 to 11 years of age, and the mechanisms of disease, symptoms, and treatment are similar to those for adults.

Impairment of Digestion, Absorption, and Nutrition

1. CF is an inherited fibrocystic disease that involves mucosal chloride and sodium ion channels in many organs, including the GI tract and pancreas; CF causes pancreatic enzyme deficiency with maldigestion.
2. CD is caused by hypersensitivity to gluten protein, with autoimmune injury and loss of the villous epithelium. It results in malabsorption and growth failure.
3. Pediatric malnutrition is an imbalance between nutrient requirements and intake that results in energy, protein, and micronutrient deficits, which impair growth and development.
4. Kwashiorkor is a severe protein deficiency. Marasmus is a deficiency of all dietary nutrients, including carbohydrates.
5. Faltering growth, or FTT, is a multifactorial condition that includes biologic, psychosocial, and environmental contributions. It may or may not be related to illness, and it results in inadequate physical growth and development of a child.
6. NEC is an ischemic, inflammatory disorder in neonates, particularly premature infants, thought to result from immaturity, infection, stress, and anoxia of the bowel wall.

Diarrhea

1. Diarrhea in infants and children is three or more watery or loose stools in 24 hours. It may last up to 4 weeks in acute cases, or longer in chronic cases. It is commonly caused by viral or bacterial enterocolitis.
2. Primary lactose intolerance is the inability to digest milk sugar because of a lack of the enzyme lactase, resulting in osmotic diarrhea.

Disorders of the Liver

1. Physiologic jaundice of the newborn is caused by mild hyperbilirubinemia that subsides in 1 or 2 weeks. Pathologic jaundice is caused by severe hyperbilirubinemia and can cause brain damage (kernicterus).
2. Biliary atresia is a congenital malformation of the bile ducts that obstructs bile flow and causes jaundice, cirrhosis, and liver failure.

3. Acute hepatitis is usually caused by a virus, and hepatitis A is the most common form of childhood hepatitis. Chronic hepatitis B or C usually occurs by maternal transmission.

4. Cirrhosis is fibrotic scarring of the liver and is rare in children, but it can develop from most forms of chronic liver disease.

5. The most common metabolic disorders or inborn errors of metabolism that cause liver damage in children are galactosemia, fructosemia, and Wilson disease. All three are inherited as genetic traits and allow toxins to accumulate in the liver and other body tissues.

KEY TERMS

Anorectal malformation (ARM), 920
Atresia, 917
Biliary atresia (BA), 928
Celiac crisis, 924
Celiac disease (CD), 923
Cirrhosis, 929
Cleft lip (CL), 916
Cleft palate (CP), 916
Cystic fibrosis (CF), 922
Diarrhea, 927
Distal intestinal obstruction syndrome (DIOS), 919
Eosinophilic esophagitis (EoE), 921

Esophageal atresia (EA), 917
Faltering growth, 926
Fructosemia, 929
Galactosemia, 929
Gastroesophageal reflux (GER), 920
Gastroesophageal reflux disease (GERD), 920
Hepatitis A virus (HAV), 928
Hepatitis B virus (HBV), 928
Hepatitis C virus (HCV), 929
Hepatitis D virus (HDV), 928
Hirschsprung disease, 920
Infantile hypertrophic pyloric stenosis (IHPS), 918

Intestinal malrotation, 919
Intussusception, 921
Jaundice (icterus), 927
Kernicterus, 928
Kwashiorkor, 925
Lactose intolerance, 927
Lactose malabsorption, 927
Marasmus, 925
Meckel diverticulum, 919
Meconium, 919
Meconium ileus (MI), 919
Meconium plug syndrome (MPS), 919
Necrotizing enterocolitis (NEC), 926

Nonceliac gluten sensitivity (GS), 924
Nonsyndromic (isolated) CP, 916
Pathologic jaundice, 928
Physiologic jaundice (hyperbilirubinemia) of the newborn, 927
Protein-energy malnutrition (PEM), 925
Rotavirus, 927
Syndromic CLP, 916
Tracheoesophageal fistula (TEF), 917
Wilson disease, 929

REFERENCES

1. Arosarena OA: Cleft lip and palate, *Otolaryngol Clin North Am* 40(1):27-60, 2007.
2. National Institute of Dental and Craniofacial Research (NIDCR): Prevalence (number of cases) of cleft lip and palate, updated October 13, 2011. Available at www.nidcr.nih.gov/DataStatistics/FindDataByTopic/CraniofacialBirthDefects/PrevalenceCleft+LipCleftPalate.htm. Last reviewed July 2018.
3. Dixon MJ, et al: Cleft lip and palate: understanding genetic and environmental influences, *Nat Rev Genet* 12(3):167-178, 2011.
4. Leslie EJ, Marazita ML: Genetics of cleft lip and cleft palate, *Am J Med Genet C Semin Med Genet* 163C(4):246-258, 2013.
5. Molina-Solana R, et al: Current concepts on the effect of environmental factors on cleft lip and palate, *Int J Oral Maxillofac Surg* 42(2):177-184, 2013.
6. Mossey PA, et al: Cleft lip and palate, *Lancet* 374(9703):1773-1785, 2009.
7. Farronato G, et al: How various surgical protocols of the unilateral cleft lip and palate influence the facial growth and possible orthodontic problems? Which is the best timing of lip, palate and alveolus repair? Literature review, *Stomatologija* 16(2):53-60, 2014.
8. Jayaram R, Huppa C: Surgical correction of cleft lip and palate, *Front Oral Biol* 16:101-110, 2012.
9. Shaye D: Update on outcomes research for cleft lip and palate, *Curr Opin Otolaryngol Head Neck Surg* 22(4):255-259, 2014.
10. Lee S: Basic knowledge of tracheoesophageal fistula and esophageal atresia, *Adv Neonatal Care* 18(1):14-21, 2018.
11. van der Zee DC, Tytgat SHA, van Herwaarden MYA: Esophageal atresia and tracheo-esophageal fistula, *Semin Pediatr Surg* 26(2):67-71, 2017.
12. El-Gohary Y, et al: Pyloric stenosis: an enigma more than a century after the first successful treatment, *Pediatr Surg Int* 34(1):21-27, 2018.
13. Langer JC: Intestinal rotation abnormalities and midgut volvulus, *Surg Clin North Am* 97(1):147-159, 2017.
14. Lin XK, et al: Clinical characteristics of Meckel diverticulum in children: a retrospective review of a 15-year single-center experience, *Medicine (Baltimore)* 96(32):e7760, 2017.

15. Sathe M, Houwen R: Meconium ileus in Cystic Fibrosis, *J Cyst Fibros* 16(Suppl 2):S32-S39, 2017.
16. Butler Tjaden NE, Trainor PA: The developmental etiology and pathogenesis of Hirschsprung disease, *Transl Res* 162(1):1-15, 2013.
17. Wester T, Granström AL: Hirschsprung disease—bowel function beyond childhood, *Semin Pediatr Surg* 26(5):322-327, 2017.
18. Cairo SB, et al: Challenges in transition of care for patients with anorectal malformations: a systematic review and recommendations for comprehensive care, *Dis Colon Rectum* 61(3):390-399, 2018.
19. Mousa H, Hassan M: Gastroesophageal reflux disease, *Pediatr Clin North Am* 64(3):487-505, 2017.
20. Adamiak T, Plati KF: Pediatric esophageal disorders: diagnosis and treatment of reflux and eosinophilic esophagitis, *Pediatr Rev* 39(8):392-402, 2018.
21. Applegate KE: Intussusception in children: evidence-based diagnosis and treatment, *Pediatr Radiol* 39(Suppl 2):S140-S143, 2009.
22. Tate JE, et al: Intussusception rates before and after the introduction of rotavirus vaccine, *Pediatrics* 138(3):2016.
23. Gray MP, et al: Recurrence rates after intussusception enema reduction: a meta-analysis, *Pediatrics* 134(1):110-119, 2014.
24. Sathe MN, Freeman AJ: Gastrointestinal, pancreatic, and hepatobiliary manifestations of cystic fibrosis, *Pediatr Clin North Am* 63(4):679-698, 2016.
25. Leonard MM, et al: Celiac disease and nonceliac gluten sensitivity: a review, *JAMA* 318(7):647-656, 2017.
26. Barbaro MR, et al: Recent advances in understanding non-celiac gluten sensitivity, *F1000Res* 7:Faculty Rev-1631, 2018.
27. Beer SS, et al: Pediatric malnutrition: putting the new definition and standards into practice, *Nutr Clin Pract* 30(5):609-624, 2015.
28. Fergusson P, Tomkins A: HIV prevalence and mortality among children undergoing treatment for severe acute malnutrition in sub-Saharan Africa: a systematic review and meta-analysis, *Trans R Soc Trop Med Hyg* 103(6):541-548, 2009.
29. Prieto MB, Cid JL: Malnutrition in the critically ill child: the importance of enteral nutrition, *Int J Environ Res Public Health* 8(11):4353-4366, 2011.

30. Million M, Diallo A, Raoult D: Gut microbiota and malnutrition, *Microb Pathog* 106:127-138, 2017.
31. Kane AV, Dinh DM, Ward HD: Childhood malnutrition and the intestinal microbiome malnutrition and the microbiome, *Pediatr Res* 77(0):256-262, 2015.
32. Maida JM, et al: Pediatric ophthalmology in the developing world, *Curr Opin Ophthalmol* 19(5):403-408, 2008.
33. Kismul H, et al: Diet and kwashiorkor: a prospective study from rural DR Congo, *PeerJ* 2:e350, 2014.
34. Homan GJ: Failure to thrive: a practical guide, *Am Fam Physician* 94(4):295-299, 2016.
35. Müller MJ, Paul T, Seeliger S: Necrotizing enterocolitis in premature infants and newborns, *J Neonatal Perinatal Med* 9(3):233-242, 2016.
36. Hackam D, Caplan M: Necrotizing enterocolitis: pathophysiology from a historical context, *Semin Pediatr Surg* 27(1):11-18, 2018.
37. Scharf RJ, Deboer MD, Guerrant RL: Recent advances in understanding the long-term sequelae of childhood infectious diarrhea, *Curr Infect Dis Rep* 16(6):408, 2014.
38. Hojsak I: Probiotics in Children: what is the evidence?, *Pediatr Gastroenterol Hepatol Nutr* 20(3):139-146, 2017.
39. Berni Canani R, et al: Diagnosing and treating intolerance to carbohydrates in children, *Nutrients* 8(3):157, 2016.
40. Muchowski KE: Evaluation and treatment of neonatal hyperbilirubinemia, *Am Fam Physician* 89(11):873-878, 2014.
41. Bhutani VK, Wong RJ, Stevenson DK: Hyperbilirubinemia in preterm neonates, *Clin Perinatol* 43(2):215-232, 2016.
42. Zagory JA, Nguyen MV, Wang KS: Recent advances in the pathogenesis and management of biliary atresia, *Curr Opin Pediatr* 27(3):389-394, 2015.
43. Klevens RM, et al: The evolving epidemiology of hepatitis A in the United States: incidence and molecular epidemiology from population-based surveillance, 2005-2007, *Arch Intern Med* 170(20):1811-1818, 2010.
44. Centers for Disease Control and Prevention (CDC): Viral hepatitis–hepatitis A information, overview and statistics. Available at https://www.cdc.gov/hepatitis/

hav/havfaq.htm#vaccine. Page last reviewed May 8, 2019.

45. Karnsakul W, Schwarz KB: Hepatitis B and C, *Pediatr Clin North Am* 64(3):641-658, 2017.

46. Komatsu H, Inui A: Hepatitis B virus infection in children, *Expert Rev Anti Infect Ther* 13(4):427-450, 2015.

47. El-Guindi MA: Hepatitis C viral infection in children: updated review, *Pediatr Gastroenterol Hepatol Nutr* 19(2):83-95, 2016.

48. Moy L, Levine J: Autoimmune hepatitis: a classic autoimmune liver disease, *Curr Probl Pediatr Adolesc Health Care* 44(11):341-346, 2014.

49. Cordova J, Jericho H, Azzam RK: An overview of cirrhosis in children, *Pediatr Ann* 45(12):e427-e432, 2016.

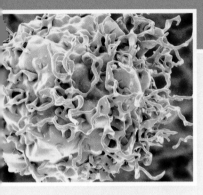

40

Structure and Function of the Musculoskeletal System

Geri C. Reeves

EVOLVE WEBSITE

CHAPTER OUTLINE

The way an individual functions in daily life, moves about, or manipulates objects physically depends on the integrity of the musculoskeletal system. The musculoskeletal system is actually two systems: (1) the skeleton composed of bones and joints and (2) soft tissues (skeletal muscles, tendons, and ligaments). Each system contributes to mobility. The skeleton supports the body and provides leverage to the skeletal muscles so that movement of various parts of the body is possible. Contraction of the skeletal muscles and bending or rotation at the joints facilitate movements of the various body parts.

STRUCTURE AND FUNCTION OF BONES

Bones give form to the body, support tissues, and permit movement by providing points of attachment for muscles. Many bones meet in movable joints that determine the type and extent of movement possible. Bones also protect many of the body's vital organs. For example, the bones of the skull, thorax, and pelvis are hard exterior shields that protect the brain, heart and lungs, and reproductive and urinary organs, respectively.

Within certain bones, the marrow cavities serve as storage sites for the hematopoietic stem cells that form both blood and immune cells. In adults, blood cells originate exclusively in the marrow cavities of the skull, vertebrae, ribs, sternum, shoulders, and pelvis. The development of blood cells is discussed in Chapter 22. Bones also have a crucial role in mineral homeostasis (storing minerals [i.e., calcium, phosphate, carbonate, magnesium] that are essential for the proper performance of many delicate cellular mechanisms), have a role in hormone homeostasis, and assist in maintaining normal immunologic function.

Elements of Bone Tissue

Mature bone is a rigid connective tissue consisting of cells; fibers; a homogenous, gelatinous medium termed **ground substance**; and large amounts of crystallized minerals, mainly calcium, that give bone its rigidity. Ground substance consists of proteoglycans and hyaluronic acid secreted by chondroblasts. The structural elements of bone are summarized in Table 40.1.

Bone cells enable bone to grow, repair itself, change shape, and continuously synthesize new bone tissue and **resorb** (dissolve or digest) old tissue. The fibers in bone are made of collagen, which gives bone its tensile strength (the ability to hold itself together). Ground substance acts as a medium for the diffusion of nutrients, oxygen, metabolic wastes, biochemicals, and minerals between bone tissue and blood vessels.

Bone formation begins during embryonic development when mesenchymal stem cells begin differentiating into either chondrocytes or preosteoblasts. In mature bone, the formation of new tissue begins with the production of an organic matrix by the bone cells. This **bone matrix** consists of ground substance, collagen, and other proteins (see Table 40.1) that take part in bone formation and maintenance.

The next step in bone formation is **calcification**, in which minerals are deposited and then crystallize. Minerals bind tightly to collagen fibers, producing tensile and compressional strength in bone and allowing it to withstand pressure and weightbearing.

Bone Cells

Bone contains three types of cells: osteoblasts, osteocytes, and osteoclasts (Fig. 40.1). Both osteoblasts and osteocytes originate from osteoprogenitor

TABLE 40.1   Structural Elements of Bone

Structural Elements	Function
Bone Cells	
Osteoblasts	Synthesize collagen and proteoglycans, mineralize osteoid matrix; produce receptor activator of nuclear factor-κB ligand (RANKL), which in turn stimulates osteoclast resorption of bone; also produce osteoprotegerin (OPG), which inhibits osteoclast formation by binding to RANKL
Osteoclasts	Resorb bone; major role in bone homeostasis
Osteocytes	Transform osteoblasts trapped in osteoid; signal both osteoblasts and osteoclasts; maintain bone matrix; mechanosensory receptors to reduce or augment bone mass; produce sclerostin (SOST), which inhibits bone growth
Bone Matrix	
Bone morphogenic proteins (BMPs)	Subfamily of transforming growth factor-β (TGF-β) cytokine growth factors; induce and regulate bone and cartilage formation; affect all other organ systems
BMP-1	Unrelated to other BMPs (is a metalloprotease); key role in extracellular matrix (ECM) formation
BMP-2	Promotes chondrogenesis, bone formation; clinically used to enhance bone formation in spine surgery
BMP-3 (osteogenin)	Inhibits bone formation
BMP-4	Osteoblast differentiation; involved in cartilage repair, endochondral bone formation; enhances chondrogenesis
BMP-6	Found in human plasma; promotes osteoblast differentiation from mesenchymal stem cells (MSCs)
BMP-7	Osteogenic cell formation from MSCs; enhances bone formation in spine surgery; induces formation of brown fat
BMP-9	Promotes osteoblast formation from MSCs
BMP-13	Inhibits bone formation by reducing calcium mineralization
Collagen fibers	Lend support and tensile strength
Proteoglycans	Control transport of ionized materials through matrix
Glycoproteins	
Albumin	Transports essential elements to matrix; maintains osmotic pressure of bone fluid
α-Glycoproteins	Promote calcification
Laminin	Stabilizes basement membranes in bones
Osteocalcin	Vitamin K–dependent protein present in bone; inhibits calcium phosphate precipitation (attracts calcium ions to incorporate into hydroxyapatite crystals); serum osteocalcin is a sensitive marker of bone formation
Osteonectin	Binds calcium in bone; necessary for normal bone formation
Sialoprotein	Promotes calcification, osteoblast formation
Minerals	
Calcium	Crystallizes, providing bone rigidity and compressive strength
Phosphate	Balance of organic and inorganic phosphate required for proper bone mineralization; regulates vitamin D, promoting mineralization
Alkaline phosphatase	Promotes mineralization
Vitamins	
Vitamin D	Assists with differentiation, mineralization of osteoblasts
Vitamin K	Increases bone calcification; reduces serum osteocalcin

cells found in the mesenchymal stem cell lineage. Osteoclasts originate from hematopoietic stem cells. Osteoblasts are the bone-forming cells. Osteocytes, the most numerous cells within bone, are osteoblasts that have become imprisoned within the mineralized bone matrix. They have multiple important duties in maintaining bone homeostasis, including synthesizing new bone matrix molecules and initiating osteoclast function. Osteoclasts primarily resorb (remove) bone during processes of growth and repair.

Osteoblasts. Originating from mesenchymal stem cells (MSCs), osteoblasts are the primary bone-producing cells, and are involved in many functions related to the skeletal system (see Table 40.1). Osteoblasts are responsive to parathyroid hormone (PTH) and produce osteocalcin when stimulated by 1,25-dihydroxy-vitamin D_3. Osteoblasts are active on the outer surfaces of bones, where they form a single layer of cells. Osteoblasts initiate new bone formation by their synthesis of osteoid (nonmineralized bone matrix). Osteoblasts also mineralize newly formed bone matrix. Stimulation of new bone formation and orderly mineralization of bone matrix occur by concentrating some of the plasma proteins (growth factors) found in the bone matrix and by facilitating the deposit and exchange of calcium and other ions at the site. Enzymes, signaling proteins, and growth factors, including bone morphogenic proteins (BMPs) and other members of the transforming growth factor-beta (TGF-β) superfamily, are critical components of bone formation, maintenance, and remodeling (Table 40.2).

Osteoblasts use intercellular calcium signaling to include osteoclastic activity. One of the most important discoveries linking osteoblast and

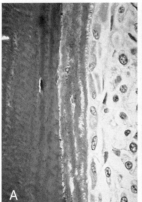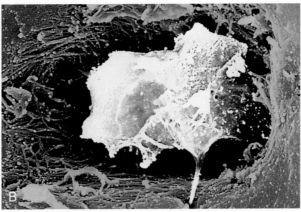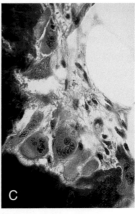

FIGURE 40.1 Bone Cells. A, Osteoblasts are responsible for the production of collagenous and noncollagenous proteins that compose osteoid. Active osteoblasts are aligned on the osteoid. Note the eccentrically located nuclei. **B,** Electron photomicrograph of an osteocyte. Osteocytes reside within the lacunae of compact bone. **C,** Osteoclasts actively resorb mineralized tissue. The scalloped surface in which the multinucleated osteoclasts rest is termed *Howship lacuna.* (**A** and **C** from Damjanov I, Linder J, editors: *Anderson's pathology,* ed 10, St Louis, 1996, Mosby; **B** from Wikimedia Commons, courtesy Robert M. Hunt.)

osteoclast function is the cytokine **receptor activator nuclear factor κ-B ligand,** or RANKL (discussed later). RANKL is expressed by osteoblasts and osteocytes and is necessary for forming osteoclasts[1-3] (see the Osteoclasts section). Thus, the cells of the osteoblastic lineage (osteoblasts, osteocytes) form a network of cells in bone that sense the shape and structure of bone and determine where it is appropriate that bone be formed or resorbed, according to the Wolff law (bone is shaped according to its function).

Osteoblasts synthesize and secrete osteoid when active, and in the resting state they are termed *satellite cells.* If appropriately stimulated, however, the resting osteoblasts are capable of resuming activity.

Osteocytes. Osteocytes, the most abundant cells in bone, are transformed osteoblasts trapped or surrounded in osteoid as it hardens because of minerals that enter during calcification (see Fig. 40.1, *B*). The osteocyte is within a space in the hardened bone matrix called a lacuna. Osteocytes are the most abundant cells found in bone and have numerous functions, including acting as mechanoreceptors and synthesizing certain matrix molecules, playing a major role in controlling osteoblast differentiation and production of growth factors, and maintaining bone homeostasis.

As the major source of sclerostin, RANKL, and osteoprotegerin, osteocytes are thought to be key regulators of both bone formation and bone resorption.[4-6] They also help concentrate nutrients in the matrix. Osteocytes obtain nutrients from capillaries in the canaliculi, which contain nutrient-rich fluids. Through exchanges among these cells, hormone catalysts, and minerals, optimal levels of calcium, phosphorus, and other minerals are maintained in blood plasma.

One of the osteocyte's primary functions is to act as a mechanoreceptor, responding to changes in weight bearing or other stressors ("loading") on bone. Lying within the lacunae are the osteocyte's primary cilia, which are likely the primary mechanoreceptors in bone. Once changes in bone, such as mechanical stress, hormonal imbalance, loading, or unloading, are detected by the osteocyte's mechanoreceptors, multiple molecular signals are produced and the process of bone remodeling begins. Remodeling is described in the Maintenance of Bone Integrity section.

Osteoclasts. Osteoclasts are large (typically 20 to 100 μm in diameter), multinucleated cells that develop from the hematopoietic monocyte-macrophage lineage. Osteoclasts are the major resorptive cells of bone. They migrate over bone surfaces to resorption areas that

have been prepared and stripped of osteoid by enzymes, such as collagenases produced by osteoblasts in the presence of PTH, which is necessary for the resorptive process. Osteoclasts travel over the prepared bone surfaces, creating irregular, scalloped cavities known as *Howship lacunae* or *resorption bays,* as they resorb bone areas and then acidify hydroxyapatite to dissolve it.

A specific area of the cell membrane forms adjacent to the bone surface and develops multiple infoldings to permit intimate contact with the resorption bay. These infoldings, known as the **ruffled border,** greatly increase the surface areas of cells under their scalloped or ruffled borders. Osteoclasts resorb bone by secretion of hydrochloric acid, acid proteases (such as cathepsin K), and matrix metalloproteinases (MMPs) that help digest collagen, along with the action of cytokines (see Table 40.2). Osteoclasts also resorb bone through the action of lysosomes (digestive vacuoles) filled with hydrolytic enzymes in their mitochondria.

Osteoclasts bind to the bone surfaces through attachments called **podosomes,** which are footlike structures that cluster together along a sealing membrane that forms a "belt" containing multiple proteins, enzymes, and **integrin** receptors. Once resorption is complete, the osteoclasts retract and loosen from the bone surface under the ruffled border through the action of calcitonin. Calcitonin binds to receptor areas of the osteoclasts' cell membranes to effectively loosen the osteoclasts from the bone surfaces. Once resorption is completed, osteoclasts disappear by the process of degeneration, either by reverting to the form of their parent cells or by undergoing cell movements away from the site, in which the osteoclast becomes an inactive or a resting osteoclast.

In addition to resorption of bone, osteoclasts assist the endocrine and renal systems in maintaining appropriate serum calcium and phosphorus levels. Osteoclasts also appear to have a role in the body's immune response.

OPG/RANKL/RANK System

Osteoprotegerin (OPG), a glycoprotein belonging to the tumor necrosis factor superfamily, inhibits bone remodeling and resorption, inhibiting osteoclast formation. Numerous cells, including osteoblasts and osteocytes, produce it. OPG is the key to the interaction between osteoblasts and osteoclasts. Osteoblasts and osteoclasts cooperate (a process called *coupling*) to maintain normal bone homeostasis. RANKL is an essential cytokine needed for the formation and activation of osteoclasts. Like an automobile's accelerator, RANKL increases bone loss. OPG, similar

TABLE 40.2 Selected Factors Affecting Bone Formation, Maintenance, and Remodeling

Factor	Function
Transforming growth factor-beta (TGF-β)	Superfamily of polypeptides; regulates bone formation, many other cellular processes through signaling
Platelet-derived growth factor (PDGF)	Increases number of osteoblasts
Fibroblast growth factor (FGF)	FGF-2 increases osteoblast population, but not function; inhibits alkaline phosphatase activity, osteocalcin, type I collagen, and osteopontin
Insulin-Like Growth Factor (IGF)	
IGF-1	Increases peak bone mass during adolescence; decreases osteoblast apoptosis; maintains bone matrix
IGF-2	Increases BMP-9–induced endochondral ossification
Smad proteins	Mediate signaling cascade of TGF-β, especially in embryonic bone development; play role in crosstalk between BMP/TGF-β and Wnt signaling pathways
Bone morphogenic proteins (BMPs)	Members of TGF-β superfamily of polypeptides; have many functions outside skeletal system; stimulate endochondral bone and cartilage formation and function, promote osteoblast maturation; augment bone remodeling by affecting both osteoblasts and osteoclasts
Tumor necrosis factors (TNFs)	Superfamily of cytokines; play major role in regulating bone metabolism, especially osteoclast function
Osteoprotegerin (OPG)	Inhibits bone remodeling/resorption; produced by several cells, including osteoblasts; is a decoy receptor for RANKL (binds to RANKL, inhibiting RANK/RANKL interactions, suppressing osteoclast formation and bone resorption); also may directly interfere with ability of osteoclasts' podosomes to attach to bone matrix
Receptor activator of nuclear factor-κB (RANK)	Stimulates differentiation of osteoclast precursors; activates mature osteoclasts
Receptor activator of nuclear factor-κB ligand (RANKL)	Promotes osteoclast differentiation/activation; inhibits osteoclast apoptosis
BMP antagonists	Prevent BMP signaling
Noggin	Binds BMP-2 and -4, reducing osteoblast function
Gremlin	Multiple effects in and out of skeletal system, but also binds BMP-2, -4, and -7, thus reducing BMP signaling; may play role in development of osteoporosis
Twisted gastrulation	Acts as either a BMP agonist or a BMP antagonist
Activin (a BMP-related protein)	Affects both osteoblasts and osteoclasts; may promote bone formation and fracture healing; expressed by both osteoblasts and chondrocytes; helps regulate bone mass
Annexins	Class of calcium-binding proteins; help mineralize matrix vesicles; may influence bone formation
Inhibin	Dominant over activin and BMPs; helps regulate bone mass and strength by affecting formation of osteoblasts and osteoclasts
Leptin	Plays role in bone formation and resorption
Wnt Antagonists	
Dickkopf family (Dkk)	Disrupt Wnt signaling, leading to reduced bone mass
Sclerostin	A protein secreted by osteocytes, osteoblasts, and osteoclasts; binds to BMP-6 and BMP-7; interferes with Wnt signaling pathway, inhibiting bone formation by osteoblasts
Transcription Factors	
β-Catenin pathway	Protein with multiple functions; one of most important is activation of genetic transcription factors; balance between Wnt/β-catenin signaling promotes normal bone formation/resorption
Wnts (complex signaling pathway)	Important in differentiating osteoblasts, bone formation; has overlapping effects with BMPs, helps regulate bone formation and remodeling; crosstalks with other signaling pathways
Nuclear factor of activated B cells (NF-κB)	Affects embryonic osteoclastogenesis; plays role in certain osteoclast, osteoblast, and chondroblast functions
Matrix Metalloproteinases (MMPs)	
Family of endopeptidases (enzymes) that includes collagenases, gelatinases, stromelysins, matrilysins	Help maintain equilibrium of extracellular matrix (ECM); breakdown almost all components of ECM
A disintegrin and metalloproteinase (ADAM)	Proteolytic enzymes; also have cell-signaling functions, usually linked to cell membrane
A disintegrin and metalloproteinase with thrombospondin motifs (ADAMTs)	Similar to ADAMs but are secreted into circulation, are found around cells; various subgroups affect multiple tissues
Cysteine protease	Cathepsin K expressed by osteoclasts; assists in bone remodeling by cleaving proteins, such as collagen type I, collagen type II, and osteonectin
Mmp Inhibitors	
Tetracyclines (especially doxycycline), bisphosphonates	Block enzymatic function of MMPs
Tissue inhibitors of metalloproteinases (TIMPs)	Balance effect of MMPs in maintaining ECM equilibrium

From Boyce BF et al: *Ann N Y Acad Sci* 1192:367-375, 2010; Genetos DC et al: *PLoS One* 9(9):e107482, 2015; Kim Y-S et al: *J Korean Med Sci* 25:985-991, 2010; Norrie JL et al: *Dev Biol* 393 (2):270-281, 2014; Stewart A et al: *J Cell Physiol* 223(3):658-666, 2010; Wang RN et al: *Genes Dis* 1(1):87-105, 2014; Zhao H et al: *Cytokine* 71(2):199-206, 2014.

to an automobile's brakes, reduces bone loss because when it is activated, it promotes bone formation. When RANKL binds to its receptor (i.e., receptor activator nuclear factor κ-B [RANK]) on osteoclast precursor cells, it triggers their proliferation and increases bone resorption. OPG is secreted by osteoblasts and B lymphocytes and serves as a decoy by binding to RANK, preventing RANKL from binding to RANK and thus preventing bone resorption. Therefore, the overall balance between RANKL and OPG determines the amount of bone loss. The balance between RANKL and OPG is regulated by cytokines and hormones. Alterations of the RANKL/RANK/OPG system can lead to dysregulation and pathologic conditions, including primary osteoporosis, immune-mediated bone diseases, malignant bone disorders, and inherited skeletal diseases (see Fig. 40.5).

Bone Matrix

Bone matrix is made of the *extracellular elements* of bone tissue, specifically collagen fibers, structural proteins (e.g., proteoglycans and certain glycoproteins), carbohydrate-protein complexes, ground substance, and minerals.

Collagen fibers. Collagen fibers make up the bulk of bone matrix. They are formed in this way:

1. Osteoblasts synthesize and secrete type I collagen and osteocalcin.
2. Collagen molecules assemble into three thin chains (alpha chains) to form fibrils.
3. Fibrils organize into the staggered pattern, with each fibril overlapping its nearest neighbor by about one fourth its length. This creates gaps into which mineral crystals are deposited.
4. After mineral deposition, fibrils interlink and twist to form rope-like fibers.
5. The fibers join to form the framework that gives bone its tensile and supportive strength.

Proteoglycans. Proteoglycans are large complexes of numerous polysaccharides attached to a common protein core. They strengthen bone by forming compression-resistant networks between the collagen fibers. Proteoglycans also control the transport and distribution of electrically charged particles (ions), particularly calcium, through the bone matrix, thereby playing a role in bone calcium deposition and calcification. Proteoglycans are important constituents of ground substance.

Glycoproteins. Glycoproteins are carbohydrate-protein complexes that control the collagen interactions that lead to fibril formation. They also may function in calcification. Four glycoproteins are present in bone: sialoprotein, which binds easily with calcium; osteocalcin, which binds preferentially to crystallized calcium; bone albumin, which is identical to serum albumin and possibly transports essential nutrients to and from bone cells and maintains the osmotic pressure of bone fluid; and alpha-glycoprotein (α-glycoprotein), which probably plays a significant role in calcification and also may facilitate bone resorption by activating osteoclasts (see Table 40.1).

Bone Minerals

After collagen synthesis and fiber formation, the final step in bone formation is mineralization. Mineralization has two distinct phases: (1) formation of the initial mineral deposit (initiation) and (2) proliferation or accretion of additional mineral crystals on the initial mineral deposits (growth). The majority of the minerals in the body are an analog of the naturally occurring mineral hydroxyapatite (HAP). The HAP crystals then penetrate the matrix vesicle membrane and enter into the extracellular space.

As the calcium and phosphorus concentrations increase in the bone matrix, the first precipitate to form is dicalcium phosphate dihydrate (DCPD). Once DCPD precipitation begins, the remaining phases of

bone crystal formation proceed until insoluble HAP is produced, with approximately 80% to 90% of the HAP incorporated into the collagen fibers. Amorphous calcium phosphate is distributed throughout the bone matrix.

Types of Bone Tissue

Bone is composed of two types of bony (osseous) tissue: compact bone (cortical bone) and spongy bone (cancellous bone) (Fig. 40.2). Cortical bone is about 85% of the skeleton; cancellous bone makes up the remaining 15%. Both types of bone tissue contain the same structural elements, with a few exceptions. In addition, both compact tissue and spongy tissue are present in every bone. The major difference between the two types of tissue is the organization of the elements.

Compact bone is highly organized, solid, and extremely strong. The basic structural unit in compact bone is the haversian system (Fig. 40.3). Each haversian system consists of:

- A central canal, called the haversian canal
- Concentric layers of bone matrix, called lamellae (sing., lamella)
- Tiny spaces (lacunae) between the lamellae
- Bone cells (osteocytes) within the lacunae
- Small channels or canals, called canaliculi (sing., canaliculus)

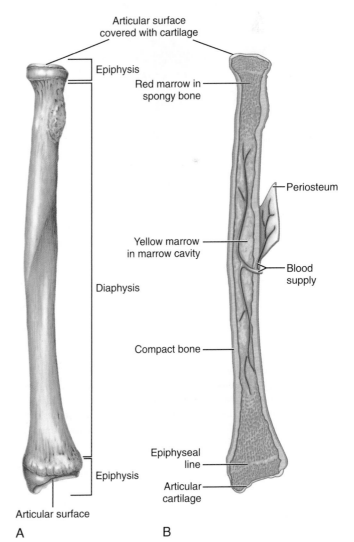

FIGURE 40.2 Anatomy of the Bone. A, External anatomy of a long bone. B, Internal structure of a long bone showing spongy (cancellous) and compact bone. (From Solomon E: *Introduction to human anatomy and physiology*, ed 4, St Louis, 2016, Saunders.)

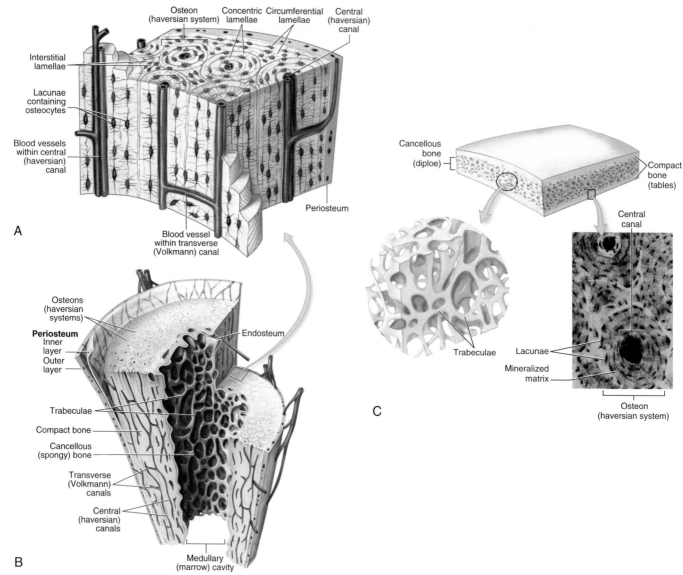

FIGURE 40.3 Structure of Compact and Cancellous Bone. A, Magnified view of compact bone. **B,** Longitudinal section of a long bone showing both cancellous and compact bone. **C,** Section of a flat bone. Outer layers of compact bone surround cancellous bone. Fine structure of compact and cancellous bone is shown in the electron photomicrograph. (From Patton KT, Thibodeau GA: *Anatomy & physiology*, ed 9, St Louis, 2016, Mosby. Photo courtesy Dennis Strete.)

Spongy bone is less complex and lacks haversian systems. In spongy bone, the lamellae are not arranged in concentric layers but in plates or bars termed **trabeculae** (sing., **trabecula**) that branch and unite with one another to form an irregular meshwork. The pattern of the meshwork is determined by the direction of stress on the particular bone. The spaces between the trabeculae are filled with red bone marrow. The osteocyte-containing lacunae are distributed between the trabeculae and interconnected by canaliculi. Capillaries pass through the marrow to nourish the osteocytes.

All bones are covered with a double-layered connective tissue called the **periosteum.** The outer layer of the periosteum contains blood vessels and nerves, some of which penetrate to the inner structures of the bone through channels called *Volkmann canals* (Fig. 40.3). The inner layer of the periosteum is anchored to the bone by collagenous fibers (Sharpey fibers) that penetrate the bone. Sharpey fibers also help hold or attach tendons and ligaments to the periosteum of bones.

Characteristics of Bone

The human skeleton consists of 206 bones that constitute the axial skeleton and the appendicular skeleton. The axial skeleton consists of 80 bones that make up the skull, vertebral column, and thorax. The appendicular skeleton consists of 126 bones that make up the upper and lower extremities, the shoulder girdle (pectoral girdle), and the pelvic girdle (os coxae) (Fig. 40.4). The skeleton contributes approximately 14% of an adult's body weight.

Bones can be classified by shape as long, flat, short (cuboidal), or irregular. Long bones are longer than they are wide and consist of a narrow tubular midportion (diaphysis) that merges into a broader neck (metaphysis) and a broad end (epiphysis) (see Fig. 40.2).

The diaphysis consists of a shaft of thick, rigid compact bone that is able to tolerate bending forces. Contained within the diaphysis is the elongated marrow (medullary) cavity. The marrow cavity of the diaphysis

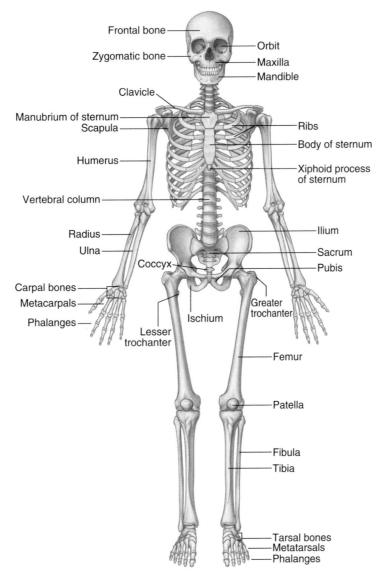

FIGURE 40.4 Anterior View of the Skeleton. (From Drake R, et al: *Gray's atlas of anatomy*, ed 2, Phila-delphia, 2015, Churchill Livingstone.)

contains primarily fatty tissue, which is referred to as *yellow marrow.* The yellow marrow assists red bone marrow in hematopoiesis only during times of stress. The yellow marrow cavity of the diaphysis is continuous with marrow cavities in the spongy bone of the metaphysis and diaphysis. The marrow contained within the epiphysis is red because it contains primarily blood-forming tissue (see Chapter 22). A layer of connective tissue, the endosteum, lines the outer surfaces of both types of marrow cavity.

The broadness of the epiphysis allows weight bearing to be distributed over a wide area. The epiphysis is made up of spongy bone covered by a thin layer of compact bone. In a child, the epiphysis is separated from the metaphysis by a cartilaginous growth plate (epiphyseal plate). After puberty, the epiphyseal plate calcifies and the epiphysis and metaphysis merge. By adulthood, the line of demarcation between the epiphysis and metaphysis is undetectable.

In flat bones, such as the ribs and scapulae, two plates of compact bone are nearly parallel to each other. Between the compact bone plates is a layer of spongy bone. Short bones, such as the bones of the wrist or ankle, are often cuboidal. They consist of spongy bone covered by a thin layer of compact bone.

Irregular bones, such as the vertebrae, mandibles, or other facial bones, have various shapes that include thin and thick segments. The thin part of an irregular bone consists of two plates of compact bone surrounding spongy bone. The thick part consists of spongy bone surrounded by a layer of compact bone.

Maintenance of Bone Integrity
Remodeling

The internal structure of bone is maintained by remodeling, a three-phase process in which existing bone is resorbed and new bone is laid down to replace it. Clusters of bone cells, termed basic multicellular units, implement remodeling. The basic multicellular units are made up of bone precursor cells that differentiate into osteoclasts and osteoblasts. Precursor cells are located on the free surfaces of bones and along the vascular channels (especially the marrow cavities).

In phase 1 (activation) of the remodeling cycle, a stimulus (e.g., hormone, drug, vitamin, physical stressor) activates the cytokine system, particularly the tumor necrosis factor (TNF) superfamily, to form osteoclasts. Osteoclasts attach to the bone matrix by actin microfilaments and multiple other proteins that form footlike structures called *podosomes.*

Once attached, the osteoclasts' integrin receptors anchor its microfilaments to the extracellular matrix, thus providing receptor pathways between the osteocyte and bone matrix. Lysosomal enzymes produced by osteoclasts "digest" bone; the osteoclasts then release the degraded bone products into the vascular system. After bone is resorbed, the osteoclast leaves behind an elongated cavity termed a *resorption cavity*. The resorption cavity in compact bone follows the longitudinal axis of the haversian system, whereas the resorption cavity in spongy bone parallels the surface of the trabeculae.

New bone formation begins as osteoblasts lining the walls of the resorption cavity express osteoid and alkaline phosphatase, forming sites for calcium and phosphorus deposition. As the osteoid mineralizes, new bone is formed. Successive layers (lamellae) in compact bone are laid down, until the resorption cavity is reduced to a narrow haversian canal around a blood vessel. In this way, old haversian systems are destroyed and new haversian systems are formed. New trabeculae are formed in spongy bone. The formation phase takes 4 to 6 months in humans.

Repair

The remodeling process can repair microscopic bone injuries, but gross injuries, such as fractures and surgical wounds (osteotomies), heal by the same stages as soft tissue injuries, except that new bone, instead of scar tissue, is the final result (see Chapter 6). The stages of bone healing are listed here and shown in Fig. 40.5:

1. Hematoma formation
2. Procallus formation
3. Callus formation
4. Replacement (basic multicellular units of the callus are replaced with lamellar or trabecular bone)
5. Remodeling (periosteal and endosteal surfaces of the bone are remodeled to the size and shape of the bone before injury)

The speed with which bone heals depends on the severity of the bone disruption; the type and amount of bone tissue that need to be replaced (spongy bone heals faster); the blood and oxygen supply available at the site; the presence of growth and thyroid hormones, insulin, vitamins, and other nutrients; the existence of systemic disease; the effects of aging (see the Osteoporosis section in Chapter 41); and the availability of effective treatment, including immobilization and the prevention of complications such as infection. In general, however, hematoma formation occurs within hours of fracture or surgery, formation of procallus by osteoblasts within days, callus formation within weeks, and replacement and contour modeling within years—up to 4 years in some cases.

✔ QUICK CHECK 40.1
1. Name the different types of bone cells.
2. What are the major cells involved in bone resorption?
3. What are the stages of bone wound healing?
4. Briefly describe the process of remodeling.

STRUCTURE AND FUNCTION OF JOINTS

The site where two or more bones are attached is called a **joint**, or an **articulation** (Fig. 40.6). The primary function of joints is to provide stability and mobility to the skeleton. A joint's function depends on both its location and its structure. Generally, joints that stabilize the skeleton have a simpler structure than those that enable the skeleton to move. Most joints provide both stability and mobility to some degree.

Joints are classified based on the degree of movement they permit or on the connecting tissues that hold them together. Based on movement, a joint is classified as a **synarthrosis (immovable joint)**, an **amphiarthrosis** (slightly movable joint), or a **diarthrosis (freely movable joint)**. From connective structures, joints are classified broadly as fibrous, cartilaginous, or synovial. Each of these three structural classifications can be subdivided according to the shape and contour of the articulating surfaces (ends) of the bones and the type of motion the joint permits.

Fibrous Joints

A joint in which bone is united directly to bone by fibrous connective tissue is called a **fibrous joint**. These joints have no joint cavity and allow little, if any, movement.

Fibrous joints are further subdivided into three types: sutures, syndesmoses, and gomphoses. A **suture** has a thin layer of dense fibrous tissue that binds together interlocking flat bones in the skulls of young children. Sutures form an extremely tight union that permits no motion. By adulthood, the fibrous tissue has been replaced by bone. A **syndesmosis** is a joint in which the two bony surfaces are united by a ligament or membrane. The fibers of ligaments are flexible and stretch, permitting a limited amount of movement. The paired bones of the lower arm (radius and ulna) and the lower leg (tibia and fibula) and their ligaments are syndesmotic joints. A **gomphosis** is a special type of fibrous joint in which a conical projection fits into a complementary socket and is held in place by a ligament. The teeth held in the maxilla or mandible are gomphosis joints.

Cartilaginous Joints

There are two types of cartilaginous joints: symphyses and synchondroses. A **symphysis** is a cartilaginous joint in which bones are united by a pad or disk of fibrocartilage. A thin layer of hyaline cartilage usually covers the articulating surfaces of these two bones, and the thick pad of fibrocartilage acts as a shock absorber and stabilizer. Examples of symphyses are the symphysis pubis, which joins the two pubic bones, and the intervertebral disks, which join the bodies of the vertebrae. A **synchondrosis** is a joint in which hyaline cartilage, rather than fibrocartilage, connects the two bones. The joints between the ribs and the sternum are synchondroses. The hyaline cartilage of these joints is called *costal cartilage*. Slight movement at the synchondroses between the ribs and the sternum allows the chest to move outward and upward during breathing.

Joint (Articular) Capsule

The **joint (articular) capsule** is fibrous connective tissue that covers the ends of bones where they meet in a joint; Sharpey fibers firmly attach the proximal and distal capsule to the periosteum, and ligaments and tendons also may reinforce the capsule. It is composed of parallel, interlacing bundles of dense, white fibrous tissue richly supplied with nerves, blood vessels, and lymphatic vessels. Nerves in and around the joint capsule are sensitive to rate and direction of motion, compression, tension, vibration, and pain.

Synovial Membrane

The **synovial membrane** is a smooth, delicate inner lining of joint capsule found in the nonarticular portion of the synovial joint and any ligaments or tendons that traverse this cavity. It is composed of two layers: the vascular subintima and the thin cellular intima. The vascular subintima merges with the fibrous joint capsule and is composed of loose fibrous connective tissue, elastin fibers, fat cells, fibroblasts, macrophages, and mast cells; the cellular intima consists of rows of synovial cells embedded in fiber-free intercellular matrix and contains two types of cells—A and B. **A cells (macrophages)** ingest and remove (phagocytose) bacteria and particles of debris in the joint cavity; **B cells (fibroblasts)** are the most numerous and secrete hyaluronate, which gives synovial fluid its viscous quality. The synovial membrane is richly

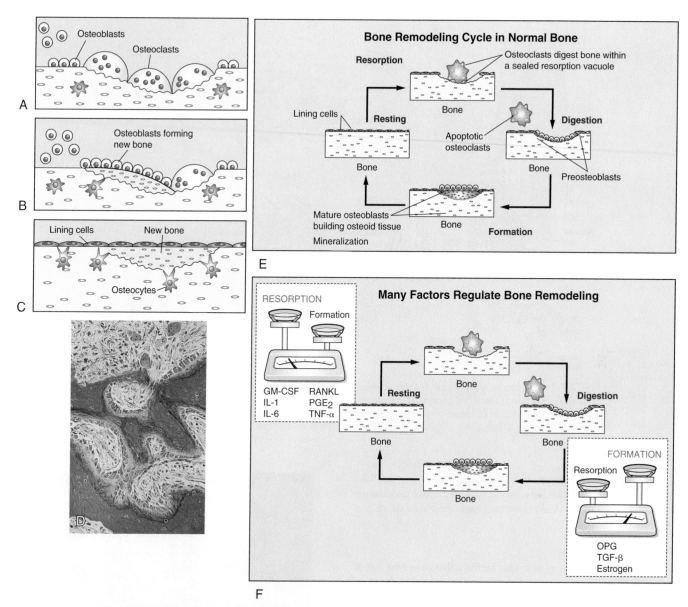

FIGURE 40.5 Bone Remodeling. All bone cells participate in bone remodeling. In the remodeling sequence, bone sections are removed by bone-resorbing cells (osteoclasts) and replaced with a new section laid down by bone-forming cells (osteoblasts). Bone remodeling is necessary because it allows the skeleton to respond to mechanical loading, maintains quality control (repair and prevent microdamage), and allows the skeleton to release growth factors and minerals (calcium and phosphate) stored in bone matrix to the circulation. The cells work in response to signals generated in the environment (see **F**). Only the osteoclastic cells mediate the first phase of remodeling. They are activated, scoop out bone (**A**), and resorb it; then the work of the osteoblasts begins (**B**). They form new bone that replaces bone removed by the resorption process (**C**). The sequence takes 4 to 6 months. **D,** Micrograph of active bone remodeling seen in the settings of primary or secondary hyperparathyroidism. Note the active osteoblasts surmounted on red-stained osteoid. Marrow fibrosis is present. **E,** Bone remodeling cycle in normal bone with (**F**). Numerous signaling factors are necessary for remodeling. Factors most important for resorption include granulocyte macrophage-colony stimulating factor (GM-CSF), interleukin-1 (IL-1) and IL-6, receptor activator for nuclear factor-κB ligand (RANKL), prostaglandin E_2 (PGE$_2$), and tumor necrosis factor-alpha (TNF-α). Important factors for bone formation include osteoprotegerin (OPG), transforming growth factor-beta (TGF-β), and estrogen. (Adapted from Nucleus Medical Art. D from Damjanov I, Linder J, editors: *Anderson's pathology,* ed 10, St Louis, 1996, Mosby.)

supplied with blood and lymphatic vessels and is capable of rapid repair and regeneration.

Joint (Synovial) Cavity

The joint (synovial) cavity is an enclosed, fluid-filled space between articulating surfaces of two bones, also called *joint space*. It enables two bones to move "against" one another and is surrounded by synovial membrane and filled with synovial fluid.

Synovial Fluid

Synovial fluid is superfiltrated plasma from blood vessels that lubricates the joint surfaces, nourishes the pad of the articular cartilage, and

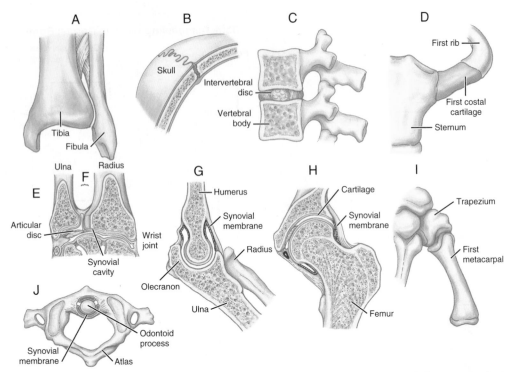

FIGURE 40.6 Various Kinds of Joints. *Fibrous:* **A,** Syndesmosis (tibiofibular); **B,** suture (skull). *Cartilaginous:* **C,** Symphysis (vertebral bodies); **D,** synchondrosis (first rib and sternum). *Synovial:* **E,** Condyloid (wrist); **F,** gliding (radioulnar); **G,** hinge or ginglymus (elbow); **H,** ball and socket (hip); **I,** saddle (carpometacarpal of thumb); **J,** pivot (atlantoaxial). (From Dorland: *Dorland's medical illustrated dictionary,* ed 32, St Louis, 2012, Saunders.)

covers the ends of the bones. Hyaluronic acid in the synovial fluid gives it important biomechanical properties. It also contains free-floating synovial cells and various leukocytes that phagocytose joint debris and microorganisms.

Articular Cartilage

Articular cartilage is a layer of hyaline cartilage that covers the end of each bone; it may be thick or thin, depending on the size of the joint, the fit of the two bone ends, and the amount of weight and shearing force the joint normally withstands. The function of articular cartilage is to reduce friction in the joint and to distribute the forces of weight-bearing. Articular cartilage is composed of chondrocytes (cartilage cells) (about 2% of the tissue) and an intercellular matrix consisting of type II collagen (about 10% to 30% of weight), proteoglycans (about 5% to 10% of weight), and water. The water content ranges from 60% to almost 80% of the net weight of the cartilage.

At the surface of articular cartilage, the collagen fibers run parallel to the joint surface and are closely compacted into a dense, protective mat. In the middle layer (the proliferative zone) of the cartilage, the fibers are arranged tangential to the surface, which allows them to deform and absorb some of the weight-bearing (Fig. 40.7). In the bottom layer (the hypertrophic zone) of the cartilage, the fibers are perpendicular to the joint surface, allowing them to resist shear forces, and are embedded in a calcified layer of cartilage called the *tidemark*. The tidemark anchors the collagen fibers to the underlying (subchondral) bone. Collagen fibers are important components of the cartilage matrix because they account for approximately 60% of the dry weight and because they (1) anchor the cartilage securely to underlying bone, (2) provide a taut framework for the cartilage, (3) control the loss of fluid from the cartilage, and (4) prevent the escape of protein polysaccharides (proteoglycans) from the cartilage. The proteoglycans give articular cartilage its stiff quality

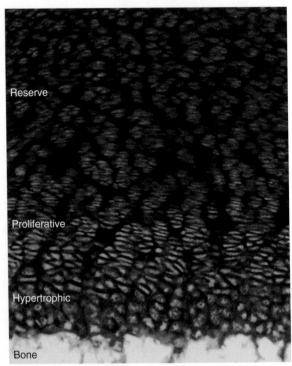

FIGURE 40.7 Collagen Zones. The three collagen zones (reserve, proliferative, and hypertrophic) are distinctly shown in a growth plate. (From Hjorten R et al: *Bone* 41[4]:535, 2007.)

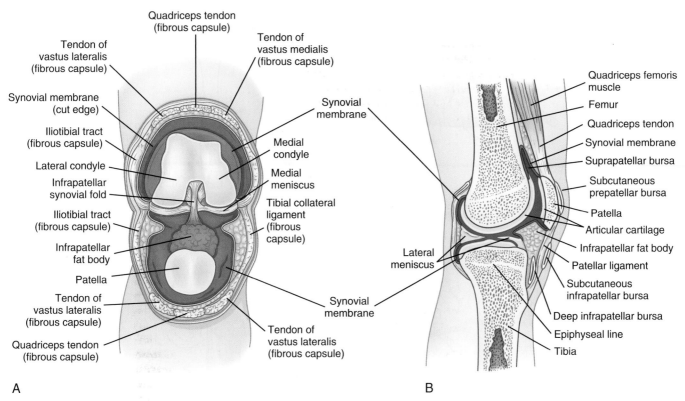

FIGURE 40.8 Knee Joint (Synovial Joint). A, Frontal view. **B,** Lateral view.

and regulate the movement of synovial fluid through the cartilage. The proteoglycans are macromolecules consisting of proteins, carbohydrates (glycosaminoglycans), and hyaluronic acid.

Synovial Joints
Structure of Synovial Joints

Synovial joints (diarthroses) are the most movable and the most complex joints in the body (Fig. 40.8).

Movement of Synovial Joints

Synovial joints are described as uniaxial, biaxial, or multiaxial according to the shapes of the bone ends and the type of movement occurring at the joint (Fig. 40.9). Usually, one of the bones is stable and serves as an axis for the motion of the other bone. The body movements made possible by various synovial joints are either circular or angular (Fig. 40.10).

✔ QUICK CHECK 40.2

1. How do these joints differ from each other: synarthrosis, amphiarthrosis, and diarthrosis?
2. Name at least two characteristics of each of the joints in the previous question that either facilitate or hinder movement.
3. Name three functions of articular cartilage.

STRUCTURE AND FUNCTION OF SKELETAL MUSCLES

Skeletal muscles arise from mesodermal precursor cells that then form myoblasts, or embryonic cells, which become muscle cells. The millions of individual fibers of skeletal muscle contract and relax to perform the work necessary to move the body (Fig. 40.11). Muscle constitutes

40% of an adult's body weight and 50% of a child's weight. Muscle is 75% water, 20% protein, and 5% organic and inorganic compounds. Thirty-two percent of all protein stores for energy and metabolism are contained in muscle. Between the ages of 30 and 60, muscle mass decreases by about 0.5 pound of muscle each year. For each 0.5 pound of muscle lost, almost 1 pound of fat typically is gained.

Whole Muscle

There are more than 350 named muscles in the body. The body's muscles vary dramatically in size and shape. They range from 2 to 60 cm in length and are shaped according to function. Fusiform muscles are elongated muscles shaped like straps that can run from one joint to another. The biceps brachii and psoas major are examples of fusiform muscles. Pennate muscles are broad, flat, and slightly fan shaped, with fibers running obliquely to the muscle's long axis. The multipennate deltoid muscle, which flexes and extends the arm, is a good example of a muscle shaped according to its function.

Each skeletal muscle is a separate organ, encased in a three-part connective tissue framework called fascia. The layers of connective tissue protect the muscle fibers, attach the muscle to bony prominences, and provide a structure for a network of nerve fibers, blood vessels, and lymphatic channels. The layers are:

1. The outermost layer, the epimysium, which is located on the surface of the muscle and tapers at each end to form the tendon (Fig. 40.12; also see the Tendons and Ligaments section for a discussion of tendons). Tendons allow short muscles to exert power on a distant joint, whereas a thick muscle would interfere with the joint's mobility.
2. The perimysium, which further subdivides the muscle fibers into bundles of connective tissue, or fascicles.
3. The endomysium, which surrounds the muscle. It is the smallest unit of muscle visible without a microscope.

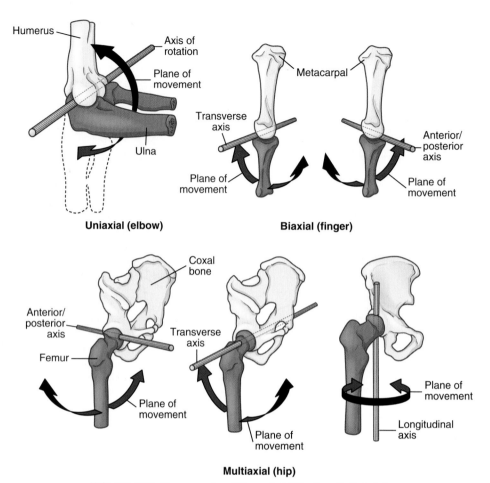

FIGURE 40.9 Movements of Synovial (Diarthrodial) Joints.

The ligaments, tendons, and fascia are made up of connective tissue that also buffers the limbs from the effects of sudden strains or changes in speed. The rapid recovery necessary for strenuous exercise is supported by the elastic property of muscle and its connective tissue.

Skeletal muscle has been designated as voluntary (controlled directly by the nervous system), striated (has a striped pattern when viewed under a light microscope), or extrafusal (to distinguish from other contractile fibers in the sensory organ of the muscle). Components that are visible on gross inspection of the whole muscle include the motor and sensory nerve fibers. These function together with the muscle, innervating portions of it and providing the electrical impulses needed for motor function.

Motor Unit

From the anterior horn cell of the spinal cord, the axons of motor nerves branch to innervate a specific group of muscle fibers. Each anterior horn cell, its axon (part of the lower motor neuron; see Chapter 14), and the muscle fibers innervated by it are called a motor unit (Fig. 40.13). The motor units are composed of lower motor neurons, which extend to skeletal muscles. Often termed the *functional unit* of the neuromuscular system, the motor unit behaves as a single entity and contracts as a whole when it receives an electrical impulse.

The whole muscle may be controlled by several motor nerve axons. These branch to innervate many motor units within the muscle. The whole muscle then may be made up of many motor units. The number of motor units per individual muscle varies greatly. In the calf, for example, 1 motor axon innervates approximately 2000 muscle fibers, out of a total of 1.2 million muscle fibers. This is a high innervation ratio of muscle fibers to axons, and it contrasts markedly with the low innervation ratio found in laryngeal muscles, where two to three muscle fibers constitute each motor unit and the innervation ratio can be of great functional significance. The greater the innervation ratio of a particular organ, the greater its endurance. Higher innervation ratios prevent fatigue, whereas lower innervation ratios allow for precision of movement.

Sensory receptors. Although muscles function as effector organs, they also contain sensory receptors and are involved in sending different signals to the central nervous system. Among these are the muscle spindles and Golgi tendon organs. Spindles are mechanoreceptors that lie parallel to muscle fibers and respond to muscle stretching. Golgi tendon organs are dendrites that terminate and branch to tendons near the neuromuscular junction. The muscle spindles, Golgi tendon organs, and free nerve endings provide a means of reporting changes in length, tension, velocity, and tone in the muscle. This system of afferent signals is responsible for the muscle stretch response and maintenance of normal muscle tone.

Muscle fibers. Each muscle fiber is a single muscle cell that is cylindrical in structure and surrounded by a membrane capable of excitation and impulse propagation. The muscle fiber contains bundles of myofibrils, the fiber's functional subunits, in a parallel arrangement along the longitudinal axis of the muscle (Fig. 40.14). At birth, the muscle fibers have completed development from precursor cells called *myoblasts*. All voluntary muscles are derived from the mesodermal layer of the embryo. Genetic transcription factors, most notably MyoD, induce skeletal muscle differentiation. Myoblasts are the main cells responsible for muscle growth and regeneration. Myoblasts are termed *satellite cells* when in a dormant state. Satellite cells are crucial in muscle growth, maintenance, repair, and regeneration. Once muscle is injured,

Arm/hand

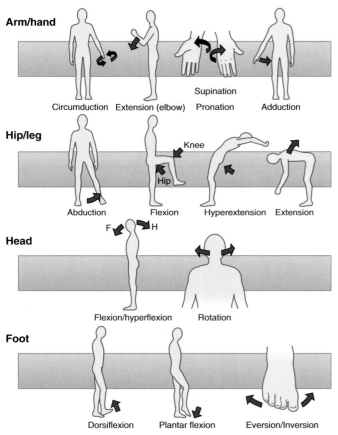

Circumduction Extension (elbow) Supination Pronation Adduction

Hip/leg

Knee

Hip

Abduction Flexion Hyperextension Extension

Head

F H

Flexion/hyperflexion Rotation

Foot

Dorsiflexion Plantar flexion Eversion/Inversion

FIGURE 40.10 Body Movements Made Possible by Synovial (Diarthrodial) Joints.

satellite cells become activated and increase the number of transcriptional factors necessary to form myoblasts and assist in repair.

The type of peripheral nerve influences the muscle fiber and motor unit considerably. Whether motor nerves are fast or slow determines the type of muscle fibers in the motor unit. White muscle (type II fibers [white fast-twitch fibers]) is innervated by relatively large type II alpha motor neurons with fast conduction velocities. These fibers rely on a short-term anaerobic glycolytic system for rapid energy transfer. Red muscle (type I fibers [slow-twitch fibers]) depends on aerobic oxidative metabolism. Table 40.3 describes the specific characteristics of type I and type II fibers.

The overlap of muscle fibers that appears with staining gives a checkerboard appearance to muscle biopsy specimens. This overlap provides an equal distribution of fiber types throughout the muscle and also helps to compensate for muscle fiber loss and fatigue of individual motor units during activity. Despite this, some muscles contain proportionally more of one fiber type than another. Postural muscles have more type I fibers, allowing them the high resistance to fatigue that is necessary to maintain the same position for extended periods. The ocular muscles have more type II muscle fibers, allowing them to respond rapidly to visual changes.

The number of muscle fibers varies according to location. Large muscles, such as the gastrocnemius, have more fibers (1.2 million) than smaller muscles, such as the lumbrical muscles in the hand (10,000). The diameter of muscle fibers also varies. The closely packed polygons are small (10 to 20 µm) until puberty, when they attain the normal adult diameter of 40 to 80 µm. Women usually have smaller diameter fibers than men. Small muscles, such as the ocular muscles, are 15 µm in diameter; larger, more proximal muscles are 40 µm in diameter. Fiber size can have functional significance, such as the association of larger fiber diameter with the generation of greater forces.

TABLE 40.3   Characteristics of Human Skeletal Muscle Fibers

Characteristics	Type I (Red) (Oxidative Fibers [OFs])	Type II (White) Type II-1A (Fast Oxidative Glycolic Fibers [FOGs])
Anatomic location	Deep axial portion of muscle	Surface portion of muscle
Fiber diameter	Small	Large
Motor neuron size	Small	Large
Contraction speed	Slow	Fast
Motor neuron type	Type I, α	Type II-A, II-B, II-X, and II-D II-A: fatigue resistant; II-B: fast fatigable; II-X and II-D: intermediate fatigability
Glycogen content (at rest)	Low	High
Oxidative capacity	High	High (for short periods)
Myosin-ATPase activity	Low	High
Metabolism	Oxidative (also most effective in removing glucose from bloodstream)	Some oxidative pathways, mostly glycolysis
Used for	Maintaining body posture, skeletal support, aerobic activity	Short, intense activity (e.g., sprinting)
Aerobic metabolic capacity	High	Low
Fatigue resistance	High	Intermediate to low
Myoglobin content	High	Low
Capillary supply	Profuse	Intermediate to low
Mitochondria	Many	Few
Intensity of contraction	Low	High
Example (most muscles are mixed)	Soleus muscle	Laryngeal
Satellite cell content	High	Low

From Schiaffino S, Reggiani C: *Physiol Rev* 91:1447-1531, 2011; Verdijk LB et al: *Age* 36(2):545-547, 2014.

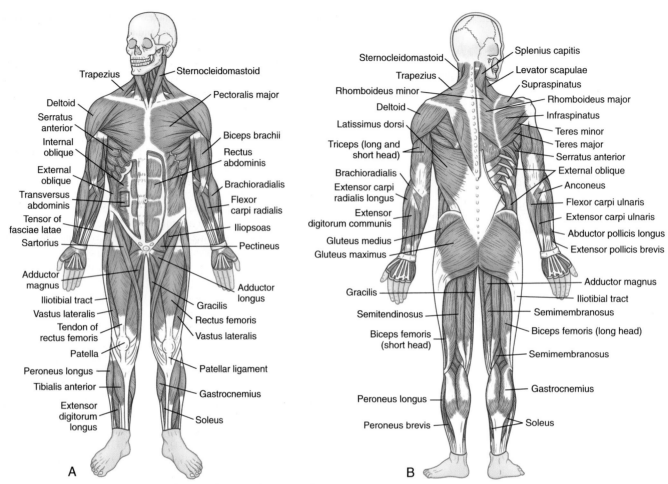

FIGURE 40.11 Skeletal Muscles of the Body. A, Anterior view. **B,** Posterior view.

The major components of the muscle fiber include the muscle membrane, sarcoplasm, mitochondria, sarcotubular system, and myofibrils (see Fig. 40.14). The muscle membrane is a two-part membrane. It includes the sarcolemma, which contains the plasma membrane of the muscle cell, and the cell's basement membrane. The sarcolemma is 7.5 μm thick and is capable of propagating electrical impulses to initiate contraction. At the motor nerve end plate, where the nerve impulse is transmitted, the sarcolemma forms the highly convoluted synaptic cleft. The sarcolemma is made up of lipid molecules and protein systems. The protein systems perform special functions, such as transport of nutrients and protein synthesis. They also provide the sodium-potassium pump and include the cell's cholinergic receptor. The basement membrane is 50 μm thick and is composed primarily of proteins and polysaccharides. It also serves as the cell's microskeleton and maintains the shape of the muscle cell. The basement membrane also may function to restrict further diffusion of electrolytes once they have crossed the sarcolemma.

The sarcoplasm is the cytoplasm of the muscle cell and contains myoglobin plus the intracellular components that are common to all cells (see Chapter 1). Myoglobin is a protein found primarily in skeletal and heart muscle. Related to hemoglobin in the blood, myoglobin stores oxygen and iron in the muscle. The sarcoplasm is an aqueous substance that provides a matrix that surrounds the myofibrils. It contains numerous enzymes and proteins that are responsible for the cell's energy production, protein synthesis, and oxygen storage. The mitochondria house enzyme systems for energy production, particularly those that regulate processes such as the citric acid cycle and adenosine triphosphate (ATP) formation.

Many other structures are present in the sarcoplasm. The ribosomes are composed of primarily ribonucleic acid (RNA) and participate in protein synthesis. The cell nucleus, satellite cells, glycogen granules, and lipid droplets are suspended in the sarcoplasmic matrix. Blood vessels, nerve endings, muscle spindles, and Golgi tendon organs are also directly located within this structure.

Unique to the muscle is the sarcotubular system, a network that includes the transverse tubules and the sarcoplasmic reticulum, which crosses the interior of the cell. The sarcoplasmic reticulum is constructed like the endoplasmic reticulum in other cells. The sarcoplasmic reticulum is composed of tubules that run parallel to the myofibrils. The longitudinal tubules are termed sarcotubules. In muscle cells, the sarcoplasmic reticulum contains a network of intracellular receptors known as ryanodine receptors (RyRs). In response to a nerve impulse, RyR1 (found in skeletal muscle cells) releases intracellular calcium and initiates muscle contraction at the sarcomere, a portion of the myofibril. The transverse tubules, which also contain calcium release channels and are closely associated with the sarcotubules, run across the sarcoplasm and communicate with the extracellular space. Together, the tubules of this membrane system allow for uptake and regulation of intracellular calcium, release of calcium during muscle contraction, and storage of calcium during muscle relaxation.

Myofibrils. Myofibrils, the most abundant subcellular muscle component (85% to 90% of the total volume), are the functional units of muscle contraction. Each myofibril contains sarcomeres, which appear at intervals (see Fig. 40.14). Sarcomeres are composed of several proteins. The two most abundant are actin and myosin, but three other giant,

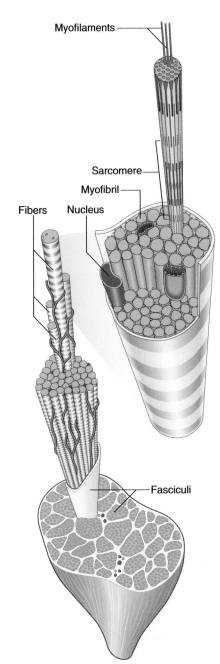

Myofilaments

Sarcomere

Myofibril

Fibers   Nucleus

Fasciculi

FIGURE 40.12 Levels of Organization Within a Skeletal Muscle Showing Muscle Fibers and Their Coverings. (From Standring S: *Gray's anatomy,* ed 40, Edinburgh, 2008, Churchill Livingstone.)

muscle-specific proteins (titin, nebulin, and obscurin) play important roles in myofibril formation and function (see Table 40.4).

On cross section, they are seen to be irregular polygons with a mean diameter of less than 1 μm. Each myofibril is composed of serially repeating sarcomeres, separated by Z bands, which give the muscle its striped, cross-striated appearance. Each sarcomere has a dark A band and is flanked by two light I bands (Fig. 40.15). The A band is 1.5 to 1.6 μm long and contains the thick myosin filaments. Included in the A band is a lighter zone called the *H band,* and in the center of the H band is the dark *M band,* or *M line.* The *I band,* which contains actin, is divided at the midpoint of each sarcomere by the *Z band.* Its length varies with the start of muscle contraction. The *Z disk* (made up of different layers of Z bands, depending on muscle type) marks the boundaries of the sarcomere.

Myofibrils are composed of myofilaments. Each myofilament is structured in a closely packed hexagonal arrangement, with two thin filaments for every thick filament. The thick filament, along with C protein and M line protein, is made up of myosin. Myosin has two subunits—heavy and light meromyosin, which resemble twisted golf club shafts. The thin filaments are twisted double strands consisting of actin, troponin, and tropomyosin (see Chapter 25 and Fig. 25.11).

Muscle proteins. A multitude of muscle proteins have been identified and their functions are still being discovered. Table 40.4 summarizes the location and function of some of the important muscle proteins.

Nonprotein constituents of muscle. Nitrogen, creatine, creatinine, phosphocreatine, purines, uric acid, and amino acids all serve in the complex process of muscle metabolism. Energy is provided by glycogen and its derivatives.

Creatine metabolism and creatinine metabolism have been used to measure muscle mass. Plasma creatine is taken up by muscle and converted into the high-energy phosphate compound phosphocreatine by the enzyme creatine kinase. Creatinine is formed in muscle from creatine at a constant rate of 2% per day. Creatine excretion is increased in muscle wasting. This change reflects the reduction in total body creatine stores and the loss of muscle mass.

Inorganic compounds, anions (phosphate, chloride), and cations (calcium, magnesium, sodium, potassium) are important in the regulation of protein synthesis, muscle contraction, and enzyme systems, as well as in the stabilization of cell membranes. The total body potassium (TBK) level, measured by the K40 method, has been used to measure muscle mass, also called *lean body mass.* TBK levels reflect changes in muscle mass seen during growth, malnutrition, and muscle wasting.

Components of Muscle Function

The ultimate function of muscle is to accomplish work. Although variously expressed in such measures as foot-pounds or kilogram-meters, work usually refers to the amount of energy liberated or force exerted over a distance (Work = Force × Distance). Muscles usually

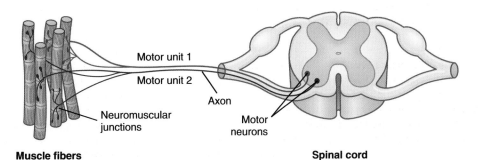

Motor unit 1

Motor unit 2

Neuromuscular junctions

Axon

Motor neurons

Muscle fibers

Spinal cord

FIGURE 40.13 Motor Units of a Muscle. Each motor unit consists of a motor neuron and all the muscle fibers (cells) supplied by the neuron and its axon branches.

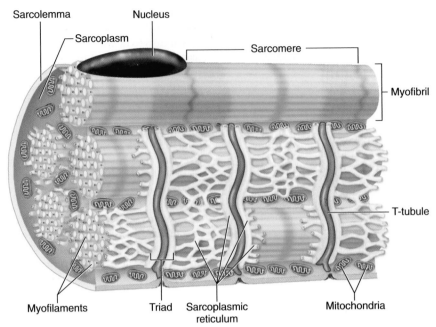

FIGURE 40.14 Myofibrils of a Skeletal Muscle Fiber (Cell) and Overall Organization of Skeletal Muscle. (From Patton KT, Thibodeau GA: *Anatomy & physiology*, ed 9, St Louis, 2016, Mosby.)

TABLE 40.4   Contractile Proteins of Skeletal Muscle Sarcomere

Protein	Location	Function
Actinin	Z disk	Attaches actin to Z disks; helps coordinate sarcomere contraction; cross-links thin filaments in adjacent sarcomeres
Actin	I band (thin filaments)	Contraction; activates myosin-ATPase; interacts with myosin
α-Actin	Z disk	Main ligand of titin; links and controls filament length
β-Actin	Z disk	Regulatory and structural function; links filaments, controls filament length
Myosin	A band (thick filament)	Contraction force; two distinct types: myosin heavy chain (MyHC) and myosin light chain (MyLC); hydrolyzes ATP and develops tension
Titin*(largest and third most abundant muscle protein)	Half of sarcomere (from Z disk to M band)	Coordinates assembly of proteins that comprise sarcomere; regulates resting length of sarcomere; important for myofibril assembly, stabilization, and maintenance
Nebulin*	I band (with α-actin)	Interacts with myosin to produce contraction; binding site for actin, desmin, titin, other proteins; stabilizes and regulates length of actin filaments; plays role in assembly, structure, and maintenance of Z disks
Obscurin*	Surrounds sarcomere (mainly at Z disk and M band)	May mediate interaction of sarcoplasmic reticulum and myofibrils; plays role in muscle response to injury; has role in formation and stabilization of M bands and A band

*Also may function as molecular scaffolds for myofibril formation.
ATP, Adenosine triphosphate; *ATPase*, adenosinetriphosphatase.
Data from Herzog JA et al: *Mol Cell Biomech* 11(1):1-17, 2014; Luther PK: *J Muscle Res Cell Motil* 30:171-185, 2009; Pappas CT et al: *J Cell Biol* 189(5):858-870, 2010; Schiaffino S, Reggiani C: *Physiol Rev* 91:1447-1531, 2011.

contract or tense while doing work. Muscle contraction occurs on the molecular level and leads to the observable phenomenon of muscle movement.

Muscle Contraction at the Molecular Level

The four steps of muscle contraction are (1) excitation, (2) coupling, (3) contraction, and (4) relaxation. The process involves the electrical properties of all cells and the movement of ions across the plasma membrane (see Chapter 1). The muscle fiber is an excitable tissue. At rest, an electrical charge of −90 mV is continually maintained across the sarcolemma. This resting potential, generated by the separation of positive and negative charges on either side of the membrane, creates an electrochemical equilibrium caused by the selective permeability of the sarcolemma to electrolytes in the intracellular and extracellular fluids, particularly potassium and sodium.

Excitation, the first step of muscle contraction, begins with the spread of an action potential from the nerve terminal to the neuromuscular junction. The rapid depolarization of the membrane initiates an electrical impulse in the muscle fiber membrane called the muscle fiber action potential. As the action potential advances along the sarcolemmal membrane, it spreads to the transverse tubules. A receptor on the transverse tubule opens, allowing calcium to enter the cell.

The second stage, coupling, follows the depolarization of the transverse tubules. This triggers the release of calcium ions from the sarcoplasmic reticulum through RyR1 channels into the sarcoplasm. The calcium then binds to a protein on the actin filament. (Calcium affects

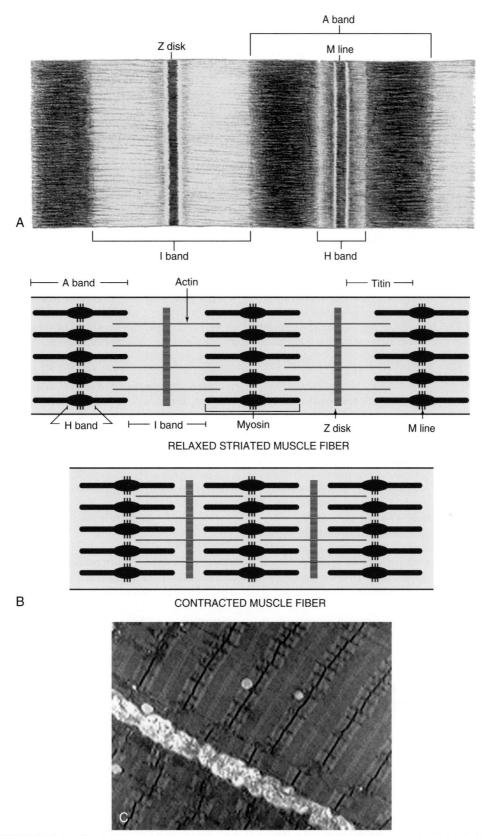

FIGURE 40.15 Muscle Fibers. A, The Z disks define the end of an individual sarcomere. The M line (which lies within the H band) is made of cross-connecting elements of the cytoskeleton. **B,** Actin is the primary protein of the I band (thin filament). Nebulin also extends along the I band and contains binding sites for actin and myosin. Myosin (thick filament) extends through the A band. Titin extends from the Z disk to the M band, binding with myosin; strong titin anchoring within the I band is necessary for proper muscle function. During contraction, the I bands and H bands shorten, moving the Z disks closer together. **C,** Electron photomicrograph of human muscle tissue corresponding to schematics in **A** and **B**. (**A** modified from Thompson JM et al: *Mosby's clinical nursing,* ed 5, St Louis, 2002, Mosby; **C** courtesy Louisa Howard.)

troponin and tropomyosin, muscle proteins that bind with actin when the muscle is at rest.) In the presence of calcium, however, both these proteins are attracted to calcium ions, leaving the actin free to bind with myosin. The release of intracellular calcium ions is the critical link between a nerve impulse (electrical excitation) and muscle contraction.

Contraction begins as the calcium ions combine with troponin, a reaction that overcomes the inhibitory function of the troponin-tropomyosin system. Myosin binds to actin, forming cross-bridges. The myosin heads attach to the exposed actin-binding sites, pulling actin (the thin filament) inward. The thin filament, actin, then slides toward the thick filament, myosin. The two ends of the myofibril shorten after contraction when the myosin heads attach to the actin molecules, forming a cross-bridge that constitutes an actin-myosin complex. ATP, located on the actin-myosin complex, is released when the cross-bridges attach. Contraction was first described by A.F. Huxley in the 1950s. It is commonly known as the cross-bridge theory because the actin and myosin proteins form cross-bridges as they contract. The useful distance of contraction of a skeletal muscle is approximately 25% to 35% of the muscle's length.

The last step, relaxation, begins as calcium ions are actively transported back into the sarcoplasmic reticulum, removing ions from interaction with troponin. The cross-bridges detach, and the sarcomere lengthens. (The cross-bridge theory of muscle contraction is discussed in Chapter 25.)

Muscle Metabolism

Skeletal muscle requires a constant supply of ATP and phosphocreatine. These substances are necessary to fuel the complex processes of muscle contraction, driving the cross-bridges of actin and myosin together and transporting calcium from the sarcoplasmic reticulum to the myofibril. Other internal processes of the muscular system that require ATP include protein synthesis, which replenishes muscle constituents and accommodates growth and repair. The rate of protein synthesis is related to hormone levels (particularly insulin), the presence of amino acid substrates, and overall nutritional status. At rest, the rate of ATP formation by oxidation of glucose or acetoacetate is sufficient to maintain internal processes, given normal nutritional status. During activity, the need for ATP increases 100-fold. The metabolic pathways for muscle activity in Table 40.5 show reactions to the immediate need for increased ATP caused by contraction. Activity lasting longer than 5 seconds expends the available stored ATP and phosphocreatine.

Stored glycogen and blood glucose are converted anaerobically to sustain brief activity without increasing the demand for oxygen. Anaerobic glycolysis is much less efficient than aerobic glycolysis, using six to eight times more glycogen to produce the same amount of ATP. With increased activity, such as intense exercise, or with ischemia, an increase in the amount of lactic acid occurs because of the breakdown of glycogen, thus causing a shift in muscle pH (see Table 40.5). This short-term mechanism buys time by allowing ATP formation in spite of inadequate energy stores or oxygen supply. When the anaerobic threshold is reached and more oxygen is required, physiologic changes occur, including an increase in lactic acid level and increases in oxygen consumption, heart rate, respiratory rate, and muscle blood flow.

Strenuous exercise requires oxygen, which activates the aerobic glycogen pathway for ATP formation. During maximal exercise, free fatty acid mobilization and the aerobic glycogen pathways provide ATP over an extended time. These pathways require oxygen both to maintain maximal activity and to return the muscle to the resting state. Maximal exercise increases oxygen uptake by 15 to 20 times over the resting state. When this system becomes exhausted or inadequate to respond to the need for ATP, fatigue and weakness finally force the muscle to reduce activity, with a resultant buildup of lactic acid in muscle fibers.

Sustaining maximal muscular activity accumulates an oxygen debt, which is the amount of oxygen needed to oxidize the residual lactic acid, convert it back to glycogen, and replenish ATP and phosphocreatine stores. For example, after running at maximal speed for 10 seconds, the average person has consumed 1 L of oxygen. At rest, oxygen consumption for the same period is approximately 40 ml. As the person recovers, the measured oxygen debt is 4 L greater than the amount used during activity.

Oxygen consumption is measured to calculate the metabolic cost of activity in normal and diseased muscle. It is an indirect measure of energy expenditure, along with timed tests of activity, heart rate, and respiratory quotient (ratio of carbon dioxide to expired oxygen consumed). Energy expenditure is measured directly by heat production, because heat is released whenever work is accomplished.

Another factor that changes energy requirements is muscle fiber type. Type II fibers rely on anaerobic glycolytic metabolism and fatigue readily. Type I fibers can resist fatigue for longer periods because of their capacity for oxidative metabolism.

Muscle Mechanics

Muscle contraction cannot be viewed in isolation. Several factors determine how force is transmitted from the cross-bridges on individual muscle fibers to accomplish whole-muscle contraction. First, when a motor unit responds to a single nerve stimulus, it develops a phasic contraction, also called a *twitch*. Because the motor unit contracts in an all-or-nothing manner, the contraction that is generated will be a maximal contraction. The central nervous system smoothly grades the force generated by recruiting additional motor units and varying the discharge frequency of each active motor unit. This adding of motor units within the muscle is called repetitive discharge.

Recruitment and repetitive discharge of motor units allow the muscle to activate the number of motor units needed to generate the desired force. The total force developed is the sum of the force generated by each motor unit. If the motor units are stimulated again and the muscle unit has not been able to relax between stimulation and the next contraction, the second contraction will fuse with the first, causing physiologic tetanus (not to be confused with the disease tetanus).

Other variables, such as fiber type, innervation ratio, muscle temperature, and muscle shape, influence the efficiency of muscular contraction. The two muscle fiber types differ in their responses to electrical activity. Tetanus and duration of phasic contractions, which take microseconds to accomplish, are achieved more rapidly in type II (white fast-twitch) than in type I (red slow-twitch) muscle fibers. Low innervation ratios promote control and coordination, whereas high ratios promote strength and endurance. Muscles work best at normal body

TABLE 40.5	**Energy Sources for Muscular Activity**	
Sources	**Reactions**
Short-term (anaerobic) sources	$ATP \rightarrow ADP + P_i + Energy$
	$Phosphocreatine + ADP \rightleftharpoons Creatine + ATP$
	$Glycogen/glucose + P_i + ADP \rightarrow Lactate + ATP$
Long-term (aerobic) sources	$Glycogen/glucose + ADP + P_i + O_2 \rightarrow H_2O + CO_2 + ATP$
	$Free\ fatty\ acids + ADP + P_i + O_2 \rightarrow H_2O + CO_2 + ATP$
	Creatine kinase catalyzes reversible reaction of ATP to ADP:
	$Creatine\ phosphate + ATP \underset{}{\overset{Creatine\ Kinase}{\rightleftharpoons}} Creatine + ATP$

ADP, Adenosine diphosphate; *ATP,* adenosine triphosphate; *CO2,* carbon dioxide; *H2O,* water; *O2,* oxygen; *Pi,* inorganic phosphate
From Spence AP, Mason EE: *Human anatomy and physiology,* ed 4, St Paul, Minn, 1992, West Publishing.

temperature, or 37° C (98.6° F). Finally, muscles with a large cross-sectional area, such as the fan-shaped pennate muscles, develop greater contractile forces than smaller diameter muscles. The initial length of a muscle and the range of shortening that occur when the muscle contracts also determine the force it can generate. The long fusiform muscles have a greater range of shortening and can contract up to 57% of their resting length. A certain amount of elongation is necessary to generate sufficient tension and muscular force. The elongation that occurs during the swing of a golf club or tennis racket is an example of how stretch improves contractile force.

Types of Muscle Contraction

During isometric (or static) contraction, the muscle maintains constant length as tension is increased (Fig. 40.16). Isometric contraction occurs, for example, when the arm or leg is pushed against an immovable object. The muscle contracts, but the limb does not move. Isometric contraction is also called static (holding) contraction.

During dynamic (formerly known as isotonic) contraction, the muscle maintains a constant tension as it moves. Isotonic contractions can be eccentric (lengthening) or concentric (shortening). Positive work is accomplished during concentric contraction, and energy is released to exert force or lift a weight. In contrast, during an eccentric contraction the muscle lengthens and absorbs energy (e.g., extending the elbow while lowering a weight). Eccentric contraction requires less energy to accomplish and has been said to result in the development of pain and stiffness after unaccustomed exercise.

Movement of Muscle Groups

Muscles do not act alone but in groups, often under automatic control. When a muscle contracts and acts as a prime mover, or agonist, its reciprocal muscle, or antagonist, relaxes. To illustrate this, hold the right arm in the horizontal position in front of the body and bend the elbow; use the other hand to feel the biceps on the top and the triceps on the bottom of the arm. When the elbow is bent, the biceps are firm, and the triceps are soft. As the arm is extended, the muscles change. When the elbow is completely extended, the biceps is soft and the triceps firm. Completing this movement causes the agonist and antagonist to change automatically; only the movement is commanded, not the alternate contraction and relaxation of the specific muscle groups.

Other associated actions occur with walking; as the foot leaves the ground, the paravertebral and gluteal muscles on the opposite sides of the body contract to maintain balance. Paralysis offsets this process and decreases balance.

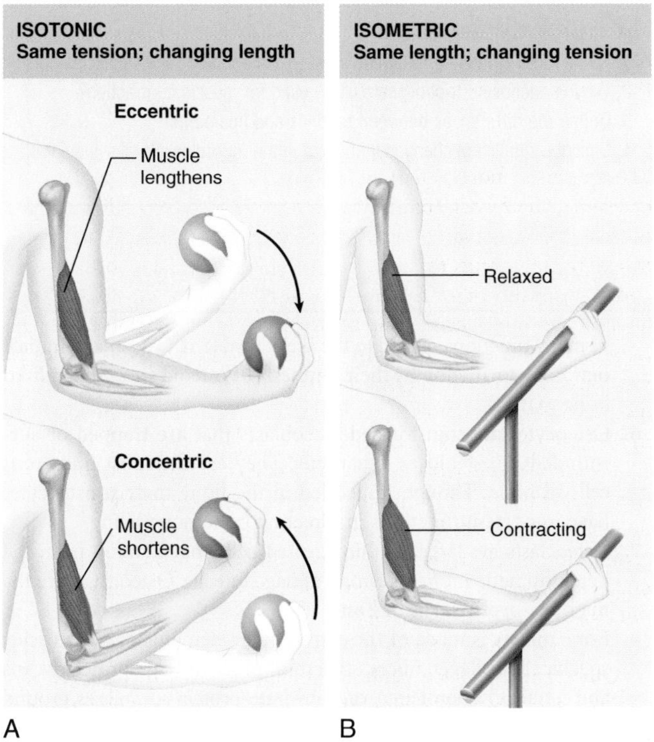

Tendons and Ligaments

Tendons are important musculoskeletal structures that attach muscle to bone at a site called an enthesis. Ligaments attach bone to bone, helping to form joints, as well as stabilizing them against excessive movement. Both tendons and ligaments are primarily composed of types III, IV, V, and VI collagen and fibroblasts (called tenocytes in tendons).

The fibroblasts in tendons are arranged in parallel rows; fibroblasts appear less organized in ligaments. Collagen fibers and fibroblasts form fascicles, with multiple fascicles then forming a whole tendon or ligament. In the proteoglycan matrix of tendons, collagen oligomeric matrix protein (COMP) assists in providing gliding and viscoelastic properties. Compared with tendons, ligament fibers typically contain a greater proportion of elastin.

Two main functions of tendons are (1) transferring forces from muscle to bone and (2) as a type of biologic spring for muscles to enable additional stability during movement. Ligaments stabilize joints by restricting movement. Although both tendons and ligaments can withstand significant distraction (stretching) force, they tend to buckle when compressive force is applied.

Both tendons and ligaments have complex structures at the attachment site of two dissimilar tissues. These complex structures and differences in mechanical and structural characteristics (either tendon and bone or ligament and bone) make healing and repair of damaged tissue complicated (see Did You Know? Tendon and Ligament Repair).

FIGURE 40.16 Isotonic and Isometric Contraction. A, In isotonic contraction, the muscle shortens, producing movement. B, In isometric contraction, the muscle pulls forcefully against a load but does not shorten. (From Patton KT, Thibodeau GA: *Structure & function of the body*, ed 15, St Louis, 2016, Mosby.)

DID YOU KNOW?
Tendon and Ligament Repair

Injury of tendons and ligaments is one of the greatest challenges in musculoskeletal rehabilitation. When these types of structures are damaged, attempts to engineer suitable tissue replacements have proved disappointing. The structures and intricate protein composition of tendons and ligaments are the basis for their complex biomechanical properties. One reason for a poor clinical outcome in synthetic tendon structures has been the inability to replicate any material that can bear the high mechanical stresses that occur at the interface between two dissimilar materials (i.e., either tendon and bone or ligament and bone). One promising area of investigation is finding or engineering a biodegradable material, or "scaffold," implanted with specific cells that would regenerate into normal tendon or ligament. The scaffold must be strong enough to withstand the forces at the tissue/bone interface and then gradually break down as it is completely replaced by new cells. Currently, investigators are using synthetic polymers, silk, and collagen as scaffolds, with tendon or ligament fibroblasts and mesenchymal stem cells as the implanted cells. Once these biochemical hurdles have been overcome, the repair of damaged tendons and ligaments will be revolutionized.

Data from Jahr H et al: *Curr Rheumatol Rep* 17(3):22, 2015.

AGING & THE MUSCULOSKELETAL SYSTEM

Aging of Bones

Aging is accompanied by the loss of bone tissue. Bones become less dense, less strong, and more brittle with aging. The bone remodeling cycle takes longer to complete, and the rate of mineralization also decelerates. With aging, women experience loss of bone density, accelerated by rapid bone loss during early menopause from increased osteoclastic bone resorption, fewer osteocytes, and decreased numbers of osteoblasts. By age 70 years, susceptible women have, on average, lost 50% of their peripheral cortical bone mass (see Chapter 41). Bone mass losses can lead to deformity, pain, stiffness, and high risk for fractures. Men also experience bone mass loss but at later ages and much slower rates than women. Also, initial bone mass in men is approximately 30% higher than in women; therefore bone loss in men causes less risk of disability than that found in women. Men's peak bone mass is related to race, heredity, hormonal factors, physical activity, and calcium intake during childhood. Bone loss in both sexes is related to smoking, calcium deficiency, alcohol intake, and physical inactivity. Bone mass can be gained in healthy young women up to the third decade through participation in physical activity, intake of dietary calcium and other minerals, and use of oral contraceptives. Height is also lost with aging because of intervertebral disk degeneration and, sometimes, osteoporotic spinal fractures.

Stem cells in the bone marrow perform less efficiently with aging, predisposing older persons to acute and chronic illnesses. Such illnesses cause weakness and confusion in older persons and may increase the risk of injury or falling.

Aging of Joints

With aging, cartilage becomes more rigid, fragile, and susceptible to fraying because of increased cross-linking of collagen and elastin, decreased water content in the cartilage ground substance, and reduced concentrations of glycosaminoglycans. Decreased range of motion of the joint is related to the changes in ligaments and muscles. Bones in joints develop evidence of osteoporosis, with fewer trabeculae and thinner, less dense bones, making them prone to fractures. Intervertebral disk spaces decrease in height. The rate of loss of height accelerates at age 70 years and beyond. Tendons shrink and harden.

Aging of Muscles

The function of skeletal muscle depends on many influences that are affected by cellular factors, such as reduced mitochondrial volume associated with aging. Other influences include the nervous, vascular, and endocrine systems. In the young child, the development of muscle tissue depends greatly on continuing neurodevelopmental maturation. Muscle loss begins at about age 50; however, muscle function remains trainable even into advanced age. Maintaining musculoskeletal fitness at any age can improve overall health.

Age-related loss in skeletal muscle is referred to as sarcopenia and is a direct cause of the age-related decrease in muscle strength. As the body ages, muscle mass and strength decline slowly; thus, strength is maintained through the fifth decade, with a slow decline in dynamic and isometric strength evident after age 70. The amount of type II fibers also decreases. There is reduced synthesis of RNA, loss of mitochondrial function, and reduction in the size of motor units. The regenerative function of muscle tissue remains normal in aging persons. As much as 30% to 40% of skeletal muscle mass and strength may be lost from the third to ninth decades. Muscle fatigue also may contribute to loss of function with aging. Sarcopenia is thought to be secondary to progressive neuromuscular changes and diminishing levels of anabolic hormones. There is an age-related decline in the synthesis of mixed proteins, myosin heavy chains, and mitochondrial protein. Changes in these muscle proteins are related to reduced levels of insulin-like growth factor-1 (IGF-1), testosterone, and dehydroepiandrosterone (DHEA) sulfate.

Maximal oxygen intake declines with age. The basal metabolic rate is reduced, and lean body mass decreases in the aged population.

> ✔ **QUICK CHECK 40.3**
> 1. Name three differences between slow-twitch and fast-twitch muscle fibers.
> 2. Why is adenosine triphosphate (ATP) used for muscle contraction?
> 3. Define the differences between tendons and ligaments.
> 4. Describe significant changes that occur in the musculoskeletal system with aging.

▮ SUMMARY REVIEW

Structure and Function of Bones

1. Bones provide support and protection for the body's tissues and organs and are important sources of minerals and blood cells. Bones permit movement by providing points of attachment for muscles.

2. Mature bone is a rigid connective tissue consisting of cells (growth, repair, synthesis, and resorption of old tissue); collagen fibers (tensile strength); a homogenous gelatinous medium called *ground substance* (diffusion); and large amounts of crystallized minerals, mainly calcium (rigidity).

3. Bone formation begins with the production of an organic matrix by bone cells. Bone minerals crystallize in and around collagen fibers in the matrix, called *calcification*, giving bone its characteristic hardness and strength.

4. Bone contains three types of cells: osteoblasts, osteocytes, and osteoclasts. These allow bone tissue to be continuously synthesized, remodeled, and resorbed.

5. Osteoblasts are cells derived from osteogenic mesenchymal stem cells; they are the primary bone-producing cells and are involved

in many functions related to the skeletal system. Osteoblasts initiate new bone formation by their synthesis of osteoid (nonmineralized bone matrix).

6. Osteocytes are transformed osteoblasts that are trapped or surrounded in osteoid as it hardens. They are the most numerous cells in bone. Though imbedded in the bone matrix, osteocytes have important functions in directing bone remodeling.

7. Osteoclasts are large, multinucleated cells that develop from the hematopoietic monocyte-macrophage lineage. Osteoclasts are the major resorptive cells of bone.

8. Bone matrix is made of the extracellular elements of bone tissue, specifically collagen fibers, structural proteins (e.g., proteoglycans and certain glycoproteins), carbohydrate-protein complexes, ground substance, and minerals.

9. Bones in the body are made up of compact (cortical) bone tissue and spongy (cancellous) bone tissue.

10. Compact bone is highly organized, solid, and extremely strong. The basic structural units are the haversian systems that consist of concentric layers of crystallized matrix called *lamellae*, surrounding

a central canal that contains blood vessels and nerves. Dispersed throughout the concentric layers of crystallized matrix are small spaces, called *lacunae,* containing osteocytes. Smaller canals, called *canaliculi,* interconnect the osteocyte-containing spaces.

11. The crystallized matrix in spongy bone is arranged in bars or plates called *trabeculae.* Spaces containing osteocytes are dispersed between the bars or plates and interconnected by canaliculi.

12. There are 206 bones in the body, divided into the axial skeleton and the appendicular skeleton. Bones are classified by shape as long, short, flat, or irregular. Long bones have a broad end (epiphysis), broad neck (metaphysis), and narrow midportion (diaphysis) that contains the medullary cavity.

13. The internal structure of bone is maintained by remodeling, a process in which existing bone is resorbed and new bone is laid down to replace it. Clusters of bone precursor cells, called *basic multicellular units,* implement remodeling.

14. Bone injuries are repaired in stages: (1) hematoma formation occurs within hours of fracture or surgery, (2) procallus formation by osteoblasts occurs within days, (3) callus formation occurs within weeks, and (4) replacement and (5) remodeling occur within years. Remodeling restores the original shape and size to the injured bone.

Structure and Function of Joints

1. A joint, or articulation, is the site where two or more bones attach. Joints provide stability and mobility to the skeleton. Joints help move bones and muscle.

2. Joints are classified as synarthroses (immovable), amphiarthroses (slightly moveable), or diarthroses (freely movable), depending on the degree of movement they allow.

3. Joints are also classified by the type of connecting tissue holding them together. Fibrous joints are connected by dense fibrous tissue, ligaments, or membranes. Cartilaginous joints are connected by fibrocartilage or hyaline cartilage. Synovial joints are connected by a fibrous joint capsule that contains a small fluid-filled space. The fluid in the space nourishes the articular cartilage that covers the ends of the bones meeting in the synovial joint.

4. Articular cartilage is a highly organized system of collagen fibers and proteoglycans. The fibers firmly anchor the cartilage to the bone, and the proteoglycans control the loss of fluid from the cartilage.

Structure and Function of Skeletal Muscles

1. *Myoblasts* are precursor cells that become muscle cells.

2. Whole muscles vary in size (2 to 60 cm) and shape (fusiform, pennate). They are encased in a three-part connective tissue framework, called *fascia,* that protects the muscle fibers, attaches the muscle to bone, and provides a structure for a network of nerve fibers, blood vessels, and lymphatic channels.

3. The fundamental concept of muscle function is the motor unit, defined as the muscle fibers innervated by a single motor nerve, its axon, and anterior horn cell.

4. Satellite cells are dormant myoblasts; however, when activated, they can regenerate muscle.

5. Skeletal muscle is made up of millions of individual muscle fibers, each of which is a single, cylindrical muscle cell. Muscle fibers contain bundles of myofibrils arranged in parallel along the longitudinal axis and include the muscle membrane, myofibrils, sarcotubular system, sarcoplasm, and mitochondria.

6. There are two types of muscle fibers, type I and type II, determined by motor nerve innervation.

7. Myofibrils and myofilaments contain the major muscle proteins actin and myosin, which interact to form cross-bridges during muscle contraction. The nonprotein muscle constituents provide an energy source for contraction and regulate protein synthesis and enzyme systems, as well as stabilize cell membranes.

8. Muscle contraction includes (1) excitation, (2) coupling, (3) contraction, and (4) relaxation.

9. Skeletal muscle requires a constant supply of ATP and phosphocreatine to fuel muscle contraction and for growth and repair. ATP and phosphocreatine can be generated aerobically or anaerobically.

10. Motor units contract in an all-or-nothing manner, so the contraction generated will be the maximal contraction. Efficiency of muscle contraction is affected by muscle fiber type, innervation ratio, temperature, and muscle shape.

11. There are two types of muscle contraction. In isometric (static) contraction, the muscle maintains a constant length as tension is increased. In dynamic (formerly called isotonic) contraction, the muscle maintains a constant tension as it moves, either lengthening (eccentric contraction) or shortening (concentric contraction).

12. Muscles act in groups. When a muscle contracts and acts as a prime mover, or agonist, its reciprocal muscle, or antagonist, relaxes.

13. Tendons attach muscle to bone at sites called *entheses.* Ligaments attach bone to bone, helping to form joints and stabilizing them against excessive movement. Both tendons and ligaments are mostly composed of types III, IV, V, and VI collagen and fibroblasts (called tenocytes in tendons).

Aging & the Musculoskeletal System

1. Bones become less dense, less strong, and more brittle with aging. The bone remodeling cycle takes longer to complete, and the rate of mineralization also decelerates.

2. With aging, cartilage becomes more rigid, fragile, and susceptible to fraying. Decreased range of motion of the joint is related to the changes in ligaments and muscles.

3. The regenerative function of muscle tissue and the trainability of muscle function remains normal in elderly persons.

4. Sarcopenia, or age-related loss of skeletal muscle, is a direct cause of decrease in muscle strength. A slow decline in dynamic and isometric strength is evident after age 70 years.

5. As much as 30% to 40% of skeletal muscle mass and strength may be lost from the third to ninth decades. Muscle fatigue also may contribute to loss of function with aging. A reduced basal metabolic rate and decreased lean body mass are also noted in the elderly population.

KEY TERMS

A cell (macrophage), 940
Agonist, 951
Alpha-glycoprotein (α-glycoprotein), 937
Amphiarthrosis (slightly movable joint), 940

Antagonist, 951
Appendicular skeleton, 938
Articular cartilage, 942
Axial skeleton, 938
B cell (fibroblast), 940
Basement membrane, 946

Basic multicellular unit, 939
Bone albumin, 937
Bone fluid, 937
Bone matrix, 933
Calcification, 933
Canaliculus (pl., canaliculi), 937

Chondrocyte, 942
Collagen fiber, 937
Compact bone (cortical bone), 937
Concentric (shortening) contraction, 951

REFERENCES

1. Jimi E, Fukushima H: NF-κB signaling pathways and the future perspectives of bone disease therapy using selective inhibitors of NF-κB, *Clin Calcium* 26(2):298-304, 2016.
2. Atkins GJ, Findlay DM: Osteocyte regulation of bone mineral: a little give and take, *Osteoporos Int* 23(8):2067-2079, 2012.
3. Honma M, et al: Regulatory mechanisms of RANKL presentation to osteoclast precursors, *Curr Osteoporos Rep* 12(1):115-120, 2014.
4. Bellido T: Osteocyte-driven bone remodeling, *Calcif Tissue Int* 94:25-34, 2014.
5. Komori T: Functions of the osteocyte network in the regulation of bone mass, *Cell Tissue Res* 352:191-198, 2013.
6. Sapir-Koren R, Livshits G: Osteocyte control of bone remodeling: is sclerostin a key molecular coordinator of the balanced bone resorption-formation cycles?, *Osteoprors Int* 25:2685-2700, 2014.

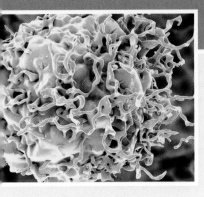

41

Alterations of Musculoskeletal Function

Benjamin A. Smallheer

EVOLVE WEBSITE

CHAPTER OUTLINE

Musculoskeletal injuries include fractures, dislocations, sprains, and strains. Metabolic disorders, infections, inflammatory or noninflammatory diseases, or tumors may cause alterations in bones, joints, and muscles. The most common disease affecting bone is osteoporosis; much attention and debate has been focused on its risk factors and pathophysiology. Soft tissue disorders—including muscle, tendon, and ligament injuries; tumors; and metabolic derangements—also affect the musculoskeletal system.

MUSCULOSKELETAL INJURIES

Trauma is referred to as the "neglected disease." It is the leading cause of death in people ages 1 to 44 years of all races and socioeconomic levels. Each year, more than 120,000 persons in the United States die from unintentional injuries.[1]

Musculoskeletal injuries have a major impact on the affected individuals, families, and society in general because of the physical and psychological effects of limitation on mobility and daily activities, pain, and decreased quality of life. In addition, there are direct costs of diagnosis and treatments, and indirect economic costs related to loss of employment and decreased productivity.

Skeletal Trauma

Fractures

A fracture is a break in the continuity of a bone. A break occurs when force is applied that exceeds the tensile or compressive strength of the bone. The incidence of fractures varies for individual bones according to age and sex with the highest incidence of fractures in young males (between the ages of 15 and 24 years) and older persons (65 years of age or older). Fractures of healthy bones, particularly the tibia, clavicle, and lower humerus, tend to occur in young persons as the result of trauma. Fractures of the hands and feet are often caused by accidents in the workplace. The incidence of fractures of the upper femur, upper humerus, vertebrae, and pelvis is highest in older adults and often is associated with osteoporosis (see the Osteoporosis section). Hip fractures, the most serious outcome of osteoporosis, have a wide variation in geographic occurrence.

Classification of fractures. There are numerous classification systems for various types of fractures, but the simplest systems describe the basic features of the broken bone. Fractures can be classified as complete or incomplete and as open or closed (Fig. 41.1). In a complete fracture the bone is broken entirely, whereas in an incomplete fracture the bone is damaged but is still in one piece. Complete and incomplete fractures also can be called open (formerly referred to as compound) if the skin is open and closed (formerly called simple or incomplete) if it is not. A fracture in which a bone breaks into more than two fragments is termed a comminuted fracture. Fractures are also classified according to the direction of the fracture line. A linear fracture runs parallel to the long axis of the bone. An oblique fracture occurs at a slanted angle to the shaft of the bone. A spiral fracture encircles the bone, and a transverse fracture occurs straight across the bone.

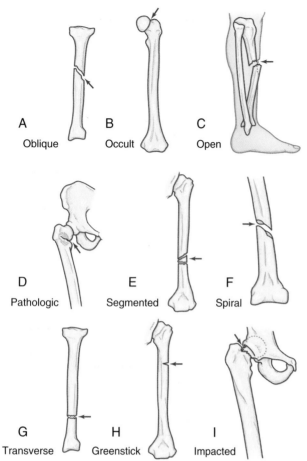

FIGURE 41.1 Examples of Types of Bone Fractures. A, *Oblique:* Fracture at oblique angle across both cortices. *Cause:* Direct or indirect energy, with angulation and some compression. **B,** *Occult:* Fracture that is hidden or not readily discernible. *Cause:* Minor force or energy. **C,** *Open:* Skin broken over fracture; possible soft tissue trauma. *Cause:* Moderate to severe energy that is continuous and exceeds tissue tolerance. **D,** *Pathologic:* Transverse, oblique, or spiral fracture of bone weakened by tumor pressure or presence. *Cause:* Minor energy or force, which may be direct or indirect. **E,** *Segmented:* Fracture with two or more pieces or segments. *Cause:* Direct or indirect moderate to severe force. **F,** *Spiral:* Fracture that curves around cortices and may become displaced by twist. *Cause:* Direct or indirect twisting energy or force with distal part held or unable to move. **G,** *Transverse:* Horizontal break through bone. *Cause:* Direct or indirect energy toward bone. **H,** *Greenstick:* Break in only one cortex of bone. *Cause:* Minor direct or indirect energy. **I,** *Impacted:* Fracture with one end wedged into opposite end of inside fractured fragment. *Cause:* Compressive axial energy or force directly to distal fragment. (Redrawn from Mourad L: Musculoskeletal system. In Thompson JM et al, editors: *Mosby's clinical nursing,* ed 7, St Louis, 2002, Mosby.)

Incomplete fractures tend to occur in the more flexible, growing bones of children. The three main types of incomplete fractures are greenstick, torus, and bowing fractures. A **greenstick fracture** perforates one cortex and splinters the spongy bone. The name is derived from the damage sustained by a young tree branch (a green stick) when it is bent sharply. The outer surface is disrupted, but the inner surface remains intact. Greenstick fractures typically occur in the metaphysis or diaphysis of the tibia, radius, and ulna. In a **torus fracture,** the cortex buckles but does not break. **Bowing fractures** usually occur when longitudinal force is applied to bone. This type of fracture is common

TABLE 41.1   **Types of Fractures**

Type of Fracture	Definition
Typical Complete Fractures	
Closed	Noncommunicating wound between bone and skin
Open	Communicating wound between bone and skin
Comminuted	Multiple bone fragments
Linear	Fracture line parallel to long axis of bone
Oblique	Fracture line at an angle to long axis of bone
Spiral	Fracture line encircling bone (as a spiral staircase)
Transverse	Fracture line perpendicular to long axis of bone
Impacted	Fracture fragments pushed into each other
Pathologic	Fracture at a point where bone has been weakened by disease, for example, by tumors or osteoporosis
Avulsion	Fragment of bone connected to a ligament or tendon detaches from main bone
Compression	Fracture wedged or squeezed together on one side of bone
Displaced	Fracture with one, both, or all fragments out of normal alignment
Extracapsular	Fragment close to joint but remains outside joint capsule
Intracapsular	Fragment within joint capsule
Typical Incomplete Fractures	
Greenstick	Break in one cortex of bone with splintering of inner bone surface; commonly occurs in children and elderly persons
Torus	Buckling of cortex
Bowing	Bending of bone
Stress	Microfracture
Transchondral	Separation of cartilaginous joint surface (articular cartilage) from main shaft of bone

in children and usually involves the paired radius-ulna or the fibula-tibia. A complete diaphyseal fracture occurs in one of the bones of the pair, which disperses the stress sufficiently to prevent a complete fracture of the second bone, which bows rather than breaks. A bowing fracture resists correction (**reduction**) because the force necessary to reduce it must be equal to the force that bowed it. Treatment of bowing fractures is also difficult because the bowed bone interferes with reduction of the fractured bone. Types of fractures are summarized in Table 41.1.

Fractures may be further classified by cause as pathologic, stress, or transchondral fractures. A **pathologic** (also known as **insufficiency** or **fragility**) **fracture** is a break at the site of a preexisting abnormality, resulting from force that would not fracture a normal bone. In any bone that lacks normal ability to deform and recover, these fractures can occur with normal weight bearing or activity. Rheumatoid arthritis, osteoporosis, Paget disease, osteomalacia, rickets, hyperparathyroidism, and radiation therapy all cause bone to lose its normal ability to deform and recover. Pathologic fractures are generally a result of bone weakness caused by another disease, such as cancer, metabolic bone disorders, or infection. Although usually considered insufficiency fractures, breaks in the bone attributable to osteoporosis can also be referred to as pathologic fractures. Any disease process that weakens a bone (especially the cortex) predisposes the bone to pathologic fracture.

During activities that subject a bone to repeated strain, such as certain types of sports, a **stress fracture** can occur in normal or abnormal bone. The forces placed on the bone are cumulative, eventually causing a fracture. A **fatigue fracture** is caused by repetitive, sometimes abnormal stress or torque applied to a bone with a normal ability to deform and recover. Fatigue fractures usually occur in individuals who engage in a new or different activity that is both strenuous and repetitive (e.g., joggers, skaters, dancers, military recruits). Because gains in muscle strength occur more rapidly than gains in bone strength, the newly developed muscles place exaggerated stress on the bones that are not yet ready for the additional stress. The imbalance between muscle and bone development causes microfractures to develop in the cortex. If the activity is controlled and increased gradually, new bone formation catches up to the increased demands and microfractures do not occur.

A **transchondral fracture** consists of fragmentation and separation of a portion of the articular cartilage. (Joint structures are defined in Chapter 40.) Single or multiple sites may be fractured, and the fragments may consist of cartilage alone or cartilage and bone. Typical sites of transchondral fracture are the distal femur, the ankle, the patella, the elbow, and the wrist. Transchondral fractures are most prevalent in adolescents.

PATHOPHYSIOLOGY   Fracture healing is a complex process that occurs primarily in one of two ways: direct or indirect healing.[2] Both types of healing require integration of cells, signaling pathways, and various molecules. In **direct** (or **primary**) **healing,** intramembranous bone formation occurs when adjacent bone cortices are in contact with one another, such as when surgical fixation devices are used. No callus formation occurs with direct bone healing. **Indirect** (or **secondary**) **healing** involves both intramembranous and endochondral bone formation, development of callus, and eventual remodeling of solid bone. Bone formation that begins with an underlying cartilage scaffold is termed **endochondral bone formation.**

A hallmark of indirect fracture healing is the formation of callus. Indirect fracture healing is most often observed when a fracture is treated with a cast. When a bone is broken, the periosteum and blood vessels in the cortex, marrow, and surrounding soft tissues are disrupted. Bleeding occurs from the damaged ends of the bone and from the neighboring soft tissue. A clot (hematoma) forms within the medullary canal, between the fractured ends of the bone, and beneath the periosteum (Fig. 41.2). Bone tissue immediately adjacent to the fracture dies. This dead tissue (along with any debris in the fracture area) stimulates vasodilation, exudation of plasma and leukocytes, and infiltration by inflammatory leukocytes, growth factors, and mast cells that simultaneously decalcify the fractured bone ends. Within 48 hours after injury, vascular tissue from surrounding soft tissue and the marrow cavity invades the fracture area, and blood flow to the entire bone increases. Bone-forming cells in the periosteum, endosteum, and marrow are activated to produce subperiosteal procallus along the outer surface of the shaft and over the broken ends of the bone (Fig. 41.2). Osteoblasts within the procallus synthesize collagen and matrix, which becomes mineralized to form callus. As the repair process continues, remodeling occurs, during which unnecessary callus is resorbed and trabeculae are formed along lines of stress as the repair tissues align with the tissue cells of the host (Fig. 41.3).

CLINICAL MANIFESTATIONS   The signs and symptoms of a fracture include unnatural alignment (deformity), swelling, muscle spasm, tenderness, pain and impaired sensation, and decreased mobility. The position of the broken bone segments is determined by the pull of attached muscles, gravity, and the direction and magnitude of the force that caused the fracture.

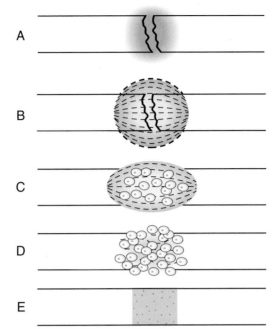

FIGURE 41.2 Schematic of Bone Healing. A, Bleeding at broken ends of the bone with subsequent hematoma formation. **B,** Organization of hematoma into fibrous network. **C,** Invasion of osteoblasts, lengthening of collagen strands, and deposition of calcium. **D,** Callus formation; new bone is built while osteoclasts destroy dead bone. **E,** Remodeling is accomplished while excess callus is reabsorbed and trabecular bone is deposited. (From Monahan FD et al: *Phipps' medical-surgical nursing: health and illness perspectives,* ed 8, St Louis, 2007, Mosby.)

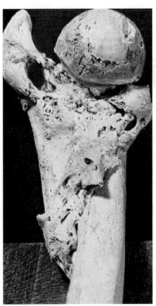

FIGURE 41.3 Exuberant Callus Formation After Fracture. (From Rosai J: *Ackerman's surgical pathology,* ed 8, St Louis, 1996, Mosby.)

Immediately after a bone is fractured, there often is numbness at the fracture site because of trauma to the nerve or nerves at the injury site. The numbness may last several minutes, during which time the injured person can continue to use the fractured bone. However, once the numbness dissipates, the subsequent pain is quite severe and may be incapacitating until relieved with medication and treatment of the fracture. Pain can be caused by muscle spasms at the fracture site, overriding of the fracture segments, or damage to adjacent soft tissues.

Pathologic fractures can cause angular deformity, painless swelling, or generalized bone pain. Stress fractures are painful because of accelerated remodeling; initially, pain occurs during activity and is usually relieved by rest. Stress fractures also cause local tenderness and soft tissue swelling. Transchondral fractures may be entirely asymptomatic or may be painful during movement. Range of motion in the joint is limited, and movement may evoke audible clicking sounds (crepitus).

EVALUATION AND TREATMENT Adequate immobilization with a splint or cast is often all that is required for healing of fractures that are *not* misaligned. Treatment of a displaced fracture involves realigning the bone fragments (reduction) close to their normal or anatomic position and holding the fragments in place (immobilization) so that bone union can occur. Several methods are available to reduce a fracture: closed manipulation, traction, and open reduction. Many displaced fractures can be reduced by closed manipulation and reduction. The bone is moved or manipulated into place without opening the skin. Closed reduction is used when the contour of the bone is in fair anatomic alignment and can be manually placed into normal alignment, and then maintained with immobilization. Splints and casts are used to immobilize and hold a closed reduction in place.

Traction may be used to accomplish or maintain reduction. When bone fragments are displaced (not in their anatomic position), weights may be used to apply firm, steady traction (pull) and countertraction to the long axis of the bone. Traction stretches and fatigues muscles that have pulled the bone fragments out of place, more readily allowing the distal fragment to align with the proximal fragment. Traction can be applied to the skin (skin traction) or directly to the involved bone (skeletal traction). Skin traction is used when only a few pounds of pulling force are needed to realign the fragments or when the traction will be used only for a brief time, such as before surgery or, for children with femoral fractures, for 3 to 7 days before a cast is applied. In skeletal traction, a pin or wire is drilled through the bone distal to the fracture site, and a traction bow, rope, and weights are attached to the pin or wire to apply tension and to provide the pulling force required to overcome the muscle spasm and help realign the fracture fragments. More often, surgical repair (open reduction and internal fixation) or external fixation devices are used to realign displaced fractures.

Open reduction is a surgical procedure that exposes the fracture site; the fragments are then manipulated into alignment under direct visualization. Some form of hardware, such as a screw, plate, nail, or wire, is used to maintain the reduction (internal fixation). External fixation, a procedure in which pins or rods are surgically placed into uninjured bone near the fracture site and then stabilized with an external frame of bars, is another method used to treat fractures that would not be adequately stabilized with a cast. Bone grafts—using donor bone from the individual (autograft), a cadaver (allograft), or bone substitutes (ceramic composites, bioactive cement)—can fill voids in the bone.

Improper reduction or immobilization of a fractured bone may result in nonunion, delayed union, or malunion. Nonunion is failure of the bone ends to grow together. The gap between the broken ends of the bone fills with dense fibrous and fibrocartilaginous tissue instead of new bone. Occasionally, the fibrous tissue contains a fluid-filled space that resembles a joint and is termed a *false joint*, or *pseudoarthrosis*. Delayed union is union that does not occur until approximately 8 to 9 months after a fracture. Malunion is the healing of a bone in an incorrect anatomic position.

Dislocation and Subluxation

Dislocation and subluxation are usually caused by trauma. Dislocation is the displacement of one or more bones in a joint in which the opposing joint surfaces entirely lose contact with one another. If contact between the opposing joint surfaces is only partially lost (partial dislocation), the injury is called a subluxation.

Dislocation and subluxation are most common in persons younger than 20 years of age and are generally associated with fractures. However, they also may be the result of congenital or acquired disorders that cause (1) muscular imbalance, seen with congenital dislocation of the hip; (2) incongruities in the articulating surfaces of the bones, as occur with rheumatoid arthritis (see the Rheumatoid Arthritis section); or (3) joint instability.

The joints most often dislocated or subluxated are the joints of the shoulder, elbow, wrist, finger, hip, and knee. The shoulder joint most often injured is the glenohumeral joint. Finger dislocations are common injuries in contact sports such as basketball, football, and rugby.

Traumatic dislocation of the elbow joint is common in the immature skeleton ("nursemaid's elbow"). In adults, an elbow dislocation is usually associated with a fracture of the ulna or head of the radius. Traumatic dislocation of the wrist usually involves the distal ulna and carpal bones. Any one of the eight carpal bones can be dislocated after an injury. Dislocation in the hand usually involves the metacarpophalangeal and interphalangeal joints.

Considerable trauma is needed to dislocate the hip. Anterior hip dislocation is rare in healthy persons; it is caused by forced abduction; for example, when an individual lands on his or her feet after falling from an elevated height. Posterior dislocation of the hip can occur as a result of an automobile accident in which the flexed knee strikes the dashboard, causing the head of the femur to be pushed posteriorly from the hip joint.

The knee is an unstable weight-bearing joint that depends heavily on the soft tissue structures around it for support. It is exposed to many different types of motion (flexion, extension, rotation) and is one of the most commonly injured joints. A knee dislocation can be anterior, posterior, lateral, medial, or rotary. It is often the result of an injury that occurs during contact sports activities, such as soccer, lacrosse, or football.

PATHOPHYSIOLOGY Dislocations and subluxations are often accompanied by fracture because stress is placed on areas of bone not usually subjected to stress. In addition, as the joint loses its normal congruity, there may be bruising or tearing of adjacent nerves, blood vessels, ligaments, supporting structures, and soft tissue. Dislocations of the shoulder may damage the shoulder capsule and the axillary nerve. Damage to axillary nerves can cause anesthesia or dysesthesia in the sensory distribution of the nerve and paralysis of the deltoid muscle. Dislocations also may disrupt circulation, leading to ischemia and possibly even permanent disability of the affected extremity tissues.

CLINICAL MANIFESTATIONS Signs and symptoms of dislocations or subluxations include pain, swelling, limitation of motion, and joint deformity. Pain may be caused by effusion of inflammatory exudate into the joint or by associated tendon and ligament injury. Joint deformity is typically caused by muscle contractions that exert pull on the dislocated or subluxated joint. Limitation of motion results from effusion into the joint or the displacement of bones.

EVALUATION AND TREATMENT Evaluation of dislocations and subluxations is based on clinical manifestations and radiographic evaluation. Treatment consists of reduction and immobilization for 2 to 6 weeks to allow healing of damaged structures, followed by exercises to restore normal range of motion in the joint. Depending on the joint and severity of injury, complete healing can take months to sometimes years.

Support Structures
Sprains and Strains of Tendons and Ligaments

Tendons and ligaments support the bones and joints and either facilitate or limit motion, respectively. Either structure can be completely separated from bone at its points of attachment, torn, lacerated, or ruptured. Tendon and ligament injuries often accompany fractures and dislocations. A tendon is fibrous connective tissue that attaches skeletal muscle to either bone or another structure; the area of attachment on a bone is called an enthesis. Functionally, muscles and tendons work together as a single, integrated unit allowing motion. A ligament is a band of fibrous connective tissue that connects bones where they meet in a joint. The structural composition of tendons and ligaments are similar. The primary difference between tendons and ligaments is their anatomic function and location.

Tearing or stretching of a muscle or tendon is commonly known as a strain. Major trauma can tear or rupture a tendon at any site in the body. The tendons most commonly injured are those of the hands and feet, the knee (patellar), the upper arm (biceps and triceps), the thigh (hamstring), the ankle, and the heel (Achilles).

Ligament tears are commonly known as sprains. Ligament tears and ruptures can occur at any joint but are most common in the wrist, ankle, elbow, and knee joints. A complete separation of a tendon or ligament from its bony attachment site is known as an avulsion and is commonly seen in young athletes, especially sprinters, hurdlers, and distance runners.

Strains and sprains are classified as first degree (mild), second degree (moderate), and third degree (severe). In first-degree injuries, the fibers are stretched but the muscle (strain) or joint (sprain) remains stable. In second-degree strains or sprains, there is more tearing of the tendon or ligament fibers, resulting in muscle weakness or some joint instability and incomplete tearing of fibers. Third-degree strains and sprains result in a full tearing of fibers, creating an inability to contract the muscle normally (strain) or cause significant joint instability (sprain).

PATHOPHYSIOLOGY   When a tendon or ligament is torn, an inflammatory exudate develops between the torn ends. Within 4 to 5 days after the injury, collagen formation begins. As the collagen fibers interweave and connect with preexisting tendon fibers, they become organized parallel to the lines of the musculotendinous unit. Eventually vascular fibrous tissue fuses the new and surrounding tissues into a single mass. Collagen fibers reconnect the tendon and bone, forming a new enthesis. It may take more than 3 months for the new enthesis to achieve mechanical stability of a joint. If powerful muscle contractions occur during healing, the tendon or ligament ends may separate again, which causes the tendon or ligament to heal in a lengthened shape or with an excessive amount of scar tissue, resulting in poor tendon or ligament function.

CLINICAL MANIFESTATIONS   Tendon and ligament injuries are painful and are usually accompanied by soft tissue swelling, changes in tendon or ligament contour, and dislocation or subluxation of bones. Pain is generally sharp and localized, and tenderness persists over the distribution of the tendon or ligament. Movement or weight bearing increases pain. Even with prompt treatment, depending on the tendon or ligament involved, significant injuries may result in decreased mobility, instability, and weakness of the affected joints.

EVALUATION AND TREATMENT   Evaluation is based on the mechanism of injury and the clinical manifestations. Stress radiography, arthroscopy, or arthrography also may be considered. Initial treatment consists of protection, rest, ice, compression, and elevation (PRICE) for the first 48 to 72 hours. Once swelling and acute pain subside, in most cases support of the affected tendon or ligament with a compression dressing or brace will provide appropriate reinforcement while the tissues heal. Rehabilitation is crucial to regaining a good functional outcome. In severe (third-degree) injuries, treatment may include surgical intervention to suture the tendon or ligament ends in close approximation with one another or the enthesis. If this is not feasible because of the extent of damage, tendon or ligament grafting may be necessary. Prolonged, functional rehabilitation programs help ensure return of near-normal functioning, but recovery may be complicated by posttraumatic arthritis.

Tendinopathy, Epicondylopathy, and Bursitis

Trauma also can cause painful inflammation of tendons (tendinopathy [tendonitis]) and bursae (bursitis). Other causes of damage to tendons include reduced tissue perfusion, mechanical irritation, crystal deposits, postural misalignment, and hypermobility of a joint. Thus, *tendinopathy* is a more accurate term than *tendonitis* in most cases. Microvascular and increased nerve growth often occur to these areas which increases the body's transmission of pain sensations.

The histopathology of common conditions, such as lateral epicondylopathy ("tennis elbow") or medial epicondylopathy ("golfer's elbow"), is a degenerative process[3] (Fig. 41.4). A bony prominence at the end of a bone where tendons or ligaments attach is termed an epicondyle.

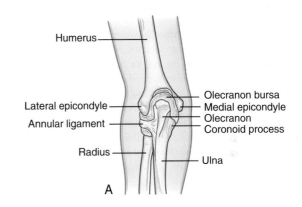

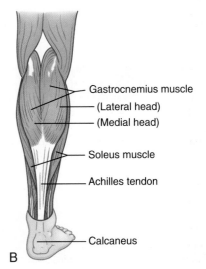

FIGURE 41.4 Epicondylopathy and Tendinopathy. A, Lateral and medial epicondyles of the distal humerus, sites of tennis elbow (lateral) and golfer's elbow (medial). B, Achilles tendon, common site of tendinopathy.

When force is sufficient to cause microscopic tears (microtears) in tissue, the result is known as tendinopathy or epicondylopathy. Microtears in the tendon, the presence of disorganized collagen fibers, and neovascularization indicate incomplete tissue repair. Initial inflammatory changes cause thickening of the tendon sheath, limited movements, and pain. Microtears cause bleeding, edema, and pain in the involved tendon or tendons.

Lateral epicondylopathy (tennis elbow) is caused by irritation and overstretching of the extensor carpi radialis brevis (ECRB) tendon and forearm extensor muscles, resulting in tissue degradation, loss of grip strength, and pain. Medial epicondylopathy (golfer's elbow) is the result of similar forces affecting the forearm muscles responsible for forearm flexion and pronation (see Fig. 41.4). Repetitive load-bearing activities or acute injuries that involve flexion, extension, pronation, or supination of the elbow and forearm can lead to either lateral or medial elbow symptoms.

Clinical manifestations of epicondylopathy are usually localized to one side of the joint. In general, there is local tenderness and more pain with active motion than with passive motion. With tendinopathy or tendonitis, the pain is localized over the involved tendon. Stressing the tendon with simple activities, such as lifting even a few pounds of weight, can increase pain. Pain and sometimes weakness limit joint movement.

Bursae are small sacs lined with synovial membrane and filled with synovial fluid that are located between bony prominences and soft tissues such as tendons, muscles, and ligaments (Fig. 41.5). Bursae can be either "constant" (those formed during embryologic development) or "adventitious" (bursae that develop as a result of chronic friction and degeneration of fibrous tissue between adjacent structures). The primary function of a bursa is to separate, lubricate, and cushion these structures. When irritated or injured, these sacs become inflamed and swell. Because most bursae lie outside joints, joint movement is rarely compromised with bursitis. Acute bursitis occurs primarily during middle age and is caused by trauma. Chronic bursitis can result from repeated trauma. Septic bursitis is caused by wound infection or bacterial infection of the skin overlying the bursae. Bursitis commonly occurs in the shoulder, hip, knee, and elbow but also can affect the spine, wrist, foot, and ankle.

PATHOPHYSIOLOGY Bursitis usually is an inflammation that is reactive to overuse or excessive pressure but also can be caused by infection, autoimmune diseases, crystal deposition, or acute trauma. The inflamed bursal sac becomes engorged, and the inflammation can spread to adjacent tissues. The inflammation may decrease with rest, ice, and aspiration of the fluid. (Inflammation is discussed in Chapter 6.)

CLINICAL MANIFESTATIONS Joint motion is rarely limited in bursitis, except by pain. Shoulder pain may impair arm abduction. Bursitis in the knee produces pain when climbing stairs, and crossing the legs is painful in bursitis of the hip. Lying on the side of the inflamed trochanteric bursa is also very painful. Signs of infectious bursitis may include the presence of pain, warmth and erythema, severe inflammation, or an adjacent source of infection, such as from total joint replacement surgery. Prior corticosteroid injections or evidence of a puncture site at the joint increases the potential for infectious bursitis.

EVALUATION AND TREATMENT The diagnosis of tendinopathy, epicondylopathy, and bursitis is primarily based on the clinical history and physical examination. Other imaging techniques, such as ultrasound or magnetic resonance imaging (MRI), may be used to evaluate the severity of the problem. Treatment may include temporary immobilization of the joint with a sling, splint, or cast; administration of systemic analgesics; application of ice or heat; or local injection of an anesthetic, a corticosteroid, platelet-rich plasma (PRP), or a combination local anesthetic/corticosteroid. Physical therapy to prevent loss of function begins after acute inflammation subsides (*Did You Know?* Managing Tendinopathy).

Muscle Strains

Muscle strain is a general term for local muscle damage. Mild injury, such as muscle strain, is usually seen after traumatic or sports injuries. It is often the result of sudden, forced motion causing the muscle to become stretched beyond normal capacity. Strains often involve the tendon as well. Penetrating injuries, such as knife and gunshot wounds, can cause traumatic rupture (see Chapter 4). The incidence of muscle rupture is greater in young people. However, tendon rupture occurs with greater frequency in the older population. Muscle strain may be chronic when the muscle is repeatedly stretched beyond its usual capacity. Tissue biopsy of a muscle experiencing chronic strain reveals evidence of tissue disruption with subsequent signs of muscle regeneration and connective tissue repair. Hemorrhage into the surrounding tissue and signs of inflammation also may be present.

Muscle healing occurs in three phases:

1. Destruction, in which the myofibers of the damaged muscle contract and necrose, beginning an inflammatory reaction. The gap between torn fibers is filled by a hematoma.
2. Repair, which begins with monocytes phagocytizing the dead tissue and activating satellite cells, which become myoblasts. The myoblasts infiltrate the scar tissue, and new capillary formation begins at the site of injury. The first two phases occur within a week of injury.
3. Remodeling occurs as the myofibers mature, form contractile tissue, and attach to the ends of scar tissue. Regeneration may take up to 6 weeks, and the affected muscle should be protected during that time.

Degrees of acute muscle strain, together with their manifestations and treatment, are summarized in Table 41.2.

A late complication of some muscle injuries is myositis ossificans, also known as heterotopic ossification (HO). Although it is not completely understood, evidence suggests the pathophysiology of HO is related to the inability of mesenchymal cells to differentiate into osteoblastic stem cells, resulting in an inappropriate differentiation of fibroblasts into bone-forming cells. Though uncommon, HO also may be associated with burns, joint surgery, and trauma to the musculoskeletal system or central nervous system. HO may involve the muscle or tendons,

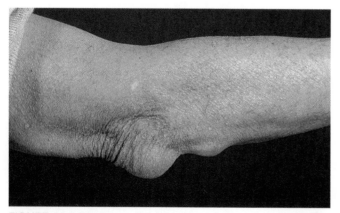

FIGURE 41.5 Olecranon Bursitis. Note swelling at the point of the elbow (olecranon). A smaller, rheumatoid nodule also is present. (From Hochberg MC et al: *Rheumatology*, ed 6, Philadelphia, 2015, Elsevier.)

DID YOU KNOW?

Managing Tendinopathy

Tennis and golfer's elbow, Achilles tendinopathy, and other tendon problems account for a large percentage of sports-related overuse injuries. Successful treatment of these conditions is challenging because of the mechanisms of tendon healing, as well as inconsistent results, with many interventions still not completely understood. Chronic pain is common and may be the result of ingrowth of nerves that accompanies ingrowth of new blood vessels during the healing process. Recent studies suggest that the traditional approach of corticosteroid injections is helpful only for the short term. Other therapies that show promise include the following:

Prolotherapy: An irritant such as glucose or lidocaine is injected into the affected tendon, inducing an inflammatory response, thereby stimulating the growth of new tendon fibers.

Eccentric exercises: The tendon is "prestretched," increasing its resting length and resulting in less strain during movement. The load on the tendon is gradually increased, causing the tendon itself to strengthen.

Extracorporeal shockwave therapy (SWT): External acoustic or sonic waves are focused on the affected area. The shockwaves stimulate soft tissue healing and inhibit pain receptors.

Needling: This treatment involves multiple insertions of a sterile needle into affected tissue. It is thought the pain sensation is reduced by stimulating A-nerve fibers. This technique is often referred to as "dry needling" since no fluid is introduced.

Platelet-rich plasma: This autologous source of concentrated platelets is obtained by centrifugation of plasma. The resulting solution contains high concentrations of cytokines and growth factors, such as platelet-derived growth factor (PDGF) and transforming growth factor-beta (TGF-β), which are thought to promote the growth of new, healthy tissue.

Autologous tenocyte injections: Autologous injection of tenocytes at the site of tendinopathy is thought to provide necessary mediators of tissue healing.

From Andarawis-Puri N et al: *J Orthop Res* 33(6):780-784, 2015; Krey D et al: *Phys Sportsmed* 43(1):80-86, 2015; Langer PR: *Clin Podiatr Med Surg* 32(2):183-193, 2015; Mautner K, Kneer L: *Phys Med Rehabil Clin North Am* 25(4):865-880, 2014; Wang A et al: *Am J Sports Med* 43(7):1775-1783, 2015.

TABLE 41.2 Muscle Strain

Type	Manifestations	Treatment
First degree (example: bench press in untrained athlete)	Muscle overstretched, pain but no muscle deformity	Ice should be applied 5 or 6 times in first 24-48 hr; gradual resumption of full weight bearing after initial rest for up to 2 weeks. Exercises individualized to specific injury
Second degree (example: any muscle strain with bruising and pain)	Muscle intact with some tearing of fibers, swelling, pain	Treatment similar to that for first-degree strains
Third degree (example: traumatic injury)	Caused by tearing of fascia, marked weakness, deformity	Surgery to approximate ruptured edges; immobilization and non–weight bearing status for 6 weeks

ligaments, or bones near the muscle, causing stiffness or deformity of an extremity. Radiographic evidence of HO may be seen as soft tissue calcification on plain radiographs.

Rhabdomyolysis

Once used interchangeably with the term *myoglobinuria,* rhabdomyolysis is the rapid breakdown of muscle that causes the release of intracellular contents, including the protein pigment myoglobin, into the extracellular space and bloodstream. Physical interruptions in the sarcolemma membrane, called *delta lesions,* are the route by which muscle constituents are released. (The sarcolemma membrane, the plasma membrane of the muscle cell, is described in Chapter 40.) Myoglobinuria refers to the presence of the muscle protein myoglobin in the urine.

PATHOPHYSIOLOGY The term rhabdomyolysis is sometimes incorrectly used interchangeably with *crush injury* (a description of injuries resulting from crushing of a body part), *compartment syndrome* (the consequences of increased intracompartmental pressures of a muscle), or *crush syndrome* (the systemic pathophysiologic events caused by rhabdomyolysis, primarily involving the kidneys and coagulation syndrome).[4] Rhabdomyolysis has many causes (Box 41.1) and can result in serious complications, including acute renal failure and electrolyte imbalances from the release of intracellular contents into the circulation (e.g., hyperkalemia and hyperphosphatemia), compounded by renal impairment, acid-base derangement, and cardiac dysrhythmias. The most clinically significant complication is acute renal failure, because myoglobin

precipitates in the tubules, obstructing flow of ultrafiltrate through the nephron and producing injury).[5] Other complications include disseminated intravascular coagulation (DIC), likely caused by activation of the clotting cascade by sarcolemma damage and the release of intracellular components from the damaged muscles.

CLINICAL MANIFESTATIONS A *classic triad* of muscle pain, weakness, and dark urine is considered typical of rhabdomyolysis. Abnormally dark urine caused by myoglobinuria may be the first and only symptom; however, the presence of myoglobin in urine alone is not a reliable test to diagnose rhabdomyolysis. The renal threshold for myoglobin is low (approximately 0.5 mg/dl of urine); therefore, only 200 g of muscle need to be damaged to cause visible changes in the urine. Myoglobin is rapidly cleared, and levels may return to normal within 24 hours of injury. Along with the release of myoglobin, creatine kinase (CK) and other serum enzymes are released in massive quantities (normal CK levels are 5 to 25 international units/L for women and 5 to 35 international units/L for men). The efflux of intracellular proteins and enzymes includes loss of potassium, phosphate, nucleotides, creatinine, and creatine. Serum hypocalcemia is seen early in the course of myoglobinuria and is followed by late hypercalcemia. The risk of renal failure increases proportionately to the increase in the levels of serum CK, potassium, and phosphorus.

EVALUATION AND TREATMENT The most important and clinically useful measurement in rhabdomyolysis is the serum CK level. A level

BOX 41.1   Selected Causes of Rhabdomyolysis

Direct Trauma

Blunt trauma or crush injury (motor vehicle crashes, collapsed buildings)

Burns (thermal)

Electrical injury

Excessive compression (from immobility attributable to stroke, alcohol or drug intoxication)

Drugs

Alcohol

Amphetamines

Anesthetic and paralytic agents (halothane, propofol, succinylcholine—malignant hyperthermia syndrome)

Antihistamines (diphenhydramine, doxylamine)

Antihyperlipidemic agents (statins, clofibrate, bezafibrate)

Antipsychotics and antidepressants (amitriptyline, doxepin, fluoxetine, haloperidol, lithium, protriptyline, perphenazine, promethazine, chlorpromazine, trifluoperazine, venlafaxine)

Caffeine

Cocaine

Corticosteroids

Fibrinates (antilipid agents: bezafibrate, ciprofibrate, clozfibrate, clofibrate, ezetimibe, gemfibrozil)

Heroin

HIV integrase inhibitor (raltegravir)

Hypnotics and sedatives (benzodiazepines, barbiturates)

LSD (lysergic acid diethylamide)

Methadone

Methamphetamine

Methylenedioxymethamphetamine (MDMA; "ecstasy")

Miscellaneous medications (amphotericin B, azathioprine, ε-aminocaproic acid, quinidine, penicillamine, salicylates, theophylline, terbutaline, thiazides, vasopressin)

Phencyclidine

Protease inhibitors

Statins (atorvastatin, fluvastatin, lovastatin, pravastatin, rosuvastatin, simvastatin)

Miscellaneous drugs (amphotericin B, arsenic, azathioprine, halothane, naltrexone, quinidine, penicillamine, propofol, salicylates, succinylcholine, theophylline, terbutaline, thiazides, vasopressin)

Excessive Muscular Contraction

Status epilepticus

Delirium tremens

Acute psychosis

Severe dystonia

Sporadic strenuous exercise (e.g., marathons, squats)

Tetanus

Infectious Agents

Bacteria (group B streptococci, *Streptococcus pneumoniae, Staphylococcus epidermidis, Borrelia burgdorferi, Escherichia coli, Clostridium perfringens, Clostridium tetani, Streptococcus viridans; Bacillus, Brucella, Legionella, Listeria, Leptospira, Mycoplasma, Plasmodium, Rickettsia, Salmonella,* and *Vibrio* species)

Fungal organisms (*Aspergillus, Candida* species)

Viruses (influenza types A and B, coxsackievirus, dengue, Epstein-Barr, HIV, cytomegalovirus, parainfluenza, varicella-zoster, West Nile)

Toxins

Carbon monoxide

Envenomation (black widow spider, Africanized honey bees, vipers)

Hemlock

Methanol

Toluene

Hereditary Enzyme Disorders (Rare)

McArdle disease (myophosphorylase deficiency)

Tarui disease (type VII glycogen storage disease)

Phosphoglycerate mutase deficiency (glycogen storage disease type X)

Carnitine palmitoyltransferase deficiency (CPT1 deficiency)

Miscellaneous Causes

Diabetic ketoacidosis

Endocrinopathy

Heatstroke

Hypothermia

Nonketotic hyperosmolar coma

Polymyositis

Severe electrolyte disorders (near-drowning or water intoxication, severe vomiting or diarrhea)

Data from Cervellin G et al: *Clin Chem Lab Med* 48(6):749-756, 2010; Croche F et al: *Int J STD AIDS* 21(11):783-785, 2010; Halpern P et al: *Hum Exp Toxicol* 30(4):259-266, 2011; Keltz E et al: *Muscles Ligaments Tendons J* 3(4):303-312, 2014; Torres PA et al: *Ochsner J* 15(1):58-69, 2015; Zutt R et al: *Neuromuscul Disord* 24(8):651-659, 2014.

5 to 10 times the upper limit of normal (about 1000 units/L) is used to identify rhabdomyolysis.[5] Once CK levels exceed 15,000 units/L, acute renal failure is likely. Other laboratory tests may include hyperkalemia, which can cause life-threatening cardiac arrhythmias, and a decreased blood urea nitrogen to creatinine ratio, caused by a release of creatine from damaged muscle being converted to creatinine. Additional laboratory tests—such as measurement of the hemoglobin, hematocrit, and platelet levels and determination of the activated partial thromboplastin time—may be indicated in the presence of other trauma or suspected bleeding. A recent study evaluated the ultrasonographic appearance of rhabdomyolysis in damaged muscle from earthquake victims and found abnormalities in muscle texture and subcutaneous tissue, as well as liquid collections in the damaged tissue.[6]

Maintaining adequate urinary flow and prevention of kidney failure are goals of treatment. Rapid intravenous hydration maintains adequate kidney perfusion. Other complications, such as hyperkalemia, may require temporary hemodialysis. Treatments such as using mannitol to cause an osmotic diuresis or bicarbonate to alkalinize the urine have not been shown to consistently improve outcomes.

Compartment Syndrome

Compartment syndrome is the result of increased pressure within a muscle compartment. Several layers of fibrous fascia surround skeletal muscles. These compartments are not able to expand. Increased pressure within these compartments creates increased pressure on the muscle tissue, leading to diminished capillary blood flow which results in local tissue hypoxia and necrosis. Causes of compartment syndrome include conditions that increase the contents of the compartment (such as bleeding or interstitial edema after an injury), a decrease in the compartment's volume (e.g., a tight bandage or cast), or a combination of these two conditions that results in a disturbance of the muscle's microvasculature[7-9] (Box 41.2). Any condition that disrupts the vascular

BOX 41.2 Factors Affecting the Development of Compartment Syndrome

Increased Intracompartmental Pressure
Fracture (open or closed)
Traction
Crush syndrome
Vigorous exercise or nonroutine activity/overuse in nonathletes
High-energy soft tissue injury (blast injuries, blunt force trauma)
Fluid infusion
Arterial puncture
Ruptured abdominal aortic aneurysm
Ruptured ganglion/other cyst
Envenomation (venomous snakes, black widow spiders)
Nephrotic syndrome
Viral myositis
Acute hematogenous osteomyelitis
Orthopedic procedures (e.g., osteotomy, joint replacement)
Seizures
Tetany

Reduced Compartment Volume
Burns
Repair of muscle herniation
Circumferential dressings
Casts that are too tight

Conditions That Disturb Microcirculation
Diabetes
Hypothyroidism
Bleeding disorders (hemophilia, von Willebrand disease, leukemia, vitamin K deficiency, viral hemorrhagic fevers [dengue])
Excessive anticoagulation
Malignancies

Data from Raza H, Mahapatra A: *Adv Orthop* 2015:543412, 2015; Shadgan B et al: *Can J Surg* 53(5):329-334, 2010.

supply to an extremity (such as severe burns, bleeding disorders, crush injury, snake or insect bites, extremely tight bandages, or casts) can cause increased pressure within the muscle compartments.

PATHOPHYSIOLOGY The weight of a limb extremity can generate enough pressure to produce muscle ischemia (Figs. 41.6 and 41.7). This causes edema, rising compartment pressure, and tamponade that lead to muscle infarction and neural injury and eventually result in cell loss.

CLINICAL MANIFESTATIONS Compartments often affected are the anterior and deep posterior tibial compartments in the leg, the forearm, the gluteal compartments in the buttocks, and the abdominal wall. Diagnosis is initiated by the clinical examination. The "6 Ps" of compartment syndrome are *p*ain (out of proportion to the injury), *p*ressure (swelling and rigidity of the affected area), *p*allor (pale appearance), *p*aresthesia (impaired or altered sensations to the area, or both), *p*aresis (impaired function of the involved extremity), and *p*ulselessness (loss of a pulse to the area). None of these signs is truly dependable, although pain with passive extension of the fingers or toes in the affected extremity and paresthesia tend to be most suggestive of compartment syndrome.[7,10]

A condition known as Volkmann ischemic contracture can develop when compartment syndrome goes unrecognized or is not adequately treated. Irreversible neurovascular damage can occur. Contracture deformities of the fingers, hand, and wrist can lead to partial or complete disability of the affected limb.

EVALUATION AND TREATMENT Direct measurement of intracompartmental pressure, using a manometer or an electronic transducer, is beneficial to confirm the diagnosis. However, the individual's history and physical examination findings alone can provide significant information to make the diagnosis of compartment syndrome. Laboratory tests, ultrasonography, and imaging studies may help exclude other conditions but generally are not helpful in diagnosing compartment syndrome. Once a diagnosis of compartment syndrome has been made or intracompartmental pressures reach 30 mm Hg, surgical intervention is warranted to relieve pressure within the compartment.

Surgical intervention consists of performing a fasciotomy of the affected area to decompress the compartment and allow the return of a normal blood supply. Skin grafts are often required to close the resultant opening, but vacuum-assisted wound closure devices also have been used successfully in accelerating wound closure.

Malignant Hyperthermia

Malignant hyperthermia (MH) is an autosomal dominant inherited muscle disorder characterized by a hypermetabolic reaction to certain volatile anesthetics or certain depolarizing muscle relaxants (e.g., succinylcholine) that activate a prolonged release of intracellular calcium from the sarcoplasmic reticulum. Researchers have described at least six forms of malignant hyperthermia susceptibility, which are caused by mutations in different genes.[11] Variations of the calcium voltage-gated channel subunit alpha 1 S (*CACNA1S*) and ryanodine receptor of skeletal muscle (*RYR1*) genes increase the risk of developing malignant hyperthermia.[11] These mutations result in a release of uncontrolled amounts of calcium from the sarcoplasmic reticulum into the cytoplasm, causing continuous muscle contraction. This process also causes hypermetabolism, with extremely high body temperature, muscle rigidity, rhabdomyolysis, and death if not quickly treated with an infusion of the skeletal muscle relaxant dantrolene.[12]

Though reported in all countries, ages, and sexes, young males tend to be more susceptible to MH. Common signs and symptoms are respiratory acidosis (with an elevated end tidal carbon dioxide), tachycardia, masseter muscle and skeletal muscle spasm, and elevated body temperature.

EVALUATION AND TREATMENT Careful and thorough preoperative assessment should alert the anesthesiologist to the possibility of an individual being susceptible to malignant hyperthermia. A family history of anesthetic problems and previous untoward anesthetic experiences (muscle cramping, unexplained fevers, dark urine) are criteria that require further clarification before administration of a volatile anesthetic, such as halothane, or the muscle relaxant succinylcholine. The caffeine halothane muscle contracture test is considered the most sensitive and definitive predictor of an individual developing MH. A muscle biopsy is obtained from the individual and then separately exposed to standardized amounts of halothane and caffeine. If the muscle bundles exhibit a contracture at specified limits, the individual is considered susceptible to MH.

Priorities in the treatment of MH include identifying and treating the underlying disorder and preventing life-threatening renal failure. MH and myoglobinuria can be treated by infusing dantrolene sodium (Dantrium). Secondary problems include electrolyte imbalance, volume depletion, acidosis, hyperuricemia, hyperkalemia, and calcium imbalance; these need specific treatment. Short-term dialysis also may be necessary.

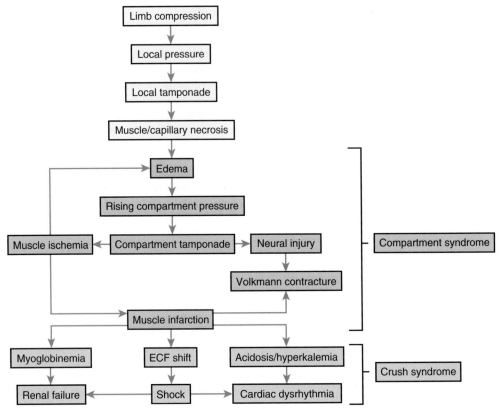

FIGURE 41.6 Pathogenesis of Compartment Syndrome and Crush Syndrome Caused by Prolonged Muscle Compression. *ECF,* Extracellular fluid.

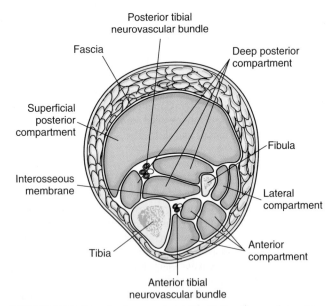

FIGURE 41.7 Muscle Compartments of the Lower Leg. (From Mohahan FD et al: *Phipps' medical-surgical nursing: health and illness perspectives,* ed 8, St Louis, 2007, Mosby.)

> ✔ **QUICK CHECK 41.1**
> 1. How are fractures classified?
> 2. What is the primary pathology of epicondylopathy?
> 3. What are some causes of compartment syndrome?
> 4. Why is myoglobinuria a dangerous complication of rhabdomyolysis?

DISORDERS OF BONES

Metabolic Bone Diseases

Metabolic bone disease is characterized by abnormal bone strength caused by abnormalities of minerals, vitamin D, bone mass, or bone structures. Individuals of all ages may be affected by this disease. Causes of these conditions are attributed to genetics, poor diet, or hormone influence leading to altered or inadequate biochemical reactions.

Osteoporosis

Osteoporosis, or porous bone, is generally described as decreased bone mineral density (BMD) and an increased risk of fractures because of alterations in bone microarchitecture. It is a complex, multifactorial, chronic disease that often progresses silently for decades until fractures occur. It is the most common disease that affects bone but is not a consequence of the aging process. The World Health Organization (WHO) has defined osteoporosis as "a systematic skeletal disease characterized by low bone density and microarchitectural deterioration of bone tissue with a consequent increase in bone fragility."[13]

Old bone is removed (resorption) and new bone is added (formation) to the skeleton throughout an individual's lifetime. In osteoporosis, old bone is being resorbed faster than new bone is being formed, causing the bones to lose density, becoming thinner and more porous. A progressive loss of bone mass may continue until the skeleton is no longer strong enough to support itself. Eventually, bones can fracture spontaneously. As bone becomes more fragile, falls or bumps that would not have caused a fracture previously now cause bone to break, referred to as a *fragility fracture*. The most common sites for osteoporosis-related fractures are the spine, femoral neck, and wrist.[14]

Bone tissue can be normally mineralized in osteoporosis, but the density of bone is decreased and the structural integrity of trabecular bone is impaired. Cortical bone becomes more porous and thinner, making bone weaker and prone to fractures (Figs. 41.8 and 41.9).

Skeletal homeostasis depends on a narrow range of plasma calcium and phosphate concentrations, which are maintained by the endocrine system. Therefore, endocrine dysfunction ultimately can cause metabolic bone disease. Hormones most commonly associated with osteoporosis are parathyroid hormone, cortisol, thyroid hormone, and growth hormone. (Endocrine function is discussed in Chapters 19 and 20.)

Other factors that can adversely affect normal bone homeostasis include multiple medications (e.g., glucocorticoids, proton pump inhibitors, thiazolidinediones, antiseizure medications, aromatase inhibitors, selective serotonin reuptake inhibitors [SSRIs], and anticoagulants), vitamin D deficiency, underlying diseases (rheumatoid disease, Paget disease, cancer, diabetes), low physical activity, and abnormal body mass index.[15-19]

During childhood and the teenage years, new bone is added faster than old bone is removed. Consequently, bones become larger, heavier, and denser. Bone formation continues at a pace faster than resorption until **peak bone mass**, or maximum bone density and strength, is reached, around age 30. Up to 90% of peak bone mass is obtained by age 20. After age 30, bone resorption slowly exceeds bone formation. In women, bone loss is most rapid in the first years after menopause but persists throughout the postmenopausal years. In 2011, the U.S. Preventive Services Task Force (USPSTF) issued a new recommendation that women age 65 or older be routinely screened for osteoporosis.[20] The major complications for persons with osteoporosis are fractures (*Did You Know?* Osteoporosis Facts and Figures at a Glance). Fractures are the major complication of osteoporosis. It is estimated that over 90% of all fractures occur as a result of falls.[21] Hip fractures, in particular, can have devastating effects on an individual's life. In addition to direct medical costs, studies have shown decreased quality of life, as well as excess loss of life-years for those experiencing hip or osteoporotic fractures.[22,23]

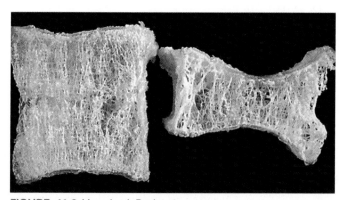

FIGURE 41.8 Vertebral Body. Osteoporotic vertebral body *(right)* shortened by compression fractures compared with a normal vertebral body. Note that the osteoporotic vertebra has a characteristic loss of horizontal trabeculae and thickened vertical trabeculae. (From Kumar V et al: *Robbins & Cotran pathologic basis of disease*, ed 9, Philadelphia, 2015, Saunders.)

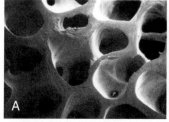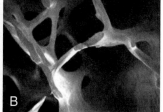

FIGURE 41.9 Electron Microscopic Comparison of Normal and Osteoporotic Bone. A, Normal trabecular structure. B, Osteoporotic bone; note the loss of supporting trabeculae. (From Golob AL, Laya MB: *Med Clin North Am* 99[3]:587-606, 2015.)

DID YOU KNOW?

Osteoporosis Facts and Figures at a Glance

- Osteoporosis is the most common bone disease of adults and the foremost cause of fractures in the elderly.
- Nearly 10 million Americans have osteoporosis (T-score ≥ 2.5 SD below normal peak bone mass) and nearly 43.1 million have low bone density (T-score 1.5 to 2.5 SD below normal peak bone mass).
- The National Osteoporosis Foundation (NOF) estimates that only about 40% of individuals with a hip fracture return to their prefracture level of functioning.
- Hip fractures account for only 14% of fractures in osteoporosis but are responsible for 72% of fracture costs.
- Osteoporosis-related fractures result in approximately 180,000 nursing home admissions, more than 432,000 hospital admissions, and nearly 2.5 million medical office visits annually.
- By 2025, fractures are estimated to increase to 3 million annually, with medical costs escalated to $25.3 billion.
- It is estimated that 1 in 2 white women and 1 in 5 white men will experience a hip, spine, or wrist fracture sometime in their lives. See discussion below for other ethnic groups see discussion below.
- By 2025, Hispanics are predicted to account for 20% of fractures in Arizona and California, with Asians and other nonwhite ethnic groups sustaining 27% of fractures in New York.

Data from National Osteoporosis Foundation: *Clinician's guide to prevention and treatment of osteoporosis,* Washington, DC, 2014, Author.

Vertebral fractures tend to occur in the later years of life; however, they are more difficult to ascertain because people may be unaware of the fracture. The degree of compression necessary to define a vertebral fracture is not standardized, although attempts have been made to standardize the definition and diagnosis of vertebral fractures. Thus, the true prevalence is unknown but fractures do increase in frequency by the sixth and seventh decades. Approximately 1 in 6 women and 1 in 12 men will sustain a vertebral fracture.[24]

Age-related loss of bone density and osteoporosis is most common in white women but affects all races. Asian and black women have only about half the fracture rate of whites, but that percentage is expected to increase with improved life expectancy.[25] In spite of a lower incidence, mortality in black women after a hip fracture is higher than among white women. Other factors may include a lower calcium intake, a high percentage of lactose intolerance, and increased prevalence of diseases such as sickle cell disease and lupus that increase the risk of developing osteoporosis.[26] Both black women and black men have generally been undertreated for osteoporosis.

Fracture prevention is a primary goal of osteoporosis treatment. Measuring the BMD by using dual x-ray absorptiometry (DXA) to calculate an individual's T-score continues to be the most common method of evaluating bone health and predicting fracture risk. Unfortunately, the technology to perform DXA scans is not available in all areas of the world. As a result, several tools that do not require BMD testing have been developed and validated to predict future fracture risk. These tools are summarized in Table 41.3. When BMD measurement is not available, fracture prediction using the Internet-based FRAX tool is similar to the use of other tools, such as the Osteoporosis Self-assessment Tool, or OST.[27]

Bone quality is not defined by bone mass alone (as measured by BMD) but also by the microarchitecture of the bone. Thus, other variables

TABLE 41.3 Comparison of Fracture Risk Assessment Tools Not Using Bone Mineral Density

Risk Factor	FRAX	SCORE	OSIRIS	ORAI	OST
Age	X	X	X	X	X
Weight	X	X	X	X	X
Previous low-energy fracture	X	X	X		
Estrogen therapy		X	X	X	
Rheumatoid arthritis	X	X			
Height	X				
Parental hip fracture	X				
Smoking	X				
Alcohol	X				
Glucocorticoid therapy	X				
Secondary osteoporosis	X				
Sex	X				
Ethnicity		X			

FRAX, World Health Organization's "Fracture Risk Assessment Tool"; *ORAI*, osteoporosis risk assessment instrument; *OSIRIS*, osteoporosis index of risk; *OST*, osteoporosis self-assessment tool; *SCORE*, simple calculated osteoporosis risk estimation.
Chart from Rubin KH et al: *Bone* 56:18, 2013.

include crystal size and shape, brittleness, vitality of bone cells, structure of the bone proteins, integrity of the trabecular network, and the ability to repair tiny cracks. Because bone density relates to the *quantity* of bone, the *quality* of bone is not accurately identified by bone density testing alone. As a result, bone density testing may not accurately identify those who will eventually be susceptible to fractures.

Postmenopausal osteoporosis is bone loss that occurs in middle-aged and older women. It can occur because of estrogen deficiency, as well as from estrogen-independent age-related mechanisms (e.g., secondary causes such as hyperparathyroidism and decreased mechanical stimulation). Estrogen deficiency can also increase with stress, excessive exercise, and low body weight. Postmenopausal changes result in a substantial increase in bone turnover—that is, a remodeling imbalance between the activity of osteoclasts (bone destroyers) and osteoblasts (bone formers). Increased formation and activity of osteoclasts causes removal or resorption of bone and results in a cascade of proinflammatory cytokines. In addition, estrogen helps osteoclast apoptosis (programmed cell death) so a decrease in estrogen levels is associated with *survival* of the bone-removing osteoclasts. Biologically, these processes involve the receptor activator nuclear factor κB ligand, osteoprotegerin signaling pathways, and insulin-like growth factor (IGF) (see Fig. 41.10; also see Chapter 40 and Fig. 40.5). Other causes may include a combination of inadequate dietary calcium intake and lack of vitamin D (and possibly decreased magnesium), lack of exercise, low body mass, and family history. IGF is known to help in fracture healing and collagen synthesis and improves conditions for bone mineralization. IGF levels significantly decline by age 60. Excessive phosphorus intake, chiefly through the intake of highly processed foods, hampers the calcium/phosphorus balance by interfering with parathyroid hormone and fibroblast growth factor 23 (FGF-23).[28,29]

Sex hormones, particularly estradiol (estrogen), are major determinants of bone density in both females and males. Androgens (i.e., testosterone and dihydrotestosterone) have long been recognized as stimulants of bone formation. Increasing age in both men and women

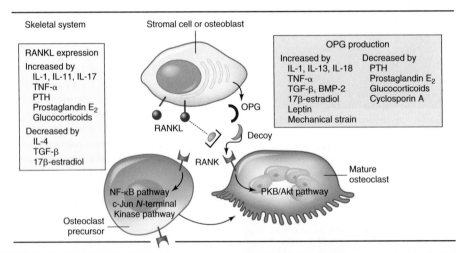

FIGURE 41.10 OPG/RANKL/RANK System. Expression of RANKL, a cytokine and part of the TNF family, and OPG, a glycoprotein receptor antagonist, is modulated by various cytokines, hormones, drugs, and mechanical strains (see inserts). In bone RANKL is expressed by both stromal cells and osteoblasts. RANKL stimulates the receptor RANK on osteoclast precursor cells and mature osteoclasts and activates intracellular signaling pathways to promote osteoclast differentiation and activation, as well as cytoskeletal reorganization and survival (PKB/Akt pathway), which increase resorption and bone loss. OPG, secreted by stromal cells and osteoblasts, acts as a "decoy" receptor and blocks RANKL binding to and activation of RANK. *BMP*, Bone morphogenic protein; *IL*, interleukin; *OPG*, osteoprotegerin; *PTH*, parathyroid hormone; *RANK*, receptor activator nuclear factor κB; *RANKL*, receptor activator nuclear factor κB ligand; *TGF-β*, transforming growth factor-beta; *TNF-α*, tumor necrosis factor-alpha. (Adapted from Hofbauer LC, Schoppet M: *JAMA* 292[4]:490-495, 2004.)

is associated with declining levels of estradiol and androgen, leading to losses in BMD. Other factors, such as inadequate dietary calcium intake, decreases in weight-bearing exercise, and sarcopenia, also are associated with osteoporosis. Other risk factors are identified in *Risk Factors: Osteoporosis*.

RISK FACTORS

Osteoporosis

Genetic	Lifestyle
Family history of osteoporosis	Sedentary
White race	Smoker
Greater age	Alcohol consumption (excessive)
Female sex	Low-impact fractures as an adult
	Inability to rise from a chair without
Anthropometric	using one's arms
Small stature	
Fair or pale skinned	**Concurrent**
Thin build	Hyperparathyroidism
Low bone mineral density	
	Illness and Trauma
Hormonal and Metabolic	Renal insufficiency, hypocalciuria
Early menopause (natural or	Rheumatoid arthritis
surgical)	Spinal cord injury
Late menarche	Systemic lupus erythematosus
Nulliparity	
Obesity	**Liver Disease**
Hypogonadism	Marrow disease (myeloma, masto-
Gaucher disease	cytosis, thalassemia)
Cushing syndrome	
Weight below healthy range	**Drugs**
Acidosis	Corticosteroids
	Dilantin
Dietary	Gonadotropin-releasing hormone
Low dietary calcium and vitamin D	agonists
Low endogenous magnesium	Loop diuretics
Excessive protein*	Methotrexate
Excessive sodium intake	Thyroid medications
Anorexia	Heparin
Malabsorption	Cyclosporin
	Medroxyprogesterone acetate
	(Depo-Provera)
	Retinoids

*Low levels of protein intake also have been reported.

Insufficient intake or malabsorption of dietary minerals is a factor in the development of osteoporosis. Calcium absorption from the intestine decreases with age, and studies of individuals with osteoporosis show that their calcium intake is lower than that of age-matched controls. Other mineral deficiencies, including magnesium, also may be important. Vitamin deficiencies, particularly vitamin D, as well as either deficiencies or excesses of protein also contribute to bone loss. Decreased serum levels of trace elements (zinc, copper, iron, magnesium, and manganese) have been associated not only with lower peak bone mass in developing bone, but also with later development of osteoporosis.[30-32] Excessive intake of caffeine, phosphorus, alcohol, and nicotine, along with low body fat (weight less than 125 pounds [56.7 kg]) has been shown to lower bone mineral density.[33-35] Secondary osteoporosis is osteoporosis caused by other conditions, including hormonal imbalances (endocrine disease, diabetes, hyperparathyroidism, hyperthyroidism), medications

(e.g., heparin, corticosteroids, phenytoin, barbiturates, lithium), and other substances (e.g., tobacco, ethanol). Other conditions, including rheumatoid disease, human immunodeficiency virus (HIV), malignancies, malabsorption syndrome, and liver or kidney disease, also increase the risk for developing osteoporosis[36] (see *Risk Factors:* Osteoporosis).

Secondary osteoporosis sometimes develops temporarily in individuals receiving large doses of heparin by reducing osteoblast formation and increasing bone resorption by reducing OPG and, thus, increasing osteoclast formation.[19] Osteoporosis caused by heparin therapy usually resolves when therapy stops. Other medications that increase the risk of osteoporosis include glucocorticoids, proton pump inhibitors, aromatase inhibitors, lithium, methotrexate, anticonvulsants, cyclophosphamide, thiazolidinediones, and cyclosporine.

Regional osteoporosis—osteoporosis confined to a segment of the appendicular skeleton—often has no known cause. Classic regional osteoporosis is associated with disuse or immobilization of a limb because of fractures or bone or joint inflammation. A negative calcium balance develops early and continues throughout the period of immobilization. After 8 weeks of immobilization, significant osteoporosis is present. One result of weightlessness has been a uniform distribution of osteoporosis observed in astronauts and in individuals treated with air suspension therapy.

Transient regional osteoporosis has no known etiology and is characterized by bone marrow edema and, sometimes, severe pain. Transient regional osteoporosis is usually self-limiting and tends to occur in middle-aged men, as well as in women during their late second or third trimester of pregnancy.[37] Bone marrow edema can be seen on magnetic resonance imaging (MRI) and areas of localized bone demineralization are seen in plain radiographs. The lower extremity is most often affected but other areas also can be involved. Treatment is primarily symptomatic, and the condition usually resolves spontaneously over 3 to 6 months, with no long-term adverse effects.

PATHOPHYSIOLOGY   Osteoporosis develops when the remodeling cycle (coupling)—bone resorption and bone formation—is disrupted, leading to an imbalance in the coupling process. Osteoclasts are differentiated cells that function to resorb bone. The explosion of new information in the field of bone biology has led to new understanding of osteoclast biology and bone pathophysiology. Of primary importance is the osteoclast differentiation pathway, which is dependent on various processes, including proliferation, maturation, fusion, and activation. These processes, in turn, are dependent on the availability of stem cells to allow differentiation to occur and are controlled by hormones, cytokines, and paracrine stromal cell interactions. Thus, proper intracellular communication within bone among its molecular regulators is necessary for normal bone homeostasis. Numerous interleukins, tumor necrosis factor (TNF), TGF-β, prostaglandin E_2, and hormones interact to control osteoclasts (Fig. 41.10). Staggering in its importance to understanding osteoclast biology is the cytokine receptor activator of nuclear factor κB ligand (RANKL); its receptor activator nuclear factor κB (RANK); and its decoy receptor osteoprotegerin (OPG), a glycoprotein (see Chapter 40 and Fig. 40.5).

Glucocorticoid-induced osteoporosis (e.g., prednisone, cortisone) is the most common type of secondary osteoporosis. Glucocorticoids have a direct impact on bone quality by improving osteoclast survival, inhibiting osteoblast formation and function, and increasing osteocyte apoptosis.[38,39] Glucocorticoids increase RANKL expression and inhibit OPG production by osteoblasts. Overall, these alterations result in decreased thickness of the bone cortex and fewer, thinner, and more widely spaced trabeculae in the marrow.

Age-related bone loss begins in the third to fourth decade. The cause remains unclear, but it is known that decreased serum growth hormone (GH) and IGF-1 levels, along with increased binding of RANKL and decreased OPG production, affect osteoblast and osteoclast function. Loss of trabecular bone in men proceeds in a linear fashion with thinning of trabecular bone rather than complete loss, as is noted in women (Fig. 41.11). Men have approximately 30% greater bone mass than women, which may be a factor in their later involvement with osteoporosis (Fig. 41.12). In addition, men have a more gradual decrease in the levels of testosterone and estradiol (and possibly progesterone), thereby maintaining their bone mass longer than women. Reduced physical activity in older persons is also a likely factor.

CLINICAL MANIFESTATIONS The specific clinical manifestations of osteoporosis depend on the bones involved. The most common manifestations, however, are pain and bone deformity because of fracture. These manifestations more often occur in an advanced disease state. Fractures are likely to occur because the trabeculae of spongy bone become thin and sparse, and compact bone becomes porous. As the bones lose volume, they become brittle and weak and may collapse or become misshapen. Vertebral collapse causes **kyphosis** (**hunchback**) and diminishes height (Fig. 41.13). Fractures of the long bones (particularly the femur), distal radius, ribs, and vertebrae are most common. Fracture of the neck of the femur tends to occur in older women with osteoporosis. Fatal complications of fractures include fat or pulmonary embolism, pneumonia, hemorrhage, and shock. Approximately 20% of persons may die as a result of surgical complications. Osteoporosis in men, as in women, also may be related to hypogonadism, with estradiol levels

being more clinically important than testosterone levels in both sexes. Adequate dietary intake of calcium, vitamin D, magnesium, and other trace minerals (*Did You Know?* Calcium, Vitamin D, and Bone Health); adherence to a regular regimen of weight-bearing exercise; and avoidance of alcoholism, tobacco, and glucocorticoids help to prevent primary osteoporosis.

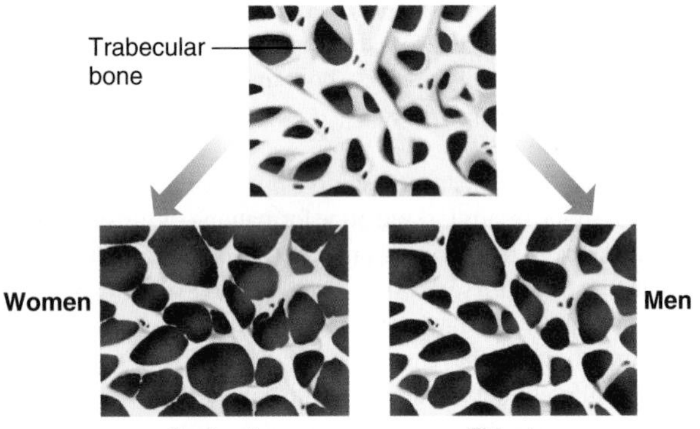

EVALUATION AND TREATMENT In general, osteoporosis is detected radiographically as increased radiolucency of bone. By the time abnormalities are detected by radiologic examination, up to 25% to 30% of bone tissue may have been lost.

Dual x-ray absorptiometry (DXA) is the current gold standard for detecting and monitoring osteoporosis; however, bone density is not necessarily indicative of bone quality. The utility of DXA in predicting fracture risk has recently been enhanced by the development of a trabecular bone score (TBS). The TBS evaluates pixel variations in the gray-level areas of lumbar spine images from DXA scans and has been shown to correlate with high-resolution peripheral quantitative computed tomography (HRpQCT) and be a reliable predictor of fractures.[40-42] High-resolution imaging techniques, such as quantitative computed tomography (QCT) scans and HRpQCT imaging, show changes in the trabecular and cortical microarchitecture. Newer MRI techniques also show promise for providing more detailed information about cortical and trabecular bone and have the added safety of no radiation exposure.[43] Other evaluation procedures include measurement of serum and urinary biochemical markers to monitor bone turnover (Box 41.3).

The goals of osteoporosis treatment are risk reduction and the prevention of fractures. Bisphosphonates are first-line medications for treating osteoporosis; they primarily work by inhibiting hydroxyapatite breakdown, reducing bone resorption. New medications formulated to prevent or treat osteoporosis are currently being prescribed and evaluated. There are new treatments that help rebuild the skeleton (*Did You Know?* New Treatments for Osteoporosis). Selective steroid agents (e.g., raloxifene) also may be prescribed. Regular, moderate weight-bearing

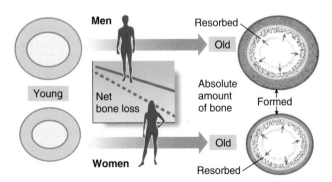

FIGURE 41.11 Mechanism of Loss of Trabecular Bone in Women and Trabecular Thinning in Men. Bone thinning predominates in men because of reduced bone formation. Loss of connectivity and complete trabeculae predominates in women.

FIGURE 41.12 Bone Loss in Men and Women. With aging, the absolute amount of bone resorbed on the inner bone surface and formed on the outer bone surface is greater in men than in women.

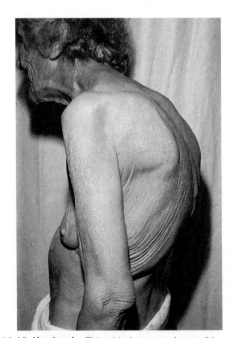

FIGURE 41.13 Kyphosis. This elderly woman's condition was caused by a combination of spinal osteoporotic vertebral collapse and chronic degenerative changes in the vertebral column. (From Kamal A, Brocklehurst JC: *Color atlas of geriatric medicine,* ed 2, St Louis, 1992, Mosby.)

Calcium, Vitamin D, and Bone Health

An adequate calcium intake is essential for developing and maintaining normal bone structure, but one question remains a topic of discussion and research: "What is an adequate calcium intake?" Calcium is the most abundant mineral in the body and plays a role in maintaining muscle function, hormonal secretion, neurotransmission, and vascular health. Recent conflicting evidence about the effect of calcium on heart disease, for example, has been hotly debated in the medical literature. The conflicting reports about extraskeletal health benefits of vitamin D also were reviewed by the Institute of Medicine (IOM) and were found to lack enough evidence to be considered reliable.

The role of vitamin D in bone health is unquestioned; the clinical effects of inadequate vitamin D (osteomalacia, rickets) have been well known for many years. Vitamin D is essential for absorbing and maintaining calcium homeostasis in the body. Recently, vitamin D has been postulated to be involved in many extraskeletal functions, such as reducing cancer risk, improving cognitive function in the elderly, preventing autoimmune diseases, improving resistance to infection, providing cardiovascular support, stabilizing posture, and inhibiting metabolic syndrome. Some of these potentially beneficial effects are from data gleaned from the National Health and Nutrition Examination Survey III (NHANES III), whereas other descriptions are based on observational or small studies. Vitamin D levels are evaluated by measuring serum 1,25-dihydroxy-vitamin D levels. There is still disagreement about what constitutes an "optimal" vitamin D level, but many sources indicate it should be at least 30 to 32 ng/ml. Based on these levels, it has been estimated that nearly 75% of the adult population in the United States have low vitamin D levels.

The IOM evaluated and summarized clinical evidence and literature reviews regarding the roles of calcium and vitamin D in disease reduction and other health outcomes in North America. Review of these findings resulted in updates of the recommended daily intake of both nutrients. In general, daily calcium intakes of 500 mg for ages 1 through 3, 800 mg for ages 4 through 8, 1100 to 1300 mg for ages 9 to 13, and 800 to 1000 mg for ages 14 through adulthood are adequate for maintaining proper bone health. Recommended dietary allowances for vitamin D vary from 400 to 600 international units (IU) a day for all ages. Additionally, the IOM found that once calcium intake exceeds more than 2000 mg a day or vitamin D intake is more than 4000 IU per day, there is increased risk for harm.

Data from Adams JS, Hewison M: *J Clin Endocrinol Metab* 95(2):471-478, 2010; Annweiler C et al: *J Neuroeng Rehabil* 7:50, 2010; Binkley N et al: *Endocrinol Metab Clin North Am* 39(2):287-301, 2010; Bolland MJ et al: *BMJ* 341:3691, 2010; Dawson-Hughes B: *BMJ* 341:4993, 2010; Grove ML, Book D: *BMJ* 342:5003, 2010; Heiss G et al: *BMJ* 342:4995, 2010; National Institutes of Health (NIH) Office of Dietary Supplements (no authors listed): *Vitamin D fact sheet for health professionals,* November 2014; Newberry SJ et al: *Vitamin D and calcium: a systematic review of health outcomes (update), evidence report/technology assessment no. 217,* prepared by the Southern California Evidence-based Practice Center under contract no. 290-2012-00006-1, AHQR Publication No. 14-E004-EF, Rockville, Md, 2014, Agency for Healthcare Research and Quality.

BOX 41.3 Biochemical Markers of Bone Turnover

Biochemical markers of bone turnover are useful in monitoring osteoporosis treatment. Markers of resorption include urinary N-telopeptide (NTx), C-telopeptide (CTx), and deoxypyridinoline. Markers of bone formation include bone-specific alkaline phosphatase (BSAP) and osteocalcin. However, these tests have diurnal variability within the same individual, so there must be significant changes in levels to indicate a difference in bone turnover.

exercise can slow the rate of bone loss and, in some cases, reverse demineralization because the mechanical stress of exercise stimulates bone formation. An exercise program to enhance strength and balance has the added benefits of reducing the risk of falls and promoting bone quality.

New Treatments for Osteoporosis

Although bisphosphonates remain the first line of osteoporosis therapy, not all individuals are able to tolerate them, and side effects can include bisphosphonate-related osteonecrosis of the jaw (BRONJ), atrial fibrillation, and fractures. Zoledronic acid, a third-generation bisphosphonate, is given as an annual intravenous infusion and has demonstrated efficacy in treating glucocorticoid-associated osteoporosis, in addition to reducing vertebral and nonvertebral fractures in women and men. However, it can cause an acute phase response in recipients and still carries some risk of BRONJ. Several new treatment options promise progress in treating osteoporosis and may be better tolerated than bisphosphonates.

Denosumab is a commercially available human monoclonal antibody for the treatment of osteoporosis. It binds to the receptor activator nuclear factor κB ligand (RANKL) (see Chapter 40) preventing activation of osteoclasts. By reducing osteoclast activity, bone density is increased and bone resorption is reduced, thus lessening the incidence of fractures. Because denosumab is not cleared by the kidneys (as are bisphosphonates), it has the potential to be useful in those with chronic kidney disease. It is given every 6 months as a 60-mg subcutaneous injection.

Raloxifene, a selective estrogen receptor modulator (SERM), has been in use for several years to treat postmenopausal osteoporosis. It has been effective in reducing vertebral fractures but not hip or other nonspinal fractures. Newer SERMs, including lasofoxifene (which is not approved for use in the United States), have been shown to reduce both vertebral and nonvertebral fractures. Bazedoxifene, in combination with estrogen, has been designated as a tissue-selective estrogen complex (TSEC), and is approved for use in Japan and Europe. It has been shown to reduce both vertebral and nonvertebral fractures in postmenopausal women. Neither of these agents, given as daily oral doses, stimulates endometrial or breast tissue.

Other biologic agents for treating osteoporosis include odanacatib, a cathepsin K inhibitor. By affecting this enzyme (produced by osteoclasts), bone density is increased. It is given as a once weekly oral agent. Agents directed at signaling pathways of bone formation and homeostasis are another target of osteoporosis intervention. One of the main signaling targets is the Wingless/Integrated (Wnt) pathway. Wnt stimulates osteoblast function and bone formation but is blocked by sclerostin (which is produced by the osteocyte gene *SOST*). Parathyroid hormone (PTH) inhibits sclerostin expression, which may result in increased numbers of osteoblasts. The development of monoclonal antibodies to sclerostin may provide another means to increase bone formation and density.

Data from Bone HG et al: *Osteoporosis Int* 26(2):699-712, 2015; Choi HJ: *J Menopausal Med* 21(1):1-11, 2015; Reid IR: *Nat Rev Endocrinol* 11(7):418-428, 2015; Reyes C et al: *J Cell Biochem* 117(1):20-28, 2016; Suresh E, Abrahamsen B: *Cleve Clin J Med* 82(2):105-114, 2015.

The anabolic or bone-building drug parathyroid hormone (PTH) has been widely studied and is a major regulator of calcium homeostasis. PTH acts directly on osteocytes, stimulates bone formation, and promotes migration of progenitor bone cells from the marrow into the bloodstream, increasing the production of osteoblasts when intermittently administered (see *Did You Know? New Treatments for Osteoporosis*).

Osteomalacia

Osteomalacia is a metabolic disease characterized by inadequate and delayed mineralization of osteoid in mature compact and spongy bone. In osteomalacia, the remodeling cycle proceeds normally through osteoid formation, but mineral calcification and deposition do not occur. Bone volume remains unchanged, but the replaced bone consists of soft osteoid instead of rigid bone. Rickets is similar to osteomalacia in pathogenesis, but it occurs in the growing bones of children, whereas osteomalacia occurs in adult bone. (Rickets is described in Chapter 42.)

Both osteomalacia and rickets are relatively rare in the United States and Western Europe but are significant health problems in Great Britain, Ethiopia, Pakistan, Iran, and India. Concomitant diseases, such as HIV, chronic kidney or liver disease, certain cancers, and impaired nutrient absorption from bariatric surgery, can result in vitamin D deficiency and secondary osteomalacia.[44] In the United States, other causes include prematurity with very low birth weight and adherence to a rigid macrobiotic vegetarian diet. Breast-fed black infants who do not receive vitamin D supplementation have been shown to be at risk for developing nutritional rickets.[45,46]

Many factors contribute to the development of osteomalacia, but the most important is a deficiency of vitamin D. The major risk factors in vitamin D deficiency are diets deficient in vitamin D, decreased endogenous production of vitamin D, intestinal malabsorption of vitamin D, renal tubular diseases, certain types of tumors (particularly of mesenchymal origin), and anticonvulsant therapy. Classic vitamin D deficiency is rare in the United States because of the addition of synthetic vitamin D to dairy products and bread.

Disorders of the small bowel, hepatobiliary system, and pancreas are causes of vitamin D deficiency in the United States. In malabsorptive disease of the small bowel, both vitamin D and calcium absorption are decreased, so vitamin D is lost in feces. Liver disease interferes with the metabolism of vitamin D to its more active form, and diseases of the pancreas and biliary system cause a deficiency of bile salts, which are necessary for normal intestinal absorption of vitamin D.

PATHOPHYSIOLOGY Crystallization of minerals in osteoid requires adequate concentrations of calcium and phosphate. When the concentrations are too low, crystallization (and hence ossification) does not proceed normally.

Vitamin D deficiency disrupts mineralization because vitamin D normally regulates and enhances the absorption of calcium ions from the intestine. A lack of vitamin D causes the plasma calcium concentrations to fall. Low plasma calcium levels stimulate increased synthesis and secretion of PTH. Although the increase in circulating PTH level raises the plasma calcium concentration, it also stimulates increased renal clearance of phosphate. When the concentration of phosphate in the bone decreases below a critical level, mineralization cannot proceed normally. Newer research has identified a complex interplay of matrix proteins, hormones, metallopeptidases, and certain proteins as also being involved in the development of osteomalacia.

Abnormalities occur in both spongy and compact bone. Trabeculae in spongy bone become thinner and fewer, whereas haversian systems in compact bone develop large channels and become irregular. Because osteoid continues to be produced but not mineralized, abnormal quantities of osteoid accumulate, coating the trabeculae and the linings of the haversian canals. Excessive osteoid also can accumulate in areas beneath the periosteum. The excess of osteoid leads to gross deformities of the long bones, spine, pelvis, and skull.

CLINICAL MANIFESTATIONS Osteomalacia causes varying degrees of diffuse muscular and skeletal pain and tenderness. Pain is noted particularly in the hips, and the individual may be hesitant to walk.

Muscular weakness is common and may contribute to a waddling gait. Facial deformities and bowed legs or "knock-knees" may be present. Bone fractures and vertebral collapse occur with minimal trauma. Low back pain may be an early complaint, but pain may also involve ribs, feet, other areas of the vertebral column, and other sites. Fragility fractures may occur. Uremia may be present in renal osteodystrophy.

EVALUATION AND TREATMENT Laboratory data may include elevated blood urea nitrogen (BUN) and creatinine levels, normal or low serum calcium levels, and a serum inorganic phosphate level that is usually more than 5.5 mg. Alkaline phosphatase and PTH levels are usually elevated. Radiographic findings may show symmetric bowing deformities and fractures with callus formation, particularly in the lower extremities. These types of fractures, known as *pseudofractures*, along with radiolucent bands perpendicular to the surface of involved bones can help differentiate osteomalacia from fragility fractures that are seen in osteoporosis. A bone biopsy is used to obtain information on bone structure and remodeling and evaluate the presence of subclinical renal osteodystrophy to determine bone architecture, turnover, and even aluminum deposits.

Treatment of osteomalacia may vary, depending on its etiology, but these general principles are followed:

- Adjustment of serum calcium and phosphorus levels to normal
- Suppression of secondary hyperthyroidism
- Chelation of bone aluminum if needed
- Administration of calcium carbonate to reduce hyperphosphatemia
- Administration of vitamin D supplements (oral or infusion)
- Administration of bisphosphonate
- Implementation of renal dialysis, if indicated

Paget Disease

Paget disease of bone (PDB, or osteitis deformans), the second most common bone disease after osteoporosis, is a state of increased metabolic activity in bone characterized by localized abnormal and excessive bone remodeling. Chronic accelerated remodeling eventually enlarges and softens the affected bones, causing bowing deformity, fracture, or neurologic problems. This process can occur in any bone but most often affects the vertebrae, skull, sacrum, sternum, pelvis, and femur. The disease process may occur in one or more bones without causing significant clinical manifestations.

Paget disease occurs with equal frequency in men more than 55 years of age and women older than 40 years of age. It is often symptomless and the diagnosis is often suspected when an elevated serum alkaline phosphatase level or abnormal x-ray film is noted. Radioisotope bone scan, x-rays, and CT are used to confirm the diagnosis. Serum plasma procollagen-1 N-peptide (PINP) is another serum marker that may provide a more accurate diagnosis.[47] Autopsy data from England and Germany indicate that approximately 3% to 4% of the population older than 40 years of age has Paget disease. It is most prevalent in Australia, Great Britain, New Zealand, and the United States. Paget disease affects several members of the same family in 5% to 25% of individuals.

The cause of PDB is not yet fully known, but studies have implicated both genetic and environmental factors. Implicated environmental factors include viruses, particularly the paramyxovirus family (that includes mumps, parainfluenza, and measles viruses), but no definitive microorganism has yet been identified.[48] Researchers have identified variations in three genes associated with PDB: *SQSTM1*, *TNFRSF11A*, and *TNFRSF11B*.[49] Interaction between genetic and environmental factors appears to increase osteoclast activity in PDB.

PATHOPHYSIOLOGY Paget disease begins with excessive resorption of spongy bone and deposition of disorganized bone. The trabeculae diminish, and bone marrow is replaced by extremely vascular fibrous tissue. The resorption phase of Paget disease is followed by the formation of abnormal new bone at an accelerated rate. The collagen fibers are disorganized, and glycoprotein levels in the matrix decrease. Mineralization may extend into the bone marrow. Bone formation is excessive around partially resorbed trabeculae, causing them to thicken and enlarge. The net result of this accelerated remodeling process is increased bone fragility and an increased risk for bone tumors.

CLINICAL MANIFESTATIONS   In the skull, abnormal remodeling is first evident in the frontal or occipital regions; then it encroaches on the outer and inner surfaces of the entire skull. The skull thickens and assumes an asymmetric shape. Thickened segments of the skull may compress areas of the brain, producing altered mentation and dementia. Impingement of new bone on cranial nerves can cause sensory abnormalities, impaired motor function, deafness from compression of the auditory nerve, atrophy of the optic nerve, and obstruction of the lacrimal duct. Headache also is commonly noted.

Extensive alterations of the facial bones are rare except in the jaw, where sclerosis and thickening of the maxilla and mandible displace teeth and produce malocclusion. In long bones, resorption begins in the subchondral regions of the epiphysis and extends into the metaphysis and diaphysis. Occasionally, Paget disease affects both ends of a tubular bone. In the femur, Paget disease produces an exaggerated lateral curvature. In the tibia, anterior curvature is also exaggerated. Stress fractures are common in the lower extremities.

Clinical manifestations of Paget disease in the vertebral column depend on the level of involvement and are caused by compression of adjacent structures. In the cervical spine, cord compression can lead to spastic quadriplegia. Approximately 1% of persons with Paget disease develop osteogenic sarcoma.

EVALUATION AND TREATMENT   Evaluation of Paget disease is made on the basis of radiographic findings of irregular bone trabeculae with a thickened and disorganized pattern. Early disease is detected by bone scanning that shows increased uptake of bone radionuclides. Plasma alkaline phosphatase and urinary hydroxyproline levels are elevated.

Many individuals require no treatment if the disease is localized and does not cause symptoms. Treatment during active disease is for relief of pain and prevention of deformity or fracture. Bisphosphonates are the treatment of choice; a one-time infusion of zoledronic acid can provide long-term reduction of biochemical markers and even remission. Several new agents have been approved for the treatment of PDB.

Infectious Bone Disease: Osteomyelitis

Osteomyelitis is a bone infection most often caused by bacteria; however, fungi, parasites, and viruses also can cause bone infection (Fig. 41.14).

Multiple classification systems have been used to describe osteomyelitis; the simplest refers to the mode of infection. A bone infection caused by pathogens carried through the bloodstream is called hematogenous osteomyelitis. Acute hematogenous osteomyelitis is more often seen in children and is characterized by fever, pain, and voluntary immobility of the affected limb. (Osteomyelitis in children is discussed in Chapter 42.) Contiguous osteomyelitis occurs when infection spreads to an adjacent bone and is often caused by open fractures, penetrating wounds, or surgical procedures. Other causes of osteomyelitis include metabolic and vascular diseases (diabetes, peripheral vascular disease), lifestyle risks (smoking, alcohol or drug abuse), and advanced age. In infants, incidence rates among males and females are approximately equal. In children and older adults, however, males are most commonly affected. A new category of autoimmune, noninfectious osteomyelitis, known as chronic nonbacterial osteomyelitis (CNO), has recently been identified as a cause of chronic bone pain in children.[50]

Staphylococcus aureus remains the primary microorganism responsible for osteomyelitis. Other microorganisms include group B streptococcus, *Haemophilus influenzae, Salmonella,* and gram-negative bacteria. Group B streptococcus and *H. influenzae* tend to infect young children; *Salmonella* infection is associated with sickle cell anemia; and gram-negative infections are most common in older adults and immunocompromised individuals with impaired immunity. Mycobacterial, viral, and fungal infections occur in immunocompromised individuals.

Cutaneous, sinus, ear, and dental infections are the primary sources of bacteria in hematogenous bone infections. Soft tissue infections, disorders of the gastrointestinal tract, infections of the genitourinary system, and respiratory tract infections are also sources of bacterial contamination. In addition, infections that occur after total joint replacement procedures are sometimes the cause. The vulnerability of specific bone depends on the anatomy of its vascular supply.

In adults, hematogenous osteomyelitis is more common in the spine, pelvis, and small bones. Microorganisms reach the vertebrae through arteries, veins, or lymphatic vessels. The spread of infection from pelvic organs to the vertebrae is well documented. Vaginal, uterine, ovarian, bladder, and intestinal infections can lead to iliac or sacral osteomyelitis.

Superficial animal or human bites inoculate local soft tissue with bacteria that later spread to underlying bone. Deep bites can introduce microorganisms directly onto bone. The most common infecting organism in human bites is *Staphylococcus aureus*. In animal bites, the most common infecting organism is *Pasteurella multocida,* which is part of the normal mouth flora of cats and dogs.

Direct contamination of bones with bacteria can also occur in open fractures or dislocations with an overlying skin wound. Intervertebral disk surgery and operative procedures involving implantation of large foreign objects, such as metallic plates or artificial joints, are associated with contiguous osteomyelitis. Osteomyelitis of the arm and hand bones

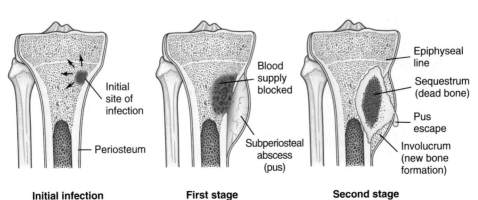

Initial site of infection

Periosteum

Blood supply blocked

Subperiosteal abscess (pus)

Epiphyseal line

Sequestrum (dead bone)

Pus escape

Involucrum (new bone formation)

Initial infection   **First stage**   **Second stage**

FIGURE 41.14 Osteomyelitis Showing Sequestration and Involucrum.

tends to occur in persons who abuse drugs. In general, persons who are chronically ill, have diabetes or alcoholism, or are receiving large doses of steroids or immunosuppressive drugs are particularly susceptible to chronic osteomyelitis or recurring episodes of this disease.

PATHOPHYSIOLOGY   Regardless of the source of the pathogen, the pathologic features of bone infection are similar to those in any other body tissue (see Chapter 6). First, the invading pathogen provokes an intense inflammatory response. *S. aureus*, in addition to producing toxins that destroy neutrophils, also forms colonies of microorganisms, called *biofilms*, that adhere to surfaces (such as implants) and increase antibiotic resistance. Biofilms also can reduce the duration of osteoblast activity while enhancing osteoclast activity and promoting inflammation (also see Chapter 9). Primarily through activation of the cytokine pathway, the biofilm and inflammation alter the normal balance between osteoblast and osteoclast activity.[51]

Once inflammation is initiated, the small terminal vessels thrombose and exudate seals the bone's canaliculi. Inflammatory exudate extends into the metaphysis and the marrow cavity and through small metaphyseal openings into the cortex. In children, exudate that reaches the outer surface of the cortex forms abscesses that lift the periosteum of underlying bone. Lifting of the periosteum disrupts blood vessels that enter bone through the periosteum, which deprives underlying bone of its blood supply. This leads to necrosis and death of the area of bone infected, producing **sequestrum**, an area of devitalized bone. Lifting of the periosteum also stimulates an intense osteoblastic response. Osteoblasts lay down new bone that can partially or completely surround the infected bone. This layer of new bone surrounding the infected bone is called an **involucrum** (Fig. 41.15). Openings in the involucrum allow the exudate to escape into surrounding soft tissue and ultimately through the skin by way of sinus tracts.

In adults, this complication is rare because the periosteum is firmly attached to the cortex and resists displacement. Instead, infection disrupts and weakens the cortex, which predisposes the bone to pathologic fracture.

CLINICAL MANIFESTATIONS   Clinical manifestations of osteomyelitis vary with the age of the individual, the site of involvement, the initiating

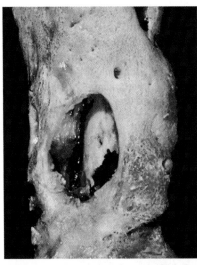

FIGURE 41.15 Resected Femur in a Person With Draining Osteomyelitis. The drainage tract in the subperiosteal shell of viable new bone (involucrum) reveals the inner native necrotic cortex (sequestrum). (From Kumar V et al: *Robbins & Cotran pathologic basis of disease*, ed 9, Philadelphia, 2015, Saunders.)

event, the infecting organism, and the type of infection—acute, subacute, or chronic. Osteomyelitis is generally considered acute if diagnosed within 2 weeks after symptom onset and is associated with an abrupt onset of inflammation (see Fig. 41.15). Subacute osteomyelitis is disease that has been present for 1 to several months, and chronic disease is that which has been present for many months to even years.[52]

If an acute infection is not completely eliminated, the disease may become subacute or chronic. In subacute osteomyelitis, signs and symptoms are usually vague. In the chronic stage, infection is silent between exacerbations. The microorganisms persist in small abscesses or fragments of necrotic bone and produce occasional exacerbations of acute osteomyelitis. The progression from acute to subacute osteomyelitis may be the result of inadequate or inappropriate therapy, or the development of drug-resistant microorganisms.

In the adult, hematogenous osteomyelitis has an insidious onset. The symptoms are usually vague and include fever, malaise, anorexia, weight loss, and pain in and around the infected areas. Edema may or may not be evident. Recent infection (urinary, respiratory, cutaneous) or instrumentation (catheterization, cystoscopy, myelography, diskography) usually precedes onset of symptoms.

Single or multiple abscesses (Brodie abscesses) characterize subacute or chronic osteomyelitis. Brodie abscesses are circumscribed lesions 1 to 4 cm in diameter that are found usually in the ends of long bones and surrounded by dense ossified bone matrix. The abscesses are thought to develop when the infectious microorganism has become less virulent or the individual's immune system is resisting the infection somewhat successfully.

In contiguous osteomyelitis, signs and symptoms of soft tissue infection predominate. Inflammatory exudate in the soft tissues disrupts muscles and supporting structures and forms abscesses. Low-grade fever, lymphadenopathy, local pain, and swelling usually occur within days of contamination by a puncture wound.

EVALUATION AND TREATMENT   Laboratory data show an elevated white cell count and an elevated level of noncardiac C-reactive protein (CRP). Radiographic studies include radionuclide bone scanning, CT, functional imaging using a combination of radionuclide scanning (using fluorodeoxyglucose [FDG]) and single photon emission computed tomography (SPECT), positron emission tomography (PET), and MRI. MRI scanning with gadolinium contrast shows both bone and soft tissue, providing more accurate assessment of infection. MRI also shows early changes of bone marrow edema. FDG-SPECT imaging is highly sensitive for evaluating osteomyelitis of the extremities.[53]

Treatment of osteomyelitis includes bone biopsy to identify the causative organism, use of antimicrobial agents, and débridement of infected bone. Biodegradable antibiotic-impregnated bioabsorbable beads have also benefited many individuals; newer therapies include the promise of injectable scaffolds impregnated with antibiotics and other antimicrobial substances.[54] Chronic conditions may require surgical removal of the inflammatory exudate followed by continuous wound irrigation with antibiotic solutions in addition to systemic treatment with antibiotics. The optimal antibiotic regimen for treating osteomyelitis is still unclear. **Hyperbaric oxygen therapy** of 100% oxygen may stimulate healing by suppressing proinflammatory cytokines and prostaglandins. Implants for total joint replacements may need to be removed to treat the infected joint more thoroughly.

✔ **QUICK CHECK 41.2**
1. What are the causes associated with osteoporosis in women and men?
2. How does osteoporosis differ from osteomalacia? Name three differences.
3. What are the risk factors for osteomyelitis?

DISORDERS OF JOINTS

The American College of Rheumatology (ACR) recognizes several groups of joint disease (arthropathies). Most of these disorders can be placed into two major categories: noninflammatory joint disease and inflammatory joint disease. With the improvement in detection methods, however, inflammatory pathways are now being identified in conditions previously classified as noninflammatory, such as osteoarthritis.

Osteoarthritis

Osteoarthritis (OA) is the most common, age-related disorder of synovial joints. Affecting the entire joint, OA is characterized by local areas of loss and damage of articular cartilage, inflammation, new bone formation of joint margins (osteophytosis), subchondral bone changes, variable degrees of mild synovitis, and thickening of the joint capsule (Fig. 41.16). Pathology centers on load-bearing areas. Advancing disease shows narrowing of the joint space, attributable to cartilage loss, bone spurs (osteophytes), and sometimes changes in the subchondral bone. OA

can arise in any synovial joint but is commonly found in the knees, hips, hands, and spine. It is less common in people younger than 40 years of age, and its prevalence increases with age. Although the exact causes of OA are unclear, obesity and trauma are well-known risk factors. Recent research has identified specific microRNAs that affect gene expression in chondrocytes, and that may play a role in the development of OA. OA involves a complex interaction of transcription factors, cytokines, growth factors, matrix molecules, the immune system, mechanical stresses on joints, and enzymes (see the Pathophysiology section). Emerging understanding of synovitis and inflammation in OA has led to the recognition of the role played by the body's immune system in OA.

Although incidence rates are quite similar in men and women, after age 50, women typically are more severely affected. OA usually occurs in those persons who put exceptional stress (or joint loading) on joints (e.g., obese persons, gymnasts, long-distance runners or marathoners); persons participating in such sports as basketball, soccer, or football have been shown to develop osteoarthritis at earlier ages than usual.

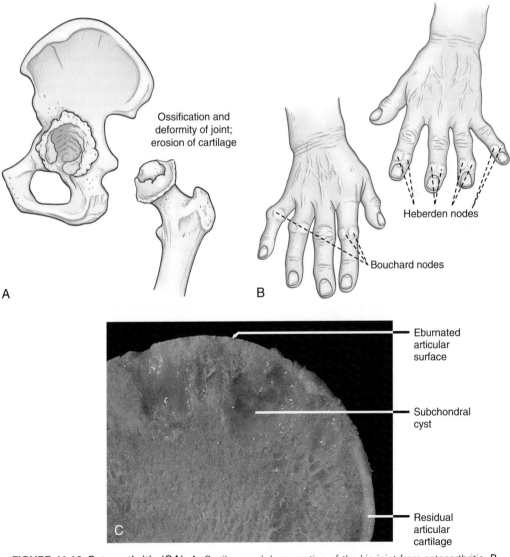

FIGURE 41.16 Osteoarthritis (OA). A, Cartilage and degeneration of the hip joint from osteoarthritis. **B,** Heberden nodes and Bouchard nodes. **C,** Severe osteoarthritis with small islands of residual articular cartilage next to exposed subchondral bone. (**C** from Kumar V et al: *Robbins & Cotran pathologic basis of disease,* ed 9, Philadelphia, 2015, Saunders.)

Obesity itself is an independent risk factor for developing OA of the knee. A previously torn anterior cruciate ligament or meniscectomy increases the risk for accelerated osteoarthritis of the knee.

Types of Osteoarthritis

PATHOPHYSIOLOGY The primary defect in OA is loss of articular cartilage. The chondrocytes of the articular cartilage become damaged early in the disease process because of atypical load bearing, as well as both genetic/epigenetic and biochemical factors (Fig. 41.17).

Early in the disease process, the articular cartilage loses its glistening appearance, becoming yellow-gray or brownish gray. As the disease progresses, surface areas of the articular cartilage flake off and deeper layers develop longitudinal fissures (fibrillation). The cartilage becomes thin and may be absent over some areas, leaving the underlying bone (subchondral bone) unprotected. Consequently, the unprotected subchondral bone becomes sclerotic (dense and hard). Cysts sometimes develop within the subchondral bone and communicate with the longitudinal fissures in the cartilage. Pressure builds in the cysts until the cystic contents are forced into the synovial cavity, breaking through

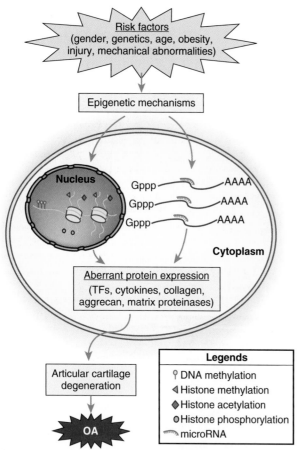

FIGURE 41.17 Working Model Epigenetic Changes in the Pathophysiology of Oa. From the proposed effects of risk factors, chondrocytes experience epigenetic events of deoxyribonucleic acid (DNA) methylation and histone modifications that occur in the nucleus and microRNAs (miRNAs) which function in the cytoplasm. Overall, these factors result in aberrant expression of transcription factors (TFs), cytokines, collagen, aggrecan, and matrix proteinases. Altered expression of these factors may disrupt the fine balance of anabolic and catabolic activity and affect cartilage homeostasis, resulting in articular cartilage degradation and the development of OA. (Adapted from Zhang M, Wang J: *Genes Dis* 2[1]:69-75, 2015.)

the articular cartilage on the way. As the articular cartilage erodes, cartilage-coated osteophytes grow outward from the underlying bone and alter the bone contours and joint anatomy. These spurlike bony projections enlarge until small pieces, called *joint mice,* break off into the synovial cavity. If osteophyte fragments irritate the synovial membrane, synovitis and joint effusion result. Joint pain, however, may be more related to inflammation of the synovium than subsequent cartilage damage or the radiographic extent of arthritis.[55,56] The joint capsule also becomes thickened and at times adheres to the deformed underlying bone, which may contribute to the limited range of motion of the joint (see Fig. 41.16).

Articular cartilage is lost through a cascade of signaling, cytokine, and anabolic growth factor pathways. Enzymatic processes (including matrix metalloproteinases) assist in breaking the macromolecules of proteoglycans, glycosaminoglycans, and collagen into large, diffusible fragments. Then the fragments are taken up by the cartilage cells (chondrocytes) and digested by the cell's own lysosomal enzymes. (Processes of cellular uptake and lysosomal digestion are described in Chapter 1.)

Enzymatic destruction of articular cartilage begins in the matrix, with destruction of proteoglycans and collagen fibers. Enzymes, particularly stromelysin and acid metalloproteinases, affect proteoglycans by interfering with assembly of the proteoglycan subunit or the proteoglycan aggregate (see Chapter 40). Changes in the conformation of proteoglycans disrupt the pumping action that regulates movement of water and synovial fluid into and out of the cartilage. Cartilage imbibes too much fluid and becomes less able to withstand the stresses of weightbearing. With aging, the proteoglycan content is decreased, and water content in cartilage can be increased by as much as 8%, affecting the strength of the cartilage. Disruptions in cellular signaling pathways, particularly the TGF-β superfamily, play a significant role in the development of OA. Other studies indicate that cytokines, such as interleukin-1 (IL-1) and TNF (see Chapter 6 for discussion of cytokines), play a major role in cartilage degradation[57] as a result of release and activation of proteolytic and collagenolytic enzymes associated with an imbalance of cell responses to growth factor activity.[58,59]

Cell-signaling proteins, particularly adipokines, such as adiponectin and collagenases (enzymes that degrade collagen), contribute to collagen breakdown in cartilage.[60] Collagen breakdown destroys the fibrils that give articular cartilage its tensile strength and exposes the chondrocytes to mechanical stress and enzyme attack. The osteochondral junction formed by cartilage and its underlying subchondral bone allows alterations in one tissue to affect the adjacent one (biomechanical coupling). When articular cartilage is damaged, abnormal subchondral bone remodeling occurs. Thus, a cycle of destruction begins that involves all the components of a joint: cartilage, bone, and the synovium.

CLINICAL MANIFESTATIONS Clinical manifestations of OA typically appear during the fifth or sixth decade of life; although often asymptomatic, articular surface changes are common after the age of 40 years. Pain in one or more joints—usually with weight bearing, use of the joint, or load bearing—is the first and most predominant symptom of the disease. Resting the joint often relieves pain. If present, nocturnal pain is usually not relieved by rest and may be accompanied by paresthesias (numbness, tingling, or prickling sensations). Sometimes pain is referred to another part of the body, such as severe pain in the back of the thigh along the course of the sciatic nerve. OA in the lower cervical spine may cause brachial neuralgia (pain in the arm) and is aggravated by movement of the neck. Osteoarthritic conditions in the hip cause pain that may be referred to the lower thigh and knee area. Sleep deprivation adds to the stress of the chronic pain of OA. Physical examination of the person with OA usually shows general involvement of both peripheral and central joints. Peripheral joints most often involved are in the hands, wrists, knees, and feet. Central joints most often afflicted are in the lower cervical spine, lumbosacral spine, shoulders, and hips.

Joint structures are capable of generating a limited number of signs and symptoms. The primary signs and symptoms of osteoarthritic joint disease are pain, stiffness, enlargement or swelling, tenderness, limited range of motion, muscle wasting, partial dislocation, and deformity (*Risk Factors: Osteoarthritis*).

RISK FACTORS
Osteoarthritis

- Trauma, sprains, strains, joint dislocations, and fractures
- Long-term mechanical stress—athletics, ballet dancing, repetitive physical tasks, and obesity
- Inflammation in joint structures
- Joint instability from damage to supporting structures
- Neurologic disorders (e.g., diabetic neuropathy, Charcot neuropathic joint) in which pain and proprioceptive reflexes are diminished or lost
- Congenital or acquired skeletal deformities
- Hematologic or endocrine disorders, such as hemophilia, which causes chronic bleeding into the joints, or hyperparathyroidism, which causes bone to lose calcium
- Drugs (e.g., colchicine, indomethacin, steroids) that stimulate the collagen-digesting enzymes in the synovial membrane

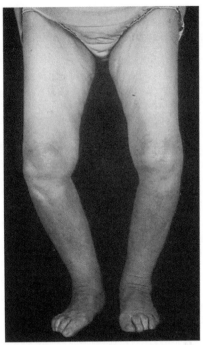

FIGURE 41.18 Typical Varus Deformity of Knee Osteoarthritis. (From Doherty M: *Color atlas and text of osteoarthritis*, London, 1994, Wolfe.)

The origin of joint stiffness is unknown. Joint stiffness is generally defined as difficulty initiating joint movement, immobility, or a loss of range of motion. The stiffness usually occurs as joint movement begins, and it dissipates rapidly after a few minutes. Stiffness lasting longer than 30 minutes is uncommon in OA. Enlargement and bulging of bone contour, commonly described as swelling, may be caused by bone enlargement or the proliferation of osteophytes around the margins of the joint. In the hands, these areas are called Heberden and Bouchard nodes, where they are typical features of OA (see Fig. 41.16). Inflammation of the joint lining, known as *synovitis*, is thought to be initiated by the release of cartilage extracellular matrix into the joint, which then activates the body's complement system. Swelling also occurs if inflammatory exudate or blood enters the joint cavity, thereby increasing the volume of synovial fluid. This condition, termed joint effusion, is caused by (1) the presence of osteophyte fragments in the synovial cavity, (2) drainage of cysts from diseased subchondral bone, or (3) acute trauma to joint structures, resulting in hemorrhage and inflammatory exudation into the synovial cavity (see Fig. 41.16, *C*).

Range of motion is limited to some degree, depending on the extent of cartilage degeneration. Frequently, joint motion is accompanied by sounds of crepitus, creaking, or grating. Abnormal knee alignment (either varus or valgus) has been shown to be a risk factor for and can increase progression of the disease.[61,62]

As OA of the lower extremity progresses, the person may begin to noticeably limp (Fig. 41.18). Having a limp is distressing because it affects the person's independence and ability to perform usual activities of daily living. The affected joint is also more symptomatic after use, such as at the end of a period of strenuous activity.

EVALUATION AND TREATMENT   Evaluation consists primarily of clinical assessment and radiologic studies. More expensive studies, including CT scan, arthroscopy, and MRI, are rarely needed. Newer imaging technologies, such as compositional MRI, are showing promise

in identifying structural changes in cartilage; improvements in technology may also allow better monitoring of OA treatment.

Treatment is either conservative or surgical. Conservative treatment includes both pharmacologic and nonpharmacologic therapies. Both exercise and weight loss have been shown to be two of the most important nonpharmacologic treatments in improving knee OA symptoms. Exercise can reduce pain and improve physical function in people with knee OA.[63,64] Exercises to improve muscle tone, range of motion, and balance; stretch the joint capsule; and reduce the fear of falling also have shown promise in reducing OA symptoms. Braces and foot orthoses may help correct biomechanical abnormalities, thereby reducing pain and improving mobility. Dietary and nutritional supplements can sometimes also improve symptoms. Nutraceuticals, such as chondroitin and glucosamine, have shown success in relieving OA pain in some individuals.[65] Other nonsurgical therapies include analgesic and antiinflammatory drug therapy to reduce swelling and pain. Acetaminophen was once considered first-line treatment, but it has been shown to be less effective than nonsteroidal antiinflammatory drugs (NSAIDs), such as ibuprofen. However, prolonged use significantly increases the risk of serious associated side effects that are common.[66] Intra-articular injection of corticosteroids and high-molecular-weight viscose supplements, such as hyaluronic acid, also decreases knee pain with OA.[67] Recently, because of its high concentration of growth factors, PRP also has been injected into osteoarthritic knee joints with some success in reducing pain and markers of inflammation.[68] Current evidence does not support low-level laser therapy for knee osteoarthritis.[69] Newer agents, including inhibitors of cytokines, matrix metalloproteinases (MMPs), and leptin, are under investigation and may prove more effective in treating OA. Surgery is used to improve joint movement, correct deformity or malalignment, or create a new joint with artificial implants. However, emerging evidence, based on systematic reviews,[70] cautions against the use of arthroscopy in nearly all persons with degenerative knee disease (*Did You Know? Evidence Against the Use of Arthroscopy for Nearly All Patients with Degenerative Knee Disease*).

Evidence Against the Use of Arthroscopy for Nearly All Patients With Degenerative Knee Disease

An international expert panel provided recommendations on the role of arthroscopic surgery in degenerative disease. These recommendations were based on a recent randomized trial of patients with a degenerative medial meniscus tear; the panel found that knee arthroscopy was no better than exercise therapy alone for these patients.[1] This study adds to the growing evidence that the benefits of arthroscopy may not outweigh the burdens and risks.[2,3] The panel made a strong recommendation against arthroscopy for degenerative knee disease.[4] This recommendation applies to patients with or without imaging evidence of osteoarthritis, mechanical symptoms, or sudden symptom onset. Here, the term *degenerative knee disease* included patients with knee pain, particularly if they are greater than 35 years old, with or without imaging evidence of osteoarthritis, meniscal tears, locking, clicking, or other mechanical symptoms. However, degenerative knee disease did not include patients with persistent locked knee, patients with acute or subacute onset of symptoms, or patients with major knee trauma and acute onset of joint swelling (e.g., hemarthrosis).[4] The international panel included orthopedic surgeons, a rheumatologist, physiotherapists, a general practitioner, general internists, epidemiologists, methodologists, and patients who had experienced degenerative knee disease. Characteristics of patients and trials included in this systemic review were as follows: 13 trials were examined; 12 of 13 trials were free of industry funding; 1668 patients were followed (median age 54.8 years); symptom duration was 3 months (12 months median, 52 months maximum); percent of women studied was 49.2; mean BMI was 27; no patients were involved in designing or conducting trials. In addition, 12 observational studies for complications (>1.8 million patients) were reviewed. In general, it takes 2 to 6 weeks to recover from arthroscopy. Patients may experience pain, swelling, and limited function. Most patients cannot bear full weight on the leg (i.e., they may need crutches) in the first week after surgery, and physical activity and driving are limited during the recovery period. Degenerative knee disease is a chronic condition and symptoms fluctuate. Pain, on average, tends to improve with time after the patient sees a physician,[5,6] and delaying knee replacement is encouraged when possible.[7]

References

1. Kise NJ, et al: Exercise therapy versus arthroscopic partial meniscectomy for degenerative meniscal tear in middle aged patients: randomised controlled trial with two-year follow-up, *BMJ* 354:i3740, 2016.
2. Khan M, et al: Arthroscopic surgery for degenerative tears of the meniscus: a systematic review and meta-analysis, *CMAJ* 186(14):1057-1064, 2014.
3. Thorlund JB, et al: Arthroscopic surgery for degenerative knee: systematic review and meta-analysis of benefits and harms, *BMJ* 350:h2747, 2015.
4. Siemieniuk RAC, et al: Arthroscopic surgery for degenerative knee arthritis and meniscal tear: a clinical guideline, *BJM* 357:j1982, 2017.
5. Brignardello-Peterson R, et al: Knee arthroscopy versus conservative management in patients with degenerative knee disease: a systematic review, *BMJ Open* 7(5):e016114, 2017.
6. de Roolij M, et al: Prognosis of pain and physical functioning in patients with knee osteoarthritis: a systematic review and meta-analysis, *Arthritis Care Res (Hoboken)* 68(4):481-492, 2016.
7. McGrory B, et al: American Academy of Orthopaedic Surgeons evidence-based clinical practice guideline on surgical management of osteoarthritis, *J Bone Joint Surg Am* 98(8):688-692, 2016.
Sihvonen R, et al: Arthroscopic partial meniscectomy versus sham surgery for a degenerative meniscal tear, *N Eng J Med* 369:2515-2524, 2013.
Howard DH: Trends in the use of knee arthroscopy in adults, *J Am Med Assoc Intern Med* 178(11):1557-1558, 2018.

Some researchers have estimated that 1 in 4 individuals has a lifetime risk of developing symptomatic OA of the hip.[71] More than 280,000 total hip and more than 600,000 total knee replacement surgeries are performed yearly in the United States, most of which are related to OA.[72]

Classic Inflammatory Joint Disease

Inflammatory joint disease is commonly called arthritis. Inflammatory joint disease is characterized by inflammatory damage or destruction in the synovial membrane or articular cartilage and by systemic signs of inflammation (fever, leukocytosis, malaise, anorexia, hyperfibrinogenemia).

Inflammatory joint disease can be infectious or noninfectious. Infectious inflammatory joint disease is caused by invasion of the joint by bacteria, mycoplasmas, viruses, fungi, or protozoa. These agents can invade the joint through a traumatic wound, surgical incision, or contaminated needle, or they can be delivered by the bloodstream from sites of infection elsewhere in the body—typically bones, heart valves, or blood vessels. Noninfectious inflammatory joint disease, the most common form, is caused by immune reactions or the deposition of crystals of monosodium urate in and around the joint. Rheumatoid arthritis, psoriatic arthritis, and ankylosing spondylitis are noninfectious inflammatory diseases caused by immune reactions and possibly hypersensitivity reactions; gouty arthritis is a noninfectious inflammatory disease caused by crystal deposition.

Rheumatoid Arthritis

Rheumatoid arthritis (RA) is a chronic, systemic, inflammatory autoimmune disease distinguished by joint swelling and tenderness and destruction of synovial joints leading to disability. (Autoimmune disease is described in Chapter 8.) RA can cause inflammation of several other tissues. The first joint tissue to be affected is the synovial membrane, which lines the joint cavity (see Chapter 40, Fig. 40.9). The two primary types of synovial cells are fibroblast-like synovial cells and macrophage-like synovial cells. Though the initiating mechanism of RA is still unknown, its pathology is fairly well understood. Some factor activates the synovial fibroblasts (SFs) that line the joint cavity.[73,74] The SFs undergo significant changes and develop an exaggerated immune response. Once activated, both types of SF abnormally proliferate and produce proinflammatory cytokines, enzymes, and prostaglandins that perpetuate the inflammatory process and thicken the synovial tissue.[75] This thickened synovial tissue, called "pannus," invades the bone and acts like a localized tumor, where other factors (including increased osteoclast activity) cause bone destruction. Some of the most significant synovial changes involve altered signaling pathways for immune reactions, where SFs attach to articular cartilage and attack it, causing more inflammation; the release of enzymes, such as MMPs, inflammatory chemokines, and cytokines (interleukins and TNF); and ingrowth of blood vessels. Increased blood vessel formation improves the opportunity for activated SFs to enter the bloodstream and affect other joints.[76] Eventually, inflammation spreads to the fibrous joint capsule and surrounding ligaments and tendons, causing pain, joint deformity, and loss of function (Fig. 41.19). The joints most commonly affected are in the fingers, feet, wrists, elbows, ankles, and knees, but the shoulders, hips, and cervical spine also may be involved, as well as the tissues of the lungs, heart, kidneys, and skin.

The incidence and prevalence of RA have decreased over the past five decades; RA now affects about 1% of the adult population in developed countries.[77] The frequency of RA increases with age. Besides inflammation and destruction of the joints, RA can cause fever, malaise,

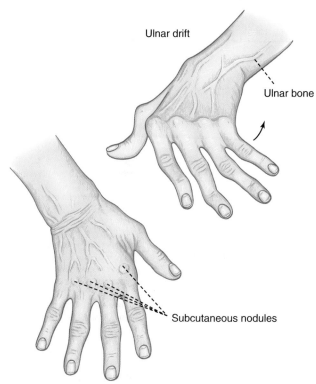

FIGURE 41.19 Rheumatoid Arthritis of the Hand. Note the swelling from chronic synovitis of metacarpophalangeal joints, marked ulnar drift, subcutaneous nodules, and subluxation of metacarpophalangeal joints with extension of proximal interphalangeal joints and flexion of distal joints. Note also deformed position of thumb. Hand has wasted appearance. (From Mourad LA: *Orthopedic disorders*, St Louis, 1991, Mosby.)

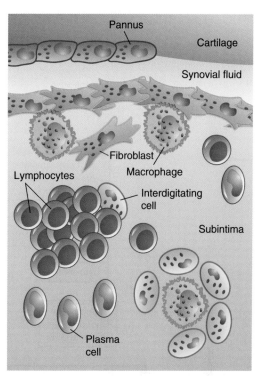

FIGURE 41.20 Synovitis. Inflamed synovium showing typical arrangements of macrophages and fibroblastic cells.

rash, lymph node or spleen enlargement, and Raynaud phenomenon (transient lack of circulation to the fingertips and toes).

Despite intensive research, the exact cause of RA remains obscure. It is likely a combination of genetic factors interacting with inflammatory mediators. There is a strong genetic predisposition to developing RA. The chronic inflammation characteristics of RA result from an intricate interplay of chemokines that are powerful mediators of inflammation. Chemokines attract T cells and produce inflammatory changes.[1] A key genetic element has been localized to the human leukocyte antigen (HLA) areas of the major histocompatibility complex in all ethnic groups. Recent research reveals the possibility of specific amino acid malpositions in the HLA molecule as a major factor in developing rheumatic diseases.[78] A surprising new discovery is the presence of T-cell abnormalities in individuals with RA. With long-term or intensive exposure to the antigen, normal antibodies (immunoglobulins [Igs]) become autoantibodies—antibodies that attack host tissues (self-antigens). Because they are usually present in individuals with RA, the altered antibodies are termed **rheumatoid factors (RFs).** The RFs usually consist of two classes of immunoglobulin antibodies (antibodies for IgM and IgG) but occasionally involve antibodies for IgA. Their main antigenic targets are portions of the immunoglobulin molecules. RFs bind with their target self-antigens in blood and synovial membrane, forming immune complexes (antigen-antibody complexes). (See Chapter 7 for a discussion about antigen-antibody binding in the immune response.)

Environmental factors, including geographic area of birth, diet, socioeconomic status, and especially smoking, have been identified as risk factors for developing and having higher disease activity of RA. RA and other autoimmune diseases have a higher prevalence among women. Additionally, because disease symptoms lessen during pregnancy

and are increased again in the postpartal period, researchers are including hormonal involvement in their studies.

PATHOPHYSIOLOGY Although no specific events (e.g., trauma, illness, or environmental conditions) have been identified that would cause immune abnormalities to develop into localized tissue and joint inflammation, the pathology of RA is fairly well understood. During inflammation, arginine (an α-amino acid) can be enzymatically modified into another α-amino acid, citrulline. The citrullinated proteins can be seen as antigens by the body's immune system. Thus both T and B cells play a role in the autoimmune response. T cells express RANKL, which promotes osteoclast formation and causes bony erosion.

Cartilage damage in RA is the result of at least three processes: (1) neutrophils and other cells in the synovial fluid become activated, degrading the surface layer of articular cartilage; (2) inflammatory cytokines induce enzymatic (metalloproteinase) breakdown of cartilage and bone; and (3) T cells also interact with synovial fibroblasts, converting synovium into a thick, abnormal layer of granulation tissue known as **pannus** (see Chapter 7). Macrophages, components of pannus (Fig. 41.20), stimulate the release of IL-1, PDGF, and fibronectin. The B lymphocytes are stimulated to produce more RFs. The newly targeted self-antigens (immunoglobulins) are in relatively constant supply and can thus perpetuate inflammation and the formation of immune complexes indefinitely (Fig. 41.21).

Inflammatory and immune processes have several damaging effects on the synovial membrane. Along with the swelling caused by leukocyte infiltration, the synovial membrane undergoes hyperplastic thickening as its cells proliferate and abnormally enlarge. As synovial inflammation progresses to involve its blood vessels, small venules become occluded by hypertrophied endothelial cells, fibrin, platelets, and inflammatory cells, which decrease vascular flow to the synovial tissue. Compromised circulation, coupled with increased metabolic needs as a result of hypertrophy and hyperplasia, causes hypoxia and metabolic acidosis.

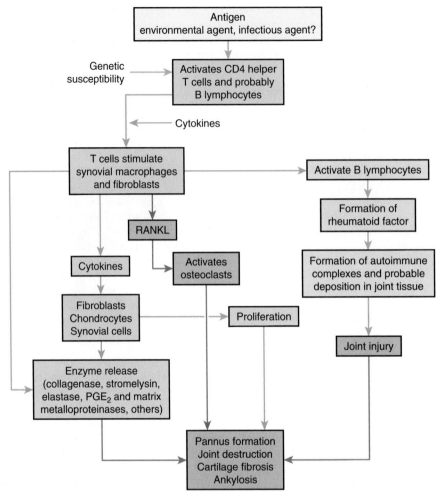

FIGURE 41.21 Emerging Model of Pathogenesis of Rheumatoid Arthritis. Rheumatoid arthritis is an autoimmune disease of a genetically susceptible host triggered by an unknown antigenic agent. A chronic autoimmune reaction with activation of CD4+ helper T cells and possibly other lymphocytes and the local release of inflammatory cytokines and mediators eventually destroy the joint. T cells stimulate cells in the joint to produce cytokines that are key mediators of synovial damage. Apparently, immune complex deposition also plays a role. Tumor necrosis factor (TNF) and interleukin-1 (IL-1), as well as some other cytokines, stimulate synovial cells to proliferate and produce other mediators of inflammation, such as prostaglandin E_2 *(PGE₂)*, matrix metalloproteinases, and enzymes that all contribute to destruction of cartilage. Activated T cells and synovial fibroblasts also produce receptor activator of nuclear factor κB ligand *(RANKL)*, which activates the osteoclasts and promotes bone destruction. Pannus is a mass of synovium and synovial stroma with inflammatory cells, granulation tissue, and fibroblasts that grows over the articular surface and causes its destruction.

Acidosis stimulates the release of hydrolytic enzymes from synovial cells into the surrounding tissue, initiating erosion of the articular cartilage and inflammation in the supporting ligaments and tendons. Pannus formation does not lead to synovial or articular regeneration but rather to formation of scar tissue that immobilizes the joint.

CLINICAL MANIFESTATIONS The onset of RA is usually insidious, although as many as 15% of cases have an acute onset. RA begins with general systemic manifestations of inflammation, including fever, fatigue, weakness, anorexia, weight loss, and generalized aching and stiffness. Local manifestations also appear gradually over a period of weeks or months. Typically, the joints become painful, tender, and stiff. Pain early in the disease is caused by pressure from swelling. Later in the disease, pain is caused by sclerosis of subchondral bone and new bone formation. Pain and inability to perform normal functions are the main reasons people seek medical help. Stiffness usually lasts for about 1

hour after rising in the morning and is thought to be related to synovitis. Initially the joints most commonly involved are the metacarpophalangeal (MCP) joints, proximal interphalangeal (PIP) joints, and wrists, with later involvement of larger weightbearing joints.

Widespread, symmetric joint swelling is caused by increasing amounts of inflammatory exudate (leukocytes, plasma, plasma proteins) in the synovial membrane, hyperplasia of inflamed tissues, and formation of new bone. On palpation, the swollen joint feels warm and the synovial membrane feels boggy. The skin over the joint may have a ruddy, cyanotic hue and may look thin and shiny.

An inflamed joint may lose some of its mobility. Even mild synovitis can lead to reduced range of motion, which becomes evident after inflammation subsides. Extension becomes limited and is eventually lost if flexion contractures develop. Limited range of motion can progress to permanent deformities of the fingers, toes, and limbs, including ulnar deviation of the hands, boutonnière and swan neck deformities of the finger joints, plantar subluxation of the metatarsal heads of the foot, and hallux valgus (angulation of the great toe toward the other toes). Flexion contractures of the knees and hips are also common.

Joint deformities cause the physical limitations experienced by persons with RA (see Fig. 41.19). Loss of joint motion is quickly followed by secondary atrophy of the surrounding muscles. With secondary muscle atrophy, the joint becomes unstable, which further aggravates joint pathology.

Two complications of chronic RA are caused by excessive amounts of inflammatory exudate in the synovial cavity. One complication is the formation of cysts in the articular cartilage or subchondral bone. Occasionally, these cysts communicate with the skin surface (such as in the sole of the foot) and can drain through passages called *fistulae*. The second complication is rupture of a cyst or of the synovial joint itself, usually caused by strenuous physical activity that places excessive pressure on the joint. Rupture releases inflammatory exudate into adjacent tissues, thereby spreading inflammation.

Extrasynovial rheumatoid nodules, seen in up to 30% of individuals with RA, are the most common extra-articular manifestations. Each nodule is a collection of inflammatory cells surrounding a central core of fibrinoid and cellular debris. Nodules are most often found in subcutaneous tissue over the extensor surfaces of elbows and fingers. Less common sites are the scalp, back, feet, hands, buttocks, and knees.

Rheumatoid nodules also may invade the skin, cardiac valves, pericardium, pleura, lung parenchyma, and spleen. These nodules are identical to those encountered in some individuals with rheumatic fever and are characterized by central tissue necrosis surrounded by proliferating connective tissue. Also noted are large numbers of lymphocytes and occasional plasma cells. Acute glaucoma may result with nodules forming on the sclera. Pulmonary involvement may result in diffuse pleuritis or multiple intraparenchymal nodules. Together, the occurrence of pulmonary nodules and pneumoconiosis (chronic inflammation of the lungs from inhalation of dust) creates the syndrome called Caplan syndrome. Diffuse pulmonary fibrosis may occur because of immunologically mediated immune complex deposition.

Rheumatoid nodules within the heart may cause valvular deformities, particularly of the aortic valve leaflets, and pericarditis. Lymphadenopathy of the nodes close to the affected joints may develop. Rheumatoid nodules within the spleen result in splenomegaly. Changes in skeletal muscle are often noted in the form of nonspecific atrophy secondary to joint dysfunction. Involvement of blood vessels results in an acute necrotizing vasculitis, characteristic of that noted in other immunologic/inflammatory states. Thromboses of such involved vessels may lead to myocardial infarctions, cerebrovascular occlusions, mesenteric infarction, kidney damage, and vascular insufficiency in the hands and fingers (Raynaud phenomenon). Fortunately, the development of vascular changes (particularly systemic vasculitis) is decreasing in frequency as more effective RA treatments are becoming available.

EVALUATION AND TREATMENT The diagnosis of RA relies on clinical evaluation of joint swelling; however, limitation of movement and control of pain often prevent identification of individuals who would benefit from treatment in early stages of the disease. Early treatment can be effective in preventing the systemic and joint abnormalities of chronic disease. Autoantibodies, RF, and anticitrullinated protein antibody (ACPA) can be present for years to decades before synovial or radiographic involvement becomes apparent.[79] Compared with RF, ACPA is a much more specific serum marker for RA. The ACR and the European League Against Rheumatism (EULAR) revised their RA classification criteria in 2010 to better identify the early stage of RA.[80] These new criteria are shown in Table 41.4. The clinical examination and history are the mainstays of RA diagnosis, but new imaging techniques show promise for earlier diagnosis, leading to earlier treatment, with a better chance for avoiding disability and joint destruction.

Early treatment of RA begins with disease-modifying antirheumatic drugs (DMARDs), such as methotrexate (MTX), azathioprine, sulfasalazine, hydroxychloroquine, leflunomide, and cyclosporine. These agents have been shown to slow the progression of RA and may prevent complications such as joint deformities and extra-articular complications. MTX remains the first line of treatment. More recently, targeted treatment for RA has involved use of agents aimed at interrupting the pathogenesis of the disease. Known as biologic DMARDs (bDMARDs), these medications affect specific processes in the development of RA and include tumor necrosis factor inhibitors, such as etanercept, adalimumab, and infliximab. They have been augmented by the monoclonal antibodies golimumab and certolizumab. Other agents interfere with cytokine function (anakinra inhibits IL-1 function and tocilizumab targets IL-6), inhibit T-cell activation (abatacept), or deplete B cells (rituximab).

Education for individuals with RA is fundamental to treatment. Other treatments and therapies include nonsteroidal antiinflammatory drugs (NSAIDs), glucocorticoids, intra-articular steroid injections, physical and occupational therapy with therapeutic exercise, and use of assistive devices. Surgery is used to treat deformities or mechanical deficiencies of joints and can include synovectomy or joint replacement surgery.

Ankylosing Spondylitis

Ankylosing spondylitis (AS) is the most common of a group of inflammatory arthropathies known as *spondyloarthropathies* (SpAs). The Assessment of SpondyloArthritis International Society (ASAS) has recommended classifying spondyloarthropathies to include individuals who do not have visible radiographic changes of the skeleton, as well as those who do. There would then be two subgroups: (1) mainly axial disease, including AS; and (2) peripheral SpA.[81]

AS is a chronic, inflammatory joint disease characterized by stiffening and fusion (ankylosis) of the spine and sacroiliac joints. Like RA, ankylosing spondylitis is a systemic, autoimmune inflammatory disease. Although inflammation is the primary pathologic process in both RA and AS, the two diseases differ in the primary site of inflammation and the end result. In RA, the primary site of inflammation is the synovial membrane, resulting in the destruction and instability of synovial joints. In AS, excessive bone formation occurs. The primary pathologic site is the enthesis (the point at which ligaments, tendons, and the joint capsule are inserted into bone), and the end result is fibrosis, ossification, and fusion of the joint, primarily the sacroiliac joints and the vertebral column (axial skeleton).

AS occurs worldwide, with the lowest prevalence in South Asian countries and highest in North America and Europe; it affects men more often than women.[82] In women, AS may affect the peripheral joints of the appendicular skeleton rather than the axial skeleton, progress less rapidly, and cause less dramatic spinal changes. Primary AS usually develops in late adolescence and young adulthood, with a peak incidence at about 20 years of age. Secondary AS affects older age groups and is often associated with other inflammatory diseases (e.g., psoriatic arthropathy, inflammatory bowel disease, Reiter syndrome).

PATHOPHYSIOLOGY The exact cause of ankylosing spondylitis is unknown, but its high association with histocompatibility antigen human leukocyte antigen (HLA-B27) has been known for decades. The disease process begins with inflammation of fibrocartilage in cartilaginous joints. In men, the sacroiliac joint is often affected first, usually before any damage can be radiographically detected. Knee pain may be the initial symptom in women. Inflammatory cells infiltrate the fibrous tissue of the joint capsule, the cartilage that surrounds intervertebral

TABLE 41.4 The 2010 American College of Rheumatology/European League Against Rheumatism Classification Criteria for Rheumatoid Arthritis

Target population to be tested:
1. Persons who have at least one joint with definite clinical synovitis (swelling)[a]
2. Persons who have synovitis not better explained by another disease[b]
Classification criteria for rheumatoid arthritis (RA) (score-based algorithm): Add scores of categories A to D; a score of ≥6/10 is needed for positive RA diagnosis[c]

Clinical Finding	Score
A. Joint involvement[d]	
1 large joint[e]	0
2-10 large joints	1
1-3 small joints (with or without involvement of large joints)[f]	2
4-10 small joints (with or without involvement of large joints)	3
>10 joints (at least 1 small joint)[g]	5
B. Serology (at least 1 test result is needed for classification)[h]	
Negative RF *and* negative ACPA	0
Low-positive RF *or* low-positive ACPA	2
High-positive RF *or* high-positive ACPA	3
C. Acute-phase reactants (at least 1 test result is needed for classification)[i]	
Normal CRP *and* normal ESR	0
Abnormal CRP *or* abnormal ESR	1
D. Duration of symptoms[j]	
<6 weeks	0
≥6 weeks	1

[a]The criteria are aimed at classification of newly presenting persons. In addition, persons with erosive disease typical of rheumatoid arthritis (RA) with a history compatible of prior fulfillment of the 2010 criteria should be classified as having RA. Persons with longstanding disease—including those whose disease is inactive (with or without treatment) and who, based on retrospectively available data, have previously fulfilled the 2010 criteria—should be classified as having RA.
[b]Differential diagnoses vary among persons with different presentations, but may include conditions such as systemic lupus erythematosus, psoriatic arthritis, and gout. If it is unclear about the relevant differential diagnoses to consider, an expert rheumatologist should be consulted.
[c]Although persons with a score <6/10 are not classifiable as having RA, their status can be reassessed and the criteria might be fulfilled cumulatively over time.
[d]Joint involvement refers to any *swollen* or *tender* joint on examination, which may be confirmed by imaging evidence of synovitis. Distal interphalangeal joints, first metacarpophalangeal joints, and first metatarsophalangeal joints are *excluded from assessment*. Categories of joint distribution are classified according to the location and number of involved joints, with placement into the highest category possible based on the pattern of joint involvement.
[e]"Large joints" refer to shoulders, elbows, hips, knees, and ankles.
[f]"Small joints" refer to the metacarpophalangeal joints, proximal interphalangeal joints, second through fifth metatarsophalangeal joints, thumb interphalangeal joints, and wrists.
[g]In this category, at least one of the involved joints must be a small joint; the others can include any combination of large and additional small joints, as well as other joints not specifically listed elsewhere (e.g., temporomandibular, acromioclavicular, sternoclavicular).
[h]Negative refers to international unit (IU) values that are less than or equal to the upper limit of normal (ULN) for the laboratory and assay; low-positive refers to values that are higher than the ULN but ≤3 times the ULN for the laboratory and assay; high-positive refers to IU values that are >3 times the ULN for the laboratory and assay. Where rheumatoid factor (RF) information is only available as positive or negative, a positive result should be scored as low-positive for RF. *ACPA,* Anticitrullinated protein antibody.
[i]Normal/abnormal is determined by local laboratory standards. *CRP,* C-reactive protein; *ESR,* erythrocyte sedimentation rate.
[j]Duration of symptoms refers to individual's self-report of the duration of signs and symptoms of synovitis (e.g., pain, swelling, tenderness) of joints that are clinically involved at the time of assessment, regardless of treatment status.
Data from Aletaha D et al: *Arthritis Rheum* 62(9):2574, 2010.

disks, the entheses, and the periosteum. As inflammatory cells (chiefly macrophages) and lymphocytes infiltrate and erode bone and fibrocartilage in joint structures, repair begins. Repair of cartilaginous structures begins with the proliferation of fibroblasts. Fibroblasts synthesize and secrete collagen. The collagen becomes organized into fibrous scar tissue that eventually undergoes calcification and ossification. With time, all the cartilaginous structures of the joint are replaced by ossified scar tissue, causing the joint to fuse, or lose flexibility.

Repair of eroded bone begins with osteoblast activation and proliferation. Osteoblasts lay down new bone (callus), which is remodeled and replaced by compact, lamellar bone. Bone repair changes the contour of the bone's surface because the new bone grows outward (outside the normal border of unaffected bone) to form a new enthesis with the end of the eroded ligament. The new enthesis, which forms on top of the old one, is called a syndesmophyte. As calcification of the spinal ligaments progresses, the vertebral bodies lose their concave anterior contour and appear square. The spine assumes the classic bamboo spine appearance of ankylosing spondylitis.

CLINICAL MANIFESTATIONS   The most common signs and symptoms of early AS are low back pain and stiffness. Typically, the individual with primary disease develops low back pain during the early twenties. The pain is at first insidious but progressively becomes persistent. It is often worse after prolonged rest and is alleviated by physical activity.

Early morning stiffness usually accompanies the low back pain, and the individual typically has difficulty sitting up or twisting the spine. Forward flexion, rotation, and lateral flexion of the spine are restricted and painful. Early pain and resultant loss of motion are caused by the underlying inflammation and reflex muscle spasm rather than by soft tissue or bony fusion.

As the disease progresses, the normal convex curve of the lower spine (lumbar lordosis) diminishes and concavity of the upper spine (kyphosis) increases. The individual becomes increasingly stooped. The thoracic spine becomes rounded, the head and neck are held forward on the shoulders, and the hips are flexed (Fig. 41.22).

Inflammation in the tendon insertions of the many costosternal and costovertebral muscles can cause pleuritic chest pain and restricted chest movement. The pain is usually worse on inspiration. Movement of the diaphragm is normal and full. Pressure on the anterior chest wall over the sternum, ribs, and costal cartilages may cause tenderness. Tenderness over the pelvic brim may cause discomfort at night and interfere with sleep because turning onto the iliac crests causes pain. Tenderness over the ischial tuberosities may make sitting on hard seats unbearable. Tenderness in the heels may contribute to a limp or cautious placement of the feet during walking.

Along with low back pain and sacroiliac pain, inflammation of the bowels, anterior uveitis, aortic regurgitation, fibrosis of the upper lobes of the lung, Achilles tendonitis, and immune-related (IgA) kidney disease frequently accompany AS. Elevated sedimentation rate (ESR) and elevated level of CRP also are common.

EVALUATION AND TREATMENT   The diagnosis of AS is based on specific criteria. One of the previous problems with diagnosing AS has been a requirement for radiographic (x-ray) evidence of sacroiliitis; MRI can discover sacroiliitis an average of 7.7 years before there is evidence on x-rays.[83] Both MRI and plain radiographic findings are important in detecting early disease and for evaluating individuals younger than 45 years of age with back pain of at least 3 months' duration.[84]

In addition to sacroiliitis being present on imaging, one or more of these features allow a diagnosis of SpA: inflammatory back pain, arthritis, anterior uveitis, heel pain, dactylitis, psoriasis, Crohn disease or ulcerative colitis, good response to NSAIDs, family history of SpA, positive HLA-B27 result, or elevated CRP. If the individual has a positive HLA-B27 result, at least two of the previously mentioned items must be present, along with sacroiliitis on MRI or radiographic imaging, to make a diagnosis.[85]

Treatment of individuals with AS consists of education about the disease, as well as physical therapy to maintain skeletal mobility and prevent the natural progression of contractures. Prevention of deformity and maintenance of mobility require a continuous program of physical therapy. Supervised group exercises have been shown to reduce pain and to maintain and improve chest expansion and respiratory function, spine mobility, and complete range of motion in the proximal joints.

NSAIDs often provide temporary symptom relief within 48 hours. Analgesic medications are prescribed to suppress some of the pain and stiffness and to facilitate exercise. The medications do not prevent disease progression, but they do provide relief from symptoms. Biologic response modifying agents, such as TNF inhibitors (certolizumab, golimumab) or B-cell depleting agents (rituximab), are increasingly being used to treat AS. Newer agents that target cytokines of Th17 and small nano particles that alter certain inflammatory pathways are showing promise in treating AS.[86,87] Surgical procedures, such as osteotomy, total hip replacement, and cervical spinal fusion, and radiation therapy are sometimes used to provide relief for individuals with end-stage disease or intolerable deformity. Individuals should stop smoking to lessen pulmonary problems.

Gout

Gout is an inflammatory response to excessive quantities of uric acid in the blood (hyperuricemia) and in other body fluids, including synovial fluid. These elevated levels lead to the formation of monosodium urate (MSU) crystals in and around joints. The result of crystallization in synovial fluid is acute, painful inflammation of the joint. This inflammatory response triggers macrophages that phagocytose MSU crystals. Altogether they form a protein scaffold known as an *inflammasome*. Inflammasomes convert inactive interleukins into their active forms. Prolonged accumulation results in joint damage, a condition known as **gouty arthritis**. Urate crystal deposits also cause oxidative stress reactions in other tissues. With time, crystal deposition in subcutaneous tissues causes the formation of small, white nodules, or **tophi**, that are visible through the skin. Tophi are associated with joint damage and an increased death rate, primarily because of cardiovascular events. Hyperuricemia is associated with hypertension, heart disease, type 2 diabetes, kidney disease, and metabolic syndrome.

Although hyperuricemia is essential for the development of gout, it is not the only factor. Other factors include age (rare before 30 years), genetic predisposition (X-linked alteration of the enzyme hypoxanthine-guanine phosphoribosyltransferase [HGPRT]), excessive alcohol consumption, obesity, certain drugs (especially thiazides), and lead toxicity. Dietary intake of purine-rich foods, such as organ meats, pork, some fish, and beer, also has been shown to contribute to the incidence of gout. Additionally, evidence exists identifying the contributory nature of foods high in fructose and sugar-sweetened soft drinks. Conversely, dairy products, coffee, and vitamin C have been shown to have a protective effect against gout.

Gout is rare in children and premenopausal women and is uncommon in males younger than 30 years. Male sex, increasing age, and high intake of alcohol, red meat, and fructose are all risk factors for gout. The peak age of onset in males is between 40 and 50 years. The risk of developing gouty arthritis is similar in males and females for a particular

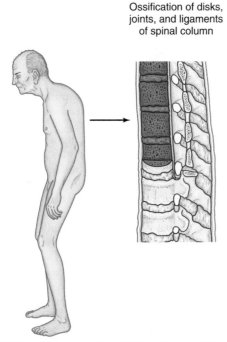

Ossification of disks, joints, and ligaments of spinal column

FIGURE 41.22 Ankylosing Spondylitis. Characteristic posture and primary pathologic sites of inflammation and resulting damage. (Redrawn from Mourad LA: *Orthopedic disorders*, St Louis, 1991, Mosby.)

TABLE 41.5 Mean Urate Concentrations by Age and Sex

Characteristic	Mean Urate Levels (mg/dl)
Prepuberty	3.5
Males (at puberty)	Steep rise to 5.2
Females (puberty to after premenopause)	Slow rise to ≈ 4
Females (after menopause)	4.7
Hyperuricemia	
Males	7
Females	6

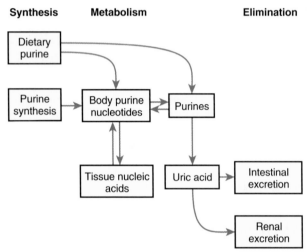

FIGURE 41.23 Uric Acid Synthesis and Elimination. Uric acid is derived from purines ingested or synthesized from ingested foods, as well as being recycled after cell breakdown. Uric acid then is eliminated through the kidneys and gastrointestinal tract. (Redrawn from Klippel JH, Dieppe PA, editors: *Rheumatology*, ed 2, St Louis, 1998, Mosby.)

urate concentration. Females tend to have an onset at a later age and have greater use of diuretics, more coexisting diseases (hypertension, renal insufficiency), more frequent involvement of other joints, and fewer recurrent episodes. The plasma urate concentration is the single most important determinant of the risk of developing gout (Table 41.5).

Uric acid is a weak acid that is ionized at normal body pH and thus occurs in the blood or tissues in the form of urate ion. When ionized, uric acid can form salts with various cations, but 98% of extracellular uric acid is in the form of monosodium urate (uric acid salt). At any time the proportion of uric acid or urate is pH dependent, so the ratio of these two forms varies considerably in urine.

The solubility of urate and uric acid is critical to the development of crystals. Urate is more soluble in plasma, synovial fluid, and urine than in aqueous solutions. The solubility of uric acid in urine rises dramatically as the pH increases. There is little change, however, in the solubility of urate within the normal pH range that exists in the plasma, synovial fluid, and other tissues. The pH can be 5 in the collecting tubules of the kidney, thus favoring the formation of uric acid. Decreasing temperatures cause both urate and uric acid solubility to fall. The pathways of production of uric acid are shown in Fig. 41.23.

PATHOPHYSIOLOGY The pathophysiology of gout is closely linked to purine metabolism (or cellular metabolism of purines) and kidney function. At the cellular level, purines are synthesized to purine

nucleotides, which are used in the synthesis of nucleic acids, ATP, cyclic adenosine monophosphate (cAMP), and cyclic guanosine monophosphate (cGMP). Uric acid is a breakdown product of purine nucleotides (urate synthesis and elimination are illustrated in Fig. 41.24).

Individuals with gout may have an accelerated rate of purine synthesis accompanied by an overproduction of uric acid. Other individuals break down purine nucleotides at an accelerated rate, also resulting in an overproduction of uric acid. A deficiency of the enzyme HGPRT (see earlier) can lead to an increased production of uric acid. A complete absence of HGPRT is uncommon but can occur in the X-linked Lesch-Nyhan syndrome, with males at risk for hyperuricemia, neurologic alterations, and sometimes gouty arthritis. The majority of individuals with gout, however, have an unknown metabolic defect, referred to as **primary gout.** When the etiology is known, it is called **secondary gout.**

Most uric acid is eliminated from the body through the kidneys. Urate is filtered at the glomerulus and undergoes both reabsorption and excretion within the renal tubules. In primary gout, urate excretion by the kidneys is sluggish; this may be the result of a decrease in glomerular filtration of urate or acceleration in urate reabsorption. In addition, MSU crystals deposited in renal tubules can cause acute nephropathy. (Kidney function is described in Chapter 31.)

MSU crystals can stimulate and continue the inflammatory response (see Fig. 41.24, *A* and *B*). The presence of the crystals triggers the acute inflammatory response, and initiation of the complement system activates cytokines and interleukins. which draw neutrophils out of the circulation to begin phagocytizing the crystals. Tissue damage ensues with the release of neutrophils. As the process continues, numerous microtophi may be present on the synovial membrane (see Fig. 41.24, *C*).

Use of advanced technology, including high-resolution ultrasound, dual-energy computed tomography (DECT), and MRI, can assess the presence of MSU crystals before joint, tendon, or ligament damage occurs.[88] Imaging modalities also can be used when joints cannot be aspirated to look for MSU crystals microscopically. Earlier identification allows timely as well as ongoing evaluation of treatment.[89]

CLINICAL MANIFESTATIONS Gout is manifested by (1) an increase in the serum urate concentration (hyperuricemia); (2) recurrent attacks of monoarticular arthritis (inflammation of a single joint); (3) deposits of MSU monohydrate (tophi) in and around the joints; (4) renal disease involving glomerular, tubular, and interstitial tissues and blood vessels; and (5) the formation of renal stones. These manifestations appear in three clinical stages:

1. **Asymptomatic hyperuricemia.** The serum urate level is elevated but arthritic symptoms, tophi, and renal stones are not present; this stage may persist throughout life.
2. **Acute gouty arthritis.** Attacks develop with increased serum urate concentrations; tends to occur with sudden or sustained increases of hyperuricemia but also can be triggered by trauma, drugs, and alcohol.
3. **Tophaceous gout.** The chronic stage of the disease; can begin as early as 3 years or as late as 40 years after the initial attack of gouty arthritis. Progressive inability to excrete uric acid expands the urate pool until MSU crystal deposits (tophi) appear in cartilage, synovial membranes, tendons, and soft tissue.

Trauma is the most common aggravating factor of an acute gouty exacerbation. Attacks of gouty arthritis occur abruptly, usually in a peripheral joint (see Fig. 41.24, *C*). The primary symptom is severe pain. Approximately 50% of the initial attacks occur in the metatarsophalangeal joint of the great toe (a condition known as *podagra*). The other 50% can occur in almost any joint, but most often involve the heel, ankle, instep of the foot, knee, wrist, or elbow. The pain is usually noted at night. Within a few hours the affected joint becomes hot, red,

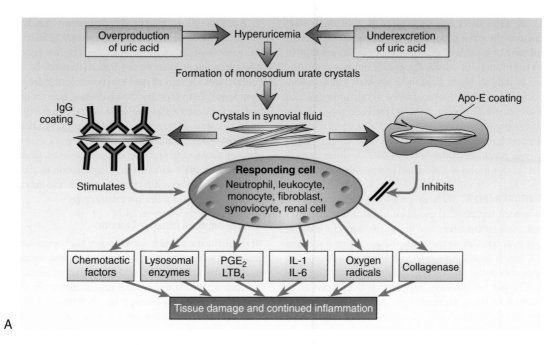

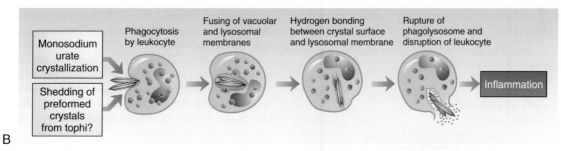

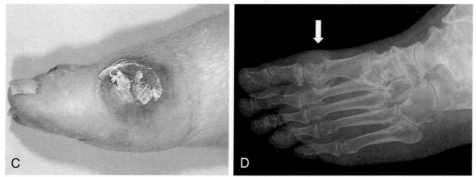

FIGURE 41.24 Pathogenesis of Acute Gouty Arthritis. **A,** Depending on the urate crystal coating, a variety of cells may be stimulated to produce a wide range of inflammatory mediators. **B,** Sequence of events in the production of the inflammatory response to urate crystals. **C,** Gouty tophus on right foot. **D,** Bone destruction of first metatarsal because of gout. *Apo-E,* Apolipoprotein E; *IgG,* immunoglobulin G; *IL,* interleukin; *LTB₄,* leukotriene B₄; *PGE₂,* prostaglandin E₂. (**C** from Dieppe PA et al: *Arthritis and rheumatism in practice,* London, 1991, Gower. **D** from Chhana A, Dalbeth N: *Rheum Dis Clin North Am* 40[2]:291-309, 2014.)

and extremely tender and may be slightly swollen. Lymphangitis and systemic signs of inflammation (leukocytosis, fever, an elevated sedimentation rate) are occasionally present. Untreated, mild attacks usually subside in several hours but may persist for 1 or 2 days. Severe attacks may persist for several days or weeks. When the individual recovers, the symptoms resolve completely.

Tophaceous deposits produce irregular swellings of the fingers, hands, knees, and feet. The helix of the ear is the most common site of tophi, which are the characteristic diagnostic lesions of chronic gout. Tophi

also may develop along the ulnar surface of the forearm, the tibial surface of the leg, the Achilles tendon, olecranon bursa, or other areas. Tophi may produce marked limitation of joint movement and can eventually cause grotesque deformities of the hands and feet (see Fig. 41.24, *C*). Although the tophi themselves are painless, they often cause progressive stiffness and persistent aching of the affected joint. Tophi in the extremities can cause nerve compression—carpal tunnel syndrome in the wrists, tarsal tunnel syndrome in the ankles. Tophi also may erode and drain through the skin.

Renal stones are 1000 times more prevalent in individuals with primary gout than in the general population. The stones can be the size of a grain of sand or a piece of gravel, or they can accumulate in massive deposits called *staghorn calculi*. They range in color from pale yellow to brown to reddish black, depending on their composition. Some stones consist of pure MSU; others consist of calcium oxalate or calcium phosphate. Renal stones can form in the collecting tubules, pelvis, or ureters, causing obstruction, dilation, and atrophy of the more proximal tubules and leading eventually to acute renal failure. Stones deposited directly in renal interstitial tissue initiate an inflammatory reaction that leads to chronic renal disease and progressive renal failure.

EVALUATION AND TREATMENT   The diagnosis of gout is made from the individual's history and physical examination; also included may be blood tests, possible joint aspiration, and the use of diagnostic imaging. The goals of gout treatment are to terminate the acute gouty attack as promptly as possible; reduce serum uric acid levels; avoid recurring attacks; prevent or reverse complications associated with urate deposits in the joints, soft tissues, and kidneys; and prevent the formation of kidney stones. Numerous drugs are used to prevent or abort attacks of arthritis. Nonpharmacologic treatment includes the application of ice to relieve pain and inflammation of the joint. Weight bearing on the involved joint is avoided until the acute attack subsides. Reducing body weight, avoiding alcohol, and changing dietary practices may reduce recurrent gouty episodes.

QUICK CHECK 41.3

1. How does noninflammatory joint disease differ from inflammatory joint disease? Describe two principal features of each.
2. How does rheumatoid arthritis affect the skin, heart, lungs, and kidneys?
3. How do monosodium urate crystals cause gout to develop?

DISORDERS OF SKELETAL MUSCLE

Muscle diseases (myopathies) encompass many entities. Muscle weakness and muscle fatigue are common symptoms. In many cases, neural, traumatic, and psychogenic causes provide an adequate explanation for the failure to generate force (weakness) or sustain force (fatigue) seen in myopathies. The pathophysiologic mechanisms in some of the metabolic and inflammatory muscle diseases have been explored, but the cause of many of the myopathies remains obscure. The complex interaction between muscles and nerves affects muscular function as well. Only inherited and acquired disorders of skeletal muscles are discussed here.

Secondary Muscular Dysfunction

Muscular symptoms arise from a variety of causes unrelated to the muscle itself. Secondary muscular phenomena (contracture, stress-related muscle tension, immobility) are common disorders that influence muscular function.

Contractures

Contractures are the lack of full passive range of motion of a joint because of muscle, or other soft tissue limitations and can be *pathologic* or *physiologic*. A physiologic muscle contracture occurs in the absence of a muscle action potential in the sarcolemma. Muscle shortening is explained on the basis of failure of the calcium pump in the presence of plentiful ATP. A physiologic contracture is seen in McArdle disease (muscle myophosphorylase deficiency) and malignant hyperthermia. The contracture is usually temporary if the underlying pathology is reversed.

A pathologic contracture is a permanent muscle shortening caused by muscle spasm or weakness. Heel cord (Achilles tendon) contractures are examples of pathologic contractures. They are associated with plentiful ATP and occur in spite of a normal action potential. The most common contractures are seen in stroke, neuromuscular diseases (e.g., muscular dystrophy), Charcot-Marie-Tooth disease, amyotrophic lateral sclerosis, and central nervous system (CNS) injury. Lower extremity contractures are more common than those in the upper extremity. Prolonged splinting in a single position or an imbalance between agonist-antagonist muscles also can cause joint stiffness and contractures. Contractures also may develop secondary to scar tissue contraction in the flexor tissues of a joint, as in scarring of burned tissues in the antecubital area of the forearm, leading to a flexion contracture.

Stress-Induced Muscle Tension

Abnormally increased muscle tension has been associated with chronic anxiety, as well as a variety of stress-related muscular symptoms, including neck stiffness, back pain, and headache. Abnormalities in the CNS, reticular activating system, and autonomic nervous system (ANS) have been implicated. For example, as an individual progressively relaxes, the amplitude of the knee jerk reflex diminishes. Conversely, individuals with absent reflexes increase tension by such maneuvers as clenching the teeth or strengthening the handgrip. The underlying pathophysiology may be related to the fact that as a muscle contracts, the muscle spindle is activated. This gamma feedback system produces a series of impulses that are transmitted to the brain by the sensitive 1A afferent fibers. Unconscious tension is thought to increase the activity of the reticular activating system as well, which stimulates firing of the efferent loop of the gamma fibers, produces further muscle contraction, and increases muscle tension. ANS function that regulates increased blood flow to the muscle during sympathetic activity may be related to increased muscle contraction tension.

Various forms of treatment have been used to reduce the muscle tension associated with stress. Progressive relaxation training, yoga, meditation, and biofeedback are examples of stress reduction therapies.

Fibromyalgia

Fibromyalgia (FM) is a chronic musculoskeletal syndrome characterized by diffuse joint and muscle pain, fatigue, and increased sensitivity to touch, called tender points. The absence of systemic or localized inflammation, and the presence of fatigue and nonrestorative sleep, anxiety, and depression also are common. Individuals with FM report widespread tenderness in all body regions and an increased sensitivity to numerous stimuli, including heat, cold, and electrical stimuli. Another emerging factor is a sensitivity to light and sound. New research continues to support the possible role of inflammation in the development of FM.[90] A common misdiagnosis in the past has been chronic fatigue syndrome; there is overlap between these two conditions. Of affected individuals, 80% to 90% are women, and the peak age is 30 to 50 years. The ACR has identified new criteria for the diagnosis of FM. A tender point evaluation is no longer required; instead, the use of a widespread pain index (WPI) and symptom severity inventory (SSI) is recommended.[91]

The etiology of FM is unknown but is thought to include both genetic susceptibility and environmental exposure that triggers alterations in gene expression (epigenetics). Despite much debate on the classification and pathophysiology of FM, it now is recognized as a disorder.

PATHOPHYSIOLOGY   FM has an unclear pathophysiology. Genetic factors are increasingly being suggested as important in the development of FM. Relatives of individuals with FM have an increased risk of developing FM. Studies of genetic factors have implicated alterations in genes affecting serotonin, catecholamines, and dopamine—all of these substances are involved in neuroendocrine and stress-response alterations (see Chapter 10). In spite of these studies, the role of genetic factors has not yet been fully identified in FM. External stressors, such as infection, psychosocial stress, and physical or emotional trauma, have been proposed as mechanisms precipitating FM. These relationships continue to be researched.

Functional magnetic resonance imaging (fMRI) and PET scans of the brains of individuals with FM have shown activity in areas of the brain different from those seen in healthy individuals exposed to painful stimuli.[92] These functional abnormalities within the CNS are shown in Fig. 41.25. Other pathophysiologic evidence suggests hypothalamic-pituitary axis alterations that show an impaired response to stress. Cytokines also are involved in the pathogenesis of FM.

CLINICAL MANIFESTATIONS The prominent symptom of fibromyalgia is diffuse, chronic pain. Pain often begins in one location, especially the neck and shoulders, but then becomes more generalized. Fatigue is most notable when arising from sleep and during the midafternoon. Headaches, symptoms of irritable bowel syndrome, and excess sensitivity to cold (Raynaud-like) are reported in 50% of individuals. Fatigue is profound. The effect on everyday life is considerable. Almost 25% of individuals seek psychological support for depression. Anxiety, particularly with regard to the diagnosis and future, is almost universal.

EVALUATION AND TREATMENT Because the manifestations of chronic, generalized pain and fatigue are present in many musculoskeletal (e.g., rheumatic) disorders, these disorders should be considered in the differential diagnosis of FM (Tables 41.6 and 41.7). In an effort to simplify and more accurately diagnose FM, the ACR expanded the diagnostic criteria to include a WPI definition as "axial pain, left- and right-sided pain, and upper and lower segment pain…"[93] and a symptom severity (SS) score. The SS score includes symptoms such as fatigue, waking unrefreshed, and cognitive difficulty. The WPI and SS scores are then tabulated to identify or exclude the diagnosis of FM in individuals who also meet these criteria:

- Symptoms have been present at a similar level for at least 3 months.
- The individual does not have a disorder that would otherwise explain the pain.[93]

The 2010 FM classification criteria were further updated in 2011 so that FM can be classified solely by patient report using a questionnaire

and scale.[94] Treatment should be highly individualized and can include mind-body interventions (e.g., biofeedback), movement therapies, and relaxation techniques, as well as medication.[95] No one regimen or medication has proved successful for FM. Current recommendations outline a combination of pharmacologic and nonpharmacologic therapies. The most effective approach is a combination of modalities, including education, medication, exercise, and cognitive behavioral therapy. Box 41.4 lists some of these modalities.

Chronic Fatigue Syndrome

Chronic fatigue syndrome (CFS), also known as myalgic encephalomyelitis (ME), is a chronic debilitating disease characterized by profound fatigue, musculoskeletal pain, cognitive impairment, unrestful sleep (major hallmark), impaired neurologic energy production, and immune impairments. Individuals also may experience sore throat, headache, and tender lymph nodes. Research emphasis is directed toward the immune and adrenal systems, genetics, and biopsychosocial involvement. As a result, CFS/ME is believed to be less of a musculoskeletal disorder and more related to hypersensitivity of the CNS, a condition known as *central sensitization* of the CNS.

Disuse Atrophy

The term disuse atrophy describes the pathologic reduction in normal size of muscle fibers after prolonged inactivity from bed rest, trauma (casting), or local nerve damage, as can be seen with spinal cord trauma

---

BOX 41.4 Educating and Providing Reassurance for Individuals With Fibromyalgia

- Stress that the illness is real, not imagined.
- Explain that fibromyalgia is presumably not caused by infection.
- Explain that fibromyalgia is not a deforming or deteriorating condition.
- Explain that fibromyalgia is neither life-threatening nor markedly debilitating, although it is an irritating presence.
- Discuss the role of sleep disturbances and the relationship of neurohormones to pain, fatigue, abnormal sleep, and mood.
- Reassure that although the cause is unknown, some information is known about the physiologic changes responsible for the symptoms.
- Use muscle "spasms" and, perhaps, "low muscle blood flow" to lay the groundwork for exercise recommendations.
- Assist the individual to use aerobic exercise to reduce stress and increase rapid eye movement (REM) sleep.

TABLE 41.6 Differential Diagnosis of Fibromyalgia

Differential Diagnosis	Helpful Differential Features
Rheumatoid arthritis*	Synovitis, serologic tests, elevated erythrocyte sedimentation rate (ESR)
Systemic lupus erythematosus	Dermatitis, serositis (renal, central erythematosus,*nervous system, etc.)
Polymyalgia rheumatica*	Elevated ESR, older adults, response to corticosteroids
Myositis	Increased muscle enzymes, weakness more than pain
Hypothyroidism*	Abnormal thyroid function tests
Neuropathies	Clinical and electrophysiologic evidence of neuropathy

*Fibromyalgia may also more commonly coexist with these conditions.
Data from Klippel JH, Dieppe PA, editors: *Rheumatology*, ed 2, London, 1998, Mosby-Wolfe.

TABLE 41.7 Concomitant Conditions With Fibromyalgia

Concomitant Condition	Relationship to Fibromyalgia
Depression	Present in 25%–60% of fibromyalgia cases
Irritable bowel syndrome	Present in 50%–80% of fibromyalgia cases
Migraine	Present in 50% of fibromyalgia cases
Chronic fatigue syndrome (CFS)	70% of CFS cases meet criteria for fibromyalgia
Myofascial pain	May be a localized form of fibromyalgia

Data from Klippel JH, Dieppe PA, editors: *Rheumatology*, ed 2, London, 1998, Mosby-Wolfe.

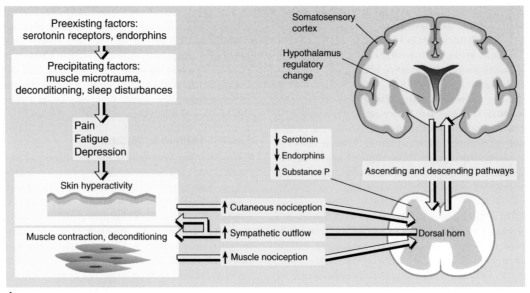

A

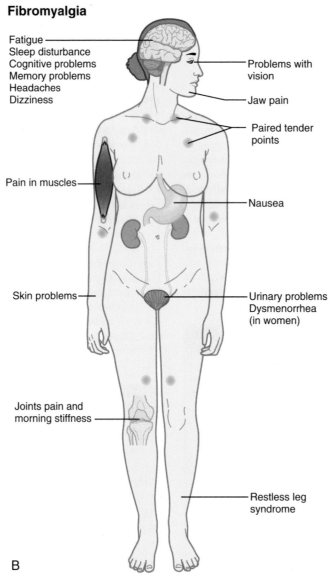

B

FIGURE 41.25 Theoretic Pathophysiologic Model of Fibromyalgia. **A,** Location of specific tender points for fibromyalgia. **B,** The 18 tender points (9 pairs) tend to be painful when pressed, and the pain may spread to other body parts. (**B** from https://www.spineuniverse.com.)

or poliomyelitis. Decreased muscle activity reduces muscle mass through both decreased muscle protein synthesis and increased muscle protein breakdown.[96] Reduced protein synthesis is primarily responsible for muscle atrophy. The effects of muscular deconditioning associated with lack of physical activity may be apparent in a matter of days. A normal individual prescribed bed rest loses muscle strength from baseline levels at a rate of 3% per day. Bed rest also is associated with cardiovascular, skeletal, and other organ system changes. Likewise, as people age, their muscles atrophy and become weaker (sarcopenia).

Measures to prevent atrophy include frequent forceful isometric muscle contractions and passive lengthening exercises. Artificial gravity (through the use of a *human centrifuge*) has shown benefit in maintaining muscle strength. One of the simplest ways to improve disuse atrophy is to restore a load to the muscle, such as returning to walking, starting active motion to a limb, and adding resistance to movements.[97] If reuse is not restored within 1 year, regeneration of muscle fibers becomes impaired.

Muscle Membrane Abnormalities

Two defects of the muscle membrane (plasma membrane of the muscle fiber) have been linked to clinical syndromes: the hyperexcitable membrane seen in myotonic disorders and the intermittently unresponsive membrane seen in periodic paralyses. Although these are rare disorders, research into their pathologic processes has led to an improved understanding of cell membrane channelopathies (ion channels are described in Chapter 14).

Skeletal Muscle Channelopathies

Skeletal muscle channelopathies can be divided into two primary groups: (1) myotonia (nondystrophic myotonias) and (2) those associated with episodes of weakness (periodic paralysis). In myotonic channelopathies, muscle relaxation is delayed after voluntary contractions, such as handgrip or eye closure, leading to a disabling muscle stiffness or weakness, or both. Periodic paralysis is an autosomal dominant disorder in which depolarization of the sarcolemma is severe enough that the muscle cannot be *fired* again, resulting in paralysis or even myotonia. Myotonia can be reproduced by removing extracellular chloride, thus reducing chloride conductance across the plasma membrane. The delicate balance in which sodium diffuses into the intracellular fluid, potassium diffuses out of the intracellular fluid, and chloride is in flux, is interrupted. Because the normal diffusion processes (described in Chapter 5) stabilize the membrane, the shift in chloride ions is thought to increase membrane excitability. The chloride abnormality may explain the resting membrane hyperexcitability, but it does not explain the delayed relaxation present in myotonia and has not been detected in human myotonia. Myotonia is noted in several disorders: myotonia congenita, paramyotonia congenita, myotonic muscular dystrophy, and some forms of periodic paralysis. Most are inherited disorders and are mild in symptomatology, with the exception of myotonic muscular dystrophy. Myotonia is treated by drugs that reduce muscle fiber excitability, such as sodium channel blocking agents (mexiletine, procainamide) and phenytoin.

Central core disease (CCD) is another inherited channelopathy that involves mutations in ryanodine receptors (RyR1) and affects calcium channels. In CCD, RyR1 channels are defective, and either too much or too little calcium is released from the cell's sarcoplasmic reticulum, resulting in symmetrical proximal muscle weakness. This weakness, however, is usually not progressive in nature. Classified as a neuromuscular disorder, CCD typically manifests during infancy as decreased muscle tone, delayed motor development, muscle weakness (particularly around the hip girdle), and other skeletal deformities, such as scoliosis.

Periodic Paralysis

Periodic paralysis (PP) includes a rare group of muscle diseases characterized by episodes of flaccid weakness. Most are hereditary (autosomal dominant) and the genetic mutations cause calcium, sodium, or potassium channel abnormalities. PP is usually transient, and during an attack of PP the muscle membrane is unresponsive to neural stimuli. PP can be either hyperkalemic or hypokalemic. The paralysis, which leaves the individual flaccid and weak, typically affects only the skeletal muscles and not the respiratory muscles. The weakness is accompanied by a change in serum potassium levels, although in most individuals the change is negligible unless a secondary underlying condition affecting potassium distribution coexists. For this reason, cardiac dysrhythmias, although not common, have been present during attacks.

Hypokalemic periodic paralysis is often triggered by thyrotoxicosis caused by alterations in potassium ion channels that are regulated by triodothyronine (T_3). Oral and intravenous potassium can relieve acute attacks. Treatment includes potassium-sparing diuretics and a high-salt diet. Long-term therapy includes medications and a low-salt diet.

Hyperkalemic periodic paralysis is episodes of extreme muscle weakness usually beginning in childhood or adolescence. These episodes most often involve a temporary inability to move muscles in the arms and legs.[98] Attacks cause severe weakness or paralysis that typically lasts hours to days. Episodes vary; some people have them almost every day, and others experience them weekly, monthly, or only rarely. Attacks can occur without warning or can be triggered by rest after exercise, a viral illness, or certain medications.[98] Often a large carbohydrate-rich meal or vigorous exercise in the evening can trigger an attack upon waking the next morning.[98] Affected individuals usually regain their strength between attacks, but repeated episodes can lead to muscle weakness later in life. Mutations in the *CACNA1S* or *SCN4A* gene can cause periodic paralysis. These genes provide instructions for making proteins that play an essential role in movement or skeletal muscles.[98] Although sufficient evidence is lacking to provide full guidelines for the treatment of people with periodic paralysis, dichlorophenamide (DCP) was effective in a large study and some evidence exists for acetazolamide or pinacidil.

Metabolic Muscle Diseases

Metabolic muscle diseases are a collection of disorders caused by a genetic mutation and endocrine abnormalities that affect a muscle's metabolism. The resulting disorders in muscle metabolism lead to diseases of energy metabolism, such as glycogen storage disease, enzyme deficiencies, and abnormalities in lipid metabolism and mitochondrial function.

Endocrine Disorders

Often the systemic effects of hormonal imbalance overshadow the individual's muscular symptoms. For example, individuals with thyrotoxicosis may have signs of proximal weakness, paresis of the extraocular muscles (exophthalmic ophthalmoplegia) and, rarely, hypokalemic periodic paralysis. Hypothyroidism is often associated with a decrease in muscle mass and strength, with weak, flabby skeletal muscles and sluggish movements.

Thyroid hormone is believed to regulate muscle protein synthesis and electrolyte balance. Alterations in muscle protein synthesis and electrolyte balance may therefore explain the changes in muscle mass and contractility seen in endocrine disorders. The muscular symptoms subside with appropriate treatment of the primary hormonal disorder.

Diseases of Energy Metabolism

Muscles rely on carbohydrates (e.g., glycogen) and lipids (free fatty acids) for energy. When stored glycogen or lipids cannot be metabolized because of lack of enzymes necessary to generate ATP for muscle contraction, the individual experiences cramps, fatigue, and exercise intolerance. Disorders of muscle metabolism can be self-limiting, such as McArdle disease and some lipid disorders, or they can cause widespread irreparable muscle destruction, as in acid maltase deficiency.

Glycogen storage disease type V. Glycogen storage disease type V (GSDV or McArdle disease) is an inherited disorder caused by an inability to metabolize glycogen. A lack of glycogen breakdown can interfere with the function of muscle cells. People with GSDV typically experience fatigue, muscle pain, and cramps during the first few minutes of exercise.[99] In affected individuals, weight lifting or jogging can trigger these symptoms. Fortunately, the discomfort is usually alleviated with rest and individuals can resume exercising with little or no discomfort, known as the "second wind."[99] Intensive or prolonged exercise can cause muscle damage and some may experience breakdown of muscle tissue (rhabdomyolysis). With severe muscle breakdown, a protein (*myoglobin*) is filtered through the kidneys and released in the urine (*myoglobinuria*). Myoglobin causes the urine to be red or brown and can damage the kidneys.[99]

The clinical manifestations of GSDV can vary. The condition typically manifests in a person's teens or twenties but can appear anytime from infancy to adulthood.[99] Over time, muscle weakness continues, but in about one-third of affected individuals it remains stable.[99] Some people with GSDV have mild or no symptoms.

Mutations in the *PYGM* gene cause GSDV.[99] This gene provides instructions for the enzyme called *myophosphorylase*. Myophosphorylase is found only in muscle cells, where it breaks down glycogen into a simple sugar. The *PYGM* mutation prevents myophosphorylase from breaking down glycogen effectively.

Pompe disease. Pompe disease is an inherited disorder caused by an accumulation of glycogen in body cells. Investigators have described three types of Pompe disease: (1) classic infantile onset, (2) nonclassic infantile onset, and (3) late onset. Mutations in the *GAA* gene cause Pompe disease. The mutation prevents alpha-glucosidase from breaking down glycogen effectively, which leads to sugar increasing to toxic levels in lysosomes. The increase in sugar causes organ and tissue damage throughout the body, particularly the muscles. Pompe disease is inherited in an autosomal recessive pattern.

The classic infantile-onset form is recognized shortly after birth by myopathy, hypotonia (poor muscle tone), hepatomegaly, and heart defects. These infants may have failure to thrive and breathing problems. If left untreated, this form of Pompe disease leads to death from heart failure. The nonclassic form of infant-onset Pompe disease typically appears by age 1. Infants have difficulty rolling over and sitting and progressive muscle weakness. The heart may be enlarged (cardiomegaly), but the infant usually does not experience heart failure.[99] With progression, the muscle weakness leads to serious breathing problems, and these children live only into early childhood.[99] Late-onset type Pompe disease occurs from later childhood, adolescence, or adulthood. Muscular symptoms are highly variable and can range from muscle cramping and weakness to varying degrees of respiratory insufficiency. The mainstay of treatment is enzyme replacement therapy, but dietary modifications also may improve the course of the disease.

Adenosine monophosphate deaminase deficiency. Adenosine monophosphate (AMP) deaminase deficiency is a condition that can affect skeletal muscles. AMP is caused by mutations in the *AMPD1* gene, which provides instructions for producing an enzyme called AMP deaminase.[100] The condition is inherited in an autosomal recessive pattern. The enzyme is found in skeletal muscle and plays a role in producing energy. For unknown reasons, many affected individuals with AMP deficiency do not have symptoms.[100] Affected individuals

have a poor capacity for sustained energy production, yet some with the condition have been able to perform as high-level athletes. The most common symptoms appear to be postexercise muscle cramping or pain, or both, and easy fatigability. The enzyme defect has been reported to be quite common, but in practice it may be rarely recognized as a cause of exercise intolerance.

Lipid deficiencies. Disorders of lipid metabolism are uncommon but account for severe changes in muscle metabolism. These disorders are caused by abnormalities in the transport and processing of fatty acids for energy. The lipid content of muscle cells consists of free fatty acids, which are oxidized in the mitochondria. These acids require carnitine and the enzyme carnitine palmitoyltransferase (CPT) to transport long-chain fatty acids to the mitochondria. There are two types of CPT deficiency: CPT I and CPT II deficiency. CPT I deficiency often appears during early childhood and is caused by mutations in the *CPT1A* gene.[101] The gene mutation creates the deficiency of the enzyme CPT IA, which is found in the liver. Individuals with CPT I deficiency are at risk for liver failure, nervous system damage, seizures, coma, and sudden death. They often exhibit hepatomegaly, liver dysfunction, and elevated blood levels of carnitine. Carnitine is a natural substance acquired mostly from diet and is used by cells to process fats and produce energy.[101] Affected individuals usually have hypoglycemia and a low level of ketones, which are produced from the breakdown of fats and used for energy. Viral infections or periods of fasting can trigger problems with CPT I deficiency, and the disorder is sometimes mistaken for Reye syndrome. Most cases of Reye syndrome are associated with the use of aspirin during viral infections.[101]

There are three main types of CPT II deficiency: a lethal neonatal form, a severe infantile hepatocardiomuscular form, and a myopathic form.[101] These three types are discussed in Table 41.8. Treatments with riboflavin, medium-chain triglycerides, oral carnitine, prednisone, and propranolol are proposed.

Inflammatory Muscle Diseases: Myositis
Viral, Bacterial, and Parasitic Myositis

Viral, bacterial, and parasitic infections of varying severity are known to produce inflammatory changes in skeletal muscle, a group of conditions collectively described by the term myositis. In tuberculosis and sarcoidosis, chronic inflammatory changes and granulomata are found in muscle as well as in other affected tissues. In the parasitic infection trichinellosis, *Trichinella* larvae reside in infected animals, such as pigs, horses, and other wildlife, including cougars and black bears. After ingestion, the parasites migrate to the intestinal mucosa and then travel to the lymphatic and circulatory systems.

Initial symptoms occur 1 to 2 days after consumption of infected meat and present as gastrointestinal distress (nausea, diarrhea, vomiting, abdominal pain). The more traditional trichinellosis symptoms generally occur 2 to 8 weeks after ingestion and include muscle pain and stiffness, fever, rash, itching, and headaches. Treatment includes administration of corticosteroids, such as prednisone, and antiparasitic agents, such as albendazole. Mebendazole also may be used, though it is not available in the United States.[102] Toxoplasmosis, a common parasitic infection, also is associated with a generalized polymyositis that responds rapidly to therapy.

In the tropics, more prevalent disorders include bacterial infections with *Staphylococcus aureus* and parasites such as cysticercus, the larva of the tapeworm *Taenia solium*. Viral infections can be associated with an acute myositis. Muscle pain, tenderness, signs of inflammation, and CK elevation are common manifestations of viral myositis. The self-limiting symptoms of muscle aches and pains during a bout of influenza may actually be a subacute form of viral myopathy.

TABLE 41.8 Types of Carnitine Palmitoyltransferase II Deficiency

Lethal Neonatal Form	Becomes apparent soon after birth
	Respiratory failure, seizures, liver failure, cardiomyopathy and dysrhythmia develop
	Affected infants have hypoglycemia and low level of ketones (hypoketonic hypoglycemia)
	The brain and kidneys may be abnormal
	Infants usually live a few days to few a few months
Severe Infantile Hepatocardiomuscular form	Affects the liver, heart and muscles
	Clinical manifestations usually appear within the first year of life
	Involves recurring episodes of hypoketotic hypoglycemia, seizures, hepatomegaly, cardiomegaly, and dysrhythmia
	Problems can be triggered by fasting or viral infections and other illnesses
	Affected infants may have liver failure, nervous system damage, coma, and sudden death
Myopathic Form	First episodes usually occur during childhood or adolescence
	Most affected individuals do not have clinical manifestations between episodes
	Include recurrent episodes of myalgia and weakness, and rhabdomyolysis
	Destruction of muscle causes the release of myoglobin by the kidneys, causing myoglobinuria
	Myoglobin causes urine to be red or brown
	Kidney failure may develop
	Myalgia and rhabdomyolysis may be triggered by exercise, stress, exposure to extreme temperatures, infections, or fasting

Data from U.S. Department of Health & Human Services, National Institutes of Health (USDHHS, NIH): *Genetics home reference: carnitine palmitoyltransferase I deficiency*, Bethesda MD, 2018, Author.

Polymyositis, Dermatomyositis, and Inclusion Body Myositis

Idiopathic inflammatory myopathy (IIM) comprises a group of disorders characterized by inflammation of skeletal muscles. There are several forms of idiopathic inflammatory myopathy, including polymyositis, dermatomyositis, and sporadic inclusion body myositis.[103] Polymyositis and dermatomyositis involve weakness of muscles such as the hips, thighs, upper arms, and neck.[103] Muscle weakness in some people may involve swallowing or breathing difficulty. Although dermatomyositis and polymyositis have similar symptoms, dermatomyositis is distinguished by a reddish or purplish rash on the eyelids (Fig. 41.26), elbows, knees, or knuckles. Sometimes, abnormal calcium deposits form hard bumps found under the skin (calcinosis).[103] Sporadic inclusion body myositis involves the muscles mostly of the wrists, fingers, and the front of the thigh. Affected individuals may stumble while walking and have difficulty with grasping items. They may also have trouble swallowing. The specific cause of the disorder is unknown and is thought to arise from both genetic and environmental factors. Most cases are sporadic, however, some individuals with idiopathic inflammatory myopathy have close relatives with autoimmune disorders.

The two approaches for treatment of myositis are medical treatment and lifestyle changes. Medical treatment may include corticosteroids

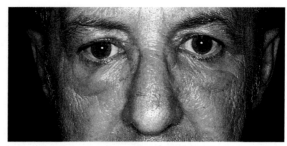

FIGURE 41.26 Dermatomyositis. Heliotrope (violaceous) discoloration around the eyes and periorbital edema. (From Habif TP: *Clinical dermatology*, ed 3, St Louis, 1996, Mosby.)

and antiinflammatories; lifestyle factors include exercise, rest, nutrition, and reduction of stress.

Myopathy

Myopathy is the term applied to a primary muscle disorder. Many pathologic processes affect muscles and cause loss of functional muscle cells. Myopathies affect muscle strength, tone, and bulk. Primary muscle disease is associated with marked weakness. The distribution of the weakness in myopathy is usually symmetrical and proximal, although occasionally the weakness is predominantly distal, such as in myotonic dystrophy. The weakness is associated with mild fatigue. Muscle tone is decreased, as are the tendon reflexes. Atrophy may be present. Some myopathies are associated with muscle hypertrophy as in cretinism and the familial progressive muscular dystrophies of childhood. Fasciculations are not present with myopathy because no denervation is present. No sensory changes are found. (Specific neurologic-associated myopathies are discussed in Chapter 16.)

Toxic Myopathies

Muscle damage caused by drugs or toxins is called toxic myopathy. A number of agents cause toxic myopathy, including corticosteroids, chloroquine, alcohol, phenytoin, azathioprine, organophosphates, and reverse transcriptase inhibitors. Other contributing agents may include lipid-lowering agents and opioids, such as heroin. Alcohol, lipid-lowering agents (fibrates and statins), antimalarial drugs, steroids, thiol derivatives, and narcotics (particularly heroin) can all cause symptoms. Additionally, many combinations of certain medications, illicit drugs, diseases, and infectious and environmental agents can cause myopathy.[104] Box 41.5 lists some of the causes of toxic myopathy.

Alcohol remains the most common cause of toxic myopathy. Two clinical syndromes are prevalent: (1) an acute attack of muscle weakness, pain, and swelling after a large consumption of alcohol; or (2) a more chronic, progressive proximal weakness associated with long-term consumption of alcohol.

Acute alcoholic myopathy can range from benign cramps and pain that resolves in a matter of hours to severe weakness and a markedly increased CK level associated with myoglobinuria and renal failure. Individuals are prone to repeated attacks after recovery. Treatment focuses on abstinence from alcohol and improved nutrition. The individual with chronic alcoholic myopathy often has coexisting peripheral neuropathy that complicates the diagnosis.

Repeated intramuscular injections also have been associated with changes in muscle fibers. Local necrosis of muscle fiber and elevated CK concentration have been reported after intramuscular injections of certain cephalosporins, lidocaine, diazepam, and digoxin; these effects were not produced with injections of saline. When drugs are injected over long periods, a chronic focal myopathy develops. Also reported is proliferation of connective tissue both in the muscle fiber and in the

BOX 41.5   Agents That Can Cause Toxic Myopathy

Drug Induced
Alcohol
Amiodarone (and others that inhibit CYP3A4 when combined with a statin)
Amphotericin B
AZT (zidovudine)
Azathioprine
Chloroquine
Clofibrate
Cocaine
Colchicine
Ethanol
Ipecac (withdrawn from U.S. markets)
3,4-Methylenedioxymethamphetamine (MDMA, "ecstasy")
Pentachlorophenol (PCP)
Statins
Steroids (especially with prolonged high doses; doses >25 mg/day; fluorinated steroids)

Endocrine Disorders
Adrenal disorders (Addison disease, Cushing disease)
Hyperparathyroidism

Hyperthyroidism (creatine kinase may be normal)
Hypothyroidism (creatine kinase may be mildly elevated)
Infectious disorders
Coxsackie A and B viruses
Human immunodeficiency virus (HIV)
Influenza
Lyme disease
Staphylococcus aureus muscle infection (frequent cause of pyomyositis)
Toxoplasmosis
Trichinosis

Miscellaneous
Licorice
Certain edible wild mushrooms
Lead poisoning
Organophosphates
Red yeast rice
European migratory quail (quail eat toxic hemlock, hellebore seeds)
Any medication that alters serum concentrations of sodium, potassium, calcium, phosphorus, or magnesium

Data from Kuncl RW: *Curr Opin Neurol* 22(5):506–515, 2009; Valiyil R, Christopher-Stine L: *Curr Rheumatol Rep* 12(3):213–220, 2010.

overlying skin and subcutaneous tissue. With time, segments of the muscles, particularly the deltoid and quadriceps, are converted into fibrotic bands. Pathophysiologic mechanisms for these changes include repeated needle trauma and infection, along with the nonphysiologic acidity and alkalinity of the injected material (see Box 41.5 for a list of some of the causes of toxic myopathy.)

QUICK CHECK 41.4
1. What is the main objective clinical finding in fibromyalgia?
2. How do metabolic muscle diseases develop? What causes them?
3. What are the main causes of toxic myopathy?

MUSCULOSKELETAL TUMORS

Bone Tumors

Many different types of tumors involve the skeleton. Although the skeleton is the major site for metastatic spread of multiple myeloma and breast, lung, and prostate cancers, primary bone tumors are relatively rare. Bone tumors may originate from bone cells, cartilage, fibrous tissue, marrow, or vascular tissue. Based on the tissue of origin, bone tumors are classified as osteogenic, chondrogenic, collagenic, or myelogenic. Table 41.9 presents the classification of primary bone tumors. Each of the types arises from one of the four stem cells that are ultimately derived from the primitive mesoderm (Fig. 41.27). In addition, bone tumors may be classified as being of histiocytic, notochordal, lipogenic, or neurogenic origin.

The mesoderm contributes the primitive fibroblast and reticulum cells. The fibroblast is the progenitor of the osteoblast and chondroblast cells. Each cell synthesizes a specific type of intercellular ground substance, and the type of ground substance produced by the cell generally characterizes the tumor derived from that cell. For example, osteogenic tumors usually contain cells that have the appearance of osteoblasts and produce an intercellular substance that can be recognized as osteoid. Chondrogenic tumors contain chondroblasts and produce an intercellular substance similar to chondroid (cartilage). Collagenic tumors contain fibrous tissue cells and produce an intercellular substance similar to the type of collagen found in fibrous connective tissue.

Tumors also are classified as benign or malignant, based on characteristics of the tumor cells (see Chapter 11). The criteria used to identify tumor cells as malignant are (1) an increased nuclear/cytoplasm ratio, (2) an irregular nuclear border, (3) an excess of chromatin, (4) a prominent nucleolus, and (5) an increase in the number of cells undergoing mitosis. However, many young, rapidly growing normal cells and cells subjected to inflammation and change in their blood supply also exhibit many of these same characteristics. (Tumor characteristics in general are described in Chapter 11.)

Epidemiology

The incidence rate of bone tumors varies with age. Osteosarcoma is the most common primary malignant bone tumor in children and young adults. Adolescents have the highest incidence of bone tumors, and adults between the ages of 30 and 35 have the lowest incidence. After age 35 years, the incidence rate slowly increases until at age 60 years it nearly equals the incidence rate in adolescents, primarily related to secondary metastatic tumors.

Patterns of Bone Destruction

The general pathologic features of bone tumors include bone destruction, erosion or expansion of the cortex, and periosteal response to changes in underlying bone. The least amount of pathologic damage occurs with benign bone tumors, which push against neighboring tissue. Because they usually have a symmetric, controlled growth pattern, benign bone tumors tend to compress and displace neighboring normal bone tissue, which weakens the bone's structure until it is incapable of withstanding the stress of ordinary use, leading to pathologic fracture. Other tumors invade and destroy adjacent normal bone tissue by producing substances that promote resorption by increasing osteoclast activity or by interfering with a bone's blood supply. Three patterns of bone

TABLE 41.9 Classification of Major Primary Tumors Involving Bone

Category and Fraction (%)	Behavior	Tumor Type	Common Locations	Age (yr)	Morphology
Hematopoietic (20)	Malignant	Myeloma, lymphoma	Vertebrae, pelvis	50-60	Malignant plasma cells or lymphocytes replacing marrow space
Cartilage forming (30)	Benign	Osteochondroma	Metaphysis of long bones	10-30	Bony excrescence with cartilage cap
		Chondroma	Small bones of hands and feet	30-50	Circumscribed hyaline cartilage nodule in medulla
		Chondroblastoma	Epiphysis of long bones	10-20	Circumscribed, pericellular calcification
		Chondromyxoid fibroma	Tibia, pelvis	20-30	Collagenous to myxoid matrix, stellate cells
	Malignant	Chondrosarcoma (conventional)	Pelvis, shoulder	40-60	Extends from medulla through cortex into soft tissue, chondrocytes with increased cellularity and atypia
Bone forming (26)	Benign	Osteoid osteoma	Metaphysis of long bones	10-20	Cortical, interlacing microtrabeculae of woven bone
		Osteoblastoma	Vertebral column	10-20	Posterior elements of vertebrae, histology similar to osteoid osteoma
	Malignant	Osteosarcoma	Metaphysis of distal femur, proximal tibia	10-20	Extends from medulla to lift periosteum, malignant cells producing woven bone
Unknown origin (15)	Benign	Giant cell tumor	Epiphysis of long bones	20-40	Destroys medulla and cortex, sheets of osteoclasts
		Aneurysmal bone cyst	Proximal tibia, distal femur, vertebrae	10-20	Vertebral body, hemorrhagic spaces separated by cellular, fibrous septae
	Malignant	Ewing sarcoma	Diaphysis of long bones	10-20	Sheets of primitive small round cells
		Adamantinoma	Tibia	30-40	Cortical, fibrous, bone matrix with epithelial islands
Notochordal (4)	Malignant	Chordoma	Clivus, sacrum	30-60	Destroys medulla and cortex, foamy cells in myxoid matrix

From Kumar V et al: *Robbins & Cotran pathologic basis of disease,* ed 9, Philadelphia, 2015, Saunders. Adapted from Unni KK, Inwards CY: *Dahlin's bone tumors,* ed 6, Philadelphia, 2010, Lippincott Williams & Wilkins; by permission of Mayo Foundation.

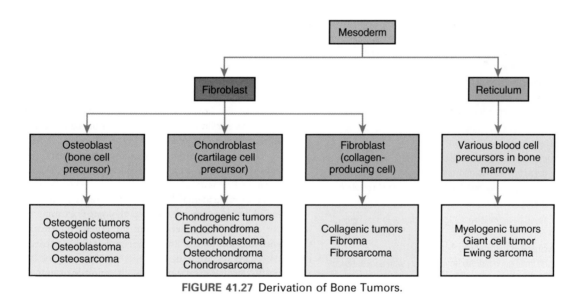

FIGURE 41.27 Derivation of Bone Tumors.

destruction by bone tumors have been identified: (1) the geographic pattern, (2) the moth-eaten pattern, and (3) the permeative pattern (Table 41.10).

Tumors that erode the cortex of the bone usually stimulate a periosteal response; that is, new bone formation at the interface between the surface of the bone and the periosteum. Slow erosion of the cortex usually stimulates a uniform periosteal response. Additional layers of bone are added to the exterior surface of the bone to buttress the cortex. Eventually, the additional layers expand the bone's contour. Aggressive penetration of the cortex, often seen with malignant tumors, usually elevates the periosteum and stimulates erratic patterns of new bone

formation. Examples of erratic patterns include concentric layers of new bone; a sunburst pattern, in which delicate rays of new bone radiate toward the periosteum from a single focus on the underlying surface; and rays of new bone that grow perpendicularly, creating a brush or bristle pattern.

DIAGNOSIS A malignant bone tumor must be identified early to allow survival of the individual and preservation of the affected limb. However, individuals often have only vague symptoms that may be attributed to minor trauma, degenerative changes, or inflammatory conditions. In addition, other conditions may obscure the diagnosis.

Thorough diagnostic studies are needed to determine the exact type and extent of bone tumor present, which also helps determine the optimal treatment regimen. Staging of any bone tumor is critical to determine future treatment and results. The American Joint Committee on Cancer (AJCC) staging system (also known as the Enneking, or TNM, staging system) is the most commonly used arrangement (Table 41.11). This system classifies tumors according to grade (G), tumor site (T), and metastasis (M). Benign tumors are given a numeric value of zero, whereas malignant tumors are low grade (G1) or high grade (G2). Serum alkaline phosphatase levels are elevated in bone lytic tumors and significantly elevated in osteosarcoma and Ewing sarcoma. Radiologic studies, including plain radiographic films, technetium-99 bone scan, CT scan, and MRI, have become the examinations of choice for the local staging of bone tumors, especially the staging of peripheral osteosarcomas (see Table 41.11).

Additional diagnostic studies done for specific bone tumors include a complete blood count and erythrocyte sedimentation rate (to rule out infection or myeloma) and measurement of serum levels of calcium and phosphorus to detect hypercalcemia. Serum glucose levels may be elevated in chondrosarcoma. Bone-specific alkaline phosphatase is elevated when there is bone metastasis. Acid phosphatase level may be moderately elevated in bone metastases, multiple myeloma, and advanced Paget disease. Serum protein electrophoresis and immuno-electrophoresis are performed to exclude other diseases. To determine the exact tumor type, core needle biopsy is usually done at the time of surgery.

Types

A large number of lesions are classified as bone tumors. Bone tumors are typically classified according to their origin—osteogenic, chondrogenic, collagenic, and myelogenic tumors.

Osteogenic tumors: osteosarcoma. Osteogenic (bone-forming) tumors are characterized by the formation of bone or osteoid tissue with a sarcomatous tissue. The tissue can have the appearance of compact or spongy bone. The most common malignant bone-forming tumor is osteosarcoma (Fig. 41.28), which is typically found in the bone marrow. Osteosarcoma occurs mostly in adolescents and young adults; 60% of osteosarcomas occur in those younger than 20 years, and it has a slightly higher incidence in males. A secondary peak incidence for osteosarcoma occurs in the 60 and older age group, primarily in individuals with a history of radiation therapy several years previously for pelvic or other malignancies.

Osteosarcoma is aggressive and has a moth-eaten pattern of bone destruction. The borders of the tumor are indistinct and merge into adjacent normal bone. Osteosarcomas contain osteoid and callus produced by anaplastic stromal cells, which are atypical, abnormal cells not seen in normal developing bone; they are neither normal nor embryonal. Many tumors are heterogeneous; for example, the osteosarcoma also may contain chondroid (cartilage) (chondroblastic sarcoma) and fibrinoid tissue (fibroblastic sarcoma) that may form the bulk of the tumor. The osteoid is deposited as thick masses or "streamers," which infiltrate the normal compact bone, destroy it, and replace it with masses of osteoid. Bone tissue produced by osteosarcomas never matures to compact bone.

Ninety percent of osteosarcomas are located in the metaphyses of long bones, especially the distal femoral metaphysis, with 50% around the knee area. The tumor typically impregnates the cortex, lifts the periosteum, and forms a soft tissue mass that is not covered by a smooth shell of new bone. Lifting of the periosteum stimulates bizarre patterns of new bone formation, called a *periosteal reaction*. Distinct osteosarcomas occur on the surface of long bones, called *parosteal*, *periosteal*, and *high-grade surface osteosarcomas*; dedifferentiated parosteal and central osteosarcomas also occur.

The most common initial symptoms are pain and swelling. The pain is initially slight and intermittent, but increases in severity and duration. Pain is usually worse at night and gradually requires medication. Often, a coincidental history of trauma is noted. Occasionally, the individual may present with a pathologic fracture.

Systemic chemotherapy and surgery are the treatments of choice, with the location of the tumor and its size, grade, and pattern of metastasis dictating the type and extent of surgery. Preoperative chemotherapy has greatly increased the number of individuals qualifying

TABLE 41.10 Patterns of Bone Destruction Caused by Bone Tumors

Type	Features
Geographic pattern	Least aggressive type
	Generally indicative of slow-growing or benign tumor
	Well-defined margins on tumor, easily separated from surrounding normal bone
	Uniform and well-defined lytic area in bone
	Margin smooth or irregular, demarcated by short zone of transition between normal and abnormal bone tissue
Moth-eaten pattern	Characteristic of rapidly growing, malignant bone tumors
	More aggressive pattern
	Tumor margin less defined or demarcated; cannot easily be separated from normal bone
	Areas of partially destroyed bone adjacent to completely lytic areas
Permeative pattern	Caused by aggressive malignant tumor with rapid growth potential
	Margins of tumor poorly demarcated
	Abnormal bone merges imperceptibly with normal bone

TABLE 41.11 The Enneking Surgical Staging System for Malignant Bone Tumors

Stage	Grade	Site (T)	Metastasis (M)
IA	Low (G$_1$)	Intracompartmental (T$_1$)	None (M$_0$)
IB	Low (G$_1$)	Extracompartmental (T$_2$)	None (M$_0$)
IIA	High (G$_2$)	Intracompartmental (T$_1$)	None (M$_0$)
IIB	High (G$_2$)	Extracompartmental (T$_2$)	None (M$_0$)
IIIA	Low (G$_1$)	Intracompartmental or extracompartmental (T$_1$ or T$_2$)	Regional or distant (M$_1$)
IIIB	High (G$_2$)	Intracompartmental or extracompartmental (T$_1$ or T$_2$)	Regional or distant (M$_1$)

Data from National Comprehensive Cancer Network: Recent updates to NCCN clinical practice guidelines in oncology: bone cancer, Version 1, Fort Washington PA, 2013, Author.

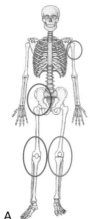
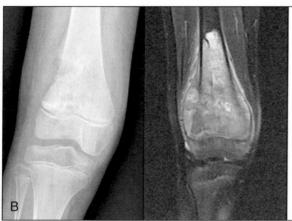

FIGURE 41.28 Osteosarcoma. **A,** Common locations of Ewing sarcoma and osteosarcoma. *Blue,* osteosarcoma; *red,* Ewing sarcoma. **B,** Comparison of plain radiograph, magnetic resonance imaging, and nuclear bone scan appearances of osteosarcoma of the distal femur. Note destruction of the bone cortex and soft tissue component. (**A** adapted from Bontrager KL, Lampignanno JP, editors: *Textbook of radiographic positioning and related anatomy,* St Louis, 2013, Elsevier. **B** from HaDuong JH et al: *Pediatr Clin N Am* 62:179-200, 2015.)

for limb salvage surgery. Other agents under investigation include monoclonal antibodies, hormone antagonists, gene therapy, and other biologic agents.

Chondrogenic tumors: chondrosarcoma. Chondrogenic (cartilage-forming) tumors produce cartilage or chondroid, a primitive cartilage or cartilage-like substance. The most common chondrogenic tumor is chondrosarcoma.

Chondrosarcoma is the second most common primary malignant bone tumor. It is a tumor of middle-aged and older adults, with incidence peaks in the sixth decade of life. The tumor is found more commonly in men than in women. Chondrosarcomas that develop from a preexisting benign bone lesion (e.g., an enchondroma) are known as secondary chondrosarcomas. Individuals with certain conditions, such as multiple osteochondromas, may be at greater risk for developing secondary chondrosarcoma. Secondary chondrosarcomas are rare, occurring most often in young adults between 20 and 30 years of age, and are more common in men.

A chondrosarcoma is a large, ill-defined malignant tumor that infiltrates trabeculae in spongy bone. It produces cartilage-forming cells, without ossification, that occurs normally in bone formation. It occurs most often in the metaphysis or diaphysis of long bones, especially the femur or proximal humerus, and in the bones of the pelvis (Fig. 41.29). Chondrosarcomas typically implant in surrounding tissue *(seeding).*

Symptoms associated with a chondrosarcoma have an insidious onset. Local swelling accompanied by a dull, intermittent pain is the usual presenting symptom. The pain gradually intensifies and becomes constant, awakening the person at night.

Diagnostic studies include radiographs, which must be reviewed carefully for an accurate diagnosis. Biopsy is done at the time of surgery. Performing a bone biopsy prior to surgery can result in seeding of tumor cells and metastasis. Additionally, sufficient tumor material must be obtained to facilitate an accurate diagnosis.

Surgical excision is generally regarded as the treatment of choice because chemotherapy and radiation seem to have little effect.[105] Many surgically treated individuals demonstrate recurrences, thus amputation becomes one treatment of choice.

Collagenic tumors: fibrosarcoma. Collagenic (collagen-forming) tumors produce fibrous connective tissue. Fibrosarcoma is the most common collagenic tumor and can affect bone or soft tissue.

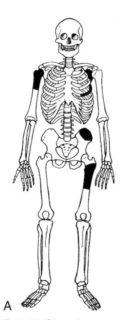
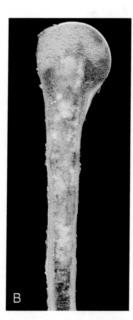

FIGURE 41.29 Chondrosarcoma. **A,** Common locations of chondrosarcoma. **B,** Chondrosarcoma of humerus. (From Damjanov I, Linder J, editors: *Anderson's pathology,* ed 10, St Louis, 1996, Mosby.)

Fibrosarcomas come from fibroblasts that originate from mesenchymal stem cells; they represent 4% of primary malignant bone tumors. The incidence has a broad age range, but this tumor type is most common in adults between 30 and 50 years of age. The incidence is slightly greater in females. Fibrosarcoma also may be a secondary complication of radiation therapy, Paget disease, and long-standing osteomyelitis; secondary fibrosarcoma tends to be more aggressive, with a poorer outcome.

Fibrosarcoma is a solitary tumor that most often affects the metaphyseal region of the femur or tibia. The tumor is composed of a firm, fibrous mass of tissue that contains collagen, malignant fibroblasts, and occasional osteoclast-like giant cells.

The tumor begins in the marrow cavity of the bone and infiltrates the trabeculae. It demonstrates a permeative growth pattern, destroys the cortex, and extends into the soft tissue. Metastasis to the lung is common.

Symptoms associated with the tumor have an insidious onset, which delays diagnosis. Pain and swelling are the usual presenting symptoms and usually indicate that the tumor has infiltrated the cortex. Local tenderness, a palpable mass, and limitation of motion also may be present. A pathologic fracture in the affected bone is often the reason for seeking medical help. Diagnostic studies include radiographs and MRI.

Radical surgery and amputation are the treatments of choice for fibrosarcoma. Radiation therapy is generally considered ineffective treatment for this tumor.

Myelogenic Tumors

Myelogenic tumors originate from various bone marrow cells. Two types of myelogenic tumors are giant cell tumor and myeloma. Myeloma is discussed in Chapter 23.

Giant cell tumor. Giant cell tumor (GCT) is the sixth most common primary bone tumor, accounting for 4% to 5% of bone tumors. GCTs have a wide age distribution; however, they are rare in persons younger than 10 years or older than 70 years. Most GCTs are found in persons between 20 and 40 years of age. Unlike most other bone tumors, GCTs affect females more often than males.

The GCTs are generally benign, solitary, circumscribed tumors that cause extensive bone resorption because of their osteoclastic origin. There is a high rate of recurrence, but metastasis is rare. A GCT is typically located in the epiphyseal regions of the femur, tibia, radius, or humerus. The tumor has a slow, relentless growth rate, and it is usually contained within the original contour of the affected bone. Aggressive bone resorption causes pathologic fractures. However, it may extend into the articular cartilage. When the tumor extends, it is usually covered by periosteum or periosteal bone growth; it may extend into surrounding soft tissue.

The most common symptoms associated with GCT are pain, local swelling, and limitation of movement. Diagnostic studies include radiographs, CT, and MRI. Cryosurgery and resection of the tumor with the use of adjuvant polymethylmethacrylate (PMMA) for bone grafts reduce recurrence and are more successful treatments than curettage and radiation.[106] Amputation may be necessary but is not common.

Muscle Tumors

Rhabdomyoma

Rhabdomyoma is an extremely rare benign tumor of striated muscle that generally occurs in the tongue, neck muscles, larynx, uvula, nasal cavity, axilla, vulva, and heart. These tumors are usually treated by surgical excision and typically do not recur. When malignant, these tumors are called *rhabdomyosarcomas*.

Rhabdomyosarcoma

Rhabdomyosarcoma is a rare malignant tumor of striated muscle. It is the most common soft tissue sarcoma in children and adolescents; 50% of all soft tissue sarcomas and 10% of all malignant tumors occur in children. These tumors are highly malignant and metastasize rapidly. Rhabdomyosarcomas are located in the muscle tissue of the head, neck, and genitourinary tract in 75% of cases, with the remainder found in the trunk, extremities, and urinary tract.

Three types of rhabdomyosarcoma are differentiated on pathologic section: anaplastic (formerly known as pleomorphic), embryonal, and alveolar. Each type differs from the other molecularly; they are all aggressive tumors and are typically more resistant to therapy. Although rare, the anaplastic (spindle cell) type is considered one of the most highly malignant tumors of the extremities seen in adulthood. Microscopically, embryonal tumors resemble a tadpole or tennis racquet and are most often seen in infancy and childhood. Alveolar-type tumors have a latticelike appearance, similar to lung tissue alveoli, and are more often found in adolescents and adults.

The diagnosis and staging of rhabdomyosarcoma are made by the history, physical examination, serologic testing, CT, and MRI. The diagnosis is confirmed by incisional biopsy with surgical resection and by examination of the specimen by a pathologist.[107] Staging is based on the site of origin, residual disease, lymph node involvement, and distant metastases.[107]

Treatment consists of a combination of surgical excision, systemic chemotherapy, and adjunct radiation therapy. The overall survival of childhood rhabdomyosarcoma has improved over the past decades, but adult survival remains poor.

Other Tumors

Metastatic tumors in muscles are rare in spite of the extensive vascular supply of skeletal muscles. It is suggested that local pH or metabolic changes within muscles prevent metastatic involvement from other tumors. When adjacent carcinomas do cause muscle damage, it is usually related to the compression of tissue and resultant muscle atrophy.

✔ **QUICK CHECK 41.5**

1. From what cells do bone tumors originate?
2. Compare five major characteristics of benign bone tumors with those of malignant bone tumors.
3. How does the presence of metastatic tumors affect treatment options and prognosis of persons with osteosarcoma?

▮ SUMMARY REVIEW

Musculoskeletal Injuries

1. A fracture is a break in the continuity of a bone. A bone can be completely or incompletely fractured. A closed fracture leaves the skin intact. An open fracture has an overlying skin wound. If a bone breaks into more than two fragments it is termed a comminuted fracture. The direction of the fracture line can be linear, oblique, spiral, or transverse. Greenstick, torus, and bowing fractures are examples of incomplete fractures that occur in the more flexible, growing bones of children.
2. Pathologic fractures (also called insufficiency or *fragility fractures*) are breaks at the site of a preexisting abnormality, resulting from force that would not fracture a normal bone. Stress fractures occur in normal or abnormal bone that is subjected to repeated stress. Fatigue fractures occur in normal bone subjected to abnormal stress. Transchondral fractures are the fragmentation and separation of a portion of the articular cartilage.
3. Immobilization by realigning bone fragments and holding them in place is used to heal fractures that are not misaligned.
4. Dislocation is complete loss of contact between the articular surfaces of two bones. Subluxation is partial loss of joint contact between two bones. As a bone separates from a joint, it may damage adjacent nerves, blood vessels, ligaments, tendons, and muscle.

5. Tearing or stretching of a muscle or tendon is known as a *strain*, and ligament tears are called *sprains*. A complete separation of a tendon or ligament from its attachment is called an *avulsion*.
6. Trauma can cause painful inflammation of tendons, called *tendinopathy*. Bursitis is the inflammation and swelling of bursae, the joint sacs filled with synovial fluid.
7. Muscle strain may be caused by traumatic or sports injuries that stretch the muscle beyond normal capacity.
8. Rhabdomyolysis is the rapid breakdown of muscle that causes the release of intracellular contents and is often manifested by the presence of myoglobinuria (myoglobin in the urine). It can have life-threatening complications, including acute renal failure.
9. Compartment syndrome is the result of increased pressure within a muscle compartment that can result in local tissue hypoxia and necrosis.
10. Malignant hyperthermia is an inherited disorder characterized by a hypermetabolic reaction that activates a prolonged release of intracellular calcium, leading to continuous muscle contraction.

Disorders of Bones
1. Metabolic bone diseases, including osteoporosis, osteomalacia, and Paget disease, are characterized by abnormal bone strength.
2. Osteoporosis is a decreased density or mass of bone and an increased risk of fractures because of changes in bone microarchitecture. Osteoporosis is caused by the bone remodeling cycle being disrupted: old bone is resorbed faster than new bone is formed. It is the most common disease that affects bone but is not a consequence of the normal aging process.
3. Osteomalacia is a metabolic bone disease characterized by inadequate bone mineralization. Vitamin D deficiency is the major contributing factor to the development of osteomalacia.
4. PDB involves excessive and abnormal bone remodeling in which enlarges and softens affected bones.
5. Osteomyelitis is a bone infection caused most often by bacteria. Infection caused by bacteria from infection sites within the body is called *hematogenous osteomyelitis*. Contiguous osteomyelitis occurs when infection spreads to an adjacent bone.

Disorders of Joints
1. OA is a common, age-related disorder of synovial joints. The primary defect in OA is loss of articular cartilage. Because of improved imaging technology, inflammation has been identified as an important feature of osteoarthritis.
2. Inflammatory joint disease, commonly called *arthritis*, is characterized by inflammatory damage or destruction in the synovial membrane or articular cartilage.
3. RA is an inflammatory joint disease characterized by inflammatory destruction of the synovial membrane, articular cartilage, joint capsule, and surrounding ligaments and tendons. Rheumatoid nodules also may invade the skin, lung, and spleen and involve small and large arteries. RA is a systemic disease that affects the heart, lungs, kidneys, and skin, as well as the joints.
4. AS is a chronic, systemic autoimmune disease characterized by stiffening and fusion of the sacroiliac and spine joints.
5. Gout is a syndrome caused by defects in uric acid metabolism with high levels of uric acid in the blood and body fluids. Uric acid crystallizes in the connective tissue of a joint where it initiates inflammatory destruction of the joint.

Disorders of Skeletal Muscle
1. Muscle diseases, or myopathies, commonly produce symptoms of muscle weakness and muscle fatigue.

2. Contractures are the lack of full passive range of motion of a joint. A physiologic muscle contracture occurs in the absence of a muscle action potential in the sarcolemma. A pathologic contracture is permanent muscle shortening caused by muscle spasticity, as seen in CNS injury or severe muscle weakness.
3. Stress-induced muscle tension is presumably caused by increased activity in the reticular activating system and gamma loop in the muscle fiber. The use of progressive relaxation training and biofeedback has been advocated to reduce muscle tension.
4. FM is a chronic musculoskeletal syndrome characterized by diffuse joint and muscle pain, fatigue, and tender points. Most cases of FM involve women, and the peak age is 30 to 50 years. Genetic factors are being increasingly recognized as agents in the development of FM.
5. CFS is a chronic debilitating disease characterized by profound fatigue, musculoskeletal pain, cognitive impairment, unrestful sleep, impaired neurologic energy production, and immune impairments.
6. Disuse atrophy is the reduction in size of muscle fibers seen after prolonged inactivity. Isometric contractions and passive lengthening exercises decrease atrophy to some degree in immobilized persons.
7. Skeletal muscle channelopathies can be divided into (1) myotonia and (2) those associated with episodes of weakness (periodic paralysis).
8. In myotonic channelopathies, muscle relaxation is delayed after voluntary contractions leading to a disabling muscle stiffness or weakness, or both. It is treated with drugs that reduce muscle fiber excitability.
9. Periodic paralysis is an autosomal dominant disorder in which depolarization of the sarcolemma is severe enough that the muscle cannot be fired again, resulting in paralysis or even myotonia. Individuals usually regain their strength between attacks, but repeated episodes can lead to muscle weakness later in life.
10. Metabolic muscle diseases are caused by a genetic mutation and endocrine abnormalities that impact muscle metabolism. The resulting disorders lead to glycogen storage diseases, enzyme deficiencies, and abnormal lipid metabolism and mitochondrial function. The muscle depends on a complex system of carbohydrates and fats converted by enzymes to produce energy for the muscle cell. Abnormalities in these pathways can inhibit function or cause damage to the muscle fiber. Diseases of energy metabolism include GSDV (McArdle disease), Pompe disease, ADM deaminase deficiency, and lipid deficiencies.
11. Viral, bacterial, and parasitic infections of muscles can cause myositis—the characteristic clinical and pathologic changes associated with inflammation. These are usually treatable and self-limiting disorders. Polymyositis (generalized muscle inflammation) and dermatomyositis (polymyositis accompanied by skin rash) are characterized by inflammation of connective tissue and muscle fibers and muscle fiber necrosis. Treatment is either medical (corticosteroids and anti-inflammatories) or lifestyle related (exercise, rest, nutrition, and stress reduction).
12. Myopathies are primary muscle disorders. The most common cause of toxic myopathy is alcohol abuse, which can cause (1) an acute attack of muscle weakness, pain, and swelling after a large consumption of alcohol or (2) a more chronic, progressive proximal weakness associated with long-term consumption of alcohol. Drug administration can also lead to toxic myopathy; a needle used during an injection, secondary infection, and alterations in the acidity and alkalinity of muscle fibers can mechanically damage muscle fibers.

Musculoskeletal Tumors

1. Bone tumors originate from bone cells (osteogenic), cartilage cells (chondrogenic), fibrous tissue cells (collagenic), or vascular marrow cells (myelogenic). The most common tumors of each type are osteosarcoma, chondrosarcoma, fibrosarcoma, and myeloma, respectively. GCTs are another type of myelogenic tumor.
2. Patterns of bone destruction by bone tumors may be geographic (caused by slow-growing or benign tumors), moth eaten (caused by rapidly growing, malignant bone tumors), and permeative (caused by aggressive malignant tumor with rapid growth potential).
3. Sarcomas of muscle tissue are rare. Rhabdomyoma is a benign tumor of striated muscle and when they are malignant, they are called rhabdomyosarcomas. Rhabdomyosarcoma has a uniformly poor prognosis, particularly in adults, because of an aggressive invasion and early, widespread dissemination. The usual treatment includes surgical excision, radiation therapy, and adjunct systemic chemotherapy.

KEY TERMS

REFERENCES

1. Roeleveld DM, Koenders MI: The role of the Th17 cytokines IL-17 and IL-22 in rheumatoid arthritis pathogenesis and developments in cytokine immunotherapy, *Cytokine* 74(1):101-107, 2014.
2. Marsell R, Einhorn TA: The biology of fracture healing, *Injury* 42(6):551-555, 2011.
3. Luk JK, et al: Lateral epicondylalgia: midlife crisis of a tendon, *Hong Kong Med J* 20(2):145-151, 2014.
4. Genthon A, Wilcox SR: Crush syndrome: a case report and review of the literature, *J Emerg Med* 46(2):313-319, 2014.
5. Zutt R, et al: Rhabdomyolysis: review of the literature, *Neuromuscul Disord* 24:651-659, 2014.
6. Nassar A, et al: Rapid diagnosis of rhabdomyolysis with point-of-care ultrasound, *West J Emerg Med* 17(6):801-804, 2016. Available at: http://doi.org/10.5811/westjem.2016.8.31255.
7. Ali P, et al: Assessment and diagnosis of acute limb compartment syndrome: a literature review, *Int J Orthop Trauma Nurs* 18(4):180-190, 2014.
8. McDonald S, Bearcroft P: Compartment syndromes, *Semin Musculoskelet Radiol* 14(2):236-244, 2010.

9. Shadgan B, et al: Current thinking about acute compartment syndrome of the lower extremity, *Can J Surg* 53(5):329-334, 2010.

10. Raza H, Mahapatra A: Acute compartment syndrome in orthopedics: causes, diagnosis, and management, *Adv Orthop* 2015:2015.

11. U.S. Department of Health & Human Services, National Institutes of Health (USDHHS, NIH): *Genetics home reference: malignant hyperthermia*, Bethesda MD, 2018, Author. Available at: https://ghr.nlm.nih.gov. (Accessed 11 July 2018).

12. Correia ACC, et al: Malignant hyperthermia: clinical and molecular aspects, *Rev Bras Anestesiol* 62(6):820-837, 2012.

13. World Health Organization (WHO) Scientific Group on the Prevention and Management of Osteoporosis: WHO technical report series, no. 921, Geneva, Switzerland, 2000, Author.

14. Chen H, Kubo KY: Bone three-dimensional microstructural features of the common osteoporotic fracture sites, *World J Orthop* 5(4):486-495, 2014.

15. Dede AD, et al: Bone disease in anorexia nervosa, *Hormones (Athens)* 13(1):38-56, 2014.

16. Gonnelli S, et al: Obesity and fracture risk, *Clin Cases Miner Bone Metab* 11(1):9-14, 2014.

17. Jackuliak P, Payer J: Osteoporosis, fractures, and diabetes, *Int J Endocrinol* 2014:2014. 820615.

18. Misra M, Klibanski A: Anorexia nervosa and bone, *J Endocrinol* 221(3):R163-R176, 2014.

19. Panday K, et al: Medication-induced osteoporosis: screening and treatment strategies, *Ther Adv Musculoskel Dis* 6(5):185-202, 2014.

20. U.S. Preventive Services Task Force (USPSTF): Screening for osteoporosis: U.S. Preventive Services Task Force recommendation statement, *Ann Intern Med* 154(5):356-364, 2011.

21. Pape HC, Bischoff-Ferrari HA: How can we influence the incidence of secondary fragility fractures? A review on current approaches, *Injury* 48:S24-S26, 2017.

22. Leslie WD, Morin SN: Osteoporosis epidemiology 2013: implications for diagnosis, risk assessment, and treatment, *Curr Opin Rheumatol* 26(4):440-446, 2014.

23. Peeters CM, et al: Quality of life after hip fracture in the elderly: a systematic literature review, *Injury* 47(7):1369-1382, 2016.

24. Kendler DL, et al: Vertebral fractures: clinical importance and management, *Am J Med* 129(2):221, e1-e10, 2016.

25. Cauley JA: Defining ethnic and racial differences in osteoporosis and fragility fractures, *Clin Orthop Relat Res* 469(7):1891-1899, 2011.

26. NIH Osteoporosis and Related Bone Diseases National Resource Center: Osteoporosis and African American women, 2015. Available at www.niams.nih.gov/Health_Info/Bone/Osteoporosis/Background/default.asp. Accessed October 2017.

27. Rubin KH, et al: Comparison of different screening tools (FRAX®, OST, ORAI, OSIRIS, SCORE and age alone) to identify women with increased risk of fracture. A population-based prospective study, *Bone* 56:16-22, 2013.

28. Calvo MS, Tucker KL: Is phosphorus intake that exceed dietary requirements a risk factor in bone health?, *Ann N Y Acad Sci* 1301:29-35, 2013.

29. Calvo MS, Uribarri J: Public health impact of dietary phosphorus excess on bone and cardiovascular health in the general population, *Am J Clin Nutr* 98(1):6-13, 2013.

30. Aaseth J, et al: Osteoporosis and trace elements—an overview, *J Trace Elem Med Biol* 26(2-3):149-152, 2012.

31. Okyay E, et al: Comparative evaluation of serum levels of main minerals and postmenopausal osteoporosis, *Maturitas* 76(4):320-325, 2013.

32. Zofkova I, et al: Trace elements and bone health, *Clin Chem Lab Med* 51(8):1555-1561, 2013.

33. Body JJ, et al: Non-pharmacological management of osteoporosis: a consensus of the Belgian Bone Club, *Osteoporos Int* 22(11):2769-2788, 2011.

34. Celec P, Behuliak M: Behavioural and endocrine effects of chronic cola intake, *J Psychopharmacol* 24(10):1569-1572, 2010.

35. Hallström H, et al: Long-term coffee consumption in relation to fracture risk and bone mineral density in women, *Am J Epidemiol* 178(8):898-909, 2013.

36. Lewiecki EM: Osteoporosis: clinical evaluation. In Endotext [Internet], 2018, MDText.com, Inc. Available at https://www.ncbi.nlm.nih.gov/books/NBK279049/.

37. Cano-Marquina A, et al: Transient regional osteoporosis, *Maturitas* 77(4):324-329, 2014.

38. Henneicke H, et al: Glucocorticoids and bone: local effects and systemic implications, *Trends Endocrinol Metab* 25:97-211, 2014.

39. Seibel MJ, et al: Glucocorticoid-induced osteoporosis: mechanisms, management, and future perspectives, *Lancet Diabetes Endocrinol* 1(1):59-70, 2013.

40. Popp AW, et al: Microstructural parameters of bone evaluated using HR-pQCT correlate with the DXA-derived cortical index and the trabecular bone score in a cohort of randomly selected premenopausal women, *PLoS ONE* 9(2):e88946, 2014.

41. Silva BC, et al: Trabecular bone score: a noninvasive analytical method based upon the DXA image, *J Bone Miner Res* 29(3):518-530, 2014.

42. Ulivieri FM, et al: Utility of the trabecular bone score (TBS) in secondary osteoporosis, *Endocrine* 47(2):435-438, 2014.

43. Link YM: The founder's lecture 2009: advances in imaging of osteoporosis and osteoarthritis, *Skelet Radiol* 39:943-955, 2010.

44. Palacios C, Gonzalez L: Is vitamin D deficiency a major global public health problem?, *J Steroid Biochem Mol Biol* 144(Pt A):138-145, 2014.

45. Thacher TD, Clarke BL: Vitamin D deficiency, *Mayo Clin Proc* 86(1):50-60, 2011.

46. Unuvar T, Buyukgebiz A: Nutritional rickets and vitamin D deficiency in infants, children and adolescents, *Pediatr Endocrinol Rev* 7(3):283-291, 2011.

47. Muschitz C, et al: Diagnosis and treatment of Paget's disease of bone: a clinical guideline, *Wien Med Wochenschr* 167(1-2):2017.

48. Galson DL, Roodman GD: Pathobiology of Paget's disease of bone, *J Bone Metab* 21(2):85-98, 2014.

49. U.S. Department of Health & Human services, National Institutes of Health (USDHHS, NIH): Genetics home reference: Paget disease of bone, Bethesda MD, Nov 7 2018. Available at https://ghr.nlm.nih.gov. (Accessed 11 July 2018).

50. Stern SM, Ferguson PJ: Autoinflammatory bone diseases, *Rheum Dis Clin North Am* 39(4):735-749, 2013.

51. Sanchez CJ, Jr, et al: *Staphylococcus aureus* biofilms decrease osteoblast viability, inhibits osteogenic differentiation, and increases bone resorption in vitro, *BMC Musculoskelet Disord* 14:187, 2013.

52. Prieto-Pérez L, et al: Osteomyelitis: a descriptive study, *Clin Orthop Surg* 6(1):20-25, 2014.

53. Gotthardt M, et al: Imaging of inflammation by PET, conventional scintigraphy, and other imaging techniques, *J Nucl Med Technol* 41(3):157-169, 2013.

54. McLaren JS, et al: A biodegradable antibiotic-impregnated scaffold to prevent osteomyelitis in a contaminated in vivo bone defect model, *Eur Cell Mater* 27:332-349, 2014.

55. Hall M, et al: Synovial pathology on ultrasound correlates with the severity of radiographic knee osteoarthritis more than with symptoms, *Osteoarthritis Cartilage* 22(10):1627-1633, 2014.

56. Haugen IK, et al: Increasing synovitis and bone marrow lesions are associated with incident joint tenderness in hand osteoarthritis, *Ann Rheum Dis* 75(4):702-708, 2016.

57. Kapoor M, et al: Role of proinflammatory cytokines in the pathophysiology of osteoarthritis, *Nat Rev Rheumatol* 7:33-42, 2011.

58. Mrosewski I, et al: Regulation of osteoarthritis-associated key mediators by TNFα and IL-10; effects of IL-10 overexpression in human synovial fibroblasts and a synovial cell line, *Cell Tissue Res* 357(1):207-223, 2014.

59. Sauerschnig M, et al: Diverse expression of selected cytokines and proteinases in synovial fluid obtained from osteoarthritic and healthy human knee joints, *Eur J Med Res* 19(1):65-71, 2014.

60. Francin P-J, et al: Association between adiponectin and cartilage degradation in human osteoarthritis, *Osteoarthritis Cartilage* 22(3):519-526, 2014.

61. Felson DT, et al: Valgus malalignment is a risk factor for lateral knee osteoarthritis incidence and progression: findings from the Multicenter Osteoarthritis Study and the Osteoarthritis Initiative, *Arthritis Rheum* 65(2):355-362, 2013.

62. Stief F, et al: Effect of lower limb malalignment in the frontal plane on transverse plane mechanics during gait in young individuals with varus knee alignment, *Knee* 21(3):688-693, 2014.

63. Fransen M, et al: Exercise for osteoarthritis of the knee, *Cochrane Database Syst Rev* (1):CD004376, 2015.

64. Juhl C, et al: Impact of exercise type and dose on pain and disability in knee osteoarthritis: a systematic review and meta-regression analysis of randomized controlled trials, *Arthritis Rheumatol* 66(3):622-636, 2014.

65. Fransen M, et al: Glucosamine and chondroitin for knee osteoarthritis: a double-blind randomized placebo-controlled clinical trial evaluating single and combination regimens, *Ann Rheum Dis* 74(5):851-858, 2015.

66. Fibel KH, et al: State-of-the-art management of knee osteoarthritis, *World J Clin Cases* 3(2):89-101, 2015.

67. Bannuru RR, et al: Comparative effectiveness of pharmacologic interventions for knee osteoarthritis: a systematic review and network meta-analysis, *Arch Int Med* 162(1):46-54, 2015.

68. Sundman EA, et al: The anti-inflammatory and matrix restorative mechanisms of platelet-rich plasma in osteoarthritis, *Am J Sports Med* 42(1):35-41, 2014.

69. Huang Z, et al: Effectiveness of low-level laser therapy in patients with knee osteoarthritis: a systemic review and meta-analysis, *Osteoarthritis Cartilage* 23(9):1437-1444, 2015.

70. Siemieniuk RAC, et al: Arthroscopic surgery for degenerative knee arthritis and meniscal tear: a clinical guideline, *BMJ* 357:j1982, 2017.

71. Cooper C, Javaid MK, Arden N: Epidemiology of osteoarthritis. In *Atlas of osteoarthritis*, New York, 2014, Springer Healthcare.

72. Kurtz SM, et al: Impact of the economic downturn on total joint replacement demand in the United States: updated projections to 2021, *J Bone Joint Surg Am* 96(8):624-630, 2014.

73. Korczowska I: Rheumatoid arthritis susceptibility genes: an overview, *World J Orthop* 5(4):544-549, 2014.

74. Mohan VK, et al: Association of susceptible genetic markers and autoantibodies in rheumatoid arthritis, *J Genet* 93(2):597-605, 2014.

75. You S, et al: Identification of key regulators for the migration and invasion of rheumatoid synoviocytes through a systems approach, *Proc Natl Acad Sci USA* 111(1):550-555, 2015.

76. Lefevre S, et al: Role of synovial fibroblasts in rheumatoid arthritis, *Curr Pharm Des* 21(2):130-141, 2015.

77. Uhlig T, Moe RH, Kvien TK: The burden of disease in rheumatoid arthritis, *Pharmacoeconomics* 32(9):841-851, 2014.

78. van Heemst J, et al: Fine-mapping the human leukocyte antigen locus in rheumatoid arthritis and other rheumatic diseases: identifying causal amino acid variants?, *Curr Opin Rheumatol* 27(3):256-261, 2015.

79. Sokolove J, et al: Rheumatoid factor as a potentiator of anti–citrullinated protein antibody–mediated inflammation in rheumatoid arthritis, *Arthritis Rheumatol* 66(4):813-821, 2014.

80. Aletaha D, et al: The 2010 American College of Rheumatology/European League Against Rheumatism classification criteria for rheumatoid arthritis: an American College of Rheumatology/

European League Against Rheumatism collaborative initiative, *Arthritis Rheum* 62(9):2569-2581, 2010.

81. Raychaudhuri SP, Deodhar A: The classification and diagnostic criteria of ankylosing spondylitis, *J Autoimmun* Feb-Mar(48-19):128-133, 2014.

82. Dean L, et al: Global prevalence of ankylosing spondylitis, *Rheumatology (Oxford)* 53(4):650-657, 2014.

83. de Winter J, et al: Magnetic resonance imaging of the sacroiliac joints indicating sacroiliitis according to the Assessment of SpondyloArthritis International Society Definition in healthy individuals, runners, and women with postpartum back pain, *Arthritis Rheumatol (Hoboken, NJ)* 70(7):1042, 2018.

84. Rudwaleit M, et al: The development of assessment of SpondyloArthritis International Society classification criteria for axial spondyloarthritis (part II): validation and final selection, *Ann Rheum Dis* 68(6):777-783, 2009.

85. Golder V, Schachna L: Ankylosing spondylitis: an update, *Austral Fam Phys* 42(11):780-784, 2013.

86. Braun J, et al: Emerging drugs for the treatment of axial and peripheral spondyloarthritis, *Expert Opin Emerg Drugs* 20(1):1-14, 2015.

87. Van den Bosch F, Dodhar A: Treatment of spondyloarthritis beyond TNF-alpha blockade, *Best Pract Res Clin Rheumatol* 28(5):819-827, 2014.

88. Perez-Ruiz F, et al: A review of uric acid, crystal deposition disease, and gout, *Adv Ther* 32:31-41, 2015.

89. Chowalloor PV, et al: Imaging in gout: a review of recent developments, *Ther Adv Musculoskelet Med* 6(4):131-143, 2014.

90. Sommer C, Leinders M: Üçeyler N: inflammation in the pathophysiology of neuropathic pain, *Pain* 159(3):595-602, 2018.

91. Jahan F, et al: Fibromyalgia syndrome: an overview of pathophysiology, diagnosis and management, *Oman Med J* 27(3):192-195, 2012.

92. Cagnie B, et al: Central sensitization in fibromyalgia? A systematic review on structural and functional brain MRI, *Semin Arthritis Rheum* 44(1):68-75, 2014.

93. Wolfe F, et al: The American College of Rheumatology preliminary diagnostic criteria for fibromyalgia and measurement of symptom severity, *Arthritis Care Res (Hoboken)* 62(5):600-610, 2010.

94. Wolfe F, et al: Fibromyalgia criteria and severity scales for clinical and epidemiological studies: a modification of the American College of Rheumatology preliminary diagnostic criteria for fibromyalgia, *J Rheumatol* 38(6):1113-1122, 2011.

95. Theadom A, et al: Mind and body for fibromyalgia, *Cochrane Database Syst Rev* (4):CD001980, 2015.

96. Powers SK: Can antioxidants protect against disuse muscle atrophy?, *Sports Med* 44(Suppl 2):S155-S165, 2014.

97. Brooks NE, Myburgh KH: Skeletal muscle wasting with disuse atrophy is multi-dimensional: the response and interaction of myonuclei, satellite cells and signaling pathways, *Front Physiol* 5:99, 2014.

98. U.S. Department of Health & Human Services, National Institutes of Health National Library of Medicine (USDHHS, NIH): Genetics home reference: hypokalemic periodic analysis, Bethesda MD, December 4, 2018, Author.

99. U.S Department of Health & Human Services, National Institutes of Health (USDHHS, NIH):

Genetics home reference: glycogen storage disease type V, Bethesda MD, December 2018, Author.

100. U.S. Department of Health & Human Services, National Institutes of Health (USDHHS, NIH): Genetics home reference: adenosine monophosphate deaminase deficiency, Bethesda MD, December 4, 2018, Author.

101. U.S. Department of Health & Human Services, National Institutes of Health (USDHHS, NIH): Genetics home reference: carnitine palmitoyltransferase I deficiency, Bethesda, MD, December 4, 2018, Author.

102. Bruschi F, Dupouy-Camet J: Trichinellosis. In Bruschi F, editor: *Helminth infections and their impact on global public health*, Wien Heidelberg, New York, Dordrecht, London, 2014, Springer, pp 229-273.

103. U.S. Department of Health & Human Services. National Institutes of Health (USDHHS, NIH): Genetics home reference: idiopathic inflammatory myopathy, Bethesda, MD, December 4, 2018, Author.

104. Lahouti AH, Christopher-Stine L: Toxic myopathies. In Chinoy H, Cooper R, editors: *Myositis*, Oxford, 2017, Oxford University Printing, pp 89-97.

105. Onishi AC, Hincker AM, Lee FY: Surmounting chemotherapy and radioresistance in chondrosarcoma: molecular mechanisms and therapeutic targets, *Sarcoma* 381654:2011, 2011.

106. van der Heijden L, et al: The clinical approach toward giant cell tumor of bone, *Oncologist* 19(5):550-561, 2014.

107. Carroll SJ, Nodit L: Spindle cell rhabdomyosarcoma: a brief diagnostic review and differential diagnosis, *Arch Pathol Lab Med* 137(8):1155-1158, 2013.

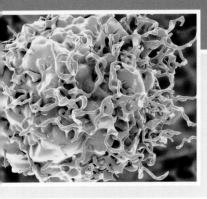

42

Alterations of Musculoskeletal Function in Children

Kathryn L. McCance

EVOLVE WEBSITE

CHAPTER OUTLINE

Musculoskeletal problems in children can be either congenital or acquired. Both pathology and treatment can cause long-term sequelae because of the growing nature of the immature skeleton. In addition, the emotional trauma of an injured or malformed child is substantial and requires that careful attention be paid to the emotional health of both the child and his or her family.

CONGENITAL DEFECTS

Clubfoot

Clubfoot describes a range of congenital foot deformities in which the foot turns inward and downward. It can affect one or both feet. Technically called talipes equinovarus (Table 42.1), the heel is positioned varus (inwardly deviated) and equinus (plantar flexed) (Fig. 42.1, *A*). The clubfoot deformity can be positional (correctable passively), idiopathic, or teratologic (as a result of another syndrome, such as spina bifida). The idiopathic clubfoot occurs in 1 in 1000 live births, with males twice as likely as females to be affected.

The clubfoot deformity can be corrected by an above-knee casting regimen popularized by Ponseti.[1] The technique involves 6 to 8 casts to be left on for 5 to 7 days each. It has revolutionized clubfoot treatment by correcting this crippling deformity without the need for surgery.

In almost 90% of idiopathic and up to 70% of teratologic clubfeet, the Ponseti method of serial casting infants' feet is effective (see Fig. 42.1, *B*). The hindfoot equinus portion of the deformity often requires lengthening of the Achilles tendon, which can be performed in a clinic with the use of a local anesthetic. Achilles tenotomy (complete transection of the tendon) can be safely performed with local anesthetic until 8 or 9 months after birth. After this age, a formal lengthening and repair procedure using a general anesthetic is required. Bracing is required until age 3.

Idiopathic feet resistant to these procedures require repeat casting or, in very rare cases, a surgical posteromedial release (PMR). The PMR includes lengthening of the Achilles, posterior tibialis, and flexor tendons and surgical release of the capsules of the ankle, subtalar, and midfoot joints. Teratologic clubfeet require surgical intervention more often than idiopathic clubfeet and more prolonged bracing, often through childhood.

Developmental Dysplasia of the Hip

Developmental dysplasia of the hip (DDH) describes imperfect development of the hip joint and can affect the femur, the acetabulum, or both (Fig. 42.2). Although most often present congenitally, dysplasia may develop later in the newborn or infant period. Like clubfoot, DDH can be idiopathic or teratologic. Teratologic hips (i.e., those attributable to another disorder such as cerebral palsy, spina bifida, or arthrogryposis) are more difficult to treat and often need operative intervention. In idiopathic DDH, 70% of cases involve the left side only and 10% to 15% are bilateral. Females are four times as likely as males to be affected. Positive family history, breech presentation, and oligohydramnios (low levels of intrauterine fluid) all predispose children to DDH. Children in these groups are considered high risk and must be carefully evaluated

TABLE 42.1 Terms Used to Describe Foot Abnormalities

Term	Definition
Position*	
Abduction	Lateral deviation away from the midline of the body
Adduction	Lateral deviation toward the midline of the body
Eversion	Twisting of the foot outward along its long axis
Inversion	Twisting of the foot inward on its long axis
Dorsiflexion	Bending of the foot upward and backward
Plantar flexion	Bending of the foot downward and forward
Abnormality	
Talipes equinovarus	Congenital abnormality of the foot (clubfoot)
Pes	Acquired deformity of the foot
Varus	Inversion and adduction of the heel and forefoot
Valgus	Eversion and abduction of the heel and forefoot
Equinus	Plantar flexion of the foot in which the heel is lower than the toes
Calcaneus	Dorsiflexion of the foot in which the heel is lower than the toes
Planus	Flattening of the medial longitudinal arch of the foot (flatfoot)
Cavus	Elevation of the medial longitudinal arch of the foot (high arch)
Equinovarus	Coexistent equinus and varus deformities
Calcaneovarus	Coexistent calcaneus and varus deformities
Equinovalgus	Coexistent equinus and valgus deformities
Calcaneovalgus	Coexistent calcaneus and valgus deformities

*NOTE: The positions listed can all be achieved by voluntary movement of the normal foot; an abnormality exists if the foot is fixed in one or more of the positions while at rest.

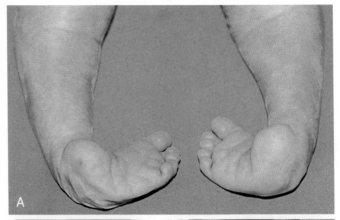
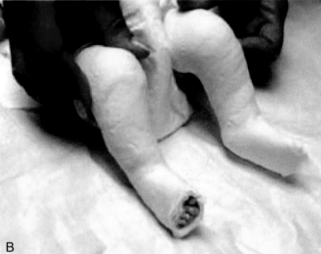

FIGURE 42.1 A, Infant With Bilateral Congenital Talipes Equinovarus. **B,** Ponseti Casting. (**A** courtesy Dr. A.E. Chudley, Section of Genetics and Metabolism, Department of Pediatrics and Child Health, Children's Hospital and University of Manitoba, Winnipeg, Manitoba, Canada. In Moore KL et al, editors: *The developing human,* ed 10, Philadelphia, 2016, Saunders. **B** from Scher, DM, *Operative Techniques in Orthopaedics,* 15(4): 345-349, 2005.)

with physical examination and, possibly, ultrasound. Variants of idiopathic DDH (see Fig. 42.2) are dislocated hip (no contact between the femoral head and acetabulum), subluxated hip (partial contact only), and acetabular dysplasia (the femoral head is located properly but the acetabulum is shallow). Idiopathic instability of the hip ranges from 3 to 7 per 1000 live births, but a true dislocation is present in only 1 of 1000 live births.

Clinical examination is the mainstay of diagnosis. The examination must be performed on a relaxed infant for accuracy. Absolute indications for treatment include a positive Barlow sign (hip reduced, but dislocatable) (Fig. 42.3, *A*) or positive Ortolani sign (hip dislocated, but reducible) (see Fig. 42.3, *B*). Other indicators for further evaluation are limitation of abduction[2] or apparent shortening of the femur (Galeazzi sign). Asymmetric skin folds at the groin also can be a clinical sign of hip pathology.

In children younger than 4 months old, bracing with a Pavlik harness is successful in 90% of DDH cases (Fig. 42.4). A Barlow positive hip is easier to treat with a Pavlik harness, and success rates approach 95% to 98%. An Ortolani positive hip must be followed closely with ultrasound and examination; the success rate with Pavlik harness is 70% in this situation. If a stable reduction is not attained within 2 to 3 weeks of treatment, the Pavlik harness should be abandoned and casting or surgery pursued instead. A partially reduced hip applies pressure on the rim of the acetabulum by the femoral head and can worsen dysplasia and make treatment more difficult. In older children (6 to 12 months), or those who failed bracing with a Pavlik harness, closed reduction of the

hip and spica casting (casting of the trunk of the body and one or both legs) performed using a general anesthetic are required. The spica cast is worn for 3 months. Children older than 12 months require surgery on the joint, the femur, or the acetabulum, or all three. The incidence of good or excellent outcome falls to only 20% by age 4, underscoring the need for early diagnosis and treatment.

Osteogenesis Imperfecta

Osteogenesis imperfecta (OI), or brittle bone disease, is a bone dysplasia related to collagen, the main component of bone and blood vessels. The Sillence classification defines six types of OI. Types I and IV are milder forms and are inherited in an autosomal dominant pattern. Types II and III are more severe and are inherited in a recessive pattern. Types V and VI are very rare and are autosomal recessive. Children with type II OI often die during infancy because of extreme bone fragility.

The classic clinical manifestations of OI are osteopenia (decreased bone mass) and an increased rate of fractures. Children can also have fatigue, pain, hearing loss, and abnormal dentition. With recurrent fractures, bone deformity (bowing) often occurs (Fig. 42.5, *A*). In type III OI, the most severe form compatible with life, children have short stature and triangular faces, possibly blue sclerae, and poor dentition. Because collagen also is the main component of blood vessels, vascular

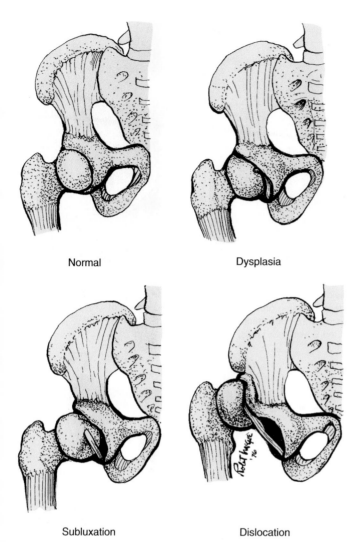

Normal   Dysplasia

Subluxation   Dislocation

FIGURE 42.2 Configuration and Relationship of Structures in Developmental Dysplasia of the Hip. (From Hockenberry MJ, Wilson DL: *Wong's nursing care of infants and children*, ed 10, St Louis, 2015, Mosby.)

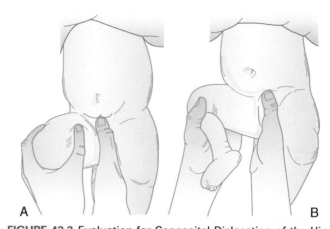

A   B

FIGURE 42.3 Evaluation for Congenital Dislocation of the Hip. **A,** Barlow maneuver *(left side)*. With one hand pressing the symphysis in front and the sacral spine in back, lateral pressure is applied to the thigh with the thumb of the other hand while pressure is applied with the palm to the knee on the side being examined. The hip that has been flexed to 90 degrees is then adducted. A positive sign is a sensation of abnormal movement, indicating dislocation of the femoral head from the acetabulum. The hands are reversed for examining the other hip. This sign and the Ortolani sign may be found only in the first weeks of life. **B,** Ortolani maneuver *(right side)*. Sign of jerking into correct position. After Barlow maneuver **(A)**, the hip should be abducted to about 80 degrees while the femur is lifted anteriorly with the fingers along the thigh. A positive sign is a sensation of a jerk or snap with reduction into the joint socket. (Adapted from Specht EE: *Am Fam Physician* 9:88-96, 1974.)

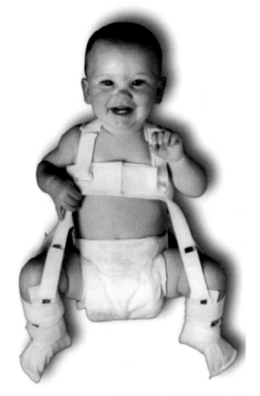

FIGURE 42.4 Pavlik Harness for Bilateral Hip Dislocation. (From Wheaton Brace Co., Carol Stream, Ill.)

deformity, such as aortic aneurysm, can occur. Type IV OI can be subtle, with the child presenting with more normal stature and with fractures often not occurring until the child is older; it can be misdiagnosed as child abuse. Analysis of skin fibroblasts is diagnostic in 85% of children with OI.

Treatment is a combination of medical and surgical approaches. For fractures and deformity, intramedullary rodding of the long bones improves position and also splints new fractures (see Fig. 42.5, *B* and *C*). Telescoping rods, which grow with the child, are improving in efficacy. Unfortunately, these children may have to undergo multiple surgeries and re-roddings with growth. The medical treatment, classically involving calcium and vitamin D supplementation, is under intense study. Pamidronate and other bisphosphates, such as alendronate (Fosamax), which decrease bone resorption by inhibiting osteoclasts, are now frequently used. A multicenter study of a bisphosphonate therapy showed promising results in type III OI, with marked improvements of bone density (up to 30%). Chronic bone pain and fatigue also are thought to be lessened with routine bisphosphonate therapy. Despite these results, there is concern that the healing of fractures and surgical intervention can be more difficult. More study is needed to address the efficacy and safety of these types of drugs. Genetic counseling for affected families should aim at primary prevention.[3]

BONE AND JOINT INFECTION

Osteomyelitis

Osteomyelitis, or bone infection, is caused by either bacterial or granulomatous (e.g., tuberculosis) infective processes (Box 42.1).

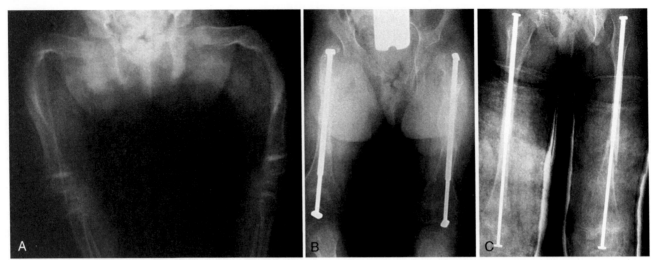

FIGURE 42.5 Osteogenesis Imperfecta Treated With Osteotomies and Telescoping Medullary Rods. **A,** Severe deformity of both femurs. **B,** Same individual after multiple osteotomies with telescoping medullary rod fixation. **C,** Same individual 4 years later demonstrating growth of femurs, no recurrence of deformity, and elongation of rods. (Plaster casts are in place for immobilization of tibial osteotomies.) (From Crenshaw AH, editor: *Campbell's operative orthopaedics,* ed 8, vol 3, St Louis, 1992, Mosby.)

BOX 42.1   Causative Microorganisms of Osteomyelitis According to Age

Newborns
Staphylococcus aureus (both methicillin-sensitive [MSSA] and methicillin-resistant [MRSA])
Group B *Streptococcus*
Gram-negative enteric rods

Infants
Staphylococcus aureus (MSSA and MRSA)
Haemophilus influenzae (decreasingly less common secondary to immunization)

Older Children
Staphylococcus aureus (MSSA and MRSA)
Pseudomonas
Salmonella
Neisseria gonorrhoeae

Adolescents and Adults
Pseudomonas
Mycobacterium tuberculosis

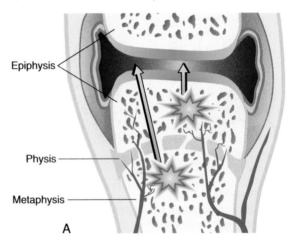

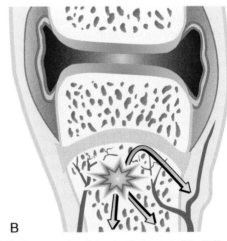

FIGURE 42.6 Pathogenesis of Acute Osteomyelitis Differs With Age. **A,** In infants younger than 1 year the epiphysis is nourished by arteries penetrating through the physis, allowing development of the condition within the epiphysis. **B,** In children up to 15 years of age, the infection is restricted to below the physis because of interruption of the vessels.

Antibiotic drugs and often surgical interventions are used to treat these infections. Morbidity and mortality resulting from osteomyelitis declined drastically until the 1980s. Unfortunately, with the escalation of methicillin-resistant *Staphylococcus aureus* (MRSA) infections, serious increases in morbidity and mortality have developed.

Acute hematogenous osteomyelitis is the most common form in children. The infection usually begins as an abscess in the metaphysis of a long bone where blood flow is sluggish and bacteria can collect. With increasing pressure, the infection will rupture out of the periosteum and spread along the diaphysis of the bone. In infants younger than 1 year old, infection may go through the physis (growth plate) and into the epiphysis (Fig. 42.6). A new shell of bone can develop under the elevated periosteum and can become an involucrum. The portion of bone that is separated from adequate blood supply by the infection can die, thereby leading to an involucrum. All three of these changes are apparent on radiograph and signify the need for surgical débridement, as well as antibiotic treatment.

These radiographic bone changes take 2 to 3 weeks to develop. Initially, osteomyelitis presents as pain, swelling, and warmth. Children often will have fever, decreased appetite, fatigue, elevated white blood cell count (50% to 70%), elevated C-reactive protein (CRP) (98%) level, and elevated erythrocyte sedimentation rate (ESR) (90%). Blood culture is positive in only 40% to 60% of cases. Without changes on plain radiograph, magnetic resonance imaging (MRI) can help define the location and extent of the infectious process. In infants, in whom osteomyelitis can be multifocal in up to 40% of cases, bone scan identifies other locations of infection that may need surgical intervention.

Treatment of osteomyelitis consists of appropriate antibiotic management for 6 weeks. If blood cultures are negative, bone aspirate must be analyzed to determine the bacterial source of the infection. With MRSA or bone changes on MRI, surgical débridement is required. MRSA often leads to more systemic illness, such as endocarditis (infection of the heart valves), organ failure, and infected thrombotic events.

Septic Arthritis

Septic arthritis is a bacterial or granulomatous infection of the joint space. This is always a surgical emergency. The bacteria, and the lysosomes created by white blood cells fighting the bacteria, can quickly destroy the articular cartilage of the joint and affect the blood supply to the epiphyseal bone nearby. Both of these complications have poor outcomes and can lead to a lifetime of disability.

Septic arthritis can occur primarily or secondary to osteomyelitis that spreads from the metaphysis of the bone into the joint space (Fig. 42.7). The metaphyses of the pediatric hip, shoulder, proximal radius, and distal lateral tibia are all located within the joint capsule, and therefore osteomyelitis in these regions must be carefully monitored for secondary septic arthritis. The most common sites for septic arthritis are knees, hips, ankles, and elbows.

Children with septic arthritis present with severe joint pain, "pseudoparalysis," or marked guarding to motion of the joint; inability to bear weight; and malaise, often with anorexia. Children appear quite ill with this diagnosis. Nonpyogenic arthritis, such as juvenile idiopathic arthritis, can be difficult to distinguish clinically from septic arthritis because both can lead to malaise and elevated ESR. The Kocher criteria are often used to distinguish septic joints from joint pain of another cause. There is a greater than 90% chance of a septic joint if three of the five following criteria are met:

1. WBC >12,000 cells/μL
2. Inability to bear weight on the joint
3. Fever >101.3° F (38.5° C)
4. ESR >40 mm/hr
5. CRP >2 mg/dl

Fever and CRP level above 2 mg/dl appear to have the most influence in the differential diagnosis.

Blood cultures are positive in 30% to 40% of cases. Joint aspirate positive for a white blood cell count of greater than 7000 per high-power field (HPF) defines the diagnosis, and culture of this fluid often determines bacterial etiology. As in osteomyelitis, *Staphylococcus aureus* is the most common bacteria; however, MRSA is now present in up to 30% of affected children.[4,5] Emerging is the understanding that *Kingella kingae* is an important pathogen, occurs in children between 6 months and 4 years of age, and can involve many joints and bone, less frequently the endocardium and other locations.[4]

After surgical débridement of the joint, antibiotics are required for 2 to 3 weeks. Long-term follow-up to assess articular or physeal damage is required.

JUVENILE IDIOPATHIC ARTHRITIS

Juvenile idiopathic arthritis (JIA) is the childhood form of rheumatoid arthritis (also see Chapter 41) and accounts for 5% of all cases of rheumatoid arthritis. JIA has three distinct modes of onset: oligoarthritis (fewer than three joints), polyarthritis (more than three joints), and Still disease (severe systemic onset) (Table 42.2). JIA differs from rheumatoid arthritis in several ways:

- Large joints are most commonly affected.
- Chronic uveitis (inflammation of the anterior chamber of the eye) is common; if the blood test for antinuclear antibody (ANA) is positive, slit lamp examination by a trained ophthalmologist is required every 6 months to avoid vision loss.
- Serum tests may be negative for rheumatoid factor (RF); RF-positive children have a worse prognosis.
- Subluxation and ankylosis may occur in the cervical spine if disease progresses.
- Rheumatoid arthritis that continues through adolescence can have severe effects on growth and adult morbidity.

Many children with oligoarthritis who are "seronegative" (blood tests negative for RF or ANA) will resolve their symptoms over time. Systemic onset, or "seropositivity," of the disease is more likely consistent with lifelong arthritis. Therefore treatment is supportive, not curative. Nonsteroidal antiinflammatory drugs (NSAIDs) are a mainstay of treatment, and methotrexate is also being used with success. The goals are to minimize inflammation and deformity.

> ✔ **QUICK CHECK 42.1**
> 1. Why is an early diagnosis of developmental dysplasia of the hip imperative?
> 2. How has MRSA changed musculoskeletal infections in children?
> 3. How does osteomyelitis develop?
> 4. How does juvenile idiopathic arthritis differ from the adult form?

OSTEOCHONDROSES

The osteochondroses are a series of avascular diseases caused by insufficient blood supply to growing bones. These childhood diseases involve areas of significant tensile or compressive stress (e.g., tibial tubercle, Achilles insertion, hip epiphysis). The pathophysiology is partial loss of blood supply, death of bone (osseous necrosis), progressive bony weakness, and then microfracture. The cause of the decreased blood supply is controversial; trauma, a change in clotting sensitivity, vascular injury, genetic predisposition, or a combination of these factors is

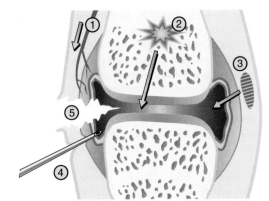

FIGURE 42.7 Routes of Infection to the Joint. *1,* Hematogenous route. *2,* Dissemination from osteomyelitis. *3,* Spread from an adjacent soft tissue infection. *4,* Diagnostic or therapeutic measures. *5,* Penetrating damage by puncture or cutting.

TABLE 42.2 Characteristics of Juvenile Idiopathic Arthritis Related to Mode of Onset

	Systemic Onset	Pauciarticular (Two or Three Subtypes)	Polyarticular (Two Subtypes)
Percentage of patients	30	45	25
Age at onset	Bimodal distribution 1-3 yr of age 8-10 yr of age	Type I: younger than 10 yr Type II: older than 10 yr	Throughout childhood and adolescence
Sex ratio (female/male)	1.5:1	Type I: almost all female Type II: 1:9	Mostly female
Joints involved	Any Only 20% have joint involvement at time of diagnosis	Usually confined to lower extremities— knee, ankle, and eventually sacroiliac; sometimes elbow	Any joint; usually symmetric involvement of small joints Hip involvement in 50% Spine involvement in 50%
Extra-articular manifestations	Fever, malaise, myalgia, rash, pleuritis or pericarditis, adenomegaly, splenomegaly, hepatomegaly Systemic signs minimal	Type I: chronic iridocyclitis; mucocutaneous lesions Type II: acute iridocyclitis; sacroiliitis common; eventual ankylosing spondylitis in many	Possible low-grade fever, malaise, weight loss, rheumatoid nodules, or vasculitis
Laboratory test results	Elevated ESR, CRP levels; RF negative; ANA rarely positive; anemia; leukocytosis	Elevated ESR, CRP levels; ANA positive Type I: HLA-DRW5 positive Type II: HLA-B27 positive Type III: HLA-TMo positive	Elevated ESR, CRP levels Type I: RF positive Type II: RF negative
Long-term prognosis	Mortality: 1%-2% of all JIA patients Joint destruction in 40%	Continuous disease; eventual remission in 60% Type I: ocular damage; functional blindness in 10% Type II: ankylosing spondylitis Type III: best outlook for recovery	Longer duration; more crippling; remission in 25% Type I: high incidence of crippling arthritis Type II: outlook good

From Hockenberry MJ, Wilson D: *Wong's nursing care of infants and children*, ed 8, St Louis, 2007, Mosby.
ANA, Antinuclear antibody; *CRP,* C-reactive protein; *ESR,* erythrocyte sedimentation rate; *HLA,* human leukocyte antigen; *JIA,* juvenile idiopathic arthritis; *RF,* rheumatoid factor.

presently considered most likely. Additionally, during the years of rapid bone growth, blood supply to the growing ends of bones (epiphyses) may become insufficient, resulting in necrotic bone, usually near joints. Because bone is normally undergoing a continuous rebuilding process, the necrotic areas can self-repair over a period of weeks or months.

Use of antiinflammatory medications, modification of activities, immobilization, and rest are recommended during active stages of the disease. Reparative correction by revascularization is the rule, although years may be required for full healing, and deformity from compression during the period of osseous necrosis can persist.

Legg-Calvé-Perthes Disease

Legg-Calvé-Perthes (LCP) disease is a common osteochondrosis of the hip usually occurring in children between the ages of 3 and 10 years, with a peak incidence at 6 years. This self-limited disease, which runs its natural course in 2 to 5 years, is presumably created by recurrent interruption of the blood supply to the femoral head. The ossification center first becomes necrotic (osteonecrosis) and then is gradually replaced by live bone.

The disorder is bilateral in 10% to 20% of children. Male children are affected five times more often than female children which is thought to be caused by males having a more poorly developed blood supply to the femoral head than do females of the same age. The role of genetics is unclear, but LCP is more common in northern European and Japanese children and rare in black children; family history is positive in 20% of cases.

PATHOPHYSIOLOGY Several causative theories have been proposed, including a generalized disorder of epiphyseal cartilage growth, thyroid hormone deficiency, trauma, infection, and blood clotting disorders. Males with a hypercoagulable state are three times more likely to acquire LCP than females with the same disorder. A study has shown the risk of LCP is five times greater in children exposed to passive smoke as opposed to children living in a smoke-free environment.[6] Increased risk has been associated with smoke from indoor use of a wood stove.

In the first stage of LCP, the soft tissues of the hip (synovial membrane and joint capsule) are swollen, edematous, and hyperemic, often with fluid present in the joint (Fig. 42.8). In the second necrotic stage, the anterior 50% or more of the epiphysis of the femoral head dies because of a lack of blood supply, and the metaphyseal bone at the junction of the femoral neck and capital epiphyseal plate is softened because of increased blood supply and decalcification. Granulation tissue (procallus) and blood vessels then invade the dead bone. The third, or regenerative healing, stage ordinarily lasts 2 to 4 years. The dead bone in the femoral head is replaced by procallus, and new bone is established (see Fig. 42.8). In the fourth, or residual, stage, remodeling takes place and the newly formed bone is organized into a live spongy bone.

CLINICAL MANIFESTATIONS Injury or trauma precedes the onset of LCP in approximately 30% to 50% of children with the disease. For several months the child complains of a limp and pain that can be referred to the knee, inner thigh, and the groin, following the path of the obturator nerve. The pain is usually aggravated by activity and relieved by rest and administration of antiinflammatory medications.

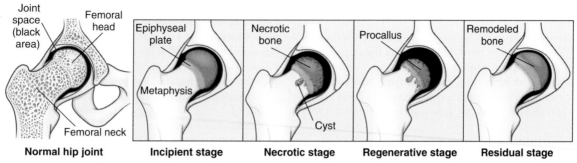

Joint space (black area) — Femoral head — Epiphyseal plate — Metaphysis — Femoral neck

Necrotic bone — Cyst — Procallus — Remodeled bone

Normal hip joint   **Incipient stage**   **Necrotic stage**   **Regenerative stage**   **Residual stage**

FIGURE 42.8 Stages of Legg-Calvé-Perthes Disease, a Form of Osteochondrosis.

The typical physical findings include spasm on rotation of the hip, limitation of internal rotation and abduction, and hip flexion–adduction deformity. If the child is walking, an early abnormal gait termed an antalgic (painful) abductor lurch, or a "Trendelenburg gait" (gluteus medius gait pattern), is apparent. If the hip pain or limp has been present for a prolonged period, muscles of the hip and thigh atrophy.

EVALUATION AND TREATMENT The goals of treatment are to preserve normal congruity of the femoral head and acetabulum and maintain spasm-free and pain-free range of motion in the hip joint. Currently, most children can be managed with antiinflammatory medications and activity modification during periods of synovitis. Serial radiographs are obtained to monitor the progress of the disease and to ensure that the femoral head remains congruent in the acetabulum. Surgery may be necessary if the femoral head becomes subluxated or incongruent with the acetabulum (Fig. 42.9). Children older than age 6 years (by bone age) have a worse prognosis attributable to poorer remodeling potential. Older children require surgery more often to avoid poor congruence of the hip. Poor congruence predisposes to early osteoarthritis, with nearly 50% requiring hip replacement surgery by age 40.

Osgood-Schlatter Disease

Osgood-Schlatter disease consists of osteochondrosis of the tibia tubercle and associated patellar (kneecap) tendonitis. Osgood-Schlatter disease occurs most often in preadolescents and adolescents who participate in sports and is more prevalent in males than in females. Osgood-Schlatter disease is one of the most common ailments reported in the 30 million children who are involved in sports.[7]

The severity of the lesion varies from mild tendonitis to a complete separation of the anterior tibial apophysis, a part of the tibial tubercle. The mildest form of Osgood-Schlatter disease causes ischemic (avascular) necrosis in the region of the bony tibial tubercle, with hypertrophic cartilage formation during the stages of repair. In more severe cases, the abnormality involves a true apophyseal separation of the tibial tubercle with avascular necrosis.

The child complains of pain and swelling in the region around the patellar tendon and tibial tubercle, just below the knee, which becomes prominent and is tender to direct pressure. The pain is most severe after physical activity that involves vigorous quadriceps contraction (jumping or running) or direct local trauma to the tibial tubercle area.

The goal of treatment for Osgood-Schlatter disease is to decrease the stress at the tubercle. Often a period of 4 to 8 weeks of restriction from strenuous physical activity, administration of antiinflammatory medications and stretching of the quadriceps muscle are sufficient. Bracing with a tubercle band can be very helpful. If the pain is not relieved, a cast or knee immobilizer is required, a situation that is particularly difficult if the condition is bilateral.

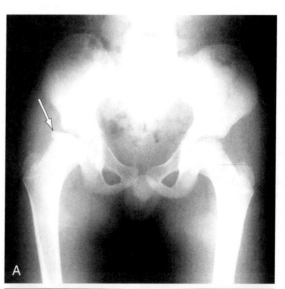
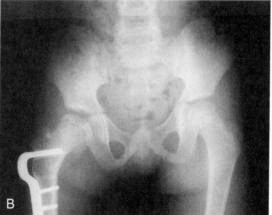

FIGURE 42.9 Pelvis of a 7-Year-Old Male With Legg-Calvé-Perthes Disease. **A,** The femoral head (*arrow*) is flat and extruded from the edge of the joint. This hip is at risk for early arthritis if left to revascularize and heal in this position. **B,** Surgical replacement of the femoral head. As the Perthes heals, the ball has assumed a round shape that matches the socket well.

Gradual resumption of activity is permitted after 8 weeks, but return to unrestricted athletic participation requires an additional 8 weeks to allow for revascularization, healing, and ossification of the tibial tubercle. With skeletal maturity and closure of the apophysis, Osgood-Schlatter disease resolves.

Sever Disease

Sever disease is like Osgood-Schlatter disease but of the calcaneus (heel bone). The insertion of the Achilles pulls on the cartilaginous apophysis of the calcaneus, causing pain. It is more common in athletic children and children who have underlying Achilles tendon tightness, for example, soccer players between the ages of 8 and 12. It is relieved by a heel lift in the shoe, rest, stretching, and antiinflammatory medications.

SCOLIOSIS

Scoliosis is a rotational curvature of the spine most obvious in the anteroposterior plane (Fig. 42.10). It can be classified as nonstructural or structural. Nonstructural scoliosis results from a cause other than the spine itself, such as posture, leg length discrepancy, or splinting from pain. Structural scoliosis is a curvature of the spine associated with vertebral rotation. Nonstructural scoliosis can become structural if the underlying cause is not found and treated.

There are three main types of structural scoliosis: idiopathic, congenital (attributable to bony deformity such as hemivertebrae), and teratologic (caused by another systemic syndrome such as cerebral palsy). Eighty percent of all scoliosis is idiopathic, which may have a genetic component. Although females and males are equally affected, once the curve becomes more than 30 degrees, females are 10 times more likely to be affected. Ninety-eight percent of curves are apex right thoracic. If a left thoracic curve appears in the adolescent with idiopathic scoliosis, MRI is performed to rule out a neurologic cause. MRI should be performed in scoliotic children with loss of abdominal reflexes and those who have exertional headaches or a congenital curve.

Idiopathic curves progress while a child is growing, and progression can be very rapid during growth spurts. When idiopathic curves progress to 25 degrees or greater, and the child is skeletally immature, bracing is required to stop or slow the progression. The total number of hours a brace is worn correlates to efficacy of treatment; 82% of children who wore the brace as prescribed had minimal progression.[8] In braced curves, 72% required no surgery compared with only 48% of those who wore no brace.[9]

Curves of more than 50 degrees will progress after skeletal maturity, so spinal fusion is required to stop progression. Bracing is the only nonoperative measure known to slow scoliotic progression. Chiropractic manipulation, physical therapy, exercise, and diet regimens have not been shown to alter natural history. Bracing is less successful in teratologic or congenital curves; therefore these conditions may require surgical intervention more often.

NEUROMUSCULAR DISORDERS

The neuromuscular disorders are a group of inherited disorders that cause progressive muscle fiber loss leading to weakness, mostly of the voluntary muscles. They cause significant disability in children resulting in lifelong neurologic, orthopedic, and pulmonary complications. Neuromuscular disorders have different inheritance patterns and different biochemical alterations that cause each specific type, and different disorders can cause disease in different stages of life. Although the classification of neuromuscular disorders has historically been based on age of onset, rate of progression, distribution of muscular involvement, findings from muscle biopsy, and patterns of inheritance, genetic testing is increasingly being used for diagnosis and classification. Common forms of neuromuscular disorders are described in Table 42.3.

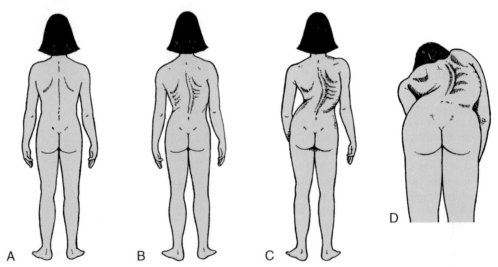

FIGURE 42.10 Scoliosis in Children. Normal spine alignment and abnormal spinal curvatures associated with scoliosis. A, Normal. B, Mild. C, Severe. D, Rotation and curvature of scoliosis.

TABLE 42.3 Major Muscular Dystrophy Syndromes

Disease	Mode of Inheritance	Age at Clinical Onset	Distribution of Weakness
Duchenne muscular dystrophy (DMD)/Becker muscular dystrophy (BMD)	X-linked, sporadic	2-3 yr/5-7 yr	Proximal with pseudohypertrophy
Facioscapulohumeral (FSH) muscular dystrophy	Autosomal dominant	Early adolescence	Face, arms, legs
Myotonic muscular dystrophy (MMD)	Autosomal dominant	Variable—birth to adulthood	Distal muscles, face

From Moxley RT III et al: Neurology 64(1):13-20, 2005.

Duchenne Muscular Dystrophy

PATHOPHYSIOLOGY   Duchenne muscular dystrophy (DMD) is X-linked, generally occurring in males, and is present in about 1 in 3500 male births. It is the most common childhood neuromuscular disorder. DMD is caused by mutations in the gene that encodes **dystrophin**, a large membrane-stabilizing protein. Dystrophin mediates anchorage of the actin cytoskeleton of skeletal muscle fibers to the basement membrane through a membrane-glycoprotein complex. Dystropin is present in normal muscle cells but absent in DMD. The lack of dystrophin causes poorly anchored fibers, which are torn apart under the repeated stress of contraction. Free calcium then enters the muscle cells, causing cell death and fiber necrosis (Fig. 42.11).

CLINICAL MANIFESTATIONS   DMD is usually identified in children at approximately 3 to 4 years of age, when the parents first notice gait abnormalities, difficulty getting up from the ground, and frequent falls. Parents also may notice enlargement of the calf muscles, which is caused by normal muscle fiber replacement with fat and connective tissue (see Fig. 42.11, *B* and *C*). Muscular weakness begins in the pelvic girdle, causing a "waddling" gait. The method of rising from the floor by "climbing up the legs" (Gower sign) is characteristic and is caused by weakness of the lumbar and gluteal muscles. The foot assumes an equinovarus position (see Fig. 42.1), and the child tends to walk on the toes because of weakness of the anterior tibial and peroneal muscles. Within 3 to 5 years, muscles of the shoulder girdle become involved.

Progressive weakness results in loss of ambulation between 12 and 15 years of age. Subsequent progression includes slowly progressive respiratory insufficiency; cardiomyopathy; and orthopedic complications, including scoliosis. Cognitive dysfunction is a common and often overlooked aspect of DMD. Full-scale IQ is 85, which is significantly lower than the average IQ of 100, although studies suggest this decrease may be caused by specific learning disabilities rather than a true decreased intelligence. As the condition progresses, constipation and incontinence of urine and stool may develop, possibly because of smooth muscle involvement. Although the life expectancy of males with DMD continues to increase, death usually occurs from respiratory tract infection and a compromised respiratory system, with the majority living into their middle twenties. Some individuals who have chosen ventilatory support live a decade or more longer. With increased survival, cardiac complications are becoming an important contributor to mortality.

EVALUATION AND TREATMENT   Diagnosis is suggested by a high blood creatine kinase (CK) level, which can be 100 times the normal level. However, a high CK level does not confirm the diagnosis because many other alterations also can increase CK. Diagnosis is confirmed by genetic testing for mutations in the dystrophin gene.

Children with DMD require a multidisciplinary approach to care, including attention to heart and breathing problems, weight loss/gain, constipation, rehabilitative/developmental problems, psychosocial needs, neurologic issues, and orthopedic problems (Fig. 42.12). Maintaining function in unaffected muscle groups for as long as possible is the primary goal of treatment. Although activity fosters maintenance of

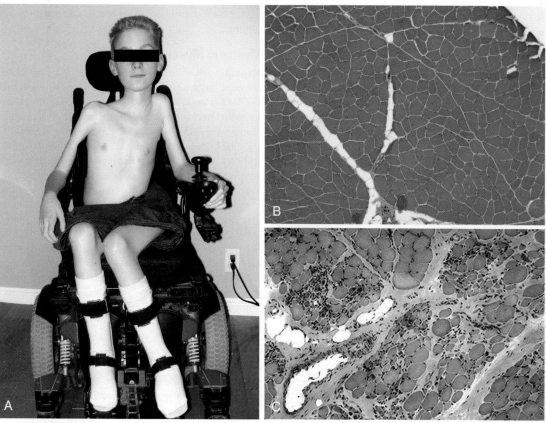

FIGURE 42.11 Duchenne Muscular Dystrophy. A, Young male with Duchenne muscular dystrophy. **B,** Transverse section of gastrocnemius muscle from a healthy male patient. **C,** Transverse section of gastrocnemius muscle from a male patient with Duchenne muscular dystrophy. Normal muscle fiber is replaced with fat and connective tissue. (From Jorde LB, Carey JC, Bamshad MJ: *Medical genetics,* ed 5, Philadelphia, 2016, Mosby.)

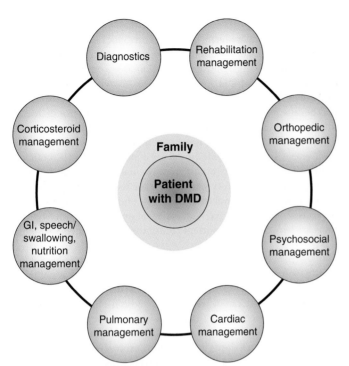

FIGURE 42.12 Multisystem Approach for Evaluation and Treatment of Duchenne Muscular Dystrophy (DMD). *GI,* Gastrointestinal. (Adapted from Bushby K: *Diagnosis and management of Duchenne muscular dystrophy part 1: diagnosis and pharmacological and psychosocial management,* 2009; Bushby K: *Diagnosis and management of Duchenne muscular dystrophy part 2: implementation of multidisciplinary care,* 2009. Available from http://www.thelancet.com/neurology. Published online November 30, 2009.)

muscle function, strenuous exercise may hasten the breakdown of muscle fibers. Range-of-motion exercises, bracing, and surgical release of contracture deformities are used to maintain normal function as long as possible. To prolong respiratory function or walking ability, or both, surgery for scoliosis is suggested when curves reach greater than 20 degrees.

Treatment with oral corticosteroids has become the standard of care and has dramatically improved outcomes. Children are able to walk an additional 2 to 5 years, and life expectancy has increased. Complications, such as compromised pulmonary function and kyphoscoliosis ("humped" upper spine combined with scoliosis), are delayed. A gene editing tool (CRISPR; Clustered Regularly Interspaced Short Palindromic Repeats) is being investigated in dogs to halt disease progression as a model for humans.

Families of children with DMD should receive genetic counseling for recurrence risk and prenatal screening. There is a chance that male siblings will have DMD and that female siblings will be carriers of the gene. Prenatal diagnosis is now possible.

Spinal Muscular Atrophy

Spinal muscular atrophy (SMA) is a common, autosomal recessive disorder characterized by degeneration of motor neurons in the spinal cord leading to progressive muscle atrophy. Children have progressive weakness and loss of motor skills. Clues to diagnosis include tongue fasciculation (involuntary muscle twitching), a bell-shaped chest in the most severely affected infants, and tremor and quadriceps atrophy in older children. Genetically, SMA is caused by a mutation in the *SMN1* gene. About 1 in 40 individuals carries the common mutation in the *SMN1* gene, making it one of the most common recessive disorders.

The severity of SMA is variable, ranging from children who are never able to independently sit to children who can walk short distances. Treatment is supportive and, like DMD, requires multidisciplinary specialty care. Gene replacement and gene modification therapies are rapidly evolving and may have a significant impact on survival and progression in coming years.

Facioscapulohumeral Muscular Dystrophy

Facioscapulohumeral (FSH) muscular dystrophy is inherited in an autosomal dominant fashion. It is more variable in presentation than DMD. FSH muscular dystrophy is usually observed in *late* childhood. Progression is usually slow and life span is normal or near normal. FSH muscular dystrophy occurs because of a deletion on chromosome 4 that is not associated with any particular gene and causes disease by still unknown mechanisms.

Muscle weakness, which is often asymmetric, usually begins in the face and is then observed in the shoulders and legs. Individuals with FSH muscular dystrophy often have weak eye closure, are not able to whistle or inflate a balloon, and have scapular winging (an abnormal protrusion of the shoulder blade).

Diagnosis is by genetic testing, although sometimes biopsies or electrodiagnostic testing may also be performed as part of the diagnostic evaluation. FSH muscular dystrophy also may be associated with mild hearing loss, retinal abnormalities, and mild cardiac problems. Unlike with DMD, children with FSH muscular dystrophy often have muscle pain, particularly in their arms and shoulders.

Treatment involves administration of NSAIDs to decrease pain and inflammation. Massage and heat treatments also may be helpful. Bracing may be performed for function; for example, dorsiflexion of the feet with ankle-foot orthotics to prevent tripping or to provide support and comfort.

Myotonic Muscular Dystrophy

Myotonic muscular dystrophy (MMD) is a multisystem disease that can occur because of mutations in either of two genes resulting in type 1 (*DMPK* gene) and type 2 (*CNBP* gene) MMD. MMD1 may demonstrate a genetic mechanism called *anticipation,* in which children born to a mother with MMD usually have a more severe form of the disease.

MMD affects the brain, skeletal and smooth muscles, eyes, heart, and endocrine system manifesting as distal muscle weakness, learning problems or intellectual disability, or both. Additionally, children can have dysphagia, constipation, cardiac dysrhythmias that if untreated may be life-threatening, diabetes, and cataracts. Males with MMD also may manifest testicular atrophy and early male pattern baldness. A hallmark of the disease is myotonia—difficulty relaxing muscles. For example, they may have difficulty relaxing their hand grip after a handshake or opening their eyes after closing them tightly.

Children with mild disease do not develop symptoms until adolescence or older and may display mild muscle weakness (usually more pronounced in the distal muscles), cataracts, and myotonia, but have normal life spans. Children with a more classic form of the disease also have onset of symptoms in the teenage years but have progressive muscle weakness, cataracts, and cardiac conduction abnormalities; they may have a shortened life span and require a wheelchair for mobility. The congenital form, the most severe, may be present at birth or become obvious over the first few years of life.

Diagnosis is made by genetic testing for the two genes known to cause MMD. In each case, an abnormal segment of deoxyribonucleic acid (DNA) causes abnormal functioning of muscle and other cells. Type 1 is more common and can present in infancy (the congenital form). Infants with MMD may have life-threatening breathing and swallowing problems and developmental delay or intellectual disability, although MMD is not observed until childhood or even adolescence.

Steroids are not useful for the treatment of MMD; however, maintaining muscle function is important, including range-of-motion exercises, bracing, and surgical release of contractures when necessary. Children need to be followed closely by neurologists and primary care providers with treatment for the various aspects of the disease, such as dysphagia, heart dysrhythmias, and constipation, as well as other problems.

✔ **QUICK CHECK 42.2**
1. What is the pathophysiology of osteochondrosis?
2. What is the difference between structural and nonstructural scoliosis?
3. What is the cause of Duchenne muscular dystrophy?
4. Discuss the clinical manifestations of Duchenne muscular dystrophy.

MUSCULOSKELETAL TUMORS

Benign Bone Tumors

The two most common forms of benign bone tumors are osteochondroma and nonossifying fibroma (Fig. 42.13).

Osteochondroma

Osteochondroma (or exostosis) can occur as a solitary lesion or as an inherited syndrome of hereditary multiple exostoses (HME). HME is an autosomal dominant condition with exostoses occurring throughout the skeleton. Osteochondromas appear as bony protuberances because of genetic anomalies near active growth plates of the proximal humerus, distal femur, or proximal tibia. The most common presentation is a palpable mass that is painful when traumatized. The lesions can lead to growth disturbance and mildly short stature. Knee valgus (knock-knee), ankle valgus, and hip problems are common. Upper extremity lesions can lead to a pronounced deformity in the forearm with a very short ulna bone. These lesions grow until skeletal maturity; growth or pain after skeletal maturity is a sign of possible malignant transformation, especially in the pelvis or scapular region. Transformation to chondrosarcoma is very rare, occurring in less than 1% of children.

Treatment involves minimizing growth disturbance, local tissue compression, and pain by resection of symptomatic lesions. The regrowth rate is 30% when lesions are removed in early childhood; therefore only symptomatic lesions should be surgically addressed in the growing child.[10]

Nonossifying Fibroma

Of all benign bone tumors, 50% are nonossifying fibromas or fibrous cortical defects. Nonossifying fibromas are sharply demarcated, cortically based lesions of fibrocytes that have replaced normal bone. The lesion can occur in any bone, at any age. Nearly 30% of all children have at least one.

Microscopically, these benign nonmetastasizing lesions appear as whorled bundles of fibroblasts and osteoclast-like giant cells. As the tumor grows, lipids make the fibroblasts foamy in appearance, and they are known as *foam cells*.

Treatment is observational only. If these lesions grow too large, however, they will compromise the biomechanical strength of the bone and lead to pathologic fractures. Curettage and bone grafting is suggested after pathologic fracture or if impending fracture (nonossifying fibroma >50% of the diameter of the bone or >3 or 4 cm) is noted radiographically.

Malignant Bone Tumors

Malignant bone tumors are uncommon tumors in childhood, accounting for fewer than 5% of childhood malignancies and occurring mostly during adolescence. The two most common malignant bone tumors are osteosarcoma and Ewing sarcoma.

Osteosarcoma

Osteosarcoma is the most common malignant bone tumor found during childhood and originates in bone-producing mesenchymal cells. It accounts for 60% of all malignant bone tumors and generally strikes between the ages of 10 and 18.

Osteosarcoma may develop as a result of rapid local growth, which increases the likelihood of mutation. It can be induced by ionizing radiation, even with relatively low doses, and can be a tragic consequence of therapeutic radiation for other forms of cancer. There also has been a link to individuals with retinoblastoma (a hereditary eye tumor). Osteosarcoma has not been linked to chemical carcinogens or viruses. No DNA or ribonucleic acid (RNA) virus has been isolated.

Molecular analysis has demonstrated deletion of genetic material on the long arm of chromosome 13, which led to the identification of a tumor-suppressor gene as being part of the mechanism for tumor development. The oncogene *src* also has been associated with osteosarcoma.

PATHOPHYSIOLOGY   Osteosarcoma occurs mainly in the metaphyses of long bones near sites of active physeal growth. The tumor most commonly occurs at the distal femur, proximal tibia, or proximal humerus. As a tumor of mesenchymal cells, osteosarcoma makes osteoid tissue.

Osteosarcoma is a bulky tumor that extends beyond the bone into a soft tissue mass. It may encircle the bone and destroy the trabeculae of the diseased area. Osteosarcoma disseminates through the bloodstream, usually to the lung. As many as 25% of children diagnosed with osteosarcoma exhibit lung metastases at diagnosis. Other sites of metastatic spread include other bones and visceral organs.

CLINICAL MANIFESTATIONS   The most common presenting complaint is pain. Night pain, awakening a child from sleep, is a particularly foreboding sign. There may be swelling, warmth, and redness caused by the vascularity of the tumor. Symptoms also may include cough, dyspnea, and chest pain if lung metastasis is present. If a lower extremity is involved, a child may limp or suffer a pathologic fracture. Although osteosarcoma is not the result of trauma, trauma may call attention to a preexisting tumor.

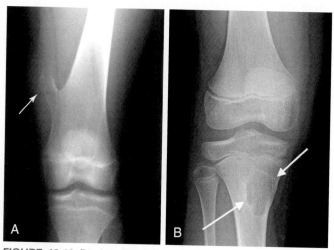

FIGURE 42.13 Benign Bone Tumors. A, Osteochondroma *(white arrow)* arising from the distal femur. **B,** Nonossifying fibroma *(white arrows)* mostly lytic.

EVALUATION AND TREATMENT   Although needle biopsy is often sufficient to establish the diagnosis, tissue biopsy confirms it. The five histologic types of osteosarcoma are determined by the predominant cell type. The tumor is graded according to degree of malignancy; the higher the grade, the worse the prognosis.

Surgery and chemotherapy are the primary treatments for osteosarcoma. If surgical excision is impossible, radiation therapy may allow local tumor control. Traditionally, surgery includes amputation at the joint above the involved bone; however, more recent limb salvage procedures have gained acceptance, and amputation may be avoided in many children.

Chemotherapy is an important component of treatment. Children routinely receive chemotherapy preoperatively; then the disease is restaged with MRI and surgical biopsy to determine rate of "tumor kill." If more than 90% of tumor cells are killed by chemotherapy, the prognosis is markedly improved. Chemotherapy is then used after surgery for any additional cell spill during surgery. The use of chemotherapy with surgery has increased the 5-year survival rate to 60% or more.[11]

A number of approaches have been used to treat pulmonary metastases. Because pulmonary metastases are generally solitary, thoracotomy with wedge resection has proven to be the most effective treatment.

Ewing Sarcoma

Ewing sarcoma is a malignant round cell tumor of bone and soft tissue and is the second most common and most lethal malignant bone tumor that occurs during childhood. The most common period of diagnosis is between 5 and 15 years of age; it is rare after age 30 years. Ewing sarcoma is slightly more common in males than females and is linked with periods of rapid bone growth.

PATHOPHYSIOLOGY   Ewing sarcoma is most commonly located in the midshaft of long bones or in flat bones. The most common sites include the femur, pelvis, and humerus.

Arising from bone marrow, Ewing sarcoma can penetrate the cortex of the bone to form a soft tissue mass (Fig. 42.14). Unlike osteosarcoma, Ewing sarcoma does not make bone and radiographically appears as a permeative, destructive lesion. Ewing sarcoma metastasizes to nearly every organ. Metastasis occurs early and is usually apparent at diagnosis or within 1 year. The most common sites are the lung, other bones, lymph nodes, bone marrow, liver, spleen, and central nervous system.

CLINICAL MANIFESTATIONS   As with osteosarcoma, the most common complaint is pain that increases in severity. A soft tissue mass is often present. Additional symptoms may include fever, malaise, and anorexia. The radiographic appearance is similar to that of infection, and diagnosis is confirmed only with biopsy.

EVALUATION AND TREATMENT   Evaluation is done with genetic testing, elevated sedimentation rate, and lactate dehydrogenase (LDH) levels. Biopsy is used to conclusively establish the diagnosis of a small round cell tumor.

Treatment includes radiation, chemotherapy, and, if possible, surgical débridement. Chemotherapy is continued for 12 to 18 months after resection. Present 5-year survival with this tritherapeutic approach is 65% to 75%;[12] however, tumors in the trunk or pelvis have a markedly worse prognosis. Metastasis at diagnosis is another poor prognostic indicator, with 5-year survival rate dropping to less than 40%.

NONACCIDENTAL TRAUMA

It is estimated that more than 1.5 million children are abused per year in the United States. Maltreatment may be psychologic, sexual, or physical.[13] Skeletal trauma is present in a significant number of abused children[14-16] (Fig. 42.15). Thirty percent of children who have been physically abused are seen by an orthopedist. Accurate and appropriate referrals to child protection agencies not only are legally mandated but also are essential for the well-being of the child. An abused child who is returned to the same situation without intervention has a 10% to 15% chance of subsequent mortality.

Fractures in Nonaccidental Trauma

Children who are not yet ambulatory and present with a long bone fracture have more than a 75% chance of that fracture being caused by nonaccidental trauma (NAT).[17] "Corner" metaphyseal fractures are nearly always from abuse but occur only 25% of the time (Fig. 42.16). Fractures at multiple stages of healing also suggest abuse; however, osteogenesis imperfecta or other causes of systemic osteomalacia must be ruled out. The most common presentation is a transverse tibia fracture. After walking age, only 2% of long bone fractures are the result of NAT.[18]

EVALUATION AND TREATMENT   NAT necessitates early consultation with child protective services. The child should undergo skeletal survey (especially if younger than 2 years of age) and have a complete physical examination to evaluate for pattern bruising, burns, or multiple soft tissue injuries. A thorough history must be obtained for all identified injuries. It is important to remember that social isolation can lead to an increased likelihood of abuse, but no social status is immune.

When the cause of injury is unclear, bone scan can be helpful in diagnosing subtle injuries, especially rib fractures. Posterior rib fractures are especially likely to be the result of abuse. MRI/computed tomography (CT) of the brain to check for subdural hematoma and retinal examination to look for hemorrhages are essential.

The treating health care provider must have a nonjudgmental attitude. The child and family involved in NAT are emotionally delicate and

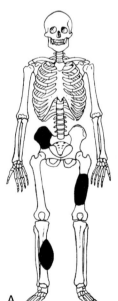
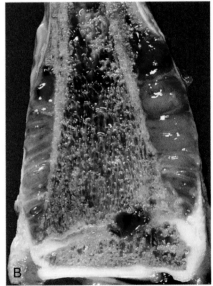

FIGURE 42.14 Ewing Sarcoma of the Distal Radius. Radiograph of an 8-year-old boy showing a permeative lesion of the distal radius. Note the loss of bone cortex on the ulnar border, suggesting an aggressive process. Bone biopsy revealed Ewing sarcoma.

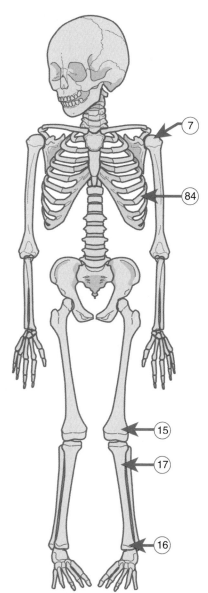

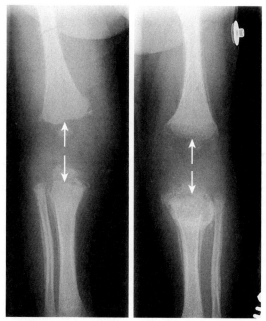

FIGURE 42.16 Corner Fracture. Bilateral knee radiograph showing healing corner fractures of bilateral proximal tibias and distal femurs. Note the varying amount of callus formation signifying fractures at different stages of healing.

require not only physical but also emotional care. Social workers need to be involved early to ensure that the child receives appropriate medical care. Fortunately, fractures tend to heal quickly for those in this age group. Neurologic injury and social disease, however, are much more difficult to cure.

✓ QUICK CHECK 42.3

1. What are the most common benign bone tumors of children?
2. How does osteosarcoma affect the respiratory system?
3. What is the most lethal bone tumor in children?
4. What is the most common orthopedic injury in NAT?

FIGURE 42.15 Rib and Metaphyseal Fractures. Rib fractures are very common and highly specific for abuse. In 31 children who died as a result of abuse, there was an extremely high incidence of rib and metaphyseal fractures. The *red arrows* indicate common sites of fracture related to abuse. (Data from Radiology Assistant Radiology Assistant Educational Site, Radiological Society of the Netherlands. Available from <www.radiologyassistant.nl/>.)

SUMMARY REVIEW

Congenital Defects

1. Clubfoot is a common deformity in which the foot is turned out of its normal shape or position. Clubfoot can be positional, idiopathic, or teratologic. Positional is correctable passively, however, idiopathic and teratologic may require casting, bracing, or surgery.
2. Developmental dysplasia of the hip (DDH) is an abnormality in the development of the femoral head, acetabulum, or both. DDH can be idiopathic or teratologic. It is a serious and disabling condition in children if not diagnosed and treated early, with best outcomes when treated before walking age.

3. Osteogenesis imperfecta (brittle bone disease) is an inherited disorder of collagen that affects primarily bones and results in serious fractures of many bones.

Bone and Joint Infection

1. Osteomyelitis is a local or generalized bacterial or granulomatous infection of bone and bone marrow. Bacteria are usually introduced by direct extension from a nearby infection, through the bloodstream, or by trauma. Infection starts in the metaphysis, then ruptures out to spread into the diaphysis.

2. Septic arthritis is a bacterial or granulomatous infection of the joint space and is a surgical emergency. It can occur on its own, or secondary to osteomyelitis in very young children in which the metaphysis is still located within the joint capsule of certain joints.

Juvenile Idiopathic Arthritis
1. Juvenile idiopathic arthritis is an inflammatory joint disorder characterized by pain and swelling. Large joints are most commonly affected.

Osteochondroses
1. Avascular diseases of the bone are collectively referred to as osteochondroses and are caused by an insufficient blood supply to growing bones.
2. Legg-Calvé-Perthes disease is characterized by the death of the epiphysis of the femoral head and degeneration of the head of the femur, followed by regeneration or recalcification. Children older than age 6 years at onset have a worse prognosis.
3. Osgood-Schlatter disease is characterized by tendonitis of the anterior patellar tendon and inflammation or partial separation of the tibial tubercle caused by chronic irritation, usually as a result of overuse of the quadriceps muscles. The condition is seen primarily in muscular, athletic adolescent males.

Scoliosis
1. Scoliosis is a rotational curvature of the spine most obvious in the anteroposterior plane and can be classified as nonstructural or structural. Nonstructural scoliosis results from a cause other than the spine itself, such as posture, leg length discrepancy, or splinting from pain. Structural scoliosis is a curvature of the spine associated with vertebral rotation.

Neuromuscular Disorders
1. The neuromuscular disorders are a group of genetically transmitted diseases characterized by progressive atrophy of skeletal muscles leading to weakness. They cause significant disability in children resulting in lifelong neurologic, orthopedic, and pulmonary complications.
2. Duchenne muscular dystrophy is characterized by the absence of the membrane-stabilizing protein dystropin in muscle cells. Weakness leads to abnormal gait, frequent falls, and eventual loss of ambulation. Respiratory, cardiac, and neurologic problems are also present, requiring a multidisciplinary approach to care.
3. Spinal muscular atrophy is characterized by degeneration of motor neurons in the spinal cord leading to progressive muscle

atrophy. Children have progressive muscle weakness and lack of motor skills.
4. Facioscapulohumeral muscular dystrophy involves asymmetric muscle weakness, starting in the face and then progressing to the shoulders and legs.
5. Myotonic muscular dystrophy classically presents with myotonia, or a difficulty relaxing muscles. It also can affect the brain, eyes, heart, and endocrine system.

Musculoskeletal Tumors
1. Musculoskeletal tumors may be benign (osteochondroma and nonossifying fibroma) or malignant (osteosarcoma and Ewing sarcoma).
2. Osteochondroma appears as a solitary bony protuberance near active growth plates of the proximal humerus, distal femur, or proximal tibia. Hereditary multiple exostoses is characterized by multiple bony protuberances throughout the skeleton.
3. Nonossifying fibromas are lesions in which fibrocytes have replaced normal bone. Treatment may be required if the lesions grow so large that they compromise the strength of the bone.
4. Osteosarcoma, the most common malignant childhood bone tumor, originates in bone-producing mesenchymal cells and is most often located near active growth plates, such as the distal femur, proximal tibia, or proximal humerus. It is a bulky tumor that creates osteoid tissue. Pain, especially night pain, is the most common presenting symptom. It commonly causes lung metastases. The primary treatments for osteosarcoma are surgery and chemotherapy.
5. Ewing sarcoma originates from cells within the bone marrow space and is most often located in the midshaft of long bones or in flat bones. The most common sites include the femur, pelvis, and humerus, and the most common presenting symptom is pain that increases in severity. Ewing sarcoma metastasizes to nearly every organ. The primary treatment for Ewing sarcoma is a combination of chemotherapy, radiation, and surgery.

Nonaccidental Trauma
1. Child abuse by nonaccidental trauma must be considered with any long bone injury in a child who is not yet walking. The health care provider is legally responsible to report suspected nonaccidental trauma.
2. The presence of soft tissue injury, corner fractures, and multiple fractures at different stages of healing is extremely helpful for making a diagnosis of nonaccidental trauma.
3. When nonaccidental trauma is suspected, a child must be evaluated radiographically for other fractures, burns, multiple soft tissue injuries, and retinal hemorrhage.

KEY TERMS

Acetabular dysplasia, 1000
Acute hematogenous osteomyelitis, 1002
Antalgic (painful) abductor lurch, 1005
Clubfoot, 999
Developmental dysplasia of the hip (DDH), 999
Dislocated hip, 1000
Duchenne muscular dystrophy (DMD), 1007
Dystrophin, 1007
Ewing sarcoma, 1010
Facioscapulohumeral (FSH) muscular dystrophy, 1008
Hereditary multiple exostoses (HME), 1009
Involucrum, 1002
Juvenile idiopathic arthritis (JIA), 1003
Legg-Calvé-Perthes (LCP) disease, 1004
Malignant bone tumor, 1009
Myotonic muscular dystrophy (MMD), 1008
Neuromuscular disorder, 1006
Nonossifying fibroma, 1009
Nonstructural scoliosis, 1006
Oligoarthritis, 1003
Osgood-Schlatter disease, 1005
Osteochondroma, 1009
Osteochondrosis, 1003
Osteogenesis imperfecta (OI; brittle bone disease), 1000
Osteomyelitis, 1001
Osteosarcoma, 1009
Polyarthritis, 1003
Scoliosis, 1006
Septic arthritis, 1003
Sever disease, 1006
Spinal muscular atrophy (SMA), 1008
Still disease, 1003
Structural scoliosis, 1006
Subluxated hip, 1000
Talipes equinovarus, 999

REFERENCES

1. Morcuende JA, et al: Plaster cast treatment of clubfoot: the Ponseti method of manipulation and casting, *J Pediatr Orthop* 3(2):161-167, 1994.
2. Jari S, et al: Unilateral limitation of abduction of the hip: a valuable clinical sign for DDH?, *J Bone Joint Surg Br* 84(1):104-107, 2002.
3. Patel RM, et al: A cross-sectional multicenter study of osteogenesis imperfecta in North America—results from the Linked Clinical Research Centers, *Clin Genet* 87(2):133-140, 2015.
4. Principi N, et al: *Kingella kingae* infections in children, *BMC Infect Dis* 15:260, 2015.
5. Vaderhave KL, et al: Community-associated methicillin-resistant *Staphylococcus aureus* in acute musculoskeletal infection in children: a game changer, *J Pediatr Orthop* 29(8):927-931, 2009.
6. Mata SG, et al: Legg-Calvé-Perthes disease and passive smoking, *J Pediatr Orthop* 20(3):326-330, 2000.
7. Cassas KJ, Cassettari-Wayhs A: Childhood and adolescent sports-related overuse injuries, *Am Fam Physician* 73(6):1014-1022, 2006.
8. Katz DE, et al: Brace wear control of curve progression in adolescent idiopathic scoliosis, *J Bone Joint Surg Am* 92:1343-1352, 2010.
9. Stuart L, et al: Effects of bracing in adolescents with idiopathic scoliosis, *N Engl J Med* 369:1512-1521, 2013.
10. Cummings JR, et al: Congenital clubfoot, *Instr Course Lect* 51:385-400, 2002.
11. Heyden JB, Hoang BH: Osteosarcoma: basic science and clinical implications, *Orthop Clin North Am* 37(1):1-7, 2006.
12. Ruyman FB, Grovas AC: Progress in the diagnosis and treatment of rhabdomyosarcoma and related soft tissue sarcomas, *Cancer Invest* 18(3):223, 2000.
13. Administration for Children and Families Children's Bureau: *Child maltreatment 2009*, Washington, DC, 2010, U.S. Department of Health and Human Services. Available at: http://www.acf.hhs.gov/programs/cb/stats_research/index.htm#can.
14. Lane WG, et al: Racial differences in the evaluation of pediatric fractures for physical abuse, *J Am Med Assoc* 288(13):1603-1609, 2002.
15. Swoboda SL, et al: Skeletal trauma in child abuse, *Pediatr Ann* 42(11):e245-e252, 2013.
16. Wood JN, et al: Evaluation for occult fractures in injured children, *Pediatrics* 136(2):232-240, 2015.
17. Rex C, Kay PR: Features of femoral fractures in nonaccidental injury, *J Pediatr Orthop* 20(3):411-413, 2000.
18. Thomas SA, et al: Long-bone fractures in young children: distinguishing accident injuries from child abuse, *Pediatrics* 88(3):471-476, 1991.

43

Structure, Function, and Disorders of the Integument

Sue Ann McCann, Sue E. Huether

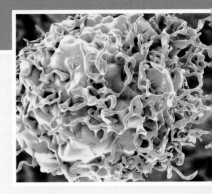

EVOLVE WEBSITE

CHAPTER OUTLINE

The skin is the largest organ of the body, accounting for about 20% of body weight. Combined with the accessory structures of hair, nails, and glands, it forms the integumentary system. The skin's primary function is environmental protection by serving as a barrier against microorganisms, ultraviolet radiation, loss of body fluids, and the stress of mechanical forces. The skin regulates body temperature and is involved in immune surveillance and the activation of vitamin D. Touch and pressure receptors provide important protective functions and pleasurable sensations. The microbiome of the skin protects against pathologic bacteria.

STRUCTURE AND FUNCTION OF THE SKIN

Layers of the Skin

The skin is formed of two major layers: (1) a superficial, or outer, layer of epidermis and (2) a deeper layer of dermis (the true skin) (Fig. 43.1). The subcutaneous layer (hypodermis) is the lowest lying layer of connective tissue that contains macrophages, fibroblasts, fat cells, nerves, fine muscles, blood vessels, lymphatics, and hair follicle roots. Each skin layer contains cells that represent progressive stages of skin cell differentiation and function. These are summarized in Table 43.1.

Dermal Appendages

The dermal appendages include the nails, hair, sebaceous glands, and the eccrine and apocrine sweat glands. The fingernails and toenails are protective keratinized plates. They are composed of (1) the proximal nail fold, (2) the eponychium (cuticle), (3) the matrix from which the nail grows and its nail root, (4) the hyponychium (nail bed), (5) the nail plate, and (6) the paronychium (lateral nail fold) (Fig. 43.2). Nail growth continues throughout life at 1 mm or less per day.

Hair color, density, grain, and pattern of distribution vary among people and depend on age, sex, and race. Hair follicles arise from the matrix (or bulb) located deep in the dermis. They extend from the dermis at an angle and have an erector pili muscle attached near the mid-dermis that straightens the follicle when contracted, causing the hair to stand up. Hair growth begins in the bulb, with cellular differentiation occurring as the hair progresses up the follicle. Hair is fully hardened, or cornified, by the time it emerges at the skin surface. Hair color is determined by melanin-secreting follicular melanocytes. Hair growth is cyclic, with periods of growth and rest that vary over different body surfaces.

The sebaceous glands open onto the surface of the skin through a canal. They are found in greatest numbers on the face, chest, and back, with modified glands on the eyelids, lips, nipples, glans penis, and prepuce. Sebaceous glands secrete sebum, composed primarily of lipids, which oils the skin and hair and prevents drying. Androgens stimulate the growth of sebaceous glands, and their enlargement is an early sign of puberty.

The eccrine sweat glands are distributed over the body, with the greatest numbers in the palms of the hands, soles of the feet, and forehead. They are important in thermoregulation and cooling of the body through evaporation. The apocrine sweat glands are fewer in number but produce significantly more sweat than the eccrine glands. They are located near

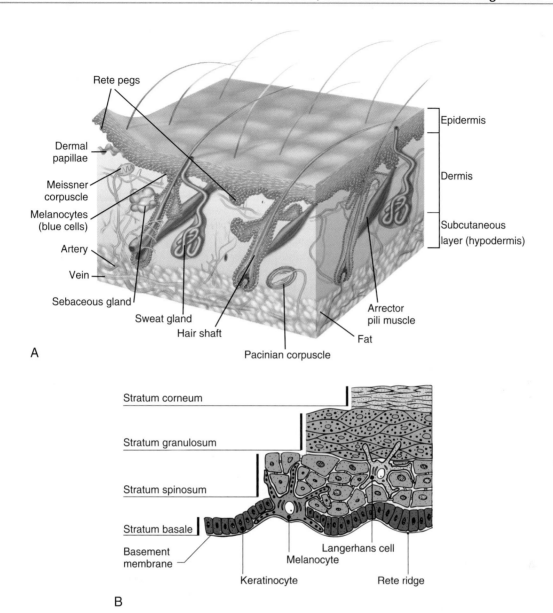

FIGURE 43.1 Structure of the Skin. A, Cross section showing major skin structures. **B,** Layers of the epidermis. (**A** from Kumar V et al: *Robbins & Cotran pathologic basis of disease,* ed 9, Philadelphia, 2015, Saunders; **B** from Gawkrodger D, Ardern-Jones M: *Dermatology,* ed 5, Philadelphia, 2012, Churchill Livingstone.)

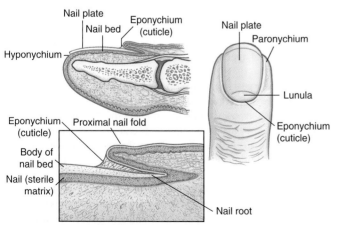

FIGURE 43.2 Structures of the Nail. (Redrawn from Thompson JM et al: *Mosby's clinical nursing,* ed 5, St Louis, 2002, Mosby.)

the bulb of hair follicles in the axillae, scalp, face, abdomen, and genital area. Their ducts open into the hair follicle. The interaction of sweat with commensal (normal) flora bacteria contributes to the odor of perspiration.

Blood Supply and Innervation

The blood supply to the skin is limited to the papillary capillaries, or plexus, of the dermis. These capillary loops are supplied by a deeper arterial plexus. Branches from the deep plexus also supply hair follicles and sweat glands. A subpapillary network of veins drains the capillary loops. Arteriovenous anastomoses in the dermis facilitate the regulation of body temperature. Heat loss is regulated by (1) variations in skin blood flow through the opening and closing of arteriovenous anastomoses and (2) the evaporative heat loss of sweat. The sympathetic nervous system regulates both vasoconstriction and vasodilation through α-adrenergic receptors in the skin. The lymphatic vessels of the skin arise in the papillary dermis and drain into larger

TABLE 43.1 Layers of the Skin

Structure	Cell Types	Characteristics
Epidermis	Keratinocytes	Most important layer of skin; normally very thin (0.12 mm) but can thicken and form corns or calluses with constant pressure or friction; includes rete pegs that extend into papillary layer of dermis
	Langerhans (dendritic) cells	Antigen presenting cells and immune functions
Stratum corneum	Keratinocytes	Tough superficial layer covering the body
Stratum lucidum	Keratinocytes	Clear layers of cells containing eleidin, which becomes keratin as cells move up to corneum layer
Stratum granulosum	Keratinocytes Melanocytes	Keratohyalin gives granular appearance to this layer
Stratum spinosum	New keratinocytes	Polygonal shaped with spinous processes projecting between adjacent keratinocytes
Stratum basale (germinativum)	Keratinocytes Melanocytes Merkel cells	Basal layer where keratinocytes divide and move upward to replace cells shed from surface Melanocytes synthesize pigment melanin Mechanoreceptors for light touch
Dermis Papillary layer (thin)	Macrophages Mast cells	Irregular connective tissue layer with rich blood, lymphatic, and nerve supply; contains sensory receptors and sweat glands (apocrine, eccrine, sebaceous), macrophages (phagocytic and important for wound healing), and mast cells (release histamine and have immune functions) (see Chapter 6)
Reticular layer (thick)	Histiocytes	Wandering macrophages that collect pigments and inflammatory debris
Subcutaneous Layer (Hypodermis)		Subcutaneous tissue or superficial fascia of varying thickness that connects overlying dermis to underlying muscle; contains macrophages, fibroblasts, fat cells, nerves, blood vessels, lymphatics, and hair follicle roots

subcutaneous trunks, removing cells, proteins, and immunologic mediators.

The structure and function of the skin change with advancing age. A summary of aging changes is included in the box *Geriatric Considerations: Aging and Changes in Skin Integrity.*

✔ QUICK CHECK 43.1
1. Describe the two layers of the skin.
2. How do the skin blood vessels and sweat glands regulate body temperature?
3. What are some changes that occur in the skin with aging?

Clinical Manifestations of Skin Dysfunction

Lesions

Identification of the morphologic structure of the skin, including differentiation between primary and secondary lesions, and assessment of the appearance of the skin in combination with obtaining a health history, are essential to identify underlying pathophysiology. Tables 43.2 and 43.3 describe and illustrate lesions of the skin. Clinical manifestations of select skin lesions are described in Table 43.4.

Pressure injury. Pressure injury is localized damage to the skin that results from unrelieved pressure, shearing forces, friction, and moisture. Pressure that consistently interrupts normal blood flow to and from the skin or underlying tissues is the most common cause. The risks for pressure injury are summarized in the box *Risk Factors: Pressure Injury.*

Pressure injuries usually develop over bony prominences, such as the sacrum, heels, ischia, and greater trochanters. Continuous pressure on tissue between the bony prominence and a resistant outside surface distorts capillaries and occludes the blood supply. Pressure injury also can occur in soft tissues from unrelieved pressure, for example, from nasal cannulas or endotracheal tubes. If the pressure is relieved within a few hours, a brief period of reactive hyperemia (redness) occurs and there may be no lasting tissue damage. If the pressure continues

unrelieved, the endothelial cells lining the capillaries become disrupted with platelet aggregation, forming microthrombi that block blood flow and cause anoxic necrosis of surrounding tissues. Shearing and friction are mechanical forces moving parallel to the skin (dragging) and can extend to the bony skeleton, causing detachment and injury of tissues. Pressure injuries are staged or graded (Fig. 43.3). One classification scheme is available from the National Pressure Advisory Panel at https://npuap.org/page/PressureInjuryStages.

Superficial damage results in a layer of dead tissue that forms as an abrasion, blister, erosion, or nonblanchable red/darkened skin or as a reddish blue discoloration when there is deeper tissue damage. Superficial lesions are more common on the sacrum as a result of shearing or friction forces (forces parallel to the skin). Deep lesions develop closer to the bone as a result of tissue distortion and vascular occlusion from pressure perpendicular to the tissue (over the heels, trochanter, and ischia). Bacteria colonize the dead tissue, and infection is usually localized and self-limiting. Proteolytic enzymes from bacteria and macrophages dissolve necrotic tissues and cause a foul-smelling discharge that resembles, but is not, pus. The necrotic tissue initiates an inflammatory response with potential pain, fever, and leukocytosis. If the lesion is large, toxicity and pain lead to a host of possible complications, including loss of appetite, debility, local/systemic infections, and renal insufficiency.

The primary goals for those at risk for pressure injury are prevention and early detection. Preventive techniques include frequent assessment of the skin, with repositioning and turning of the individual; promotion of movement; implementation of pressure reduction (type of positioning and use of specialty beds), pressure removal (positioning interval), and pressure distribution devices (positioning aids); and elimination of excessive moisture and drainage. Adequate nutrition, oxygenation, and fluid balance must be maintained.

Superficial lesions should be covered with flat, moisture-retaining but not wet dressings that cannot wrinkle and cause increased pressure or friction. Successful healing requires continued adequate relief of pressure, débridement of necrotic tissue, opening of deep pockets for

TABLE 43.2   Primary Skin Lesions

Macule

A flat, circumscribed area that is a change in the color of the skin; less than 1 cm in diameter

Examples: Freckles, flat moles (nevi), petechiae, measles, scarlet fever

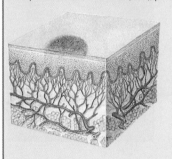
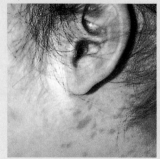

Macules[a]

Papule

An elevated, firm, circumscribed area less than 1 cm in diameter

Examples: Wart (verruca), elevated moles, lichen planus, fibroma, insect bite

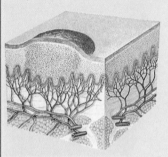
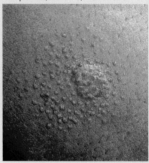

Lichen Planus[b]

Patch

A flat, nonpalpable, irregular-shaped macule more than 1 cm in diameter

Examples: Vitiligo, port-wine stains, mongolian spots, café au lait spots

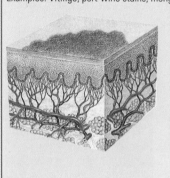
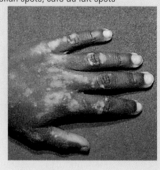

Plaque

Elevated, firm, and rough lesion with flat top surface greater than 1 cm in diameter

Examples: Psoriasis, seborrheic and actinic keratoses

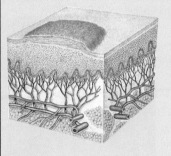
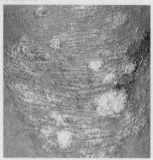

Plaque[d]

Wheal

Elevated, irregularly shaped area of cutaneous edema; solid, transient; variable diameter

Examples: Insect bites, urticaria, allergic reaction

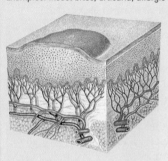
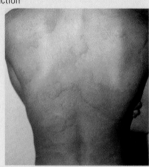

Wheal[e]

Nodule

Elevated, firm, circumscribed lesion; deeper in dermis than a papule; 1-2 cm in diameter

Examples: Erythema nodosum, lipomas

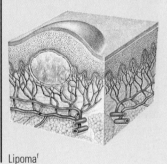
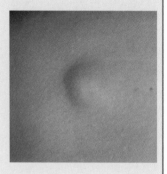

Lipoma[f]

Continued

TABLE 43.2   Primary Skin Lesions—cont'd

Tumor

Elevated, solid lesion; may be clearly demarcated; deeper in dermis; more than 2 cm in diameter

Examples: Neoplasms, benign tumor, lipoma, neurofibroma, hemangioma

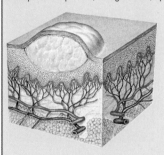 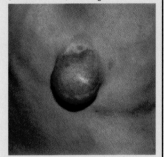

Neurofibroma[f]

Vesicle

Elevated, circumscribed, superficial; does not extend into dermis; filled with serous fluid; less than 1 cm in diameter

Examples: Varicella (chickenpox), herpes zoster (shingles), herpes simplex

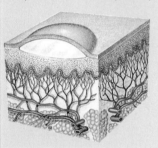 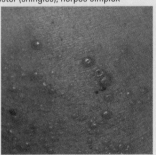

Vesicles[g]

Vesicle more than 1 cm in diameter

Examples: Blister, pemphigus vulgaris

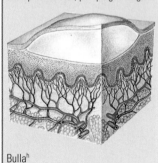 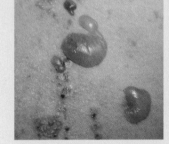

Bulla[h]

Pustule

Elevated, superficial lesion; similar to a vesicle but filled with purulent fluid

Examples: Impetigo, acne

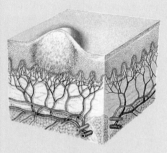 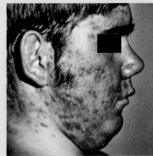

Acne[c]

Cyst

Elevated, circumscribed, encapsulated lesion; in dermis or subcutaneous layer; filled with liquid or semisolid material

Examples: Sebaceous cyst, cystic acne

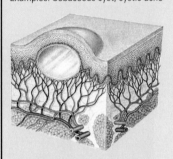 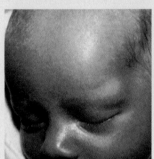

Sebaceous Cyst[c]

Telangiectasia

Fine (0.5-1 mm), irregular red lines produced by capillary dilation; can be associated with acne rosacea (face), venous hypertension (spider veins in legs), systemic sclerosis, or developmental abnormalities (port wine birthmarks)

Example: Telangiectasia in rosacea

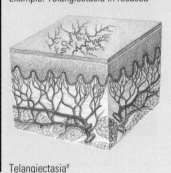 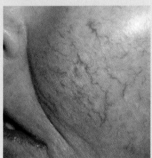

Telangiectasia[e]

[a]Farrar WE et al: *Infectious diseases*, ed 2, London, 1992, Gower.
[b]James WD et al: *Andrews' diseases of the skin*, ed 11, Philadelphia, 2011, Saunders.
[c]Weston WL, Lane AT: *Color textbook of pediatric dermatology*, ed 3, Philadelphia, 2002, Mosby.
[d]Habif TP: *Clinical dermatology: a color guide to diagnosis and therapy*, ed 5, Philadelphia, 2010, Mosby.
[e]Bolognia JL et al: *Dermatology*, ed 3, Philadelphia, 2012, Saunders.
[f]Weston WL et al: *Color textbook of pediatric dermatology*, ed 4, Philadelphia, 2007, Mosby.
[g]Black MM et al: *Obstetric and gynecologic dermatology*, ed 3, Philadelphia, 2008, Mosby.
[h]Marks JG, Miller JJ: *Lookingbill & Marks' principles of dermatology*, ed 4, London, 2006, Saunders.

TABLE 43.3   Secondary Skin Lesions

Scale
Heaped-up, keratinized cells; flaky skin; irregular shape; thick or thin; dry or oily; variation in size

Examples: Flaking of skin with seborrheic dermatitis after scarlet fever, or flaking of skin after a drug reaction; dry skin

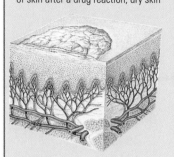
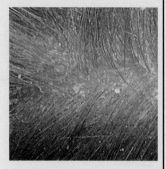

Fine Scaling[a]

Lichenification
Rough, thickened epidermis secondary to persistent rubbing, itching, or skin irritation; often involves flexor surface of extremity

Example: Chronic dermatitis

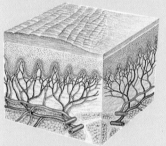
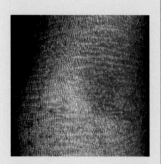

Atopic Dermatitis of Arm[b]

Keloid
Irregularly shaped, elevated, progressively enlarging scar; grows beyond boundaries of wound; caused by excessive collagen formation during healing

Examples: Keloid formation after surgery

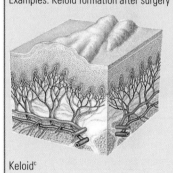
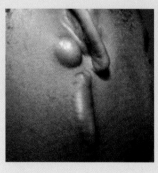

Keloid[c]

Scar
Thin to thick fibrous tissue that replaces normal skin after injury or laceration to the dermis

Examples: Healed wound or surgical incision

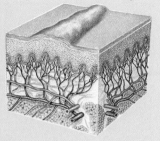
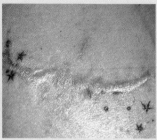

Hypertrophic Scar[d]

Excoriation
Loss of epidermis; linear, hollowed-out, crusted area

Examples: Abrasion or scratch, scabies

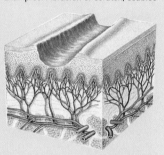
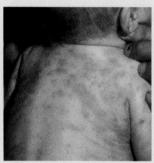

Scabies[c]

Fissure
Linear crack or break from the epidermis to the dermis; may be moist or dry

Examples: Athlete's foot, cracks at the corner of mouth, anal fissure, dermatitis

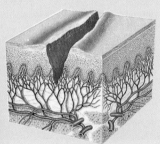
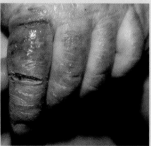

Fissures From Infected Dermatitis[c]

Continued

TABLE 43.3   Secondary Skin Lesions—cont'd

Erosion

Loss of part of the epidermis; depressed, moist, glistening; follows rupture of a vesicle or bulla or chemical injury

Example: Chemical injury

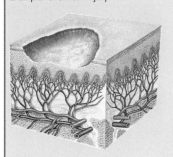 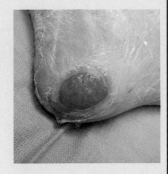

Erosion on Leg[e]

Ulcer

Loss of epidermis and dermis; concave; varies in size

Examples: Pressure ulcer, stasis ulcers

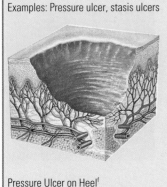

Pressure Ulcer on Heel[f]

Atrophy

Thinning of skin surface and loss of skin markings; skin appears translucent and paperlike

Examples: Aged skin, striae

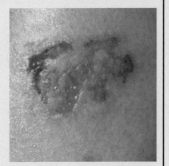 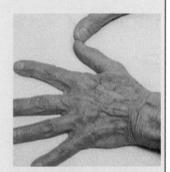

Aged Skin[g]

[a]Baran R et al: *Color atlas of the hair, scalp, and nails,* St Louis, 1991, Mosby.

[b]James WD et al: *Andrews' diseases of the skin,* ed 11, Philadelphia, 2011, Saunders.
[c]Weston WL et al: *Color textbook of pediatric dermatology,* ed 4, St Louis, 2007, Mosby.
[d]Nouri K, Leal-Khouri S: *Techniques in dermatologic surgery,* Philadelphia, 2003, Mosby.
[e]Bolognia JL et al: *Dermatology,* ed 3, Philadelphia, 2012, Saunders.
[f]Robinson JK et al: *Surgery of the skin,* ed 3, Philadelphia, 2015, Saunders.
[g]Seidel HM et al: *Seidel's guide to physical examination,* ed 8, St Louis, 2015, Mosby.

RISK FACTORS

Pressure Injury

External Factors
- Prolonged pressure or immobilization
- Prolonged moisture exposure
- Neurologic disorders (coma, spinal cord injuries, cognitive impairment, or cerebrovascular disease)
- Fractures or contractures
- Debilitation
- Pain
- Sedation
- Use of vasopressors
- Friction and shearing forces
- Coarse bed sheets used for turning by dragging, which produces friction and a shearing force

- Prolonged head of bed elevation greater than 30 degrees.
- Inadequate caretaking staff
- Lack of communication/education regarding pressure injury care

Disease/Tissue Factors
- Impaired mobility or sensation
- Impaired perfusion; low blood pressure, ischemia
- Fecal or urinary incontinence; prolonged exposure to moisture
- Malnutrition, dehydration
- Chronic diseases accompanied by anemia, edema, renal failure, malnutrition, peripheral vascular disease, or sepsis
- Previous history of pressure injury
- Thin skin associated with aging or prolonged use of steroids

Data from Cox J, Roche S, Murphy V: *Adv Skin Wound Care* 31(7):328-334, 2018; Raetz JG, Wick KH: *Am Fam Physician* 92(10):888-894, 2015.

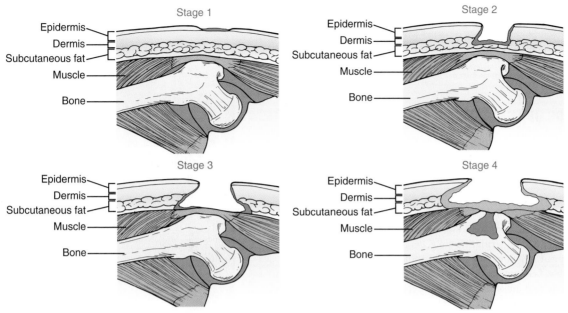

FIGURE 43.3 Stages of Pressure Ulcers. Stage 1—nonblanchable intact dermis. Stage 2—partial thickness skin loss into the dermis. Stage 3—full thickness skin loss through the dermis with visible adipose tissue. Stage 4—full thickness with exposure of muscle and bone. (From *Buck's Step-by-Step Medical Coding*, 2020 Edition, ed 1, St. Louis, 2020, Elsevier.)

TABLE 43.4	**Clinical Manifestations of Select Skin Lesions**
Type	**Clinical Manifestation**
Comedone	Plug of sebaceous and keratin material lodged in opening of hair follicle; open comedone has dilated orifice (blackhead) and closed comedone has narrow opening (whitehead)
Burrow	Narrow, raised, irregular channel caused by parasite
Petechiae	Circumscribed area of blood less than 0.5 cm in diameter
Purpura	Circumscribed area of blood greater than 0.5 cm in diameter
Telangiectasia	Dilated, superficial blood vessels

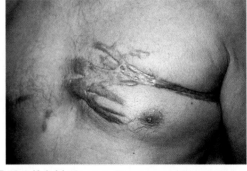

FIGURE 43.4 Keloid. (Courtesy Department of Dermatology, University of Utah School of Medicine, Salt Lake City, Utah.)

drainage, and repair of damaged tissue by construction of skin flaps for large, deep ulcers. Infection requires treatment with antibiotics, and pain should be controlled.[1]

Keloids and Hypertrophic Scars

Keloids are rounded, firm elevated scars with irregular clawlike margins that extend beyond the original site of injury (Fig. 43.4). They are most common in darkly pigmented skin types and generally appear weeks to months after a stable scar has formed. Hypertrophic scars are elevated erythematous fibrous lesions that do not extend beyond the border of injury. Hypertrophic scars appear within 3 to 4 months after injury and usually regress within 1 year. Both lesions are caused by abnormal wound healing with excessive fibroblast activity and collagen formation, and loss of control of normal tissue repair and regeneration. Genetic susceptibility is likely.

Excessive or poorly aligned tension on a wound, introduction of foreign material into the skin, infection, and certain types of trauma (e.g., burns) are all provocative factors. Those parts of the body at risk include shoulders, back, chin, ears, and lower legs.

Various treatments are available for the management of keloids and hypertrophic scars.[2]

Pruritus

Pruritus, or itching, is a symptom associated with many primary skin disorders, such as eczema, psoriasis, or insect infestations, or it can be a manifestation of systemic disease (e.g., chronic renal failure, cholestatic liver disease, thyroid disorders, iron deficiency, neuropathies, or malignancy) or the use of opiate drugs. It may be acute or chronic (neuropathic itch), localized or generalized, and migratory (moves from one location to another). Multiple stimuli can produce itching, and there is interaction between itch and pain sensations. There are many itch mediators, including histamine, serotonin, prostaglandins, bradykinins, neuropeptides, acetylcholine, interleukin-2 (IL-2), and IL-31. Small unmyelinated type C nerve fibers transmit itch sensations, and specific spinal pathways carry itch sensations to the brain.

Management of pruritus is challenging and depends on the cause; the primary condition must be treated. Both topical and systemic therapies are used.[3]

DISORDERS OF THE SKIN

Disorders of the skin may be precipitated by trauma, abnormal cellular function, infection, immune responses and inflammation, and systemic diseases.

Inflammatory Disorders

The most common inflammatory disorders of the skin are eczema and dermatitis. Eczema and dermatitis are general terms that describe a particular type of inflammatory response in the skin and can be used interchangeably. Eczematous disorders are generally characterized by pruritus, lesions with indistinct borders, and epidermal changes. These lesions can appear as erythema, papules, or scales; they can present in an acute, subacute, or chronic phase. Edema, serous discharge, and crusting occur with continued irritation and scratching. In chronic eczema, the skin becomes thickened, leathery, and hyperpigmented from recurrent irritation and scratching. Eczematous inflammations need to be differentiated from other epidermal rashes and dermatoses, particularly psoriasis.

Allergic Contact Dermatitis

Allergic contact dermatitis is a common form of T-cell–mediated or delayed hypersensitivity (see Chapter 8 for different types of allergic responses). The response is an interaction of skin barrier function, reaction to irritants, and neuronal responses, such as pruritus. Genetic susceptibility involves several genes including loss of function mutations in the gene encoding the epidermal protein filaggrin which binds keratin filaments and provides a skin barrier.

Various allergens (e.g., microorganisms, chemicals, foreign proteins, latex, drugs, metals) can form the sensitizing antigen. Contact with poison ivy is a common example (Fig. 43.5). When the allergen contacts the skin, it is bound to a carrier protein, forming a sensitizing antigen. The Langerhans cells (antigen-presenting dendritic cells) process the antigen and present it to T cells. T cells then become sensitized to the antigen, inducing the release of inflammatory cytokines, resulting in the symptoms of dermatitis. In latex allergy there is either a type IV hypersensitivity reaction to chemicals used in latex rubber processing or a type I immediate hypersensitivity reaction with immunoglobulin E (IgE) antibodies formed in response to latex rubber protein.[4]

In delayed hypersensitivity (type IV), several hours pass before an immunologic response is apparent. The T cells play an important role because they differentiate and secrete lymphokines that affect macrophage (Langerhans cells) movement and aggregation, coagulation, and other inflammatory responses (see Chapter 8). Sensitization usually develops with the first exposure to the antigen, and symptoms of dermatitis occur with reexposure.

The manifestations of allergic contact dermatitis include erythema and swelling with pruritic (itching) vesicular lesions in the areas of allergen contact. The pattern of distribution provides clues to the source of the antigen (e.g., hands exposed to chemical solutions or boundaries from rings and bracelets). The antigen must be removed for the inflammatory response to resolve and tissue repair to begin. Treatment may require topical or systemic steroids.

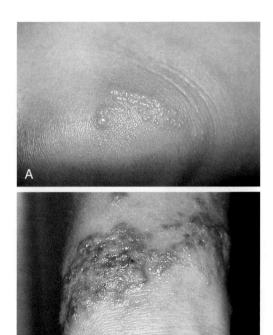

FIGURE 43.5 Poison Ivy. A, Poison ivy on knee. **B,** Poison ivy dermatitis. (Courtesy Department of Dermatology, University of Utah School of Medicine, Salt Lake City, Utah.)

Irritant Contact Dermatitis

Irritant contact dermatitis is a nonspecific inflammatory dermatitis caused by activation of the innate immune system by proinflammatory properties of chemicals. The severity of the inflammation is related to the concentration of the irritant, length of exposure, and disruption of the skin barrier. Chemical irritation from acids and prolonged exposure to soaps, detergents, and various agents used in industry can cause inflammatory lesions. The skin lesions resemble allergic contact dermatitis. Removing the source of irritation and using topical agents provide effective treatment.

Atopic Dermatitis

Atopic dermatitis (allergic dermatitis) is common in individuals with a history of hay fever or asthma and is associated with IgE antibodies. It is more common in infancy and childhood, but some individuals are affected throughout life. Specific details of this disorder are presented in Chapter 44.

Stasis Dermatitis

Stasis dermatitis usually occurs on the lower legs as a result of chronic venous stasis and edema and is associated with varicosities, phlebitis, and vascular trauma. Pooling of venous blood traps neutrophils that may release oxidants and proteolytic enzymes. Increased venous pressure widens interendothelial pores, with deposition of red blood cells, fibrin, and other macromolecules, making them unavailable for repair while promoting inflammation. Erythema and pruritus develop initially, followed by scaling, petechiae, and hyperpigmentation. Progressive lesions become ulcerated, particularly around the ankles and pretibial surface (Fig. 43.6).

Treatment includes elevating the legs as often as possible, not wearing tight clothes around the legs, and not standing for long periods. Defined infections are treated with antibiotics. Chronic lesions with ulceration are treated with moist dressings, external compression/dressings, and vein ablation surgery.[5]

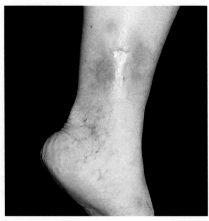

FIGURE 43.6 Stasis Ulcer. (Courtesy Department of Dermatology, University of Utah School of Medicine, Salt Lake City, Utah.)

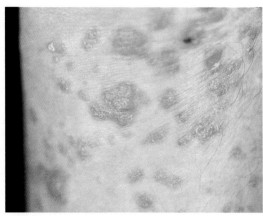

FIGURE 43.8 Psoriasis. Typical oval plaque with well-defined borders and silvery scale. (Courtesy Department of Dermatology, University of Utah School of Medicine, Salt Lake City, Utah.)

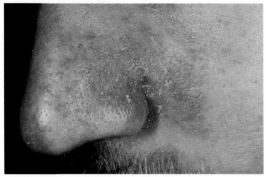

FIGURE 43.7 Seborrheic Dermatitis. (Courtesy Department of Dermatology, University of Utah School of Medicine, Salt Lake City, Utah.)

Seborrheic Dermatitis

Seborrheic dermatitis is a common chronic inflammation of the skin involving the scalp, eyebrows, eyelids, ear canals, nasolabial folds, axillae, chest, and back (Fig. 43.7). In infants it is known as *cradle cap*. The cause is unknown. Proposed theories include genetic predisposition, *Malassezia* yeast infection, immunosuppression, and epidermal hyperproliferation.[6]

The lesions develop from infancy to old age with periods of remission and exacerbation. They appear as scaly, white or yellowish inflammatory plaques with mild pruritus. Topical therapy includes antifungal shampoos, calcineurin inhibitors (immunomodulating agents that reduce inflammation), and low-dose steroids for acute flares. Corticosteroids should not be used for maintenance therapy.

Papulosquamous Disorders

Psoriasis, pityriasis rosea, lichen planus, acne vulgaris, acne rosacea, and lupus erythematosus are characterized by papules, scales, plaques, and erythema. Collectively they are described as papulosquamous disorders.

Psoriasis

Psoriasis is a chronic, relapsing, proliferative, inflammatory disorder that involves the skin, scalp, and nails and can occur at any age. The onset is generally established by 40 years of age, but it can occur in children. A family history of psoriasis is common, and the genetic mechanisms are complex. The onset of psoriasis later in life is less familial and more secondary to comorbidities, such as obesity, smoking, hypertension, and diabetes.[7]

The inflammatory cascade of psoriasis involves the complex interactions between macrophages, fibroblasts, dendritic cells, natural killer cells, T-helper cells, and regulatory T cells. These immune cells lead to the secretion of numerous inflammatory mediators, such as tumor necrosis factor-alpha (TNF-α), and other cytokines, including IL-17 and IL-23, that promote the lesions of psoriasis. These inflammatory markers are the target for several therapeutic drugs known as biologic agents.[8]

Both the dermis and the epidermis are thickened because of cellular hyperproliferation, altered keratinocyte differentiation, and expanded dermal vasculature. Epidermal shedding time escalates to 3 to 4 days from the normal of 14 to 20 days. Cell maturation and keratinization are bypassed, and the epidermis thickens and plaques form. The loosely cohesive keratin gives the lesion a silvery appearance. Capillary dilation and increased vascularization occurs to accommodate the increased cell metabolism and causes erythema. The disease can be mild, moderate, or severe, depending on the size, distribution, and inflammation of the lesions. Psoriasis is marked by remissions and exacerbations.

The types of psoriasis include plaque (psoriasis vulgaris), inverse, guttate, pustular, and erythrodermic. Plaque psoriasis is the most common. The typical plaque psoriatic lesion is a well-demarcated, thick, silvery, scaly, erythematous plaque surrounded by normal skin (Fig. 43.8). Small, erythematous papules enlarge and coalesce into larger inflammatory lesions on the face, scalp, elbows, and knees and at sites of trauma (Koebner phenomenon).

Inverse psoriasis is rare and involves lesions that develop in skin folds (i.e., the axilla or groin). In guttate psoriasis, small papules appear suddenly on the trunk and extremities (Fig. 43.9) a few weeks after a streptococcal respiratory tract infection. Guttate psoriasis may resolve spontaneously in weeks or months. Pustular psoriasis appears as blisters of noninfectious pus (collections of neutrophils), and erythrodermic (exfoliative) psoriasis is often accompanied by pruritus or pain with widespread red, scaling lesions that cover a large area of the body.

Psoriatic arthritis of the hands, feet, knees, and ankle joints develops in 5% to 30% of cases. Psoriatic nail disease can occur in all psoriasis subtypes with pitting, onycholysis, subungual hyperkeratosis, and nail plate dystrophy. A number of comorbidities are associated with the inflammatory mechanisms of psoriasis (*Did You Know?* Psoriasis and Comorbidities).

Psoriasis and Comorbidities

In addition to skin and joint manifestations, severe psoriasis is associated with inflammatory bowel disease and metabolic syndrome, which includes hypertension, insulin resistance, dyslipidemias, abdominal obesity, and non-alcoholic fatty liver disease. There is an increased risk for atherosclerosis, myocardial infarction, and stroke that is independent of traditional risk factors for these diseases. The underlying mechanisms are thought to be related to increased levels of systemic proinflammatory mediators and chemokines, which are central to the chronic inflammation, oxidative stress, and angiogenesis of psoriasis. The increased prevalence of cancer, particularly lymphoma, may be related to the pathogenesis of psoriasis or may be a consequence of immune modulation therapies. Crohn disease also is associated with psoriasis, and these two diseases have a genetic overlap. The psychosocial effects of psoriasis include depression, suicidal ideation, anxiety, and an overall reduced quality of life. Treatment considerations need to include screening, monitoring, and managing of comorbidities and assuring support systems to maintain quality of life.

Data from Hu SC, Lan CE: *Int J Mol Sci* 18(10):E2211, 2017; Pietrzak D et al: *Arch Dermatol Res* 309(9):679-693, 2017; Takeshita J et al: *J Am Acad Dermatol* 76(3):393-403, 2017.

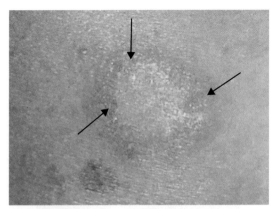

FIGURE 43.10 Pityriasis Rosea Herald Patch. A collarette pattern has formed around the margins *(arrows)*. (Courtesy Department of Dermatology, University of Utah School of Medicine, Salt Lake City, Utah.)

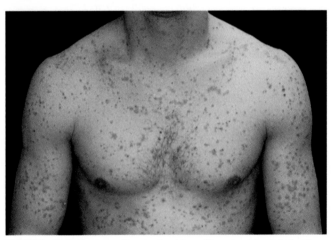

FIGURE 43.9 Guttate Psoriasis After Streptococcal Infection. Numerous uniformly small lesions may abruptly occur after streptococcal pharyngitis. (Courtesy Department of Dermatology, University of Utah School of Medicine, Salt Lake City, Utah.)

Treatment is individualized and related to maintaining skin moisture, reducing epidermal cell turnover and pruritus, and promoting immunomodulation. Mild psoriasis is treated with skin-directed therapy, such as medium- to high-strength topical corticosteroids, vitamin D analogues, emollients, and keratolytic agents (e.g., salicylic acid), and ultraviolet light therapy. Systemic therapy is indicated for moderate to severe disease or in the presence of psoriatic arthritis. Medications currently approved by the U.S. Food and Drug Administration include methotrexate, acitretin, and cyclosporine (short term). Newer FDA-approved biologics target TNF-α, IL-17, and IL-23.[9,10]

Pityriasis Rosea

Pityriasis rosea is a self-limiting inflammatory disorder that occurs more often in young adults. The cause is thought to be a herpeslike virus (e.g., human herpesvirus 6 [HHV6-roseola] and HHV7).[11] Pityriasis rosea begins as a single lesion (herald patch) that is circular, demarcated, and salmon-pink, approximately 3 to 10 cm in diameter, and usually located on the trunk. Early lesions are macular and papular. Secondary lesions develop within 14 to 21 days and extend over the trunk and upper part of the extremities (Fig. 43.10), although rarely on the face. The small, erythematous, rose-colored papules expand into characteristic oval lesions that are bilateral, symmetrically distributed, and have raised, scaly borders. The pattern of distribution on the back follows the skin lines around the trunk and resembles a drooping pine tree. The scales are sloughed from the margin of the lesions, forming a collarette pattern. Itching is the most common symptom. Occasionally headache, fatigue, or sore throat precedes the development of the lesions.

The diagnosis of pityriasis rosea follows the clinical appearance of the lesion. Secondary syphilis, psoriasis, drug eruption, nummular eczema, and seborrheic dermatitis are among the differential diagnosis considerations. The disorder is usually self-limiting and resolves in a few months with symptomatic treatment for pruritus or cosmetic concerns. Ultraviolet light (with some risk for hyperpigmentation) or systemic corticosteroids have been used to control pruritus. Acyclovir and erythromycin also may be used for treatment.[12]

Lichen Planus

Lichen planus (LP) is a benign autoimmune inflammatory disorder of the skin and mucous membranes. The age of onset is usually between 30 and 70 years. The cause is unknown, but T cells, adhesion molecules, inflammatory cytokines, perforin, and antigen-presenting cells are involved. LP also is linked to numerous drugs and to the hepatitis C virus. The disorder begins with nonscaling, purple-colored, flat-topped, polygonal pruritic papules 2 to 4 mm in size, usually located symmetrically on the wrists, ankles, lower legs, and genitalia (Fig. 43.11). New lesions are pale pink and evolve into a dark violet color. Persistent lesions may be thickened and red, forming hypertrophic lichen planus. Oral lesions (oral lichen planus) appear as lacy white rings that must be differentiated from leukoplakia or oral candidiasis. Usually, oral lesions do not ulcerate, but localized or extensive painful ulcerations can occur, and, rarely, there may be an increased risk for oral cancer. Thinning and splitting of nails are common, and part of or the entire nail may be shed.

Pruritus is the most distressing symptom. The lesions are self-limiting and may last for months or years, with an average duration of 6 to 18 months. Postinflammatory hyperpigmentation is a common consequence of the lesion. Some individuals have a recurrence. The diagnosis is made by the clinical appearance and the histopathology of the lesion. Treatment is individualized and includes topical, intralesional, or systemic

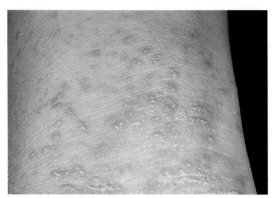

FIGURE 43.11 Hypertrophic Lichen Planus on Arms. (Courtesy Department of Dermatology, University of Utah School of Medicine, Salt Lake City, Utah.)

corticosteroids (second line for resistant LP), and systemic acitretin, with or without adjuvant light therapy. Antihistamines are given for itching, and topical or systemic corticosteroids may be used short term to control inflammation. Mucous membrane lesions are treated with topical steroids, topical retinoids or immunomodulators (or both), and systemic glucocorticoids.[13]

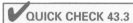

QUICK CHECK 43.3
1. Why does inflammation occur with contact dermatitis?
2. What factors are associated with atopic dermatitis?
3. What lesions are associated with papulosquamous disorders?
4. Give three examples of papulosquamous disorders.

Acne Vulgaris

Acne vulgaris is an inflammatory disorder of the pilosebaceous follicle (the sebaceous gland contiguous with a hair follicle) that usually occurs during adolescence. Acne vulgaris is discussed in Chapter 44.

Hydradenitis Suppurativa (Inverse Acne)

Hydradenitis suppurativa (inverse acne) is an inflammatory disease involving the deep sections of apocrine (sweat) glands complicated by fibrosis and draining sinus tracts. Occurring more commonly in women, the incidence and cause is unknown but may be related to genetic predisposition, altered structure of the pilosebaceous unit with bacterial infection, and an altered immune response. Aggravating factors include smoking, tight clothing, heat, perspiration, shaving of prone areas, obesity, and stress. The lesions present as deep, firm painful subcutaneous nodules, often with sinus tracts, and rupture horizontally under the skin. Sites of involvement include apocrine gland–rich areas (e.g., the axillae, groin, perianal region, and perineum). Other areas include the neck, adjacent scalp, back, buttocks, scrotum or labia, and inframammary or mammary region in women. Lesions may be minimal or severe, with multiple draining fistulas. Treatment includes topical therapy, systemic medication, and incision and drainage of nodules. Complete, spontaneous resolution is rare.

Acne Rosacea

Acne rosacea is a chronic inflammation of the skin that develops in middle-aged adults and occurs more commonly in women. There are four subtypes of lesions, and they may occur in combination: erythematotelangiectatic, papulopustular, phymatous (nodular), and ocular (eyelids and ocular surface). The exact cause is unknown. Genetic

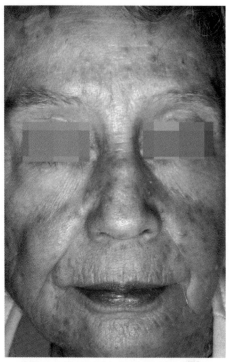

FIGURE 43.12 Granulomatous Rosacea. Pustules and erythema occur on the forehead, cheeks, and nose. (From Habif TP: *Clinical dermatology*, ed 6, Philadelphia, 2016, Saunders.)

factors, immune dysregulation, and neurovascular dysregulation are involved. Factors that trigger altered immune responses include sun exposure and damage; consumption of alcohol or hot beverages; hormonal fluctuations; and microorganisms, such as *Demodex folliculorum* [mites].[14] The most common lesions are erythema, papules, pustules, and telangiectasia. They occur in the middle third of the face, including the forehead, nose, cheeks, and chin (Fig. 43.12). Neurovascular dysregulation is associated with chronic, inappropriate vasodilation, resulting in flushing, a burning sensation, and sun sensitivity. Sebaceous hypertrophy, fibrosis, and telangiectasia may be severe enough to produce an irreversible bulbous appearance of the nose (rhinophyma). Disorders of the eye often accompany rosacea, particularly conjunctivitis and keratitis, which can result in visual impairment. Facial application of fluorinated topical steroids may increase the severity of telangiectasias.

Photoprotection (sunscreen, wide-brimmed hat) is essential, along with avoidance of other triggers. Both topical drugs (metronidazole, azelaic acid) and oral drugs (tetracyclines and doxycycline) may be effective. Surgical excision of excessive tissue may be required for rhinophyma.

Lupus Erythematosus

Lupus erythematosus is a systemic inflammatory, autoimmune disease with cutaneous manifestations (see Chapter 8). Discoid (or cutaneous) lupus erythematosus (DLE) is limited to the skin but can progress to systemic lupus erythematosus.

Discoid (cutaneous) lupus erythematosus. Discoid (cutaneous) lupus erythematosus (DLE) usually occurs in genetically susceptible adults, particularly women in their late thirties or early forties, but people of any age can be affected. Differentiation of acute, subacute, intermittent, or chronic subtypes is by physical examination, laboratory studies, histologic (skin biopsy) analysis, and antibody serology direct immunofluorescence. The lesions may be single or multiple and vary in size. Often the lesions are located on light-exposed areas of the skin, and photosensitivity is common. The face is the most common site of lesion involvement, with a butterfly pattern of distribution found over the nose and cheeks.

The cause is unknown but is related to genetic and environmental factors and an altered immune response to an unknown antigen or to ultraviolet B wavelengths. There is development of self-reactive T and B cells, a decreased number of regulatory T cells, and increased levels of proinflammatory cytokines. Autoantibodies and immune complexes cause tissue damage and inflammation (Fig. 43.13). On skin biopsy with immunofluorescent observation, there are lumpy deposits of immunoglobulins, especially IgM (lupus band test).[15,16]

The early lesion is asymmetric, a 1- to 2-cm raised red plaque with a brownish scale. The scale penetrates the hair follicle and leaves a visible follicle opening (carpet-tack appearance) when removed. The lesions persist for months and then resolve spontaneously or atrophy, causing a depressed scar. Healed lesions may have residual telangiectasia and hypopigmented scarring. Treatment options include sun protection and use of topical steroids, calcineurin inhibitors, antimalarial drugs (e.g., hydroxychloroquine sulfate), and immunosuppressants. These medications must be used with caution to prevent serious side effects.

Vesiculobullous Diseases

Vesiculobullous skin diseases share a common characteristic of vesicle, or blister, formation. Two such diseases are pemphigus and erythema multiforme.

Pemphigus

Pemphigus (meaning to blister or bubble) is a group of rare autoimmune blistering diseases of the skin and oral mucous membranes. Pemphigus vulgaris is the most common form and is caused by circulating autoantibodies directed against desmosome adhesion molecules in the epidermis. Loss of adhesion causes fluid accumulation, resulting in blister formation (Fig. 43.14). There are often painful, superficial erosions prone to infection. Pemphigus can occur in all age groups but is more prevalent in persons between 40 and 50 years of age. There

is a genetic predisposition, as well as environmental (viral infections, drug-induced, dietary intake, or physical effects, such as radiation or surgery) and endogenous (emotional or hormonal stressors) influences.

The diagnosis of pemphigus is made from the clinical and histologic findings of antibodies at the site of blister formation. The clinical course of the disease may range from rapidly fatal to relatively benign. The primary treatment for pemphigus is systemic corticosteroids in combination with adjuvant immunosuppressants.[17]

Erythema Multiforme

Erythema multiforme is a syndrome characterized by inflammation of the skin and mucous membranes caused by an immunologic reaction to a drug or microorganisms (e.g., herpes simplex virus) that targets small blood vessels in the skin or mucosa.[18] Bullous erythema multiforme involves the mucous membranes. It is relatively rare and occurs more often during the second to fourth decade of life; however, it can occur at any age. Edema develops in the superficial dermis, forming vesicles and bullae. The lesions vary in clinical presentation, involving the skin or mucous membranes, or both. Characteristically, a "bull's-eye" or "target" lesion develops on the skin surface with a central erythematous region surrounded by concentric rings of alternating edema and inflammation. The lesions usually occur suddenly in groups over a period of 2 to 3 weeks. However, urticarial plaques, 1 to 2 cm in diameter, can develop without the target lesion. A vesiculobullous form is characterized by mucous membrane lesions and erythematous plaques on the extensor surfaces of the extremities. Single or multiple vesicles or bullae may arise on a part of the plaque, accompanied by pruritus and burning. The lesions heal within 3 to 4 weeks.

Stevens-Johnson Syndrome and Toxic Epidermal Necrolysis

Stevens-Johnson syndrome (SJS) (severe mucocutaneous bullous form involving 10% of body surface area) and toxic epidermal necrolysis (TEN) (severe mucocutaneous bullous form involving more than 30% of body surface area) are the same disease with a continuum of symptoms based on clinical presentation and severity. Both of these diseases are type IV hypersensitivity reactions to drugs and are medical emergencies[18] (see Chapter 44 for pediatric considerations).

Prodromal symptoms of SJS/TEN, which include fever, headache, malaise, sore throat, and cough, develop in approximately one third of the cases. The bullous lesions form erosions and crusts when they rupture. With mucosal involvement, the mouth, air passages, esophagus, urethra,

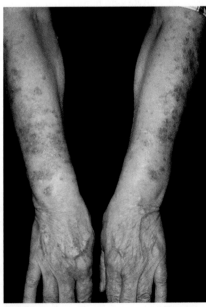

FIGURE 43.13 Subacute Cutaneous Lupus (Discoid Lupus Erythematosus). (Courtesy Department of Dermatology, University of Utah School of Medicine, Salt Lake City, Utah.)

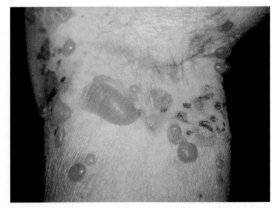

FIGURE 43.14 Bullous Pemphigoid. Generalized eruption with blisters arising from an edematous, erythematous annular base. (Courtesy Department of Dermatology, University of Utah School of Medicine, Salt Lake City, Utah.)

and conjunctiva may be affected. Blindness can result from corneal ulcerations. Difficulty eating, breathing, and urinating may develop, with severe consequences. The disease can involve the kidneys and extend from the upper respiratory passages into the lungs. Severe forms of the disease can be fatal.

Recognizing the person's medication history that preceded the target lesion and performing a skin biopsy are required to establish the diagnosis. Any ongoing drug therapy should be withdrawn and reevaluated, and underlying infections should be treated. The fluid and electrolyte balance should be monitored in severe forms of the disease, and mucous membranes should be carefully managed with a bland diet, warm saline eyewashes, topical anesthetics, or corticosteroids to maintain comfort and prevent infection. IgG and cyclosporin A are commonly used for immunosuppression, but there is lack of consensus regarding this treatment.[19] Individuals with TENS are commonly referred to a burn unit for care or receive wound care dressings comparable to burn care. Ophthalmic, kidney, and lung involvement require special care. Resolution occurs in 8 to 10 days, usually without scarring. Mucosal lesions may take 6 weeks to heal.

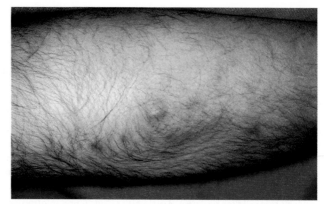

FIGURE 43.15 Furuncle of the Forearm. (Courtesy Department of Dermatology, University of Utah School of Medicine, Salt Lake City, Utah.)

>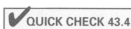
> **QUICK CHECK 43.4**
> 1. Describe the inflammatory lesion associated with lupus erythematosus.
> 2. Compare the three forms of pemphigus.
> 3. What is the characteristic lesion of erythema multiforme?

Infections

Cutaneous infections are common forms of skin disease. They generally remain localized, although serious complications can develop with systemic involvement that can be life-threatening. The types of skin infection include bacterial, viral, and fungal. The microbiome of the skin consists of aerobes, yeast, and anaerobes and often provides protection against pathogens that cause skin infections, including *Staphylococcus* and *Streptococcus*.

Bacterial Infections

Most acute bacterial skin and skin-structure infections are caused by local invasion of pathogens. Coagulase-positive *Staphylococcus aureus* and, less often, beta-hemolytic streptococci are the common causative microorganisms. Community-acquired methicillin-resistant *Staphylococcus aureus* (CA-MRSA [see Chapter 9]) also is a cause of serious skin infection, particularly skin abscesses.

Folliculitis. Folliculitis is an infection of the hair follicle. It can be caused by bacteria, viruses, or fungi, although *S. aureus* is the common culprit. The infection develops from proliferation of the microorganism around the opening and inside the follicle. Inflammation is caused by released enzymes from the bacteria. The lesions appear as pustules with a surrounding area of erythema. They are most prominent on the scalp and extremities and rarely cause systemic symptoms. Prolonged skin moisture, skin trauma (e.g., shaving hair), occlusive clothing, topical agents, and poor hygiene are associated contributing factors. Cleaning with soap and water and topical application of antibiotics are effective treatments.

Furuncles and carbuncles. Furuncles, or "boils," are abscesses of hair follicles (Fig. 43.15). They may develop after folliculitis spreads into the surrounding dermis. The invading microorganism is usually *S. aureus,* including CA-MSRA (see Chapter 9). The infecting strain may spread to the skin from the anterior nares. The initial lesion is a deep, firm, red, painful nodule 1 to 5 cm in diameter. Within a few days, the erythematous nodules change to a large, fluctuant, and tender cystic nodule accompanied by cellulitis. No systemic symptoms are present, and the lesion may drain large amounts of pus and necrotic tissue.

Carbuncles are a collection of furuncles and usually occur on the back of the neck, the upper back, and the lateral thighs. The lesion begins in the subcutaneous tissue and lower dermis as a firm mass that evolves into an erythematous, painful, swollen abscess that drains through many openings. Chills, fever, and malaise can occur during the early stages of lesion development.

Furuncles and carbuncles are treated with warm compresses to provide comfort and promote localization and spontaneous drainage. Abscess formation, recurrent infections, extensive lesions, or lesions associated with cellulitis or systemic symptoms require incision and drainage and are treated with systemic antibiotics.[20]

Cellulitis. Cellulitis is an infection of the dermis and subcutaneous tissue usually caused by *S. aureus,* CA-MRSA, or group B streptococci. Cellulitis can occur as an extension of a skin wound, as an ulcer, or from furuncles or carbuncles. The infected area is warm, erythematous, swollen, and painful. The infection is usually in the lower extremities and responds to systemic antibiotics. Cellulitis also can be associated with other diseases, including chronic venous insufficiency and stasis dermatitis.

Cellulitis must be differentiated from necrotizing fasciitis. Necrotizing fasciitis is a rare, rapidly spreading infection. It is commonly caused by *Streptococcus pyogenes,* starting in the fascia, muscles, and subcutaneous fat, with subsequent necrosis. Treatment requires antibiotics and often surgical débridement to prevent toxic shock syndrome.

Erysipelas. Erysipelas is an acute superficial infection of the upper dermis most often caused by *S. pyogenes,* beta-hemolytic streptococci, and *S. aureus.* The face, ears, and lower legs are involved. Chills, fever, and malaise precede the onset of lesions by 4 hours to 20 days. The initial lesions appear as firm, red spots that enlarge and coalesce to form a clearly circumscribed, advancing, bright red, hot lesion with a raised border. Vesicles may appear over the lesion and at the border. Pruritus, burning, and tenderness are present. Cold compresses provide symptomatic relief, and systemic antibiotics are required to arrest the infection.[21]

Impetigo. Impetigo is a superficial infection of the skin that is caused by coagulase-positive *Staphylococcus* or beta-hemolytic streptococci. The disease occurs in adults but is more common in children (see Chapter 44).

Lyme disease. Lyme disease is a multisystem inflammatory disease caused by the spirochete *Borrelia burgdorferi.* It is transmitted by the bite of the *Ixodes* tick, and it is the most frequently reported vector-borne illness. The highest incidence of Lyme disease is among children. The microorganism is difficult to culture, escapes immunodefenses, and hides in tissue. It spreads to other tissues by entering capillary beds.

Symptoms of the disease occur in three stages, although about half of infected individuals are symptom free.[22] *Localized infection* (stage 1) occurs soon after the bite (within 3 to 32 days) with erythema migrans (bull's-eye rash), a T-cell–mediated response, usually with fever. Within days to weeks after the onset of the illness, there is *disseminated infection*, with secondary erythema migrans, usually with myalgias, arthralgias, and more rarely, meningitis, neuritis, or carditis (stage 2). Post-Lyme disease syndrome, or *chronic Lyme disease*, can continue for years with arthritis, encephalopathy, polyneuropathy, or heart failure (stage 3). The diagnosis of Lyme disease is based on the clinical presentation and history of the tick bite, if known. Serologic tests are used to confirm the diagnosis, although there is a delayed antibody response and the test may be negative during the first 3 weeks after infection. Antibiotics (e.g., doxycycline [not used in children younger than 8 years or in pregnant or breast-feeding women] or amoxicillin) are used for treatment. Reinfection can occur. There is currently no vaccine for Lyme disease.

Viral Infections

Herpes simplex virus. Skin infections with herpes simplex virus (HSV) are commonly caused by two types of HSV: HSV-1 and HSV-2. Either type can occur in different parts of the body, including oral and genital locations. Their differences are distinguished by laboratory tests. HSV-1, transmitted by contact with infected saliva, is generally associated with oral infections (cold sore or fever blister) or infection of the cornea (herpes keratitis), mouth (gingivostomatitis), and orolabia (lips/labialis), but it can also cause genital herpes. With initial (primary) infection, the virus is imbedded in sensory nerve endings and it moves by retrograde axonal transport to the dorsal root ganglion, where the virus develops lifelong latency.[23] During the secondary phase, the lesions occur at the same site from reactivation of the virus. The virus travels down the peripheral nerve to the site of the original infection, where it is shed. Exposure to ultraviolet light, skin irritation, fever, fatigue, or stress may cause reactivation.

The lesions for HSV-1 appear as clusters of inflamed and painful vesicles on an erythematous base (e.g., within the mouth, over the tongue, on the lips, around the nose) (Fig. 43.16). Increased sensitivity, paresthesias, pruritus, and mild burning may occur before the onset of the lesions. The vesicles rupture, forming a crust. Lesions may last 2 to 6 weeks but usually resolve within 2 weeks. Treatment is symptomatic and includes topical or oral antiviral agents.

Genital infections are more commonly caused by HSV-2.[24] The virus is spread by skin-to-skin mucous membrane contact during viral shedding. Risk of infection is high in immunosuppressed persons or in persons who have sexual contact with infected individuals. Vertical transmission from mother to neonate is associated with significant neonatal neurologic morbidity and mortality. The initial infection is asymptomatic. With recurrent exposure, the lesions begin as small vesicles that progress to ulceration within 3 to 4 days with pain, itching, and weeping. Treatment is symptomatic and includes topical or oral antiviral agents. Long-term suppression of HSV-1 and HSV-2 may be attempted with daily antiviral dosing. Currently there is no vaccine to prevent HSV infection.

Herpes zoster and varicella. Herpes zoster (shingles) and varicella (chickenpox) are caused by the same herpesvirus—varicella-zoster virus (VZV). VZV occurs as a primary infection, followed years later by activation of the virus to cause herpes zoster. During this time, the virus remains latent in trigeminal and dorsal root ganglia.

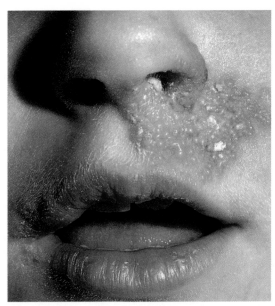

FIGURE 43.16 Herpes Simplex of the Lips (Labialis). Typical presentation with tense vesicles appearing on the lips and extending onto the skin. (From Habif TP: *Clinical dermatology: a color guide to diagnosis and therapy*, ed 4, St Louis, 2004, Mosby.)

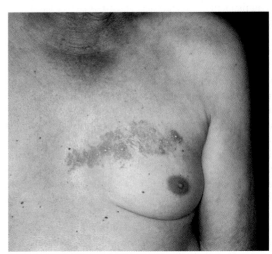

FIGURE 43.17 Herpes Zoster. Diffuse involvement of a dermatome. (Courtesy Department of Dermatology, University of Utah School of Medicine, Salt Lake City, Utah.)

Herpes zoster has initial symptoms of pain and paresthesia localized to the affected dermatome (the cutaneous area innervated by a single spinal nerve; see Chapter 14), followed by vesicular eruptions that follow a facial, cervical, or thoracic lumbar dermatome (Fig. 43.17). Local symptoms are alleviated with compresses, calamine lotion, or baking soda. Approximately 15% to 20% of individuals experience postherpetic neuralgia (pain) with reactivation of the virus. Antiviral drugs, tricyclic antidepressants, and analgesics are helpful treatments. The varicella vaccine is safe and effective in children and adults to prevent chicken pox. The herpes zoster vaccine is given to adults 60 years and older to prevent shingles.[25]

Warts. Warts (**verrucae**) are benign lesions of the skin caused by the many different types of human papillomavirus (HPV) that infect the stratified epithelium of skin and mucous membranes. The lesions can occur anywhere and are flat, round, or fusiform and elevated with a rough, grayish surface. Warts are transmitted by touch. Common warts (verruca vulgaris) occur most often in children and are usually on the fingers (Fig. 43.18). Plantar warts are usually located at pressure points on the bottom of the feet. Warts are commonly removed with cryotherapy, electrocautery, topical salicylic acid, or other topical or intralesional agents.

Condylomata acuminata (venereal warts) are caused by HPV. These warts are sexually transmitted and highly contagious. The cauliflower-like lesions occur in moist areas, along the glans of the penis, vulva, and anus. Oncogenic types of HPV are a primary cause of cervical and other types of cancer and are preventable by prophylactic vaccination[26] (see Chapter 35).

Fungal Infections

Dermatophytes are the fungi that cause superficial skin infections. These fungi thrive on keratin (stratum corneum, hair, nails). Fungal disorders are known as *mycoses*; when caused by dermatophytes, the mycoses are termed *tinea* (dermatophytosis or ringworm).

Tinea infections. Tinea infections are classified according to their location on the body. Fig. 43.19 shows the location and extension of tinea pedis. The most common sites are summarized in Table 43.5.

Tinea is diagnosed by culture, microscopic examination of skin scrapings prepared with potassium hydroxide wet mount, or observation of the skin with an ultraviolet light (Wood lamp). Cultures establish the diagnosis for a particular type of fungus. Fungi have characteristic spores and filaments, known as *hyphae*, that are more prominent when prepared in potassium hydroxide. The spores fluoresce blue-green when exposed to ultraviolet light. Treatment is related to the type of fungi and includes both topical and systemic antifungal medication.

Candidiasis. Candidiasis is caused by the yeastlike fungus *Candida albicans* and normally can be found on mucous membranes, on the skin, in the gastrointestinal tract, and in the vagina. *C. albicans* can change from a normal microorganism to a pathogen, particularly in the critically ill and those who are immunosuppressed.

Under normal circumstances, the resident bacteria on the skin, mainly cocci, inhibit proliferation of *C. albicans*. Factors that predispose to *C. albicans* infection include (1) local environment of moisture, warmth, maceration, or occlusion; (2) systemic administration of antibiotics; (3) pregnancy; (4) diabetes mellitus; (5) Cushing disease; (6) debilitated states; (7) infants younger than 6 months of age (as a result of decreased immune reactivity); (8) immunosuppressed persons; and (9) certain neoplastic diseases of the blood and monocyte/macrophage system. Candidiasis affects only the outer layers of mucous membranes and

skin and occurs in the mouth, vagina, uncircumcised penis, nail folds, interdigital areas, and large skin folds. Table 43.6 lists the points of differentiation of various sites of candidiasis habitation.

The initial lesion is a thin-walled pustule that extends under the stratum corneum with an inflammatory base that may burn or itch. The accumulation of inflammatory cells and scale produces a whitish yellow, curdlike substance over the infected area. The lesion ceases to spread when it reaches dry skin. Topical antifungal agents are commonly used for treatment.[27]

TABLE 43.5	Common Sites of Tinea Infections
Site	**Clinical Manifestations**
Tinea capitis (scalp)	Scaly, pruritic scalp with bald areas; hair breaks easily
Tinea corporis (skin areas, excluding scalp, face, hands, feet, groin)	Circular, clearly circumscribed, mildly erythematous scaly patches with slightly elevated ringlike border; some forms are dry and macular, and other forms are moist and vesicular
Tinea cruris (groin, also known as "jock itch")	Small, erythematous, and scaling vesicular patches with well-defined borders that spread over inner and upper surfaces of thighs; occurs with heat and high humidity
Tinea pedis (foot; also known as "athlete's foot")	Occurs between toes and may spread to soles of feet, nails, and skin or toes; slight scaling; macerated, painful skin, occasionally with fissures and vesiculation
Tinea manus (hand)	Dry, scaly, erythematous lesions, or moist, vesicular lesions that begin with clusters of intensely pruritic, clear vesicles; often associated with fungal infection of feet
Tinea unguium or onychomycosis (nails)	Superficial or deep inflammation of nail that develops yellow-brown accumulations of brittle keratin over all or portions of nail

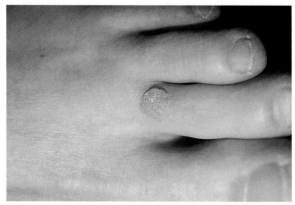

FIGURE 43.18 Verruca Vulgaris (Near Toes). (Courtesy Department of Dermatology, University of Utah School of Medicine, Salt Lake City, Utah.)

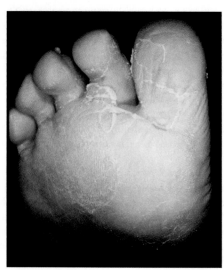

FIGURE 43.19 Tinea Pedis. Inflammation has extended from the web area onto the dorsum of the foot. (Courtesy Department of Dermatology, University of Utah School of Medicine, Salt Lake City, Utah.)

TABLE 43.6   Sites of Candidiasis

Site	Risk Factors	Clinical Manifestations	Treatment
Vagina (vulvovaginitis)	Heat, moisture, occlusive clothing Pregnancy Systemic antibiotic therapy Diabetes mellitus Sexual intercourse with infected male	Vaginal itching; white, watery, or creamy discharge Red, swollen vaginal and labial membranes with erosions Lesions may spread to anus and groin	Miconazole cream Clotrimazole tablets or cream Nystatin tablets Ketoconazole cream Loose cotton clothing
Penis (balanitis)	Uncircumcised Sexual intercourse with infected female	Pinpoint, red, tender papules and pustules on glans and shaft of penis	Any of creams listed above Topical steroids for severe inflammation
Mouth	Diabetes mellitus Immunosuppressive therapy Inhaled steroid therapy	Red, swollen, painful tongue and oral mucous membranes Localized erosions and plaques appear with chronic infection	Nystatin oral suspension Clotrimazole troches Ketoconazole

Vascular Disorders

Vascular abnormalities are commonly associated with skin diseases; they may be congenital or may involve vascular responses to local or systemic vasoactive substances. Blood vessels may increase in number, dilate, constrict, or become obliterated by disease processes.

Cutaneous Vasculitis

Vasculitis (angiitis) is an inflammation of the blood vessel wall that can result in bleeding aneurysm formation, or occlusion with ischemia or infection of surrounding tissue. The extensive vascular bed in the skin results in vasculitic syndromes that may be localized and self-limiting or generalized with multiorgan involvement. The initiating site may be the blood, the vessel wall, or the adjacent tissue. Small vessels are usually affected.

Cutaneous vasculitis develops from the deposit of immune complexes in small blood vessels as a toxic response to drugs (phenothiazines, barbiturates, sulfonamides), allergens, or streptococcal or viral infection, or as a component of systemic vasculitic syndromes. The deposits activate complement, which is chemotactic for polymorphonuclear leukocytes (neutrophils), and proinflammatory cytokines.

The disorder is also known as *cutaneous leukocytoclastic angiitis* (from the presence of leukocytes [i.e., neutrophils] in and around vessel walls). A systemic form (cutaneous systemic vasculitis) can involve other organs, including the kidneys, lungs, and gastrointestinal tract. The pattern of skin involvement includes palpable purpura in the lower legs and feet (from the leakage of blood from damaged vessels) that may progress to hemorrhagic bullae with necrosis and ulceration from occlusion of the vessel. Lesions appear in clusters and persist for 1 to 4 weeks. The disease may be self-limiting and occur as a single episode. Biopsy confirms the diagnosis.

Identifying and removing the antigen (chemical, drug, or source of infection) is the first step of treatment. Corticosteroids and immunosuppressants may be used when symptoms are severe.[28]

Urticaria

Urticaria (hives) is a circumscribed area of raised erythema and edema of the superficial dermis. Urticarial lesions are most commonly associated with type I hypersensitivity reactions to drugs (penicillin, aspirin), certain foods (strawberries, shellfish, food dyes), environmental exposure (pollen, animal dander, insect bites), systemic diseases (intestinal parasites, lupus erythematosus), or physical agents (heat or cold) (see Chapter 8). The lesions are mediated by histamine release from sensitized mast cells or basophils, or both, which causes the endothelial cells of skin blood vessels to contract. The leakage of fluid from the vessel appears as wheals, welts, or hives, and there may be few or many that may be distributed over the entire body. Most lesions resolve spontaneously within 24 hours, but new lesions may appear. All possible causes of the reaction should be removed. Antihistamines usually reduce hives and provide relief of itching. Corticosteroids and β-adrenergic agonists (e.g., epinephrine) may be required for severe attacks. Chronic urticaria (recurrent wheals for more than 6 weeks) is either induced by an external trigger or develops spontaneously from an endogenous mechanism. Both types involve inappropriate activation of mast cells.[29] Angioedema (welts or swelling deeper within the skin or mucous membranes) is associated with both groups and more commonly affects the eyes and mouth.

Scleroderma

Localized scleroderma (morphea) means sclerosis of the skin and underlying tissue. The disease is rare, more common in females, and the cause is unknown but thought to be related to an autoimmune reaction to endothelial cells and fibroblasts.[30] Genetic predisposition and an immune reaction to a toxic substance are possible initiating mechanisms of the disease. Autoantibodies are often recovered from the skin and serum of individuals with scleroderma. Impaired regulation of collagen gene expression by fibroblasts probably underlies the persistent fibrosis. There are subtypes of localized scleroderma but all involve thickening of the skin. The lesions appear as shiny patches of hardened or tightened skin or streaks on the skin. Localized scleroderma is differentiated from the systemic form of the disease by the absence of sclerodactyly (thickening and tightness of the skin of the fingers or toes) Raynaud phenomenon, or abnormalities of the nail bed capillaries. The disease is usually self-limiting, but there may be recurring lesions.

Systemic scleroderma involves the connective tissues of the skin and internal organs, including the kidneys, gastrointestinal tract, and lungs. There are massive deposits of collagen (the collagen that makes scar tissue) with progressive fibrosis accompanied by inflammatory reactions. There are vascular changes in the capillary network, with a decrease in the number of capillary loops, dilation of the remaining capillaries, formation of perivascular infiltrates, and the development of occlusion and ischemia.[31]

The clinical features of systemic scleroderma can be summarized using the CREST syndrome as a guide:

Calcinosis—calcium deposits in the subcutaneous tissue that cause pain

Raynaud phenomenon—episodes of arteriolar vasoconstriction or spasm in response to cold or stress

Esophageal changes—swallowing difficulty related to acid reflux and increased esophageal fibrosis

Sclerodactyly—tightening of skin over the fingers and toes leading to tapering of the digits with scarring and tissue atrophy

Telangiectasias—dilation of capillaries causing small (0.5 cm), weblike red marks on the skin surface

The cutaneous lesions are most often on the face and hands, the neck, and the upper chest, although the entire skin can be involved. The skin is hard, hypopigmented, taut, shiny, and tightly connected to the underlying tissue. The tightness of the facial skin projects an immobile, masklike appearance, and the mouth may not open completely. The nose may assume a beaklike appearance. The hands are shiny and sometimes red and edematous (Fig. 43.20). Progression to internal organs may occur, and death is caused by subsequent respiratory failure, renal failure, cardiac dysrhythmias, or esophageal or intestinal obstruction or perforation.

Suitable clothing and a warm environment are essential for protecting the hands. Trauma and smoking should be avoided. Treatment is individualized and based on the severity and progression of the disease.

> ✔ **QUICK CHECK 43.5**
> 1. Name two bacterial skin infections, and describe the typical lesions.
> 2. Compare herpes zoster and varicella.
> 3. What features distinguish urticarial lesions?

Benign Tumors

Most benign tumors of the skin are associated with aging. Benign tumors include seborrheic keratosis, keratoacanthoma, actinic keratosis, and moles. Lipomas (moveable fatty tumors) and ganglion cysts (fluid-filled sacs near tendons or joints) are nodular lesions that are palpable under the skin.[32]

Seborrheic Keratosis

Seborrheic keratosis is a benign proliferation of cutaneous basal cells that produces flat or slightly elevated lesions that may be smooth or warty in appearance. The pathogenesis is unknown. These benign tumors are usually seen in older people and occur as multiple lesions on the chest, back, and face. The color varies from tan to waxy yellow, flesh colored, or dark brown-black. Lesion size varies from a few millimeters to several centimeters, and they are often oval and greasy appearing with a hyperkeratotic scale (Fig. 43.21). Cryotherapy with liquid nitrogen and laser therapy are effective treatments.

Keratoacanthoma

A keratoacanthoma is a benign, self-limiting tumor of squamous cell differentiation arising from hair follicles. It usually occurs on sun-damaged skin of elderly individuals. The incidence is highest among smokers and males. The most commonly affected sites are the face, back of the hands, forearms, neck, and legs. The lesion develops in stages (proliferative, mature, and involution) over a period of 1 to 2 months with a histologic pattern resembling that of squamous cell carcinoma.

Although the lesions will resolve spontaneously, they can be removed by curettage or excision to improve the cosmetic appearance and reduce the risk of evolution to squamous cell carcinoma (SCC). A biopsy is performed to rule out SCC.

Actinic Keratosis

Actinic keratosis is a premalignant lesion composed of aberrant proliferations of epidermal keratinocytes caused by prolonged exposure to ultraviolet radiation. The prevalence is highest in individuals with unprotected, light-colored skin and rare in those with dark-colored skin. The lesions appear as rough, poorly defined papules, which may be felt more than seen. Surrounding areas may have telangiectasias. Treatment options include cryoablation, photodynamic therapy, laser surgery, and topical therapies.

Excision and biopsy may be performed. Any existing lesions should continue to be evaluated for progression to squamous cell carcinoma. Sun protection clothing and sun-blocking agents are required to prevent lesions from developing elsewhere.

Nevi (Moles)

Nevi (sing., nevus) (also known as *moles* or *birthmarks*) are benign pigmented or nonpigmented lesions. Melanocytic nevi, formed from melanocytes, may be congenital or acquired and small (less than 1 cm) or large (greater than 20 cm). Congenital melanocytic nevi are monitored and may be removed to reduce the risk of cutaneous malignant melanoma. During the early stages of nevi development, the cells accumulate at the junction of the dermis and epidermis and are macular lesions. Over time, the cells move deeper into the dermis, and the nevi become nodular and symmetric without irregular borders. Nevi may appear on any part of the skin, may vary in size, may occur singly or in groups, and may undergo transition to malignant melanoma (see Fig. 43.25). The classification of nevi is summarized in Table 43.7. Nevi irritated by clothing or trauma or large lesions may be excised. Multiple and changing moles require regular evaluation.[33]

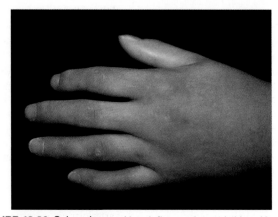

FIGURE 43.20 Scleroderma. Note inflammation and shiny skin resulting from a combination of Raynaud phenomenon and scleroderma affecting the fingers (acrosclerosis). (Courtesy Department of Dermatology, University of Utah School of Medicine, Salt Lake City, Utah.)

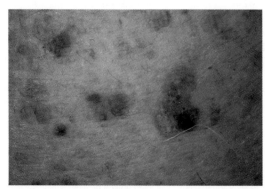

FIGURE 43.21 Seborrheic Keratosis. Typical lesion is broad and flat with a comparatively smooth surface. (Courtesy Department of Dermatology, University of Utah School of Medicine, Salt Lake City, Utah.)

Skin Cancer

Skin cancer is the most common cancer in the world. Nonmelanoma skin cancers include basal cell carcinoma and squamous cell carcinoma. Malignant melanoma is the most serious type of skin cancer and the most common cause of death from skin cancer.[34] Important trends related to skin cancer are described in Box 43.1.

Chronic exposure to ultraviolet (UV) radiation causes most skin cancers. Lesions are most common on the face, neck, hands, and other areas subject to intense, repetitive sunlight exposure. Protection from the sun and avoidance of tanning beds, particularly during childhood, significantly reduce the risk of skin cancer in later years. Genetic mutations in oncogenes and tumor-suppressor genes (see Chapter 11) are associated with skin cancers. Dark-skinned persons and those who avoid sunlight are significantly less likely to develop these malignant tumors. In dark-skinned persons, basal cells contain more of the pigment melanin, a protective factor against sun exposure.

Basal Cell Carcinoma

Basal cell carcinoma (BCC) of the skin is the most common cancer in the world. BCC is thought to be caused by UV radiation exposure and also is associated with arsenic in food or water.

BCCs have numerous subtypes, including superficial, nodular, pigmented, morpheaform, and combinations of these; thus, they can have very different clinical presentations—from superficial erythematous papules; to thick, pigmented nodules resembling melanomas; to erosive, necrotic, and ulcerating lesions (Fig. 43.22). As the tumor grows, it usually has a depressed center, a rolled border, and small blood vessels on the surface (telangiectasias). Early tumors are so small they are not clinically apparent. The lesion grows slowly, often ulcerates, develops crusts, and is firm to the touch. If left untreated, basal cell lesions invade surrounding tissues and, over months or years, can destroy a nose, eyelid, or ear (for treatment, see Box 43.1). Metastasis is rare because these tumors do not invade blood or lymph vessels.

Squamous Cell Carcinoma

Squamous cell carcinoma (SCC) of the skin is a tumor of the epidermis and is the second most common human cancer. Two

TABLE 43.7 Classification of Nevi

Type	Common Characteristics
Junctional nevus	Flat, well-circumscribed; vary in size up to 2 cm; dark-colored hairs may be present; originate in basal layer of epidermis and can eventually reach cutaneous surface; most likely to develop into melanoma
Compound nevus	Most common in adolescents; majority of pigmented lesions in children; usually 1 cm in size; hairs may be present; surface is elevated and smooth; rarely develops into melanoma;
Intradermal nevus	Small, less than 1 cm, with regular edges and bristlelike hairs; color ranges from fair skin tone to light brown; slight likelihood of developing into melanoma

BOX 43.1 Important Trends in Skin Cancer

Incidence
- Skin cancer is the most commonly diagnosed cancer in the United States. An estimated 5.4. million cases of squamous and basal cell carcinoma were diagnosed among 3.3 million people in 2012
- Malignant melanoma is the most serious form of skin cancer; it is not as common as the other forms of skin cancer; an estimated 91,270 new cases were predicted in 2018

Mortality
- Total estimated deaths from skin cancer in 2018 (excluding basal cell and squamous cell carcinomas*) were 13,460; 9320 deaths were from malignant melanoma, and 4140 were from other nonepithelial skin cancers

Risk Factors
- Excessive exposure to ultraviolet radiation from the sun or tanning salons
- Fair complexion
- Occupational exposure to coal tar, pitch, creosote, arsenic compounds, and radium
- In people of color, skin cancer is less common, is diagnosed at a more advanced stage, and has a higher morbidity and mortality than in people with light-colored skin; it is often found on the palms and soles.
- Immunosuppression

Warning Signs
- Any unusual skin condition, especially a change in the size, borders, or color of a mole or other darkly pigmented growth or spot

Prevention and Early Detection
- Avoid the sun when ultraviolet light is strongest (e.g., 10 a.m. to 3 p.m.), avoid sun tanning beds, seek shade, use sunscreen preparations, especially those containing ingredients such as para-aminobenzoic acid (PABA), and wear protective clothing
- Basal cell and squamous cell skin cancers often form a pale, waxlike pearly nodule or a red, scaly, sharply outlined patch
- Melanomas usually have a dark brown or black pigmentation; they start as small, molelike growths that increase in size, change color, become ulcerated, and bleed easily from slight injury

Treatment
- Options for treatment include surgery, electrodesiccation (tissue destruction by heat), radiation therapy, cryosurgery (tissue destruction by freezing)
- Malignant melanomas require wide and often deep excisions and removal of nearby lymph nodes; selective lymphadenectomy, immunotherapy; vaccines; oncolytic viruses; and targeted small molecules.

Survival
- For basal cell and squamous cell cancers, cure is virtually ensured with early detection and treatment; malignant melanoma, however, metastasizes quickly and accounts for a lower 5-year survival rate.

*There are no accurate estimates for basal cell and squamous cell carcinomas.
Data from American Cancer Society: *Cancer facts & figures 2018,* Atlanta, 2018, Author.

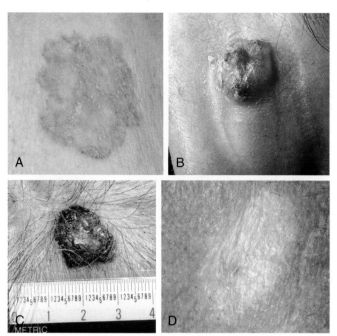

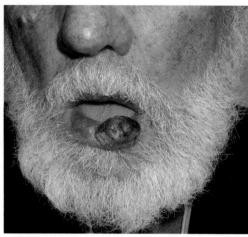

FIGURE 43.23 **Lip Cancer.** Biopsy confirmed squamous cell carcinoma. Lip vermilion shows diffuse actinic keratosis. (From Bagheri SC et al: *Current therapy in oral and maxillofacial surgery*, Philadelphia, 2012, Saunders.)

FIGURE 43.22 **Types of Basal Cell Carcinoma. A,** Superficial. **B,** Nodular. **C,** Pigmented. **D,** Morpheaform—recurrent tumor. (**A** and **D** from Bolognia JL et al: *Dermatology*, ed 3, Philadelphia, 2012, Saunders. **B** and **C** from James WD et al: *Andrews' diseases of the skin: clinical dermatology*, ed 11, Philadelphia, 2009, Saunders.)

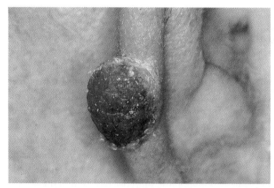

FIGURE 43.24 **Squamous Cell Carcinoma.** The sun-exposed ear is a common site for squamous cell carcinoma. (Courtesy Department of Dermatology, University of Utah School of Medicine, Salt Lake City, Utah.)

types are characterized: in situ and invasive. Ultraviolet radiation exposure causes SCC, and actinic keratosis is a precursor lesion. Other risk factors include arsenic at a higher level in drinking water, exposure to x-rays and gamma rays, immunosuppression, and light-colored skin.

Premalignant lesions include actinic keratosis, leukoplakia (whitish discolored areas), scars, radiation-induced keratosis, tar and oil keratosis, and chronic ulcers. In situ SCC is usually confined to the epidermis (intraepidermal) but may extend into the dermis. Bowen disease is a dysplastic epidermal lesion often found on unexposed areas of the body such as the penis and demonstrated by flat, reddish, scaly patches. These lesions rarely invade surrounding tissue and, although they rarely metastasize, they do so more often than BCCs. Other components of the skin (e.g., sweat glands, hair follicles) can develop into skin cancer, but this is relatively uncommon.

SCC is the most common cause of lip cancer and is more prevalent in older white men. The lower lip is the most common site. Long-term environmental exposure results in dryness, chapping, hyperkeratosis, and predisposition to malignancy. Immunosuppression, pipe smoking, and chronic alcoholism increase the risk for lip cancer. The most common lesion is termed *exophytic* and usually develops in the outer part of the lip along the vermilion border. The lip becomes thickened and evolves to an ulcerated center with a raised border (Fig. 43.23). These lesions have an irregular surface, follow cracks in the lip, and tend to extend toward the inner surface.

Invasive SCC can arise from premalignant lesions of the skin. It rarely develops from normal-appearing skin and is usually confined to the epidermis (intraepidermal), but it may extend into the reticular layer of the dermis (see Table 43.1). Invasive SCCs grow more rapidly than BCCs and can spread to regional lymph nodes. These tumors are firm and increase in both elevation and diameter. The surface may be granular and bleed easily (Fig. 43.24). Treatment includes surgical excision, radiotherapy, chemical destruction, immunotherapy, and adjuvant therapy.[35]

Cutaneous Melanoma

Cutaneous melanoma is a malignant tumor of the skin originating from melanocytes, cells that synthesize the pigment melanin and are located in the basal layer of the skin. The incidence is increasing worldwide. Risk factors include a personal or family history, or both, UV radiation exposure (including sun bed use before age 30 years), immunosuppression, fair hair, light skin with repeated sunburns, freckles, younger females and older males, geographic location, past pesticide exposure, and three or more clinically atypical (dysplastic) nevi. The risk of melanoma is lower in nonwhite people. However, they have more advanced disease and a higher death rate when diagnosed.

Cutaneous melanomas arise as a result of malignant degeneration of melanocytes located either along the basal layer of the epidermis (see Fig. 43.1) or in a benign melanocytic nevus. The clinical varieties of cutaneous melanoma include *superficial spreading melanoma* (SSM), the most common; *lentigo malignant melanoma* (LMM) (Fig. 43.25), frequently found in the elderly and confused with age spots; *primary*

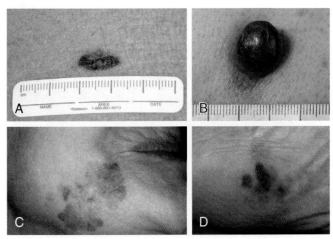

FIGURE 43.25 Types of Melanoma. A, Superficial spreading melanoma. **B,** Nodular melanoma. **C,** Lentigo malignant melanoma. **D,** Acral lentiginous melanoma on plantar surface of foot. (From Bolognia JL et al: *Dermatology essentials,* Philadelphia, 2014, Saunders.)

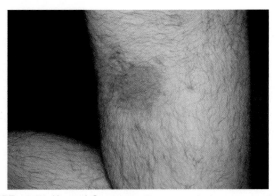

FIGURE 43.26 Kaposi Sarcoma. The purple lesion commonly seen on the skin. (Courtesy Department of Dermatology, University of Utah School of Medicine, Salt Lake City, Utah.)

nodular melanoma (PNM), an aggressive tumor. *Acral lentiginous melanoma* (ALM) is rare and aggressive and occurs on non–hair-bearing surfaces (i.e., palms of the hands and soles of the feet) and mucous membranes in African-American people. *Amelanotic* (lack of pigment) and *desmoplastic* (fibrous or connective tissue) melanomas are similar rare forms of melanoma and may be aggressive and difficult to diagnose. Melanoma also can arise in the uvea of the eye and on mucous membranes, where they are less visible.

The pathogenesis of malignant melanoma is complex. Most familial melanomas are associated with tumor-suppressor genes and proto-oncogenes. Melanomas have a high mutation rate stimulated by UV radiation. Four major genomic subtypes (*BRAF* mutant, *RAS* mutant, *NF1* mutant, and Triple wild-type) have been identified, providing guidance for targeted therapy.

The relationship between nevi and melanoma makes it important for the clinician to understand the various forms of nevi (see Table 43.7). Most nevi never become suspicious, but suspicious pigmented nevi need to be evaluated and removed. Indications for biopsy include any color change, size change, irregular notched margin, itching, bleeding or oozing, nodularity, scab formation, and ulceration or an unusual pattern of presentation. The ABCDE rule is used as a guide: **A**symmetry, **B**order irregularity, **C**olor variation, **D**iameter larger than 6 mm, and **E**levation or **E**volving, which includes raised appearance or rapid enlargement. Staging is determined by vertical lesion thickness (depth of tumor), lymph node involvement, and presence of metastasis (TNM staging).

Treatment of melanoma with no evidence of metastatic disease involves a wide surgical excision of the primary lesion site. A lymph node biopsy of the peripherally draining lymph node (sentinel node) is warranted for lesions greater than 1 mm deep. Lesions on the extremities have the best surgical prognosis. Radiation therapy, chemotherapy, and immunotherapy (checkpoint inhibitors that block proteins to stop the immune system from attacking cancer cells and signal transduction), oncolytic viruses, and targeted molecular therapy that inhibits gene mutations, in addition to vaccines, are used to treat metastatic disease and have demonstrated long-term improvement in disease outcome.[36] Early detection is critical to reducing mortality from metastatic disease.

Kaposi Sarcoma

Kaposi sarcoma (KS) is a vascular malignancy associated with immunodeficiency states and occurs among transplant recipients taking immunosuppressive drugs. Genetic and environmental cofactors determine disease progression. Four forms of the disease have been described: classic (more benign), epidemic (rapidly progressive and associated with acquired immunodeficiency syndrome [AIDS]), African endemic (associated with HPV), and iatrogenic (associated with immunosuppressant treatment, including organ transplant).[37]

The endothelial cell is thought to be the progenitor of KS. The lesions emerge as red, purple, or brown macules and develop into plaques and nodules. They tend to be multifocal rather than spreading by metastasis. The lesions initially appear over the lower extremities in the classic form (Fig. 43.26). The rapidly progressive form associated with AIDS tends to spread symmetrically over the upper body, particularly the face and oral mucosa. The lesions are often pruritic and painful. Most individuals with epidemic KS have involvement of lymph nodes, particularly in the gastrointestinal tract and lungs. Organ involvement is much less common in the classic form than in the epidemic form. The rapidly progressive form has a poor prognosis and shorter survival rates than the classic form. (See Chapter 8 for a further discussion of AIDS.)

Diagnosis is by medical history, physical examination, and skin biopsy, with a high index of suspicion for those with immunodeficiency. Chest x-ray reveals lesions in the lungs. Local lesions can be excised. Multiple disseminated lesions may be treated with a combination of α-interferon, radiotherapy, and cytotoxic drugs. Antiangiogenic agents are being tested. Individuals receiving highly active antiretroviral therapy (HAART) have a markedly reduced incidence of KS.

Primary Cutaneous Lymphomas

Primary cutaneous lymphomas are cutaneous T-cell and B-cell lymphomas present in the skin without evidence of extracutaneous disease at the time of diagnosis (see Chapter 22 for classification and general pathophysiology of lymphomas). Cutaneous lymphomas are rare but are the second most common site of extranodal non-Hodgkin lymphoma. Cutaneous lymphomas present with skin lesions and are more common in men, usually in the fifth and sixth decades.

Cutaneous lymphomas develop from clonal expansion of B cells, T-helper cells, and rarely T-suppressor cells. The most common is cutaneous T-cell lymphoma and mycosis fungoides is the most prominent subtype. **Mycosis fungoides** can present as focal or widespread erythematous patches or plaques, follicular papules, comedone-like lesions, and tumors. There may be patches of alopecia. The lesions progress over a period of months or years.

The differential diagnosis of the different types of cutaneous lymphomas is based on clinical manifestations, histologic, immunologic and cytogenetic features, and response to appropriate treatment. Treatment is based on the clinical presentation and staging of the disease and includes topical therapy, immunotherapy, chemotherapy, radiation therapy, and phototherapy.[38]

> ✔ **QUICK CHECK 43.7**
> 1. What is the most common skin cancer?
> 2. What malignancy can arise from melanocytes?
> 3. How is Kaposi sarcoma related to AIDS?

Burns

The incidence of burn injuries has declined in the past several years. Most burns occur in the home, with the highest percentage occurring in men.[39]

Burns may be caused by thermal or nonthermal sources, including chemical, electrical, or radioactive sources. Thermal injuries result from thermal contact, scalds, or radiation. Direct contact, inhalation, and ingestion of acids, alkalis, or blistering agents cause chemical burns. Electrical burns occur with the passage of electrical current through the body to the ground or electrical flames or flashes. In addition to cutaneous injury, burns can be associated with smoke inhalation and other traumatic injuries that exacerbate local and systemic responses. Ventilatory support is often needed with inhalation injury.

Burn Wound Depth

The depth of injury identifies the level of tissue destruction; the extent of injury determines clinical management, healing, and mortality. The depth of the burn is divided into four categories, summarized in Table 43.8.

First-degree burns require no treatment unless the person is elderly or an infant, in which case severe nausea and vomiting may lead to inadequate fluid intake and dehydration. Fluid therapy may be required in these cases. First-degree burns heal in 3 to 5 days without scarring.

Second-degree burns involve thin-walled, fluid-filled blisters that develop within just a few minutes after injury (Fig. 43.27). Tactile and pain sensors remain intact throughout the healing process, and wound care can cause extreme pain. Wounds heal in 3 to 4 weeks with adequate nutrition and no wound complications. Scar formation is unusual and is genetically determined.

TABLE 43.8	**Depth of Burn Injury**				
		SECOND DEGREE	**THIRD DEGREE**		**FOURTH DEGREE**
Characteristic	**First Degree**	**Superficial Partial Thickness**	**Deep Partial Thickness**	**Full Thickness**	**Full Thickness and Deeper Tissue**
Morphology	Destruction of epidermis only; local pain and erythema	Destruction of epidermis and some dermis	Destruction of epidermis and dermis, leaving only skin appendages	Destruction of epidermis, dermis, and underlying subcutaneous tissue	Destruction of epidermis, dermis, and underlying subcutaneous tissue, tendons, muscle, and bone
Skin function	Intact	Absent	Absent	Absent	Absent
Tactile and pain sensors	Intact	Intact	Intact but diminished	Absent	Absent
Blisters	Usually none or present after first 24 hr	Present within minutes; thin walled and fluid filled	May or may not appear as fluid-filled blisters; often is layer of flat, dehydrated tissue paper–like skin that lifts off in sheets	Blisters rare; usually a layer of flat, dehydrated tissue paper–like skin that lifts off easily	None
Appearance of wound after initial débridement	Skin peels at 24-48 hr; normal or slightly red underneath	Red to pale ivory, moist surface	Mottled with areas of waxy, white, dry surface	White, cherry red, or black; may contain visible thrombosed veins; dry, hard, leathery surface	Black and charred appearing wound
Healing time	3-5 days	21-28 days	30 days to many months	Will not heal; may close from edges as secondary healing if wound is small	Will not heal; requires skin grafting; may require amputation and/or reconstructive surgery
Scarring	None	May be present; low incidence influenced by genetic predisposition	Highest incidence because of slow healing rate promoting scar tissue development; also influenced by genetic predisposition	Skin graft; scarring minimized by early excision and grafting; influenced by genetic predisposition	Degree of scarring associated with reconstruction and grafting success

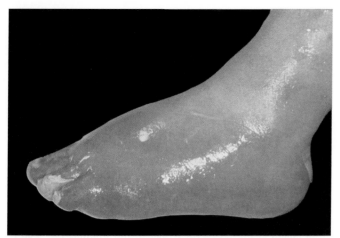

FIGURE 43.27 Superficial Partial-Thickness Burn. Scald injury after débridement of overlying blister and nonadherent epithelium. (Courtesy Intermountain Burn Center, University of Utah, Salt Lake City, Utah.)

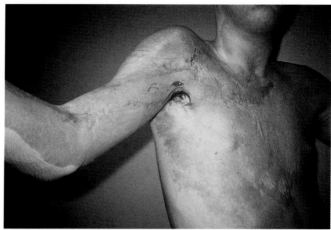

FIGURE 43.29 Axillary Burn Scar Contracture. Note the blanching of the anterior axillary fold and small ulceration from a deep partial-thickness burn, both indicating the diminished range of motion. (Courtesy Intermountain Burn Center, University of Utah, Salt Lake City, Utah.)

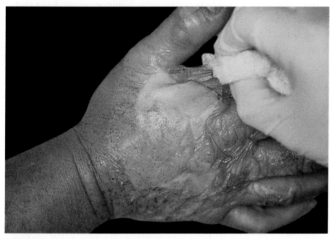

FIGURE 43.28 Deep Partial-Thickness Burn. Note pale appearance and minimal exudates. (Courtesy Intermountain Burn Center, University of Utah, Salt Lake City, Utah.)

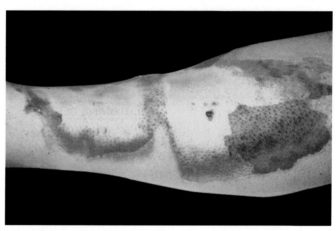

FIGURE 43.30 Full-Thickness Burn. The wound is dry and insensate. (Courtesy Intermountain Burn Center, University of Utah, Salt Lake City, Utah.)

Deep partial-thickness burns (Fig. 43.28) look waxy white and take weeks to heal. Necrotic tissue is surgically removed, and then the person's own unburned skin from another body area (autograft) is applied. Healing commonly results in hypertrophic scarring with poor functional and cosmetic results (Fig. 43.29).

Third-degree burns, or **full-thickness burns,** have a dry, leathery appearance from loss of dermal elasticity (Fig. 43.30). In areas of circumferential burns, distal circulation may be compromised from pressure caused by edema. **Escharotomies** (tissue decompression by cutting through burned skin) are performed to release pressure and prevent compartment syndrome (the compression of blood vessels, veins, muscles, or abdominal organs resulting in ischemia, necrosis, and irreversible injury). Full-thickness burns are painless because all nerve endings have been destroyed by the injury.

Fourth-degree burns require skin grafting or reconstructive surgery.

The extent of **total body surface area (TBSA)** burned is estimated using either the "Rule of Nines" (Fig. 43.31) or the modified Lund-Browder chart.[40] The severity of burn injury also considers many factors, including age, medical history, extent and depth of injury, and body area involved. The American Burn Association has defined criteria to assist health care professionals in identifying who should be referred to a specialized multidisciplinary burn center (https://ameriburn.org/public-resources/burn-center-referral-criteria/).

PATHOPHYSIOLOGY AND CLINICAL MANIFESTATIONS   Burn injury results in dramatic changes in many physiologic functions of the body within the first few minutes after the event.[41] Burns exceeding 20% of TBSA in most adults are considered to be major burn injuries and are associated with massive evaporative water losses and fluctuations of large amounts of fluids, electrolytes, and plasma proteins into the body tissues, manifested as generalized massive edema, circulatory hypovolemia, and hypotension.

The immediate (acute) systemic physiologic consequences of a major burn injury focus on the profound, life-threatening hypovolemic shock that occurs in conjunction with cellular and immunologic disruption within a few minutes of injury (Fig. 43.32). **Burn shock** is a condition consisting of a hypovolemic cardiovascular component and a cellular component.

Hypovolemia associated with burn shock results from massive fluid losses and shifts to the interstitial space from the circulating blood volume. The losses are caused by an increase in capillary permeability that occurs immediately and persists for approximately 24 hours after

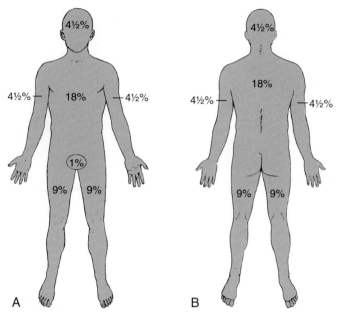

FIGURE 43.31 Estimation of Burn Injury: Rule of Nines. A commonly used assessment tool with estimates of the percentages (in multiples of 9) of the total body surface area burned. **A,** Adults *(anterior view).* **B,** Adults *(posterior view).*

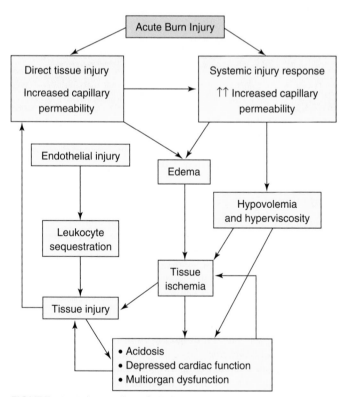

FIGURE 43.32 Immediate Cellular and Immunologic Alterations of Burn Shock.

burn injury. There is decreased cardiac contractility and decreased blood volume. Blood is shunted away from the liver, kidney, and gut—known as the "ebb phase" of the burn response. This phase persists during the first 24 to 72 hours after the burn injury and is associated with a hypometabolic state with hypodynamic circulation, decreased oxygen consumption, and hyperglycemia. Most organ systems are affected.

Decreased perfusion of the viscera can diminish gut barrier function and result in translocation of bacteria and endotoxemia with sepsis. Intravenous fluid resuscitation, often with lactated Ringer solution, is critical to restore the circulating blood volume. The rate of fluid replacement must be carefully monitored to prevent complications associated with fluid overload. Formulas are available (i.e., the Parkland formula or the modified Brooke formula) to guide calculation of the fluid volume replacement.[42]

Cellular metabolism is disrupted with the onset of the burn wound, resulting in altered cell membrane permeability and loss of normal electrolyte homeostasis. Many cytokines and inflammatory mediators in burn serum play a role in these cellular processes. Acute kidney injury is associated with hypovolemia, decreased cardiac output, the inflammatory response, and the effects of angiotensin, vasopressin, and aldosterone.

Cardiovascular and Systemic Response to Burn Injury

The clinical manifestations of burn shock are the result of multiple physiologic alterations related to burn injury and the release of inflammatory cytokines, in addition to the loss of fluid. The hallmark of burn shock is decreased cardiac contractility and diminished cardiac output with inadequate capillary perfusion in most tissues. Decreased cardiac output is related to myocardial depressant factor, as well as reduced intravascular volume.

Fluid and protein movement out of the vascular compartment results in an elevated hematocrit level and white blood cell count, and hypoproteinemia. If these are not treated immediately, profound hypovolemic shock and inadequate perfusion lead to irreversible shock and death within a few hours. Restoration of capillary integrity and renewal of a functional lymphatic system are required for resolution of the edema. Usually this occurs within 24 hours, but in extensive burns, it may take days or weeks. After the individual has reached the endpoint of burn shock, the term used to describe the person's condition is **capillary seal**.

The liver, with its metabolic, inflammatory, immune, and acute phase functions, plays a pivotal role in burn injury survival and recovery by modulating multiple metabolic pathways. Hepatic changes are common after a major burn, including fatty changes and hepatomegaly, which can influence burn wound recovery.[43] The hepatic response also alters clotting factors and contributes to a hypercoagulable state, and it can increase the risk for disseminated intravascular coagulation (systemic formation of microthrombi and abnormal bleeding).[44]

Metabolic Response to Burn Injury

A major burn injury (greater than 30% of the TBSA) initiates a systemic hypermetabolic response with an increase in the metabolic rate and a hyperdynamic circulation that begins about 48 hours after the ebb phase. This phase is known as the "flow phase" and can persist for a year or longer after a burn.[45] Metabolic responses involve the sympathetic nervous system and other homeostatic regulators. Levels of catecholamines, cortisol, glucagon, and insulin (insulin resistance) are elevated, with a corresponding increase in energy expenditure and increased gluconeogenesis, glycogenolysis, lipolysis, proteolysis, and lactic acidosis. Myocardial oxygen consumption is elevated, and there is catabolic loss of muscle mass. Hyperglycemia and insulin resistance can be prolonged in severe burns and require management with intensive insulin therapy to improve postburn morbidity and mortality.

Burn injury initiates an inflammatory response, with local activation and recruitment of inflammatory cells, such as leukocytes and monocytes, at the site of injury. These cells release inflammatory cytokines that contribute to the hypermetabolic state. The metabolic rate increases in proportion to the burn size and compensates for the profound water and heat loss associated with the burn. The inflammatory response and the release of cytokines at the wound level are magnified into a generalized systemic inflammatory response syndrome that can lead to multiple organ dysfunction.

Hypermetabolism also increases the thermal regulatory set point and core and skin temperatures. There is persistent tachycardia, hypercapnia, and body wasting. Wound healing may be impaired, contributing to increased risk for infection and sepsis. Increasing the ambient temperature and early excision and grafting can decrease resting energy expenditure and improve mortality after major burns. Inflammatory mediators circulating to the lung result in pulmonary edema that can be life-threatening.

Immunologic Response to Burn Injury

The immunologic/inflammatory response to burn injury is immediate, prolonged, and severe. The result in individuals surviving burn shock is *immunosuppression* with increased susceptibility to potentially fatal systemic burn wound sepsis. White blood cells are altered at a time when their need to inhibit sepsis is vital. Macrophages, neutrophils, lymphocytes, and platelets release large amounts of inflammatory cytokines and antibodies; their levels remain elevated for weeks after burn injury. Phagocytosis is impaired, and cellular and humoral immunity is abnormal. Individuals with altered immunocompetence or chronic disease before burn injury are at additional risk for complications, including wound sepsis.

Evaporative Water Loss

With major burn injury, there is loss of the skin's barrier function and ability to regulate evaporative water loss. Normally, the skin is the major source of insensible water loss (75%), and the lungs are minor sources (25%), with a total loss of about 600 to 800 ml/day. This increases dramatically with burns because both the skin and the lungs have increased loss of water as a result of skin injury, hypermetabolism, and hyperventilation, especially in an intubated individual. Total evaporative losses exceed many liters per day in an adult with large burn wounds. Replacement of the loss is mandatory to prevent volume deficit and shock.

EVALUATION AND TREATMENT Burn recovery is complex and prolonged, and complications are the rule rather than the exception. The severity of inhalation injury is also a significant morbidity and mortality factor. The goal of burn management is wound débridement and closure in a manner that promotes survival. Scar formation with contractures is often a consequence of healing in deep partial-thickness and third-degree burns (Fig. 43.33).

The essential elements of survival of major burn injury are (1) provision of adequate fluids and nutrition, (2) meticulous management of wounds with early surgical excision and grafting (Fig. 43.34), (3) aggressive treatment of infection or sepsis, and (4) promotion of thermoregulation. Several drugs are used for the management of severe burns, including β-adrenergic antagonists, β-adrenergic agonists, recombinant human growth hormone, insulin, androgenic steroids, and antibiotics. Burn pain is almost always acute and severe, and treatment strategies are aggressive. The risk of developing stress ulcers (Curling ulcers) is reduced with antacids or histamine H_2-receptor antagonists.

Nutritional therapy focuses on early enteral therapy to reduce gut-mediated sepsis and to reduce the catabolic state. Advancements in skin replacement procedures promote wound closure and healing. Reconstructive surgery reduces complications associated with scarring and contractures.

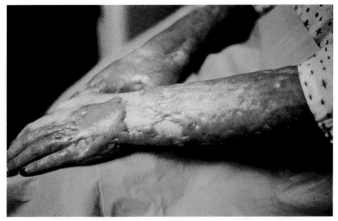

FIGURE 43.33 Hypertrophic Scarring. Deep partial-thickness thermal injury can result in extensive hypertrophic scarring. (Courtesy Intermountain Burn Center, University of Utah, Salt Lake City, Utah.)

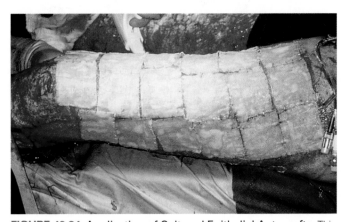

FIGURE 43.34 Application of Cultured Epithelial Autografts. Thin sheets of keratinocytes are attached to a gauze backing to allow application onto the clean, excised thigh. (Courtesy Intermountain Burn Center, University of Utah, Salt Lake City, Utah.)

Cold Injury

Exposure to extreme cold includes a spectrum of injuries[46]:

- *Frostnip*—mild and completely reversible injury characterized by skin pallor and numbness
- *Chilblains*—more serious than frostnip; violaceous skin color with plaques or nodules, pain, and pruritus, but no ice crystal formation; chronic vasculitis can develop and is usually located on the face, anterior lower leg, hands, and feet
- *Frostbite*—tissues freeze and form ice crystals at temperatures below −2° C (28° F); progresses from distal to proximal and potentially reversible
- *Flash freeze*—rapid cooling with intracellular ice crystals associated with contact with cold metals or volatile liquids

The most common areas affected are fingers, toes, ears, nose, and cheeks. Mild frostbite (frostnip) is cold exposure without tissue freezing. It causes pallor and pain, followed by redness and discomfort during rewarming, with no tissue damage. Frostbite occurs when tissues freeze slowly with ice crystal formation. Frozen skin becomes white or yellowish and has a waxy texture. There is numbness and no sensation of pain. Frostbite injury is related to direct cold injury to cells, indirect injury from ice crystal formation, and endothelial cell damage. During rewarming, there is progressive microvascular thrombosis followed by reperfusion injury with the release of inflammatory mediators (including thromboxanes, prostaglandins, bradykinins, and histamines) and with impaired circulation and anoxia to the exposed area. Cyanosis and mottling develop, followed by redness, edema, and burning pain on rewarming in more severe cases. Edema can cause capillary compression and vascular stasis. Within 24 to 48 hours, vesicles and bullae appear that resolve into crusts that eventually slough, leaving thin, newly formed skin. Frostbite may be classified by depth of injury: superficial includes partial skin freezing (first degree) and full-thickness skin freezing (second degree); deep includes full-thickness and subcutaneous freezing (third degree) and deep tissue freezing (fourth degree). Third-degree and fourth-degree frostbite result in gangrene with loss of tissue.

Immediate treatment of frostbite is to cover affected areas with other body surfaces and warm clothing. The area should not be rubbed or massaged. Rewarming for severe frostbite should occur after emergency transport. Immersion in a warm water bath (40° to 42° C [104° to 107.6° F]) until frozen tissue is thawed is the best treatment. Pain is severe and should be treated with potent analgesics. Antibiotics may be given. Vasodilators, thrombolytics, hyperbaric oxygen, and sympathectomy may improve healing responses. Débridement or amputation of necrotic tissue occurs when there is a clear line of demarcation.

DISORDERS OF THE HAIR

Alopecia

Alopecia means loss of hair from the head or body. Hair loss occurs when there is disruption in the growth phase of the hair follicle. Hair loss can be associated with systemic disorders such as hypothyroidism and iron deficiency, chemotherapy for cancer, malnutrition, compulsive hair pulling (trichotillomania), traction on hair from braiding and ponytails, use of hair treatment chemicals, hormonal alterations, and immune reactions.

Androgenic Alopecia

Androgenic alopecia, or localized hair loss, occurs in about 80% of men. It is not a disease but a genetically predisposed response to androgens that clusters in families. Within the distribution of hair over the scalp, androgen-sensitive hair follicles are on top and androgen-insensitive follicles are on the sides and back. In genetically predisposed men, the androgen-sensitive follicles are transformed into vellus follicles that grow short, thin hair. Male-pattern baldness begins with frontotemporal recession and progresses to loss of hair over the top of the scalp. Minoxidil may be used to stimulate hair growth and finasteride (a 5α-reductase inhibitor) may reduce the effect of androgens on hair follicles.

Female-Pattern Alopecia

Some genetically susceptible women in their twenties and thirties experience progressive thinning and loss of hair over the central part of the scalp, and the prevalence increases with advancing age. Contrary to male-pattern baldness, there is usually no loss of hair along the frontal hairline but the hairs are shorter and thinner (follicular miniaturization). The mechanism of hair loss is unknown but related to genetic and hormonal changes.

Alopecia Areata

Alopecia areata is an autoimmune T-cell–mediated chronic inflammatory disease directed against hair follicles and results in hair loss.[47] There is a rapid onset of hair loss in multiple areas of the scalp, usually in round patches. The eyebrows, eyelashes, beard, and other areas of body hair are rarely involved. Stressful events, cell-mediated immune cytokines, genetic susceptibility, and metabolic disorders (e.g., Addison disease, thyroid disease, and lupus erythematosus) are associated with alopecia areata.

The affected areas of skin are smooth or may have short shafts of poorly developed hair that breaks at the surface ("exclamation mark" hair). Regrowth occurs within 1 to 3 months, but hair loss may recur at the same site. Permanent regrowth of hair usually occurs. The diagnosis is made by observation of the pattern of hair loss. Biopsy may show a lymphocytic infiltrate around the follicle. There are several treatments for alopecia areata, including corticosteroids and topical immunotherapy.

Hirsutism

Hirsutism occurs in women and is the abnormal growth and distribution of hair on the face, body, and pubic area in a male pattern. There is also frontotemporal hair recession. These areas of hair growth are androgen sensitive. Variations of hair growth in women are great, and a male pattern may be normal. Women who develop hirsutism may be secreting hormones associated with polycystic ovarian syndrome, adrenal hyperplasia, or adrenal tumors; and these disorders require treatment. If no hormonal pathologic conditions exist, treatment may include cosmetic removal of hair, suppression of excessive androgen production, or blockage of peripheral androgen receptors.

DISORDERS OF THE NAIL

Paronychia

Paronychia is an acute or chronic infection of the cuticle. One or more fingers or toes may be involved. Individuals whose hands are frequently exposed to moisture are at greatest risk. The most common causative microorganisms are staphylococci and streptococci. Occasionally Candida will be present. Acute paronychia is manifested by the rapid onset of painful inflammation of the cuticle, usually after minor trauma. An abscess may develop requiring incision and drainage for relief of pain. The skin around the nail becomes more edematous and painful with progressive infection. Pus may be expressed from the proximal nail fold, and an abscess may develop. The nail plate is usually not affected, although it can become discolored with ridges. Chronic paronychia develops slowly, with tenderness and swelling around the proximal or lateral nail folds, and tends to affect more than one nail.

Treatment includes prevention by keeping the hands dry. Oral antifungals are not effective because they do not penetrate the affected tissues. Therapy includes topical application of antiinflammatory agents and antifungals, steroids, or calcineurin inhibitors.[48]

Onychomycosis

Onychomycosis (tinea unguium) is a fungal or dermatophyte infection of the nail unit. The most common pattern is a nail plate that turns yellow or white and becomes elevated with the accumulation of hyperkeratotic debris within the plate. Fungal infections of the nail are differentiated from psoriasis, lichen planus, and trauma by culture and microscopy and the absence of pitting on the nail surface, which is characteristic of psoriasis. Treatment is difficult because topical or systemic antifungal agents do not penetrate the nail plate readily. Systemic antifungal drugs are effective and topical drugs are available; when used in combination the potential for success improves. Rarely, surgical excision of the nail may be required. Education is essential to preventing recurrence.[49]

> **QUICK CHECK 43.8**
> 1. Describe the three degrees of burn injury.
> 2. What dangers accompany frostbite?
> 3. What is alopecia? Compare the different types.
> 4. What disorders of the nail are seen?

GERIATRIC CONSIDERATIONS

Aging & Changes in Skin Integrity

- Skin becomes thinner, dryer, and more wrinkled. These changes are accelerated by exposure to sunlight and air pollution.
- DNA repair of damaged skin decreases.
- Epidermal cells contain less moisture and change shape.
- The dermis thins, producing translucent, paper-thin quality that is more susceptible to tearing.
- The dermis becomes more permeable and less able to clear substances, so they accumulate and cause irritation.
- A loss of epidermal rete pegs occurs, which weakens the connection to the dermis and gives skin a smooth, shiny, and wrinkled appearance with an increased likelihood of tearing from shearing forces.
- There is a loss of elastin, contributing to wrinkling.
- There is a loss of flexibility of collagen fibers, so skin cannot stretch and regain shape as readily.
- The barrier function of the stratum corneum is diminished, increasing the risk for injury and infection.
- A significantly decreased number of Langerhans cells reduces the skin's immune response.

- The dermoepidermal border flattens, shortening and reducing the number of capillary loops.

Other Skin Changes With Aging

- Wound healing declines as a result of decreased estrogen in both men and women, decreased blood flow, and a slower rate of basal cell and fibroblast turnover.
- There are fewer melanocytes; pigmentation becomes irregular, giving decreased protection from ultraviolet radiation and leading to graying of hair.
- Atrophy of eccrine, apocrine, and sebaceous glands causes dry skin.
- Pressure and touch receptors and free nerve endings decrease in number, causing reduced sensory perception.
- With compromised temperature regulation, loss of cutaneous vasomotion, and decreased eccrine sweat production, there is an increased risk of heat stroke and hypothermia.
- The nail plate thins, and nails are more brittle.

Data from Chang AL: *J Invest Dermatol* 136(5):897-899, 2016; Newton VL et al: *G Ital Dermatol Venereol* 150(6):665-674, 2015.

SUMMARY REVIEW

Structure and Function of the Skin

1. Skin is the largest organ of the body and equals 20% of body weight. Its major functions are to provide a protective barrier and to regulate body temperature.
2. The skin has two layers—the epidermis (outermost layer) and dermis. The underlying hypodermis (subcutaneous layer) contains connective tissue, fat cells, fibroblasts, and macrophages.
3. The epidermis contains basal and spinous layers with melanocytes, keratinocytes, Langerhans cells, and Merkel cells.
4. The dermis is composed of connective tissue elements, hair follicles, sweat glands, sebaceous glands, blood vessels, nerves, and lymphatic vessels.
5. The dermal appendages include the nails, hair, sebaceous glands, and eccrine and apocrine sweat glands.
6. The papillary capillaries provide the major blood supply to the skin, arising from deeper arterial plexuses.
7. Heat loss and heat conservation are regulated by arteriovenous anastomoses that lead to the papillary capillaries in the dermis and evaporative loss of sweat.
8. Clinical manifestations of skin dysfunction include lesions, keloids and hypertropic scars, and pruritus.
9. Pressure injury is localized damage to the skin that results from unrelieved pressure and shearing forces that occlude capillary blood flow, with resulting ischemia and necrosis. Areas at greatest risk are pressure points over bony prominences, such as the greater trochanters, sacrum, ischia, and heels.
10. Keloids are sharply elevated scars that extend beyond the border of traumatized skin. Hypertrophic scars are elevated fibrous lesions that do not extend beyond the border of injury. Both are caused by excess fibroblast activity and abnormal wound healing.
11. Pruritus, or itching, is associated with many skin disorders. Itch mediators stimulate small unmyelinated type C nerve fibers to transmit itch sensation.

Disorders of the Skin

1. The most common inflammatory disorders of the skin are eczema and dermatitis. Eczema is characterized by pruritus, lesions with indistinct borders, and epidermal changes. There are multiple types of dermatitis.
2. Allergic contact dermatitis is a form of delayed hypersensitivity that develops with sensitization to allergens, such as metal, chemicals, or poison ivy.
3. Irritant contact dermatitis develops from prolonged exposure to chemicals, such as acids or soaps, with disruption of the skin barrier. Removing the source of irritation and using topical agents provide effective treatment.
4. Atopic or allergic dermatitis is associated with a family history of asthma or hay fever and is associated with elevated IgE levels. It is more common in infancy and childhood.
5. Stasis dermatitis occurs on the legs and results from chronic venous stasis and edema. Progressive lesions become ulcerated. Elevating the legs, not wearing tight clothes, and not standing for long periods are used with treatment.
6. Seborrheic dermatitis involves scaly, yellowish, inflammatory plaques of the scalp, eyebrows, eyelids, ear canals, chest, axillae, and back. The cause is unknown but a genetic predisposition, *Malassezia* yeast infection, immunosuppression, and epidermal hyperproliferation have been implicated.
7. Papulosquamous disorders are characterized by papules, scales, plaques, and erythema and include psoriasis, pityriasis rosea, lichen planus, acne vulgaris, acne rosacea, and lupus erythematosus.
8. Psoriasis is a chronic inflammatory skin disease associated with a complex inflammatory cascade involving multiple immune cells resulting in cellular proliferation of both the epidermis and the dermis; it is characterized by scaly, erythematous, pruritic plaques.
9. Pityriasis rosea is a self-limiting inflammatory disease characterized by oval lesions with scales around the edges; it is located along skin lines of the trunk and may be caused by a herpeslike virus.

10. Lichen planus is an autoimmune papular, violet-colored inflammatory lesion of unknown origin manifested by severe pruritus.

11. Acne vulgaris is an inflammation of the pilosebaceous follicle.

12. Hydradenitis suppurativa (inverse acne) is an inflammatory disease involving the deep sections of apocrine glands. The lesions present in apocrine-gland rich areas as deep, firm painful subcutaneous nodules, often with sinus tracts, and rupture horizontally under the skin.

13. Acne rosacea develops on the middle third of the face with hypertrophy and inflammation of the sebaceous glands and is associated with altered innate immune responses.

14. Discoid (cutaneous) lupus erythematosus is an autoimmune disease that can affect only the skin. The systemic form also presents cutaneous lesions. The cutaneous inflammatory lesions usually occur in sun-exposed areas with a butterfly distribution over the nose and cheeks.

15. Pemphigus is a chronic, autoimmune, blistering disease that begins in the mouth or on the scalp and spreads to other parts of the body, often with a fatal outcome.

16. Erythema multiforme is an acute inflammation of the skin and mucous membranes (bullous form) with lesions that appear target-like, with alternating rings of edema and inflammation; it is often associated with immunologic reactions to drugs.

17. Stevens-Johnson syndrome (severe mucocutaneous bullous form involving 10% of the body surface area) and toxic epidermal necrolysis (severe mucocutaneous bullous form involving more than 30% of the body surface area) are the same disease with a continuum of symptoms. Both are type IV hypersensitivity reactions to drugs and are medical emergencies.

18. Cutaneous infections generally remain localized and can be bacterial, viral, and fungal in origin.

19. Bacterial infections include (1) folliculitis, infection of the hair follicle; (2) furuncle, abscess of the hair follicle that extends to the surrounding tissue; (3) carbuncle, collection of furuncles that forms a draining abscess; (4) cellulitis, diffuse infection of the dermis and subcutaneous tissue; (5) erysipelas, superficial streptococcal infection of the skin commonly affecting the face, ears, and lower legs; (6) impetigo, a superficial infection caused by *Staphylococcus* or *Streptococcus*; and (7) Lyme disease.

20. Lyme disease is an immune response caused by the spirochete *Borrelia burgdorferi*. It is transmitted by tick bites and often shows migrating erythematous bull's eye lesions that can progress to myalgias, arthralgias, and neurologic manifestations.

21. Viral skin infections include HSV, herpes zoster and varicella, and warts.

22. HSV-1 causes cold sores but can infect the cornea, mouth, and labia. HSV-2 commonly causes genital lesions and is usually spread by sexual contact.

23. Herpes zoster (shingles) and varicella (chickenpox) are both caused by the varicella-zoster virus and can be prevented by vaccination.

24. Warts are benign, rough, elevated lesions caused by human papillomavirus. Condylomata acuminata, or venereal warts, are spread by sexual contact.

25. Tinea infections (fungal infections) can occur anywhere on the body and are classified by location (i.e., tinea pedis, tinea corporis, tinea capitis).

26. Candidiasis is a yeastlike fungal infection *(Candida albicans)* that occurs on the skin and mucous membranes and in the gastrointestinal tract and vagina.

27. Vascular abnormalities are commonly associated with skin diseases.

28. Cutaneous vasculitis is an inflammation of skin blood vessels related to immune complex deposition, with purpura, ischemia, and necrosis resulting from vessel necrosis.

29. Urticarial lesions are commonly associated with type I hypersensitivity responses and appear as wheals, welts, or hives.

30. Localized scleroderma is an autoimmune-mediated fibrosis that primarily affects the skin.

31. Systemic scleroderma is an autoimmune-mediated sclerosis of the skin that may also affect systemic organs and cause renal failure, bowel obstruction, or cardiac dysrhythmias.

32. Most benign tumors of the skin are associated with aging.

33. Seborrheic keratosis is a benign proliferation of basal cells that produces elevated, smooth, or warty lesions of varying size. It is most common among the elderly population.

34. Keratoacanthoma arises from hair follicles on sun-exposed areas. Three stages of development over a period of 1 to 2 months characterize the lesion. Lesions resolve spontaneously or can be removed.

35. Actinic keratosis is a rough, poorly defined papule that develops in sun-exposed individuals with fair skin. The lesion may become malignant in the form of a squamous cell carcinoma.

36. Nevi (moles) arise from melanocytes and may be pigmented or nonpigmented. They occur singly or in groups and may undergo transition to malignant melanoma.

37. Skin cancer is usually caused by chronic exposure to ultraviolet radiation and is the most common cancer in the world.

38. Basal cell carcinoma is the most common skin cancer and occurs most often on ultraviolet-exposed areas of the skin.

39. Squamous cell carcinoma is a tumor of the epidermis and can be localized (in situ) or invasive.

40. Cutaneous melanoma is a malignant tumor that arises from melanocytes. If it is not excised early, metastasis occurs through the lymph nodes.

41. Kaposi sarcoma is a vascular malignancy associated with immunodeficiency.

42. Primary cutaneous lymphomas are clonal expansions of T-cell and B-cell lymphocytes. Mycosis fungoides is the most common T-cell lymphoma.

43. Burns are classified according to depth and extent of injury as first-, second-, third-, or fourth-degree burns.

44. Severe burns cause profound edema and burn shock related to an inflammatory response throughout the cardiovascular system, with loss of capillary seal. Fluid resuscitation is critical to prevent shock and death.

45. Burns cause a hypermetabolic response, with increased cortisol, glucagon, and insulin levels (insulin resistance) and gluconeogenesis.

46. Immune suppression associated with inflammatory cytokine release from burned tissue increases the risk for infection and can delay wound healing.

47. Cold injury usually occurs on the face and digits, with direct injury to cells and impaired circulation.

Disorders of the Hair

1. Alopecia is loss of hair from the head or body.

2. Androgenic alopecia is an inherited form of baldness with hair loss in the central scalp and recession of the frontotemporal hairline.

3. Female-pattern alopecia is a thinning of the central hair of the scalp beginning in women at 20 to 30 years of age.

4. Alopecia areata is an autoimmune-mediated loss of hair and may be associated with stress or metabolic diseases; it is usually reversible.

5. Hirsutism is a male pattern of hair growth in women that may be normal or the result of excessive secretion of androgenic hormones.

Disorders of the Nail

1. Paronychia is an inflammation of the cuticle that can be acute or chronic. It is usually caused by staphylococci, streptococci, or fungi.
2. Onychomycosis is a fungal infection of the nail plate.

Aging & Changes in Skin Integrity

1. Skin becomes thinner, drier, and more wrinkled.
2. Wound healing decreases.
3. Fewer melanocytes means pigmentation becomes irregular, providing less protection from ultraviolet light.

KEY TERMS

Acne rosacea, 1025
Acne vulgaris, 1025
Actinic keratosis, 1031
Allergic contact dermatitis, 1022
Alopecia, 1039
Alopecia areata, 1039
Androgenic alopecia, 1039
Apocrine sweat gland, 1014
Atopic dermatitis (allergic dermatitis), 1022
Basal cell carcinoma (BCC), 1032
Bullous erythema multiforme, 1026
Burn shock, 1036
Candidiasis, 1029
Capillary seal, 1037
Carbuncle, 1027
Cellulitis, 1027
Chronic urticaria, 1030
Condylomata acuminata (venereal warts), 1029
Cutaneous melanoma, 1033
Cutaneous vasculitis, 1030
Deep partial-thickness burn, 1036
Dermal appendage, 1014
Dermatitis, 1022

Dermis, 1014
Discoid (cutaneous) lupus erythematosus (DLE), 1025
Eccrine sweat gland, 1014
Eczema, 1022
Epidermis, 1014
Erysipelas, 1027
Erythema multiforme, 1026
Erythrodermic (exfoliative) psoriasis, 1023
Escharotomy, 1036
First-degree burn, 1035
Folliculitis, 1027
Fourth-degree burn, 1036
Frostbite injury, 1038
Furuncle, 1027
Guttate psoriasis, 1023
Herald patch, 1024
Herpes simplex virus (HSV), 1028
Herpes zoster (shingles), 1028
Hirsutism, 1039
Human papillomavirus (HPV), 1028
Hydradenitis suppurativa (inverse acne), 1025
Hypertrophic scar, 1021

Impetigo, 1027
Inverse psoriasis, 1023
Irritant contact dermatitis, 1022
Kaposi sarcoma (KS), 1034
Keloid, 1021
Keratoacanthoma, 1031
Lichen planus (LP), 1024
Lip cancer, 1033
Localized scleroderma (morphea), 1030
Lupus erythematosus, 1025
Lyme disease, 1027
Mycosis fungoides, 1035
Necrotizing fasciitis, 1027
Nevus (pl., nevi), 1031
Onychomycosis (tinea unguium), 1039
Papillary capillary, 1015
Papulosquamous disorder, 1023
Paronychia, 1039
Pemphigus, 1026
Pityriasis rosea, 1024
Plaque psoriasis, 1023
Pressure injury, 1016
Primary cutaneous lymphoma, 1034
Psoriasis, 1023

Psoriatic arthritis, 1023
Psoriatic nail disease, 1023
Pustular psoriasis, 1023
Sebaceous gland, 1014
Seborrheic dermatitis, 1023
Seborrheic keratosis, 1031
Second-degree burn, 1035
Squamous cell carcinoma (SCC), 1032
Stasis dermatitis, 1022
Stevens-Johnson syndrome (SJS), 1026
Subcutaneous layer (hypodermis), 1014
Systemic scleroderma, 1030
Third-degree burn (full-thickness burn), 1036
Tinea infection, 1029
Total body surface area (TBSA), 1036
Toxic epidermal necrolysis (TEN), 1026
Urticaria (hives), 1030
Urticarial lesion, 1030
Varicella (chickenpox), 1028
Wart (verrucae), 1028

REFERENCES

1. Westby MJ, et al: Dressings and topical agents for treating pressure ulcers, *Cochrane Database Syst Rev* (6):CD011947, 2017.
2. Lee HJ, Jang YJ: Recent understandings of biology, prophylaxis and treatment strategies for hypertrophic scars and keloids, *Int J Mol Sci* 19(3):E711, 2018.
3. Nowak D, Yeung J: Diagnosis and treatment of pruritus, *Can Fam Physician* 63(12):918-924, 2017. Review: Erratum in: *Can Fam Physician* 64(2):92, 2018.
4. Burkhart C, Schloemer J, Zirwas M: Differentiation of latex allergy from irritant contact dermatitis, *Cutis* 96(6):369-371, 401, 2015.
5. Sundaresan S, Migden MR, Silapunt S: Stasis dermatitis: pathophysiology, evaluation, and management, *Am J Clin Dermatol* 18(3):383-390, 2017.
6. Dessinioti C, Katsambas A: Seborrheic dermatitis: etiology, risk factors, and treatments: facts and controversies, *Clin Dermatol* 31(4):343-351, 2013.
7. Conrad C, Gilliet M: Psoriasis: from pathogenesis to targeted rherapies, *Clin Rev Allergy Immunol* 54(1):102-113, 2018.
8. Woo YR, Cho DH, Park HJ: Molecular mechanisms and management of a cutaneous inflammatory disorder: psoriasis, *Int J Mol Sci* 18(12):E2684, 2017.
9. Liau MM, Oon HH: Therapeutic drug monitoring of biologics in psoriasis, *Biologics.* 13:127-132, 2019.
10. Ogawa E, et al: Pathogenesis of psoriasis and development of treatment, *J Dermatol* 45(3):264-272, 2018.

11. Drago F, et al: Pityriasis rosea: a comprehensive classification, *Dermatology* 232(4):431-437, 2016.
12. Mahajan K, et al: Pityriasis rosea: an update on etiopathogenesis and management of difficult aspects, *Indian J Dermatol* 61(4):375-384, 2016.
13. Arnold DL, Krishnamurthy K: *Lichen, planus, StatPearls [Internet]*, Treasure Island FL, 2018, StatPearls Publishing. Available from: http://www.ncbi.nlm.nih.gov/books/NBK526126/. Last update March 21, 2019.
14. Ahn CS, Huang WW: Rosacea pathogenesis, *Dermatol Clin* 36(2):81-86, 2018.
15. Ribero S, et al: The cutaneous spectrum of lupus erythematosus, *Clin Rev Allergy Immunol* 53(3):291-305, 2017.
16. Zhang YP, et al: Pathogenesis of cutaneous lupus erythema associated with and without systemic lupus erythema, *Autoimmun Rev* 16(7):735-742, 2017.
17. Kasperkiewicz M, et al: Pemphigus, *Nat Rev Dis Primers* 3:17026, 2017.
18. Lerch M, et al: Current perspectives on erythema multiforme, *Clin Rev Allergy Immunol* 54(1):177-184, 2018.
19. Schneider JA, Cohen PR: Stevens-Johnson syndrome and toxic epidermal necrolysis: a concise review with a comprehensive summary of therapeutic interventions emphasizing supportive measures, *Adv Ther* 34(6):1235-1244, 2017.
20. Russo A, et al: Current and future trends in antibiotic therapy of acute bacterial skin and skin-structure infections, *Clin Microbiol Infect* 22(Suppl 2):S27-S36, 2016.

21. Michael Y, Shaukat NM: *Erysipelas, StatPearls [Internet]*, Treasure Island FL, 2019, StatPearls Publishing. Available from: http://www.ncbi.nlm.nih.gov/books/NBK532247/. Last update February 3, 2019.
22. Steere AC, et al: Lyme borreliosis, *Nat Rev Dis Primers* 2:16090, 2016.
23. Miranda-Saksena M, et al: Infection and transport of herpes simplex virus type 1 in neurons: role of the cytoskeleton, *Viruses* 10(2):E92, 2018.
24. Garland SM, Steben M: Genital herpes, *Best Pract Res Clin Obstet Gynaecol* 28(7):1098-1110, 2014.
25. James SF, et al: Shingrix: the new adjuvanted recombinant herpes zoster vaccine, *Ann Pharmacother* 52(7):673-680, 2018.
26. Hancock G, Hellner K, Dorrell L: Therapeutic HPV vaccines, *Best Pract Res Clin Obstet Gynaecol* 47:59-72, 2018.
27. Dadar M, et al: Candida albicans—biology, molecular characterization, pathogenicity, and advances in diagnosis and control—an update, *Microb Pathog* 117:128-138, 2018.
28. Marzano AV, et al: Skin involvement in cutaneous and systemic vasculitis, *Autoimmun Rev* 12(4):467-476, 2013.
29. Moolani Y, Lynde C, Sussman G: Advances in understanding and managing chronic urticaria, *F1000Res* 5:2016.
30. Raker V, et al: Early inflammatory players in cutaneous fibrosis, *J Dermatol Sci* 87(3):228-235, 2017.
31. Asano Y: Systemic sclerosis, *J Dermatol* 45(2):128-138, 2018.

32. Higgins JC, Maher MH, Douglas MS: Diagnosing common benign skin tumors, *Am Fam Physician* 92(7):601-607, 2015.
33. Puig S, Malvehy J: Monitoring patients with multiple nevi, *Dermatol Clin* 31(4):565-577, 2013.
34. Linares MA, Zakaria A, Nizran P: Skin cancer, *Prim Care* 42(4):645-659, 2015.
35. Dl Stefani A, et al: Practical indications for the management of non-melanoma skin cancer patients, *G Ital Dermatol Venereol* 152(3):286-294, 2017.
36. Leonardi GC, et al: Cutaneous melanoma: from pathogenesis to therapy (review), *Int J Oncol* 52(4):1071-1080, 2018.
37. PDQ® Adult Treatment Editorial Board: PDQ Kaposi sarcoma treatment, Bethesda, MD: National Cancer Institute. Available at: https://www.cancer.gov/types/soft-tissue-sarcoma/hp/kaposi-treatment-pdq. Last updated July 27, 2018.

38. Dabaja B: Renaissance of low-dose radiotherapy concepts for cutaneous lymphomas, *Oncol Res Treat* 40(5):255-260, 2017.
39. American Burn Association: Burn incidence and treatment in the United States: 2016 fact sheet. Available at: http://ameriburn.org/resources_factsheet.php.
40. Yu CY, et al: Human body surface area database and estimation formula, *Burns* 36(5):616-629, 2010.
41. Kaddoura I, et al: Burn injury: review of pathophysiology and therapeutic modalities in major burns, *Ann Burns Fire Disasters* 30(2):95-102, 2017.
42. Cancio LC: Initial assessment and fluid resuscitation of burn patients, *Surg Clin North Am* 94(4):741-754, 2014.
43. Jeschke MG: The hepatic response to thermal injury: is the liver important for postburn outcomes?, *Mol Med* 15(9-10):337-351, 2009.

44. Glas GJ, Levi M, Schultz MJ: Coagulopathy and its management in patients with severe burns, *J Thromb Haemost* 14(5):865-874, 2016.
45. Williams FN, Herndon DN: Metabolic and endocrine considerations after burn injury, *Clin Plast Surg* 44(3):541-553, 2017.
46. Fudge J: Preventing and managing hypothermia and frostbite injury, *Sports Health* 8(2):133-139, 2016.
47. Rajabi F, et al: Alopecia areata: a review of disease pathogenesis, *Br J Dermatol* 179(5):1033-101048, 2018.
48. Leggit JC: Acute and chronic paronychia, *Am Fam Physician* 96(1):44-51, 2017.
49. Rosen T, et al: Onychomycosis: epidemiology, diagnosis, and treatment in a changing landscape, *J Drugs Dermatol* 14(3):223-233, 2015.

44

Alterations of the Integument in Children

Noreen Heer Nicol, Sue E. Huether

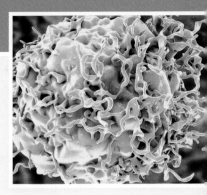

EVOLVE WEBSITE

http://evolve.elsevier.com/Huether/
Student Review Questions
Audio Key Points

Case Studies
Animations
Quick Check Answers

Children frequently develop alterations of the skin, which may be minor or severe and localized or generalized. Skin diseases in children may have different causative mechanisms and different patterns of distribution than those found in adults, although there may be similarities. Some skin diseases resolve spontaneously and require no treatment. Diagnosis is commonly made from the history, appearance, and distribution of the lesion or lesions. Common skin diseases of childhood are presented here.

ACNE VULGARIS

Acne vulgaris is the most common skin disease and occurs primarily between the ages of 12 and 25 years. Acne tends to occur in families, and genetic susceptibility may determine the severity of the disease.

Acne develops at distinctive pilosebaceous units known as *sebaceous follicles.* Located primarily on the face and upper parts of the chest and back, these follicles have many large sebaceous glands, a small vellus hair (very short, nonpigmented, and very thin hair), and a dilated follicular canal that is visible as a pore on the skin surface. Acne lesions may be noninflammatory or inflammatory (cystic) (Fig. 44.1). In noninflammatory acne, the comedones are open (blackheads) and closed (whiteheads), with the accumulated material causing distention of the follicle and thinning of follicular canal walls. Inflammatory (cystic) acne develops in closed comedones when the follicular wall ruptures, expelling sebum into the surrounding dermis and initiating inflammation. Pustules form when the inflammation is close to the surface; papules and cystic nodules can develop when the inflammation

is deeper, causing mild to severe scarring. Both types of lesions may exist in the same individual.

The pathophysiology includes (1) hyperkeratinization of the follicular epithelium; (2) excessive sebum production; (3) follicular proliferation of anaerobic *Cutibacterium acnes (C. acnes,* previously known as *Propionibacterium acnes);* and (4) inflammation and rupture of a follicle from accumulated debris and bacteria (see Fig. 44.1). *C. acnes* shifts from being symbiotic to a pathogenic strain of bacteria and from being noninflammatory to inflammatory The causal mechanism is not completely understood. Androgens (dehydroepiandrosterone sulfate and testosterone), synthesized in increasing amounts during puberty, increase the size and productivity of the sebaceous glands, which promotes proliferation of inflammatory *C. acnes* strains in susceptible individuals A diet high in simple carbohydrates and high glycemic dairy products may be associated with acne by increasing insulin/insulin-like growth factor 1 (IGF-1) that enhances signaling of androgens and overstimulates the nutrient and growth factor-sensitive kinase mechanistic target of rapamycin complex (1mTORC) in pilosebaceous units.[1,2] The result is an alteration of the skin barrier, hyperkeratinization, plugging of the pilosebaceous unit, inflammation, edema, pus formation, and breakdown of the follicle wall.[3]

The treatment of acne should be individualized according to severity. Combinations of a topical retinoid, benzoyl peroxide, and antimicrobial agents are preferred. Retinoids are anticomedogenic and comedolytic, have antiinflammatory effects, and target multiple pathogenic microorganisms associated with acne. Benzoyl peroxide is antimicrobial with some keratolytic effects. Antibiotics have antiinflammatory and

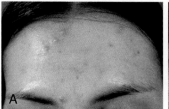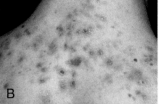

FIGURE 44.1 Acne. A, Inflammatory papules and pustules. B, Severe nodular cystic acne. (From Kliegman RM et al, editors: *Nelson textbook of pediatrics*, ed 19, Philadelphia, 2011, Saunders.)

antimicrobial effects, although stronger recommendations to limit oral antibiotic usage in acne are being made worldwide to avoid development of antibiotic resistance and to promote future effectiveness of the drugs. Use of systemic therapies, including oral antibiotics, sex hormones, corticosteroids, and isotretinoin (requires pregnancy prevention), may be limited by side effects. New drugs are available including immune modulators and inhibitors of proinflammatory cytokines.[1] Acne surgery, including comedo extraction, intralesional steroids, and cryosurgery, is useful in selected individuals. Severe scarring may be treated with dermabrasion, lasers, and resurfacing techniques. Diets should avoid high glycemic index foods. Psychologic support is important because acne negatively affects quality of life, self-esteem, and mood in adolescents and is associated with an increased risk of anxiety, depression, and suicidal ideation. Special consideration must be given to treatment for those with darker skin because they have greater risk for hyperpigmentation and keloidal scarring. Research is continuing on the development of vaccines to prevent acne.[4]

Acne conglobata is a highly inflammatory form of acne with communicating cysts and abscesses beneath the skin that can cause scarring. Remissions tend to occur during the summer, perhaps from more exposure to sunlight. This type of acne requires the use of systemic and combination therapies to prevent drug resistance.

DERMATITIS

Atopic Dermatitis

Atopic dermatitis (AD), also known as atopic eczema, is the most common cause of eczema in children. Individuals with AD may develop asthma and allergies later in life. Onset is usually from 2 to 6 months of age, and most cases develop within the first 5 years of life.

The cause of this chronic relapsing form of pruritic eczema involves an interplay of genetic predisposition; altered skin barrier function associated with filaggrin gene mutations and filaggrin deficiency (proteins that bind keratin in the epidermis); reduced ceramide (a stratum corneum lipid) levels; decreased antimicrobial peptides; altered innate immunity; and altered immune responses to allergens, irritants, and microbes. Filaggrin gene mutations also are associated with increased risk for asthma in AD and ichthyosis vulgaris (dry, scaly skin) (Fig. 44.2). There is an altered skin microbiome with formation of biofilm by *Staphylococcus aureus* that may act as super-antigens causing exacerbations of eczema.[5] Although AD is predominantly associated with type 2 immune responses, activation of T-cell cytokine pathways have been reported, resulting in new therapeutic targets using novel biologic therapy, including treatment of adults.[6]

AD has a constellation of clinical features that include severe pruritus and a characteristic eczematoid appearance with redness, edema, and scaling. The skin becomes increasingly dry, itchy, sensitive, and easily irritated because the barrier function of the skin is impaired. Itching is the hallmark of atopic dermatitis and rubbing and scratching to

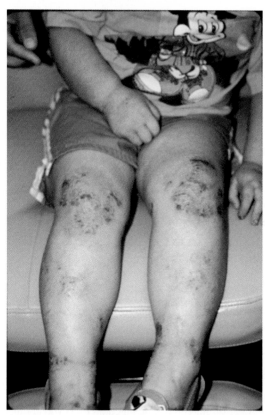

FIGURE 44.2 Atopic Dermatitis. Characteristic lesions with crusting from irritation and scratching over knees and around ankles. (Courtesy Department of Dermatology, School of Medicine, University of Utah, Salt Lake City, Utah.)

relieve the itch are responsible for many of the clinical skin changes of AD. In young children, a rash appears primarily on the face, scalp, trunk, and extensor surfaces of the arms and legs (see Fig. 44.2). In older children and adults, the rash tends to be found on the neck, antecubital and popliteal fossae, and hands and feet. Individuals with AD also tend to develop viral, bacterial, and fungal skin infections in the eczematous areas. There are no specific laboratory features of AD that can be used for diagnostic and treatment purposes. Most affected individuals show increased serum levels of immunoglobulin E (IgE) level, eosinophils (eosinophilia), and positive skin test results to a variety of common food and inhalant allergens.

Management of individuals with AD includes accurate diagnosis and comprehensive evaluation of triggers and response to treatment; management of confounding factors, including sleep disruption; and education of individuals and caregivers. Avoidance of triggers and promotion of skin hydration, including soaking baths and consistent use of an emollient moisturizer, are key to good therapy.[7] Antiinflammatory agents, such as topical corticosteroids and calcineurin inhibitors, are necessary during active flare-ups of eczema. Immunomodulator therapy and wet wrap therapy[8] are used for severe eczema. Systemic therapy for moderate to severe eczema includes the use of sedating antihistamines, antibiotics, and new biologic agents.[8]

Diaper Dermatitis

Diaper dermatitis (diaper rash) is a form of irritant contact dermatitis initiated by a combination of factors including prolonged exposure to and irritation by urine wetness and feces as well as maceration by wet diapers or airtight plastic diaper covers. Disposable diaper designs have decreased the incidence of diaper dermatitis in infants. Diapers with a meshlike, aperture topsheet may represent a better way to mitigate known causes of diaper dermatitis through their superior ability to absorb fecal matter.[9] Often, diaper dermatitis is secondarily infected with *Candida albicans.* The resulting inflammation affects the lower aspect of the abdomen, genitalia, buttock, and upper portion of the thigh.

The lesions vary from mild erythema to erythematous papular lesions and can affect overall infant health. Candidal (monilial) diaper dermatitis is usually very erythematous, with sharp margination and pustulovesicular satellite lesions (Fig. 44.3).

Treatment involves frequent diaper changes to keep the affected area clean and dry or regular exposure of the perineal area to air, use of superabsorbent diapers, and topical protection with a product containing petrolatum or zinc oxide, or both. Topical antifungal medication is used to treat *C. albicans* when present.[10]

✔ QUICK CHECK 44.1
1. What causes the inflammation of acne vulgaris?
2. What lesions are typical of atopic dermatitis in children?
3. What causes diaper dermatitis?

INFECTIONS OF THE SKIN

Infectious diseases caused by bacteria, viruses, and fungi constitute the major forms of skin disease. Breaks in the skin integrity, particularly those that inoculate pathogens into the dermis and epidermis, may cause or exacerbate infections. Most infections tend to occur superficially; however, systemic signs and symptoms develop occasionally and can be life-threatening in immunosuppressed children.

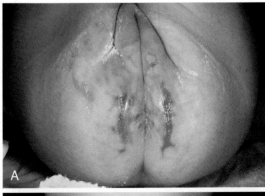

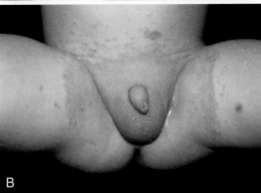

FIGURE 44.3 Diaper Dermatitis. A, Diaper dermatitis with erosions. **B,** Diaper dermatitis with *Candida albicans* secondary infection. (Courtesy Department of Dermatology, School of Medicine, University of Utah, Salt Lake City, Utah.)

Bacterial Infections
Impetigo Contagiosum

Impetigo is the most common bacterial skin infection in children 2 to 5 years of age and is highly contagious. *S. aureus* and, less commonly, *Streptococcus pyogenes* cause impetigo. The mode of transmission is by both direct and indirect contact. The disease is more common in midsummer to late summer, with a higher incidence in hot, humid climates. Impetigo is particularly infectious among people living in crowded conditions with poor sanitary facilities or in settings such as day-care facilities. It affects children in good health, but conditions such as anemia and malnutrition are predisposing factors.

Bacterial invasion occurs through minor breaks in the cutaneous surface or as a secondary infection of a preexisting dermatosis or infestation. The staphylococci produce bacterial toxins called *exfoliative toxins (ETs)* that cause a disruption in the skin barrier with blister formation. There are two types of impetigo: nonbullous and, more rarely, bullous (caused only by *S. aureus*), in which blisters enlarge or coalesce to form bullae. Both forms of impetigo begin as vesicles that rupture to form a honey-colored crust (Fig. 44.4). The lesions are often located on the face, around the nose and mouth, but the hands and other exposed areas also are involved. Impetigo is clinically characterized by crusted erosions or ulcers that may arise as a primary infection or as a secondary infection of a preexisting dermatosis or infestation.

The treatment of choice for both types of impetigo is topical antibiotics (e.g., mupirocin or fusidic acid) for uncomplicated lesions. For extensive or complicated impetigo, systemic antibiotics may be warranted but β-lactam antibiotics should be avoided if methicillin-resistant *Staphylococcus aureus* (MRSA) is suspected. Prompt treatment avoids complications, such as glomerulonephritis, necrotizing fasciitis, and septic shock syndrome. Lesions usually resolve in 2 to 3 weeks without scarring. Using good handwashing techniques and isolating the infected child's washcloth, towels, drinking glass, and linen are important for prevention.[11]

Staphylococcal Scalded-Skin Syndrome

Staphylococcal scalded-skin syndrome (SSSS), also known as Ritter disease, is considered a pediatric emergency. It is the most serious staphylococcal infection that affects the skin and usually occurs in infants within 48 hours after birth and children younger than 5 years of age. SSSS is caused by virulent group II strains of staphylococci that produce an exfoliative toxin. The toxin attacks desmoglein and keratinocyte adhesion molecules and causes a separation of the skin just below the

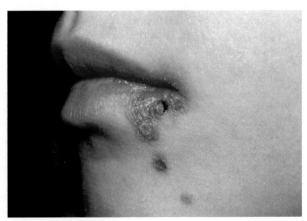

FIGURE 44.4 Impetigo. Multiple crusted and oozing lesions of impetigo. (From Kliegman RM et al, editors: *Nelson textbook of pediatrics,* ed 19, Philadelphia, 2011, Saunders.)

granular layer of the epidermis with blister formation[12] (see Fig. 43.1). The toxin is usually produced at body sites other than the skin and arrives at the epidermis through the circulatory system. Staphylococci typically are not found in the skin lesions themselves. Adults have circulating antistaphylococcal antibodies and are better able to metabolize and excrete the toxin. Neonates are at the highest risk because of their lack of immunity with no prior exposure to the toxin.

The clinical symptoms begin with fever, malaise, rhinorrhea, and irritability followed by generalized erythema with exquisite tenderness of the skin. There may be an associated impetigo, but the infection often begins in the throat or chest. The erythema spreads from the face and trunk to cover the entire body except for the palms, soles, and mucous membranes. The diagnosis is mainly clinical, based on the findings of tender erythroderma, bullae, and desquamation with a scalded appearance, especially in friction zones, periorificial scabs/crusting, positive Nikolsky sign, and absence of mucosal involvement. Within 48 hours, blisters and bullae may form, giving the child the appearance of being scalded. The pain is severe (Fig. 44.5). Fluid loss from ruptured blisters and water evaporation from denuded areas may cause dehydration. Perioral and nasolabial crusting and fissures develop. In severe cases, the skin of the entire body may slough. When secondary infection can be prevented, healing of the involved skin occurs in 10 to 14 days, usually without scarring.

Before medical intervention is initiated, culture and histologic or exfoliative cytologic studies must be performed to differentiate SSSS from *erythema multiforme* and *toxic epidermal necrolysis* (TEN), both of which are usually caused by an immune reaction to drugs (see Chapter 43). When SSSS infection is confirmed, treatment with oral or intravenous antibiotics begins. The skin should be treated in the same manner as a severe burn, with meticulous aseptic technique. Special care is required when there is involvement of the lips and eyelids. Infection control practices are important for prevention.[13]

Fungal Infections
Tinea Capitis

Tinea capitis, a fungal infection of the scalp (scalp ringworm), is the most common fungal infection of childhood. It rarely affects infants and is seen in children between 2 and 10 years of age. The primary microorganism responsible for this disease in North America is *Trichophyton tonsurans*. There is direct human transmission of *T. tonsurans* in crowded areas, the most prevalent environment of the fungus, and also from contact with infected cats and dogs.

The lesions are often circular and manifested by broken hairs 1 to 3 mm above the scalp, leaving a partial area of alopecia from 1 to 5 cm in diameter (Fig. 44.6). A slight erythema and scaling with raised borders can be observed.

Diagnosis is best confirmed by potassium hydroxide (KOH) examination, and fungal culture and dermoscopy can be helpful. Tinea capitis always requires systemic treatment because topical antifungal agents do not penetrate the hair follicle. Several oral antifungal agents are available for treatment.[14]

Tinea Corporis

Tinea corporis (ringworm) is a common superficial dermatophyte infection in children. The organisms most commonly responsible for this disease are *Microsporum canis* and *Trichophyton mentagrophytes*. As in tinea capitis, contact with kittens and puppies is a common source of the disorder. Tinea corporis preferentially affects the nonhairy parts of the face, trunk, and limbs. Lesions are often erythematous, round or oval scaling patches that spread peripherally with clearing in the center, creating the ring appearance, which is why this disease is commonly referred to as *ringworm*. The lesions are distributed asymmetrically, and multiple lesions, when present, overlap. Transmission occurs by direct contact with an infected lesion and through indirect contact with personal items used by the infected person. KOH examination of the scale from the border of the lesions confirms the diagnosis. Most lesions respond well to applications of appropriate topical antifungal medications.

Thrush

Thrush is the term used to describe the presence of *C. albicans* in the mucous membranes of the mouths of infants. It occurs less commonly in adults, and infected adults are usually immunocompromised. *C. albicans* penetrates the epidermal barrier more easily than other microorganisms because of its keratolytic proteases and other enzymes. Thrush is characterized by the formation of white plaques or spots in the mouth that lead to shallow ulcers caused by keratolytic proteases from the microorganism. The tongue may have a dense, white covering. The underlying mucous membrane is red and tender and may bleed when the plaques are removed. The disease is often accompanied by fever and gastrointestinal irritation. The infection commonly spreads to the groin, buttocks, and other parts of the body. Treatment may be difficult and includes oral antifungal washes, such as nystatin oral

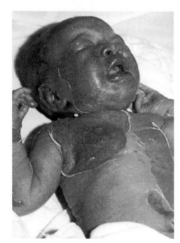

FIGURE 44.5 Staphylococcal Scalded-Skin Syndrome (SSSS). The skin lesions, showing desquamation and wrinkling of the skin margins, appeared 1 day after drainage of a staphylococcal abscess. (From Kliegman RM et al: *Nelson textbook of pediatrics*, ed 19, St Louis, 2011, Saunders.)

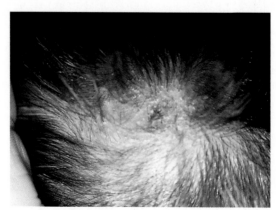

FIGURE 44.6 Tinea Capitis. (Courtesy Department of Dermatology, School of Medicine, University of Utah, Salt Lake City, Utah.)

suspension. Simultaneous treatment of a *Candida* nipple infection or vaginitis in the mother is helpful in reducing the *C. albicans* surface colonization of the infant. Feeding bottles and nipples should be sterilized to prevent reinfection. The diaper area should be kept clean and dry.

Viral Infections

Viral infections of the skin in children are caused by poxvirus, papovavirus, and herpesvirus.

Molluscum Contagiosum

Molluscum contagiosum is a common, highly contagious viral infection of the skin and, occasionally, conjunctiva that affects school-aged children, sexually active young adults, and immunocompromised individuals. The incidence is higher among children who swim or have eczema; however, the mechanism of disease is not clear.[15] The disease is transmitted by skin-to-skin contact or from autoinoculation.

Molluscum contagiosum virus (MCV) is the sole member of the *Molluscipoxvirus* genus and the causative agent of molluscum contagiosum. The poxvirus proliferates within the follicular epithelium and induces epidermal cell proliferation. The epidermis grows down into the dermis to form saccules containing clusters of virus. The characteristic molluscum body is composed of mature, immature, and incomplete viruses and cellular debris.[16]

The lesions of molluscum are discrete, slightly umbilicated, dome-shaped papules 1 to 5 mm in diameter that appear anywhere on the skin or conjunctiva. The lesions are mainly on the trunk, face, and extremities in children (Fig. 44.7). There is usually no inflammation surrounding molluscum lesions unless they are traumatized or secondary infection occurs. Scarring may occur with healing.

The three best diagnostic procedures are (1) staining smears of the expressed molluscum body, (2) examining a biopsy specimen, or (3) inoculating a molluscum suspension into cell cultures to demonstrate the cytotoxic reactions. Most lesions are self-limiting and clear in 6 to 9 months if not manipulated.

Treatment options include immunomodulatory and antiviral therapy and destructive procedures (cryotherapy, curettage, or laser ablation); however, no treatment is universally effective. KOH solution applications can be safe, effective, and inexpensive. Treatment is recommended for genital molluscum to prevent sexual transmission and autoinoculation. Measures to prevent spread of infection must be taken. Recurrences are common.[17]

Rubella (German or 3-Day Measles)

Rubella is a common communicable disease of children and young adults caused by a ribonucleic acid (RNA) virus that enters the bloodstream through the respiratory route. This disease is mild in most children. The incubation period ranges from 14 to 21 days. Prodromal symptoms include enlarged cervical and postauricular lymph nodes, low-grade fever, headache, sore throat, rhinorrhea, and cough. A faint-pink to red coalescing maculopapular rash develops on the face with spread to the trunk and extremities 1 to 4 days after the onset of initial symptoms (Fig. 44.8). The rash is thought to be the result of virus dissemination to the skin. The rash subsides after 2 to 3 days, usually without complication. Children are usually not contagious after development of the rash (Table 44.1).

Vaccination for rubella is usually combined with vaccines for mumps and measles (rubeola) (MMR). Measles is known to occur in previously immunized children. The Centers for Disease Control and Prevention vaccine recommendations are available at https://www.cdc.gov/vaccines/schedules/hcp/child-adolescent.html. Rubella has almost been eliminated in the United States because of vaccination campaigns. However, challenges to maintain elimination include large outbreaks of measles in highly traveled developed countries, frequent international travel, and clusters of U.S. residents who remain unvaccinated because of personal belief exemptions. Although MMR vaccine may rarely be associated with adverse neurologic events, studies conclude that MMR immunization does not cause autism. Lack of vaccination, however, leads to loss of herd immunity and significant morbidity and mortality with pneumonia, croup, and encephalitis being causes of death worldwide.

Women of childbearing age are immunized if their rubella hemagglutination-inhibition titer is low. Pregnancy should be avoided for

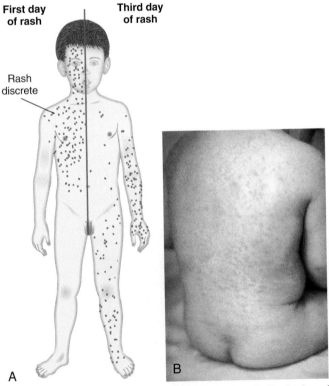

FIGURE 44.8 Rubella (3-Day Measles). **A,** Typical distribution of full-blown maculopapular rash with tendency to coalesce. **B,** Rash of rubella. (From Centers for Disease Control and Prevention: Image Bank, Figure #712. Available from <https://www.cdc.gov/rubella/about/photos.html>, accessed October 11, 2015.)

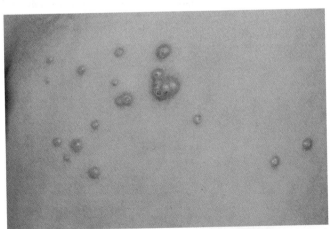

FIGURE 44.7 Molluscum Contagiosum. Waxy pink globules with umbilicated centers. (From Habif TP: *Clinical dermatology: a color guide to diagnosis and therapy,* ed 4, St Louis, 2004, Mosby.)

TABLE 44.1   Differential Presentation of Viral Diseases Producing Rashes

Viral Disease	Incubation	Prodromal Symptoms	Duration/Characteristics	Clinical Symptoms
Rubella (German measles; rubivirus)	14-21 days	1-2 days Mild fever Malaise Respiratory symptoms	1-3 days Pink-red maculopapular rash Face and trunk	Enlarged and tender occipital and periauricular lymph nodes
Rubeola (measles; paramyxovirus)	7-12 days	2-5 days Fever Cough Respiratory symptoms	3-5 days Purple-red to brown maculopapular papules Face, trunk, extremities	Koplik spots*1-3 days before rash Rash develops when fever subsides
Roseola (exanthema subitum; human herpesvirus 6 and 7)	5-15 days	2-5 days High fever	1-3 days Pink-red macular papules Neck and trunk	
Varicella (chickenpox; herpes zoster virus)	11-20 days	1-2 days Low-grade fever Cough May be asymptomatic	Red papules, vesicles, pustules in clusters	Eruption of new lesions for 4-5 days Occasional ulcerative lesion in mouth
Hand, foot, and mouth disease (coxsackie A virus)	4-6 days	Fever, sore throat, anorexia	3-7 days Gray thick-walled vesicles 3-6 mm in diameter with a red or noninflamed base, commonly on palms, soles and sides of feet, and mouth mucosa	None or fever, diarrhea, sore throat

*Koplic spots: clusters of white lesions on the lower buccal mucosa.

3 months after vaccination because the attenuated virus in the vaccine may remain viable for this period. Pregnant women who have rubella early in the first trimester may have a fetus who develops congenital defects.

There is no specific treatment for rubella. Recovery is spontaneous, although lymph nodes may remain enlarged for weeks. Supportive therapy includes rest, fluids, and use of a vaporizer. In rare cases, a mild encephalitis or peripheral neuritis may follow rubella.[18]

Rubeola (Red Measles)

Rubeola is a highly contagious, acute viral disease of childhood. Transmitted by direct contact with droplets from infected persons, rubeola is caused by an RNA-containing paramyxovirus with an incubation period of 7 to 12 days, during which there are no symptoms. The virus enters the respiratory tract and attaches to alveolar macrophages, amplifies in local lymphatic tissue, and progresses to systemic disease. Prodromal symptoms include high fever (up to 40.5° C [104.9° F]), malaise, enlarged lymph nodes, rhinorrhea, conjunctivitis, and barking cough. Within 3 to 4 days, an erythematous maculopapular rash develops over the head and spreads distally over the trunk, extremities, hands, and feet. Early lesions blanch with pressure, followed by a brownish hue that does not blanch as the rash fades. Characteristic pinpoint white spots surrounded by an erythematous ring develop over the buccal mucosa and are known as *Koplik spots*. These spots precede the rash by 1 to 2 days. The rash then subsides within 3 to 5 days.

Complications associated with measles may be caused by the primary infection or by a secondary bacterial infection. Measles encephalitis occurs rarely, and most children recover completely; only a small minority of children develop permanent brain damage or die. Bacterial complications include otitis media and pneumonia, usually caused by group A hemolytic *Streptococcus*, *Haemophilus influenzae*, or *S. aureus* infection.

Measles is prevented by vaccination. As discussed in the Rubella section, immunization is key to prevention. There is no specific treatment for measles, and supportive therapy is the same as that recommended for rubella. Antibiotic therapy is initiated if secondary bacterial infections develop.

Roseola (Exanthema Subitum)

Roseola is a human herpesviruses 6 or 7 infection of children between 6 months and 2 years of age and can be seen in children up to 4 years of age. The incubation period is 5 to 15 days, followed by the sudden onset of fever (38.9° to 40.5° C [102° to 104.9° F]) that lasts 3 to 5 days. After the fever, an erythematous macular rash that lasts about 24 hours develops primarily over the trunk and neck. Children usually feel well, eat normally, and have few other symptoms. There is usually no treatment.

Small Pox

Smallpox (variola) was a highly contagious and deadly, but also preventable, disease caused by poxvirus variolae. Smallpox was eradicated worldwide in 1977. Routine vaccination in the United States was discontinued in 1972, and a new vaccine, ACAM2000, has been produced for the U.S. Strategic National Stockpile. Information is available from the U.S. Food and Drug Administration at http://www.fda.gov/BiologicsBloodVaccines/Vaccines/QuestionsaboutVaccines/ucm078041.htm (last updated: 03/23/2018).

Chickenpox

Chickenpox (varicella) is a disease of early childhood, with 90% of unvaccinated children contracting the disease during the first decade of life. Being a highly contagious virus, chickenpox is spread by close person-to-person contact and by airborne droplets. Introduction of an infected person into a household results in a 90% possibility of susceptible persons developing the disease within the incubation period, usually 14 days. Vesicular lesions occur in the epidermis as infection occurs within keratinocytes. An inflammatory infiltrate is often present. Vesicles eventually rupture, followed by crust formation or the development of transient ulcers on mucous membranes. Children are contagious for at least 1 day before development of the lesions. Transmission of the virus may occur until approximately 5 to 6 days after the onset of the first skin lesions in healthy children. In immunocompromised children, the virus is recoverable for a longer period, but infected children must be considered contagious for at least 7 to 10 days.

Normally, children who develop chickenpox have no prodromal symptoms. The first sign of illness may be pruritus or the appearance of vesicles, usually on the trunk, scalp, or face. The rash later spreads to the extremities. Characteristically, lesions can be seen in various stages of maturation with macules, papules, and vesicles present in a particular area at the same time (Fig. 44.9). The vesicular lesions are superficial and rupture easily. New lesions will erupt for 4 to 5 days, until there are approximately 100 to 300 in different stages of development. The vesicles become crusted, and over time only the crust remains, although there may be an occasional vesicle on the palm later in the disease. Although uncommon, ulcerative lesions are sometimes seen in the mouth and, less commonly, on the conjunctiva and pharynx. Fever usually lasts 2 to 3 days, with body temperature ranging from 38.5° to 40° C (101.3° to 104° F).

Complications are rare in children but more common in adults. They can include transient hematuria (from rupture of vesicles in the bladder), epistaxis, laryngeal edema, and varicella pneumonia. One case of chickenpox produces almost complete immunity against a second attack. Rarely, the fetus may be malformed (congenital varicella syndrome) if chickenpox develops in the first half of pregnancy. Infants whose mothers have chickenpox at any stage of pregnancy have a higher risk of developing herpes zoster during the first few years of life.[19] Varicella-zoster immunoglobulin should be administered to neonates whenever the onset of maternal disease is between 5 days before and 2 days after delivery.

Uncomplicated chickenpox requires no specific therapy. Baths, wet dressings, and oral antihistamines occasionally help relieve pruritus and prevent secondary infection from developing as a result of scratching. Oral antibiotics should be given if secondary bacterial infection is present. Zoster immune globulin may be administered to immunodeficient individuals if given within 72 hours after exposure to chickenpox. Oral acyclovir may be valuable in immunosuppressed or other select groups of children. The varicella vaccine protects against varicella.[20] Herpes zoster is a vesicular eruption from a recurrence of the latent varicella virus, along the distribution of a dorsal root ganglion (see Chapter 43).

Hand, Foot, and Mouth Disease

Hand, foot, and mouth disease (HFMD) is a contagious viral disease primarily of infants and young children. It is commonly caused by coxsackievirus and enterovirus. The infection manifests as fever; vesicular ulcerous lesions in the mouth; and vesicular rashes on the hands, feet, and buttocks. A small number of children may experience severe complications, such as meningitis, encephalitis, acute flaccid paralysis, and neurorespiratory syndrome. The disease is self-limiting with supportive care. Research is in progress to develop a preventive vaccine.[21]

Erythema Infectiosum (Fifth Disease)

Erythema infectiosum (fifth disease) is cause by infection with B19 parvovirus. The infection is characterized by a mild fever, headache, sore throat, pruritus, and arthralgia followed by a blotchy, maculopopular, lacy rash on the cheeks (slapped-cheek), which spreads to the trunk and limbs and may last for up to 6 weeks. Symptoms are usually self-limiting. Diagnosis is related to symptoms and can include immunologic assays or a polymerase chain reaction test to identify the virus.[22] Treatment is symptomatic and includes nonsteroidal antiinflammatory drugs for arthralgias and antihistamines for pruritus. Infection in women less than 20 weeks pregnant can lead to miscarriage and requires special care.

> ✔ **QUICK CHECK 44.2**
> 1. Compare the cause and presentation of impetigo and staphylococcal scalded-skin syndrome.
> 2. Describe rubella and rubeola.
> 3. How are chickenpox and herpes zoster related?

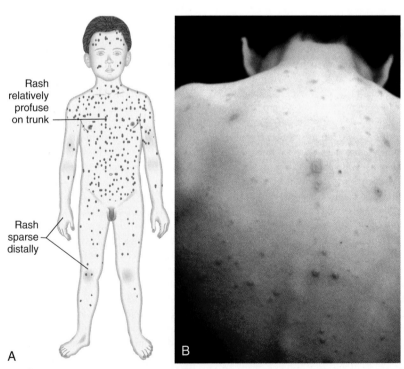

Rash relatively profuse on trunk

Rash sparse distally

A   B

FIGURE 44.9 Chickenpox. A, Pattern of generalized, polymorphous eruption. **B,** Chickenpox lesions. (From Centers for Disease Control and Prevention: Image Bank, Figure #6121. Available from <https://phil.cdc.gov/details.aspx?pid=6121>, accessed October 11, 2018.)

INSECT BITES AND PARASITES

Insect bites and infestations are common causes of skin disorders in children and adults. Skin damage occurs by various mechanisms, including trauma of bites and stings, allergic reactions, transmission of disease, injection of substances that cause local or systemic reactions, and inflammatory reactions resulting from embedded and retained insect mouth parts and scratching of the skin.

Scabies

Scabies is a contagious disease caused by the itch mite *Sarcoptes scabiei* (Fig. 44.10, *A*), which can colonize the human epidermis. It is transmitted by close personal contact and by infected clothing and bedding. Scabies is often epidemic in areas of overcrowded housing, with poor sanitation, and in children. Immunocompromised individuals are at greater risk. Scabies can facilitate *S. pyogenes* and *S. aureus* skin coinfections with systemic complications. The scabies mite has adapted mechanisms to overcome host defenses. Infestation is initiated by a female mite that tunnels into the skin, depositing eggs, and creating a burrow several millimeters to 1 cm long. Over a 3-week period, the eggs mature into adult mites, which sometimes are recognized as tiny dots at the ends of intact burrows.

Symptoms appear 3 to 5 weeks after infestation. The primary lesions are burrows, papules, and vesicular lesions, with intense pruritus that worsens at night. Pruritus is thought to be related to immune and inflammatory responses. In older children and adults, the lesions occur in the webs of fingers; in the axillae; in the creases of the arms and wrists; along the belt line; and around the nipples, genitalia, and lower buttocks. Infants and young children have a different pattern of distribution, with involvement of the palms, soles, head, neck, and face (see Fig. 44.10, *B*). Secondary infections and crusting develop as a result of scratching and eczematous changes.

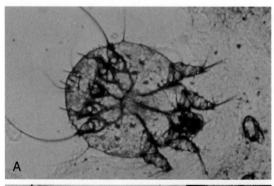

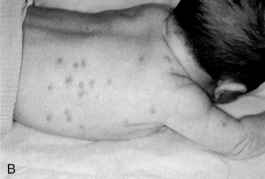

FIGURE 44.10 Scabies. A, Scabies mite, as seen clinically when removed from its burrow. **B,** Characteristic scabies bites. (Courtesy Department of Dermatology, School of Medicine, University of Utah, Salt Lake City, Utah.)

Diagnosis of scabies is made by observation of the tunnels and burrows and by microscopic examination of scrapings of the skin to identify the mite or its eggs or feces. Treatment involves the application of a scabicide, which is curative. All clothing and linens should be washed and dried in hot cycles or dry-cleaned. Development of a protective vaccine is in progress.[23]

Pediculosis (Lice Infestation)

The three known types of human lice are (1) the head louse *(Pediculus capitis),* (2) the body louse *(Pediculus corporis),* and (3) the crab or pubic louse *(Phthirus pubis).* They are parasites and survive by sucking blood. The female louse reproduces every 2 weeks, producing hundreds of nits as newly hatched lice mate with older lice. The mouthparts are shaped for piercing and sucking and are attached to the skin of the host while the louse is feeding. When piercing the skin, the louse secretes toxic saliva, and the mechanical trauma and toxin produce a pruritic dermatitis. Head and body lice are acquired directly by personal contact or indirectly by sharing of combs, brushes, or towels or contact with infested clothes, toys, furniture, carpets, or bedding. Crab lice are spread by close body contact, usually with an infected adult. Other common sources of transmission include sharing clothing or headphones.

Pruritus is the major symptom of lice infestation. With head lice, the ova attach to hairs above the ears and in the occipital region. The primary lesion caused by the body louse is a pinpoint red macule, papule, or wheal with a hemorrhagic puncture site. The primary lesion often is not seen, because it is masked by excoriations, wheals, and crusts. The crab louse is found on pubic hairs but also may be found in other body hair, such as eyelashes, mustache, beard, and underarm hair. Young children in particular may become infected with crab lice on their eyebrows or eyelashes.

The live louse, 2 to 3 mm long, is rarely observed. The ova, or nits, can be observed as oval, yellowish, pinpoint specks fastened to a hair shaft. The ova fluoresce under an ultraviolet light (Wood's lamp) and are observed best with a microscope. Nits are removed with a nit comb, and pediculicides, such as lindane shampoo or lotion, are the most effective treatment. Success or failure of therapy for ectoparasitic infestation depends on education related to the use of the topical preparation than on the type of scabicide or pediculicide used.[24]

All clothes, towels, bedding, combs, and brushes should be washed and dried in hot air or instead washed in boiling water, or clothes can be ironed to rid them of lice. Individuals who have close personal contact with the infected person also should be treated.

Fleas

Young children are very susceptible to fleabites. Bites occur in clusters along the arms and legs or where clothing is tight fitting, such as near elastic bands that circle the thigh or waist. The bite produces an urticarial wheal with a central hemorrhagic puncture (Fig. 44.11). Itching can be controlled with antihistamines.[25] Treatment includes spraying carpets, crevices, and furniture with malathion or lindane powder. Infected animals should be treated, and clothes and bedding should be washed in hot water.

Bedbugs

Bedbugs *(Cimex lectularius)* are blood-sucking parasites that live in the crevices and cracks of floors, walls, and furniture and in bedding or furniture stuffing. They are 3 to 5 mm long and reddish brown. Bedbugs are nocturnal, emerging to feed in darkness by attaching to the skin to suck blood, and are attracted by warmth and carbon dioxide. Feeding occurs for 5 to 15 minutes, and the bedbug then leaves and can survive for a year from one feeding. It will move long distances to search for food and can travel from house to house.

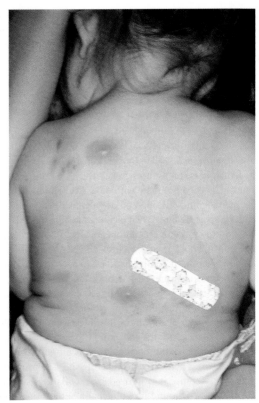

FIGURE 44.11 Fleabites. Fleabite producing a urticarial wheal with central puncture.

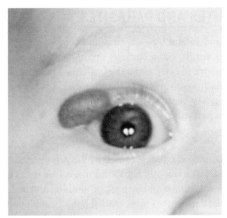

FIGURE 44.12 Superficial (Capillary) Hemangioma. (Courtesy Department of Dermatology, School of Medicine, University of Utah, Salt Lake City, Utah.)

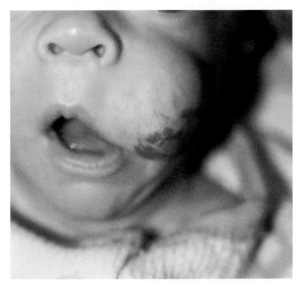

FIGURE 44.13 Deep Hemangioma. (Courtesy Department of Dermatology, School of Medicine, University of Utah, Salt Lake City, Utah.)

Immunologic reactions to bedbug saliva vary, but bites typically yield erythematous and pruritic papules. The face and distal extremities, areas uncovered by sleeping clothes or blankets, are preferentially involved. If the host has not been previously sensitized, the only symptom is a red macule that develops into a nodule, lasting up to 14 days. In sensitized children and adults, pruritic wheals, papules, and vesicles may form. Most lesions respond to oral antihistamines or topical corticosteroids, or both. Secondary infections require antibiotic treatment. Bedbugs are eliminated by inspecting and cleaning or disposing of bedding, mattresses, furniture, and other contaminated items and by using applications of approved insecticides, usually by a professional.[26]

CUTANEOUS HEMANGIOMAS AND VASCULAR MALFORMATIONS

Cutaneous vascular anomalies are frequent tumors of early infancy and are categorized as either hemangiomas or vascular malformations.

Cutaneous Hemangiomas

Cutaneous hemangiomas are benign tumors that form from the rapid growth of vascular endothelial cells, which results in formation of extra blood vessels. Hemangiomas can be superficial or deep. The etiology may be related to embolization of fetal placental endothelial cells with placental trauma or loss of placental angiogenic inhibitor of placental and maternal origin.

Superficial hemangiomas (previously known as infantile hemangiomas) are associated with expression of endothelial glucose transporter 1 (GLUT1), an erythrocyte-type glucose transporter protein. Infiltration of fat cells, fibrosis, and the rich vascular network give the lesions a

firm, rubbery feel. Female children are affected more often than male children. Some superficial hemangiomas are apparent at birth, but usually emerge 3 to 5 weeks after birth. They grow rapidly during the first few years of life and become bright red and elevated with minute capillary projections that give them a strawberry appearance. Only one lesion is usually present and is located on the head and neck area or trunk (Fig. 44.12). After the initial growth, the lesion grows at the same rate as the child and then starts to involute at 12 to 16 months of age. Most superficial hemangiomas involute by 5 to 9 years of age, usually without scarring and require no treatment. Hemangiomas located over the eye, ear, nose, mouth, urethra, or anus may require treatment because they interfere with function and have a higher risk for infection or injury.[27]

Deep hemangiomas (previously known as cavernous hemangiomas) are a rare variant of superficial hemangiomas and located deeper in the dermis or subcutaneous tissue (Fig. 44.13). They are present and fully grown at birth and are usually solitary lesions on the head or limbs that appear as a spongy purplish mass of tissue. They have larger and more mature vessels within the lesion. There are two groups of deep hemangiomas: rapidly involuting and noninvoluting. Rapidly involuting deep hemangiomas disappear by 12 months to 14 months of age, leaving an area of thin skin. Noninvoluting cavernous hemangiomas do not undergo involution.

Rapidly progressing hemangiomas are treated with a beta blocker (e.g., propranolol), with regression occurring within 2 weeks, and should be considered a first-line agent. Other therapies include systemic or intralesional steroids and ablative procedures. Interferons, vincristine, cyclophosphamide, and radiotherapy can suppress angiogenesis.

Cutaneous Vascular Malformations

Cutaneous vascular malformations are rare congenital malformations present at birth but may not be apparent for several years.[28] They grow proportionately with the child and never regress. Occasionally they expand rapidly, particularly during the hormonal changes of puberty or pregnancy and in association with trauma. Vascular malformations are classified as low flow or high flow. *Low-flow malformations* involve capillaries, veins, and lymphatics. *High-flow malformations* involve arteries. The most common capillary malformations are nevus flammeus (port-wine stains) and salmon patches (stork bite, angel kiss).

Port-wine (nevus flammeus) stains are congenital malformations of the dermal capillaries. The lesions are flat, and their color ranges from pink to dark reddish purple. They are present at birth or within a few days after birth and do not fade with age. Involvement of the face and other body surfaces is common, and the lesions may be large (Fig. 44.14). Overgrowth of underlying structures (i.e., legs, arms, facial bones) also can occur. The pulsed dye laser is the treatment of choice to successfully lighten the color and flatten the more nodular and cavernous lesions. Waterproof cosmetics may be used to cover the lesions.

Salmon patches (nevus simplex) are macular pink lesions present at birth and located on the nape of the neck, forehead, upper eyelids, or nasolabial fold region. They are a variant of port-wine stains, more superficial, and one of the most common congenital malformations in the skin. The pink color results from distended dermal capillaries, and most of the patches fade by 1 year of age. Those located at the nape of the neck may persist for a lifetime. They generally do not present a cosmetic problem.

OTHER SKIN DISORDERS

Miliaria

Miliaria is a dermatosis commonly seen in infants that is characterized by a vesicular eruption after prolonged exposure to perspiration with subsequent obstruction of the eccrine ducts. There are two forms of miliaria: miliaria crystallina and miliaria rubra. In miliaria crystallina, ductal rupture occurs within the stratum corneum and appears as 1- to 2-mm clear vesicles without erythema. They rupture within 24 to 48 hours and leave a white scale. In miliaria rubra (prickly heat), the ductal rupture occurs in the lower epidermis with inflammatory cells attracted to the site of the rupture. Miliaria rubra is characterized by 2- to 4-mm discrete erythematous papules or papulovesicles (Fig. 44.15). Both forms may become secondarily infected, requiring systemic antibiotics. The key to management is avoidance of excessive heat and humidity, which cause sweating. Light clothing, cool baths, and air conditioning assist in keeping the skin surface dry and cool.

Erythema Toxicum Neonatorum

Erythema toxicum neonatorum (toxic erythema of the newborn) is a benign, erythematous accumulation of macules, papules, or pustules that appears at birth or 3 to 4 days after birth. The lesions first appear as a blotchy, macular erythematous rash. The macules vary from 1 mm to 1 cm in diameter. When papules or pustules develop, they are light yellow or white and 1 to 3 mm in diameter. There may be a few or several hundred lesions, and any body surface can be affected, with the exception of the palms and soles, where there are no pilosebaceous follicles. The cause of the lesion is unknown but may be related to an innate immune response to the first commensal microflora with release of inflammatory mediators. It is self-limiting and resolves spontaneously within a few weeks after birth. No treatment is required.

✔ **QUICK CHECK 44.3**
1. Give two examples of insect bites or parasites that affect children. What features are observed in each?
2. Compare a superficial hemangioma with a vascular malformation.

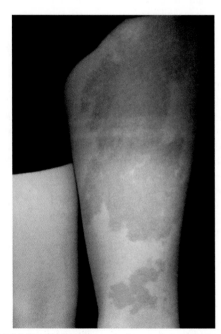

FIGURE 44.14 Port-Wine Hemangioma. Port-wine hemangioma in a child. (Courtesy Department of Dermatology, School of Medicine, University of Utah, Salt Lake City, Utah.)

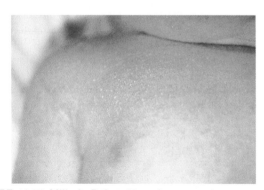

FIGURE 44.15 Miliaria Rubra. Note discrete erythematous papules or papulovesicles. (Courtesy Department of Dermatology, School of Medicine, University of Utah, Salt Lake City, Utah.)

SUMMARY REVIEW

Acne Vulgaris

1. Acne vulgaris is a common disorder related to obstruction of pilo-sebaceous follicles and proliferation of *Cutibacterium acnes*, with follicular occlusion and inflammation primarily of the face, neck, and upper trunk. It is characterized by both noninflammatory and inflammatory lesions. Treatment is dependent on severity.

Dermatitis

1. Atopic dermatitis is an alteration in the skin barrier. It occurs as red, scaly lesions on the face, cheeks, and flexor surfaces of the extremities in infants and young children. Atopic dermatitis is associated with inflammatory cytokines. Individuals may develop asthma and allergies later in life.
2. Diaper dermatitis, or diaper rash, is a type of irritant contact dermatitis that develops from prolonged exposure to urine and feces and often becomes secondarily infected with *Candida albicans*.

Infections of the Skin

1. Impetigo is a contagious bacterial disease occurring in two forms: bullous and vesicular. The toxins from the bacteria produce a weeping lesion with a honey-colored crust.
2. Staphylococcal scalded-skin syndrome (Ritter disease) is a staphylococcal skin infection that produces an exfoliative toxin with painful blisters and bullae formation over large areas of the skin, requiring emergency care and systemic antibiotic treatment.
3. Tinea capitis (scalp ringworm) and tinea corporis (ringworm) are fungal infections of the scalp and body caused by dermatophytes.
4. Thrush is a fungal infection of the mouth caused by *Candida albicans*.
5. Molluscum contagiosum is a poxvirus infection of the skin that produces pale papular lesions filled with viral and cellular debris.
6. Rubella (German or 3-day measles) is a communicable viral disease characterized by fever, sore throat, enlarged cervical and postauricular lymph nodes, and a generalized maculopapular rash that lasts 1 to 4 days.
7. Rubeola (red measles) is a viral contagious disease with symptoms of high fever, enlarged lymph nodes, conjunctivitis, and a red rash that begins on the head, spreads to the trunk and extremities, and lasts 3 to 5 days. Both bacterial and viral complications may accompany rubeola.
8. Roseola (exanthema subitum) is a benign disease of infants with a sudden onset of fever that lasts 3 to 5 days, followed by a rash that lasts 24 hours.
9. Smallpox (variola) was a highly contagious, deadly viral disease that has been eradicated worldwide by vaccination.
10. Chickenpox (varicella) is a highly contagious disease caused by the varicella-zoster virus. Vesicular lesions occur on the skin and mucous membranes. Individuals are contagious from 1 day before the development of the rash until about 5 to 6 days after the rash develops.
11. Hand, foot, and mouth disease is a contagious viral disease commonly caused by coxsackievirus and enterovirus that manifests with fever, vesicular ulcerous lesions in the mouth, and vesicular rashes on the hands, feet, and buttocks.
12. Erythema infectiousum (fifth disease) is an infection caused by B19 parvovirus that usually causes mild symptoms of fever, headache, pruritus, and arthralgias followed by a rash on the cheeks spreading to the trunk and limbs.

Insect Bites and Parasites

1. Scabies is a pruritic lesion caused by the itch mite, which burrows into the skin and forms papules and vesicles. The mite is very contagious and is transmitted by direct contact.
2. Pediculosis (lice infestation) is caused by blood-sucking parasites that secrete toxic saliva and damage the skin to produce pruritic dermatitis. Lice are spread by direct contact and are recognized by the ova or nits that attach to the shafts of body hairs.
3. Fleabites produce a pruritic wheal with a central puncture site and occur as clusters in areas of tight-fitting clothing.
4. Bedbugs are blood-sucking parasites that live in cracks of floors, furniture, or bedding and feed at night. They produce pruritic wheals and nodules.

Cutaneous Hemangiomas and Vascular Malformations

1. Cutaneous hemangiomas are benign tumors that form from the rapid growth of vascular endothelial cells and result in formation of extra blood vessels that can be superficial or deep.
2. Superficial hemangiomas involve infiltration of fat cells, fibrosis, and the rich vascular network, giving the lesions a firm, rubbery feel. Most superficial hemangiomas involute by 5 to 9 years of age.
3. Deep hemangiomas are present at birth, with larger vessels than a superficial hemangioma, and are purplish. Rapidly involuting deep hemangiomas disappear by 12 to 14 months of age, leaving an area of thin skin.
4. Cutaneous vascular malformations are rare congenital anomalies of blood vessels present at birth.
5. Port-wine stains are congenital malformations of dermal capillaries that do not fade with age.
6. Salmon patches are macular pink lesions with dilated capillaries that usually resolve by 1 year of age. They are a variant of port-wine stains.

Other Skin Disorders

1. Miliaria is characterized by a vesicular eruption that results from obstruction of the sweat duct opening in infants. In miliaria crystallina, ductal rupture occurs within the stratum corneum and appears as 1- to 2-mm clear vesicles without erythema. In miliaria rubra (prickly heat), the ductal rupture occurs in the lower epidermis, attracts inflammatory cells, and appears as 2- to 4-mm discrete erythematous papules or papulovesicles
2. Erythema toxicum neonatorum is a benign accumulation of macules, papules, and pustules that spontaneously resolves within a few weeks after birth.

KEY TERMS

REFERENCES

1. Bhat YJ, Latief I, Hassan I: Update on etiopathogenesis and treatment of acne, *Indian J Dermatol Venereol Leprol* 83(3):298-306, 2017.

2. Melnik BC: Acne vulgaris: the metabolic syndrome of the pilosebaceous follicle, *Clin Dermatol* 36(1):29-40, 2018.

3. Dréno B: What is new in the pathophysiology of acne, an overview, *J Eur Acad Dermatol Venereol* 31(Suppl 5):8-12, 2017.

4. Wang Y, et al: The anti-inflammatory activities of *Propionibacterium acnes* CAMP factor-targeted acne vaccines, *J Invest Dermatol* 138(11):2355-2364, 2018.

5. Malik K, Heitmiller KD, Czarnowicki T: An update on the pathophysiology of atopic dermatitis, *Dermatol Clin* 35(3):317-326, 2017.

6. Deleanu D, Nedelea I: Biological therapies for atopic dermatitis: an update, *Exp Ther Med* 17(2):1061-1067, 2019.

7. Fleischer DM, et al: Atopic dermatitis: skin care and topical therapies, *Semin Cutan Med Surg* 36(3):104-110, 2017.

8. Nicol NH, Boguniewicz M: Wet wrap therapy in moderate to severe atopic dermatitis, *Immunol Allergy Clin North Am* 37(1):123-139, 2017.

9. Gustin J, et al: The impact of diaper design on mitigating known causes of diaper dermatitis, *Pediatr Dermatol* 35(6):792-795, 2018.

10. Fölster-Holst R: Differential diagnoses of diaper dermatitis, *Pediatr Dermatol* 35(Suppl 1):s10-s18, 2018.

11. Nardi NM, Schaefer TJ: *Impetigo, StatPearls [Internet]*, Treasure Island FL, 2017, StatPearls Publishing. Available at: http://www.ncbi.nlm.nih.gov/books/NBK430974/.

12. Ross A, Shoff HW: *Staphylococcal scalded skin syndrome, StatPearls [Internet]*, Treasure Island FL, 2019, StatPearls Publishing. Available at: http://www.ncbi.nlm.nih.gov/books/NBK448135/. last updated June 10, 2019.

13. Leung AKC, Barankin B, Leong KF: Staphylococcal-scalded skin syndrome: evaluation, diagnosis, and management, *World J Pediatr* 14(2):116-120, 2018.

14. Gupta AK, et al: Tinea capitis in children: a systematic review of management, *J Eur Acad Dermatol Venereol* 32:2264-2274, 2018.

15. Olsen JR, et al: Epidemiology of molluscum contagiosum in children: a systematic review, *Fam Pract* 31(2):130-136, 2014.

16. Zorec TM, et al: New insights into the evolutionary and genomic landscape of molluscum contagiosum virus (MCV) based on nine MCV1 and six MCV2 complete genome sequences, *Viruses* 10(11):2018.

17. Forbat E, Al-Niaimi F, Ali FR: Molluscum contagiosum: review and update on management, *Pediatr Dermatol* 34(5):504-515, 2017.

18. Spencer JP, Trondsen Pawlowski RH, Thomas S: Vaccine adverse events: separating myth from reality, *Am Fam Physician* 95(12):786-794, 2017.

19. Smith CK, Arvin AM: Varicella in the fetus and newborn, *Semin Fetal Neonatal Med* 14(4):209-217, 2009.

20. Lo Presti C, et al: Chickenpox: an update, *Med Mal Infect* 49(1):1-8, 2019.

21. Esposito S, Principi N: Hand, foot and mouth disease: current knowledge on clinical manifestations, epidemiology, aetiology and prevention, *Eur J Clin Microbiol Infect Dis* 37(3):391-398, 2018.

22. Allmon A, Deane K, Martin KL: Common skin rashes in children, *Am Fam Physician* 92(3):211-216, 2015.

23. Arlian LG, Morgan MS: A review of *Sarcoptes scabiei*: past, present and future, *Parasit Vectors* 10(1):297, 2017.

24. Bragg BN, Simon LV: *Pediculosis humanis (lice, capitis, pubis), StatPearls [Internet]*, Treasure Island FL, 2018, StatPearls Publishing. Available at: http://www.ncbi.nlm.nih.gov/books/NBK470343/.

25. Juckett G: Arthropod bites, *Am Fam Physician* 88(12):841-847, 2013.

26. Ibrahim O, Syed UM, Tomecki KJ: Bedbugs: helping your patient through an infestation, *Cleve Clin J Med* 84(3):207-211, 2017.

27. Smith CJF, et al: Infantile hemangiomas: an updated review on risk factors, pathogenesis, and treatment, *Birth Defects Res* 109(11):809-815, 2017.

28. Slaughter KA, Chen T, Williams E, 3rd: Vascular lesions, *Facial Plast Surg Clin North Am* 24(4):559-571, 2016.

Page numbers followed by "f" indicate figures, "t" indicate tables, and "b" indicate boxes.

PREFIXES AND SUFFIXES USED IN MEDICAL TERMINOLOGY

Prefix	Meaning	Prefix	Meaning
a-	Without, not	tri-	Three; triple
acantho-	Spiny, thorny	**Suffix**	**Meaning**
af-	Toward	-al, -ac	Pertaining to
an-	Without, not	-algia	Pain
ante-	Before	-aps, -apt	Fit; fasten
anti-	Against; resisting	-arche	Beginning; origin
auto-	Self	-ase	Signifies an enzyme
bi-	Two; double	-blast	Sprout; make
blast-	Immature cell, embryonic	-centesis	A piercing
circum-	Around	-cide	To kill
co-, con-	With; together	-clast	Break; destroy
contra-	Against	-crine	Release; secrete
crine-	Secrete, separate	-cytosis	Increase in number
de-	Down from, undoing	-ectomy	A cutting out
dia-	Across; through	-emesis	Vomiting
dipl-	Twofold, double	-emia	Refers to blood condition
dys-	Bad; disordered; difficult	-flux	Flow
ecto-	Displaced, outside	-gen	Creates; forms
ef-	Away from	-genesis	Creation, production
em-, en-	In, into	-gram	Something written
endo-	Within	-graph(y)	To write, draw
epi-	Upon, above	-hydrate	Containing H2O (water)
eu-	Good	-ia, -sia	Condition; process
ex-, exo-	Out of, out from	-iasis	Abnormal condition
extra-	Outside of	-ic, -ac	Pertaining to
hapl-	Single	-in	Signifies a protein
hem-, hemat-	Blood	-ism	Signifies "condition of"
hemi-	Half	-itis	Signifies "inflammation of"
hom(e)o-	Same; equal	-lemma	Sheath, covering
hyper-	Over; above	-lepsy	Seizure
hypo-	Under; below	-lith	Stone; rock
infra-	Below, beneath	-logy	Study of
inter-	Between	-lunar	Moon; moonlike
intra-	Within	-malacia	Softening
iso-	Same, equal	-megaly	Enlargement
juxta-	Near	-metric, -metry	Measurement, length
macro-	Large	-oid	Like; in the shape of
mega-	Large; million(th)	-oma	Tumor
mes-	Middle	-opia	Vision, vision condition
meta-	Beyond, change, after	-oscopy	Viewing
micro-	Small; millionth	-ose	Pertaining to, sugar
milli-	Thousandth	-osis	Condition, process
mono-	One (single)	-ostomy	Formation of an opening
necro-	Death	-otomy	Cut
neo-	New	-penia	Lack
non-	Not	-philic	Loving
oligo-	Few, scanty	-phobic	Fearing
ortho-	Straight; correct, normal	-phragm	Partition
para-	By the side of; near	-plasia	Growth, formation
per-	Through	-plasm	Substance, matter
peri-	Around; surrounding	-plasty	Shape; make
poly-	Many	-plegia	Paralysis
post-	After	-pnea	Breath, breathing
pre-	Before	-(r)rhage, -(r)rhagia	Breaking out, discharge
pro-	First; promoting	-(r)rhaphy	Sew, suture
quadri-	Four	-(r)rhea	Flow
re-	Back again	-some	Body
retro-	Behind	-tensin, -tension	Pressure
semi-	Half	-tonic	Pressure, tension
sub-	Under	-tripsy	Crushing
super-, supra-	Over, above, excessive	-ule	Small, little
trans-	Across; through	-uria	Refers to urine condition